SURGICAL RADIOLOGY

A COMPLEMENT IN RADIOLOGY AND IMAGING
TO THE SABISTON
DAVIS-CHRISTOPHER TEXTBOOK OF SURGERY

Volume I

Edited by

J. GEORGE TEPLICK, M.D., F.A.C.R.

Professor and Director, Division of General
Diagnosis, Department of Diagnostic Radiology,
Hahnemann Medical College and Hospital, Philadelphia

MARVIN E. HASKIN, M.D., F.A.C.R., F.A.C.P.

Professor and Chairman, Department of Diagnostic Radiology,
Hahnemann Medical College and Hospital, Philadelphia

W. B. SAUNDERS COMPANY • Philadelphia • London • Toronto

W. B. Saunders Company: West Washington Square
Philadelphia, PA 19105

1 St. Anne's Road
Eastbourne, East Sussex BN21 3UN, England

1 Goldthorne Avenue
Toronto, Ontario M8Z 5T9, Canada

Library of Congress Cataloging in Publication Data

Main entry under title:

Surgical radiology.

1. Surgery.   2. Diagnosis, Radioscopic.   3. Imaging systems in medicine.   I. Teplick, J. George.   II. Haskin, Marvin E.   III. Textbook of surgery. [DNLM: 1. Surgery 2. Radiography. W0100 S9626]

RD31.S925   617'.07572   78-20730

ISBN 0–7216–8781–4 (v. 1)

SURGICAL RADIOLOGY   ISBN 0-7216-8781-4

© 1981 by W. B. Saunders Company. Copyright under the Uniform Copyright Convention. Simultaneously published in Canada. All rights reserved. This book is protected by copyright. No part of it may be reproduced, stored in a retrieval system, or transmitted in any form or by any means, electronic, mechanical, photocopying, recording, or otherwise, without written permission from the publisher. Made in the United States of America. Press of W. B. Saunders Company. Library of Congress catalog card number 78-20730.

Last digit is the print number: 9   8   7   6   5   4   3   2

To
SELMA AND PAM
for their love, patience, and encouragement

CONTRIBUTORS

Volume I

ROBERT N. BERK, M.D.

Professor and Chairman, Department of Radiology, University of California, San Diego, School of Medicine; Chief, Department of Radiology, Hospital of the University of California, San Diego, California.

Peptic Ulcer, Tumors of the Stomach, Non-Neoplastic Diseases of the Stomach, The Postoperative Stomach

JOSEPH J. BOOKSTEIN, M.D.

Professor of Radiology, University of California, San Diego, School of Medicine; Chief, Vascular Radiology, Hospital of the University of California, San Diego, California.

Gastrointestinal Hemorrhage: Angiography and Transcatheter Therapy

HARLEY C. CARLSON, M.D., Ph.D.

Professor of Radiology, Mayo Medical School and Mayo Postgraduate School of Medicine; Consultant In Diagnostic Radiology, Mayo Clinic, Rochester, Minnesota.

Tumors of the Small Intestine, Carcinoid Tumors and the Carcinoid Syndrome

JAMES L. CLEMENTS, M.D.

Professor of Radiology, Emory University School of Medicine; Radiologist, Emory University Hospital and Grady Memorial Hospital, Atlanta, Georgia.

Nonhormonal Diseases of the Pancreas

JOHN L. DOPPMAN, M.D.

Chief, Diagnostic Radiology Department, The Clinical Center, National Institutes of Health, Bethesda, Maryland.

Endocrine Tumors of the Pancreas

RONALD G. EVENS, M.D.

Elizabeth Mallinckrodt Professor and Head, Mallinckrodt Institute of Radiology, Washington University School of Medicine; Attending Radiologist, Barnes Hospital and St. Louis Children's Hospital, St. Louis, Missouri.

The Spleen

LEONARD M. FREEMAN, M.D.

Professor of Radiology and Co-Director, Divisions of Nuclear Medicine, Albert Einstein College of Medicine; Chief, Division of Nuclear Medicine, Montefiore Hospital and Medical Center, Bronx, New York.

Radioisotope Techniques

CONTRIBUTORS

MATHIS P. FRICK, M.D.

Assistant Professor of Radiology, University of Minnesota Hospitals, Minneapolis, Minnesota.

Radiology after Intestinal Bypass Surgery for Morbid Obesity

RICHARD GARDINER, M.D.

Associate Professor of Diagnostic Radiology, Rush Medical College; Senior Attending Radiologist, Presbyterian–St. Luke's Hospital; Director, Section of Gastrointestinal Radiology, Rush-Presbyterian–St. Luke's Medical Center, Chicago, Illinois.

Inflammatory Bowel Disease, Precancerous and Malignant Lesions

EUGENE GEDGAUDAS, M.D.

Professor of Radiology and Head, University of Minnesota Hospitals, Minneapolis, Minnesota.

Radiology after Intestinal Bypass Surgery for Morbid Obesity

GARY G. GHAHREMANI, M.D.

Professor of Radiology and Chairman, Department of Diagnostic Radiology, Evanston Hospital–Northwestern University, Evanston, Illinois.

Hernias

HENRY I. GOLDBERG, M.D.

Professor of Radiology, University of California, San Francisco, School of Medicine, San Francisco, California.

The Liver

ANTONIO C. GONZALEZ, M.D.

Associate Professor of Radiology, Emory University School of Medicine; Radiologist, Veterans Administration Hospital, Decatur, and Grady Memorial Hospital, Atlanta, Georgia.

Nonhormonal Diseases of the Pancreas

LAWRENCE R. GOODMAN, M.D.

Associate Professor of Diagnostic Radiology, Hahnemann Medical College and Hospital, Philadelphia, Pennsylvania.

The Acute Care Unit: Radiographic Considerations

ANTONIO F. GOVONI, M.D.

Associate Professor of Radiology, Cornell University Medical College; Associate Attending Radiologist, The New York Hospital, New York, N.Y.

The Acute Abdomen

GUERDON D. GREENWAY, M.D.

Assistant Professor of Radiology University of California, San Diego, School of Medicine; Professor of Radiology, Hospital of the University of California, San Diego, California.

Gastrointestinal Hemorrhage: Angiography and Transcatheter Therapy

MARVIN E. HASKIN, M.D., F.A.C.R., F.A.C.P.

Professor and Chairman, Department of Diagnostic Radiology, Hahnemann Medical College and Hospital, Philadelphia, Pennsylvania.

Meckel's Diverticulum

GERALD M. KLEIN, M.D.

Clinical Assistant Professor of Radiology, University of Pennsylvania Medical School; Associate Radiologist, Presbyterian–University of Pennsylvania Medical Center, Philadelphia, Pennsylvania.

Colonic Polyposis and Associated Syndromes, The Rectum and Anal Canal

ROBERT E. KOEHLER, M.D.

Associate Professor, Mallinckrodt Institute of Radiology, Washington University School of Medicine; Barnes Hospital and St. Louis Children's Hospital, St. Louis, Missouri.

The Liver, The Spleen

PATRICIA A. LAFFEY, M.D.

Assistant Professor, Hahnemann Medical College and Hospital; Chief, Section of Noninvasive Imaging, Department of Diagnostic Radiology, Hahnemann Medical College and Hospital, Philadelphia, Pennsylvania.

Ultrasound Techniques

CARL R. LARSEN, M.D.

Assistant Clinical Professor in Radiology, Boston University School of Medicine; Radiologist, New England Baptist Hospital; Departments of Diagnostic Radiology and Ultrasonography, Lahey Clinic Foundation, Boston, Massachusetts.

Acute Suppurative Cholangitis, Gallstone Ileus and Fistula, Carcinoma of the Gallbladder and Biliary Ducts

IGOR LAUFER, M.D.

Associate Professor of Radiology, University of Pennsylvania School of Medicine; Chief, Gastrointestinal Radiology Section, Hospital of the University of Pennsylvania, Philadelphia, Pennsylvania.

Tumors of the Esophagus

LETTY GOODMAN LUTZKER, M.D.

Clinical Assistant Professor of Radiology, Albert Einstein College of Medicine; Chief of Service, Division of Nuclear Medicine, Lenox Hill Hospital, New York, N.Y.

Radioisotope Techniques

HEBER MACMAHON, M.B.

Assistant Professor, Department of Diagnostic Radiology, The University of Chicago School of Medicine; Assistant Professor, Department of Diagnostic Radiology, University of Chicago Hospitals and Clinics, Chicago, Illinois.

Corrosive Strictures of the Esophagus

ALEXANDER R. MARGULIS, M.D.

Professor and Chairman, Department of Radiology, University of California, San Francisco, School of Medicine, San Francisco, California.

Small Bowel Obstruction, Regional Enteritis, Malabsorption Syndromes, Appendicitis, Radiation Enteritis

JAMES B. MASTERSON, M.B., B.CH., B.A.O., F.R.C.P.I., D.M.R.D., F.R.C.R.

Tutor, Faculty of Radiologists of the Royal College of Surgeons in Ireland; Consultant Radiologist, St. Vincent's Hospital and St. Laurence's Hospital, Dublin, Ireland.

The Abdominal Wall, Umbilicus, Peritoneum, Mesenteries, and Retroperitoneum

MORTON A. MEYERS, M.D.

Professor and Chairman, Department of Radiology, School of Medicine, State University of New York at Stony Brook, New York.

Hernias

ROSCOE E. MILLER, M.D.

Distinguished Professor of Radiology, Indiana University School of Medicine, Indianapolis, Indiana.

Disorders of Esophageal Motility, Diverticula and Miscellaneous Conditions of the Esophagus, Hiatus Hernia

CHARLES M. NICE, JR., M.D., Ph.D.

Professor and Chairman, Department of Radiology, Tulane University; Head, Department of Radiology, Tulane Medical Center, New Orleans, Louisiana.

Non-Neoplastic Lesions of the Large Bowel

DENIS J. O'CONNELL, M.R.C.P., F.R.C.R.

Clinical Teacher, University College, Dublin; Consultant Radiologist, Mater Misericordiae Hospitals and St. Mary's Hospital, Cappagh, Dublin, Ireland.

Perforation of the Esophagus

STEVEN H. OMINSKY, M.D.

Assistant Clinical Professor of Radiology, University of California, San Francisco, School of Medicine, San Francisco, California.

Small Bowel Obstruction, Regional Enteritis, Malabsorption Syndromes, Appendicitis, Radiation Enteritis

CHARLES PUTMAN, M.D.

Chairman and Professor, Department of Radiology, Duke University Medical Center, Durham, North Carolina.

The Acute Care Unit: Radiographic Considerations

FRANCIS A. PUYAU, M.D.

Professor of Medicine, Pediatrics and Radiology, Tulane University; Tulane Medical Center, New Orleans, Louisiana.

Non-Neoplastic Lesions of the Large Bowel

STUART S. SAGEL, M.D.

Professor of Radiology, Washington University School of Medicine; Director, Chest Radiology Section, Mallinckrodt Institute of Radiology; Barnes Hospital, St. Louis, Missouri.

Computed Tomography in the Diagnosis of Surgical Disorders

FRANCIS J. SCHOLZ, M.D.

Clinical Instructor in Radiology, Peter Bent Brigham Hospital and Harvard Medical School; Chairman, Department of Diagnostic Radiology, Lahey Clinic Foundation; Radiologist, New England Baptist Hospital, Boston, Massachusetts.

The Duodenum

JOVITAS SKUCAS, M.D.

Associate Professor of Radiology, University of Rochester School of Medicine and Dentistry, Rochester, New York.

Disorders of Esophageal Motility, Diverticula and Miscellaneous Conditions of the Esophagus, Hiatus Hernia

ROBERT J. STANLEY, M.D.

Professor of Radiology, Washington University School of Medicine; Director, Abdominal Radiology Section, Mallinckrodt Institute of Radiology. Barnes Hospital and St. Louis Children's Hospital, St. Louis, Missouri.

Computed Tomography in the Diagnosis of Surgical Disorders

GEORGE N. STEIN, M.D.

Professor of Radiology, University of Pennsylvania School of Medicine; Director, Department of Radiology, Presbyterian–University of Pennsylvania Medical Center, Philadelphia, Pennsylvania.

Colonic Polyposis and Associated Syndromes, The Rectum and Anal Canal

J. GEORGE TEPLICK, M.D., F.A.C.R.

Professor and Director, Division of General Diagnosis, Department of Diagnostic Radiology, Hahnemann Medical College and Hospital, Philadelphia, Pennsylvania.

Meckel's Diverticulum

STEVEN K. TEPLICK, M.D.

Associate Professor of Radiology, Hahnemann Medical College and Hospital, Philadelphia, Pennsylvania.

Biliary Tract Investigation by Imaging Modalities; Cholecystitis, Calculi, and Miscellaneous Conditions

H. STEPHEN WEENS, M.D.

Professor and Chairman of Radiology, Emory University School of Medicine; Radiologist, Emory University Hospital and Grady Memorial Hospital, Atlanta, Georgia.

Nonhormonal Diseases of the Pancreas

JOSEPH P. WHALEN, M.D.

Professor and Chairman, Department of Radiology, Cornell University Medical College; Radiologist-in-Chief, The New York Hospital, New York, N.Y.

The Acute Abdomen

ROBERT E. WISE, M.D.

Department of Diagnostic Radiology, Lahey Clinic Foundation; Chairman, Department of Radiology, New England Baptist Hospital; Clinical Professor of Radiology, Boston University School of Medicine, Boston, Massachusetts.

Acute Suppurative Cholangitis, Gallstone Ileus and Fistula, Carcinoma of the Gallbladder and Biliary Ducts

FOREWORD

This new three-volume work on surgical radiology fills a much needed role and is a very welcome addition to this field. Drs. Teplick and Haskin are to be highly commended for their comprehensive approach to all aspects of radiologic diagnosis in surgical patients. These authors have been unusually thorough in their coverage of the entire field of surgery and have included each of the surgical specialties in this impressive undertaking.

In 1967 Teplick and Haskin met a pressing need with the introduction of a two-volume work designed as a radiologic companion to the Beeson-McDermott *Textbook of Medicine*. This innovative concept added much to the famous text with which it was to be jointly used. Carefully and exhaustively illustrated, these two volumes were extremely well received; a second edition was published in 1971, and a third edition appeared in 1976. The success of these editions is a matter of record, and it is easy to predict that the new surgical companion text will also be widely used and be rapidly recognized as a timely addition to the surgical armamentarium.

Since the discovery of x-rays by Roentgen in 1895, massive strides have been made in the field of radiology. A number of subspecialties have developed and now constitute an established part of this discipline. In the first volume of this series on surgical radiology, special emphasis has been placed upon the newer aspects of radioisotope techniques in surgical diagnosis, the role of ultrasound in surgical patients, and the expanding indications for the use of computerized tomography. Each of these sections is presented in a clear and concise manner with excellent illustrations. This extensive work by Teplick and Haskin emphasizes the expanding role of the radiologist not only in *diagnostic* but also in therapeutic procedures. The passage of a variety of catheters, needles, and tubes with the use of image intensification permits a multidimensional approach to the *treatment* of a number of specific disorders. Techniques that have proved highly effective in radiologic management include removal of gallstones; biopsy of pulmonary, mediastinal, and other masses; dilatation of stenotic lesions of the arterial system; control of massive hemorrhage by selective arteriography and perfusion of vasoconstrictors; direct embolization of bleeding sites; selective chemotherapeutic and embolic infusion of neoplasms; and a variety of additional procedures. Each of these serves as an example of the ever-increasing magnitude of the radiologic sciences upon diagnosis and treatment in modern medicine.

There is little doubt that this three-volume series will be very favorably received by all members of the surgical and allied professions, and much praise is due the editors and contributors for this comprehensive and highly useful text.

David C. Sabiston, Jr.

PREFACE

These volumes are designed to provide a single source of radiologic information related to surgical conditions. In addition to preoperative radiographic diagnosis, emphasis is placed on radiographic appearances following surgery and on the radiographic findings associated with surgical complications.

In the main, this is planned to be a radiologic compendium for hospital practice, embracing knowledge unique to the hospital environment, including the emergency room, recovery room, and intensive care units. The emphasis, therefore, is quite different from that of the usual radiologic textbook. A recurring theme is comparative pre- and postoperative radiographic appearances, with appropriate attention to complications following surgery.

The explosive development of both newer techniques and the modalities in ultrasound, computed tomography, Chiba needle aspiration biopsy, and nuclear medicine has made closer cooperation between the clinician and the radiologist imperative for integrating the necessary imaging studies of surgical patients and those who are candidates for surgery. These modalities are discussed in detail and illustrated profusely throughout these volumes. In addition, special detailed sections on newer and updated imaging modalities precede the chapters on specific disorders.

The general organization will follow that of the Davis-Christopher *Textbook of Surgery,* edited by D. C. Sabiston, M.D. The numerous contributors to *Surgical Radiology* have been selected for their demonstrated interest and experience in subjects appropriate to the scope of these volumes.

Volume I comprises general abdominal conditions, including the acute abdomen and disorders of the gastrointestinal and biliary tracts, liver, pancreas, and spleen. Chapter 1 discusses radiographic considerations of the acute care unit. Contributions by 27 individual authors or collaborating groups and about 1800 illustrations are contained in Volume I. Each volume includes a separate index, and a combined index of the three volumes appears in Volume III.

Surgical Radiology should prove a most useful addition to the armamentarium of the hospital radiologist, the clinician, and the surgeon as well as the entire resident staff.

We gratefully acknowledge the assistance and guidance of John Hanley, President of the W. B. Saunders Company. We would especially like to thank Mildred Strehle for her patience, graciousness, and many kindnesses. We are also grateful for Constance Burton's fine editorial assistance.

J. GEORGE TEPLICK, M.D.

MARVIN E. HASKIN, M.D.

CONTENTS

VOLUME I

Chapter 1
THE ACUTE CARE UNIT: RADIOGRAPHIC CONSIDERATIONS 1
Lawrence R. Goodman, M.D., and Charles E. Putman, M.D.

Chapter 2
RADIOISOTOPE TECHNIQUES 23
Letty G. Lutzker, M.D., and Leonard M. Freeman, M.D.

Chapter 3
ULTRASOUND TECHNIQUES 55
Patricia A. Laffey, M.D.

Chapter 4
COMPUTED TOMOGRAPHY IN THE DIAGNOSIS OF SURGICAL DISORDERS 125
Robert J. Stanley, M.D., and Stuart S. Sagel, M.D.

Chapter 5
THE ACUTE ABDOMEN 169
Antonio F. Govoni, M.D., and Joseph P. Whalen, M.D.

Chapter 6
THE ABDOMINAL WALL, UMBILICUS, PERITONEUM, MESENTERIES, AND
RETROPERITONEUM 248
James B. Masterson, M.B., B.Ch., B.A.O., F.R.C.P.I., D.M.R.D., F.R.C.R.

Chapter 7

HERNIAS 287
Gary G. Ghahremani, M.D., and Morton A. Meyers, M.D.

Chapter 8

THE ESOPHAGUS 319

Part I

Disorders of Esophageal Motility 319
Jovitas Skucas, M.D., and Roscoe E. Miller, M.D.

Part II

Diverticula and Miscellaneous Conditions of the Esophagus 335
Jovitas Skucas, M.D., and Roscoe E. Miller, M.D.

Part III

Hiatus Hernia 348
Jovitas Skucas, M.D., and Roscoe E. Miller, M.D.

Part IV

Perforation of the Esophagus 368
Denis J. O'Connell, M.R.C.P., F.R.C.R.

Part V

Corrosive Strictures of the Esophagus 379
Heber MacMahon, M.B.

Part VI

Tumors of the Esophagus 387
Igor Laufer, M.D.

Chapter 9

PEPTIC ULCER... 419
Robert N. Berk, M.D.

Chapter 10

THE STOMACH 448
Robert N. Berk, M.D.

Part I

Tumors 448

Part II

Non-Neoplastic Diseases... 469

Part III

The Postoperative Stomach 484

Chapter 11

DUODENUM ... 502

Francis J. Scholz, M.D.

Chapter 12

THE SMALL INTESTINE ... 538

PART I

SMALL BOWEL OBSTRUCTION ... 538

Steven H. Ominsky, M.D., and Alexander R. Margulis, M.D.

PART II

REGIONAL ENTERITIS ... 550

Steven H. Ominsky, M.D., and Alexander R. Margulis, M.D.

PART III

MALABSORPTION SYNDROMES ... 562

Steven H. Ominsky, M.D., and Alexander R. Margulis, M.D.

PART IV

APPENDICITIS ... 577

Steven H. Ominsky, M.D., and Alexander R. Margulis, M.D.

PART V

RADIATION ENTERITIS ... 590

Steven H. Ominsky, M.D., and Alexander R. Margulis, M.D.

PART VI

TUMORS ... 596

Harley C. Carlson, M.D.

PART VII

CARCINOID TUMORS AND THE CARCINOID SYNDROME ... 620

Harley C. Carlson, M.D.

PART VIII

MECKEL'S DIVERTICULUM ... 625

J. George Teplick, M.D., and M. E. Haskin, M.D.

PART IX

RADIOLOGY AFTER INTESTINAL BYPASS SURGERY FOR MORBID OBESITY ... 637

Mathis P. Frick, M.D., and Eugene Gedgaudas, M.D.

Chapter 13

THE LARGE BOWEL ... 647

PART I

NON-NEOPLASTIC LESIONS ... 647

Charles M. Nice, Jr., M.D., Ph.D., and Francis A. Puyau, M.D.

PART II
Inflammatory Bowel Disease 688
Richard Gardiner, M.D.

PART III
Precancerous and Malignant Lesions 722
Richard Gardiner, M.D.

PART IV
Colonic Polyposis and Associated Syndromes 748
George N. Stein, M.D., and Gerald M. Klein, M.D.

PART V
The Rectum and Anal Canal 773
George N. Stein, M.D., and Gerald M. Klein, M.D.

Chapter 14
GASTROINTESTINAL HEMORRHAGE: ANGIOGRAPHY AND TRANSCATHETER THERAPY 789
Joseph J. Bookstein, M.D., and Guerdon D. Greenway, M.D.

Chapter 15
THE LIVER 811
Henry I. Goldberg, M.D., and Robert Koehler, M.D.

Chapter 16
THE BILIARY SYSTEM 866

PART I
Biliary Tract Investigation by Imaging Modalities 866
Steven K. Teplick, M.D.

PART II
Cholecystitis, Calculi, and Miscellaneous Conditions 913
Steven K. Teplick, M.D.

PART III
Acute Suppurative Cholangitis 963
Carl R. Larsen, M.D., and Robert E. Wise, M.D.

PART IV
Gallstone Ileus and Fistula 968
Carl R. Larsen, M.D., and Robert E. Wise, M.D.

PART V
Carcinoma of the Gallbladder and Biliary Ducts 985
Carl R. Larsen, M.D., and Robert E. Wise, M.D.

Chapter 17

THE PANCREAS 1003

   PART I

   NONHORMONAL DISEASES OF THE PANCREAS 1003
      James L. Clements, Jr., M.D., Antonio C. Gonzalez, M.D., and H. Stephen Weens, M.D.

   PART II

   ENDOCRINE TUMORS 1054
      John L. Doppman, M.D.

Chapter 18

THE SPLEEN.. 1064
   Robert E. Koehler, M.D., and Ronald G. Evens, M.D.

Index 1089

1

THE ACUTE CARE UNIT: RADIOGRAPHIC CONSIDERATIONS

LAWRENCE R. GOODMAN, M.D.
CHARLES E. PUTMAN, M.D.

INTENSIVE CARE UNIT RADIOLOGY

The intensive care unit patient presents a unique set of clinical and radiographic problems. For the radiologist, the problems are twofold: the difficulty of obtaining quality radiographs and the difficulty in sorting out the patient's numerous radiographic abnormalities. This chapter will deal very briefly with the problems of portable radiography and then discuss in some detail the radiographic evaluation of the acutely ill postsurgical patient. In this latter section, we will consider the support and monitoring devices and the cardiopulmonary disorders frequently encountered in the intensive care unit.

PORTABLE RADIOGRAPHY

Portable radiographic equipment allows one to obtain radiographs at the bedside, thereby avoiding the need to transport seriously ill patients to the x-ray department. Using modern portable equipment and careful radiographic technique, chest radiographs of diagnostic quality can usually be obtained on all but the most uncooperative or obese patients.

The advantages of portable radiography must be weighed against its numerous inherent disadvantages. Stationary equipment is capable of higher kilovoltage and milliamperage, which allows decreased exposure time and therefore less motion degradation of the radiographic image. Stationary equipment also allows more precise patient positioning, the use of grids when necessary, less geometric distortion, and a smaller radiation dosage. In addition, the overall cost is considerably lower when the film is taken in the department. Therefore, although inconvenient, radiographs should be obtained in the x-ray department if it is safe to transport the patient.

Although the radiation dose for portable chest radiography is relatively small, it is nonetheless two to four times the dose of a comparable stationary film.[17] The average portable abdominal film requires a many-fold increase in radiation exposure, yet furnishes very limited diagnostic information.

Scattered radiation from portable radiography is a potential problem for physicians, nurses, and other intensive care unit patients, but it can be almost eliminated with minimal basic precautions. At 1 meter from the patient, scattered radiation is approximately one thousandth of the patient dose.[17] A lead apron decreases exposure at least another hundredfold. Therefore, if the patient must be held, exposure will be minimized if the operator wears a lead apron and gloves and holds the patient at arm's length. Careful beam collimation should be part of basic radiographic technique.

Modern intensive care of the critically ill has evolved into a multidisciplinary approach. The patient's problems are complex and rapidly changing. To ensure optimal film interpretation, the radiologist must be aware of both the patient's clinical problems and the details of the therapy employed. Free communication between the radiologist and the referring physician is necessary for most efficient patient management.

INTRAVASCULAR CATHETERS

Although intravascular catheters for diagnostic and therapeutic purposes are invaluable in the management of critically ill patients, they have a definite mortality and morbidity. The radiograph is a valuable aid in correctly positioning these devices in order to maximize their usefulness and minimize their complications. Immediately following the insertion of a catheter (other than a peripheral venous catheter) into the vascular system, a radiograph should be obtained to ascertain catheter position and the presence of unsuspected complications.[23]

Central Venous Pressure

Regardless of the site of entry, to accurately reflect right atrial pressure a central venous pressure catheter must lie in a major intrathoracic vein beyond the valves that may damp accurate pressure readings. In both the subclavian vein and the internal jugular vein, the last venous valve is approximately 2 cm proximal to their confluence into the innominate vein.[11] This point is usually located over the anterior end of the first rib. On the radiograph, any catheter medial to this point or assuming a vertical orientation is beyond the valves. A properly placed catheter may be in the superior vena cava or innominate vein (Fig. 1–1A).[34] The catheter should be free of kinks, loops, and sharp angulation (Fig. 1–1A).

Numerous studies indicate that approximately one third of all central venous pressure catheters are initially malpositioned.[11, 12, 27] The aberrant catheter may stop short of the thorax; leave the thorax via the jugular vein, the opposite innominate vein, or the inferior vena cava; enter a small feeding vein; or enter the right atrium, right ventricle, or pulmonary artery. Poorly positioned catheters yield unreliable and unpredictable central venous pressure readings.[12] They are also more likely to cause thrombosis.

Although uncommon, complications can result from an indwelling catheter placed

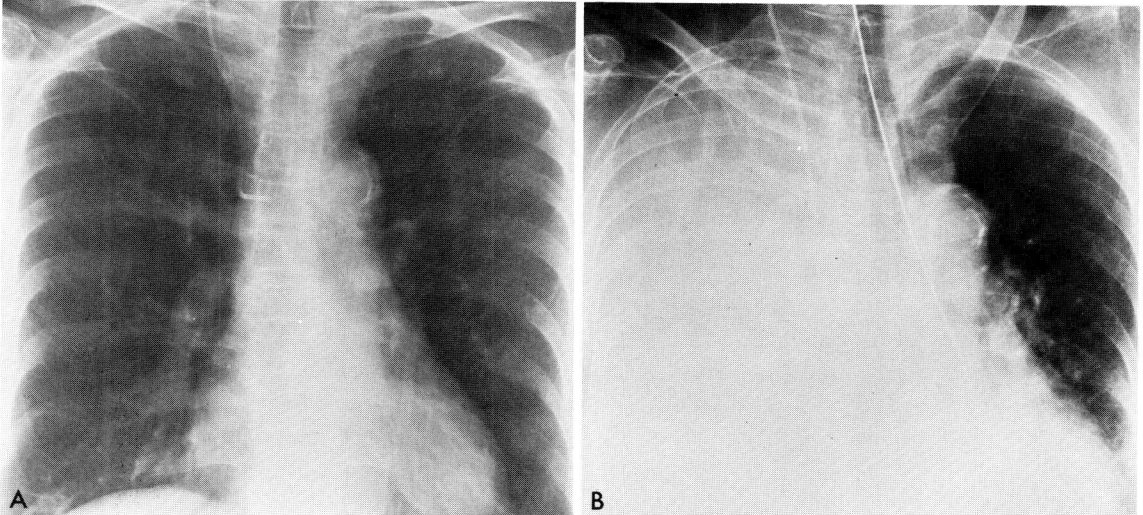

Figure 1–1. Ectopic infusion of fluid. *A,* Central venous pressure catheter has a right angle bend. *B,* Opaque hemithorax after infusion of intravenous fluid into pleural space. (*From* Goodman, L. R., and Putman, C. E.: Intensive Care Radiology: Imaging of the Critically Ill. St. Louis, The C. V. Mosby Company, 1978.)

within the right heart. The catheter can perforate the atrial or ventricular wall into the pericardial space. Perforation may be immediate or delayed, and the patient may be asymptomatic or suffer from fatal cardiac tamponade. Because the right ventricle is sensitive to mechanical irritation, catheter-induced arrhythmias are not infrequent.[11] Recognition of this phenomenon is important, because withdrawal of the catheter is usually sufficient treatment.

Following radiographic documentation of an aberrant catheter position, the catheter should be repositioned and its position checked on a follow-up radiograph. Perforation of the vein during or after insertion should be suspected whenever good venous backflow is not obtained or the radiograph demonstrates either acute mediastinal widening or pleural effusion (Fig. 1–1B). Intrapleural bleeding and ectopic infusions are especially frequent following subclavian vein catheterization and may be due to venous laceration, perivenous insertion of the catheter, or inadvertent puncture of the adjacent subclavian artery at the time of venipuncture. These fluid collections are usually self-limited and without sequelae when the cause is corrected early.[3] In patients who have had recent cardiothoracic surgery or chest trauma it may be difficult to differentiate catheter-induced fluid collections from other pathologic processes (Figs. 1–2A and 1–2B). Iodinated contrast injected through the catheter is often invaluable when the clinical diagnosis is uncertain (Fig. 1–2C).

Pneumothorax may follow subclavian vein catheterization because of the proximity of the apical pleura to the subclavian vein. An upright portable radiograph should be obtained following each subclavian vein catheterization to rule out a clinically silent pneumothorax (Fig. 1–3).[34] If the initial subclavian vein catheterization is unsuccessful, a film must be obtained prior to attempting the opposite side, to prevent the possibility of a bilateral pneumothorax. Another potentially serious complication is that of catheter emboli. The intravenous catheter may shear off and lodge in a vein, the heart, or a pulmonary artery. The emboli may cause potentially fatal cardiac arrhythmias or may serve as a delayed focus for thrombosis, embolus, infection, or perforation.[13] Because of these complications, all intravascular catheters should be radiopaque.

Owing to the mortality and morbidity associated with catheter emboli, broken catheters should be removed.[13] In peripheral cannulations, if the catheter breaks at the time of insertion, a tourniquet should be applied high in the axilla and x-rays obtained of the arm and chest in order to map out the appropriate retrieval procedure. When it is in the major thoracic veins, the heart, or the proximal pulmonary arteries, the catheter may be removed under fluoroscopic control using commercially available snares or a homemade snare fashioned out of an angiogram catheter and guide wire.[16, 24] Surgery is usually required for extravascular catheters and catheters in the more distal pulmonary vessels (Fig. 1–4).

Venous thrombosis with or without sepsis may complicate prolonged intravascular cannulation. This is especially frequent during parenteral hyperalimentation after catheterization via the femoral vein, or when local or systemic infection is present.[3] Symptoms, if present, are usually related to local thrombosis (that is, signs of obstruction) or distal effects (that is, pulmonary emboli, septic emboli, and sepsis). Although usu-

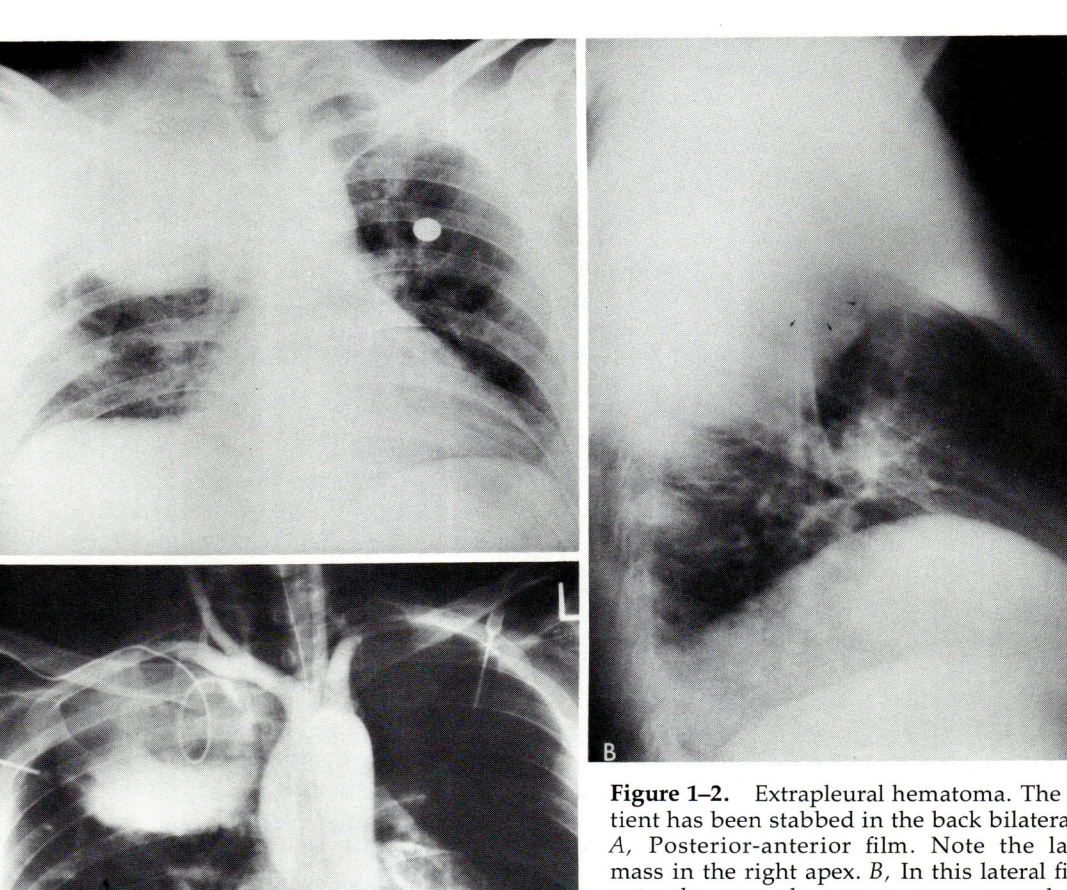

Figure 1–2. Extrapleural hematoma. The patient has been stabbed in the back bilaterally. *A*, Posterior-anterior film. Note the large mass in the right apex. *B*, In this lateral film, note the central venous pressure catheter coiled in the mass (arrows). *C*, Combined angiogram-venogram—contrast enters the mass via the extravascular venous catheter. The aortogram is normal.

THE ACUTE CARE UNIT: RADIOGRAPHIC CONSIDERATIONS — 5

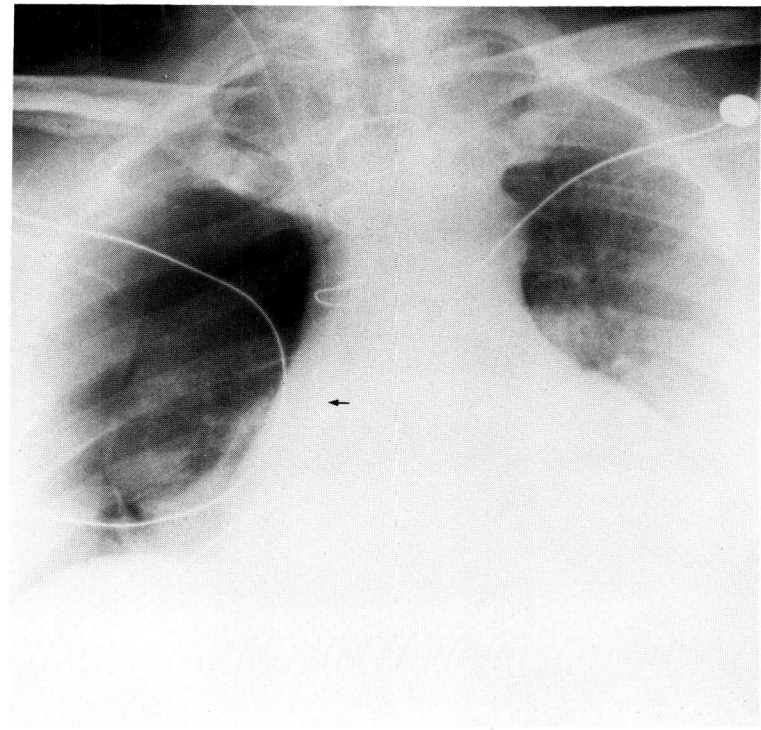

Figure 1–3. Pneumothorax. A right pneumothorax followed the insertion of a jugular venous pressure catheter in this postoperative patient with pulmonary edema. The catheter tip is in the right atrium (arrow).

ally not needed, iodinated contrast material may be injected as the catheter is withdrawn to document the extent of the thrombosis.

Pulmonary Capillary Wedge Pressure Monitoring

In both the acutely ill and the postoperative patient, central venous pressure readings do not adequately predict left ventricular end diastolic pressure.[1, 36] The flow-directed balloon tip catheter developed by Swan and Ganz allows the measurement of pulmonary capillary wedge pressure, which is used to estimate left ventricular end diastolic pressure. The catheter is inserted percutaneously and floated into the pulmonary artery with the aid of a small balloon. The balloon is then deflated and is reinflated whenever pulmonary capillary wedge pressures are being recorded.

On the radiograph, the tip of the catheter should be in a major pulmonary artery to prevent constant wedging and obstruction of a pulmonary artery. As a general rule, if the tip of the catheter is within two fingerbreadths of the lateral margin of the spine, it is in a major pulmonary vessel. Excess slack in the catheter should be avoided to prevent the catheter from migrating peripherally or coiling within the heart (Fig. 1–5A).[28] Because an initially well-positioned catheter may migrate with time, the position of the catheter should be checked on each radiograph. Since wedge pressures are not taken at the time of the radiograph, air should not be visible within the balloon (Fig. 1–5B).

The majority of complications of Swan-Ganz catheterization are due to distal mi-

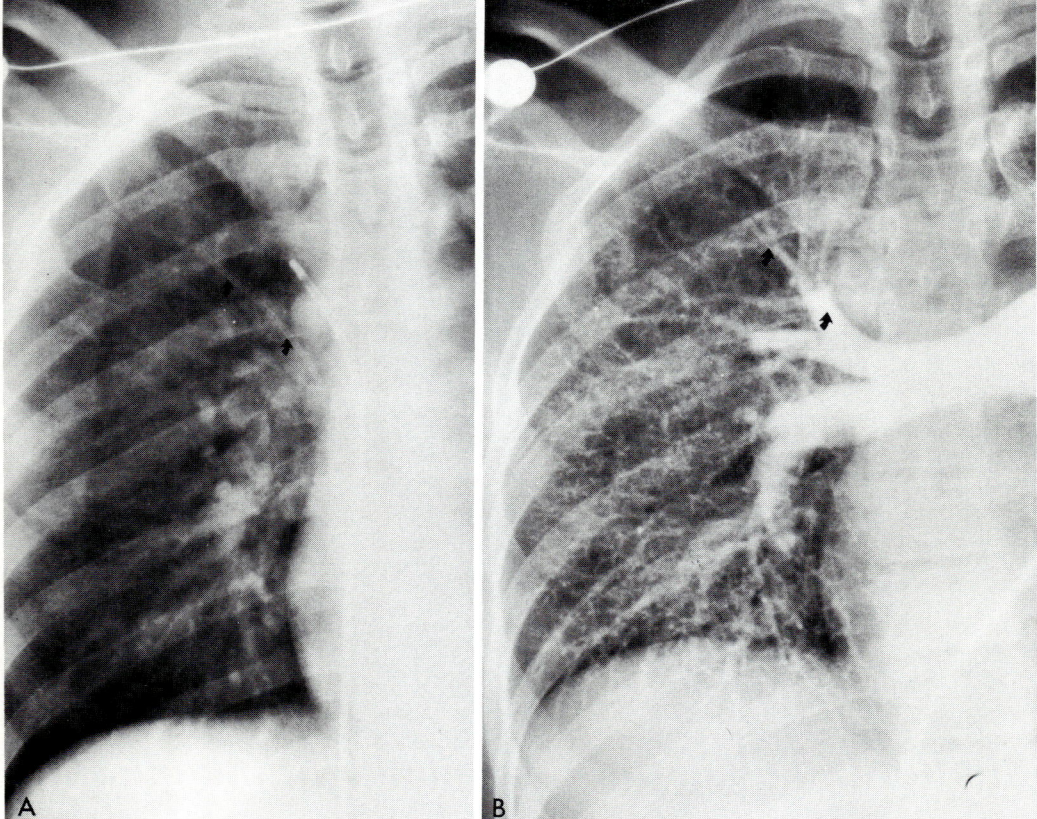

Figure 1-4. Catheter embolus. *A,* A piece of catheter (arrows) is seen in the right upper lobe. The patient is asymptomatic and was last hospitalized three years ago. An angiogram catheter is in the superior vena cava. *B,* A pulmonary angiogram demonstrates the catheter fragment (arrows) in the thrombosed apical segment artery.

gration of the catheter.[28] A catheter in a constant wedge position causes slow flow and thrombus formation. Vascular occlusion may also result from a persistently inflated balloon or clots forming in or around the catheter.[14] Should pulmonary thrombosis or embolization be followed by pulmonary infarction, the radiograph will usually demonstrate an area of alveolar infiltrate distal to the catheter in the distribution of the catheterized vessel (Fig. 1–6). Although a lung scan or angiograms confirm the suspicion of a pulmonary embolus, they are seldom required, since therapy is simply withdrawal of the catheter.

An unusual complication of peripheral positioning is pulmonary artery rupture. If the catheter is in a small vessel and the balloon is reinflated, the vessel may tear. Prolonged wedging in the vessel may also lead to vascular erosion. In either case, the patient presents with hemoptysis and rapidly spreading pulmonary alveolar infiltrates. Ventilation and perfusion scans may be abnormal in the suspected area (Fig. 1–7). The bleeding is usually self-limited, but fatal cases have been reported.[1, 36]

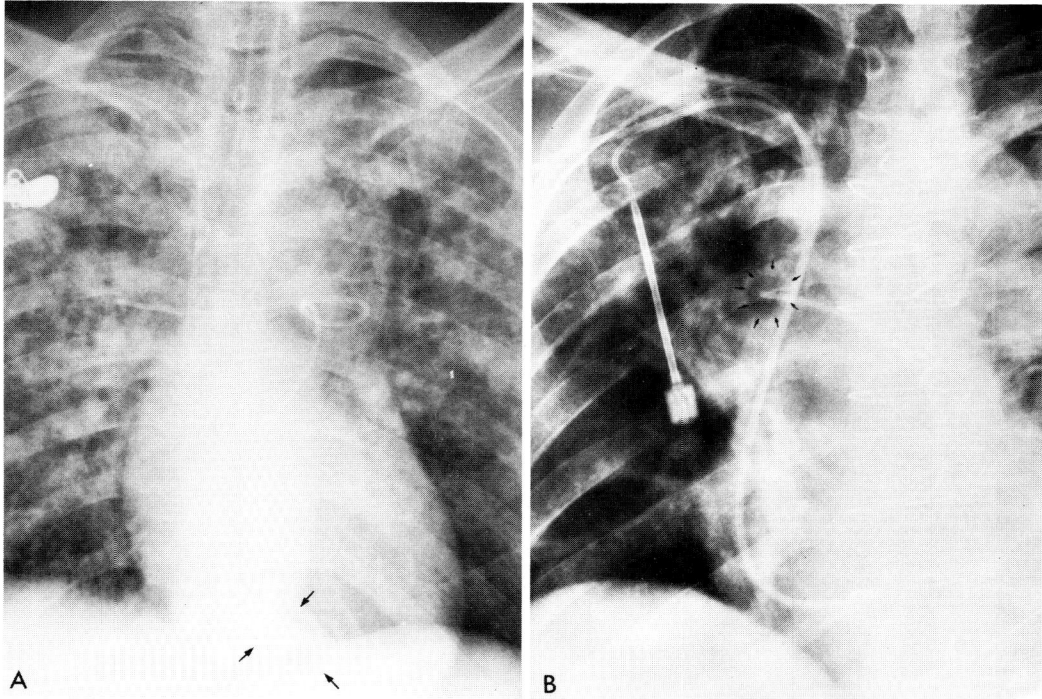

Figure 1–5. *A*, Coiled Swan-Ganz catheter. There is an extra loop in the right ventricle (arrows) and the main pulmonary artery. The patient has pulmonary fibrosis, tuberculosis, and adult respiratory distress syndrome. *B*, An inflated Swan-Ganz balloon, is a potential cause of pulmonary artery thrombosis. (Courtesy of B. Rohlfing, M.D., San Francisco.)

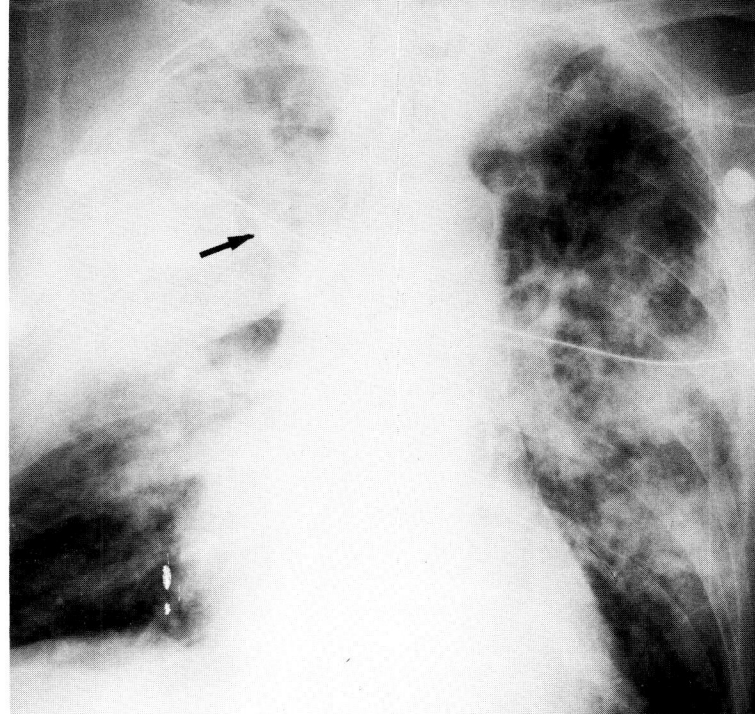

Figure 1–6. Pulmonary infarction (unproven). Consolidation of the right upper lobe following prolonged peripheral placement (arrow) of a Swan-Ganz catheter in a patient with pneumonia.

8 — THE ACUTE CARE UNIT: RADIOGRAPHIC CONSIDERATIONS

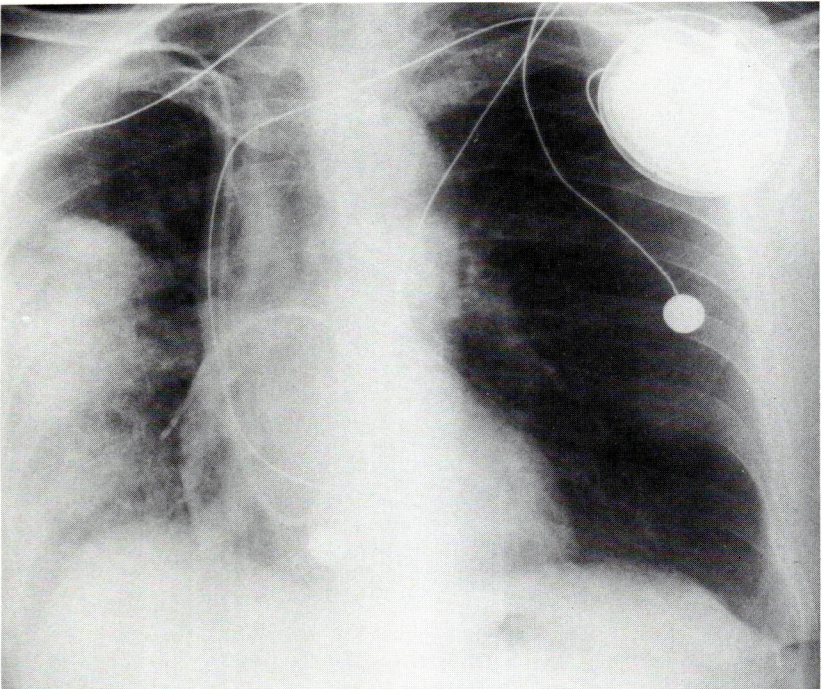

Figure 1–7. Pulmonary hemorrhage. The patient developed severe hemoptysis within hours of insertion of a Swan-Ganz catheter. The alveolar infiltrates are new and do not follow a lobar distribution. The infiltrates cleared within a few days.

INTRA-AORTIC COUNTERPULSATION DEVICES

See Chapter 26, Part X.

CARDIAC PACEMAKERS

See Chapter 26, Part IX.

RESPIRATORY SUPPORT

The endotracheal tube affords temporary support for patients requiring assistance in ventilation or protection of the trachea. The ideally located endotracheal tube is seen on the radiograph in the midtrachea, approximately 5 to 7 cm from the carina.[18] When the carina is not visible, its position may be estimated from prior portable radiographs because the carina-vertebral body relationship is relatively constant. If old films are not available, the level of the carina is approximated from the vertebral bodies. On 95 per cent of portable radiographs, the carina projects over T_5, T_6, or T_7.[18]

The position of the head and neck should also be evaluated, because flexion causes the tube to descend several centimeters and extension causes an ascent of several centimeters. In the average patient, the tube tip moves 4 cm caudally when the extended head and neck are flexed.[10] Thus, the ideally located tube is 5 to 7 cm from the carina when the neck is in the neutral position. When the neck is flexed (chin seen over T_1 or T_2), the tube should be 3 to 5 cm from the carina. When the neck is extended (chin seen over C_4), the tube should be 7 to 9 cm from the carina (Fig. 1–8).[18]

Complications of endotracheal intubation are not uncommon. Initial complications are the result of improper positioning of the tube, whereas delayed complications are most often the result of laryngotracheal injury. Perforation of the soft tissues at the time of placement of the endotracheal tube, although rare, may lead to subcutaneous emphysema, retropharyngeal edema, hematoma, infection, or abscess.[22] Complications may be immediately apparent or have a delayed presentation. A lateral soft tissue radiograph of the neck demonstrates a mass separating the trachea from the cervical spine or subcutaneous emphysema. An air-fluid level may be seen on horizontal beam radiographs. An esophagogram using a water-soluble contrast agent helps define the extent of the mass and, possibly, the site of perforation.

Errors of positioning are the most frequent radiographically demonstrated complications of intubation. As many as 10 to 15 per cent of intubations result in poor initial tube position.[40] Initially well-positioned tubes may change position with head and neck motion or may slip from their anchored position in the nose or mouth. Therefore, both the immediate postintubation radiograph and all subsequent radiographs should be checked for tube position relative to the carina.

Because the right mainstem bronchus leaves the trachea at a smaller angle than the left bronchus, accidental endobronchial intubation is almost invariably right sided. Although endobronchial intubation may be diagnosed clinically, the radiograph may be the first indicator of endotracheal tube malposition. The early radiograph after right mainstem bronchus intubation shows no aeration abnormalities. As air in the obstructed left side is resorbed, the left lung increases in density, the right lung becomes hyperlucent, and the mediastinum shifts to the left (Fig. 1–9). Overinflation of the right lung by the respirator may result in a pneumomediastinum or a right tension pneumothorax.

A tube placed too close to the vocal cords is also a potential problem. If the cuff is inflated in this location, vocal cord edema or ulceration, as well as subglottic edema, may thwart later extubation attempts (Fig. 1–10). A subglottic location may also lead

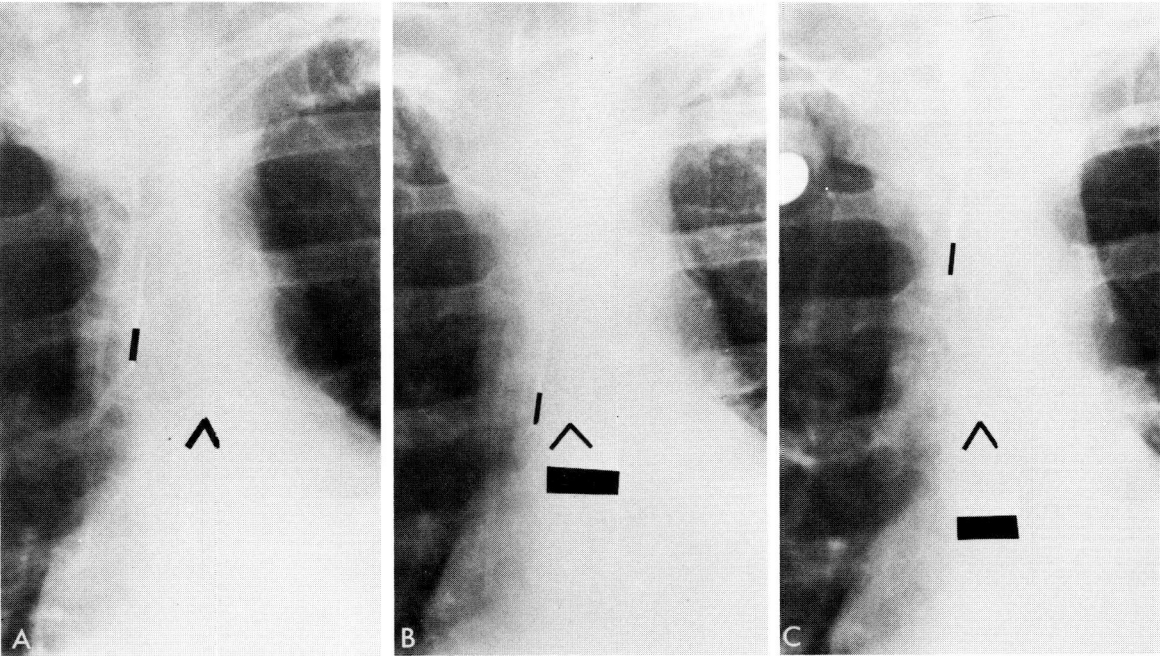

Figure 1–8. Effects of head and neck flexion and extension. *A*, In the neutral position, the endotracheal tube is 1.8 cm from the carina. *B*, Flexion causes a 2.1-cm descent into the right mainstem bronchus. *C*, Extension raises the tube to 3.5 cm above the carina.

10 — THE ACUTE CARE UNIT: RADIOGRAPHIC CONSIDERATIONS

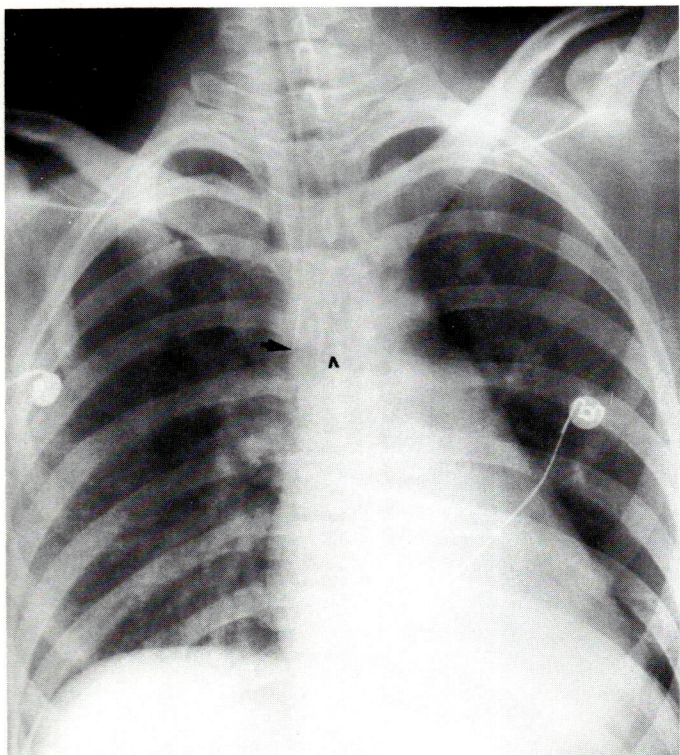

Figure 1–9. Right main stem bronchus intubation. The endotracheal tube (arrow) is just beyond the carina (∧), and the neck is extended. The left lower lobe is collapsed behind the heart, the mediastinum is shifted to the left, the diaphragm is elevated, and the descending aorta is not visible. The lobe reexpanded within 72 hours of repositioning the endotracheal tube.

Figure 1–10. Endotracheal tube in subglottic area. The opaque stripe of the tube is faintly visible beneath the respirator tubing (arrow). The patient has severe chronic obstructive pulmonary disease.

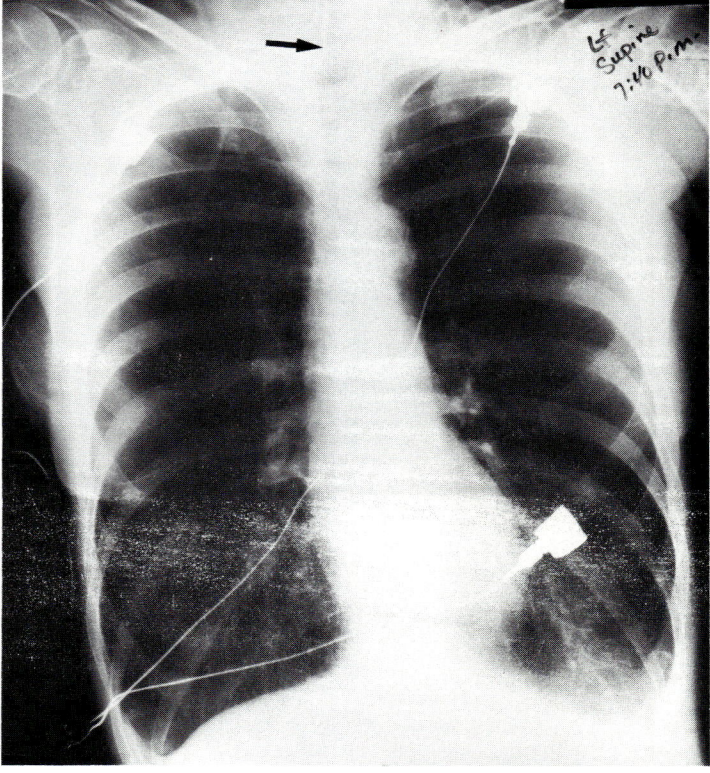

to accidental extubation with disrupted ventilation and possible aspiration of gastric contents.

Although delayed complications of short-term endotracheal intubation are uncommon with the use of low pressure–high volume cuffs, they do occur. Problems such as postintubation scarring and tracheomalacia are more frequent with tracheostomies and are discussed in Chapter 19, Part I.[26]

Tracheostomy

See Chapter 19, Part I.

VENTILATORY SUPPORT

Placing a patient on a ventilator may markedly alter the appearance of the chest x-ray. Since the radiograph is routinely exposed at the peak of inspiration, the radiograph's appearance is affected by the volume of gas delivered. Increased lung volume diminishes lung density, reverses atelectasis, and may drive water from the alveoli.[29] Thus, one is often impressed by the appearance of a dramatic improvement in the pulmonary infiltrate immediately after instituting positive-pressure therapy. Conversely, when the patient is weaned, the radiograph may return to its previous abnormal appearance in spite of obvious clinical improvement. These changes are especially pronounced with the use of positive end-expiratory pressure (PEEP) (Fig. 1–11). It is therefore necessary to know the relationship of each radiograph to the patient's assisted ventilation.[39a]

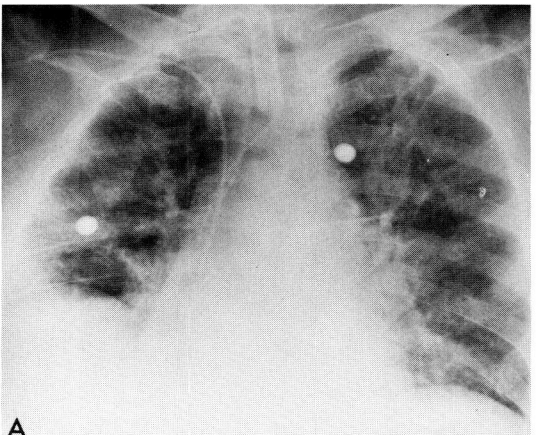
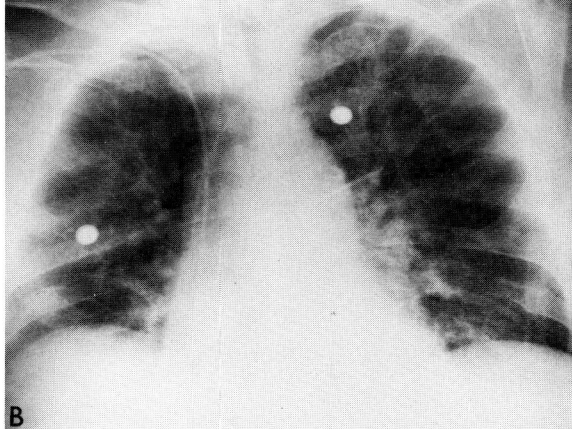
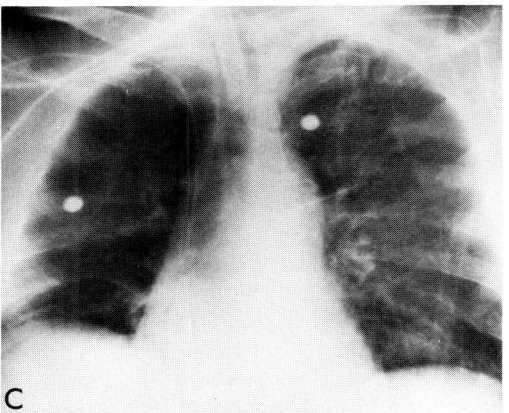

Figure 1–11. The effects of position end-expiratory pressure (PEEP). The three films were exposed within 15 minutes of one another using the identical radiographic technique. The patient is in congestive heart failure. *A,* Tidal volume (800 cc). *B,* one and one half tidal volume (1200 cc). *C,* tidal volume and PEEP (800 cc & 12 cm). (*From* Goodman, L. R., and Putman, C. E.: Intensive Care Radiology: Imaging of the Critically Ill. St. Louis, The C. V. Mosby Company, 1978.)

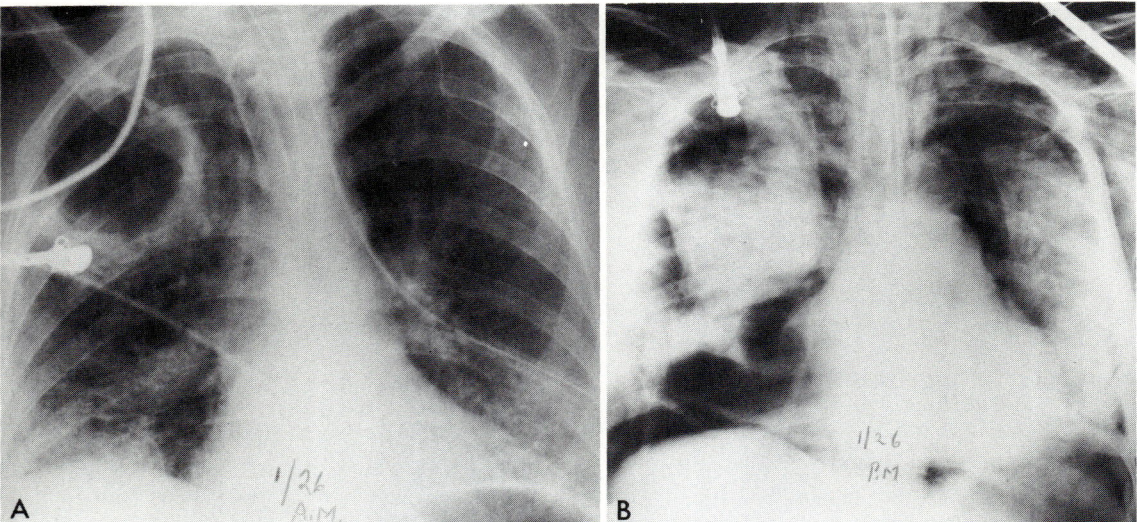

Figure 1–12. Rupture of pneumatocele. *A,* Patient with staphylococcal pneumonia. The pneumatocele in the right upper lung developed within 48 hours. *B,* Several hours later, it ruptured, causing massive pneumothorax, subcutaneous emphysema, and intraperitoneal air.

Five to fifteen per cent of patients receiving positive-pressure therapy have complications of pulmonary barotrauma. This may be due to the overexpansion and rupture of a bulla, bleb, pneumatocele, or abscess directly into the pleural space (Fig. 1–12). More frequently, pneumothorax is due to the rupture of a small airway with dissection of air along the interstitial tissues to the mediastinal space and then rupture into the pleural space. Air may also dissect into the neck or retroperitoneum (Fig. 1–13).[35] Pulmonary barotrauma may be a dramatic clinical event or an unexpected radiographic finding. Therefore, each radiograph should be carefully scrutinized for evidence of pneumothorax or pneumomediastinum, since prompt attention may prevent a potentially fatal tension pneumothorax. The radiology of extra-alveolar air is discussed in the following section.

CARDIOPULMONARY DISORDERS

It is beyond the scope of this chapter to describe in detail the radiographic spectrum of all cardiopulmonary disorders encountered in the intensive care unit. Instead, several cardiopulmonary problems frequently encountered will be discussed and references provided for further detail. Several texts are also available that provide greater depth.[15, 19] In addition, Chapters 19 and 26 discuss specific postoperative problems.

Extra-Alveolar Air

Air in the pleural, mediastinal, or pericardial space or in the subcutaneous tissues may result from invasive diagnostic and therapeutic procedures, such as tracheostomy, ventilator therapy, subclavian catheterization, transtracheal aspiration, thoracentesis, lung biopsy, and thoracic surgery (see Figs. 1–3 and 1–13). When a pneumothorax is

Figure 1–13. Barotrauma. *A,* Irregular linear and bubbly lucencies at the right lung base represent pulmonary interstitial emphysema in a ventilator patient. Air was also noted in the neck and right flank prior to the insertion of a chest tube for a concomitant pneumothorax. *B,* Decubitus view of the abdomen demonstrates a retroperitoneal air pocket (arrows) that does not change with change in position.

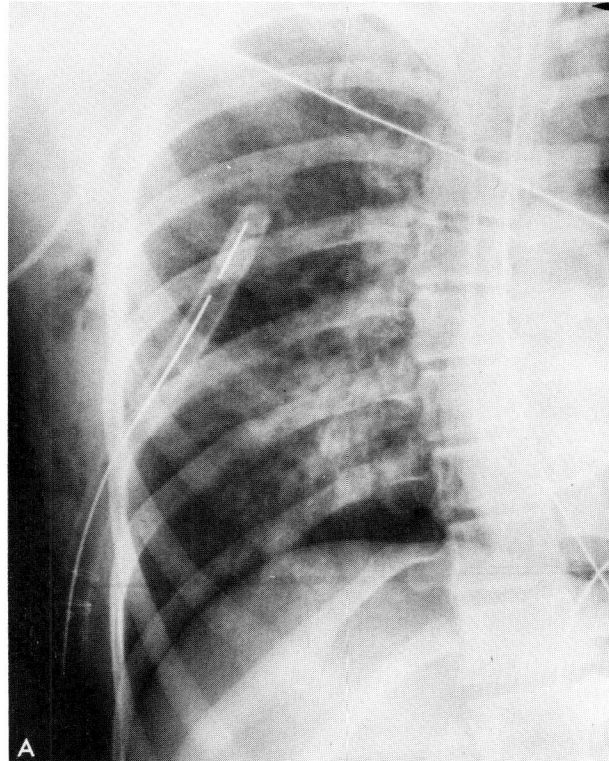

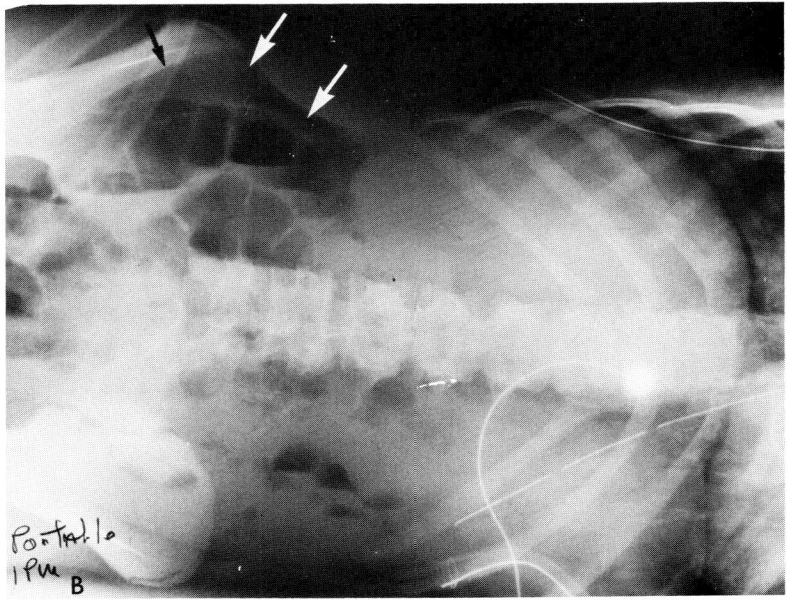

suspected, every effort must be made to obtain an upright film (expiratory, if possible), for even a moderate pneumothorax may be missed on a supine radiograph. When the patient cannot assume the upright position, a lateral decubitus film may be obtained in bed, with the side in question elevated (Fig. 1–14). The diagnosis requires the

14 — THE ACUTE CARE UNIT: RADIOGRAPHIC CONSIDERATIONS

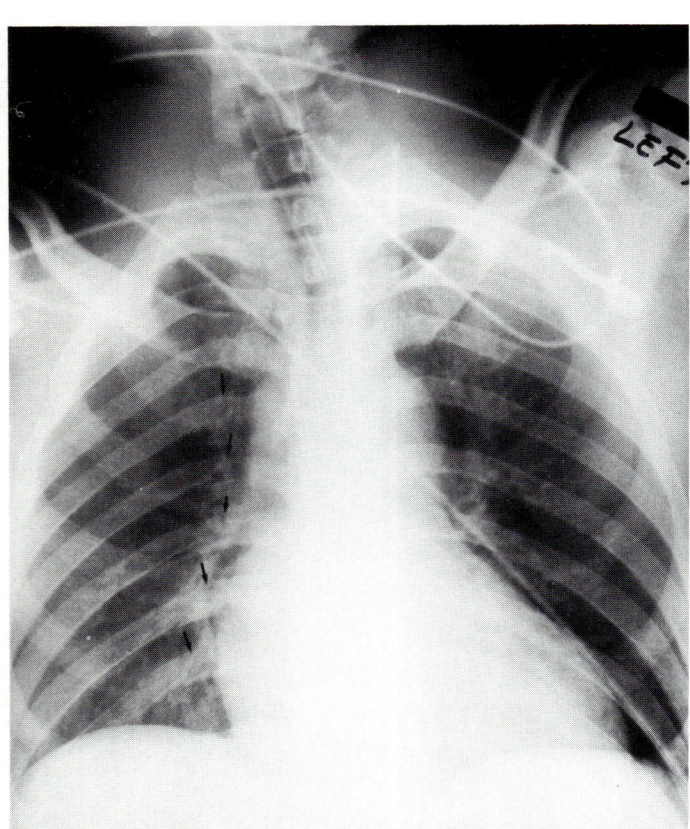
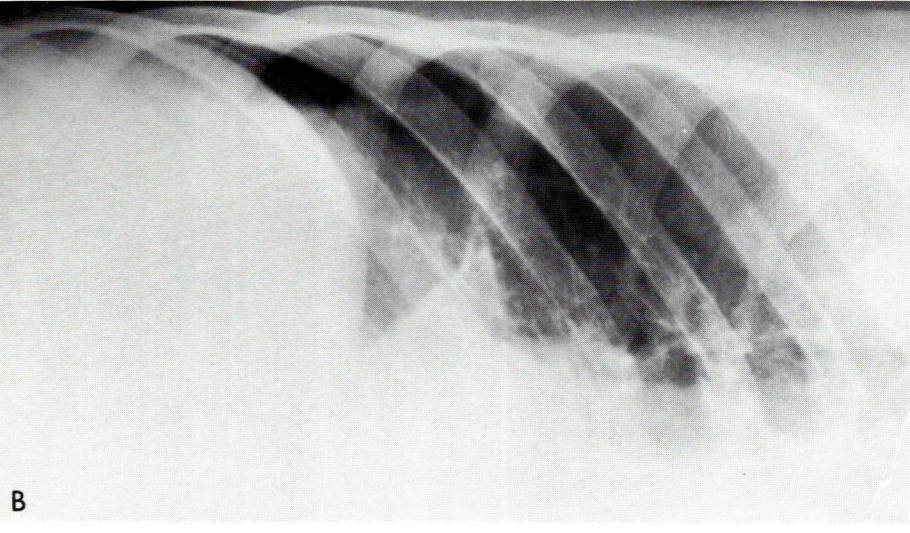

Figure 1–14. Pneumothorax. *A*, Arrows indicate multiple posterior rib fractures following trauma. No pneumothorax is seen on this supine radiograph. *B*, Left lateral decubitus film with horizontal central ray demonstrates a right pneumothorax at the costophrenic angle.

THE ACUTE CARE UNIT: RADIOGRAPHIC CONSIDERATIONS — 15

visualization of both a radiolucent zone without lung markings between the ribs and the pulmonary parenchyma *and* a thin radiodense line of the visceral pleural reflection. A horizontal-beam lateral examination of a supine patient may demonstrate air behind the sternum if a pneumothorax is present. This examination is difficult to interpret and should not be used routinely.

On supine or semi-erect radiographs or in radiographs of patients with pleural adhesions, pneumothorax may present as an atypical collection of air. It is not infrequent to see air in the costophrenic angle, between the diaphragm and the lung base, or in the pleural space along the mediastinum. The absence of air in these locations does not rule out a pneumothorax, however. Care must be taken not to confuse skin folds, tube tracks, or bullae with a pneumothorax (Fig. 1–15).

When a tension pneumothorax is suspected clinically, therapy is instituted without waiting for x-ray confirmation. Radiographic evidence of a tension pneumothorax includes a collapsed lung, a shift of the mediastinum to the opposite side (in a patient who is not rotated), and inversion of the diaphragm. Even in the presence of a tension pneumothorax, severe pulmonary consolidation or pleural adhesions may prevent complete lung collapse (Fig. 1–16).

Air in the mediastinum deflects the mediastinal pleura away from the mediastinum

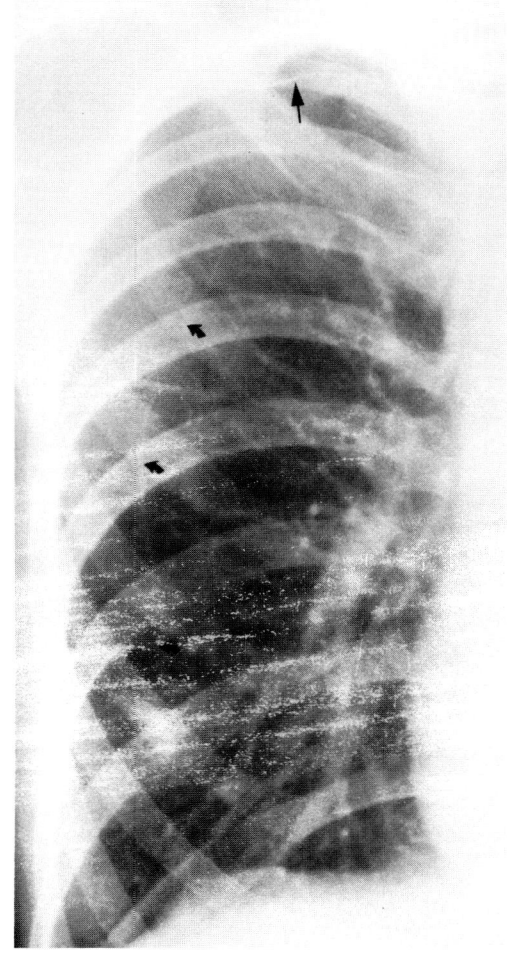

Figure 1–15. Tube tract. A white line of thickened pleura is seen parallel to the ribs (arrows). Pulmonary vessels are seen beyond the line, and a review of the previous day's radiograph showed a drainage tube in that location. A small pneumothorax is seen at the apex (upper arrow). (From Goodman, L. R., and Putman, C. E.: Intensive Care Radiology: Imaging of the Critically Ill. St. Louis, The C. V. Mosby Company, 1978.)

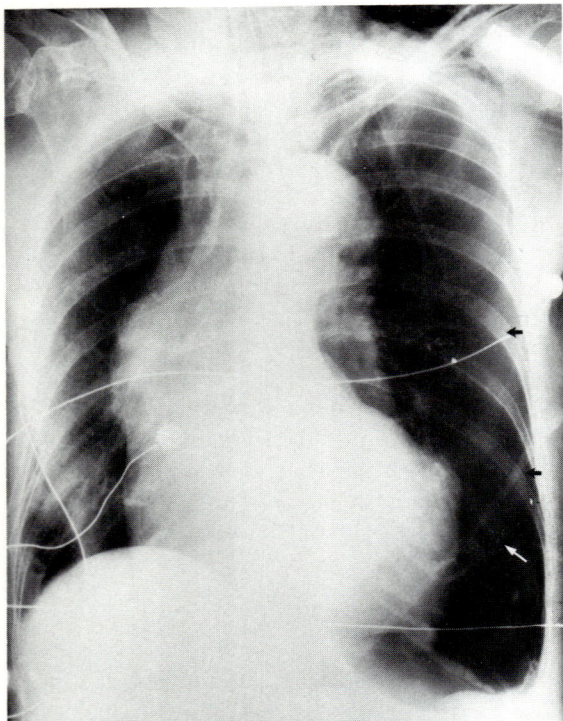

Figure 1–16. Tension pneumothorax. The diaphragm on the left is inverted and the mediastinum questionably shifted. Only the lower lung (arrows) collapsed, whereas adhesions prevented upper lobe collapse. Note the subcutaneous air in the neck. After insertion of a chest tube, the left diaphragm returned to normal.

and heart and is often associated with streaks of air in the soft tissues of the neck. The air may be homogenously lucent or bubbly in appearance and does not change with patient positioning. Subtle early signs of pneumomediastinum include a thin black crescent around the heart, aortic knob, or descending aorta. On the lateral film, the ascending aorta, great vessels, or thymus may be outlined by air.

Air in the subcutaneous tissues may be due to recent surgery, infection, or dissection from a pneumomediastinum or pneumothorax. Since the mediastinum is continuous with the soft-tissue planes in the neck and retroperitoneum, patients with pneumomediastinum may present with extrathoracic subcutaneous emphysema. Intraabdominal or retroperitoneal air may be particularly troublesome in the surgical patient because one must distinguish it from the free air of a perforated hollow viscus (see Fig. 1–13).[35] Patients with intraperitoneal or retroperitoneal air resulting from pulmonary barotrauma invariably have radiographic evidence of pneumomediastinum. Peritoneal or retroperitoneal air in the absence of a visible pneumomediastinum should not be ascribed to respirator-induced barotrauma.

Following the insertion of a chest tube, a small amount of air is normally seen in the soft tissues. This should diminish with time. A definite increase in air suggests a mechanical malfunction of the tube or the presence of a bronchopleural fistula leaking around the tube.

Atelectasis

The most frequent pulmonary abnormality in the surgical intensive care unit is atelectasis. Although varying degrees of atelectasis accompany any general anesthesia, it is most often seen following thoracic or upper abdominal surgery, in patients with preoperative lung disease, in smokers, and in obese or elderly patients.[31]

The radiographic appearance of atelectasis varies greatly. Most frequently, several irregular linear streaks of atelectasis (discoid) are visualized above the diaphragm. They vary with inspiration. Segmental or lobar consolidation or volume loss may also follow general anesthesia.[20, 31] This presents as a patchy or homogeneous infiltrate having a definite anatomic boundary. After left upper quadrant or cardiac surgery, left lower lobe atelectasis is especially common and easily overlooked behind the heart. Well-penetrated radiographs are required to visualize the infiltrate or to document elevation of the diaphragm with silhouetting of the diaphragm, retrocardiac vessels, or descending aorta (see Figs. 1–9 and 1–17).[19a, b]

Uncomplicated postoperative atelectasis usually responds dramatically to physical therapy and suctioning. The failure of radiographs to show improvement within 24 to 36 hours suggests the possibility of secondary infection or aspiration pneumonia.

Particularly vexing is the patient with severe postoperative deterioration of blood gases with evidence of shunting but with a relatively normal chest x-ray. In this instance, three major entities deserve consideration: pulmonary embolus, adult respiratory distress syndrome (ARDS), and microatelectasis.

A normal or near-normal lung scan rules out a pulmonary embolus.[33] The surgical history and subsequent physical, laboratory, and x-ray examinations confirm or rule out the presence of ARDS (see p. 20). When diagnoses of pulmonary embolus and ARDS have been excluded, microatelectasis is diagnosed. In this disorder, atelectasis is at the level of multiple peripheral airways, resulting in a relatively normal radiograph in spite of severe physiologic shunting.[20]

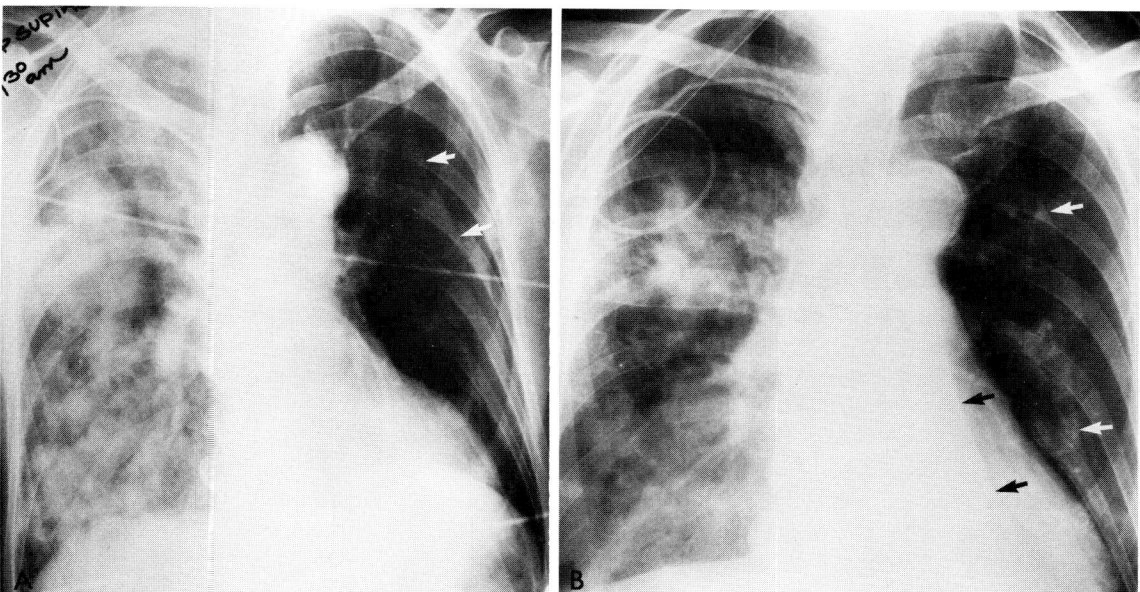

Figure 1–17. Postoperative aspiration. *A*, Radiograph approximately 12 hours after a large aspiration shows fluffy infiltrates involving the entire right lung. Note the skin fold on the left (arrows). *B*, Moderate clearing occurred over the next four days; however, the right upper and lower lobe infiltrates increased (gram negative enteric organisms stained and cultured). Note multiple skin folds on the left (white arrows) and total collapse of left lower lobe due to retained secretions (black arrows). The atelectasis cleared with suctioning and physical therapy. (From Goodman, L. R., The postoperative chest x-ray alterations following major abdominal surgery. Am. J. Roentgenol., March 1980.)

Aspiration Pneumonia

Numerous factors, such as vomiting, intratracheal intubation, nasogastric intubation, general anesthesia, and a depressed central nervous system, combine to make aspiration of gastric contents a frequent problem in the surgical intensive care unit. Gastric contents with a pH of less than 2.5 cause a chemical pneumonitis, often with dramatic clinical and radiographic features.[2, 7, 15a] As a general rule, the radiograph demonstrates a fluffy or patchy infiltrate within two to four hours of aspiration. The distribution of the infiltrate depends on the patient's position at the time of aspiration and on the volume of material aspirated. Infiltrates are most frequently seen in gravity-dependent segments. Massive aspiration may produce a diffuse, bilateral pulmonary edema, mimicking congestive heart failure; the cardiac silhouette is usually normal in size, however.

In uncomplicated aspiration pneumonia, the infiltrates often progress for the first 24 to 36 hours and then start to show progressive radiographic improvement (see Fig. 1–17A). Failure to show improvement of the infiltrate, or the recurrence of an infiltrate in that area, suggests secondary bacterial infection or retained particulate matter in that lobe or segment (see Fig. 1–17B). Retained food or foreign bodies may be silent initially and lead to local infection or abscess formation in the ensuing weeks.

Pneumonia

The diagnosis of pneumonia in the surgical patient is often difficult. Both the clinical and the radiographic appearances are often atypical, and differentiation from atelectasis, aspiration peneumonitis, edema, and so forth, may be difficult or impossible. Further complicating the diagnosis is the frequency of oropharyngeal colonization by pathogenic and nonpathogenic organisms and the presence of underlying cardiopulmonary diseases (chronic obstructive pulmonary disease [COPD], congestive heart failure [CHF], and others). Patients who acquire pneumonia while in the intensive care unit have a mortality rate as high as 50 per cent, the majority of deaths being due to gram-negative organisms.[38]

Unfortunately, there are no radiographic patterns that are specific for pulmonary infection. For a diagnosis of pneumonia to be made, a combination of fever, an increased white blood cell count, sputum rich in white blood cells, and a stable or progressive infiltrate on the chest x-ray must be observed.[6] Only by adherence to these requirements for diagnosis will the overdiagnosis of pneumonia be avoided. The radiograph is of value in monitoring the clearing of the infiltrate and checking for complications or superinfection. The radiologic clearing of the infiltrate usually lags behind the clinical resolution.

An additional problem in the intensive care unit is the compromised host. The patient's defense mechanisms may be altered by his primary disease, poor nutrition, or drug therapy. The spectrum of infection then includes both the expected pathogens and many opportunistic infections.[5, 39]

Pulmonary Edema

Exudation of fluid from the capillaries into the interstitium or alveoli of the lung is most often due to increased pulmonary venous pressure or increased capillary permeability. The most frequent cause of increased pulmonary venous pressure is left ventricular failure. Because of the effects of gravity on the pulmonary vascular circulation, every effort must be made to obtain upright films when one is evaluating for congestive heart failure. The upright film is a relatively sensitive indicator of the state of left heart function, and the radiograph correlates well with pulmonary capillary wedge pressure readings.[9, 21]

In the normal upright radiograph, the upper lobe pulmonary vessels are smaller than the lower lobe vessels and disappear in the outer third of the lung. As the pulmonary capillary wedge pressure increases into the range of 12 to 18 mm of mercury, the upper lobe vessels dilate, the lower lobe vessels decrease in size, and the pulmonary vessels appear in the outer third of the lung. As the pulmonary capillary wedge pressure increases to 18 to 22 mm of mercury, interstitial edema interferes with the normally sharp vessel-air interface, and the vessels and perihilar areas become fuzzy. Peribronchial edema thickens the bronchial walls. A further increase in wedge pressure causes fluid to enter the alveoli and presents as small, fluffy, or confluent infiltrates involving the middle and lower lung fields (see Figs. 1–3 and 1–11).[30] On the portable radiograph, pulmonary artery size, cardiomegaly, pleural effusions, and Kerley B lines are inconsistent findings and correlate poorly with pulmonary capillary wedge pressure.[9, 21] On the supine radiograph, upper lobe vascular dilatation is a normal finding and should not be confused with redistribution due to elevated left atrial pressure.

In the uncomplicated case, these criteria are reliable indicators of congestive heart failure. Under certain circumstances, pulmonary edema may have an atypical distribution, making the diagnosis difficult. Because edema is a gravity-dependent phenomenon, it may present in odd distributions in patients who have been confined to one position for a long period. Patients with disturbances of pulmonary capillary blood flow (COPD, pulmonary embolus) do not have edema in underperfused areas (Fig. 1–18).[8, 37] Noncardiogenic pulmonary edema (resulting from increased capillary perme-

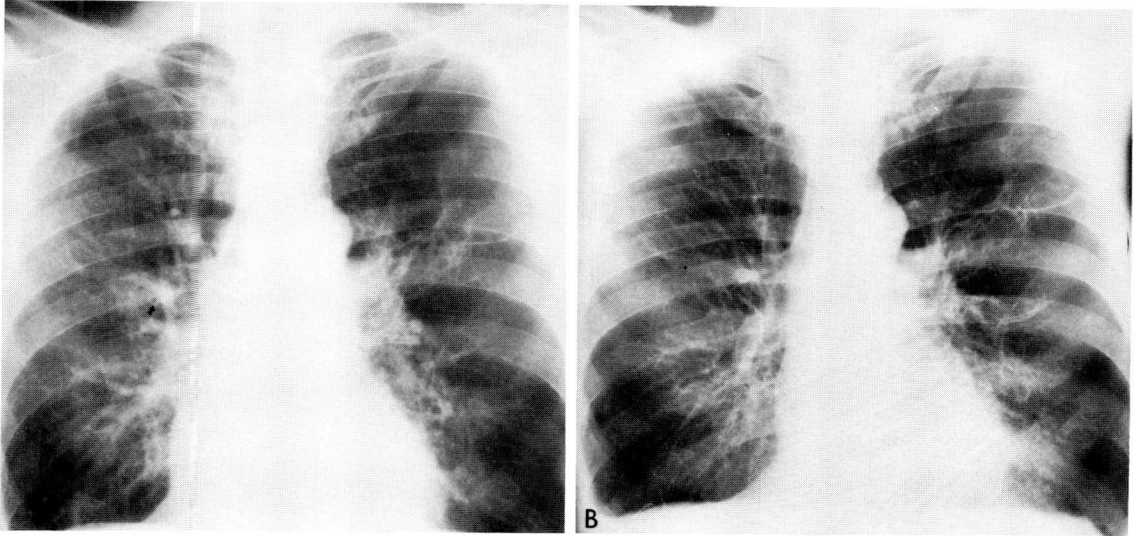

Figure 1–18. Atypical congestive heart failure (moderate). *A,* The right side demonstrates vascular redistribution, a plethora of indistinct hilar vessels, and a hazy midlung zone. There is peribronchial cuffing (arrow), and the adjacent artery is larger than the bronchus. Multiple bullae are seen on the left. The heart does not appear enlarged. *B,* Following therapy, there is marked improvement on the right and the heart is slightly smaller. The hilar vessels on the left are also more distinct.

TABLE 1–1. SYNONYMS FOR ADULT RESPIRATORY
DISTRESS SYNDROME

Shock lung
Wet lung
Post-traumatic pulmonary insufficiency
Congestive atelectasis
Progressive pulmonary insufficiency
DaNang lung
Adult hyaline membrane disease
Respirator lung
Oxygen toxicity
Pump lung

ability) may mimic many of the pulmonary changes of congestive heart failure. Vascular redistribution, pulmonary plethora, and cardiomegaly are usually absent, however. Frequent causes of noncardiac pulmonary edema include uremia, aspiration pneumonitis, sepsis, allergic reactions, fluid overload, and neurogenic disorders.[37]

Adult Respiratory Distress Syndrome

Adult respiratory distress syndrome (ARDS) refers to a characteristic combination of clinical, physiologic, and radiologic changes in the lungs following severe lung injury. Because of the greatly varying conditions that lead to adult respiratory distress syndrome, numerous names have been applied to it (Table 1–1). Thus, ARDS appears to be the final common pathway for numerous severe lung insults. Several excellent reviews of the syndrome have been published recently.[4, 25, 32] Although the radiographic changes in ARDS are nonspecific, when the temporal sequence of clinical and radiologic changes are correlated a definite picture emerges (Table 1–2). At the time of the initial systemic insult (shock, sepsis, surgery, and so forth) the lungs are normal clinically and radiologically. This is followed 24 to 36 hours later by the onset of tachypnea, dyspnea, cyanosis, and severe hypoxia. At this stage, the radiograph is still normal or demonstrates interstitial perihilar edema. Over the next 24 to 48 hours there is a further fall in oxygen saturation despite mechanical ventilation and oxygen administration (Fig. 1–19). During this period, the radiograph rapidly changes from a pattern of interstitial edema to a pattern of patchy, ill-defined alveolar infiltrates to one of confluent bilateral alveolar densities. After the development of bilateral diffuse infiltrates, the radiograph usually stabilizes and shows little change for many days.

TABLE 1–2. CONDITIONS LEADING TO ADULT RESPIRATORY
DISTRESS SYNDROME

Shock
Oxygen toxicity
Fluid overload
Emboli (fat, amniotic fluid, transfusions)
Sepsis
Chemical pneumonitis (aspiration, inhalation)
Trauma
Major surgery
Viral infection
Disseminated intravascular coagulopathy (DIC)
Bowel infarction

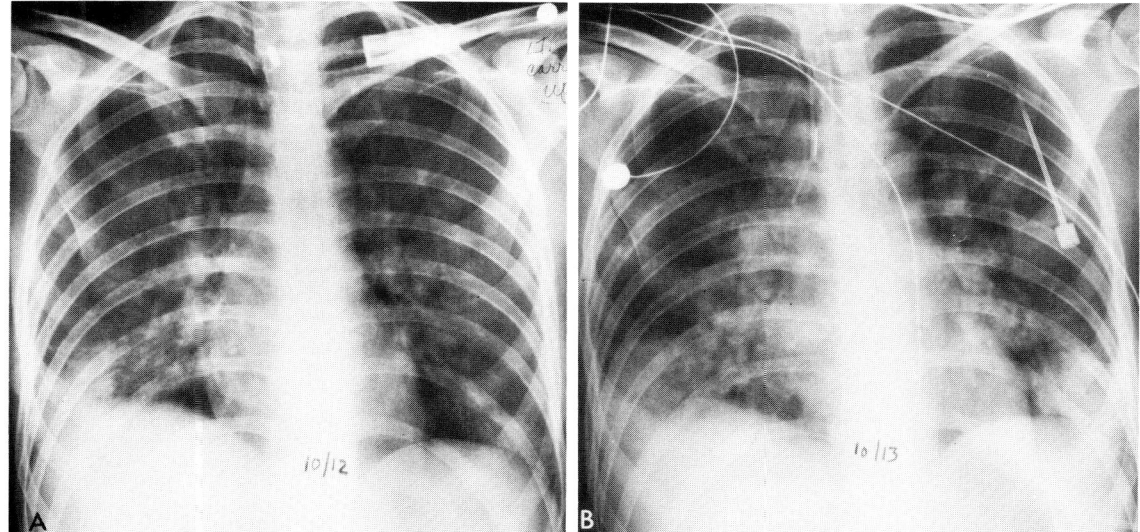

Figure 1–19. Adult respiratory distress syndrome (ARDS) developed following cesarean section. *A*, Film taken 36 to 48 hours after delivery shows bilateral perihilar edema, a right lower lobe infiltrate, and a normal-sized heart. *B*, The following day, the patchy infiltrates are more generalized. This picture remained unchanged for four days, then slowly cleared as the patient recovered.

As one follows the temporal sequence of events in ARDS, several important points emerge. During the initial stages, ARDS and massive pulmonary emboli with or without infarction are the two conditions most likely to result in dramatic symptoms and decreased oxygenation with a normal chest x-ray. A lung scan can eliminate the possibility of emboli (pulmonary embolus is discussed in detail in Chapter 20).[33] In the postanesthesia patient, microatelectasis must also be considered.

With a rapid onset of bilateral alveolar infiltrates, the radiograph may suggest left ventricular failure. However cardiomegaly and distention of the upper lobe vessels are not usually present. A pulmonary capillary wedge pressure measurement is often required to eliminate a component of congestive heart failure.

After the bilateral alveolar pattern is established on the x-ray, the bilateral pulmonary infiltrates stabilize. The relatively monotonous day-to-day radiograph is very suggestive of ARDS. Further deterioration of the chest x-ray at this point is usually the result of a secondary process, such as retained secretions, aspiration pneumonia, infection, or pulmonary barotrauma.

References

1. Archer, G., and Cobb, L. A.: Long-term pulmonary artery pressure monitoring in the management of the critically ill. Ann. Surg. *100*:747–752, 1974.
2. Bartlett, J. C., and Gorbach, S. L.: The triple threat of aspiration pneumonia. Chest *68*:560–566, 1975.
3. Bernard, R. W., and Stahl, W. M.: Subclavian vein catheterizations: a prospective study. Ann. Surg. *173*:181–190, 1973.
4. Blaisdell, F. W., and Schlobohm, R. M.: The respiratory distress syndrome: a review. Surgery *74*:251–262, 1973.
5. Blank, N., Castellino, R. V., and Shah, V.: Radiographic aspects of pulmonary infection in patients with altered immunity. Radiol. Clin. North Am. *11*:175–190, 1973.
6. Bryant, L. R., Mohin-Uddin, K., Dillon, M. L., et al.: Misdiagnosis of pneumonia in patients needing mechanical respiration. Arch. Surg. *106*:286–288, 1973.
7. Bynam, L. J., and Pierce, A. K.: Pulmonary aspiration of gastric contents. Am. Rev. Respir. Dis. *114*:1129–1136, 1976.
8. Calenoff, L. Kruglik, G. D., and Woodruff, A.: Unilateral pulmonary edema. Radiology *126*:53–56, 1978.
9. Chait, A., Cohen, H. E., Meltzer, L., et al.: The bedside chest x-ray in the evaluation of incipient congestive heart failure. Radiology *105*:563–566, 1972.

10. Conrardy, P. A., Goodman, L. R., Laing, F., et al.: Alteration of endotracheal tube position—flexion and extension of the neck. Crit. Care Med. 4:8–12, 1976.
11. Dane, T. E. B., and King, E. G.: Fatal cardiac tamponade and other mechanical complications of cardiovascular catheters. Br. J. Surg. 62:6–10, 1975.
12. Deitel, M., and McIntyre, J. A.: Radiographic confirmation of the site of central venous pressure catheters. Can. J. Surg. 14:42–52, 1972.
13. Doering, R. B., Stemmer, E. A., and Connolly, J. E.: Complications of indwelling venous catheters with particular reference to catheter embolus. Am. J. Surg. 114:259–266, 1967.
14. Foote, G. A., Schabel, S. I., and Hodges, M.: Pulmonary complications of the flow-directed balloon-tipped catheter. N. Engl. J. Med. 290:927–931, 1974.
15. Fraser, R. G., and Paré, J. A. P.: Diagnosis of Diseases of the Chest. Philadelphia, W. B. Saunders Company, 1970.
15a. Frock, J. L., Clark, T. S., et al.: Aspiration pneumonia: a ten year review. Am. Surg., 45:305–313, 1979.
16. Glickman, M.: Special procedures. In Goodman, L. R., and Putman, C. E.: Intensive Care Radiology: Imaging of the Critically Ill. St. Louis, The C. V. Mosby Company, 1978.
17. Goodenough, D., and Weaver, K.: Physical aspects of the portable radiograph. In Goodman, L. R., and Putman, C. E.: Intensive Care Radiology: Imaging of the Critically Ill. St. Louis, The C. V. Mosby Company, 1978.
18. Goodman, L. R., Conrardy, P. A., Laing, F., et al.: Radiographic evaluation of endotracheal tube position. Am. J. Roentgenol. Radium Ther. Nucl. Med. 127:433–434, 1976.
19. Goodman, L. R., and Putman, C. E.: Intensive Care Radiology: Imaging of the Critically Ill. St. Louis, The C. V. Mosby Company, 1978.
19a. Goodman, L. R.: The post-operative chest x-ray: alterations following major intrathoracic surgery. Am. J. Roentgenol. March 1980.
19b. Goodman, L. R.: The post-operative chest x-ray: alterations following abdominal surgery. Am. J. Roentgenol. March 1980.
20. Hamilton, W. K.: Atelectasis, pneumothorax and aspiration as postoperative complications. Anesthesiology 22:708–722, 1961.
21. Harrison, M. O., Conte, P. J., and Heitzman, E. R.: Radiological detection of clinically occult cardiac failure following myocardial infarction. Br. J. Radiol. 44:265–272, 1971.
22. Hawkins, D. B., Seltzer, D. C., Barnett, T. E., et al.: Endotracheal tube perforation of the hypopharynx. West. J. Med. 120:282–286, 1974.
23. Henzel, J. H., and DeWeese, M. S.: Morbid and mortal complications associated with prolonged central venous cannulation: awareness, recognition and prevention. Am. J. Surg. 121:600–605, 1971.
24. Hipona, F. A., Sciammas, F. D., and Hublitz, U. F.: Non-thoracotomy retrieval of intraluminal cardiovascular foreign bodies: Clinical and experimental aspects. Radiol. Clin. North Am. 9:583–596, 1971.
25. Joffee, N.: The adult respiratory distress syndrome. Am. J. Roentgenol. Radium Ther. Nucl. Med. 122:719–731, 1974.
26. King, K., Mandava, B., and Kamin, J. M.: Tracheal tube cuffs and tracheal dilatation. Chest 67:458–462, 1975.
27. Langston, C. S.: Aberrant central venous catheters and its complications. Radiology 100:55–59, 1971.
28. McLoud, T. C., and Putman, C. E.: Radiology of Swan-Ganz catheter and associated pulmonary complications. Radiology 116:19–22, 1975.
29. McLoud, T. C., Barash, P. G., and Ravin, C. E.: PEEP: radiographic features and associated complications. Am. J. Roentgenol. Radium Ther. Nucl. Med. 129:209–214, 1977.
30. McHugh, J. J., Forrester, J. S., Adler, L., et al.: Pulmonary vascular congestion in acute myocardial infarction. Ann. Intern. Med. 76:29–33, 1972.
31. Pierce, A. K., and Robertson, J.: Pulmonary complications of general surgery. Annu. Rev. Med. 28:211–221, 1977.
32. Putman, C. E., Minagi, H., and Blaisdell, F. W.: Roentgen appearance of disseminated intravascular coagulation. Radiology 109:12–18, 1972.
33. Putman, C. E.: Adult respiratory distress syndrome. In Goodman, L. R., and Putman, C. E.: Intensive Care Radiology: Imaging of the Critically Ill. St. Louis, The C. V. Mosby Company, 1978.
34. Ravin, C. E., Putman, C. E., and McLoud, T. C.: Hazards of the I. C. U. Am. J. Roentgenol. Radium Ther. Nucl. Med. 126:423–431, 1976.
35. Rohlfing, B., Webb, W. R., and Schlobohm, R. M.: Ventilator-related extra-alveolar air in adults. Radiology 121:25–31, 1976.
36. Swan, H. J. C., and Ganz, W.: Use of balloon flotation catheters in critically ill patients. Surg. Clin. North Am. 55:501–520, 1975.
37. Shapiro, J. H., and Hublitz, U. F.: The radiology of pulmonary edema: four decades of observation, clinical correlations, and studies of the underlying pathophysiology. CRC Crit. Rev. Clin. Radiol. Nucl. Med. 5:389–422, 1974.
38. Stevens, R. M., Teres, D., Skillman, J. J., et al.: Pneumonia in an intensive care unit. Arch. Intern. Med. 134:106–111, 1974.
39. Williams, D. M., Krick, J. A., and Remington, J. S.: Pulmonary infection in the compromised host. Am. Rev. Respir. Dis. 114:359–394, 593–628, 1976.
39a. Zimmerman, J. E., Goodman, L. R., and Shahuari, M. B. G.: Effect of mechanical ventilation and positive end expiratory pressure (PEEP) on chest radiography. Am. J. Roentgenol. 133:811–815, 1979.
40. Zwillich, C. W., Pierson, D. J., Creagh, C. T., et al.: Complications of assisted ventilation. Am. J. Med. 57:161–170, 1974.

2

RADIOISOTOPE TECHNIQUES

LETTY G. LUTZKER, M.D.
LEONARD M. FREEMAN, M.D.

Radionuclide imaging has become quite sophisticated in the last several years. With modern technology, a large variety of radiopharmaceuticals, and increasing awareness of pharmacokinetics in normal and disease states, the number of clinical applications has increased.

A radioactive tracer is introduced, usually into the patient's peripheral venous system, but occasionally into another site, such as the bladder or subarachnoid space. Tracer localization may occur by one or more of several metabolic or physical mechanisms: active transport, phagocytosis, cell sequestration, capillary blockage, simple or exchange diffusion, compartmental localization, and antigen-antibody reaction (Table 2–1). Detection of the gamma radiations emitted from the site or sites of localization provides functional information about the organ or system.

TABLE 2–1. MECHANISMS OF RADIOPHARMACEUTICAL LOCALIZATION

Active Transport
  Thyroid: isotopes of iodine, ^{99m}Tc-pertechnetate
  Salivary gland: ^{99m}Tc-pertechnetate
  Liver: ^{131}I-rose bengal, ^{99m}Tc-hepatobiliary agents
  Myocardium: ^{201}Tl, ^{43}K
  Kidney: ^{131}I-orthoiodohippurate, ^{99m}Tc-glucoheptonate, ^{99m}Tc-DmSA
  Abscess and Tumor: ^{67}Ga-citrate
  Marrow: ^{111}In-chloride
Phagocytosis
  Reticuloendothelial: ^{99m}Tc-sulfur colloid, ^{113m}In-colloid
  Thrombus or infection: labeled leukocytes
Cell Sequestration
  Spleen: Heat-damaged ^{51}Cr or ^{99}Tc-labeled red blood cells
Capillary Blockage
  Lung: ^{99m}Tc-labeled macroaggregates and microspheres
Simple or Exchange Diffusion
  Bone: ^{18}F, ^{85}Sr, ^{87m}Sr
  Brain: all common agents
  Kidney: ^{99m}Tc-DTPA
  Lung: ^{133}Xe ventilation studies
Physiochemical Adsorption
  Bone: ^{99m}Tc-labeled phosphates
  Thrombi: Radiofibrinogen, ^{99m}Tc-MAA and microspheres
Compartmental Localization
  Cardiovascular blood pool: ^{99m}Tc-labeled albumin and red cells
  First-pass flow studies: ^{99M}TcO$_4$ or ^{99m}Tc-labeled agents

TABLE 2–2. ADULT PATIENT RADIATION DOSE FROM COMMON IMAGING PROCEDURES

Procedure and Agent	Usual Administered Dose (mCi)	Radiation Dose (Rads)	
		Target Organ	*Whole Body*
BRAIN SCAN			
^{99m}Tc O$_4$	15	3 (colon)	0.2
^{99m}Tc-DTPA	15	5 (bladder)	0.2
		0.5 (kidney)	
^{99m}Tc-glucoheptonate	15	2.3 (kidney)	0.15
CISTERNOGRAPHY			
^{111}In-DTPA	1.0	6–12 (cord)	0.5–0.3
LUNG SCAN			
^{99m}Tc-mAA or microspheres	3	0.6 (lung)	0.1
^{133}Xe	10–15	0.1–0.2	0.002
CARDIOVASCULAR SCANNING			
^{201}Tl	1.5	2.2 (kidneys)	0.4
		1 (liver, thyroid)	
		0.8 (gonads)	
^{99m}Tc-HSA or RBC	20	1.0 (blood)	
^{99m}Tc-phosphates	15	0.6 (bone)	0.2
THYROID SCAN			
^{131}I uptake	.005	7.5	0.0001–0.02
scan	.05	75.0	0.001–0.2 (depending on uptake)
^{123}I uptake and scan	0.1–0.3	1.5–4.5	0.003
^{99m}Tc O$_4$	1–2	0.4	0.02
LIVER-BILIARY TRACT–SPLEEN SCAN			
^{99m}Tc-sulfur colloid	2	1 (liver)	0.06
^{51}Cr-heated red blood cells	0.1–0.3	4–10 (spleen)	0.05
^{99m}Tc-HIDA	5–10	– (biliary, liver)	
BONE SCAN			
^{99m}Tc-phosphates	15	0.6 (bone)	0.2
KIDNEY SCAN			
^{99m}Tc-DTPA	15	5 (bladder)	0.2
		0.5 (kidney)	
^{99m}Tc-glucoheptonate	15	2–3 (kidney)	0.15
^{99m}Tc-DMSA	5	6 (kidney)	0.07
^{131}I-orthoiodohippurate	0.3	0.3 (kidney)	0.01
		5 (bladder)	
TUMOR AND ABSCESS LOCALIZATION			
^{67}Ga-citrate	5	4.5 (colon)	1.0
^{67}Ga-citrate	5	2.5 (skeleton, liver, marrow, spleen)	

The emitted radiation is detected by a phosphorescent crystal which, when leaving the state of excitation to which it is raised by the entering radiation, emits light proportional in amount to the energy of the initial impinging radiation. The crystal is coupled to a number of photomultiplier tubes that increase the size of the signal exiting at the end of the series of tubes. This signal may be used to obtain an image of the initial radiation distribution on x-ray or Polaroid film or on a video screen. The information may also be collected by a computer or data processor for later retrieval and manipulation. The detector may be placed in a scanning arm, which moves across the patient until the area of interest is covered, or in a gamma camera, which is a stationary imaging device. The latter has largely replaced the rectilinear scanner as the basic radionuclide imaging instrument. There is no study the scanner can perform that cannot be done on the camera, often more quickly, and there are several studies that only the camera can do.

Static images can be obtained on either the camera or the scanner. These are pictorial displays of the distribution of radioactivity fixed to an organ or tissue, such as the liver, the skeleton, and so forth. Dynamic imaging, or scintiangiography, requires rapid-sequence images, often of a fraction of a second, during which the transit of a radioactive bolus through a vessel or organ can be monitored.

The images obtained, even under the best of technical circumstances, are of relatively low resolution compared to those of standard radiography. However, the functional information obtained is well beyond the capabilities of radiologic examinations, which supply primarily morphologic data. The examinations are most productive when the nuclear physician is an active participant in the clinical dialogue, aware of the specific information desired from the study. The specificity of radionuclide imaging is enhanced by interpretation in the total clinical context. In many cases, obtaining a normal scan may make further tests unnecessary.

The functional aspect of nuclear imaging is one of its major advantages over more anatomic modalities, such as conventional radiography and contrast studies, ultrasound, and CT scanning, all of which are complementary procedures. Another advantage is the totally noninvasive nature of these tests; allergic or toxic reactions are virtually nonexistent, and the tracer doses used do not affect normal physiologic states. A third advantage, in many instances, is the greater sensitivity of radionuclide imaging compared with other modalities in the early detection of pathologic states. With current radiopharmaceuticals, the radiation dose to the patient is low, usually the equivalent or less than that of conventional radiography, and in almost all cases less than that of contrast angiography (Table 2–2).

CENTRAL NERVOUS SYSTEM SCINTIGRAPHY

For brain scintigraphy, the renal agents ^{99m}Tc-DTPA and ^{99m}Tc-glucoheptonate are fast replacing ^{99m}Tc-pertechnetate because of better background clearance. Normally, an effective blood-brain barrier prevents entry of these radiopharmaceuticals into the brain tissue, so the study is more properly called non-brain scintigraphy. When the blood-brain barrier is compromised by neoplasm, vascular accident, arteriovenous malformation, or intra- or extracerebral hematoma, the radiopharmaceutical leaks by simple or exchange diffusion into the abnormal area and becomes visible on the scintigram.

Cerebral radionuclide angiography is rapid sequential imaging obtained immediately after bolus injection of the radiopharmaceutical, providing an index of carotid and cerebral blood flow (Fig. 2–1). With data processing, relative flow to a hemisphere or lesion can be quantitated.

The typical findings in various brain disorders are summarized in Table 2–3. The brain scan is most helpful in the initial diagnosis of vascular lesions and in the evaluation of their response to medical or surgical treatment. When the primary diagnosis is neoplasm, CT scanning is probably a more appropriate screening test.

The configuration of abnormal activity on a static image is usually not a reliable indicator of the nature of the lesion. Strokes may be as round as tumors and abscesses, although it is rare for the latter to be wedge-shaped and to reach the periphery (Fig. 2–2). Meningioma may sometimes be suspected by a typical location adjacent to the falx, sphenoid ridge, or parasagittal region. The "doughnut sign," a circle of increased activity surrounding a cold center, was once thought to be typical of a malignant glioma

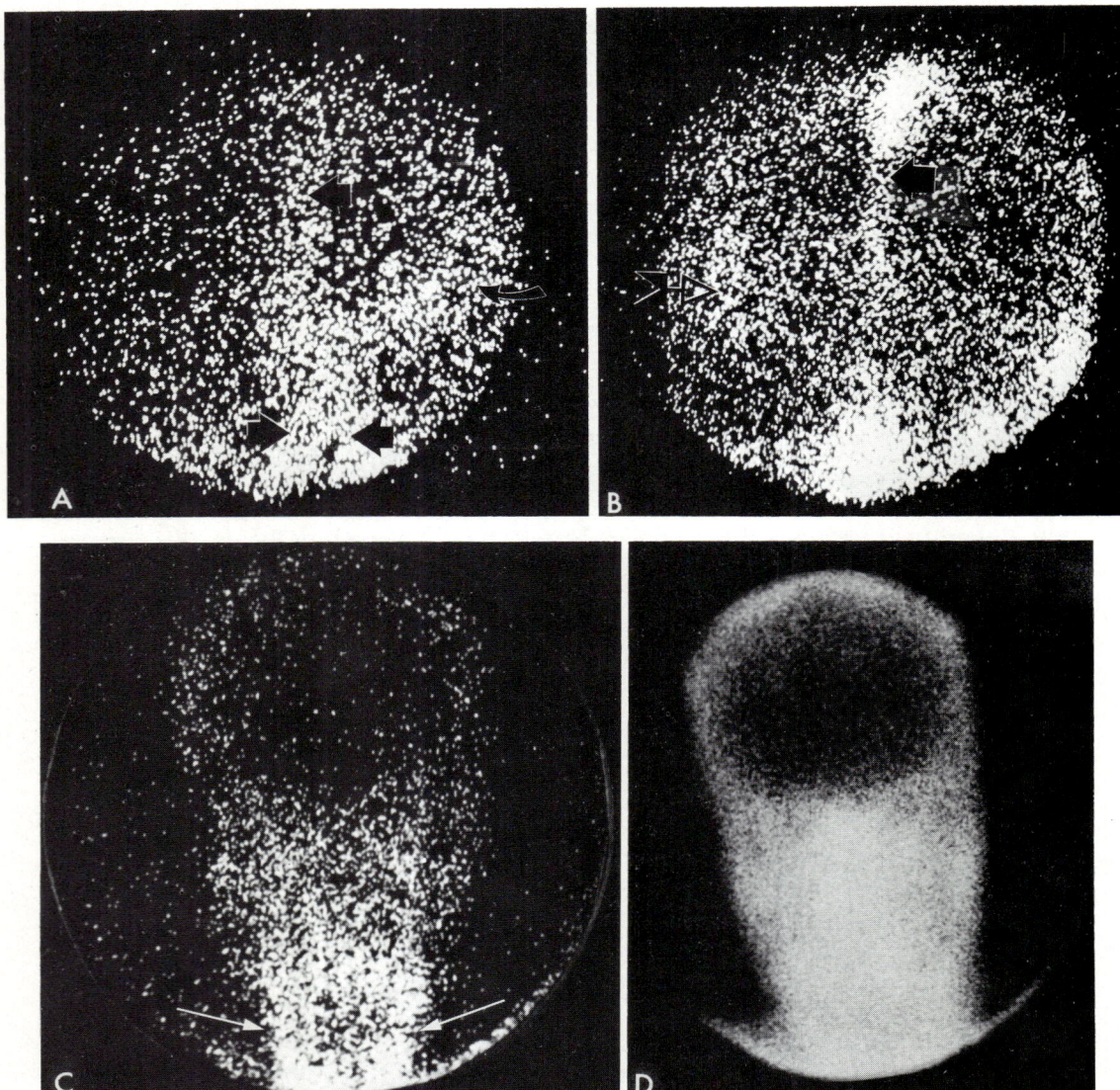

Figure 2–1. Abnormalities of cerebral blood flow. *A* and *B*, In a patient with a right-sided stroke, flow is normal in the right and left carotid arteries, left middle cerebral artery, and anterior cerebral arteries (*A*, arrows) but absent in the right middle cerebral artery in the early arterial phase. In the venous phase, normal activity is present in the sagittal sinus (*B*, closed arrow), and the left middle cerebral artery has emptied. Abnormal late filling of the right middle cerebral artery territory is the "flip-flop phenomenon" typical of cerebrovascular disease (open arrow). *C* and *D*, In brain death, carotid flow is intact bilaterally (*C*, arrows) but no intracerebral flow is seen early and no sagittal sinus return is seen even on the postdynamic static view *(D)*. In arteriovenous malformation, abnormally intense activity is seen early in the arterial phase.

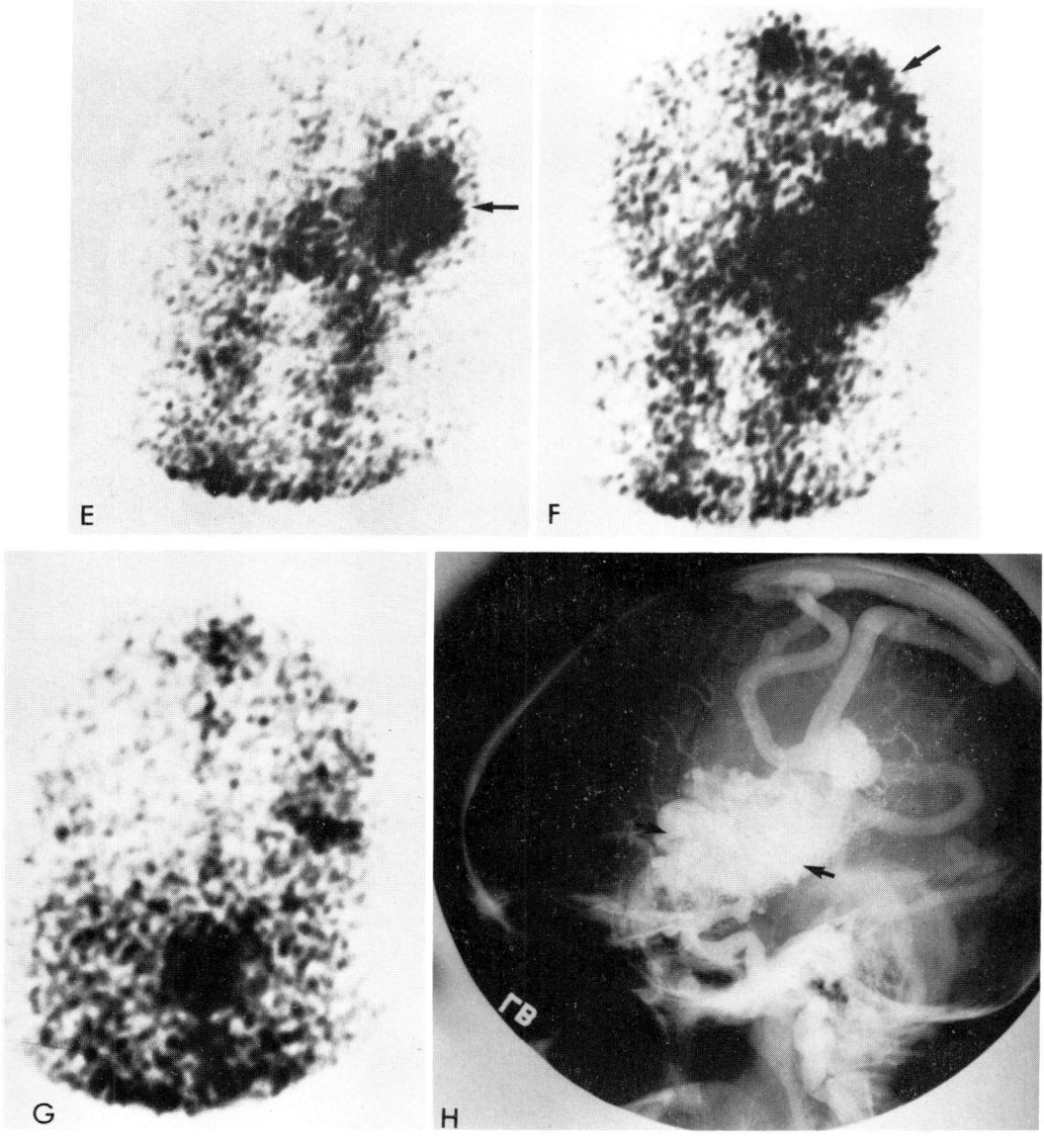

Figure 2–1 *Continued.* (*E*, arrow). Even more activity is present in the venous phase, with a large draining vein seen over the left convexity (*F*, arrow), and activity has diminished by late dynamic view (*G*). The left lateral film from the angiogram shows arteriovenous malformation (*H*, arrows).

TABLE 2–3. CHARACTERISTIC RADIOGRAPHIC FINDINGS IN BRAIN DISORDERS

	Dynamic (Flow)	Immediate Static (Activity)	Delayed Static (Activity)
Cerebrovascular accident	↓	N ↑	↑
Malignant glioma	↑	↑	↑ ↑
Astrocytoma	N	N ↑	↑
Meningioma	↑	↑	↑ ↑
Metastases	N	N ↑	↑ (multiple)
Arteriovenous malformation	↑	↑ ↑	↑ N
Abscess	N ↑	↑	↑ ↑
Extracerebral hematoma	Edge defect	Edge defect	↑ Vascular rim

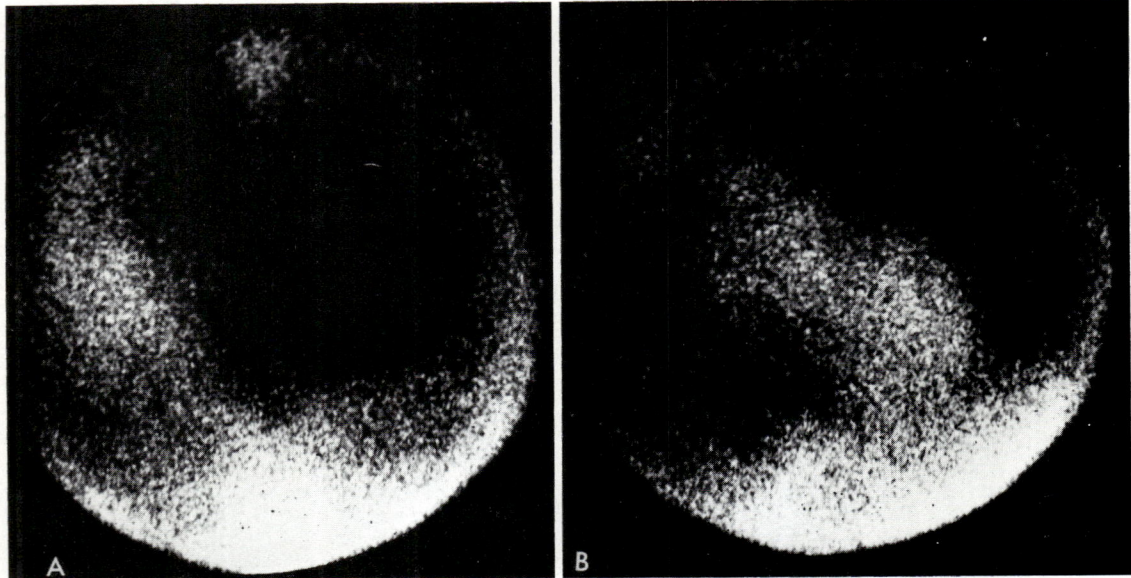

Figure 2–2. Left cerebrovascular accident. Anterior *(A)* and right lateral *(B)* images two hours after injection in the same patient as in Figure 2–1, *A* and *B*. Abnormal right parietal activity accumulates in the area of damaged blood-brain barrier.

(Fig. 2–3). However, this sign has since been observed in abscess, other tumors, infarcts, extracerebral hematomas, and postoperative skull lesions. It implies that the central portion of the lesion is less vascular than the outer portion, which may be useful information for the neurosurgeon.

The presence of multiple brain lesions in the appropriate clinical context suggests the diagnosis of metastasis. However, it is rare to find a positive brain scintigram in the absence of clinical symptoms or focal neurologic findings. The brain scintigram is

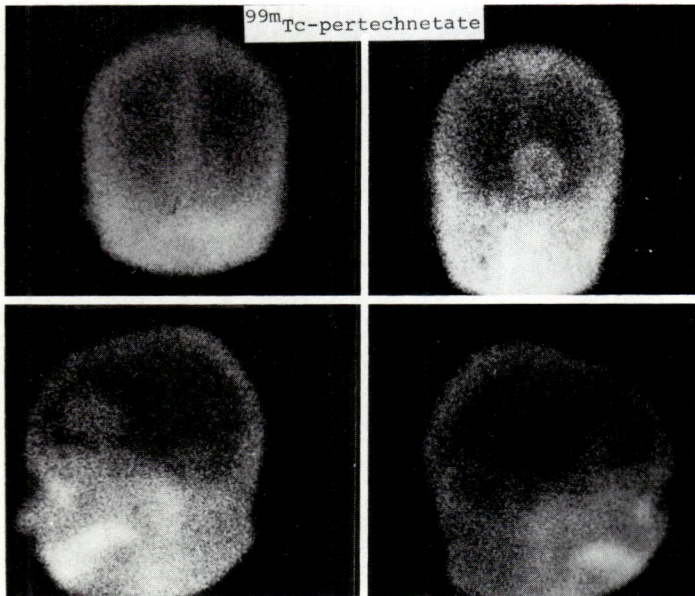

Figure 2–3. Doughnut lesion. This was a glioblastoma multiforme. Other lesions may look identical (see text).

therefore not a reasonable screening test for occult metastases, in contrast to the situation with bone and liver imaging, in which occult disease is found frequently enough to justify its use as a screening procedure.

The second radionuclide imaging procedure for evaluation of the central nervous system is radionuclide cisternography, performed after intrathecal instillation of indium-111-DTPA, which has replaced iodinated human serum albumin as the radiopharmaceutical of choice. After its introduction into the spinal subarachnoid space, the pharmaceutical ascends to the basal cisterns and around the convexities of the brain, from where it is absorbed into the blood stream. Images are obtained shortly after injection, to ensure entry into the subarachnoid rather than the epidural or subdural space, and again at 6, 24, and usually 48 hours. This procedure is useful in the localization of cerebrospinal fluid leaks and sometimes in the determination of those patients with known communicating hydrocephalus who might benefit from shunt procedures (Fig. 2–4).

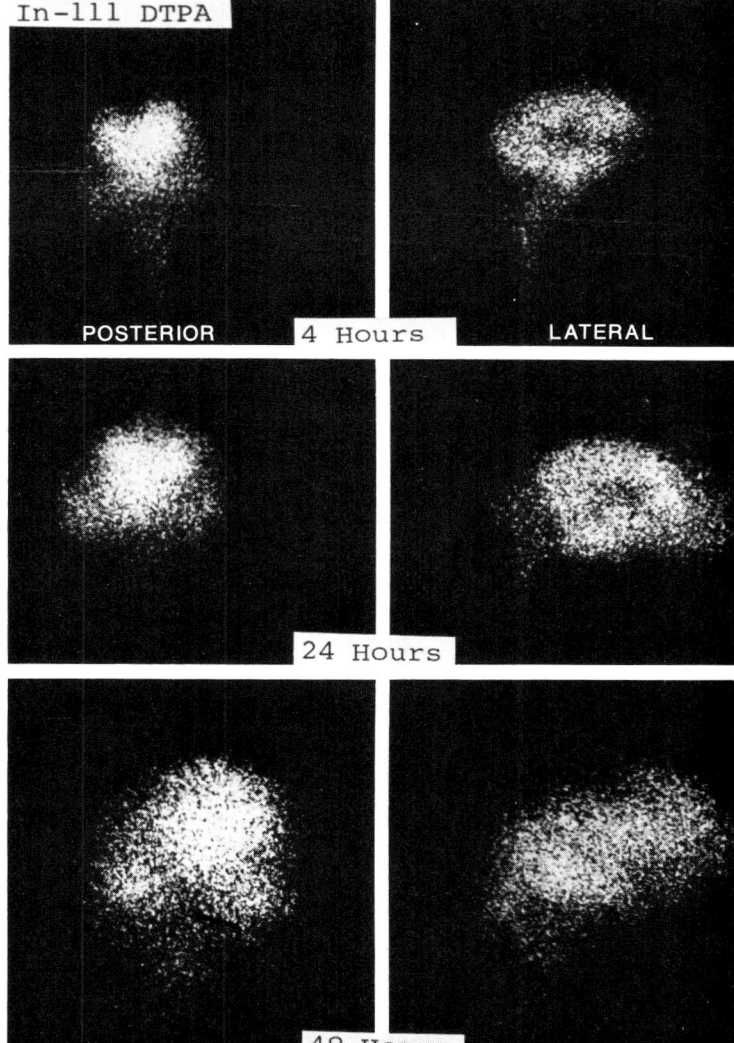

Figure 2–4. Ventricular reflux and delayed clearance on cisternogram. The lateral ventricles can be seen on both posterior and lateral images at 4 and 24 hours after instillation of radioactivity. No clearance over the convexities has occurred even by 48 hours.

THYROID IMAGING

It is possible to follow the active transport of iodide into the thyroid gland, which traps it and organifies it by binding to tyrosine residues to produce thyroid hormones. If a tracer dose of known size is administered, radioactive iodine uptake can be measured 24 hours later. The normal thyroid accumulates from 5 to 35 per cent of the administered dose. Uptakes below or above this level are abnormal but not specific for a particular disease state. Imaging can be performed while the radioactive iodine is in the thyroid gland. Today, I-123 is the agent of choice because of its more favorable dosimetry (16 mrads per μCi compared with 1500 mr per μCi for I-131). The routine use of iodine-131 for imaging can no longer be justified except for the diagnosis of functioning metastases in patients with known thyroid carcinoma, for which it is the agent of choice. ^{99m}Tc-pertechnetate is trapped but not organified by the thyroid gland and can be used for thyroid imaging when iodine uptake is low or time is short, because large doses can be administered. It is used routinely in many laboratories. However, one major problem is that some hypofunctioning nodules on iodine imaging may appear to function normally on pertechnetate imaging (discordant nodules).

The traditional rectilinear thyroid scan projects a life-size image of the gland. Technical artifacts, such as improper selection of background level, may cause the gland to appear larger or smaller than it really is. Also, nodules less than 1 cm may be invisible. Gamma camera imaging with the pinhole collimator eliminates problems of background artifact and produces images of somewhat higher resolution. Oblique views can be obtained. Glands with low uptake are more easily imaged, and a gland that is partially suppressed in the presence of a functioning nodule may still be visible on the gamma camera image, making a thyroid stimulation test unnecessary.

The major indications for thyroid imaging are (1) evaluation of masses in the neck, base of the tongue, or mediastinum; (2) assessment of thyroid nodule function; and (3) diagnosis of functioning thyroid metastases. The single most important use of the thyroid scan is the evaluation of palpable or suspected thyroid nodules. Nodules are classified as "cold" (nonfunctioning or with less activity than the surrounding gland) (Fig. 2–5), "warm" (functioning but not necessarily hotter than the surrounding gland), or "hot" (with more activity than the surrounding tissue).

Virtually all hot and warm nodules are benign, although there are occasional cases of malignancy in functioning nodules. Five to 25 per cent of hypofunctioning nodules contain malignancy, but many of these are clinically suspected; malignancy rarely occurs in the smooth, mobile, nonfixed nodule that is stable in size during a long follow-up period. Administration of T-4 or T-3 as suppressive thyroid therapy causes many benign nodules to regress in size. Continuing enlargement on therapy or the presence of tracheal or esophageal compression is an indication for surgery. Ultrasound can provide further information as to whether the lesion is cystic, and therefore most probably benign, or solid, in which case biopsy may be indicated.

In recent years, an increased incidence of thyroid carcinoma has been reported in patients who received external head and neck irradiation in childhood or adolescence for such conditions as thymus or tonsil enlargement or acne. Routine thyroid scanning has been suggested in order to find occult carcinoma in these patients. The significance of finding nonpalpable small nodules is not clear, and the role of this diagnostic modality in these patients is not established. There is as yet no convincing evidence that internal thyroid irradiation, after radioactive iodine therapy for hyperthyroidism or functioning nodules, causes thyroid cancer.

For functioning problems, correlation of the radioactive iodine uptake, scan, and serum levels of thyroid hormones and thyroid-stimulating hormone (TSH) is necessary

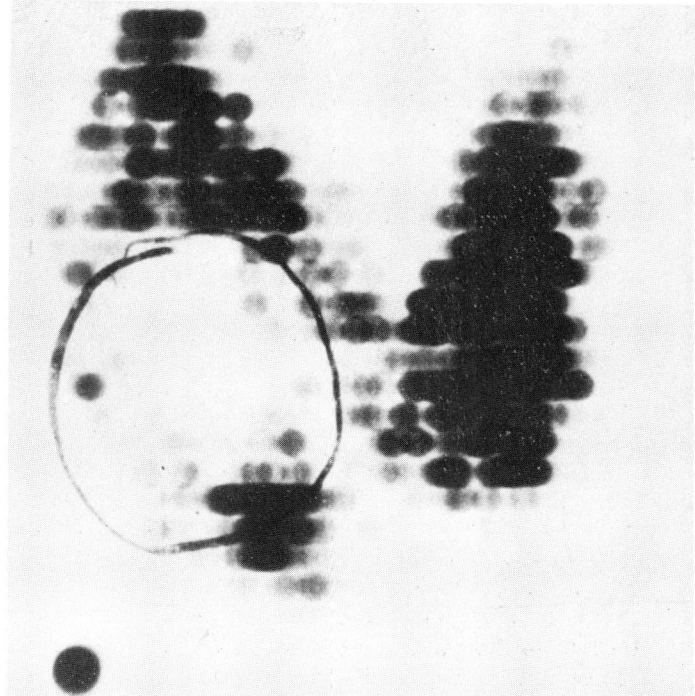

Figure 2–5. Cold thyroid nodule.

for final diagnosis. The uptake may be spuriously elevated or depressed from several causes:

1. Previous administration of iodide, of which the examiner is unaware, depresses the uptake. One of the most common offenders is radiographic contrast media. Following injection the uptake evaluation may not be valid for several weeks to several months.

2. Ongoing medication for thyroid problems with perchlorate, propylthiouracil, and thyroid hormone itself depresses the uptake.

3. Patients who suffer dietary iodine deprivation because of geographic location may have elevated radioactive iodine uptakes and clinical goiter despite being euthyroid clinically

4. In different phases of thyroiditis, radioactive iodine uptake may be low, normal, or high and out of phase with the level of serum thyroid hormone.

For the diagnosis of metastatic thyroid carcinoma, particularly of the well-differentiated follicular type, ablation of the normal thyroid and primary tumor must be accomplished first. Exogenous TSH may be administered, but some investigators rely on the endogenous TSH stimulation caused by the hypothyroid state. One to two mCi of iodine-131 are administered, and total-body imaging is performed 48 to 72 hours later (Fig. 2–6).

Radioactive iodine is used for therapy of Graves' disease or diffuse toxic goiter (in a range of 4 to 10 mCi), autonomous nodules (in a range of 20 to 30 mCi), and functioning thyroid carcinoma metastases or residual thyroid after ablation (in a range of 100 mCi).

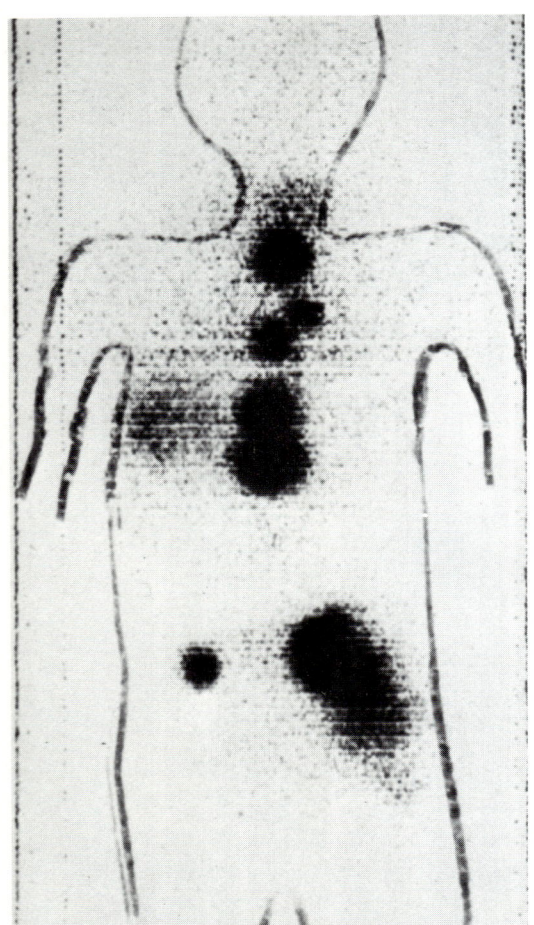

Figure 2–6. Thyroid carcinoma metastases. Seventy-two hours after administration of 1 mCi of ^{131}I, there are multiple areas of accumulation in the sternum, right lung, and pelvis as well as local extension on the neck.

CARDIOVASCULAR SCINTIGRAPHY

Cardiac Studies

Many radionuclide tests are now available for the evaluation of the heart. They fall generally into four groups: (1) dynamic "first pass" radiocardiography, (2) gated blood pool studies, (3) myocardial perfusion imaging, and (4) myocardial infarct imaging. "First pass" radiocardiography is a refinement of dynamic imaging that often requires the addition of data processing capability to the gamma camera. An early use of radiocardiography was the detection of pericardial effusion. Separation of the cardiac blood pool from lung and liver activity creates the appearance of a "halo" around the heart when fluid is present. This test has been replaced by ultrasound examination, which can detect effusions of 50 to 75 ml, as compared with 100 to 150 ml for the radionuclide test. The study may be used for the detection and quantitation of intracardiac shunts in congenital heart disease. Patients suspected of such lesions may be screened for cardiac catheterization by this method, and if cardiac catheterization has already been performed the study may be used to follow the patient noninvasively.

If a very rapid frame rate is used, such that each cycle is broken into 20 to 30 segments, the examination can quantitate left ventricular ejection fraction. This is achieved by obtaining end-diastolic and end-systolic count rates and inserting these data into the formula

$$\frac{\text{end-diastolic counts minus end-systolic counts}}{\text{end-diastolic counts}}$$

The dynamics of the right ventricle can best be studied by this method since right ventricular activity is temporally separate from left.

Blood pool studies are performed after injection of an agent that remains confined to the vascular space, usually human serum albumin or red blood cells labeled *in vivo* or *in vitro* with technetium-99m. An electrocardiographic "gate" is used to trigger the acquisition of imaging data, so that separate images of end-systole and end-diastole can be obtained, or each cardiac cycle can be broken up into a predetermined number of segments with the images from several cycles then being totaled. The data from either method can be displayed as a moving picture of the beating heart for evaluation of wall motion abnormalities. As with the first pass method, the activity levels can be counted for determination of ejection fraction. Since the radiopharmaceutical remains relatively intact for several hours, imaging can be repeated after pharmacologic intervention to improve cardiac function, without the need for a second injection. The data compare favorably with those obtained from contrast ventriculography, and the studies are obviously far less invasive and can be repeated more frequently (Fig. 2–7).

Myocardial perfusion imaging is most commonly performed with thallium-201. Thallium, a potassium analog, enters the myocardial cell via the sodium-potassium-ATPase pump but remains within the cell somewhat longer than does potassium. The amount of activity in a particular area of myocardium is proportional to its regional perfusion. Because the left ventricle receives a much higher share of coronary perfusion than the right, only the former is seen on resting thallium imaging except in cases of right ventricular overload. During exercise, both left and right ventricular perfusion is increased, and the right ventricle may be seen.

Thallium imaging is most usefully performed in conjunction with a treadmill stress test. When the patient has reached maximal exercise, 1 to 2 mCi are injected, and the

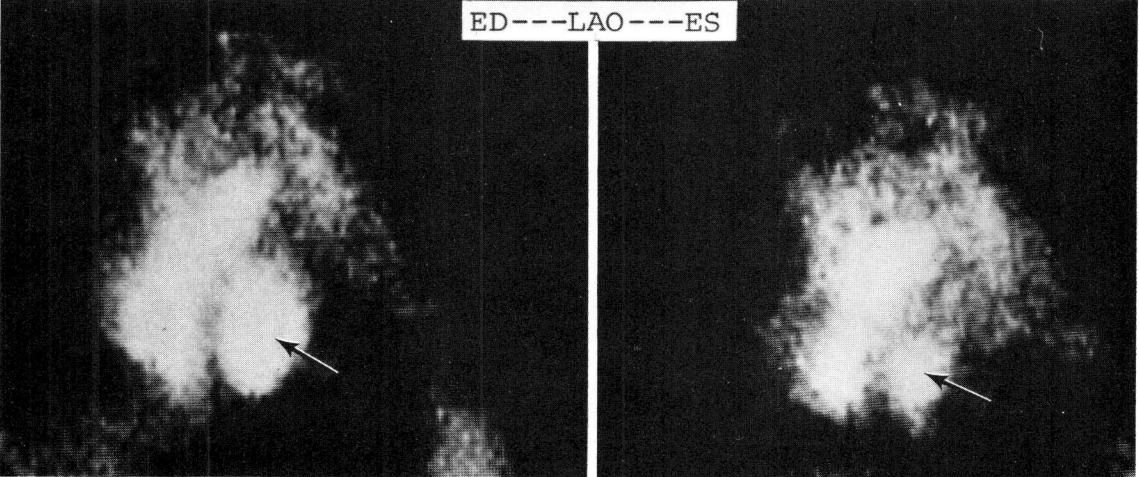

Figure 2–7. Gated blood pool images. In the left anterior oblique position, the left ventricle (arrows) is clearly separate from the right ventricle, in end-diastole (left) and end-systole (right). Computer processing can be used to calculate ejection fraction.

patient is exercised for one more minute to ensure that the initial distribution of radiotracer represents true regional perfusion. Imaging is begun immediately thereafter, in several projections, to visualize as much of the left ventricle as possible. A resting study is then performed either as a separate examination or, more economically, by reimaging the patient four hours after the stress test when myocardial redistribution has presumably occurred. The presence of a defect at the time of stress, followed by a return of activity on the resting images, suggests the presence of myocardial ischemia (Fig. 2–8). A defect present on both studies suggests previous myocardial damage from infarction.

The specificity of exercise stress testing has been greatly improved by the addition of thallium imaging. This study is used in the evaluation of symptomatic patients with suspected coronary artery disease; in patients with abnormal electrocardiograms in whom the presence of coronary artery disease is not proven; in the selection of patients for cardiac catheterization; and in the determination of graft patency in patients who have undergone coronary artery bypass surgery. Repeat coronary artery catheterization can often be postponed or the optimal time for its performance selected by following the patient with perfusion imaging. When bypass surgery is being considered, the study is helpful in demonstrating whether viable myocardium exists in the area where bypass is to be performed, so that unnecessary surgery can be avoided.

Although the diagnosis of myocardial infarction is often straightforward, in some instances equivocal symptoms, signs, electrocardiographic findings, or serum creatine phosphokinase (CPK) determinations lead to uncertainty. In some of these cases, the addition of radionuclide imaging may be of help. Infarcts may be imaged negatively or positively. The negative image is produced by a defect in the distribution of a perfusion agent, such as thallium chloride, as described previously. Almost all patients with acute myocardial infarction have a positive thallium study in the first few hours following the episode, but the defects become smaller and in many cases disappear

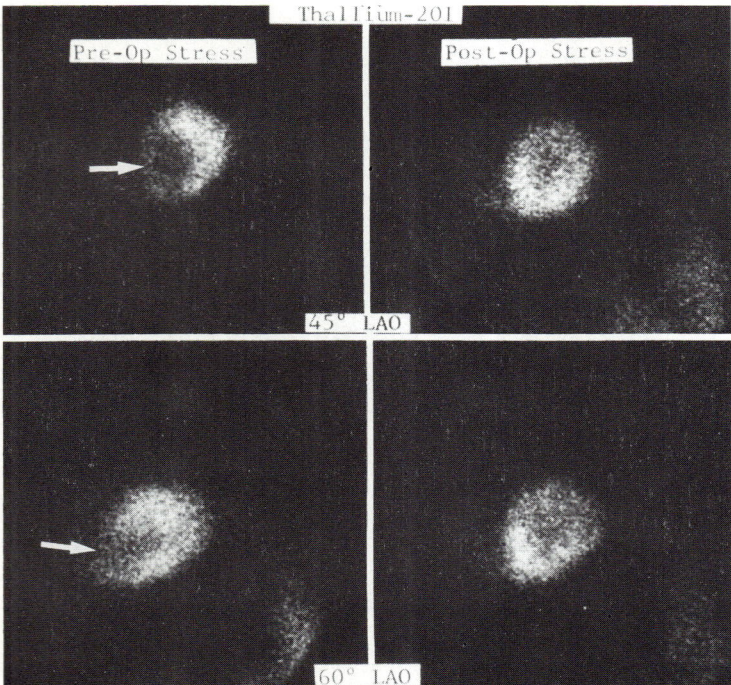

Figure 2–8. Myocardial ischemia. A defect in the septal wall is seen in the immediate poststress image in a patient with near-total left anterior descending artery occlusion and angina (arrows). After coronary artery bypass graft, perfusion is normal.

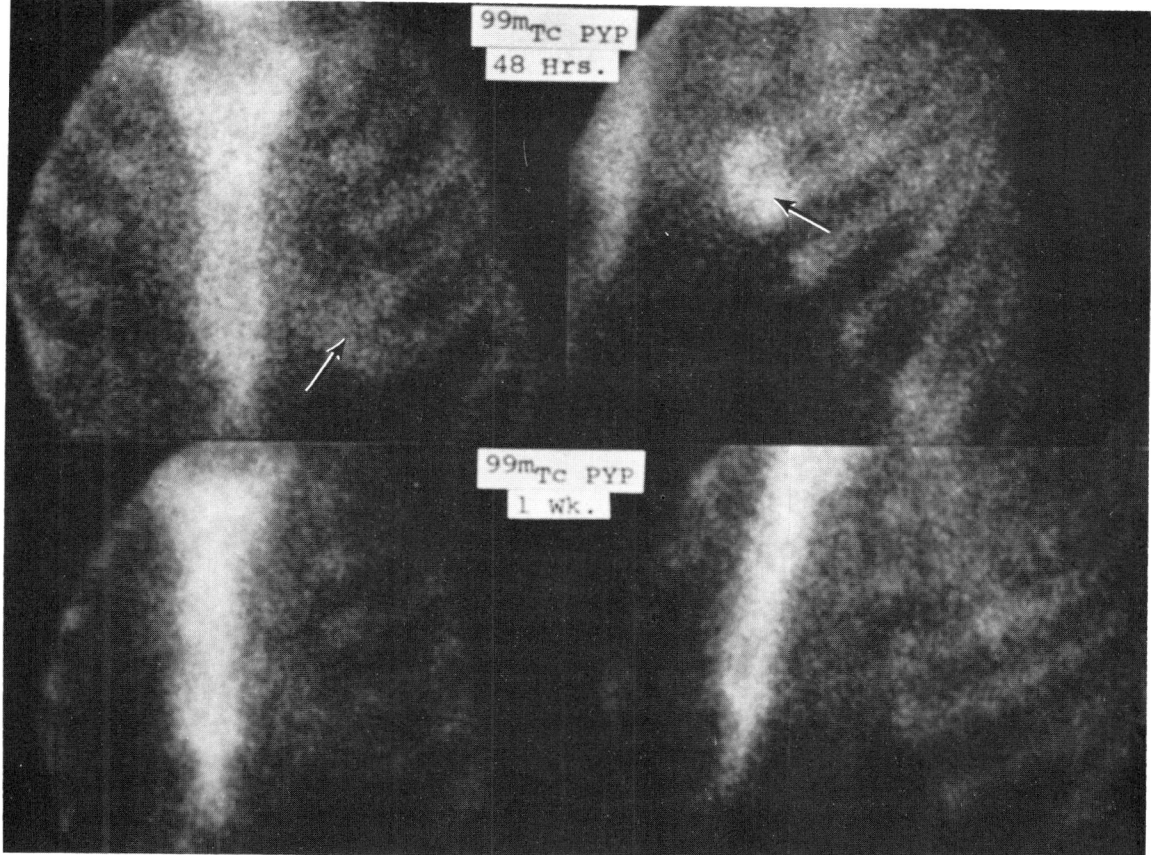

Figure 2–9. New myocardial infarct. There is focal accumulation of ^{99m}Tc pyrophosphate in the anterolateral left ventricular wall 48 hours after the acute episode (arrows). The activity has disappeared at one week.

within two to three days. This is more likely to occur with small or subendocardial infarctions, the very ones that create diagnostic problems with other tests. Nonetheless, there are circumstances in which the test may be helpful, such as perioperative infarct after surgery when the electrocardiogram may be unreliable, or in patients with left bundle branch block, in whom the electrocardiogram is unreliable in any case. In the latter instance, a septal defect is sometimes visualized even in the absence of myocardial infarction.

Infarct-avid imaging is performed after injection of ^{99m}Tc-pyrophosphate, a bone tracer that actively accumulates in areas of recent myocardial infarction, as it does in areas of skeletal muscle injury. Changes in intracellular calcium flux associated with the insult appear to play a role in phosphate localization in this area. This accumulation reliably occurs by 24 hours after the insult, peaks at 72 hours, and trails off in 5 to 7 days (Fig. 2–9). Therefore, the test is not a dependable substitute for the other methods of early infarct detection and is an unnecessary addition when the diagnosis is clear by other means. The major use of infarct imaging is in the determination of which patients need *not* remain in the coronary care unit because of equivocal findings on other tests rather than in the diagnosis of myocardial infarction *per se*. If scintigraphy is performed during the period in which it is most sensitive, a negative scan is a reasonably reliable indication of the absence of infarction when the other examinations have been normal or equivocal. Infarct-avid imaging can also detect myocardial damage after trauma. Certain false positive results, most notably in cardiomyopathy and unstable angina, can usually be distinguished by their generalized nature from the focal uptake of myocardial infarction.

Radionuclide Angiography

After the bolus injection of a radiopharmaceutical, rapid-sequence imaging facilitates the evaluation of arterial flow and tissue perfusion. Some of its applications are discussed in the sections on brain and renal imaging.

The study may be used for the noninvasive evaluation of aortic aneurysm and the patency of major arterial trunks. It therefore has applications in the evaluation of occlusive peripheral vascular disease and graft patency after surgery and of suspected arterial injury after trauma. In the presence of a mediastinal mass that might represent aneurysmal dilatation of the dorsal aorta, the study can be very helpful for biopsy or surgery. Dynamic imaging can be used in combination with static imaging to demonstrate the vascular nature of a defect seen on a liver or renal image. This was even more useful in the days before ultrasound was so widely available in the differentiation of cystic from solid lesions.

LUNG SCINTIGRAPHY

Radionuclides can be used to assess pulmonary perfusion or ventilation. The most common perfusion agents are ^{99m}Tc-albumin particles, either macroaggregates or microspheres. The mechanism of uptake is capillary blockade, the radioactive particles of 10 to 50 μ being trapped in terminal arterioles and capillaries. Only one in several thousand vessels is blocked, so that no discernible effect on pulmonary dynamics can be detected except in patients with extremely severe underlying pulmonary disease. It is in such patients that the very few morbid effects of lung imaging have occurred. Scintigraphy provides a map of pulmonary perfusion at a peripheral level that can be approached by pulmonary angiography only when superselective catheterization is used, a procedure associated with much greater morbidity than scintigraphy.

A full examination includes anterior, posterior, both lateral, and both posterior oblique projections. The most important and reliable information is the documentation of normal perfusion to both lungs, which effectively rules out any possibility of clinically significant pulmonary embolus, the most frequent clinical indication for the examination.

The classic findings of pulmonary embolus are absent perfusion to an entire lung, lobe, or well-defined pulmonary segment in the presence of a normal chest x-ray and the appropriate clinical setting (Fig. 2–10A). Perfusion defects may also be caused by emphysema, asthma, congestive heart failure, pneumonia, tumor, granuloma, cyst, or bulla; the finding of any of these conditions on the radiograph renders the scintigram indeterminate.

To increase the specificity of perfusion imaging, particularly in the presence of known or suspected ventilatory disease, ventilation imaging with radioactive gases or aerosols can be used. Xenon-133, injected or inhaled, is the most common pharmaceutical used. Xenon-127 and krypton-81m, which have more favorable physical energies, are not yet widely available. Abnormally ventilated areas fill and empty more

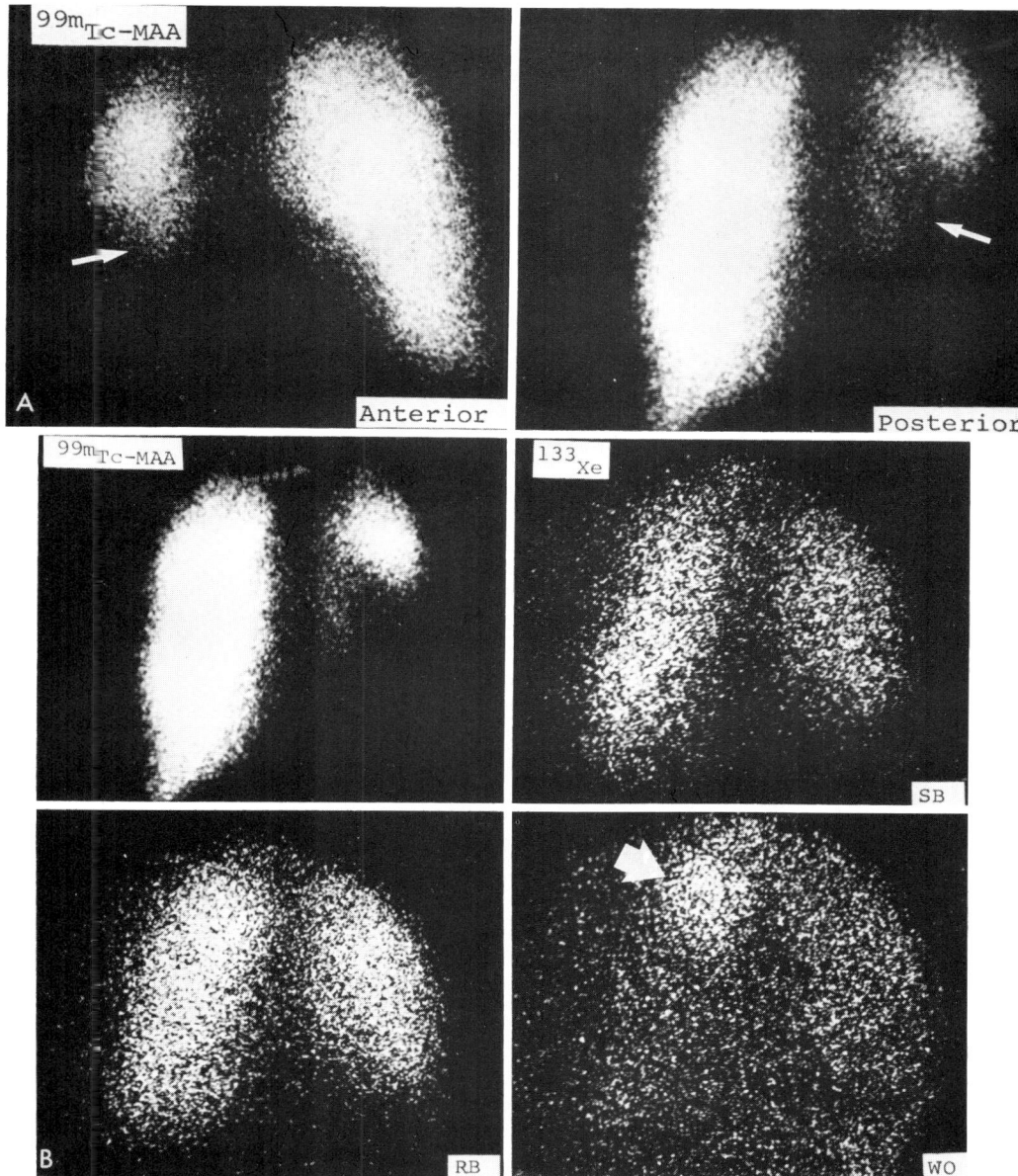

Figure 2–10. Pulmonary embolus in a patient with chronic obstructive pulmonary disease. There is no perfusion to the right lower lobe (*A,* arrows). On single-breath (SB) and rebreathing (RB) ventilation images *(B)* there is normal ventilation bilaterally, including the unperfused lung (V/Q mismatch). The washout (WO) ventilation image shows normal clearance from the right lower lobe, but abnormal retention in the left upper lobe (arrow) indicates ventilatory disease on the left and embolus on the right.

slowly than normal areas of the lung. In pulmonary embolus, the classic finding is a ventilation-perfusion mismatch (V/Q mismatch) or abnormal perfusion in an area of normal ventilation (Figure 2–10*B*). V/Q match suggests underlying ventilatory disease. However, this has been found in scattered cases of pulmonary embolus as well, especially if the study is not performed until several days after the embolic episode.

Radionuclide methods are also available for the detection of thrombophlebitis that might be responsible for pulmonary emboli (see the following section).

Applications of pulmonary imaging in other contexts are less frequent but sometimes helpful. The magnitude of right-to-left cardiac shunts can be quantitated by obtaining kidney counts after injection of labeled microspheres, multiplying by five since the kidneys receive 20 per cent of cardiac output, and comparing these counts with the lung counts. After surgically created shunts, such as the Blalock-Taussig or Waterston operation, the effectiveness of operative correction can be determined. When pneumonectomy is planned, perfusion and ventilation capacity of the contralateral lung can be assessed. If this is severely compromised, lobectomy or other more limited resection may be more feasible.

THROMBOSIS DETECTION

Venous System Scintigraphy

Radionuclide phlebography or venography is somewhat analogous to contrast venography. A lung imaging agent, ^{99m}Tc-microspheres or macroaggregates of albumin, is introduced via a 25-gauge butterfly needle inserted into a vein in the dorsum of the foot. The radioactive column can be visualized ascending in the deep and superficial veins of the lower leg, the long saphenous and superficial femoral veins in the thigh, the iliac veins, and the inferior vena cava. The findings in thrombophlebitis include (1) a cut-off of the radioactive column, (2) collateralization around an area of obstruction, and (3) accumulation of particles causing a "hot spot" in the area of thrombophlebitis, on slightly delayed images (Fig. 2–11). All but the last may be caused by old disease with chronic changes. The study has the advantage of superb visualization of the thigh and pelvic veins, areas where contrast studies may be suboptimal. The procedure is considerably more comfortable for the patient than contrast phlebography, and side effects are virtually unknown. Its main value is in detecting deep vein thrombosis above the knee, the site from which most pulmonary emboli originate. Since the lung imaging agent is used, a lung scan is always performed at the conclusion of the venogram.

Fibrinogen Uptake Test

Another method of diagnosing thrombophlebitis is the radioactive fibrinogen uptake test. Fibrinogen labeled with iodine-125 is injected into patients at risk for developing thrombophlebitis, such as those undergoing hip surgery or elderly persons who will be confined to bed for any reason. Should thrombosis occur in the lower extremity, radioactive fibrinogen will be incorporated into the forming clot. Serial counts may be obtained for several days over the lower extremities, so that the accumulation of radioactivity in a site of developing thrombosis can be detected. This is not an imaging test, for which the low energy of iodine-125 is not suitable. Owing to this low energy, the study cannot reliably detect thrombosis in the upper thighs or pelvis. In the thighs, false positive findings may be the result of hematoma related to surgery or other areas of inflammation. A modification of this procedure includes labeling fibrinogen with iodine-131, so that imaging can be obtained; this should increase the specificity of the test. However, this modification is not yet in general use. A major drawback to this type of study is that radioactive material must be injected

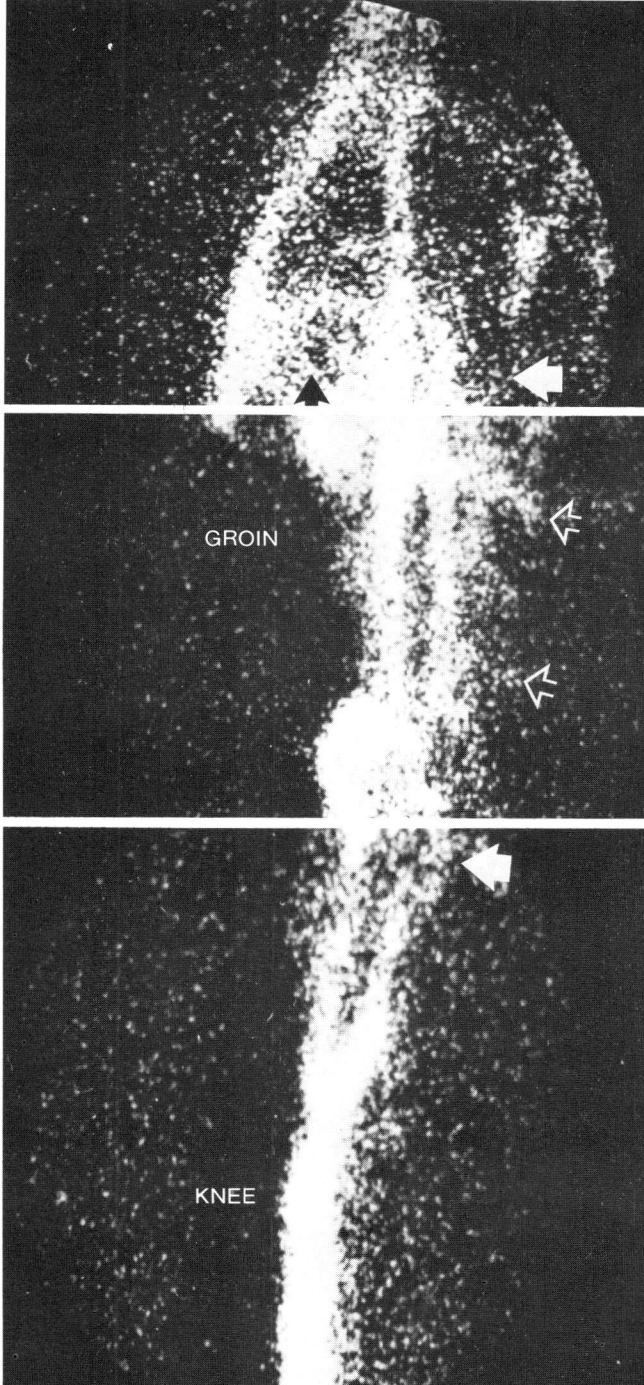

Figure 2–11. Iliofemoral thrombophlebitis. *A*, The radionuclide venogram shows obstruction in the left superficial femoral vein and groin (closed arrows), with no visualization of left iliac vein and multiple collateral veins in the thigh and pelvis (open arrows).

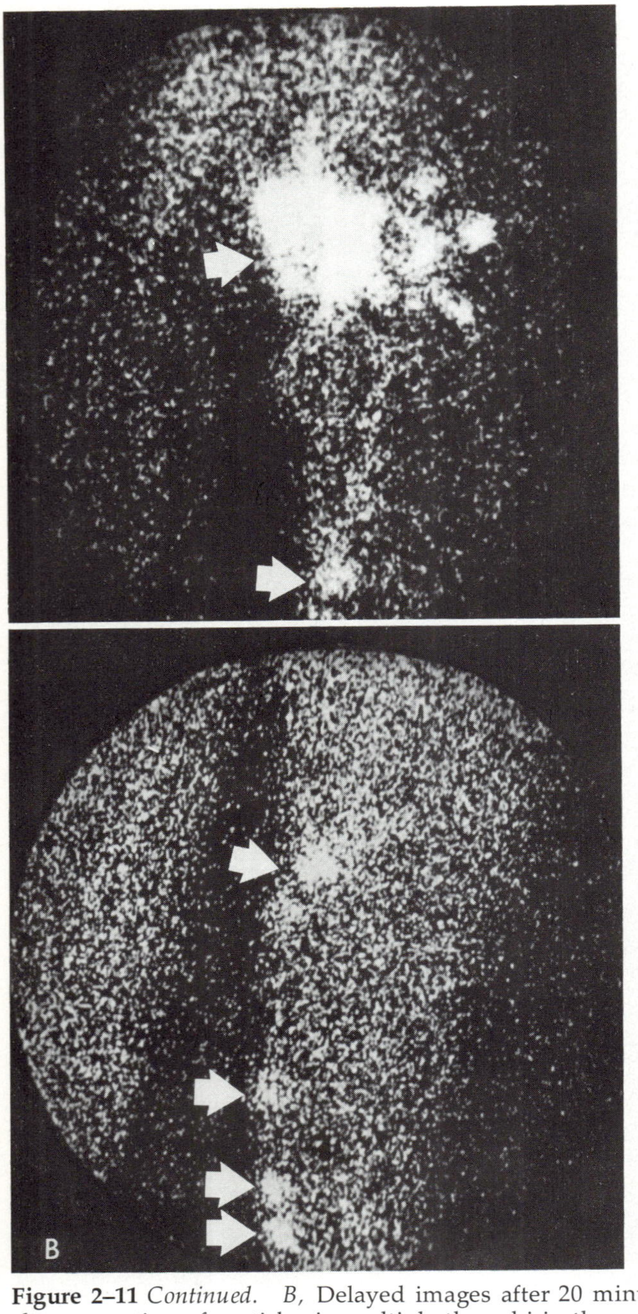

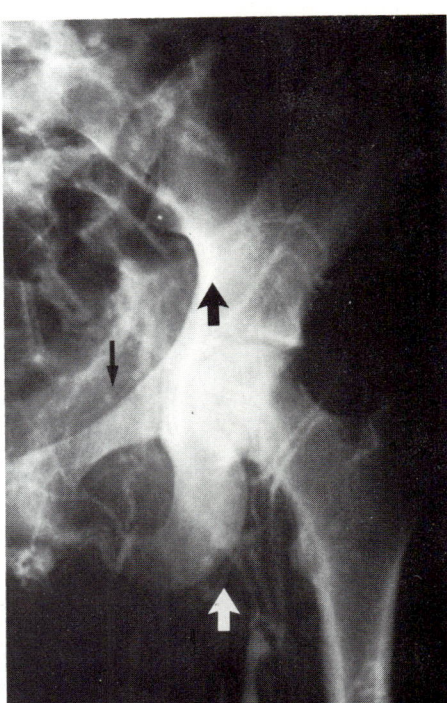
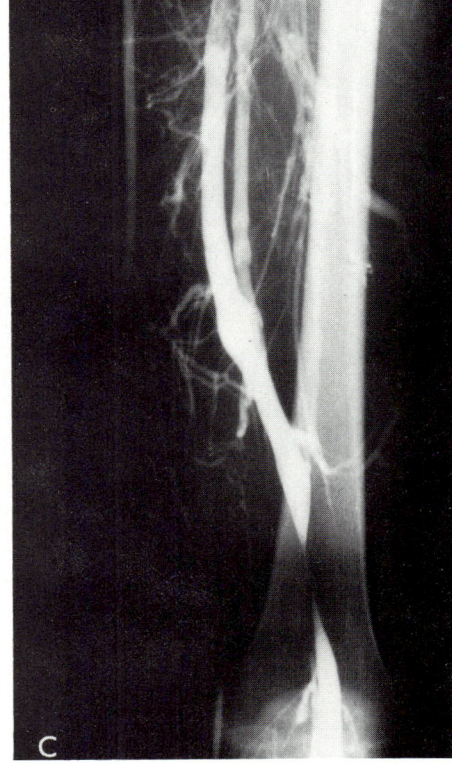

Figure 2–11 *Continued.* B, Delayed images after 20 minutes show retention of particles in multiple thrombi in the groin, thigh, and knee (arrows). C, The contrast venogram shows thrombosis in the superficial femoral vein and many collaterals, but visualization of the upper thigh and pelvic collaterals is less striking than on the scan.

before the fact, when a patient is at risk for, but not yet suspected of, harboring the pathologic state in question.

LIVER AND BILIARY TRACT SCINTIGRAPHY

Liver scintigraphy may be performed after injection of substances that either localize in the reticuloendothelial system or are concentrated by the hepatocytes and excreted into the bile. The most common reticuloendothelial imaging agent is ^{99m}Tc-sulfur colloid, injected as particles 0.1 to 0.3 μ in size. More than 90 per cent of the particles injected are sequestered by the Kupffer cells of the hepatic sinusoids, and the remainder lodge in the spleen and bone marrow. The study may be used for accurately assessing hepatic size, for evaluating questions of abnormal situs, for establishing the nature of right upper quadrant masses, and for distinguishing diaphragmatic hernia or eventration from chest masses. Space-occupying disease causes a void in the image (Fig. 2–12A). Surface lesions as small as 2 cm may be visible, but those farther from the detector must be larger to be detected. For this reason, liver imaging is performed in multiple views. Although lesions deep within the liver may go unobserved until they reach several centimeters in size, the liver scintigram is still one of the most useful screening examinations for the most common multifocal disease, metastasis. The void itself is nonspecific and may also be caused by primary tumor, cyst, abscess, or less commonly, by adenoma, hemangioma, or regenerative nodule in cirrhosis. The examination can be used to facilitate subsequent ultrasound or CT evaluation, both of which are technically less well suited for initial screening of the entire organ.

Before the introduction of gallium-67 citrate, liver imaging was combined with lung imaging for detection of subphrenic abscess. The liver-lung scan is now obsolete in the diagnosis of this problem, since it cannot distinguish subphrenic abscess from disease of the lung or pleural space and cannot evaluate the remainder of the abdomen, both of which can be done with gallium imaging 48 to 72 hours following radiocolloid

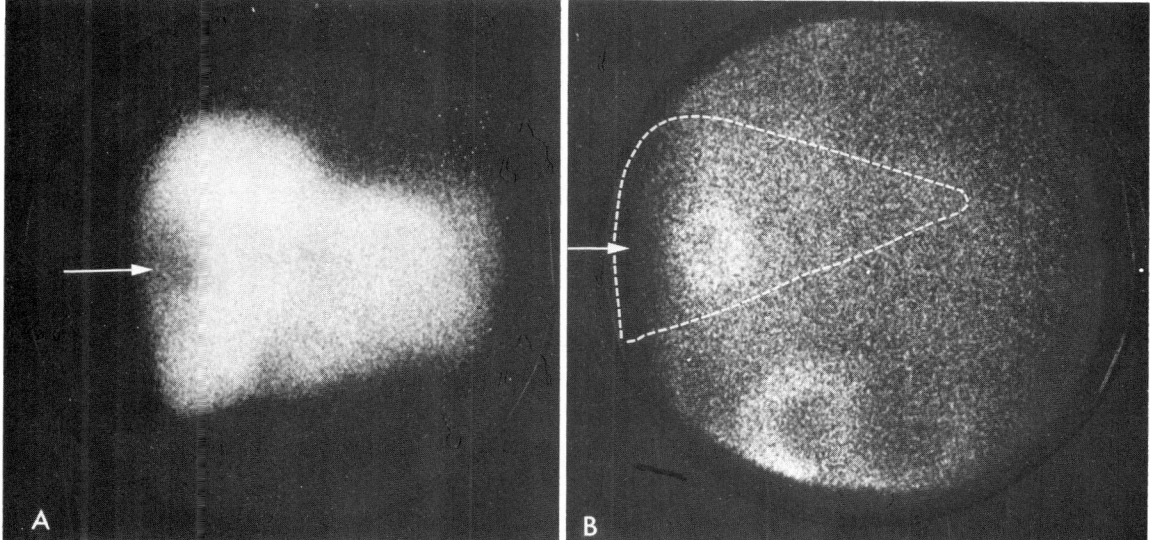

Figure 2–12. Liver abscess. Colloid image (A) shows a defect (arrow), which is hot on the gallium image (B, arrow).

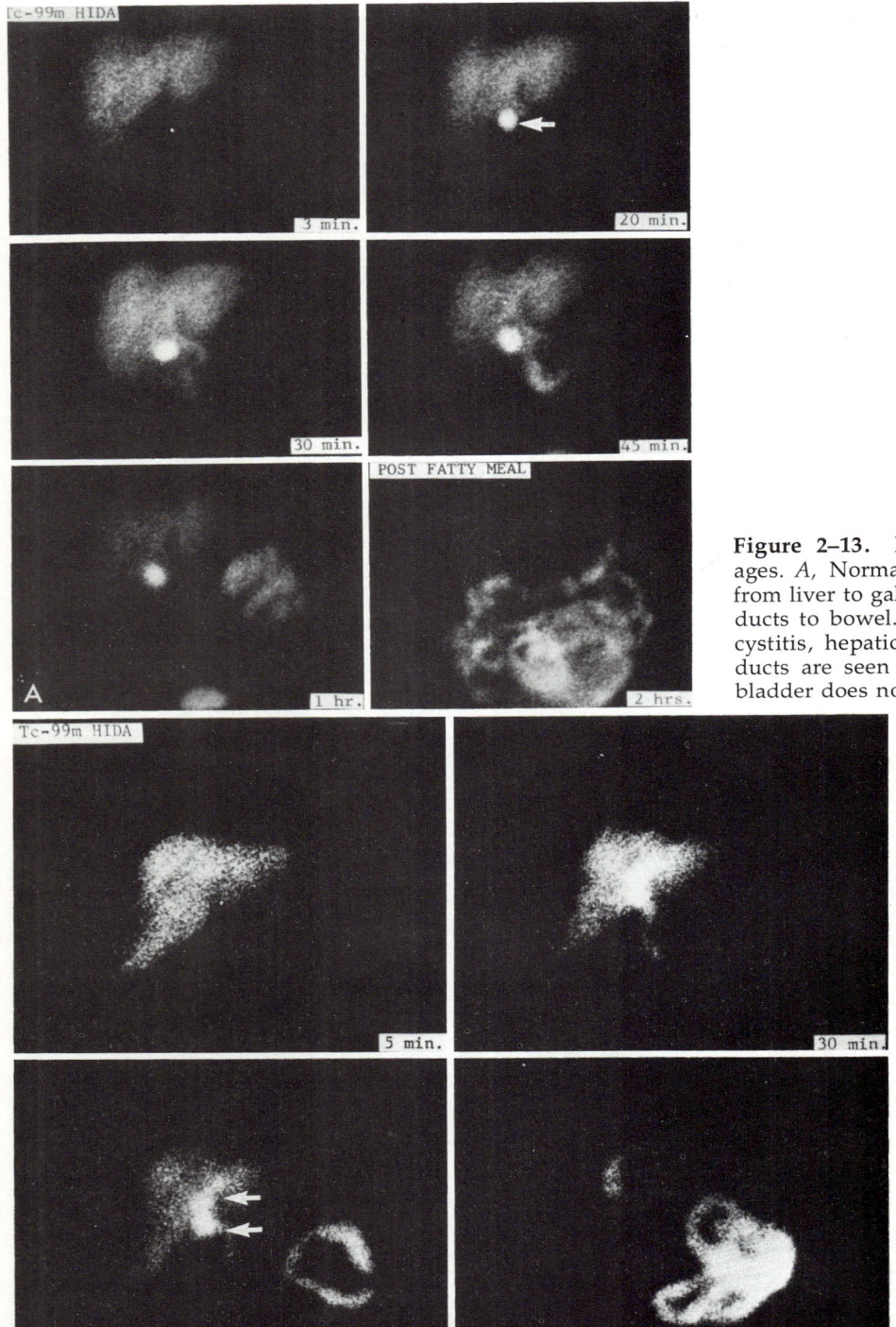

Figure 2–13. Hepatobiliary images. *A,* Normally, activity moves from liver to gallbladder (arrow) to ducts to bowel. *B,* In acute cholecystitis, hepatic and common bile ducts are seen (arrows), but gallbladder does not fill.

imaging. The accumulation of radiogallium focally within or around the liver in the appropriate clinical context suggests abscess (Fig. 2–12B). Radiogallium accumulates in hepatoma with equal avidity, so clinical context is important. It is also necessary to be aware of the patient's operative history, since surgical incisions accumulate gallium citrate. However, such activity decreases during the first few weeks, so that repeat images in equivocal cases may still be useful.

Diffuse parenchymal disease, such as cirrhosis or hepatitis, causes decreased radiocolloid uptake and "colloid shift" to the spleen and marrow, which appear more intense than usual. The liver may be large or small, depending on the stage of disease. Splenic size is often increased. Liver imaging in diffuse disease helps detect the coexistence of focal disease, which may affect the choice of biopsy site.

The original agent developed for hepatobiliary imaging was I-131 rose bengal, a radioiodinated fluorescein dye that is cleared by the polygonal cells, as is Bromsulphalein (BSP). After representative background counts over the head are obtained at 5 and 20 minutes after injection, a "radioactive BSP test" can be performed for estimation of hepatic clearance. Repeat imaging over the abdomen demonstrates early appearance of a hepatic image, which gradually disappears as activity enters the bowel. Although this examination is capable of distinguishing hepatic disease from obstruction, it was never widely used for this purpose except for the distinction between neonatal hepatitis and biliary atresia.

New technetium-labeled forms of iminodiacetic acid and Schiff's bases (^{99m}Tc-HIDA—technetium-99m dimethyl acetanilide iminodiacetic acid) are coming into use. These provide far superior delineation of the liver itself in the early part of the study and of the biliary tract in the later part. In the fasting patient, the gallbladder is always visualized within 30 to 60 minutes after injection if the cystic duct is patent, so the test *can rule out the presence of acute cholecystitis with virtually complete reliability* (Fig. 2–13).[8a] The biliary tree can be visualized at serum levels of bilirubin higher than those needed for radiographic visualization. Another important use is in the evaluation of bile flow after biliary tract bypass procedures and in the detection of bile leaks, for which the examination is exquisitely sensitive.

The use of imaging in liver trauma is discussed in the following section on spleen scintigraphy.

SPLEEN SCINTIGRAPHY

The spleen is also imaged with ^{99m}Tc-sulfur colloid. Since the spleen appears on every radionuclide liver examination, the test is more accurately considered a liver-spleen scintigram. An exception is functional asplenia, most commonly seen in sickle cell crisis, when a palpably large spleen is not visualized because blockage of the splenic sinusoids by sickled red cells prevents entry of the radiocolloid. This phenomenon has been reported, although rarely, in cases of metastatic disease to the spleen.

Because the spleen is often mobile, a palpable organ may not be truly large. Scintigraphy is the most accurate method of determining splenic size. To localize the spleen for radiotherapy, marks can be placed on the skin at the time of imaging. Space-occupying lesions are less common in the spleen than in the liver but also produce defects in the scan.

Liver-spleen imaging has replaced angiography as the initial and definitive diagnostic modality for the evaluation of trauma. The sensitivity of the examination is equal to or better than that of angiography, and the morbidity of the procedure is nil. Fracture, hematoma, or contusion cause a round, linear, or wedge-shaped defect in activity (Fig. 2–14). Subcapsular lesions flatten the border. The size of the defect does

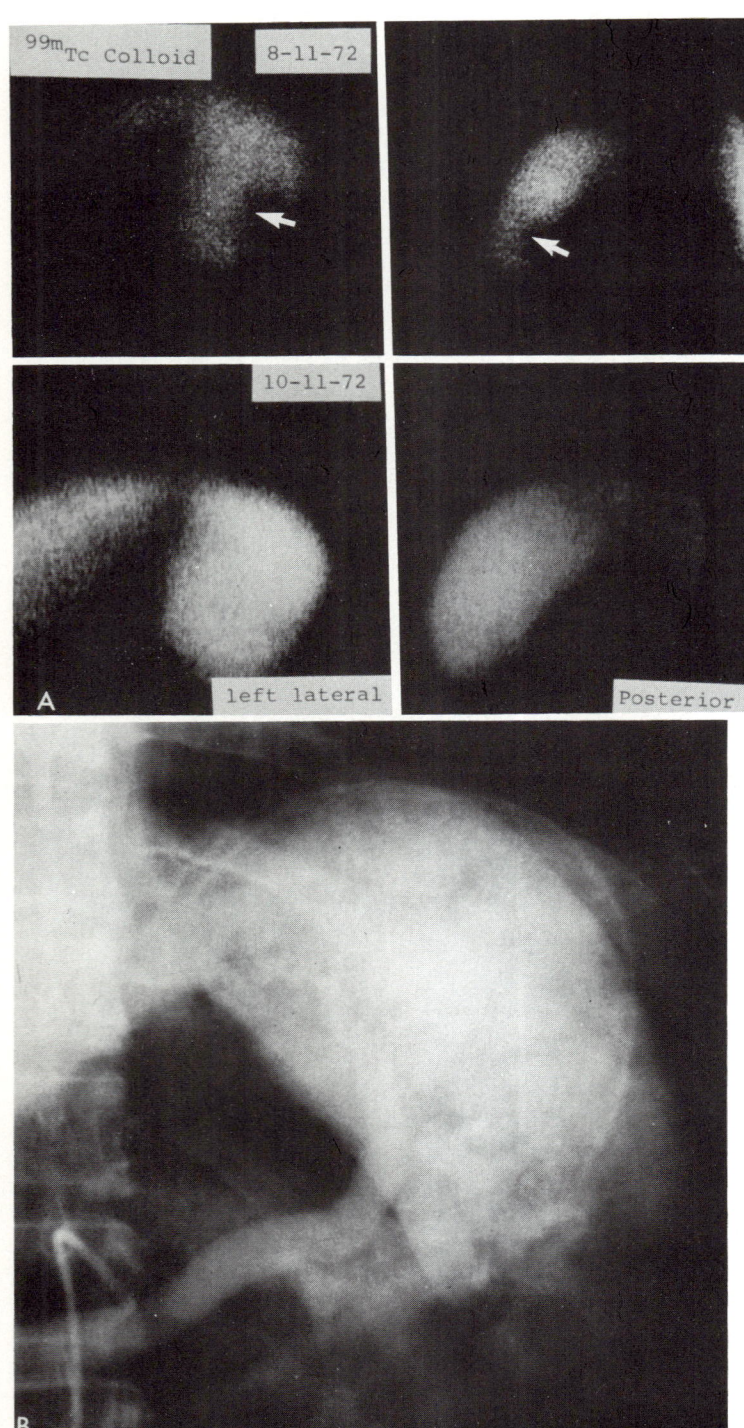

Figure 2–14. Splenic injury with resolution. *A*, A posteriorly situated hematoma is seen on lateral and posterior views immediately after injury (arrows) but has resolved without surgery two months later. *B*, An angiogram was done in the standard anterior view and was normal at the time of initial injury.

not correlate with the severity of the injury, which must be determined clinically. Until recently, the discovery of a definite splenic defect in patients with a low or falling hematocrit was sufficient indication for immediate surgery. However, pediatric surgeons are now much more conservative in advocating immediate splenectomy for trauma because of the increased incidence of overwhelming sepsis in children who are splenectomized at an early age. Scintigraphy can be used to follow the progressive resolution of a splenic injury. The danger of delayed rupture or occult enlargement of splenic hematoma is mitigated if repeat scans are performed; this danger appears less than was thought in the days before repeat imaging was available. It is quite likely that this approach may be feasible for the liver as well, but only a small amount of data has been accumulated.

In the search for splenosis or polysplenia, the spleen parenchyma may be imaged after injection of heat-damaged red blood cells, in which case an image of the spleen alone may be obtained. However, because the pharmaceutical is time consuming to prepare, ^{99m}Tc-sulfur colloid is used for most indications.

In the evaluation of hematologic disorders, sequential counts may be obtained over the spleen after reinjection of the patient's own labeled undamaged red cells to determine if sequestration is present, a possible reason for splenectomy.

GENITOURINARY TRACT SCINTIGRAPHY

Radionuclide methods can be used for the assessment of renal function, vesicoureteral reflux, and scrotal imaging.

Renal scintigraphy may be helpful in several clinical contexts: (1) in the determination of renal presence, size, shape, position, and function when visualization with contrast urography is difficult or impossible; (2) in the evaluation of functional status in obstructive uropathy; (3) in the evaluation of some space-occupying lesions; (4) in the study of renal vascular supply and perfusion in trauma, infarction, and hypertension; (5) in the evaluation of renal transplants; and (6) in the diagnosis of inflammatory disease. Renal scintigraphy is actually a function test; the activity in the kidneys is easily quantitated. Such quantitative evaluation of differences in radiographic density on intravenous urography is impossible. The kidney can be visualized with as little as 10 per cent of renal function, and gas or feces in the abdomen do not interfere with satisfactory visualization at scintigraphy.

Many radiopharmaceuticals are available. The traditional agent is I-131 orthoiodohippurate or iodohippuran, which is virtually completely excreted by the normal kidney, 80 per cent by tubular secretion and 20 per cent by glomerular filtration. Because of the I-131 label, only small doses can be administered. For evaluation of cortical morphologic status and uptake, ^{99m}Tc-labeled agents, such as DMSA (dimercaptosuccinate) and GHA (glucoheptonate), provide information about functioning tubular cortex Technetium 99m-DTPA (diethylene triamine penta-acetic acid) is a rapidly excreted agent that may yield information about perfusion, morphologic condition, and excretion (Fig. 2–15). None of these agents imposes an osmotic load. All may safely be administered to patients with cardiovascular problems, diabetes, multiple myeloma, dehydration, or allergy to contrast media.

Serial scintiphotography and renography performed with ^{131}I-hippuran or ^{99m}Tc-labeled agents can be used to monitor function in patients with obstructive uropathy during passage of a calculus or after surgical correction. Repeat urograms become unnecessary.

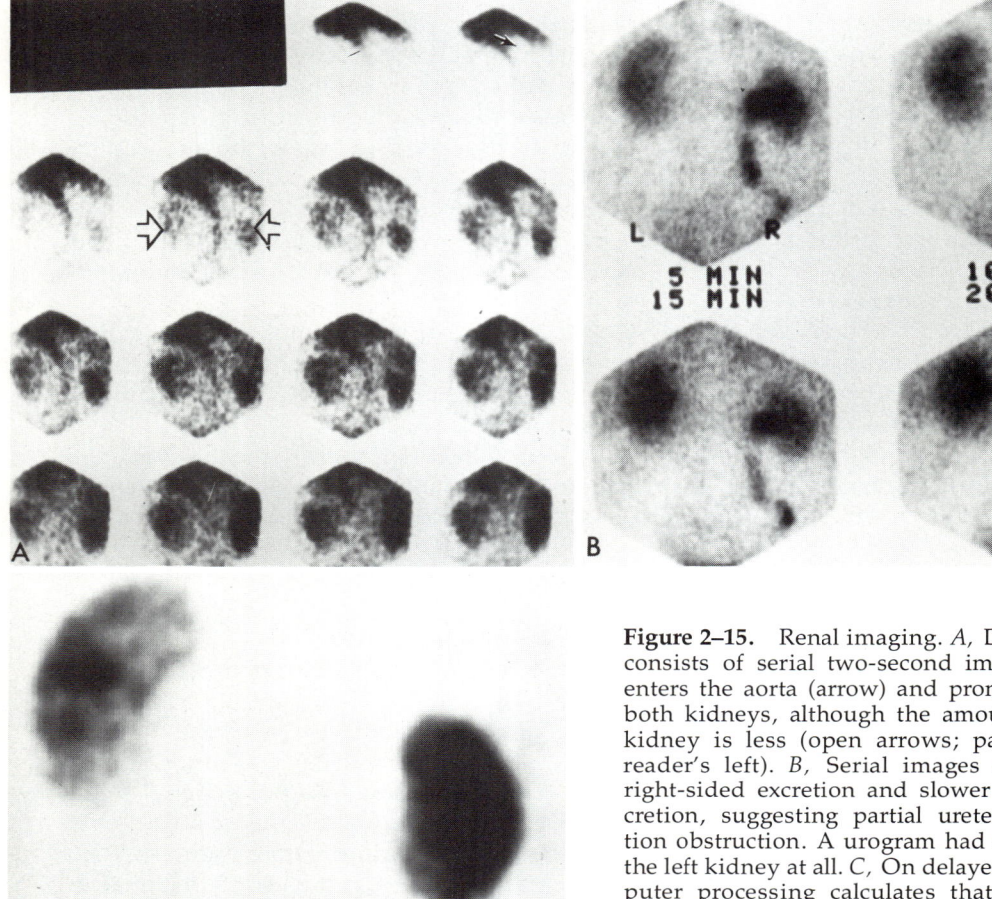

Figure 2–15. Renal imaging. *A,* Dynamic study consists of serial two-second images. Activity enters the aorta (arrow) and promptly perfuses both kidneys, although the amount in the left kidney is less (open arrows; patient's left is reader's left). *B,* Serial images show prompt right-sided excretion and slower left-sided excretion, suggesting partial ureteropelvic junction obstruction. A urogram had not visualized the left kidney at all. *C,* On delayed images computer processing calculates that the compromised left kidney is contributing 39 per cent of total renal function.

When the urogram demonstrates splayed calyces, the scintigram can reliably distinguish hypertrophied renal column from a space-occupying lesion. Virtually no abnormal renal mass, benign or malignant, can accumulate a renal cortical isotopic agent.

In the traumatized patient, the demonstration of early perfusion and cortical activity on dynamic renal scintigraphy is proof that the main renal artery is not occluded or severed and that immediate angiography and surgery may not be necessary. Contusion, infarction, and fracture can readily be seen on cortical imaging. Extravasation may be seen on excretory images. Serial studies can differentiate contusion (transient defect) from infarction (persistent defect); since medical management usually suffices in either case, it is not necessary to distinguish these two at the time of injury.

For evaluation of renal transplant function, iodohippuran is superior to the technetium-labeled agents, although the latter are often used for evaluation of early per-

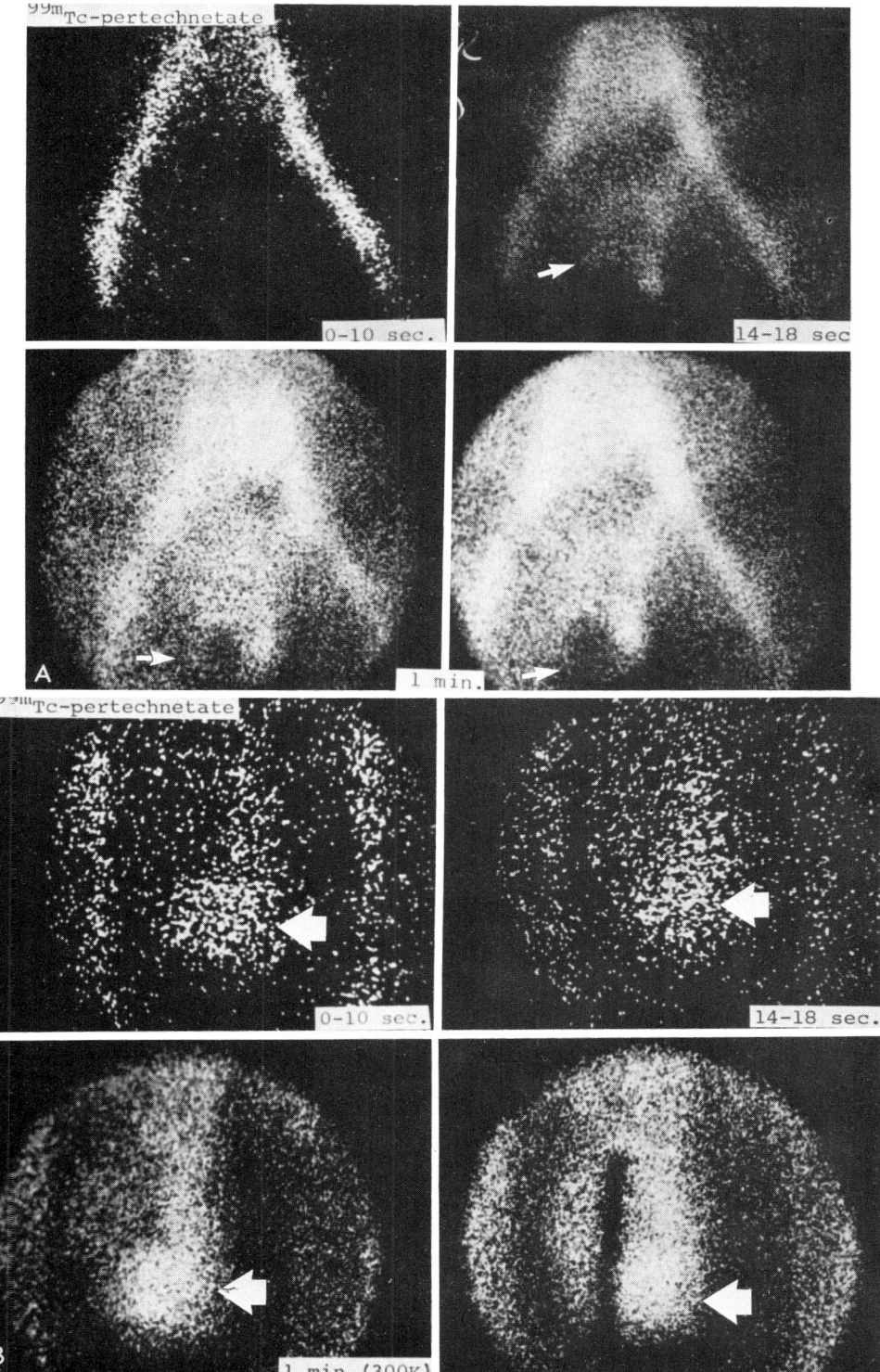

Figure 2–16. Scrotal imaging. *A*, In testicular torsion, a cold area representing nonperfusion is seen in the dynamic vascular phase and the static tissue phase, representing the devascularized testis (arrows). *B*, In epididymitis, early and late activity is increased compared with the normal side (arrows).

fusion. Acute tubular necrosis, rejection, obstruction, lymphocele, and arterial compromise can be detected.

Pyelonephritis causes well-defined focal defects in the renal cortex as well as general diminution of activity. The scintigraphic findings are generally more striking than those seen on urography. Radiogallium also accumulates in pyelonephritis. Scintigraphically, pyelonephritis and renal abscess may have the same findings. The distinction is made noninvasively with ultrasound; if there is no mass lesion in an area of abnormally decreased renal activity or abnormally increased gallium activity, the diagnosis of pyelonephritis is virtually assured.

The presence of vesicoureteral reflux can be determined after instillation of 500 μCi or less of pertechnetate into the bladder, followed by a saline infusion to bladder capacity. The entire filling and voiding phases are monitored, a complete observation not permissible with standard fluoroscopic voiding cystourethrography. The actual volume of urine refluxed can be quantitated, as can the bladder volume at which reflux occurs. Residual volume can be determined at the end of a radionuclide VCU or an antegrade renal radionuclide study. Radionuclide cystography is useless, however, for evaluation of the male urethra.

Dynamic and immediate static imaging over the scrotum can distinguish acute torsion from epididymo-orchitis in a patient with an inflamed hemiscrotum. During the first few hours of clinical presentation, the latter causes increased flow and tissue hyperemia, whereas the former demonstrates decreased flow and a cold defect representing the avascular testis (Fig. 2–16). The study can be used to avoid unnecessary surgical exploration.

BONE SCINTIGRAPHY

Most bone imaging is currently done with ^{99m}Tc-labeled phosphates: pyrophosphate, diphosphonate, and methylene diphosphonate. These are best suited to the gamma camera, least expensive, and most widely available. Scintigraphy can begin within two hours of injection, and the entire body can be imaged in less than one-half hour. Special magnification collimators can be used for better evaluation of the hips and of the small bones of children.

The ^{99m}Tc-phosphates accumulate in areas of reactive bone formation, either by chemadsorption to the hydroxyapatite crystal or by incorporation into immature collagen. This accumulation is an index of metabolic activity, *not* of mineral content, and the study may therefore be equally positive in radiographically lucent or sclerotic lesions. Although the presence of increased activity is itself nonspecific and is caused by a variety of insults to the bone, the pattern of activity, interpreted in the clinical context and with correlative x-rays when appropriate, may facilitate specific diagnosis.

For the evaluation of multifocal bone disease, the scintigram is the appropriate screening examination in most cases. Radiographic assessment of the skeleton requires multiple views of most areas for complete evaluation. A more productive approach is to perform radionuclide imaging and then to obtain coned-down radiographs in multiple views of positive areas if necessary.

By pointing to metabolically active areas, the most suitable sites for histologic evaluation, the imaging examination aids in the selection of a biopsy site for both benign and malignant lesions. Inactive lesions, benign or malignant, may appear dense on a radiograph and be negative on the scan.

The original, and still most common, indication for bone scintigraphy is the search

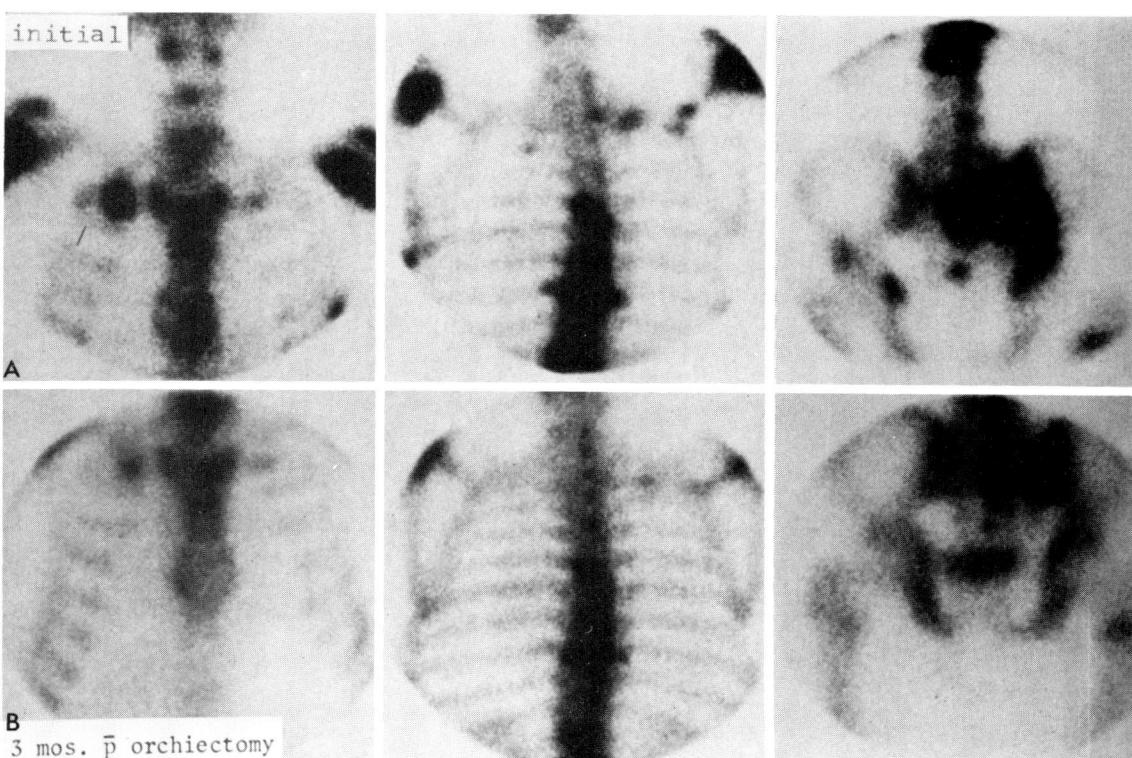

Figure 2–17. Bone metastases. In a patient with prostatic carcinoma, multiple abnormal hot foci are present *(A)*. These have decreased in extent and intensity after orchiectomy *(B)*.

for occult metastatic disease, the detection of which obviously affects the choice of therapy. Radiography misses approximately 25 to 50 per cent of occult lesions in most carcinomas and lymphoma, whereas scintigraphy misses about 5 per cent (Fig. 2–17). A glaring exception is multiple myeloma, which causes little or no reactive bone formation, and is therefore often missed scintigraphically when lytic lesions are readily apparent radiographically.

In the presence of acute osteomyelitis, the radiograph does not usually become positive for 10 to 14 days. The bone scintigram, however, usually becomes abnormal within one to two days. The pattern of activity can usually be distinguished from cellulitis and arthritis. The addition of imaging with gallium-67 citrate, more specific for active infection than reactive bone formation, assists in finding acute or persistent infection sites in areas of chronic osteomyelitis, distinguishing osteomyelitis from diabetic osteoarthropathy, and in evaluating the efficacy of antibiotic therapy.

Scintigraphy is more sensitive than radiography for diagnosing acute fractures of the vertebral bodies or processes, hairline stress fractures of the extremities, and fractures at bone-cartilage interfaces, such as the costochondral and costovertebral junctions. The study may help evaluate post-traumatic complications, such as nonunion, osteonecrosis, motion of orthopedic appliances, and infection, all of which cause early scintigraphic changes.

Some lesions are "cold" on imaging, with less-than-normal activity. If the radiograph is normal, absent tracer activity indicates vascular compromise. This finding can lead to early diagnosis of Legg-Perthes disease as well as early detection of sickle

50 — RADIOISOTOPE TECHNIQUES

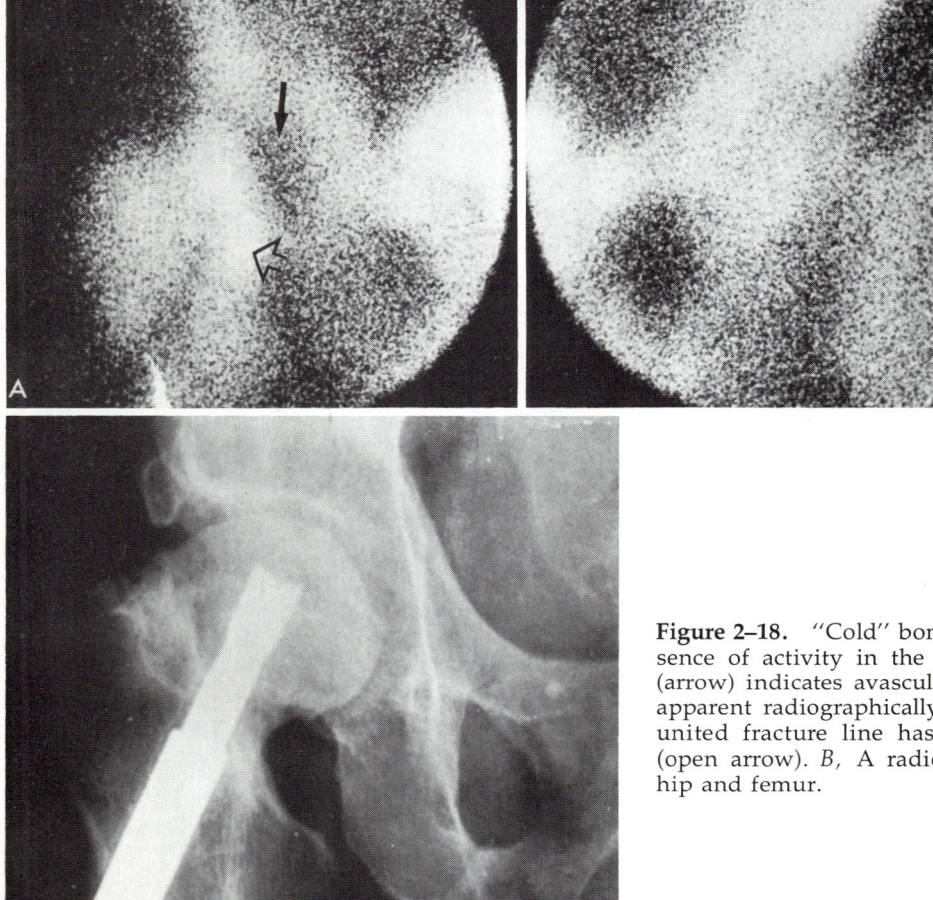

Figure 2–18. "Cold" bone lesion. *A,* An absence of activity in the right femoral head (arrow) indicates avascular necrosis, not yet apparent radiographically. The incompletely united fracture line has increased activity (open arrow). *B,* A radiograph of the right hip and femur.

cell infarcts, devitalized femoral head after subcapital fracture, the level at which vital bone remains in gangrenous extremities, and the presence of viable bone at sites of nonunion (Fig. 2–18).

In certain soft tissue lesions, such as myositis ossificans, activity appears earlier than radiographic ossification and persists as long as the process is active. This can help determine the optimal time for surgical intervention.

TUMOR AND ABSCESS IMAGING

Gallium-67 citrate has been mentioned in the sections on liver, kidney, and bone imaging. Although this pharmaceutical was initially developed as a tumor-tracing agent, it quickly became obvious that it accumulated in areas of active infection as well. Today it is probably more widely used in the latter context than in the evaluation of neoplasm. It can be useful in the evaluation of unexplained postoperative fever, inflammatory bowel disease, gallbladder empyema, urinary tract infection, and fever of unknown origin. In general, if a specific organ site is suspected of harboring infection or abscess, the imaging agent specific for that organ should be used first: radiocolloid for the liver, technetium phosphates for bone, renal agents for the kidney, and so forth. When such studies are unproductive, or when they demonstrate defects whose nature requires elucidation, gallium imaging may be added (see Fig. 2–12).

After injection, gallium citrate is bound to transferrin. Any cause of hyperferremia, which decreases iron-binding capacity by saturating transferrin, severely compromises gallium imaging. This can be a problem in some hematologic disorders and, more commonly, in patients who have had chemotherapy or total-body irradiation. In tissue, gallium is strongly bound to lactoferrin or to another gallium-binding protein found in the lysosomal fraction of cell cytoplasm. Normal distribution includes the liver, lacrimal and salivary glands, bone marrow, and colon. Because the latter often compromises the quality of the image, many practitioners use routine bowel preparations.

In the evaluation of chest disease, gallium reliably localizes in most primary untreated lung carcinomas of the squamous cell type and may be used to determine the extent of mediastinal involvement. It also accumulates in many inflammatory processes, including active pulmonary tuberculosis, pneumoconiosis, pulmonary abscess, and bacterial pneumonia. Inactive tuberculosis is virtually always negative, so the study can be used to evaluate the success of therapy. Some investigators use the examination to differentiate pulmonary embolus from pneumonia, since the former does not concentrate the radiopharmaceutical in most cases.

Although gallium imaging cannot be reliably used to diagnose lymphoma, it can be used to advantage in staging the disease, evaluating therapeutic success, and searching for recurrence.

MISCELLANEOUS EXAMINATIONS

Radionuclide Dacryocystography

The initial images following instillation of a drop of technetium pertechnetate, containing only a few hundred microcuries of activity or less, over the punctum of the lacrimal gland satisfactorily delineate the drainage of the lacrimal duct and identify sites of obstruction. The radiation dose is less than that required for contrast dacryocystography, and no catheterization is required.

Pancreas and Parathyroid Imaging

Selenium-75-selenomethionine is incorporated into proteins and accumulates at sites of protein synthesis. This radiopharmaceutical has been used for imaging the pancreas and parathyroid gland. These examinations are hampered by the proximity of a large protein-producing organ in both cases—the liver and the thyroid gland. Complicated subtraction techniques are necessary, and many studies are technically suboptimal. Pancreas imaging has been largely replaced by ultrasound and CT scanning.

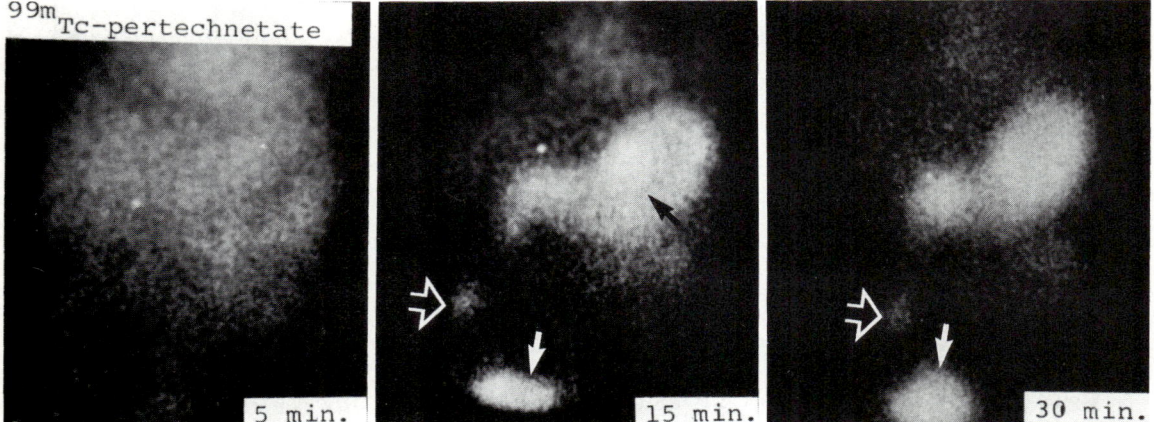

Figure 2–19. Meckel's diverticulum. Activity should be present only in the stomach (closed arrow), but an abnormal focus is seen in the right lower quadrant (open arrow). Activity in urine depicts the bladder (closed white arrows).

Imaging of Gastric Mucosa

Secretion of pertechnetate by gastric mucosa has been helpful in the detection of Meckel's diverticulum, since the ectopic gastric mucosa in many diverticula accumulates the radiopharmaceutical. Because its sensitivity is in the range of 70 per cent, this examination should be the initial diagnostic modality when this question arises (Fig. 2–19). Ectopic gastric mucosa in any other site, such as bowel duplication and Barrett's esophagus, can also be diagnosed as well as retained gastric antrum in the duodenal stumps of patients who have undergone Billroth II procedures and continue to have ulcer symptoms. Pertechnetate sometimes accumulates in areas of other bowel disease without gastric mucosa, such as intussusception, inflammatory bowel disease, and vascular malformations.

Gastric Function and Malfunction Imaging

Gastroesophageal reflux can be diagnosed by repeated imaging after the patient drinks radiocolloid particles. The test is more sensitive than barium studies and less distasteful to the patient.

Gastric emptying time is easily monitored noninvasively by obtaining repeated images or counts over the stomach after introduction of a known amount of radioactivity. Hypotonic gastric states, in conditions such as diabetes mellitus, and effectiveness of therapy may be easily followed by serial studies.

Adrenal Imaging

Compounds of cholesterol labeled with radioactive iodine can be used to image the adrenal cortex. The radiation dose from iodine-131–labeled agents is considerable, but newer agents labeled with iodine-123 are being developed. Although still in the experimental state, these agents hold significant promise for evaluation of known adrenal disease in certain situations:

1. In secondary Cushing's syndrome caused by excess ACTH, both adrenal glands can be visualized with greater-than-normal uptake.
2. In adrenal cortical carcinoma, the destroyed involved gland may be nonvisualized, and increased steroid secretion may suppress the contralateral gland.
3. After "total" adrenalectomy, when symptoms of Cushing's syndrome persist, residual functioning tissue can be observed.
4. In primary aldosteronism caused by tumor, the tumor can be visualized and will not suppress after dexamethasone administration, while the normal contralateral gland will.
5. Aldosteronism resulting from bilateral hyperplasia is characterized by complete suppression of uptake after dexamethasone administration.

Adrenal medullary tumors, such as pheochromocytoma and neuroblastoma, compress the adrenal cortex, eventually causing nonvisualization of adrenal cortical agents. Compounds of dopamine labeled with radioactive carbon are being developed for direct medullary visualization.

Bone Marrow Imaging

Radiocolloid or indium-111 chloride can be used to label the bone marrow. Colloid particles are accumulated by the reticuloendothelial cells of the marrow, while indium chloride is handled similarly to iron and reflects the erythropoietic component. Studies with both types of agent are hampered by uptake in the liver, which masks a portion of the ribs and vertebral column. In most cases, reticuloendothelial and erythropoietic activity are coincident, but in some patients reticuloendothelial activity may remain in areas where no blood cells are being produced. Clinical applications of this study are limited. If bone marrow biopsy is contemplated in patients with known marrow compromise, particularly after chemotherapy or radiotherapy, it may be useful to perform the scan first, so that biopsy can be directed to an area where active marrow persists. The study may also be used in patients with sickle cell disease to map the sites of marrow infarcts.

Placental Imaging

Blood pool counting with ^{131}I-radioactive iodinated serum albumin (RISA) was replaced by imaging studies with ^{99m}Tc-albumin for demonstration of placental location in cases of suspected placenta previa or abruptio placentae. Although the fetal radiation dose was acceptably small, the advent of ultrasound, which gives no ionizing radiation, has made the radionuclide evaluation obsolete.

Salivary Gland Imaging

Pertechnetate can be used to demonstrate salivary gland function, since the ion is concentrated and secreted by these glands. Uptake is increased in acute inflammation. Both concentration and excretion may be compromised in Sjögren's syndrome, chronic inflammation, or chronic obstruction.

Lymphography

With new microcolloids, it is possible to visualize the nodes in a particular drainage area after subcutaneous injection at the appropriate site. Correlation with contrast lymphangiography is excellent.

References

1. Freeman, L. M., and Blaufox, M. D. (eds.): Radionuclide Studies of the Genitourinary System. II. New York, Grune & Stratton, 1974.
2. Freeman, L. M., and Blaufox, M. D. (eds.): Radionuclide Studies in Evaluation of Trauma. New York, Grune & Stratton, 1974.
3. Freeman, L. M., and Blaufox, M. D. (eds.): Benign Bone Disorders. New York, Grune & Stratton, 1976.
4. Freeman, L. M., and Blaufox, M. D. (eds.): Thrombosis Detection. New York, Grune & Stratton, 1977.
5. Freeman, L. M., and Blaufox, M. D. (eds.): Gallium-67 Citrate. New York, Grune & Stratton, 1978.
6. Freeman, L. M., and Johnson, P. M. (eds.): Clinical Scintillation Imaging. Ed. 2. New York, Grune & Stratton, 1975.
7. Gottschalk, A., and Potchen, E. J. (eds.): Diagnostic nuclear medicine. *In* Golden's Diagnostic Radiology. Section 20. Baltimore, The Williams & Wilkins Company, 1976.
8. Howman-Giles, R., Gilday, D. L., Venugopal, S., et al.: Splenic trauma—nonoperative management and long-term follow-up by scintiscan. J. Pediatr. Surg. *13*:121–126, 1978.
8a. Weissmann, H. S., Frank, M. S., Bernstein, L. H., et al.: Rapid and accurate diagnosis of acute cholecystitis with ^{99m}Tc-HIDA cholescintigraphy. Am. J. Roentgenol. *132*:523–528, 1979.
9. Willerson, J. T. (ed.): Nuclear Cardiology. Philadelphia, F. A. Davis Company, 1979.

3

ULTRASOUND TECHNIQUES

PATRICIA A. LAFFEY, M.D.

Ultrasound is a noninvasive imaging modality employing high-frequency acoustic waves. The information provided about the nature, location, and size of internal structures is useful in diagnosis and treatment planning as well as in the postoperative management of the patient. Visualization is independent of organ function, and studies can be performed rapidly, safely, and with a minimum of patient preparation. Unlike conventional x-rays, ultrasound can distinguish between different types of soft tissue, i.e., cystic versus solid components, based on their differential transmission and reflection of sound waves.[12]

GENERAL CONSIDERATIONS

Physical Principles

Ultrasound waves are generated by electrical stimulation of a piezo-electric crystal, one that will vibrate at a high frequency as a result of such stimulation. Diagnostic studies are generally performed using short pulses of ultrasound in the 1 to 10 megahertz (MHZ) range. The crystal is mounted in a transducer that also acts as a receiver to record echoes reflected back from the body. The transducer is applied directly to the skin surface using mineral oil or water-soluble gel as a surface couplant. As the ultrasound waves pass through the body, they are reflected, transmitted, and attenuated to a varying degree dependent on the acoustic properties of the tissues through which they travel. Reflections occur whenever two adjacent tissues have different acoustic impedances (the product of the density of the material and velocity of the sound passing through it). The strength of the echo depends on the size of that difference, so that at a water-tissue interface, strong reflections are produced, whereas within a solid tissue mass, with only small internal differences in composition, the reflections generated are weak.

The reflections returning to the transducer are displayed on an oscilloscope that shows their level of intensity as well as the position in the body from which they arose. A-mode scanning permits a reading at a single point, with the amplitude of the deflection on the oscilloscope a function of the strength of the echo (Fig. 3–1A).

Bistable or B-mode scanning consists of a series of readings displayed as dots of brightness (Fig. 3–1B). A storage oscilloscope enables one to build up a series of such readings in the scanning plane, so that each complete picture is a tomographic section. By coupling the oscilloscope to a scan converter, the information can be displayed in varying shades of gray, corresponding to different levels of intensity. Gray-scale scanning, a relatively recent development in ultrasound, has greatly enhanced the diagnostic capability by enabling a display of the small-scale internal structural anatomy (Fig. 3–1C).

In M-mode scanning, the baseline rather than the transducer is moved, so that a recording of the position of structures in a single plane over a specified time is obtained. This is particularly useful in echocardiography for recording valve motion and diagnosis of diseases involving the cardiac valves and chambers. A more recent development is the "real-time" scanner. Unlike M-mode, which permits a single-sweep recording of structures at a specific point, real-time scanning provides continuous recording of a wide anatomic sector, similar to a video tape x-ray study. These units are useful not only for echocardiography but also for recording normal and abnormal motion of such structures as the abdominal aorta, kidneys, and fetal heart in addition to aiding in the positive identification of small vessels.

Fluid-filled structures show strong interfaces at their borders, no internal echoes, and good through-transmission of the sound waves (Fig. 3–2A). Solid structures show internal echoes of variable intensity and attenuate the sound beam so that the posterior margin is less sharply defined than the anterior and only a portion of the beam is

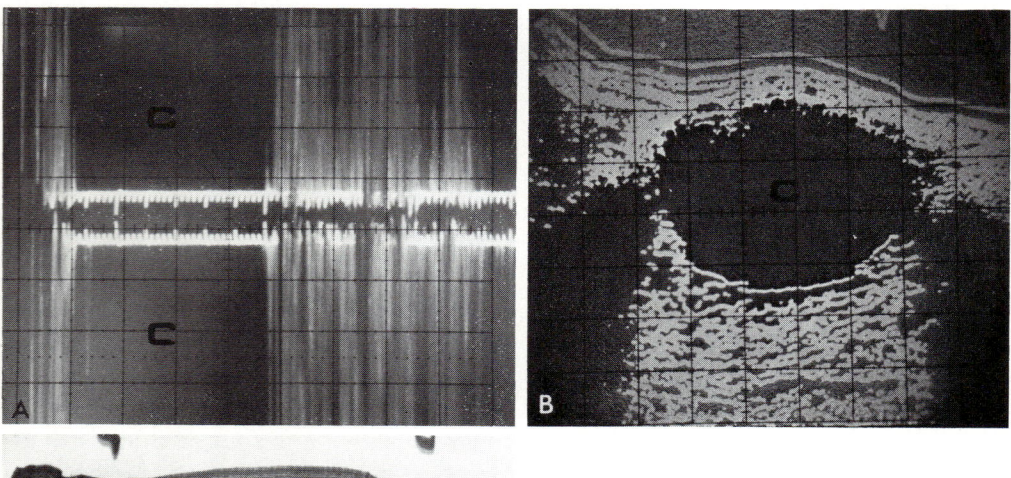

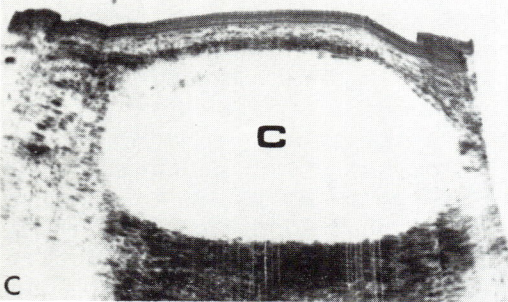

Figure 3–1. Ultrasound display modes of a cystic mass (C). *A,* A-mode recording at low- and high-gain settings. *B,* Bistable image. *C,* Gray-scale image.

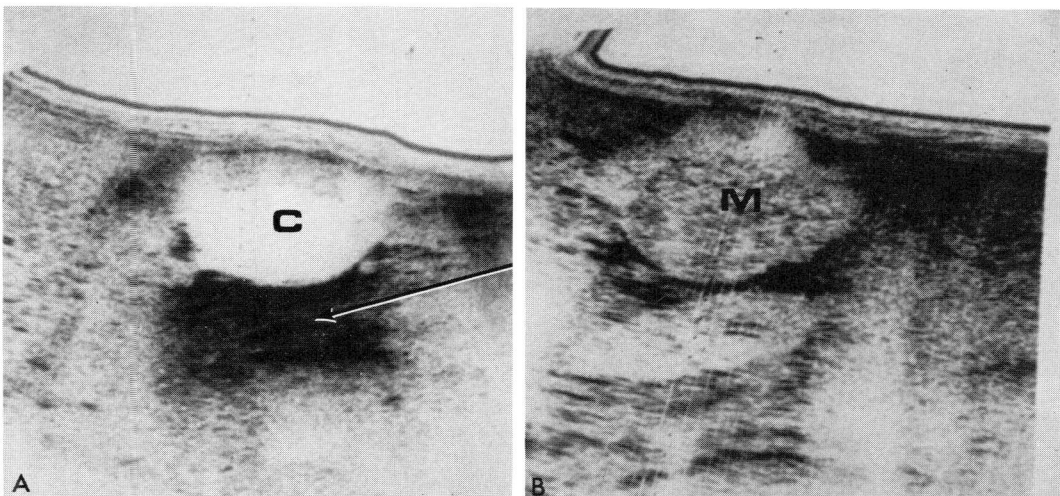

Figure 3–2. *A*, Gray-scale image of a cyst (C) showing an echo-free mass with high through-transmission, yielding considerable echo recording posterior to the mass (arrow). *B*, Scan of a solid mass (M) shows echoes recorded from within the tumor. The resulting attenuation yields considerably less echo recording posterior to the mass compared with the cyst.

transmitted (Fig. 3–2B).[12, 28] The characteristic appearance of the echo pattern of a tissue structure is altered by a change in tissue character, such as an increase in the fluid (edema, cyst formation) or in the solid (fibrosis, infiltrative disease, tumor) content as well as change in size.[93]

Limitations of Ultrasound

The major limitations of ultrasound are (1) acoustic "barriers," such as air, bone, and barium, and (2) the need for contact scanning. Air reflects virtually all of the ultrasound beam, making structures beneath it inaccessible. Barium may produce considerable artifacts and spurious masses.[104] Bone reflects a variable degree of the sound, depending on its thickness. This barrier limitation can be partially overcome by instructing the patient to avoid gas-producing foods and carbonated beverages and to fast immediately prior to the study and by performing the scan before or not less than 48 hours after a barium study. The use of simethicone and similar agents has been suggested, but it is only occasionally helpful. A full bladder aids in studies of the pelvis by displacing gas-filled bowel and rendering the pelvic organs accessible to view. Changes in scanning technique and position are also used to circumvent these barriers.

The second limitation is encountered primarily in the postoperative patient. Since the transducer must be in direct contact with the skin, the presence of overlying dressings, retention sutures, drains, and open wounds prevents scanning in these areas. Although angulation of the transducer or scanning in small sectors frequently yields information, an adequate study may be extremely difficult or impossible to obtain in these patients.

Safety

An important feature of diagnostic ultrasound is its safety. Studies to date have determined no untoward effects on the mammalian tissues at the intensity levels currently employed in diagnostic ultrasound.[3] Studies can be performed without the risk of exposure incurred in conventional radiographic studies. Ultrasound is an ideal modality for studies of children and pregnant women[74] and for serial examinations when the risks of radiation exposure are of particular concern.

Resolution

It is difficult to specify an absolute limit of resolution because of the many factors that can affect it. A theoretical limit is imposed by the equipment and is basically a function of transducer design and selection. Resolution improves with higher frequency transducers, which have a shorter wave length. Unfortunately, high-frequency transducers have low penetrating power, and the selection of a transducer for a given study is a compromise between resolution and depth penetration. Other factors affecting resolution are the attenuation of a lesion relative to surrounding structures and the location of the lesion from the scanning surface. A small cyst within a solid organ may be easily imaged, whereas a large lesion that has very little difference in attenuation with respect to surrounding structures may escape detection. As a practical guide, the approximate limit of resolution for cystic lesions is 1 cm, and that for solid lesions is 2 cm. Reports in the literature regarding the resolution and accuracy of ultrasound in the diagnosis of many conditions have until recently been based on A-mode and bistable B-mode scanning. The improvements afforded by the development of gray-scale and real-time scanning are reflected in more current studies.

Indications for Ultrasound Examination

PREOPERATIVE STUDIES. Ultrasound is useful in the preoperative evaluation of a wide variety of disorders affecting virtually all intra-abdominal contents, except for internal lesions of the gastrointestinal tract. It is also valuable in the study of a number of extra-abdominal and retroperitoneal lesions.[34, 75]

Ultrasound is a primary or adjunctive modality for the detection and characterization of masses for tumor staging,[18, 19] for imaging of major blood vessels, for detection of inflammatory disorders and abscess, and for diagnosis of obstruction of the biliary and urinary tracts. Specific areas of application are discussed in the following sections.

POSTOPERATIVE STUDIES. The management of the patient and the detection of complications can be greatly facilitated by ultrasound.[34] It is a simple and safe study that allows for early diagnosis; in many instances it is the only modality that can determine the presence and nature of an abnormality. Some of the more frequent applications are listed in Table 3–1. Specific entities are discussed in the following sections.

As indicated earlier, the major limitation of ultrasound is interference from overlying dressings, retention studies, and so forth. Although this does not necessarily prevent a specific study from being obtained, it is a significant problem and must be kept in mind determining the usefulness or reliability of an ultrasound study.

LIVER

Examination of the liver has been greatly enhanced by the use of gray-scale technique, which provides details of the small-scale internal anatomy as well as the organ outline. The normal liver has a relatively homogeneous pattern of internal echo with visible portal and hepatic veins (Fig. 3–3).[22]

TABLE 3–1. USE OF ULTRASOUND IN POSTOPERATIVE COMPLICATIONS

Clinical Situation	Ultrasound Used to Detect
Infection	Abscess formation[35, 45, 82, 94, 105, 129, 172]
Jaundice	Obstruction of biliary system[26, 116] Pancreatitis[36] Common duct stones[143]
Renal failure	Obstructive uropathy[14, 141, 170] Renal size

Renal transplant	Transplant size[5, 100]
	Parenchymal changes with rejection[171]
	Hydronephrosis[91, 134]
	Extrarenal mass[5, 91, 115, 122]
	    Abscess
	    Lymphocele
	    Hematoma
	    Urinoma

Abdominal distention
Drop in hematocrit
	Ascites[124]
	Hematoma
	    retroperitoneal, rectus
	    sheath[82, 84, 86, 107]

Hyperamylasemia	Pancreatitis[36] Pancreatic pseudocyst[102]
Vascular surgery	False aneurysm[59, 98] Hematoma formation
Recurrent mass	Recurrent tumor versus other mass (abscess, lymphocele, urinoma)[6, 16]

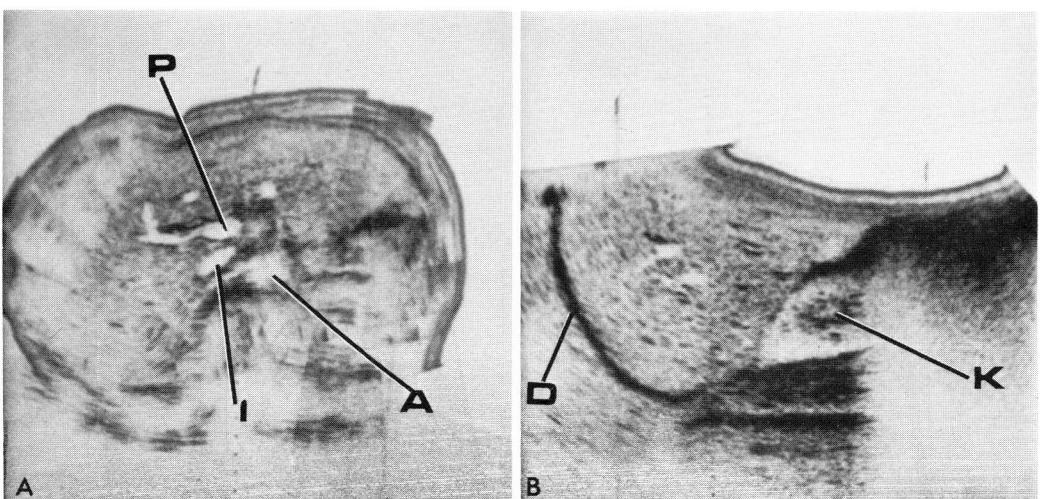

Figure 3–3. Normal liver. *A,* Transverse scan in the upper abdomen shows the liver at the level of the portal vein (P) bifurcation. The aorta (A) and inferior vena cava (I) can be seen posteriorly. *B,* Longitudinal scan through the right lobe shows the normal ultrasonic appearance of the liver with portal and hepatic veins. A portion of the right kidney (K) is seen inferiorly and the diaphragm (D) superiorly.

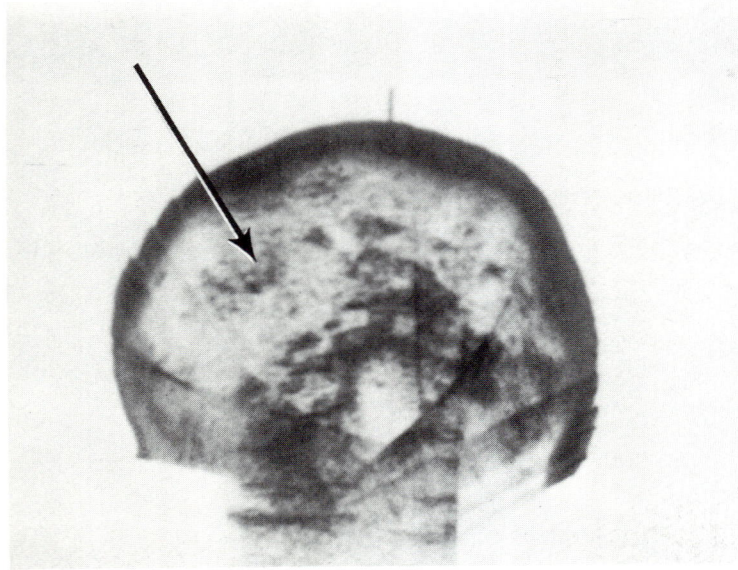

Figure 3–4. Metastases. The transverse scan on this patient with hepatomegaly and a primary colon carcinoma shows numerous echogenic metastases with a large metastatic deposit in the right lobe (arrow).

Tumors

Tumors of the liver may be either more or less echogenic areas than normal liver tissue (Fig. 3–4). Some authors have suggested that certain metastases, particularly adenocarcinoma, are more commonly echogenic.[144] There is no consistent relationship between histologic appearance or vascularity and the ultrasonic appearance.[61] A change

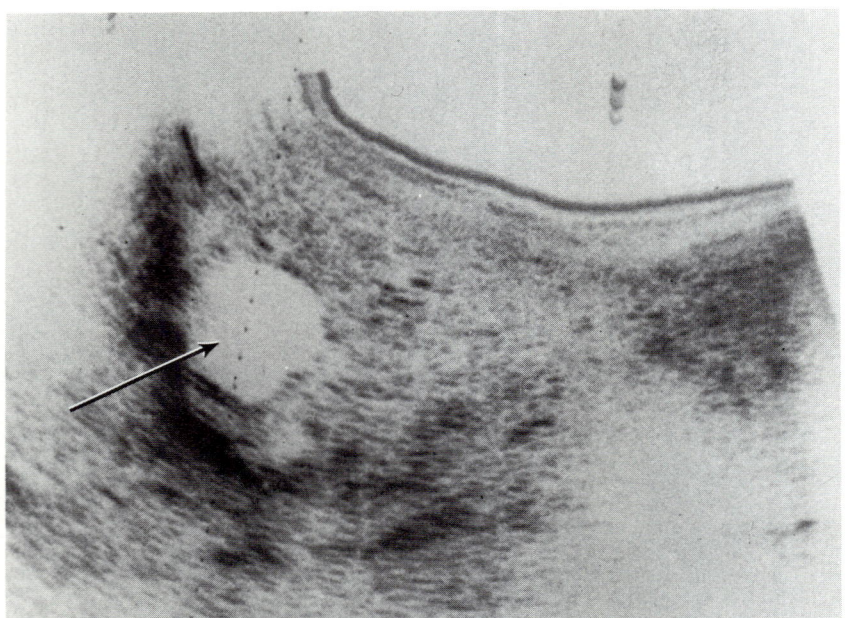

Figure 3–5. Liver cyst. A large cyst (arrow) is seen posteriorly in the right lobe on this longitudinal scan. Hepatomegaly was discovered on a routine physical examination, and a filling defect was seen on the isotope scan. No renal cysts were evident.

in echographic appearance during treatment has been noted. Primary tumors of the liver, although they can be localized by ultrasound, do not have a distinctive pattern that distinguishes them from other neoplastic diseases.

Radionuclide scanning with 99m Tc sulphur colloid remains the procedure of choice for initial evaluation and screening, since it can provide a rapid evaluation of the entire organ and requires little operator expertise. Ultrasonography is particularly useful for (1) clarification of abnormalities seen on isotope scans, i.e., cystic versus solid, intrinsic versus extrinsic;[46, 152] (2) investigation of equivocal areas on isotope scans, particularly in the porta hepatis;[66] and (3) further evaluation in cases in which there is a strong clinical suspicion of focal liver disease in the presence of a normal isotope scan.[157] It can also be helpful in guiding percutaneous biopsy for diagnosis of a solitary mass lesion (see Aspiration-Biopsy Techniques). The overall accuracy in detection of tumors by ultrasound is approximately 90 per cent.[155]

Cysts

Cysts are the most easily detected lesions because of the large difference in attenuation, with sharp contrast provided between the sonolucency of the cysts and the echo pattern of surrounding tissue (Fig. 3–5). Simple cysts, polycystic liver disease, and hydatid cysts[88] have been imaged with an accuracy approaching 100 per cent.

Abscesses

Abscesses of the liver generally appear as circular lesions with irregular borders, internal fluid, and varying amounts of internal debris (Fig. 3–6). They are usually single and may be uniloculated or multiloculated. Amebic abscesses are often multiple. Studies employing ultrasound for diagnosis have shown uniformly high accuracy.[162] The

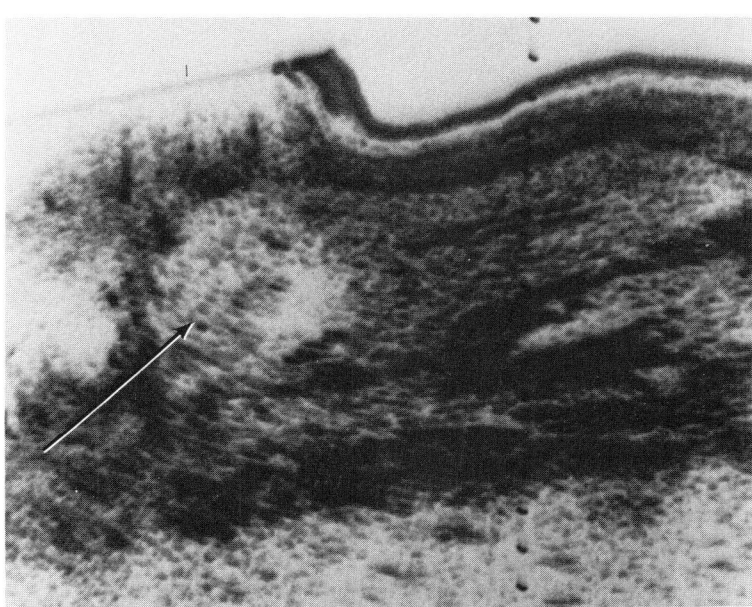

Figure 3–6. Liver abscess. A longitudinal scan through the left lobe of the liver shows a poorly marginated mass (arrow) with both fluid and solid components. Percutaneous aspiration using ultrasonic guidance yielded positive cultures, and a definitive drainage procedure was performed.

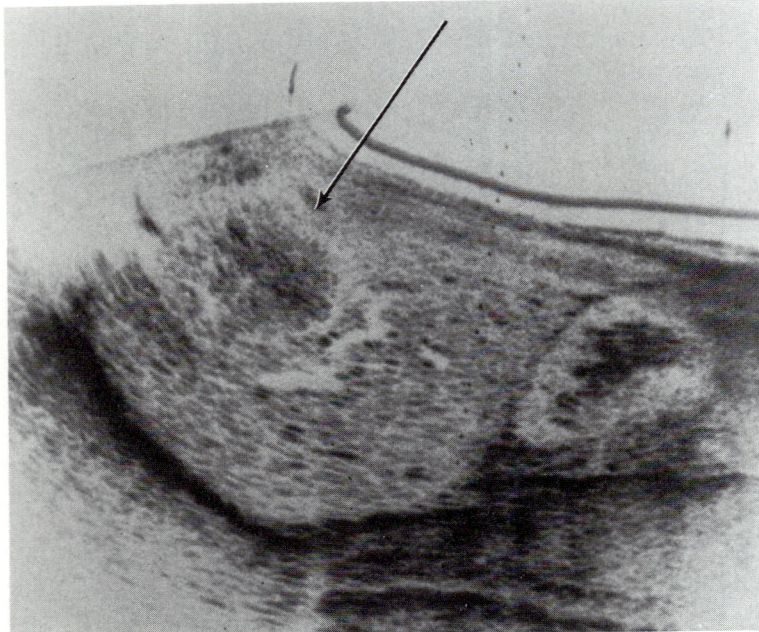

Figure 3–7. Necrotic metastasis. The development of necrosis and fluid within a metastasis may produce an appearance similar to that of an abscess. Clear fluid was obtained in the aspirate of this lesion (arrow), although no malignant cells could be identified cytologically. Resection of the lesion demonstrated anaplastic carcinoma.

primary ultrasonic differential diagnosis includes intrahepatic hematoma and necrotic metastases (Fig. 3–7). Percutaneous aspiration and even catheterization for drainage and instillation of therapeutic agents has been safely accomplished using ultrasound for localization and guidance (see Aspiration-Biopsy Techniques).

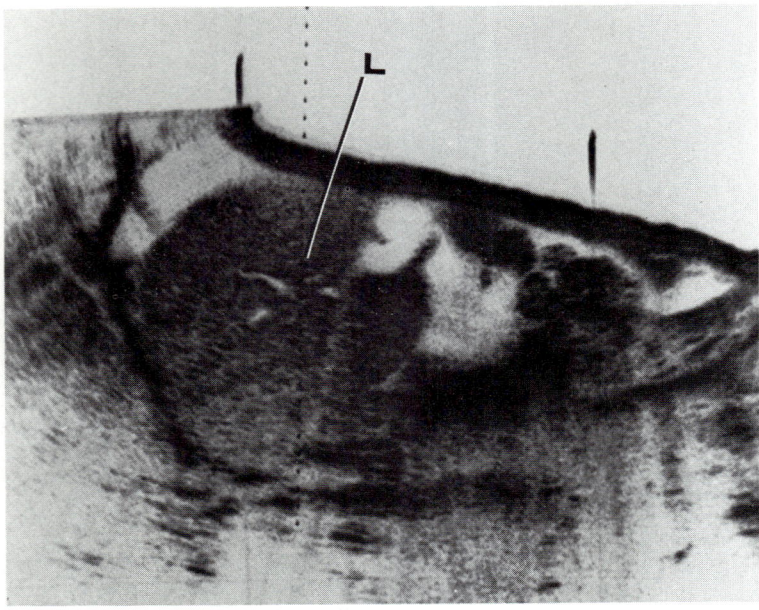

Figure 3–8. Cirrhosis with ascites. This longitudinal scan shows an abnormally dense pattern of echo within the liver (L), which is surrounded by ascitic fluid.

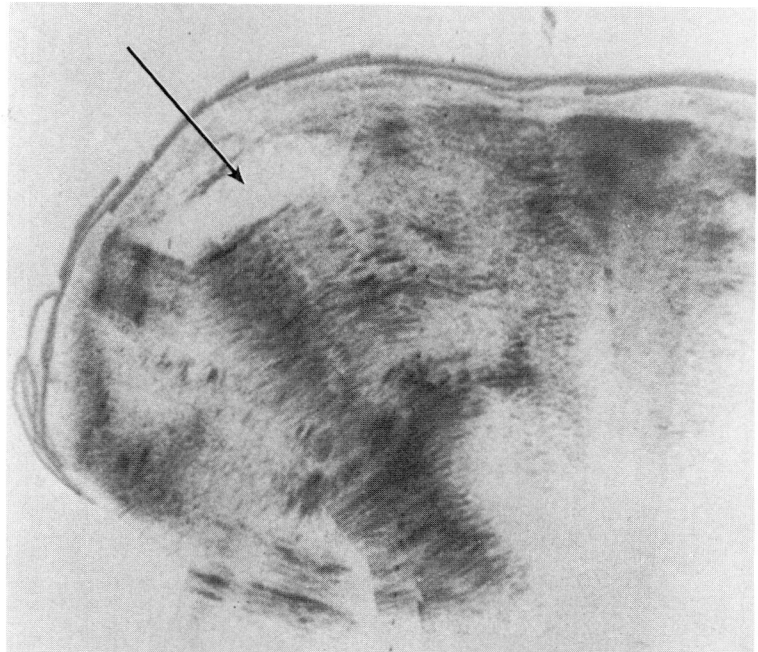

Figure 3–9. Subcapsular hematoma. A collection of fluid (arrow) is seen along the anterolateral liver surface on this transverse scan. The patient developed right upper quadrant pain following a liver biopsy.

Cirrhosis

The changes in the echographic appearance secondary to fibrosis occur only in the late stages of cirrhosis, so that ultrasound is not useful for early diagnosis. The presence of ascites, however, can be easily detected (Fig. 3–8). Measurements of the width of the portal vein and splenic vein may be helpful in evaluating portal hypertension.

Trauma

Ultrasonography can be used to evaluate subcapsular and intrahepatic hematomas following trauma. A subcapsular hematoma appears as a crescentic echo-free collection surrounding all or a portion of the hepatic parenchyma and conforming to the hepatic outline (Fig. 3–9). Intracapsular hematomas, like hematomas elsewhere, have a variable appearance, ranging from cystic to a mixed echo pattern with variable amounts of internal echo. The pattern depends upon the amount of clot formation and the degree of liquefaction. Although occasionally it resembles an intrahepatic abscess, the clinical picture will help in differentiation.

Postoperative Studies

Ultrasound can be used to detect intrahepatic abscess and hematoma formation as well as collections in the subphrenic or subhepatic regions (Fig. 3–10). Volumetric changes in liver size following portacaval shunting can be monitored.[126] Recent studies have demonstrated the ability to visualize portacaval shunts; evaluation of flow dy-

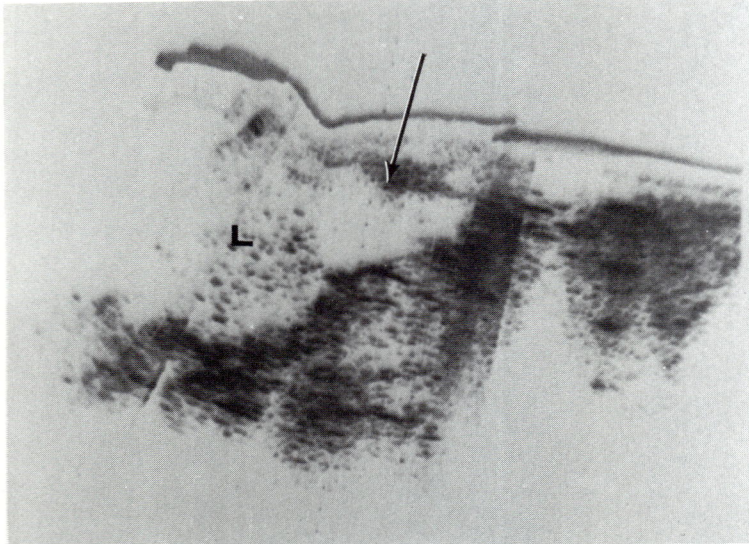

Figure 3–10. Subhepatic abscess. This longitudinal scan on a patient with sepsis following an appendectomy shows an irregular fluid collection (arrow) inferior to the right lobe of the liver (L).

namics by observing changes in size during the Valsalva maneuver determines patency.[52]

BILIARY SYSTEM

Cholecystitis and Calculi

Oral cholecystography is the procedure of choice for initial evaluation of the gallbladder, since it can provide information regarding function and diagnose lesions not ordinarily seen with ultrasound. These include polyps and the cholecystoses.

Ultrasound is an excellent tool for investigation of the nonvisualized gallbladder, since imaging is independent of function. It has an accuracy of 90 per cent or greater in the diagnosis of stones.[4, 103, 160] Ideally, ultrasound should be performed in all cases of nonvisualization on single-dose oral cholecystography. Double-dose oral cholecystography should be reserved for those cases in which ultrasound studies are inadequate. Despite a high rate of accuracy, false normal oral cholecystograms may occur in patients with calculi and those with acalculous cholecystitis.[40] Ultrasound can be used as a supplemental procedure to look for calculi in those patients with normal oral studies and a strong clinical suspicion of biliary disease. It is also useful as the initial study in patients with suspected acute cholecystitis or jaundice and in pregnant females and patients who are hypersensitive to the contrast media.[4, 9]

The gallbladder is best imaged in fasting patients (Fig. 3–11). Calculi produce discrete internal echoes and significantly attenuate the beam, producing an "acoustic shadow" distally (Fig. 3–12). In the case of a scarred, contracted gallbladder with stones, a very dense echo and acoustic shadow are seen in the plane of the gallbladder with no visible lumen or fluid component (Fig. 3–13). Inability to image the gallbladder in a fasting patient, unless the gallbladder is inaccessible owing to a high position under the right rib cage, is highly suggestive of disease. It has much the same significance as nonvisualization by oral cholecystography. With visualization, size can easily be determined, although there is a wide variation. A transverse dimension of greater than

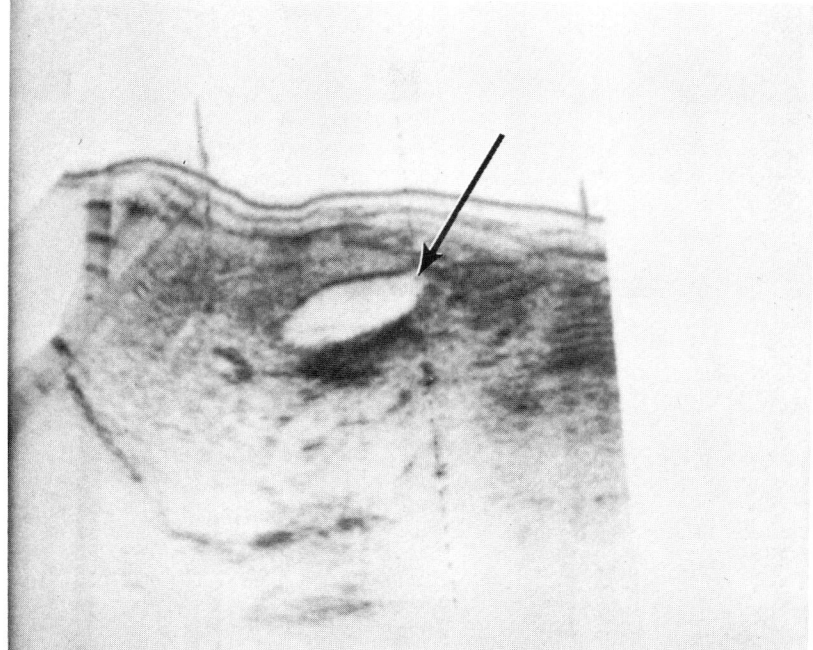

Figure 3–11. Normal gallbladder. The gallbladder appears as a well-delineated fluid-filled structure (arrow) on this longitudinal scan.

4 cm is indicative of dilatation.[49] Comparative scans can be performed following fatty meal ingestion or cholecystokinin injection to assess the degree of contraction.

Thickening of the walls secondary to inflammation has been noted, although not consistently (Fig. 3–14).[80] It may be seen in both acute and chronic cholecystitis. An

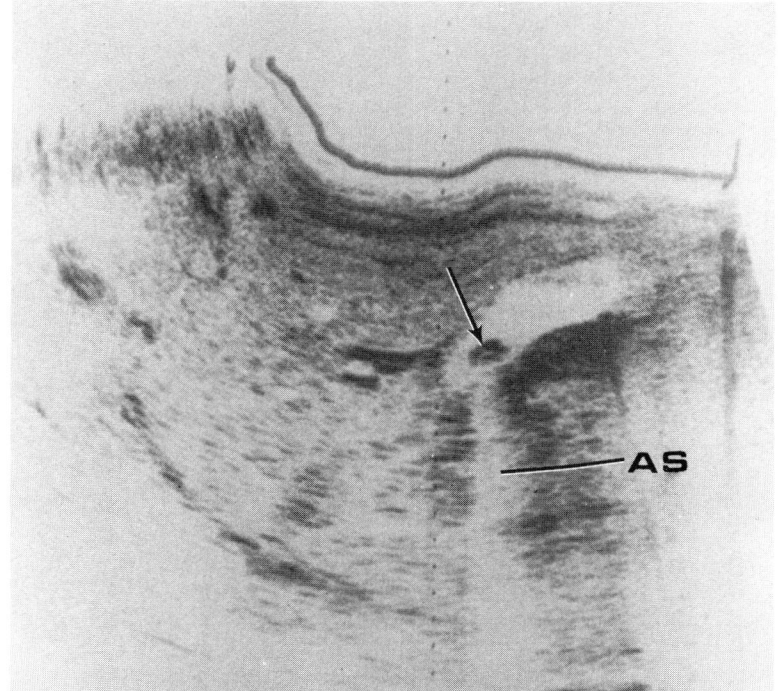

Figure 3–12. Gallstone. A strong echo is recorded from the calculus (arrow), and there is an absence of echo recording or "acoustic shadow" (AS) posterior to it.

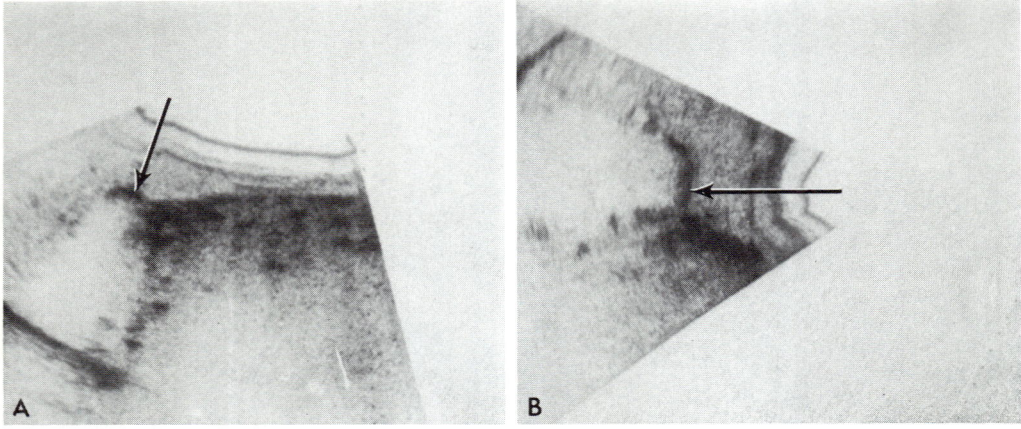

Figure 3–13. Gallstones. Longitudinal (A) and decubitus (B) scans demonstrate a dense band of echoes and acoustic shadow limited to the region of the gallbladder (arrows). The gallbladder itself is not seen as a fluid-filled structure; a scarred contracted gallbladder with multiple calculi was removed surgically.

abnormal echo pattern may occur in the adjacent liver with acute suppurative cholecystitis. This is a result of reactive inflammation and pericholecystic abscess formation. Ultrasound is helpful in depicting collections secondary to perforation or fistula formation.[9] It is not particularly useful for the diagnosis of carcinoma of the gallbladder or bile ducts, although abnormal configurations or accompanying ductal dilatation may be apparent.[32]

Jaundice

Ultrasound should be the initial study for the investigation of obstructive jaundice, since it can be performed rapidly, simply, and with a high degree of accuracy. Recent studies have disclosed an accuracy as high as 97 per cent in distinguishing obstructive

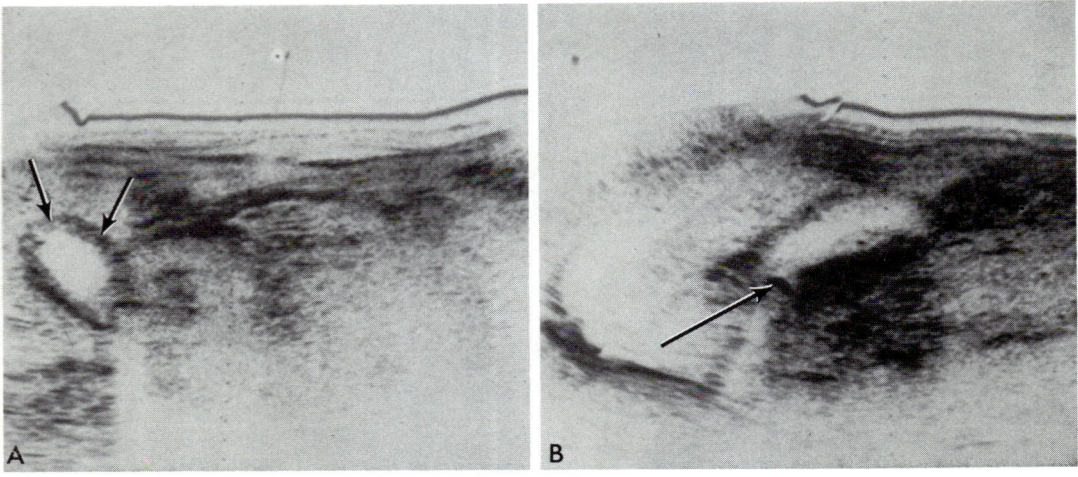

Figure 3–14. Cholecystitis with cholelithiasis. A, Thickening of the gallbladder wall (arrows) is evident on this transverse scan. B, A calculus is seen on the longitudinal scan (arrow).

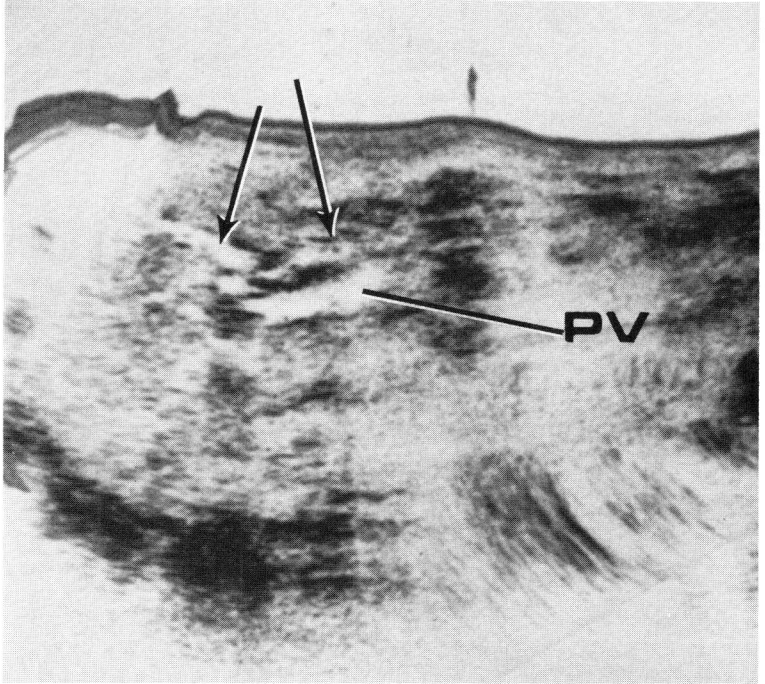

Figure 3–15. Obstructive jaundice. Dilated bile ducts (arrows) are seen along the anterior edge of the portal vein (PV) in the porta hepatis. As the major branches of the biliary tract dilate, they approach the size of the portal veins that they accompany, producing a "parallel channel," or double-track sign.

from nonobstructive jaundice; failures are usually found in cases of minimal duct dilatation.[116, 156] The normal intrahepatic bile ducts are not usually seen on scans.

Recent studies employing more flexible real-time scanners have reported frequent visualization of the normal main bile duct, which ranges from 4 to 8 mm in diameter.[167] Particular attention to the junction of the right and left biliary ducts permits early diagnosis in cases of minimal dilatation (Fig. 3–15).[26] With more advanced degrees of obstruction, the peripheral ducts are also visible (Fig. 3–16). Frequently, the exact level

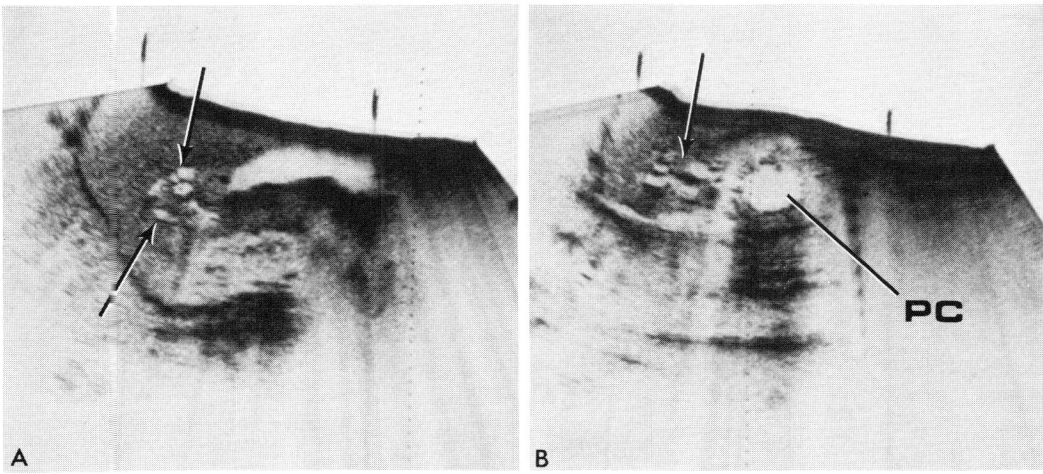

Figure 3–16. Dilated biliary radicles secondary to pancreatic pseudocyst. *A*, A longitudinal scan through the right lobe of the liver shows dilated biliary radicles (arrows) as well as an enlarged gallbladder. *B*, A more medial scan through the level of the inferior vena cava shows a pseudocyst (PC) in the head of the pancreas as well as dilated intrahepatic bile duct (arrow).

68 — ULTRASOUND TECHNIQUES

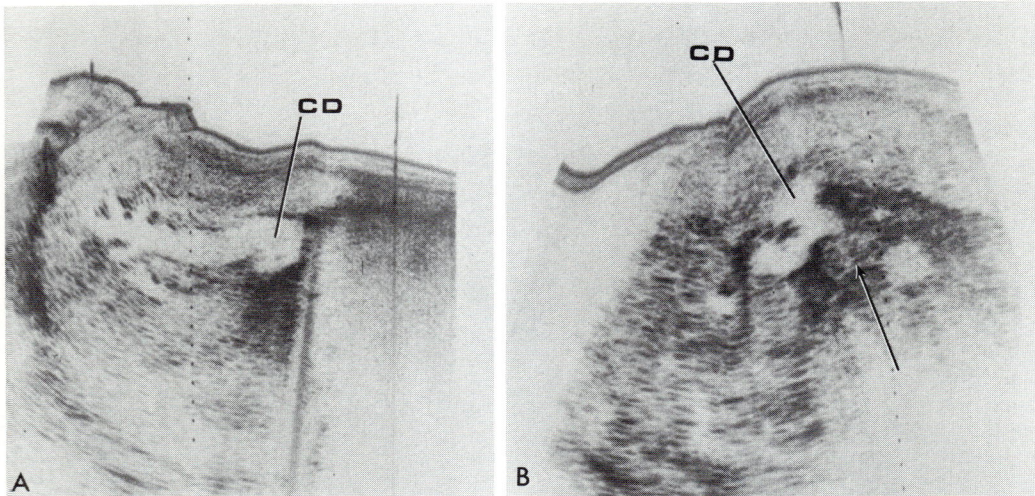

Figure 3–17. Pancreatic carcinoma with obstructive jaundice. *A,* A markedly dilated common duct (CD) is evident on the longitudinal scan. *B,* Transversely, a small mass (arrow) in the head of the pancreas can be seen at the distal portion of the dilated common duct (CD).

and cause of the obstruction, e.g., tumors or cysts in the head of the pancreas, tumors involving the porta hepatis, or choledocholithiasis, can also be determined, thus expediting further investigations (Fig. 3–17).

Choledochal cysts have also been imaged with ultrasound.[41] Difficulty sometimes arises in distinguishing this entity from other cystic masses occurring in the right upper quadrant, such as pancreatic pseudocysts, although demonstration of a common

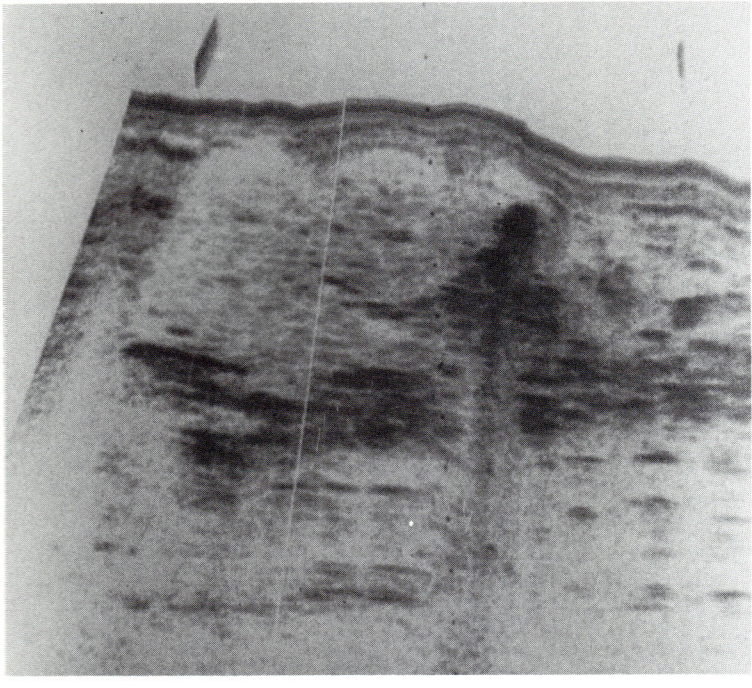

Figure 3–18. Biliary atresia. Longitudinal scan on a one-month-old jaundiced infant shows no evidence of a gallbladder or dilated ducts. A microcystic pattern of ducts may occur; areas of dilatation can be detected.

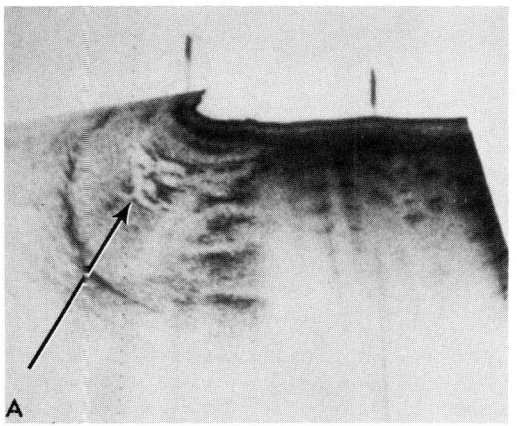 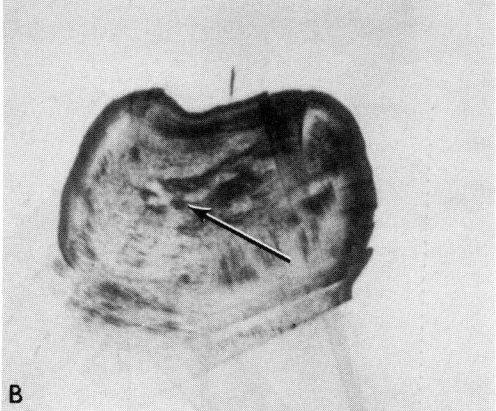

Figure 3–19. Choledocholithiasis. This patient with previous cholecystectomy presented with jaundice. *A,* The longitudinal scan shows multiple dilated ducts (arrow). *B,* On the transverse view, a calculus (arrow) can be seen in the distal common duct.

bile duct entering the cyst permits a specific diagnosis. Ultrasound can also be used to look for the presence of a gallbladder in cases of suspected biliary atresia (Fig. 3–18).[153]

Postoperative Studies

Ultrasound can be used to reliably distinguish between obstructive and nonobstructive jaundice in the postoperative patient. Attempts should be made to define residual common duct stones to exclude the possibility of a tumor overlooked at surgery (Fig. 3–19).[143] Ligation of the common duct or stricture formation is not evident on ultrasound scans.

Abscesses may be identified in the subphrenic or subhepatic regions. Pancreatitis and pancreatic pseudocysts can be documented.

PANCREAS

Gray-scale scanning, in contrast to bistable studies, results in visualization of the normal pancreas in the majority of patients.[168] The pancreas appears as a relatively homogeneous echogenic structure ranging from 1 to 3 cm in thickness.[70] The splenic vein, which courses along its posterior surface, serves as a useful landmark for identification (Fig. 3–20).[42] The pancreatic head often lies inferior to the splenic vein and the rest of the gland. Because of bowel gas in the left upper quadrant, scanning in the prone position is usually required in order for the tail to be visualized just anterior to the left kidney. Ultrasound has proven useful for both acute inflammatory and neoplastic diseases of the pancreas.

Pancreatitis

Acute pancreatitis produces an enlargement of the gland, with a decrease in the number of internal echoes and an increase in the transmission of ultrasound due to

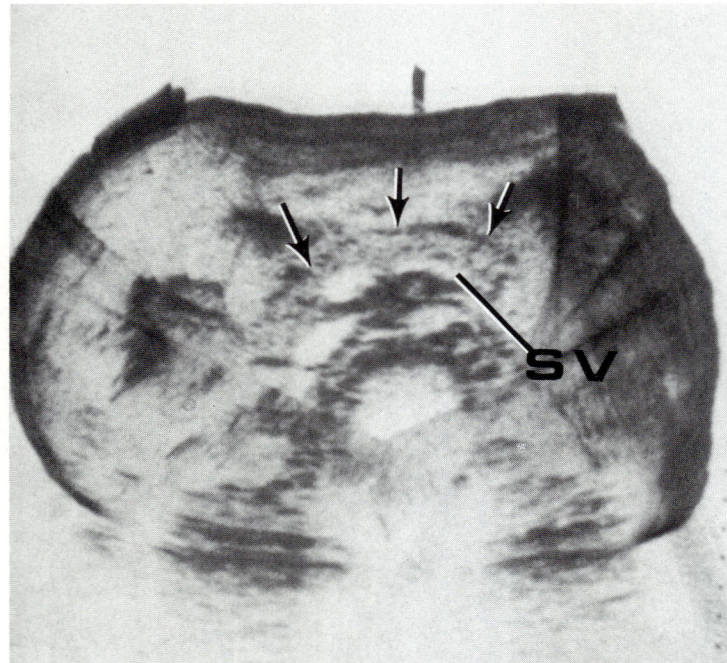

Figure 3–20. Normal pancreas. The splenic vein (SV) is seen along the posterior surface of the pancreas (arrows). The pancreas normally has more internal echo than the adjacent liver.

the increased fluid content (Fig. 3–21). While an elevation of serum amylase is a good clinical indicator of pancreatitis, the ultrasound findings persist longer and are useful for confirming the diagnosis and for investigating patients with chronic renal failure and hyperamylasemia who may have associated pancreatitis.[36]

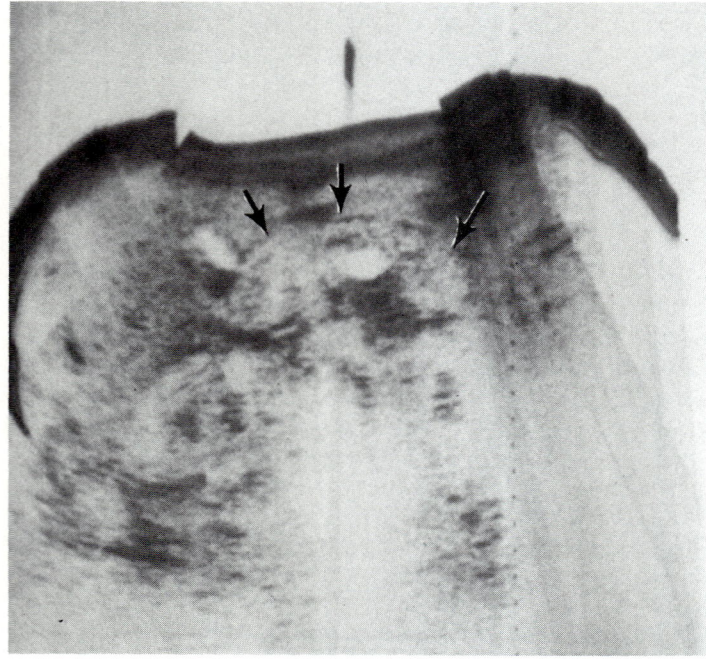

Figure 3–21. Acute pancreatitis. The typical findings are an enlarged pancreas (arrows) and a decrease in the internal echoes.

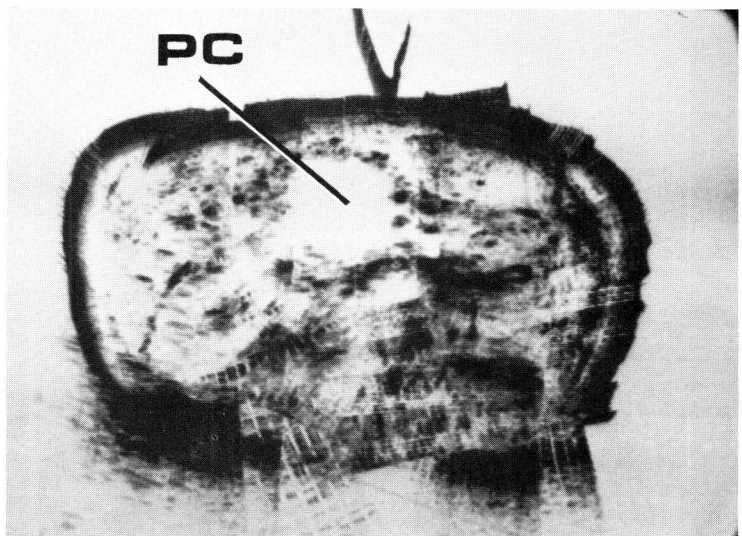

Figure 3–22. Pancreatic pseudocyst. A large cyst (PC) is seen in the head of the pancreas in this patient with acute and chronic pancreatitis.

The findings in chronic pancreatitis are related to the fibrosis produced by the disease. The gland often has a diffuse increase in the number of internal echoes and may be difficult to outline. Calcifications may produce strong echoes within the gland and acoustic shadowing behind them.

Pseudocyst

Ultrasound is a definitive study for the diagnosis of pancreatic pseudocysts and has an accuracy rate approaching 100 per cent.[58, 102] These pseudocysts may be unilocular or multilocular (Fig. 3–22). Occasionally, there are multiple cysts. Rarely, they may appear in unusual locations, such as the mediastinum or pelvis, and they may occasionally involve the spleen or kidney directly.[27] The majority of pseudocysts are echo-free, although a small amount of necrotic debris may be seen. Significant amounts of solid tissue within the cyst should alert the surgeon to the possibility of cystadenocarcinoma and suggest biopsy sites. Serial studies provide a simple method of following the progress of the cyst (Fig. 3–23). An increase in size, spontaneous resolution, or rupture can be easily documented. A 20 per cent incidence of spontaneous resolution was noted in one series.[58] Although attempts have been made to measure the wall thickness, this cannot be reliably estimated by ultrasound.[17]

Tumor

Pancreatic carcinoma can be detected ultrasonically with an accuracy of approximately 85 per cent. This is far higher than the accuracy of barium contrast studies and isotope scanning and is comparable to the confirmatory studies of angiography and endoscopic retrograde cannulation.[163] Since the ultrasonic examination can be performed simply and without risk to the patient, it should be the initial study in suspected pancreatic carcinoma. These tumors appear most often as focal areas of enlargement with fewer internal echoes than the surrounding tissue (Fig. 3–24). These masses

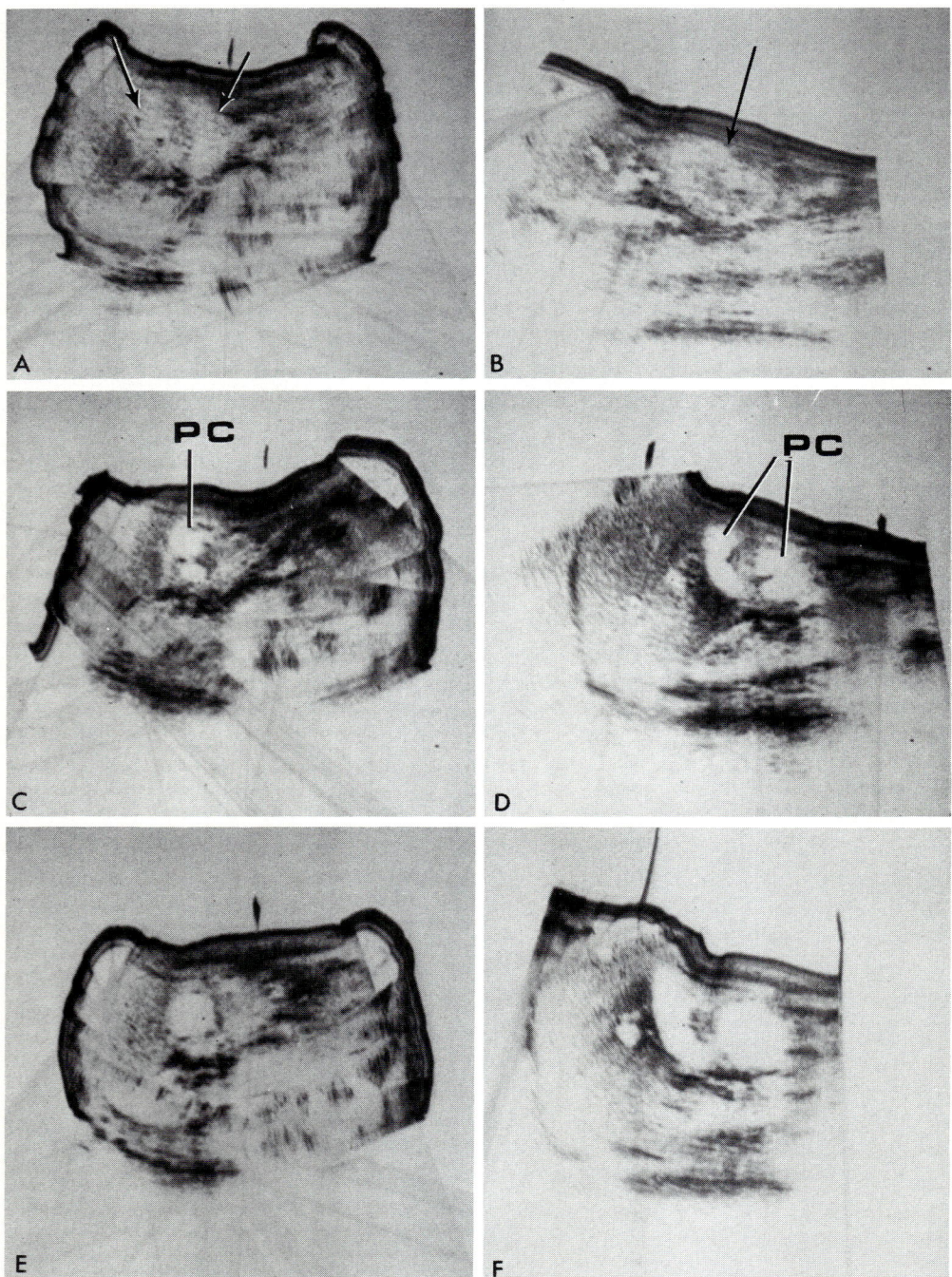

Figure 3–23. Pancreatic pseudocyst. Serial scans on this patient demonstrate the development and progression of pancreatic pseudocyst. *A* and *B*, The initial transverse and longitudinal scans show enlargement and edema of the head of the pancreas (arrows). *C* and *D*, Three weeks later, two cysts (PC) have developed. *E* and *F*, Scans at six weeks demonstrate further enlargement. The transverse view *(E)* is a section through the inferior cyst. The cysts were subsequently drained surgically.

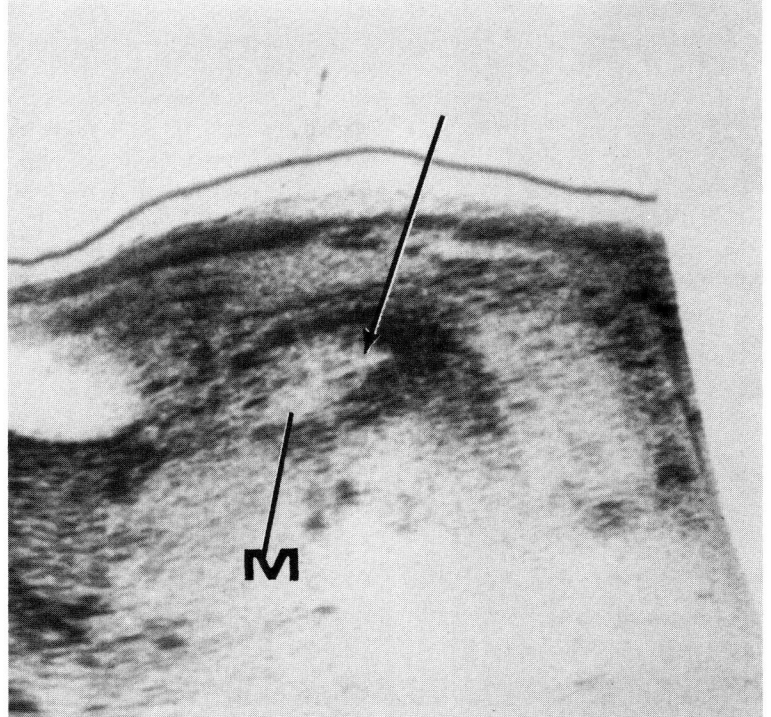

Figure 3–24. Pancreatic carcinoma. There is a relatively sonolucent or echo-free mass (M) in the head of the pancreas with dilatation of the pancreatic duct (arrow).

are acoustically dense and often attenuate a great deal of the sound beam, making it difficult to define their posterior margins. Metastases to the pancreas are indistinguishable in appearance from primary pancreatic carcinoma.

Retroperitoneal lymphoma in this region may mimic pancreatic tumor, although

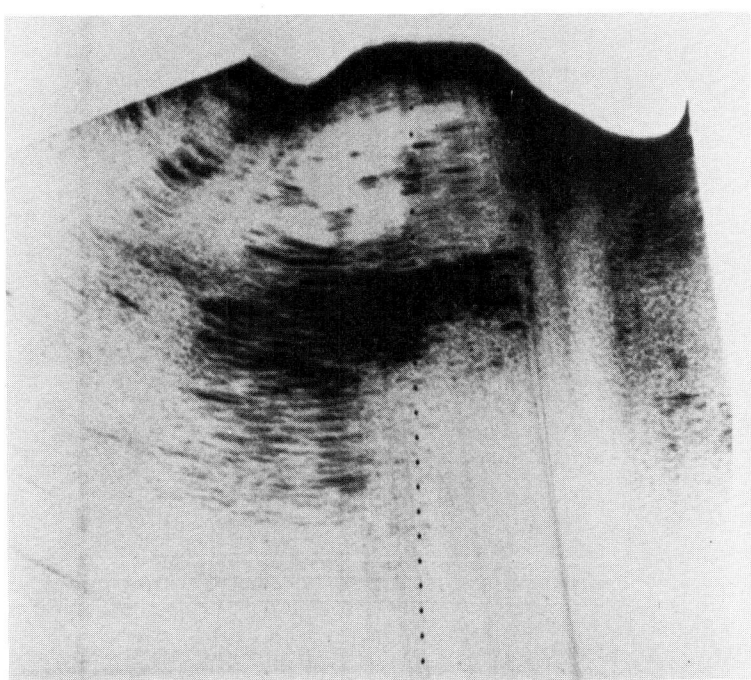

Figure 3–25. Pancreatic cystadenocarcinoma. This longitudinal scan just to the right in a middle-aged female with a palpable mass shows the typical appearance, with well-defined cysts and solid stroma.

lymphomas usually show better sound transmission, i.e., appear sonolucent. Localization of a mass posterior to the splenic vein and extension posteriorly along the paravertebral areas are helpful in identifying the mass as nonpancreatic retroperitoneal tumor. Chronic pancreatitis, which may produce focal abnormalities, may be indistinguishable from pancreatic carcinoma. The most difficult lesions to diagnose ultrasonically are small islet cell tumors and tumors of the tail of the pancreas. The latter may be obscured by gas in the left upper quadrant. Prone scans are helpful in identifying this area of the pancreas.

Cystadenoma and cystadenocarcinoma have a typical, although not pathognomonic, appearance owing to their cystic nature (Fig. 3–25).[173] Necrotic carcinomas and cystic islet cell tumors must be considered in the differential diagnosis. The most important distinction is between pancreatic pseudocysts and cyst-containing tumors. Careful scans of all apparent cysts should be made in a search for solid areas or atypical features that might suggest a neoplastic lesion.

KIDNEY

Ultrasound is an ideal tool for study of the kidneys, and its use and indications are rapidly expanding.[33] Scans of the kidney are usually performed with the patient in the prone position. This places the kidney closer to the transducer, increasing the resolution and eliminating the problems of overlying bowel gas that hinder supine examinations, particularly of the left kidney (Fig. 3–26). Supine and decubitus scans may provide additional information. The increased resolution afforded by recent technical advances permits differentiation of the cortex and medulla based on identification of the arcuate vessels.[30] The renal arteries and veins can often be identified on supine scans.

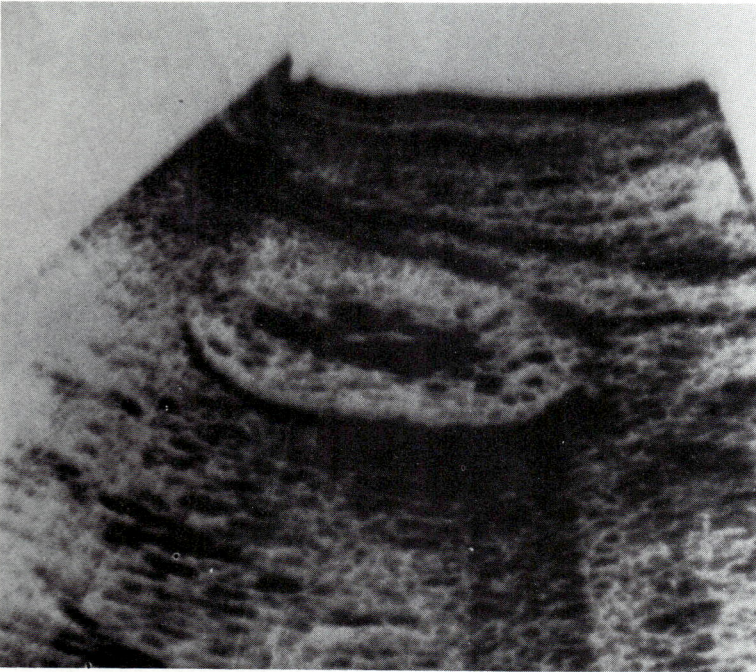

Figure 3–26. Normal kidney. The normal kidney shows strong echoes arising centrally from the collecting system with low-level echoes in the parenchyma.

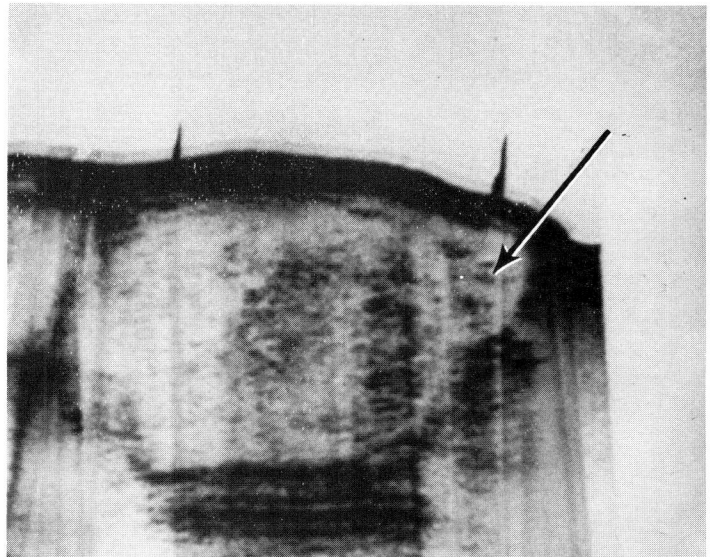

Figure 3-27. Hypernephroma. A large solid mass occupies the upper pole of the left kidney and left upper quadrant. The remaining normal kidney (arrow) is seen along the inferior edge.

Renal Mass

Ultrasound is particularly useful in the evaluation of a renal mass detected on an intravenous urogram (Fig. 3-27). The urogram should precede the ultrasound examination in cases of suspected mass, although ultrasonography may be used as the initial study in patients with a history of contrast allergy. It may also be useful to periodically monitor patients with a known risk of development of a renal tumor. Ultrasonography has the obvious advantage of avoiding radiation exposure and contrast reactions, although its effectiveness in such situations has not yet been evaluated.

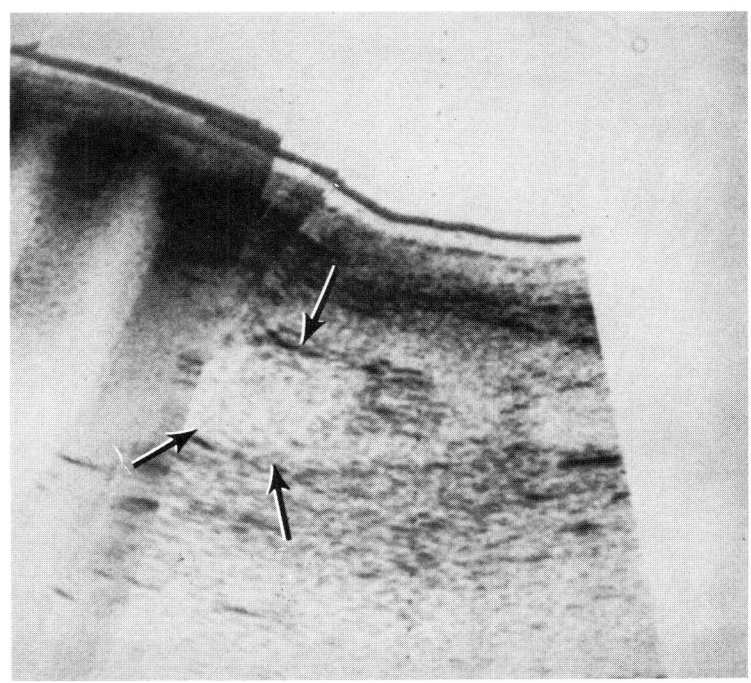

Figure 3-28. Hypernephroma. A solid mass (arrows) with relatively few internal echoes and poor through-transmission is seen in the upper pole of the kidney.

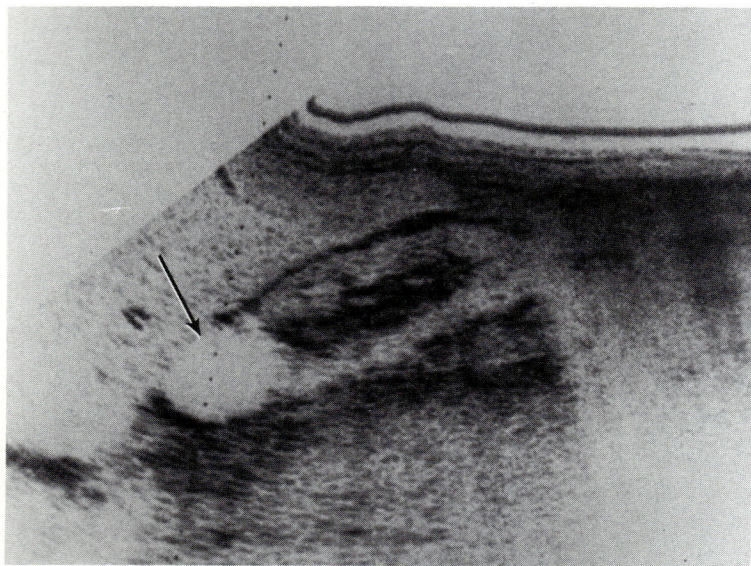

Figure 3–29. Renal cyst. A well-defined echo-free cyst (arrow) is demonstrated in the upper pole of the right kidney.

Solid or complex lesions can be differentiated from cysts (Fig. 3–28). A tumor thrombus from hypernephromas can sometimes be identified in the renal vein and inferior vena cava. Cysts can be localized with an accuracy of 98 per cent (Fig. 3–29).[150] The ultrasonic diagnosis of a cyst is 95 per cent reliable; the diagnosis can be confirmed by cyst puncture performed with ultrasound localization (see Aspiration-Biopsy Techniques).

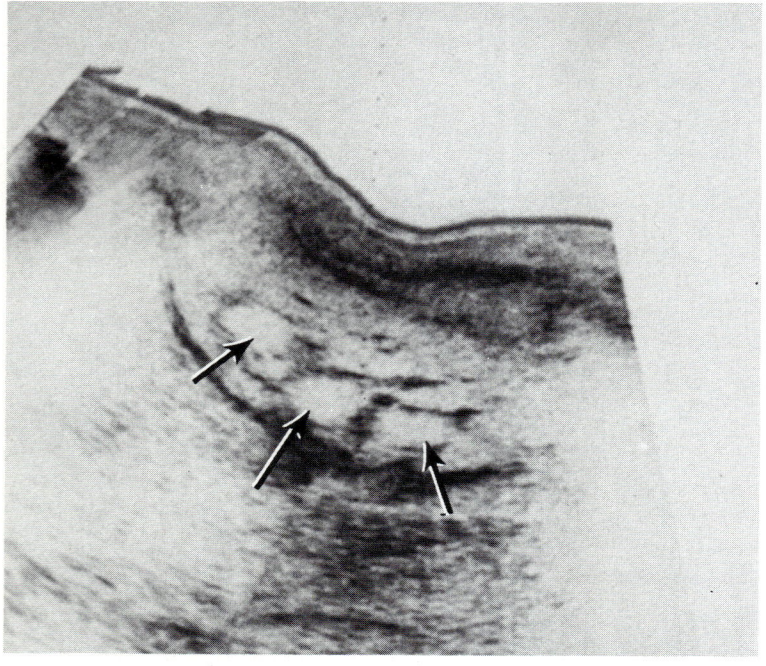

Figure 3–30. Hydronephrosis. Dilated fluid-filled calices have replaced the normal linear collecting system echoes.

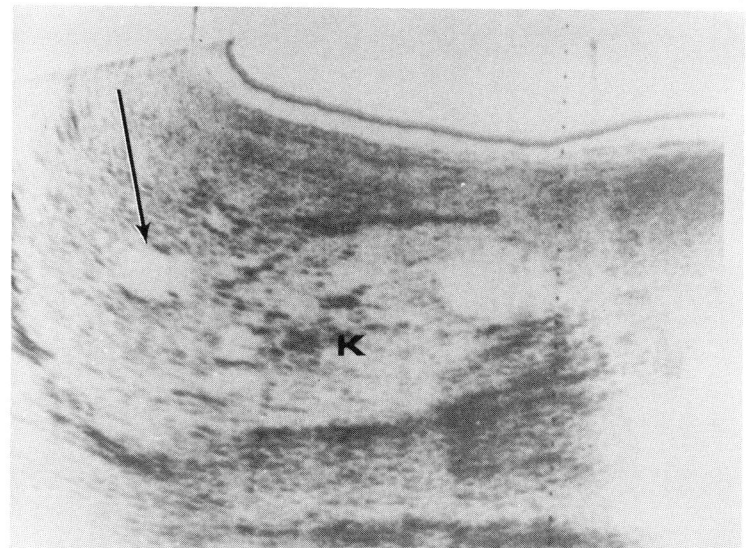

Figure 3–31. Polycystic disease. This longitudinal scan shows an enlarged right kidney (K) with numerous cysts. A cyst (arrow) is also seen in the liver.

Renal Failure — Nonvisualizing Kidney

Since ultrasound imaging does not require renal function, it can be used to assess the status of the kidneys in both acute and chronic renal failure and may obviate the need for invasive studies, such as retrograde pyelography and angiography.[14, 141, 170] Scans are used to determine the size, presence, and location of the kidneys. Hydronephrosis, cystic disease, and tumors can be identified (Fig. 3–30). Obstructive uropathy, which may be amenable to surgical intervention, can be distinguished from nonobstructive disease. Visualization of abnormally small kidneys indicates that the renal failure is probably secondary to chronic infection or vascular disease. Polycystic disease produces a characteristic pattern. Scans may reveal polycystic disease of the liver, which occurs in approximately one third of the cases (Fig. 3–31).[87]

Ultrasound is also of value in the study of a unilateral nonvisualizing kidney, when it may obviate or supplement retrograde pyelography.

Renal Calculi

The acoustic properties of calculi cause a strong echo reflection and prevent transmission of the sound beam, producing an acoustic shadow (Fig. 3–32). This allows localization of both opaque and nonopaque calculi[38] and distinction between stones and other causes of filling defects of the renal pelvis.[123]

Infection

Alterations in the renal parenchyma have been detected in a variety of inflammatory conditions.[63, 132] The findings are not specific and do not provide a definitive diagnosis, although scans can be used for confirmation. Perinephric abscesses cause a complex perirenal mass with both cystic and solid components (Fig. 3–33).

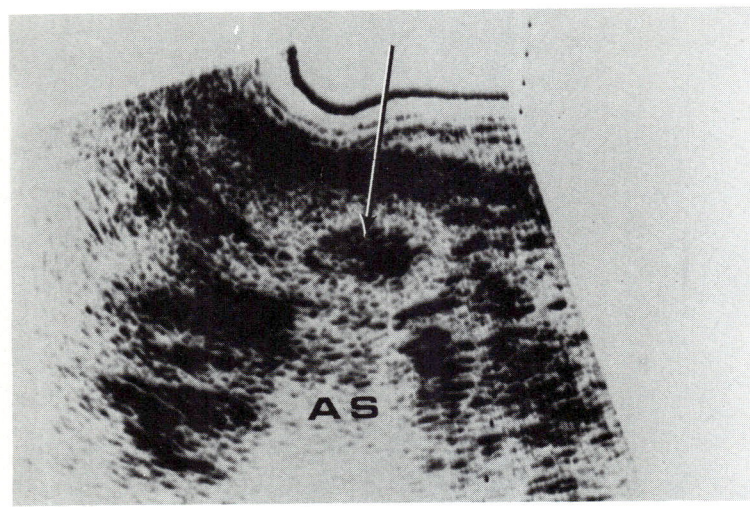

Figure 3–32. Renal calculus. A strong central echo is recorded from a staghorn calculus (arrow). The resulting attenuation produces an "acoustic shadow" (AS) distally, similar to that seen with gallbladder calculi.

Trauma

Ultrasound is not a primary tool in the investigation of traumatic renal lesions. It can be used to confirm the presence of intrarenal and perirenal hematoma and provides an excellent tool for serial evaluation when surgery is not contemplated.

Postoperative Studies

Scans in postoperative patients can be used to evaluate the kidneys and nephric space when development of hematoma, lymphocele, urinoma, or perinephric abscess is suspected (Fig. 3–34). Ultrasound is helpful in the investigation of renal failure and particularly in the early diagnosis of urinary tract obstruction.[170]

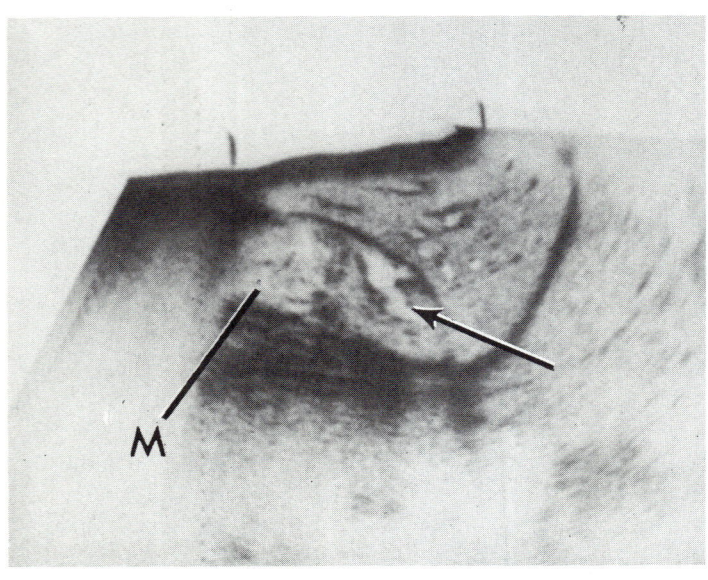

Figure 3–33. Perinephric abscess. A mass (M) with both fluid and solid components is seen along the lower pole of the right kidney. The proximal ureter was obstructed, and dilated calices are seen (arrow).

Figure 3–34. Nephric space collection. A collection of fluid (arrow) is seen in the right nephric space following a radical nephrectomy for hypernephroma.

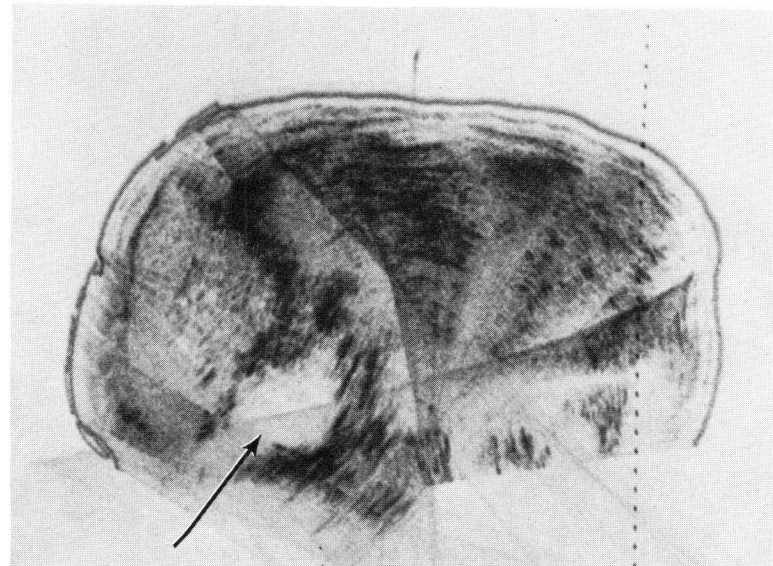

Transplant Kidney

Ultrasound has proved to be a very useful study in the evaluation of the transplanted kidney (Fig. 3–35). It may not only confirm the clinical suspicion of rejection but, more importantly, detect extrarenal collections and hydronephrosis that may mimic rejection (Fig. 3–36).[5, 91, 122, 134] Routine serial scanning in the postoperative period provides an objective assessment of size[100] and permits identification of extrarenal collections before they become symptomatic or clinically apparent.[115]

In cases of rejection there is an increase in allograft size. In the acute phases, an increased transmission may be evident secondary to edema.[171] Subacute and chronic rejection produce an alteration in the intrarenal architecture with increased echogenicity and a loss of normal anatomic distinctions (Fig. 3–37).

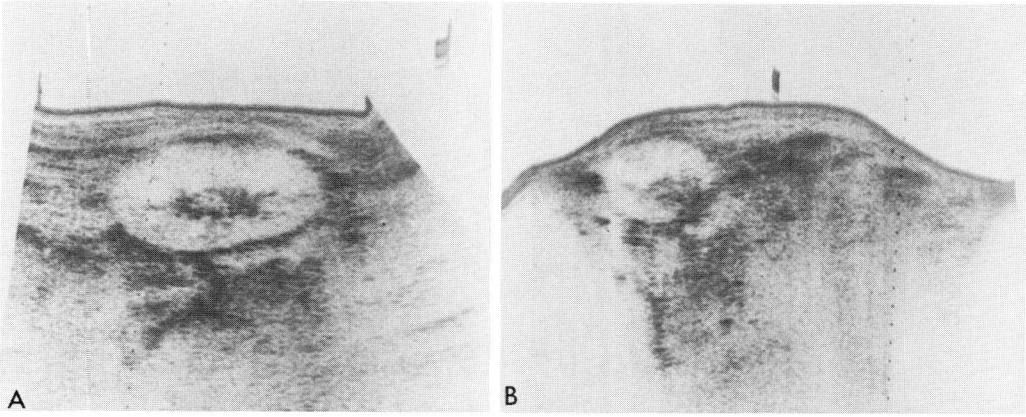

Figure 3–35. Renal transplant. Longitudinal (A) and transverse (B) scans show the normal appearance of a transplanted kidney in the right iliac fossa.

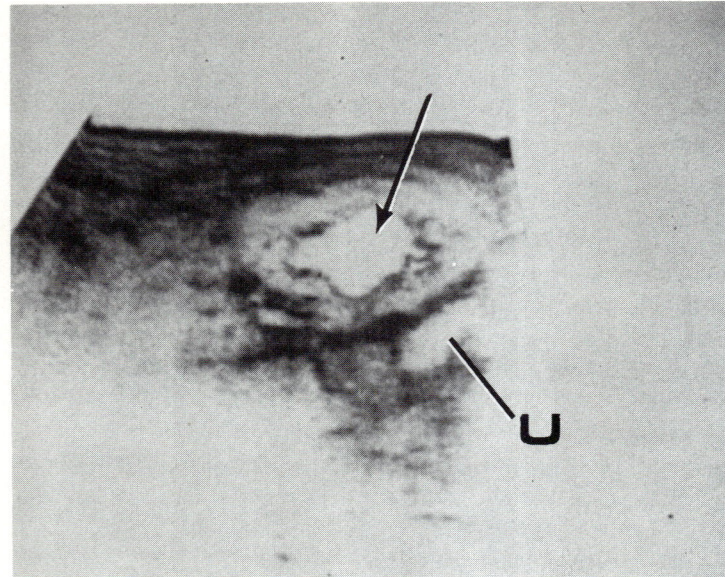

Figure 3–36. Transplant hydronephrosis. There is marked dilatation of the renal pelvis (arrow) as well as of the proximal ureter (U).

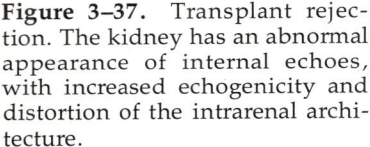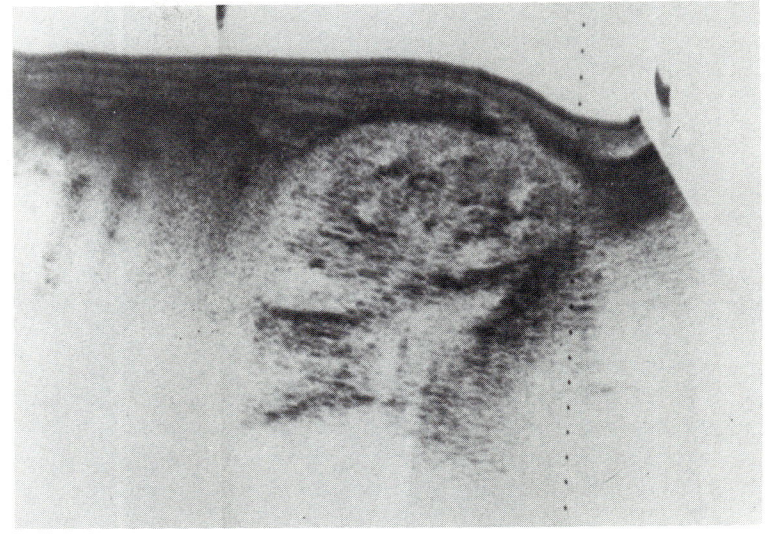

Figure 3–37. Transplant rejection. The kidney has an abnormal appearance of internal echoes, with increased echogenicity and distortion of the intrarenal architecture.

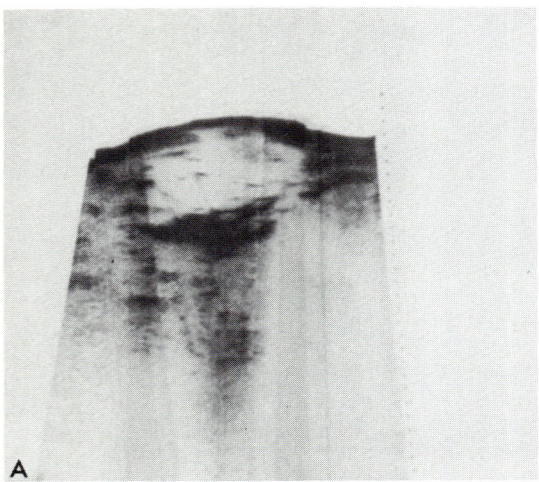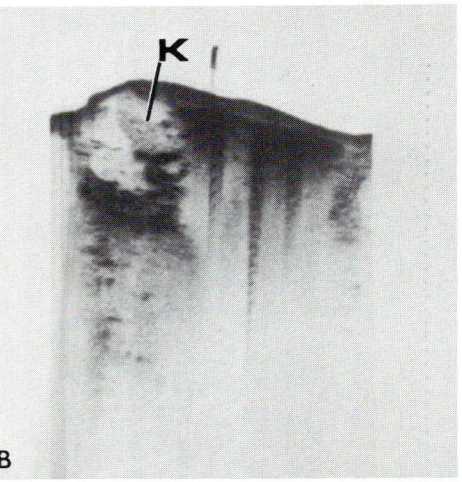

Figure 3–38. Lymphocele. *A,* A longitudinal scan along the lateral margin of the transplant shows a large extrarenal fluid collection. *B,* Transversely, the fluid is seen along the lateral and inferior borders of the transplanted kidney (K).

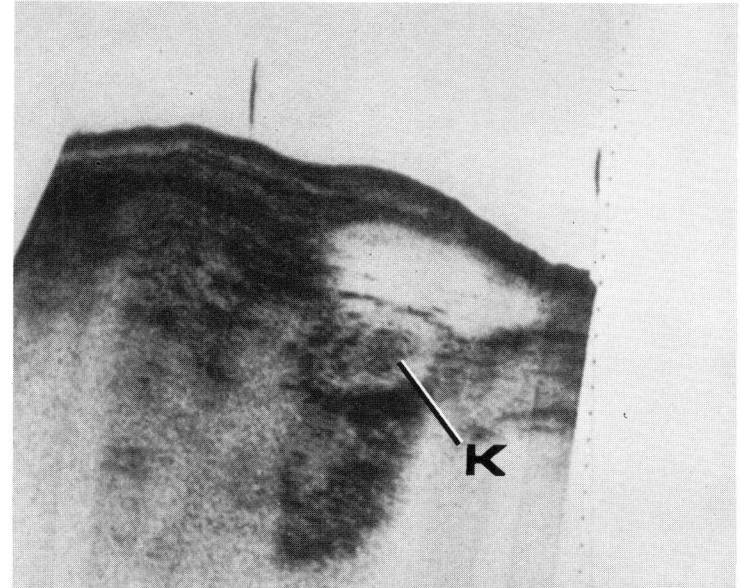

Figure 3–39. Abscess. A fluid collection is seen along the anterolateral aspect of the transplanted kidney (K). The clinical picture of fever and leukocytosis suggested abscess as the most likely diagnosis; the abscess was drained surgically.

Extrarenal collections that occur include lymphoceles, urinomas, hematomas, and abscesses (Fig. 3–38). Although there is considerable overlap in the ultrasonic appearance of these entities, the clinical situation may help make the distinction (Fig. 3–39). The fact that these collections are usually not detectable by other studies makes ultrasound a particularly valuable tool. When incisional wound abscesses or collections occur, ultrasound may be used to confirm their presence, to determine depth and extent, and to provide localization for percutaneous aspiration and drainage (Fig. 3–40).

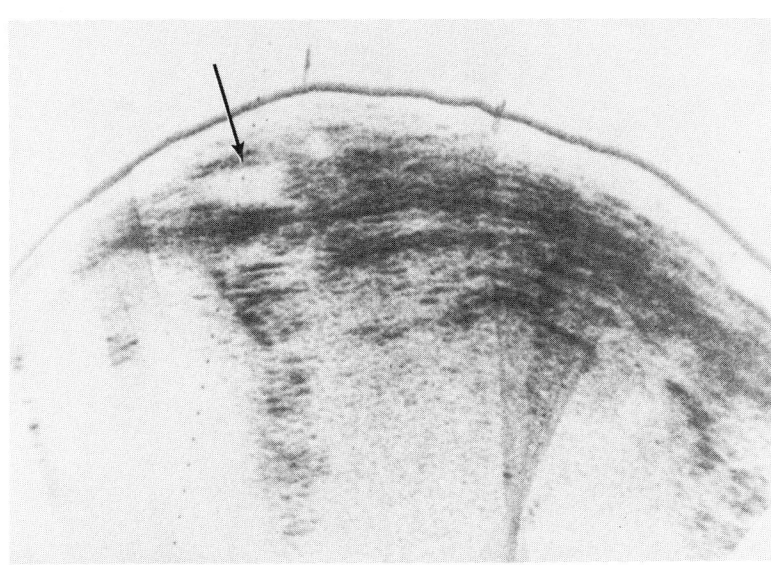

Figure 3–40. Wound abscess. This transverse scan of a patient with fever and graft tenderness shortly after transplantation shows a small fluid collection (arrow) in the subcutaneous space, which was successfully treated by percutaneous drainage.

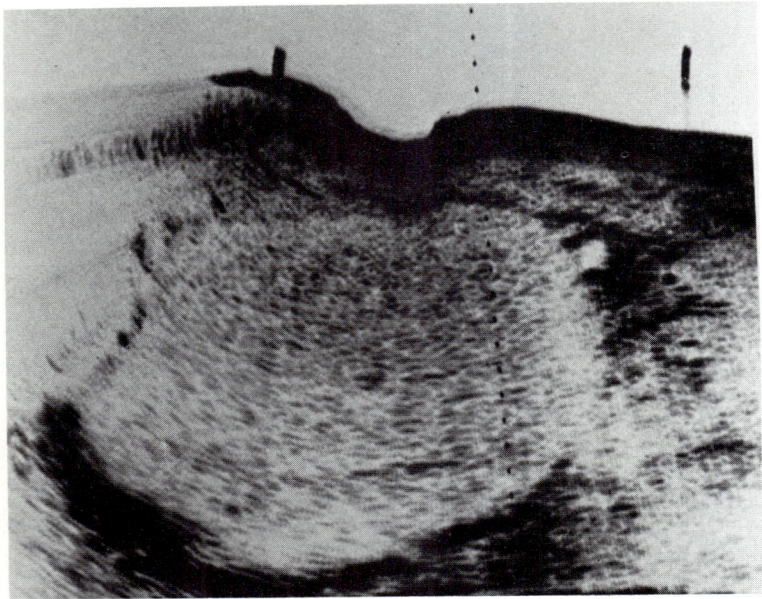

Figure 3–41. Splenomegaly. A longitudinal scan on the left side demonstrates an enlarged spleen with an increase in internal echo in a patient with myelofibrosis.

SPLEEN

Ultrasound can depict splenomegaly (Fig. 3–41) and can be used to determine spleen size using either the volumetric[125] or the cross-sectional area method.[92] As in other organs, it is useful in characterizing focal lesions (Fig. 3–42); splenic cysts, in particular, can be diagnosed quite accurately.[11] Cases of suspected spleen ruptures secondary to blunt trauma have been subjected to ultrasound.[2] Although the diagnosis can sometimes be made on the basis of changes in size and contour, the study appears to be most useful in identifying a normal spleen in suspected cases.

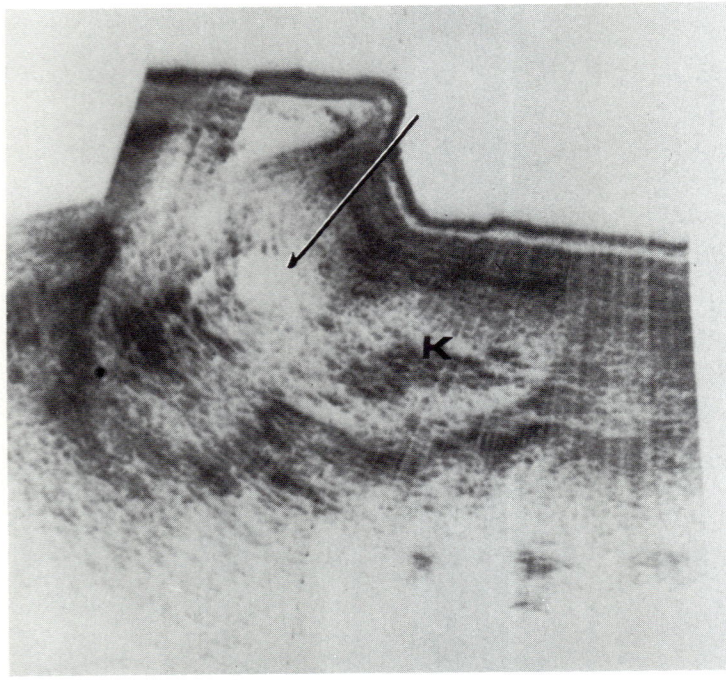

Figure 3–42. Splenic abscess. An abscess with a large cystic component (arrow) is seen in the anterior half of the spleen in this patient with subacute bacterial endocarditis and a filling defect in the spleen on the radionuclide scan. The left kidney (K) is seen inferiorly.

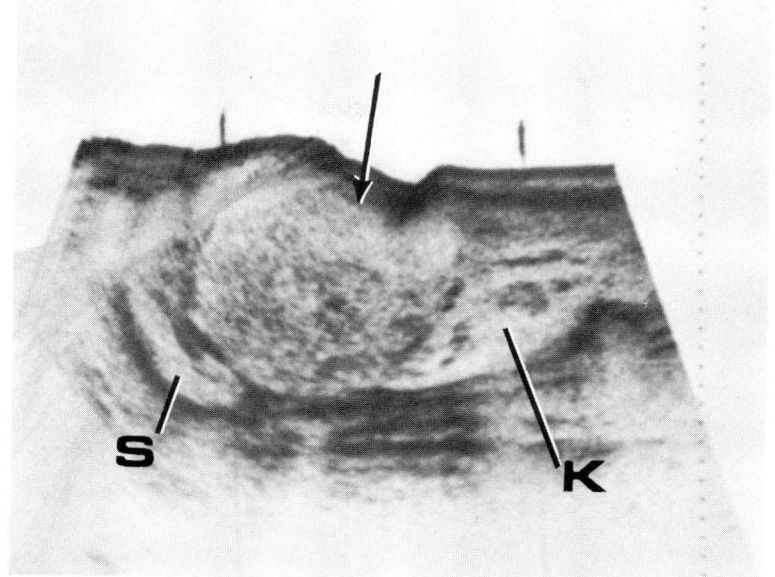

Figure 3–43. Pheochromocytoma. A large solid tumor (arrow) between the left kidney (K) and spleen (S) is seen on this longitudinal scan.

ADRENAL GLANDS

Because of their location and relatively small size, the normal adrenals are difficult to identify, although a recent series has reported an identification success rate of 85 per cent.[136] Changes in configuration and size produced by various lesions facilitate their recognition. One of the more commonly seen lesions is an adrenal cyst. Not infrequently, this may show a complex pattern owing to calcification or particulate matter within the cyst. The appearance of hematoma varies with the degree of liquefaction. A variety of solid lesions, including pheochromocytomas (Fig. 3–43), cortical

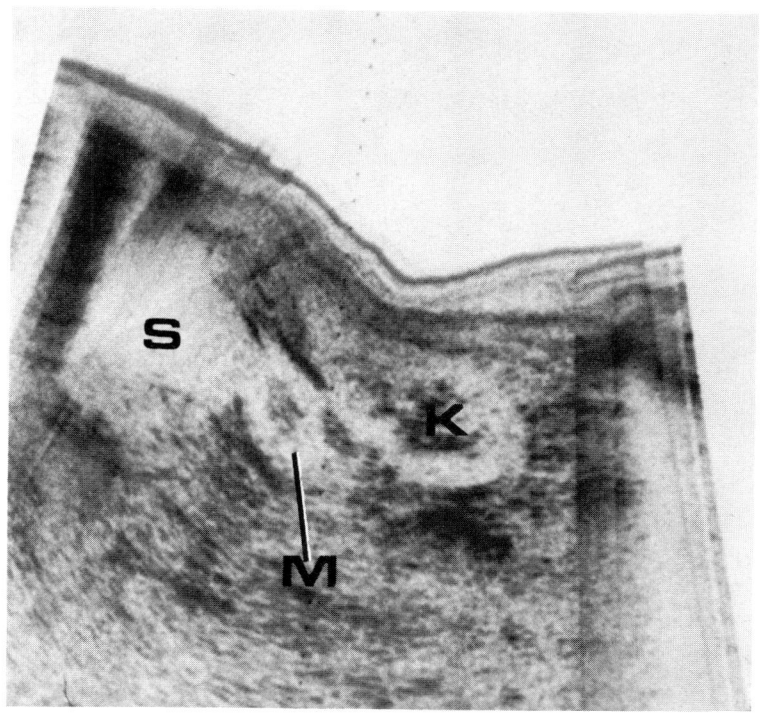

Figure 3–44. Adrenal metastasis. A solid adrenal mass (M) along the anterior surface of the upper pole of the left kidney (K) is demonstrated on this patient with bronchogenic carcinoma. The spleen (S) is seen superiorly.

carcinomas, metastases (Fig. 3–44), and adrenal hyperplasia have been identified.[174, 175] Although it is difficult to identify lesions less than 3 cm in diameter, tumors as small as 1.5 cm have been successfully imaged. Ultrasound is a useful screening tool in patients with a strong clinical suspicion of adrenal lesions and in those at risk of adrenal metastases.[10]

RETROPERITONEUM AND LYMPH NODES

The retroperitoneum is a difficult area to evaluate with conventional radiographic studies. Intravenous urography and barium studies provide only indirect evidence based on organ or viscera displacement, and a lesion can grow to considerable size before its presence is evident. Ultrasound provides exact delineation of masses, their consistency, and their relationship to other retroperitoneal structures, particularly the spleen, kidneys, and blood vessels.

Retroperitoneal Mass

The most common tumors identified in the retroperitoneal space are lymphomas and sarcomas. Lymphomas appear as sonolucent masses. Sarcomas generally have a cystic component of variable size. Liposarcomas have a typical ultrasonic appearance with very dense internal echoes associated with good through transmission, allowing preservation of detail of the posterior margins and surrounding structures (Fig. 3–45). This marked echogenicity is characteristic and may be seen with other fat-containing tumors, such as myelolipomas (Fig. 3–46).

Hematoma and Abscess Formation

Both abscess and hematoma may be similar ultrasonically, showing a fluid collection with variable amounts of solid debris and irregular margins. They are usually

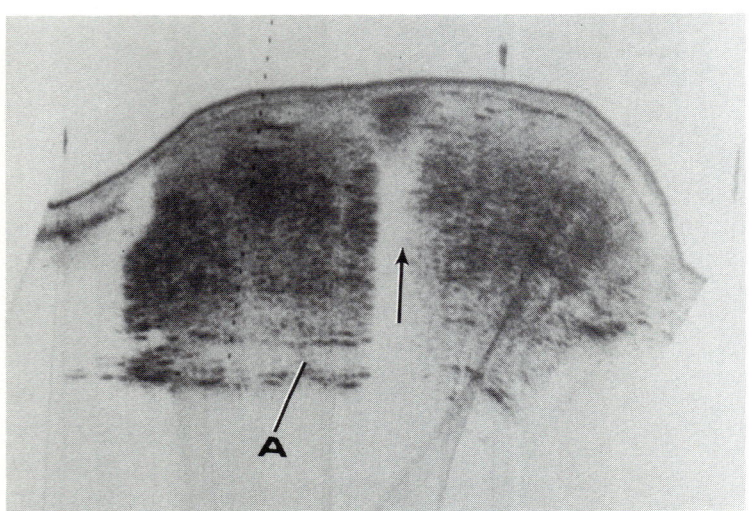

Figure 3–45. Liposarcoma. This massive tumor, which arose in the retroperitoneum, fills the abdominal cavity. The arteriogram showed an avascular mass consistent with cyst or lipoma. The marked echogenicity is characteristic of a fatty tumor. The acoustic shadow (arrow) is produced by anteriorly displaced gas-filled bowel. The aorta (A) is seen posteriorly.

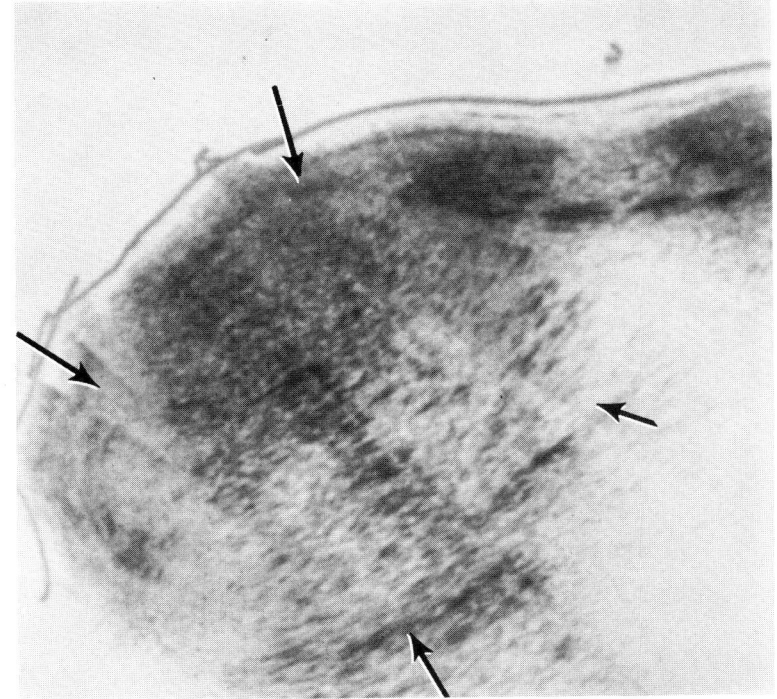

Figure 3–46. Myelolipoma. A large left upper quadrant mass was noted in this patient a few weeks after abdominal trauma. This transverse scan in the prone position shows a large, highly echogenic mass (arrows) situated above the left kidney.

somewhat elliptic in configuration and frequently follow the course of the psoas margin. The clinical picture is usually helpful in making the distinction.[107] Ultrasound is particularly useful in patients with dropping hematocrit and possible concealed hemorrhage (Fig. 3–47).

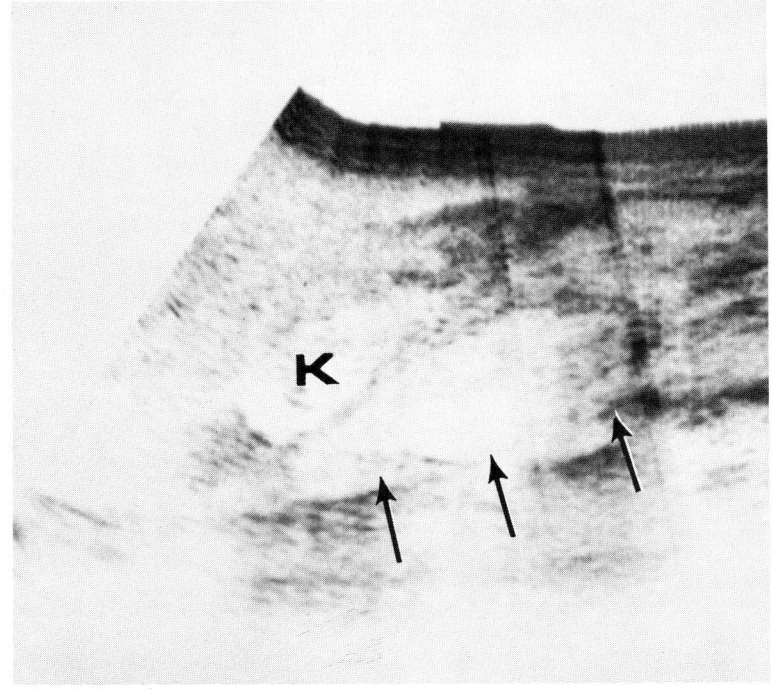

Figure 3–47. Retroperitoneal hematoma. A sudden drop in hematocrit occurred in this elderly patient taking anticoagulation drugs. The longitudinal scan shows a relatively sonolucent mass along the right psoas (arrows). The right kidney (K) is displaced anteriorly.

86 — ULTRASOUND TECHNIQUES

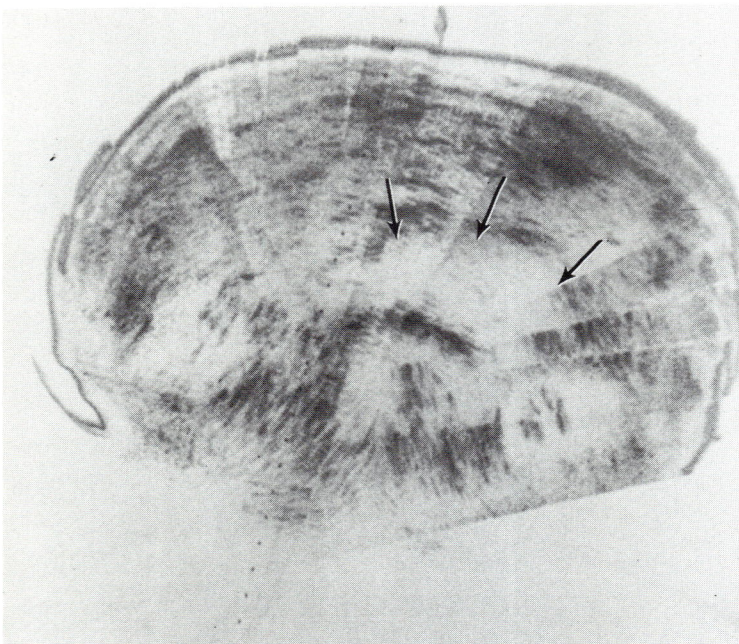

Figure 3–48. Histiocytic lymphoma. A lobulated, relatively sonolucent mass (arrows) is seen in the prevertebral area.

Lymphoma and Retroperitoneal Lymphadenopathy

Lymphoma is one of the more common retroperitoneal tumors and appears ultrasonically as a relatively sonolucent solid mass. Enlarged lymph nodes appear as a lobulated, acoustically homogeneous mass draped over the prevertebral vessels (Fig. 3–48). A cluster of involved nodes may appear as a bulky septate mass that can obscure the anterior margin of the aorta. The aorta and vena cava may be displaced anteriorly

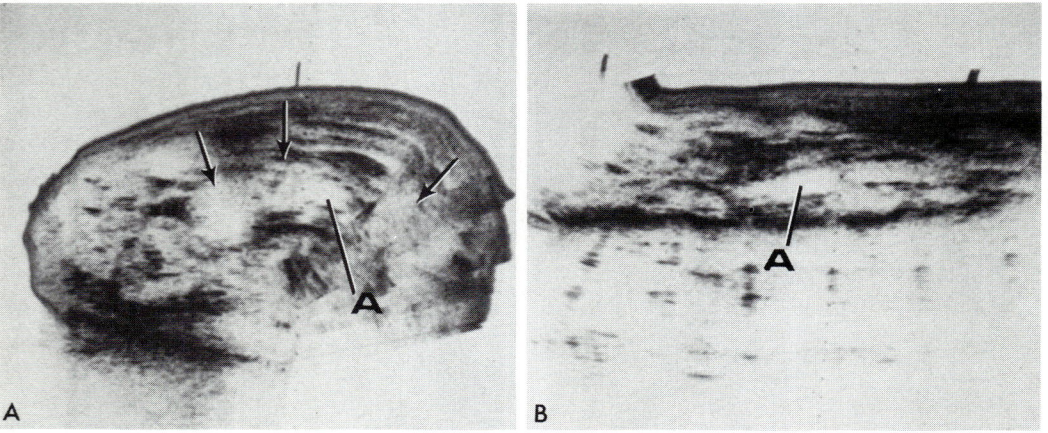

Figure 3–49. Retroperitoneal lymphadenopathy. This patient presented with recurrence of symptoms six months after resection of a pheochromocytoma (see Fig. 3–43). A, The transverse scan in the midabdomen shows extensive para-aortic lymphadenopathy (arrow). The aorta is to the left of the midline. B, On the longitudinal scan, the aorta (A) is surrounded by nodes and is displaced forward.

(Fig. 3–49). Lymphadenopathy in the porta hepatis and splenic hilus can also be identified.[90]

Lymphangiography remains the procedure of choice for the evaluation of lymph node involvement, since nodes that may be diseased but are not significantly enlarged are not always detectable by ultrasound or computed tomography. However, ultrasound has proved valuable for evaluation of the higher para-aortic nodes or those outside the para-aortic chain that are not opacified on lymphangiogram.[19, 130] It can also be used for examination of suspicious areas detected by lymphangiography and lymph node scan and for serial evaluations of the nodes during the course of therapy.

BLADDER AND MALE GENITAL SYSTEM

Scans of the pelvic organs can be performed either by contact scanning on the skin surface or by transrectal scanning with a transducer mounted on the endoscopic arm. Adequate filling of the bladder is essential to the study of internal pelvic organs.

Bladder

Intraluminal masses including tumors, stones, and clots can be detected (Fig. 3–50). Ultrasound is not as sensitive for the diagnosis of bladder tumor as are cystoscopy and cytology. It is, however, a very accurate method for staging, having an overall accuracy of 80 per cent; this is surpassed only by angiographic examinations employing perivesical and endovesical gas.[108] Ultrasound is useful for determining the presence of residual urine and for providing direct guidance for suprapubic aspiration.[121] Variability in bladder configuration does not allow quantitative estimates of residual urine, although a calibration graph can be constructed for an individual patient using instillation of known volumes via catheter.

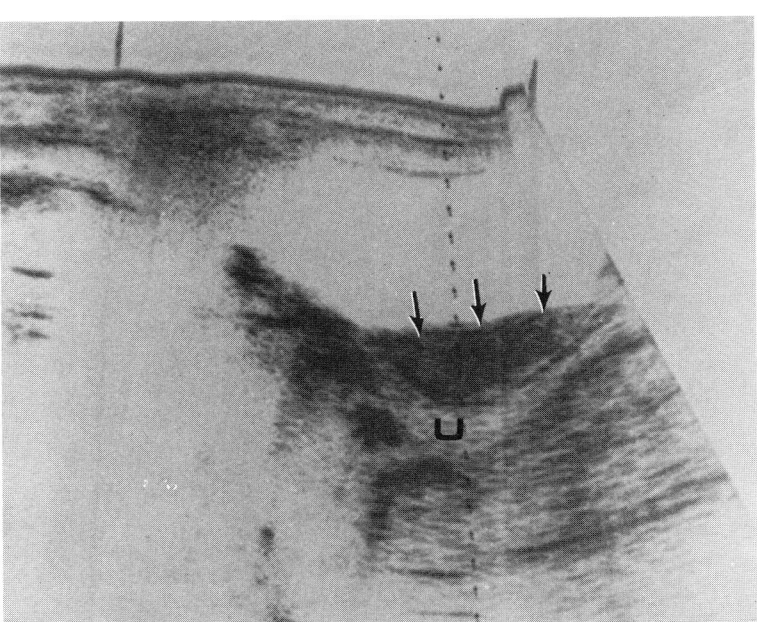

Figure 3–50. Cystitis. The longitudinal scan shows a thick layer of echogenic material (arrows) along the base of the bladder. A deposit of sludge-like material and necrotic debris was seen at cystoscopy. The uterus (U) can be seen posteriorly.

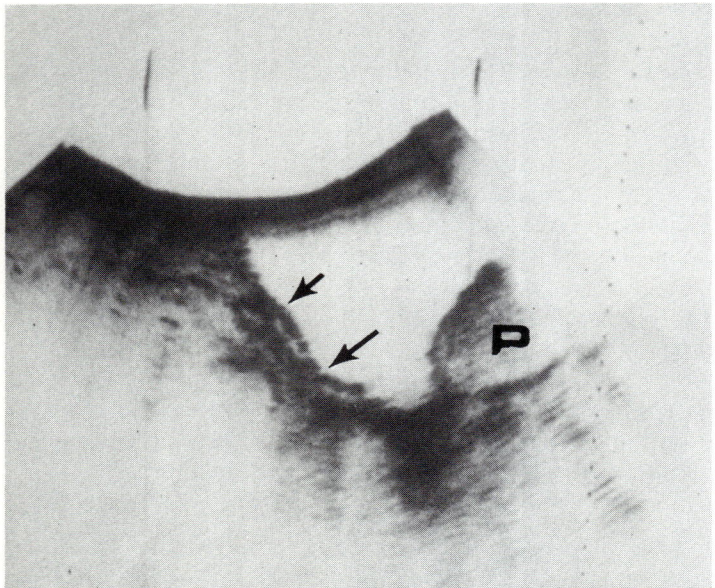

Figure 3–51. Prostatic enlargement. This anterior longitudinal scan shows an enlarged prostate (P) at the base of the fluid-filled bladder as well as thickening of the bladder wall (arrows).

Male Genitals

Studies of the prostate using transrectal scanning have demonstrated an 80 per cent accuracy in the diagnosis of carcinoma, with the rate of false negative results comparable to that of needle biopsy.[166] Scans are helpful in planning surgical staging and may indicate areas of extension that are not palpable at surgery.[16] Size can be evaluated using either abdominal or transrectal scanning, and size estimates have proved more accurate than clinical examination or urography (Fig. 3–51).[110] Cysts of the seminal vesicles, prostate, and müllerian duct anlagen have also been detected.[164]

The scrotum can be studied using direct-contact superficial scanning. Recent studies have showed a differentiation in the testicular and epididymal regions that allowed precise determination of the origin of abnormality in 80 per cent of cases of chronic scrotal swelling.[137] Cystic and solid masses can be distinguished. Hydroceles, hernias, varicoceles, tumors, hematomas, and abscesses have been identified.[111, 145]

Postoperative complications of radical pelvic surgery, such as lymphocyst,[6] abscess, and urinoma, can be detected. Scans are also useful on a long-term basis for monitoring tumor recurrence.[16]

FEMALE GENITAL SYSTEM

Scans of the female pelvis are used for direct imaging of normal anatomic structures as well as for investigation of masses. It is essential that these studies be performed with a well-distended urinary bladder, which serves as a reference cystic structure and displaces the bowel gas from the pelvis, rendering the pelvic organs accessible for scanning.

Current uses of ultrasound in gynecology include confirmation of a mass suggested by physical examination; evaluation of pelvic structures in obese or pediatric patients; localization of IUD's;[15] detection of pelvic abscess;[161] and investigation of suspected ectopic pregnancy[106] and trophoblastic disease.[44] It has been helpful in the evaluation of patients with ambiguous genitalia and precocious puberty.[69]

Pelvic Mass

The aim of ultrasound in the study of pelvic masses is to confirm the existence of the mass and to determine its size, location, and consistency. This can be accomplished with an accuracy of 90 per cent.[97] The information provided allows for differential diagnosis based on location and consistency as well as clinical history and is useful in planning radiation treatment fields. Serial studies provide an objective assessment of the response to therapy.

Tumors may be classified ultrasonically as cystic, predominantly cystic with solid pole or projections, solid, and predominantly solid with cystic spaces caused by mucin production or necrosis.[78] Ovarian cysts as small as 1 cm in diameter can frequently be identified. Loculations within larger cysts are evident. Ascites, if present, can be demonstrated. Cystic masses in the pelvis are almost always extrauterine in origin. Difficulty may arise in distinguishing a large solid ovarian mass from leiomyomas of the uterus if the uterus is sufficiently displaced and compressed so that it cannot be visualized as a separate structure.

Serous cystadenomas, cystadenocarcinomas, and dermoid cysts appear as predominantly cystic masses with definable soft tissue pole or projections (Fig. 3–52). A solid appearance is seen with any of the benign or malignant solid tumors, including serous carcinomas, fibroma, thecoma, and granulous cell tumor (Fig. 3–53). Cystic spaces may be evident if the tumor undergoes necrosis. Pseudomucinous cystadenomas and cyst-

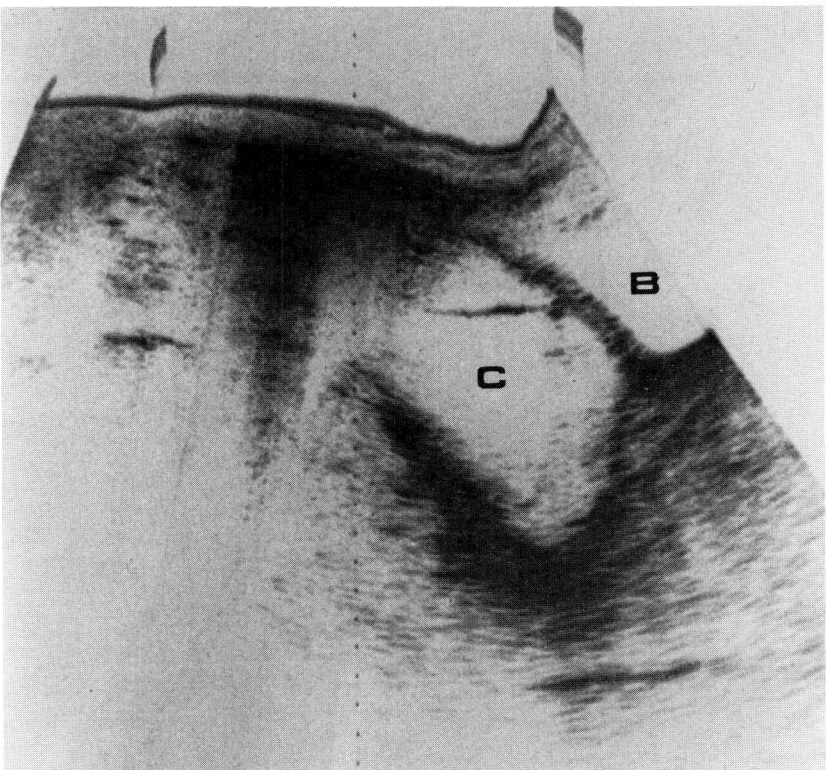

Figure 3–52. Ovarian cystadenoma. A complex mass (C) with a large fluid component, septation, and solid tissue is seen posterior to the urinary bladder (B) on longitudinal scan.

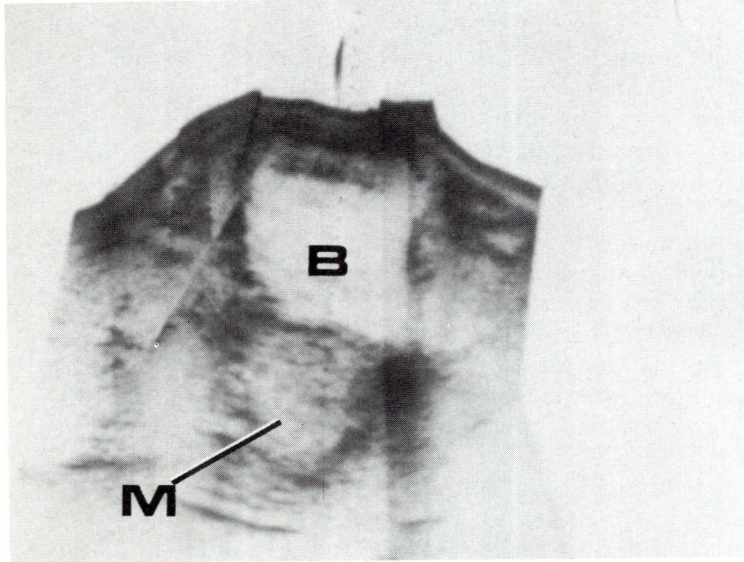

Figure 3–53. Granulosa cell tumor. This transverse scan shows a solid mass (M) behind the bladder (B) and extending toward the right.

adenocarcinomas have a characteristic appearance, with multiple internal septations (Fig. 3–54).

The most frequently imaged uterine mass is the leiomyoma, which has a characteristic, although not pathognomonic, appearance (Fig. 3–55). Areas of necrosis can be visualized within the mass. These tumors may be difficult or impossible to define with ultrasound in the presence of a large amount of calcification.

Trophoblastic disease often presents with a characteristic appearance owing to its vascular nature, although a spectrum of sonographic patterns has been seen.[44] Incom-

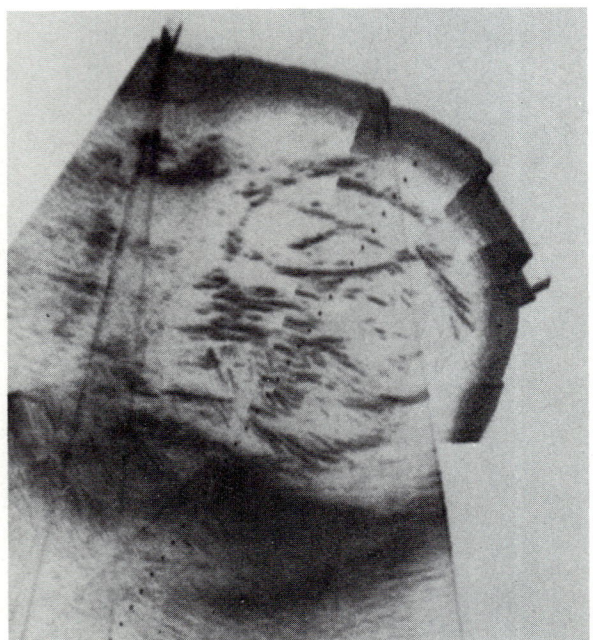

Figure 3–54. Pseudomucinous cystadenocarcinoma. This cystic mass with numerous internal septa has a characteristic appearance.

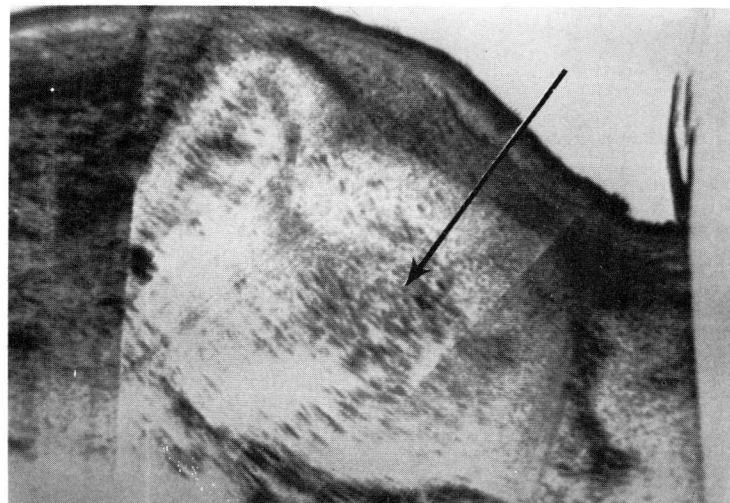

Figure 3–55. Uterine fibroids. A dense central clump of echoes (arrow) originating from a necrotic area is seen in this large solid uterine mass.

plete abortion may mimic a hydatid mole sonographically. Concomitant theca lutein cysts may be evident.

Pelvic Infection

Pelvic inflammatory disease may produce considerable distortion of pelvic anatomy, making it difficult to define the uterus and anexa. Tubo-ovarian abscesses appear as predominantly cystic masses with irregular margins (Fig. 3–56). They may be multiloculated. The irregularity of the walls is an important feature in differentiating them from other cystic adnexal masses. A chronic ectopic pregnancy may be indistinguish-

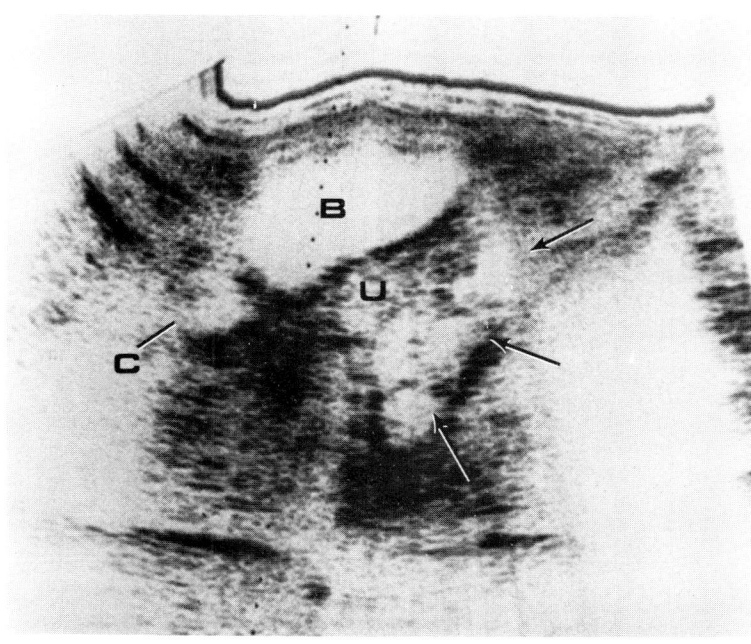

Figure 3–56. Pelvic inflammatory disease. The uterus (U) is seen to the left of the midline behind the bladder (B) and is surrounded on its lateral margin by a left tubo-ovarian abscess (arrows). A small fluid collection (C) with irregular margins is seen in the right adnexa. Endometriosis can also produce anatomic distortion and multiple fluid collections, although the margins are usually more sharply defined.

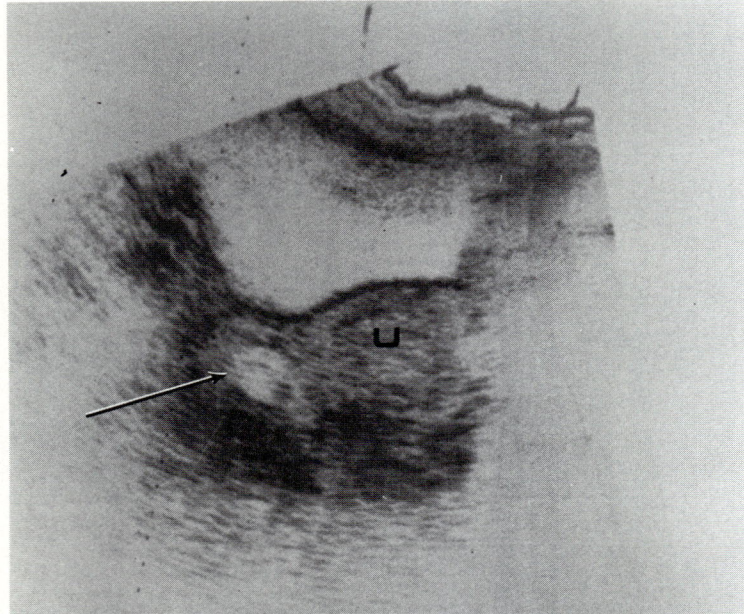

Figure 3–57. Ectopic pregnancy. This transverse scan demonstrates an intact gestational sac (arrow) in the right adnexa adjacent to a slightly enlarged uterus (U).

able. Abscesses can often be seen in the cul-de-sac. Localization and characterization of the abscess can be helpful in judging the approach of drainage procedures and can be used to follow the response to therapy.[161] Hydrosalpinx may be evident in cases of chronic pelvic inflammatory disease. The ultrasound examination is of particular help in excluding the possibility of a mass in patients with fibrosis and adhesions.

Ectopic Pregnancy

The diagnosis of ectopic pregnancy is generally based on a series of presumptive findings: an enlarged uterus without evidence of intrauterine pregnancy and an ex-

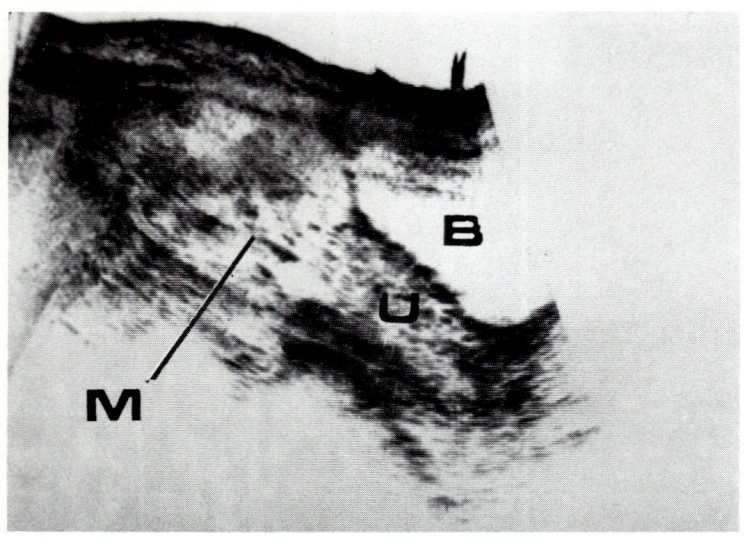

Figure 3–58. Ruptured ectopic pregnancy. This chronic ruptured ectopic pregnancy appears as a mass (M) with both solid and cystic components above the uterus (U) and bladder (B). A large tubo-ovarian abscess may be identical in appearance.

trauterine pelvic mass with irregular echoes and cystic areas. Hematoma formation may be seen in the cul-de-sac. Visualization of an extrauterine gestational sac or fetal parts is diagnostic, but this is the exception (Fig. 3–57). Hemorrhage into an ovarian cyst may mimic an ectopic gestational sac. Distinction between a chronic ruptured ectopic abscess and a pelvic abscess may not be possible on the ultrasonic appearance alone (Fig. 3–58).[106, 131]

Despite the difficulty in diagnosis, ultrasound remains an important tool in the investigation of suspected ectopic pregnancies. Frequently, the clinical picture is due to an ovarian cyst complicating a normal intrauterine pregnancy. This can easily and quickly be identified by ultrasound. The nature of the noninvasive study allows the clinician to investigate a case in which there is suspicion of ectopic pregnancy without posing a risk to the mother or fetus.[74]

Complications of Pregnancy

Since it does not employ ionizing radiation or present any risk to the development of the fetus, ultrasound can be used to study complications of pregnancy in the abdomen and retroperitoneum as well as in the pelvic (Fig. 3–59). It provides an alternative to radiographic procedures, particularly in evaluating the gallbladder and kidney (Fig. 3–60).

Postoperative Studies

Postoperatively, scans are helpful in detecting complications of surgery and in monitoring the patient for tumor recurrence.

Lymphoceles, hematomas, abscesses, and urinomas may occur following radical pelvic surgery (Fig. 3–61).[6] The role of ultrasound is in the detection of the mass and

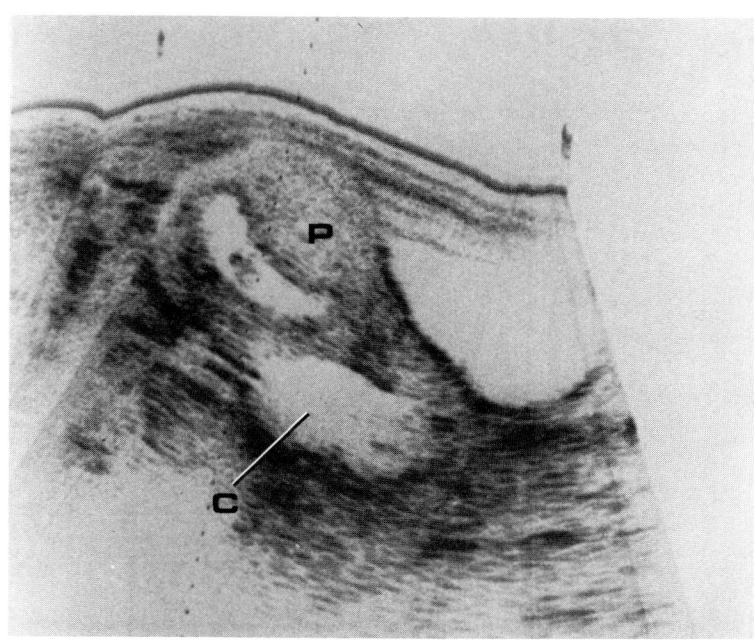

Figure 3–59. Pregnancy with hemorrhagic corpus luteum cyst. A gestational sac of 12 weeks, with placental tissue (P) and echoes arising from a fetal extremity, is present within the uterus. Posterior to the lower uterine segment is a large cyst (C). Its position and size necessitated surgical removal.

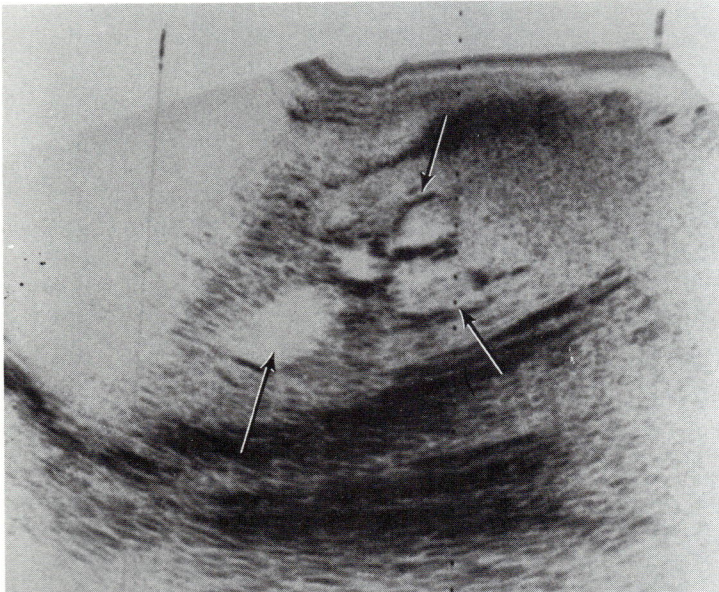

Figure 3–60. Hydronephrosis. This primigravida presented in midtrimester with severe right upper quadrant pain. This longitudinal scan shows hydronephrosis of the right kidney with dilated calices (arrows). Calcifications were present in the region of the proximal ureter; the obstruction was relieved with a ureteral catheter.

identification of its extent, particularly its relationship to the anterior wall and cul-de-sac (Fig. 3–62). While the clinical history and the presence of typical features on ultrasound examination may indicate the nature of the collection, there is an overlap in the appearance of the various fluid collections; aspiration may be required to establish the specific diagnosis.

Studies for tumor recurrence are greatly aided by a baseline postoperative scan. A full bladder is critical to adequate examination, so that studies of deep pelvic contents are often impossible following cystectomy.

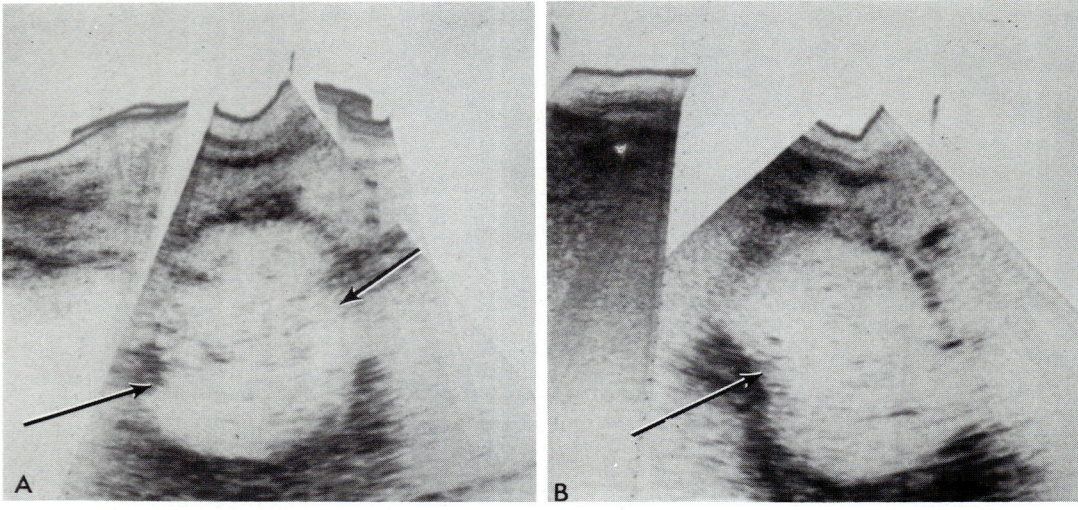

Figure 3–61. Pelvic abscess. Transverse *(A)* and longitudinal *(B)* scans of a patient with sepsis following a radical hysterectomy for ovarian tumor show a large pelvic abscess (arrow).

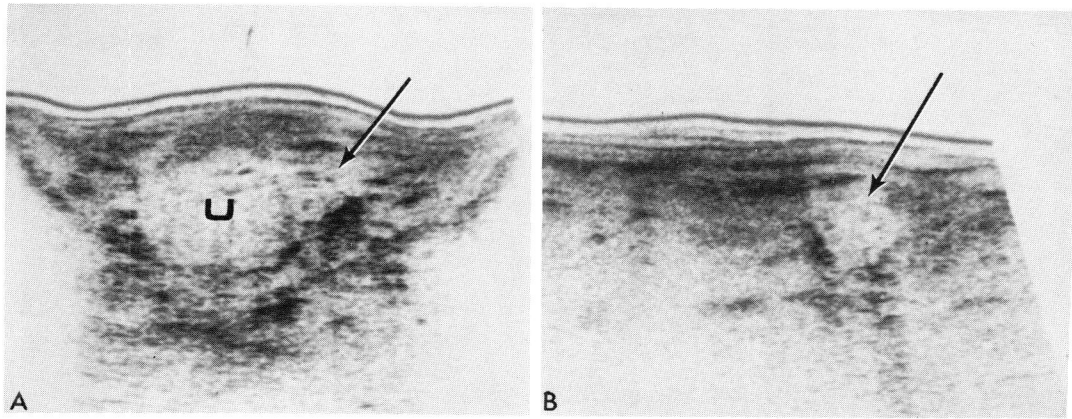

Figure 3–62. Abscess. This patient developed fever one week following a tubal ligation. The transverse *(A)* and longitudinal *(B)* scans show a collection with fluid and solid components in the left adnexa (arrow) adjacent to an enlarged uterus (U).

BLOOD VESSELS

Aorta

The abdominal aorta is easily evaluated by ultrasound (Fig. 3–63). Ideally, the studies should be performed prior to angiography to confirm the diagnosis and assess the appearance of an aneurysm. The size of the aneurysm is most accurately determined by ultrasound, and the presence of organized thrombus is evident (Fig. 3–64). It is often possible to evaluate the relationship of the aneurysm to the renal vessels, although statistically the latter are rarely involved.[98] Dissection of the aorta is suggested in cases showing dilatation with a double lumen. The characteristic feature is visualization of an intimal flap. Real-time or M-mode scanning shows an abnormal pattern of aortic wall pulsation.[169]

Ultrasound is also useful for serial evaluation when surgical intervention is not contemplated.[118] It has also been suggested that serial screening studies in the older, high-incidence age group may be helpful in earlier identification of aneurysms.

Frequently, a pulsatile aorta of normal size in a thin patient clinically mimics an

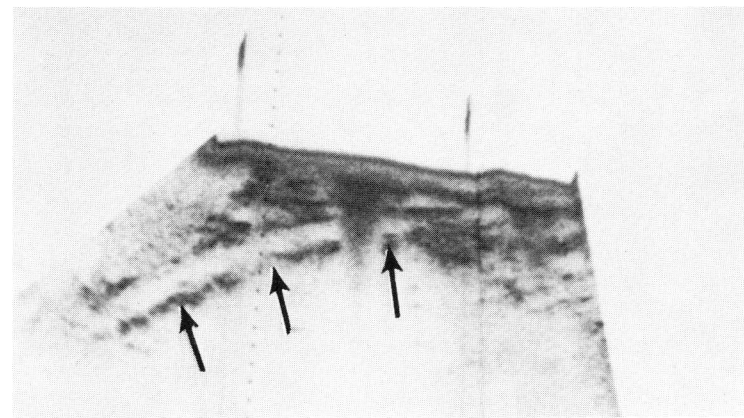

Figure 3–63. Normal aorta. This longitudinal midline scan shows the normal course and caliber of the abdominal aorta (arrows).

96 — ULTRASOUND TECHNIQUES

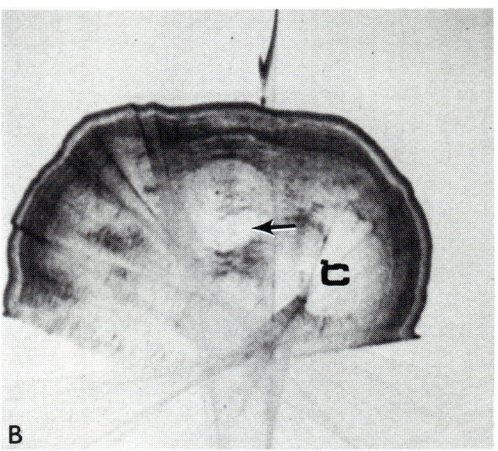

Figure 3–64. Aortic aneurysm. *A,* The longitudinal scan demonstrates a large aneurysm with thrombosis seen anteriorly (arrows). *B,* Transversely, the lumen (arrow) is seen posteriorly and to the left. A left renal cyst (C) is also present.

aneurysm; demonstration of a normal aorta eliminates the need for further studies. Similarly, ultrasound can detect a variety of masses, especially lymphomas and carcinomas of the pancreas, which may simulate an aneurysm clinically (Fig. 3–65).[99]

Studies of the thoracic aorta are hampered because of interference from the spine and posterior ribs. The dilated aneurysm or aorta usually presents lateral to the spine, and scans in the posterior rib interspace can sometimes be used to determine size.[50] Because of interference from the ribs, it is not possible to obtain a complete profile of the thoracic aorta.

Intra-abdominal Arteries

Both the superior mesenteric artery and the renal arteries can be seen in the majority of patients (Fig. 3–66).[101] The celiac artery is occasionally identified, but the

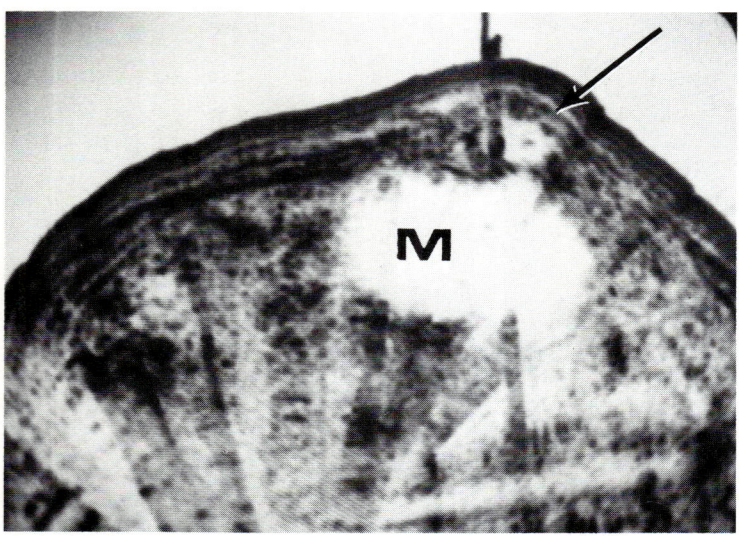

Figure 3–65. Lymphoma. This patient had a pulsatile abdominal mass thought clinically to be an aneurysm. The transverse scan shows a large, relatively echo-free mass (M) invading the abdominal wall (arrow).

ULTRASOUND TECHNIQUES — 97

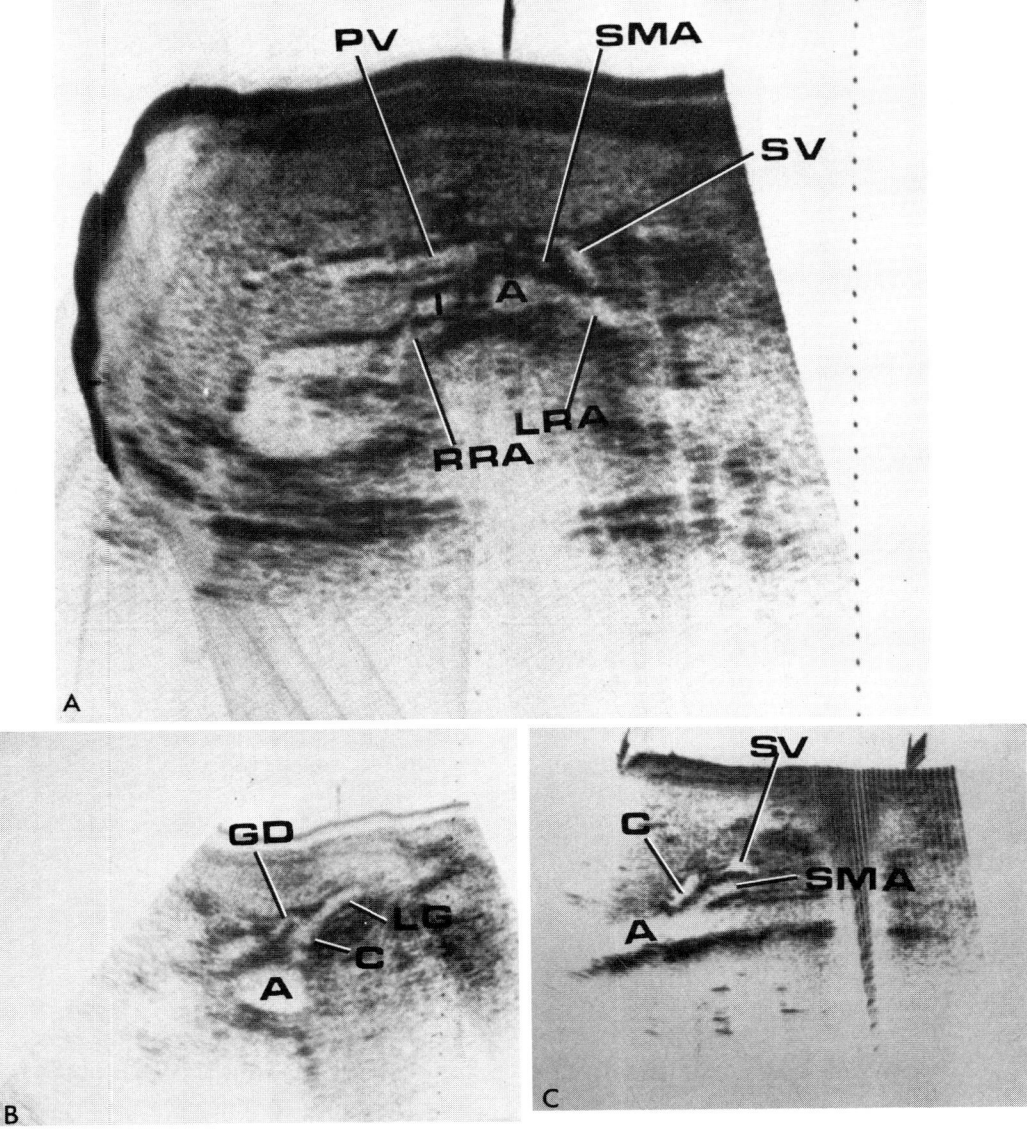

Figure 3–65. Normal vessels. These transverse (*A* and *B*) and longitudinal (*C*) scans demonstrate the normal vasculature in the upper abdomen: aorta (A), inferior vena cava (I), superior mesenteric artery (SMA), celiac axis (C), left renal artery (LRA), right renal artery (RRA), splenic vein (SV) and portal vein (PV). The gastroduodenal (GD) and left gastric (LG) branches of the celiac axis are infrequently identified.

inferior mesenteric is rarely depicted. Identification of these vessels is primarily useful in localization of intra-abdominal structures, particularly the pancreas. Aneurysms involving the hepatic, renal,[62] and superior mesenteric arteries have been identified with ultrasound.[43] Studies of the aortic–superior mesenteric angle have been made; changes in this angle are helpful in determining the site of origin of masses.[53]

The iliac vessels are difficult to identify because of overlying gas in the lower bowel. However, aneurysms of the aorta extending into the iliac frequently produce sufficient dilatation to make these vessels visible (Fig. 3–67).

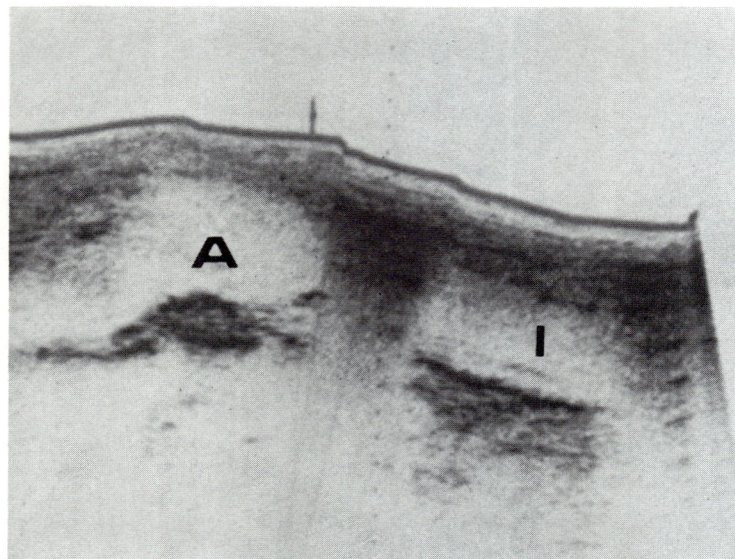

Figure 3–67. Iliac artery aneurysm. This longitudinal scan shows a large aneurysm of the abdominal aorta (A) and right iliac (I). The actual point of bifurcation is obscured by overlying bowel gas.

Peripheral Arteries

Doppler studies of peripheral vessels are helpful in determining flow patterns and areas of stenosis.[39] Direct visualization of the popliteal[33] and carotid[13] arteries can be performed (Fig. 3–68). These are helpful not only in confirmation of the clinical diagnosis but in detection of clinically occult aneurysms.[147]

Veins

The inferior vena cava is easily identified (Fig. 3–69).[140] The most commonly observed abnormalities in the inferior vena cava are extrinsic pressure from retroperitoneal or intraperitoneal masses and displacement (Fig. 3–70).[60, 154] Tumor thrombus from hypernephromas has been seen in the inferior vena cava as well as in the renal vein.[64] Leiomyosarcomas of the inferior vena cava have been identified with ultrasound.

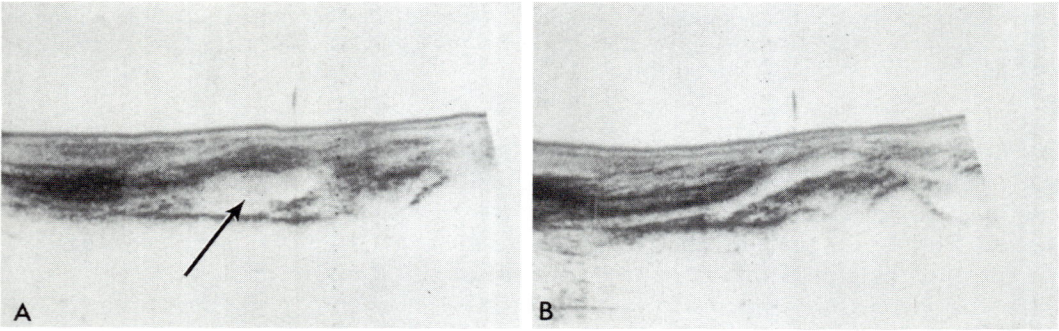

Figure 3–68. Popliteal artery aneurysm. *A*, There is a 2.5-cm aneurysm of the left popliteal artery (arrow). *B*, The right side is normal. Popliteal aneurysms frequently occur bilaterally.

ULTRASOUND TECHNIQUES — 99

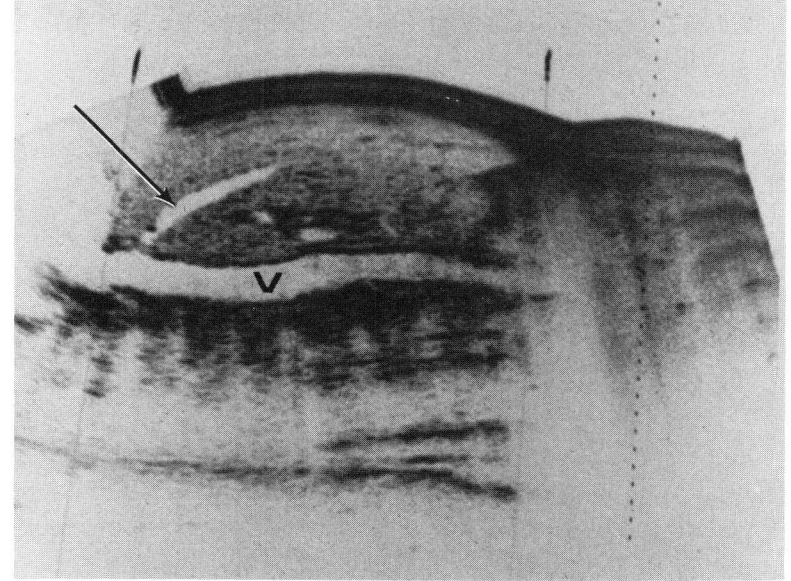

Figure 3–69. Inferior vena cava. This longitudinal scan shows the normal course of the inferior vena cava (V). A hepatic vein (arrow) is seen entering superiorly.

The portal vein is easily identified, and the enlargement occurring with an increase in right ventricular pressure or portal hypertension can be objectively measured (Fig. 3–71). The splenic vein can also be identified in most cases.

Postoperative Studies

Postoperative changes in the retroperitoneum may distort the sonographic changes of false aneurysm and retroperitoneal hemorrhage; it is therefore helpful to have a baseline scan for comparison (Fig. 3–72).[98] Confusion can be avoided if the ultrason-

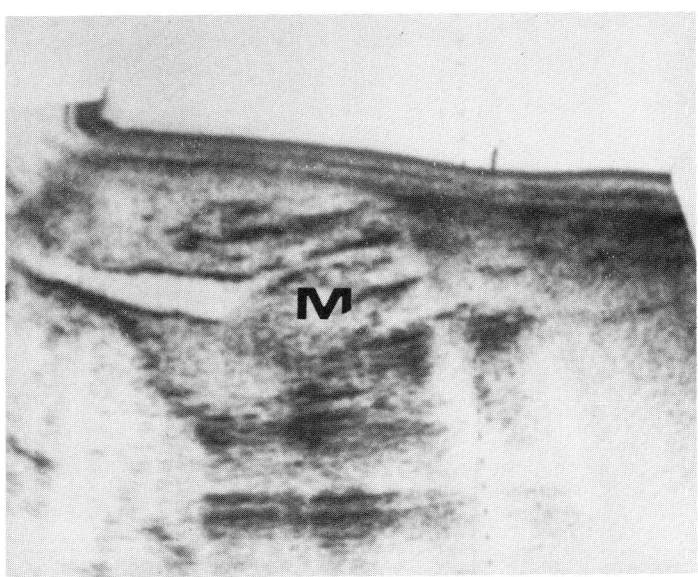

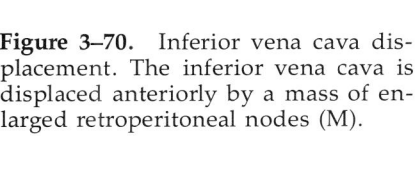

Figure 3–70. Inferior vena cava displacement. The inferior vena cava is displaced anteriorly by a mass of enlarged retroperitoneal nodes (M).

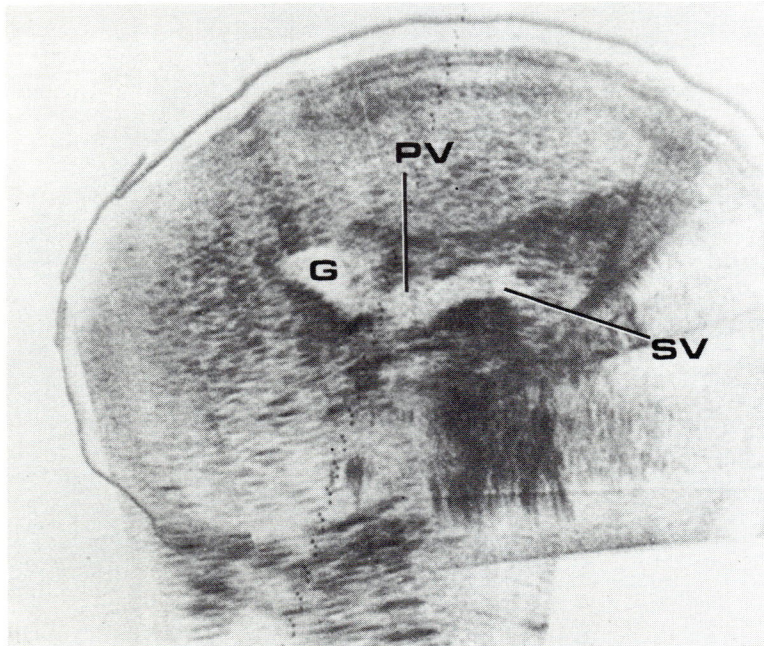

Figure 3–71. Portal hypertension. Enlargement of the splenic (SV) and main portal veins (PV) is seen in this patient with cirrhosis. A portion of the gallbladder (G) is seen to the right.

ographer is aware of the details of the surgical procedure (i.e., whether the aneurysm was resected, the type of anastomosis, and the presence of retroperitoneal hematoma initially). Ultrasound can also be used for evaluation of peripheral arteries and A-V shunts and may be particularly helpful in distinguishing between hematoma and false aneurysm as the cause of postoperative swelling.[59]

Indications for postoperative studies of the venous structures are largely limited to imaging of the inferior vena cava and evaluation of portacaval shunts (see Postoperative Studies of the Liver).[52] Umbrellas in the inferior vena cava can also be localized with gray-scale scan.

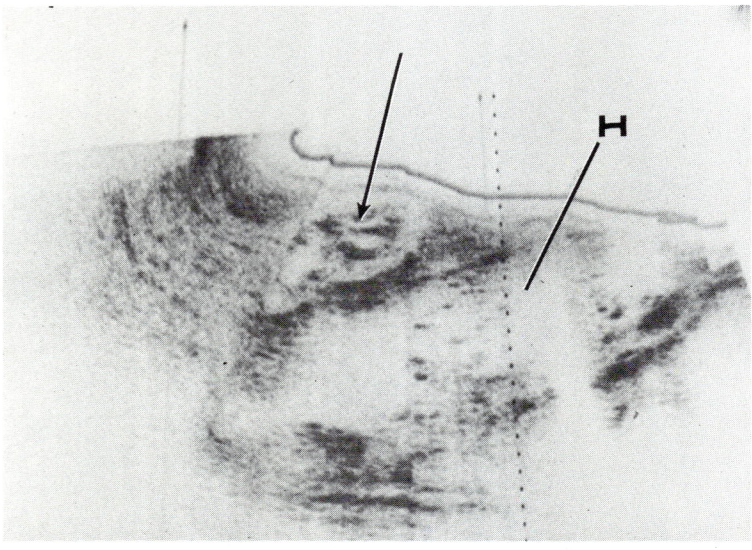

Figure 3–72. Retroperitoneal hematoma. A scan following repair of a ruptured aneurysm shows a large hematoma (H) along the left psoas. The left kidney is displaced anteriorly and is hydronephrotic, with dilatation of the collecting system (arrow). The hematoma subsequently became infected and was drained surgically.

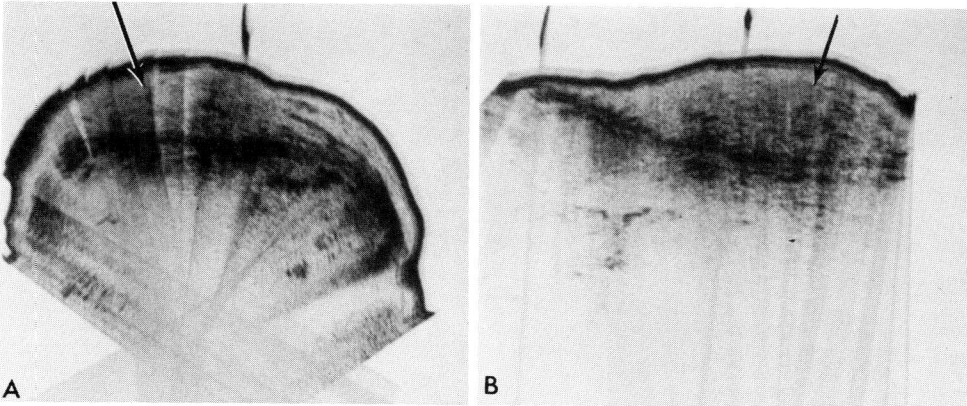

Figure 3–73. Rectus sheath hematoma. *A,* The transverse scan shows a large hematoma (arrow) involving the rectus sheath on the right side. This developed spontaneously in a patient on anticoagulant therapy. *B,* The longitudinal scan shows the typical ovoid or spindle-shaped mass along the rectus sheath (arrow). This hematoma shows somewhat more internal echoes than usual, although the echogenicity is variable.

ABDOMINAL WALL AND MESENTERY

Delineation of the subcutaneous and muscular layers of the abdominal wall makes it possible to determine whether masses are arising in or invading the abdominal wall. Rectus sheath hematomas, frequently occurring as a result of anticoagulation, can be diagnosed and serially monitored (Fig. 3–73).[84] Of the solid tumors, lipomas have a typical ultrasonic appearance, showing a dense pattern of internal echo.[93] Sarcomas involving the abdominal wall usually appear as complex lesions with cystic areas and homogeneous solid tissue components (Fig. 3–74).[20] The fluid nature of cysts arising from the mesentery or omentum can be easily documented with ultrasound, and solid lesions that may mimic cysts can be readily distinguished.[68, 114] The site of origin cannot usually be ascertained, so that cystic masses of other origins must be included in the differential diagnosis.

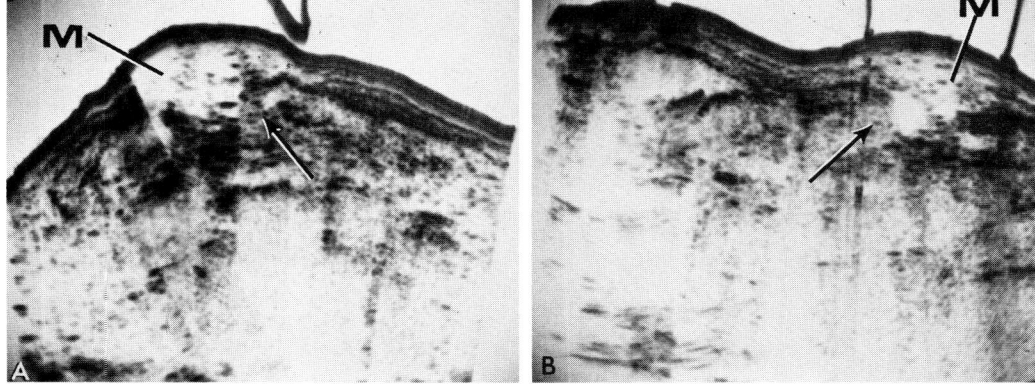

Figure 3–74. Leiomyosarcoma of the abdominal wall. Transverse *(A)* and longitudinal *(B)* scans show an abdominal wall mass (M) with both cystic and solid components. There is invasion of the peritoneum with disruption of the peritoneal reflection (arrows).

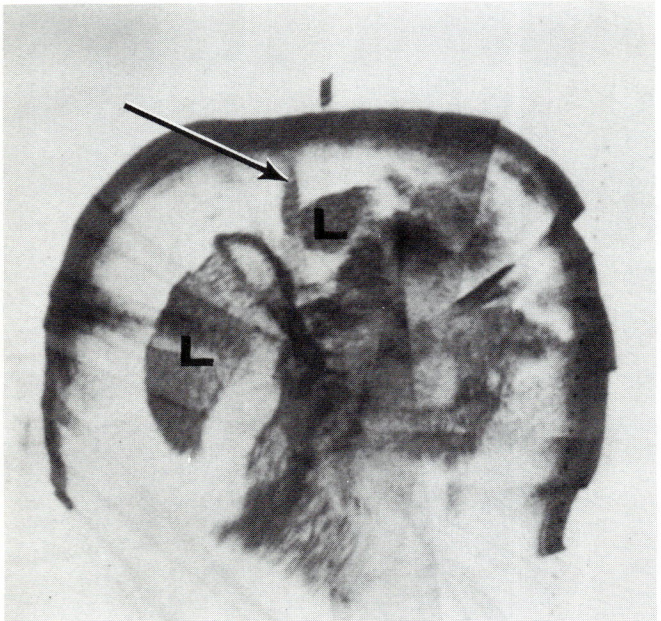

Figure 3–75. Ascites. A large amount of ascitic fluid surrounds the liver (L). The falciform ligament (arrow) is seen anteriorly (arrow).

ASCITES AND OTHER INTRA-ABDOMINAL FLUID COLLECTIONS

Ascites

Ascitic fluid is easily detected and appears as large, echo-free, trans-sonic areas filling the flanks and surrounding the lateral and anterior margins of the liver (Fig. 3–75). Loculated collections may occur and must be distinguished from cystic masses.[176] Bowel loops are seen displaced from the flanks and floating centrally, in distinction to the lateral displacement produced by large cystic masses. It has been suggested that the presence of adhesions with fixation of bowel loops is indicative of malignant as-

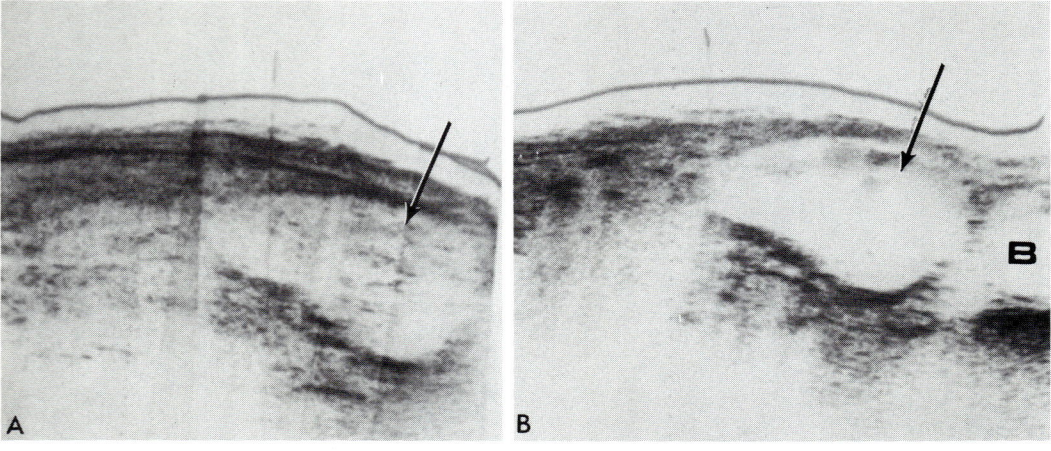

Figure 3–76. Hematoma. *A*, The longitudinal scan shows a large mass with scattered internal echoes in the lower abdomen (arrow). *B*, A repeat scan 24 days later shows a more cystic quality to the hematoma (arrow), which lies just above the urinary bladder (B).

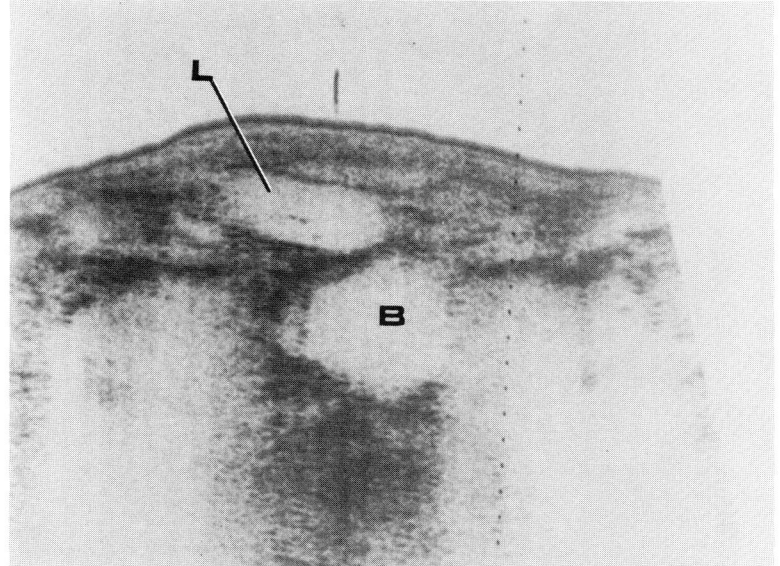

Figure 3–77. Lymphocele. This lymphocele (L), which developed following renal transplantation, appears as a cystic mass anterior to the urinary bladder (B).

cites, although inflammation can produce the same findings The smallest amount of ascitic fluid detectable by gray-scale scanning has not been established. The amount probably exceeds the 100 cc detected experimentally with A-mode scan,[48] but the technique is more sensitive than physical examination or radiography.[124]

Hematoma

The appearance of a hematoma varies with the degree of liquefaction (Fig. 3–76). There may be a significant component of internal echo owing to clot formation. The shape is dependent on its location. Ultrasound is the study of choice in patients with a drop in hematocrit and no obvious bleeding site. Scans should be directed particularly to the retroperitoneum, which is a common site of spontaneous hematoma formation (see Fig. 3–47). Hematomas can be monitored with serial scans for progression and resolution.[86]

Lymphocele

Lymphoceles can occur following renal transplantation and any radical pelvic procedure and are included in the differential diagnosis of postoperative pelvic masses (Fig. 3–77). Ultrasound conclusively demonstrates the fluid nature of the mass, although the appearance is not specific for lymphocele. Typically, they are ovoid, unilocular, cystic masses with no internal echoes. Spontaneous regression may occur and can be documented with serial scans.[6]

Other Fluid Masses

Other fluid collections that may be detected include urinoma (Fig. 3–78) and cerebrospinal fluid pseudocysts following ventricular peritoneal shunts.[57] These usually

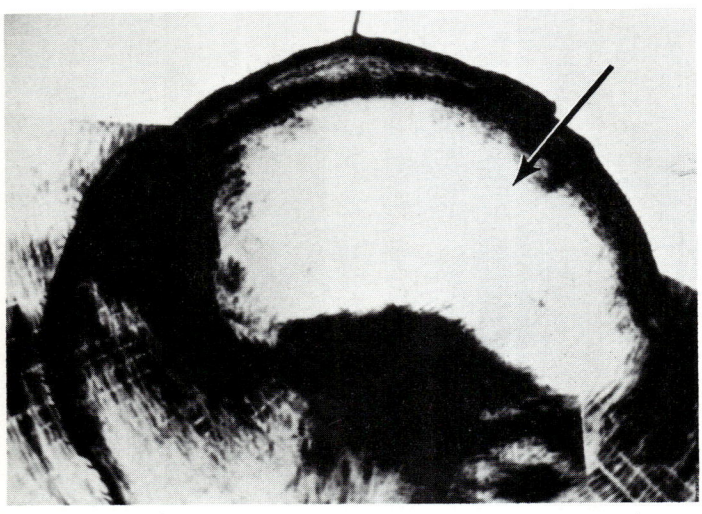

Figure 3–78. Urinoma. A large cystic mass (arrow) is seen in this patient who presented with abdominal distention several weeks after abdominal aortic surgery.

appear as sharply marginated cystic masses. The nature of the fluid contained in a cystic mass cannot be determined by ultrasound and must be identified on the basis of the clinical history or by percutaneous aspiration of the fluid.

ABSCESS

The diagnosis of abscess formation is a difficult clinical problem and one that is greatly aided by the use of ultrasound.[35, 45, 82] The ultrasonographer must be aware of possible sites and multiplicity as well as various other structures and masses that may mimic abscess.[37] A specific diagnosis must also incorporate clinical and laboratory findings.

Abscesses appear as fluid collections with variable amounts of internal echo, owing to necrotic debris, and irregular borders. This pattern is common to all fluid collections that may have associated cellular material or clot formation, including hematoma and necrotic tumor. Unlike cystic tumors, abscesses usually have an irregular, ragged appearance. Difficulty occasionally arises in attempting to distinguish a fluid-filled distended bowel loop from abscess, although configuration is a helpful distinguishing feature.[37] Abscesses usually have an elliptic shape. Dilated small bowel loops appear as multiple circular masses of similar size. The colon may simulate abscess on transverse views, but its continuity with the bowel above and below as a long tubular segment can be seen on longitudinal scans. In questionable cases, comparison of the area of abnormality on scans with its appearance on abdominal radiographs may be helpful.

Ultrasound can also be used as a complement to gallium scans. Since gallium accumulates in areas of inflammation and at recent surgical sites as well as in frank abscesses, ultrasound can be used to determine if there is a significant fluid component that can be drained.[139]

Subphrenic Abscess

A right subphrenic abscess appears as a crescentic collection along the posterior-superior surface of the liver (Fig. 3–79). Observation of the diaphragmatic motion during scanning is helpful in distinguishing between abscess and pleural effusion.[96]

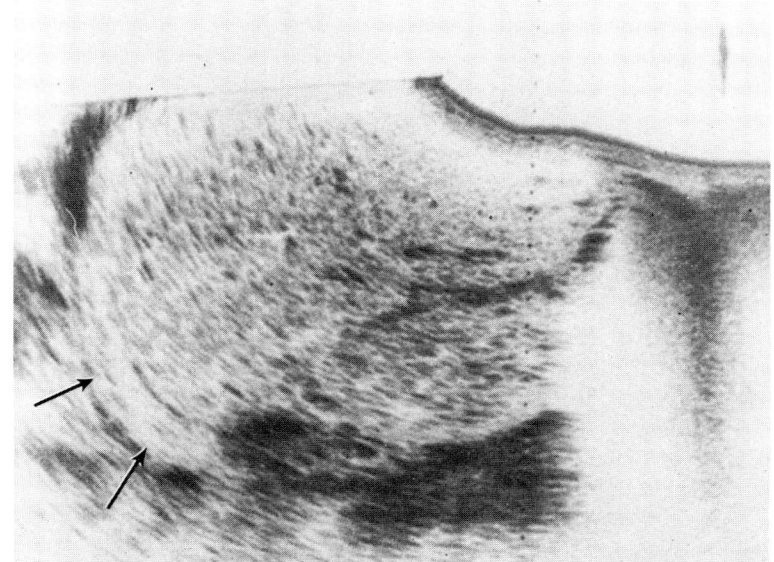

Figure 3–79. Subphrenic abscess. A thin collection of fluid (arrows), with scattered internal echoes due to debris, is seen between the posterior surface of the liver and the right hemidiaphragm.

Left subphrenic collections are more difficult to diagnose because of bowel gas in the left upper quadrant, although the bowel loops are frequently displaced in the presence of an abscess. Another source of difficulty in this region is a fluid-filled stomach, which may mimic an abscess. This confusion can be avoided by having the patient fast or by using nasogastric suction.

Subhepatic Abscess

Subhepatic abscesses are usually elliptic in contour and may be interposed between the liver and the kidney (see Fig. 3–10). Care must be taken not to confuse a distended gallbladder or cyst arising anteriorly from the upper pole of the kidney.

Intra-abdominal Abscess

Abscesses elsewhere in the abdomen may be secondary to perforation of the colon, as in diverticulitis, colitis, and appendicitis, or may be a complication of abdominal surgery (Fig. 3–80). They are usually ovoid or elliptic in shape and may be multiple. Scans should attempt to define the extent of the abscess, the presence of loculation, and the involvement of extraperitoneal tissues (Fig. 3–81).[45]

Visceral Abscess

Abscesses that form within solid organs usually have a spherical shape and, like abscesses elsewhere, show an internal fluid component (see Fig. 3–6). The irregular margins distinguish these collections from cysts.

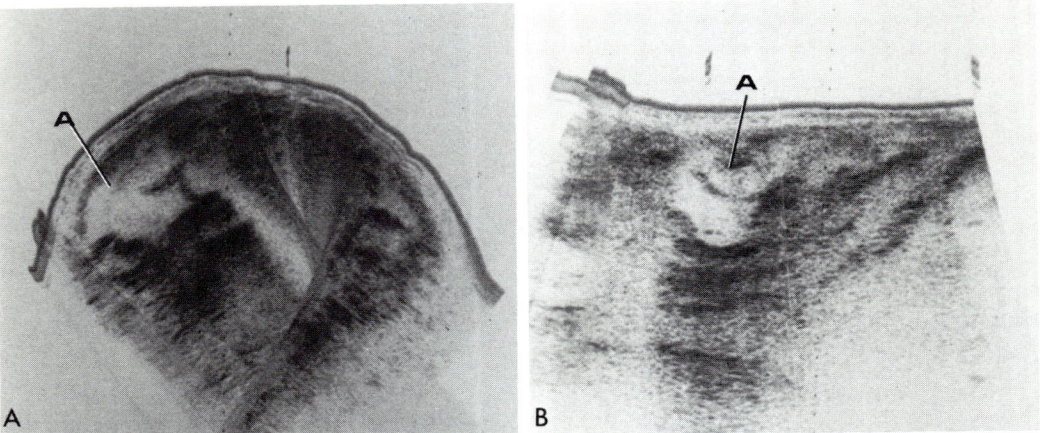

Figure 3–80. Intra-abdominal abscess. *A,* Transverse scan of this young female with Crohn's disease shows an abscess collection in the right flank (A). *B,* A longitudinal scan on the right side shows a large fluid component within the abscess (A).

Retroperitoneal and Perinephric Abscess

Retroperitoneal abscesses often follow the course of the psoas and appear as irregular-shaped masses with internal echoes (Fig. 3–82). Anterior displacement of the kidney is frequently evident.[94]

Diagnosis of a perinephric abscess extending along the course of the kidney usually presents no difficulty. Perinephric hematoma may appear similar; the clinical picture is usually helpful in distinguishing the two. A perinephric abscess may also present as a relatively localized mass (see Fig. 3–33). The fluid content differentiates it from most other renal or perirenal masses, although it may mimic a necrotic tumor.

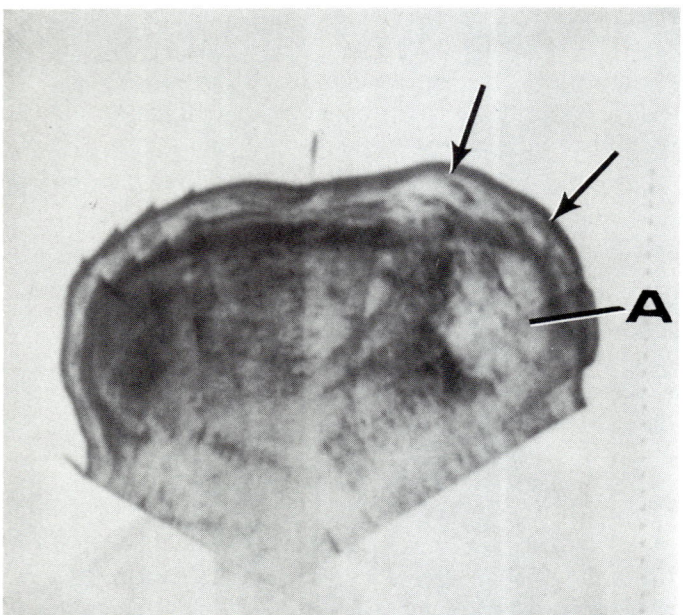

Figure 3–81. Diverticular abscess. This abscess (A), which developed secondary to diverticulitis and perforation, involves the abdominal wall (arrows).

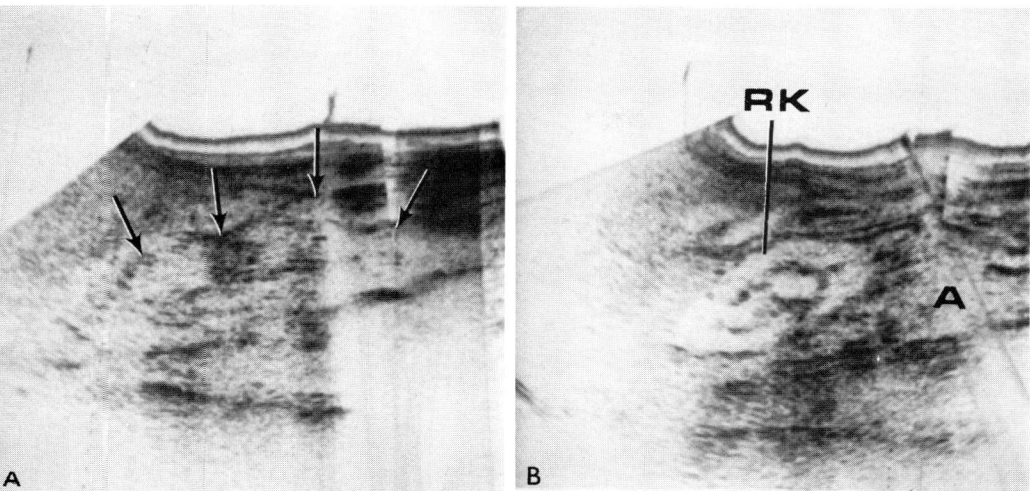

Figure 3-82. Retroperitoneal abscess. *A,* This longitudinal scan on a patient who developed sepsis following a partial colectomy shows a mass (arrows) along the course of the right psoas. *B,* A more medial scan shows elevation and partial obstruction of the right kidney (RK) as well as the abscess (A).

Pelvic Abscess

The patient's bladder should be full before a scan of the pelvis is performed in order to avoid confusion between a cystic mass and a partially distended bladder. Abscesses in this area must be distinguished from chronic ectopic pregnancy and hematoma. Abscesses secondary to a ruptured appendix can extend into the pelvis and may be indistinguishable from tubo-ovarian abscesses (Fig. 3–83). Scans should define the relationship of the abscess to the other pelvic structures and may be helpful in determining whether a colpotomy or anterior approach is required for adequate drainage.

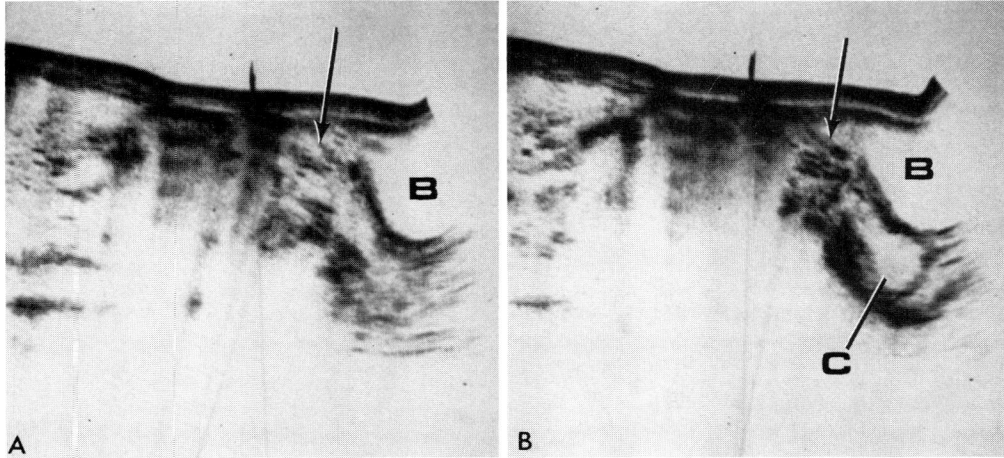

Figure 3-83. Pelvic abscess following appendiceal rupture. *A,* Longitudinal scan to the right of midline in this young male shows a mass (arrow) above the urinary bladder (B). *B,* A more medial scan shows a collection of fluid deep in the pelvis (C) and continuous with the mass (arrow).

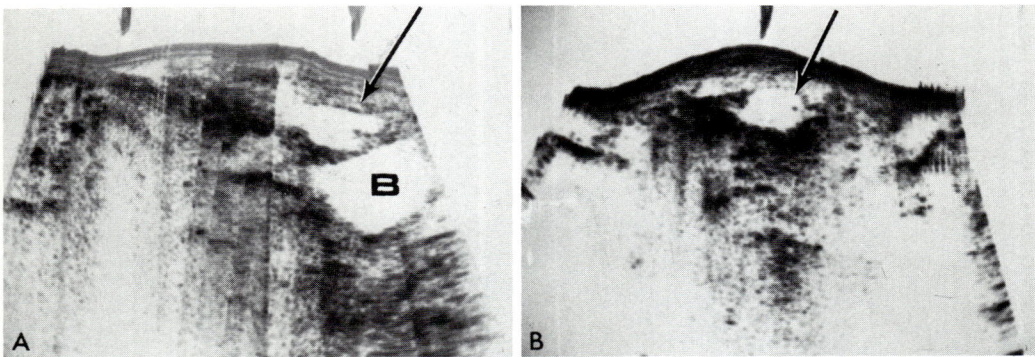

Figure 3–84. Wound abscess. This patient presented with fever and suprapubic tenderness two weeks after abdominal hysterectomy. *A,* The longitudinal scan shows a mass with a predominant fluid component (arrow) along the lower margin of the incision and anterior to the bladder (B). *B,* The transverse scan shows the anterior abscess (arrow), which was successfully treated by percutaneous drainage.

Wound Abscess

Ultrasound is helpful in distinguishing between edema of subcutaneous tissues and a distinct fluid collection within the wound (Fig. 3–84). Scans can be used to demonstrate the size and extent of the collection, to guide percutaneous aspiration, and to evaluate the completeness of drainage.[172]

THYROID AND PARATHYROID GLANDS

The echographic appearances of thyroid lesions are independent of function (i.e., hot versus cold) or histologic findings (i.e., benign versus malignant). Scans have been employed most frequently to evaluate nodules that are cold on isotope scans.[113] Those that are cystic and may be amenable to percutaneous aspiration can be differentiated from solid or complex lesions (Fig. 3–85).[83] Although ultrasound cannot distinguish between benign and malignant solid lesions, results have suggested some typical pat-

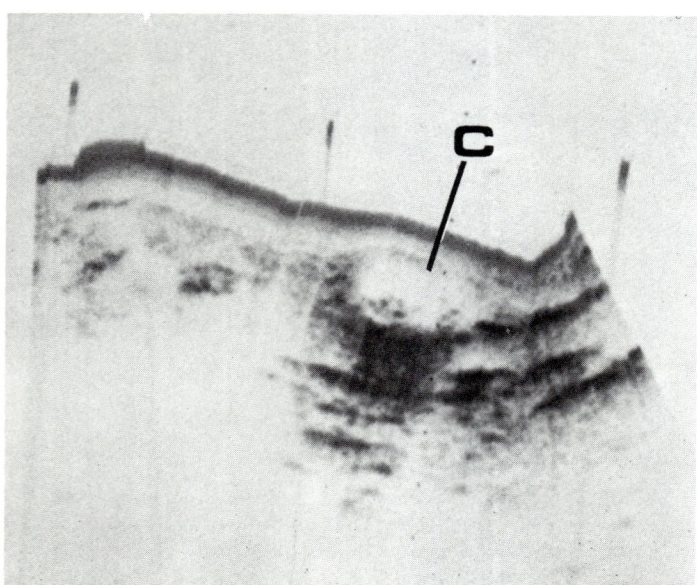

Figure 3–85. Hemorrhagic cyst. This longitudinal scan through the right lobe shows a predominantly cystic nodule (C) with a few foci of internal echoes layered along the posterior wall.

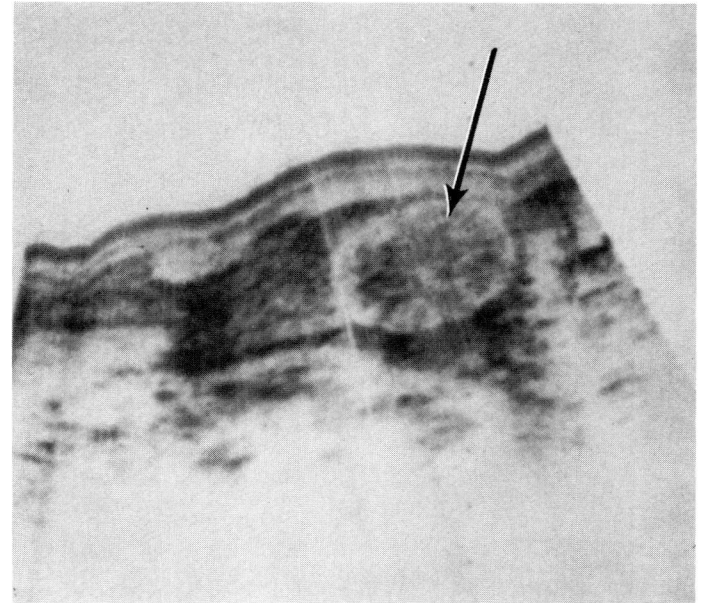

Figure 3–86. Thyroid adenoma. This nodule (arrow) is well demarcated and is surrounded by a thin echo-free zone, or "halo." This appearance is frequently seen with adenoma but is not diagnostic of a benign lesion.

terns, particularly for thyroid adenoma, which frequently appears as a well-demarcated homogeneous solid nodule with a surrounding echo-free rim or "halo" (Fig. 3–86).

Diseases that produce diffuse enlargement also have some typical features.[135] Graves' disease produces a homogeneous solid pattern, while a nodular goiter shows areas of inhomogeneity, and subacute thyroiditis has diffusely diminished echoes. While these patterns are not diagnostic, the ultrasound scan may be confirmatory. Scans can also be used to confirm the location of suspected extrathyroidal lesions.

Recent studies have shown success in visualization of parathyroid adenomas, indicating that ultrasound may be a useful screening procedure in patients with hypercalcemia or other clinical evidence of parathyroid disease (Fig. 3–87).[138]

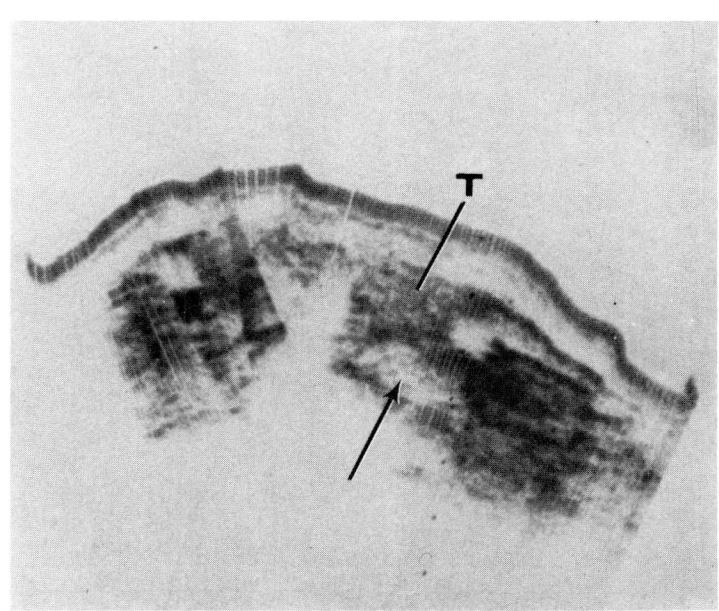

Figure 3–87. Parathyroid adenoma. This transverse scan shows a parathyroid adenoma (arrow) along the posteroinferior aspect of the left lobe of the thyroid (T).

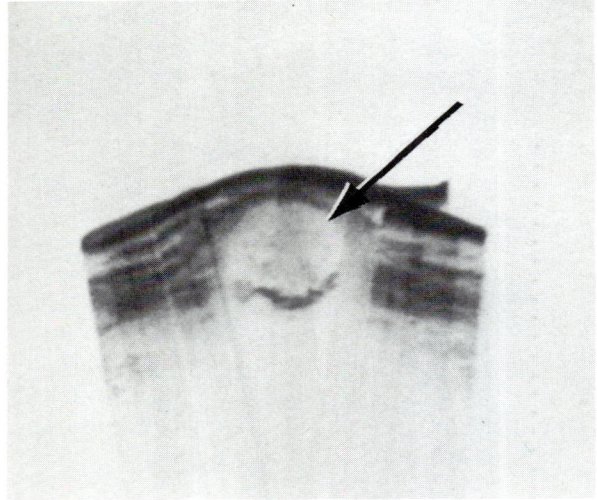

Figure 3–88. Soft tissue tumor. This patient presented with a soft tissue mass anterior to the sternum that had been present for several years. Ultrasound showed a solid mass (arrow) arising between the bone and the subcutaneous tissue. Pathologic diagnosis was metastatic follicular carcinoma.

SUPERFICIAL MASSES

A wide variety of superficial masses have been subjected to ultrasonic evaluation.[117] Their superficial location permits the use of relatively high-frequency, high-resolution transducers. In general, ultrasound is most helpful in distinguishing cystic from solid lesions, permitting identification of those lesions that are amenable to percutaneous puncture, and in determining the exact margins and depths of the lesion (Fig. 3–88).[47] Determination of a lesion's relationship to surrounding structures, particularly blood vessels, is often helpful in surgical planning. More frequently examined areas include the neck and popliteal space (Fig. 3–89).[23, 59] In many instances, scans have proved useful in detecting clinically occult lesions. In patients with bilateral lesions the scan may uncover an occult contralateral lesion.

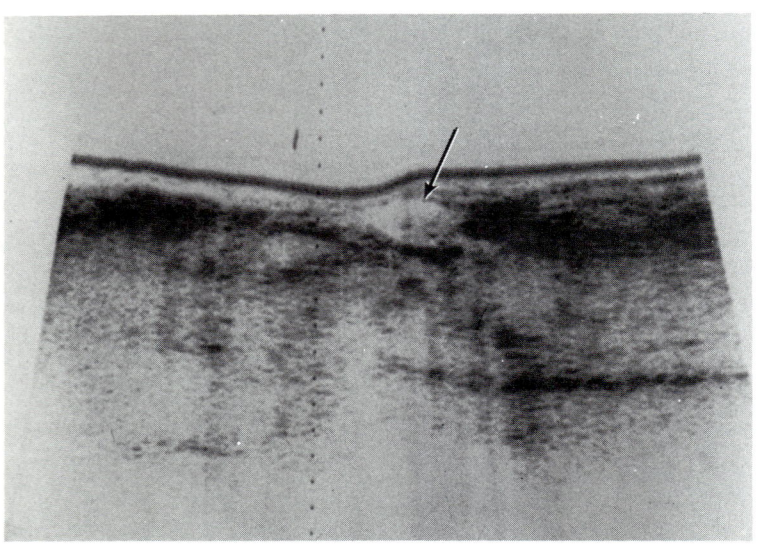

Figure 3–89. Baker's cyst. Ultrasound examination of the popliteal fossa in this middle-aged male presenting with thrombophlebitis shows an ovoid cyst inferomedially (arrow). This was subsequently confirmed by arthrography.

BREAST

Ultrasound has been used primarily as an adjunctive method for the study of breast lesions.[7] Its efficacy as a primary screening device is being investigated.[159] It is useful for the study of palpable masses 1 cm or larger. Cysts can be easily identified and localized for puncture. Accuracy of 80 to 90 per cent in the diagnosis of carcinoma has been achieved by some investigators.[89]

ORBITS

The eye and orbit are readily examined by 0ultrasound.[109] The superficial location permits the use of high-frequency, high-resolution transducers. Ultrasound is particularly useful when direct visualization is limited by opacification of the ocular media. Retinal detachments, foreign bodies, and tumors can be localized. The study is also useful for ocular biometry. Orbital mass lesions and inflammatory changes can be demonstrated.

THORAX

Chest lesions are amenable to scanning only if they are in direct contact with the chest wall, since any intervening air prevents imaging. Scans are most frequently used in the study of pleural opacities, when they can determine the nature of pleural densities and guide attempts at thoracentesis by providing accurate localization and depth estimates (Fig. 3–90).[67, 142] Loculated fluid collections as small as 5 cc have been successfully localized and aspirated using ultrasound guidance.[128]

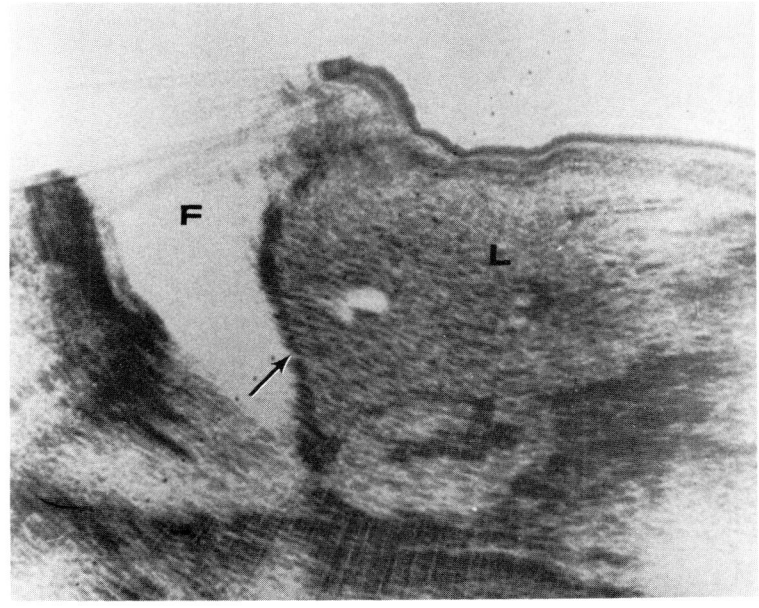

Figure 3–90. Pleural effusion. This patient presented with opacification of the lower half of the right hemithorax on chest x-ray. Attempts at thoracentesis were unsuccessful. This supine scan shows fluid (F) loculated anteriorly just above the right hemidiaphragm (arrow) and liver (L).

PEDIATRIC CONSIDERATIONS

The basic principles of ultrasound and general application do not differ i the pediatric patient. There are, however, some obvious distinctions: The age and size of the patient requires special technical considerations, and the diagnostic possibilities of specific symptoms or findings differ.

The patient's smaller size and the lessened depth penetration required permit the use of higher frequency, higher resolution transducers. The study is painless, and the majority of infants and children are cooperative; occasionally mild sedation may be required to obtain a diagnostic study in the restless or squirming infant.

The specific areas to be evaluated and the interpretation of findings on scans are affected by the presence of congenital abnormalities, developmental anomalies, and disease entities peculiar to childhood. Ultrasound is frequently employed in the evaluation of an abdominal mass;[14] Solid and cystic masses can be differentiated (Fig. 3–91). The majority of these masses are renal in origin. A moderate degree of hydronephrosis can be distinguished from a multicystic or dysplastic kidney;[8] in severe hydronephrosis, the appearance of all of these entities is similar (Fig. 3–92). Since it provides direct imaging, ultrasound may better display the full extent of a solid tumor than urography.[81] There are no specific features allowing distinction between the histologic types of solid tumors.

Another useful application is the evaluation of the kidneys in renal failure or nonvisualization on intravenous urography (Fig. 3–93).[14, 146] The scan can verify the absence of a kidney or assess the structural state of the kidney if one is present. In renal agenesis, care must be taken not to confuse a posteriorly placed splenic flexure for a dysplastic kidney.[158]

The evaluation of the jaundiced infant may be aided by ultrasound examination.[153] If the scan shows dilated ducts or obstructive jaundice, a careful search should be made for a choledochal cyst.[41] Scans may also be helpful in determining the presence or

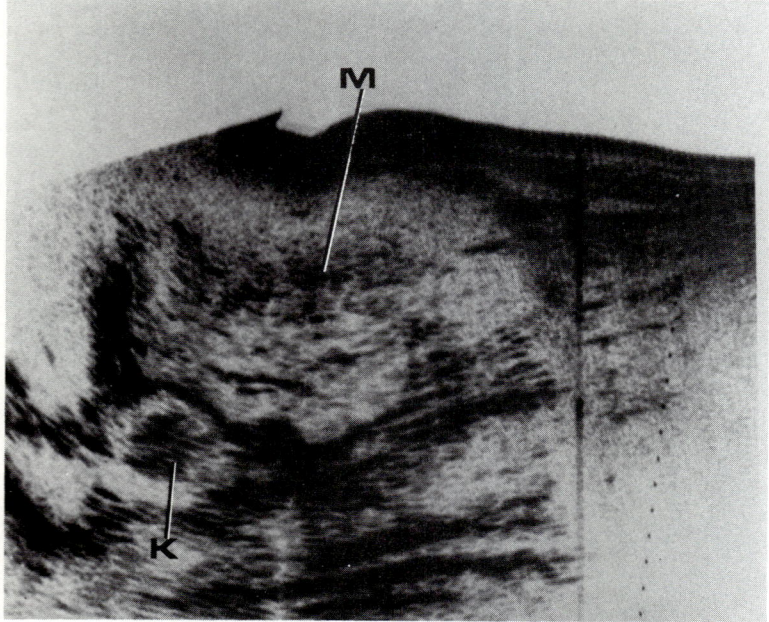

Figure 3–91. Neuroblastoma. A large solid mass (M) is seen in the left upper quadrant anterior to the left kidney (K).

ULTRASOUND TECHNIQUES — 113

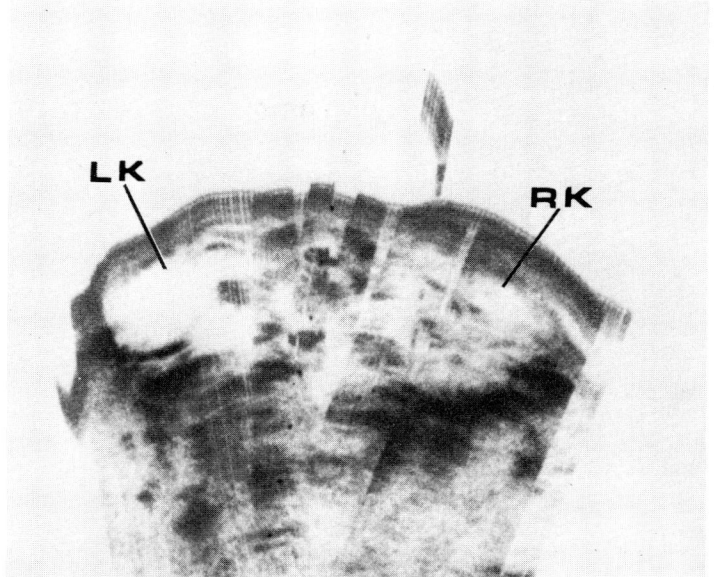

Figure 3–92. Multicystic kidney. This transverse prone scan on an infant with an enlarged left kidney shows multiple cysts in the left kidney (LK). The right kidney (RK) is normal.

absence of the gallbladder as well as ductal dilatation in cases of suspected biliary atresia (see Fig. 3–18).[153]

Ultrasound can also be used to evaluate and obtain measurements of ventricular size in neonates and young children (Fig. 3–94). This is particularly useful in monitoring the degree of ventricular dilatation both before and after ventricular shunting procedures. The examination can be performed rapidly and easily with both contact B-scanners and real-time instruments, obviating the need for repeated computed tomography (CT) examinations and thus reducing the risk of radiation exposure as well as the need for repeated sedation or anesthesia often required to obtain adequate CT examinations. Recent studies comparing the accuracy of ultrasound and CT measure-

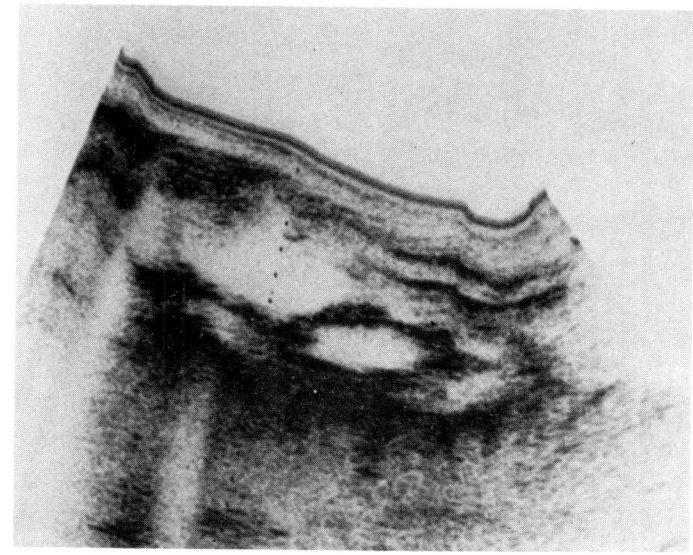

Figure 3–93. Hydronephrosis. This young boy with renal failure had an enlarged hydronephrotic left kidney. The right kidney was absent. Vesicoureteral reflux was demonstrated on cystography.

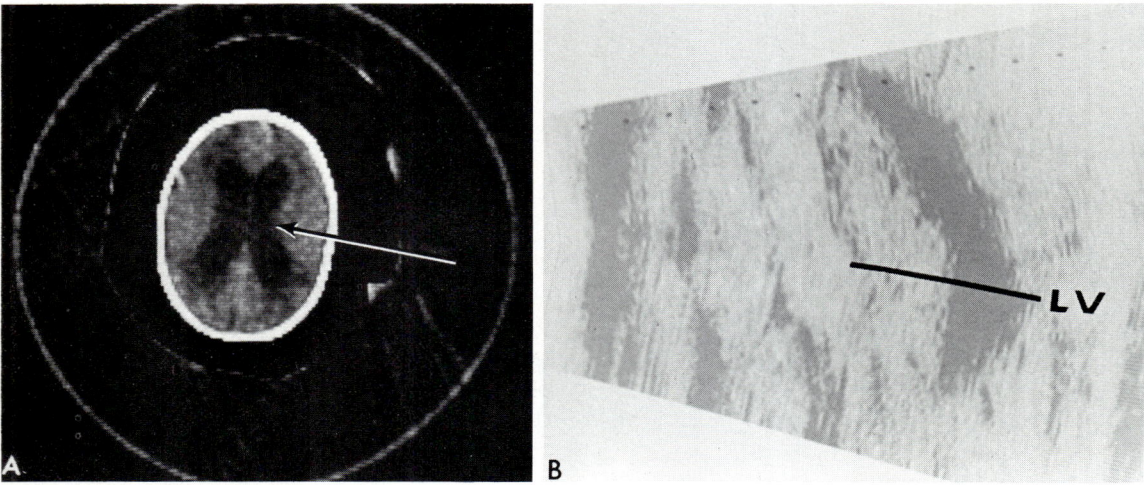

Figure 3–94. Hydrocephalus. ;1A,;2 A CT scan shows evidence of enlargement of the lateral ventricles (arrow). ;1B,;2 An ultrasound scan at approximately the same level shows a similar degree of hydrocephalus of the lateral ventricles (LV). The biventricular width as measured on both studies is identical at 2.6 cm. The lateral ventricular-cranial ratio as calculated by ultrasound is 40 per cent; by CT it is 38 per cent.

ments show excellent correlation, with biventricular width varying by less than 0.5 cm in 85 per cent and less than 1 cm in 95 per cent of cases.[147a]

Other particularly useful applications include evaluation of lymphadenopathy; residual urine determinations;[72] peripheral mass evaluation, particularly in the neck region (Fig. 3–95); diagnosis of appendiceal abscess (see Fig. 3–83); and pelvic studies in the evaluation of ambiguous genitalia and precocious puberty.[69]

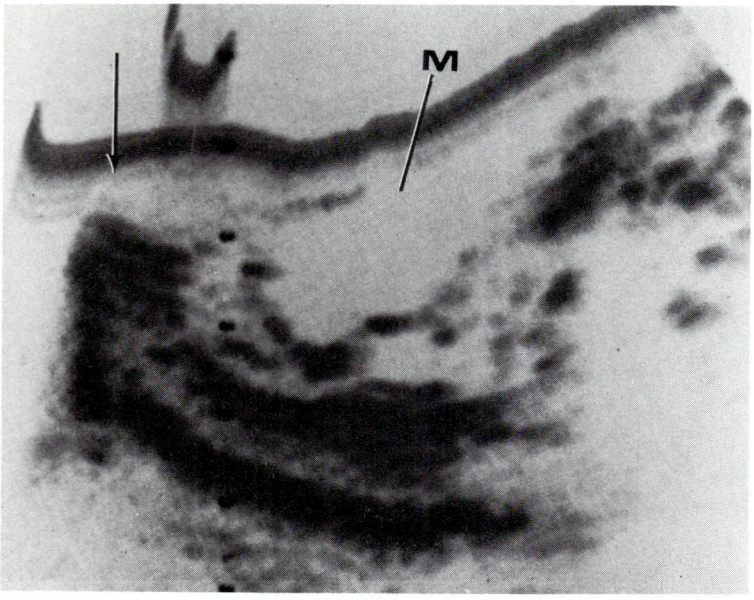

Figure 3–95. Cystic hygroma. Scan of a neck mass in a neonate shows a multiloculated cystic mass (M) that does not extend below the level of the clavicle (arrow).

TABLE 3–2. DIAGNOSTIC AND THERAPEUTIC PROCEDURES USING ULTRASOUND GUIDANCE

Abscess
    Diagnostic aspiration and drainage[29, 65, 148]
Cyst aspiration[55, 71, 83]
Nephrostomy[119]
Obstetric procedures
    Amniocentesis[112]
    Fetoscopy and fetal blood sampling[76, 77]
    Intrauterine transfusion[31]
    Placental aspiration[85]
Paracentesis
Pericardiocentesis[54]
Renal biopsy[15, 177]
Suprapubic bladder aspiration[51]
Thoracentesis[128, 142]
Transhepatic portography[21]
Tumor biopsy[24, 79, 127, 149]

ASPIRATION BIOPSY PROCEDURES

The direct visualization of a lesion and surrounding tissues provided by ultrasound can be used to guide needle placement for aspiration and biopsy techniques. Specially designed transducers with a central lumen allow continuous monitoring of needle placement and depth.[56] The technique has been employed for aspiration of cysts and abscesses[148] as well as for aspiration biopsies of solid lesions.[79] It can also be used for instillation of therapeutic agents and placement of drainage catheters.[65] Scans are also helpful to assess the adequacy of drainage and to detect postbiopsy complications.

The risks and complications of various aspiration or biopsy procedures employing ultrasound guidance are no greater than in other techniques.[73, 95, 128] The procedures in which ultrasound guidance has proved useful are listed in Table 3–2. Some of the more frequently employed procedures are discussed in the following section.

Renal Cyst Aspiration

This is a relatively simple procedure that can be performed on an outpatient basis. The depth and approximate volume of the cyst can be obtained from the initial scan (Fig. 3–96). The site is cleansed and draped, and local anesthetic is applied. A thin-gauge needle is then inserted into the sterilized transducer and placed over the prepared site. The position of the needle tip within the cyst can be monitored during the aspiration.[55] Cyst fluid is obtained for cytologic testing and biochemical analysis (Fig. 3–97). Contrast material can then be injected for fluoroscopic examination of the cyst following the procedure. The technique carries a very minimal risk, and in experienced hands the rate of major complications is less than 1 per cent.[95]

Renal Biopsy

Ultrasound guidance is particularly useful in patients with nonfunctioning kidneys in whom fluoroscopic guidance after contrast injection is not possible.[15] The major disadvantage in the biopsy of a solid mass as opposed to a cystic structure is the

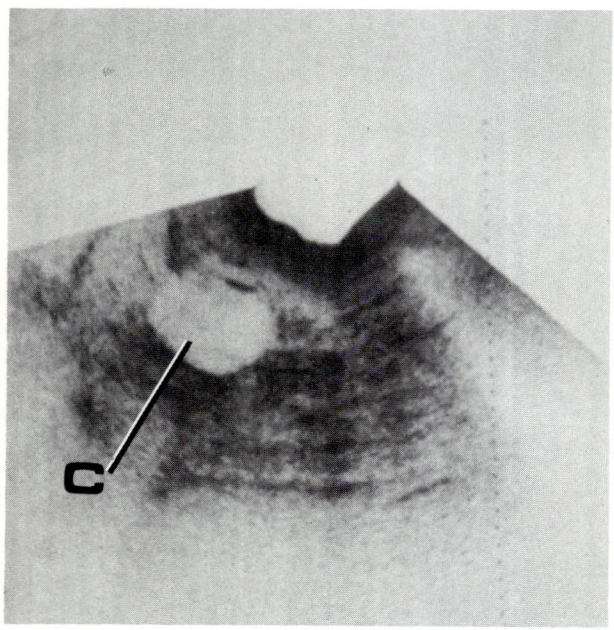

Figure 3–96. Renal cyst. This well-defined cyst (C) in the upper pole of the left kidney was identified and localized prior to aspiration. The aspirated fluid was clear; the results of cytologic examination were negative for malignancy. A contrast agent and air injected following aspiration provided radiographic visualization of the cyst interior.

inability to visualize the needle tip within the mass using currently available transducers. Adaptation of real-time transducers may improve the situation as well as provide continuous monitoring of renal position during inspiration and expiration.[120] Follow-up scans can be performed following biopsy by this or any other method to detect perinephric hematoma formation (Fig. 3–98).

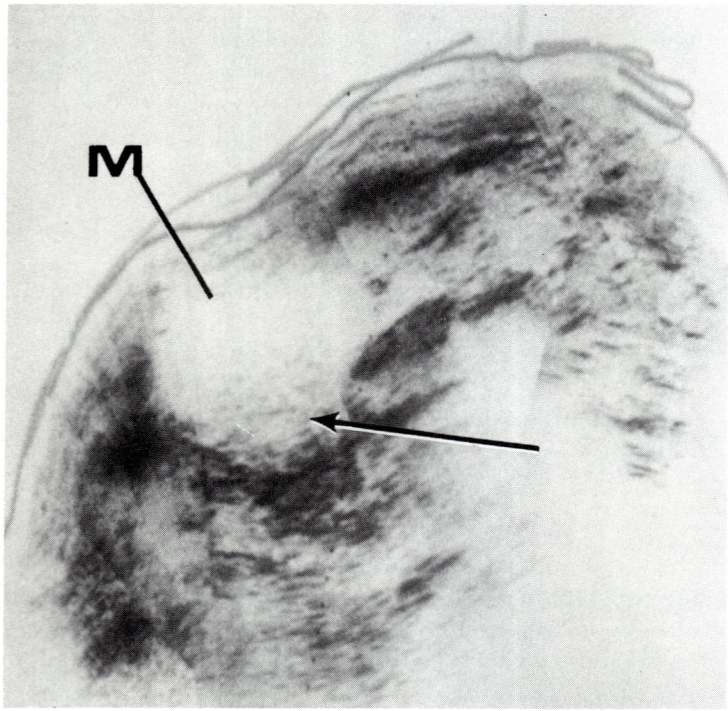

Figure 3–97. Renal tumor with cyst. Scans of this renal mass (M) show a predominantly fluid-filled mass with an irregular contour and low-level echoes in the dependent portion (arrow), suggesting infected cyst or necrotic tumor. Aspiration under ultrasound guidance yielded bloody fluid and malignant cells.

ULTRASOUND TECHNIQUES — 117

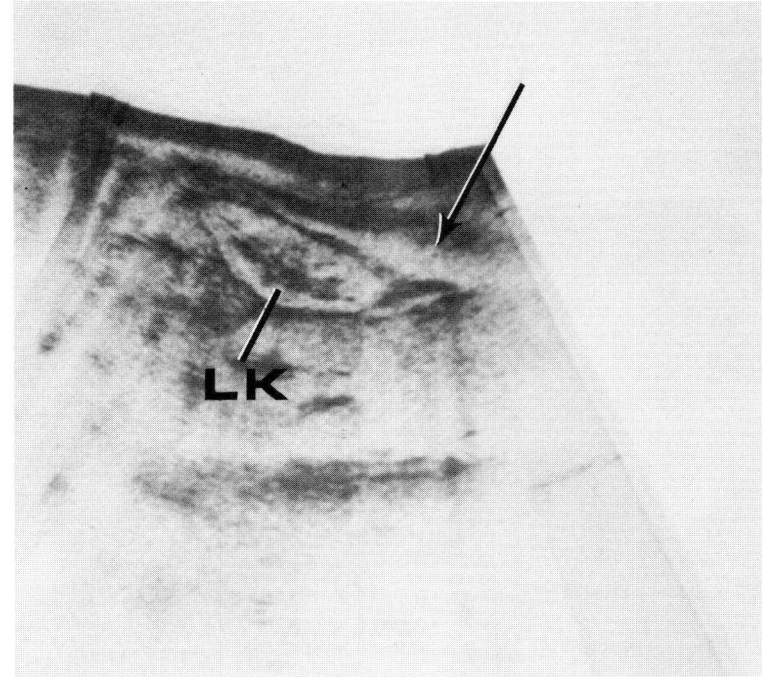

Figure 3–98. Perinephric hematoma. This longitudinal scan following a closed renal biopsy shows a collection of fluid (arrow) along the posterior aspect of the left kidney (LK).

Pancreas

A recent and potentially valuable application is the aspiration of pancreatic masses.[149] Despite its retroperitoneal location, the pancreas is relatively close to the abdominal wall and pancreatic masses tend to grow anteriorly (Fig. 3–99). Biopsy under

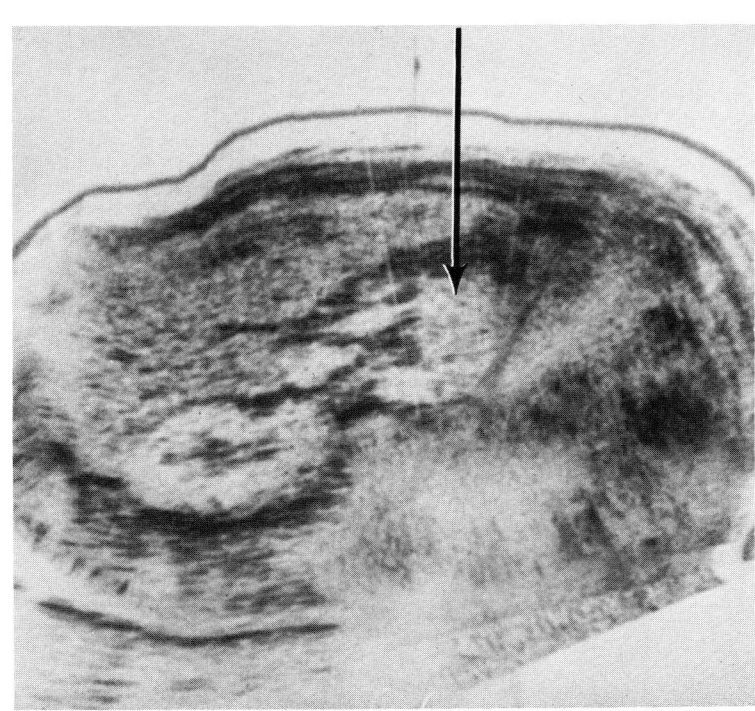

Figure 3–99. Pancreatic carcinoma. The transverse scan shows a mass (arrow) involving the distal pancreas. Arteriography indicated vascular involvement and unresectability. Percutaneous aspiration with a fine-gauge needle provided cytologic confirmation of malignancy prior to therapy.

118 — ULTRASOUND TECHNIQUES

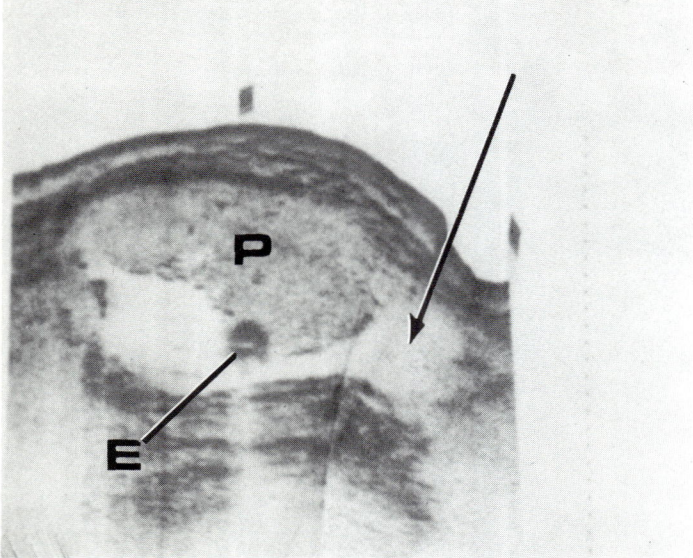

Figure 3–100. Amniocentesis. This longitudinal scan of a gravid uterus shows an appropriate site for amniocentesis (arrow) below the inferior margin of the placenta (P). The location of the fetus is medial to this plane; a fetal extremity (E) is seen beneath the placenta.

direct imaging provides a comparatively simple and safe method of obtaining histologic confirmation when the diagnosis is in question or when the patient is a poor surgical risk.

Amniocentesis

The use of ultrasound eliminates the need for blind placement of the needle, with the attendant risk to the mother and fetus, and the problem of unsuccessful or bloody

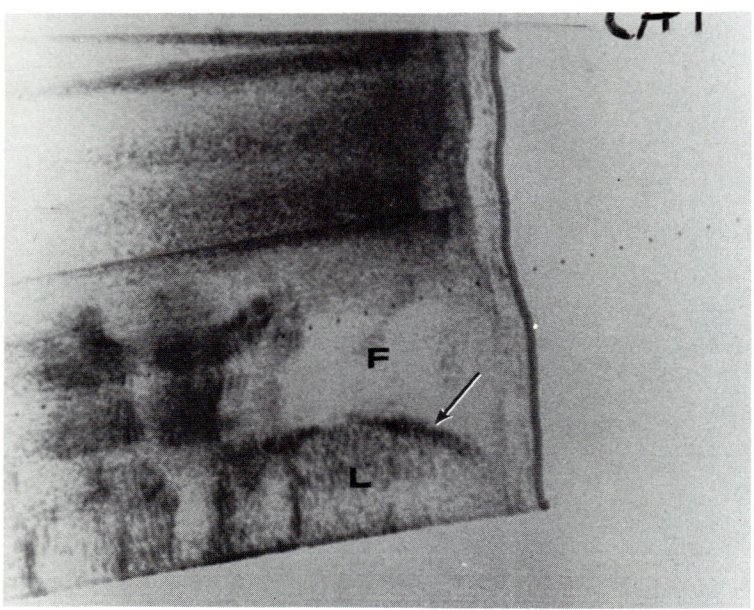

Figure 3–101. Pleural effusion. Attempts at thoracentesis in this patient with radiographic findings consistent with pleural effusion were unsuccessful. The ultrasound scan in the exact position shows fluid (F) along the lateral margin of the right hemithorax, which was successfully aspirated. The liver (L) and diaphragm (arrow) are seen below. Scans posteriorly in the area of attempted thoracentesis showed no evidence of fluid.

taps.[73, 112] Scans can localize the position of the placenta and fetus and help to determine the optimal site for an aspiration (Fig. 3–100). Since fetal position is not constant, the procedure should ideally be done with ultrasound monitoring. Ultrasound guidance can also be used for a variety of other obstetric procedures, including intrauterine transfusion,[31] fetoscopy,[76] fetal blood sampling,[77] and placental aspiration.[85]

Thoracentesis

Ultrasound is helpful in localizing loculated fluid collections as well as in determining the relationship of the proposed aspiration site to the spleen or liver below (Fig. 3–101).[128] It is not possible to determine from the ultrasound appearance the consistency of the fluid or the likelihood of successful drainage.

References

1. Anderson, J. M., Lee, T. G., and Nagel, N.: Ultrasound diagnosis of non-obstetric disease during pregnancy. Obstet. Gynecol. 48:359–362, 1976.
2. Asher, W. M., Parvin, S., Virgilio, R. W., et al.: Echographic evaluation of splenic injury after blunt trauma. Radiology 118:411–415, 1976.
3. Baker, M. L., and Dalrymple, G. V.: Biologic effects of diagnostic ultrasound: a review. Radiology 126:479–483, 1978.
4. Bartrum, R. J., Crow, H. C., and Foote, S. R.: Ultrasonic and radiographic cholecystography. N. Engl. J. Med. 296:538–540, 1977.
5. Bartrum, R. J., Smith, E. H., D'Orsi, C. J., et al.: Evaluation of renal transplants with ultrasound. Radiology 118:405–410, 1976.
6. Basinger, G. T., and Gittes, R. F.: Lymphocyst: ultrasound diagnosis and urologic management. J. Urol. 114:740–745, 1975.
7. Baum, G.: Ultrasound mammography. Radiology 122:199–205, 177.
8. Bearman, S. B., Hine, P. L., and Sanders, R. C.: Multicystic kidney: a sonographic pattern. Radiology 118:685–688, 1976.
9. Berger, M., Smith, E., Holm, H. H., et al.: The utility of ultrasound in the differential diagnosis of acute cholecystitis. Arch. Surg. 112:273–275, 1977.
10. Bernardino, M. E., Goldstein, H. M., and Green, B.: Gray scale ultrasonography of adrenal neoplasms. Am. J. Roentgenol. 130:741–744, 1978.
11. Bhimji, S. D., Cooperberg, P. L., Naiman, S., et al.: Ultrasound diagnosis of splenic cysts. Radiology 122:787–789, 1977.
12. Birnholz, J. C.: Sonic differentiation of cysts and homogeneous solid masses. Radiology 108:699–702, 1973.
13. Blue, S. K., McKinney, W. M., Barnes, R., et al.: Ultrasonic B-mode scanning for study of extracranial vascular disease. Neurology 22:1079–1085, 1972.
14. Boineau, F. G., Rothman, J., and Lewy, J. E.: Nephrosonography in the evaluation of renal failure and masses in infants. J. Pediatr. 87:195–201, 1975.
15. Bolton, W. K., Tully, R. J., Lewis, E. J., et al.: Localization of the kidney for percutaneous biopsy. Ann. Intern. Med. 81:159–164, 1974.
16. Boyce, W. H., McKinney, W. M., Resnick, M. I., et al.: Ultrasonography as an aid in the diagnosis and management of surgical diseases of the pelvis. Ann. Surg. 184:477–489, 1976.
17. Bradley, E. L., and Clements, J. L.: Implications of diagnostic ultrasound in the surgical management of pancreatic pseudocysts. Am. J. Surg. 127:163–173, 1974.
18. Brascho, D. J.: Tumor, localization and treatment planning with ultrasound. Cancer 39:697–705, 1977.
19. Brascho, D. J., Durant, J. R., and Green, L. G.: The accuracy of retroperitoneal ultrasonography in Hodgkin's disease and non-Hodgkin's lymphoma. Radiology 125:485–487, 1977.
20. Bree, R. L., and Green, B.: The gray scale sonographic appearance of intra-abdominal mesenchymal sarcomas. Radiology 128:193–197, 1978.
21. Burcharth, F., and Rasmussen, S. N.: Localization of the porta hepatis by ultrasonic scanning prior to transhepatic portography. Br. J. Radiol. 47:598–600, 1974.
22. Carlsen, E. N., and Filly, R. A.: Newer ultrasonographic anatomy in the upper abdomen: I. The portal and hepatic venous anatomy. J. Clin. Ultrasound 4:85–90, 1976.
23. Carpenter, J. R., Hattery, R. R., Hunter, G. G., et al.: Ultrasound evaluation of the popliteal space: comparison with arthrography and physical examination. Mayo Clin. Proc. 51:498–503, 1976.

24. Chandrasekhar, A. J., Reynes, C. J., and Churchill, R. J.: Ultrasonically guided percutaneous biopsy of peripheral pulmonary masses. Chest 70:627–630, 1976.
25. Cochrane, W. J., and Thomas, M. A.: The use of ultrasound B-scanning in the localization of intrauterine contraceptive devices. Radiology 104:623–627, 1977.
26. Conrad, M. R., Landay, M. J., and Janes, J. O.: Sonographic "parallel channel" sign of biliary tree enlargement in mild to moderate obstructive jaundice. Am. J. Roentgenol. 130:279–286, 1978.
27. Conrad, M. R., Landay, M. J., and Khoury, M.: Pancreatic pseudocysts: unusual ultrasound features. Am. J. Roentgenol. 130:265–268, 1978.
28. Conrad, M. R., Sanders, R. C., and James, A. E.: The sonolucent "light bulb" sign of fluid collections. J. Clin. Ultrasound 4:409–415, 1976.
29. Conrad, M. R., Sanders, R. C., and Mascardo, A. D.: Perinephric abscess aspiration using ultrasound guidance. Am. J. Roentgenol. 128:459–464, 1977.
30. Cook, J. H., Rosenfield, A. T., and Taylor, K. J. W.: Ultrasonic demonstration of intrarenal anatomy. Am. J. Roentgenol. 129:831–835, 1977.
31. Cooperberg, P. L., and Carpenter, C. W.: Ultrasound as an aid in intrauterine transfusion. Am. J. Obstet. Gynecol. 128:239–241, 1977.
32. Cunningham, J. J.: Atypical cholesonograms in primary and secondary malignant disease of the biliary tract. J. Clin. Ultrasound 5:264–266, 1977.
33. Davis, R. P., Neiman, H. L., Yao, J. S., et al.: Ultrasound scan in diagnosis of peripheral aneurysms. Arch. Surg. 112:55–58, 1977.
34. Doust, B. D.: The use of ultrasound in the diagnosis of gastroenterological disease. Gastroenterology 70:602–610, 1976.
35. Doust, B. D., and Doust, V. L.: Ultrasonic diagnosis of abdominal abscess. Am. J. Dig. Dis. 21:569–576, 1976.
36. Doust, B. D., and Pearce, J. D.: Gray scale ultrasonic properties of the normal and inflamed pancreas. Radiology 120:653–657, 1976.
37. Doust, B. D., Queroz, F., and Stewart, J. M.: Ultrasonic distinction of abscesses from other intra-abdominal fluid collections. Radiology 125:213–218, 1977.
38. Edell, S., and Zegel, H.: Ultrasonic evaluation of renal calculi. Am. J. Roentgenol. 130:261–263, 1978.
39. Felix, W. R., Sigel, B., and Popky, G. L.: Doppler ultrasound in the diagnosis of peripheral vascular disease. Semin. Roentgenol. 10:315–321, 1975.
40. Fiegenschuh, W. H., and Loughry, C. W.: The false normal oral cholecystogram. Surgery 81:239–242, 1977.
41. Filly, R. A., and Carlsen, E. N.: Choledochal cyst: report of a case with specific ultrasonographic findings. J. Clin. Ultrasound 4:7–10, 1976.
42. Filly, R. A., and Carlsen, E. N.: Newer ultrasonographic anatomy in the upper abdomen: II. The major systemic veins and arteries with a special note on localization of the pancreas. J. Clin. Ultrasound 4:91–96, 1976.
43. Filly, R. A., and Freimanis, A. K.: Thrombosed hepatic artery aneurysm. Radiology 97:629–630, 1970.
44. Fleischer, A. C., James, A. E., Krause, D. A., et al.: Sonographic patterns in trophoblastic disease. Radiology 126:215–220, 1978.
45. Friday, R. O., Barriga, P., and Crummy, A. B.: Detection and localization of intra-abdominal abscesses by diagnostic ultrasound. Arch. Surg. 110:335–337, 1975.
46. Garrett, W. J., Kossoff, G., Uren, R. F., et al.: Gray scale ultrasonic investigation of focal defects on ^{99}Tc-sulfur colloid liver scanning. Radiology 119:425–428, 1976.
46a. Gerzhof, S. G., Robbins, A. H., Birkett, D. H., et al.: Percutaneous catheter drainage of abdominal abscesses guided by ultrasound and computed tomography. Am. J. Roentgenol. 133:1–8, 1979.
47. Goldberg, B. B.: Ultrasonic evaluation of superficial masses. J. Clin. Ultrasound 3:91–94, 1975.
48. Goldberg, B. B., Goodman, G. A., and Clearfield, H. R.: Evaluation of ascites by ultrasound. Radiology 96:15–22, 1970.
49. Goldberg, B. B., Harris, K., and Brooker, W.: Ultrasonic and radiographic cholecystography: a comparison. Radiology 111:405–409, 1974.
50. Goldberg, B. B., and Lehman, J. S.: Aortosonography: ultrasound measurement of the abdominal and thoracic aorta. Arch. Surg. 100:652–655, 1970.
51. Goldberg, B. B., and Meyer, H.: Ultrasonically guided suprapubic urinary bladder aspiration. Pediatrics 51:70–74, 1973.
52. Goldberg, B. B., and Patel, J.: Ultrasonic evaluation of portocaval shunts. J. Clin. Ultrasound 5:304–306, 1977.
53. Goldberg, B. B., and Perlmutter, G.: Ultrasonic evaluation of the superior mesenteric artery. J. Clin. Ultrasound 5:185–187, 1977.
54. Goldberg, B. B., and Pollack, H. M.: Ultrasonically guided pericardiocentesis. Am. J. Cardiol. 31:490–492, 1973.
55. Goldberg, B. B., and Pollack, H. M.: Ultrasonically guided renal cyst aspiration. J. Urol. 109:5–7, 1973.
56. Goldberg, B. B., and Pollack, H. M.: Ultrasonic aspiration-biopsy transducer. Radiology 108:667–671, 1973.
57. Goldfine, S. L., Turetz, F., Beck, A. R., et al.: Cerebrospinal fluid intraperitoneal cyst: an unusual abdominal mass. Am. J. Roentgenol. 130:568–569, 1978.

58. Gonzalez, A. C., Bradley, E. L., and Clements, J. L.: Pseudocyst formation in acute pancreatitis: ultrasonographic evaluation of 99 cases. Am. J. Roentgenol. 127:315–317, 1976.
59. Gooding, G. A. W., Herzog, K. A., Laing, F. C., et al.: Ultrasonographic assessment of neck masses. J. Clin. Ultrasound 5:248–252, 1977.
60. Gosink, B. B.: The inferior vena cava: mass effects. Am. J. Roentgenol. 130:533–536, 1978.
61. Green, B., Bree, R. L., Goldstein, H. M., et al.: Gray scale ultrasound evaluation of hepatic neoplasms: patterns and correlations. Radiology 124:203–208, 1977.
62. Green, W. M., King, D. L., and Casarella, W. J.: A reappraisal of sonolucent renal masses. Radiology 121:163–171, 1976.
63. Green, W. M., and King, D. L.: Diagnostic ultrasound of the urinary tract. J. Clin. Ultrasound 4:55–64, 1976.
64. Greene, D., and Steinbach, H. L.: Ultrasonic diagnosis of hypernephroma extending into the inferior vena cava. Radiology 115:679–680, 1975.
65. Grønvall, J., Grønvall, S., and Hegedus, V.: Ultrasound-guide drainage of fluid-containing masses using angiographic catheterization techniques. Am. J. Roentgenol. 129:997–1002, 1977.
66. Grossman, Z. D., Wistow, B. W., Bryan, P. J., et al.: Radionuclide imaging, computed tomography and gray-scale ultrasonography of the liver: a comparative study. J. Nucl. Med. 18:327–332, 1977.
67. Gryminski, J., Krakowka, P., and Lypacewicz, G.: The diagnosis of pleural effusions by ultrasonic and radiologic techniques. Chest 70:33–37, 1976.
68. Haller, J. O., Schneider, M., Kassner, E. G., et al.: Sonographic evaluation of mesenteric and omental masses in children. Am. J. Roentgenol. 130:269–274, 1978.
69. Haller, J. O., Schneider, M., Kassner, E. G., et al.: Ultrasonography in pediatric gynecology and obstetrics. Am. J. Roentgenol. 128:423–429, 1977.
70. Hancke, S.: Ultrasonic scanning of the pancreas. J. Clin. Ultrasound 4:223–230, 1976.
71. Hancke, S., and Pedersen, J. F.: Percutaneous puncture of pancreatic cysts guided by ultrasound. Surg. Gynecol. Obstet. 142:551–552, 1976.
71a. Handler, S. J.: Ultrasound of gallbladder wall thickening and its relation to cholecystitis. Am. J. Roentgenol. 132:581–585, 1979.
72. Harrison, N. W., Parks, C., and Sherwood, T.: Ultrasound assessment of residual urine in children. Br. J. Urol. 47:805–814, 1975.
73. Harrison, R., Campbell, S., and Craft, I.: Risks of feto-maternal hemorrhage resulting from amniocentesis with and without ultrasound placental localization. Obstet. Gynecol. 46:389–391, 1975.
74. Hellman, L. M., Duffus, G. M., Donald, I., et al.: Safety of diagnostic ultrasound in obstetrics. Lancet 1:1133–1134, 1970.
75. Hill, B. A., Yamaguchi, K., Flynn, J. J., et al.: Diagnostic sonography in general surgery. Surgery 110:1089–1094, 1975.
76. Hobbins, J. C., and Mahoney, M. J.: Experience with fetal blood drawing. Lancet 2:107–109, 1975.
77. Hobbins, J. C., Mahoney, M. J., and Goldstein, L. A.: New method of intrauterine evaluation by the combined use of fetoscopy and ultrasound. Am. J. Obstet. Gynecol. 118:1069–1072, 1974.
78. Hobbins, J. C., and Winsberg, F.: Ultrasonography in Obstetrics and Gynecology. Baltimore, The Williams & Wilkins Company; 1977, pp. 146–158.
79. Holm, H. H., Pedersen, J. F., Kristensen, K., et al.: Ultrasonically guided percutaneous puncture. Radiol. Clin. North Am. 13:493–503, 1975.
80. Hublitz, U., Kahn, P., and Sell, L.: Cholecystosonography: an approach to the non-visualized gallbladder. Radiology 103:645–649, 1972.
81. Hunig, R., and Kinser, J.: Ultrasonic diagnosis of Wilm's tumor. Am. J. Roentgenol. 117:119–127, 1973.
82. Jensen, F., and Pedersen, J. F.: The value of ultrasonic scanning in the diagnosis of intra-abdominal abscesses and hematomas. Surg. Gynecol. Obstet. 139:326–328, 1974.
83. Jensen, F., and Rasmussen, S. N.: The treatment of thyroid cyst by ultrasonically guided fine needle aspiration. Acta Chir. Scand. 142:209–211, 1976.
84. Kaftore, J. K., Rosenberger, P., Pollack, S., et al.: Rectus sheath hematoma: ultrasonic diagnosis. Am. J. Roentgenol. 128:283–285, 1977.
84a. Kamin, P. D., Bernardino, M. E., and Green, B.: Ultrasound manifestations of hepatocellular carcinoma. Radiology 131:459–461, 1979.
85. Kan, Y. W., Valenti, C., Guidotti, R., et al.: Fetal blood sampling in utero. Lancet 1:79–80, 1974.
86. Kaplan, G. N., and Sanders, R. C.: B-scan ultrasound in the management of patients with occult abdominal hematomas. J. Clin. Ultrasound 1:5–13, 1973.
87. Kelsey, J. A., and Bowie, J. D.: Gray scale ultrasonography in the diagnosis of polycystic kidney disease. Radiology 122:791–795, 1977.
88. King, D. L.: Ultrasonograph of echinococcal cysts. J. Clin. Ultrasound 1:64–67, 1973.
89. Kobayashi, T.: Gray scale echography for breast cancer. Radiology 122:207–214, 1977.
90. Kobayashi, T., Takatani, O., and Kimura, K.: Echographic patterns of malignant lymphoma. J. Clin. Ultrasound 4:181–186, 1976.
91. Koehler, P. R., Kanemoto, H. H., and Maxwell, J. G.: Ultrasonic "B" scanning in the diagnosis of complications in renal transplant patients. Radiology 119:661–664, 1976.
92. Koga, T., and Morikawa, Y.: Ultrasonographic determination of splenic size and its usefulness in various liver diseases. Radiology 115:157–162, 1975.

93. Kosoff, G., Garrett, W. J., Carpenter, D. A., et al.: Principles and classification of soft tissues by gray scale echography. Ultrasound Med. Biol. 2:89–105, 1976.
94. Laing, F. C., and Jacobs, R. P.: Value of ultrasonography in the detection of retroperitoneal inflammatory masses. Radiology 123:169–172, 1977.
95. Lang, E. K.: Renal cyst puncture and aspiration: a survey of complications. Am. J. Roentgenol. 128:723–727, 1977.
96. Landay, M., and Harless, M.: Ultrasonic differentiation of right pleural effusion from subphrenic fluid on longitudinal scans of the right upper quadrant: importance of recognizing the diaphragm. Radiology 123:155–158, 1977.
97. Lawson, T. L., and Albarelli, J. N.: Diagnosis of gynecologic pelvic masses by gray scale ultrasonography: analysis of specificity and accuracy. Am. J. Roentgenol. 128:1003–1006, 1977.
98. Lee, K. R., Walls, W. J., Martin, N. L., et al.: A practical approach to the diagnosis of abdominal aortic aneurysms. Surgery 78:195–201, 1975.
99. Lee, T. G., and Henderson, S. C.: Ultrasonic aortography: unexpected findings. Am. J. Roentgenol. 128:273–276, 1977.
100. Leopold, G. R.: Renal transplant size measured by reflected ultrasound. Radiology 95:687–689, 1970.
101. Leopold, G. R.: Gray scale ultrasonic angiography of the upper abdomen. Radiology 117:665–671, 1975.
102. Leopold, G. R.: Pancreatic echography: a new dimension in the diagnosis of pseudocyst. Radiology 104:365–369, 1972.
103. Leopold, G. R., Amberg, J., Gosink, B. B., et al.: Gray scale ultrasonic cholecystography: a comparison with conventional radiographic techniques. Radiology 121:445–448, 1976.
104. Leopold, G. R., and Asher, W. M.: Deleterious effects of gastrointestinal contrast material on abdominal echography. Radiology 98:637–640, 1971.
104a. Leopold, G. R., Woo, V. L., Scheible, W., et al.: High resolution ultrasonography of scrotal pathology. Radiology 131:719–722, 1979.
105. Maklad, N. F., Doust, B. D., and Baum, J. K.: Ultrasonic diagnosis of post-operative intra-abdominal abscess. Radiology 113:417–422, 1974.
106. Maklad, N. F., and Wright, C. H.: Gray scale ultrasonography in the diagnosis of ectopic pregnancy. Radiology 126:221–225, 1978.
106a. Maklad, N. F., Wright, C. H., and Rosenthal, S. J.: Gray scale ultrasonic appearances of renal transplant rejection. Radiology 131:711–717, 1979.
107. McCullough, D. L., and Leopold, G. R.: Diagnosis of retroperitoneal fluid collections by ultrasonography: series of surgically proved cases. J. Urol. 115:656–659, 1976.
108. McLaughlin, I. S., Morley, P., Deane, R. F., et al.: Ultrasound in the staging of bladder tumors. Br. J Urol. 47:51–56, 1975.
109. McQuown, D. S.: Ocular and orbital echography. Radiol. Clin. North Am. 13:523–541, 1975.
110. Miller, S. S., Garvie, W. H. H., and Christie, A. D.: The evaluation of prostate size by ultrasonic scanning: a preliminary report. Br. J. Urol. 45:187–191, 1973.
111. Mishkin, M. M., Buckspan, M., and Bain, J.: Ultrasonographic evaluation of scrotal masses. J. Urol. 117:185–188, 1977.
112. Mishkin, M., Doran, T. A., Rudd, N., et al.: Use of ultrasound for placental localization in genetic amniocentesis. Obstet. Gynecol. 43:872–877, 1974.
113. Mishkin, M., Rosen, I., and Walfish, P. G.: B-mode ultrasonography in assessment of thyroid gland lesions. Ann. Intern. Med. 79:505–510, 1973.
114. Mittelstaedt, C.: Ultrasonic diagnosis of omental cysts. Radiology 117:673–676, 1975.
115. Morley, P., Barnett, E., Bell, P. R. F., et al.: Ultrasound in the diagnosis of fluid collections following renal transplantation. Clin. Radiol. 26:199–207, 1975.
116. Neiman, H. L., and Mintzer, R. A.: Accuracy of biliary duct ultrasound: comparison with cholangiography. Am. J. Roentgenol. 129:979–982, 1977.
117. Neiman, H. L., Phillips, J. F., Jacques, D. A., et al.: Ultrasound of the parotid gland. J. Clin. Ultrasound 4:11–13, 1976.
117a. Neiman, H. L., Yao, J. S. T., and Silver, T. M.: Gray scale ultrasound diagnosis of peripheral arterial aneurysms. Radiology 130:413–416, 1979.
118. Neisbaum, J. W., Freimanis, A. K., and Thomford, N. R.: Echography in the diagnosis of abdominal aortic aneurysm. Arch. Surg. 102:385–388, 1971.
119. Pedersen, J. F.: Percutaneous nephrostomy guided by ultrasound. J. Urol. 112:157–159, 1974.
120. Pedersen, J. F.: Percutaneous puncture guided by ultrasonic multitransducer scanning. J. Clin. Ultrasound 5:175–177, 1977.
121. Pedersen, J. F., Bartrum, R. J., and Grytter, C.: Residual urine determination by ultrasonic scanning. Am. J. Roentgenol. 125:474–478, 1975.
122. Petrek, J., Tilney, N. L., Smith, E. H., et al.: Ultrasound in renal transplantation. Ann. Surg. 185:441–447, 1977.
123. Pollack, H. M., Arger, P. H., Goldberg, B. B., et al.: Ultrasonic detection of nonopaque renal calculi. Radiology 127:233–237, 1978.
124. Proto, A. V., Lane, E. J., and Marangola, J. P.: A new concept of ascitic fluid distribution. Am. J. Roentgenol. 126:974–980, 1976.

125. Rasmussen, S. N., Christensen, B. E., Holm, H. M., et al.: Spleen volume determination by ultrasonic scanning. Scand. J. Haematol. *10*:298–304, 1973.
126. Rasmussen, S. N., Kardel, T., and Jorgensen, B. J.: Liver volume estimated by ultrasonic scanning before and after portal decompression surgery. Scand. J. Gastroenterol. *10*:25–28, 1975.
127. Rasmussen, S. N., Holm, H. H., Kristensen, J. K., et al.: Ultrasonically guided liver biopsy. Br. Med. J. *2*:500–502, 1972.
128. Ravin, C. E.: Thoracentesis of loculated pleural effusions using gray scale ultrasonic guidance. Chest *71*:666–668, 1977.
129. Robinson, S. H., Hayt, D. B., Reynold, B., et al.: Gray scale ultrasound: utility pre-operatively and post-operatively in a patient with obstructive jaundice. Arch. Surg. *112*:1135–1138, 1977.
130. Rochester, D., Bowie, J. D., Kunzman, A., et al.: Ultrasound in the staging of lymphoma. Radiology *124*:483–487, 1977.
131. Rogers, W. F., Staub, M., and Wilson, R.: Chronic ectopic pregnancy: ultrasonic diagnosis. J. Clin. Ultrasound *5*:257–273, 1977.
132. Rosenfield, A. T., Taylor, K. J. W., Crade, M., et al.: Anatomy and pathology of the kidney by gray scale ultrasound. Radiology *128*:737–744, 1978.
133. Rosenfield, A. T., and Taylor, K. J. W.: Gray scale nephrosonography: current status. J. Urol. *117*:2–6, 1977.
134. Rosenfield, A. T., and Taylor, K. J. W.: Obstructive uropathy in the transplanted kidney: evaluation by gray scale sonography. J. Urol. *116*:101–102, 1976.
135. Sackler, J. P., Passalaqua, A. M., Blum, M., et al.: A spectrum of diseases of the thyroid gland as imaged by gray scale water bath sonography. Radiology *125*:467–472, 1977.
136. Sample, W. F.: A new technique for evaluation of the adrenal gland with gray-scale ultrasonography. Radiology *124*:463–469, 1977.
137. Sample, W. F., Gottesman, J. E., Skinner, D. G., et al.: Gray scale ultrasound of the scrotum. Radiology *127*:225–228, 1978.
138. Sample, W. F., Mitchell, S. P., and Bledsoe, R. C.: Parathyroid ultrasonography. Radiology *127*:485–490, 1978.
139. Sanders, A. D., and Sanders, R. C.: The complementary use of ultrasound and radionuclide imaging techniques. J. Nucl. Med. *18*:205–220, 1976.
140. Sanders, R. C., Conrad, M. R., and White, R. I.: Normal and abnormal upper abdominal venous structures as seen by ultrasound. Am. J. Roentgenol. *128*:657–662, 1977.
141. Sanders, R. C., and Jeck, D. L.: B-scan ultrasound in the evaluation of renal failure. Radiology *119*:199–202, 1976.
142. Sandweiss, D. A., Hanson, J. C., Gosink, B. B., et al.: Ultrasound in the diagnosis, localization and treatment of loculated pleural empyema. Ann. Intern. Med. *82*:50–53, 1975.
143. Sapala, M. A., Steel, W. B., RestoSoto, A. D., et al.: Ultrasonic scanning in post-cholecystectomy stones. Surgery *82*:420–424, 1977.
144. Scheible, W., Gosink, B. B., and Leopold, G. R.: Gray scale echographic patterns of hepatic metastatic disease. Am. J. Roentgenol. *129*:983–987, 1977.
145. Shawker, T. H.: B-mode ultrasonic evaluation of scrotal swellings. Radiology *8*:417–419, 1976.
146. Shkolnik, A.: B-mode ultrasonic and the nonvisualizing kidney in pediatrics. Am. J. Roentgenol. *128*:121–125, 1977.
147. Silver, T. M., Washburn, R. L., Stanley, J. C., et al.: Gray scale ultrasound evaluation of popliteal artery aneurysms. Am. J. Roentgenol. *129*:1003–1006, 1977.
147a. Skolnick, M. L., Rosenbaum, A. E., Matzuk, T., et al.: Detection of dilated cerebral ventricles in infants: a correlative study between ultrasound and computed tomography. Radiology *131*:447–451, 1979.
148. Smith, E. H., and Bartrum, R. J.: Ultrasonically guided percutaneous aspiration of abscesses. Am. J. Roentgenol. *122*:308–312, 1974.
149. Smith, E. H., Bartrum, R. J., Chang, Y. C., et al.: Percutaneous aspiration biopsy of the pancreas under ultrasound guidance. N. Engl. J. Med. *292*:825–828, 1975.
150. Smith, E. H., and Bennett, A. H.: The usefulness of ultrasound in the evaluation of renal masses in adults. J. Urol. *113*:525–529, 1975.
151. Stuber, J. L., Leonidas, M. C., and Holden, T. M.: Abdominal ultrasonography in pediatrics. Am. J. Dis. Child. *129*:1096–1101, 1975.
152. Sullivan, D. C., Taylor, K. J. W., and Gottschalk, A.: The use of ultrasound to enhance the diagnostic utility of the equivocal liver scintigraph. Radiology *128*:727–732, 1978.
153. Suruga, K., Hirai, Y., Nagashimi, K., et al.: Ultrasonic echo examination as an aid in diagnosis of congenital bile duct lesions. J. Pediatr. Surg. *4*:452–456, 1969.
154. Taylor, K. J. W.: Ultrasonic investigation of inferior vena cava obstruction. Br. J. Radiol. *48*:1024–1026, 1975.
155. Taylor, K. J. W., Carpenter, D. A., Hill, D. A., et al.: Gray scale ultrasound imaging: the anatomy and pathology of the liver. Radiology *119*:415–423, 1976.
156. Taylor, K. J. W., and Rosenfield, A. T.: Gray scale ultrasound in the differential diagnosis of jaundice. Arch. Surg. *112*:820–825, 1977.
157. Taylor, K. J. W., Sullivan, D., Rosenfield, A. T., et al.: Gray scale ultrasound and isotope scanning: complementary techniques for imaging the liver. Am. J. Roentgenol. *128*:277–281, 1977.

158. Teele, R. L., Rosenfield, A. T., and Freedman, G. S.: The anatomic splenic flexure: an ultrasonic renal impostor. Am J. Roentgenol. *125*:115–120, 1977.
159. Texidor, H. S., and Kazam, E.: Combined mammographic-sonographic evaluation of breast masses. Am. J. Roentgenol. *128*:409–417, 1977.
160. Thal, E. R., Weigelt, J., Landay, M., et al.: Evaluation of ultrasound in the diagnosis of acute and chronic biliary tract disease. Arch. Surg. *113*:500–503, 1978.
161. Uhrich, P. C., and Sanders, R. C.: Ultrasonic characteristics of pelvic inflammatory masses. J. Clin. Ultrasound *4*:199–204, 1976.
162. Vicary, F. R., Cusick, G., Shirley, I. M., et al.: Ultrasound and amoebic liver abscess. Br. J. Surg. *64*:113–114, 1977.
163. Walls, W. J., Gonzalez, G., Martin, N. L., et al.: B scan ultrasound evaluation of the pancreas. Radiology *114*:127–134, 1975.
164. Walls, W. J., and Lin, F.: Ultrasonic diagnosis of a seminal vesicle cyst. Radiology *114*:693–694, 1975.
165. Walls, W. J., Roberts, F. F., and Templeton, A. W.: B scan diagnostic ultrasound in the pediatric patient. Am. J. Roentgenol. *120*:431–437, 1974.
166. Watanabe, H., Igari, D., Tanahashi, Y., et al.: Transrectal ultrasonography of the prostate. J. Urol. *114*:734–739, 1975.
167. Weill, F., Eisenscher, A., and Zeltner, F.: Ultrasonic study of the normal and dilated biliary tree. Radiology *127*:221–224, 1978.
168. Weill, F., Schraub, A., Eisenscher, A., et al.: Ultrasonography of the normal pancreas. Radiology *123*:417–423, 1977.
169. Winsberg, F., Cole-Beuglet, C., and Mulder, D. S.: Continuous ultrasound "B" scanning of abdominal aortic aneurysms. Am. J. Roentgenol. *121*:626–633, 1974.
170. Winston, M., Pritchard, J., and Paulin, P.: Ultrasonography in the management of unexplained renal failure. J. Clin. Ultrasound *6*:23–27, 1978.
171. Winterberger, A. R., Palma, L. D., and Murphy, G. P.: Ultrasonic testing in human renal allografts. J.A.M.A. *219*:475–479, 1972.
172. Wolson, A. H.: Ultrasound diagnosis of pelvic and wound abscess after an appendectomy. Surg. Gynecol. Obstet. *144*:376–380, 1977.
173. Wolson, A. H., and Walls, W. J.: Ultrasonic characteristics of cystadenoma of the pancreas. Radiology *119*:203–205, 1976.
174. Yeh, H. C., Mitty, H. A., Rose, J., et al.: Ultrasonography of adrenal masses: unusual manifestations. Radiology *127*:475–483, 1978.
175. Yeh, H. C., Mitty, H. A., Rose, J., et al.: Ultrasonography of adrenal masses: usual features. Radiology *127*:467–474, 1978.
176. Yeh, H. C., and Wolf, B. S.: Ultrasonography in ascites. Radiology *124*:783–789, 1977.
177. Zeis, P. M., Spigos, D., Samyoa, C., et al.: Ultrasound localization for percutaneous renal biopsy in children. J. Pediatr. *89*:263–265, 1976.

4

COMPUTED TOMOGRAPHY IN THE DIAGNOSIS OF SURGICAL DISORDERS

ROBERT J. STANLEY, M.D.
STUART S. SAGEL, M.D.

GENERAL PRINCIPLES OF COMPUTED TOMOGRAPHY (CT)

Computed tomography, in existence since 1972, is a revolutionary imaging technique that involves (1) the acquisition of x-ray attenuation data, (2) the integration of this data in mathematical terms by the use of a computer, and (3) the conversion of this data into either a numeric print-out or a cross-sectional image of the parts studied.[25] The visual display is accomplished by the assignment of vaying shades of gray to the individual picture elements according to their relative attenuation values (black indicates low attenuation, white, high attenuation).

In step 1, an x-ray beam from a conventional x-ray tube, mounted opposite an array of crystal or ionization chamber detectors, undergoes attenuation as it passes through the body. The original EMI scanner employed a rotate-translate motion, a single x-ray beam, and a single detector system and required over four minutes for a complete scan. The subsequent use of a fan-shaped x-ray beam and multiple detectors reduced the scan time to less than 20 seconds, partially overcoming problems of body and organ motion.[35, 58] Recently, rotation-only scanners have made it possible to scan in two to five seconds.[82]

In step 2, the x-ray beam that has interacted with the detectors is measured and then transmitted in the form of electric signals. These data enter a computer and are mathematically manipulated. The matrix-solving calculations performed by the computer result in a discrete numeric attenuation value for each picture element within the mosaic of elements composing the total scan image.

In step 3, the mosaic can be represented as a print-out of the actual numeric attenuation values or as a picture on a cathode ray tube (television) screen. These pictures are viewed as if one were looking at the cross-sectional images from below. As in conventional radiographs, the patient's right side is displayed on the viewer's left. Because the scintillation detectors used in CT are far more sensitive to slight differences in beam attenuation than conventional radiographic film and screen systems, tissue densities are more accurately represented with CT. Tissue density differences of 1 per cent can be detected. Conventional screen-film combinations need differences of at least 5 per cent to be seen.

In conventional linear tomography, structures outside the plane of interest produce blurred shadows on the radiograph. In CT the x-ray beams traverse only the specific plane of interest. All the x-ray photons detected provide information concerning this plane, and scattered radiation is reduced to a minimum. Thus, subtle contrasts are preserved.

This discussion of general principles of CT is, of necessity, simplistic. Numerous articles relating to the physics, computer technology, and system specifications are available for the interested reader.[7, 25, 26, 82]

TECHNIQUE

Techniques for performing CT examinations of the chest and abdomen have evolved during the past few years owing to both increasing experience and technical improvements in instrumentation.[71] The principle of tailoring the examination to the specific clinical problem should underlie all scanning techniques. This requires clear communication with the radiologist regarding the reason for performing the examination. Supervision and monitoring during the examination results in the greatest service to the patient and the referring clinician.

Some form of preliminary scout film is used before initiating the CT scan, for localization purposes, the detection of potentially interfering high-density material (barium, metallic clips, electrodes), and correlation with the CT images. An overlying lead grid or spaced lead markers corresponding to easily identifiable topographic landmarks on the patient's chest or abdomen provide reasonably accurate reference points for starting the scan of a particular organ or area. Recently introduced scout-imaging techniques, employed while the patient is in the CT scanner and using the imaging system of the scanner, show promise of a more rapid and accurate localization approach to the initiation of the CT scan.

It is helpful to employ a dilute oral contrast agent for the visual identification of the lumen of the gastrointestinal tract in scans of the abdomen. A dilute solution (3 to 4 per cent) of an iodinated water-soluble contrast agent, such as Gastrografin, provides sufficient enhancement of the density of the luminal contents to allow distinction between loops of bowel and solid structures within the abdomen. The use of the oral contrast agent is particularly helpful in the evaluation of the pancreas and retroperitoneum. The more slender a patient is the greater is the need for an oral contrast agent, since there is less body fat to outline the organ. If CT units with scanning times of 18 seconds or longer are used, intravenous glucagon (0.5 to 1.0 mg) is generally recommended to diminish peristaltic activity and eliminate motion artifacts.[51] With more rapid scans performed within two to six seconds, glucagon may not be needed.

Intravenous iodinated renal contrast agents have proved useful in the evaluation of both the thorax and the abdomen. Scanning during the intravenous infusion of a contrast agent differentiates vascular from nonvascular structures and is especially valuable in mediastinal scanning. In any situation in which greater differentiation is needed between a structure that has a normal or increased blood supply and a structure that contains little or no flowing blood, the use of intravenous contrast agents is appropriate.[10, 19, 37, 74] Intravenous contrast agents have also proved useful for differential enhancement in the assessment of lesions of the liver, spleen, pancreas, kidneys, and great vessels of the abdomen. Whether a single bolus injection or a steady infusion should be employed depends upon the organ or organs under study and the specific nature of the clinical problem. In situations in which one desires enhancement of blood vessels, such as the splenic vein or vena cava, scanning during a rapid infusion has proved more useful than the single-bolus technique. In most examinations of the kidney in which the differential enhancement of benign cysts or solid tumor is sought, a bolus injection generally suffices.

The number, sequence, and degree of contiguity of the scans vary with the organ or the area studied. Careful evaluation of the pancreas, for example, may require contiguous or overlapping scans. Similarly, small lesions of the kidney may require overlapping scans to ensure complete coverage. A combination of evenly spaced survey scans and contiguous or overlapping scans in the region of interest frequently provides the best approach.

Whereas most patients are scanned in the supine position, the prone or decubitus position may be required for the evaluation of certain anatomic areas or for the placement of a percutaneous aspiration or biopsy needle.

NORMAL ANATOMY

Thorax

Cross-sectional CT scans provide a unique perspective of the mediastinum, and it is often possible to identify structures that cannot be separated out by conventional radiographic techniques.[24, 28] The aorta is usually easily seen, separated from other mediastinal structures by a thin band of fat. In the elderly, it is often outlined by a rim of calcium. If the identification of the aorta is in question, the intravenous injection of iodinated contrast will clearly opacify the vessel lumen. The other great vessels may be similarly profiled. The esophagus is difficult to evaluate, as it blends with the other mediastinal structures. A small amount of air may be seen within the lumen in approximately 50 per cent of normal patients. In the hilar areas the pulmonary artery, veins, and major airways are clearly depicted.

In order to see the lungs, a different window width and level are necessary on the viewing console. It is possible to demonstrate the intrapulmonary vessels, moderate-sized bronchi, and some of the pulmonary parenchyma. As on the standard erect chest radiograph, there is preferential pulmonary blood flow to the dependent portion of the lung. On the CT scan performed with the patient in the usual supine position, one can see that the dorsal portion of the lung receives the most blood.

At the present time, little clinical information can be obtained about intracardiac anatomy owing to the motion of the heart during the scanning cycle. Certain innovations in CT equipment (limited angle reconstruction, gating, and so forth) may allow more precise demonstration of the cardiac structures and the study of dynamic physiologic changes.[61]

Abdomen

The upper abdominal organs that may be well studied with CT include the liver, spleen, pancreas, kidneys, and adrenal glands.[36, 54] Although the stomach, duodenum, proximal small bowel, transverse colon, and colic flexures are included in these levels, intrinsic abnormalities of these structures are better sought with conventional barium studies than with CT. Of course, the recognition of normal bowel structures is important in the correct interpretation of the upper abdominal scans.

The normal liver occupies nearly all of the space within the right upper quadrant of the abdomen (Fig. 4–1). A concavity on the posterior surface of the right lobe accommodates the right kidney and its surrounding cone of fat. The inferior vena cava is immediately contiguous to the posteromedial surface of the liver and runs vertically in a groove or sulcus on the posterior surface of the caudate lobe. As the inferior vena cava moves anteriorly in its course to the right atrium, it can become almost entirely surrounded by hepatic parenchyma and may be difficult to discern, unless there is an appreciable difference in the attenuation value of the flowing blood and the surrounding hepatic tissue. The aorta does not come into direct contact with the liver. At the level of the aortic hiatus, it is separated from the posterior surface of the liver only by the thickness of the right crus of the diaphragm.[72, 75]

The anterior wall of the stomach is contiguous to the posterior surface of the left lobe of the liver. The low-density fluid and gas contents of the stomach or the use of oral contrast media generally distinguish it from the adjacent hepatic parenchyma. The normal liver and spleen usually do not have a common interface, but exceptions can

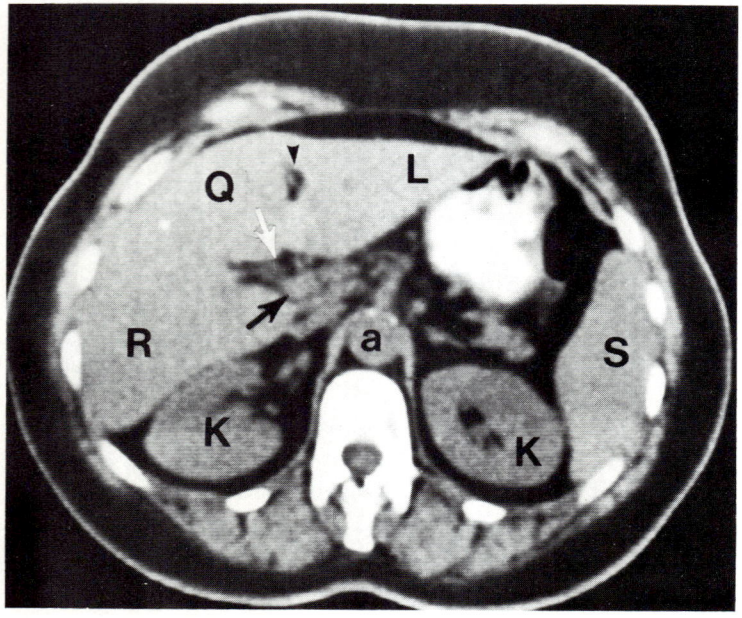

Figure 4–1. Normal anatomy of the liver at the level of the porta hepatis. a = aorta; L = lateral segment of left lobe; Q = quadrate lobe (medial segment of left lobe); R = right lobe; K = kidney; S = spleen; common hepatic duct (white arrow); portal vein (black arrow); ligamentum teres within fat-containing cleft (black arrowhead). An incidental calcified granuloma is noted in the anterolateral aspect of the right hepatic lobe.

occur, especially in patients with a horizontally oriented spleen positioned high beneath the left hemidiaphragm.

Two fat-containing clefts are visible on the surface of the liver extending toward the hilus. The vertically oriented cleft is the falciform ligament, which contains the ligamentum teres (obliterated umbilical vein) in its free border. The horizontally oriented cleft enters from the medial surface, just anterior to the aorta. This is the porta hepatis through which pass the main portal vein, the proper hepatic artery, and the common hepatic duct. If there is sufficient fat within the porta hepatis, these individual structures can be identified.

If the lobar anatomy of the liver is based on the main divisions of the hepatic artery, the portal vein, and the biliary tree, the right and left lobes of the liver are roughly equal in size and weight. A vertical plane passing through the fossa of the gallbladder and the sulcus for the inferior vena cava divides the liver approximately into the anatomic right and left lobes. The cleft formed by the falciform ligament subdivides the left lobe into the medial and lateral segments. The medial segment lies between the fossa of the gallbladder and the falciform ligament and is also known as the quadrate lobe. The lateral segment of the left lobe lies to the left of the falciform ligament. The caudate lobe, which lies posterior to the porta hepatis and anterior to the inferior vena cava, is anatomically part of the medial segment of the left lobe.

The hepatic parenchyma has a uniform density that is usually slightly higher than that of the other intra-abdominal organs.[46] The uniform density of the liver substance is broken up by linear and circular areas of slightly lower density produced by the portal and hepatic veins. The portal venous structures are best seen at the level of the bifurcation of the main portal vein into its left and right branches. At this level these vascular structures are at their greatest diameter. The more cephalad the scans, the more the tributaries of the hepatic veins increase in diameter. The hepatic veins are at their greatest diameter before their entry into the inferior vena cava just beneath the diaphragmatic hiatus.

The normal peripheral intrahepatic biliary tree is of insufficient caliber to be visualized by current CT scanners. Even when enhanced with iodinated contrast agents, only the larger, more central portions of the biliary tree can be clearly identified. When sufficient fat is present within the hilus of the liver, the unenhanced common hepatic duct can be identified as a discrete, rounded, water-density structure with a diameter of approximately 5 to 6 mm. It usually lies anterolateral to the adjacent portal vein. As the bile duct is followed inferiorly, it diverges slightly from the course of the portal vein and enters the head of the pancreas, where it terminates in the ampulla, at the interface of the lateral border of the pancreatic head and the medial border of the second portion of the duodenum (Fig. 4–2).

The gallbladder lies on the inferior surface of the liver. Its fossa demarcates the junction of the right and left lobes. It appears as a round or oval structure containing water-density bile. The long axis of the gallbladder extends anterolaterally toward the right. When the gallbladder extends beyond the inferior margin of the liver, it may appear as an isolated water-density structure surrounded by perivisceral fat and lying adjacent to the right hepatic flexure or second portion of the duodenum. When the normal gallbladder is profiled with a free margin, its wall thickness is virtually imperceptible.[23]

The spleen occupies a posterolateral position in the left upper quadrant. The tail of the pancreas and splenic arteries and veins extend into the hilus. The interface of the spleen with the kidney is usually sharply defined. The stomach is the other structure in apposition to the spleen over a large area. The contours of both the liver and the spleen are usually well defined, regardless of the amount of perivisceral fat. The density of the spleen is generally equal to or slightly less than that of the liver. The

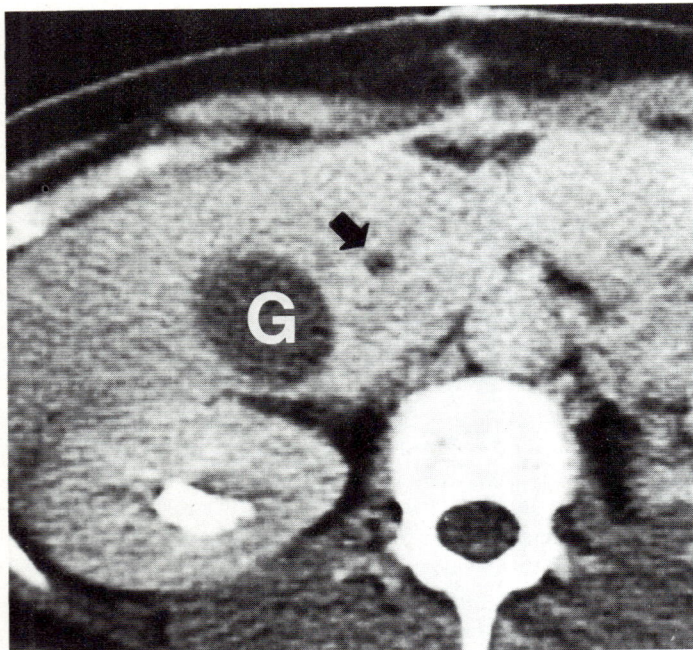

Figure 4–2. A normal-caliber common bile duct (arrow) is seen end-on. The larger, water-density gallbladder (G) lies more laterally. The visibility of the 5-mm duct is improved by the enhancement of surrounding liver and pancreatic parenchyma with an intravenous renal contrast agent. (From Margulis A. R. et al.: Alimentary Tract Radiology. Vol 3. St. Louis, The C. V. Mosby Company, 1979, p. 166. Reproduced by permission.)

range of variation in the size of the normal spleen is wide, and absolute figures for the determination of normality on a CT scan are not yet established.

The nomal pancreas is identified as a structure of relatively uniform density in the upper midabdomen (Fig. 4–3). Its head lies anterior to the inferior vena cava, its body lies anterior to the aorta and the superior mesenteric vessels, and its tail lies anterior to the left adrenal gland and the upper pole of the left kidney on its course to the hilus of the spleen. The splenic vein can commonly be seen posterior and parallel to the body and tail of the pancreas. A fat plane separates the normal pancreas from the posteriorly located vascular structures in all but the leanest patients. In addition to the plane of fat that separates the pancreas from the superior mesenteric artery and inferior vena cava, a thin plane of fat may also be seen separating the pancreas and the splenic vein. This thin linear area of diminished attenuation should not be confused with the main pancreatic duct, which lies more anterior within the substance of the gland. At the level of the uncinate process of the pancreas the superior mesenteric artery and vein are seen on end, medial and slightly anterior to this extension of the head of the pancreas, which occasionally extends in a hooklike fashion posterior to these vessels.

A gradual decrease in the anteroposterior diameter of the gland is usually seen without abrupt alterations in site or contour from the head to the tail. Infrequently, the tail of the normal pancreas may be thicker than the body. The diameter of the pancreatic head is measured perpendicular to the long axis of the gland. The ratio of this diameter to the transverse diameter of the adjacent lumbar vertebral body varies from 0.5 to 1.0, with that of the majority of normal patients being close to 0.7. When the ratio is 1.0, one must carefully assess other factors before excluding the possibility of tumor, since at this ratio the normal overlaps the abnormal. In cases in which a tumor is present in the head of a pancreas in patients with a pancreatic vertebral ratio of 1.0, an abrupt alteration in the contour of the gland is generally present and the head appears disproportionately large when compared with the body and the tail. The surface contour of the normal pancreas occasionally appears lobulated rather than smooth.

The third and fourth portions of the duodenum also run transversely across the midline in a fashion similar to that of the pancreas. In distinction to the pancreas, however, the third and fourth portions of the duodenum pass between the aorta and the superior mesenteric vessels. The use of an oral contrast agent clarifies the relationship of the duodenum and the proximal small bowel to the pancreas.

Normal kidneys are easily recognizable. All but the leanest patients have sufficient perinephric fat to provide sharp definition of the renal contours. The hilus of the kidney faces anteromedially, and the renal arteries and veins can usually be distinguished. The veins lie anterior to the arteries. The left renal vein is significantly longer in its course, passing anterior to the aorta before entering the inferior vena cava. The right renal vein is short and more direct in its entry into the inferior vena cava. At this level the inferior vena cava is often elliptic in contour, being narrowest in its anteroposterior diameter. The renal arteries can sometimes be traced to their origin in the aorta.

Renal sinus fat is occasionally abundant enough to define portions of the renal pelvis and calyces without the aid of intravenous contrast agents. Scans obtained after the administration of intravenous urographic contrast media usually show discrete calyceal and infundibular structures.

The shape of the renal pelvis in cross section is similar to its frontal appearance on excretory urograms. Normal variations in the collecting systems and the position of the kidneys are as commonly appreciated in CT as in conventional urography.

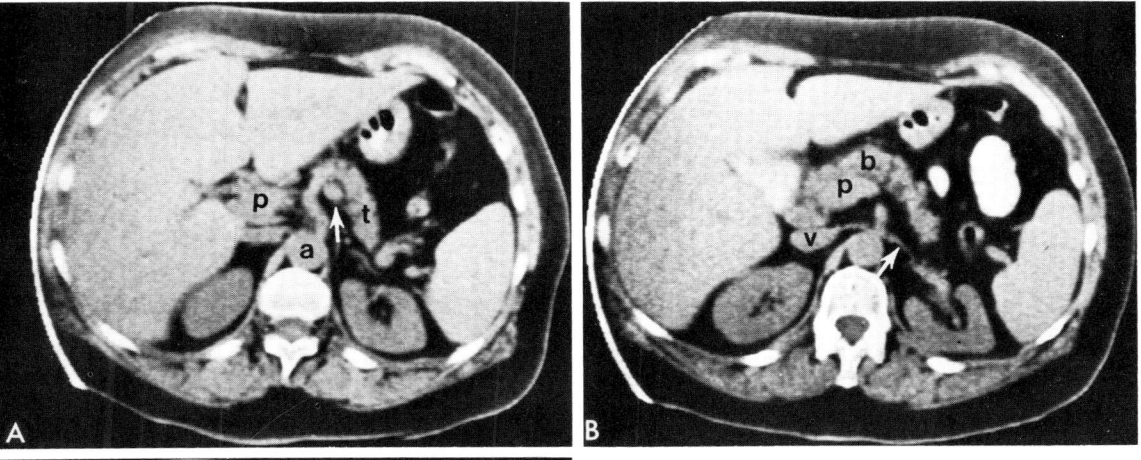
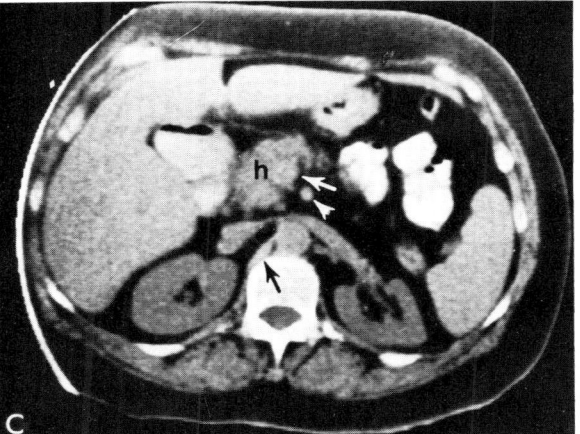

Figure 4–3. Normal anatomy of the pancreas. Note that several levels must be scanned in order to study all portions of the pancreas in their entirety. A, t = tail of the pancreas; p = portal vein; a = aorta. A portion of the splenic vein is seen end-on (white arrow). The S-shaped structure arising from the anterior surface of the aorta is the celiac axis. B, Level of the pancreatic body and tail. b = body of pancreas; p = portal vein at confluence of splenic vein; v = inferior vena cava. The superior edge of the left renal vein (white arrow) is seen crossing the aorta and entering the vena cava. Note that the neck of the pancreas, just anterior to the portal vein, is thinner in its anteroposterior dimension than the body or head (C) of the pancreas. If the portal vein is not clearly identified, it can be mistaken for part of the pancreas, making the neck region appear abnormally thick. C, Level of the pancreatic head. h = head of pancreas. The superior mesenteric artery is seen end-on (white arrowhead) anterior to the aorta and the prominent left renal vein. Superior mesenteric vein (white arrow) is partly obscured by the contiguous pancreatic parenchyma. The continuation of the crus of the right hemidiaphragm along the anterior surface of the lumbar vertebrae (black arrow) should not be confused with an enlarged lymph node.

Abundant perinephric fat has been found by CT to account for unusually lateral positions of one or both kidneys or for prominently bowed ureters; this obviates the need to use more invasive studies to exclude the possibility of the presence of a mass. The contrast-enhanced ureter usually can be traced to its junction with the bladder.

Normal adrenal glands can almost always be demonstrated.[8, 30, 50] The right adrenal gland lies directly posterior to the inferior vena cava and usually anterior, medial, and superior to the upper pole of the right kidney. A normal amount of perivisceral fat allows sharp definition of the caret-shaped (inverted V-shaped) adrenal gland, the vertex of which is directed anteromedially. Occasionally, at a higher level the adrenal appears linear or slightly S-shaped.

The left adrenal gland is at a comparable level behind the splenic vein and the pancreas, at approximately the junction of the body and the tail, just lateral to the aorta. It too is caret-shaped and oriented in the same anteromedial direction.

Below the level of the kidneys the aorta and the vena cava are the most prominent retroperitoneal structures seen. Normal retroperitoneal lymph nodes, less than 10 mm in diameter, are commonly seen surrounding these vascular structures. Portions of the colon are commonly encountered, the ascending and descending sections being the most consistent in their locations. A definite haustral pattern may be seen in the horizontal portions of the transverse colon. Random loops of collapsed or fluid-filled small bowel complete the high density structures usually encountered at these levels. The paired psoas muscles become larger in diameter as more caudal scans are obtained. Smaller vascular structures are occasionally seen coursing through the mesenteric fat.

In contrast to those of the upper abdomen, many of the important pelvic structures are paired and the symmetry can be evaluated (Fig. 4–4). The internal and external iliac vessels and accompanying lymph nodes can be assessed in most patients. Alterations in the symmetry of the pelvic musculature frequently indicates the lateral extension of a pelvic tumor or the presence of an intrinsic lesion, such as a soft tissue neoplasm or an inflammatory process.

In the male, the prostate gland, the seminal vesicles, and the urinary bladder can be identified, especially if the urinary bladder is filled with urine or with a contrast medium. The normal prostate is round and midline in location. It usually has a slightly higher density than muscle. The seminal vesicles are paired and extend from the pos-

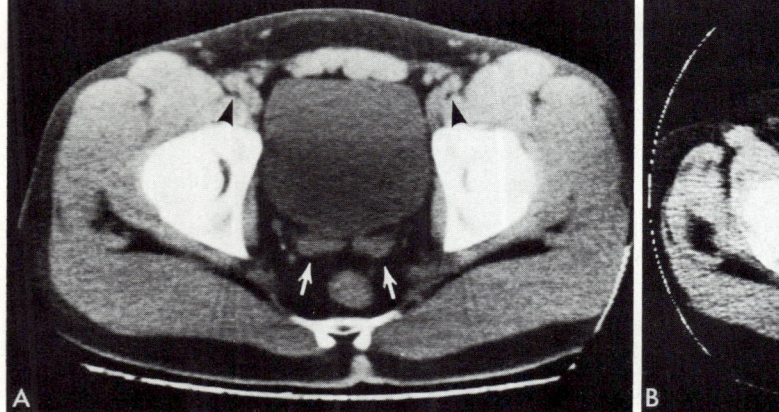
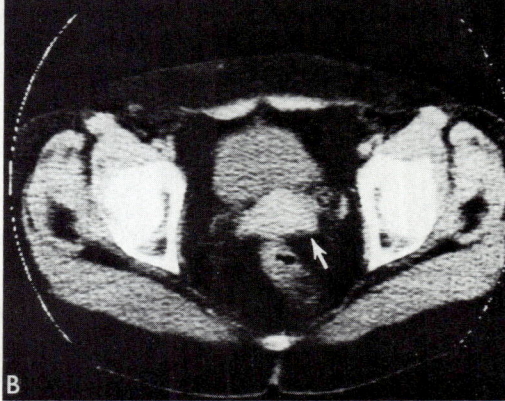

Figure 4–4. *A*, Normal male pelvis. Paired seminal vesicles (arrows) lie posterior to the urine-filled bladder. Femoral vascular structures (arrowheads) lie anteromedial to the thigh muscles. *B*, Normal female pelvis. The muscle-density uterus (arrow) lies between the bladder (anteriorly) and the gas-containing rectum. Parts of adnexal structures are suggested on either side of the uterus.

terior aspect of the prostate in a posterolateral direction to the left and right. Although the prostate lies at the base of the bladder, the anterior portion of the urinary bladder may lie on the same level as the prostate when the patient is scanned in the supine position.

Abundant pelvic fat generally allows clear visualization of the rectum and portions of the sigmoid colon as it rises out of the pelvis. Finer structures, such as the spermatic cord, may also be identified at lower levels through the inguinal region. The presacral space and the ischiorectal fossa can also be easily studied with CT.

In the female, the uterus is usually evident between the urinary bladder and the colon (Fig. 4–4). Portions of the broad ligaments can also be seen frequently but the normal ovaries, which lie close to the uterus, are rarely identifiable with any degree of confidence.

PATHOLOGY

Thorax

The relatively inexpensive and universally available standard chest roentgenogram continues to serve well as the initial radiologic evaluator of patients with suspected chest disease. Thoracic CT is used most often as a supplementary technique when the nature of an abnormality demonstrated on or suggested by the plain chest radiograph cannot be determined by conventional noninvasive radiologic methods (for example, fluoroscopy, decubitus views, or laminography). The superior ability of CT scanning to distinguish specific tissue densities and to display the mediastinum and lungs in the transverse plane makes it a unique and useful diagnostic tool.[11, 13, 24, 28, 32, 49, 56]

MEDIASTINUM. The recognition of the precise attenuation value of a mediastinal mass using CT may permit a definitive noninvasive diagnosis. Lesions that present with attenuation values characteristic of benign fatty tissue (–80 to –90 Hounsfield units) include a pericardial fat pad and lipomatous herniations through the foramen of Morgagni or Bochdalek. In such cases, the CT diagnosis is usually conclusive, and no further diagnostic work-up is indicated. Most benign cysts (for example, pericardial or bronchogenic) have a water-equivalent density (Fig. 4–5), but sometimes these cystic lesions are filled with thick, viscid secretions and the attenuation value is higher. In the case of an attenuation density of more than 20 Hounsfield units, the diagnosis of neoplasm cannot be excluded, and further evaluation is indicated (Fig. 4–6). Although CT may be valuable in determining the extent or the origin of a soft tissue mass and its relationship to other mediastinal structures, histologic diagnosis is not possible.

When mediastinal widening is detected on the plain chest radiograph, the cause may be a normal variant (such as abundant fat deposition), vascular ectasia, aneurysm (Fig. 4–7), or solid neoplasm. In problem cases, CT often can define the precise cause, obviating the need for such invasive procedures as mediastinoscopy or aortography. Also, when the cause of paraspinal line widening seen on a plain chest radiograph cannot be determined by conventional radiologic techniques (for example, a barium esophagogram or detailed spine views), CT may be used with excellent results. Enlarged lymph nodes, abnormal vessels, and omental fat herniation through the esophageal hiatus can be readily differentiated (Fig. 4–8).

Generally, conventional laminography (often in the 55 degree posterior oblique projection) can adequately differentiate a hilar mass (enlarged lymph nodes or a neoplasm) from an enlarged pulmonary artery. When such techniques fail, however, CT is usually helpful in this determination. Furthermore, in patients with myasthenia

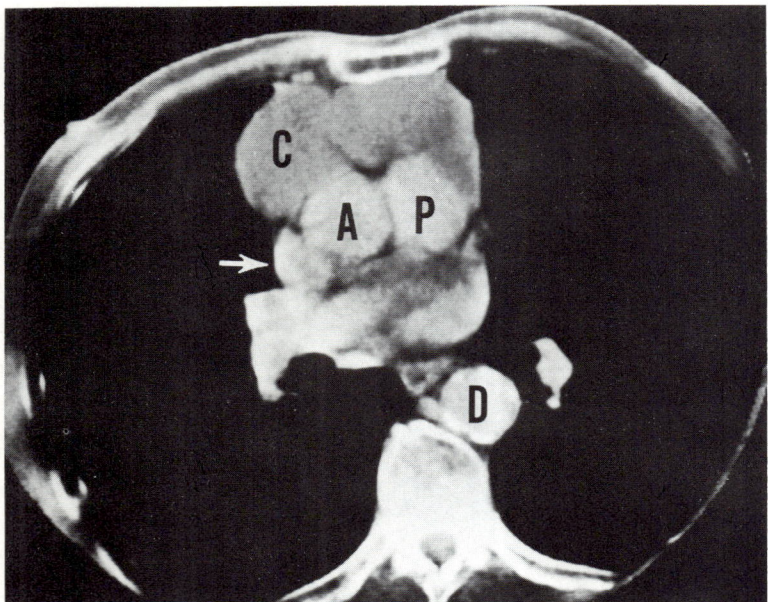

Figure 4–5. A near water-density noncontrast enhancing mass (C) is shown anterior to the ascending aorta (A) and the main pulmonary artery (P), findings consistent with a duplication cyst. D = descending aorta. The superior vena cava (white arrow) lies just lateral to the ascending aorta.

gravis and a normal or suspicious plain chest roentgenogram, the detection of a thymoma may be possible with CT.[49]

LUNG. CT may provide a more sensitive method for evaluating lung lesions (such as small pulmonary nodules) that are undetectable or poorly demonstrated by standard chest radiography and tomography. A major limitation, however, is that CT usually cannot adequately differentiate small metastatic nodules from benign healed granu-

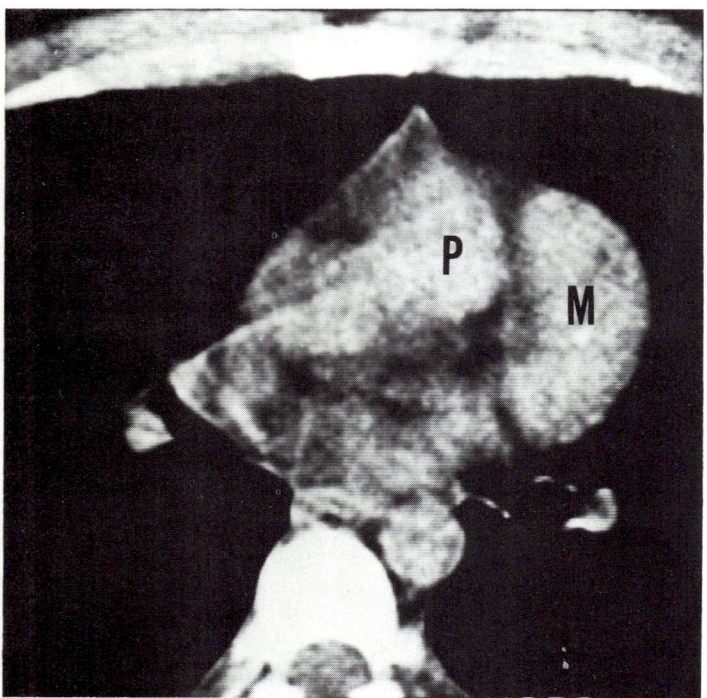

Figure 4–6. Thymoma. CT scan performed at the level of the pulmonary outflow tract to determine the nature of a mass inseparable from the pulmonary outflow tract on conventional roentgenography. A soft tissue (muscle)–density mediastinal mass (M) is shown to be separate from the pulmonary outflow tract (P).

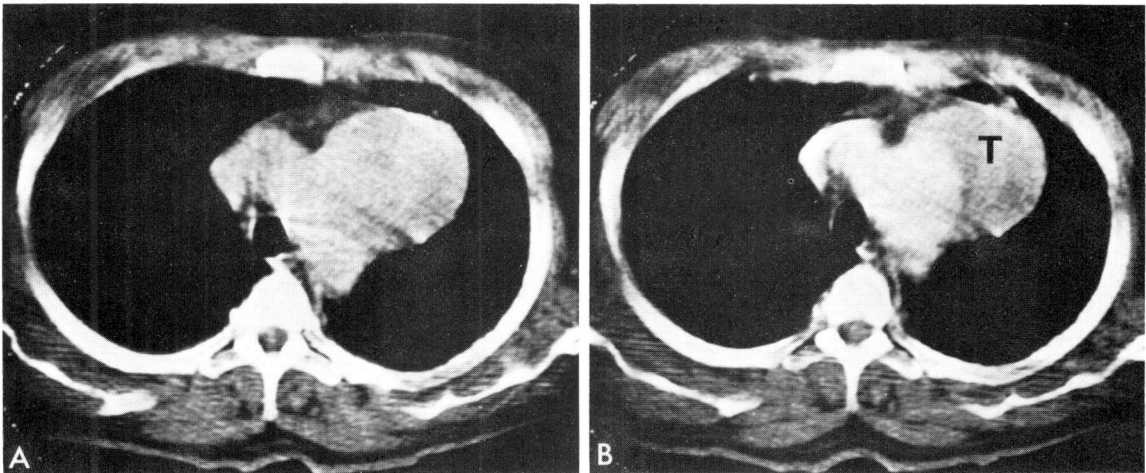

Figure 4–7. Aortic aneurysm. *A,* The preinfusion scan shows a large left anterior mediastinal mass continuous with the aortic arch. *B,* Intravenous contrast media enhances the lumen of the aortic aneurysm; the remainder of the mass consists of nonenhancing thrombus (T). The appearance is characteristic of an aneurysm of the aortic arch.

lomas. Although the precise role of CT in screening for occult lung metastases requires further investigation, CT can be valuable in the case of patients in whom extensive surgery is planned for a known primary neoplasm with a high propensity for lung metastases (for example, osteosarcoma or testicular neoplasm) or those with an apparent solitary lung metastasis in whom resection is planned. In such cases, the recognition through CT of otherwise occult pulmonary metastases may alter the planned surgical management. Also, in the patient with a positive sputum cytologic test and with no lesions demonstrable by chest radiography or fiberoptic bronchoscopy, CT may be able to detect a primary lung tumor.[28, 52, 65]

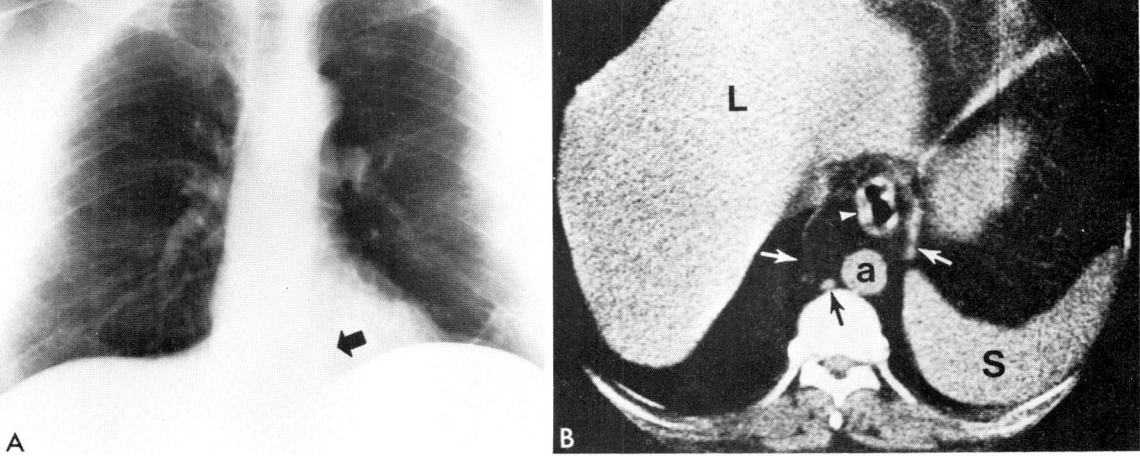

Figure 4–8. Omental fat herniation. *A,* A mass (arrow) projects to the left behind the heart at the level of the esophageal hiatus. A barium swallow showed a small hiatus hernia but did not account for the entire soft tissue mass. *B,* The CT scan shows, in addition to the small esophageal hiatus hernia (arrowhead), a large amount of herniated omental fat bulging through the esophageal hiatus (white arrows). S = spleen, L = liver. A normal-sized azygous vein (black arrow) lies to the right of the aorta (a).

The definitive evaluation of a solitary pulmonary nodule demonstrated on a plain chest radiograph is a common clinical problem. Low-kilovoltage spot films or conventional tomograms or both are first employed to discover calcification and determine its pattern within the nodule. When such studies are indeterminate (for example, in the case of a well-circumscribed nodular density without definite calcification) CT may provide conclusive evidence of diffuse calcification within the nodule and thus permit conservative clinical management (Fig. 4–9). Because of current technical problems with partial volume averaging, however, precise calculation for the presence of calcification usually requires the nodule to be at least 1.5 cm in diameter. In the near future, CT sections obtained rapidly with thin collimation may afford more precise data about smaller lesions.

CT may provide new information about the extent of intrathoracic spread of bronchogenic carcinoma. Enlarged lymph nodes in the mediastinum (especially in the azygoesophageal recess and the internal mammary chain) may be more easily demonstrated by CT than by standard radiography. With CT it may be possible to differentiate neoplastic disease that invades a structure from disease that is merely contiguous. The demonstration of direct mediastinal or pleural invasion may influence the decision against thoracotomy.[11, 13, 28]

PLEURA AND CHEST WALL. The extent of a disease process, especially neoplasm, involving the extrapulmonary space generally can be well defined by CT. Bony, muscular, and subcutaneous tissue invasion can be detected as well as intrusion of a mass into the thoracic cavity or spinal canal.[32] The clinical detection of such soft tissue extension is usually not possible unless the disease extends outward from the chest wall.

The presence, localization, and extent of any parenchymal lung abnormality underlying obscuring pleural disease (effusion or thickening) may be assessed. Addi-

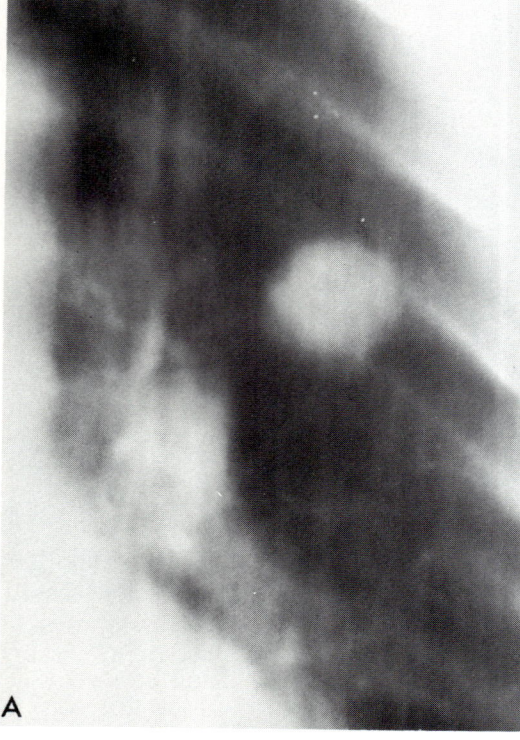

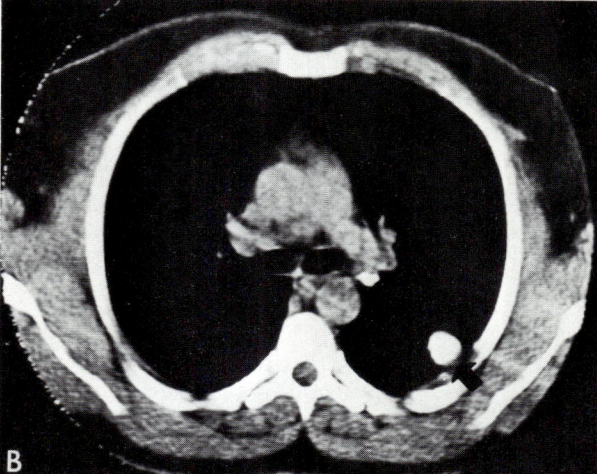

Figure 4–9. Calcified pulmonary nodule. *A,* Plain film tomogram of a left midlung field nodule. Calcification cannot be identified with confidence. Hilar calcification is present. *B,* Diffuse calcification is present throughout the nodule (arrow) on the CT scan.

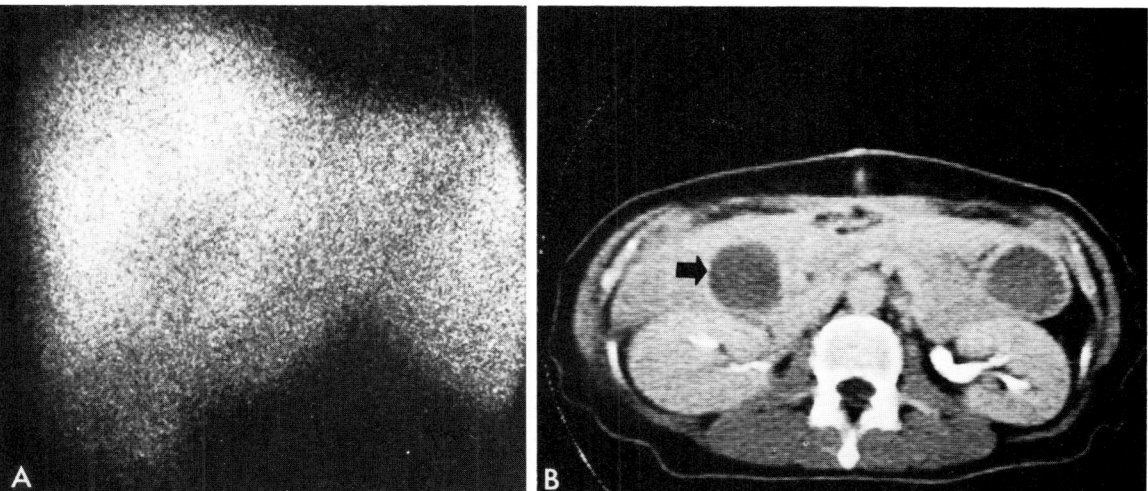

Figure 4–10. *A,* A central focal defect on the radionuclide liver scan in a patient with weight loss and night sweats. *B,* The central defect is shown to be a prominent gallbladder fossa (arrow).

tionally, the use of CT may be valuable in the distinction of a peripheral pulmonary nodule from localized pleural thickening (plaque). This may be especially important in patients with asbestos exposure.[35]

PERCUTANEOUS NEEDLE BIOPSY. When fluoroscopic direction is inadequate (for example, in the case of certain mediastinal masses or a pulmonary lesion low in the costovertebral angle or beneath the scapula) CT may permit guidance of the needle tip into the mass for tissue sampling.

Liver and Biliary Tree

Radionuclide imaging is currently the first choice for screening patients suspected of having focal liver lesions.[5] CT is used to clarify the nature of focal defects detected with a radionuclide study.[67, 72, 75] At present these two imaging methods display similar sensitivity in the detection of lesions. CT has the added capability of clarifying the nature of the defect, however, and with CT one can distinguish a benign cyst, an abscess, a solid tumor, a variant of normal anatomy simulating replaced parenchyma (for example, a thin left lobe or an intrahepatic gallbladder) (Fig. 4–10), and an extrinsic mass compressing hepatic parenchyma. In addition, subcapsular and intrahepatic hematomas can be clearly demonstrated. The distinction between these focal lesions is based primarily on the measured attenuation value. Benign cysts have a density close to that of water. The density of tumors is variable, that of most lesions being slightly less than the density of normal parenchyma (Fig. 4–11). When necrosis or cystic change occurs in a neoplastic mass, the lesion has an attenuation value midway between water density and the density of normal hepatic parenchyma. Some tumors, including hepatomas and adenomas are isodense, but postcontrast scans frequently reveal their presence. At other times, an alteration in the surface contour of the liver is the only clue to the presence of an isodense tumor. When a primary tumor is identified on CT in another upper abdominal organ (for example, the pancreas), close scrutiny of the liver for metastases should be performed.

Hepatic abscesses have an attenuation value intermediate between those of cyst and tumor and can usually be differentiated from tumor. In the spectrum of densities

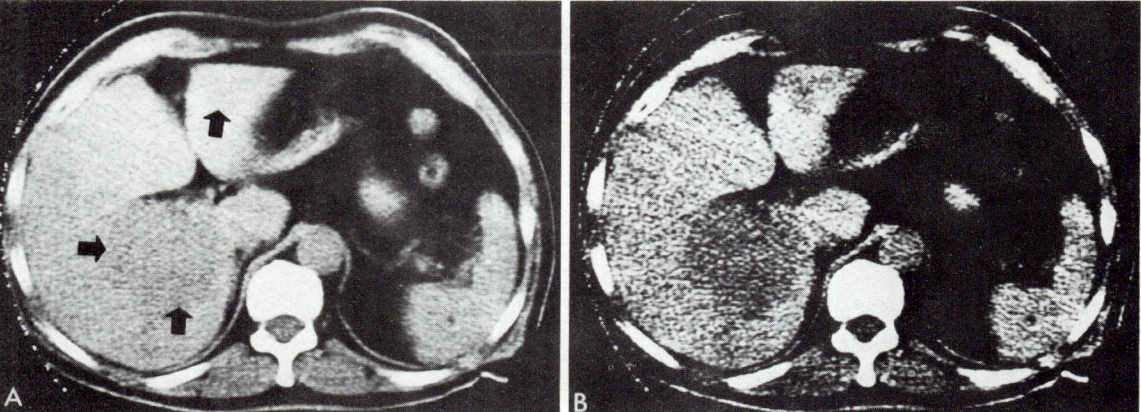

Figure 4–11. Liver metastases. *A,* A large metastasis is present in the right lobe, and a smaller one is visible in the lateral segment of the left lobe (arrows). The density of the tumor is only slightly less than that of the normal parenchyma. *B,* A narrow window-width view of the same scan accentuates the small difference in densities and causes the tumors to be more visible.

of lesions within the liver, however, a definite overlap exists between the densities of abscesses and low-density necrotic tumors. CT-guided aspiration biopsy of these indeterminate lesions can accurately differentiate them, if the clinical distinction is not obvious.[15, 18]

Errors in interpretation of focal liver lesions can arise from confusing portal or hepatic veins on end with metastases. Scanning during an infusion of iodinated contrast medium identifies the enhanced vascular structures. Small metastases (1 cm or smaller) especially those with a true attenuation value of only 6 to 12 Hounsfield units less than that of the normal hepatic parenchyma may be undetectable owing to the partial volume effect. In this situation, the Z-axis of the picture elements in the area of the small tumor includes both normal parenchyma and tumor tissue. The resultant attenuation value is an average of the values of both tissues and is very close to the attenuation value of the normal parenchyma.[75] A similar loss of information occurs when respiratory motion causes the lesion in question to move in and out of the cross-sectional region being scanned.[2] Narrower collimation, resulting in slice thicknesses of 2 to 6 mm and rapid scanning times (two to five seconds), tends to diminish the problems presented by small spheric lesions and by motion. Recent examinations with the most advanced CT instrumentation, incorporating the aforementioned features, support this concept.

The problems related to the imaging of small or moving lesions in the liver occur also in the evaluation of the pancreas, adrenal glands, and kidneys. Since these organs are smaller in relation to the lesions they contain, however, and since all are usually surrounded by fat, interpretive difficulties arise less frequently.

The early differentiation of medical from surgical forms of jaundice can be made with CT.[22, 41, 72] Moderately dilated intrahepatic portions of the biliary tree produce linear, branching, or end-on water density structures that increase in diameter as the main central ducts are approached (Fig. 4–12). When the intrahepatic bile ducts are only minimally dilated, it may be necessary to use an intravenous iodinated renal contrast agent to improve their visibility. The attenuation value of the surrounding contrast-enhanced hepatic parenchyma increases significantly; the value of the bile within the slightly dilated ducts remains unchanged. By increasing the difference between the attenuation values of the hepatic parenchyma and the bile, the detectability of the low-density ducts is improved.

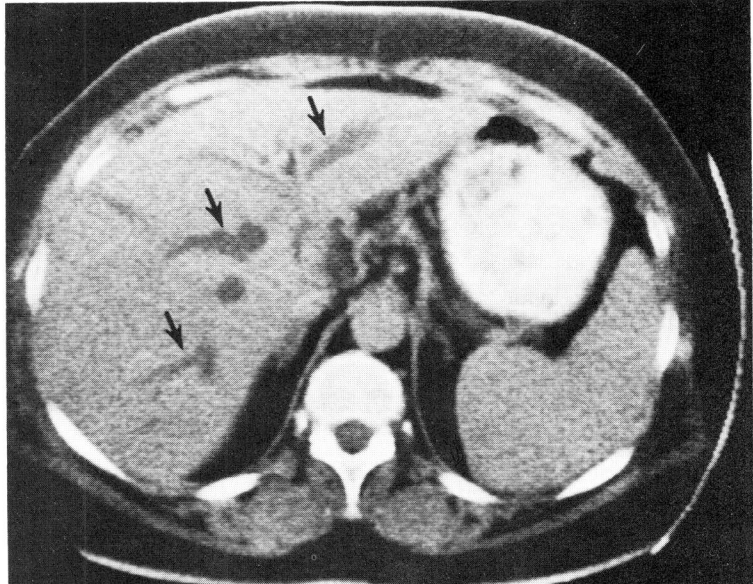

Figure 4–12. Branching water-density structures (arrows) within the liver represent dilated bile ducts in a patient with an obstructing tumor of the pancreatic head. Compare the density of the bile ducts with the blood in the aorta.

In mildly jaundiced patients with partial distal common bile duct obstruction by stone, inflammation, or tumor, the intrahepatic bile ducts may remain normal in caliber. Only the common bile duct itself may become dilated. Thus, careful attention must be directed to the extrahepatic course of the common duct. It can be defined in its intrapancreatic portion as a water-density cylinder, seen on end, with a diameter not exceeding 6 to 7 mm in the normal state. Contrast enhancement of the surrounding pancreatic parenchyma aids in its visualization. A duct that measures 8 to 10 mm in diameter should be regarded with suspicion. If the diameter of the common duct exceeds 10 mm in a patient whose gallbladder is present, it is considered abnormally dilated and the presumption of obstruction is made (Fig. 4–13).

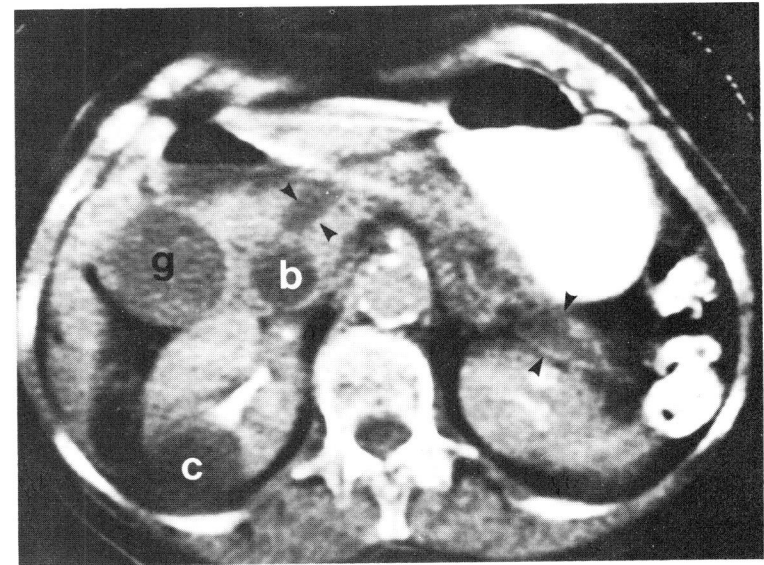

Figure 4–13. Ampullary tumor. A scan at the level of the head of the pancreas shows dilatation of the common bile duct (b) and main pancreatic duct (arrowheads) extending into the tail of the pancreas. Note the distended gallbladder (g) laterally. An incidental right renal cyst (c) is also present. A small tumor of the ampulla was found at operation.

In most instances, the level and the cause of obstruction (for example, calculus in the distal common bile duct or tumor in the head of the pancreas) can be determined by CT. The capability of CT to provide critical preoperative information has obviated to a large extent the use of endoscopic retrograde pancreaticocholangiography (ERPC) and percutaneous transhepatic cholangiography (PTC). In some cases, however, PTC and ERPC may still be necessary to provide detailed anatomic information when the nature or the level of obstruction remains unclear.

Pancreas

CARCINOMA. The radiologic diagnosis of carcinoma of the pancreas, once considered to be almost exclusively the province of the angiographer, is now accurately achieved with two noninvasive methods—CT and ultrasound. The role of ultrasound in the evaluation of the pancreas is briefly discussed in another section (Chapter 17, Part I). In this section, the CT findings in cases of pancreatic neoplasm are described and illustrated.

With CT one is able to image the entire gland with a clarity unmatched by any other radiologic technique. The absence of perivisceral fat and the inability to restrain motion are the two factors that may limit the quality of the study. The framing of the margins of the lean patient's pancreas by opacifying the lumen of the contiguous stomach, duodenum, and proximal jejunum with a dilute oral contrast agent largely alleviates the first problem. The administration of intravenous glucagon to inhibit peristaltic activity and its attendant artifacts and more rapid scanning times minimize the image-degrading effect of biologic motion.

Two thirds of cases of carcinoma occur in the head of the pancreas. An abrupt alteration in the surface contour of the gland due to focal enlargement of the head disproportionate to the thickness of the body and tail is the most common CT finding (Fig. 4–14).[16, 70, 73] Careful attention must be directed to the uncinate process, the small hooklike extension of the head that passes lateral and posterior to the superior mes-

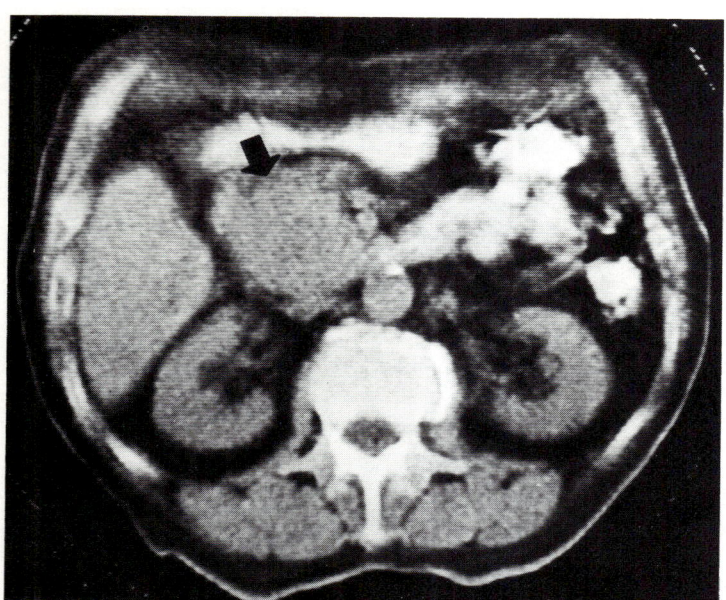

Figure 4–14. Carcinoma of the head of the pancreas. A large mass is present in the head of the pancreas (arrow), displacing contiguous vascular structures. Most pancreatic head carcinomas present in this fashion on a CT scan.

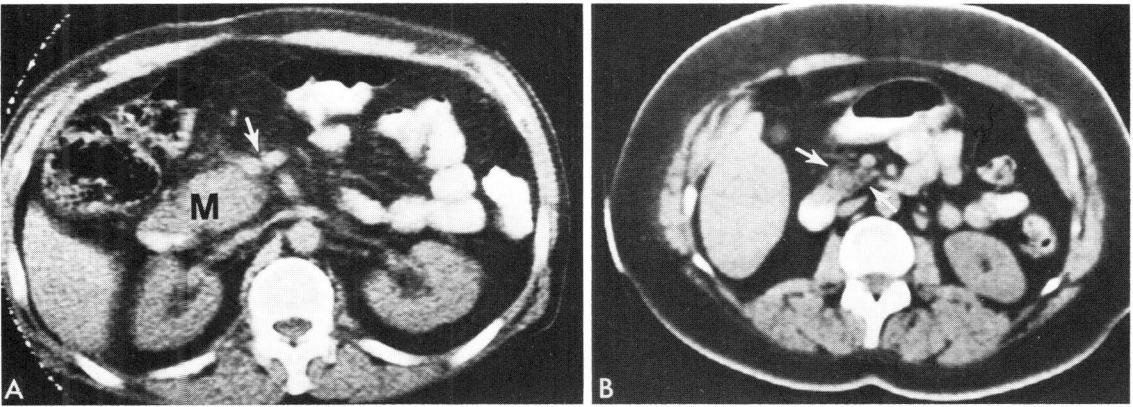

Figure 4–15. Carcinoma in the uncinate process of the pancreas. *A,* This patient with a 10-day history of epigastric pain, normal serum bilirubin and alkaline phosphatase, and a slightly elevated serum amylase is shown by CT to have a mass arising in the uncinate process of the pancreas (M). Note the anterior position of the superior mesenteric vein and artery (arrow). *B,* For comparison, note the size and shape of this normal uncinate process (arrows) and its relationship to the superior mesenteric vessels, which lie anterior and medial to it.

enteric vein and artery. A round or oval shape to this normally slender portion of the pancreas should be viewed with suspicion (Fig. 4–15). Some of the smallest detectable tumors within the head of the pancreas have been diagnosed because of this change in shape.

Frequently associated with a mass in the head is dilatation of the biliary tree and, unfortunately, even at the time of initial evaluation, metastases within the liver. The main pancreatic duct is also capable of measurable dilatation and occasionally presents, much like the dilated bile ducts, as a linear or end-on water-density structure running the length of the pancreas, proximal to the obstructing tumor (see Fig. 4–13). The intravenous infusion of an iodinated contrast agent helps to define the dilated duct by increasing the density difference between the water-density duct and the contrast-enhanced pancreatic parenchyma. The technique is identical to that employed for the improved detection of mildly dilated intrahepatic bile ducts.

In a few cases, an apparent reduction in the diameter of the body and tail accompanies tumor of the head, suggesting atrophy of the uninvolved portion of the gland. Pseudocyst formation can also occur proximal to an obstructing tumor in patients without a clinical history of pancreatitis. In such a case, the presence of a tumor may be ignored and the patient's clinical findings attributed to the pseudocyst, a possibility that again emphasizes the danger of interpreting the CT scans without clinical correlation.

Small tumors of the head may produce no appreciable change in the appearance of the gland and dilatation of the biliary tree or the main pancreatic duct or both may be the only detectable finding. In the absence of calculi, isolated dilatation is almost invariably associated with a tumor of the head, and a presumptive diagnosis can be made. Unfortunately, the attenuation value of solid tumors of the pancreas differs little, if at all, from the attenuation value of the normal pancreatic parenchyma, and if a focal mass is not present the tumor goes unrecognized. Areas of diminished density, related to necrosis or cystic change, have been seen in scans of some pancreatic cancers, but in all instances to date a focal mass was obvious.

When invasion of the posterior peripancreatic fat plane occurs, contiguous struc-

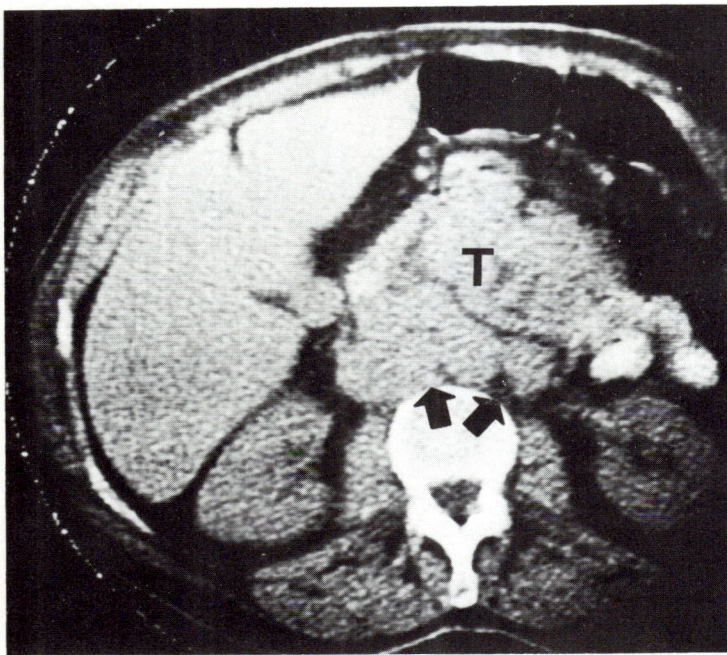

Figure 4–16. Pancreatic carcinoma. A bulky tumor (T) is present in the body and tail of the pancreas. Multiple enlarged para-aortic and paracaval nodes (arrows) reflect the advanced stage of metastatic disease.

tures, such as the superior mesenteric artery, the splenic vein or the inferior vena cava, may become enveloped by tumor and lose their definition. This generally occurs in association with sizable tumors.

Tumors in the body and tail are often larger than those in the head at the time of initial evaluation, possibly owing to a longer asymptomatic growth period. As in the case of tumor in the head, a focal mass is the common finding, with obliteration of the posterior fat plane being a frequent accompaniment. Enlarged nodes containing metastatic tumor are occasionally seen in a para-aortic location directly posterior to the body and tail (Fig. 4–16).

One must be careful not to confuse an apparent mass formed by contiguous loops of fluid-filled small bowel with a true mass lesion of the tail. The use of an oral contrast agent eliminates this source of false positive studies.

PANCREATITIS. The alterations in the morphologic condition and density of the inflamed pancreas vary from none to marked diffuse enlargement with diminished density, which is a reflection of edema and obliteration of the normal peripancreatic fat planes. Associated obscuration of the anterior portion of the perinephric (Gerota's) fascia on the left side is a common finding as fluid and tissue response extends laterally in the anterior pararenal space (Fig. 4–17).

CT is seldom utilized in the diagnosis of uncomplicated acute pancreatitis when clinical and biochemical data support that diagnosis. In the face of clinically unexplained severe upper abdominal pain, however, CT may aid diagnosis by demonstrating diffuse enlargement of the pancreas or a complication of unrecognized acute pancreatitis, such as a pseudocyst. When the symptoms of a patient with known acute pancreatitis are unusually protracted or the patient's condition is deteriorating despite supportive care, CT may reveal the presence of a complicating pseudocyst, abscess, or peripancreatic hemorrhage (Fig. 4–18).

Most pseudocysts appear as circular or oval masses having a density close to that of water and a measurably thick wall (Fig. 4–19). Variations in the density of the fluid

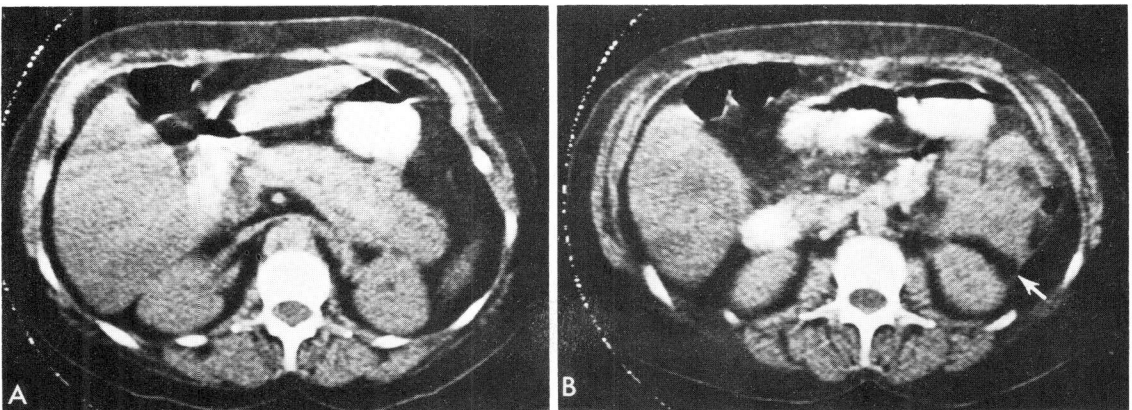

Figure 4–17. Acute pancreatitis. *A*, Diffuse enlargement of the body and tail of the pancreas is evident in this patient with acute pancreatitis. *B*, The lateral aspect of the anterior pararenal space, which normally contains fat, is filled with higher density inflammatory tissue, reflecting the marked peripancreatic tissue response. Note the sharp demarcation of the perinephric space and the thickening of Gerota's fascia (arrow). (*From* Wilson, G. H.: Current Radiology. Vol. 2. Boston, Houghton, Mifflin Company, 1979, p. 93. Reproduced by permission.).

relate to its composition. The more suspended cellular debris and proteinaceous content, the higher is the density. An abscess may resemble a pseudocyst. Generally, the attenuation value of the abscess material is higher than that of the fluid within a pseudocyst. Although an abscess may appear round or oval, it may also extend along or through adjacent tissue planes, conforming to the shape of the cavity into which it has dissected. Although it may be difficult to differentiate the pancreatic abscess from pseudocyst during certain stages of its development using the CT scan alone, clinical information usually suggests the appropriate diagnosis. Hemorrhage as a complication

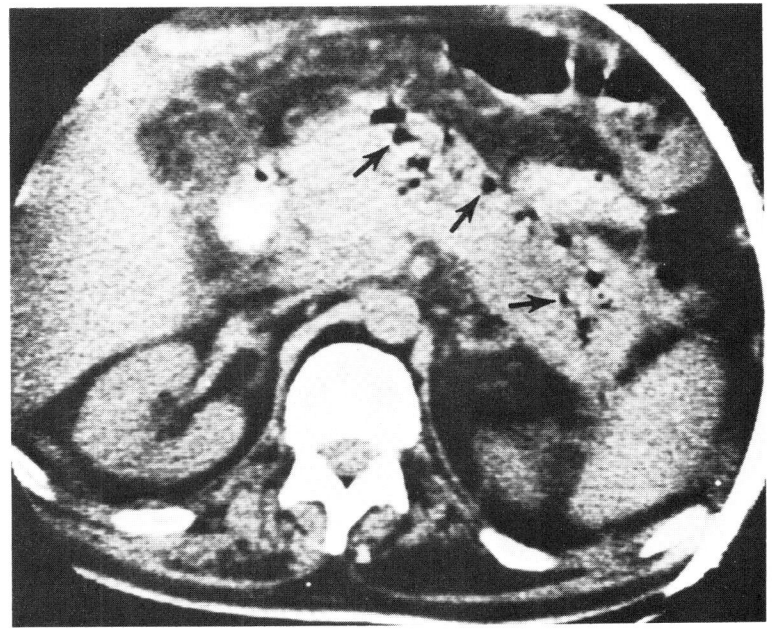

Figure 4–18. Multiple gas bubbles (arrows) are seen within the dense inflammatory tissue anterior to the enlarged, poorly marginated pancreas. The findings are consistent with a complication of acute pancreatitis, namely an abscess with gas-forming organisms. Note the increased density of the fat in the lesser sac just posterior to the stomach, compared with the lower density perinephric and subcutaneous fat. This increase in density is commonly seen in fat that is contiguous to an inflammatory process.

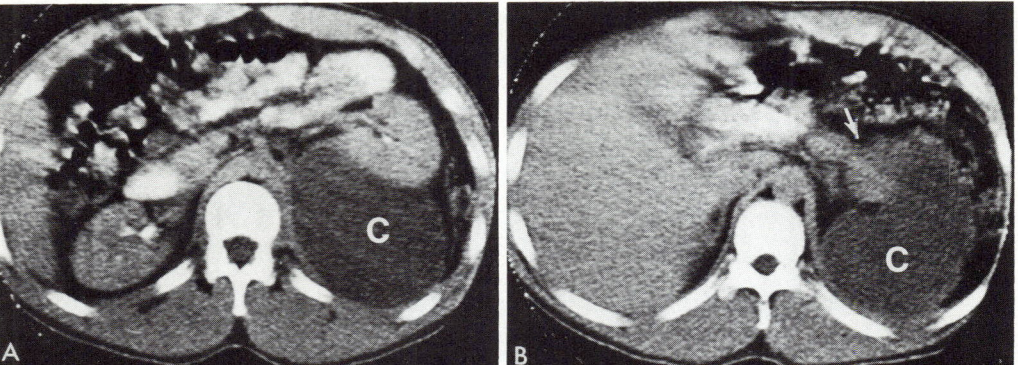

Figure 4–19. Unusual extension of surgically proven pancreatic pseudocyst into the perinephric space. *A,* Dissection of pseudocyst (C) into the posterior perinephric space produces anterior displacement of the left kidney. *B,* Scan at a more cephalic level reveals that the low-density, thick-walled pseudocyst (C) arises from the tail of the pancreas (arrow). (*From* Radiol. Clin. North Am. *16*:110, 1979. Reproduced by permission.)

of pancreatitis may result in the rapid development of a poorly marginated mass with a density equal to or higher than that of the pancreatic parenchyma. If it is possible to obtain follow-up scans, one can see a gradual change in the attenuation value of the mass as the hematoma becomes a lower density seroma.

In chronic pancreatitis, pancreatic calcification can sometimes be demonstrated by CT at an earlier stage than it can on a plain radiograph. Calcification has been seen in the wall of pseudocysts and, rarely, in neoplasms as well. Intraductal calculi may be associated with visible dilatation of the main pancreatic duct.

Atrophy of the pancreas is a late sequela of chronic pancreatitis. A decrease in the size of the pancreas has been noted in the elderly without any history of pancreatitis, however. Thus, correlation of the CT findings with the patient's age and clinical history must be made when postinflammatory atrophy is suspected.

At times, pancreatitis may present as a focal inflammatory mass rather than as diffuse enlargement. There are no absolute CT criteria for distinguishing such an inflammatory mass from a neoplasm. When the presence of neoplasm is considered unlikely, follow-up scans may prove the benign inflammatory nature of the mass (Fig. 4–20).

As stated earlier, pseudocysts can also develop in association with a carcinoma of the pancreas, presumably secondary to obstruction with focal dilatation and disruption of the pancreatic duct. In such cases, a history of pancreatitis is lacking, and the tumor itself may be visible as a separate focal mass.

A pseudocyst can be mimicked in its CT appearance by cystic tumors of the pancreas, such as cystadenoma and cystadenocarcinoma (Fig. 4–21). Areas of hemorrhage or necrosis within a tumor may also resemble pseudocyst. The margins are usually not as well defined, however, and the tumor has a thicker, irregular wall.

Kidney

Diagnostic problems related to the kidneys that CT has proved remarkably useful in clarifying include (1) the detection and clarification of renal or pararenal masses; (2) the determination of the extent of renal carcinoma metastases to lymph nodes, major draining veins and perinephric space; (3) the detection of postoperative tumor recur-

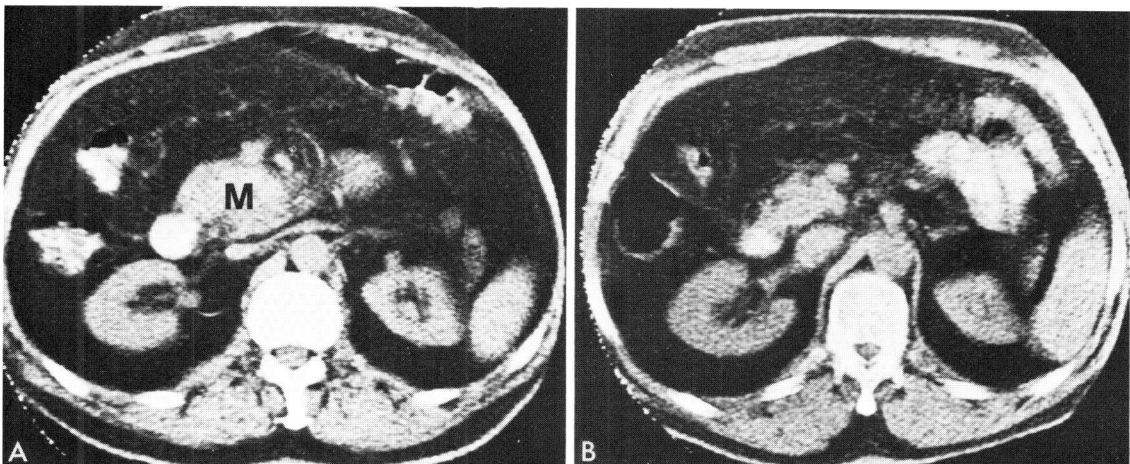

Figure 4–20. Acute focal pancreatitis. *A*, An apparent focal mass (M) is present in this patient with signs and symptoms more consistent with pancreatitis than with carcinoma of the pancreas. Note the similarity to Figure 4–15*A*. The body and tail of the pancreas were not enlarged. *B*, Follow-up CT scan four weeks later at approximately the same level shows a marked reduction of the size of the uncinate process of the pancreas, which is now within normal limits. The findings are consistent with the evolution of an acute focal pancreatitis.

rence; (4) the assessment of renal trauma; (5) the determination of the presence, degree, and cause of obstruction; and (6) the evaluation of inflammatory lesions of the kidney and adjacent tissue.[21, 60] Additionally, CT can be used to distinguish a radiographically nonopaque calculus from a soft tissue tumor of the uroepithelium when other diagnostic techniques fail to permit distinction. Despite the lack of obvious calcification on a radiograph, the attenuation value of these calculi is significantly higher than that of soft tissue (120 to 240 Hounsfield units versus 20 to 40). Renal size, shape, and location can be accurately determined with CT, which is especially useful when function is severely diminished or absent.

CT has proved highly reliable in the differentiation of benign renal cysts from

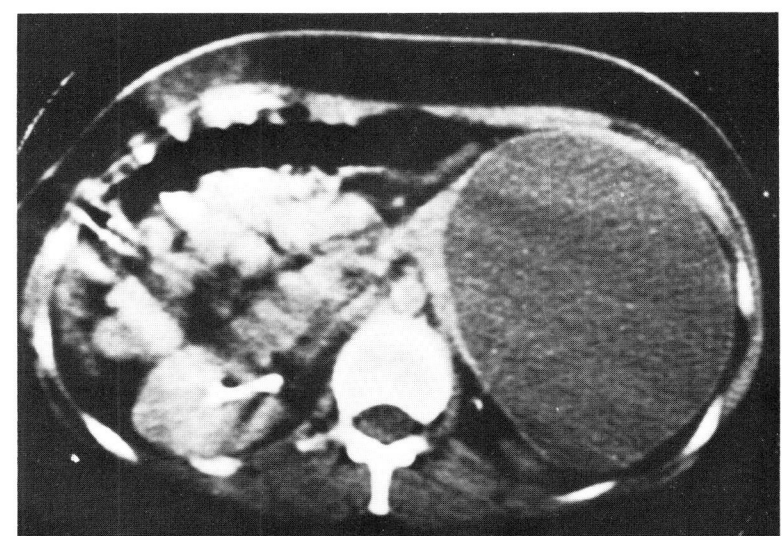

Figure 4–21. Cystadenoma of the pancreas. A large, near-water density mass, 11 cm in diameter, with a perceptible wall thickness arises from the tail of the pancreas. The patient had no history of pancreatitis. The differential diagnosis included pseudocyst of the pancreas and cystadenoma. A benign cystadenoma was resected. (*From* Radiol. Clin. North Am. *16*:110, 1979. Reproduced by permission.)

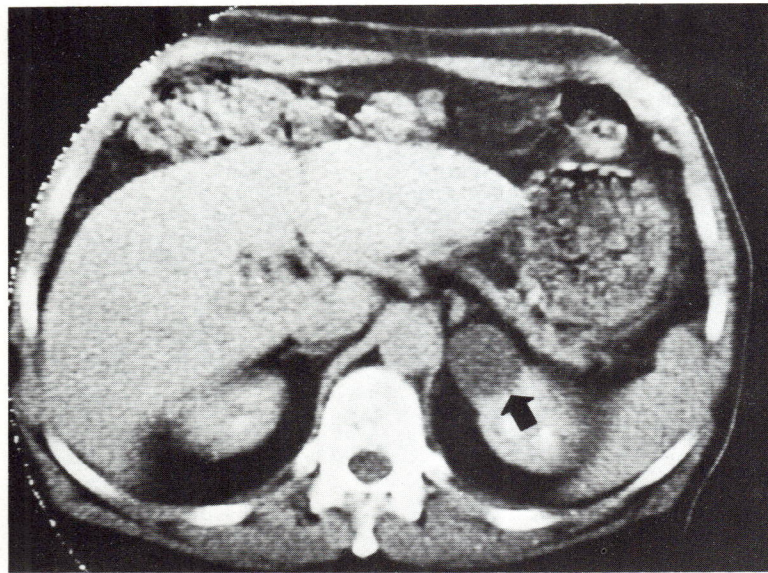

Figure 4–22. Renal cyst. A postcontrast CT scan of the kidney. A typical benign cyst (arrow) arises from the anteromedial surface of the left upper pole in a location difficult to evaluate with ultrasound

renal tumor. Renal cysts, as seen with CT, display a uniform water density, imperceptible wall thickness (if a portion of the cyst projects beyond the surface contour of the kidney), and nonenhancement following the intravenous administration of iodinated contrast medium (Fig. 4–22). If these three criteria are met, the diagnosis of benign cyst is established and nothing further needs to be done. In equivocal cases, in which thickness is perceptibly increased or the attenuation value of the mass is more than 16 Hounsfield units greater than water value, additional diagnostic tests, including percutaneous needle aspiration and selective arteriography should be considered (Fig. 4–23). Lesions that may morphologically resemble a benign serous cyst on CT scans include inflammatory cyst, abscess, hemorrhagic cyst, neoplasm with cystic or necrotic

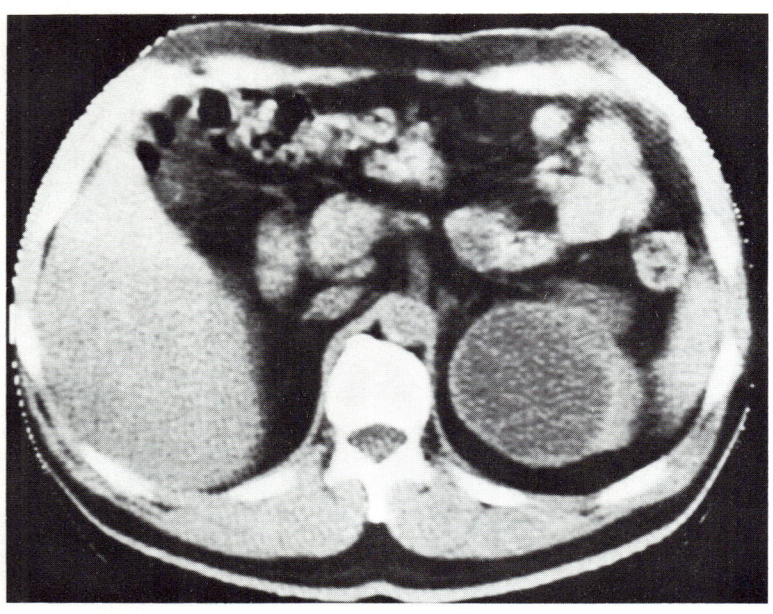

Figure 4–23. Renal abscess. A rounded, low-density mass with a measurably thickened wall arises from the upper pole of the left kidney. The attenuation value of the center of the mass is 10 EMI units, a value that would be unusually high for benign cyst fluid. This indeterminate mass was found at operation to be a thick-walled sterile abscess.

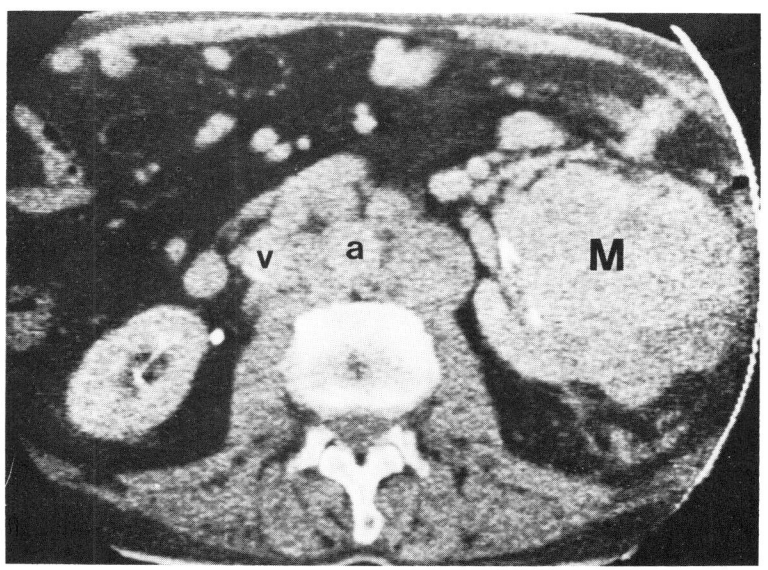

Figure 4–24. Renal cell carcinoma with lymph node metastases. On a post-intravenous contrast CT scan, a large mass (M) is seen arising from the lateral aspect of the left kidney. Although the attenuation value of the mass is somewhat inhomogeneous, reflecting focal areas of necrosis, overall the density is similar to renal parenchyma. Multiple enlarged lymph nodes secondary to metastatic renal tumor surround the aorta (a) and vena cava (v), which are visible owing to their greater enhancement from the intravenous contrast medium.

portions, and contiguous cystic lesion arising in another organ. If careful attention is paid to the three characteristics cited earlier, diagnostic errors can be avoided.

Renal tumor differs from cyst in that it has a higher attenuation value closer to that of the renal parenchyma (Fig. 4–24). The density of large neoplasms may be inhomogeneous, reflecting focal areas of necrosis, hemorrhage, or cystic change. All but necrotic and cystic tumors are enhanced after the intravenous injection of iodinated contrast. The characteristically thick walls of cystic and necrotic tumors, which usually can be enhanced, serve to distinguish these less common tumors from cysts (Fig. 4–25).

Local extension of neoplasm beyond the renal capsule can be defined. When gross extension into the main renal vein and inferior vena cava occurs, the changes in the shape and enhancing characteristics of these structures are apparent on the CT scan (Fig. 4–26).[74]

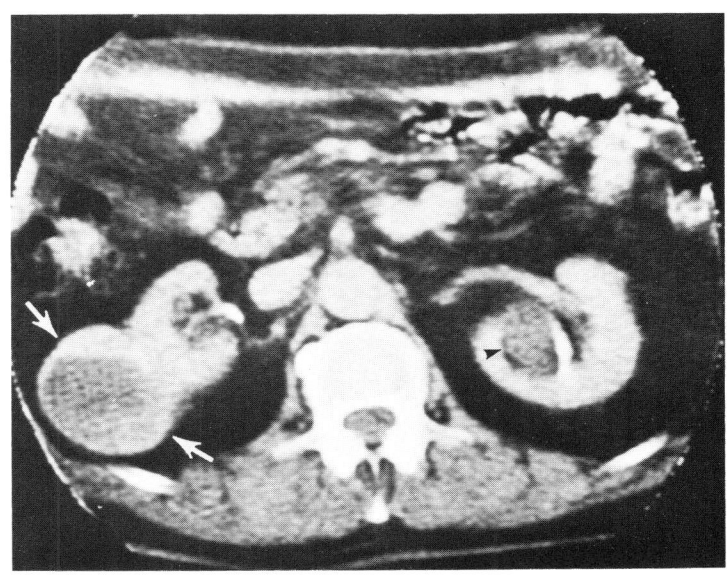

Figure 4–25. Renal carcinoma. A thick-walled mass (arrows) with a lower density center projects from the lateral surface of the right kidney. The interface with the renal parenchyma is not well defined. The findings are typical of centrally necrotic renal cell carcinoma. An incidental water-density peripelvic cyst is present on the left (arrowhead).

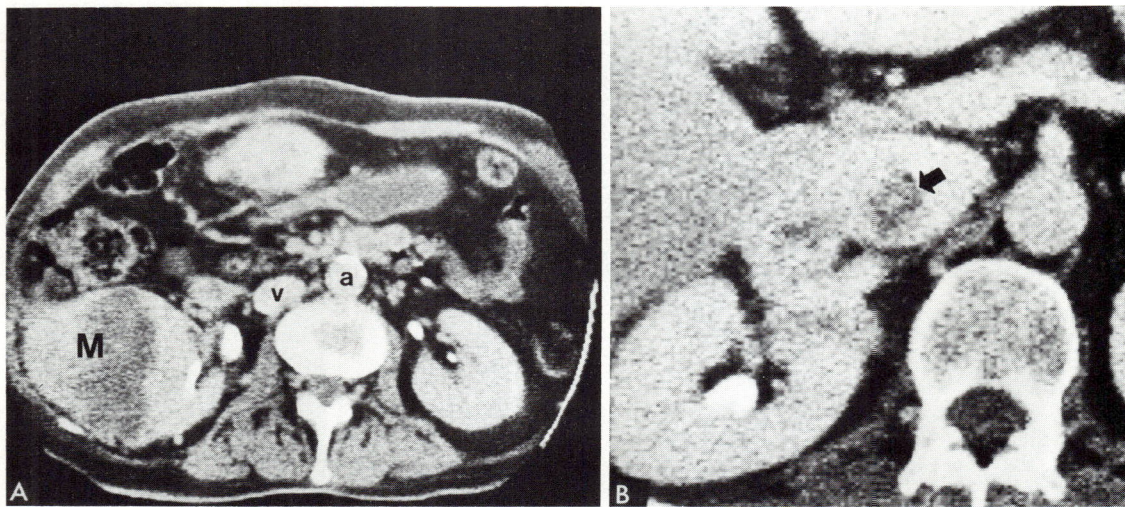

Figure 4–26. Renal cell carcinoma with venous involvement. *A,* A large, partially necrotic neoplastic mass (M) arises from the lateral aspect of the right kidney. The lumen of the inferior vena cava (v) appears patent at this level. Compare with the appearance of the lumen of the aorta (a). *B,* A detail view of the renal vein and vena cava, at a slightly higher level in the abdomen, demonstrates thrombus (arrow) within the lumen of the distended vena cava. Thrombus can also be seen within the dilated renal vein, which is entering the vena cava at this level. The increased diameter of the renal vein and vena cava is partly related to the large volume of blood shunting through this vascular tumor.

Certain inflammatory masses, such as xanthogranulomatous pyelonephritis, are indistinguishable from neoplasm on CT scans.[60] Benign cystic lesions containing fluid with a high attenuation value, such as blood, may also be mistaken for tumors. Large arteriovenous malformations, which may be clinically suspected, can be distinguished from a neoplasm on CT scans only if the highly enhanceable lesion is studied during the infusion of a contrast agent. Otherwise, the resemblance to a solid tumor is marked (Fig. 4–27).

The non–contrast enhanced collecting system in the unobstructed kidney is barely perceptible as a water-density structure surrounded by the renal sinus fat. After the injection of contrast, a urogram effect is obtained, and sharply marginated calyces and renal pelvis can be seen.

In the presence of partial obstruction a visibly dilated collecting system can be seen, often without the use of a contrast agent. The enhancement provided by an iodinated contrast agent improves the visualization of the collecting system and the confidence of the diagnosis, however. By following the ureter(s) caudally, the level and cause of obstruction often can be identified (Fig. 4–28). When obstruction is complete and little or no renal function remains, CT can clearly display the rim of residual renal parenchyma surrounding the markedly dilated collecting system as well as the dilated ureter if the level of obstruction is below the pelviureteric junction.

The perinephric space as well as the anterior and posterior pararenal spaces is clearly defined by CT scanning. Perinephric abscess, hematoma, and urinoma can be identified and their extent assessed (Fig. 4–29). A process such as a retroperitoneal tumor or abscess can be shown to lie outside of Gerota's fascia when intrinsic renal involvement is suggested by excretory urography. When the excretory urogram shows distortion of the axis or displacement of a kidney or ureter, the CT image can differentiate between a pathologic condition, such as lymphadenopathy, and simple asymmetric distribution of normal retroperitoneal fat (Fig. 4–30).

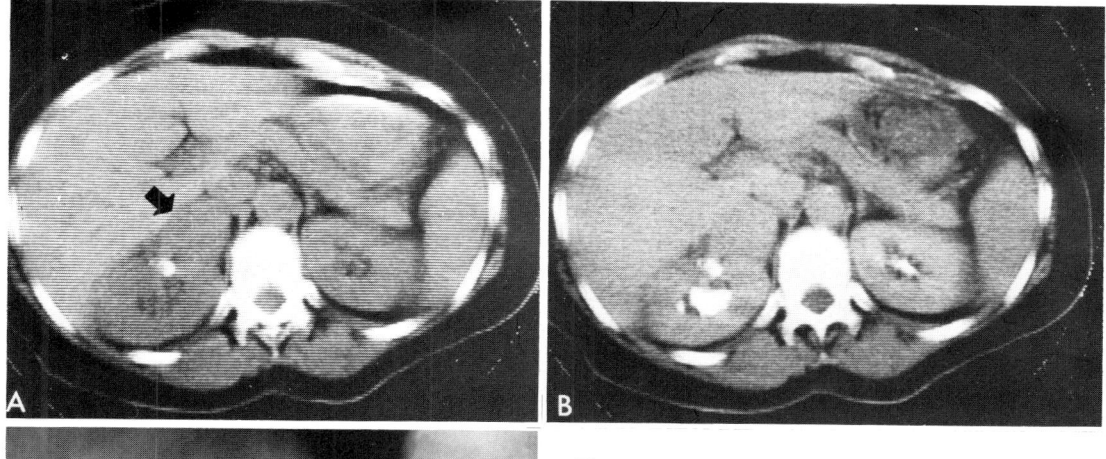

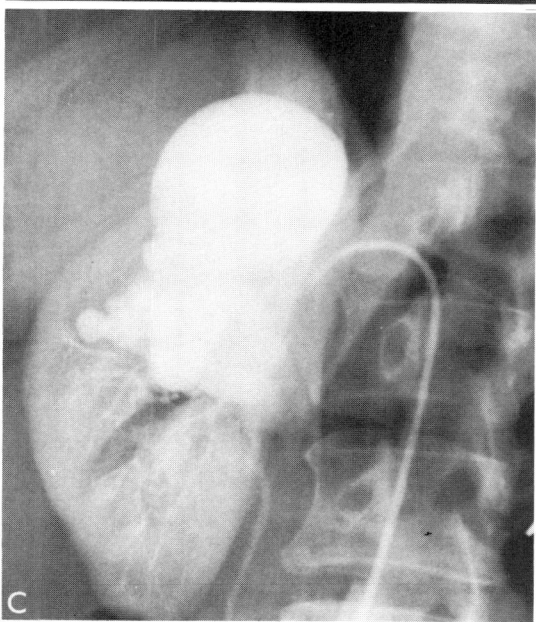

Figure 4–27. Renal arteriovenous fistula. *A,* The precontrast scan reveals the presence of an oval mass (arrow), equal in density to renal parenchyma, arising from the anterior surface of the right upper pole. A focus of calcification lies at the base of the mass. *B,* A CT scan taken several minutes after a single intravenous bolus of contrast medium shows the enhancement of the mass to be approximately equal to that of the renal parenchyma. These CT features suggest a solid renal tumor. *C,* A large arteriovenous fistula, demonstrated by a selective renal arteriogram, accounts for the mass seen on CT. The calcification was in the wall of an intrarenal artery aneurysm. Demonstration of this lesion on CT would require precise timing in order to show that the enhancement of the mass was equal to the aorta during the period of 12 to 18 seconds after the bolus injection of contrast medium. Current technology provides this capability.

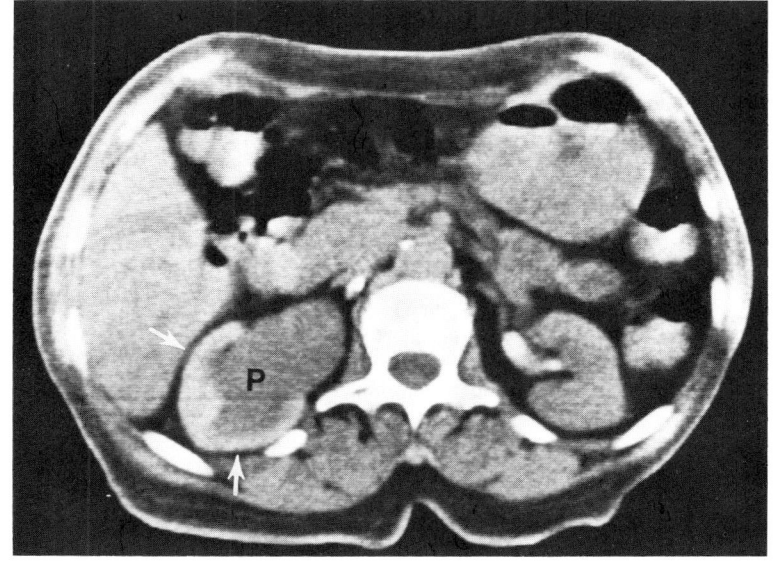

Figure 4–28. Unilateral hydronephrosis. A 4-hour post-intravenous contrast medium CT scan shows the characteristic features of marked hydronephrosis. An attenuated rim of renal parenchyma (arrows) with a persisting obstructive nephrogram surrounds the markedly dilated pelvicalyceal system (P). Note that no contrast medium is being excreted into the collecting system on the right. Excretion is continuing on the left. A dilated ureter could be traced to the obstructing lesion deep in the pelvis.

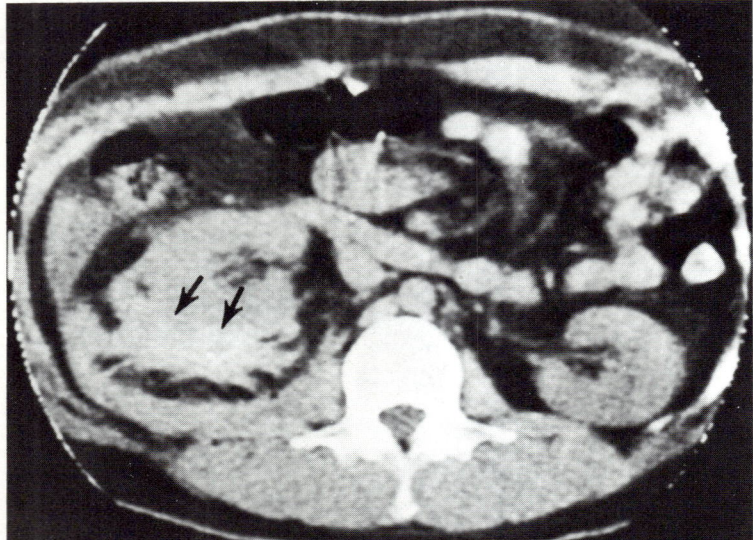

Figure 4–29. Post-renal biopsy hematoma. Twenty-four hours after renal biopsy, the hematocrit dropped from 45 per cent to 40 per cent. A large perinephric hematoma extends from the posterior surface of the right kidney (arrows). Note that the density of the fresh clot is greater than that of the unenhanced renal parenchyma. Increased density is characteristic of fresh hematomas. (*From* Kidney Int. *14*:87–92, 1978. Reproduced by permission.)

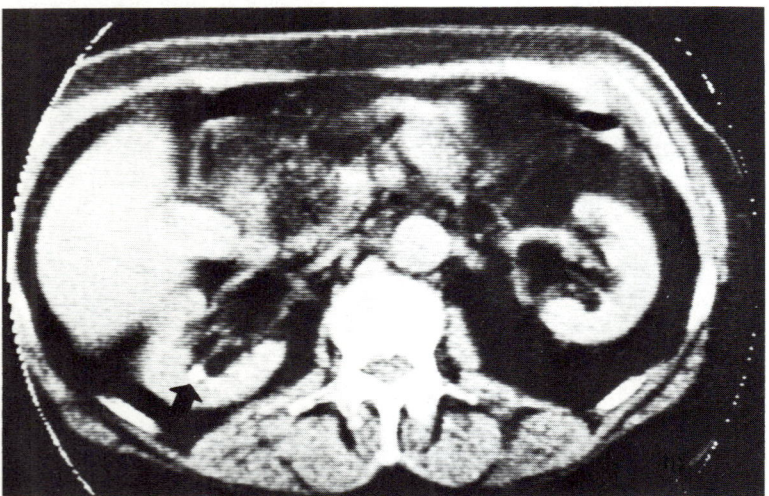

Figure 4–30. Retroperitoneal fat displacing kidney. Excretory urography suggested lateral displacement of the left kidney by a retroperitoneal mass. The CT scan shows asymmetric distribution of normal retroperitoneal fat, which accounts for the renal position. An incidental calyceal stone is visible on the right (arrow).

Adrenal Glands

Computed tomography is an accurate radiologic method of imaging both the normal and the abnormal adrenal gland. The normal adrenal gland can be seen in approximately 95 per cent of patients.[8, 30, 50] With the exception of bilateral minimal enlargement related to adrenal hyperplasia, virtually all pathologic conditions involving the adrenal gland can be confidently identified with CT. Although the morphologic condition of the normal adrenal glands may vary, the margins of the normal gland are always straight or concave. In no instance are the borders externally convex, nor is the normal gland ever spherical. The maximal anteroposterior diameter is almost always less than 2.5 cm and the maximal mediolateral thickness never exceeds 1 cm. Although more difficult to assess exactly, the vertical length of the normal adrenal gland, as determined by contiguous 1-cm scans, rarely exceeds 4 cm.

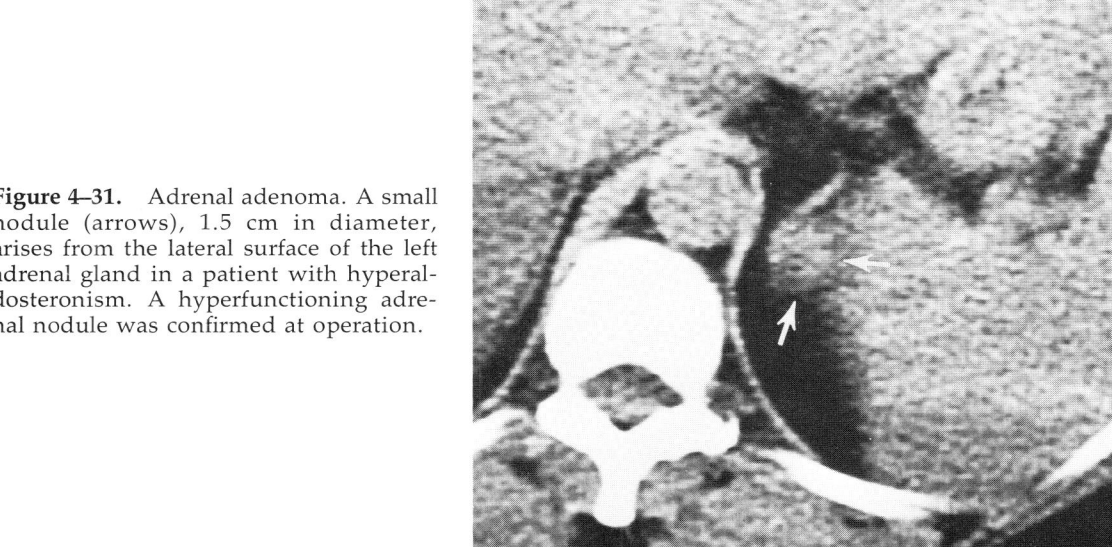

Figure 4–31. Adrenal adenoma. A small nodule (arrows), 1.5 cm in diameter, arises from the lateral surface of the left adrenal gland in a patient with hyperaldosteronism. A hyperfunctioning adrenal nodule was confirmed at operation.

CT scans are capable of displaying tumors of the adrenal gland as small as 1 cm in diameter.[30, 62] Such small lesions appear as localized masses with convex borders arising from a portion of an otherwise normal gland (Fig. 4–31). The adrenal tumor becomes more easily recognizable as it increases in size, until the size of the lesion results in its crossing contiguous anatomic boundaries. At this point, it may be difficult to differentiate a large adrenal mass from an upper pole renal mass. Although biochemical evidence of adrenal hyperfunction may resolve this diagnostic problem in many cases, it may be necessary to obtain further confirmation of these anatomic relationships from either an excretory urogram or an ultrasound scan.

A wide variety of benign and malignant tumors of the adrenal gland can be precisely defined by CT. In the case of benign cysts and myelolipoma, a rare tumor composed of varying proportions of fat and bone marrow, a specific pathologic diagnosis can be rendered on the basis of the characteristic low attenuation value. In other instances in which a mass lesion has been identified within the adrenal gland, clinical correlation with biochemical data and other pertinent historical and physical findings must be made in order to establish a correct diagnosis (Fig. 4–32).[66] Primary adenocarcinomas, pheochromocytomas, functioning and nonfunctioning adenomas, metastatic involvement (Fig. 4–33), hyperplasia, and granulomatous disease have all been identified by CT. Unilateral adrenal enlargement is caused most commonly by a pheochromocytoma or a cortical adenoma or carcinoma. Mild symmetric bilateral enlargement in the hyperfunctioning syndromes suggests hyperplasia, whereas bilateral mass lesions are more indicative of adrenal metastases, although bilateral pheochromocytomas have also been encountered.

In addition to displaying the primary tumor, the CT scan may also detect retroperitoneal lymph node involvement, tumoral extension into the inferior vena cava, or metastases to the liver.

Of considerable value is the ability of CT to exclude the diagnosis of adrenal disease by the demonstration of a normal adrenal gland when other radiologic proce-

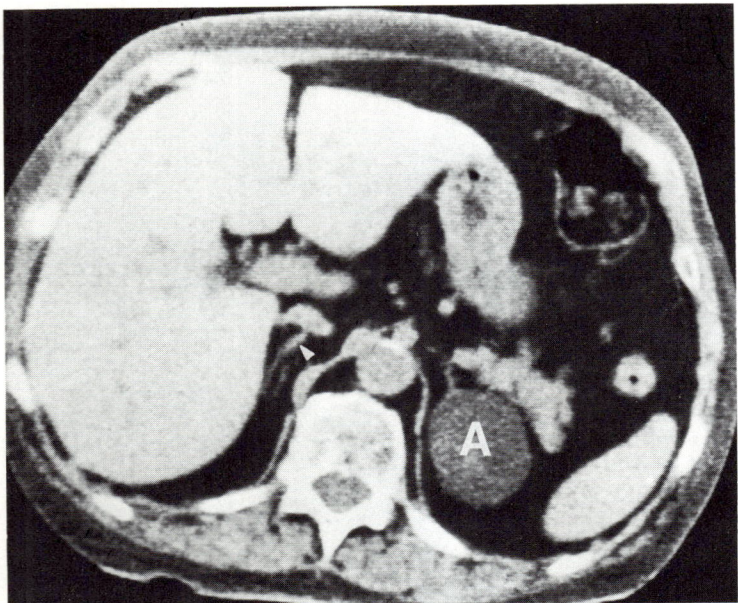

Figure 4–32. Adrenal adenoma. A low-density mass 4.5 cm in diameter (A) arises from the posterior aspect of the left adrenal gland. A portion of the tail of the pancreas is seen just anterior to the adenoma. A normal right adrenal gland (arrowhead) can be clearly seen directly posterior to the vena cava. The low density of many adrenal adenomas is related to a high lipid content. A benign adrenal adenoma was removed at operation.

dures have suggested the possibility of a mass in this region. Pseudomasses, such as a prominent splenic lobulation or a loop of bowel, occasionally present diagnostic problems.[30] It was sometimes necessary in the past to use more invasive procedures, such as arteriography, to resolve these difficulties.

Although excretory urography with tomography, ultrasound, and radionuclide imaging may play a role in the evaluation of the adrenal glands, CT has proven remarkably useful, reliable, and rapid in its precise display of the normal or pathologic adrenal gland.[30, 60] The merits of other radiologic imaging methods are discussed in a later section of this chapter (p. 163).

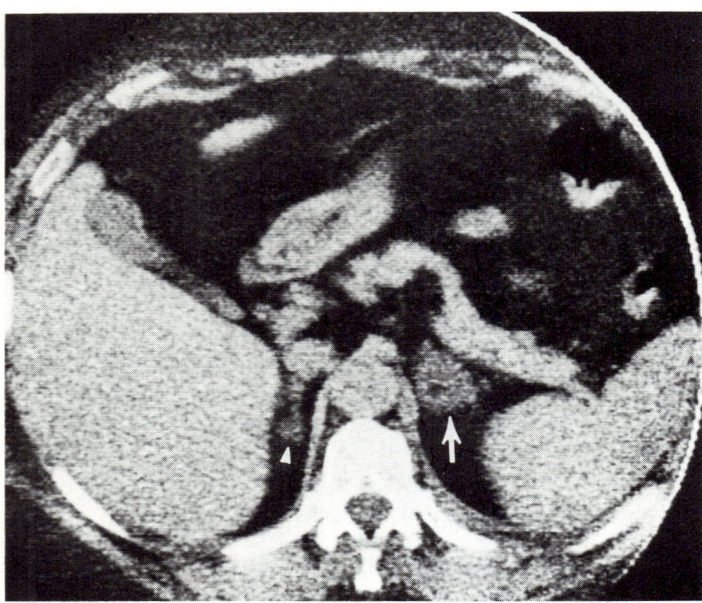

Figure 4–33. Metastatic melanoma to the left adrenal gland produces a nodule 2 cm in diameter (arrow). A smaller focus of metastatic disease can be seen altering the contour of the posterior aspect of the right adrenal gland (arrowhead). The findings were confirmed at operation.

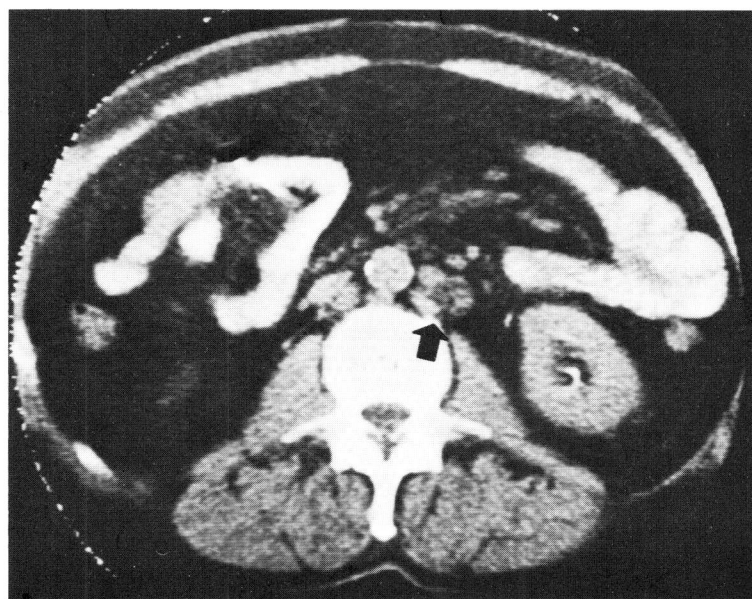

Figure 4–34. Nodular sclerosing Hodgkin's disease—early involvement. A focus of discrete nodal enlargement (arrow) is visible to the left of the aorta in this patient with nodular sclerosing Hodgkin's disease. The involvement was confirmed at staging laparotomy. Although the lymph nodes measure in the range of 1 to 1.5 cm in diameter, theoretically within normal limits, such a cluster of visible nodes should be viewed with great suspicion in a patient with Hodgkin's disease.

Retroperitoneum and Peritoneal Cavity

LYMPHADENOPATHY. CT has proven to be a useful diagnostic tool in detecting intra-abdominal and pelvic nodal involvement by lymphoma.[1, 6, 20, 34, 38, 64, 77] In all but the leanest patients, the midline retroperitoneal landmarks—the aorta and inferior vena cava—are clearly visible owing to the presence of surrounding retroperitoneal fat. Normal lymph nodes, ranging in size from 3 to 10 mm, can be seen in the usual para-aortic and paracaval sites as well as contiguous to the iliac vessels extending into the pelvis. Abdominal lymph nodes are considered abnormal if they exceed 2 cm in diameter. An isolated lymph node 1 to 2 cm in size is regarded as a suspicious finding. The presence of numerous lymph nodes of this size is considered pathologic, however (Fig. 4–34).

The spectrum of changes in the lymphomatous retroperitoneal nodes ranges from isolated nodal enlargement in one or more areas to huge, confluent, nodal masses that obscure the aorta and the inferior vena cava by obliteration of the surrounding fat planes and displacement of these structures (Fig. 4–35). In addition, enlarged nodes in areas not normally opacified by a bipedal lymphangiogram, including the hepatic, splenic, and renal hilar nodes and nodes in the mesentery (Fig. 4–36) and retrocrural regions,[9] are equally well displayed with CT. Extensive involvement of the mesenteric nodes is more common in the non-Hodgkin's lymphomas, and CT has been most helpful in defining the extent of this involvement.

Computed tomography does not differentiate between benign and malignant causes of lymph node enlargement; it merely displays the enlarged nodes. The attenuation values of benign hyperplastic lymph nodes and lymphomatous nodes are similar. Thus, diffuse lymph node enlargement secondary to viral or granulomatous disease cannot be differentiated from lymphoma or metastatic tumor based on CT findings alone. In the staging of a patient with known lymphoma, this inability to differentiate is not a practical problem. Additionally, lymph node masses 3 cm or more in diameter, a not uncommon finding in lymphoma, are exceedingly unusual in the benign reactive inflammatory conditions.

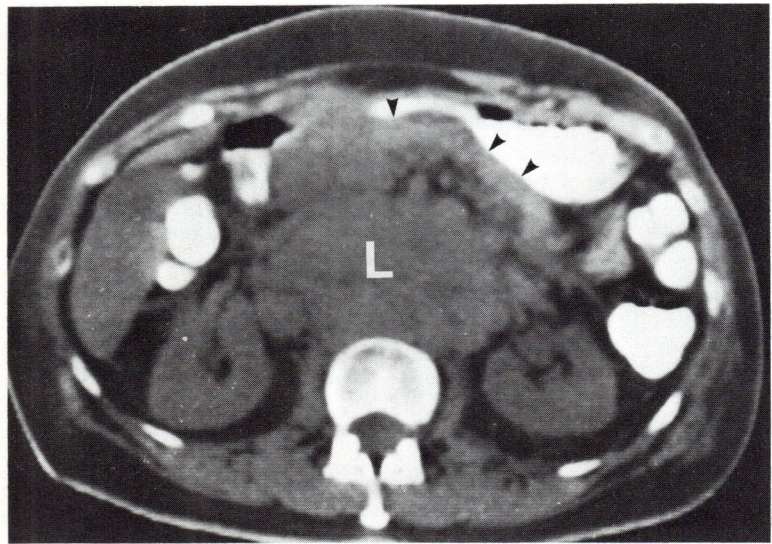

Figure 4–35. Lymphocytic lymphoma. A huge confluent mass of lymphomatous para-aortic and paracaval nodes (L) obscures the normal retroperitoneal structures and rotates the right kidney along its long axis. The pancreas (arrowheads) is displaced far anteriorly by the mass. However, the distinction between retropancreatic disease and primary pancreatic disease is easily made in this scan.

The major cause of a false negative CT examination in the staging of lymphoma patients is the inability to recognize normal-sized but abnormal nodes that are involved with tumor. Fortunately, in most instances, lymphomatous nodes are enlarged. In 5 to 10 per cent of patients with Hodgkin's disease, however, para-aortic and paracaval nodes are involved with tumor but not enlarged. These nodes appear normal on CT. In such a circumstance, lymphangiography is helpful in defining the abnormal nodal architecture. Thus, sound clinical judgment must enter into the interpretation of a "normal" CT scan.

Although there has been good correlation between lymphangiography and CT scans of the same retroperitoneal nodal chains, CT has been found to be superior to lymphangiography in demonstrating abnormal nodes in the upper para-aortic (or re-

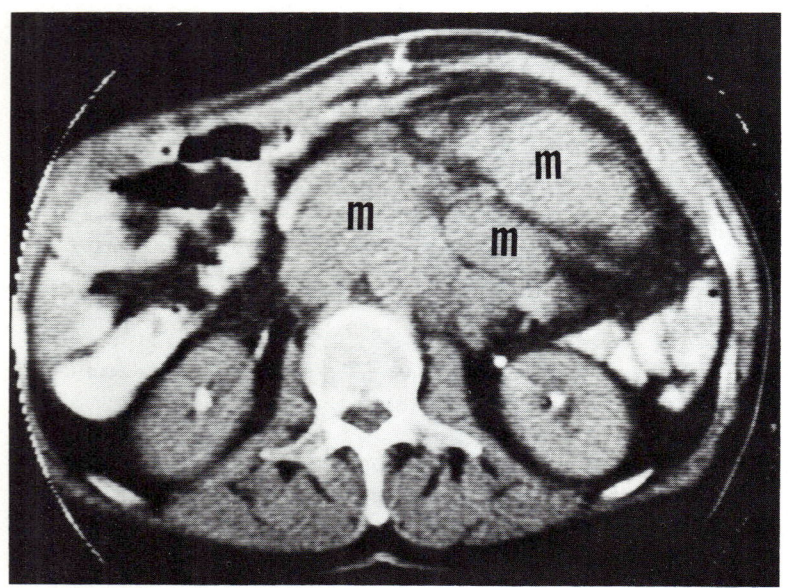

Figure 4–36. Histiocytic lymphoma. Massive enlargement of mesenteric lymph nodes (m) produces a soft, palpable mass in the left midabdomen. The para-aortic and paracaval nodes are involved to a lesser degree. Mesenteric involvement is common in the non-Hodgkin's lymphomas.

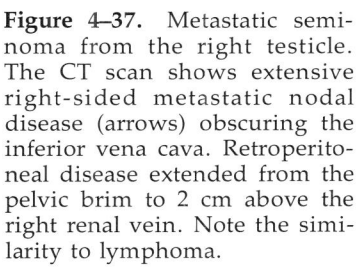

Figure 4–37. Metastatic seminoma from the right testicle. The CT scan shows extensive right-sided metastatic nodal disease (arrows) obscuring the inferior vena cava. Retroperitoneal disease extended from the pelvic brim to 2 cm above the right renal vein. Note the similarity to lymphoma.

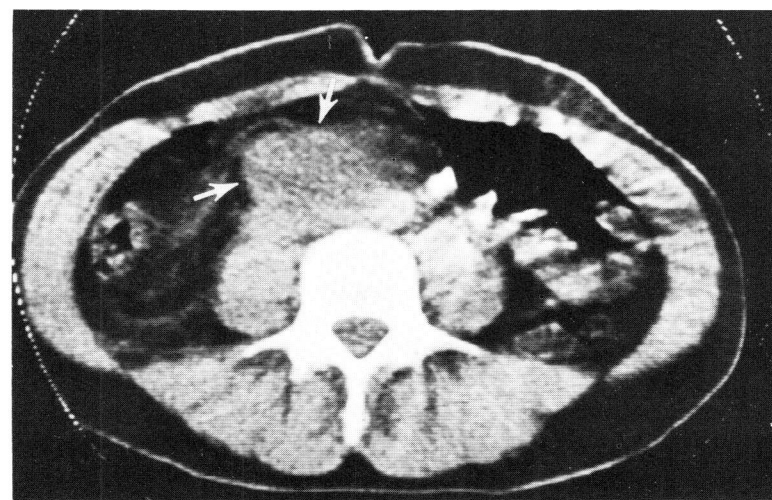

trocrural), mesenteric, renal, splenic, and hepatic hilar areas, which are not normally opacified during lymphangiography. When failure to opacify intra-abdominal lymph nodes is the result of lymphatic obstruction or unanticipated consumption of all of the opaque oil by markedly enlarged pelvic nodes, CT is most helpful in evaluating the nonopacified node-bearing areas. The exact extent of tumor mass is better delineated with CT, which often shows that the abnormality demonstrated on a lymphangiogram represents only a small portion of the tumor mass and that much more extensive disease is actually present. This is a matter of considerable importance in radiation therapy treatment planning.[38, 53]

The false negative and false positive rate is gratifyingly low, and CT serves as an excellent technique for staging lymphoma patients, obviating the need for using lymphangiography on the majority of patients. In a recent review of surgically proven patients, the overall accuracy of CT was 90 per cent.[38]

In the evaluation of pelvic and abdominal lymph nodes for the presence of metastatic neoplasms, such as carcinomas arising in the pelvic organs, the normal-appearing, or "negative," CT scan has less value owing to the prevalence of normal-sized, totally replaced lymph nodes. In this category of disease, only the positive CT scan has clinical merit.[40] Although the application of CT scanning to the staging of pelvic malignancies and other tumors known to metastasize to the retroperitoneum is evolving, it nevertheless lags in value behind its use in the evaluation of lymphoma patients.

An exception to this general statement is the use of CT in the staging of testicular tumors.[27, 40] The usual lymphatic drainage of the testicle is directly to nodes at the level of the renal veins. These nodes frequently escape detection, since they are normally not opacified at bipedal lymphangiography. When seminoma, the most common testicular tumor, metastasizes to lymph nodes, the nodes often enlarge and are readily detectable on CT (Fig. 4–37). Enlarged nodes involved by other testicular tumors, including embryonal cell carcinomas, teratocarcinomas, and tumors of mixed cellularity, have also been detected with CT. A positive CT scan may obviate the need for lymphangiography. Lymphangiography still plays an important role in the detection of involved normal-sized nodes, however, and in the evaluation of unusually lean patients who are not good candidates for study with CT.

PRIMARY TUMORS. The primary tumors arising in the retroperitoneum or from the peritoneal lining include a wide variety of benign and malignant soft tissue lesions.[76] Sarcomas of varied cell origin appear on CT scans as soft tissue masses displacing, compressing, or invading adjacent organs. Provided that some perivisceral and retroperitoneal fat is present, the size and extent of the tumor can be defined with accuracy.

Lipomas appear as localized masses with an attenuation value equal to that of normal fat. Liposarcomas have an attenuation value higher than that of fat and often higher than that of water, owing to the presence of myxoid tissue and other cellular components, which differ in their density from adult fat cells. A few liposarcomas have contained areas of normal-density fat, but contiguous higher density tumor tissue indicates the complex nature of the lesion, making the diagnosis of a simple lipoma unlikely.[76, 77]

Some large, muscle-density leiomyosarcomas studied with CT contain discrete rounded areas of necrosis and hemorrhage that are not enhanced following the intravenous infusion of iodinated contrast. Generally these tumors displace contiguous organs. Clear planes of separation cannot always be seen, however, a fact that precludes the determination of whether the tumor has actually invaded the adjacent organ. In most instances, predictions about resectability are unwise. Some tumors that seem the least resectable on CT have proved to be easily manageable at operation.

METASTATIC TUMOR OF THE PERITONEAL SURFACE AND MESENTERY. Computed tomography can be utilized in the direct evaluation of metastatic implants on the peritoneal surface.[45] Prior to the existence of CT and ultrasound, diagnosis relied upon indirect evidence obtained with gastrointestinal contrast studies. CT currently detects only gross involvement of the mesentery and peritoneal surfaces. Diffuse studding of the peritoneal cavity and omentum with small metastases, 1 to 9 mm in size, may easily go unrecognized owing to partial volume averaging or to a paucity of surrounding fat. In some cases, it may be difficult to separate a primary tumor from its contiguous metastases (for example, carcinoma of the pancreatic head from surrounding celiac node metastases). In such a case, only the primary tumor is described in the CT interpretation.

In cases diagnosed with CT, the neoplastic involvement appears as a mass of soft tissue (muscle) density. Involvement of the omentum produces a large, anteriorly placed mass, often extending inferiorly directly into the pelvis. The mass is the thickened omentum diffusely infiltrated with tumor nodules (Fig. 4–38). On occasion, isolated parietal peritoneal implants may be visible against a background of ascitic fluid.

Involvement of the mesentery with metastases from lymphoproliferative disease commonly results in clusters of round soft tissue masses surrounded by mesenteric fat (see Fig. 4–36). These masses represent enlarged lymphomatous mesenteric nodes. When a carcinoma, such as ovarian, breast, or colon cancer, metastasizes to the mesentery, a single, large, well-defined, soft tissue–density mass most often results.

ABSCESS. The detection and localization of an abdominal abscess is a common clinical problem. Conventional radiographic methods often fail to detect the presence of an abscess and are less dependable in the determination of the absence of one. Computed tomography, however, has proved useful in the evaluation of abscess.[3, 15, 18] The ability to define the location and the extent of an abscess has been greatly improved since the introduction of CT. The clear demonstration of a normal peritoneal cavity and retroperitoneal space by CT virtually excludes the possibility of a surgically treatable abscess in the area under study. Although CT can be used as the initial diagnostic method for evaluating the possibility of an intra-abdominal abscess, it is often used to clarify a positive gallium scan.[41] The application of gallium scanning to the detection of abscess is discussed in another section (p. 164).

The CT appearance of abdominal abscesses varies with their location, extent, and contents. Most commonly, the abscess appears as a mass with a low attenuation value—usually between 10 and 30 Hounsfield units; the mass may or may not have a higher density peripheral rim (Fig. 4–39). Although the rim may become enhanced following

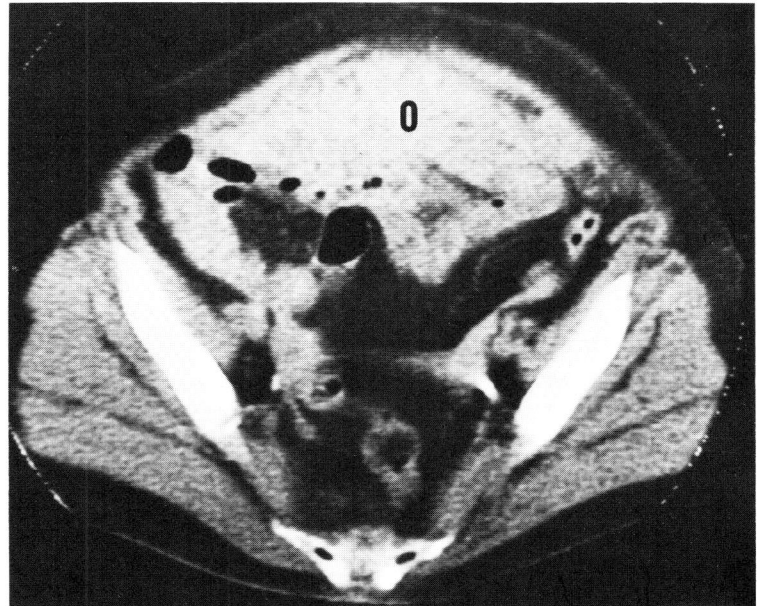

Figure 4–38. Omental metastases from ovarian cancer. A large omental metastasis (O) is shown to be enhancing in this postcontrast CT scan. The findings are typical of metastatic disease from ovarian adenocarcinoma to the omental surface.

the intravenous infusion of iodinated contrast, the center of an abscess does not. If small pockets of gas or an air-fluid level are present and the mass is clearly outside of the gastrointestinal tract, an unequivocal diagnosis of abscess can be made. If gas is absent in the low-density mass, other diagnostic possibilities, including simple cyst, hematoma, seroma, lymphocele, urinoma, necrotic neoplasm, and unusual anatomic variant, must be considered.

Additional CT findings include thickening or obliteration of adjacent fascial planes and displacement of normal surrounding structures. Abscesses that are not located within a solid organ, such as the liver or kidney, commonly derive their configuration from the fascial planes or the peritoneal compartment surrounding them. This feature

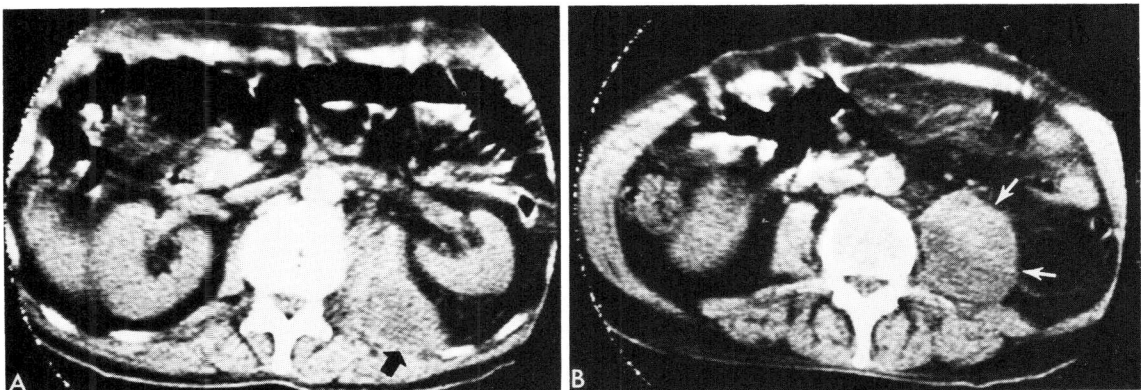

Figure 4–39. Psoas abscess. *A,* CT scan at the level of the kidneys shows displacement of the left kidney laterally by an enlarged left psoas muscle. Note the central area of lower density (arrow). *B,* At a lower level, the psoas is greatly expanded (arrows) by the same process. The density of the center is intermediate between that of water and muscle and is characteristic of abscess material.

may serve to differentiate an abscess from a necrotic tumor, which tends to maintain its own rounded or ovoid configuration regardless of its surroundings.

Needle aspiration for diagnosis and catheter placement for definitive drainage can be greatly assisted by the precise guidance of the CT scan.[15, 17] With this technique, complete drainage of deep-seated abscesses has been accomplished in selected high-risk surgical patients.

HEMORRHAGE. The detection of hemorrhage into the extraperitoneal space by conventional radiographic methods is limited to inferential signs and is lacking in sensitivity. The loss of a psoas shadow, the displacement of bowel or solid organ, and an "ileus pattern" may all suggest hemorrhage on a plain roentgenogram. These signs are frequently absent, however, and when present may be due to other causes, including variants of normal anatomy.

Retroperitoneal hemorrhage is detectable with CT, appearing as an abnormal soft tissue density with attenuation values ranging from 20 to 60 Hounsfield units; the higher values occur in the most acute collections.[59, 63] The shape of the hemorrhage (or hematoma) depends upon the location of the bleeding and the organ or structures involved. Spontaneous hemorrhage into the retroperitoneal space dissects along fascial planes and displaces adjacent fat and organs. If the hemorrhage is large enough, it may extend semicircularly in the extraperitoneal space from back to front but rarely crosses the midline.

Perinephric hematomas (following renal biopsy, for example) generally remain within the perirenal fascial cone. Extravasated blood from a rupturing aortic aneurysm may initially be concentric but eventually dissects laterally in the anterior and posterior pararenal spaces (Fig. 4–40). Hemorrhages (especially those related to anticoagulant therapy) may occur within a muscle, such as the psoas or anterior rectus muscle, resulting in obvious asymmetry of the muscle groups (Fig. 4–41).

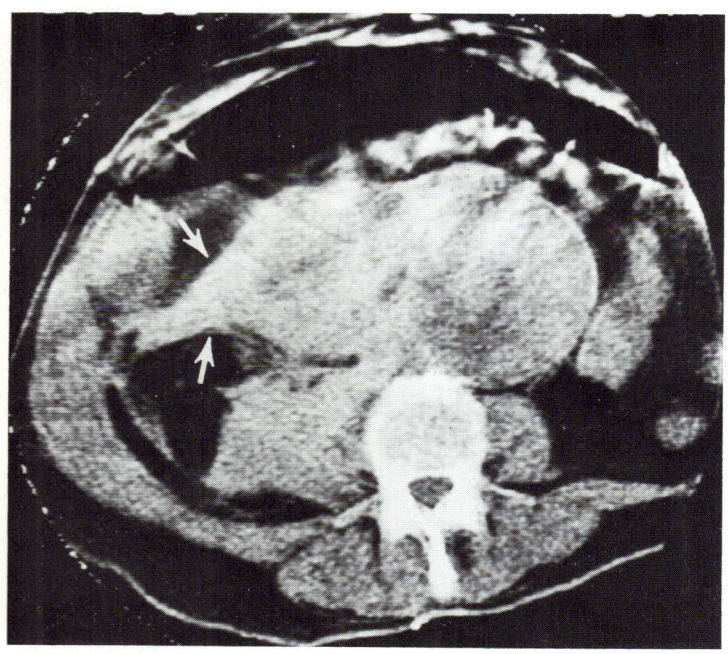

Figure 4–40. Ruptured aortic aneurysm in a patient with an indeterminate clinical presentation. A large hematoma dissects laterally into the right anterior pararenal space (arrows) and posteriorly into the fascial compartment of the psoas muscle. Note the large amount of bowel gas anteriorly, which may have compromised an ultrasound examination.

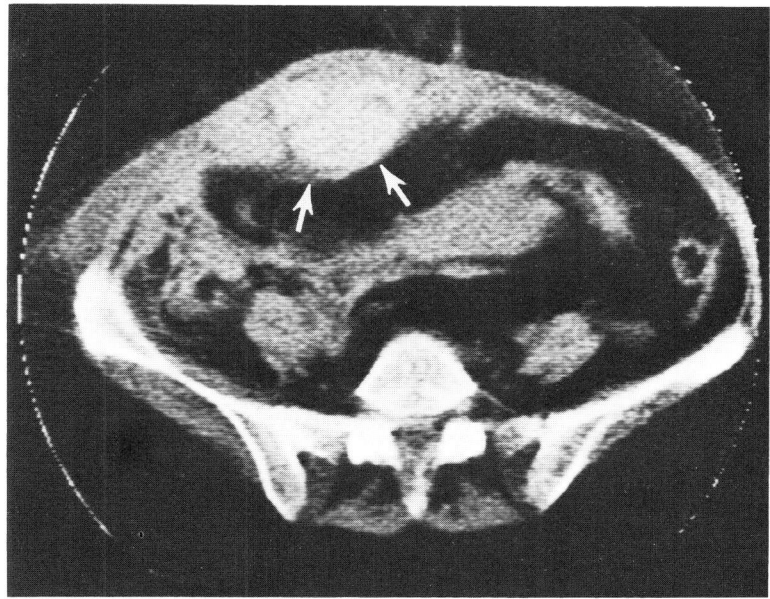

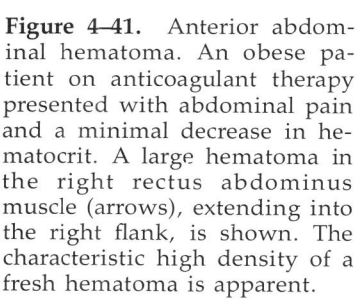

Figure 4–41. Anterior abdominal hematoma. An obese patient on anticoagulant therapy presented with abdominal pain and a minimal decrease in hematocrit. A large hematoma in the right rectus abdominus muscle (arrows), extending into the right flank, is shown. The characteristic high density of a fresh hematoma is apparent.

If a hematoma is studied serially over the course of several weeks, the attenuation value will be found to decrease gradually to the level of a seroma (12 to 24 Hounsfield units), and presuming no further bleeding occurs, the size of the mass will also decrease.[33] The changing size and decreasing attenuation value are reassuring signs that the diagnosis of hematoma is correct when the clinical circumstances at the time of the initial scan do not necessarily support that impression.

VASCULAR DISEASE. The abdominal aorta and inferior vena cava are clearly imaged by CT. Larger branches and tributaries, such as the iliac arteries and veins, the superior mesenteric artery and vein, the celiac axis, and the renal artery and vein, can also be seen. Obstruction of the vena cava by tumor, involvement of the renal veins by intraluminal tumor, aneurysm of the abdominal aorta or its branches, and hemorrhage secondary to the rupture of an aneurysm (see Fig. 4–40) are some of the pathologic processes that can be shown by CT.

Ultrasound is generally the imaging method of choice for evaluating the abdominal aorta when the presence of aneurysm is suspected, since it can rapidly display the aorta both longitudinally and cross-sectionally. In addition, it can differentiate the lumen of the aorta from the surrounding wall of clot and grumous material. When obesity or marked ileus accompanied by excessive gas in the small and large bowel results in an uninterpretable ultrasound examination, or when the presence of aneurysm is clinically unsuspected, CT is effective in showing the size and the extent of the aneurysm. The flowing blood within the lumen is enhanced with the intravenous infusion of contrast medium, thus allowing differentiation of the lumen from the surrounding wall. Extravasated blood into the adjacent retroperitoneal space from a slowly leaking aneurysm can also be identified, clarifying a confusing clinical situation and alerting the surgeon to the gravity of the patient's condition.

Primary tumors of blood vessels have been identified with CT, although there is nothing characteristic about the CT appearance of these mass lesions to differentiate them from other retroperitoneal tumors.

Pelvis

Certain aspects of pelvic anatomy are advantageous for CT evaluation. The pelvic organs, muscle groups, blood vessels, and lymph nodes are either in the midline or bilaterally symmetric. Tissue planes and organs are normally well defined by contiguous peripelvic fat. Anatomic relationships are kept constant by the confines of the bony pelvis, and respiratory motion is rarely a problem in pelvic CT scans.[43]

If sufficient pelvic fat is present, pelvic vessels and associated lymph nodes can be identified. Vessels and lymph nodes appear as clusters of round, soft tissue densities on the CT scans. Arteries can often be identified by calcification within the wall, but the relationship of veins to adjacent lymph nodes is not constant, so that it is difficult to differentiate between these normal structures. There are no absolute criteria for the size of normal lymph nodes on pelvic scans, but nodes greater than 10 mm in diameter should be considered suspect. Lymph nodes generally are smaller than adjacent vessels and of similar size bilaterally.

CT can be utilized to evaluate mass lesions that are both extrinsic and intrinsic to the genitourinary organs. Based upon the attenuation value and the clinical history, it has been possible to identify and usually to differentiate abscesses, hematomas, lymphoceles, and cystic lesions within the pelvis. Since overlap exists in the attenuation values of abscess, hematoma, and necrotic tumor, differentiation of these entities may not be possible if the clinical history is complex.

In the evaluation of presacral masses, CT may be used to confirm their presence as well as to characterize their tissue composition. The presence of fat- or water-density material within a presacral mass not only helps to differentiate it from a solid tumor but also may suggest its specific histologic nature (for example, that of a dermoid cyst containing fat-density material). CT is also useful in showing that no presacral mass exists when the opposite possibility has been suggested by physical examination or another radiographic study.

Pelvic lipomatosis may mimic a presacral or pelvic mass by producing displacement and straightening of the rectosigmoid on a barium-contrast study of the colon. Although the diagnosis may be suggested on the barium enema examination, the tissue characterization on the CT scan is definitive.[14, 43]

CT has been used both to define the initial extent of biopsy-proven soft tissue

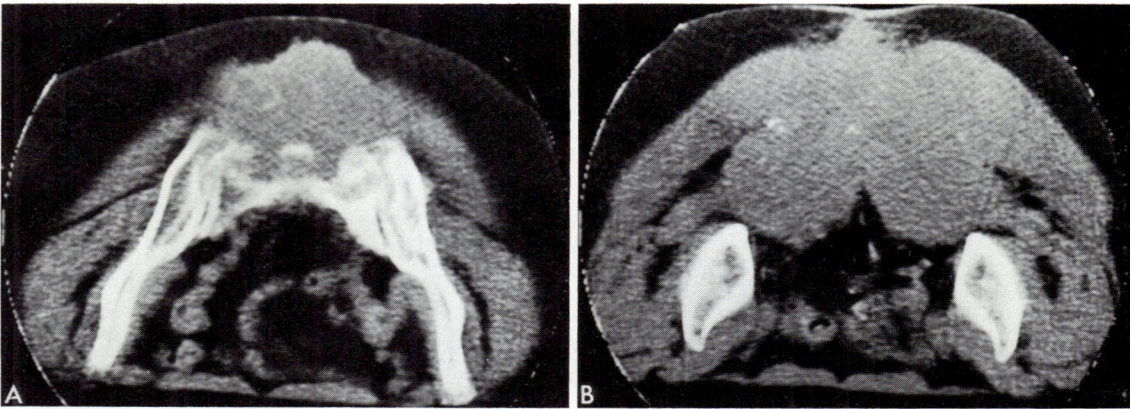

Figure 4–42. Recurrent chordoma. *A,* The destruction of the sacrum and a large posterior extension of recurrent chordoma are well demonstrated at the sacroiliac joint level on this prone scan. *B,* A scan several centimeters caudad reveals unanticipated massive intrapelvic extension of the tumor, a finding of considerable importance in the planning of radiation therapy.

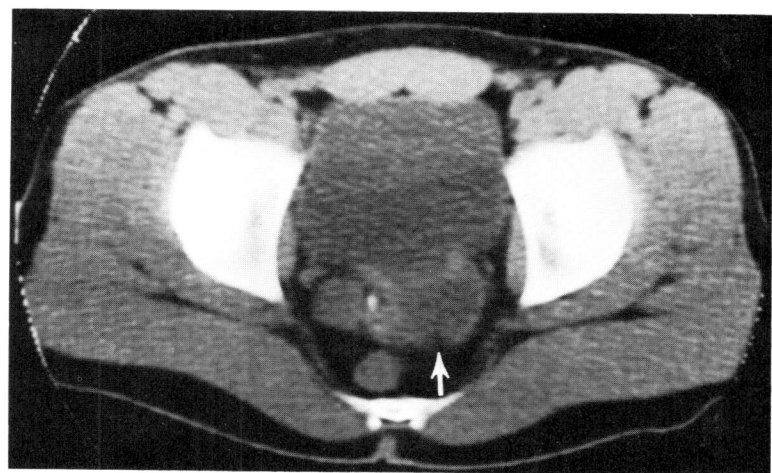

Figure 4–43. This CT scan demonstrates cystic dilatation of the left seminal vesicle (arrow). An adjacent calcific density represents a phlebolith. The right seminal vesicle appears normal. (*From* Semin. Roentgenol. 13:193–200, 1978. Reproduced by permission.)

tumors of the pelvis and to follow the therapeutic response of these tumors, thereby obviating the need for more invasive procedures.[39] CT is able to define the extent of soft tissue involvement by primary and metastatic tumors of the pelvic bones (Fig. 4–42). The plain radiographic film findings in some cases of pelvic bone tumor fail to demonstrate the extent of extraosseous involvement.[12, 48, 68]

CT is occasionally valuable in assessing disease within the pelvic genitourinary organs. Mass lesions within the uterus, ovary, prostate gland, or seminal vesicle can be detected when the lesion produces either an alteration in the normal size and shape of the organ or a focal change in the attenuation value of the organ (Fig. 4–43). If such morphologic changes are lacking, CT is unable to detect the lesion. Moreover, the information provided by CT does not allow differentiation between benignancy and malignancy if the mass in question is well circumscribed.

CT can be used to localize an undescended testicle in the teenaged or adult male. At present, two invasive techniques, water-soluble contrast herniography and selective gonadal venography, are the only other radiologic approaches to this clinical problem. If the testicle does not lie in the inguinal canal, little if any information concerning its size can be obtained by these two techniques prior to surgical exploration. Computed tomography may be successful in imaging the normal-sized undescended testicle if it lies close to the internal inguinal ring within the peritoneal cavity (Fig. 4–44). An enlarged undescended testicle involved with tumor (Fig. 4–45) is more easily demonstrated.

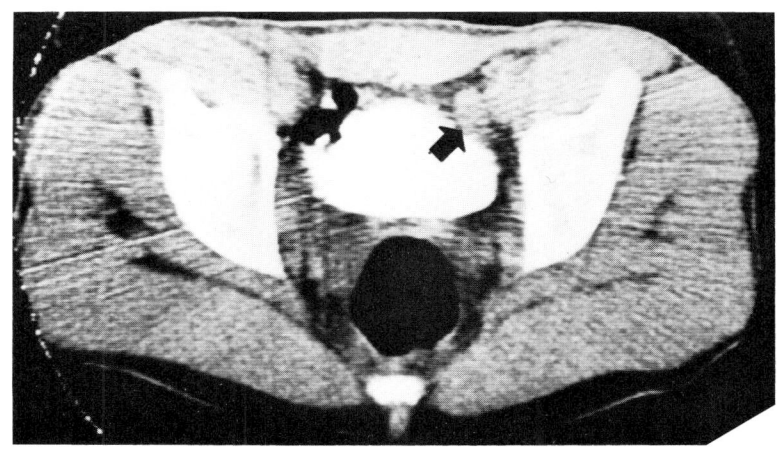

Figure 4–44. A normal-sized undescended left testicle (arrow) is shown lying along the course of the vas deferens proximal to the internal inguinal ring.

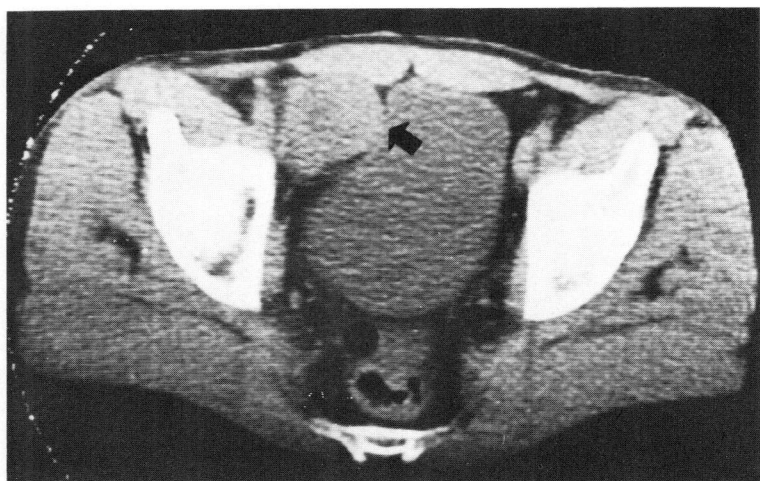

Figure 4–45. An embryonal cell carcinoma enlarges this right-sided undescended testicle (arrow). The central low density corresponds to focal necrosis. (*From* Curr. Radiol. 2:100, 1979. Reproduced by permission.)

CT has been found useful in the staging of genitourinary neoplasms.[69] The lateral spread of tumor from the bladder, prostate gland, or cervix into the peripelvic fat as far as the lateral pelvic wall is seen on CT scans as a poorly marginated soft tissue density extending from the organ involved by the neoplasm.[43] Metastases to pelvic lymph nodes can also be suspected if these lymph nodes are shown to be enlarged.[40] Tumor staging with CT has limitations, however. It has been of little value in determining whether there is minimal extension of prostatic cancer through its capsule. Also, CT is unable to detect metastases to pelvic lymph nodes if the lymph nodes are not enlarged by the metastatic deposit. Despite the presence of a normal-appearing plane of perivisceral fat surrounding the prostate gland, bladder, or uterine cervix, microscopic spread of tumor can be present. Only gross extension of the pelvic neoplasm is identifiable by CT.

Musculoskeletal System

In the examination of the musculoskeletal system, CT may be used to define the nature and extent of clinically unexplained soft tissue masses (Fig. 4–46).[12, 47, 80, 81] In

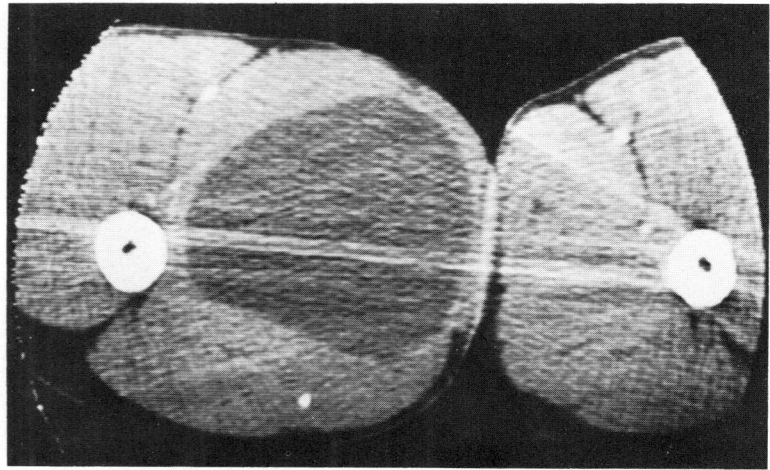

Figure 4–46. Chronic thigh hematoma. A 22-year-old hemophiliac with a mass in the medial aspect of the right thigh for two years was sent for evaluation because of a recent enlargement of the mass. Following the injection of intravenous contrast medium, the scan reveals a homogeneous, low-density (10 EMI units) mass with a slightly enhancing rim consistent with an old hematoma (seroma) and fibrous pseudocapsule. Thin brown fluid was drained at operation.

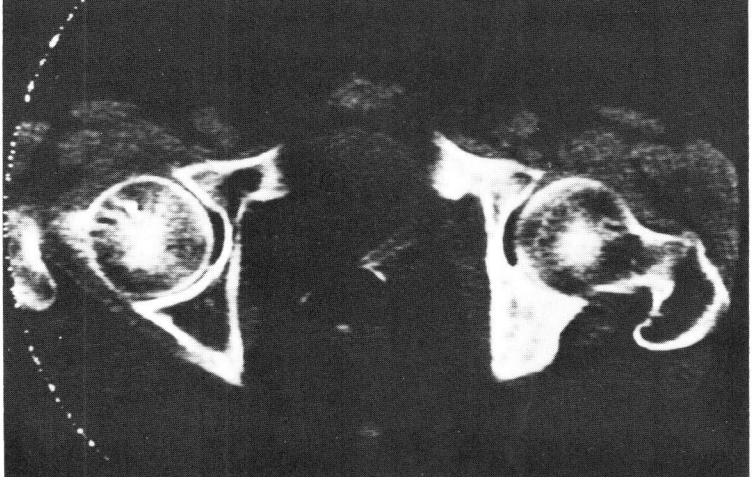

Figure 4–47. Metastatic prostate cancer. A marked increase in density of the left ischium compared with the right is shown in this high window-level view of the pelvis. Increased bone density could not be appreciated, even retrospectively, on plain radiographs of the pelvis.

the evaluation of a primary bone tumor, the use of CT may be indicated if there is a need to determine the soft tissue extent (especially valuable in the investigation of neoplasms of the pelvic bones) or the intramedullary extent of a neoplasm.[4, 68] Additionally, CT can be valuable in the early detection of recurrent tumor in the soft tissues.

CT is rarely of value in the detection or differential diagnosis of primary bone tumors. It may help to distinguish between a parosteal sarcoma and its occasional "look alike," myositis ossificans, however.[29] The CT demonstration of a large soft tissue component may suggest that a chondrosarcoma, rather than an osteochondroma, is present. CT may also reinforce the conventional radiographic impression of a benign bone cyst.

In patients with tumors that are known to metastasize to bone, a careful survey of the bones at the appropriate window settings while scanning the patient for other reasons may reveal one or more unexpected bony metastases (Fig. 4–47). Rarely, in patients with a positive radionuclide bone scan and negative conventional radiographs, CT may demonstrate a lesion compatible with metastatic tumor.

CT has been utilized to show nonunion of a fracture. The anatomic relationships of facial or spinal fractures as well as encroachment of bony spurs on the caliber of the spinal canal may be better and more easily demonstrated on the cross-sectional CT images than on conventional radiologic studies.[48]

CT may also permit an earlier radiologic diagnosis of osteomyelitis.[4] The demonstration of an increase in the density of the marrow space on the CT scan may precede any visible change on a conventional radiograph. The unique cross-sectional view can help distinguish soft tissue inflammation from bony disease. In addition, pure cortical involvement may be differentiated from another process involving the medullary cavity.

RELATIONSHIP OF CT TO RADIONUCLIDE IMAGING AND ULTRASOUND

Other chapters have covered the role of radionuclide imaging and ultrasound in the evaluation of surgical disease (see Chapters 2 and 3). What follows is a brief discussion of the relationships of radionuclide imaging and ultrasound to CT. It should be emphasized that the definition of the clinical role of the new imaging method, CT, has resulted in the constant reassessment of the appropriate uses of the various tests. This state of flux precludes dogmatic statements about which imaging method is most efficacious. Recent experience indicates that these imaging studies are complementary or supplementary, rather than competitive or redundant.[5, 42, 44]

At present, most applications of radionuclide imaging to the thorax, including radiocolloid lung scanning, myocardial imaging, and cardiac function tests, are not competitive with CT. Except in echocardiography and for the localization of pericardial and pleural space fluid collections, ultrasound has a limited role in the examination of the thorax. Therefore, this section primarily concerns abdominal and musculoskeletal considerations.

Radionuclide Imaging

The radionuclide liver scan, which demonstrates labeled colloidal agents accumulated by the reticuloendothelial system, is a sensitive screening test for suspected focal liver disease. Its specificity is low, however. Anatomic variants, primary and secondary tumors, benign cysts, abscesses, regenerating nodules, and a variety of other focal lesions can all produce focal defects of similar appearance. Computed tomography has been most useful in clarifying the nature of these focal defects.[5, 72]

At present, radionuclide imaging plays a minor role in the evaluation of jaundiced patients. Newer hepatobiliary radiopharmaceuticals, such as technetium-labeled pyridoxylidene-glutamate and the imidodiacetic acid derivatives, are being evaluated in laboratory and clinical trials in an effort to define their clinical roles. Although they may prove helpful in the diagnosis of acute cholecystitis, there is little evidence to suggest that they are as effective as CT, ultrasound, percutaneous transhepatic cholangiography, or endoscopic retrograde cholangiography in the critical separation of hepatocellular from surgical jaundice and in defining the cause of the latter.[57]

Gallium scanning has been shown to provide a reliably sensitive survey of the patient with suspected abscess. Its role in tumor detection is less well defined. The gallium scan has the advantage of providing a whole-body survey and is not confined to a specific organ or area. It is a nonspecific test, however, and positive results (persisting focal accumulation of the radionuclide) can be obtained in scans of a variety of inflammatory conditions, such as acute pyelonephritis, ascending cholangitis, ulcerative colitis, and radiation proctitis as well as scans of frank abscess formation and neoplasm. The activity within healing wounds and the prolonged retention of the radionuclide within the colon—its normal route of excretion—can also cause confusion. The test requires a minimum delay of 24 hours following injection, and follow-up scans at 48 and 72 hours are frequently required.

A recent review of patients suspected of having an abscess and evaluated with CT and gallium scans indicated a complementary, rather than competitive, role for these two imaging methods.[44] According to the results of this study, patients with suspected abscess fall into two categories: those with focal or localizing findings and those without. CT provides the most rapid and direct assessment of those patients with focal findings. At a less emergent pace, the gallium scan localizes the inflammatory process in those patients with few, if any, focal signs and symptoms, thereby providing a target for clarification with CT.

At present, renal CT is primarily concerned with the demonstration of morphologic change. On the other hand, morphologic findings are usually incidental on the function-oriented radionuclide renal scan. Thus, the indications for these two tests rarely overlap.

Radionuclide bone scanning provides a complete skeletal survey, which is most often followed up with conventional radiography when the results of the scan suggest metastases or other causes of abnormal bone metabolism. CT normally does not compete with the radionuclide bone scan but may incidentally display a clinically unsuspected bone metastasis. The primary role of CT in the investigation of musculoskeletal disorders is to define the extent of disease rather than to detect or diagnose the process definitively.

Owing to the limited availability of the imaging agents ^{131}I-19-iodocholesterol and ^{131}I-6-β-NOR-iodomethylcholesterol (NP59), scanning of the adrenal glands has not had a major impact on the surgical management of adrenal disease. A minimum delay of 72 hours postinjection is required to obtain a valid scan. Adrenal scintigraphy has been shown to be useful in the diagnosis of adrenal cortical hyperfunctioning states, especially Cushing's disease.[78, 79] A diagnostic accuracy approaching 100 per cent may be achieved in cases of functioning adenoma. The results are not as good in cases of adrenal hyperplasia and carcinoma, but concomitant biochemical studies may strongly implicate bilateral hyperplasia as the cause of the syndrome. Adrenal scintigraphy has an accuracy rate of 80 per cent in the diagnostic evaluation of autonomous hypersecretion of aldosterone (Conn's syndrome) but yields both false positive and false negative results.

When CT cannot definitively distinguish between an adenoma and bilateral hyperplasia, scintigraphy may be helpful. CT is capable of imaging both the normal and the abnormal adrenal gland with considerably greater consistency than the radionuclide method, it involves no delay, and disease processes other than hyperfunctioning cortical tumors (for example, pheochromocytoma and metastatic tumor) can be imaged. The precise demonstration of morphologic detail possible with CT should make it the screening test of choice.[30, 60]

Ultrasound

Considerable overlap exists in the clinical indications for the use of CT and ultrasound to examine the abdomen. General considerations, related to body habitus, amount of gas in the bowel, overlying bone, and clinical expertise, enter into the choice of the initial imaging technique. Air and bone greatly impede the transmission of sound, and abundant fat has a similar, but less pronounced, effect. Thus, an obese patient with gaseous distention of the small and large bowel is a poor candidate for ultrasound evaluation of the pancreas. The same patient can be successfully studied with CT. The marked absence of body fat makes interpretation of abdominal scans more difficult, since the clear delineation of anatomic structures within the abdomen depends to a large extent on the presence of adequate perivisceral fat. An asthenic patient is generally better studied with ultrasound.

Biologic motion (respiratory, cardiac, peristaltic) has a degrading effect on the CT scan, resulting in volume averaging and motion artifacts. This factor assumes less importance as newer CT units, with scanning times of 2 to 5 seconds, have emerged.

Assuming that the study of the organ or area can be technically accomplished, ultrasound and CT show nearly equal capabilities in the evaluation of the liver, pancreas, and kidneys. Ultrasound currently provides more information on the major abdominal blood vessels, owing to its multiplane capability. However, CT has an advantage in the evaluation of the entire retroperitoneum (for example, the assessment of lymph nodes), since bowel gas does not interfere with the quality of the image. Although the adrenal gland can be imaged with ultrasound, CT provides a rapid and precise delineation of the normal and the pathologic adrenal gland in nearly all cases, and it is much more easily accomplished; it should be the first choice of imaging method, except for the patient with a very thin body habitus.

Ultrasound has unique obstetric applications, and CT does not compete in this area. However, ultrasound is of little use in the evaluation of lesions contiguous to the lateral pelvic walls, such as enlarged lymph nodes, or of the lateral spread of prostatic or cervical carcinoma.

Large fluid collections, including ascites, cysts and pseudocysts of various organs, abscesses, hematomas, urinomas, and lymphoceles, are equally well imaged with ultrasound and CT. Because it does not use ionizing radiation, ultrasound should be the primary imaging technique in these cases. Clinical conditions such as persisting ileus, interfering wound dressings, or a location beneath the ribs frequently eliminate ultrasound as the imaging technique of choice.

As experience broadens with the use of both imaging methods, appropriate patterns of utilization will evolve that will capitalize on the complementary aspect of each.

References

1. Alcorn, F. S., Mategrano, V. C., Petasnick, J. P., et al.: Contributions of computed tomography in the staging and management of malignant lymphoma. Radiology 125:717–723, 1977.
2. Alfidi, R. J., MacIntyre, W. J., and Haaga, J. R.: The effects of biological motion on CT resolution. Am. J. Roentgenol. 127:11–15, 1976.
3. Aronberg, D. J., Stanley, R. J., Levitt, R. G., et al.: The evaluation of abdominal abscess with computed tomography. J. Comput. Assist. Tomogr. 2:384–387, 1978.
4. Berger, P. E., and Kuhn, J. P.: Computed tomography of tumors of the musculoskeletal system in children. Radiology 127:171–175, 1978.
5. Biello, D. R., Levitt, R. G., Siegel, B. A., et al.: Computed tomography and radionuclide imaging of the liver. A comparative evaluation. Radiology 127:159–164, 1978.
6. Breiman, R. S., Castellino, R. A., Harell, G. S., et al.: CT—pathologic correlations in Hodgkin's disease and non-Hodgkin's lymphoma. Radiology 126:159–166, 1978.
7. Brooks, R. A., and DiChiro, G.: Theory of image reconstruction in computed tomography. Radiology 117:561–572, 1975.
8. Brownlie, K., and Kreel, L.: Computer assisted tomography of normal suprarenal glands. J. Comput. Assist. Tomogr. 2:1–10, 1978.
9. Callen, P. W., Korobkin, M., and Isherwood, I.: Computed tomographic evaluation of the retrocrural prevertebral space. Am. J. Roentgenol. 129:907–910, 1977.
10. Carter, B. L., and Ignatow, S. B.: Neck and mediastinal angiography by computed tomography scan. Radiology 122:515–516, 1977.
11. Crowe, J. K., Brown, L. R., and Muhm, J. R.: Computed tomography of the mediastinum. Radiology 128:75–87, 1978.
12. deSantos, L. A., Goldstein, H. M., Murray, J. A., et al.: Computed tomography in the evaluation of musculoskeletal neoplasms. Radiology 128:89–94, 1978.
13. Emami, B., Melo, A., Carter, B. L., et al.: Value of computed tomography in radiotherapy of lung cancer. Am. J. Roentgenol. 131:63–67, 1978.
14. Gerson, E. S., Gerzof, S. G., and Robbins, A. H.: CT confirmation of pelvic lipomatosis. Am. J. Roentgenol. 119:338–340, 1977.
15. Haaga, J. R., Alfidi, R. J., Havrilla, T. R., et al.: CT detection and aspiration of abdominal abscesses. Am. J. Roentgenol. 128:465–474, 1977.
16. Haaga, J. R., Alfidi, R. J., Havrilla, T. R., et al.: Definitive role of CT scanning of the pancreas. Radiology 124:723–730, 1977.
17. Haaga, H. R., Reich, N. E., Havrilla, T. R., et al.: Interventional CT scanning. Radiol. Clin. North Am. 15:449–456, 1977.
18. Haaga, J. R., Baldwin, G. N., Reich, N. E., et al.: CT detection of infected synthetic grafts: preliminary report of a new sign. Am. J. Roentgenol. 131:317–320, 1978.
19. Hacker, H., and Becker, H.: Time controlled computed tomography angiography. J. Comput. Assist. Tomogr. 1:405–409, 1977.
20. Harell, G. S., Breiman, R. S., Glatstein, E. J., et al.: Computed tomography of the abdomen in the malignant lymphomas. Radiol. Clin. North Am. 15:391–400, 1977.

21. Hattery, R. R., Williamson, B., Stephens, D. H., et al.: Computed tomography of renal abnormalities. Radiol. Clin. North Am. *15*:401–418, 1977.
22. Havrilla, T. R., Haaga, J. R., Alfidi, R. J., et al.: Computed tomography and obstructive biliary disease. Am. J. Roentgenol. *128*:765–768, 1977.
23. Havrilla, T. R., Reich, N. E., Haaga, J. R., et al.: Computed tomography of the gallbladder. Am. J. Roentgenol. *130*:1059–1067, 1978.
24. Heitzman, E. R., Goldwin, R. L., and Proto, A. V.: Radiologic analysis of the mediastinum utilizing computed tomography. Radiol. Clin. North Am. *15*:309–329, 1977.
25. Hounsfield, G. N.: Computerized transverse axial scanning (tomography). I. Description of system. Br. J. Radiol. *46*:1016–1022, 1973.
26. Hounsfield, G. N.: Picture quality of computed tomography. Am. J. Roentgenol. *127*:3–9, 1976.
27. Javadpour, N., Doppman, J. L., Bergman, S. M., et al.: Correlation of computed tomography and serum markers in metastatic retroperitoneal testicular tumor. J. Comput. Assist. Tomogr. *2*:176–180, 1978.
28. Jost, R. G., Sagel, S. S., Stanley, R. J., et al.: Computed tomography of the thorax. Radiology *126*:125–136, 1978.
29. Kagan, A. R., and Steckel, R. J.: Heterotopic new bone formation myositis ossificans versus malignant tumor. Am. J. Roentgenol. *130*:773–776, 1978.
30. Karstaedt, N., Sagel, S. S., Stanley, R. J., et al.: CT of the adrenal gland. Radiology *129*:723–730, 1978.
31. Kirkpatrick, R. H., Wittenberg, J., Schaffer, D. L., et al.: Scanning techniques in computed body tomography. Am. J. Roentgenol. *130*:1069–1075, 1978.
32. Kollins, S. A.: Computed tomography of the pulmonary parenchyma and chest wall. Radiol. Clin. North Am. *15*:297–308, 1977.
33. Korobkin, M., Moss, A. A., Callen, P. W., et al.: Computed tomography of splenic subcapsular hematomas: a clinical and experimental study. Radiology *129*:441–445, 1978.
34. Kreel, L.: The EMI whole body scanner in the demonstration of lymph node enlargement. Clin. Radiol. *27*:421–429, 1976.
35. Kreel, L.: Computerized tomography using the EMI general purpose scanner. Br. J. Radiol. *50*:2–14, 1977.
36. Kreel, L., Haertel, M., and Katz, D.: Computed tomography of the normal pancreas. J. Comput. Assist. Tomogr. *1*:290–299, 1977.
37. Kressel, H. Y., Korobkin, M., Goldberg, H. I., et al.: The portal venous tree simulating dilated biliary ducts on computed tomography of the liver. J. Comput. Assist. Tomogr. *1*:169–175, 1977.
38. Lee, J. K. T., Stanley, R. J., Sagel, S. S., et al.: Accuracy of computed tomography in detecting intra-abdominal and pelvic adenopathy in lymphoma. Am. J. Roentgenol. *131*:311–315, 1978.
39. Lee, J. K. T., Levitt, R. G., Stanley, R. J., et al.: The utility of computed body tomography in the clinical follow-up of abdominal masses. J. Comput. Assist. Tomogr. *2*:607–611, 1978.
40. Lee, J. K. T., Stanley, R. J., Sagel, S. S., et al.: Accuracy of CT in detecting intraabdominal and pelvic lymph node metastases from pelvic lymph node metastases from pelvic cancers. Am. J. Roentgenol. *131*:675–679, 1978.
41. Levitt, R. G., Sagel, S. S., Stanley, R. J., et al.: Accuracy of computed tomography of the liver and biliary tree. Radiology *124*:123–128, 1977.
42. Levitt, R. G., Geisse, G., Sagel, S. S., et al.: Complementary use of ultrasound and computed tomography in studies of the pancreas and kidney. Radiology *126*:149–152, 1978.
43. Levitt, R. G., Sagel, S. S., Stanley, R. J., et al.: Computed tomography of the pelvis. Semin. Roentgenol. *13*:193–200, 1978.
44. Levitt, R. G., Biello, D. R., Sagel, S. S., et al.: Role of computed tomography and Ga-67 citrate radionuclide imaging in the evaluation of suspected abdominal abscess. Am. J. Roentgenol. *132*:529–534, 1979.
45. Levitt, R. G., Sagel, S. S., and Stanley, R. J.: Detection of neoplastic involvement of the mesentery and omentum by computed tomography. Am. J. Roentgenol. *131*:835–838, 1978.
46. Mategrano, V. C., Petasnick, J., Clark, J., et al.: Attenuation values in computed tomography of the abdomen. Radiology *125*:135–140, 1977.
47. McLeod, R. A., Gisvold, J. J., Stephens, D. H., et al.: Computed tomography of soft tissues and breast. Semin. Roentgenol. *13*:267–275, 1978.
48. McLeod, R. S., Stephens, D. H., Beabout, J. W., et al.: Computed tomography of the skeletal system. Semin. Roentgenol. *13*:235–247, 1978.
49. Mink, J. H., Bein, M. E., Sukor, R., et al.: Computed tomography of the anterior mediastinum in patients with myasthenia gravis and suspected thymoma. Am. J. Roentgenol. *130*:239–246, 1978.
50. Montagne, J. P., Kressel, H. Y., Korobkin, M., et al.: Computed tomography of the normal adrenal glands. Am. J. Roentgenol. *130*:963–966, 1978.
51. Moss, A. A., Kressel, H. Y., Korobkin, M., et al.: The effect of Gastrografin and glucagon on CT scanning of the pancreas: a blind clinical trial. Radiology *126*:711–714, 1978.
52. Muhm, J. R., Brown, L. R., and Crowe, J. K.: Use of computed tomography in the detecting of pulmonary nodules. Mayo Clin. Proc. *52*:345–348, 1977.
53. Munzenrider, J. E., Pilepich, M., Rene-Ferrero, J. B., et al.: Use of body scanner in radiotherapy treatment planning. Cancer *40*:170–179, 1977.
54. Petasnick, J. P.: Normal anatomy as seen on the abdominal computed tomogram. Crit. Rev. Diagn. Imag. *10*:291–323, 1978.

55. Pistolesi, G. F., Marzoli, G. P., Colosso, P. Q., et al.: Computed tomography in surgical pancreatic emergencies. J. Comput. Assist. Tomogr. 2:165–169, 1978.
56. Rohlfing, B. M., Korobkin, M., and Hall, A. D.: Computed tomography of intrathoracic omental herniation and other mediastinal fatty masses. J. Comput. Assist. Tomogr. 1:181–183, 1977.
57. Ronai, P. M.: Hepatobiliary radiopharmaceuticals: defining their clinical role will be a galling experience. J. Nucl. Med. 18:488–490, 1977.
58. Sagel, S. S., Stanley, R. J., and Evens, R. G.: Early clinical experience with motionless whole body computed tomography. Radiology 119:321–330, 1976.
59. Sagel, S. S., Siegel, M. J., Stanley, R. J., et al.: Detection of retroperitoneal hemorrhage by computed tomography. Am. J. Roentgenol. 129:403–407, 1977.
60. Sagel, S. S., Stanley, R. J., Levitt, R. G., et al.: Computed tomography of the kidney. Radiology 124:359–370, 1977.
61. Sagel, S. S., Weiss, E. S., Gillard, R. G., et al.: Gated computed tomography of the human heart. Invest. Radiol. 12:563–566, 1977.
62. Sample, W. F., and Sarti, D. A.: Computed tomography and grey scale ultrasonography of the adrenal gland: a comparative study. Radiology 128:377–383, 1978.
63. Schaner, E. G., Balow, J. E., and Doppman, J. L.: Computed tomography in the diagnosis of subcapsular and perirenal hematoma. Am. J. Roentgenol. 129:83–88, 1977.
64. Schaner, E. G., Head, G. L., Doppman, J. L., et al.: Computed tomography in the diagnosis, staging and management of abdominal lymphoma. J. Comput. Assist. Tomogr. 1:176–180, 1977.
65. Schaner, E. G., Chang, A. E., Doppman, J. L., et al.: Comparison of computed and conventional whole lung tomography in detecting pulmonary nodules: a prospective radiologic-pathologic study. Am. J. Roentgenol. 131:51–54, 1978.
66. Schaner, E. G., Dunnick, N. R., Doppman, J. L., et al.: Adrenal cortical tumors with low attenuation coefficients: a pitfall in computed tomography diagnosis. J. Comput. Assist. Tomogr. 2:11–15, 1978.
67. Scherer, V., Rainer, R., Eisenburg, J., et al.: Diagnostic accuracy of CT in circumscript liver disease. Am. J. Roentgenol. 130:711–714, 1978.
68. Schumacher, T., Genant, H. K., Korobkin, M. T., et al.: Computerized tomography: its use in space-occupying lesions of the musculoskeletal system. J. Bone Joint Surg. 60:600–607, 1978.
69. Seidelmann, F. E., Cohen, W. N., and Bryan, P. J.: Computed tomographic staging of bladder neoplasms. Radiol. Clin. North Am. 15:419–440, 1977.
70. Sheedy, P. F., Stephens, D. H., Hattery, R. R., et al.: Computed tomography in the evaluation of patients with suspected carcinoma of the pancreas. Radiology 124:731–737, 1977.
71. Stanley, R. J., Sagel, S. S., and Levitt, R. G.: Computed tomography of the body: early trends in application and accuracy of the method. Am. J. Roentgenol. 126:53–67, 1976.
72. Stanley, R. J., Sagel, S. S., and Levitt, R. G.: Computed tomography of the liver. Radiol. Clin. North Am. 15:331–348, 1977.
73. Stanley, R. J., Sagel, S. S., and Levitt, R. G.: Computed tomography of the pancreas. Radiology 124:715–722, 1977.
74. Steele, J. R., Sones, P. J., and Heffner, L. T.: The detection of inferior vena caval thrombosis with computed tomography. Radiology 128:385–386, 1978.
75. Stephens, D. H., Sheedy, P. F., Hattery, R. R., et al.: Computed tomography of the liver. Am. J. Roentgenol. 128:579–590, 1977.
76. Stephens, D. H., Sheedy, P. F., Hattery, R. R., et al.: Diagnosis and evaluation of retroperitoneal tumors by computed tomography. Am. J. Roentgenol. 129:395–402, 1977.
77. Stephens, D. H., Williamson, B., Sheedy, P. F., et al.: Computed tomography of the retroperitoneal space. Radiol. Clin. North Am. 15:377–390, 1977.
78. Troncone, L., Galli, G., Salvo, D., et al.: Radioisotopic study of the adrenal glands using ^{131}I-19-iodocholesterol. Br. J. Radiol. 50:340–349, 1977.
79. Wahner, H. W., Northcutt, R. C., and Salassa, R. M.: Adrenal scanning: usefulness in adrenal hyperfunction. Clin. Nucl. Med. 2:253–264, 1977.
80. Weinberger, G., and Levinsohn, E. M.: Computed tomography in the evaluation of sarcomatous tumors of the thigh. Am. J. Roentgenol. 130:115–118, 1978.
81. Wilson, J. S., Korobkin, M., Genant, H. K., et al.: Computed tomography of musculoskeletal disorders. Am. J. Roentgenol. 131:55–61, 1978.
82. Zatz, L. M.: Basic principles of computed tomography. In Korobkin, M. (ed.): Computed Tomography, Ultrasound and X-ray: An Integrated Approach. San Francisco, University of California Press, 1978, pp. 27–43.

5

THE ACUTE ABDOMEN

ANTONIO F. GOVONI, M.D.
JOSEPH P. WHALEN, M.D.

The radiographic examination and the interpretation of radiographic evidence in the clinical setting of the acute abdomen are challenging. Many specific diagnoses may be made on a plain radiograph, whereas others may require further investigation by contrast studies with barium, ultrasound, arteriography, and CT scans. In some causes of an acute abdomen the radiologic examination is of no benefit. This chapter will attempt to formulate an approach to the interpretation of the plain radiographs of the abdomen as well as suggest other radiologic procedures that may help in the difficult differential diagnosis.

For adequate interpretation of a plain radiograph of the abdomen, knowledge of the basic anatomy and the interrelationships of organ systems is essential. Many times the clinical presentation and the radiologic appearance of a disease process in one organ system is overshadowed by abnormalities of adjacent systems. For instance, an acute abdominal process may give clinical and radiologic manifestations of an extraperitoneal disease. In the past, anatomy has been taught by means of a dissectional approach, separating the organ systems; there exists, however, a relationship between the intra- and extraperitoneal organs that explains the confusing clinical and radiologic picture. Consequently, the anatomy of the abdomen will be shown (Fig. 5–1), followed by a discussion of how this anatomy is reflected on a plain radiograph (Fig. 5–2).

This chapter will deal first with the acute abdomen as it presents in a "virgin" abdomen. Second, the more difficult problem of postoperative complications as a result of either progressive disease or surgical intervention will be discussed.

170 — THE ACUTE ABDOMEN

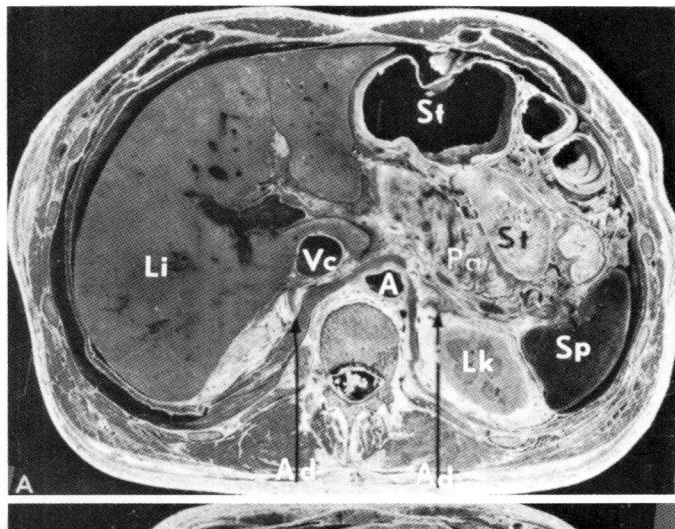

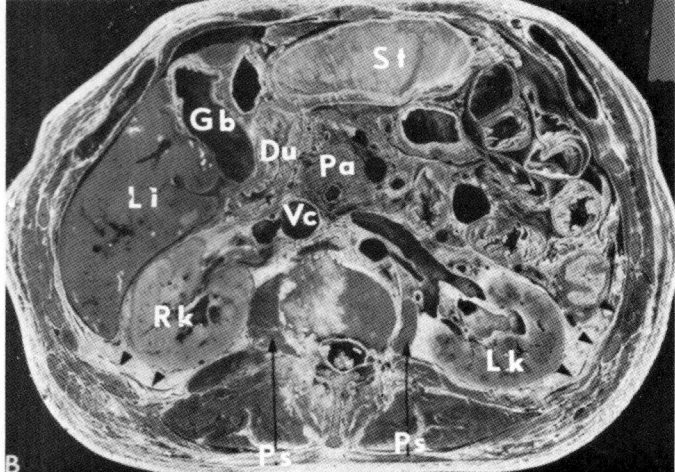

Figure 5–1 *A,* Horizontal section at the level of the hilus of the spleen (Sp). Perirenal fat separates it from the left kidney (Lk). The pancreas (Pa) is anterior to the left kidney and in close contact with the posterior wall of the stomach (St). Note the left and right adrenal glands (Ad arrows) within the rich extraperitoneal fat. Li = liver; A = aorta; Vc = vena cava. *B,* This section is at the level of the junction of the duodenal bulb and pancreas (Pa). The visceral surface of the liver surrounds the lateral surface of the right kidney (Rk). The renal fascia (arrowheads) divides the extraperitoneal space into the perirenal space, which surrounds the kidney, and the pararenal space, external to the renal fascia. The extraperitoneal fat surrounds the kidneys (Rk, Lk) and the psoas muscles (Ps arrows). The gallbladder (Gb) lies anterior and lateral to the descending duodenum (Du). Medial to the duodenum is the head of the pancreas (Pa). The inferior vena cava (Vc) is medial and posterior to the descending duodenum. The stomach (St) lies in the anterior portion of the abdomen. (*From* Whalen, J. P.: Radiology of the Abdomen. An Anatomic Approach. Philadelphia, Lea & Febiger, 1976. Reproduced by permission.)

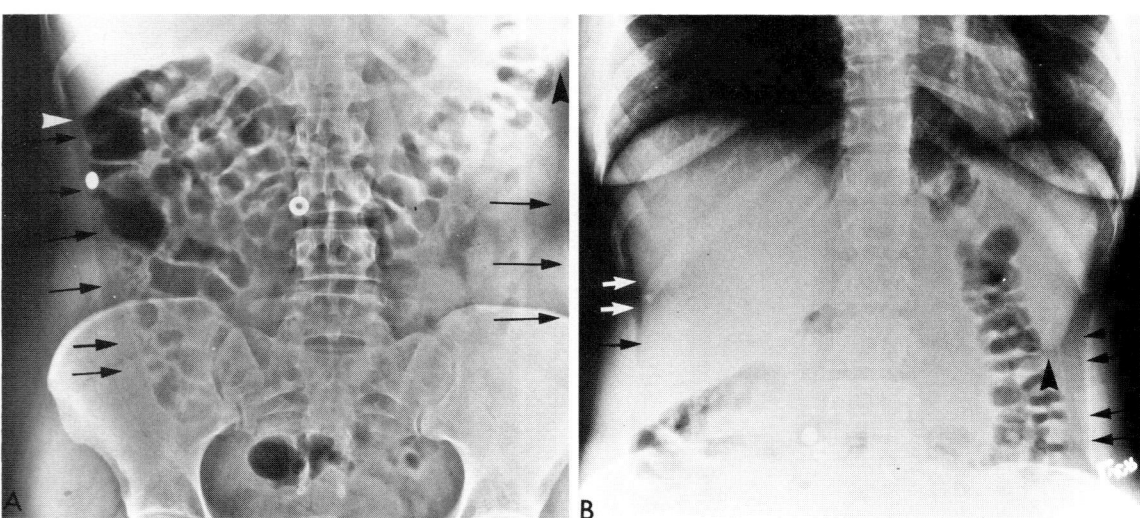

Figure 5–2. Supine *(A)* and upright *(B)* radiographs of the abdomen showing the hepatic angle (white arrowhead), the properitoneal fat stripes (arrows), and the splenic angle (black arrowhead).

ANATOMIC CONSIDERATIONS

Figure 5–1 illustrates organ relationships as they appear in horizontal sections of the abdomen. The peritoneal cavity is not entirely anterior, and there are portions of the extraperitoneal (retroperitoneal) space extending far ventrally. Conversely, the liver and the posterior portion of the spleen are quite far posterior and are as intimately related to the extraperitoneal fat as are the kidneys and the psoas muscles. Further, the pancreas, though an extraperitoneal organ, is very far ventral and has a relationship to the duodenum, the stomach, and the transverse colon. The gallbladder, an intraperitoneal structure, is lateral to the descending duodenum and much more anterior than the posterior portion of the liver or the kidney. The ureters course laterally and ventrally to the psoas muscle but are in close relationship to the ileum, the appendix, and the pelvic structures. The transverse mesocolon (Fig. 5–3) separates processes that are above and below the mesocolon. The realization that certain organs are above the mesocolon and others below it allows a rational approach to the localization of pathologic processes arising from infra- and supramesocolic structures.

Moreover, the intraperitoneal space is separated into various compartments by ligamentous structures. In and around the liver there are multiple spaces that we have separated into those related to the visceral space of the liver (subhepatic) and those above the liver and below the diaphragm (subphrenic).

In the left upper quadrant, the attachment of the stomach to the liver, the spleen, and the pancreas divides the peritoneal cavity into a gastrohepatic recess, a gastrosplenic recess, and a splenorenal recess. The lesser sac is located behind the gastrohepatic recess and medial to the splenorenal recess. Below the mesocolon, the mesentery of the small bowel separates the right half of the abdomen from the left. The ascending colon, which is not on a mesentery, separates the right paracolic gutter from the inframesocolic space medially, as the descending colon separates the left inframesocolic portion from the left paracolic gutter. The phrenicocolic ligament on the left separates the left paracolic gutter from the subphrenic space, while on the right side the paracolic gutter is confluent with the right subphrenic space (Fig. 5–4). The subhepatic (visceral) space of the liver is confined superiorly by the inferior coronary ligament, medially by the descending duodenum, and inferiorly by the transverse mesocolon. Ventrally, the visceral surface of the liver is the anterior border of the right subhepatic space. These compartments of the peritoneal cavity are illustrated in Figures 5–5 through 5–10—drawings of sagittal sections of the abdomen. Figure 5–11 is a plain radiograph of the abdomen with the superimposed anatomic compartments drawn in.

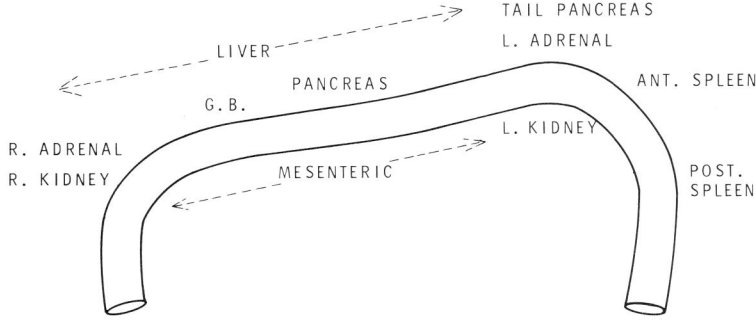

Figure 5–3. Diagrammatic representation of the relationship of the major organs of the abdomen to the colon. (*From* Whalen, J. P.: Radiology of the Abdomen. An Anatomic Approach. Philadelphia, Lea & Febiger, 1976. Reproduced by permission.)

172 — THE ACUTE ABDOMEN

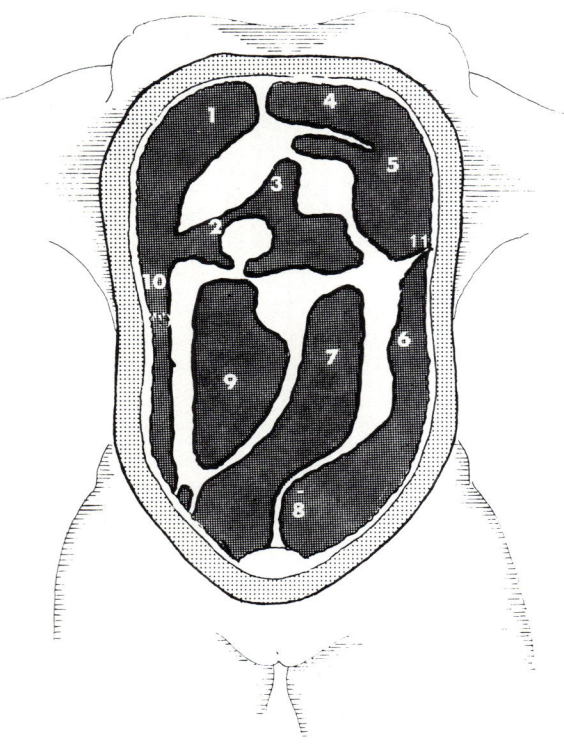

Figure 5–4. Diagram of the peritoneal spaces. *Supramesocolic:* 1. right subphrenic; 2. right subhepatic (visceral); 3. lesser sac; 4. left subphrenic; 5. perisplenic. *Inframesocolic:* 6. Left paracolic; 7. left infracolic; 8. pelvic; 9. right infracolic; 10. right paracolic; 11. phrenicocolic ligament. (*From* Whalen, J. P.: Radiology of the Abdomen. An Anatomic Approach. Philadelphia, Lea & Febiger, 1976. Reproduced by permission.)

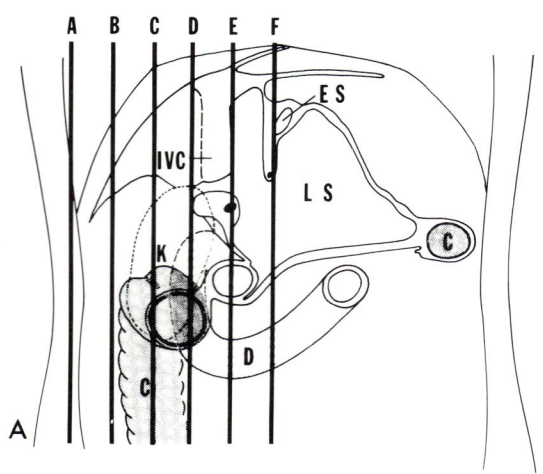
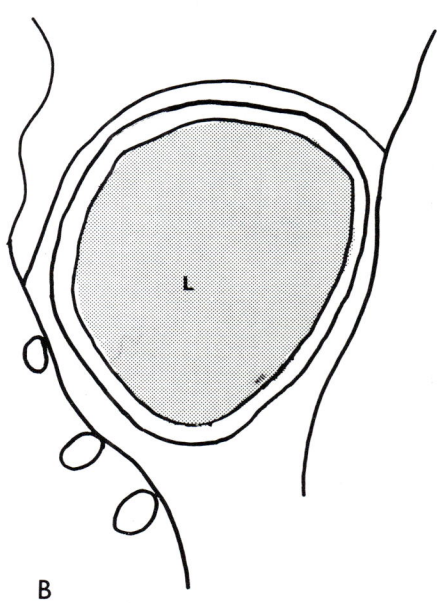

Figure 5–5. *A,* Diagram of peritoneal reflections of the upper abdomen. ES = esophagus; IVC = inferior vena cava; LS = lesser sac; C = colon; D = duodenum; K = right kidney. Lines A through F correspond to the drawings of sagittal sections illustrated in Figures 5–5B to 5–10, respectively. *B,* Drawing of a sagittal section through the liver (L) lateral to the right triangular ligament. Note the confluence of the subhepatic (visceral) and subphrenic spaces. (*From* Whalen, J. P.: Radiology of The Abdomen. An Anatomic Approach. Philadelphia, Lea & Febiger, 1976. Reproduced by permission.)

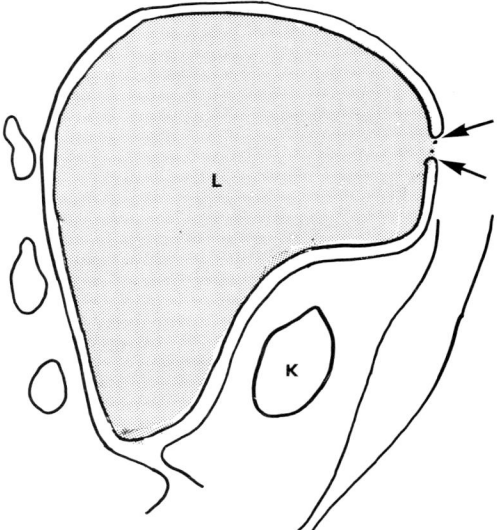

Figure 5–6. Drawing of sagittal section B through the lateral aspect of the right kidney (K). Demonstrated is the attachment of the posterior portion of the liver (L) by the superior and inferior coronary ligaments (arrows). (*From* Whalen, J. P.: Radiology of The Abdomen. An Anatomic Approach, Philadelphia, Lea & Febiger, 1976. Reproduced by permission.)

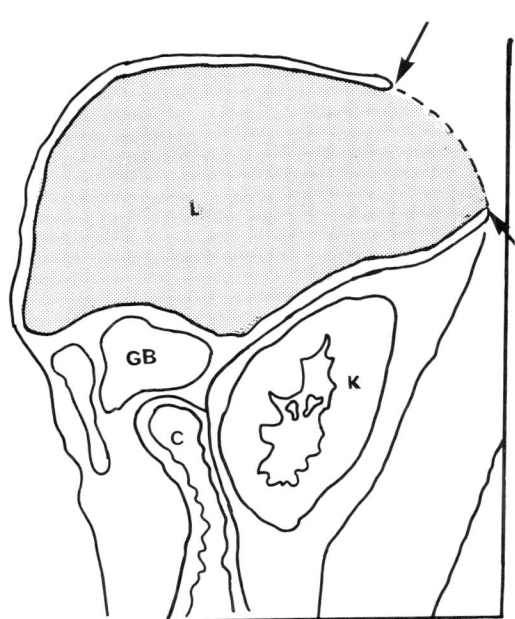

Figure 5–7. Shown in sagittal section C are the coronary ligaments (arrows) and the bare area of the liver (L) between the ligaments. Their separation is at the expense of the posterior subphrenic space. Note the indentation on the visceral surface of the liver produced by the kidney (K) and, anterior to the kidney, the colon (C) and gallbladder (GB). (*From* Whalen, J. P.: Radiology of The Abdomen. An Anatomic Approach. Philadelphia, Lea & Febiger, 1976, Reproduced by permission.)

Figure 5–8. This drawing of section D through the medial aspect of the left kidney shows the descending duodenum (D) interposed between the transverse colon (C) and the kidney (K). The bare area of the liver (L) is between the arrows. P = psoas muscle. (*From* Whalen, J. P.: Radiology of The Abdomen. An Anatomic Approach. Philadelphia, Lea & Febiger, 1976. Reproduced by permission.)

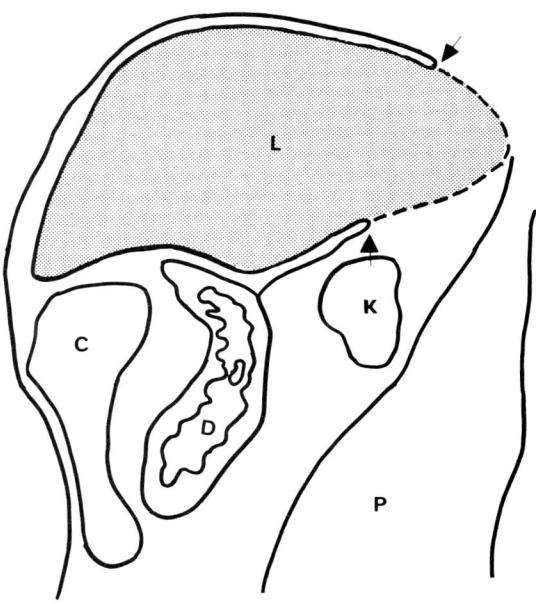

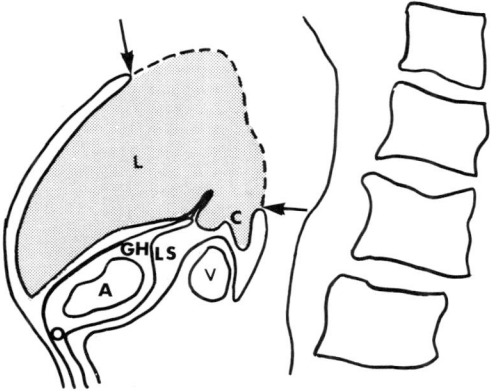

Figure 5–9. This drawing of sagittal section E through the lesser sac demonstrates the wider separation of the superior and inferior coronary ligaments (arrows) and essentially no posterior subphrenic space. A = antrum of the stomach; GH = gastrohepatic ligament (lesser omentum); LS = lesser sac; C = caudate lobe of liver (L); V = portal vein; O = greater omentum. (*From* Whalen, J. P.: Radiology of The Abdomen. An Anatomic Approach. Philadelphia, Lea & Febiger, 1976. Reproduced by permission.)

The extraperitoneal space has abundant fat and extends more anteriorly than portions of the peritoneal cavity. The extraperitoneal space is divided into three compartments. The first is the *perirenal space,* which is around the kidney fat, marginated by the renal capsule (tightly adherent to the kidney) and the renal fascia. Anterior to the renal fascia and behind the parietal peritoneum is the *anterior pararenal space.* This contains the ascending and descending colon, the entire duodenum, and the pancreas. Behind the posterior renal fascia and anterior to the transversalis fascia is the *posterior pararenal space.* This contains the great vessels, nerves, fat, and muscle.

Visualization of structures consistently seen on a plain abdominal radiograph because of fat–soft tissue interface is almost entirely due to the extraperitoneal fat. This fat comes in contact with both intra- and extraperitoneal structures. The peritoneal fat, although occasionally abundant, is not uniform and is not responsible for the visualization of structures. Consequently, only the posterior portion of the liver and the posterior portion of the spleen are visualized directly on a plain radiograph of the abdomen. The same fat that outlines the liver and the spleen also outlines the kidneys

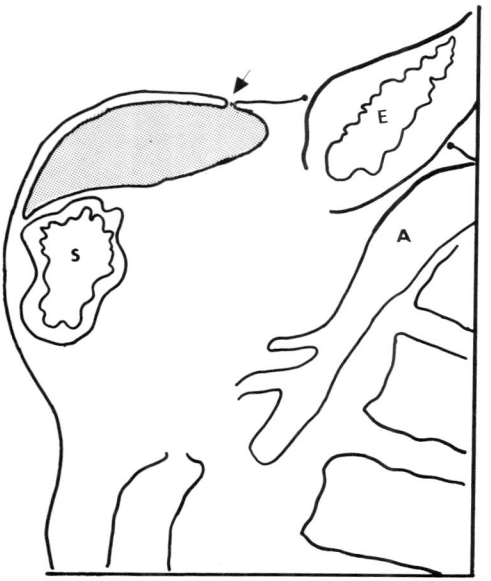

Figure 5–10. Drawing of section F through the left superior and inferior coronary ligaments demonstrating the superior attachment of the liver to the coronary ligaments (arrow) rather than the posterior attachment, as on the right side. E = esophagogastric junction; A = aorta; S = stomach. (*From* Whalen, J. P.: Radiology of the Abdomen. An Anatomic Approach. Philadelphia, Lea & Febiger, 1976. Reproduced by permission.)

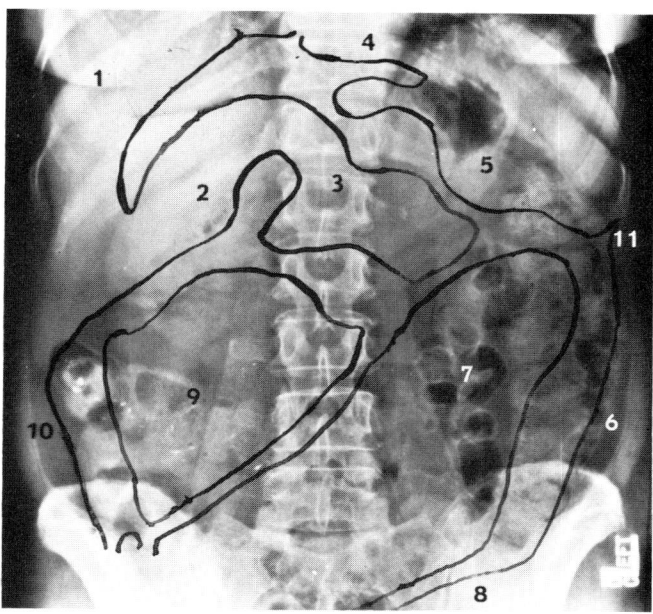

Figure 5–11. Diagram of peritoneal spaces on radiograph of the abdomen. *Supramesocolic:* 1. right subphrenic; 2. right subhepatic (visceral); 3. lesser sac; 4. left subphrenic; 5. perisplenic. *Inframesocolic.* 6. left paracolic; 7. left infracolic; 8. pelvic; 9. right infracolic; 10. right paracolic; 11. phrenicocolic ligament. (*From* Whalen, J. P.: Radiology of the Abdomen. An Anatomic Approach. Philadelphia, Lea & Febiger, 1976. Reproduced by permission.)

and the psoas muscles. The more anterior structures, which are in the anterior pararenal space (for example, the pancreas), and the more anterior portions of the intraperitoneal cavity (for example, the anterior edge of the liver and the anterior edge of the spleen) are beyond the extraperitoneal fat and are not seen on the plain radiograph. Their position and size, however, may be determined when air is contained within the more anterior stomach, transverse colon, and loops of small bowel.

For the interpretation of the plain abdominal radiograph it is necessary to know the mechanism by which the renal shadows, the psoas muscles, and the visualized portions of the spleen and liver are seen. Visualization of the upper half of the psoas muscles and the kidneys is made possible by perirenal fat. Visualization of the lower half of the psoas muscles is made possible by pararenal fat. The hepatic and splenic angles are seen because of their interface with the lateral aspects of the perirenal fat. The flank fat stripe is visualized (see Fig. 5–2) because of the posterior pararenal fat in its anterior and lateral extensions. This posterior pararenal space is continuous ventrally on both sides and fuses anteriorly. The anterior pararenal fat is not significant in the visualization of structures on the plain radiograph of the abdomen.

The clinician and the radiologist must be aware both of the structures contained in each anatomic compartment and of which portions of these structures are visualized. If a structure can no longer be visualized because of replacement of fat by either phlegmon or abscess, the differential diagnosis should be anatomically localized because of the alterations affecting the structures contained within that space. For example, if the upper portion of the psoas muscle is lost, a perirenal process should be suspected. If the medial aspect of the hepatic angle is lost, a perirenal abscess localized to the lateral portion of the perirenal space is probable. If the flank fat stripe is altered, the problem can probably be localized to the posterior pararenal space extending laterally and anteriorly. Alternatively, a process in the intraperitoneal space may have violated the parietal peritoneum and extended into the posterior pararenal fat (Fig. 5–12*B*).

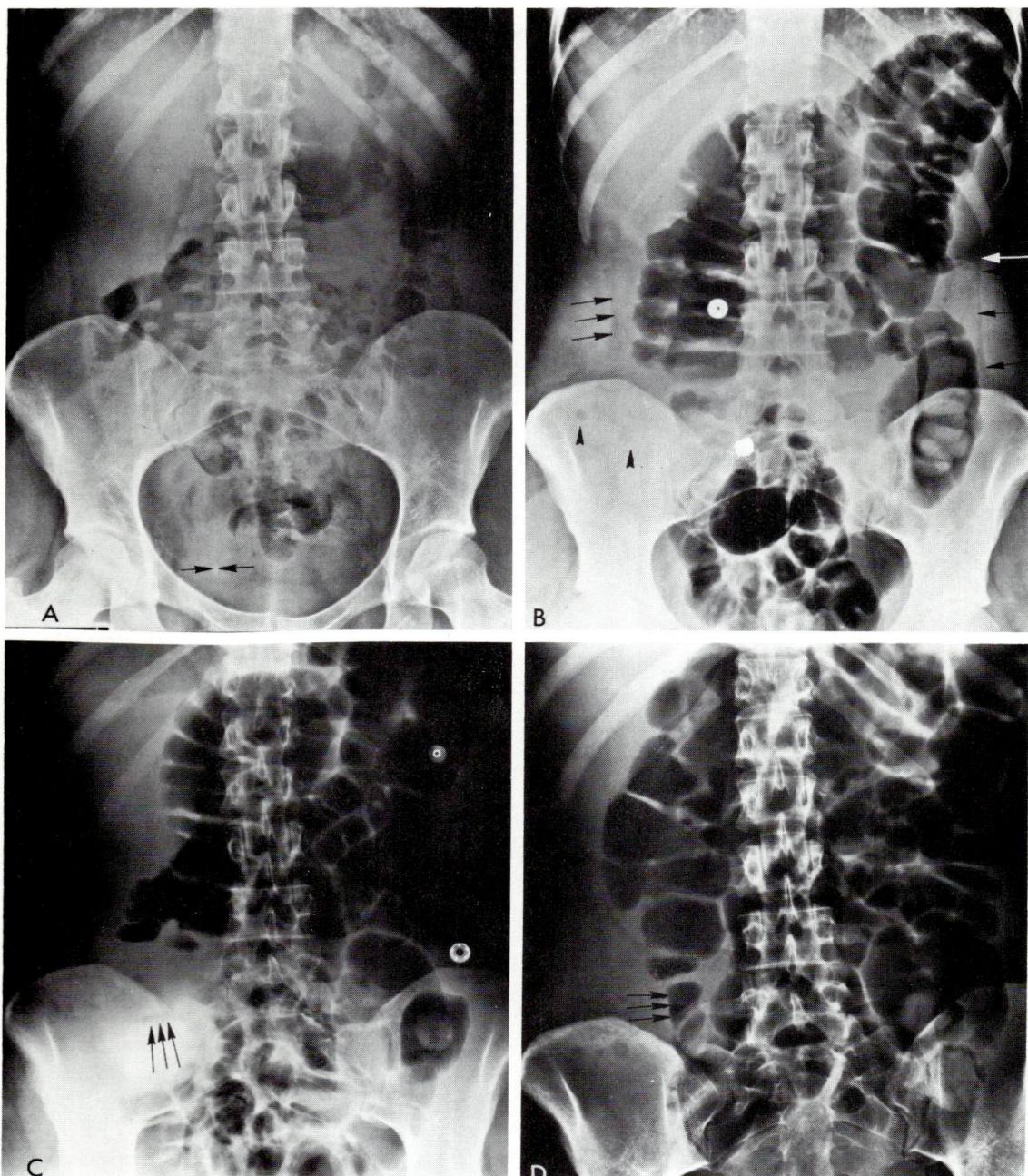

Figure 5–12. Acute appendicitis: postoperative abscess. A 21-year-old female presented with acute right lower quadrant pain. *A,* The supine radiograph of the abdomen shows a small calcific shadow in the right pelvic area (arrows). There are adjacent ill-defined loops of bowel filled with fluid. The diagnosis of acute appendicitis was confirmed at surgery. *B,* An abdominal survey was performed four days after surgery because of sudden fever and abdominal discomfort. The supine radiograph shows loss of the lower third of the properitoneal fat stripe, clearly seen in its superior third and on the left side (arrows). There are also ill-defined gas shadows in the right lower quadrant (arrowheads). *C,* The upright radiograph now shows an air-fluid level in the same area (arrows). *D,* Five days after surgery the gas collection has increased, and the mass displaces the colon medially (arrows). The abscess was confirmed at surgery and drained.

RADIOLOGIC APPROACH

The Acute Abdomen in the Emergency Room

Radiologic monitoring of the abdomen should be tailored to the clinical setting. In general, the approach is to begin with a supine and an upright radiograph of the abdomen (Table 5–1). These are carefully observed for abnormality and, depending upon the clinical setting and the findings on the initial radiographs, additional studies are obtained. These may include decubitus or lateral radiographs. In general, the position of the patient should be dictated by the effort to use gravity in the ascent of air, so that air outlines the area of suspected disease. If, for example, a distended transverse colon is demonstrated in the supine film, placing the patient in the prone position allows gas, if it is not obstructed at the splenic flexure, to move to the descending colon. If gas does not fill the entire transverse colon in the supine position, a right side–down lateral decubitus projection may be helpful in excluding a mechanical cause of obstruction in the distal transverse colon. In addition, contrast material may be introduced either by rectum or by mouth. Other procedures such as ultrasonography or CT scan also may be done. Finally, it is important to remember that organs alter their relationships with changes in the patient's position. That is, with a right side–down lateral abdominal radiograph the organs on the left side of the abdomen fall forward, while on the left side–down lateral radiograph the organs on the right side fall forward. It is therefore important to interpret the lateral radiograph in light of the patient's position.

TABLE 5–1. ACUTE ABDOMEN: RADIOLOGIC ABDOMINAL SURVEY

1. Supine radiograph of the abdomen that includes the pelvic floor.
2. Upright radiograph of the abdomen taken after the patient has been in the sitting position for a few minutes. This allows free air to rise to the diaphragm.
3. Lateral decubitus radiographs. The left lateral decubitus projection is particularly useful in cases of a questionable obstructive lesion in the rectosigmoid area because it facilitates passage of gas into the distal segments, thereby eliminating or confirming the presence of obstruction.
4. Lateral radiograph of the abdomen (cross-table, right, or left) to include the diaphragm.
5. Prone radiograph for reversal of gas and fluid pattern of the colon compared with the supine radiograph.
6. Posteroanterior or anteroposterior and lateral chest radiographs. These show supra- and subdiaphragmatic changes.

The Acute Postoperative Abdomen

The postoperative abdomen is more difficult to interpret than the preoperative abdomen, since the effects of surgery on the anatomy and physiology of structures may simulate more serious complications. In general, the patients are more ill, and the technical quality of the radiographs is not as good. Our usual study consists of a supine and an upright radiograph; again, however, the examination must be tailored to the clinical situation. The same radiographic examinations are carried out as those performed on the emergency room patient. Ultrasonography is important postoperatively, especially in the diagnosis of abscess. CT is still being evaluated.

PATHOLOGIC ENTITIES: THE EMERGENCY ROOM

General Radiologic Findings

LOSS OF VISUALIZATION OF STRUCTURES NORMALLY SEEN. The initial radiographs (supine and upright) are observed to determine the integrity of the renal and the psoas muscle shadows, the presence of the hepatic and splenic angles, and the gas pattern within the stomach and the small and large bowel. The mucosal pattern of the loops of bowel may also be evaluated if there is air within the lumen. In addition, the position of the air-filled structures is evaluated to detect the enlargement of organs or the presence of masses. The distribution of the small and large bowel should be observed to detect an abnormal location that would suggest hernia.

In the supine position the transverse colon and the sigmoid are more anterior than the descending colon, so that in the anteroposterior radiograph most of the gas in the large bowel resides in the transverse colon. The rectum and the ascending and descending colon, being more posterior, tend to be filled with fluid. The supine radiograph may then simulate obstruction of the distal transverse colon when its appearance is merely a gravity phenomenon. In the prone position there is a reversal of fluid and gas: the fluid occupies the more dependent transverse colon, and air ascends to the more superior ascending and descending colon and the rectum. Knowledge of the patient's position is vital in the interpretation of the gas pattern of the abdominal radiograph.

INTRAPERITONEAL FREE AIR. Recognition of free intraperitoneal air is important in the diagnosis of peptic ulcer disease and other entities causing perforation. In the supine position, free air rises anteriorly and many times is obscured in this projection. Since the small bowel and the transverse colon are anterior, air may occasionally outline their outer walls, a useful sign of intraperitoneal air (Fig. 5–13A). In addition, since the falciform ligament is an anterior structure and may be surrounded by

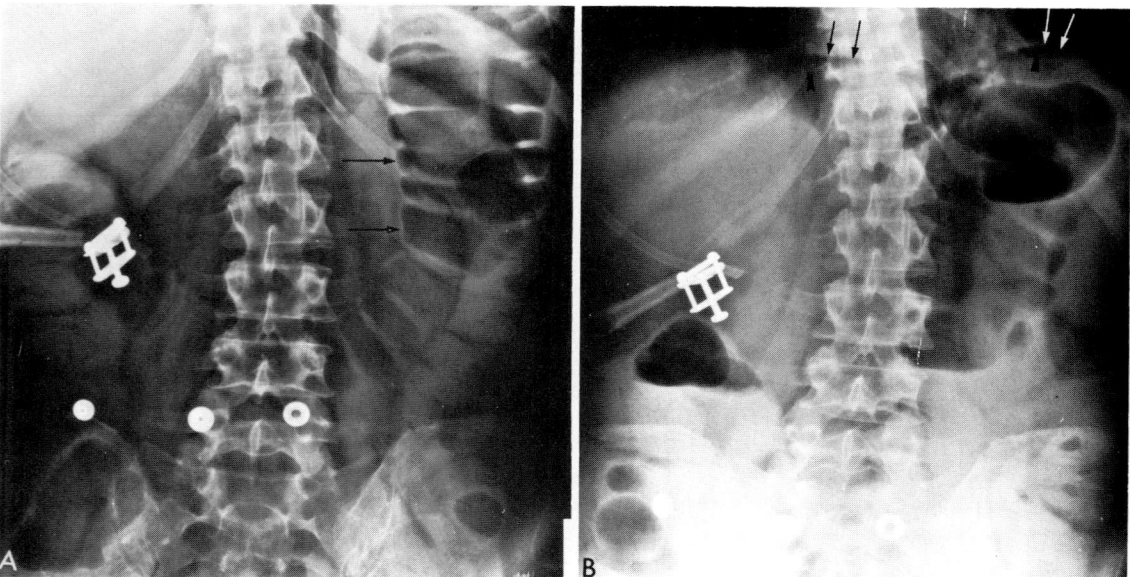

Figure 5–13. Perforated duodenal ulcer. A 50-year-male was admitted with acute upper abdominal pain and shock. The supine radiograph (A) shows air outlining the serosal surface of the bowel (arrows). The upright radiograph (B) demonstrates free air (arrowhead) beneath the diaphragm (white arrows) and, in particular, under the central tendinous portion (black arrows).

Figure 5–14. Intraperitoneal air. Supine (A) and upright (B) films of a 72-year-old man five days after surgery for sigmoidectomy. The falciform ligament (arrowheads) is outlined by free residual air. D = diaphragm.

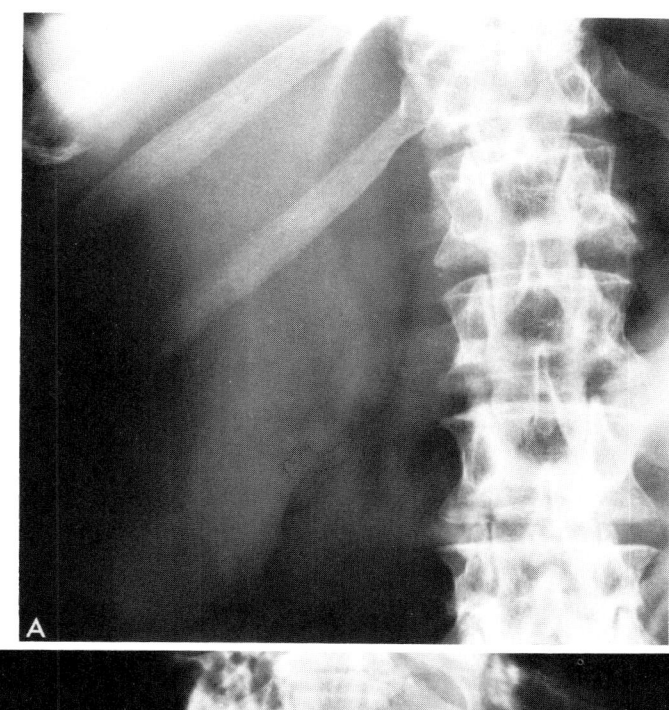
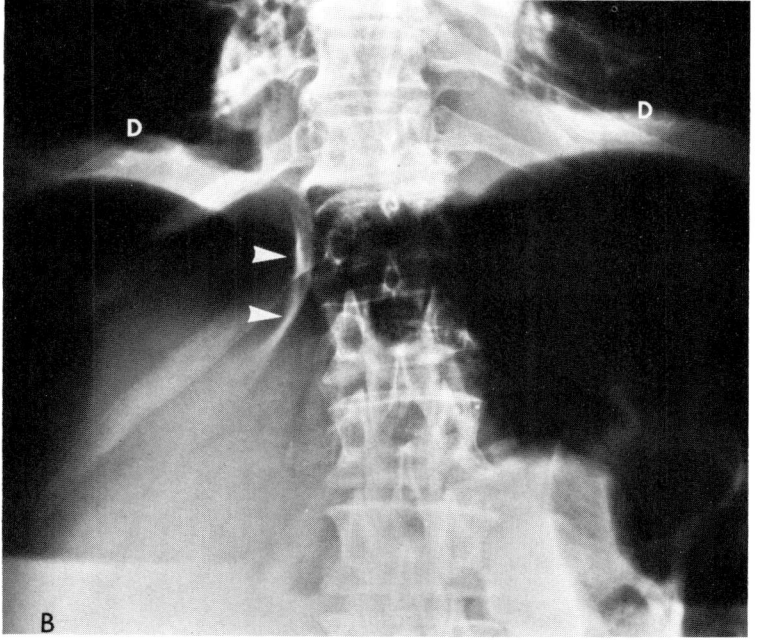

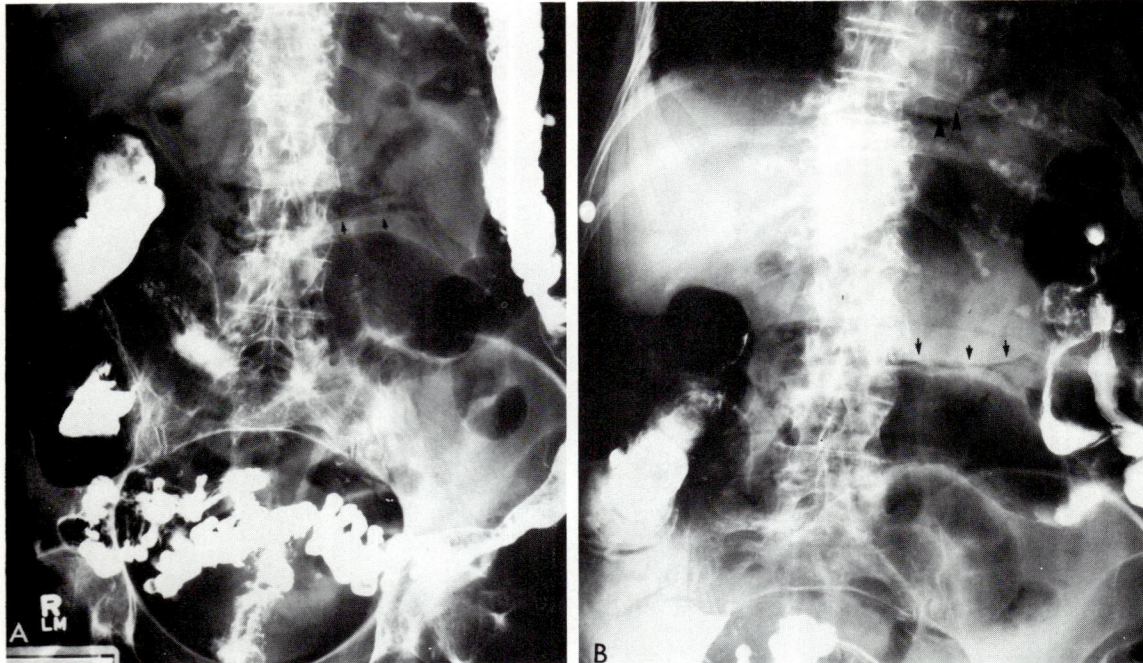

Figure 5–15. Perforated diverticulitis. A 62-year-old female with a long history of diverticular disease presented with acute onset of left lower quadrant pain. *A,* The supine radiograph of abdomen after a barium enema shows a narrow band of gas (arrows) not corresponding to the intraperitoneal space. *B,* The same gas shadow in the upright radiograph is fixed (arrows). In addition, free air is present beneath the diaphragm (arrowheads) in the peritoneal cavity. A diagnosis of diverticulitis with perforation into the intra- and extraperitoneal spaces was made.

air (Fig. 5–14), its visualization should alert the observer to the presence of free air. The upright position is the most helpful in the detection of free air (Figs. 5–13B and 5–14B). At times the upright chest radiograph may be more valuable than the abdominal radiograph because of the greater contrast between air and the surrounding diaphragm and liver. In the upright position, air ascends to the highest portions of the abdomen—the domes of the diaphragm and under the central tendinous portion, which is anterior (Fig. 5–15B; see Fig. 5–96D). Air in the lesser sac localizes behind the stomach but may be confused on a frontal radiograph with air beneath the central tendon. A lateral radiograph is essential in differentiating these two localizations: lesser sac air will be behind the stomach and air beneath the central tendinous area will be anterior to the stomach. If there is doubt, the decubitus radiograph may be of value.

INTRAPERITONEAL EFFUSION. Detection of intra- or retroperitoneal fluid is often the key to the diagnosis of acute abdomen. Intraperitoneal effusions usually first collect in the pelvis, which is the most dependent portion. The fluid then ascends up the paracolic gutters on the right and left sides. On the right side it may then progress unimpeded to the subphrenic space or, more commonly, to the more dependent portion of the upper intraperitoneal cavity, Morrison's pouch. On the left side it ascends along the paracolic gutter and is usually thwarted by the phrenicocolic ligament.

THE ACUTE ABDOMEN — 181

An early roentgen sign of intraperitoneal effusion is fluid density in the pelvis (Fig. 5–16). This requires approximately 200 cc of fluid. As the amount of fluid increases, it displaces the right and left colon medially, separating them from their respective flank fat stripes (Fig. 5–17). As fluid increases further, it collects around the hepatic angle (posterior portion of the liver) and floats the liver out of the extraperitoneal fat, causing loss of visualization of the hepatic angle (Fig. 5–18). The same changes occur on the left side of the abdomen, similarly obscuring the splenic angle, but to a lesser extent because of the protection afforded by the phrenicocolic ligament. As even more fluid collects, loops of small bowel, which are anterior, become separated. At this point the psoas and renal shadows are intact, but as greater amounts of fluid collect and greater distention occurs the flank fat stripes are thinned laterally (Fig. 5–19); combined with increased scatter radiation, eventually even the renal outlines and the psoas muscles are lost. Table 5–2 lists the radiographic findings of intraperitoneal effusion.

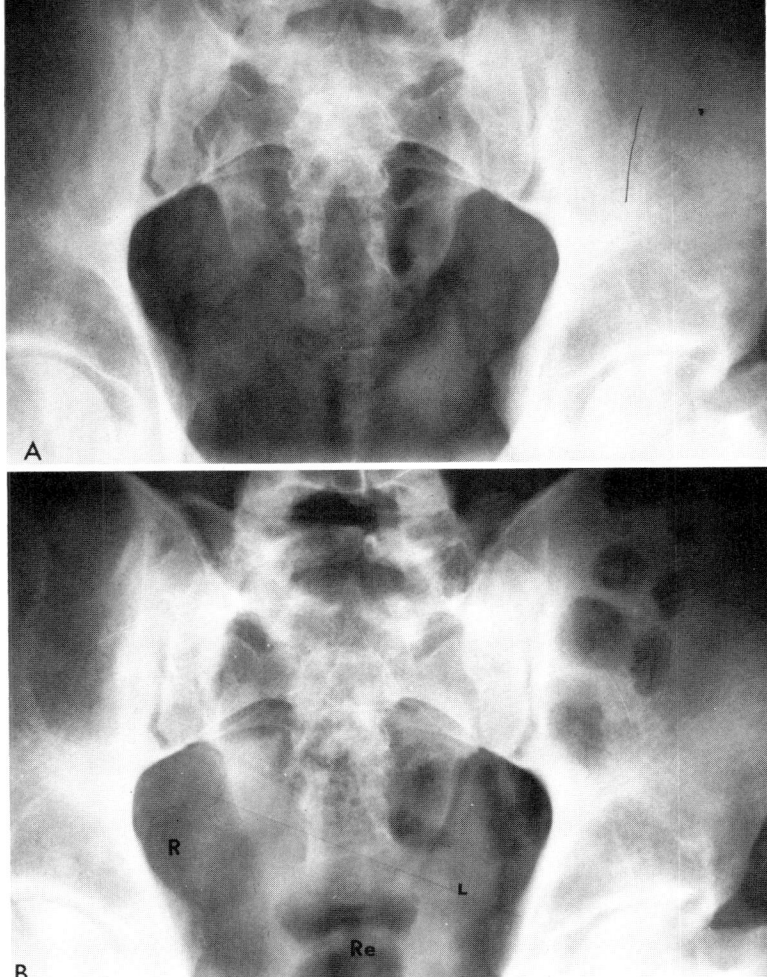

Figure 5–16. Intraperitoneal blood. *A,* An adult male with normal pelvic shadows. *B,* The supine radiograph of the same patient following filling of the most dependent pararectal fossae (R,L) by blood. Re = rectum outlined by gas. (*From* Whalen, J. P.: Radiology of The Abdomen. An Anatomic Approach. Philadelphia, Lea & Febiger, 1976. Reproduced by permission.)

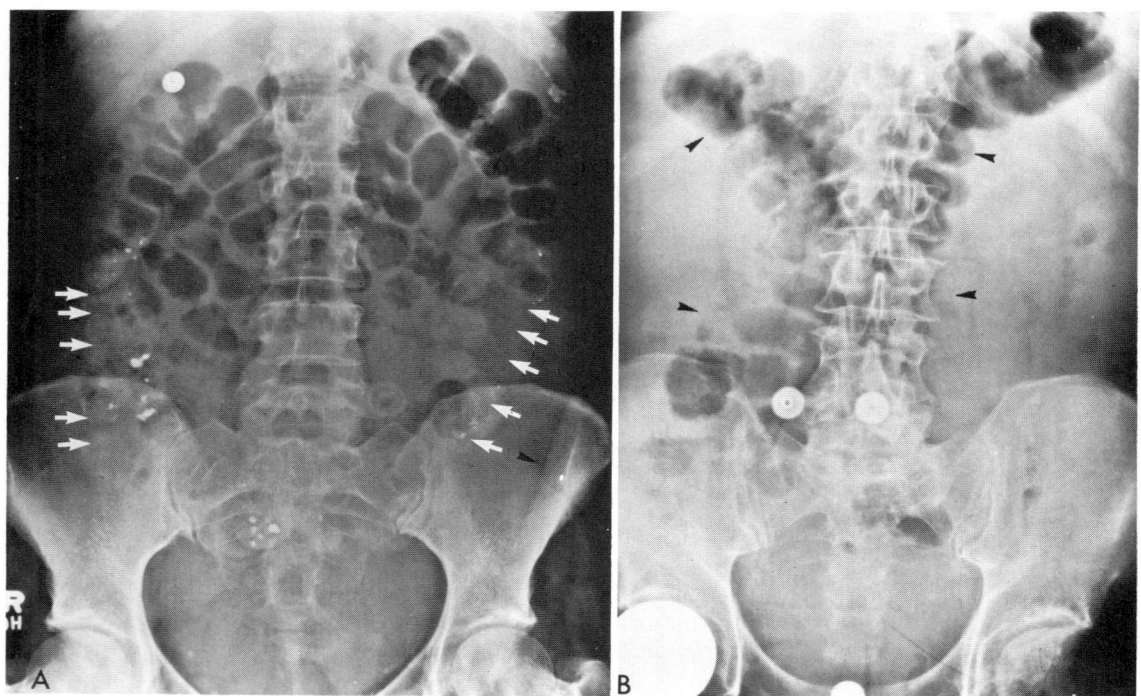

Figure 5–17. Ascites. *A,* A 53-year-old female with a history of ethanol abuse presented with symptoms suggesting diverticulitis. (A previous barium enema had shown diverticular disease of the left colon.) The supine radiograph demonstrates a moderate degree of ascites with slight medial displacement of the ascending and descending colon (arrows), thinning of the properitoneal fat stripes (arrowhead), and fluid in the pelvic floor. *B,* A 62-year-old male with cirrhosis was admitted with abdominal distress and vomiting. The supine radiograph of the abdomen shows ascites and marked medial displacement of the gas-filled colon by the fluid (arrowheads). There is loss of the properitoneal fat stripes.

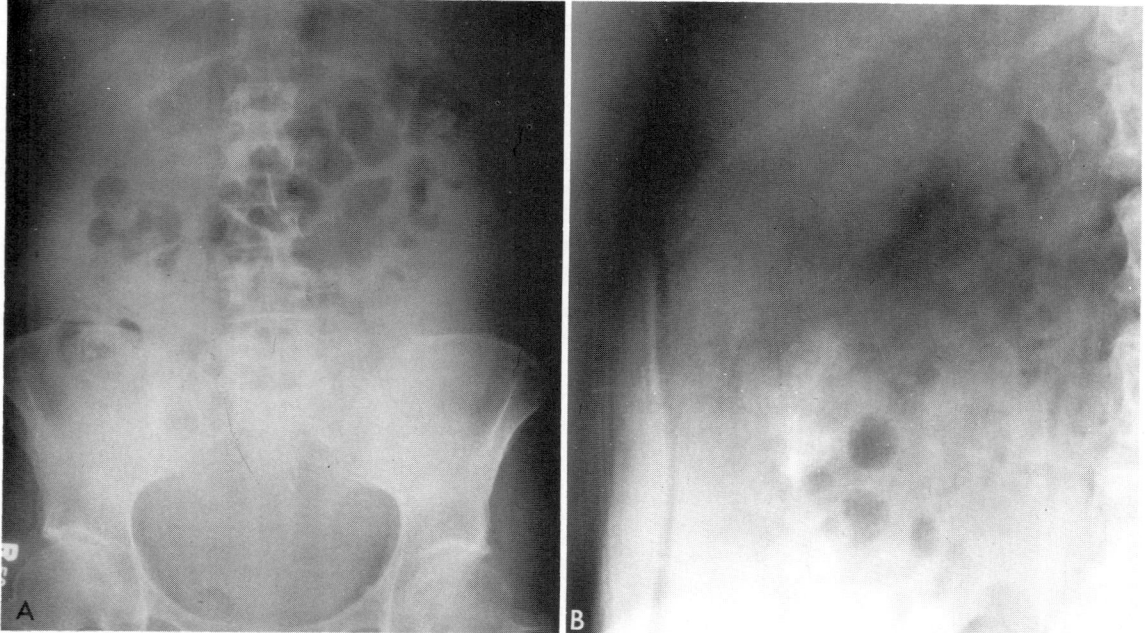

Figure 5–18. *A,* The supine radiograph in a patient with massive ascites. Note bulging of the flanks and loss of the hepatic angle. *B,* The coned radiograph demonstrates the thinned properitoneal fat stripe and the loss of the hepatic angle. (*From* Whalen, J. P., and Berne, A. S.: The extraperitoneal perivisceral fat pad. II. Alterations. Radiology *92:*473, 1969. Reproduced by permission.)

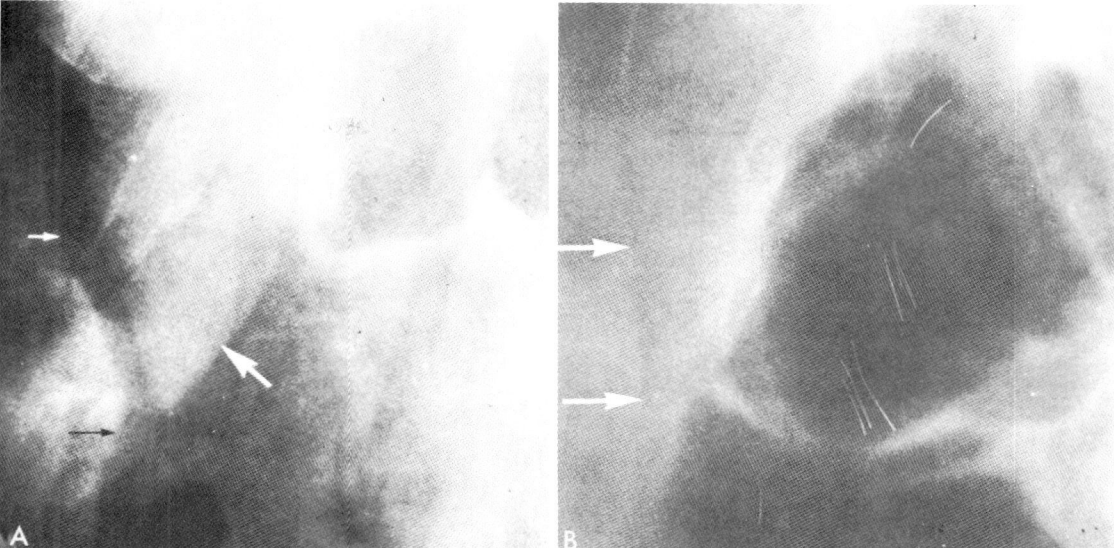

Figure 5-19. Intraperitoneal fluid. *A*, Supine radiograph of the right upper quadrant of the abdomen. Shown are the medial contour of the hepatic angle (large arrow) and normal properitoneal fat outlining the lateral aspect of the liver (small arrows). *B*, Same patient and same projection after accumulation of minimal amount of intraperitoneal fluid. There is loss of the medial contour of the hepatic angle and thinning of the properitoneal fat stripe (arrows). (*From* Whalen, J. P., and Berne, A. S.: The extraperitoneal perivisceral fat pad. II. Roentgen interpretation of pathological alterations. Radiology 92:473, 1969. Reproduced by permission.)

TABLE 5-2. RADIOGRAPHIC FINDINGS IN INTRAPERITONEAL EFFUSION

Anatomic Feature	Radiographic Appearance
Pelvic floor	"Dog ears"
Flank fat stripe	Intact or thinned
Psoas muscle margin	Intact, unless massive effusion
Kidney outline	Intact, unless massive effusion
Kidney position	Unaltered
Hepatic or splenic angle	Lost
Descending duodenum or duodenojejunal junction	Unaltered
Ascending or descending colon	Possibly displaced medially
Small intestine	Loops separated by fluid

EXTRAPERITONEAL EFFUSION. As stated previously the extraperitoneal space is divided into three compartments. If fluid collects in the anterior pararenal space, little is observed on the plain radiograph in terms of alteration of the normal fat and soft tissue densities (Fig. 5-20). As more fluid collects, there may be displacement of the more anterior structures, such as stomach and colon. In effusion from pancreatitis, the renal shadows and psoas muscles are intact, as are the liver and the hepatic angle. If effusion occurs in the perirenal space, there is loss of the upper portion of the psoas muscle if the collection is medial, or loss of the hepatic angle (Fig. 5-21) or splenic angle if the collection is lateral. Portions of the renal outline will also be lost, again depending on the location of the effusion. Effusions in the posterior pararenal space cause little loss of roentgen outlines except when they extend inferiorly and obliterate the lower portion of the psoas muscle. If the fluid extends laterally and anteriorly it will interfere with visualization of the lateral aspect of the liver or of the spleen and obliterate the flank fat stripe (Fig. 5-22). These findings are summarized in Table 5-3.

Text continued on page 187.

184 — THE ACUTE ABDOMEN

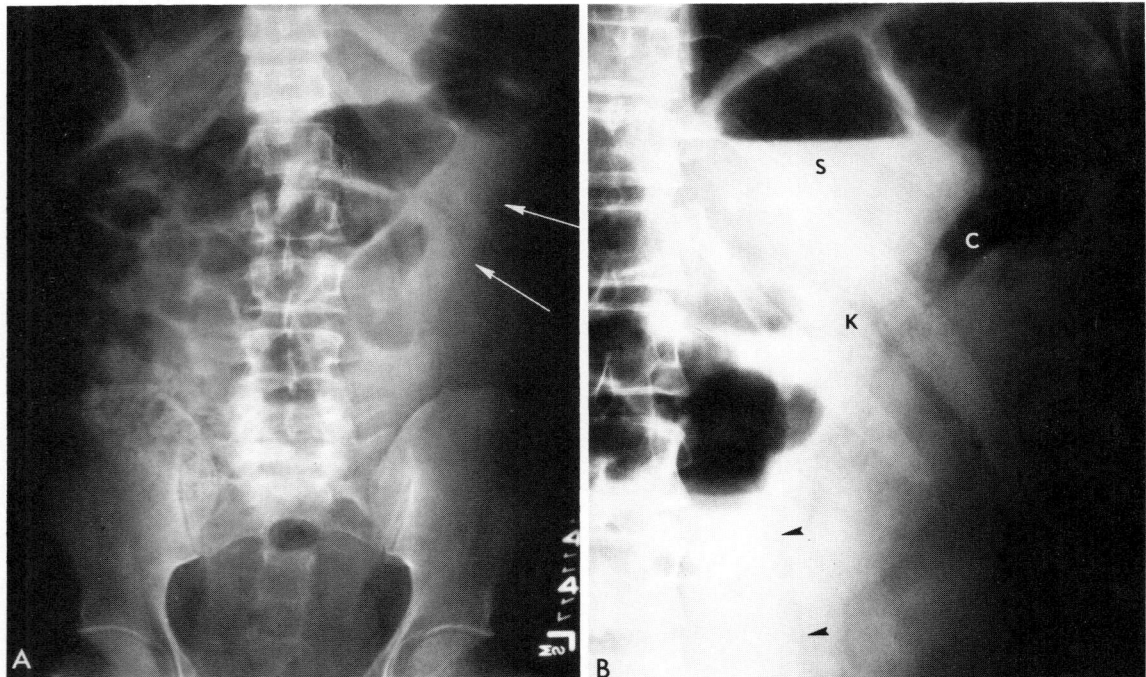

Figure 5–20. Post-traumatic fluid collection in the anterior pararenal space. *A,* The supine radiograph shows a soft tissue density in the left upper quadrant extending to the pelvis. The kidneys maintain a normal position (arrows). *B,* The upright radiograph shows the descending colon (C) narrowed in the area of the fluid collection. The kidney (K) and spleen (S) maintain a normal relationship. The psoas muscle is also intact (arrowheads). (*From* Whalen, J. P.: Radiology of The Abdomen. An Anatomic Approach. Philadelphia, Lea & Febiger, 1976. Reproduced by permission.)

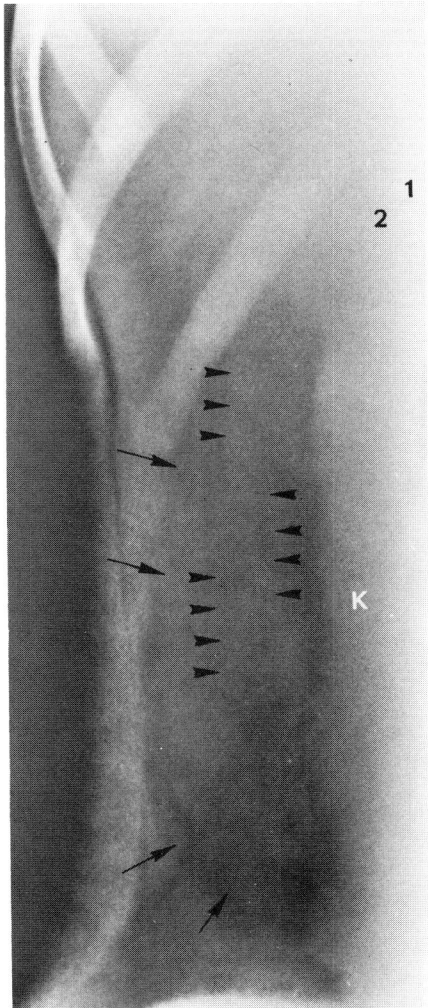

Figure 5–21. A young patient following traumatic contusion of the right kidney with subcapsular and perirenal hematoma. A coned supine radiograph of the right upper quadrant shows the flattened kidney (K), the ill-defined contours of the subcapsular collection (arrowheads), and the perinephric fluid contrasted with the remainder of the extraperitoneal space (arrows). The margins of the attachment of the perirenal (1) and subcapsular (2) component are marked. (*From* Whalen, J. P.: Radiology of The Abdomen. An Anatomic Approach. Philadelphia, Lea & Febiger, 1976. Reproduced by permission.)

186 — THE ACUTE ABDOMEN

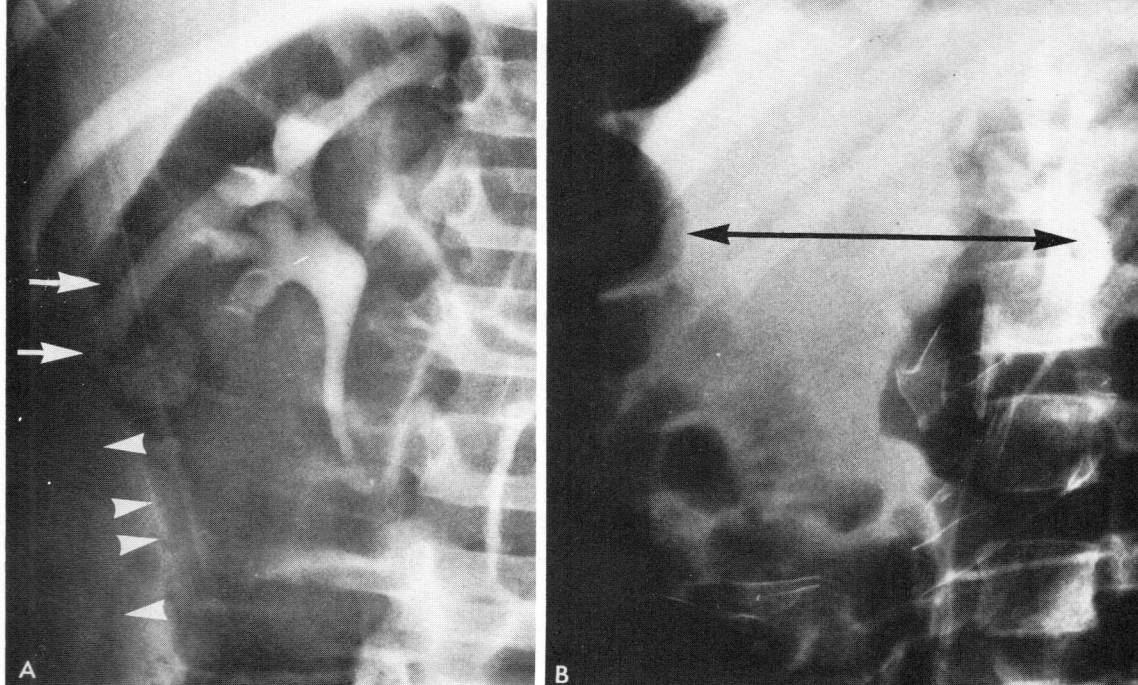

Figure 5–22. Trauma to the right flank. Hematoma in right perirenal and posterior pararenal spaces. *A,* A supine radiograph obtained during emergency intravenous urography demonstrates loss of the hepatic angle (arrows). The properitoneal fat line is widened and irregularly effaced (arrowheads). *B,* The left lateral view shows the separation of the right kidney from the gas-filled colon. (*From* Whalen, J. P., and Berne, A. S.: The extraperitoneal perivisceral fat pad. II. Roentgen interpretation of pathological alterations. Roentgenology 92:473, 1969. Reproduced by permission.)

TABLE 5–3. RADIOGRAPHIC SIGNS OF EFFUSION IN THE EXTRAPERITONEAL SPACES

Area of Interest	Anterior Pararenal Space	Perirenal	Posterior Pararenal
Flank fat stripe	Not involved	May be thinned	Obliterated with lateral extension of effusion
Psoas muscle margin	Not involved	Obliterated in upper third	Obliterated if involved medially
Kidney outline	Not involved	Not demonstrable	Normal
Kidney position	Affected by massive effusion	Anteriorly if the collection is medial. There is also lateral displacement	Anterior
Hepatic or splenic angle	Unaffected except in massive effusion	Normal if collection is medial; obliterated if lateral	Obliterated if collection is lateral
Descending duodenum or duodenojejunal junction	Anteriorly displaced or narrowed	Anterior position	Displaced anteriorly
Ascending or descending colon	Anteriorly displaced or constricted	Superior segments displaced anteriorly and medially	Displaced anteriorly and medially
Small intestine	Anteriorly displaced	Not involved	Displaced anteriorly

ABNORMAL GAS PATTERN. In the adult, varying amounts of gas and stool are seen in the large bowel, and minimal amounts of gas are seen in the small bowel. One of the most difficult problems in interpreting abdominal radiographs is to differentiate an ileus from a mechanical obstruction.[21] In some instances the history and physical findings are clear. In others, however, they are less certain, and diagnosis depends to a great extent on the radiographic findings.

The radiologic diagnosis of mechanical large or small bowel obstruction is dependent upon the finding of dilatation of bowel to a point beyond which there is collapse of bowel. All other findings are secondary to this. Again, the diagnosis of mechanical ileus is based upon the observation of a sharp transition at the point of obstruction where dilated bowel meets collapsed bowel. Unfortunately, in many cases this sharp transition is not always discernible. Further, a mechanical obstruction may be complicated by a reflex ileus, which alters the appearance of the primary pathologic process. The postoperative abdomen is particularly difficult to interpret, since the intrinsic trauma of surgery is superimposed on any complication secondary to the surgical procedure. Consequently, postoperative mechanical obstruction may be masked by a postoperative ileus pattern. Table 5-4 lists the radiologic criteria for the differentiation of adynamic from dynamic ileus of the small bowel. Since the colon is usually involved in an ileus pattern, the greater the collapse of the colon and the greater the dilatation of the small bowel, the more likely the presence of mechanial obstruction. The roentgen signs of mechanical colonic obstruction are listed in Table 5-5.[14]

TABLE 5-4. RADIOGRAPHIC FINDINGS IN PLAIN RADIOGRAPHS OF THE ABDOMEN IN SMALL BOWEL ILEUS

Adynamic Ileus	Dynamic Ileus
Gas and fluid distend segments of the jejunum and ileum without any preferred location.	Distended loops containing gas and fluid occupy mainly the midabdomen.
Because of retained fluid in several loops, these segments appear as sausage-like shadows of water density.	Segments of small bowel containing only fluid with a sausage-like appearance are seen.
Thick mucosal folds are present.	There is demonstration of folds, mostly in loops of jejunum, at times with the typical coiled appearance of the valvulae conniventes.
Long fluid levels are found in long loops. In the arch-like loops, the fluid levels are at the same height in each limb.	In the upright or decubitus radiographs, inverted U-shaped loops are demonstrated, with fluid levels at a different height in each limb.
There is no stepladder arrangement of distended loops.	There is a stepladder arrangement of distended loops.
The string-of-beads sign is absent or rare.	Small, rounded obliquely directed gas shadows are present, resembling a string of beads and produced by small collections of gas retained between folds of jejunum.
No significant interval change in the gas pattern is seen in subsequent abdominal surveys.	A change of gas pattern occurs in subsequent abdominal surveys, usually demonstrable between four and six hours later.
The colon is distended by gas, and fluid levels are demonstrable.	A minimal amount of gas is present in the colon, without fluid levels. If the large bowel is dilated the haustral pattern can still be recognized.

188 — THE ACUTE ABDOMEN

TABLE 5–5. ROENTGEN SIGNS OF COLONIC OBSTRUCTION DEMONSTRABLE IN PLAIN RADIOGRAPHS OF THE ABDOMEN

Closed-loop obstruction with competent ileocecal valve	Colon dilated to the level of obstruction Distention of cecum Minimal or no dilatation of distal ileal coils
Closed-loop obstruction with competent ileocecal valve and obstruction patterns in small bowel	Colon dilated to level of obstruction Marked dilatation of loops of small bowel proximal to cecum In this type of obstruction the cecum may become markedly dilated, and perforation is more common
Closed-loop obstruction with incompetent ileocecal valve	Colon dilated to level of obstruction Moderately distended loops of ileum Fluid levels in colon and small bowel Moderately dilated cecum

ORGAN ENLARGEMENT. The clue to the cause of an acute abdomen may be enlargement of an organ that is detectable radiographically. That is, an enlarged kidney may reflect an obstructed ureter, or an enlarged spleen after trauma may suggest the diagnosis of subcapsular hematoma (Figs. 5–23 and 5–24). Analysis of organ size is essential in evaluating the acute abdomen.

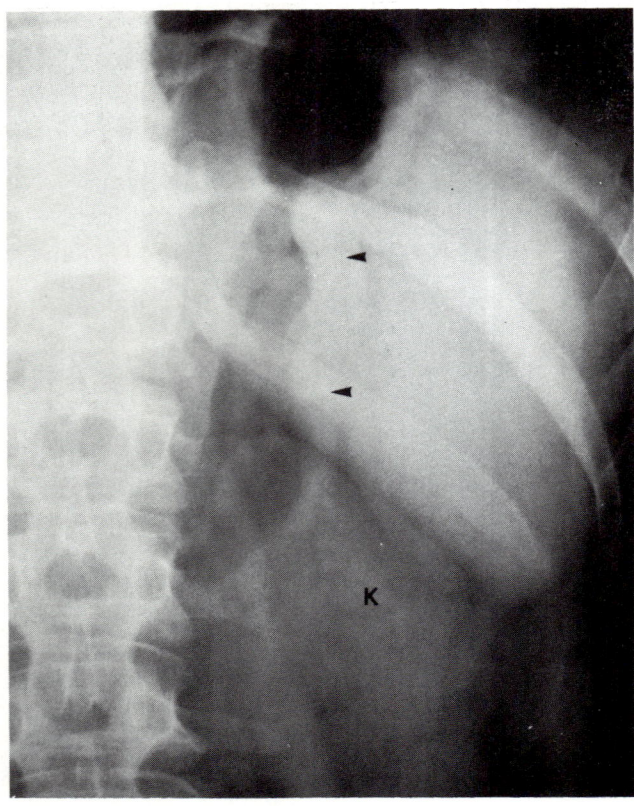

Figure 5–23. Splenic hematoma. A 35-year-old male sustained an injury to the left upper abdomen in an automobile accident. The supine radiograph shows an enlarged splenic shadow displacing the kidney (K) inferiorly and the stomach medially (arrowheads). The findings suggested subcapsular splenic hematoma. No intraperitoneal fluid was detected on the radiograph.

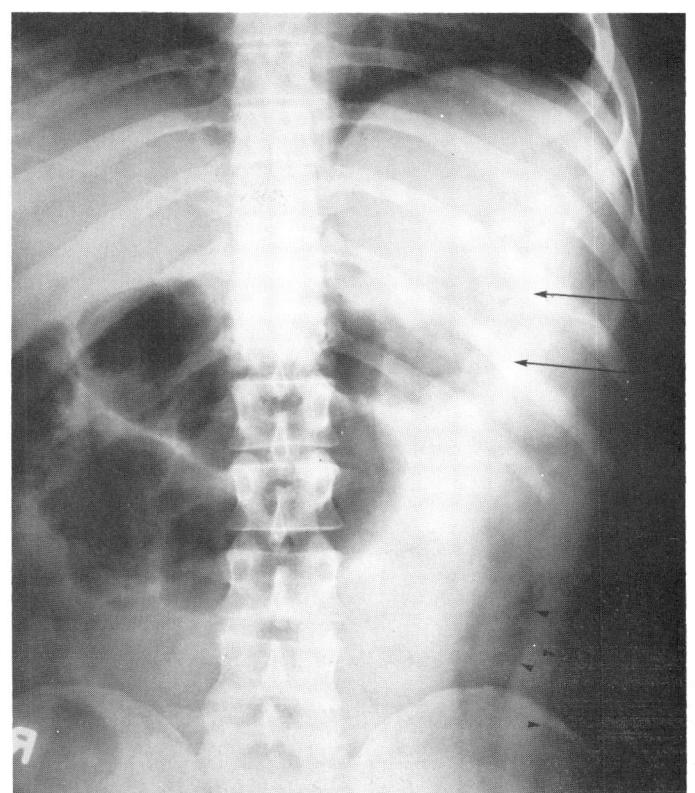

Figure 5–24. Splenic subcapsular hematoma. A 30-year-old male had fallen six feet from a ladder. There is tense pain in the left quadrant of the abdomen. The plain anteroposterior radiograph of the abdomen shows findings suggesting splenic subcapsular hematoma, with medial displacement of the stomach (arrows) and inferior displacement of the kidney. There is also fluid separating the descending colon, which is displaced medially, from the properitoneal fat line (arrowheads).

MASS. The presence of mass densities within the abdomen should be carefully investigated (Fig. 5–25). It is well known that patients with acute pancreatitis may have large pseudocysts that can be detected by displacement of gas-containing structures such as stomach (see Fig. 5–53), colon, or loops of small bowel. Hydrops of the gallbladder may present acutely and characteristically displaces the descending duodenum (Fig. 5–26) and the more anterior portion of the hepatic flexure (Fig. 5–27). Perforations may be followed by abscess and consequent formation of a mass density.

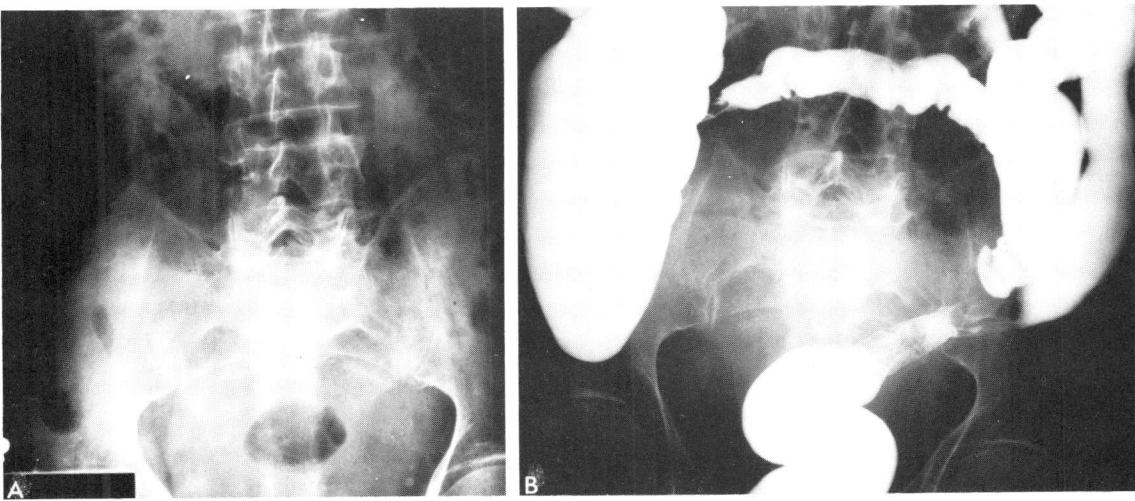

Figure 5–25. The patient is a 79-year-old male with severe acute lower abdominal pain and a palpable mass. *A,* The supine radiograph shows a mass in the pelvis. *B,* A barium enema verified draping of the ileum and colon around a mass, which was shown at cystoscopy to be an enlarged urinary bladder.

190 — THE ACUTE ABDOMEN

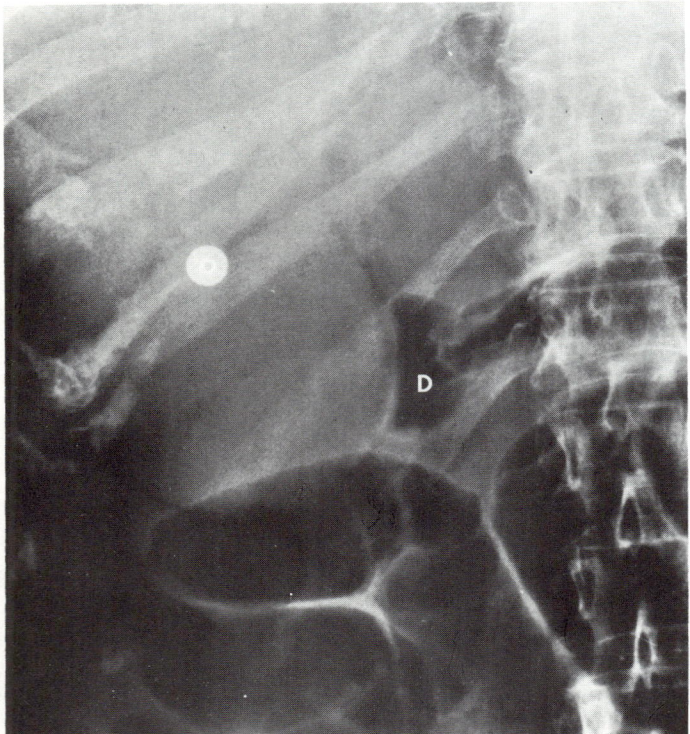

Figure 5–26. Hydrops of gallbladder. A 63-year-old female with acute onset of right upper quadrant pain and a palpable mass. The plain radiograph shows a mass effect on the duodenal bulb (D) and the anterior portion of the hepatic flexure of the colon. A diagnosis of acute obstructive cholecystitis (hydrops of gallbladder) was made.

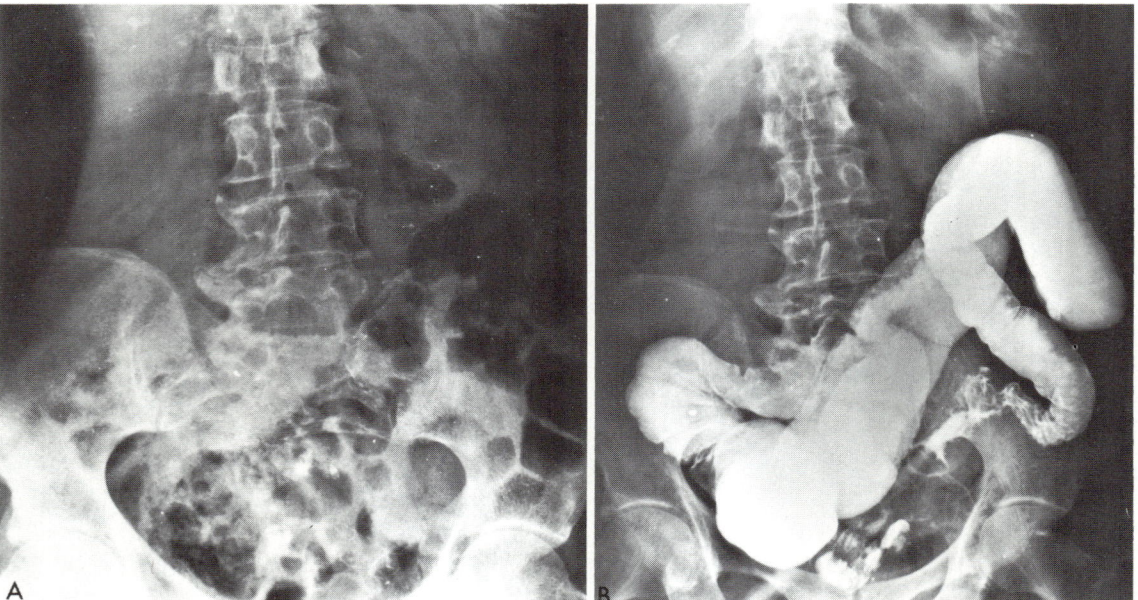

Figure 5–27. Gallbladder mass. An 80-year-old female with a three week history of right upper quadrant pain and acute exacerbations of pain with vomiting. *A*, A supine radiograph of the abdomen shows a large mass in the right upper quadrant depressing the colon. *B*, A barium enema demonstrates the supramesocolic position of the mass. The roentgen diagnosis was hydrops of the gallbladder. The pathologic diagnosis was carcinoma of the gallbladder.

THE ACUTE ABDOMEN — 191

ABNORMAL GAS COLLECTIONS. Careful search should be made for abnormal gas collections. No gas should appear beyond the normal anatomic confines of the stomach and the small and large bowel. Caution should be observed, however, because variations such as interposition of colon between liver and diaphragm may simulate free air and be misleading (Figs. 5–28 to 5–30). Occasionally, abundant fat in various areas (Fig. 5–31), especially beneath the diaphragm, may simulate free air in the peritoneum (Fig. 5–32). Because the supine radiograph does not always show small amounts of air, upright and decubitus radiographs are required. When air is identified, its distribution and mobility are essential in its localization to the peritoneal free space, to compartments within the peritoneum (such as the renal, or lesser sac), or to the extraperitoneal space (perirenal, anterior pararenal, or posterior pararenal) (see Figs. 5–13 and 5–15; Fig. 5–33).

Gas may also be localized rather than free and may point to a specific diagnosis. For example, communication of a gallstone with the duodenum causes passage of air into the biliary system (Fig. 5–34). Gas may also arise from gas-forming organisms within an abscess, as in emphysematous cholecystitis (Figs. 5–35 and 5–36).

Text continued on page 196.

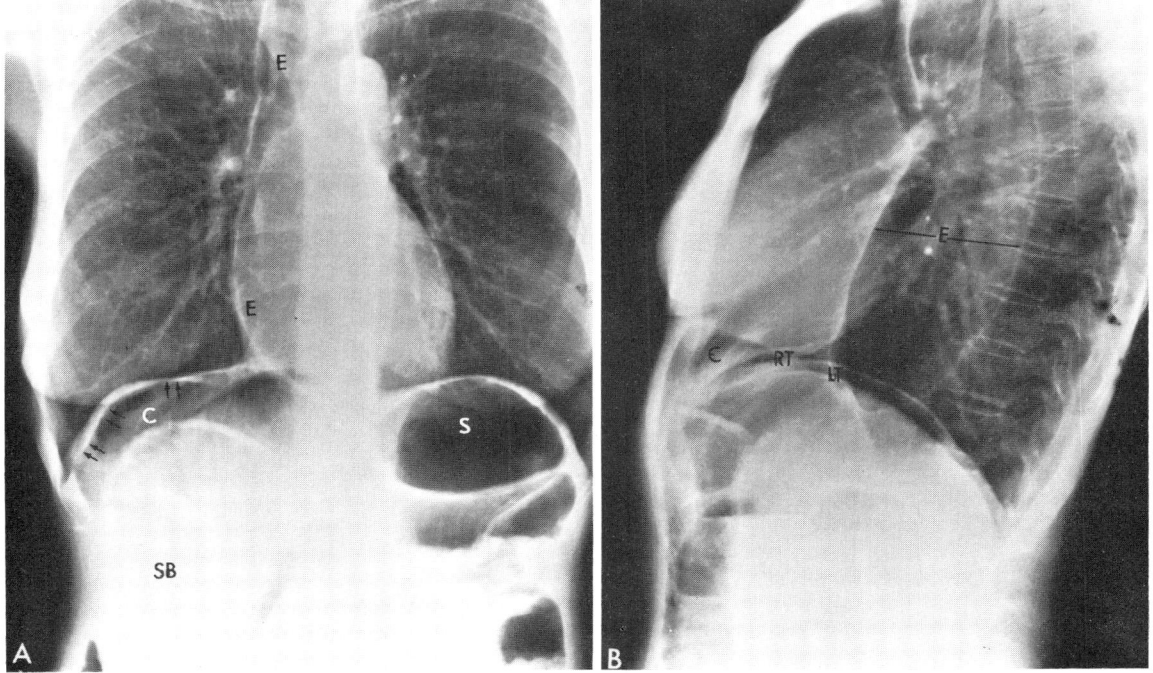

Figure 5–28. Scleroderma. *A* and *B*. Posteroanterior and left lateral chest radiographs of a 52-year-old female with a history of scleroderma. The colon (C) is interposed between the liver and the right hemidiaphragm (arrows). There is dilatation of the esophagus (E), stomach (S), and small bowel (SB). This constellation of findings confirms the diagnosis of scleroderma. RT = right hemidiaphragm; LT = left hemidiaphragm.

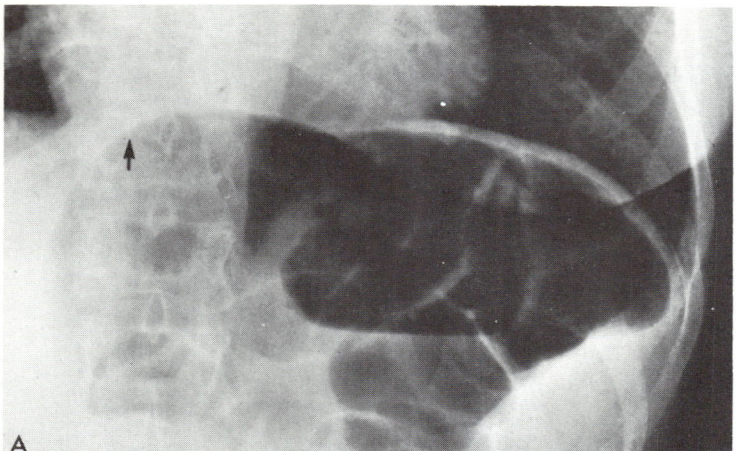

Figure 5–29. High colon simulating free air. Anteroposterior (A) and lateral (B) radiographs of chest show air beneath the diaphragm, particularly in the area of the central tendinous portion (arrow), due to a high colon, not free air. See Figure 5–13B, in which free air occupies this space.

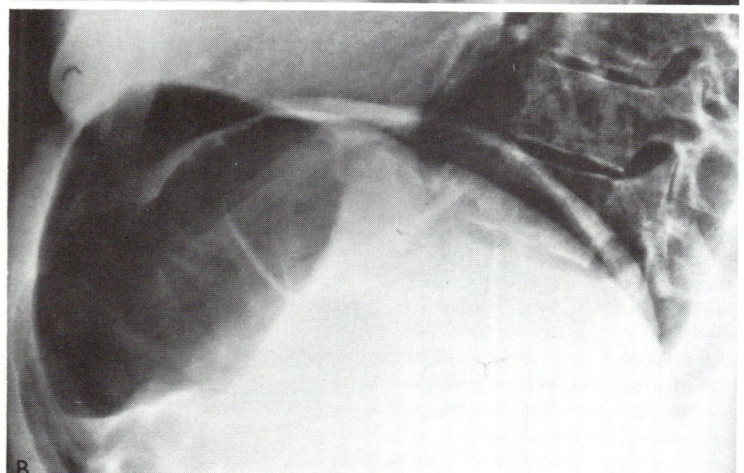

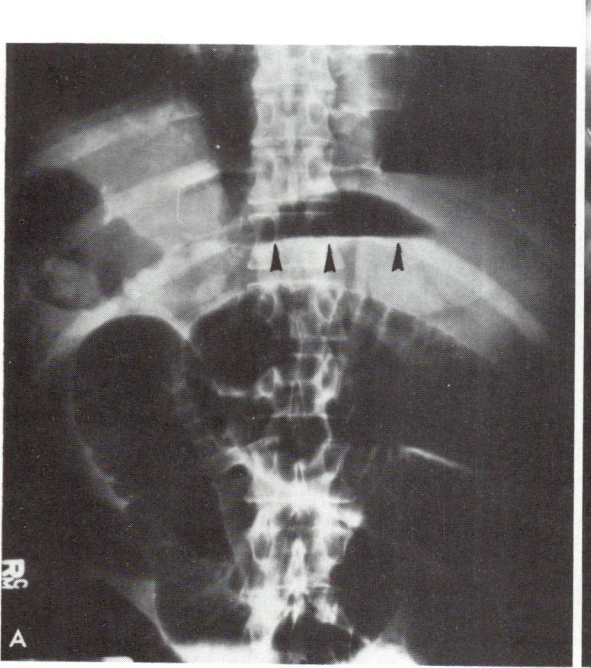
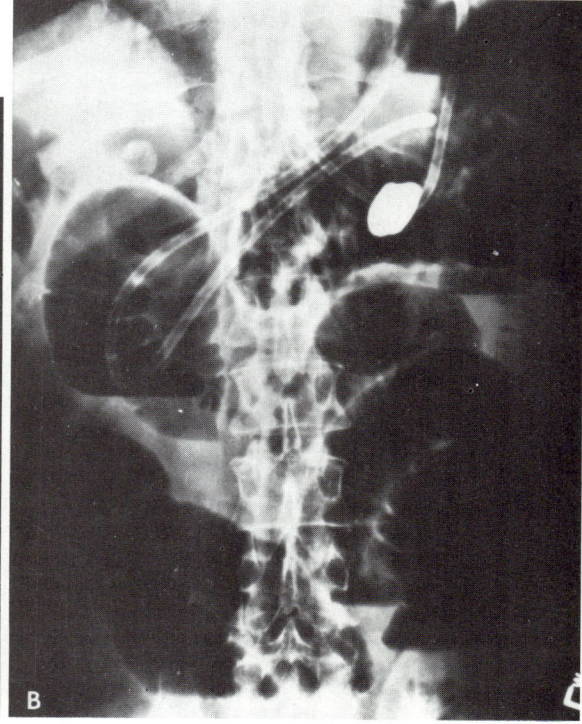

Figure 5–30. (Below) A 66-year-old male with small bowel obstruction secondary to adhesions. A, An upright radiograph taken nine days postoperatively shows gas beneath the central tendinous portion of the diaphragm (arrowheads), raising the possibility of free air. B, After a Cantor tube was placed, the gas collection was demonstrated to be a distended stomach.

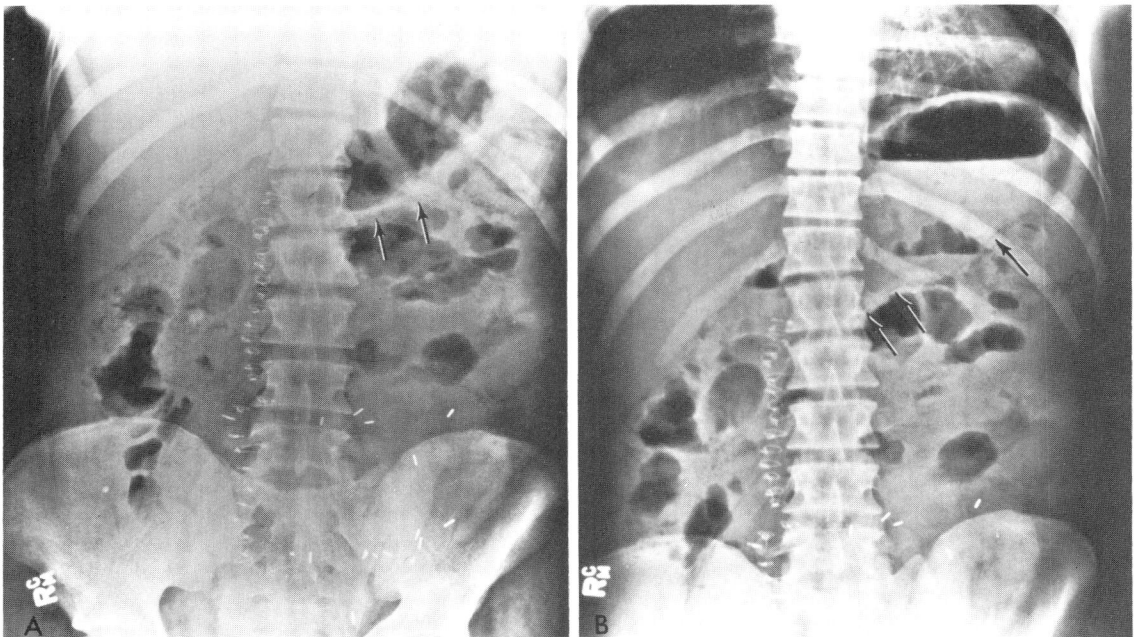

Figure 5–31. Pericolonic fat simulating pneumatosis. A 21-year-old male two weeks after renal transplant experienced increasing abdominal pain, distention, and rigid abdomen. *A,* The supine radiograph shows a lucent band paralleling the small bowel (arrows). *B,* The finding is constant on the upright radiograph. The radiologic diagnosis was subserosal air with necrosis. At surgery no abnormality was found. The roentgen appearance was caused by abundant fat.

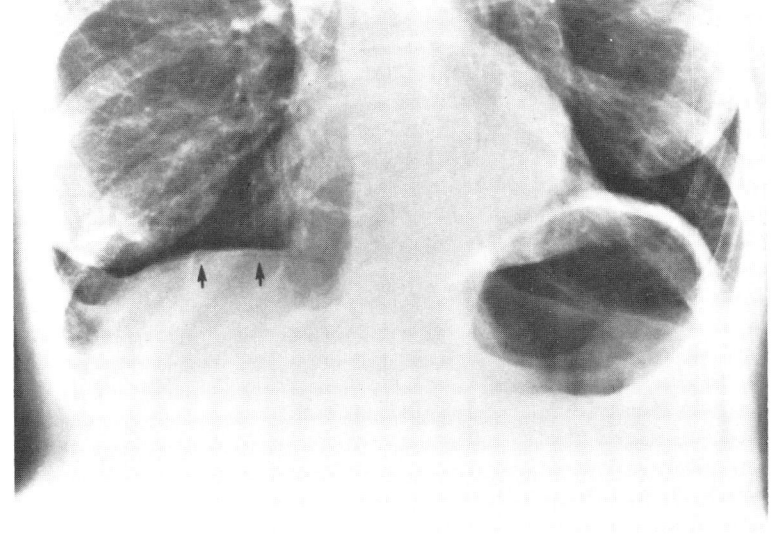

Figure 5–32. A 68-year-old female with acute abdominal pain. An upright chest radiograph demonstrates fat beneath the diaphragm (arrows), simulating pneumoperitoneum.

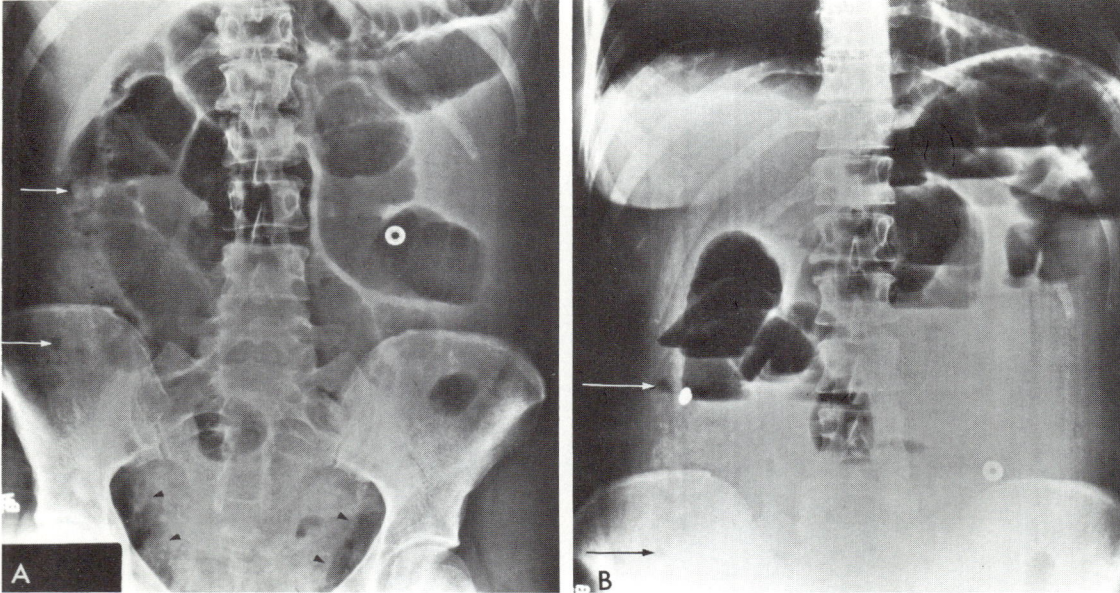

Figure 5–33. Paracolic abscess. A 36-year-old female developed fever and abdominal pain two days after surgery for ectopic pregnancy. *A,* A supine radiograph shows distended loops of small bowel, collapsed colon, gas in the extraperitoneal spaces in the pelvis (arrowheads), and fluid and air lateral to the right colon in the peritoneal cavity (arrows). *B,* The upright radiograph demonstrates small bowel air-fluid levels and fixation of the intraperitoneal gas (arrows). Noninfected postoperative extraperitoneal air and right paracolic abscess were diagnosed.

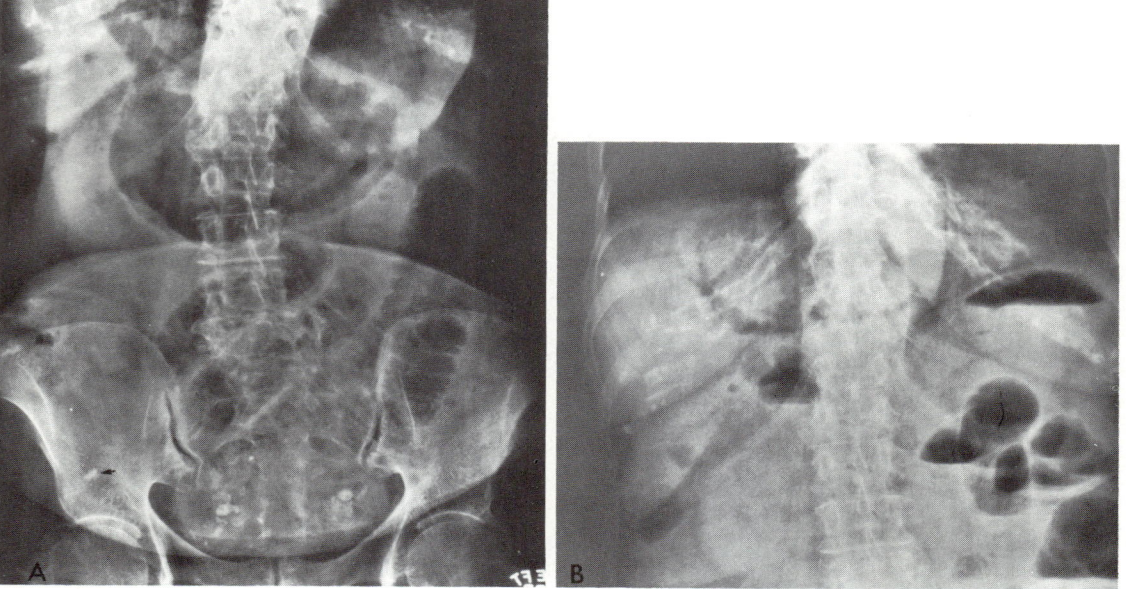

Figure 5–34. Gallstone ileus. A 91-year-old female with nausea, vomiting, and upper abdominal pain of two days' duration. *A,* The supine radiograph shows a radiopaque calculus in the right lower quadrant (arrow) and small bowel obstruction. *B,* The upright radiograph clearly shows air in the biliary tree and air-fluid levels in the obstructed small bowel.

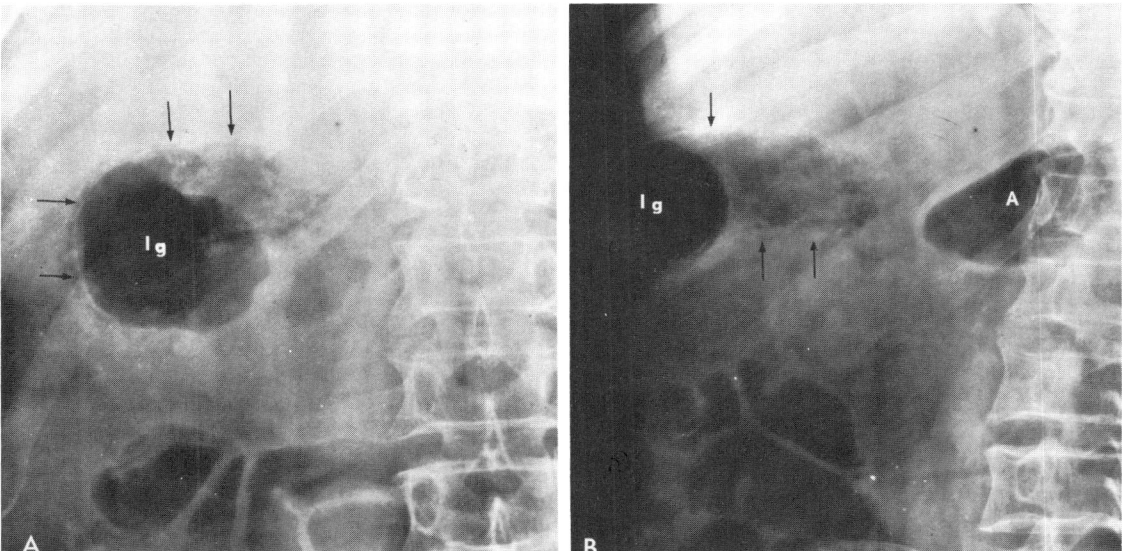

Figure 5–35. Emphysematous cholecystitis. A 63-year-old male with fever, vomiting, and abdominal pain. Radiographs of the abdomen in the anteroposterior (A) and slight right posterior oblique projections (B) show the gallbladder outlined by intramural gas (arrows) and intraluminal gas (Ig). A = antrum.

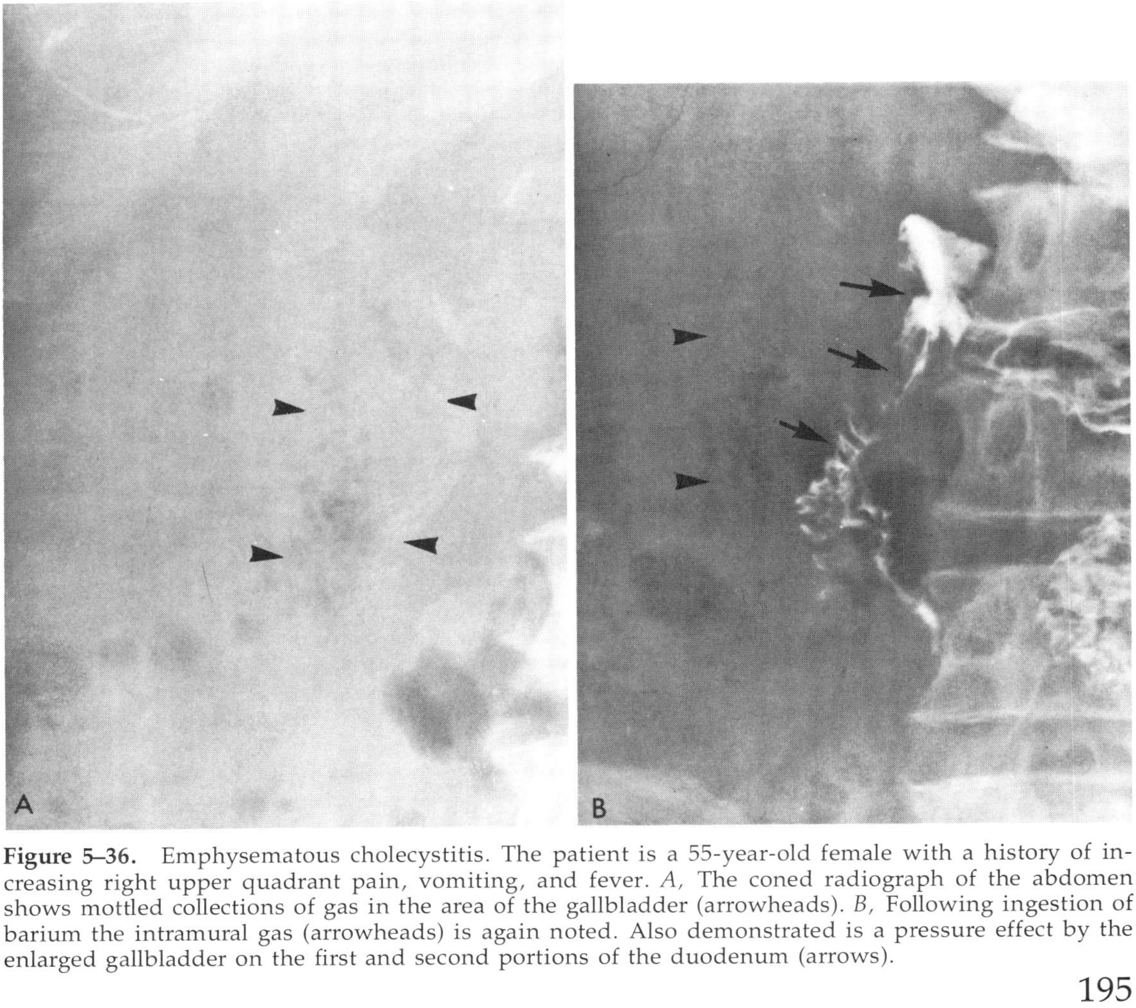

Figure 5–36. Emphysematous cholecystitis. The patient is a 55-year-old female with a history of increasing right upper quadrant pain, vomiting, and fever. A, The coned radiograph of the abdomen shows mottled collections of gas in the area of the gallbladder (arrowheads). B, Following ingestion of barium the intramural gas (arrowheads) is again noted. Also demonstrated is a pressure effect by the enlarged gallbladder on the first and second portions of the duodenum (arrows).

195

196 — THE ACUTE ABDOMEN

ABNORMAL CALCIFICATION. Abdominal calcifications have multiple causes (Figs. 5–37 to 5–43). Certain calcifications are of diagnostic importance in the assessment of an acute abdomen. For example, the demonstration of appendicoliths in the presence of acute abdominal pain has a high degree of correlation with acute appendicitis (see Fig. 5–12A; Figs. 5–44 and 5–45). Table 5–6 lists those calcifications that may be important in the diagnosis of the acute abdomen.

Text continued on page 201.

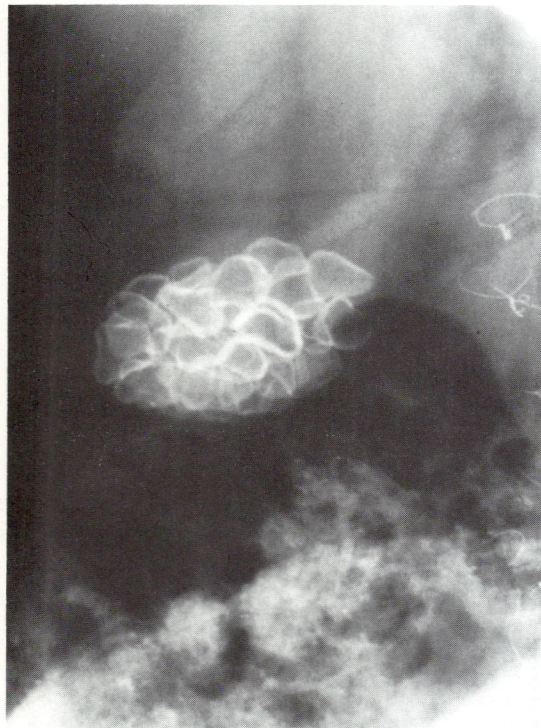

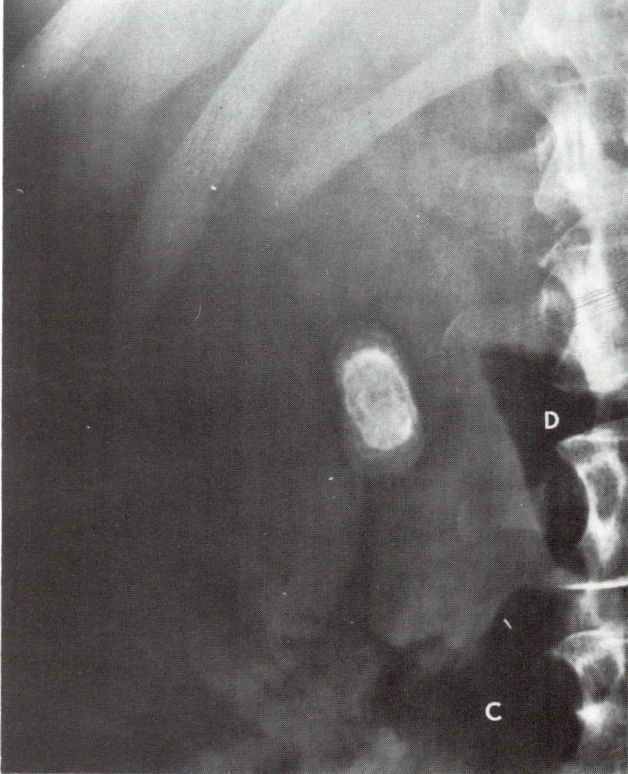

Figure 5–37. Acute and chronic cholecystitis and cholelithiasis. A 62-year-old female with a long history of gallbladder disease presented with acute right upper quadrant pain. Oral cholecystography showed faint visualization of the gallbladder and multiple calculi.

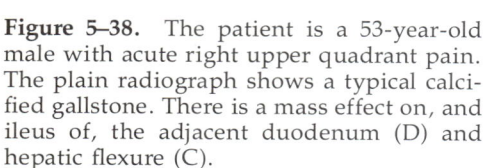

Figure 5–38. The patient is a 53-year-old male with acute right upper quadrant pain. The plain radiograph shows a typical calcified gallstone. There is a mass effect on, and ileus of, the adjacent duodenum (D) and hepatic flexure (C).

THE ACUTE ABDOMEN — 197

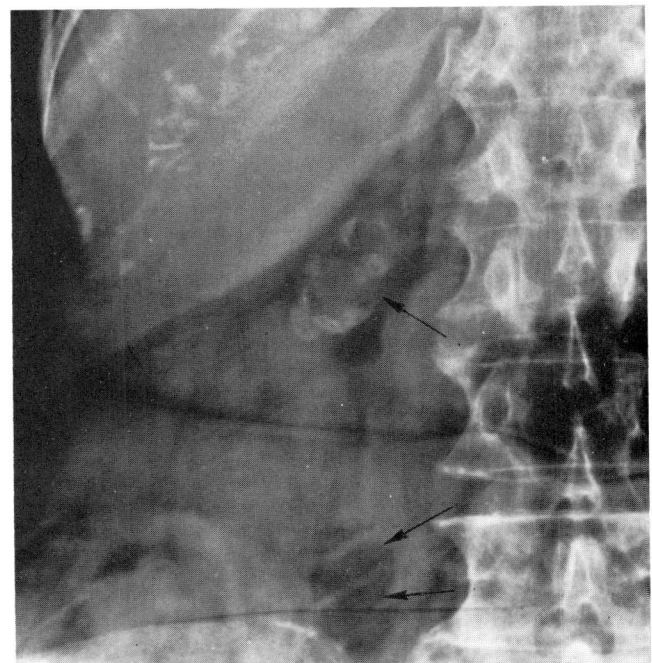

Figure 5–39. A 65-year-old female with acute upper abdominal pain, fever, chills, and elevated leukocyte count. The plain radiograph shows a calculus of the gallbladder (upper arrow) and an ileus of the duodenum (lower arrows).

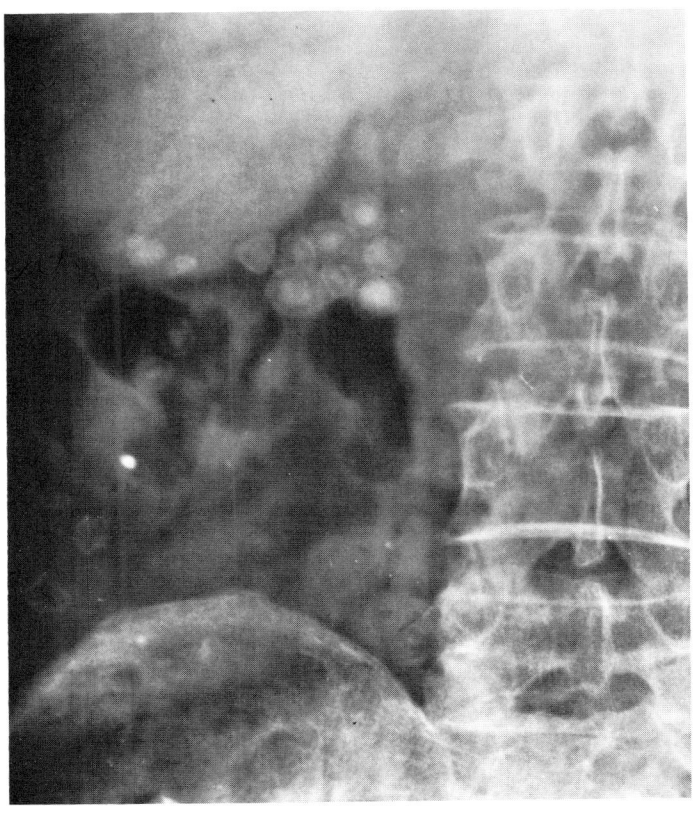

Figure 5–40. Renal colic. A 74-year-old male with acute right upper quadrant pain medially and to the back, associated with vomiting. The plain film shows multiple calculi, which appear to be in the gallbladder. An oral cholecystogram was normal. Intravenous urography showed renal calculi.

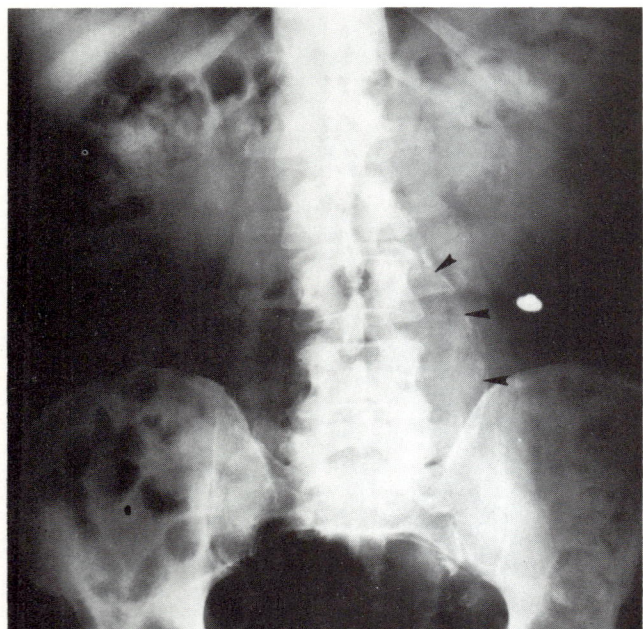

Figure 5-41. Aortic aneurysm simulating a urologic disorder. A 74-year-old male with symptoms suggesting renal colic. The plain radiograph of the abdomen shows a large aortic aneurysm with a calcified wall (arrowheads). Emergency urography was within normal limits.

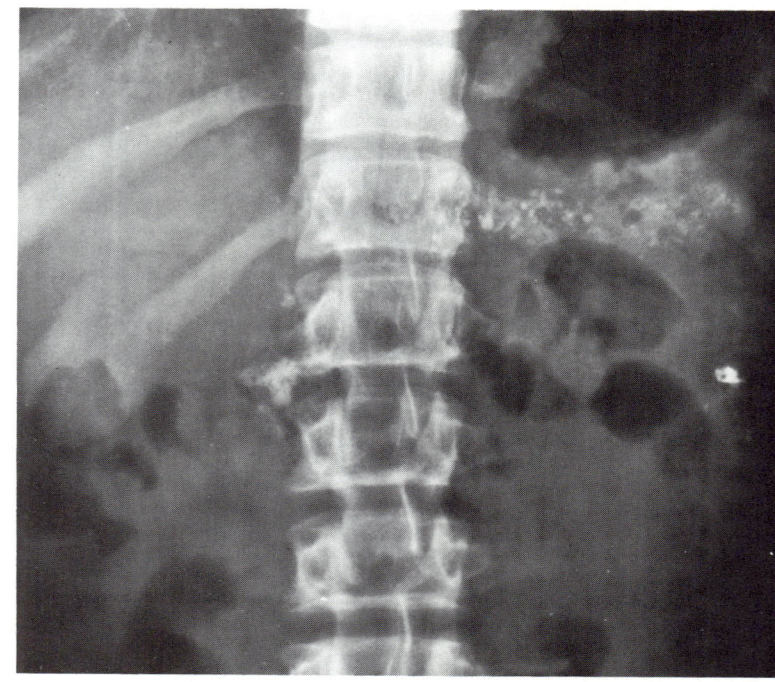

Figure 5-42. Calcific pancreatitis. A 44-year-old male with subacute abdominal pain. Oral cholecystography performed the following day showed faint opacification of the gallbladder. Note the extensive calcific pancreatitis.

THE ACUTE ABDOMEN — 199

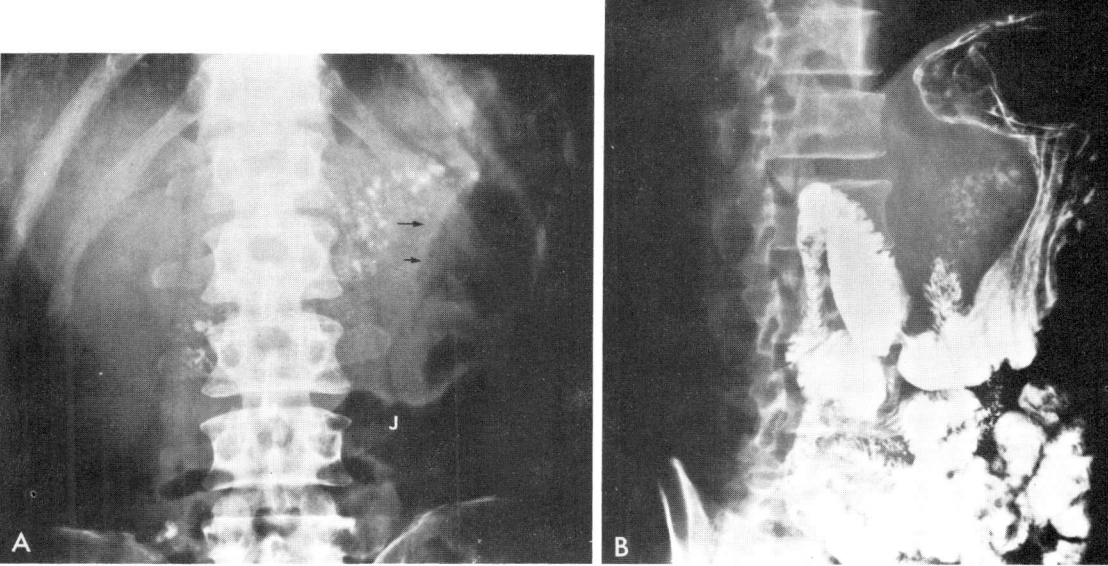

Figure 5–43. Pancreatitis. A 47-year-old male with acute abdominal pain. *A*, A plain radiograph shows extensive calcifications in the pancreas with an ileus of the distal transverse colon (arrows) — cut-off sign — and of the proximal jejunal (J). *B*, Three weeks later, when the patient was asymptomatic, an upper, gastrointestinal series showed resolution of the ileus and a mass in the tail of the pancreas indenting the posterior wall of the stomach.

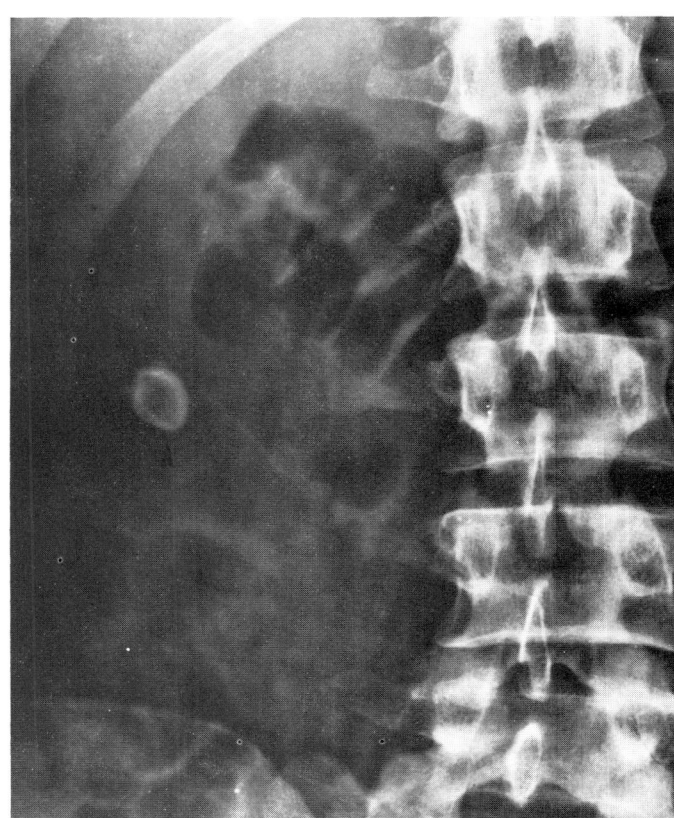

Figure 5–44. Appendicitis in a high retrocecal appendix with appendicolith. A 40-year-old male with acute onset of right upper quadrant pain. There were fever and guarding on palpation.

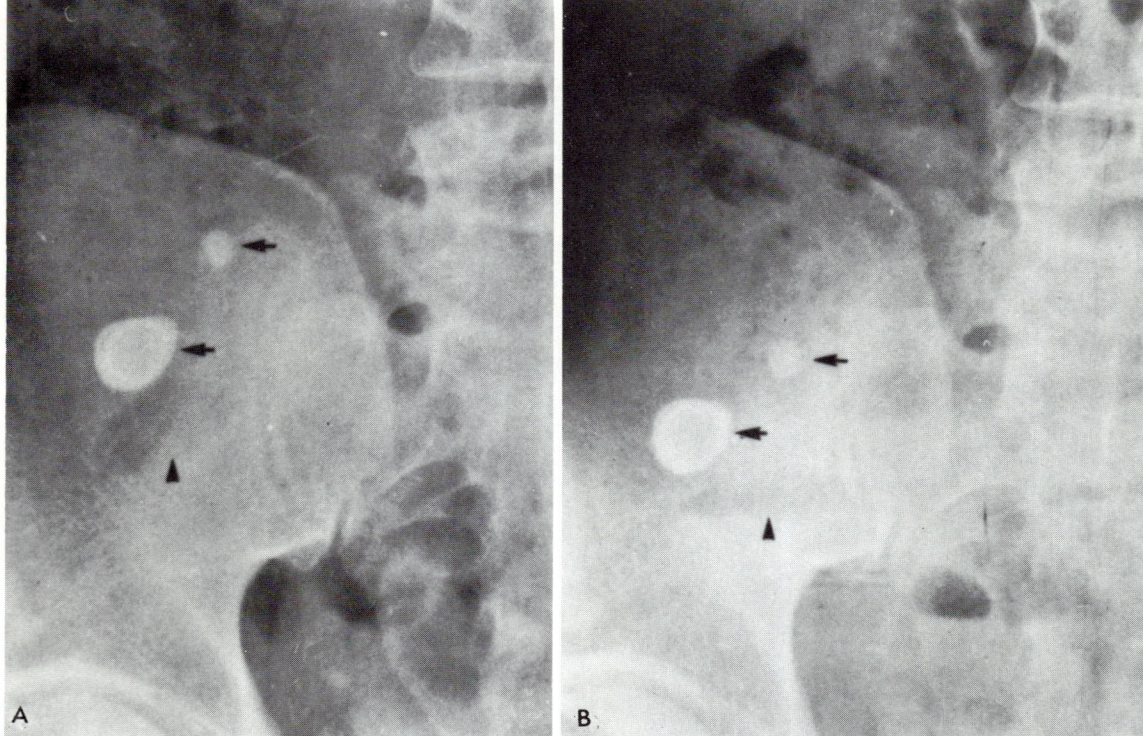

Figure 5–45. Appendiceal abscess and appendicoliths in acute appendicitis. A 32-year-old male with right lower quadrant pain, which had increased in intensity for one week prior to admission. Fever and localized tenderness were present. Coned views of the right lower quadrant in the supine (A) and upright (B) positions show two lamellated calculi (arrows) in the area of the appendix and a soft tissue mass containing air (arrowhead, A), causing an air-fluid level in the upright position (arrowhead, B).

TABLE 5–6. ABDOMINAL CALCIFICATIONS IN AN ACUTE ABDOMEN

Calculi of the gallbladder
Calcified plaques in walls of gallbladder
Milk of calcium bile
Calculus in common bile duct, recognizable by its location just lateral to transverse processes of L_1 to L_3
Abnormal location of a gallbladder calculus—gallstone ileus
Atheromatous plaques in aneurysm of abdominal aorta
Atheromatous plaques in aneurysm of hepatic and splenic artery
Abnormal size, shape, and position of other vascular shadows
Appendicoliths—seen in about 10 per cent of patients with acute abdomen
Calcific deposits in appendiceal mucocele, either amorphous or ringlike, surrounding the mucocele
Ribbonlike calcifications in Meckel's diverticulum—seen more frequently in the right lower quadrant
Pancreatic calculi
Ureteral calculus
Calcium deposits in dermoid cyst

INTRAPERITONEAL PATHOLOGIC ENTITIES

Perforated Gastric and Duodenal Ulcer

Perforation of a duodenal or gastric ulcer usually presents dramatically. Statistically, perforation of a gastric ulcer is more common than that of a duodenal ulcer. The radiologic finding of free air in the peritoneal cavity is the most helpful sign in confirming this diagnosis. Commonly, the gas collects beneath the diaphragm (Fig. 5–46) if perforation is secondary to an ulcer of the duodenal bulb or of the anterior wall of the stomach. Gas in the subhepatic space is usually due to a duodenal ulcer (Fig. 5–47). If perforation is from the posterior wall of the stomach behind the gastrohepatic ligament, air is present in the lesser sac. The importance of obtaining a lateral radiograph cannot be overemphasized in differentiating gas collections in front of the gastrohepatic ligament in the gastrohepatic recess from those collections behind the stomach in the lesser sac.

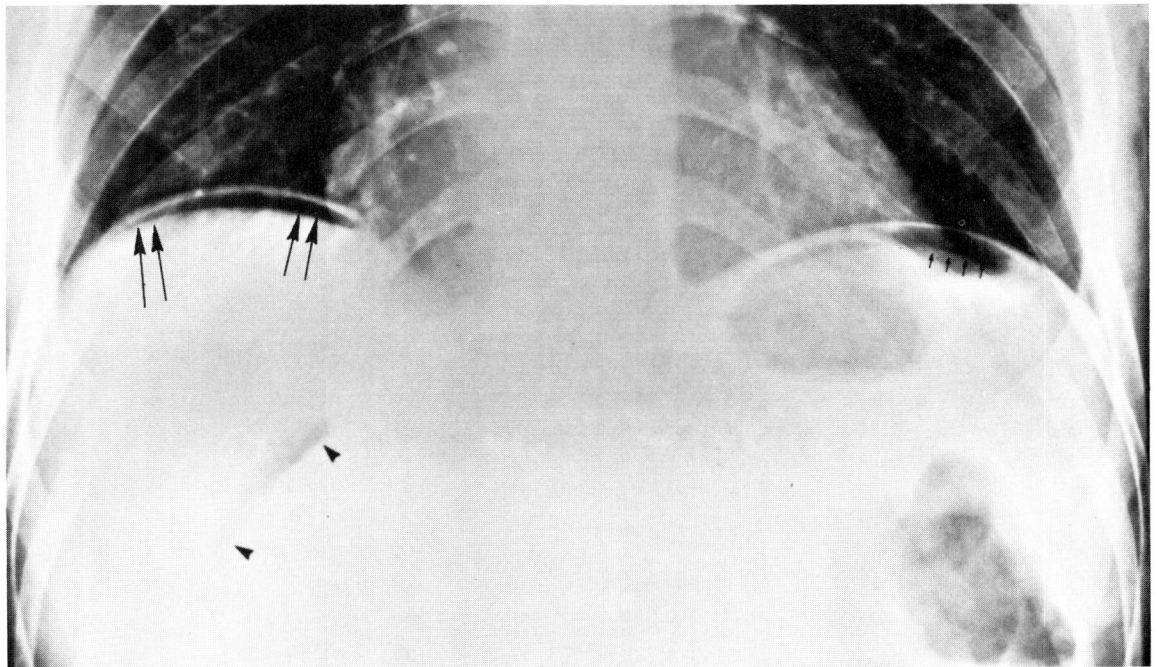

Figure 5–46. Perforated ulcer. A 46-year old male was admitted with acute stabbing pain in the epigastrium and vomiting. The upright radiograph shows free air in the peritoneal cavity (arrows) and in the subhepatic area (arrowheads). At surgery a perforated duodenal ulcer was found.

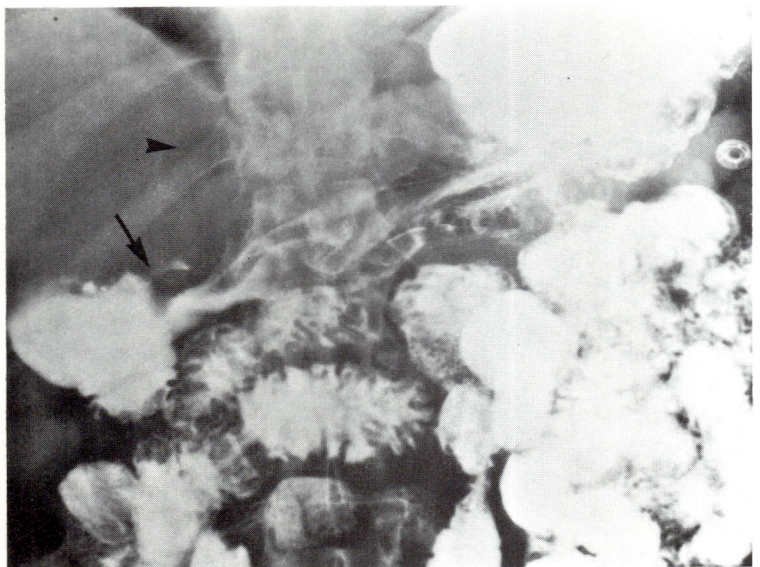

Figure 5–47. Perforated peptic ulcer. A 48-year-old male with a long history of peptic ulcer disease presented with severe epigastric pain. An abdominal survey was unremarkable. An emergency upper gastrointestinal series shows perforation (arrow) and extravasation of contrast medium. A collection of air is seen in the visceral space of the liver (arrowhead), which was not demonstrated on the preliminary plain radiographs.

Biliary Tract

The presentation of acute biliary tract disease is usually in the form of acute cholecystitis or acute obstruction of the common bile duct. Acute cholecystitis is often associated with a calculus obstructing the gallbladder. Occasionally it may be a nonobstructive acute cholecystitis. There may be enlargement of the gallbladder with obstruction, in which case hydrops of the gallbladder occurs and a mass may be discernible on the radiograph by virtue of displacement of the adjacent gas-filled structures (see Figs. 5–26 and 5–27). There may be ileus of structures adjacent to the gallbladder, such as the duodenum and the proximal portion of the transverse colon (Fig. 5–48). Intravenous cholangiography may be required to make the diagnosis of obstruction of the cystic duct; it may also be useful in separating acute pancreatitis, a nonsurgical emergency, from acute obstructive cholecystitis, a surgical emergency. Ultrasound examination may be definitive, demonstrating the presence of calculi, gallbladder size, and thickening of the gallbladder wall. If the cholecystitis is caused by bacteria capable of gas formation, it may present radiologically as intraluminal gas outlining the wall of the viscus or gas within the lumen (see Figs. 5–35 and 5–36). The most common organisms presenting in this manner are *Escherichia coli*, *Bacillus aerogenes*, *Proteus*, and *enterococci*. Gas may also appear in the biliary tree following the passage of a gallstone into the gastrointestinal tract (see Fig. 5–34; Fig. 5–49).

The demonstration of a radiopaque calculus of the gallbladder occurs in approximately 15 per cent of cases. The calculi may be lamellated or of mixed types (see Fig. 5–38) and either solitary or multiple (see Fig. 5–37). The calcifications in the right upper quadrant may occasionally take the form of calcific deposits in the wall of the gallbladder (see Fig. 5–39).

The findings of acute cholecystitis, then, may be a mass effect, gas within the biliary system, calculi, or ileus of the adjacent viscera. Caution should be observed in diagnosing air in the biliary system, since gas in the portal venous system may simulate air in the biliary tree. The peripheral location and characteristic branching of the portal venous system make the differentiation (Fig. 5–50). In addition, after passage of a

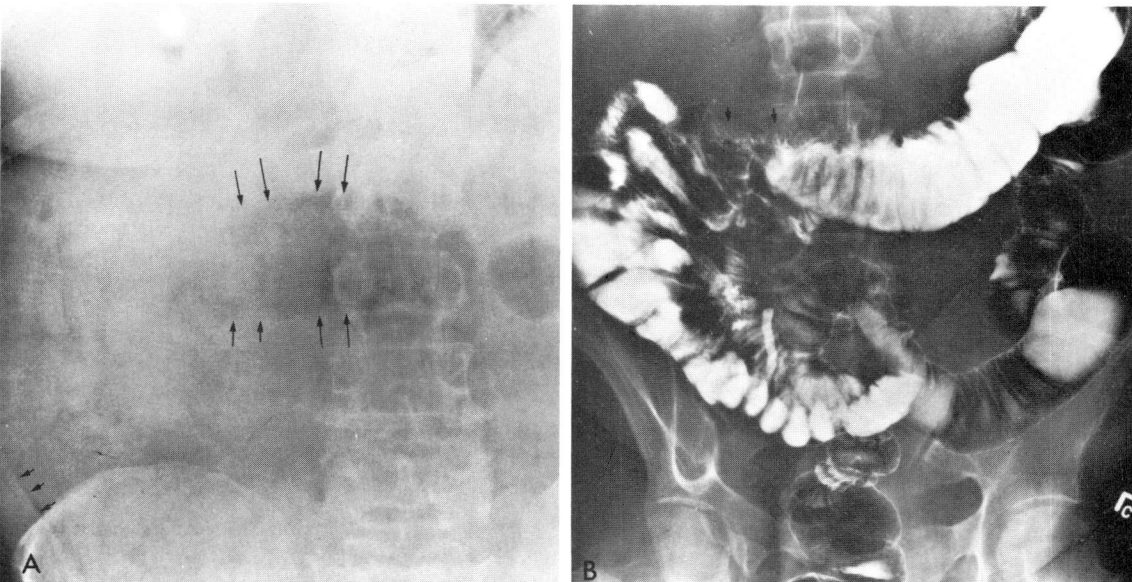

Figure 5–48. Acute cholecystitis. A 63-year-old female was admitted with acute right upper quadrant pain, vomiting, and diarrhea. *A,* The plain radiograph of the abdomen shows an ileus of the proximal transverse colon (long arrows) and flattening of the flank stripe (smallest arrows), suggesting intraperitoneal fluid. *B,* Barium enema shows an extrinsic defect of the transverse colon with some tethering in the area of the gallbladder (arrows). The roentgen diagnosis of acute cholecystitis, with the gallbladder adherent to the transverse colon, and fluid in the peritoneal cavity was confirmed at surgery.

common bile duct calculus causing incompetence of the sphincter of Oddi, gas may be present in the biliary tree. Also, fat in and around the liver and its ligaments and around the common bile duct may at times simulate gas. Ultrasound gray-scale studies or CT examinations may give highly important and frequently diagnostic information.

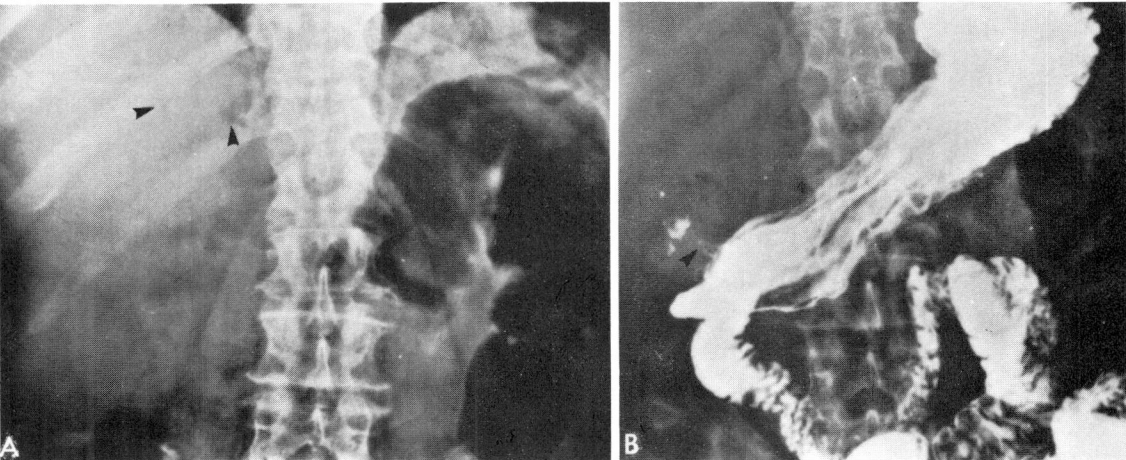

Figure 5–49. Cholecystoduodenal fistula. A 50-year-old male with acute right upper quadrant pain and slightly elevated bilirubin. *A,* A plain radiograph of the abdomen suggests air in the biliary tree (arrowheads). *B,* An upper gastrointestinal series shows a fistula (arrowhead) communicating to the gas shadow seen on the plain radiograph. The diagnosis was cholecystoduodenal fistula secondary to perforated gallbladder by a gallstone.

204 — THE ACUTE ABDOMEN

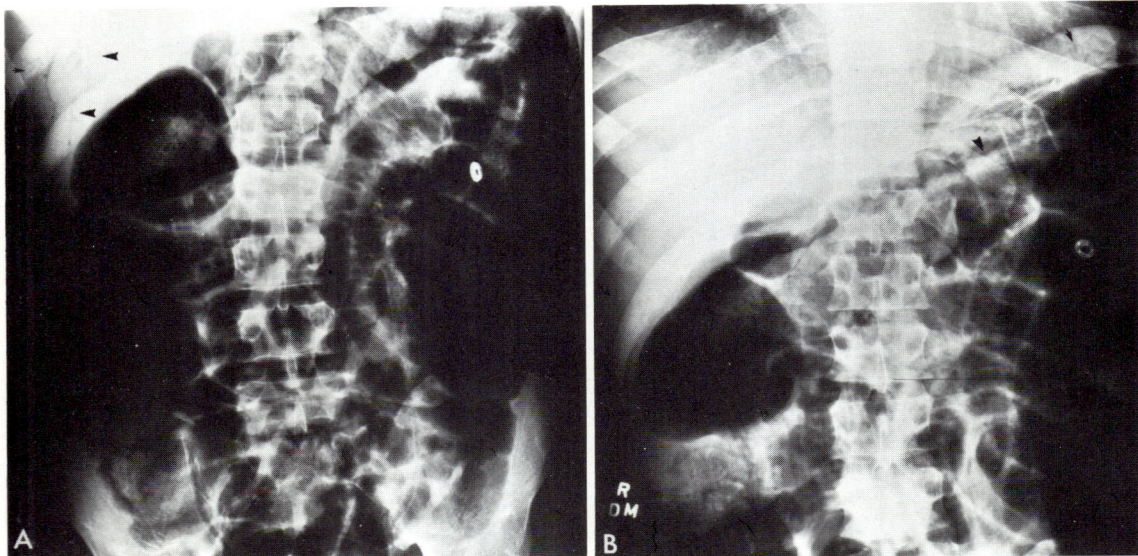

Figure 5–50. Small bowel ischemia. A 28-year-old male on dialysis, experienced sudden onset of severe, diffuse abdominal pain. Abdominal distention and tenderness were present. A clinical diagnosis of small bowel obstruction was made. *A,* A plain radiograph of the abdomen shows gas in the portal vein system (arrowheads) and dilated loops of small and large bowel. *B,* The upright radiograph shows gas in the walls of the small bowel (arrowheads). The radiologic diagnosis was ischemia of the small bowel with infarction and gas along the walls and in the portal venous system as well as secondary ileus. These findings were confirmed at surgery.

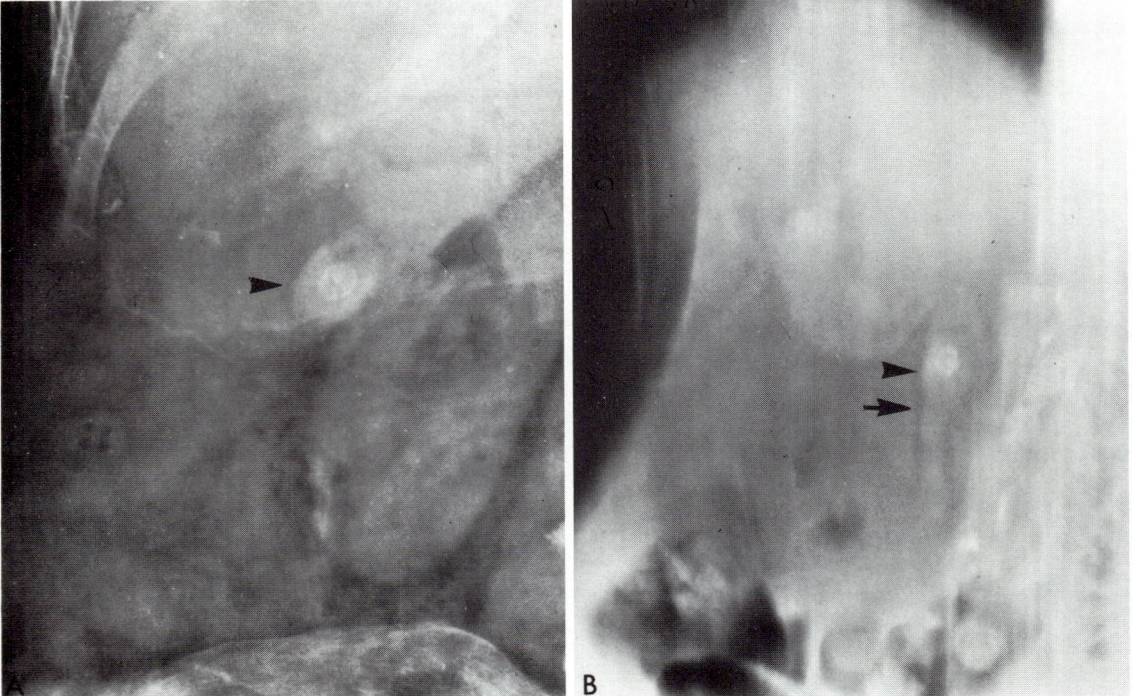

Figure 5–51. Common duct stone. A 74-year-old male was admitted with sudden severe right upper quadrant pain and vomiting. *A,* A radiograph of the right upper quadrant taken 16 months previously showed a gallbladder calculus (arrowhead). An abdominal survey suggests that the calculus is now in the common bile duct. *B,* An emergency intravenous cholangiogram confirmed its location (arrowhead) and also demonstrated partial obstruction and dilatation of the common bile duct (arrow).

Common bile duct obstruction may present as an acute abdomen and is difficult to separate from an inflammatory or obstructive process in an adjacent area. Radiographic findings of common duct obstruction are usually absent. Occasionally, however, a calculus may be seen in the location of the common duct (Fig. 5–51). Intravenous cholangiography will demonstrate the obstruction. Ultrasonography and CT studies may be of help in showing dilatation of the common bile duct to the level of the calculus.

Pancreatitis

Acute pancreatitis is at times a difficult radiologic diagnosis to make. The radiographic signs of acute pancreatitis[1] are a pseudocyst, calcifications, mass effect of the pancreas, gas in the pancreas, or ileus of the adjacent structures (see Figs. 5–41 and 5–43; Figs. 5–52 to 5–55). The inflammation may extend into the gastrocolic ligament, into the paraduodenal area, or outside the peritoneum, following the route of the mesentery of the small bowel. The inflammatory process may involve the entire anterior pararenal space. Table 5–7 lists the radiologic findings of acute pancreatitis. Ultrasound or CT scans may show enlargement of the pancreas as well as the presence of a pseudocyst or abscess.

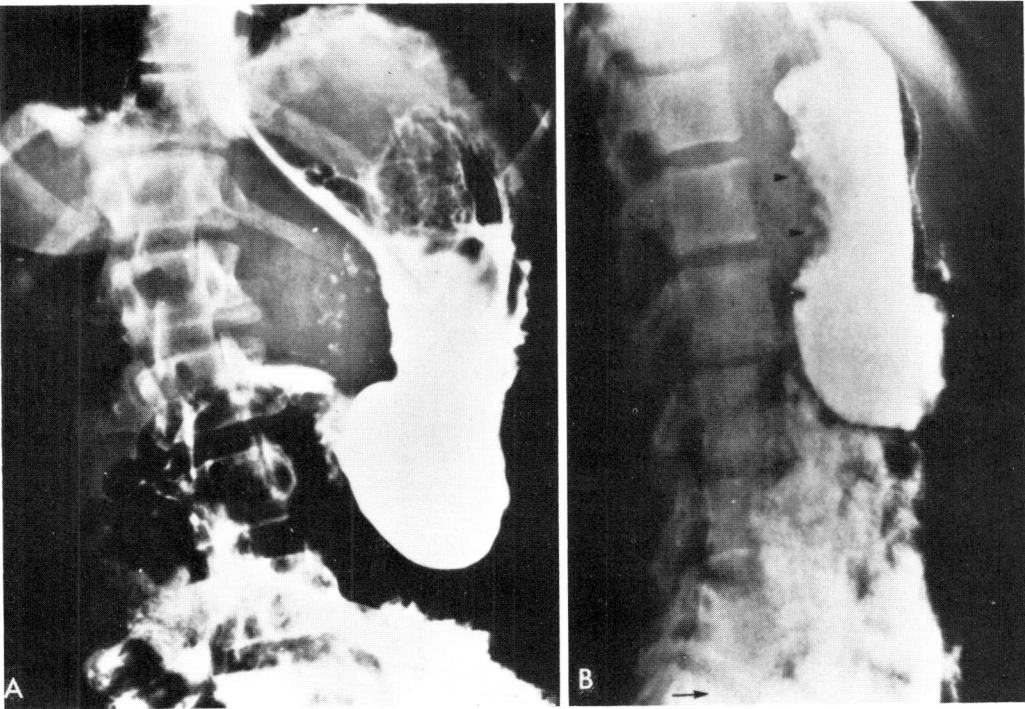

Figure 5–52. Pancreatitis. *A* and *B*, A 39-year-old female with a history of chronic alcoholism and onset of severe abdominal pain. In the differential diagnosis were peptic ulcer disease or pancreatitis. An upper gastrointestinal series shows evidence of chronic calcific pancreatitis and cystic formation adherent to the posterior gastric wall (arrowheads). No ulcer is seen. The diagnosis was acute and chronic pancreatitis.

206 — THE ACUTE ABDOMEN

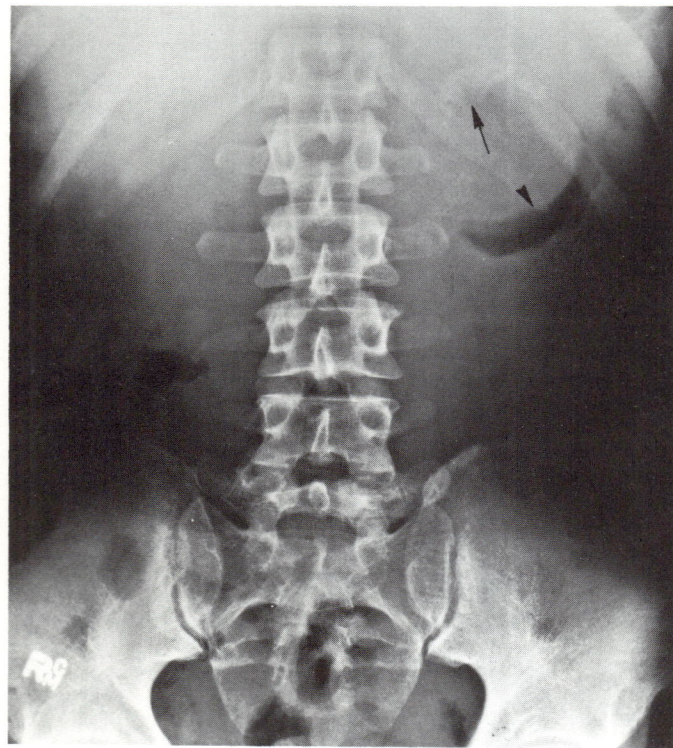

Figure 5–53. Pancreatic cyst. A 35-year-old male with a history of alcoholic abuse was admitted with increasing abdominal pain of several days duration. A plain radiograph of the abdomen shows a crescent type of calcium deposition in the upper contour of a pancreatic cyst (arrow) and a pressure effect by the lower pole of the cyst on the stomach (arrowhead).

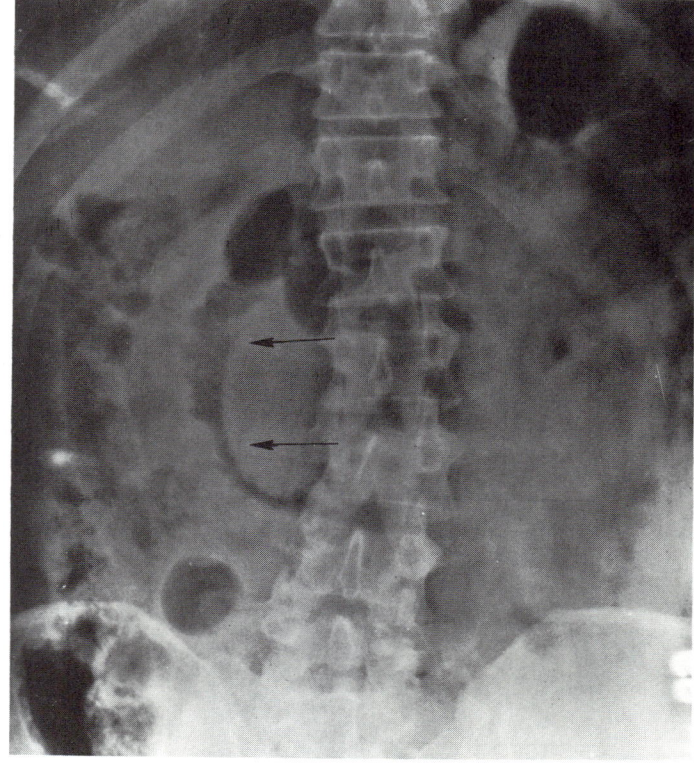

Figure 5–54. Acute pancreatitis. The patient is a 41-year-old male with acute epigastric pain showing a mass effect (arrows) on the medial aspect of the descending duodenum secondary to enlargement of the head of the pancreas.

THE ACUTE ABDOMEN — 207

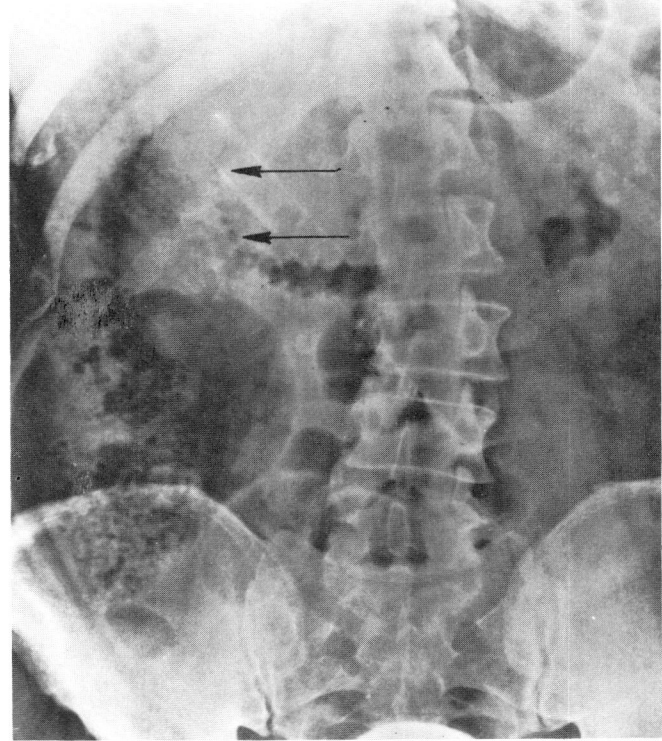

Figure 5–55. Acute pancreatitis. A 48-year-old male with acute abdominal pain and elevated amylase. The supine radiograph shows an ileus of the descending duodenum (arrows) and of the portion of the colon related to the head of the pancreas.

TABLE 5–7. RADIOGRAPHIC SIGNS OF ACUTE PANCREATITIS DEMONSTRABLE IN PLAIN RADIOGRAPHS OF THE ABDOMEN

Most Common Findings

Dilated and atonic first and second portions of the duodenum
Adynamic ileus with dilatation of several loops of small bowel, usually on the left (sentinel loop), but frequently bilateral
Dilatation of large bowel—the ascending and transverse colon to the splenic flexure (colon cut-off sign)
Sentinel loop in right lower quadrant proximal to dilated distal ileal coil

Less Specific Findings

Loss of visualization of the psoas margins if effusion extends to posterior pararenal space
Increased interspace between stomch and transverse colon (greater than 3 cm)
Displacement and abnormal appearance of greater curvature of stomach
Numerous mottled radiolucent shadows seen in the region of the pancreas, produced by fat necrosis
Pancreatic calcifications

Blunt Trauma to the Abdomen

The radiographic findings of blunt abdominal trauma are related to hemorrhage (see Fig. 5–22), enlargement of organs (see Figs. 5–23 and 5–24), or air within the abdominal cavity due to perforation of a hollow viscus.

Careful scrutiny should be made for evidence of free fluid (blood) in the peritoneal cavity (see Table 5–2), or in the extraperitoneal space (see Table 5–3). There may be a

208 — THE ACUTE ABDOMEN

localized ileus of structures adjacent to the traumatized organ. A subcapsular hematoma of the liver or spleen may manifest radiographically as enlargement with evidence of free fluid. Enlargement localized to a portion of an organ is suspicious. Gas in the intraperitoneal cavity may reflect laceration of those portions of hollow viscus that have intraperitoneal relationships. Gas in the extraperitoneal space also reflects rupture of a hollow viscus located in the extraperitoneal space (Fig. 5–56). The radiologic findings of hepatic rupture are illustrated in Table 5–8 and those of splenic rupture are listed in Table 5–9.[15, 16] Splenic rupture may be diagnosed by radioisotope studies.

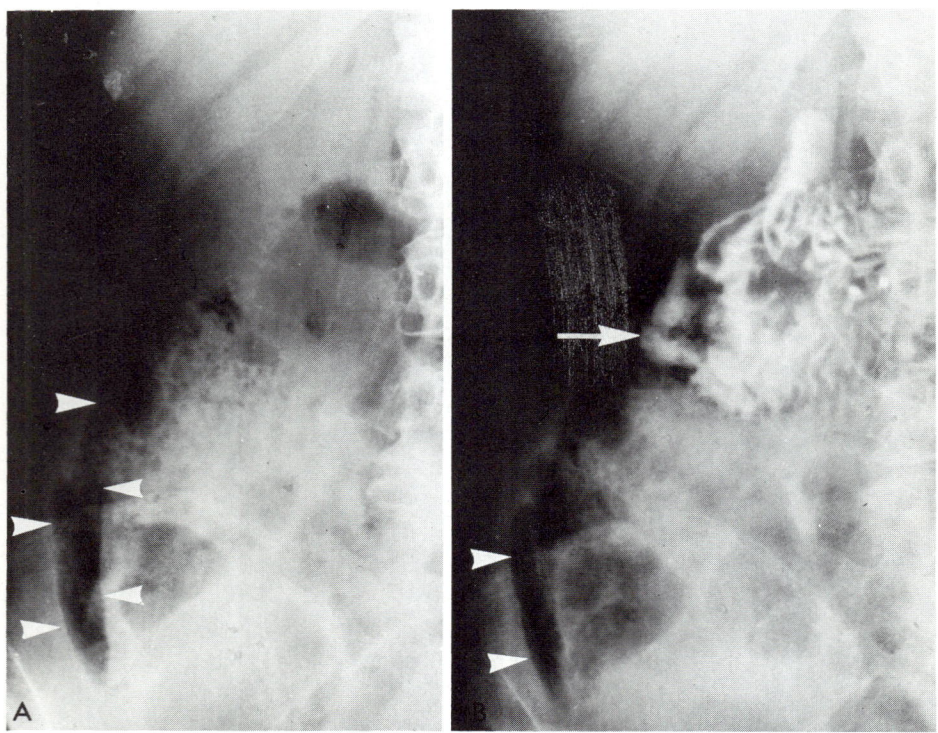

Figure 5–56. Ruptured duodenum. A, A supine radiograph of the abdomen of a young adult following a seatbelt injury. There is absence of the hepatic angle and gas (arrowheads) lying in the anterior pararenal space (properitoneal fat region). B, Following the introduction of contrast material, the stomach and duodenum are outlined, rupture (arrow) of the descending duodenum with extravasation into the anterior pararenal space is demonstrated. (*From* Whalen, J. P., and Berne, A. S.: The extraperitoneal perivisceral fat pad. II. Roentgen interpretation of pathological alterations. Radiology *92*:473, 1969. Reproduced by permission.)

TABLE 5–8. ROENTGEN SIGNS OF HEPATIC RUPTURE IN PLAIN RADIOGRAPHS OF THE ABDOMEN

Loss of visualization of hepatic angle
Enlarged liver shadow
Hepatic flexure and proximal transverse colon displaced downward and laterally
Stomach displaced to left and posteriorly
Fluid in peritoneal cavity
Fractures of right lower ribs

TABLE 5–9. ROENTGEN SIGNS OF SPLENIC RUPTURE IN PLAIN RADIOGRAPHS OF THE ABDOMEN

Enlargement of splenic shadow
Dilatation of air-filled stomach
Prominent gastric rugal folds along the greater curvature
Left pleural reaction
Separation of fundus of stomach from left dome of diaphragm
Increased distance between stomach and ribs on a left lateral decubitus radiograph
Fractures of lower left ribs
Fluid in peritoneal cavity

Rupture of the stomach is extremely rare and results in free air within the peritoneal cavity. The duodenum may rupture in its intraperitoneal portion, although laceration of its extraperitoneal segment is more common. The radiographic findings of traumatic rupture of duodenum, small bowel, and colon are listed in Table 5–10.[7, 15]

Laceration of the pancreas may also occur. The radiographic findings include fluid in the anterior pararenal space. If extensive spread occurs to the posterior pararenal space, pseudocysts may become evident during convalescence, but generally masses do not occur in acute rupture of the pancreas. However, there may be secondary effects on adjacent anatomic structures;[7] these findings are listed in Table 5–11.

TABLE 5–10. ROENTGEN FINDINGS IN TRAUMATIC PERFORATION OF DUODENUM, SMALL BOWEL, AND COLON DEMONSTRABLE IN PLAIN RADIOGRAPHS OF THE ABDOMEN

Duodenum

A. Intraperitoneal laceration

   1. Signs of intraperitoneal effusion (see Table 5–2)
   2. Pneumoperitoneum
   3. Paralytic ileus of small and large intestine

B. Retroperitoneal laceration

   1. Signs of extraperitoneal effusion (see Table 5–3)
   2. Mottled gas, relatively fixed in the anterior pararenal space
   3. Gas in the perirenal space if the anterior renal fascia ruptures

C. Intramural hemorrhage

   1. Distended segment of duodenum with cut-off sign
   2. Distorted outline of involved segment of duodenum, at times with thumbprinting appearance

Small Bowel

1. Thickened, irregular folds (hemorrhage and exudate), with involved segment at times ending in a beaklike manner
2. Moderately dilated stomach, duodenum, and segment of jejunum proximal to the laceration
3. Fractures of pelvic bones or lumbar vertebrae
4. Pneumoperitoneum, rarely

Large Bowel

Pneumoperitoneum and signs of peritonitis (most commonly involved: cecum, ascending colon, descending colon, and sigmoid)

210 — THE ACUTE ABDOMEN

TABLE 5–11. ROENTGEN FINDINGS IN BLUNT TRAUMA TO THE PANCREAS

Dilatation and atony of dueal sweep and most proximal segment of jejunum
Widening of duodenal loop
Generalized paralytic ileus
Pressure effect on the posterior or posterolateral wall of stomach
Pressure effect on transverse colon and jejunal loops
Loss of visualization of the left psoas (if there is involvement of posterior pararenal space)
Colon cut-off sign
Signs of intraperitoneal effusion (see Table 5–2)
Left pleural reaction with poor diaphragmatic excursions

Small Bowel

In evaluating small bowel dilatation, mechanical obstruction must be distinguished from adynamic ileus. If small bowel obstruction is present, a number of differential causes should be considered, the most likely being postoperative adhesions. Primary tumors of the small bowel may occasionally present as an acute abdomen with complete or near-complete obstruction. Of the malignant tumors of the small bowel, carcinoma is the most likely to produce obstruction.

The character of the wall of the small bowel may help to establish the diagnosis of an acute abdomen. Tumor may efface the air-filled loops of bowel (Fig. 5–57). On occasion, Crohn's disease presents as an acute abdomen. The radiographic appearance

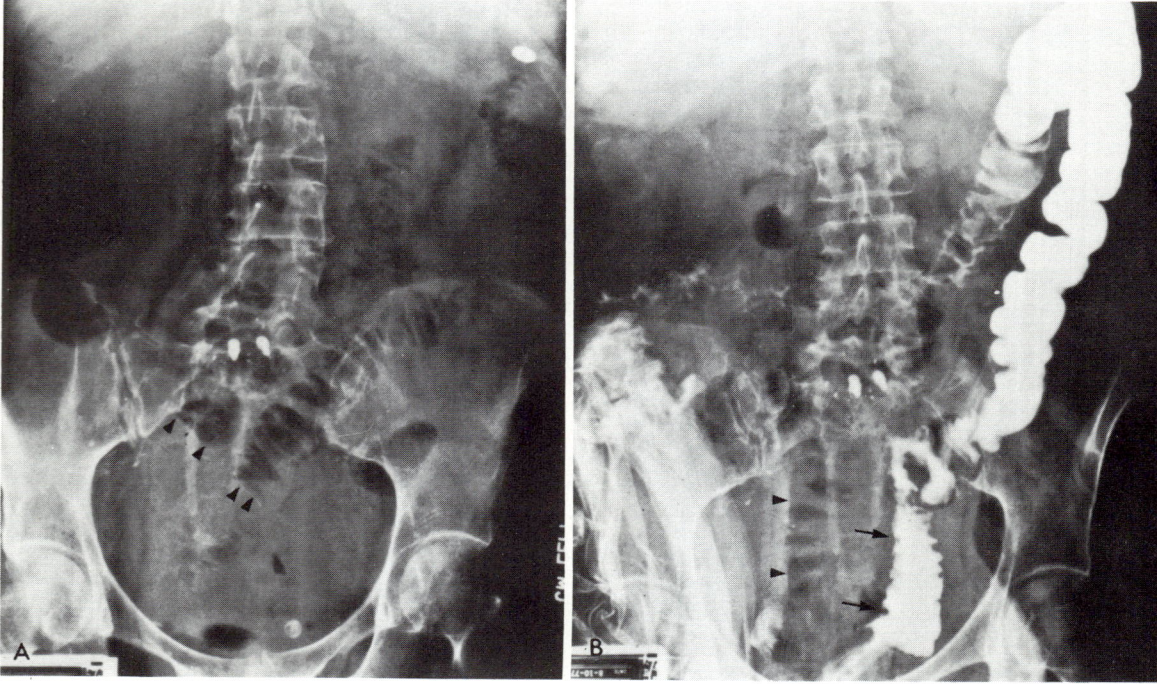

Figure 5–57. Lymphosarcoma. A 71-year-old female with acute onset of lower abdominal pain where a mass was palpable. *A*, The plain radiograph shows dilated loops of small bowel displaced by a mass in the right lower quadrant (arrowheads). *B*, A barium enema verified the mass effect displacing the rectum and sigmoid to the left (arrows). The trapped loop of air-filled small bowel is seen within the mass (arrowheads). Roentgen diagnosis: tumor mass presenting as small bowel obstruction. Pathologic diagnosis: lymphosarcoma.

THE ACUTE ABDOMEN — 211

of large and small bowel may suggest the diagnosis (Fig. 5–58), but contrast studies may be required for verification.

Acute ischemia of the bowel alters the appearance of the wall of the involved segment of intestine, causing thickening of the wall; characteristically there are submucosal filling defects (thumbprinting). At times gas is present in the wall of the small bowel and even in the portal venous system (see Fig. 5–50). The radiologic findings of ischemia of the small bowel are listed in Table 5–12.[17]

The diagnosis of Meckel's diverticulum is extremely difficult because it cannot usually be demonstrated on plain radiographs. Even with contrast studies, the diagnosis of Meckel's diverticulum is seldom made roentgenologically. However, it may be visualized on plain abdominal films (Fig. 5–59) if gas is present within the diverticulum.

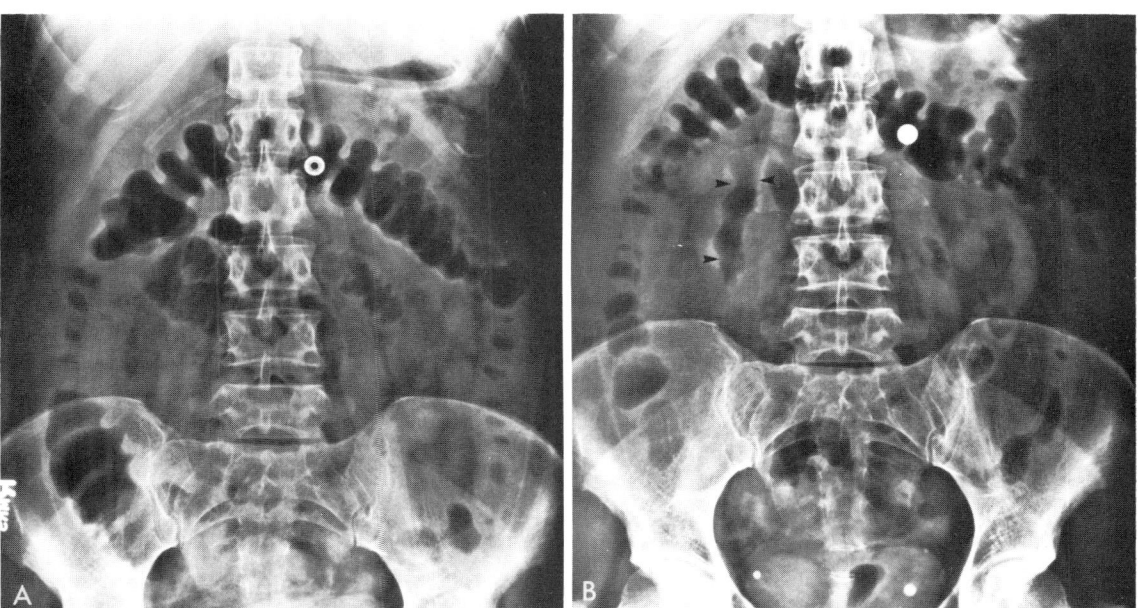

Figure 5–58. Granulomatous ileocolitis. A 40-year-old female with acute right quadrant pain. Standard radiographs of the abdomen were performed at admission and two days later. A, The initial study shows an abnormal right colon with a pseudo–small bowel appearance. B, The second radiograph two days later shows an amorphous appearance of a segment of small bowel (arrowheads). The diagnosis of granulomatous ileocolitis was confirmed by examination with contrast media.

TABLE 5–12. ROENTGEN SIGNS OF ISCHEMIC SMALL BOWEL DISEASE DEMONSTRABLE IN PLAIN RADIOGRAPHS OF THE ABDOMEN

Specific Signs
Thickening of bowel walls
Obliteration of mucosal pattern
Thumbprinting due to hemorrhage in the submucosa
Intramural air (cystlike or thin lucent bands parallel to bowel wall)
Gas in the portal venous system

Nonspecific Signs
Adynamic ileus
Pseudo-obstruction pattern
Airless abdomen
Small bowel obstruction pattern (if hemorrhage occludes a loop)

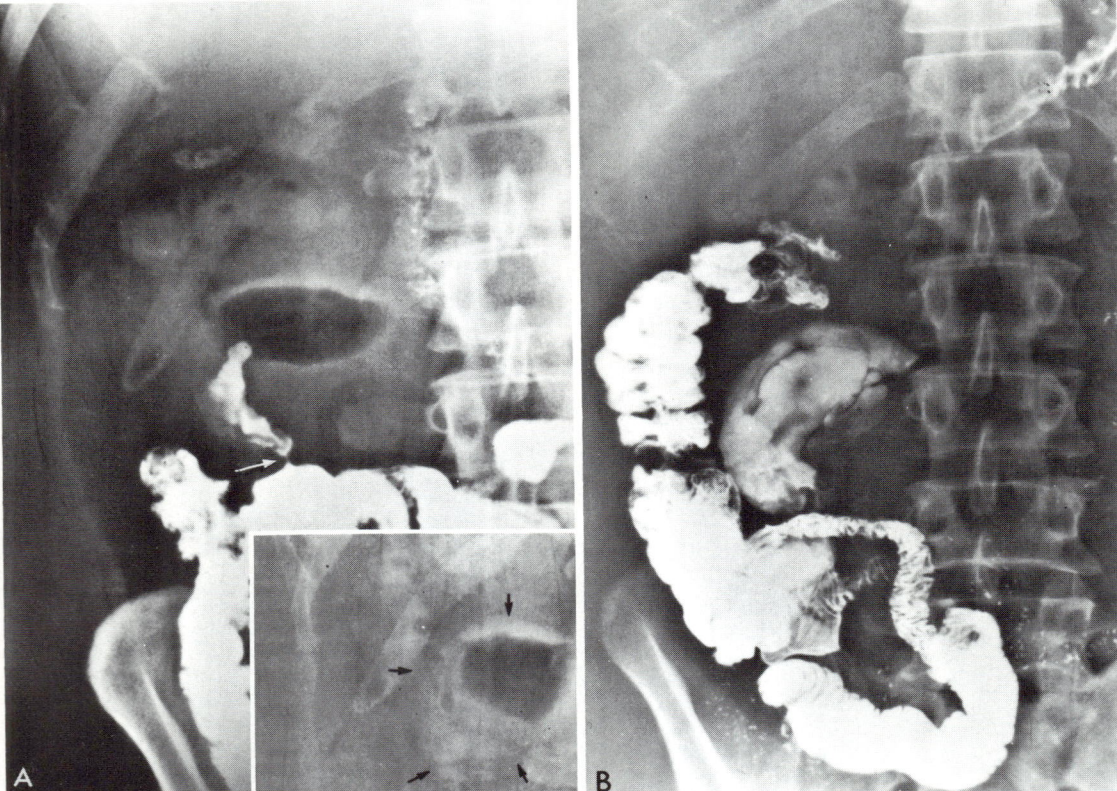

Figure 5–59. Meckel's diverticulitis. A 55-year-old male with a history of intermittent rectal bleeding and vague right-sided abdominal discomfort was admitted with acute onset of crampy abdominal pain. *A*, Inset shows evidence of a gas collection (arrows) just below the twelfth rib. Following ingestion of barium, a narrow tract (white arrow) was displaced in one of the distal ileal coils leading into the gas collection seen in the plain radiograph of the abdomen. *B*, Later, the gas collection is replaced by barium. The roentgen diagnosis of Meckel's diverticulum was confirmed at surgery.

Intussusception of small bowel presents radiographically as a mechanical obstruction; at times the intussusceptum is outlined by gas.

Volvulus of the small bowel is a rare occurrence that may present as a closed loop obstruction (Fig. 5–60). This appearance, which has been likened to that of a coffee bean, is caused by the twisted loop of bowel distended by gas and only partially closed. At times the involved segment of small bowel is completely closed and distended by fluid; it then appears in the supine radiograph as a dense mass—the pseudotumor sign (Fig. 5–61).

Internal hernias of small bowel may occur in multiple sites and may require special views for demonstration. Inguinal hernias may be diagnosed by a gas-containing loop of obstructed bowel in the area of the inguinal canal. Ventral hernias may require cross-table lateral radiographs to show the entrapped loops of small intestine.

An uncommon cause of mechanical obstruction, although one that may be specifically diagnosed, is gallstone ileus (see Fig. 5–34). The findings of this entity are listed in Table 5–13.[6]

THE ACUTE ABDOMEN — 213

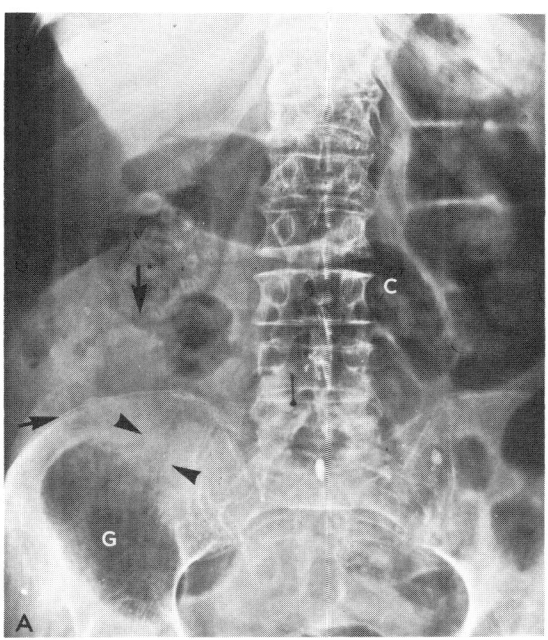

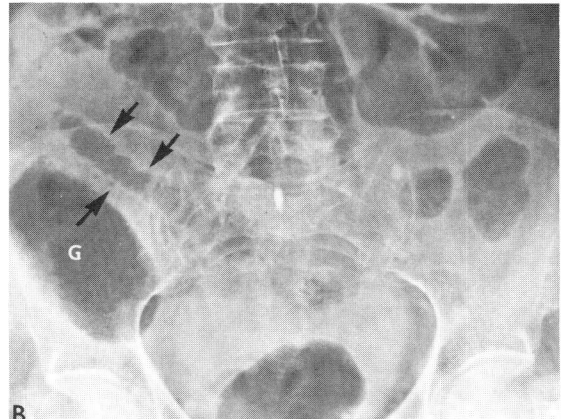

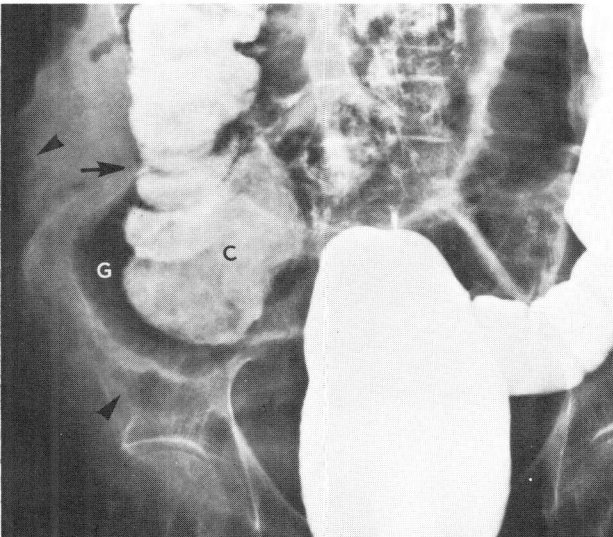

Figure 5–60. Gangrenous closed loop obstruction. A 72-year-old woman with a ten-day history of nausea and vomiting. *A,* There is an ill-defined mass (arrows) in the right lower quadrant, with a rounded (G) and linear gas collection (arrowheads) below. *B,* A few hours later, a solitary edematous loop of ileum (arrows) is overlying the mass. *C,* Gas (G) is seen outside the cecum (C) and in adjacent ileal loops (arrowheads). Some mass pressure is apparent on the lateral aspect of the ascending colon (arrow). These changes were due to closed loop obstruction and gangrene of a segment of ileum. (Courtesy of A. Vasilas, M.D., Beckman-Downtown Hospital, New York, N.Y.)

TABLE 5–13. ROENTGEN SIGNS OF GALLSTONE ILEUS

Partial or total small bowel obstruction
Larger amount of fluid in distended loops than is seen in simple small bowel obstruction
Abnormal location of a gallstone
Gas within gallbladder and bile ducts

214 — THE ACUTE ABDOMEN

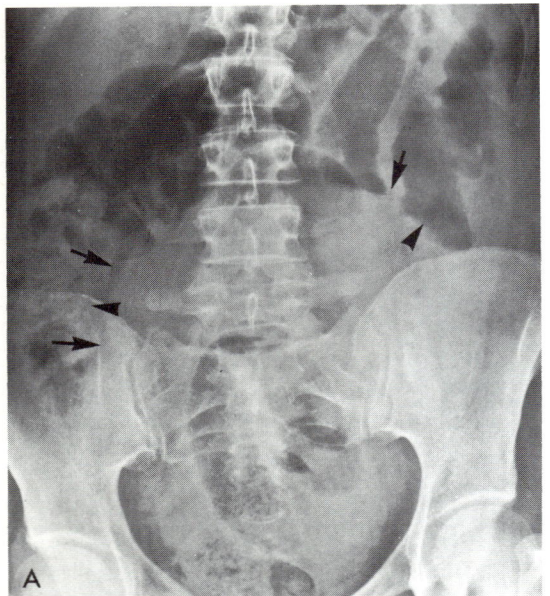

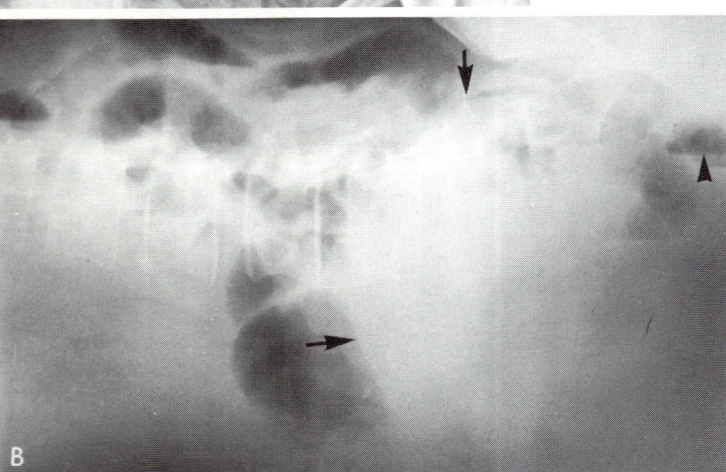

Figure 5–61. Volvulus of small bowel: Pseudotumor. A 44-year-old female was admitted with a chief complaint of severe lower abdominal cramps for the past 36 hours, progressive pain, nausea, and vomiting. A, The plain radiograph of the abdomen demonstrates a well-defined water-density mass over the mid- and lower abdomen (arrows) displacing loops of small bowel and ascending colon (arrowheads). There is also dilatation of several loops of small bowel in the left upper quadrant of the abdomen. B, The right lateral decubitus radiograph shows no significant change in the appearance of the mass (arrows). Fluid levels are seen in loops of small bowel (arrowhead). The findings suggesting volvulus of the small bowel with "pseudotumor" sign were confirmed at surgery. (Courtesy of A. Vasilas, M.D., Beekman-Downtown Hospital, New York, N.Y.)

Large Bowel

As with the small bowel, differentiation of mechanical obstruction from adynamic ileus in the colon is important. Both the colon and the small bowel may be involved in a total ileus pattern. At other times the ileus of the large bowel may predominate (Figs. 5–62 and 5–63). This occurs in the diseases listed in Table 5–14.[5] Localized ileus of the large bowel can be explained by the anatomic relationship of the adjacent inflammatory process. The ascending and descending colon are in the anterior pararenal spaces, while the transverse colon and sigmoid, having a mesentery, are intraperitoneal. The location of a segmental colonic ileus may therefore be a clue to the location of the primary pathologic process. The normal diameter of the cecum, the most distensible portion of the colon, is less than 9 cm. Dilatation greater than this should warn the physician of possible impending perforation.

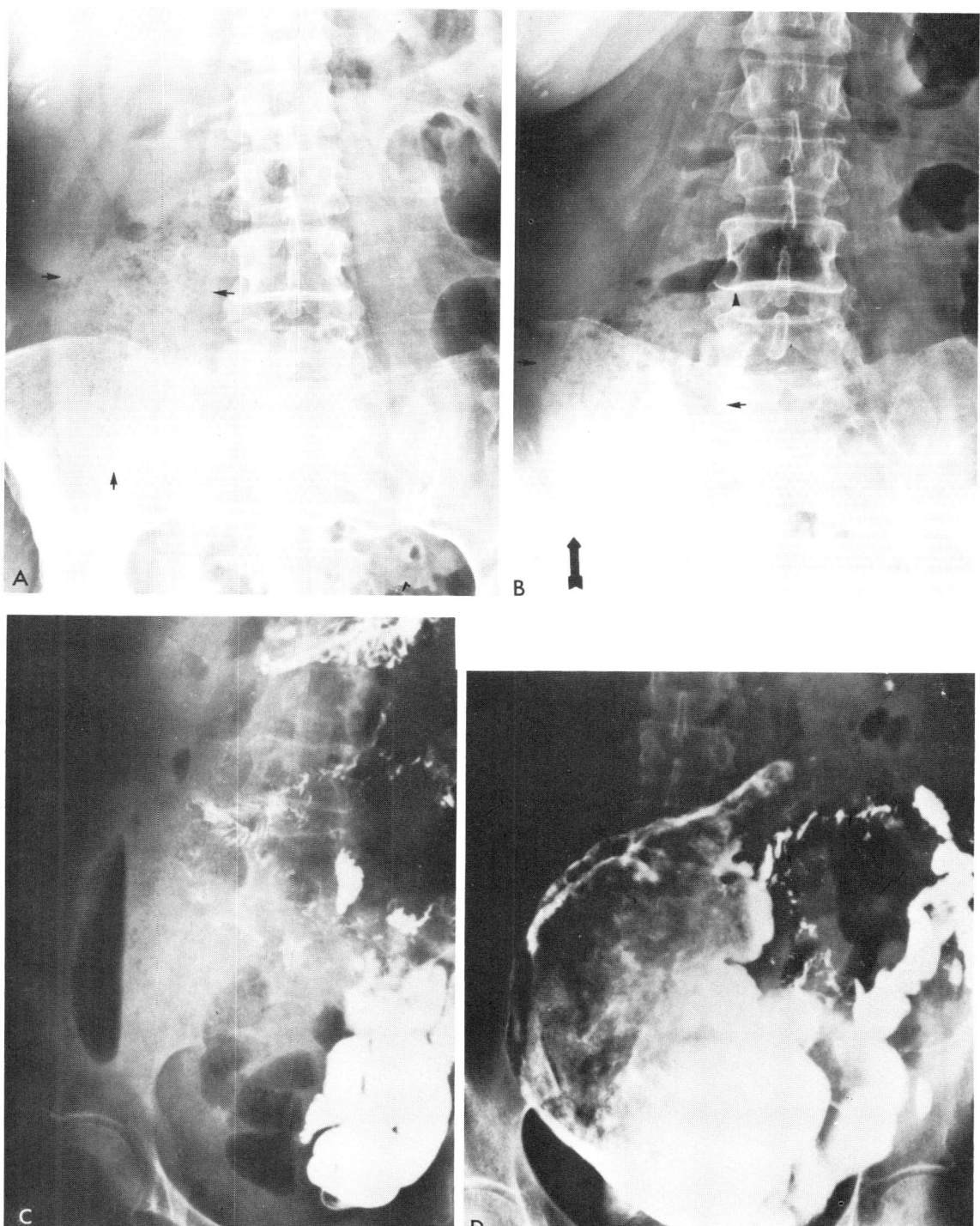

Figure 5–62. Ileus of the right colon simulating abscess. Five days after transverse colon resection for carcinoma a 64-year-old female presented with pain, low-grade fever, a palpable mass, constipation, and diminished bowel sounds. *A,* The supine radiograph shows a mottled gas collection in the right middle and lower quadrants (arrows). *B,* An upright radiograph shows an air-fluid level in same area (arrowhead). *C,* A left lateral decubitus radiograph, taken after ingestion of barium, confirms the large collection of air and fluid. *D,* In a delayed radiograph, the collection is shown to be a markedly distended right colon.

216 — THE ACUTE ABDOMEN

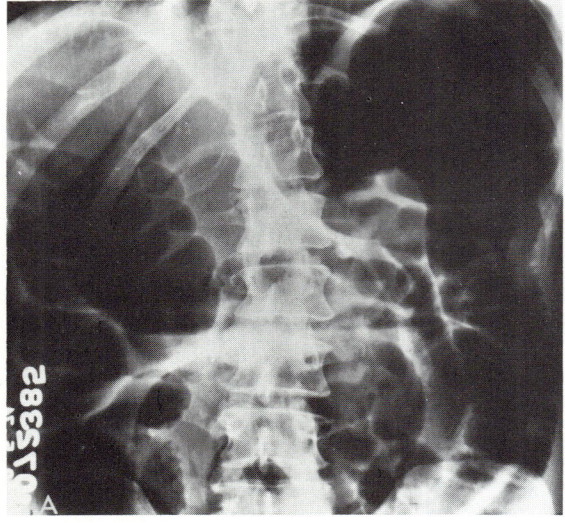

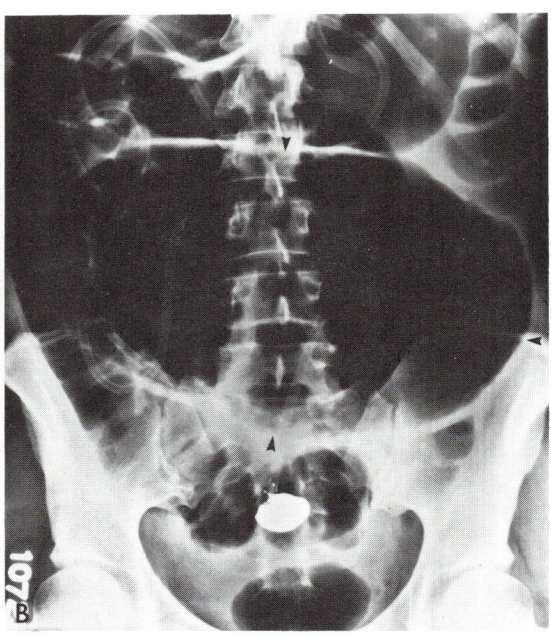

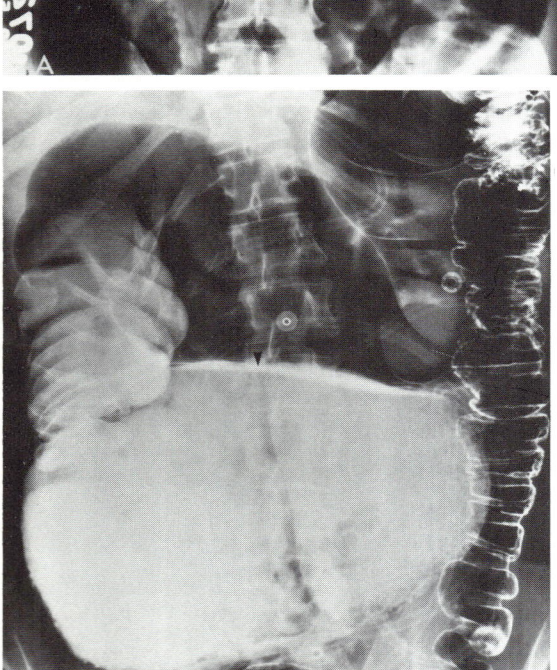

Figure 5–63. Cecal bascule. An 55-year-old female one week after surgery with progressive abdominal distention. *A,* The supine radiograph shows marked dilatation of the large bowel and some dilatation of the small bowel. *B,* A large, centrally located, gas-containing structure (arrowheads) is thought to be a distended cecum. *C,* This is confirmed by barium enema. The diagnosis was cecal bascule or a flaplike cecum.

TABLE 5–14. MOST COMMON CAUSES OF COLONIC ILEUS

Acute appendicitis
Acute cholecystitis
Acute pancreatitis
Congestive heart failure
Idiopathic
Low serum potassium concentration
Low spinal and cauda equina lesions
Inferior mesenteric thrombosis
Morphine overdosage
Peritonitis
Pelvic postsurgical states
Renal failure
Urinary calculus

THE ACUTE ABDOMEN — 217

Mechanical obstruction of the large bowel is most commonly caused by a primary carcinoma. On occasion this obstruction is the first sign of disease, and the patient presents with an acute abdomen. The mass may be visualized on a plain radiograph (Fig. 5–64).

Diverticulitis may also present with an obstruction. It is more common, however, to see either signs of localized ileus in the area of the diverticulitis or a partial large bowel obstruction. Gas collections, localized or generalized, outside the lumen of the large bowel may also be seen (see Fig. 5–15).

Volvulus of the large bowel occurs in the cecum, the sigmoid, and, rarely, the transverse colon. A mechanical closed-loop large bowel pattern is present. In sigmoid volvulus the distended loops of bowel point to the pelvis (Figs. 5–65 and 5–66). De-

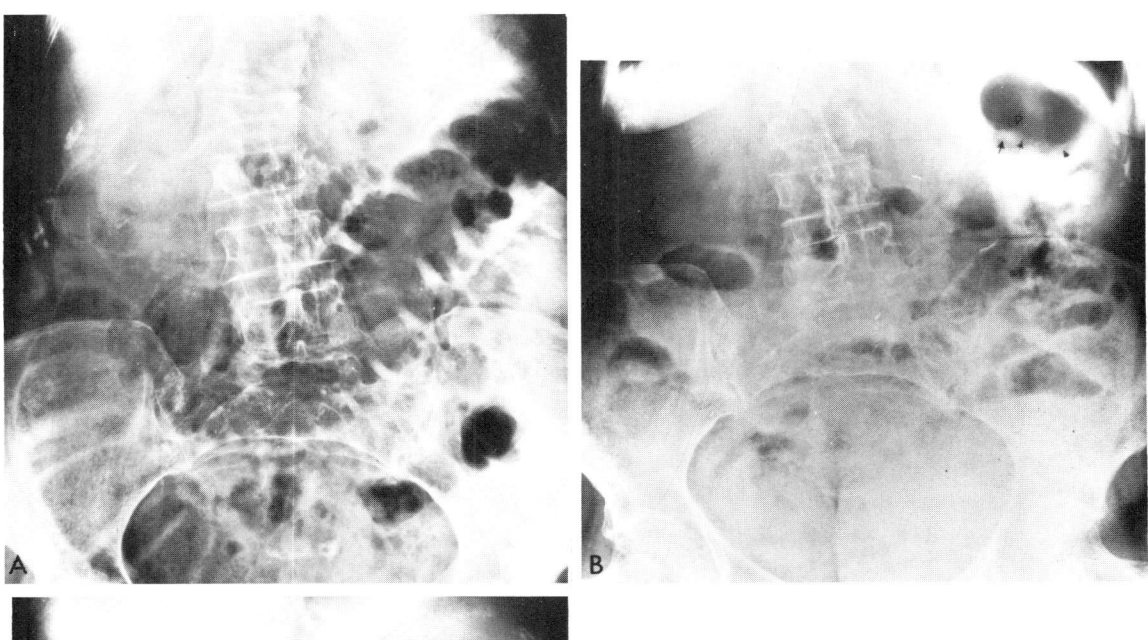

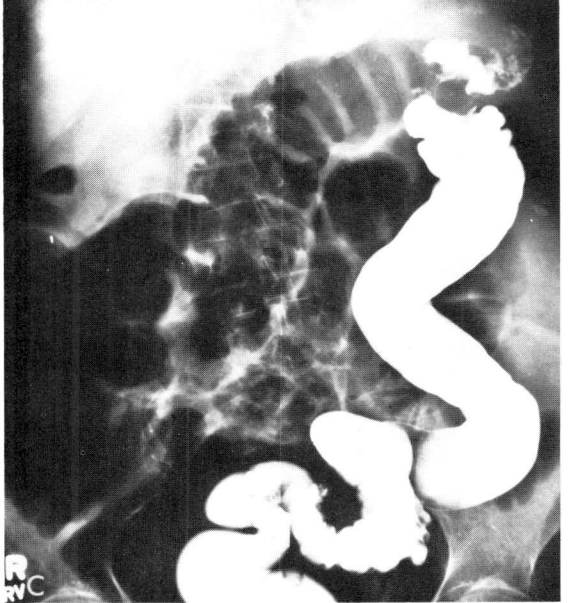

Figure 5–64. Carcinoma of the transverse colon. A 65-year-old female with left upper quadrant pain and abdominal distention. *A,* The supine radiograph shows dilatation of the colon to the level of the distal transverse colon. *B,* The upright radiograph suggests a soft tissue intraluminal mass (arrows) outlined by colonic gas. *C,* Barium enema demonstrates an annular carcinoma of the distal transverse colon.

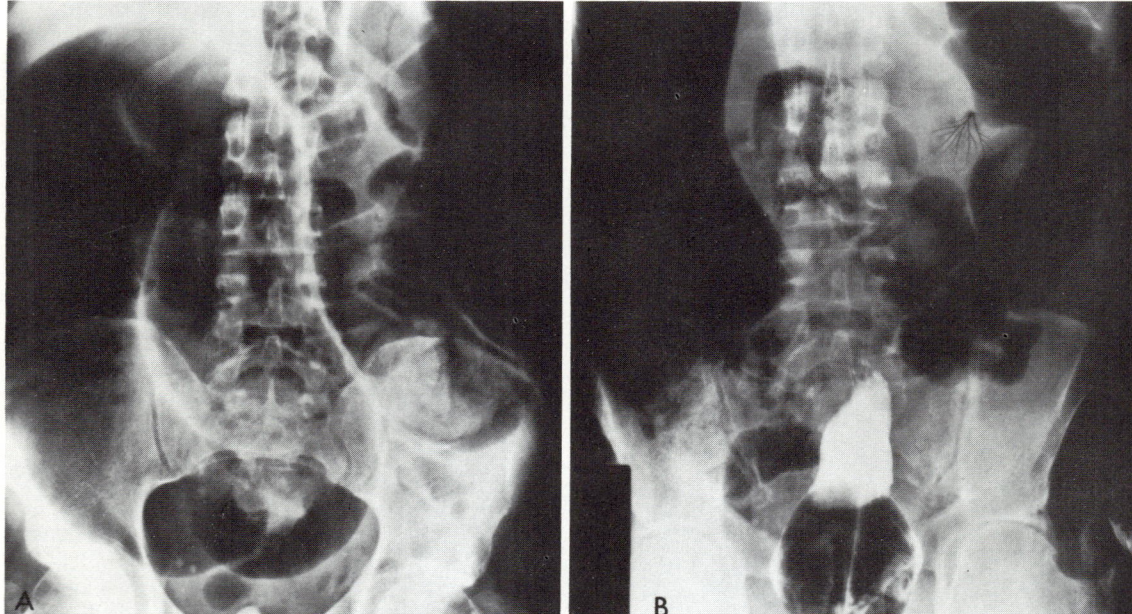

Figure 5–65. Sigmoid volvulus. A 56-year-old male with acute abdominal pain and distention. *A*, A plain radiograph shows marked dilatation of the colon with a dilated loop pointing to the pelvis. *B*, Barium enema demonstrates a beaklike obstruction of the distal sigmoid colon.

pending upon the patency of the ileocecal valve, a secondary obstruction to the volvulus may cause distention of the cecum alone or extend into the small bowel. Volvulus of the cecum presents with a collapsed distal colon. The gas shadows of the limbs of the volvulus appear in the middle or left upper quadrant of the abdomen (Figs. 5–67 and 5–68). Air in the small bowel may not be present, again depending upon the patency of the ileocecal valve. A variation of cecal volvulus occurs when the cecum bends anteriorly on the ascending colon, resulting in marked angulation and a "flap valve" occlusion to the emptying of the cecum (see Fig. 5–63).[3] This is termed pseudovolvulus or cecal bascule.[19]

Intussusception can sometimes be specifically diagnosed by a plain radiograph. In the adult it is usually secondary to a leading tumor of either colon or terminal ileum. In pediatric patients, tumor is a less frequent cause. If the intussusception begins in the small bowel, it may be visualized anywhere throughout the large bowel, but it is usually seen in the right or transverse colon. The mechanical obstruction is then visible on the radiograph; occasionally the leading tumor of the intussusception may be outlined by colonic gas (Fig. 5–69).

Ischemia most commonly occurs in the older age group and is associated with arteriosclerotic cardiovascular disease. The findings may be heralded by an ileus, sometimes of the small bowel (Figs. 5–70 and 5–71). The key to this diagnosis is clinical suspicion and certain radiographic findings, which are summarized in Table 5–15.[22]

Hemorrhage into the lumen of the large bowel may present as an acute abdomen. The possible causes of this include trauma, vasculitis, or bleeding tendencies from hematologic disorders in anticoagulant use. The radiographic signs of hemorrhage into the large bowel are submucosal filling defects outlined by gas within the lumen. An ileus and, rarely, a partial obstruction may occur.

Inflammatory disease of the large bowel may present as an acute abdomen. The radiologic diagnosis of the cause of the acute abdomen is more difficult in the presence

THE ACUTE ABDOMEN — 219

of chronic colitis. The radiographic findings attributable to colitis as the cause of the acute abdomen are hard to separate from the changes of colitis not associated with acute symptoms. Also, other causes of abdominal complaints may be masked by the coexistence of ulcerative colitis. The plain radiographic findings are listed in Table 5–16 (Figs. 5–72 to 5–74). Occasionally (particularly in granulomatous colitis) the diagnosis may not be apparent clinically, and the initial presentation may be that of an acute abdomen. Nonspecific or infective colitis may show no radiographic changes. Viral gastroenteritis also has no specific roentgen signs.

Text continued on page 224.

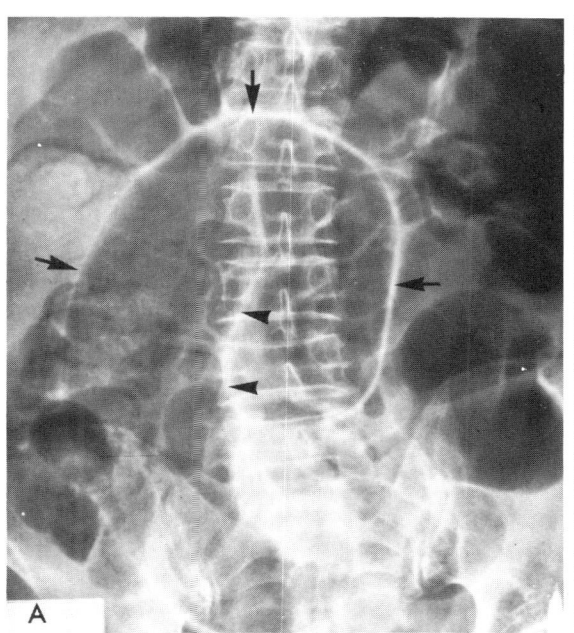

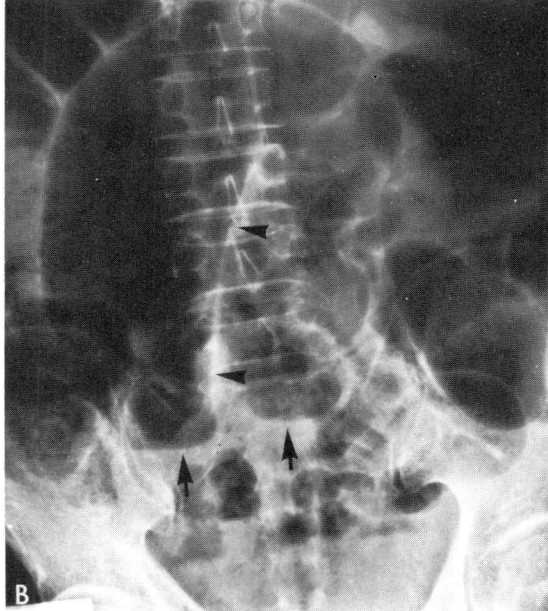

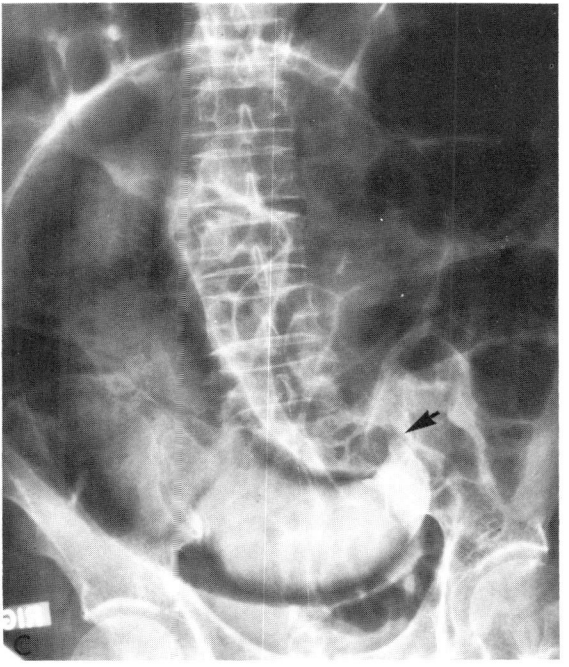

Figure 5–66. Volvulus of sigmoid. A 77-year-old man was admitted with constipation of one week's duration. The abdomen was distended, soft, and nontender. Bowel sounds were active. *A,* In the supine radiograph an abdominal survey shows a markedly distended sigmoid reaching up to the body of L_1, located mainly over the midline and to the right and clearly outlined by a denser contour (arrows). A dense line is noted between the two segments of sigmoid closed together (arrowheads) and pointing downward toward the point of torsion. *B,* In the upright radiograph, fluid levels are seen in the distended segments of the sigmoid (arrows) and again noted in the midline dense band (arrowheads). *C,* A barium enema was attempted, and this showed the column of barium stopped at the level of torsion with the typical tapered, beaklike appearance of the loop at the point of torsion (arrow). (Courtesy of A. Vasilas, M.D., Beekman-Downtown Hospital, New York, N.Y.)

220 — THE ACUTE ABDOMEN

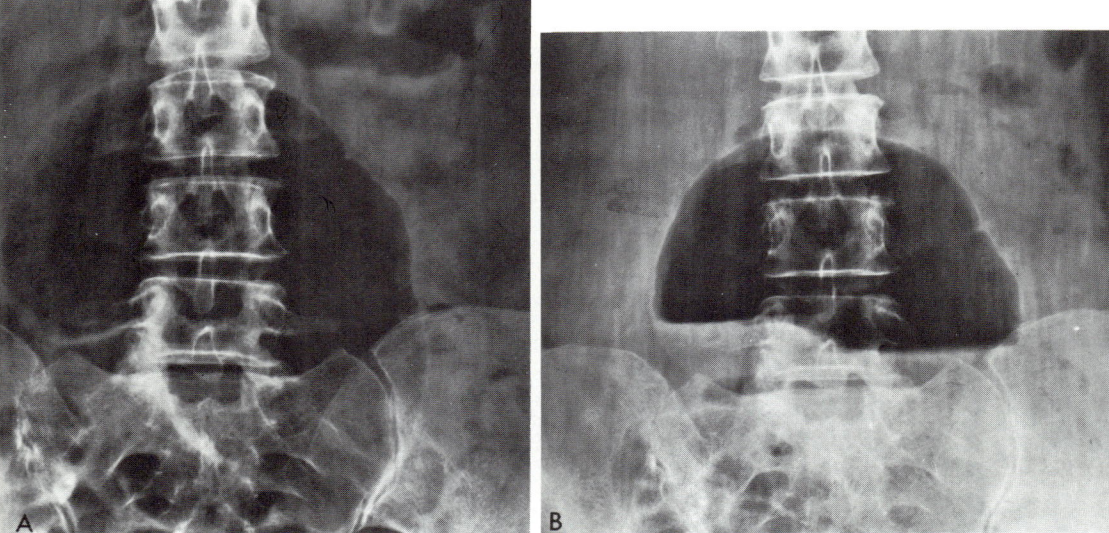

Figure 5–67. Cecal volvulus. A 57-year-old male with acute onset of lower abdominal pain. *A*, The supine radiograph shows a central distended loop of bowel. *B*, In the upright radiograph two separate air-fluid levels are seen in the dilated loop.

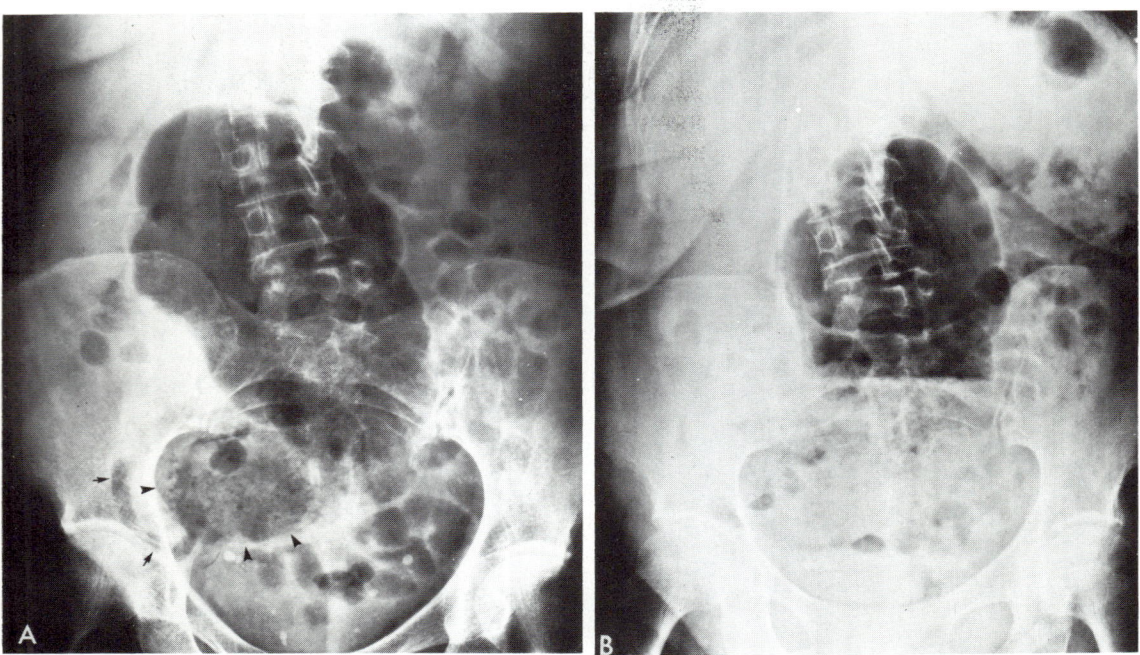

Figure 5–68. Cecal volvulus. A 69-year-old female with progressive symptoms of small bowel obstruction. There is abdominal distention with a tympanitic mass over the midquadrant of the abdomen. *A*, The supine radiograph shows a markedly distended cecum and proximal ascending colon with retained feces (arrowheads) and normal distal ileal coils (arrows). *B*, In the upright radiograph a large single air-fluid level is noted in the cecum.

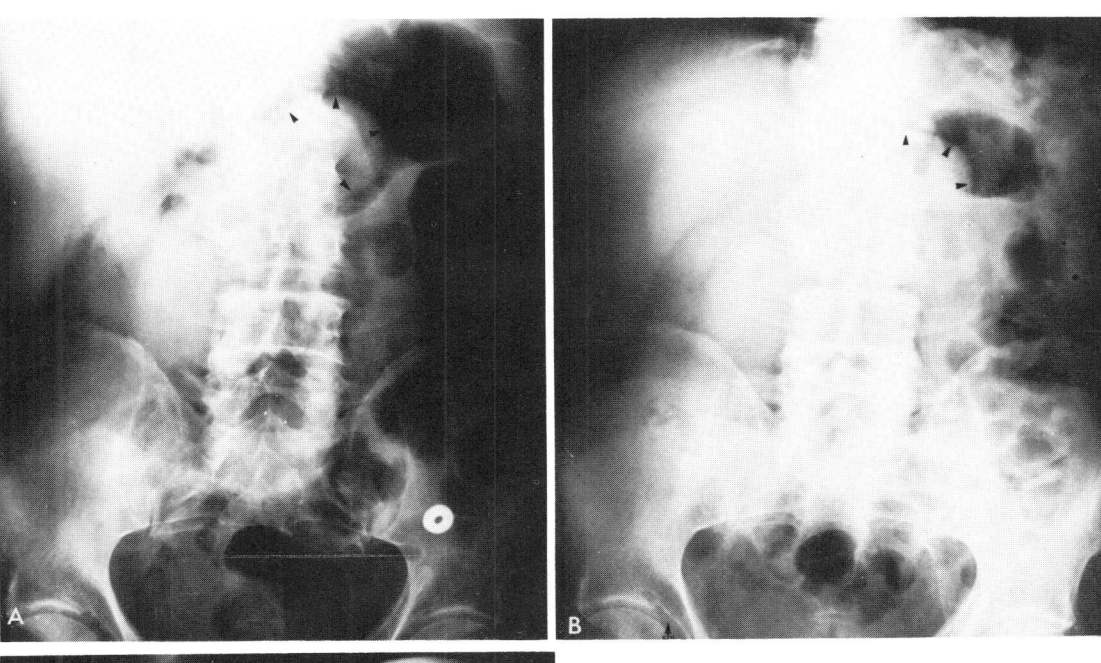
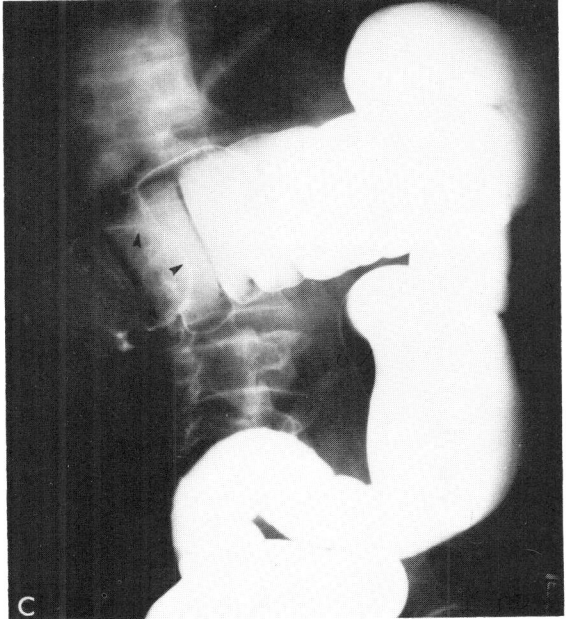

Figure 5–69. Intussusception of colon. An 83-year-old male with a three week history of diffuse abdominal discomfort and recent onset of acute upper abdominal pain. A, The supine radiograph shows a gasless right colon, a soft tissue mass in the distal transverse colon (arrowheads), and some dilatation of the small bowel. B, In the upright radiograph these findings remain consistent. C, Barium enema demonstrates the mass (arrowhead), which was partially reducible, completely obstructing the retrograde flow of barium. The diagnosis was intussuscepting lipoma of the right colon causing mechanical obstruction.

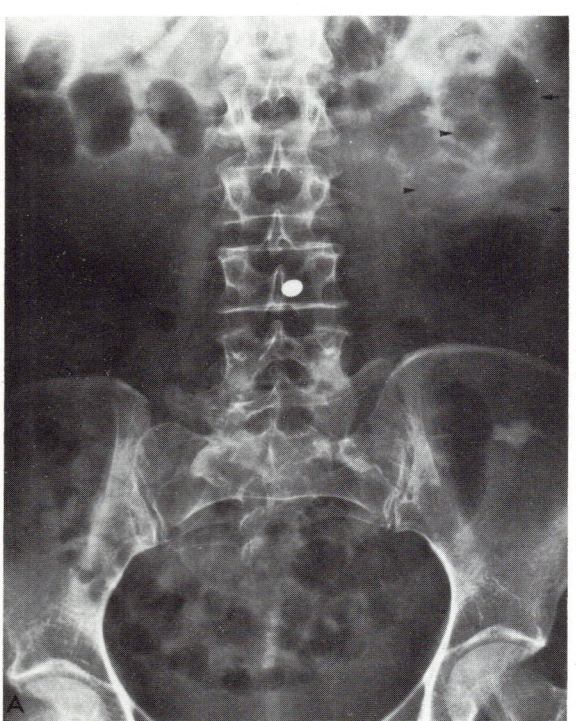
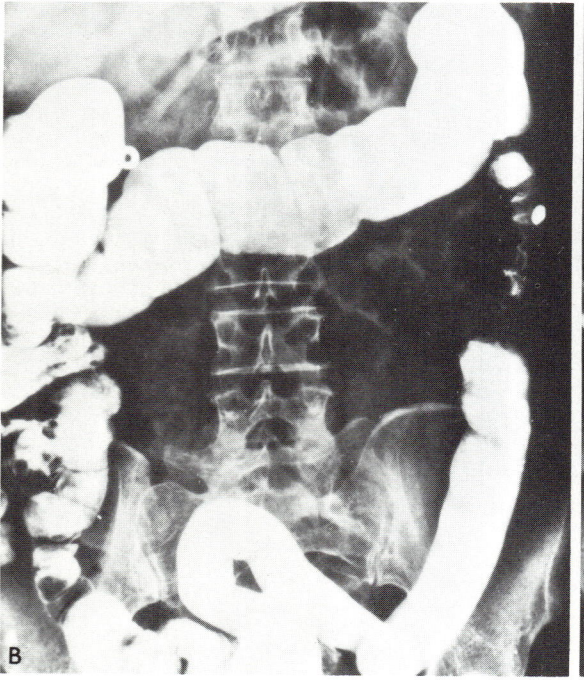
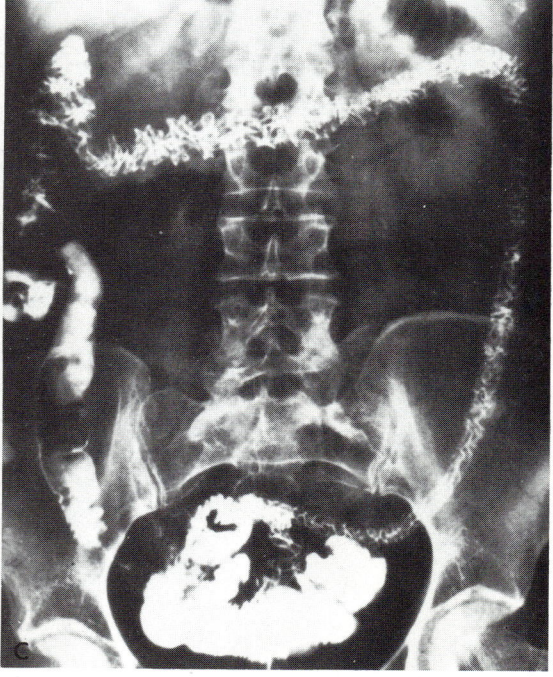

Figure 5–70. Ischemic colitis. A 67-year-old woman with a long history of heart disease presented with acute abdominal pain and rectal bleeding. *A,* The supine radiograph shows a localized ileus in the left upper quadrant (arrowheads) and the suggestion of thumbprinting in the proximal descending colon (arrows). *B,* A barium enema confirms the thumbprinting in the descending colon. *C,* A barium enema performed two weeks later shows normal mucosa in the area of the previous thumbprinting.

THE ACUTE ABDOMEN — 223

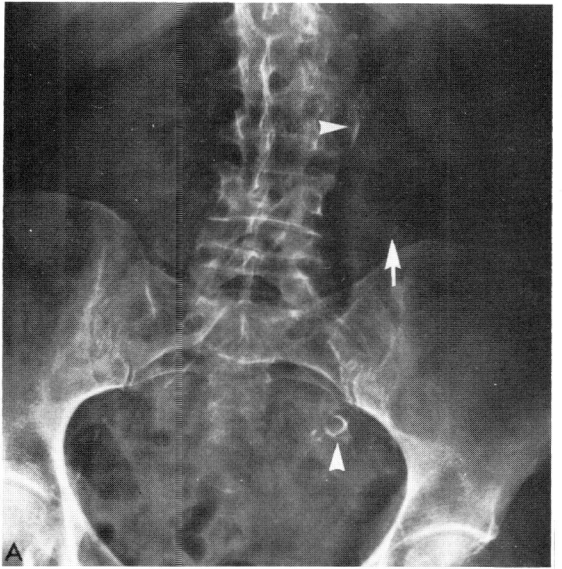

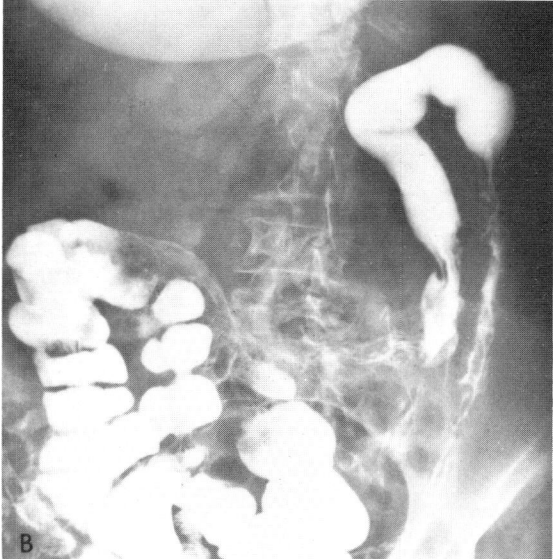

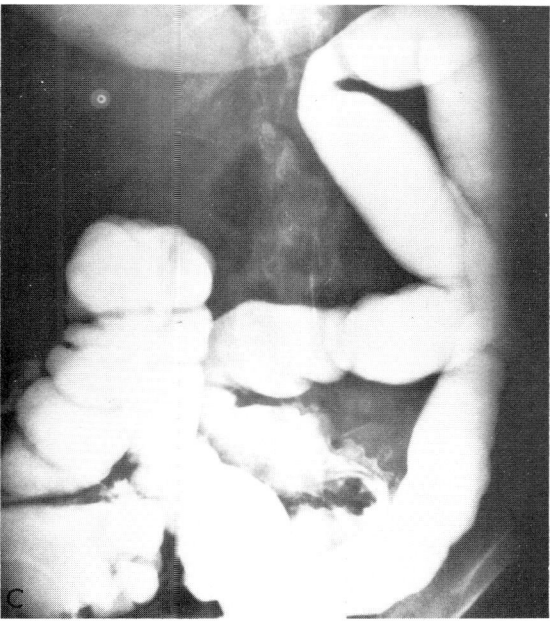

Figure 5–71. Ischemic colitis. A 72-year-old female presented with acute left abdominal pain. *A,* A plain radiograph shows calcific deposits in the aorta (horizontal arrowhead) and in the left iliac artery (vertical arrowhead) as well as a localized ileus (arrow). *B,* Barium enema performed the same day shows submucosal thickening (thumbprinting) in the descending colon. *C,* Eight days after onset of pain the patient was asymptomatic, and the area of abnormality was restored to normal.

TABLE 5–15. ROENTGEN SIGNS OF ISCHEMIC COLITIS

Most Common Findings

Thumbprinting, produced by submucosal hemorrhage
Transverse ridging, produced by multiple parallel lucent bands crossing the involved segment of colon
Thickened and blunted mucosal folds
Loss of haustral pattern
Slight to moderate distention of small and large intestine

Rare Complications

Development of intramural gas
Gas in portal veins
Megacolon

224 — THE ACUTE ABDOMEN

TABLE 5–16. ROENTGEN SIGNS OF ULCERATIVE COLITIS

Signs of an Acute Process

Distention of colon, particularly of the transverse segment (if more than 5.5 cm, toxic megacolon should be suspected)[13]
Free air in peritoneal cavity secondary to perforation

Signs of a Less Acute or Chronic Process

Nodularities of mucosa, with ragged, irregular contour of bowel lumen
Loss of haustration
Thickened walls
Shortening of colon
Associated moderate small bowel distention

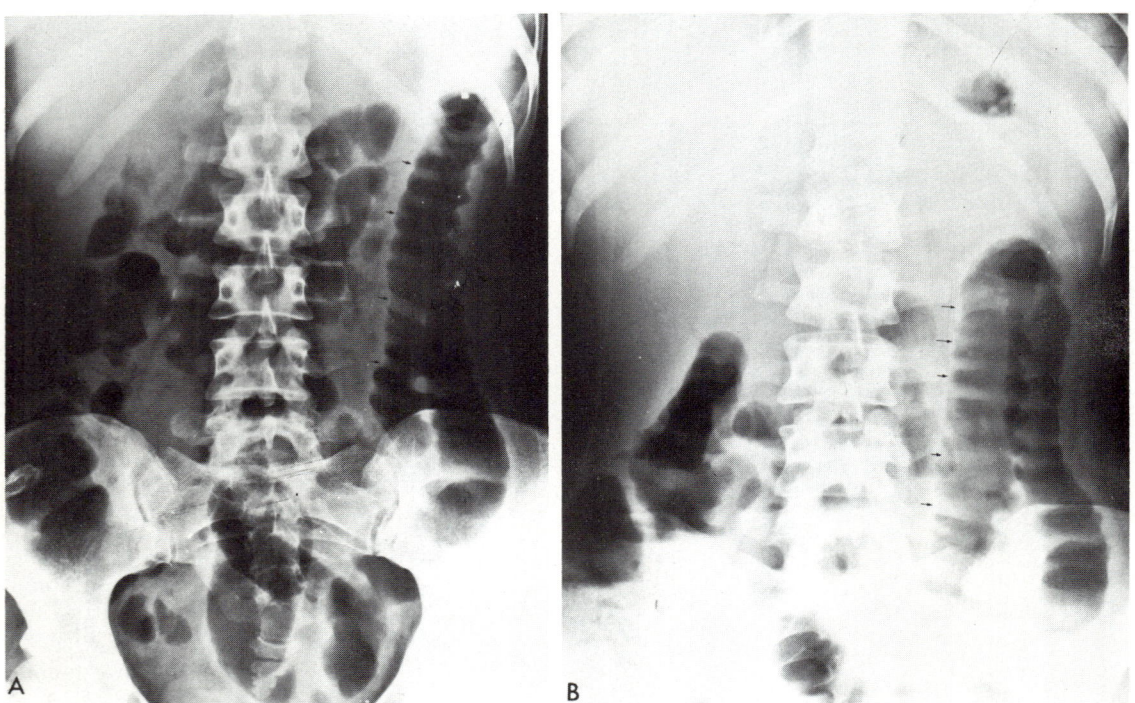

Figure 5–72. Ulcerative colitis. A 35-year-old female with abdominal pain, diarrhea, and slight fever. Supine (A) and upright (B) radiographs of the abdomen show thickened walls of large bowel (arrows) with a pseudo–small bowel appearance.

Appendicitis is extremely common. Table 5–17 lists the plain film radiographic findings of appendicitis, and Figures 5–44, 5–45, 5–75, and 5–76 illustrate some of these manifestations. The radiologic signs result from inflammatory change and an associated ileus or, as the disease progresses, perforation and abscess formation. The latter results in an ileus of the cecum with indentation on its medial border, while the diffuse inflammation permeates the adjacent fat (properitoneal) and causes indistinctness of its lower third and also loss of the lower psoas muscle shadow. The inflammatory process may also produce small bowel obstruction if several loops of distal ileum become matted together. The high correlation between the presence of a calculus in the appendix and appendicitis has been documented by Soter.[18] Air may be a normal finding in the appendix, particularly if it is high and retrocecal (Fig. 5–77). However, if air does not homogeneously distend the appendix, appendicitis must be suspected.

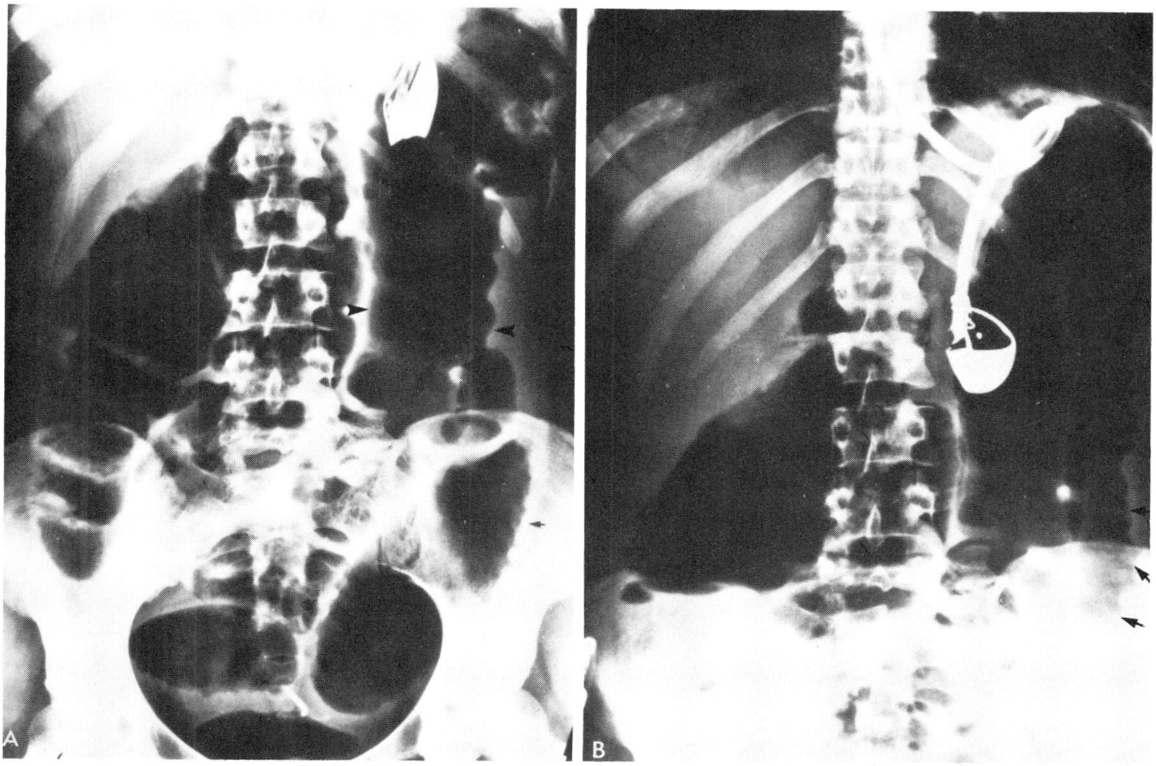

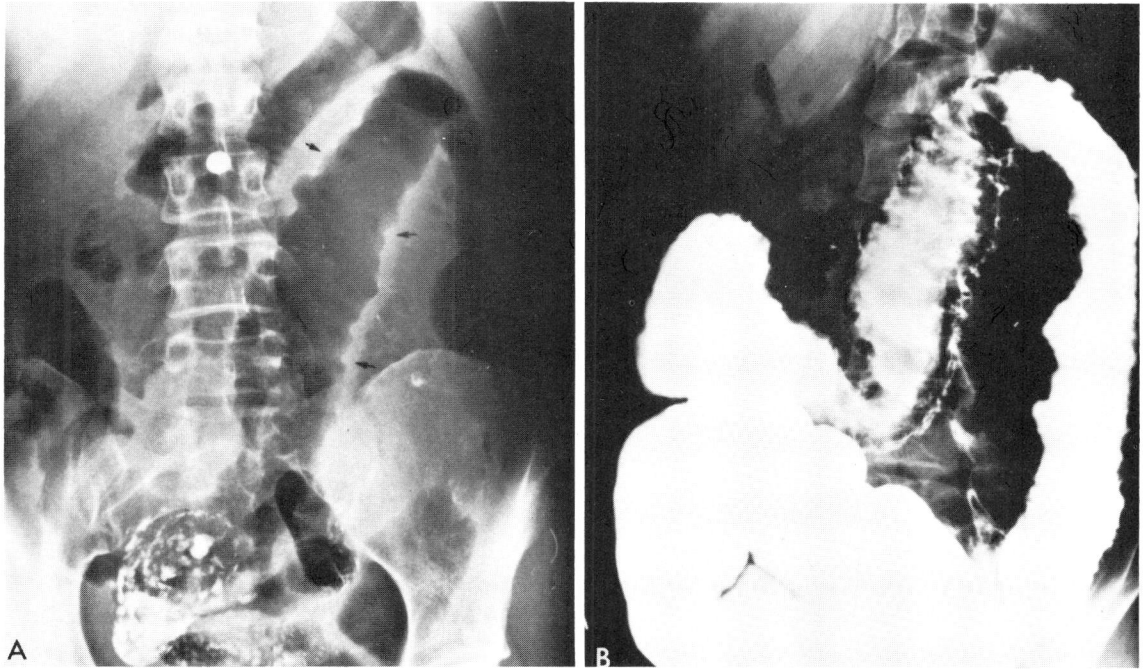

Figure 5–73. Toxic megacolon. A 23-year-old female with fever, acute diffuse abdominal pain, rectal bleeding and a history of ulcerative colitis. *A*, A supine radiograph shows dilatation of the large bowel (arrowheads) and mucosal thickening (arrow). *B*, The upright radiograph shows air-fluid levels and mucosal thickening (arrows).

Figure 5–74. Ulcerative colitis. A 24-year-old female with ulcerative colitis presented with diarrhea, rectal bleeding, and diffuse abdominal pain. *A*, The plain radiograph shows marked thickening of the bowel walls and mucosal edema (arrows). *B*, Barium enema confirms the typical changes of ulcerative colitis.

226 — THE ACUTE ABDOMEN

TABLE 5–17. RADIOLOGIC SIGNS OF APPENDICITIS IN PLAIN RADIOGRAPHS OF THE ABDOMEN

Primary Signs
Atonic distal ileum with fluid levels
Dilated cecum (especially with a long fluid level)
Appendiceal ileus
Fluid in the pericecal area
Appendicolithiasis. The calculi range from a few mm to several cm and may appear homogeneous or have concentric layers.
Air in an appendix, not homogeneously distended (gas is often seen in normal cases, particularly if the appendix is high and retrocecal)
Mass (abscess) indenting the cecum

Secondary Signs
Loss of peritoneal fat line. Occasionally the increased space between this line and the colon is filled by gas if there is a retrocecal appendix.
Loss of lower third of psoas muscle
Scoliosis to right of lumbar spine
Distention of small bowel
Free air in peritoneal cavity (unusual)

Pneumatosis intestinalis may at times present clinically as an acute abdomen. The plain film findings are characterized by numerous collections of noncommunicating, gas-filled cysts that project along the outer border of the colon, particularly the sigmoid colon (Fig. 5–78A). The diagnosis, however, should be confirmed by barium enema, which will outline the air-filled cysts (Fig. 5–78B). Free air in a relatively asymptomatic patient may also be due to pneumatosis intestinalis.

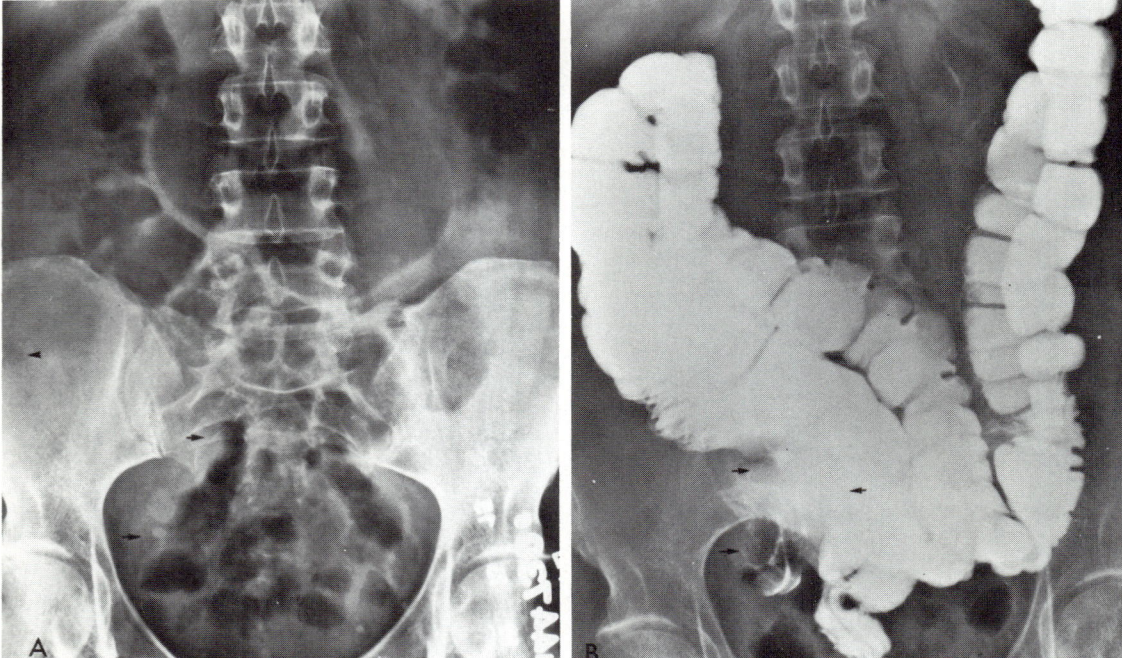

Figure 5–75. Appendiceal abscess. A 52-year-old female with intermittent right lower quadrant pian, rebound, and a palpable mass. A, The supine radiograph shows a soft tissue mass in the right lower abdomen displacing the cecum medially (arrows). There is loss of the normal properitoneal fat stripe (arrowhead). B, Barium enema confirms the mass effect on the cecum (arrows).

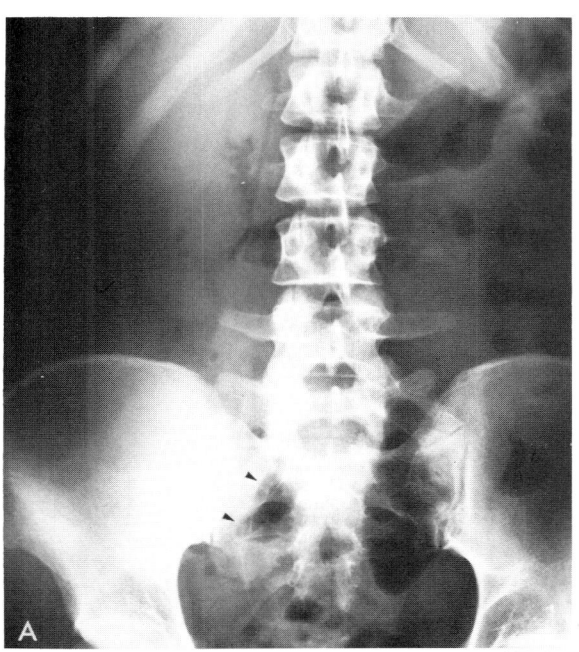
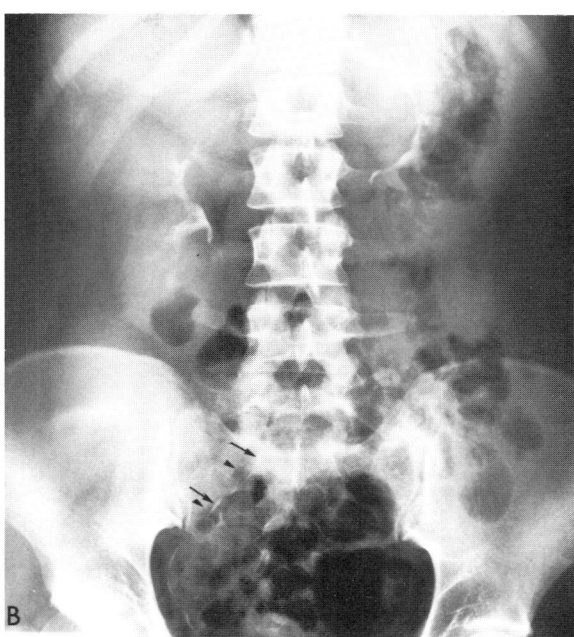
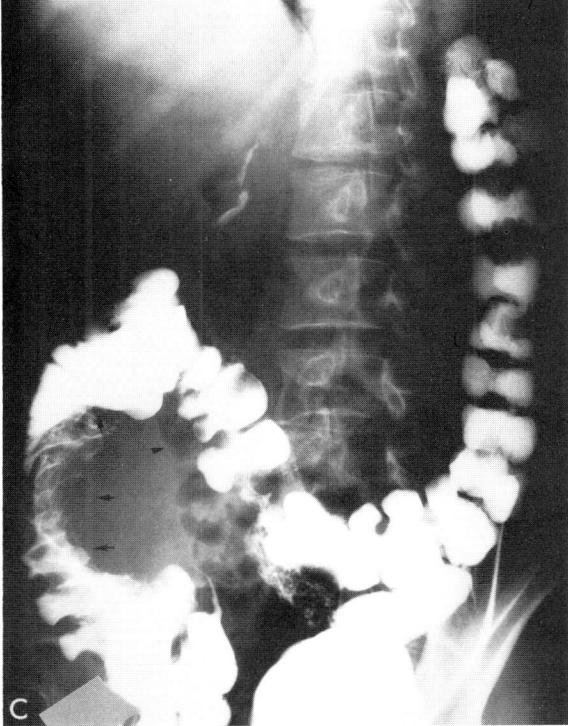

Figure 5–76. Appendiceal abscess. A 26-year-old female with a ten day history of right lower quadrant pain and fever. Physical examination revealed right lower quadrant tenderness and fullness and rectal tenderness. *A,* The plain radiograph shows a soft tissue mass in the right lower quadrant displacing loops of bowel (arrowheads). *B,* Intravenous urography demonstrates medial displacement and compression of the distal right ureter (arrows) and, again, compression, and displacement of bowel (arrowheads). *C,* Barium enema verifies the mass and its pressure effect on the distal ileum (arrowhead) and on the medial aspect of the ascending colon (arrows). The appendix is only partially opacified but shows a tapered distal portion pointing to the mass.

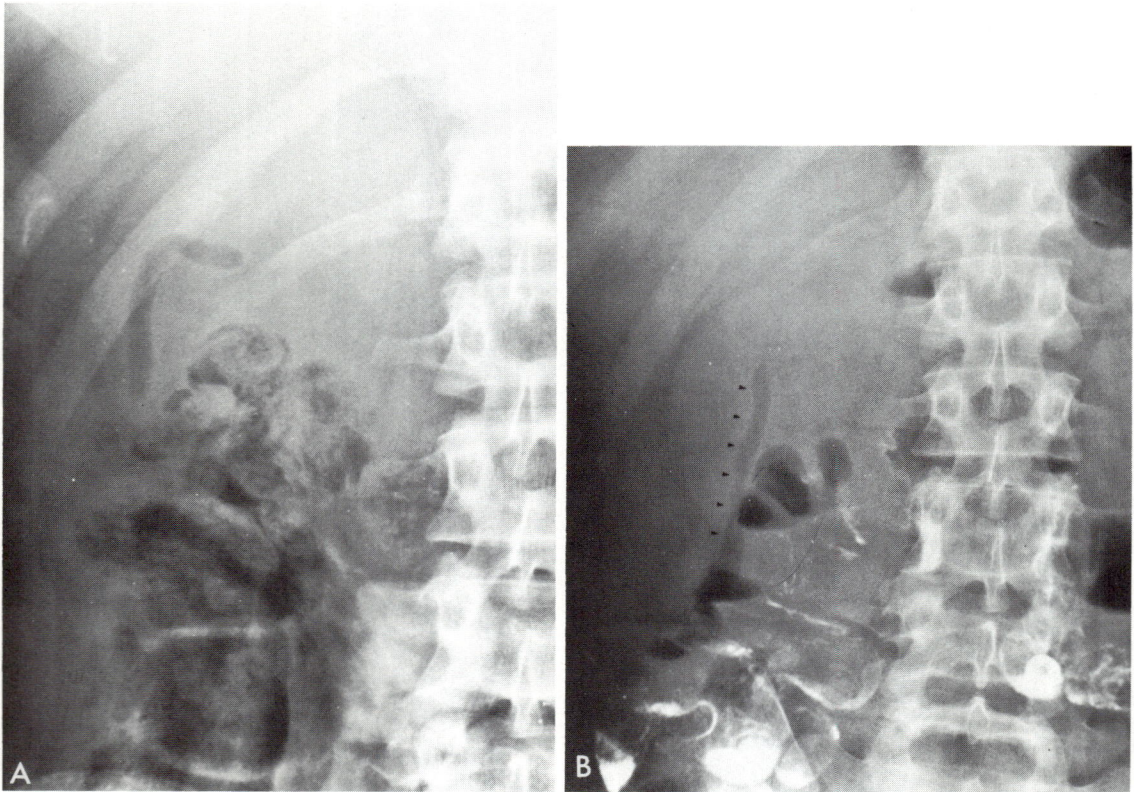

Figure 5–77. Retrocecal appendix. *A,* Radiograph of the right upper quadrant of the abdomen shows a linear gas collection. *B,* In an upright radiograph following barium enema, the gas collection (arrowheads) proves to be the appendix. The diagnosis was gas-filled, retrocecal, subhepatic appendix.

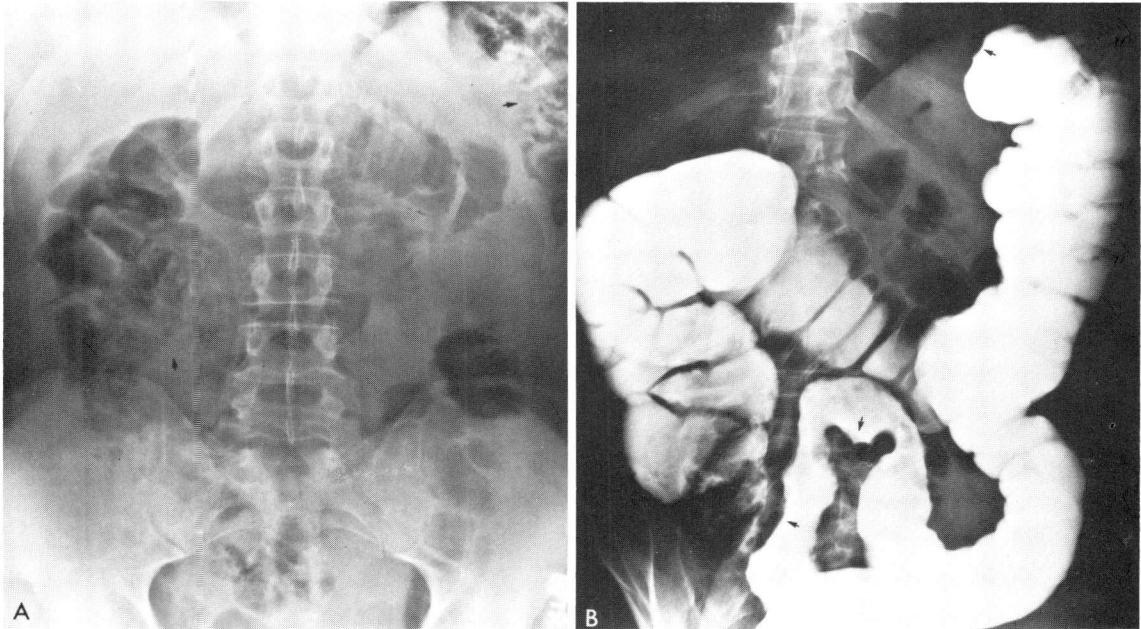

Figure 5–78. Pneumatosis intestinalis. A 45-year-old male with a history of diarrhea and abdominal distress. *A,* The plain abdominal radiograph shows gas shadows with a typical extraluminal appearance (arrows). *B,* Barium enema shows filling defects in the sigmoid and descending colon corresponding to the gas collections (arrows).

Gynecologic Disorders

The radiographic findings in gynecologic disorders are caused by abnormalities in the area of the pelvis or are secondary signs within the peritoneal cavity, such as fluid or an ileus adjacent to the pathologic process. Ovarian tumors may cause obstruction of loops of bowel in the pelvis and present as an acute abdomen.

The diagnosis of ectopic pregnancy is usually clinically suspected and verified by laboratory examination. In the early stages, before fetal parts can be discerned, the radiologic diagnosis is difficult; ultrasonography may be of value at this time. Later on, if ectopic pregnancy develops and ossification of fetal parts occurs, the position or lie of the fetus may be apparent on the abdominal radiograph. Commonly, however, the ectopic pregnancy presenting as an acute abdomen merely gives suggestive radiologic signs of a pathologic process in the area of the ectopia.

Ovarian cysts may present as acute abdominal processes if twisting with subsequent infarction occurs. Radiologically, a mass in the pelvis and its associated adjacent inflammatory changes may be identified. Enlargement of the ovaries is easily detected by ultrasound or CT scan. A dermoid cyst may be suggested radiographically if the cyst contains fat or calcifications. Again, the associated finding of fluid in the peritoneal cavity may be supportive evidence of torsion or infarction of an ovarian cyst. Rupture of the cyst may occur and present with fluid (blood) in the pelvic floor, in the pouch of Douglas. Larger amounts of fluid may extend along the paracolic gutters and displace the colon medially.

Clinically, it may be difficult to separate salpingitis from other inflammatory diseases in and around the pelvis. The radiographic findings of salpingitis are similar to those of other inflammatory processes, such as appendicitis, in which loops of small bowel may be slightly distended by gas, with air-fluid levels located in the area of the pelvic floor. If these changes occur in the left lower quadrant, differentiation from diverticulitis may be difficult. In general, either clinical correlation or further studies, such as ultrasonography, are required to exclude other processes simulating acute salpingitis.

The radiologic changes of endometriosis demonstrable on the abdominal plain film are all secondary to involvement of loops of small and large bowel. This may cause obstruction, or the implant may actually result in filling defects in the bowel wall, which are visualized because of the presence of intraluminal air. A barium enema, however, is required to verify the presence of these implants.

EXTRAPERITONEAL PATHOLOGIC ENTITIES

The diagnosis of acute processes in the extraperitoneal space and their differentiation from processes in the intraperitoneal space may be difficult. As stated previously, the extraperitoneal area is divided into pararenal and perirenal compartments. Pancreatitis, which occurs in the anterior pararenal space, has been included with the intraperitoneal processes already discussed. In general, however, the observer is required not only to localize the pathologic process by means of the criteria already reviewed but also to attempt to separate those processes within the various extraperitoneal compartments. For instance, if effusion is seen in the anterior pararenal space, the differential diagnosis is between processes affecting the pancreas, a ruptured descending duodenum, or a ruptured ascending or descending colon. If the diagnostic criteria indicate a lesion in the perirenal space, considerations are different. Likewise, the posterior pararenal space involves the great vessels; therefore, involvement of this space suggests different pathologic processes.

Obstructive uropathy commonly presents with acute abdominal pain. According to Frimann-Dahl,[10] 40 per cent of patients admitted with ureteral obstruction are admitted with the diagnosis of acute abdomen. The calculi of the urinary tract most often producing acute symptoms are those lodged in the ureter at any point from the ureteropelvic to the ureterovesical junction. The plain radiograph may show the calculus, which may be small and at times difficult to distinguish from a phlebolith. The latter, however, can generally be recognized because of its radiolucent center. Other radiographic findings may be lumbar scoliosis concave toward the side of the obstruction. There may also be a sentinel loop or localized ileus in the area (Figs. 5–79 and 5–80). The renal outline may be enlarged, and there may even be some loss of the normal fat around the kidney and effacement of that portion of the psoas muscle that relates to the kidney itself. An intravenous urogram is usually required to establish the diagnosis and delineate the point of obstruction. Ultrasonography also may be helpful in demonstrating dilatation of the collecting system proximal to the site of obstruction.

Emphysematous pyelonephritis, a condition that occurs in patients with uncontrolled diabetes mellitus or obstructive uropathy, may be recognized in the plain abdominal radiograph by the presence of bubbles of gas in the kidney and perirenal space. The gas is distributed along the renal tubules in a unique lacework arrangement.[9] Similarly, the presence of gas in the walls of the bladder and ureters indicates the presence of acute fulminating renal papillary necrosis.

Uriniferous perirenal pseudocysts secondary to trauma may also be diagnosed on plain abdominal radiographs by the presence of an elliptically shaped mass directed medially and inferiorly. There is also an associated upward displacement of the kidney with lateral deviation of its lower pole.

Extraperitoneal hemorrhage manifests the radiologic signs described previously for extraperitoneal effusion. Table 5–3 lists the radiographic signs of extraperitoneal

THE ACUTE ABDOMEN — 231

Figure 5–79. Ureteral calculus and ileus. A 56-year-old male with acute onset of left lower abdominal pain. A radiograph of the abdomen shows dilated large and small bowel loops and a ureteral calculus (arrow).

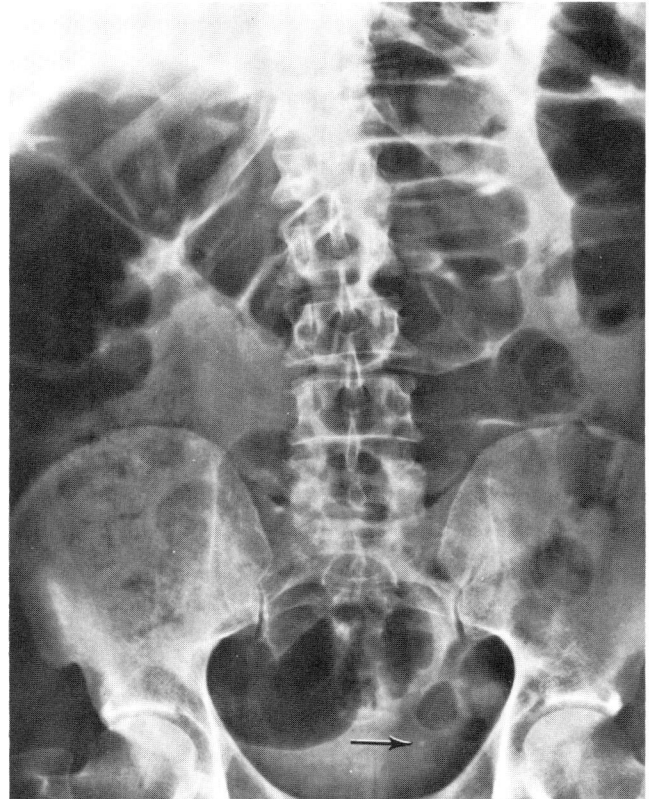

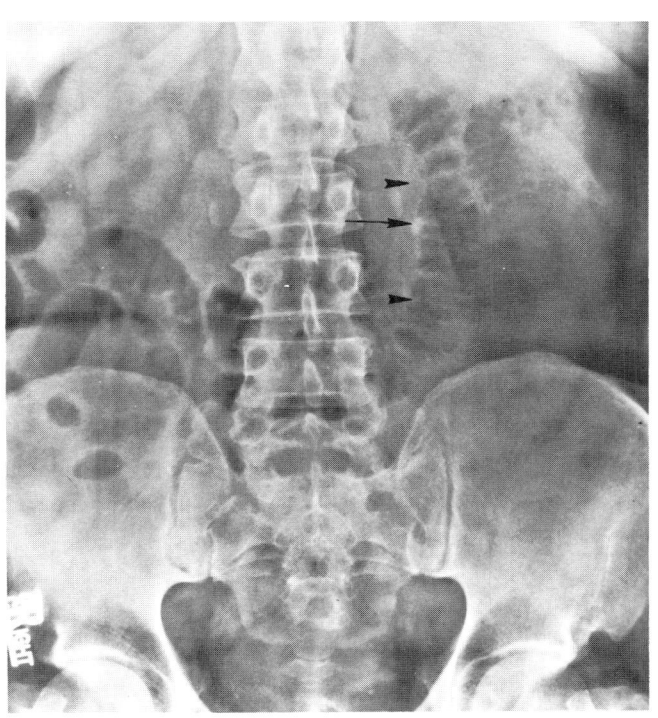

Figure 5–80. Ureteral calculus and associated localized ileus. A 59-year-old male with severe left-sided abdominal pain. The clinical impression was diverticulitis. The radiograph shows a localized ileus (arrowheads) as well as a ureteral calculus (arrow).

232 — THE ACUTE ABDOMEN

hemorrhage in the various compartments. Among the most common causes of spontaneous hemorrhage (Table 5–18) is rupture of the abdominal aorta. Aneurysms of the abdominal aorta may be suggested if hemorrhage occurs extensively and fills the compartments of the extraperitoneal space. Occasionally, the plain radiograph may show the atheromatous plaques in the walls of the aneurysm and a soft tissue mass lateral to it (Figs. 5–81 and 5–82). Ultrasonography is now the procedure used to establish the diagnosis of abdominal aneurysm and extraperitoneal hematoma. Trauma is the most common cause of extraperitoneal hemorrhage. The criteria for its radiographic diagnosis are the same as those for a ruptured aneurysm. Clinical correlation is required for specific diagnosis. Arteriography demonstrates the etiology of the hematoma.

Abscesses in the extraperitoneal space are dignosed by observation of the normal dense and gas-filled structures of the peritoneal cavity. The radiographic signs of extraperitoneal abscesses are listed in Table 5–19. If an abscess can be localized to a specific compartment in the extraperitoneal space, a knowledge of the structures in

TABLE 5–18. MOST COMMON CAUSES OF RETROPERITONEAL HEMORRHAGE

Anticoagulant medication
Fractures of pelvis, ribs, lumbar vertebrae
Pancreatitis
Trauma to segments of urinary tract
Trauma to gastrointestinal tract—duodenum, colon, rectum
Laceration of the abdominal aorta
Rupture of an aneurysm of the abdominal aorta

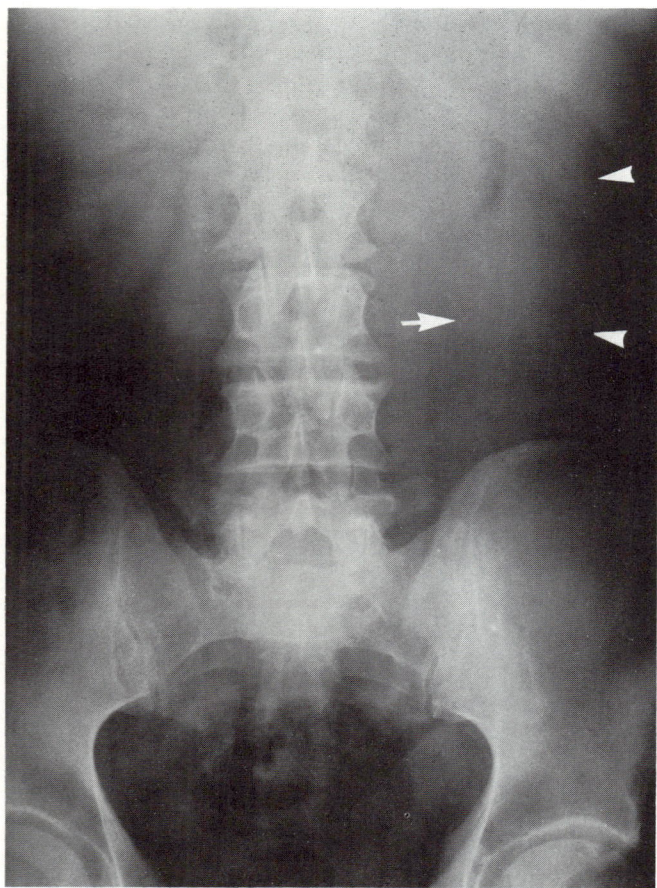

Figure 5–81. Ruptured aneurysm. A 65-year-old female known to have an atheromatous abdominal aorta presented with a history of increasing abdominal pain, which had begun suddenly in the left quadrant of the abdomen. The patient was in shock. The plain radiograph of the abdomen shows a mass in the left quadrant (arrowheads). There is nonvisualization of the left kidney and psoas muscle and a faintly outlined calcified linear band (arrow). The diagnosis of a ruptured aortic aneurysm was confirmed at surgery. (Courtesy of A. Vasilas, M.D., Beekman-Downtown Hospital, New York, N.Y.)

THE ACUTE ABDOMEN — 233

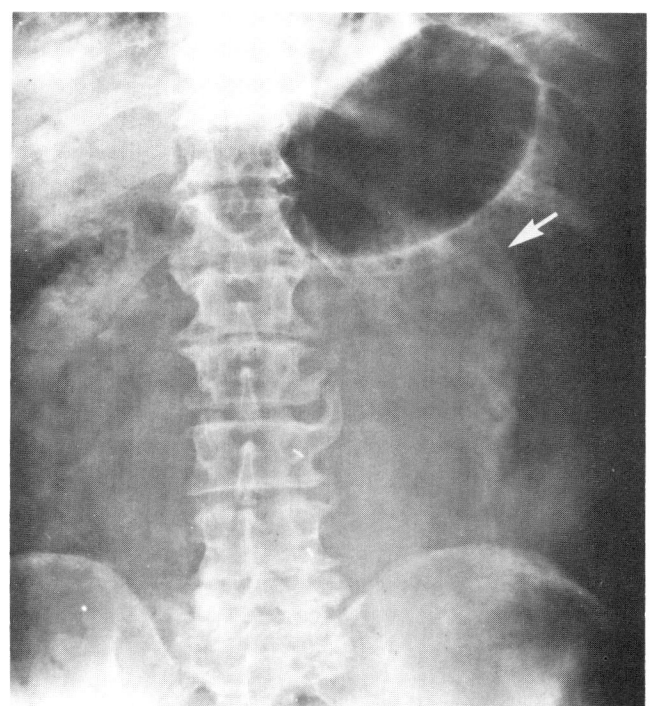

Figure 5–82. Ruptured aneurysm. A 78-year-old man was admitted in shock with a history of rather dull and unsevere abdominal pain of slow onset. A plain radiograph of the abdomen shows a left quadrant water-density mass, well defined in its upper and outer contours (arrow) and fading in its lower third. There is no visualization of the left kidney shadow and effacement of the left psoas muscle. The diagnosis of ruptured abdominal aortic aneurysm was confirmed at surgery. (Courtesy of A. Vasilas, M.D., Beekman-Downtown Hospital. New York, N.Y.)

each of these compartments will afford a more precise differential diagnosis. If gas is seen in the anterior pararenal space, an emphysematous pancreatitis may be suspected. If gas is seen in the posterior pararenal space, a paravertebral abscess extending into the posterior pararenal space may be suspected. Ultrasound and CT scan have an increasingly significant and frequently definitive role in the diagnosis of abscess.

TABLE 5–19. RADIOGRAPHIC SIGNS OF EXTRAPERITONEAL ABSCESS DEMONSTRABLE ON PLAIN RADIOGRAPHS

Area of Interest	Anterior Pararenal Space	Perirenal Space	Posterior Pararenal Space
Flank stripe	Intact	Intact, may be thinned	Lost with lateral extension
Psoas muscle outline	Intact	Lost in upper third if collection is medial; lower two thirds intact	Lost throughout if medial
Renal outline	Intact	Lost	Intact
Renal position	Unaffected unless massive	Anterior if collection is medial; lateral displacement	Anterior
Hepatic or splenic angle	Intact unless massive	Intact if collection is medial; lost if collection is lateral	Lost if lateral
Descending duodenum or duodenojejunal junction	Anterior displacement or constriction	Anterior position	Anterior position
Ascending or descending colon	Anterior displacement or constriction	Anterior and medial displacement in superior portions	Anterior and medial displacement
Small bowel	Anterior displacement	Unaffected	Anterior displacement

PATHOLOGIC ENTITIES AND DIFFERENTIAL DIAGNOSIS IN THE POSTOPERATIVE ABDOMEN

Intraperitoneal

The same general criteria for detecting abnormalities on plain abdominal radiographs of the preoperative acute abdomen apply to the postoperative acute abdomen. However, because of the surgical alterations the diagnostic criteria are more difficult to interpret. Specifically, postoperative ileus may simulate an obstruction, although in general diagnostic differentiation uses the same parameters that obtain in the preoperative abdomen (Figs. 5–83 to 5–88).

Of particular importance in the radiographic analysis of the postoperative abdomen is a knowledge of the incidence, significance, and persistence of pneumoperitoneum.[2, 4, 12] The following factors should be considered: (1) the type of surgical intervention, (2) whether the pneumoperitoneum involves the upper or lower abdomen, (3) body habitus, and (4) type of anesthesia. Generally, a large amount of residual free intraperitoneal air is found in patients who have had surgery of the upper abdomen (gastric surgery), pelvic surgery (see Fig. 5–14), or abdominal laparotomy. Usually, more air remains trapped in asthenic patients than in obese ones and is absorbed at a faster rate in younger individuals. Although free residual air tends to be greater following general anesthesia, there is no significant relationship between the type of anesthetic agent and the amount of free residual air.

In almost all cases the residual air tends to collect under the right diaphragm; less frequently it is bilateral; even less often it collects only under the left diaphragm. It should be noted that unilateral residual air has a greater tendency to be caused by complications.

The absolute amount of free residual air is difficult to assess and varies between 100 cc and over 1000 cc. Absorption is, of course, related to the amount present, but generally complete absorption takes place within five to ten days (Fig. 5–89). In all cases an increase in the free residual air suggests leakage (Fig. 5–90).

An anastomotic leak is a common cause of increased intraperitoneal air and fluid.

Text continued on page 239.

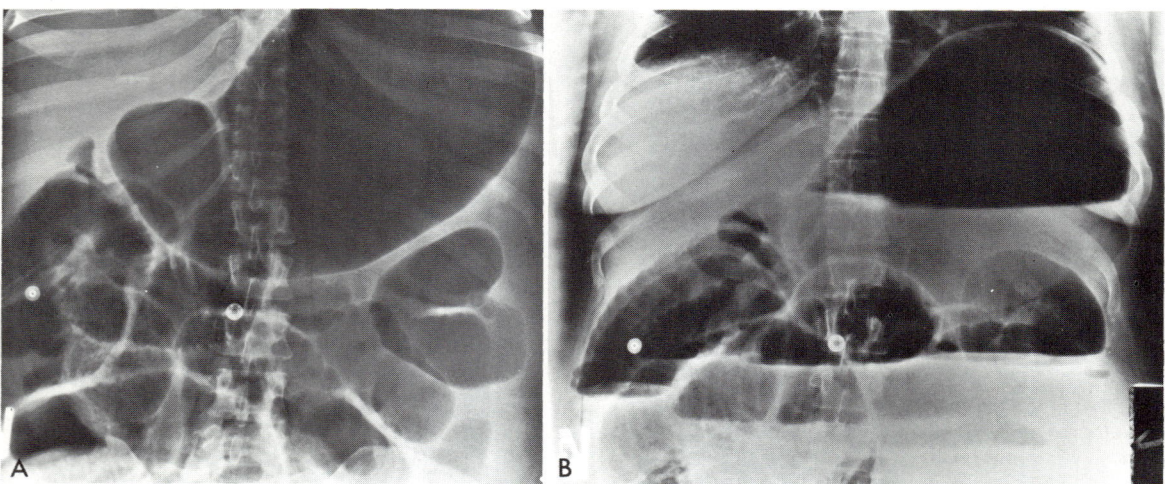

Figure 5–83. Paralytic ileus. A 29-year-old female four days following surgery for cesarian section developed abdominal distention. The radiographs in the supine *(A)* and upright *(B)* positions show marked dilatation of the small and large bowel without differentiated fluid levels.

THE ACUTE ABDOMEN — 235

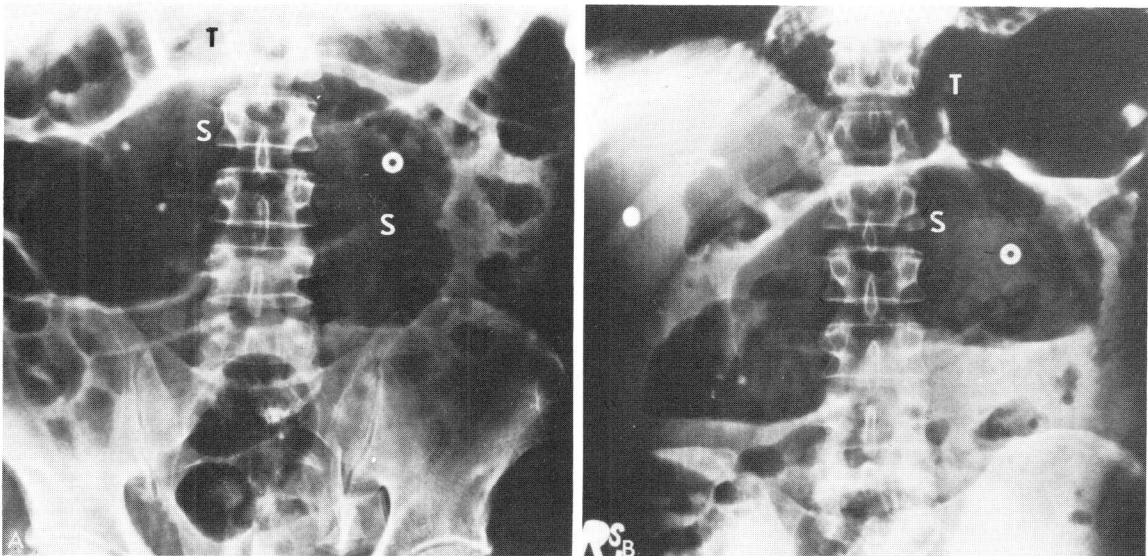

Figure 5–84. Colonic ileus. A 54-year-old male three days after surgical removal of a left ureteral calculus. The patient developed abdominal distention. Supine (A) and upright (B) radiographs of the abdomen demonstrated marked dilatation of the transverse (T) and sigmoid (S) colon. Conservative treatment resulted in improvement. The diagnosis was colonic ileus simulating mechanical obstruction.

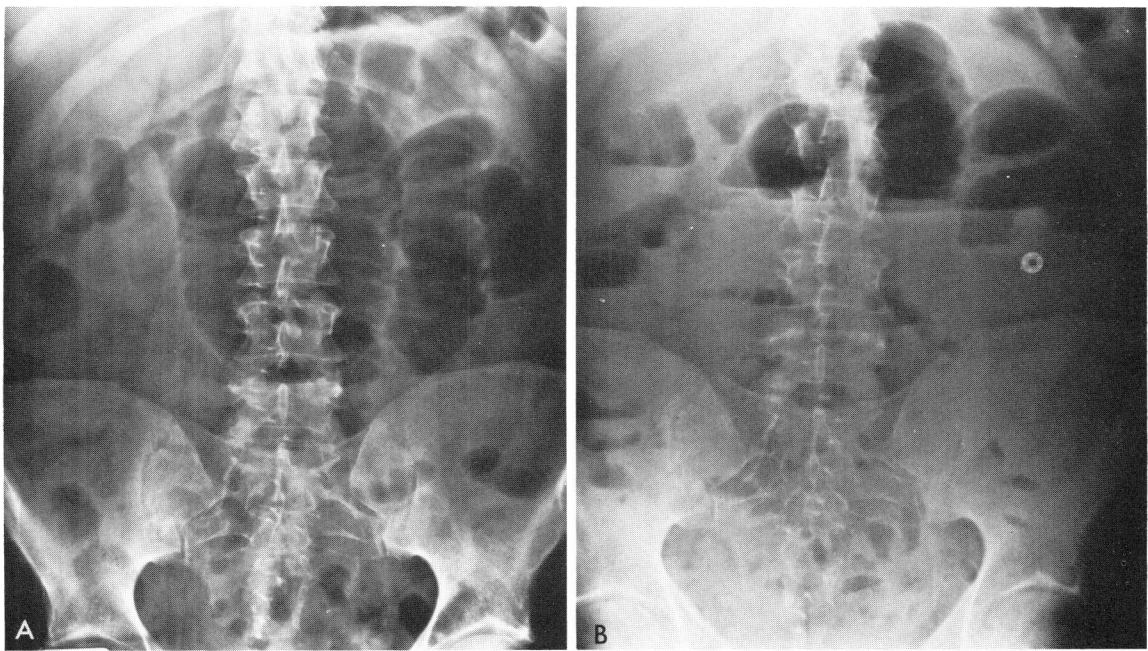

Figure 5–85. Small bowel ileus. A 53-year-old male developed abdominal distention three days after surgery. A, The supine radiograph shows dilatation of proximal loops of jejunum simulating obstruction. B, The upright radiograph shows air-fluid levels in the dilated loops but of undifferentiated type.

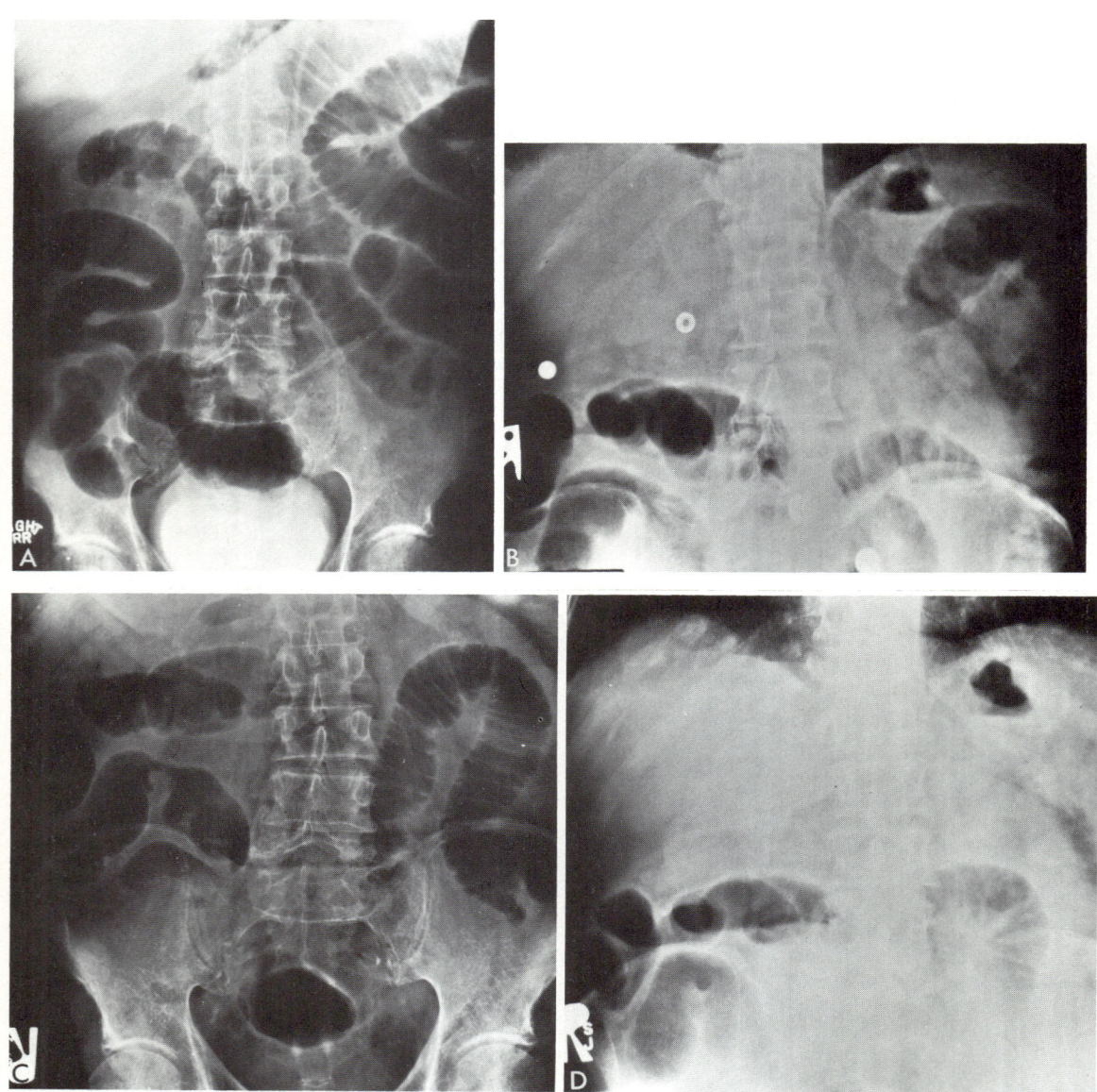

Figure 5–86. Paralytic ileus. A 73-year-old male with metastatic lung disease who developed abdominal distention five days following craniotomy. *A* and *B,* Radiographs show slight dilatation of loops of small bowel, but without significant fluid levels. *C* and *D,* Radiographs taken seven days following surgery. The small bowel pattern shows no significant interval changes.

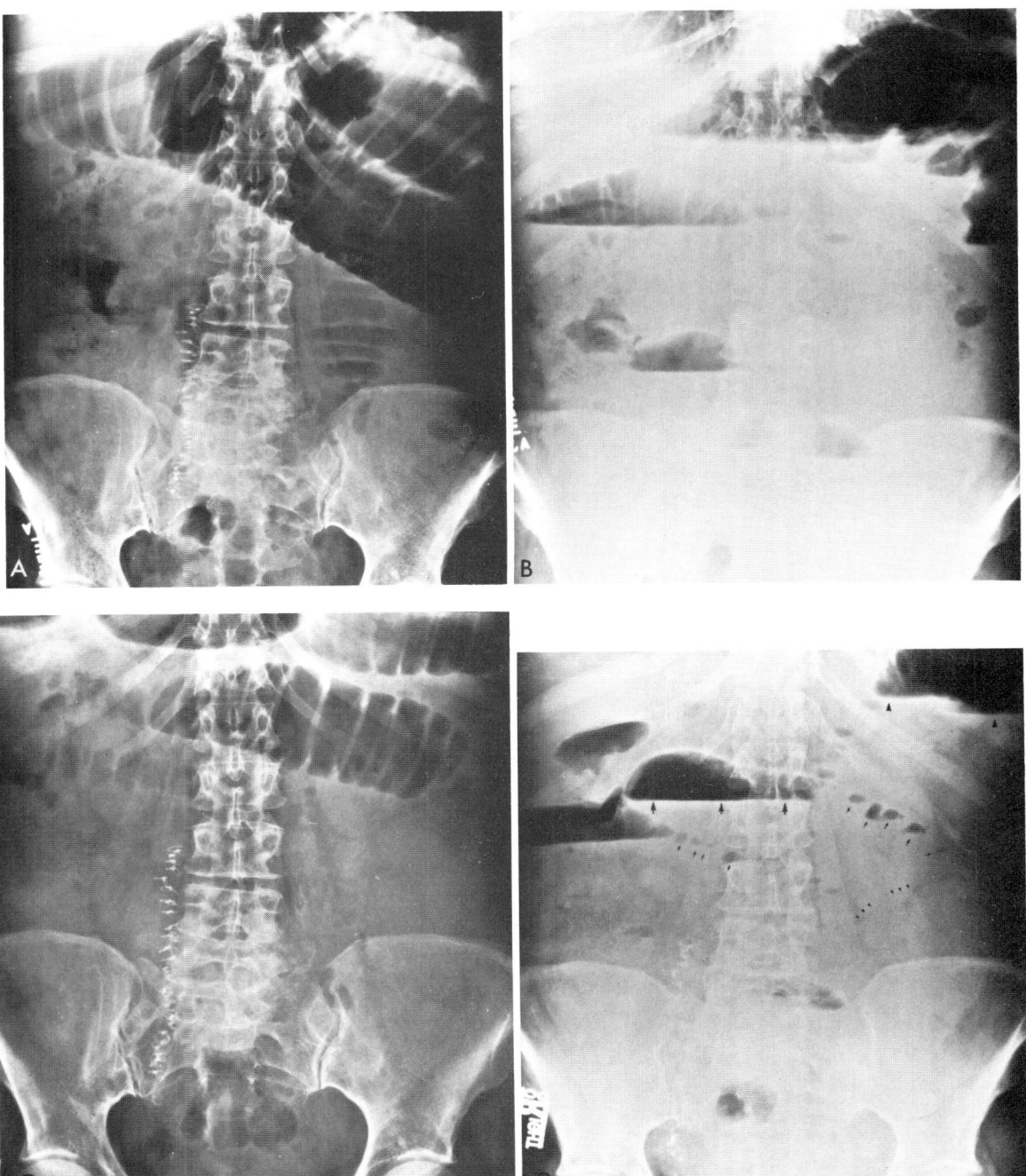

Figure 5–87. Small bowel obstruction. A 48-year-old female complained of pain and abdominal distention six days after surgery. There had been no bowel movements and there were high-pitched bowel sounds. Supine (A) and upright (B) radiographs show marked dilatation of the small bowel loops with long and differentiated fluid levels. There is stool in the right colon (C and D). An abdominal survey made 36 hours later shows a change in the appearance of the distended loops of small bowel. There is now much fluid (arrows and arrowheads) replacing the air. Adhesions were found at surgery.

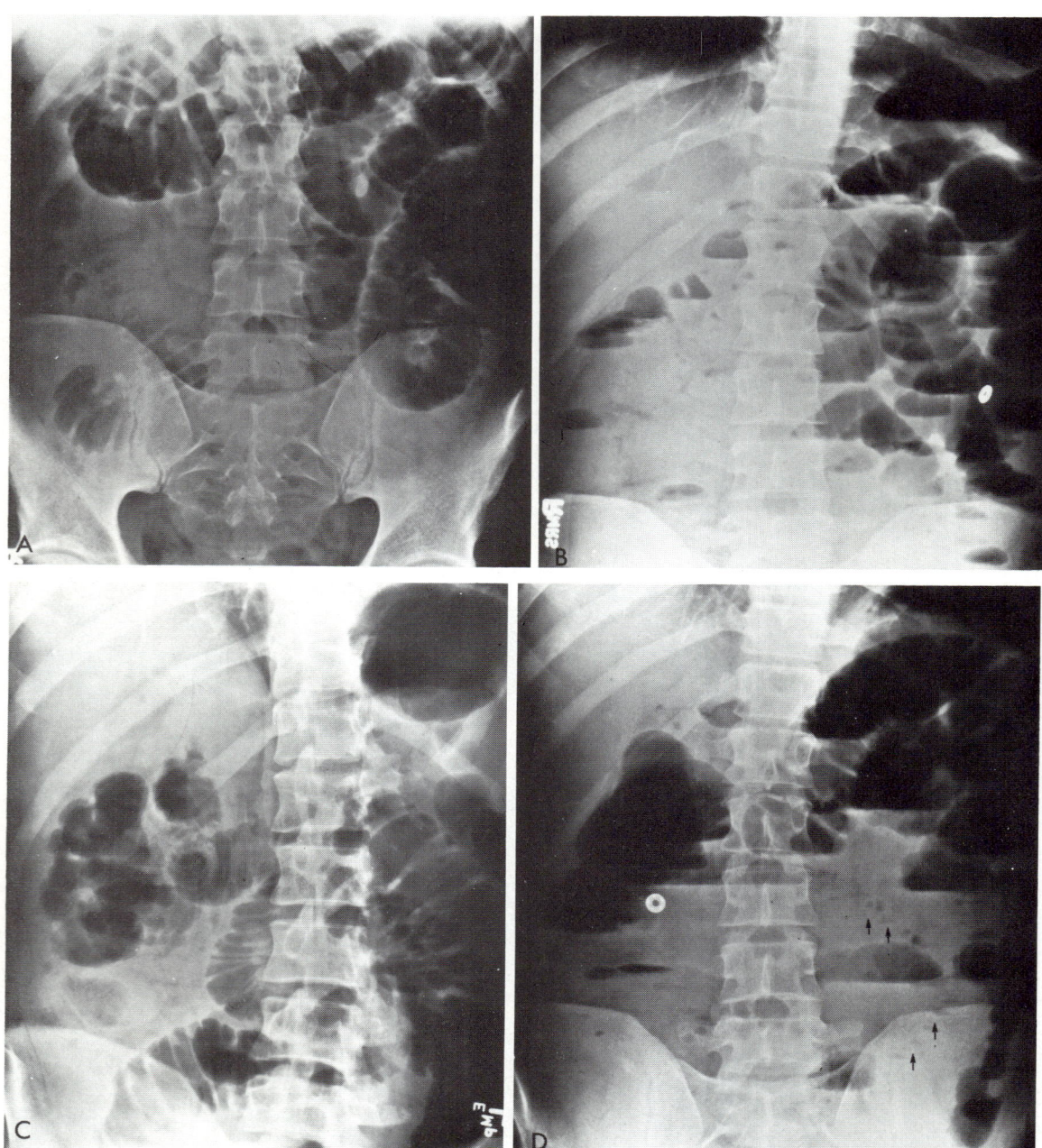

Figure 5–88. Small bowel obstruction. A 45-year-old female with a one-week history of abdominal pain. Physical examination revealed abdominal rebound in the right lower quadrant and high-pitched bowel sounds. The patient had had an appendectomy 13 years prior to admission. *A* and *B*, A radiograph shows marked distention of the small bowel and multiple differentiated air-fluid levels. *C* and *D*, Four days later the distention of small bowel persists but with a different pattern and multiple beading (arrows). Again, there is no distention of the large bowel. The diagnosis of mechanical obstruction of the distal small bowel, secondary to adhesions, was proved at surgery.

Figure 5–89. *A*, A radiograph taken two days following surgery shows intraperitoneal air. *B*, Six days after surgery the upright radiograph shows clearing of the intraperitoneal residual air.

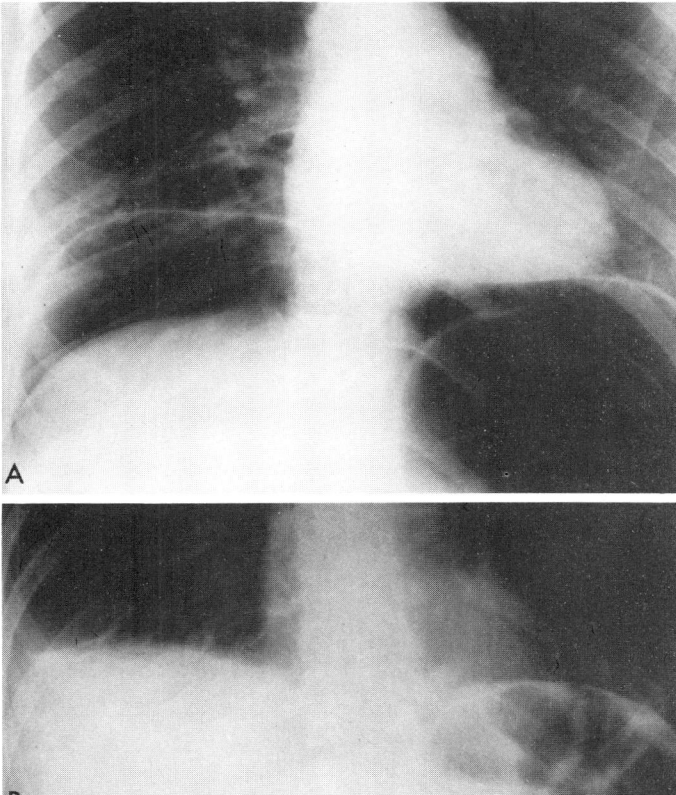

Depending upon the location of the anastomosis, air and fluid may collect within a compartment of the peritoneal cavity and lead to abscess formation. Radiographic evidence of air or abscess should be sought in the area of previous surgery.[20]

Fistulas may develop postoperatively as primary complications of the surgical procedure. Generally, fistulous tracts are not demonstrable on plain radiographs, but areas of ileus may be present adjacent to the fistula. Occasionally, gas in the sinus tract may be observed, but its demonstration requires introduction of a contrast agent through a catheter into the fistulous tract.

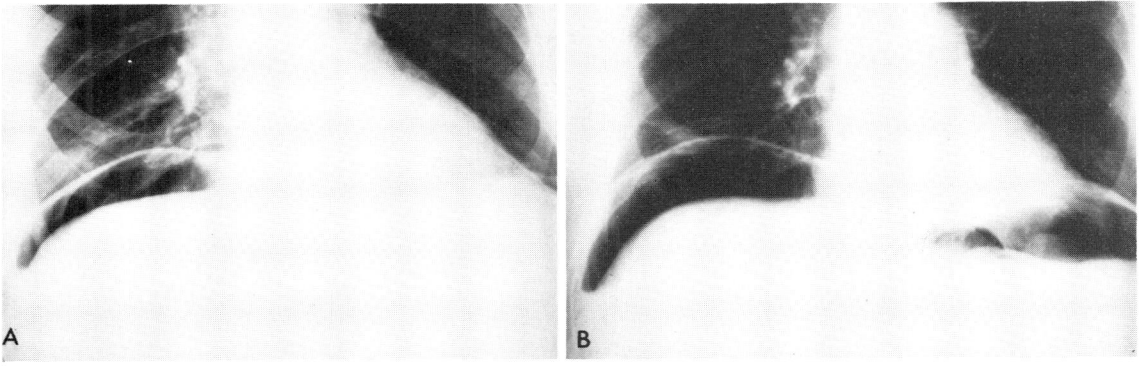

Figure 5–90. Anastomotic leakage. *A*, A 53-year-old male acquired postoperative residual air three days following sigmoidectomy. *B*, Eight days later the amount of intraperitoneal air is increased. An anastomotic leak was diagnosed.

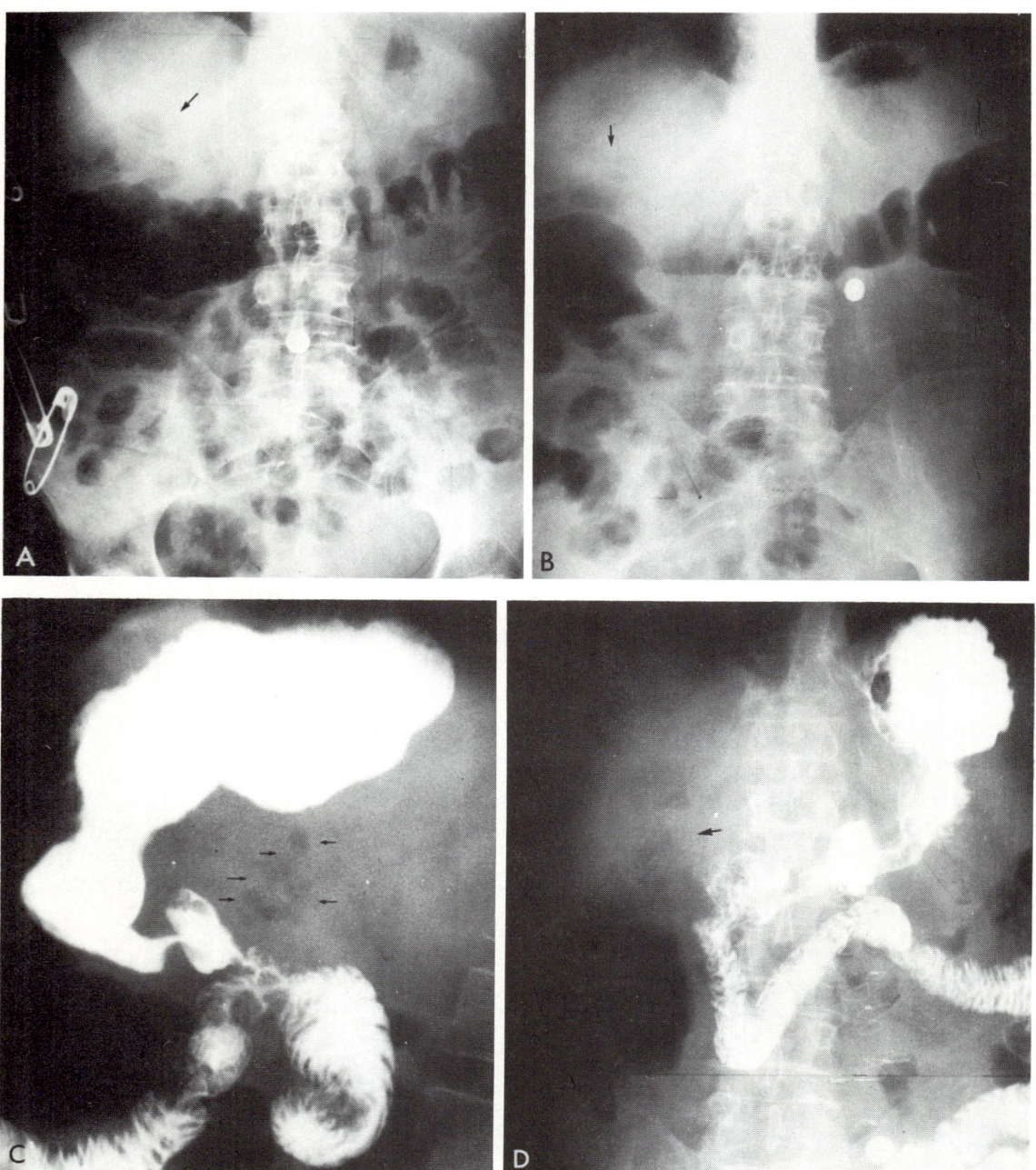

Figure 5–91. Abscess. A 76-year-old female developed fever, nausea, and vomiting ten days postcholecystectomy. *A,* The supine radiograph shows gas in right upper quadrant (arrow). *B,* The upright radiograph shows no change in position of the gas shadow (arrow). *C,* The lateral radiograph localizes the abscess to the subhepatic (midvisceral) space (arrows). *D,* The left lateral decubitus film shows constancy of the gas shadow (arrow), lateral to the duodenum. Abscess was confirmed at surgery.

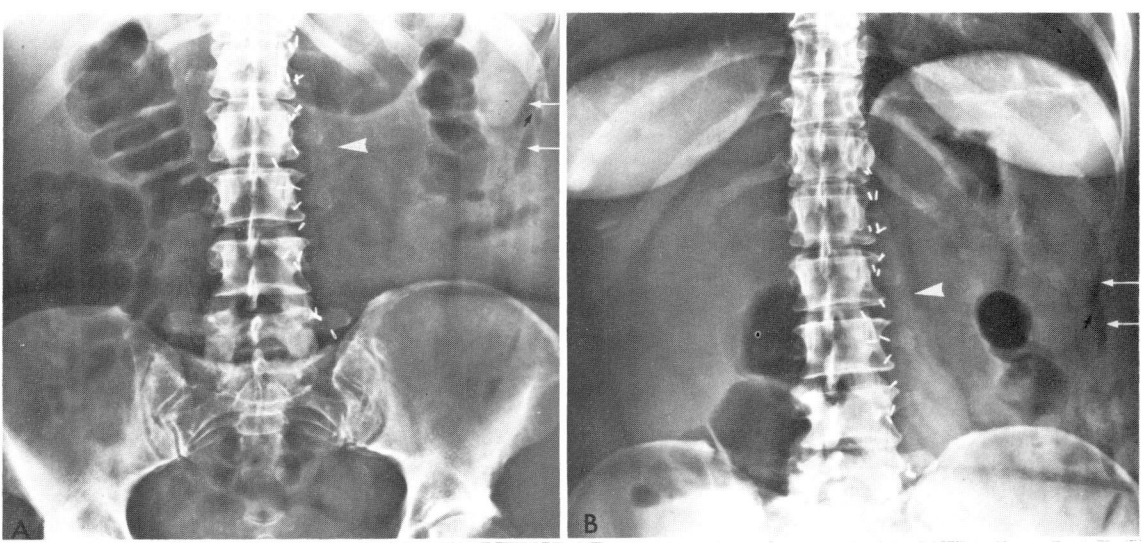

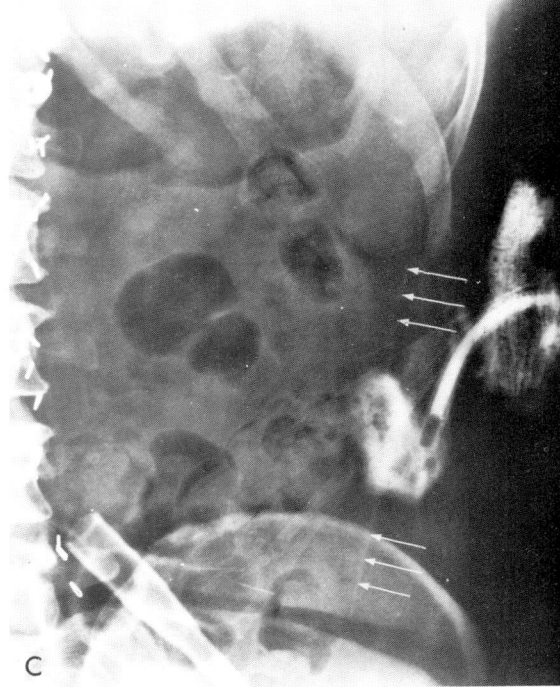

Figure 5–92. Pararenal abscess. A 45-year-old female developed fever and left flank pain five days following lumbar sympathectomy. Supine (A) and upright (B) radiographs show loss of the left lower two thirds of the psoas margin (arrowhead). There is extraperitoneal gas in the flanks (white arrows) outlining the extraperitoneal fascia. The black arrow points to the phrenicocolic ligament. C, A radiograph taken after drainage of the abscess in the flank and injection of a contrast agent shows the properitoneal stripes (arrows). Posterior pararenal abscess was diagnosed.

Abscesses have been discussed previously. In general, surgery is one of the most common causes of intraperitoneal abscesses (Figs. 5–91 to 5–94). The operation itself may be the sole cause of the abscess. Surgical procedures that often result in this complication are partial gastrectomy, cholecystectomy for chronic gallbladder disease, and splenectomy. Dineen and McSherry,[8] in a series of 63 subphrenic abscesses, found that operation on the stomach (25 cases) and the biliary tract (13 cases) accounted for the majority of the abscesses. Perforated ulcers tend to involve all spaces, but duodenal ulcers produce abscesses primarily on the right side (Fig. 5–95), whereas ruptured gastric ulcers produce abscesses on the left side. Table 5–21 lists the most common direct and indirect findings of intra-abdominal abscesses. Table 5–20 lists the roentgen findings of intra-abdominal pseudoabscesses.

Text continued on page 244.

242 — THE ACUTE ABDOMEN

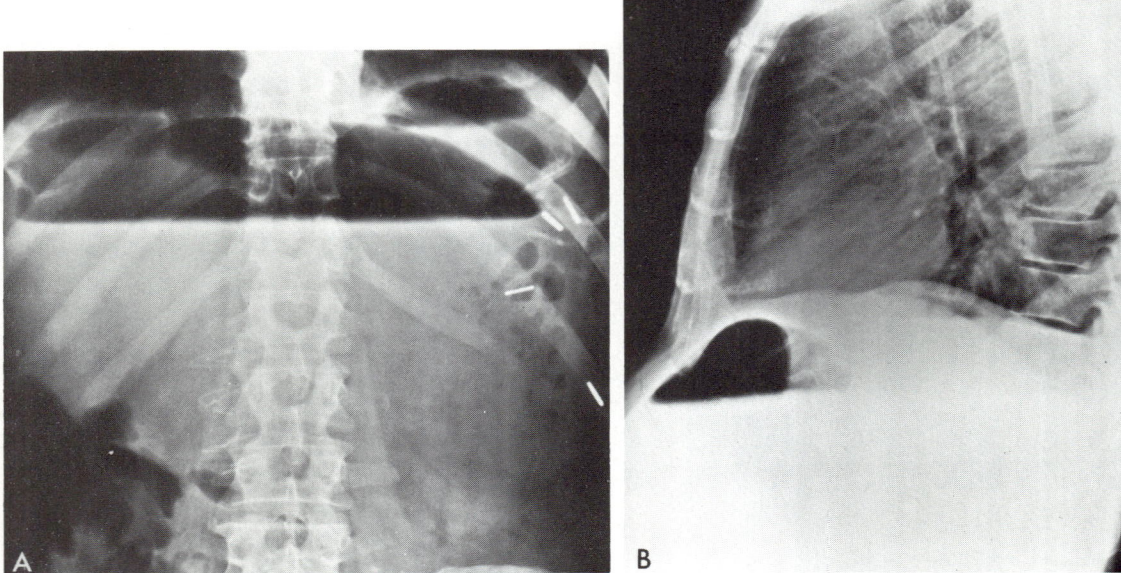

Figure 5–93. Intraperitoneal abscess. A 64-year-old female with fever and abdominal distention three days after right hemicolectomy and removal of the distal ileum. *A,* The upright radiograph of the abdomen shows a large air-fluid level in the upper abdomen. *B,* The lateral radiograph demonstrates the anterior location of the air-fluid level corresponding to the peritoneal cavity. The diagnosis was intraperitoneal abscess involving the entire free intraperitoneal (subphrenic and subhepatic) space. At surgery, 2500 cc of fluid were removed from a 5000 cc cavity.

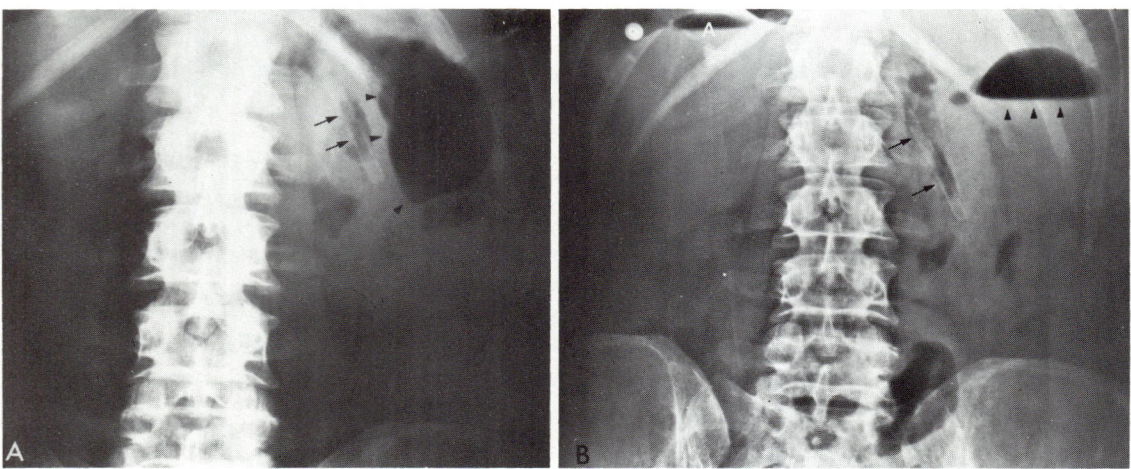

Figure 5–94. Subdiaphragmatic abscess. A 74-year-old male five days following resection of the distal esophagus and fundus of the stomach for carcinoma. *A* and *B,* Supine and upright radiographs show a collection of the gas with an air-fluid level (arrowheads) lateral to the stomach, which can be identified by a nasogastric tube (arrows). There is residual free air *(A)* under the right diaphragm.

Illustration and legend continued on the following page.

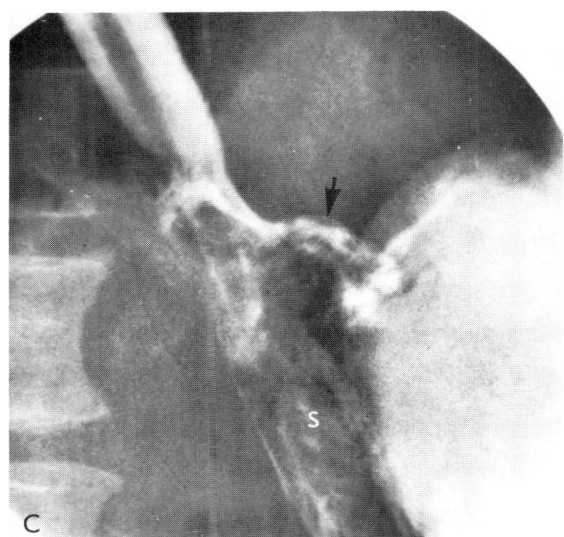
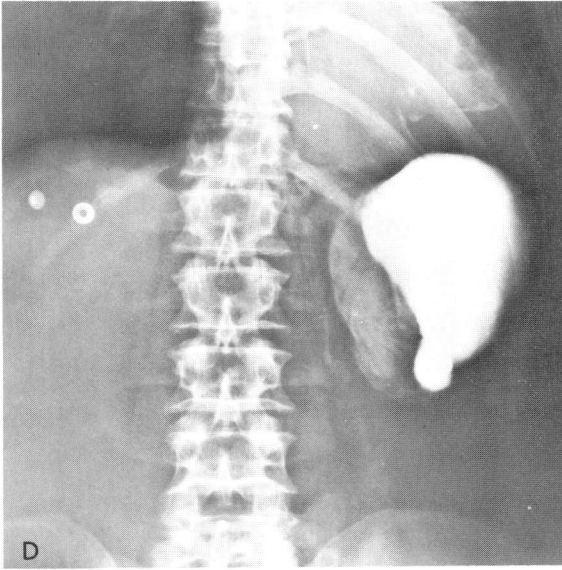
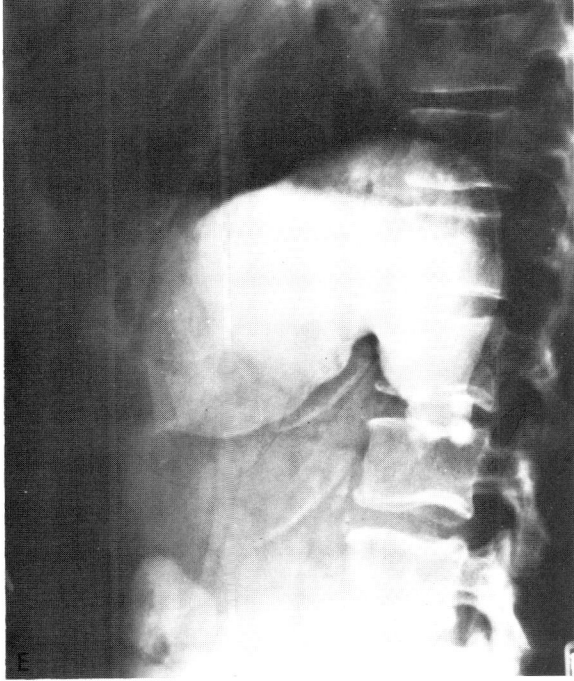

Figure 5–94 *Continued.* *C*, Barium swallow demonstrates communication (arrow) of stomach with a huge subdiaphragmatic collection. The stomach (S) is posterior and only minimally filled. *D* and *E*, Anteroposterior cross-table lateral radiographs show the barium filling the large cavity. The diagnosis was anastomotic leak and secondary abscess.

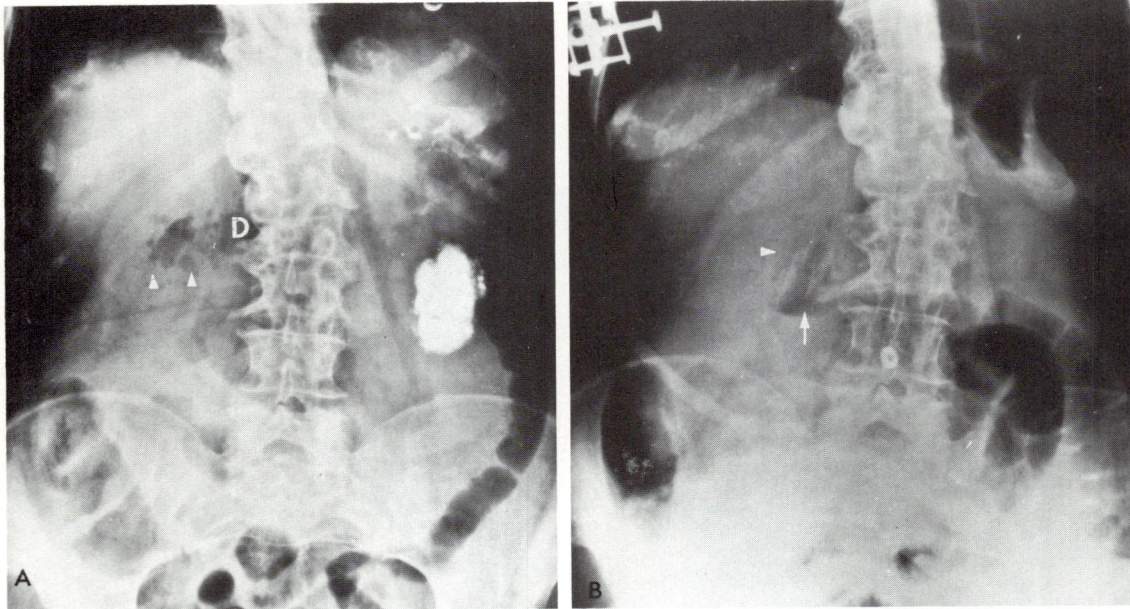

Figure 5–95. Abscess. A 71-year-old female with a diagnosis of pyloric obstruction. There was a long history of peptic ulcer disease. Six days after admission, pain developed in the right upper quadrant with fever and a leukocyte count of 36,000. *A,* The supine radiograph demonstrates a mottled gas collection (arrowheads) outside and lateral to the duodenum (D). *B,* The upright radiograph shows an air-fluid level (arrow) in the same area where the cluster of gas is still noted (arrowhead). The diagnosis of anterior visceral abscess was proved at surgery.

Hemorrhage in the postoperative patient is radiologically demonstrable by the presence of fluid within the peritoneal cavity (see Table 5–2).

The signs of ischemia in the postoperative state are the same as in the preoperative state. That is, there are thickened walls of bowel with some constriction and occasionally an ileus of bowel adjacent to the ischemic area. The ischemia may be secondary to postoperative complications or to interruption of the blood supply (Fig. 5–96) during surgery.

Postoperatively, the roentgen findings of perforated stress ulcers are usually less specific in terms of free air than preoperatively. The superimposition of the findings of slowly resolving intraperitoneal air, ileus, and fluid in the peritoneal cavity may suggest the diagnosis. However, these findings can be confused with many other postoperative conditions. The use of contrast agents to visualize perforation may be required to make the radiologic diagnosis. Angiography is the definitive modality if bleeding is active.

TABLE 5–20. INTRA-ABDOMINAL PSEUDOABSCESS

Hepatodiaphragmatic interposition of colon—Chilaiditi syndrome
Subhepatic appendix
Pneumatosis cystoides intestinalis
Subdiaphragmatic extraperitoneal fat pad

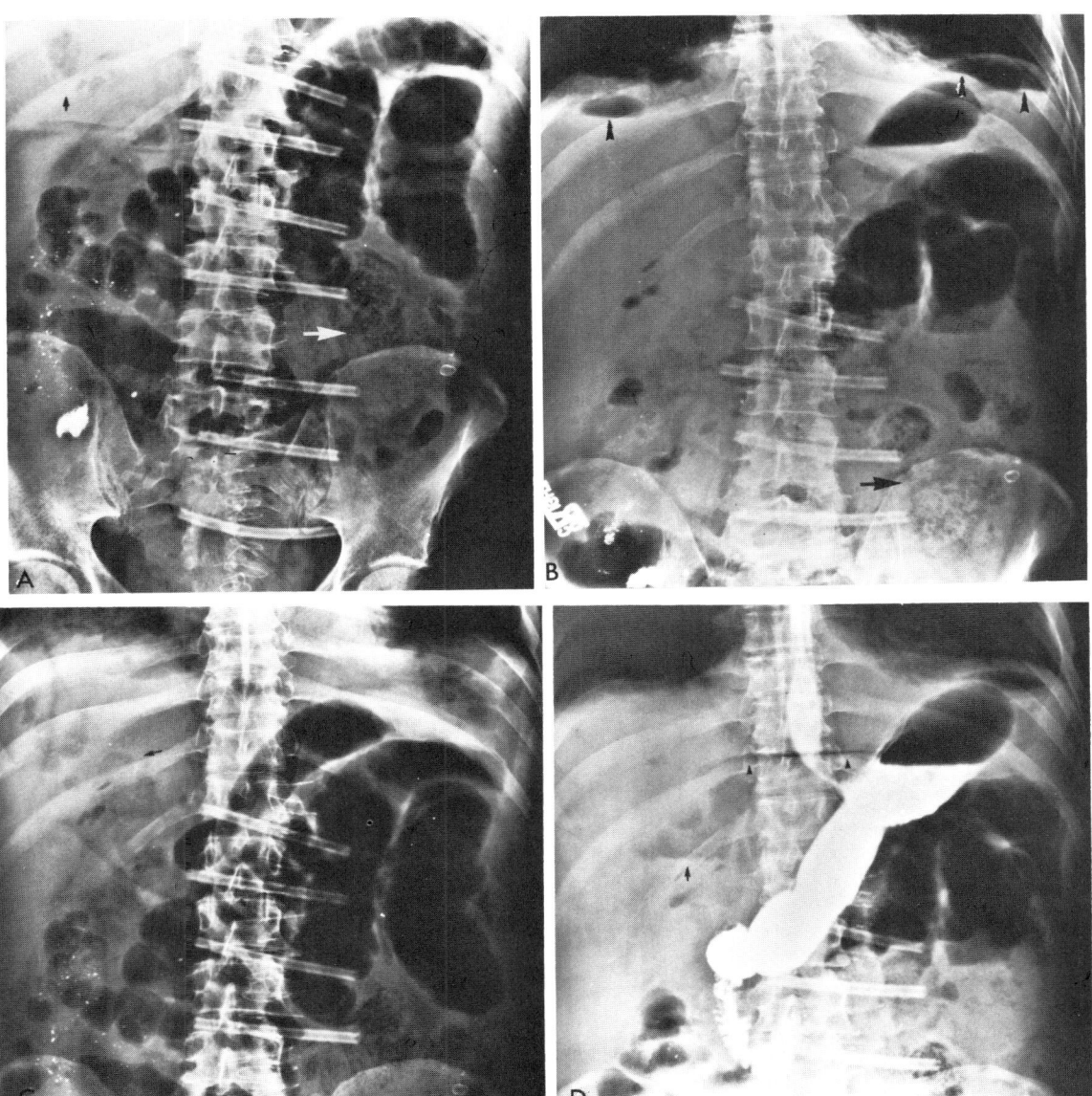

Figure 5–96. Perforation of small bowel infarction. A 60-year-old male following surgery for infarction of the small bowel. On the eleventh postoperative day there was sudden, acute, diffuse abdominal pain and signs of peritonitis. *A,* The supine radiograph shows an extraluminal gas collection (black arrow) and submucosal air in the small bowel (white arrow). *B,* The upright radiograph shows intraperitoneal air-fluid levels (arrowheads) and, again, the submucosal air (arrow). *C,* A supine radiograph taken 30 minutes later shows an increase in the amount of intraperitoneal air (arrow). *D,* A barium study of the stomach performed soon after shows a further increase of free air (arrow) now also seen under the central tendinous portion of the diaphragm (arrowheads). The diagnosis of small bowel infarction with perforation was confirmed at surgery.

Extraperitoneal

Obstruction of a ureter can be a complication of intra- or extraperitoneal surgery. The plain radiograph may demonstrate enlargement of the renal shadow or, occasionally, an ileus associated with the area of obstruction. An ileus is less likely to occur from a surgically ligated ureter than from a calculus. In addition, calculi may form in the postoperative state, and the classic findings of calculous ureteral obstruction may be demonstrated. In general, however, ultrasound or intravenous urography is required to confirm the diagnosis and delineate the site of obstruction.

Hemorrhage may be a complication of surgery involving the extraperitoneal space. In general its localization is the same as in the preoperative abdomen (see Table 5–3) and requires separating the compartments of the extraperitoneal space into the anterior pararenal, perirenal, and posterior pararenal spaces. In the postoperative patient, the radiologist must look for integrity of the intra-abdominal structures, the loss of which may raise the suspicion of postoperative hemorrhage.

Abscesses may occur in the extraperitoneal space after surgery and, again, the signs of localization are the same as in the preoperative patient (Table 5–19). Specifically, evidence of abscess may be manifested by fluid collection, gas collection, or loss of the structures normally seen. Fluid in gas collections corresponding to the extraperitoneal compartments should therefore raise the suspicion of an abscess.

TABLE 5–21. ROENTGEN SIGNS OF INTRA-ABDOMINAL ABSCESS DEMONSTRABLE IN STANDARD ABDOMINAL SERIES

Most Common Direct Signs	Comment
Soft tissue mass	Because of different degrees of density, the mass may be well or poorly defined
Pathologic collection of extraluminal gas	Cluster of small, round, bubblelike lucencies, or lucent bands, usually following a fascial plane or outlining an anatomic space; or homogeneous, rounded, well-outlined gas collection
Ill-defined appearance, or loss of normally demonstrable anatomic structures	Produced by the inflammatory process on adjacent organs, fascial planes, or muscle outline
Mobility of certain anatomic structures	Fixation of a viscus, such as sigmoid or transverse colon, by a periabscessual inflammatory process on the normal mobile mesenteric portions of the colon. Similarly, a kidney that does not descend by changing the position of the patient from supine to upright should raise the question of a perinephric abscess.
Most Common Indirect Signs	**Comment**
Displacement of a viscus	By pressure effect
Lumbar spine	Scoliosis concave toward the site where the abscess is located
Diaphragm	Elevation or splinting of a hemidiaphragm
Ileus	A localized ileus or a sentinel loop may be the early roentgen sign of the formation of an abscess. An obstruction pattern indicates occlusion either by pressure from the abscess on a loop of bowel or by formation of adhesions.
Pulmonary changes	A subphrenic abscess is often associated with supradiaphragmatic discoid atelectases, pleural reaction, or both

References

1. Balthazar, E. J., and Lutzker, S.: Radiological signs of acute pancreatitis. CRC Crit. Rev. Clin. Radiol. Nucl. Med. 8:199–242, 1976.
2. Bevan, P. G.: Incidence of postoperative pneumoperitoneum and its significance. Br. Med. J. 2:605–609, 1961.
3. Bobroff, L. M., Messinger, N. N. H., Subbarao, K., et al.: The cecal bascule. Am. J. Roentgenol. 115:249–252, 1972.
4. Bryant, L. R., Wiot, J. G., and Kloecher, R. J.: A study of the factors affecting the incidence and duration of the postoperative pneumoperitoneum. Surg. Gynecol. Obstet. 117:145–150, 1963.
5. Bryk, D., and Soong, K. Y.: Colonic ileus and its differential roentgen diagnosis. Am. J. Roentgenol. 101:329–337, 1967.
6. Bryk, D., Silverman, M. J., Venucopale, M. K., et al.: Fluid filled small bowel loops in gallstone ileus: clinical and experimental observations. Invest. Radiol. 12:357–363, 1977.
7. Burell, M., Toffler, R., and Lowman, R.: Blunt trauma to the abdomen and gastrointestinal tract. Plain film and contrast study. Radiol. Clin. North Am. 11:561–578, 1973.
8. Dineen, P., and McSherry, C. K.: Subdiaphragmatic abscess. Ann. Surg. 115:506–517, 1962.
9. Elkin, M.: Emergency uroradiology for the nontraumatized patient. Radiol. Clin. North Am. 16:135–146, 1978.
10. Frimann-Dahl, J.: Roentgen Examinations in Acute Abdominal Diseases. Ed. 3. Springfield, Illinois, Charles C Thomas, Publisher, 1974.
11. Govoni, A. F., and Whalen, J. P.: La dimostrazione radiografica di ascesso abdominale di origine postoperatoria: "abscess series." Radiol. Med. 63:1041–1047, 1977.
12. Harrison, I., Litwer, H., and Gerwig, W. H., Jr.: Studies on the incidence and the duration of postoperative pneumoperitoneum. Ann. Surg. 145:591–594, 1957.
13. Jones, J. H., and Chapman, M.: Definition of megacolon in colitis. Gut 10:562–564, 1969.
14. Love, L.: Large bowel obstruction. Semin. Roentgenol. 8:299–322, 1973.
15. McCort, J.: Radiographic Examination in Blunt Abdominal Trauma. Philadelphia, W. B. Saunders Company, 1966.
16. Myers, R. A. M., Andrew, W., and Wilkinson, A. E.: Reappraisal of the left lateral decubitus x-ray in splenic rupture. Br. J. Surg. 64:482, 1977.
17. Nelson, S. W.: Extraluminal gas collections due to diseases of the gastrointestinal tract. Am. J. Roentgenol. 115:225–248, 1972.
18. Soter, C. S.: The contribution of the radiologist to the diagnosis of acute appendicitis. Semin. Roentgenol. 8:375–388, 1975.
19. Weinstein, M.: Volvulus of the cecum and ascending colon. Ann. Surg. 107:248–259, 1938.
20. Whalen, J. P.: Radiology of the Abdomen. An Anatomic Approach. Philadelphia, Lea & Febiger, 1976.
21. Whalen, J. P., and Berne, A. S.: The extraperitoneal perivisceral fat pad. II. Roentgen interpretation of pathological alterations. Radiology 92:473–480, 1969.
22. Wittenberg, J., Athanasoulis, C. A., Williams, L. F., et al.: Ischemic colitis. Radiology and pathophysiology. Am. J. Roentgenol. 123:287–300, 1975.

6

THE ABDOMINAL WALL, UMBILICUS, PERITONEUM, MESENTERIES, AND RETROPERITONEUM

JAMES B. MASTERSON, M.B., B.Ch., B.A.O.,
F.R.C.P.I., D.M.R.D., F.R.C.R.

THE ABDOMINAL WALL

Congenital Abnormalities

Although most congenital anomalies of the abdominal wall are clinically obvious, radiology often plays an important role in assessing whether an associated abnormality exists. The closure of the embryo body is accomplished by the ventral coalescence of four folds. The failure of the formation of any of the folds results in a hernia of the anterior abdominal wall, or celosomia.

The failure of the formation of the cephalic fold results in anterior chest wall and diaphragmatic defects, with apparent ectopia cordis, omphalocele, and commonly, cardiovascular malformations. The dextroposition of the heart is invariable, and ventricular and atrial septal defects and pulmonary stenosis are frequently present. There is an anterior defect of the diaphragm, and the pericardial and peritoneal cavities communicate. Twenty per cent of cases show a left ventricular diverticulum extending into the peritoneal cavity. Chest x-rays show dextrocardia, with the lateral displacement of the anterior rib ends and the absence of the lower sternal segments. The deficient anterior chest wall simulates ectopia cordis clinically, but radiographically the heart is shown to maintain its position relative to the lungs and diaphragm. Roentgenographic features of the associated cardiac anomalies may be evident. Abdominal films show the omphalocele, the main portion of which is in the epigastrium. Malrotation, with intestinal obstruction, may be present.

The failure of the formation of the lateral folds results in an umbilical defect or omphalocele. The prolapsed abdominal viscera are covered by a membrane composed of amnion and peritoneum. The sac varies enormously in size and may contain most of the abdominal cavity contents, including the liver, spleen, pancreas, and genital organs. Preoperative films may demonstrate evidence of obstruction but are usually not necessary. Because the mesentery is usually fixed only by the superior mesenteric artery, duodenal bands and malrotation may occur postoperatively; evidence of these may be detected on films of the abdomen.

The failure of the development of the caudal fold results in exstrophy of the bladder. This is a complex defect, associated with an omphalocele and frequently with neural arch defects, including sacral meningomyelocele, a cutaneous presentation of the colon that ends blindly, and bifid genitalia. Plain films of the abdomen show the deficient pubis and the spinal anomalies, if present. Excretion urography may demonstrate the frequent urinary tract anomalies, which include absent or ectopic kidneys. Gastrointestinal tract examination may reveal malrotation, localized stenosis, or reduplication and shows the site at which the small bowel exits onto the abdominal wall. Absorbable-contrast examination of the blindly ending colon should also be performed if surgical reconstruction is being considered.

Gastroschisis stems from a failure of the development of a lateral fold and results in a defect adjacent to, but not involving, the umbilicus. Preoperative plain films to detect obstruction due to a bowel atresia are sufficient, since associated anomalies are not common in this condition.

AGENESIS (PRUNE BELLY SYNDROME).[7] This triad of abnormalities—absent abdominal muscle, undescended testes, and urinary tract anomalies—is thought to be due to a developmental failure at the sixth to tenth week of intrauterine life. The absence of abdominal walls has occurred in females, but the condition is far more common in males.

The urinary tract anomalies affect the following:

1. *The kidneys.* These are usually small but are often hydronephrotic.
2. *The ureters and bladder.* There is a reduction of muscle in the walls of these structures with dilatation and tortuosity of the ureters, which show diminished peristalsis. The bladder is large and may have a urachal diverticulum.
3. *The posterior urethra.* This is dilated and elongated and narrows abruptly at the junction with the membranous urethra.

Excretion urography and micturating cystography are all that are required to demonstrate the extent of urinary tract anomalies (Fig. 6–1).

OMPHALOMESENTERIC DUCT AND URACHAL ANOMALIES. The omphalomesenteric duct and the allantoic canal may remain patent throughout their length or at either end, or they may persist as a fibrous cord that contains cysts (Fig. 6–2). If the omphalomesenteric duct remains patent throughout its length, it forms an ilioumbilical

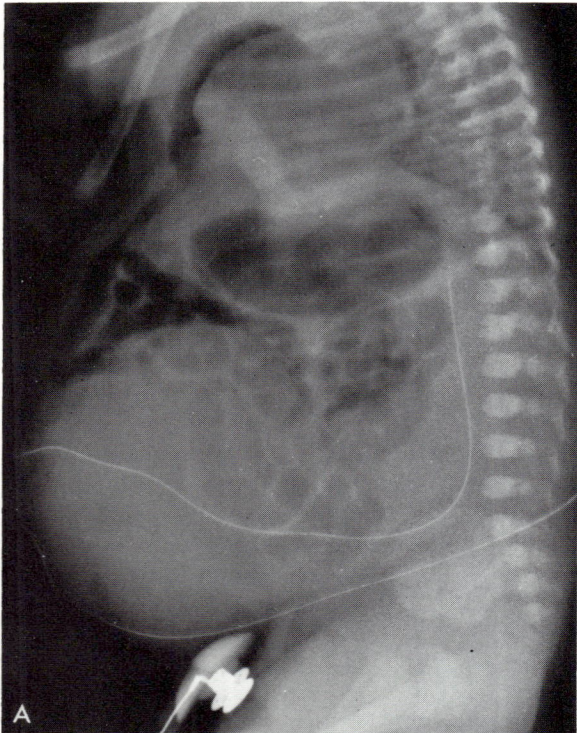

Figure 6–1. Prune belly syndrome. *A,* Deficient musculature of the abdomen. Note the large soft tissue density anteriorly, which was shown on cystography *(B* and *C)* to be due to a highly distended bladder. Free reflux into hydronephrotic renal collecting systems and ureters is also shown. Note the dilated elongated posterior urethra (arrow). Such renal tract abnormalities are common in this syndrome.

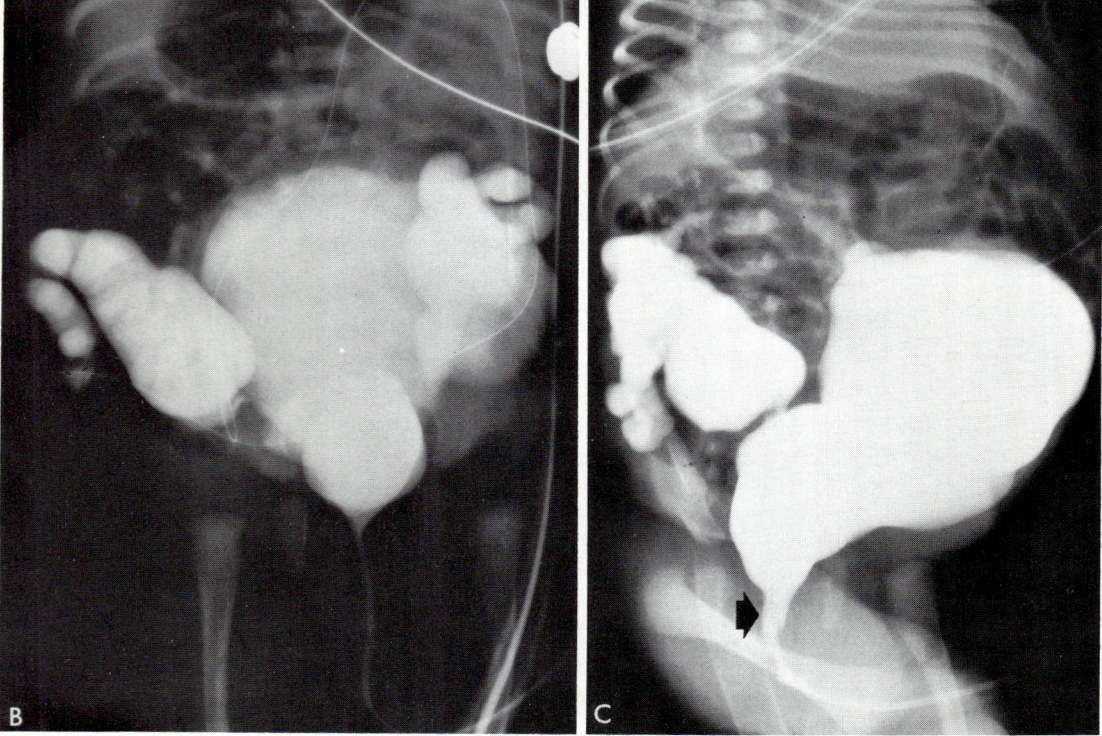

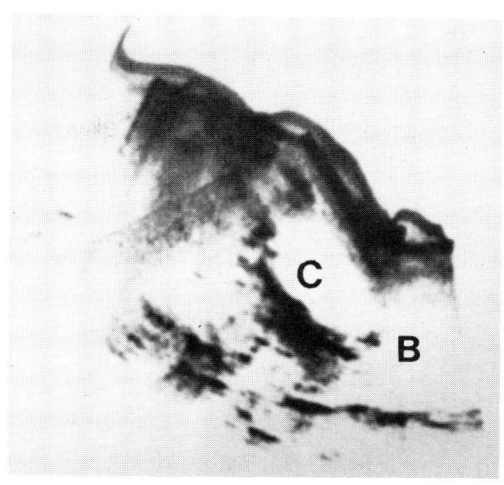

Figure 6–2. Midline longitudinal ultrasound scan showing an oval cystic mass, the result of a urachal cyst (C) deep to the abdominal wall between the umbilicus and the bladder (B).

fistula; if the allantoic canal is patent throughout, it forms a vesicoumbilical fistula. This situation may lead to the discharge of feces or urine at the umbilicus. Occasionally, only a short segment of the duct remains patent at its umbilical end, and this may also lead to an umbilical discharge. At times, the only evidence of the patency of one of the structures is a raised area of mucosa or granulation tissue at the umbilicus. Patency at the visceral end of the ducts gives rise to Meckel's diverticulum, in the case of the omphalomesenteric duct, or to a urachal diverticulum—a tonguelike projection of the anterior surface of the bladder up toward the umbilicus—in the case of the allantoic canal (Figs. 6–3 to 6–5). A common presenting feature in anomalies of the ducts is umbilical discharge.

In the initial radiographic investigation of patients with anomalies of the umbilical region, an attempt is made to cannulate a sinus or fistula and outline it by the injection

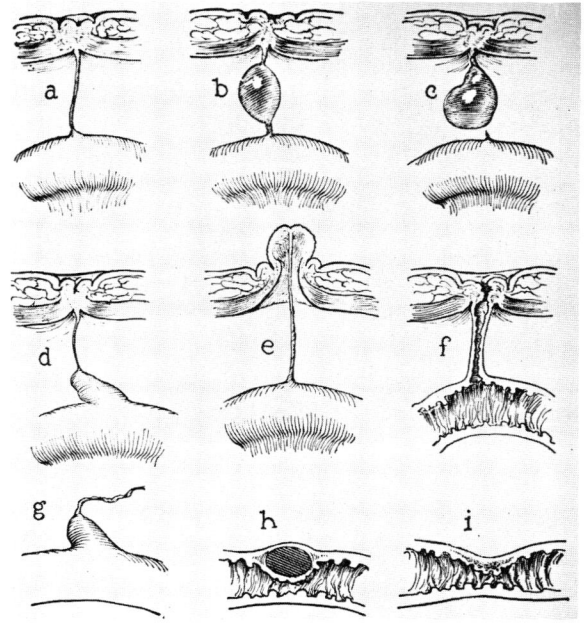

Figure 6–3. Schematic drawings of congenital malformations that may result from persistence of the omphalomesenteric duct. a. persistent cord between ileal wall and closed umbilicus; b. cyst in this same cord; c. cyst anchored at the umbilical end of the cord but free at the ileal end; d. Meckel's diverticulum attached to closed umbilicus by closed cord; e. everted mucocele of the umbilicus with cord attachment to ileal wall; f. fecal fistula open at both umbilical and ileal ends; g. Meckel's diverticulum open at ileal end but blind at umbilical end, which is unattached; h. intramural cystic diverticulum; i. local stenosis of the ileum at the site of the mouth of a persistent omphalomesenteric duct. (*From* Caffey, J., Pediatric X-Ray Diagnosis. Chicago, Year Book Medical Publishers, Inc., 1973. Reproduced by permission.)

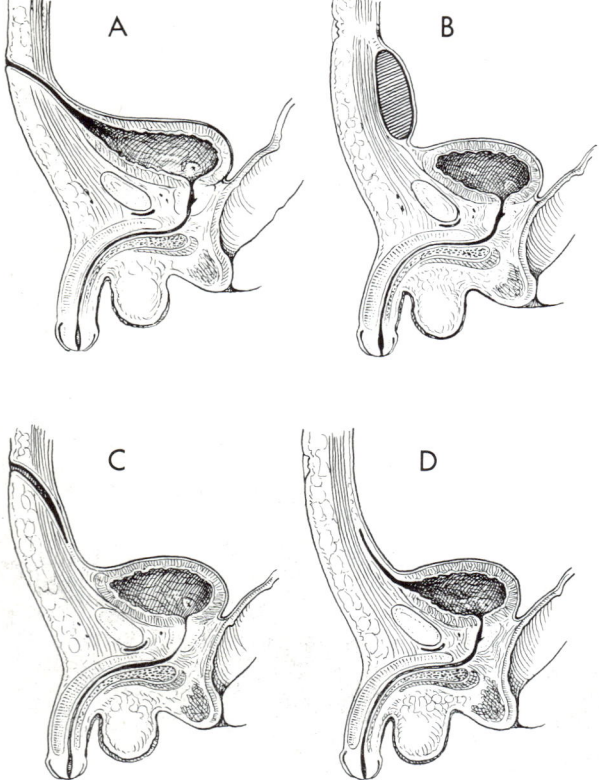

Figure 6–4. Patency of the urachus and urachal remnant. *A,* Patent urachal canal connecting the umbilicus and bladder; *B,* Urachal cyst with both ends of the urachal canal closed and the lumen dilated with epithelial exudate; *C,* Urachal remnant open at the umbilicus and closed at the vesical end; *D,* Urachal remnant open at the vesical end and closed at the umbilicus. (*From* Caffey, J.: Pediatric X-Ray Diagnosis. Chicago, Year Book Medical Publishers, Inc., 1973. Reproduced by permission.)

of contrast medium. Since it is occasionally impossible to distinguish among an omphalomesenteric duct, a patent urachus, and an umbilical vein, only water-soluble contrast medium suitable for intravascular injection should be used, and the technique of cannulation and injection should be sterile. A duct is patent when contrast injection demonstrates the length of the duct, to the distal ileum in the case of the omphalomesenteric duct or to the bladder in the case of the urachal duct. If no umbilical orifice is detectable, contrast examination of the small bowel and urinary tract may reveal urachal or omphalomesenteric duct anomalies.

Patency of the visceral end of an omphalomesenteric duct is the most common congenital anomaly; it is present in 1.5 per cent of the population. The patent visceral end communicates with the distal ileum as a Meckel's diverticulum. It varies enormously in size. The diverticulum may contain heterotopic gastric mucosa and may be the site of peptic ulceration and bleeding. Meckel's diverticulum is notoriously difficult to detect on barium examination of the small bowel. If gastric mucosa is present in the diverticulum, technetium 99m scanning may demonstrate it; the technetium is excreted by the gastric mucosa. Ultrasound examination of the abdomen may reveal urachal or omphalomesenteric cysts.

The induction of a nitrous oxide pneumoperitoneum, followed by a single horizontal-beam radiograph with the patient in the supine position, has been used to demonstrate urachal and omphalomesenteric duct anomalies. It is most useful in the investigation of the persistence of either duct. The technique is less likely to be successful in a search for Meckel's diverticulum, as only a small proportion of these diverticula maintain a connection with the umbilicus.

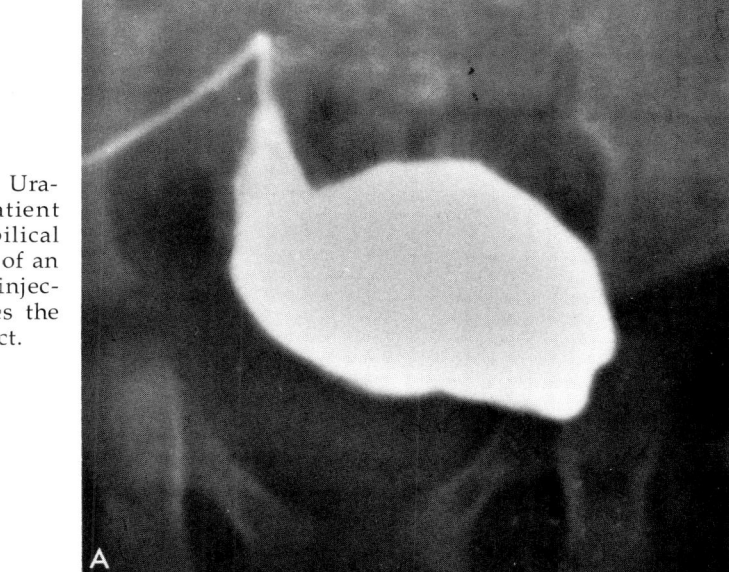

Figure 6–5. *A* and *B*, Urachal anomaly. The patient had a persistent umbilical discharge. Cannulation of an umbilical sinus with injection of contrast outlines the bladder and urachal duct.

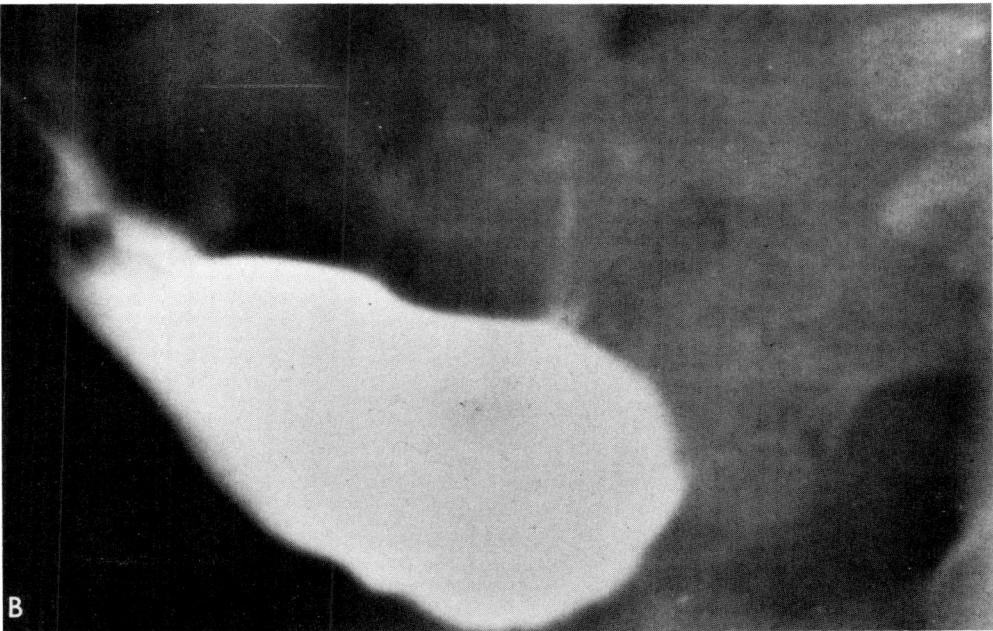

Tumors

Most tumors of the anterior abdominal wall are clinically obvious. Ultrasound examination is often useful in delineating the extent of the tumor and giving information on its internal characteristics. It is chiefly in the matter of staging that radiologic investigation plays a role. In the case of the thick musculoskeletal structures of the posterior abdominal wall, however, radiologic examination can aid in the diagnosis and delineation of tumor. The most common primary malignant tumors of the abdominal wall are, in order of frequency, sarcomas, neurogenic sarcomas, spindle cell sarcomas, synoviomas, and rhabdomyosarcomas.

Metastases from sarcomas and carcinomas are not uncommon. Osseous metastases to the spine and pelvis are by far the most common tumors of the body wall. These are usually considered separately with their primary tumors—breast, prostate, lung, and so forth.

RADIOLOGIC FINDINGS. The usual radiologic finding is a mass displacing or destroying adjacent structures. The plain abdominal film may reveal an area of increased density, with displacement or obliteration of the psoas shadow. As the mass enlarges it may displace other retroperitoneal structures, such as the kidney, the spleen, or even the liver (Fig. 6–6). Involvement of the spine with destruction of transverse processes, pedicles, or even vertebral bodies may be seen (Fig. 6–7). Further enlargement may lead to the displacement of bowel loops by the mass.

Contrast examinations, including barium studies, excretion urography, and venacavography, may provide additional information regarding the size of the tumor. More direct information on the extent of the mass may be obtained by ultrasound examination. Radionuclide studies using tumor-seeking agents, such as gallium, may outline the tumor and its metastases. Computerized axial tomography can usually delineate these tumors with considerable accuracy and is particularly useful in demonstration of the involvement of the spine, which may be undetectable by other radiologic means. Arteriography is particularly helpful in the demonstration of a tumor's vascular supply when its surgical removal is contemplated. Additional studies, such as myelography, may be indicated in specific instances.

The most appropriate modality for the postoperative follow-up of these tumors depends upon their site and other factors, such as whether the tumor takes up gallium.

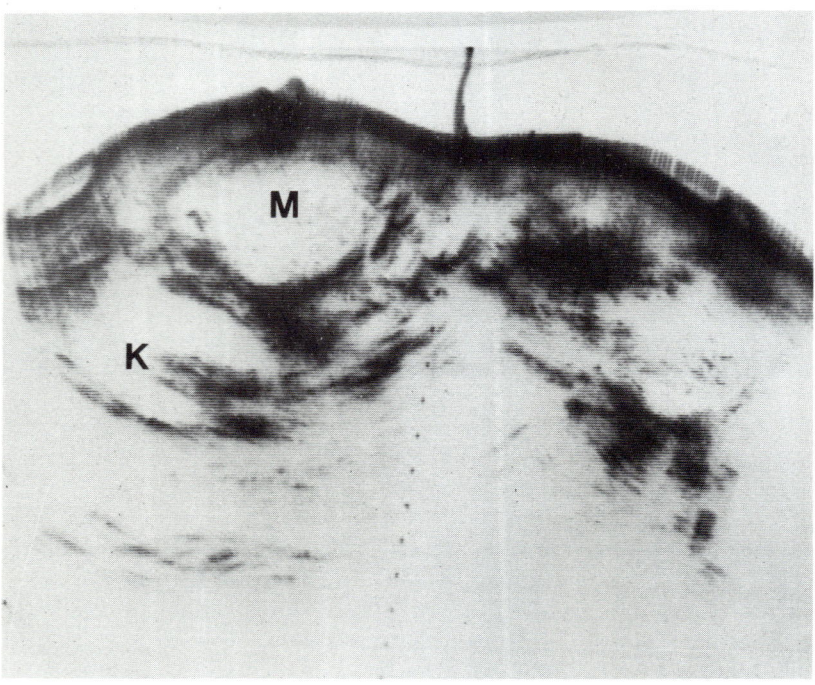

Figure 6–6. Transverse ultrasound scan with the patient prone shows a large mass in the left paraspinal muscles. The mass (M) extends to the spine medially and displaces the left kidney (K) anteriorly. The appearances are those of a solid tumor (note the internal echoes in this high-frequency scan) of the posterior body wall. The differential diagnosis includes sarcoma, lipoma, and metastasis.

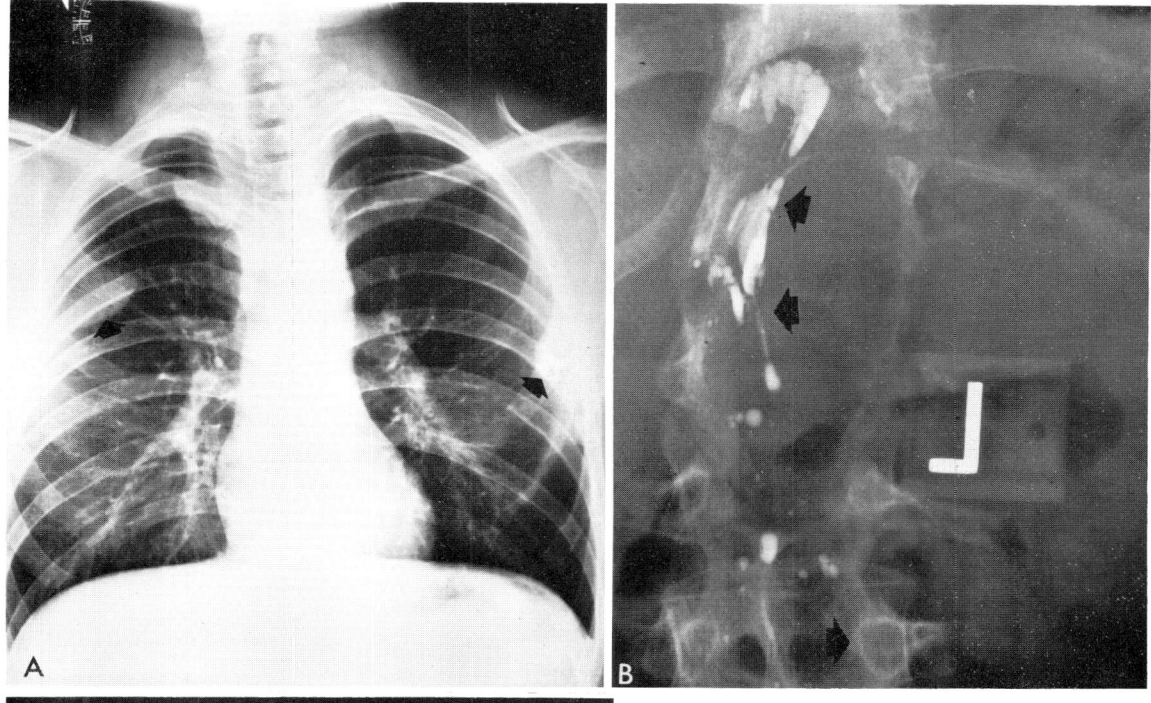

Figure 6–7. *A,* Neurofibromatosis showing soft tissue masses of neurofibromas along the ribs (arrows). *B,* Malignant degeneration with extensive destruction of vertebrae from T_{11} to L_2. Note the absence of pedicles of T_{12}, L_1, and L_2 on the left side compared with the normal pedicle on L_3 (arrow pointing right). Displacement of the spinal subarachnoid with contrast medium contained by extradural mass (arrows pointing left) is shown. Destruction of the twelfth left rib is also demonstrated. *C,* CT scan reveals mass (arrow) and destruction of the posterior vertebra. S = spleen; L = liver.

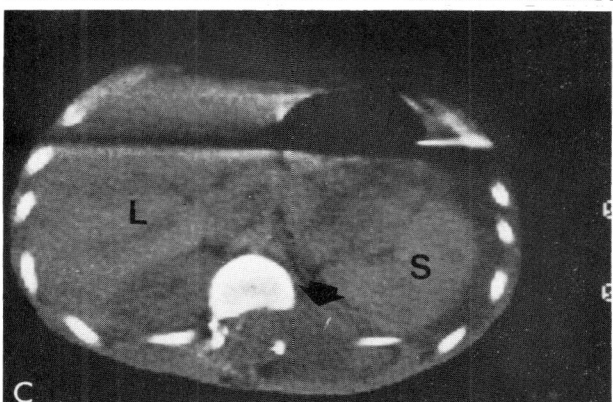

Rectus Sheath Hematoma

The clinical importance of this fairly uncommon condition is in its ability to simulate an acute abdomen. The hematoma is most often due to the rupture of the muscle or bleeding from the inferior epigastric artery or vein and is most often on the right side. It may be traumatic or spontaneous in origin. Traumatic causes include blows, falls, heavy lifting, and shock therapy. The spontaneous causes include bleeding disorders, obesity, pregnancy, atherosclerotic and hypertensive vascular disease, and severe coughing. The signs and symptoms are the sudden onset of severe lower abdominal pain and a lower quadrant tender mass.

RADIOLOGIC FINDINGS. Tangential films using soft tissue technique may reveal a spindle-shaped swelling in the rectus sheath. Chronic hematomas may show rim calcification. The investigative method of choice, however, is ultrasonography, which demonstrates the hematoma within the abdominal wall (Fig. 6–8).

256 — THE ABDOMINAL WALL AND RELATED STRUCTURES

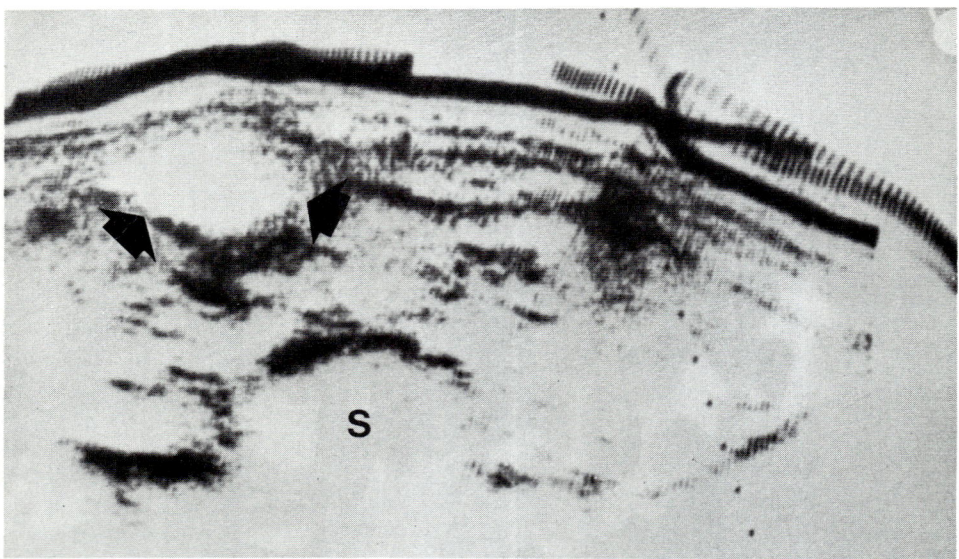

Figure 6–8. Transverse ultrasound scan a little above the symphysis pubis showing an oval transonic area in the right abdominal wall (arrows) (S = spine). The patient's history of severe abdominal pain following a paroxysm of coughing and the finding of an extremely tender mass in the right lower abdominal wall suggested the diagnosis of rectus sheath hematoma, confirmed by examination.

Pneumoperitoneum[9, 17, 19, 21, 28]

Although the demonstration of free peritoneal gas is of great value in the diagnosis of a perforated abdominal viscus, other important causes exist:

1. From within the lumen of the gastrointestinal tract
    a. Perforated peptic ulcer
    b. Other perforative diseases
    c. Blunt and penetrating trauma to the abdomen
    d. Endoscopic instrumentation
    e. Anesthesia
2. From outside the lumen of the gastrointestinal tract
    a. Surgery
    b. Diagnostic examinations
        (1) Rubin test
        (2) Pneumoperitoneography
    c. Therapy (e.g., peritoneal dialysis)
    d. Penetrating trauma
    e. Pneumatosis cystoides intestinalis
3. Idiopathic

DEMONSTRATION OF INTRAPERITONEAL GAS. Large amounts of gas within the peritoneal cavity may be detectable on supine films of the abdomen by the demonstration of a large central oval lucency in the abdomen due to the collection of the free gas in the uppermost part of the peritoneal cavity beneath the abdominal wall (Fig. 6–9); by the demonstration of both sides of the wall of a hollow viscus (Fig. 6–10), the wall being outlined by gas; or by the demonstration of normally invisible structures,

THE ABDOMINAL WALL AND RELATED STRUCTURES — 257

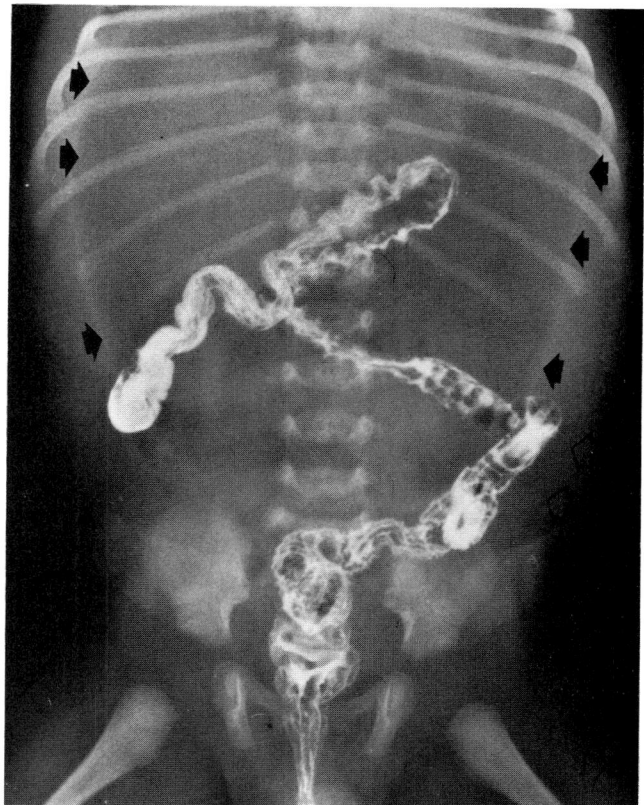

Figure 6–9. Pneumoperitoneum following spontaneous gastric perforation. In this supine film the free gas occupies the uppermost part of the abdominal cavity to form an oval lucency, the so-called football sign (closed arrows). Note that the colon is displaced away from the properitoneal fat line, indicating the presence of ascites (open arrows).

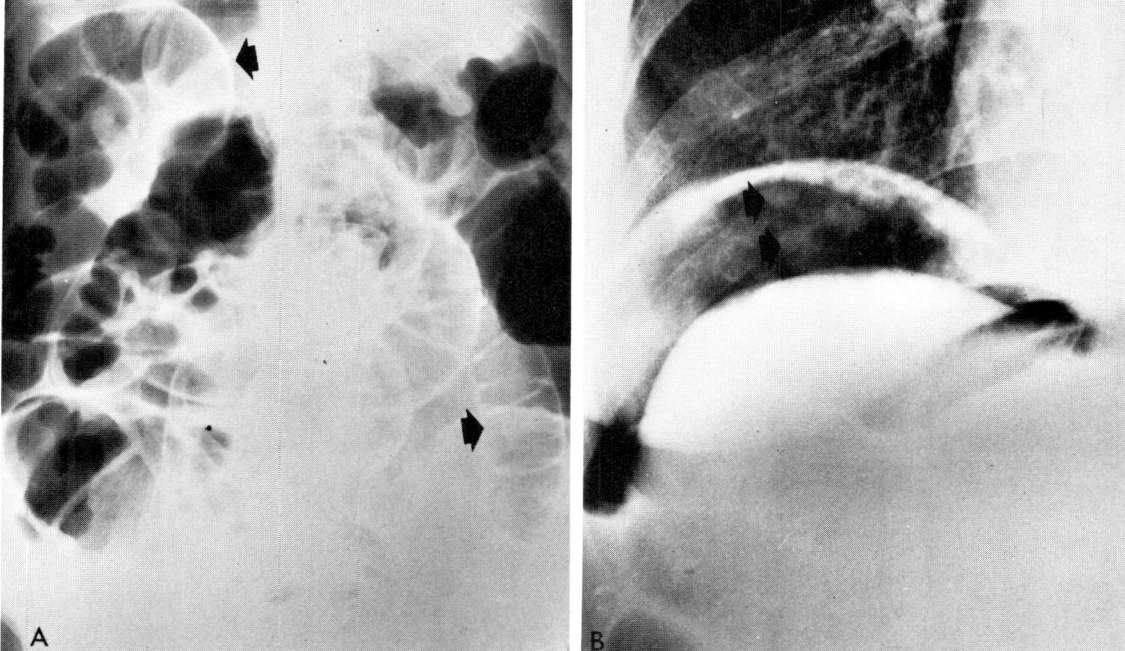

Figure 6–10. A, Pneumoperitoneum in a patient with extensive serosal metastases. Air both within and outside the bowel wall enables the bowel wall to be clearly seen (arrows). B, The diaphragm is clearly demonstrated by contrast with the air above and below it. There is clear demonstration of the nodular densities caused by multiple serosal metastases (arrows).

such as the falciform ligament (Fig. 6–11), urachus, lateral umbilical ligaments, liver, or spleen (Fig. 6–12). The demonstration of small amounts of free gas demands more specialized techniques, however.

A radiologic routine devised by Miller and Nelson may enable demonstration of as little as 1 cc of free intraperitoneal air.[21] The patient is placed in the left lateral decubitus position for 10 to 20 minutes to allow free gas to make its way to the right flank. The gas then settles between the abdominal wall and the bowel in the iliac fossa or between the liver and the diaphragm. A left lateral decubitus film is taken. With the right side uppermost the patient is moved into the erect position and a chest film is taken. An erect abdominal film is also exposed. The final film is a supine view of the abdomen.

On the erect chest film small amounts of free peritoneal gas between the liver and the right hemidiaphragm are readily detected. In some cases the left lateral decubitus view may show gas not demonstrated on the erect film if the liver is bound to the diaphragm by adhesions, and it also allows gas to egress from the lesser sac, a site where free gas is difficult to demonstrate. Free gas may be demonstrated in more than 80 per cent of patients with a perforated bowel, but its absence does not preclude a perforation. Frequently no free air is demonstrable in the presence of a perforated diverticulum or appendix.

SPECIFIC TYPES OF PNEUMOPERITONEUM. Perforated peptic ulcer (Fig. 6–13) is

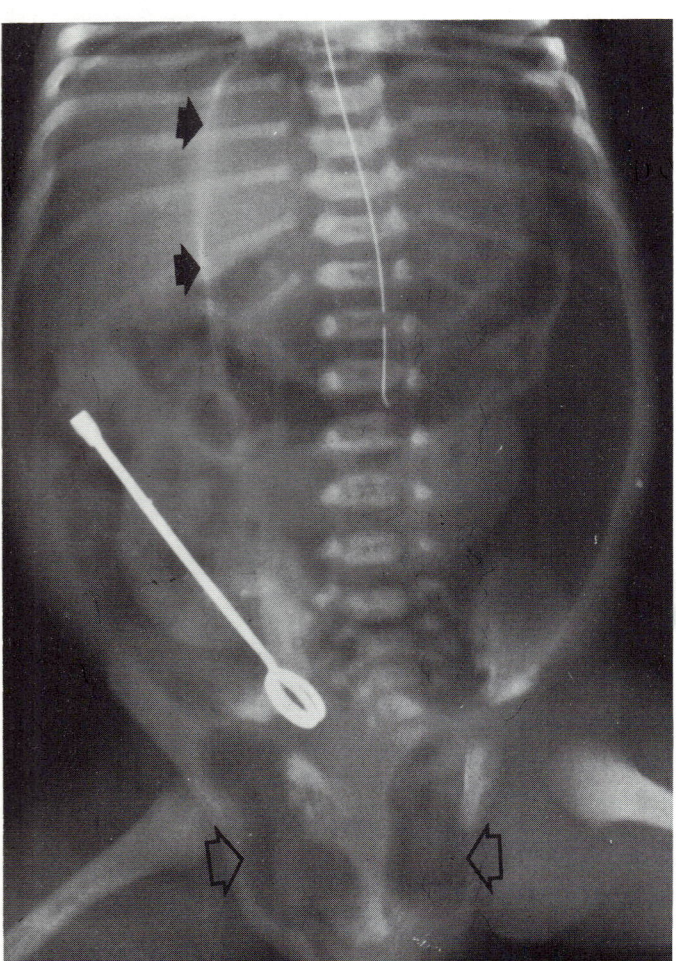

Figure 6–11. Pneumoperitoneum due to spontaneous lesser curvature perforation in a neonate. Tracking of air along tunica vaginalis to scrotum (open arrows) is demonstrated. Air is present between the liver and the diaphragm, and the falciform ligament is outlined by air.

THE ABDOMINAL WALL AND RELATED STRUCTURES — 259

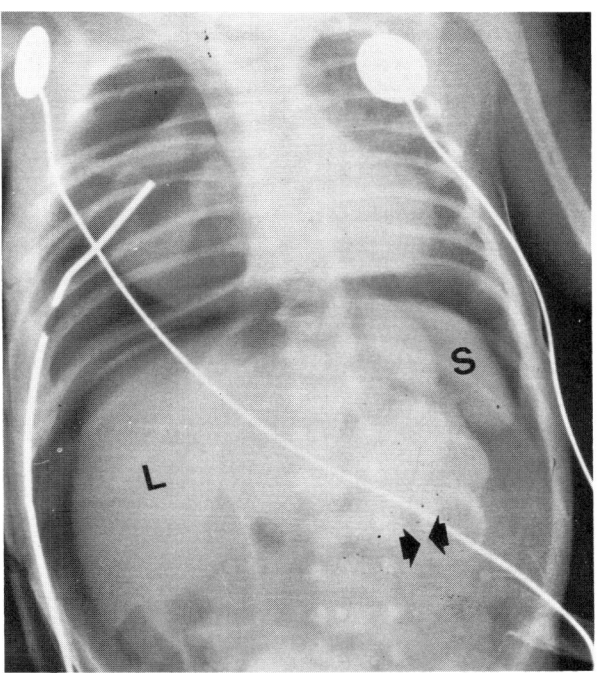

Figure 6–12. Film of the chest and abdomen of a neonate following operation for tracheoesophageal fistula showing pneumothorax and pneumoperitoneum. The occurrence of pneumoperitoneum following anesthesia is well documented, although its mechanism is incompletely understood. The upper surfaces of both liver (L) and spleen (S) are displayed. Both the inner and the outer wall of a loop of bowel are shown, the bowel wall outlined by air inside and outside of it (arrows).

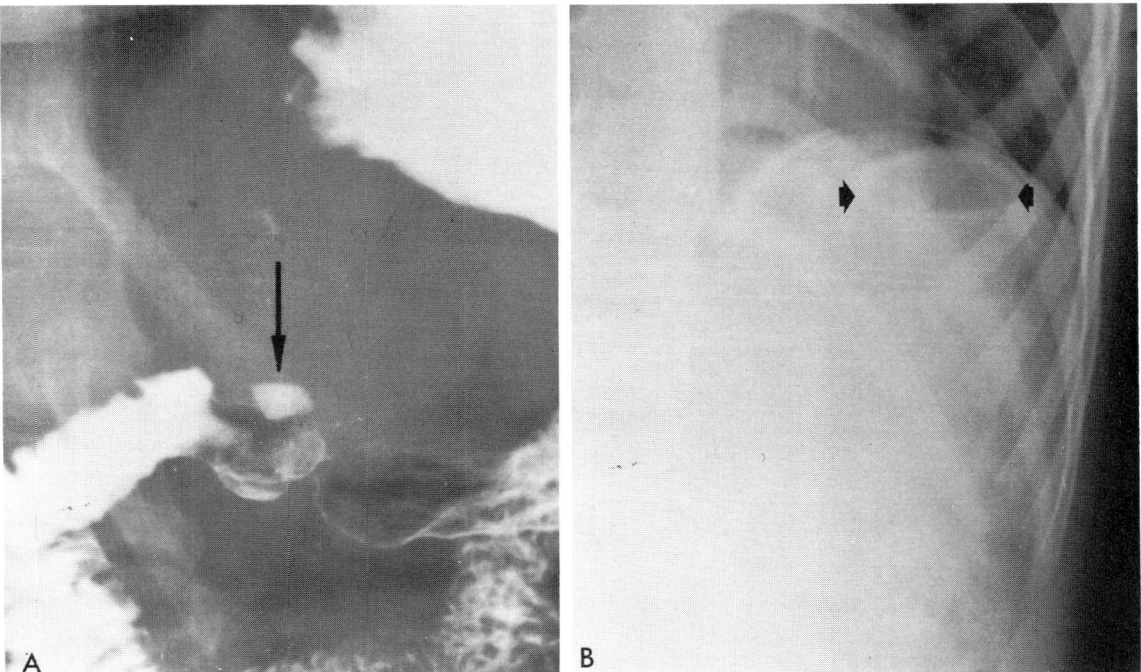

Figure 6–13. Perforated duodenal ulcer (A) with pneumoperitoneum (B). The gastric air bubble (arrows) is shown below the thin rim of free peritoneal air. Perforated peptic ulcer is the most common disease causing pneumoperitoneum.

the most frequent disease process causing pneumoperitoneum. Thirty-three per cent show no evidence of pneumoperitoneum, however, either because of rapid sealing by the omentum or because the perforation occurred into a solid viscus, such as the head of the pancreas. Another cause may be the absence of air in the stomach or duodenum at the time of perforation. The time lapse from occurrence of the perforation may alter the findings. Small amounts of peritoneal air may be absorbed fairly rapidly. It is often possible to demonstrate a suspected perforated peptic ulcer by a contrast examination, using a water-soluble contrast medium. Blunt and penetrating abdominal trauma may cause pneumoperitoneum; in the former case this results from the rupture of a hollow viscus, and in the latter from air entering either through the abdominal wound or from the perforation of a hollow viscus. Differentiation between the latter two may require contrast studies.

DIAGNOSTIC PNEUMOPERITONEUM. Very occasionally, air is introduced into the abdominal cavity for the radiologic investigation of the abdominal viscera, the diaphragm, and the female pelvic organs. This technique has been largely superseded by ultrasound and computer-assisted tomography. However, it is still occasionally useful in the delineation of possible diaphragmatic tumors, bladder wall tumors, and serosal abnormalities, such as serosal metastases. An induced pneumoperitoneum is also used to confirm the diagnosis of ventral hernia, whether congenital or acquired. More detailed information can sometimes be acquired by the instillation of a small amount of water-soluble contrast medium with the gas (usually carbon dioxide or nitrous oxide because they are rapidly absorbed and are less likely to cause air embolism if injected intravenously by accident) to enable a double-contrast examination of the peritoneum.

Pneumoperitoneum may follow the insufflation of the fallopian tubes by carbon dioxide as part of the Rubin test.

POSTOPERATIVE PNEUMOPERITONEUM. Pneumoperitoneum is common after abdominal surgery, occurring in 58 per cent of patients. It is more frequent and more marked in asthenic patients. The absorption of the air requires from 1 to 24 days, and the rate depends only upon the amount of air trapped within the peritoneal cavity. An apparent increase in the amount of postoperative peritoneal air has no significance unless the films are taken in strictly comparable conditions. It must be remembered that air may occasionally enter the peritoneal cavity via abdominal drainage tubes, and almost always after peritoneal dialysis.

ACCIDENTAL PNEUMOPERITONEUM. Gastroscopy, sigmoidoscopy, and colonoscopy may occasionally be followed by the development of pneumoperitoneum. In most cases this is thought to result from the leakage of air through the thinned-out wall of the distended segment of the gut. Frank bowel perforation resulting from instrumentation is rare.

Gas-forming organisms in the peritoneum may occasionally cause a pneumoperitoneum. Most frequently there is a localized bubbly appearance owing to small locules of gas in the abscess, but occasionally sufficient gas is produced to be visible underneath the diaphragm in an erect abdominal film.

POSTANESTHETIC PNEUMOPERITONEUM. Marked gastric dilatation, with the development of a pneumoperitoneum without frank peritonitis (see Fig. 6–12), may occur during anesthesia or resuscitation. Tracheal injury during anesthesia may allow gas to enter from the mediastinum and to dissect downward into the extraperitoneal tissues and then rupture into the peritoneal sac. Although these mechanisms undoubtedly operate in some cases, the pathogenesis of free peritoneal air during anesthesia is poorly understood.

IDIOPATHIC AND ACCIDENTAL PNEUMOPERITONEUMS. Pneumoperitoneum has occurred following vaginal douching and in the postpartum period. Undoubtedly, the female genital tract may occasionally be the route of entry of air into the peritoneum.

OTHER TYPES. Pneumatosis cystoides intestinalis, which may be idiopathic or associated with chronic respiratory disease or inflammatory bowel disease, may occasionally give rise to pneumoperitoneum. Colon interposed between the liver and the diaphragm (Chilaiditi's syndrome) is occasionally mistaken for free peritoneal air. In doubtful cases, a right-side-up decubitus film or barium examination of the colon enables differentiation.

PERITONEOGRAPHY. Delineation of hernial sacs by the injection of small amounts of water-soluble contrast medium into the peritoneal cavity is useful in assessing the hernial orifices. In children, the failure of the processus vaginalis to close may result in an indirect inguinal hernia. These are often bilateral, making the assessment of both inguinal canals helpful when the repair of an inguinal hernia is contemplated.

ABNORMALITIES OF PERITONEUM[4, 11, 14]

Intraperitoneal Fluid

With the patient supine, free peritoneal fluid tends to pool in the more dependent pelvic fossae and paracolic gutters. In the pelvis the fluid may collect in the lower peritoneal fossae above a distended bladder, producing the "dog-ears" densities. Fluid in the paracolic gutters causes the separation of the colon, which can often be identified by its fecal and gas contents, from the lateral abdominal wall and the layer of fat that lies between the parietal peritoneum, and the transverse abdominal muscle (Fig. 6–14).

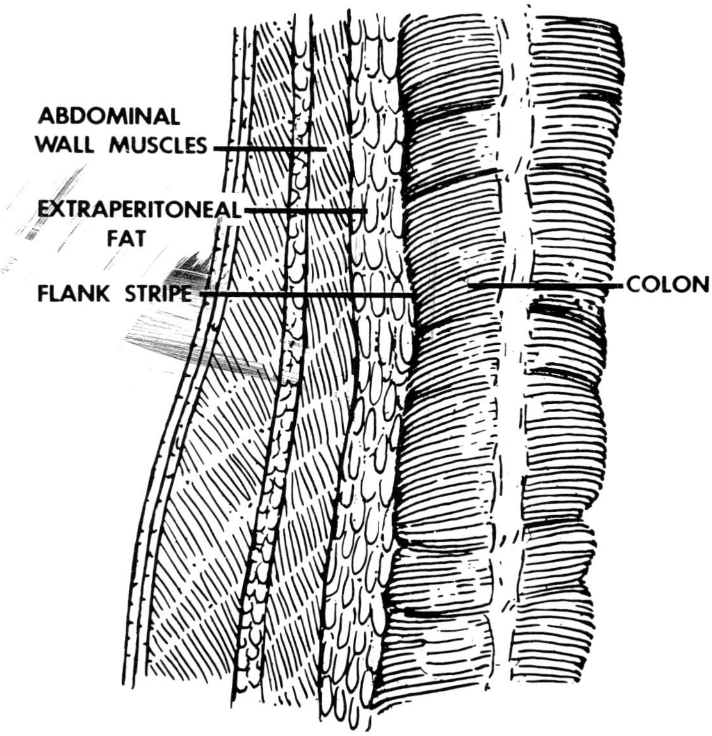

Figure 6–14. Diagrammatic representation of the normal close relationship of the colon to the flank stripe and extraperitoneal fat. (*From* O'Keefe, E. J., Ciaghardi, R. A., and Pfister, R. C.: The roentgenographic evaluation of ascites. Am. J. Roentgenol. *101*:388–396, 1967. Reproduced by permission.)

Normally, the space between the colon and the properitoneal fat line should not exceed 2 mm (Fig. 6–15). An exception to this rule can occur on the left side, where fluid-filled loops of small bowel may become interposed between the colon and the parietal peritoneum.

As the amount of intraperitoneal fluid increases, the width of the density separating the colon and the properitoneal fat increases and the flanks bulge laterally. The loops of bowel containing air tend to float on top of the fluid and move toward the center of the abdominal cavity, which is uppermost when the patient is supine. Sometimes fluid accumulates between the loops, widening the space between them. In the erect position air-fluid levels are often seen within the bowel. Although large amounts of fluid in the peritoneal cavity may produce an overall haziness, peritoneal fluid does not obliterate the psoas or renal outlines, since these depend only upon the presence of surrounding retroperitoneal fat for visualization (Fig. 6–16).

The separation of the liver density from the lateral abdominal wall by the slightly less dense ascitic fluid is a sign likely to be seen only in the case of large effusions. More often, the shadow of the lower liver edge is obliterated, since there is a tendency for fluid to accumulate behind the liver.

Ultrasound (Fig. 6–17) and computerized axial tomography are both capable of detecting smaller amounts of intraperitoneal fluid than can be detected by other radiographic means; as little as 100 ml is demonstrable by these modalities. CT scanning has the additional capability of distinguishing between ascites and hemoperitoneum on the basis of fluid-density differences.

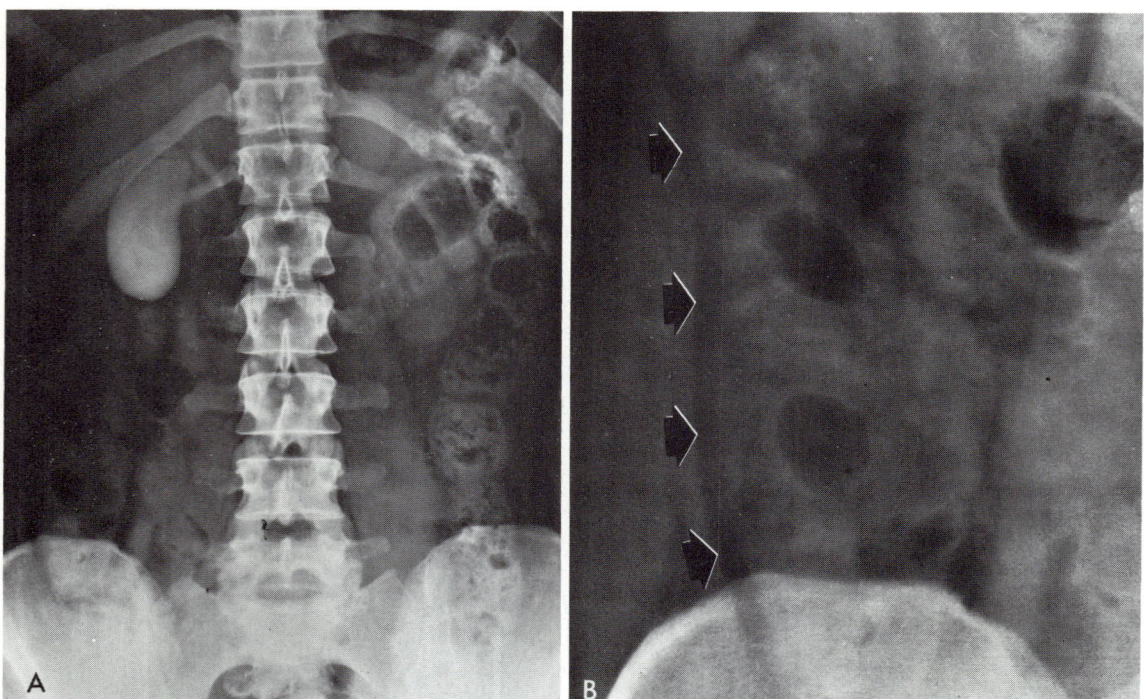

Figure 6–15. *A*, Oral cholecystogram showing the gallbladder and common bile duct outlined by contrast medium. Contrast medium mixed with feces is shown in the ascending colon. *B,* An enlarged picture shows the normal relationship of the ascending colon to the properitoneal fat line (arrows). The distance between the two should not normally exceed 2 mm. Distances greater than this indicate ascitic fluid in the paracolic gutter separating the two.

THE ABDOMINAL WALL AND RELATED STRUCTURES — 263

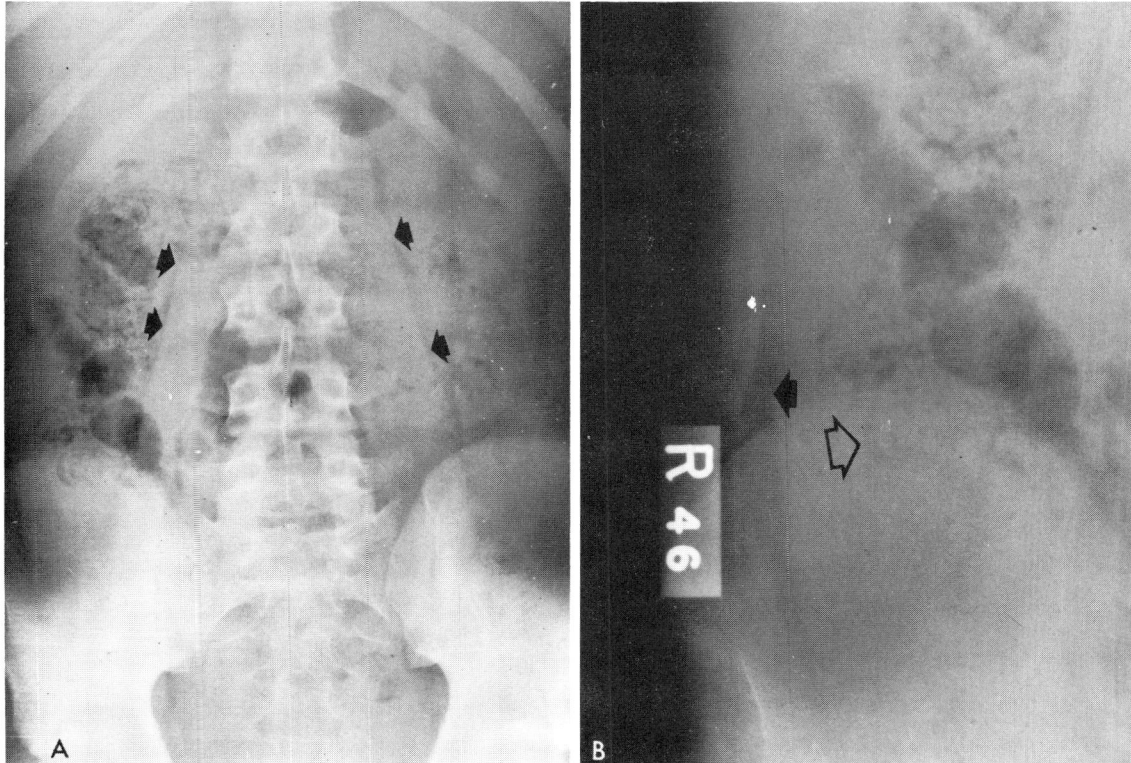

Figure 6–16. Ascites. Separation of the ascending colon (B, open arrow) from the properitoneal fat line (B, closed arrow), indicating the presence of ascites in the paracolic gutter. Note the psoas shadows (A, arrows) are intact. The presence of fluid in the peritoneal cavity has no effect on the contrast between the psoas shadows and their surrounding fat, because they are retroperitoneal structures.

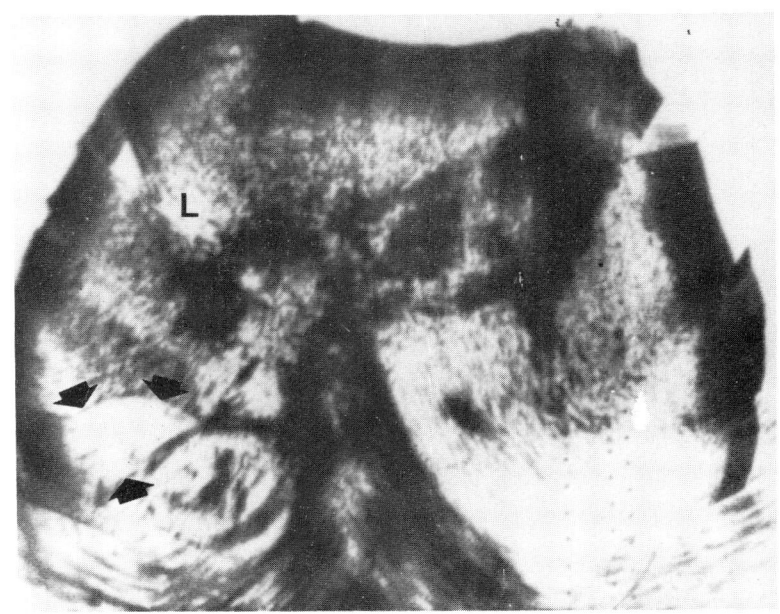

Figure 6–17. Transverse scan of the upper abdomen shows hepatosplenomegaly with ascites (arrows) giving a transonic area behind the liver (L) in a patient with cryptogenic cirrhosis.

Plain abdominal radiography may disclose other abnormalities suggestive of the source of the intraperitoneal fluid.

Peritonitis[6, 8, 13, 15, 18, 22, 23, 25, 29]

Many agents can cause peritoneal inflammation. Acute peritoneal inflammation with exudation of fluid into the peritoneal cavity is usually associated radiographically with ileus. A more chronic case of peritonitis may be unsuspected until it is manifested by signs of adhesion with or without bowel obstruction.

SIMPLE PERITONITIS. The radiologic signs may be minimal. Multiple small fluid levels in localized dilated loops of small bowel may be seen, and small amounts of peritoneal fluid may be detectable. Often, an ileus of small and large bowel is seen.

TUBERCULOUS PERITONITIS. This is now rarely seen in the Western Hemisphere. It is characterized radiologically by scattered loops of distended bowel often with fluid levels. Barium studies (Fig. 6–18) show accelerated or delayed transit time. The bowel wall may be rigid or even narrowed and may show deformities from adhesions. The small bowel is often displaced upward out of the pelvis. Spasm of the cecum (Sterlin's sign) may be present. Often, no radiographic abnormalities are present. In more than 50 per cent of cases the site of primary infection is never found.

MECONIUM PERITONITIS. Meconium may reach the peritoneal cavity through one or more intestinal perforations during pregnancy or shortly after delivery. An intense peritoneal reaction ensues either locally or generally, with the formation of dense adhesions, fibrosis, and calcifications (Fig. 6–19). Adhesions may later cause bowel obstruction. Plain films of the abdomen may show evidence of adhesions, intestinal obstruction, and peritoneal calcification.

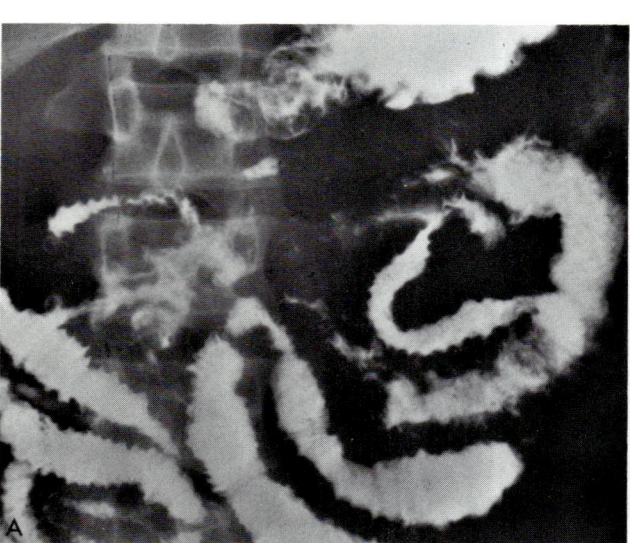
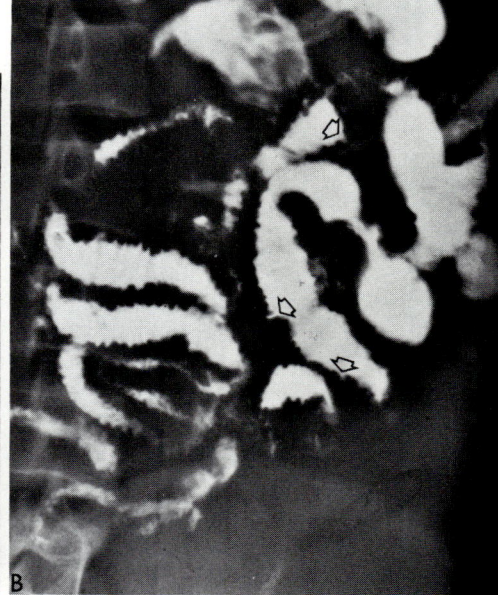

Figure 6–18. *A* and *B*, Tuberculous peritonitis. Separation of bowel loops and marked irregularity of bowel wall, with ulceration (open arrows) and thickening of mucosal folds, are evidence of both enteritis and peritonitis.

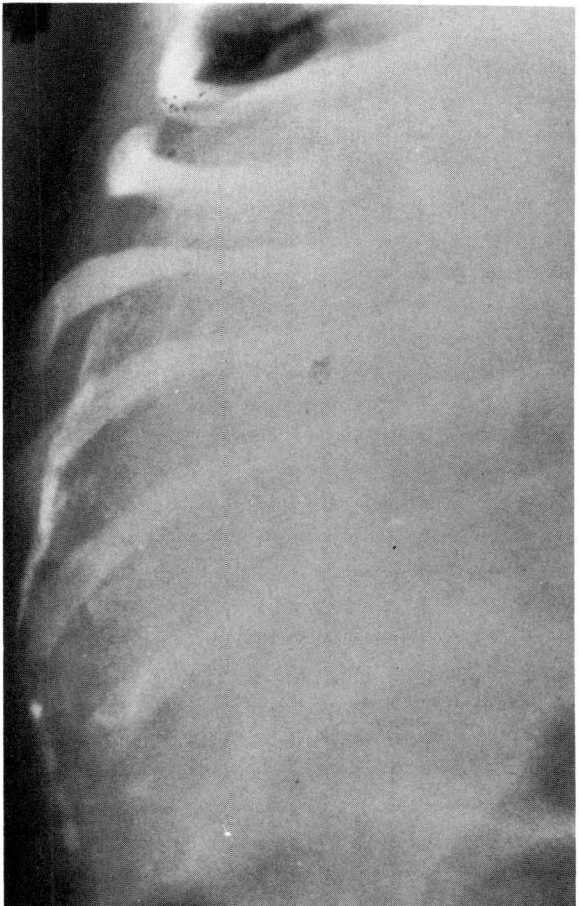

Figure 6–19. Meconium peritonitis. Note the fine irregular calcification of the peritoneum that is characteristic of this condition.

IATROGENIC PERITONITIS. Radiation, surgery, and more recently, the beta-adrenergic blocking drug practolol have all been shown to cause peritonitis. Direct peritoneal exposure to oil, starch, or barium may also cause a peritonitis. The clinical history is usually helpful in elucidating the origin (Figs. 6–20 and 6–21).

In the immediate postoperative period, it may be difficult to differentiate prolonged postoperative ileus from bowel obstruction due to adhesions. If the clinical findings suggest obstruction, a barium enema or a small bowel contrast examination may be helpful in determining the cause.

FIBROUS PERITONITIS. A severe or prolonged insult to the peritoneum results in the deposition of fibrous tissue, with adhesion of the visceral to the parietal peritoneum and of adjacent loops of bowel to one another. A wide variety of etiologic agents may evoke this response, including infection, surgery, a perforated viscus, radiation, intraperitoneal hemorrhage, or a foreign body, such as talc, lipid, barium, or practolol, which is used in the treatment of patients with angina pectoris, hypertension, thyrotoxicosis and cardiac arrhythmias. As the fibrous tissue contracts, it may bind bowel loops together and distort or even obstruct the bowel lumen.

RADIOLOGIC FINDINGS. Signs of complete or incomplete obstruction may be present, with dilated loops of bowel, which may contain air-fluid levels on erect films. The plain abdominal film may show a mass effect owing to the matting together of loops of bowel.

266 — THE ABDOMINAL WALL AND RELATED STRUCTURES

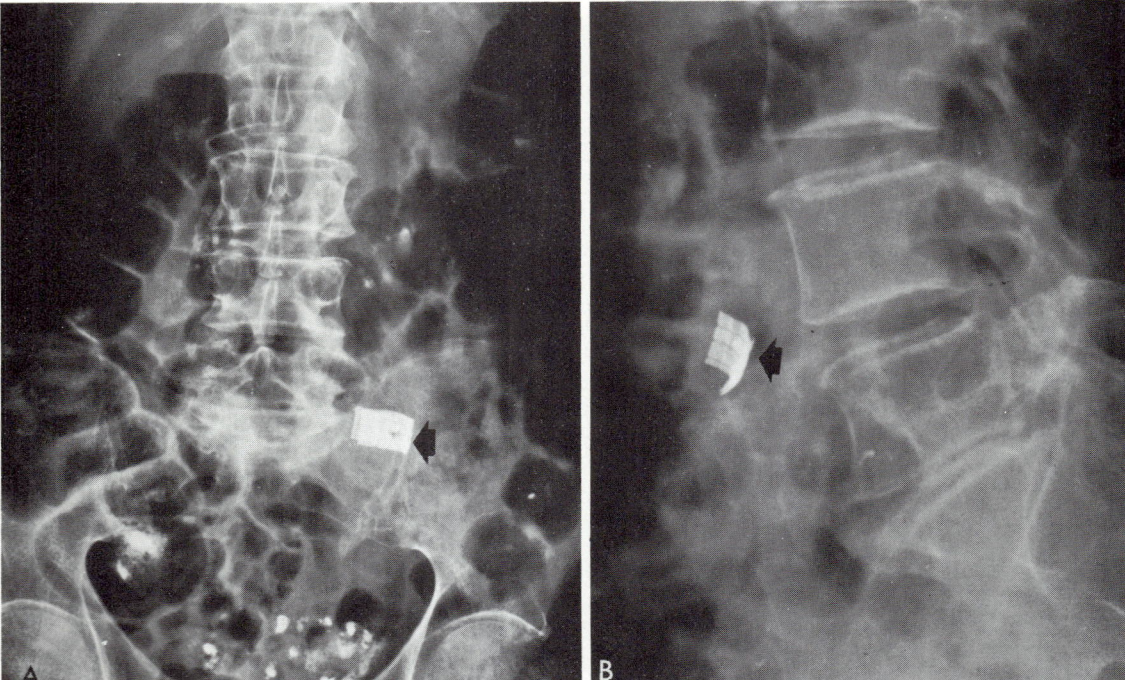

Figure 6–20. *A* and *B*, Persistent fever following a staging laparotomy caused these films to be obtained. The metal marker (arrow) is the surgical sponge within the patient's abdomen. Uneventful recovery followed retrieval of the sponge.

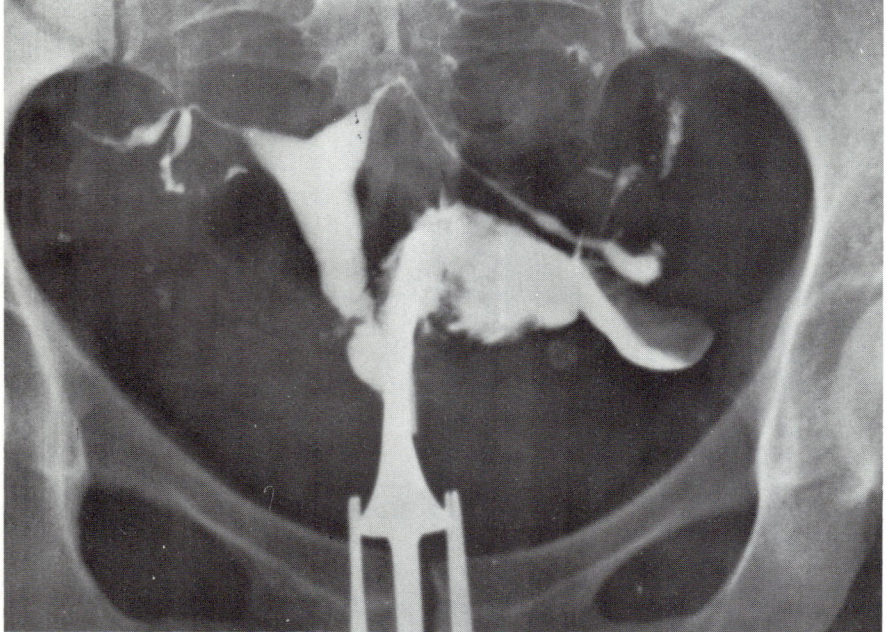

Figure 6–21. Perforation of the uterine cervix by a cannula during hysterosalpingography. Note the spillage of contrast medium into the peritoneal cavity.

Barium examination of the small bowel shows dilatation, and abnormal kinking and angulation of loops of bowel; in other areas the bowel may show areas of stretching or straightening, with loss of the normal serpiginous course of the bowel (Fig. 6–22). The mucosa may appear stretched and even spiculated at its margins. There may be rigidity of the bowel wall and separation of loops of bowel, with abnormal peristalsis and prolonged transit time. Barium examination of the colon may show obstruction resulting from compression by bands of fibrous tissue.

Primary Tumors of Peritoneum, Mesentery, and Omentum

With the exception of lymphoma, primary tumors of these structures are rare, usually presenting as abdominal masses that displace the surrounding bowel. Mesenteric cysts may be developmental (cystic lymphangiomas) or acquired after surgical injury to the lymphatics (lymphocele). They are sharply marginated masses, displacing adjacent viscera, usually the small bowel. Occasionally, wall calcification is seen.

RADIOLOGIC FEATURES. The findings, those of a space-occupying lesion, are nonspecific. The mass, which may appear as a density on plain films and barium examination, shows the displacement of the surrounding bowel (see Fig. 6–32).

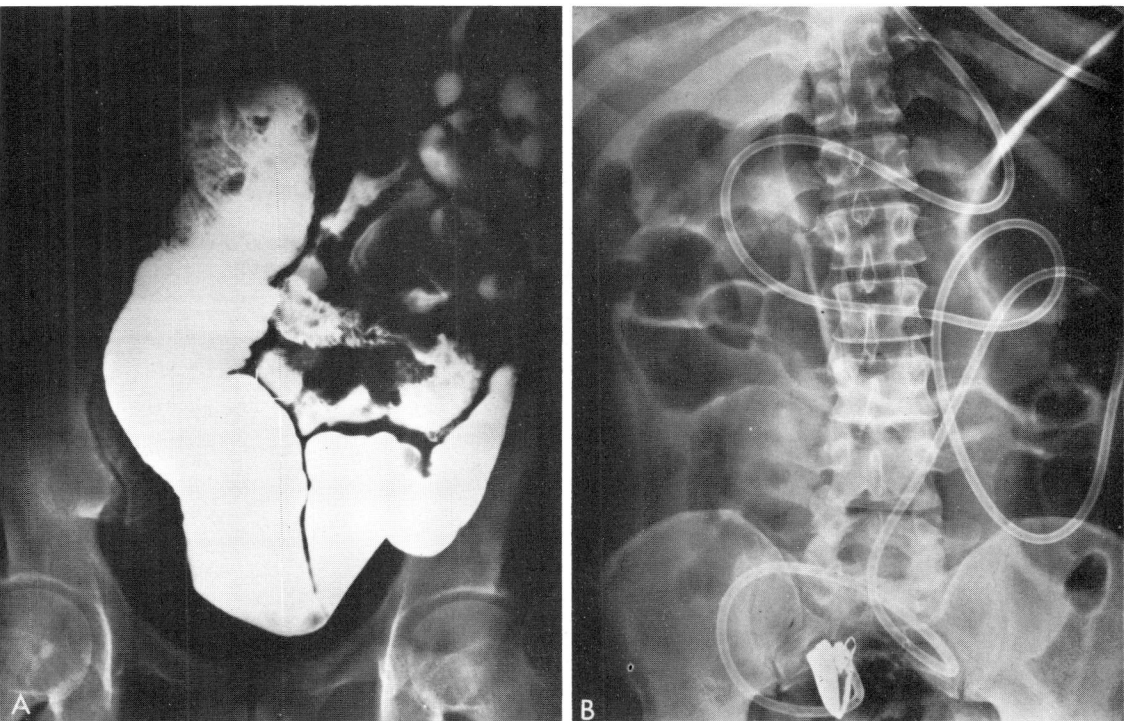

Figure 6–22. *A,* Adhesions causing partial small bowel obstruction with marked dilatation of loops of bowel. There is sharp angulation of the bowel loops, with irregularity of the outline of the bowel replacing the normal smoothly coiled configuration. *B,* A plain film following attempted decompression by Cantor tube shows massive dilation of loops of small bowel in the left upper quadrant. Barium examination of the colon was normal in this case of chronic small bowel dilatation due to adhesions.

Lymphoma, cyst, mesothelioma, and sarcoma may all produce large peritoneal masses, but radiologic differentiation among them is rarely possible. Abdominal ultrasonography (Fig. 6–23), CT scanning, and lymphography may all be helpful in elucidating the nature of an intra-abdominal mass, particularly whether it is solid or cystic.

Secondary Tumors of Peritoneum, Mesentery, and Omentum

These account for the vast majority of tumors. The most common primary tumors causing metastatic peritoneal seeding are from the ovary, pancreas, stomach and colon. The sites of preference are (1) the pouch of Douglas, (2) the right lower quadrant, (3) the left lower quadrant along the superior border of the mesocolon and colon, and (4) the right paracolic gutter.

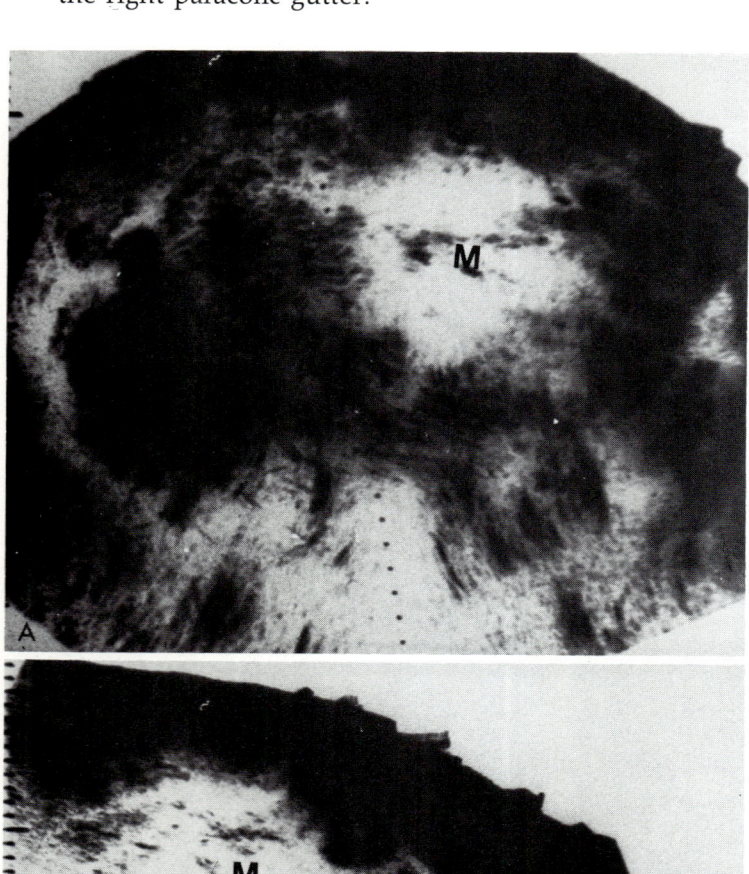

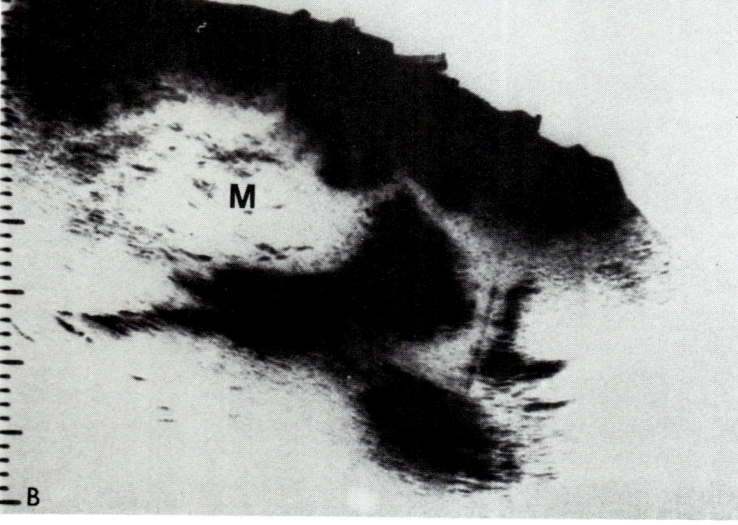

Figure 6–23. *A*, Transverse ultrasound scan of abdomen below the umbilicus showing a lobulated, largely transonic mass with scattered internal echoes (M). *B*, A sagittal scan 3 cm to the left of the midline again demonstrates the mass (M). The mass was the result of intraperitoneal lymphoma. Any intraperitoneal or mesentery tumor might have a similar appearance.

THE ABDOMINAL WALL AND RELATED STRUCTURES — 269

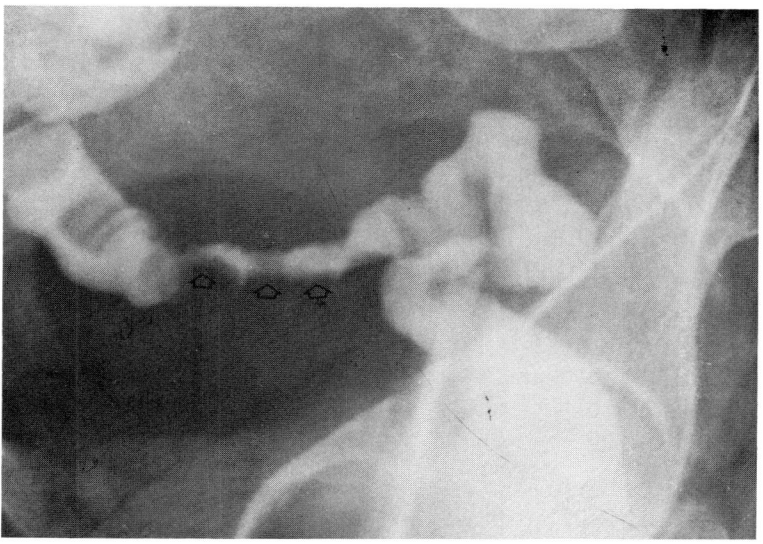

Figure 6–24. Encasement and indentation of the sigmoid colon by serosal metastases from carcinoma of breast. Note the rigid narrowing of the bowel lumen and the nodular impressions on the barium column by the metastases.

RADIOLOGIC FEATURES. The plain film of the abdomen often shows evidence of the associated malignant ascites. Barium examination shows the indentation of the wall of the bowel by the serosal metastases (Fig. 6–24). Metastases in the pouch of Douglas may cause extrinsic impressions shown by barium examination of the colon and may become sufficiently large to simulate rectal cancer. There is often separation of the bowel loops, many of which show an abnormal, angulated appearance (Fig. 6–25).

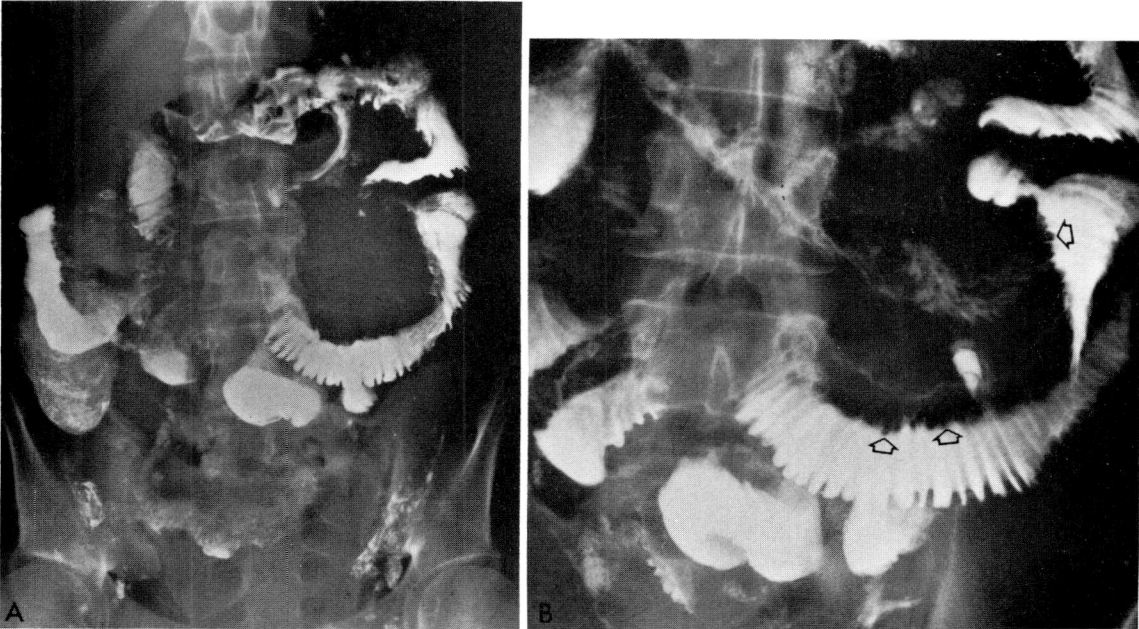

Figure 6–25. *A* and *B*, Extensive serosal and mesenteric metastases in a patient with carcinoma of the uterine cervix. Note the wide separation of bowel loops with gross distortion of the normal serpiginous course of the small bowel. There is marked widening of the loops, some of which show sharp angulations. Nodularity of the bowel wall, consistent with serosal metastases, is shown in some areas. In other areas the mucosa is distorted, spiculated, and bound down by adhesions (arrows).

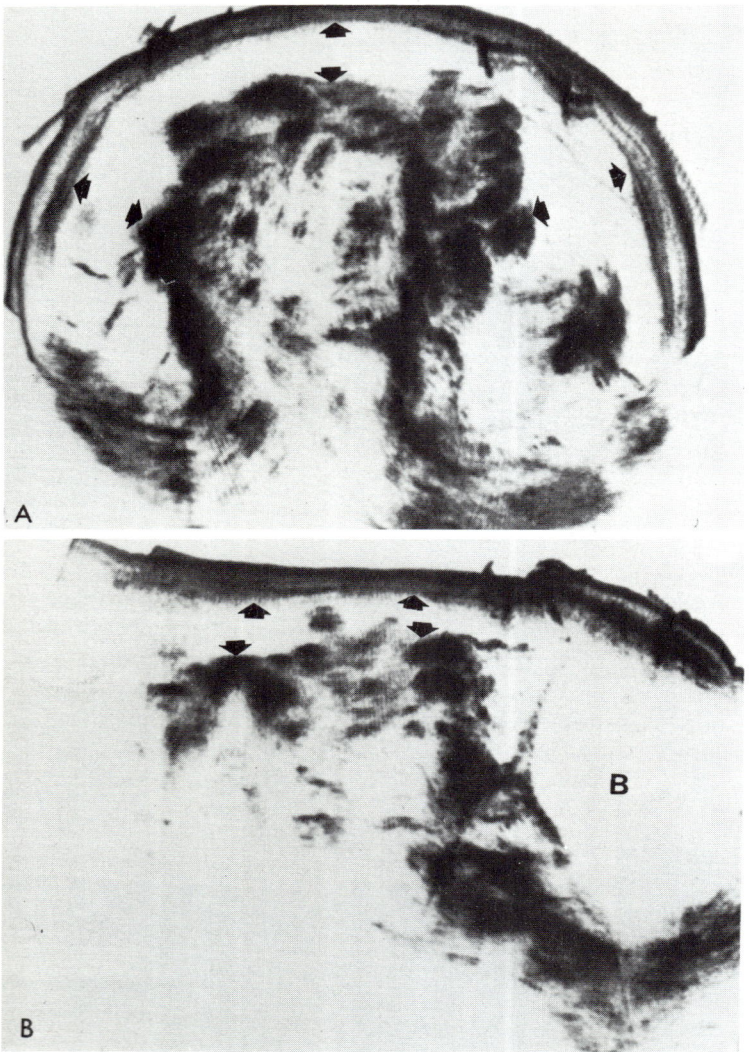

Figure 6–26. Malignant ascites and tumor infiltration of the mesentery. *A,* A transverse ultrasound scan of the abdomen at the level of the umbilicus shows retraction of the bowel away from the abdominal wall as a result of tumor infiltration of the mesentery. There is separation of the bowel from the abdominal wall by a considerable amount of ascitic fluid (arrows). The fact that loops of bowel do not float on the ascitic fluid, thus coming in contact with the abdominal wall in the midline as they do in simple ascites, indicates that the bowel loops are matted together, in this case by extensive infiltration of the mesentery by metastases. *B,* A sagittal scan 2 cm to the right of the midline shows the bowel separated from the abdominal wall by ascites (arrows). The large sonolucent area to the right is the bladder (B).

Serosal metastases may show a characteristic pattern on ultrasonography if there is associated ascites. Instead of floating on top of the ascitic fluid as they do in cases of simple ascites, the bowel loops are bound down in front of the spine and separated from the anterior abdominal wall by a layer of ascitic fluid (Fig. 6–26). Adhesions and mesenteric infiltration are thought to cause the clumping of the bowel in front of the spine.

ABNORMALITIES OF RETROPERITONEUM[2, 5, 16, 20]

Radiology plays a unique role in the diagnosis of abnormalities of the retroperitoneal space and contents, which lie deep within the body and are usually inaccessible to physical examination. Plain radiography, contrast examinations, and the recent techniques of nuclear medicine, ultrasound, and computer-assisted tomography have done much to throw light on the complex diagnostic problems of this area. The radiology of specific retroperitoneal structures and organs, such as the pancreas, kidneys, and aorta, is dealt with elsewhere in these volumes. In this chapter retroperitoneal fibrosis and primary extravisceral tumors are considered.

Retroperitoneal Tumors

By far the most common primary retroperitoneal tumors are in the lymphoma group; liposarcoma and a large heterogeneous group of other tumors have the next highest incidence. Many benign tumors, including fibroma, lipoma and teratodermoid tumors, occur in the retroperitoneal space. Metastases to retroperitoneal nodes, especially from tumors of the genitourinary tract, are fairly common.

RADIOLOGIC FINDINGS. The plain abdominal film may be normal, or it may show a mass, with or without displacement or distortion of surrounding structures (Figs. 6–27 and 6–28). The psoas or renal outlines may be displaced or disrupted (Fig. 6–29). There may be bone destruction of the spine or pelvis. If the mass is sufficiently large, the adjacent bowel may be displaced (Fig. 6–30). Areas of radiolucency may be detectable within a liposarcoma or teratodermoid (see Fig. 6–28), and fragments of tooth or bone or curvilinear calcification may also be seen in the latter. Splenomegaly may occur in lymphomatous disease or if the splenic vein is compromised.

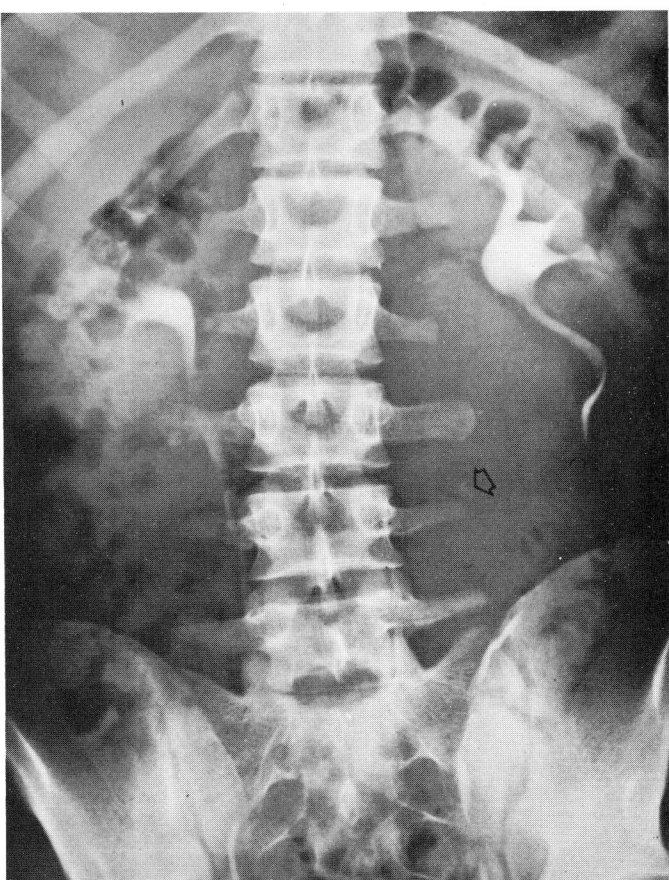

Figure 6–27. Large retroperitoneal teratoma displacing the left kidney upward and laterally. There is absence of the psoas shadow. A tooth fragment (arrow) is shown within the mass, confirming the diagnosis.

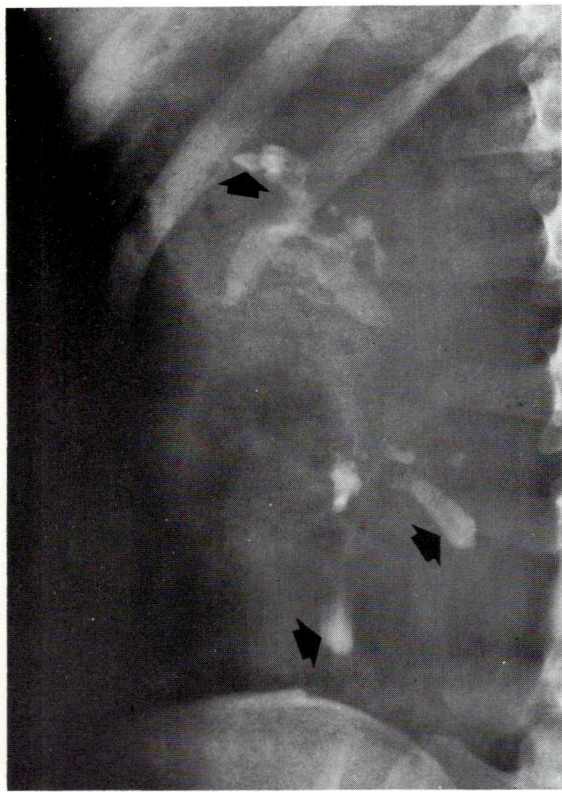

Figure 6–28. Retroperitoneal teratodermoid. Note the well-formed teeth (arrows) and the varying density of the mass reflecting the presence of fat, water-density tissue, and calcification in the heterogenous tissue types within the tumor.

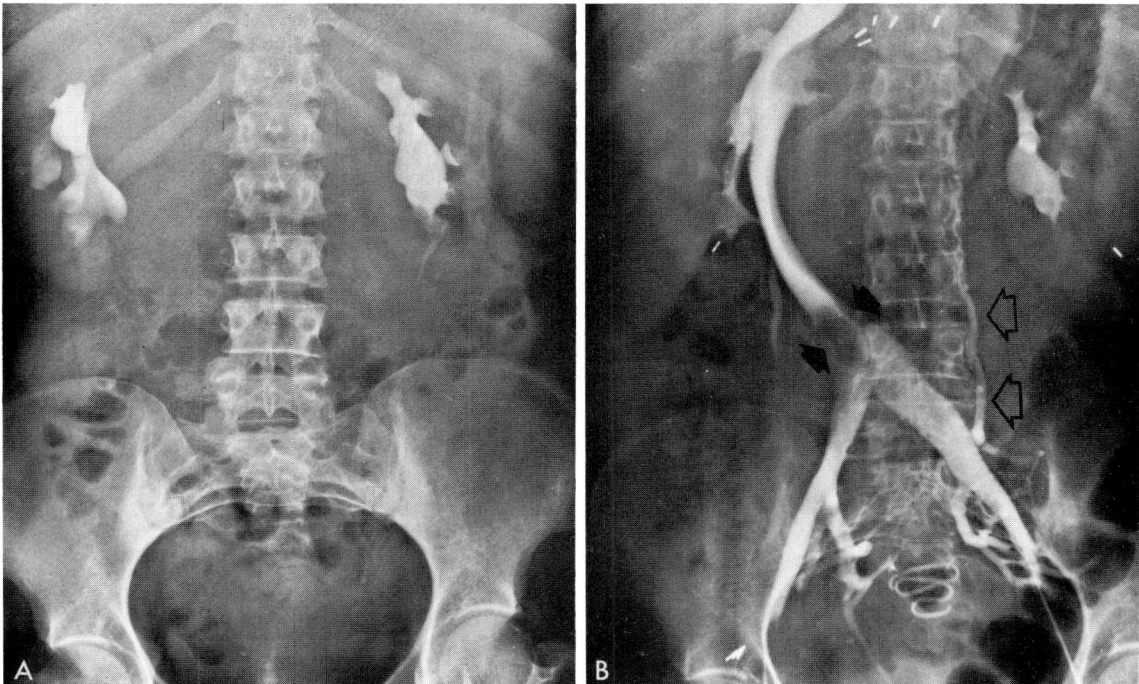

Figure 6–29. *A,* Excretion urography showing lateral displacement of both kidneys, with some rotation of the right kidney by huge masses of nodes in this patient with lymphoma. *B,* Anterior and lateral displacement of the inferior vena cava by large mass of retroperitoneal nodes in lymphoma. Note the partial occlusion of the vena cava near its bifurcation (closed arrows) with filling of the paravertebral collaterals (open arrows).

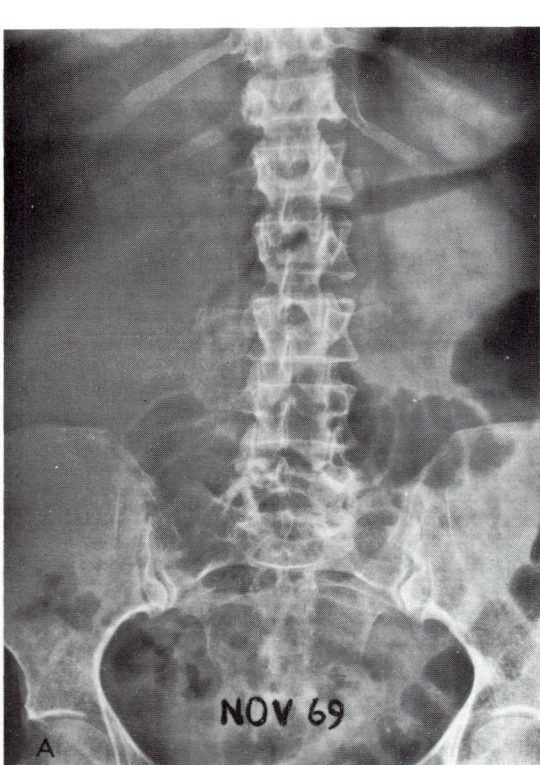
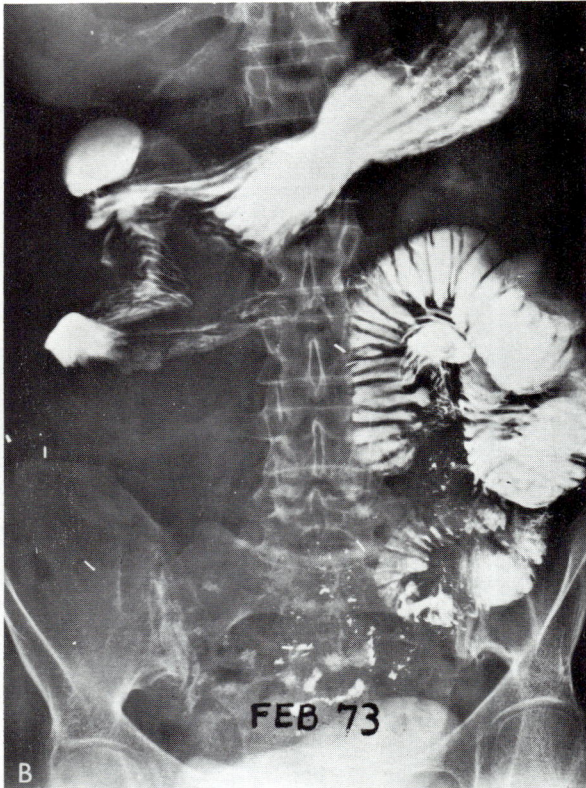
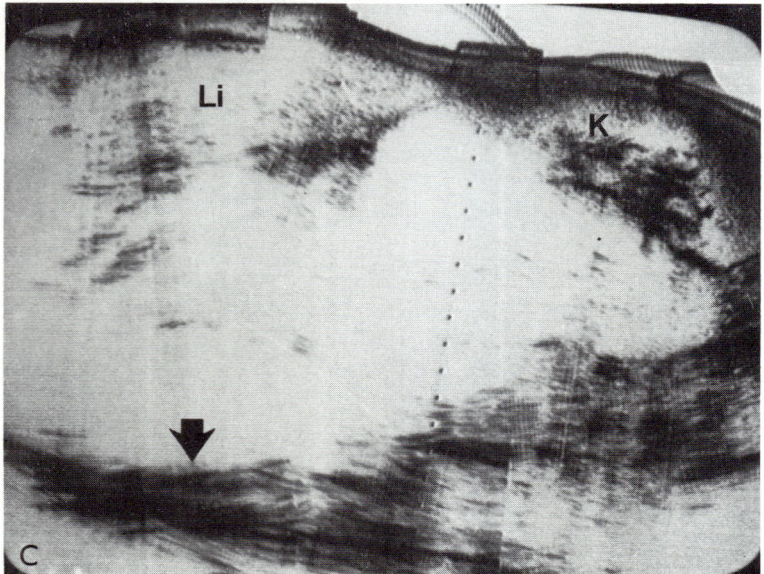

Figure 6–30. *A,* Right retroperitoneal mass with displacement of the bowel downward and to the left from the right upper quadrant. There is loss of all retroperitoneal landmarks, such as the renal outline or the psoas shadow. Some small areas of lucency within the tumor mass suggest contained fat. The tumor was resected. Histologic studies showed it to be a liposarcoma. The patient remained well for three years but returned complaining of abdominal distention. *B,* A barium examination shows regrowth of the tumor with displacement of the bowel by the mass. *C,* Sagittal abdominal ultrasound examination shows a huge retroperitoneal liposarcoma displacing the liver (Li) anteriorly and compressing it against the anterior abdominal wall. The kidney (K) is displaced downward and anteriorly to lie immediately behind the anterior abdominal wall. The position of the diaphragm is indicated by the arrow.

Excretion urography may demonstrate ureteral obstruction or deviation or renal displacement or compression. Excretion urography is also important in the presurgical examination of patients with retroperitoneal tumors to assess renal function in case a kidney must be sacrificed at operation. Serial excretion urography may also be helpful in assessing the effect of therapy.

The wide range of normal positions of the ureter makes excretion urography almost useless in the detection of glandular enlargement in known cases of lymphoma. Venacavography may demonstrate indentation, obstruction, or displacement of the contrast-filled vena cava, indicative of adjacent tumor (see Fig. 6–29B). Lymphography, abdominal ultrasound, and computer-assisted tomography, together with gallium scanning, have largely replaced other methods of detecting retroperitoneal involvement by lymphoma (Fig. 6–31).

Ultrasonography may reveal relatively sonolucent masses of enlarged nodes, or their presence may be inferred from the loss of the normal interfaces between such structures as the inferior vena cava and the aorta. Masses of nodes may also be demonstrated by computed tomography, and their anatomic relationships may be better seen with enhancement by intravascular contrast material (Fig. 6–32).

Gallium-67 citrate scanning detects the presence of disease in 70 per cent of patients with lymphoma. In the abdomen, problems of bowel excretion reduce its sensitivity to about 50 per cent but it is still a most useful adjunct to other diagnostic modalities in staging of lymphoma. Gallium scanning is more sensitive in the detection of nodal than of extranodal involvement and in the detection of histiocytic lymphoma than of other forms of lymphoma. The role of gallium scanning in the diagnosis of other retroperitoneal tumors has not yet been fully established.

LYMPHOGRAPHY.   Since its introduction in 1952 the use of lymphography in the staging of lymphoma and other malignancies has become well established. The cannulation of a lymphatic vessel in each foot, with the injection of an oily contrast medium such as Ultrafluid Lipiodol, allows the demonstration of the lymphatic vessels of the leg, groin, and iliac and para-aortic vessels; abdominal and pelvic films taken 24 hours after infusion outline the anatomy of the lymph nodes in these regions.

Abnormal radiologic findings include evidence of the blockage of lymphatics; failure of a group of nodes to fill; and enlargement of nodes, with disruption of the normal appearance of the internal architecture either by discrete filling defects or by a more diffuse abnormality, such as the "soap-bubble" appearance of Hodgkin's disease (see Fig. 6–31). Glandular masses may be outlined, and simultaneous excretion urography is often helpful in demonstrating the relationship of the ureters to gland masses.

Apart from its relatively high sensitivity in detecting unsuspected abdominal disease in cases of lymphoma, lymphography is helpful in delineating abnormal glands for biopsy; postsurgical films indicate whether the abnormal glands were included in the biopsy specimen. The contrast medium remains in the glands for up to two months following lymphography, and post-treatment films can help assess the response to therapy.

Abdominal ultrasound is often valuable in the assessment of retroperitoneal tumors or effusions (see Fig. 6–30). Delineation of the mass, demonstration of its anatomic relationships, and information regarding its internal characteristics (whether it is solid or cystic) may enable a more accurate diagnosis (Figs. 6–33 and 6–34).

Computer-assisted tomography can demonstrate similar findings and may give additional information regarding the radiodensity of the mass (Figs. 6–35 and 6–36). It is especially valuable in the detection of early bone involvement when such involvement is not demonstrated by skeletal radiography.

Arteriography may help in confirming the presence of a suspected vascular lesion, such as a leaking aortic aneurysm. It may delineate the mass, demonstrate vascular involvement or displacement, and disclose the presence of tumor vessels. Other techniques, such as retroperitoneal air insufflation (Fig. 6–37), have largely been superseded by the newer imaging techniques.

Text continued on page 284.

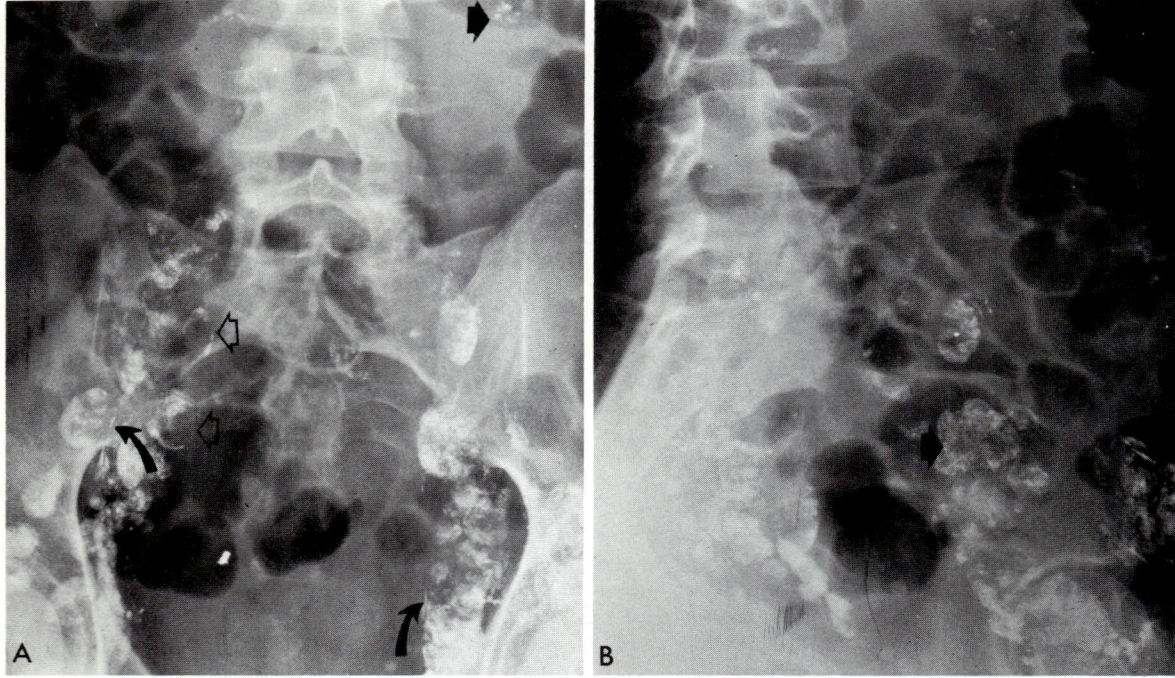

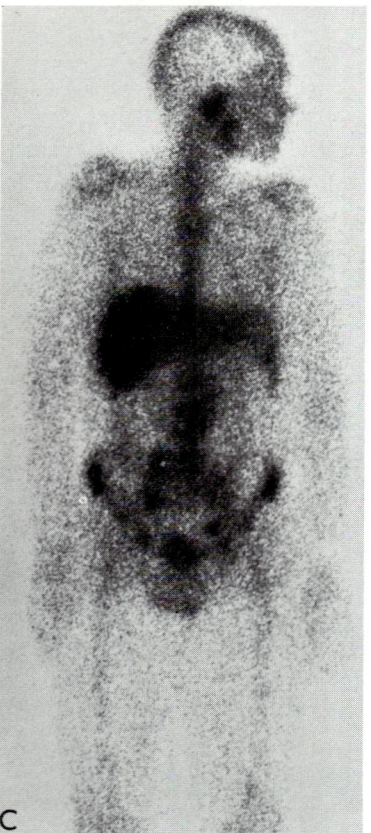

Figure 6–31. *A* and *B,* Lymphography in a patient with lymphoma showing enlargement of nodes, some of which show discrete filling defects (*A,* open arrows) and some which show a "foamy" pattern (*B,* arrow) typical of lymphoma. There is incomplete filling of the para-aortic nodes and some nodes that are visualized are displaced outside the normal lateral limit of para-aortic nodes shown by lymphography—the tips of the transverse processes of the vertebrae (*A,* closed arrow). Stasis is seen within obstructed lymph vessels in the pelvis (*A,* curved arrows). Peripheral filling defects in lymph nodes is always abnormal. Care must be taken in the interpretation of central filling defects and careful correlation made with the filling films to avoid confusion with the normal defect due to afferent and efferent vessels. *C,* A gallium ^{67m}citrate scan in the same patient showing tracer accumulation in the pelvic iliac and para-aortic glands.

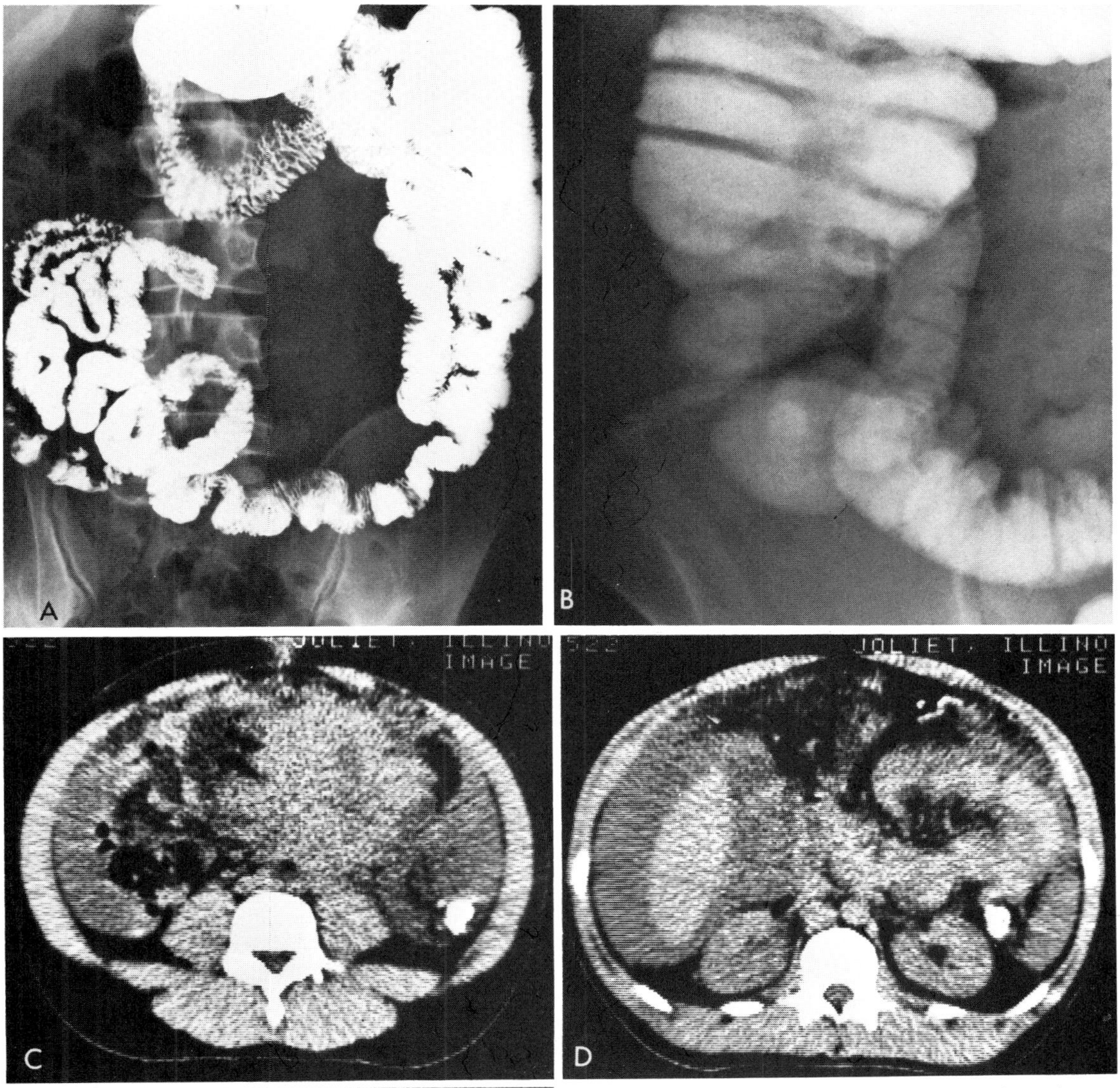

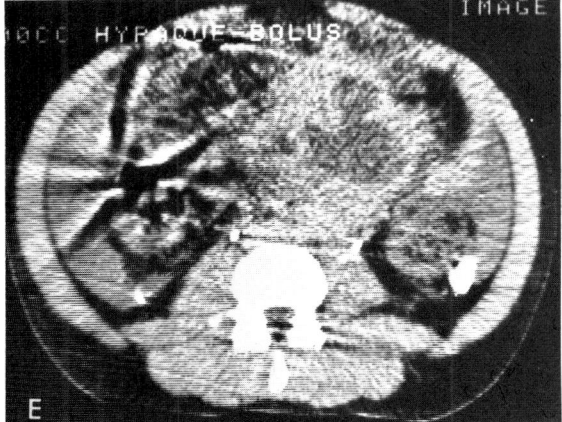

Figure 6–32. *A*, This patient with lymphoma presented with a large abdominal mass. Barium examination of the small bowel shows displacement of the bowel around a large upper abdominal mass. *B*, The presence of ascites is shown by displacement of the ascending colon from the properitoneal fat line. *C*, This CT scan of the abdomen shows a large irregular mass slightly to the left of the midline. Collections of ascitic fluid are shown behind the liver, and the spleen, and the posterior abdominal wall. *D*, A section higher in the abdomen shows the mass to be separate from the kidneys and lying in an intraperitoneal situation. The relative radiolucency of the center of the mass suggests that its center is necrotic. *E*, This impression is confirmed by enhancement of the tumor periphery following contrast infusion while the center remains radiolucent.

278 — THE ABDOMINAL WALL AND RELATED STRUCTURES

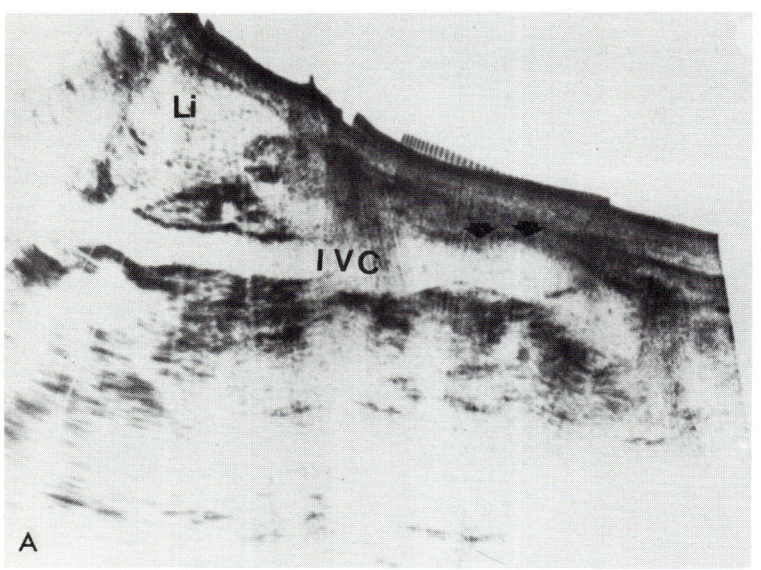

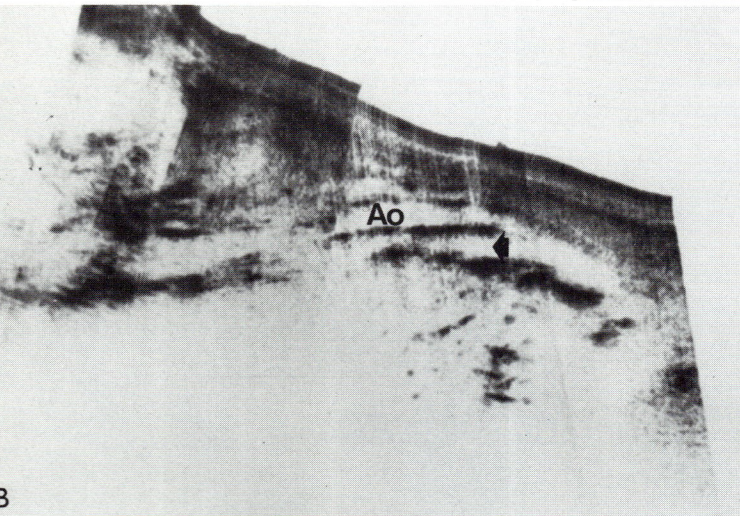

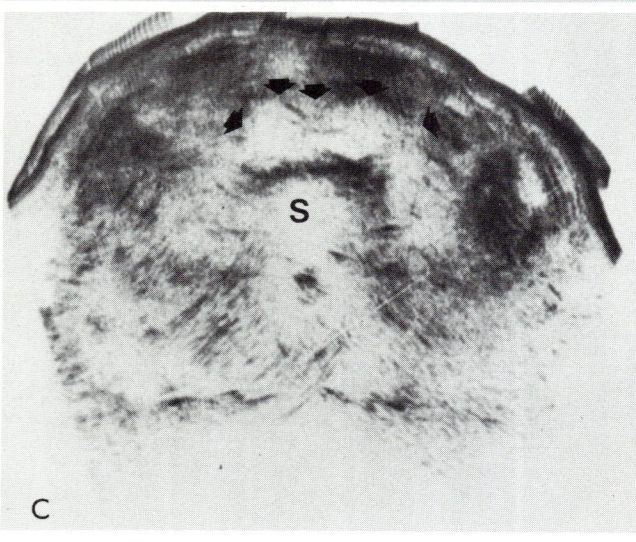

Figure 6–33. *A*, A sagittal scan of the abdomen in a patient with lymphoma shows lymph node masses anterior to the inferior vena cava. *B*, A similar scan to the left of the midline shows the aorta displaced anteriorly from the spine by retroaortic lymph node masses (arrow). *C*, A transverse scan shows a large mass of nodes straddling the spine (arrows). It is not possible to identify the aorta or vena cava within the mass. This is a common appearance in lymphoma. Li = liver; IVC = inferior vena cava; Ao = aorta; S = spine.

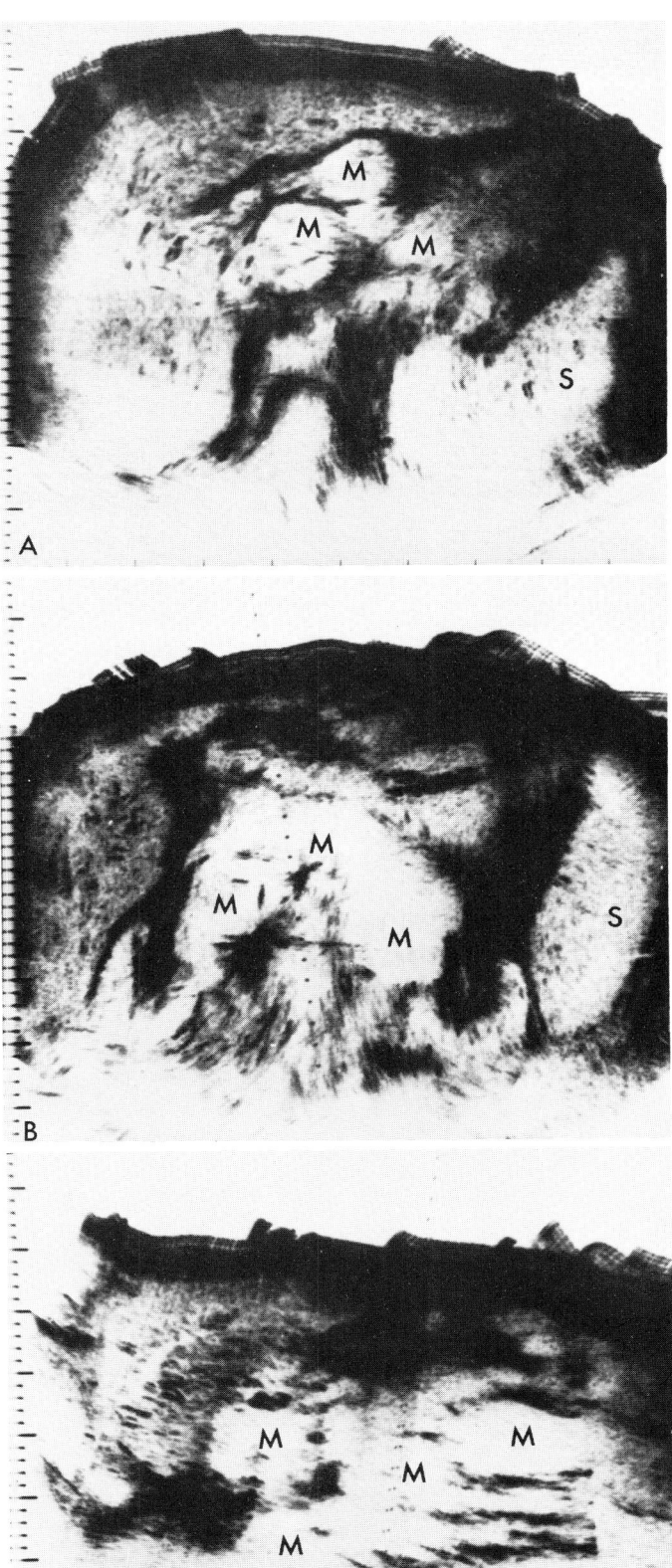

Figure 6–34. Extensive abdominal lymphoma. *A,* Extensive lobular masses (M) with irregular contained echoes and good sound transmission properties. There is considerable splenomegaly (S). It is not possible to identify the major vessels with any certainty, as their outlines have been obscured by adjacent gland masses. These appearances are typical of lymphoma. *B,* A mantle of enlarged glands (M) is draped over the great vessels. They have almost certainly been displaced anteriorly by enlarged glands between them and the spine. Splenomegaly is again demonstrated. *C,* A longitudinal scan redemonstrates large masses. Some are in the mesentery, but it is not possible to state accurately which are definitely retroperitoneal and which are intraperitoneal. The inferior vena cava is seen over only a short segment and is displaced anteriorly by retrocaval nodes.

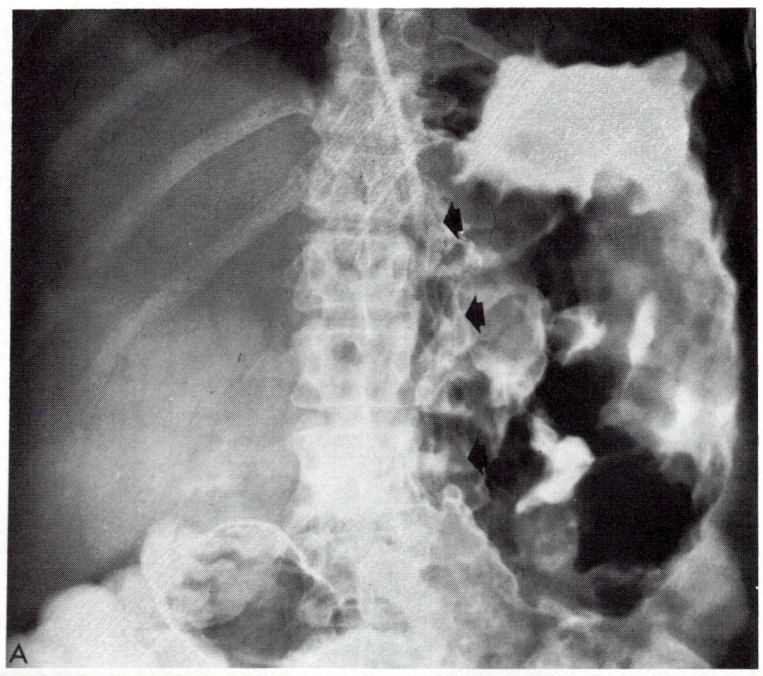
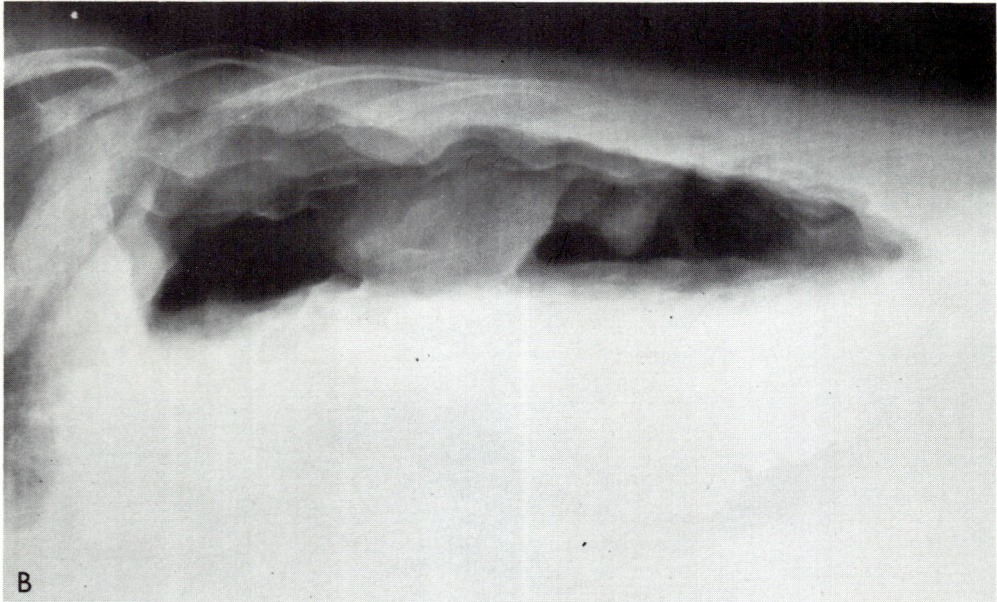

Figure 6–35. *A*, A huge retroperitoneal leiomyosarcoma has cavitated and communicated with the stomach. The stomach is displaced medially and downward (arrows), and a nasogastric tube has been passed through the communication into the tumor cavity. *B*, Note the markedly irregular walls of the cavity shown on the right lateral decubitus film. Large nubbins of tumor hang from the wall of the cavity.

Illustration and legend continued on opposite page.

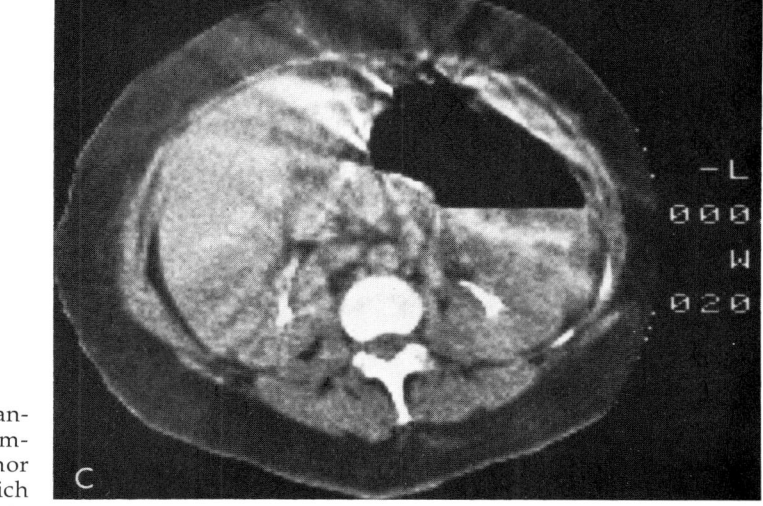

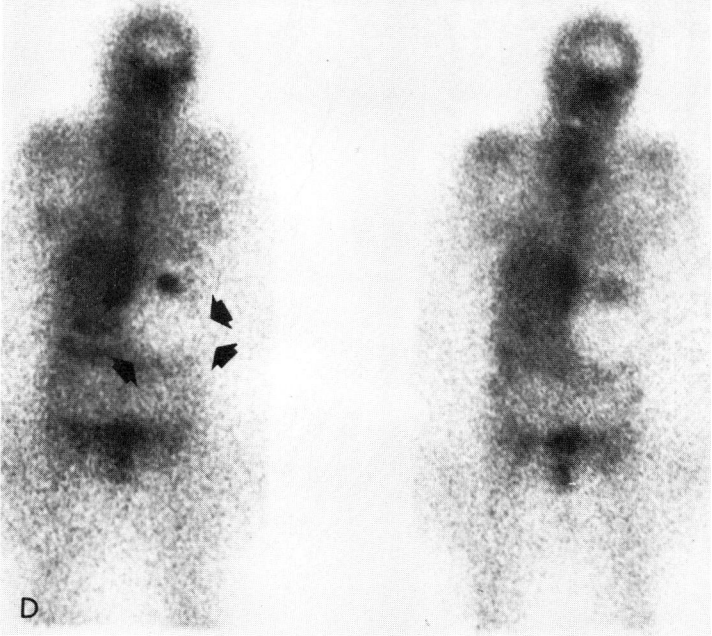

Figure 6–35 *Continued. C,* The anterior extent of the tumor is well demonstrated on this CT scan. The tumor extends back to the left kidney, which appears intact. *D,* A gallium ^{67m}citrate scan shows a round area of decreased activity below the left lobe of the liver with a peripheral rim of increased activity (arrows). Gallium scans frequently show this rim effect in tumors that are centrally necrotic.

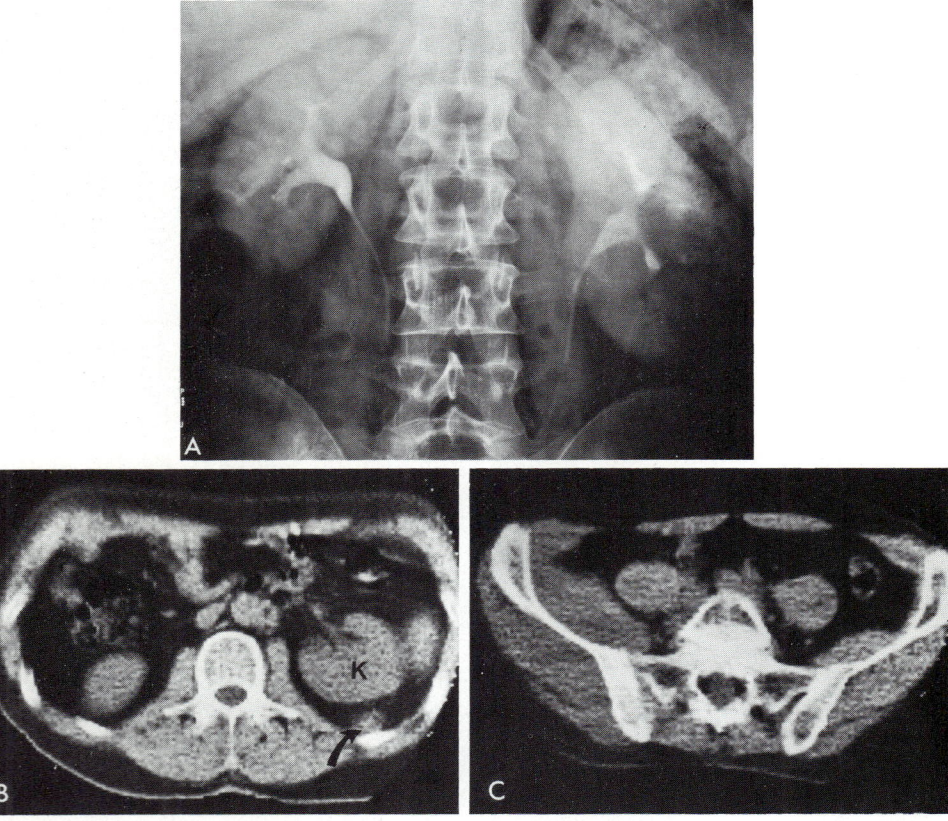

Figure 6–36. *A,* Excretion urography in this patient complaining of right buttock pain revealed distortion of the lower pole of the left kidney, with splaying of the calyces in the middle and lower parts of the kidney. This was thought to be due to an intrarenal tumor, possibly a metastasis. *B,* CT scanning, however, revealed a retrorenal mass (arrow) displacing the kidney (K) anteriorly. *C,* CT scan in the pelvis reveals increased soft tissue anterior and posterior to the wing of the right ilium but no evidence of bone destruction. Biopsy revealed a fibrous histiocytoma.

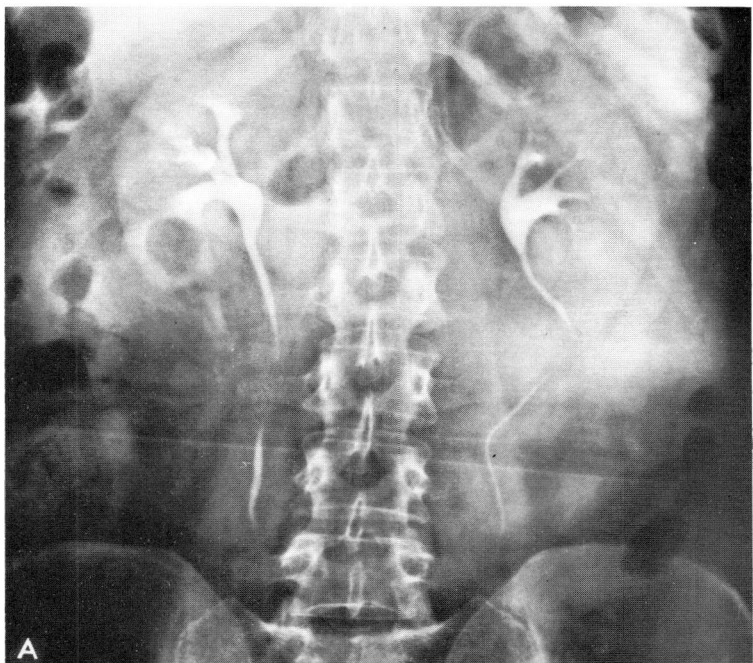
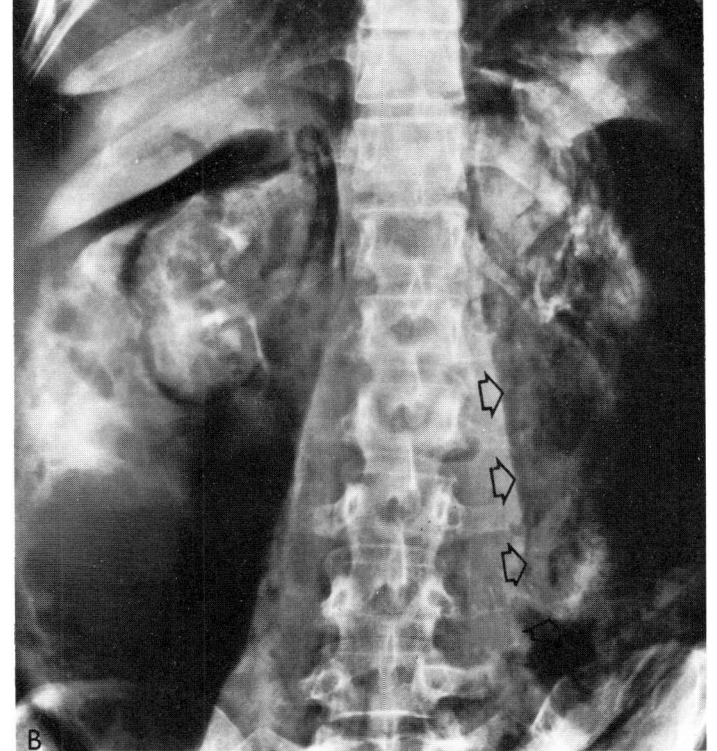

Figure 6–37. *A*, Lateral displacement of the lower pole of the left kidney and upper left ureter by retroperitoneal reticulum cell sarcoma. Note loss of outline of the lower pole of the left kidney. *B*, Retroperitoneal air insufflation delineates a long tumor mass extending from the lower pole of the left kidney to near the posterior iliac crest (arrows). This technique has been superseded by ultrasound, CT, gallium scintigraphy, and angiography.

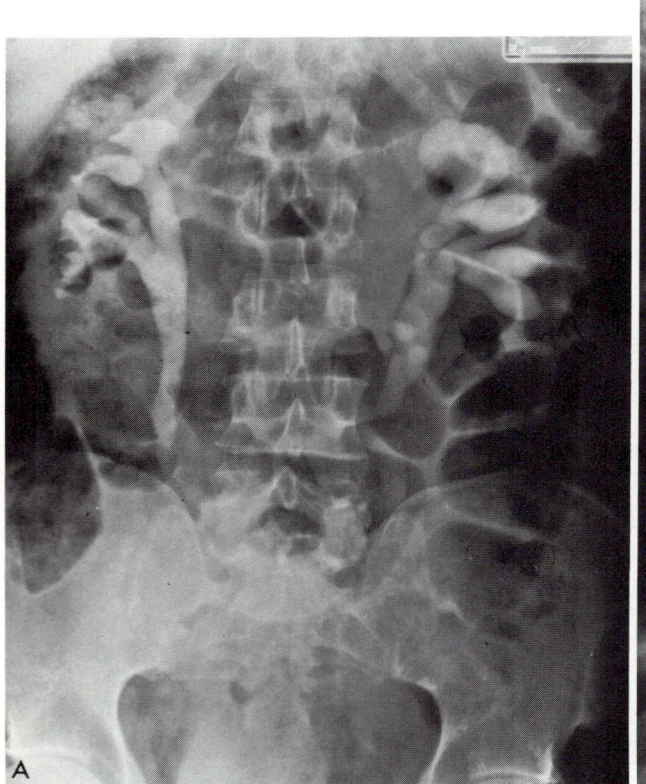
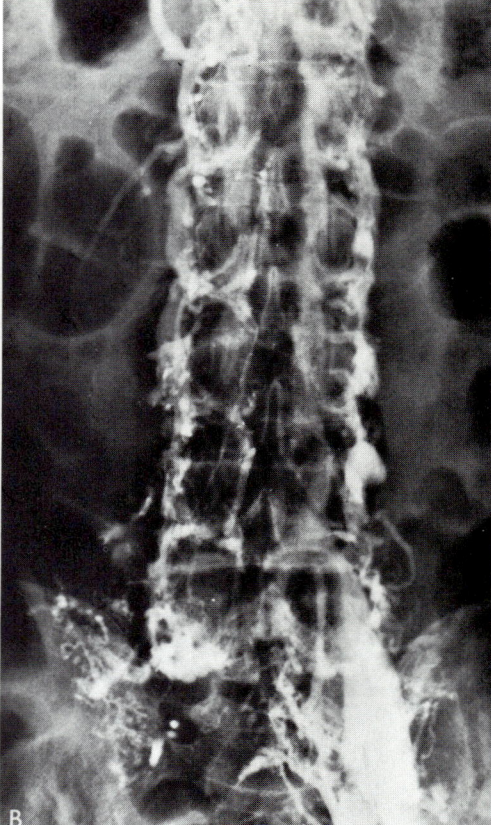
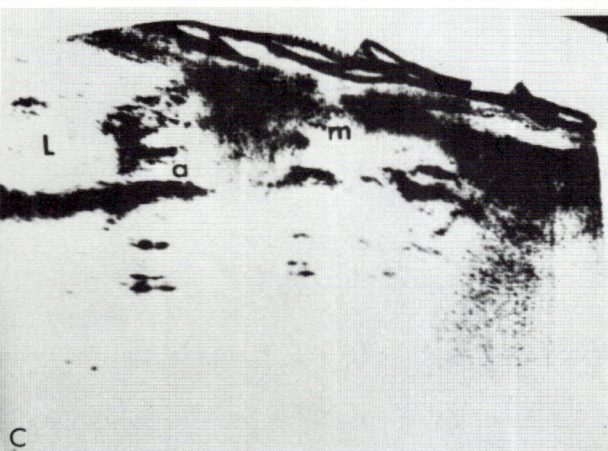

Figure 6–38. *A,* Excretion urography in retroperitoneal fibrosis showing partial obstruction of ureters at the level of the pelvic brim with proximal hydronephrosis. *B,* Ascending venography in the same patient showing obstruction of the inferior vena cava at its bifurcation with extensive collateral filling of the paravertebral veins. *C,* Midline sagittal sonogram showing the mass of fibrous tissue (m) anterior to the aorta. The anterior wall of the aorta (a) is not identified as it passes through the mass. L = liver. (*C* from Bowie, J. D., and Bernstein, J. R.: Retroperitoneal fibrosis: ultrasound findings and case report. J. Clin. Ultrasound 4:435–437, 1976. Reproduced by permission.)

Retroperitoneal Fibrosis[3, 26, 27]

This is a disease characterized by the development of a plaque of fibrous tissue in the retroperitoneum. Etiologic factors include methysergide (an ergot derivative) therapy, prostatovesiculitis, retroperitoneal hemorrhage, and intense desmoplastic response to retroperitoneal malignancy. The idiopathic form, however, is the most common.

In the majority of cases the fibrosis starts at about the level of L_5 and may extend for a variable distance upward toward the kidneys or more rarely, downward into the pelvis. In most cases, both ureters are encased in the fibrous tissue and as it contracts they are usually drawn toward the midline and their lumen is narrowed. Any of the retroperitoneal vascular structures may be similarly involved and compromised, including the inferior vena cava, iliac veins, lymphatics, and aorta. Cases involving the gallbladder and bowel have also been described. Ureteric involvement is most often bilateral but one ureter is frequently more severely affected than the other.

Retroperitoneal fibrosis may be associated with mediastinal fibrosis.

RADIOLOGIC FEATURES. The abdominal film is usually normal, but the loss of the psoas and renal outlines may be observed. Excretion urography shows delayed excretion, with hydronephrosis and hydroureter above the obstruction. If the complete obstruction of a ureter occurs, nonfunction of the corresponding kidney may result. The level of obstruction is most commonly at the pelvic brim but may be at any level. There is medial deviation of the ureter at the level of obstruction, and the ureter is frequently irregular and tapered above the obstruction (Fig. 6–38).

Venography may show involvement of the iliac veins or vena cava, with obstruction and collateral flow. Lymphography may demonstrate delay in the passage of contrast material through the para-aortic nodes and vessels, with dilatation of the lymph vessels and blockage of flow. The occurrence of filling defects in the para-aortic nodes has been described. Ultrasonography may demonstrate the plaque of fibrous tissue.

References

1. Adler, S., Parthasorothy, K. L., Bakshi, S. P., et al.: Gallium[67] citrate scanning for the localization and staging of lymphomas. J. Nucl. Med. *16*:255–259, 1975.
2. Bowie, J. D., and Bernstein, J. R.: Retroperitoneal fibrosis: ultrasound findings and case report. J. Clin. Ultrasound *4*:435–437, 1976.
3. Budin, E., and Jacobson, G.: Roentgenographic diagnosis of small amounts of intraperitoneal fluid. Am. J. Roentgenol. *99*:62–70, 1967.
4. Caffey, J.: Pediatric X-ray Diagnosis. Chicago, Year Book Medical Publishers, 1973.
5. Castellino, R. A., Fuks, Z., Bland, N., et al.: Roentgenologic aspects of Hodgkin's disease: Repeat lymphangiography. Radiology *109*:53–58, 1973.
6. Cohen, W. N., and Safare-Sharazi, S.: Starch granulomatous peritonitis. Am. J. Roentgenol. *117*:334–339, 1973.
7. Cremin, B. J.: The urinary tract anomalies associated with agenesis of the abdominal walls. Br. J. Radiol. *44*:767–772, 1971.
8. Dayalan, N., and Ramakrishnan, M. S.: Meconium peritonitis: postneonatal intestinal distention. J. Pediatr. Surg. *9*:243–244, 1974.
9. Felson, B., and Wiot, J. F.: Another look at pneumoperitoneum. Semin. Roentgenol. *4*:437–443, 1973.
10. Franken, E. A.: Anomalies of the anterior abdominal wall: classification and roentgenology. Am. J. Roentgenol. *112*:58–67, 1971.
11. Goldberg, B. B., Goodman, G. A., and Clearfield, H. R.: Evaluation of ascites by ultrasound. Radiology *96*:15–22, 1970.
12. Herzan, F. A.: Roentgenologic diagnosis of rectus sheath hematoma. Am. J. Roentgenol. *101*:397–405, 1967.
13. Huckman, M. S., and Fisher, M. S.: Roentgenographic signs of tumors of the greater omentum. Cancer *33*:1526–1530, 1974.
14. Keeffe, E. J., Gagliardi, R. A., and Pfister, R. C.: The roentgenographic evaluation of ascites. Am. J. Roentgenol. *101*:388–396, 1967.
15. Lee, R. E. J., Baddeley, H., Marshall, A. J., et al.: Practolol peritonitis. Clin. Radiol. *28*:119–128, 1977.
16. Lawman, R. M., Grnja, V., Peck, D. R., et al.: The angiographic patterns of the primary retroperitoneal tumors. Radiology *104*:259–268, 1972.
17. Macbeth, R. A., and MacKenzie, W. C.: The abdominal wall, umbilicus, peritoneum, mesenteries, and retroperitoneum. *In* Sabiston, D. C., Jr. (ed.): Davis-Christopher Textbook of Surgery. Ed. 10. Philadelphia, W. B. Saunders Co., 1974, p. 773.

18. Meyers, M. A.: Distribution of intra-abdominal malignant seeding: dependency on dynamics of flow of ascitic fluid. Am. J. Roentgenol. *119*:198–206, 1973.
19. Meyers, M. A.: Peritoneography, normal and pathologic anatomy. Am. J. Roentgenol. *117*:353–365, 1973.
20. Meyers, M. A., Whalen, J. P., Reele, K., et al.: Radiologic features of extraperitoneal effusions. Radiology *104*:249–257, 1972.
21. Miller, R. E., and Nelson, S. W.: The roentgenologic demonstration of tiny amounts of free intraperitoneal gas: experimental and clinical studies. Am. J. Roentgenol. *112*:574–585, 1971.
22. Pear, B. L., and Boyden, F. M.: Intraperitoneal lipid granuloma. Radiology *89*:47–51, 1967.
23. Sacks, B., Jaffe, M., and Harris, N.: Isolated mesenteric desmoids (mesenteric fibromatosis). Clin. Radiol. *29*:95–100, 1978.
24. Shackelford, G. D., and McAlister, W. H.: Pneumoperitoneography in the evaluation of congenital anomalies in the umbilical region. Radiology *104*:361–363, 1972.
25. Stassa, G.: Tuberculous peritonitis. Am. J. Roentgenol. *101*:409–413, 1967.
26. Webb, A. J., and Dawson-Edwards, P.: Malignant retroperitoneal fibrosis. Br. J. Surg. *54*:506–508, 1967.
27. Webb, A. J., and Dawson-Edwards, P.: Non-malignant retroperitoneal fibrosis. Br. J. Surg. *54*:508–518, 1967.
28. Weiner, C. I., Diaconis, J. N., and Dennis, J. M.: The "Inverted V": a new sign of pneumoperitoneum. Radiology *107*:47–48, 1973.
29. Yannopoulos, K., and Stout, A. P.: Primary solid tumors of the mesentery. Cancer *16*:914–927, 1963.

7

HERNIAS

GARY G. GHAHREMANI, M.D.
MORTON A. MEYERS, M.D.

An external abdominal hernia is best defined as an opening in the encompassing wall of the abdominal cavity through which the viscera may protrude beyond their normal area of confinement. In contrast, the term "internal abdominal hernia" designates an aperture in the mesentery or peritoneum permitting protrusion and encapsulation of a viscus in another compartment within the otherwise intact abdominal cavity.[17] In both instances the causative hernial orifice or ring may be a pre-existing anatomic structure, such as the esophageal hiatus of the diaphragm or the foramen of Winslow. The hernia ring may also represent a pathologic defect of congenital or acquired origin.

Abdominal hernias are quite common, considering the fact that they occur in approximately 1.5 per cent of the population and account for nearly half a million operations per year in the United States.[37] The great majority of these hernias involve the groin and anterior abdominal wall so that their diagnosis can be made easily by inspection and palpation. In such cases, roentgen examinations are used mainly for preoperative delineation of the hernial content and evaluation of suspected complications, such as mechanical bowel obstruction. The more important contribution of radiologic studies as a primary diagnostic measure is in the evaluation of diaphragmatic and internal hernias.[6, 12, 14, 17, 52]

Most abdominal hernias include a peritoneal sac that passes through the hernial orifice and receives the eventrated viscera. The greater omentum and various segments of the small or large intestine usually compose the contents of the external hernial sac, whereas other abdominal organs are only occasionally involved.

It is important to note that the nomenclature of specific hernias is determined by the location of the hernial ring and not by the eventual position of the protruding viscera.[17, 54] The following classification is therefore based upon anatomic regions where the relatively common types of hernias with distinctive clinical and radiographic findings occur:

1. External abdominal hernias

    a. Diaphragmatic hernias
        (1) Esophageal hiatus
        (2) Foramen of Bochdalek
        (3) Foramen of Morgagni
        (4) Acquired diaphragmatic defects

     b. Hernias of the groin and pelvic regions
        (1) Inguinal (indirect, direct, sliding, combined)
        (2) Femoral
        (3) Obturator
        (4) Sciatic
     c. Abdominal wall hernias
        (1) Umbilical
        (2) Ventral (epigastric, spigelian, lumbar, incisional)
  2. Internal abdominal hernias
     a. Paraduodenal
     b. Foramen of Winslow
     c. Pericecal
     d. Intersigmoid
     e. Transmesenteric
     f. Retroanastomotic

EXTERNAL ABDOMINAL HERNIAS

Diaphragmatic Hernias

HERNIA THROUGH THE ESOPHAGEAL HIATUS. The most common site for diaphragmatic hernia in adults is the esophageal hiatus.[14] The sliding type occurs about ten times more frequently than paraesophageal herniation. In infants, 25 per cent of diaphragmatic hernias involve the esophageal hiatus and may be associated with a congenitally short esophagus.[42]

The clinical and radiologic features of hiatus hernias are described in detail elsewhere (see Chapter 8, Part III). Briefly, the correct diagnosis requires a careful evaluation of the esophagogastric junction by barium contrast study. Herniation of a large portion of the stomach may also be recognizable on plain chest radiographs as a retrocardiac mass, usually containing an air-fluid level. The herniated stomach can undergo volvulus within the mediastinum (Fig. 7–1). Long-standing herniations of the fundus or the entire stomach frequently result in incarceration, but strangulation is very rare.[4, 16]

HERNIA THROUGH THE FORAMEN OF BOCHDALEK. This entity represents the most common type of diaphragmatic hernia in the pediatric age group.[6, 8, 14, 18, 42] It results from a congenital anomaly of the posterolateral portion of the diaphragm.

Most Bochdalek hernias (80 to 90 per cent) occur on the left side, mainly because a similar defect in the right hemidiaphragm is protected by the liver.[42] The defect may be only a few centimeters in diameter or large enough to occupy most of a hemidiaphragm. Therefore, the time of onset and the severity of clinical symptoms depend upon the extent of herniated viscera into the pleural space and the resultant pulmonary collapse and mediastinal shift.[6, 14]

Small, asymptomatic Bochdalek hernias, which are often incidental findings on chest radiographs, present as localized bulges on the posterolateral aspect of the diaphragm.[14] These usually contain retroperitoneal fat, portions of the greater omentum or transverse colon, and, rarely, the upper pole of a kidney (Fig. 7–2).

At times, an initially small Bochdalek hernia remains clinically silent until adulthood, when gradual enlargement of the diaphragmatic defect results in progressive herniation of the abdominal viscera (Fig. 7–3). Without surgical intervention there may be the added danger of incarceration and strangulation of the intrathoracically displaced intestinal loops.[8, 14, 25]

HERNIAS — 289

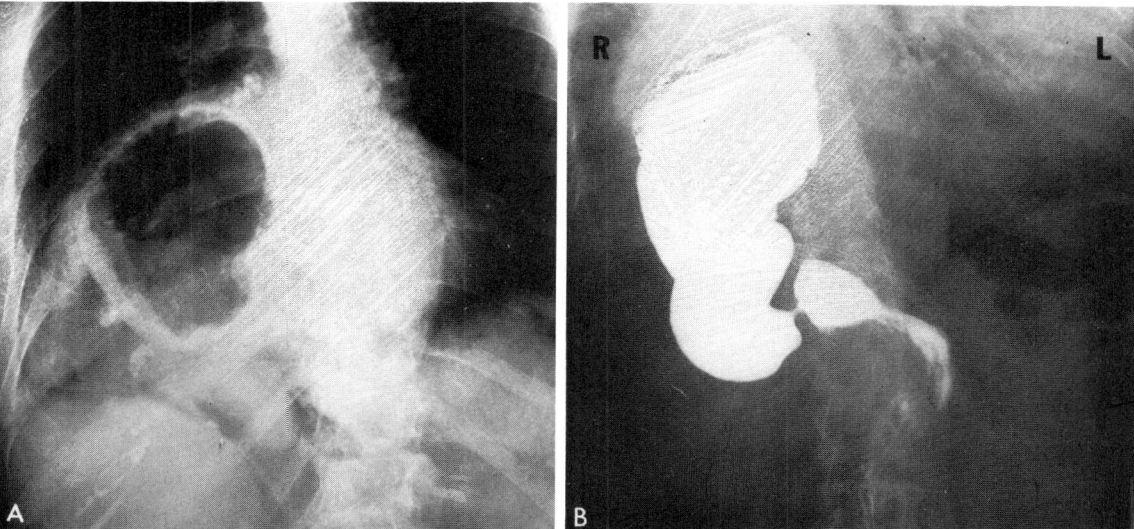

Figure 7–1. Large hiatus hernia with torsion of the intrathoracic stomach and duodenal bulb. *A,* Chest radiograph shows the gas-filled stomach within the posterior mediastinum and the right hemithorax. *B,* Barium-contrast examination reveals 180 degree anterior organoaxial torsion of the stomach and duodenal bulb. Note the location of the greater curvature on the right side and the reversed direction of the duodenal bulb. There is slight narrowing of the postbulbar duodenum at the hiatus.

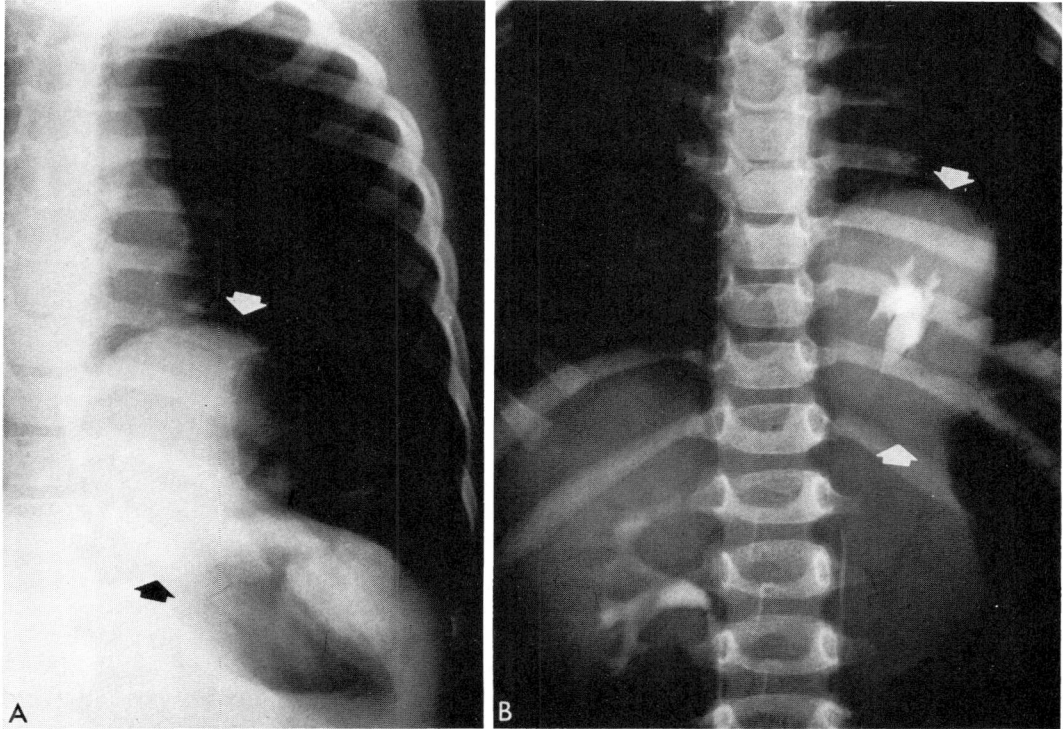

Figure 7–2. Bochdalek hernia in a child. *A,* Chest radiograph demonstrates a retrocardiac mass projecting above the left hemidiaphragm. *B,* Excretory urogram documents intrathoracic herniation of the left kidney (arrows) through the foramen of Bochdalek.

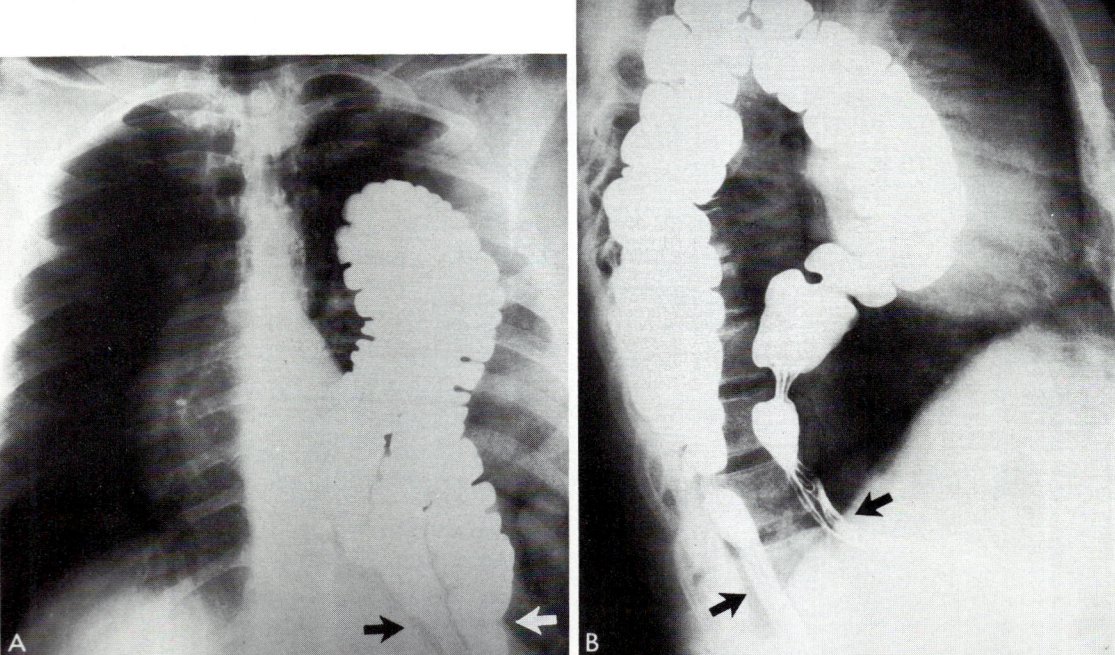

Figure 7–3. Large Bochdalek hernia in an adult. A and B, Chest radiographs obtained during a barium enema examination illustrate herniation of the colon into the left pleural space. The posterior location of the foramen of Bochdalek (arrows) is best seen on the lateral view.

Large Bochdalek hernias usually cause acute respiratory distress soon after birth, when the herniated intestine fills with gas and food. There is usually no confining hernial sac, so that a free communication exists between the abdomen and the thorax. Therefore, the stomach or the entire abdominal contents may occupy the pleural cavity, thereby interfering with maturation of the lung.[6, 14] The clinical findings include progressive dyspnea, cyanosis, absent respiratory sounds on the affected side, and a scaphoid abdomen. Chest radiographs demonstrate gas-filled intestinal loops in the pleural space, collapse of the ipsilateral lung, and mediastinal shift to the opposite side. These findings are often associated with partial or complete absence of intestinal gas pattern within the abdomen.[8, 42]

Barium contrast studies of the gastrointestinal tract are seldom necessary for the diagnosis of Bochdalek hernias, and the size of the diaphragmatic defect cannot be accurately predicted from such studies. However, barium examination may be useful for differentiation of Bochdalek hernias from cystic disease of the lungs and pneumatocele, as well as for preoperative evaluation of the thoracic stomach with respect to the length of the esophagus. In one study, twenty-three per cent of children with congenital diaphragmatic hernias had associated cardiovascular abnormalities, such as congenital heart disease, cardiac malposition, and abnormal pulmonary circulation.[13]

HERNIA THROUGH THE FORAMEN OF MORGAGNI. The foramina of Morgagni represent embryologic defects in the fusion of the sternal and costal portions of the diaphragm and are located just posterior to the sternum on either side of the midline. The foramen on the left side is protected by the heart, so that the majority of Morgagni hernias occur on the right. They account for nearly 10 per cent of congenital diaphragmatic hernias.[42]

In contrast to Bochdalek hernias, in a Morgagni hernia a true membranous sac confines the protruding viscera. The usual content is the greater omentum, but liver and intestinal loops may also be involved.[8, 14, 42] In most cases the hernia remains asymptomatic, but obstruction and strangulation of the intestinal loops have been reported as a complication in 10 to 15 per cent of these patients.[14] Furthermore, an associated defect may be present in the diaphragmatic portion of the pericardium. This permits displacement of the abdominal contents into the pericardial sac, producing severe cardiorespiratory symptoms that necessitate prompt corrective surgery.[46]

The diagnosis of a Morgagni hernia is usually first made on a routine chest radiograph.[14, 27] The typical appearance is that of a well-defined soft tissue mass or gas-containing loop in the right cardiophrenic angle (Fig. 7–4). An upper gastrointestinal series, a barium enema, and a radionuclide scan of the liver may be used to confirm the diagnosis and identify the hernial contents. In rare cases of herniations extending into the pericardial sac, the gas-containing bowel may be seen anterior to the cardiac shadow.[14, 43] Such patients may also have associated congenital cardiovascular anomalies, so that preoperative evaluation by cardiac angiography may be required.[18]

HERNIA THROUGH ACQUIRED DIAPHRAGMATIC DEFECTS. Approximately 5 per cent of all diaphragmatic hernias develop through tears of the diaphragm caused by blunt abdominal trauma (for example, in a car accident or fall) or by direct penetrating

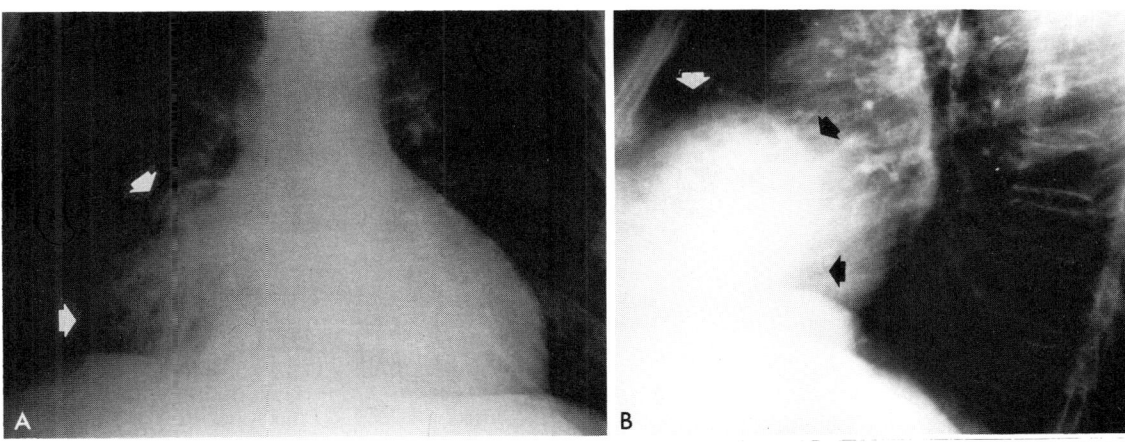

Figure 7–4. Morgagni hernia. A and B, Radiographs of the chest demonstrate a gas-containing soft tissue mass (arrows) in the right cardiophrenic angle. C, Barium enema study shows the transverse colon protruding through the foramen of Morgagni.

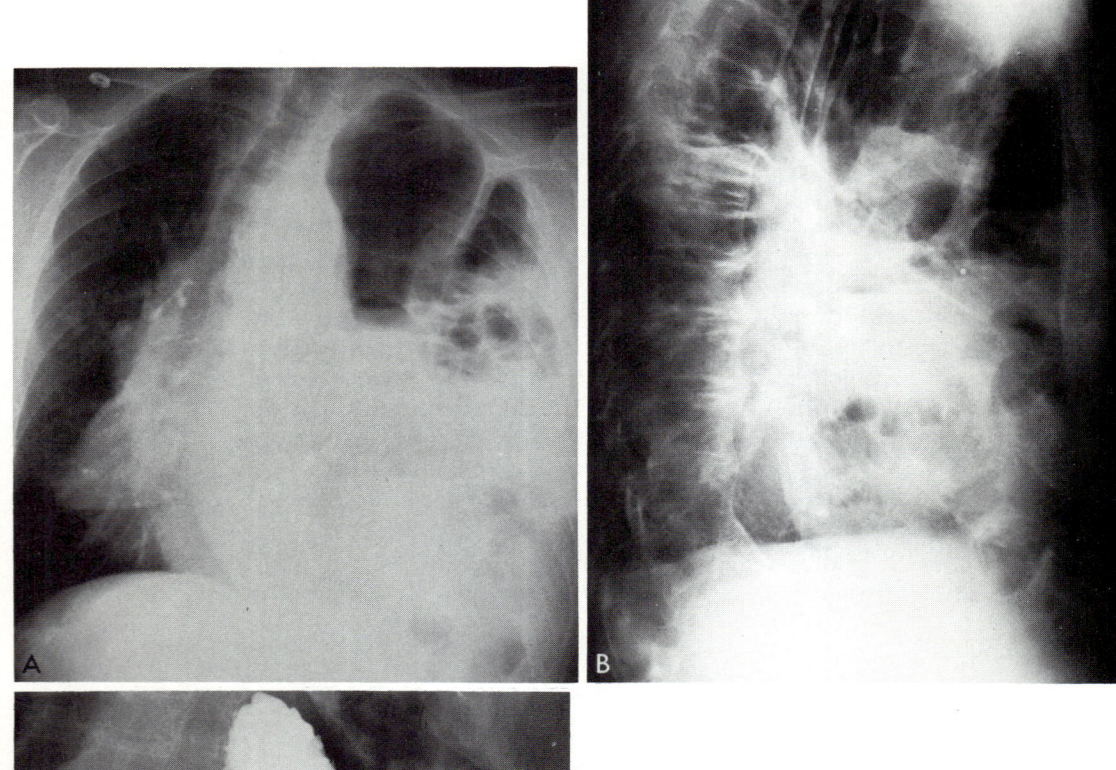
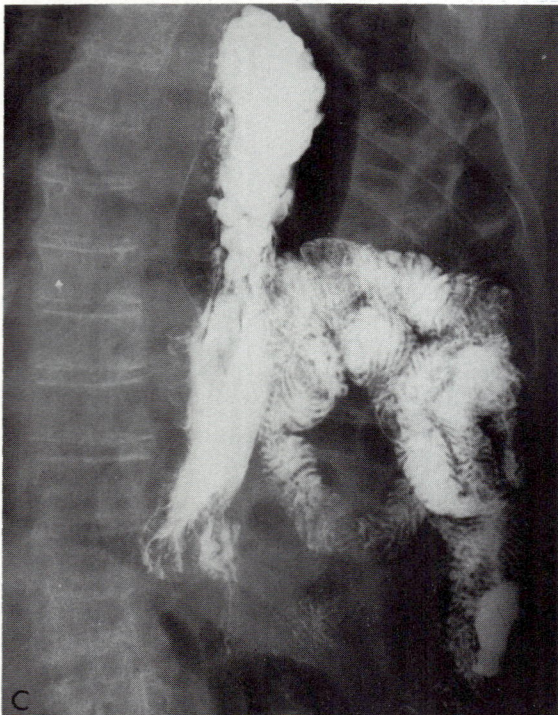

Figure 7–5. Traumatic diaphragmatic hernia. *A* and *B*, Chest radiographs show multiple air- and fluid-filled intestinal loops occupying the left pleural space. The heart and mediastinum are shifted to the right, and the left hemidiaphragm is no longer visible. There are old compression fractures of the lower thoracic vertebrae. *C*, Upper gastrointestinal series shows massive herniation of the stomach and small intestine through a large defect of the left hemidiaphragm.

injuries of the thorax or upper abdomen (gunshot, stab wounds, and so forth).[11, 12] Rarely, such hernias represent a complication of severe vomiting, transdiaphragmatic perforation of subphrenic abscess or empyema, or dehiscence of diaphragmatic suture lines following transthoracic hiatus hernia repair.[3, 14]

More than 90 per cent of these traumatic hernias occur on the left side and involve the central or posterior portions of the hemidiaphragm.[11]

Despite a relatively low incidence, traumatic hernias of the diaphragm have considerable clinical significance because of diagnostic difficulties and associated complications. First, the severity of injuries to other organs may initially obscure the diagnosis of diaphragmatic rupture. On the other hand, a tear can result from a blow to the chest or abdomen that is so minor that a complete radiologic evaluation is not performed at the time of the accident. Second, the absence of a limiting peritoneal sac may permit major herniations of abdominal content into the thorax, producing acute respiratory distress or intestinal obstruction sufficient to endanger the patient's life. In fact, 90 per cent of all strangulated diaphragmatic hernias are traumatic in origin.[25]

In many instances, a clinically unsuspected traumatic hernia of the diaphragm is first recognized on chest radiographs obtained several months or years after the causal injury.[12, 14] Usually, air- and fluid-containing intestinal loops are seen to protrude into the left pleural space, and the outline of the affected hemidiaphragm cannot be traced. The hernial contents may include the greater omentum, stomach, various segments of the small and large intestine, and occasionally, the left kidney and spleen.[3, 11, 12, 14] Rupture of the right hemidiaphragm can produce upward herniation of the liver, which then presents as a mushroom-like mass within the right hemithorax.

Differentiation of a large Bochdalek hernia from a traumatic hernia of the diaphragm is at times difficult. Bochdalek hernia is usually recognized at an earlier age because of its congenital origin, and the defect is located in the posterolateral portion of the diaphragm. Furthermore, the development of the hernia during fetal life frequently allows intrathoracic displacement of the left kidney, the ascending or descending colon, and the duodenal loop prior to their retroperitoneal fixation (Figs. 7–2 and 7–3). In contrast, it is not uncommon to find the stomach displaced inferiorly into the pelvis.[14] Traumatic hernias, however, commonly contain the stomach and the intraperitoneally mobile intestinal loops. Furthermore, the defect is in the central or posterior portion of the left hemidiaphragm (Fig. 7–5). Association with fractures of the lower ribs or vertebrae, bullet fragments adjacent to the diaphragm, or an accompanying hemothorax is particularly suggestive of a traumatic hernia when the clinical history is not readily available.

Hernias of the Groin and Pelvis

INGUINAL HERNIA. Nearly 75 per cent of all abdominal hernias occur in the inguinal region and predominantly affect males.[37, 54] The signs and symptoms of these inguinal hernias are usually sufficiently characteristic to permit a diagnosis to be made by inspection and palpation. Therefore, radiologic studies are primarily performed for evaluation of complicated inguinal hernias or when preoperative delineation of the herniated viscera is desirable.

INDIRECT INGUINAL HERNIA. In this type of hernia the sac protrudes at the internal inguinal ring and passes down the course of the inguinal canal anterior to the structures of the spermatic cord. If sufficiently large, it then emerges through the external inguinal ring and may actually extend into the scrotum (Fig. 7–6). In females, the hernial sac follows the course of the round ligament of the uterus into the labium majus.

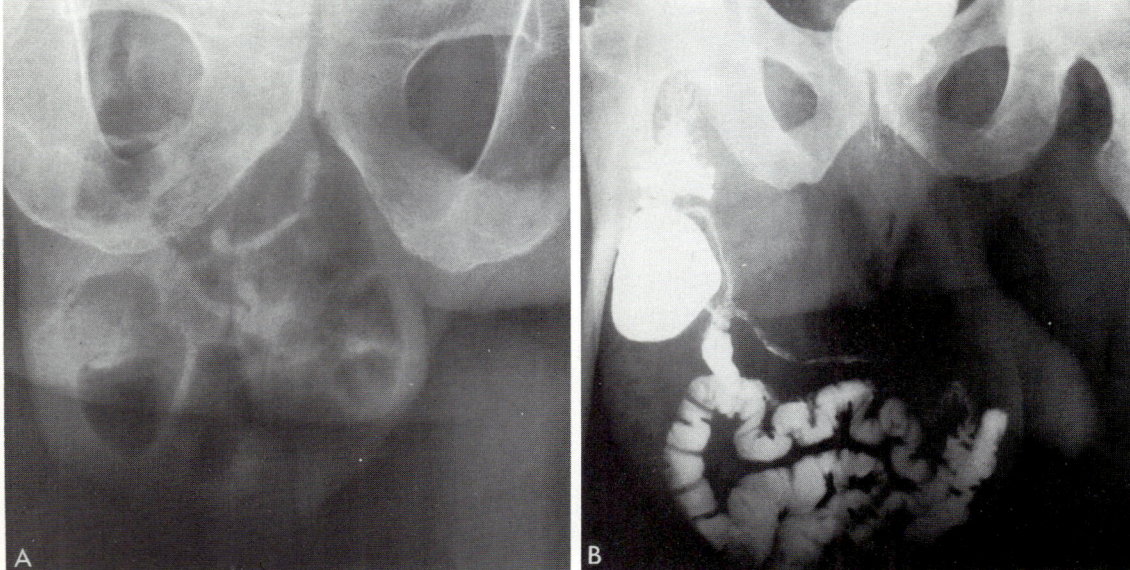

Figure 7–6. Large indirect inguinal hernia. *A*, Radiograph shows the gas-filled intestinal loops within the scrotum and over the right obturator foramen. *B*, Spot film from barium enema examination demonstrates the herniated ileal loops, cecum, and appendix.

Approximately 40 per cent of children older than two years of age with inguinal hernias have a patent vaginal process in the opposite groin.[38, 48] In about half this group, a contralateral hernia develops sometime during life.[44] Therefore, many pediatric surgeons prefer to routinely explore the apparently normal opposite groin during surgical repair of a unilateral hernia or hydrocele.[33, 44, 48] In such cases, an alternative method for evaluation of the inguinal regions is preoperative positive-contrast peritoneography or herniography.[2, 38, 48] This safe and easily performed procedure permits identification of patent vaginal processes, hernias, communicating hydroceles, and undescended testes. For this purpose, a relatively small volume of a water-soluble iodinated contrast material (2 ml per kg) is injected intraperitoneally, and the entire inferior border of the peritoneal cavity is then evaluated on serial radiographs (Fig. 7–7). The absence of a patent vaginal process as documented by herniography indicates that an inguinal hernia is neither present nor likely to develop. Therefore, the need for exploration of the opposite groin is precluded when only a unilateral hernia is clinically apparent.[2, 38, 48]

The contents of indirect inguinal hernias are usually the greater omentum and small bowel. Other viscera that are encountered less frequently include the cecum, appendix, Meckel's diverticulum, sigmoid, urinary bladder, testes, and female adnexa (Figs. 7–8 to 7–10). Inflammation of the organs occupying the sac, particularly appendicitis, or involvement by primary and metastatic tumors may also occur.[54]

SLIDING INGUINAL HERNIA. This term is used when partially extraperitoneal structures, such as the bladder, ascending colon, or descending colon, form a portion of the wall of the sac (Fig. 7–11). About 3 per cent of inguinal hernias are of the sliding type, and the left side is involved four or five times as often as the right.[54] Patients with inguinal or femoral hernia who present with urinary symptoms should have an excretory urogram, including an erect view of the pelvis and upper thighs, to detect herniations of the bladder or ureter (Fig. 7–12).[41]

Indirect inguinal hernias are well recognized as a major cause of intestinal obstruction and strangulation.[47, 54] Volvulus and perforation of the herniated loops may further complicate the process (Fig. 7–13).

Radiologic studies of the abdomen are not only important in establishing the diagnosis of intestinal obstruction, but often can localize the site and define the cause of obstruction. The examination should include supine and either upright or lateral decubitus films of the abdomen. Care must be taken that the pelvis and, particularly, the upper thighs are included. The following radiologic findings are particularly useful in the plain film diagnosis of incarcerated and strangulated hernias of the groin.

1. The massively distended small bowel loops appear to converge toward the region of herniation (Fig. 7–14). The afferent loop of the hernia may be recognized as tapering toward the groin and showing relatively fixed position on serial films.

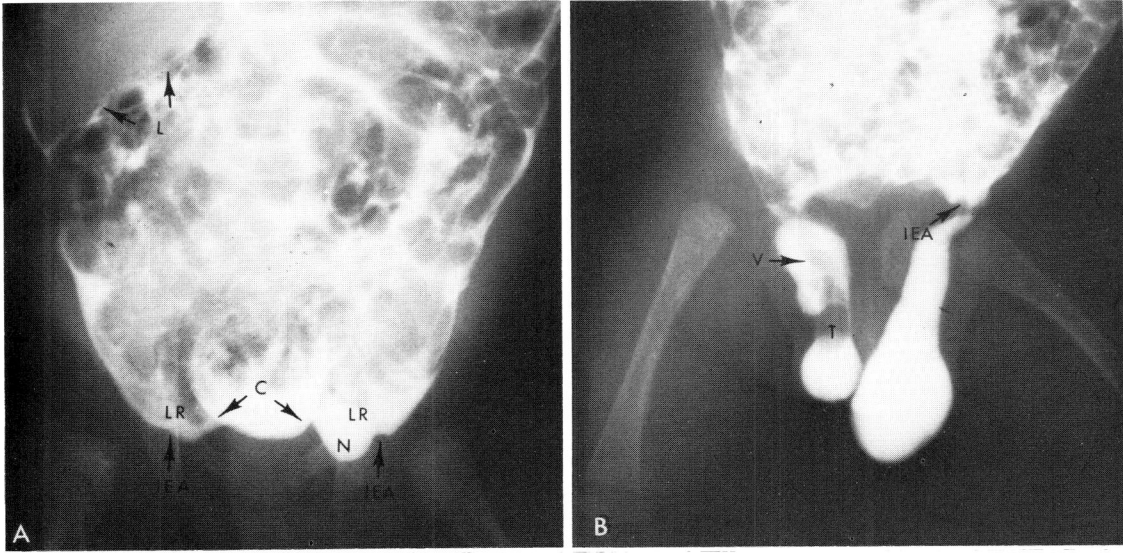

Figure 7–7. Positive-contrast herniography. *A*, In this normal study the opacification of the peritoneal cavity outlines the liver edge (L), cul-de-sac (C), and lateral recesses (LR). The notch created by the inferior epigastric artery (IEA) and the normal peritoneal pouch medial to it (N) are well demonstrated. *B*, This five-week-old boy had the clinical diagnosis of a right inguinal hernia. However, herniography documented large bilateral communicating hydroceles (potential hernia sacs) that required bilateral surgical repair. The right testicle (T), vas deferens (V), and left inferior epigastric artery are visualized. *C*, A left inguinal hernia was clinically diagnosed in this infant. The herniogram reveals bilateral indirect inguinal hernias (arrows) and the normal appearance of the cul-de-sac (C). (*From Swischuk, L. E., and Stacy, T. M.: Herniography: radiologic investigation of inguinal hernia. Radiology 101:139–146, 1971.*)

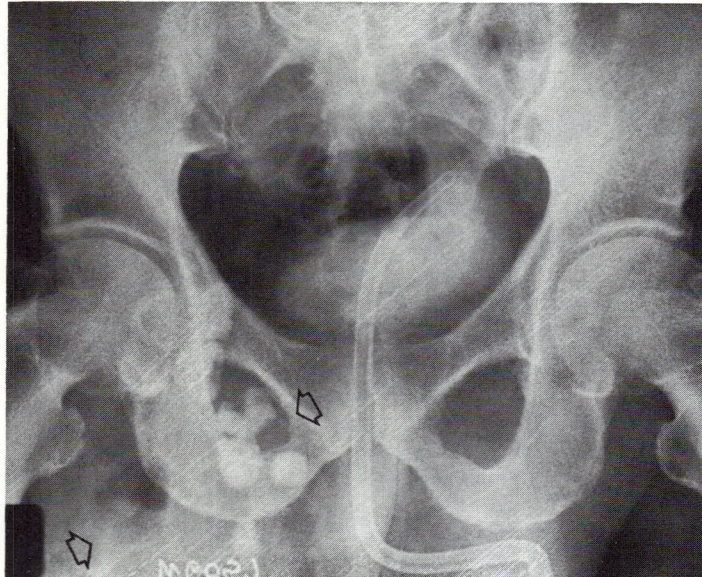

Figure 7–8. Indirect right inguinal hernia (arrows) containing calcified mesenteric lymph nodes and a gas-filled intestinal loop.

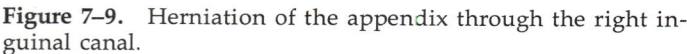

Figure 7–9. Herniation of the appendix through the right inguinal canal.

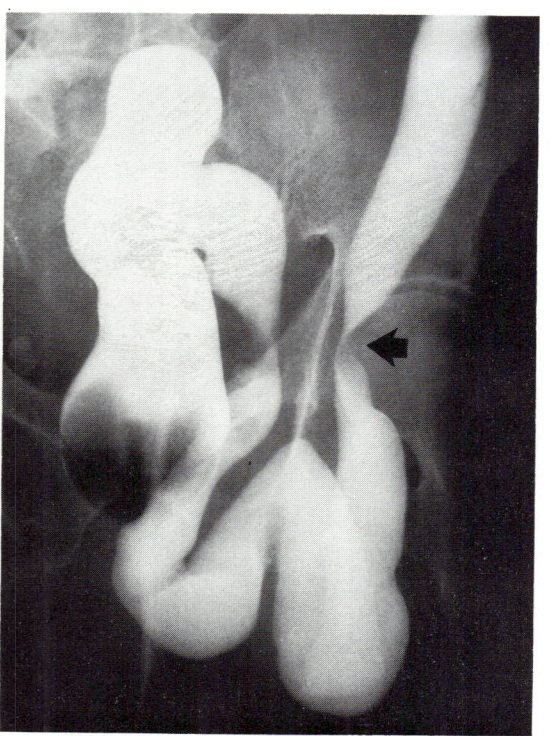

Figure 7–10. Barium enema examination shows a large indirect left inguinal hernia containing the sigmoid colon. There is narrowing of the lumen of both sigmoid loops at the hernial orifice (arrow).

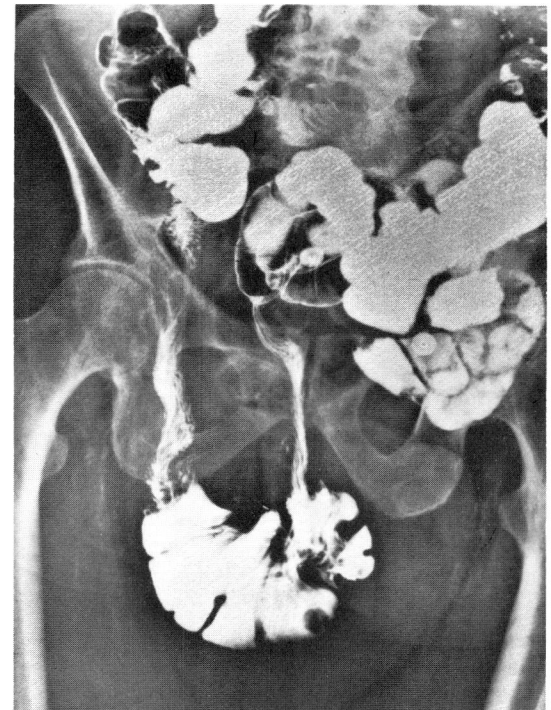

Figure 7–11. Sliding right inguinal hernia. In this patient, the ascending colon constitutes the lateral wall of the sac, and the cecum and terminal ileum are within the scrotal hernia.

2. On lateral films of the abdomen the incarcerated inguinal hernia may be seen as a bulging groin mass containing a low gas-fluid level (Fig. 7–15).

3. A gas-filled loop overlying the obturator foramen and associated bowel distention indicate the presence of an incarcerated inguinal hernia (Fig. 7–16). However, when the obturator foramen on the affected side is occupied by a soft-tissue mass of higher density than that of the opposite side, a strangulation must be suspected.

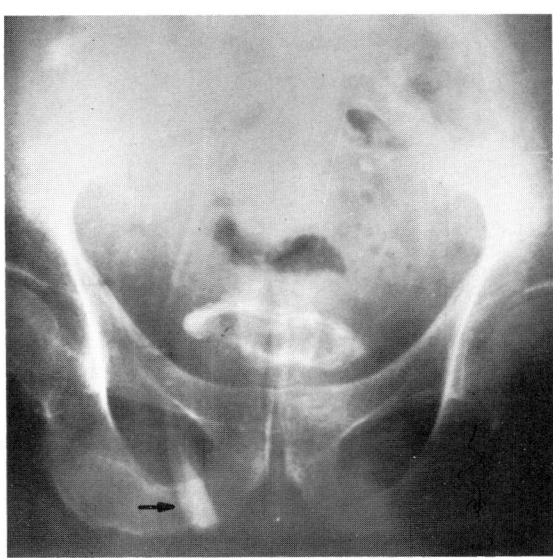

Figure 7–12. Erect view of the pelvis obtained during excretory urography shows a herniated distal ureter (arrow) in a patient with a sliding right inguinal hernia. (*From* Pollack, H. M., Popky, G. L., and Blumberg, M. L.: Hernias of the ureter. An anatomic-roentgenographic study. Radiology *117*:275–281, 1975.)

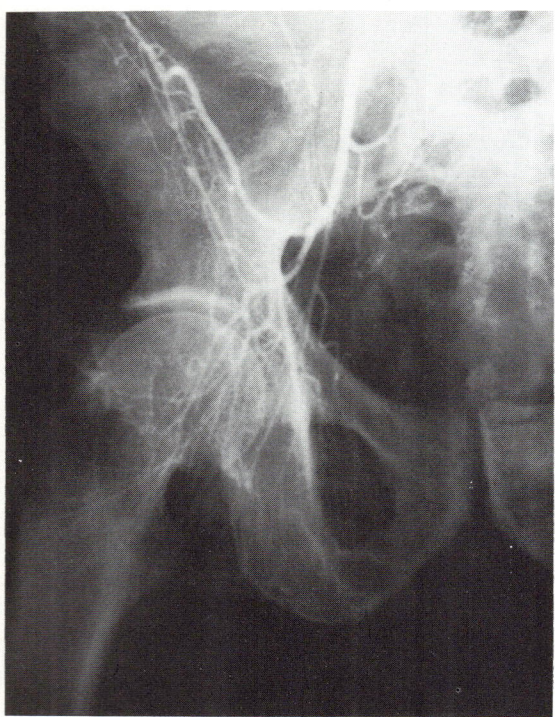

Figure 7–13. Superior mesenteric arteriogram in this patient with an incarcerated right inguinal hernia shows diminished blood flow to the herniated loops. Ischemic changes and volvulus of the involved ileum were found at surgery.

DIRECT INGUINAL HERNIA. Direct inguinal hernia is a protrusion directly through the posterior wall of the inguinal canal medial to the inferior epigastric vessels. It may present through the external inguinal ring and manifest itself as a rounded swelling of limited size. Direct hernias rarely occur in children and are very uncommon in females.[37, 54] Strangulation is seldom a complication because of the blunt and diffuse character of the protrusion. The close proximity of the internal and external inguinal

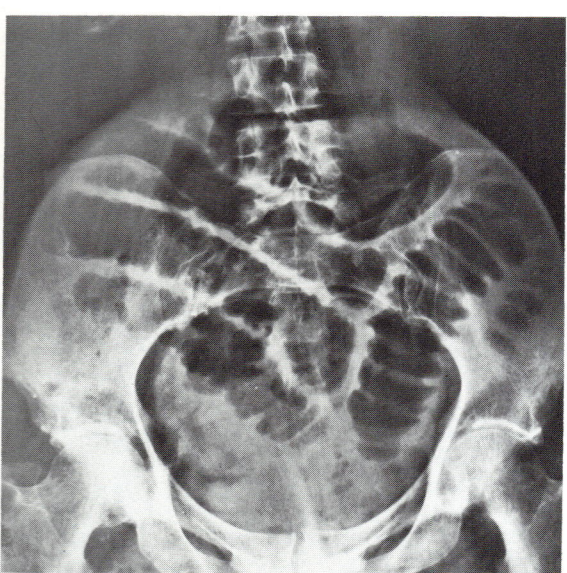

Figure 7–14. Strangulated left inguinal hernia in an adult. Note that the massively distended small bowel loops converge toward the left inguinal region, and the colon is free of gas.

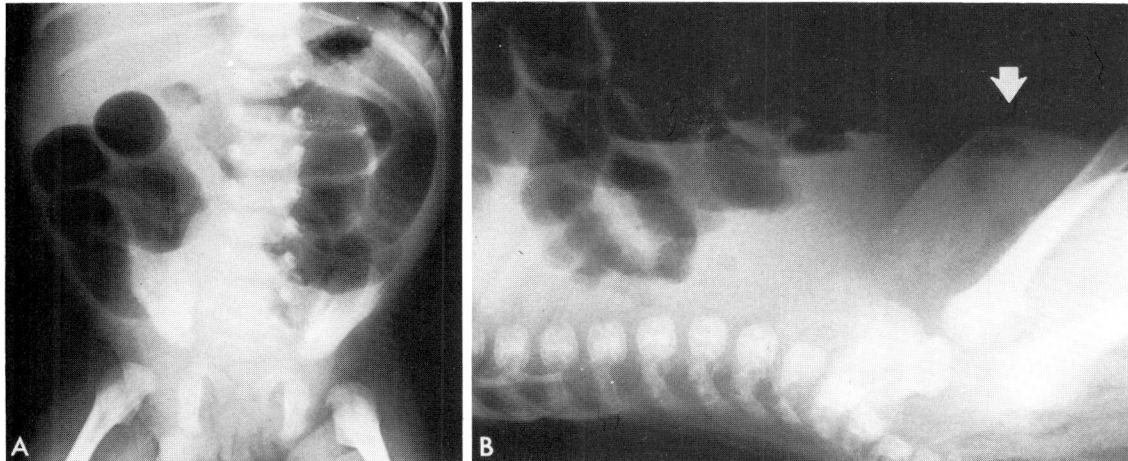

Figure 7–15. Strangulated left inguinal hernia in a child. *A*, Supine film of the abdomen shows marked distention of the small bowel. *B*, Cross-table lateral view clearly illustrates a bulging mass with an air-fluid level in the left groin (arrow). The small intestine proximal to the herniated ileal loop contains many air-fluid levels.

rings on frontal projection makes radiologic differentiation between direct and indirect inguinal hernia very difficult.[41] The obliquely elongated tubular course of the indirect hernias and their frequent extension into the scrotum are useful diagnostic features, however.

COMBINED INGUINAL HERNIA. Also referred to as pantaloon or saddlebag hernia, this designates the simultaneous presence of direct and indirect hernia in the same

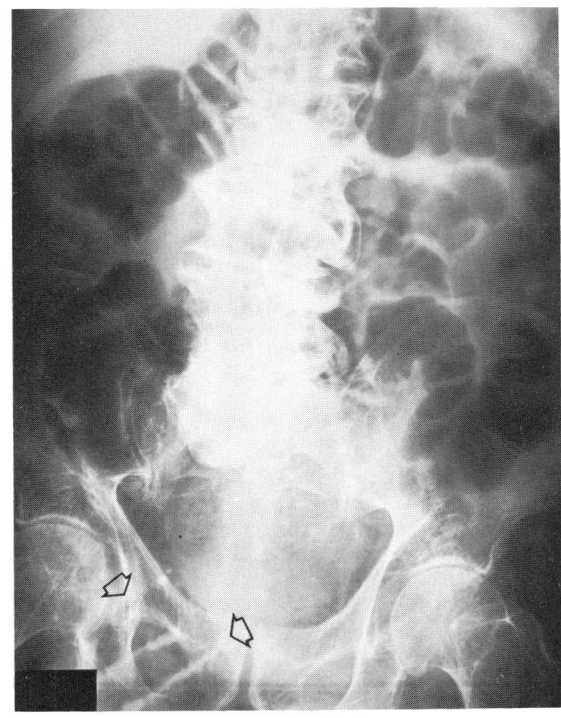

Figure 7–16. Incarcerated right inguinal hernia. A supine abdominal radiograph shows several gas-filled loops (arrows) overlying the right obturator foramen. There is evidence of mechanical obstruction of the distal small bowel.

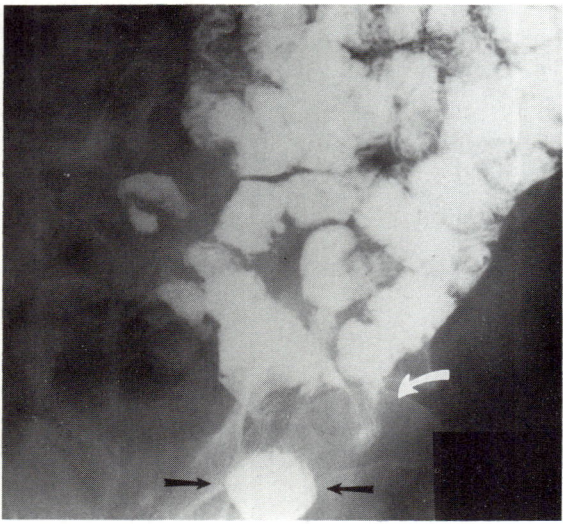

Figure 7–17. This radiograph from a small bowel series demonstrates an indirect inguinal hernia (black arrows) as well as a small femoral hernia (white arrow) on the left side. Both hernial rings are very narrow, but no intestinal obstruction is produced.

inguinal region. The separation of the two hernial sacs by the inferior epigastric vessels accounts for the bilocular appearance of such combined herniations.[54]

FEMORAL HERNIAS. This hernia enters the femoral canal at the femoral ring. Femoral hernias account for 34 per cent of all hernias in women. The incidence in men is three or four times less, and children are rarely affected.[54] The hernial content is usually preperitoneal fat, omentum, and small bowel (Figs. 7–17 and 7–18). Strangulation in femoral hernias occurs 8 to 12 times as frequently as it does in inguinal

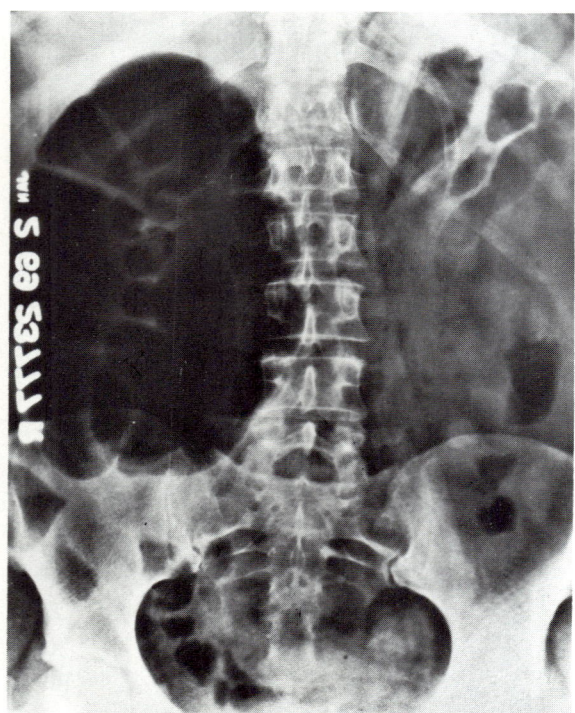

Figure 7–18. Incarceration of the greater omentum in a right femoral hernia. The transverse colon is pulled toward the right lower abdomen, and there is distention of the proximal colon.

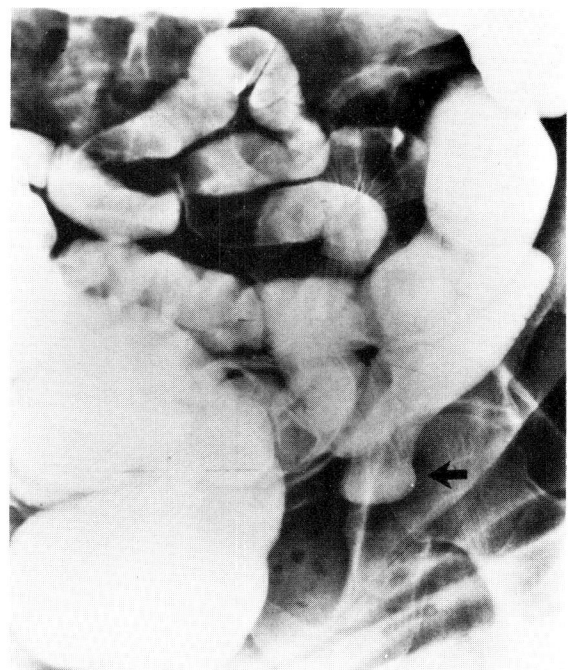

Figure 7–19. Richter's type of inguinal hernia (arrow). Only a portion of the antimesenteric wall of an ileal loop protrudes through the hernial ring, so that the intestinal lumen remains patent.

hernias. The high incidence of this complication (25 to 40 per cent) is the result of small, firm, unyielding margins of the femoral ring.[54]

RICHTER'S HERNIA. One form of femoral hernia that is particularly prone to strangulation is Richter's hernia. This contains only a portion of the antimesenteric wall of the bowel, so that the intestinal lumen may remain patent despite strangulation of a portion of its wall (Fig. 7–19).[37, 54] Therefore, Richter's hernia should be suspected in any patient presenting with nausea, vomiting, and abdominal pain but with no apparent intestinal obstruction evidenced by either radiographic examination or by the presence of normal bowel movements. Approximately 90 per cent of these hernias are found in the femoral region, but the condition can also be seen in other locations.[54]

LITTRE'S HERNIA. This is an unusual entity in which a preformed diverticulum, notably Meckel's, is the herniated content.[37, 54] Of these hernias, 50 per cent present through the inguinal orifice, 30 per cent at the umbilicus, and a smaller percentage in the femoral region.[50] The term "partial enterocele" is also used to describe both Richter's and Littre's hernias.[54] Since only a portion of the bowel wall protrudes through the hernial ring, there is usually no occlusion of the intestinal lumen and no external hernial mass is palpable.

HESSELBACH'S HERNIA OR EXTERNAL FEMORAL HERNIA. The sac of this rare hernia passes below the inguinal ligament and protrudes lateral to the femoral vessels. It may occur in combination with an indirect inguinal hernia on the same side.[37]

OBTURATOR HERNIA. This is a rare type of herniation along the fibro-osseous canal through which pass the obturator vessels and nerve. In view of the depth at which it lies, the preoperative diagnosis of an obturator hernia is extremely difficult. The only local symptom may be pain radiating down the inner side of the thigh along the distribution of the obturator nerve (the Howship-Romberg sign). Rectal or vaginal examination may permit the palpation of a tender mass in the region of the obturator canal.[26, 37, 54]

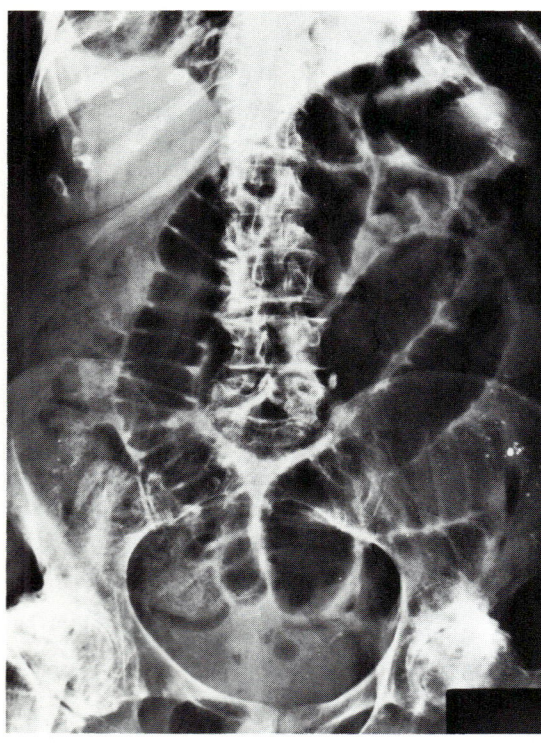

Figure 7–20. Strangulated right obturator hernia. Preoperative supine radiograph of the abdomen shows the massively distended small bowel loops converging toward the right obturator foramen.

These hernias occur predominantly in elderly women, probably owing to the enlargement of the obturator canal associated with relaxation of the pelvic peritoneum after multiple pregnancies and aging. The hernia usually consists of a peritoneal sac and may contain the small or large intestine or the pelvic organs. A Richter type of partial enterocele is commonly found in patients with a strangulated obturator hernia. The radiologic findings are those of mechanical bowel obstruction, but the hernia itself is rarely recognized preoperatively (Fig. 7–20).[16]

SCIATIC HERNIA. These hernias pass through the greater, or less frequently, through the lesser, sciatic notch. They present under the inferior border of the gluteus maximus muscle in the posteromedial aspect of the thigh.[37, 54] When the sciatic hernia is small, its preoperative clinical or radiologic diagnosis is as difficult as that of an obturator hernia. The presence of pain in the distribution of the great sciatic nerve and a tender bulge in the posteromedial aspect of the thigh are helpful diagnostic clues.[37] These local findings, together with radiologic evidence of mechanical intestinal obstruction, indicate strangulation of the hernial contents.

Abdominal Wall Hernias

UMBILICAL HERNIA. Umbilical hernia is a defect at the umbilical ring through which the viscera protrude. Although the congenital form, or omphalocele, is often included among umbilical hernias, this is not, strictly speaking, a typical hernia, since the viscera never enter the abdomen in this condition.

Umbilical hernia of childhood is commonly found prior to the age of three years. The vast majority of these often small hernias are asymptomatic and may disappear spontaneously. Incarceration or strangulation is seldom a complication.[37, 54]

Umbilical hernias in adults account for 4 per cent of all hernias.[54] They occur predominantly in middle-aged females and are often associated with obesity and a history of multiple pregnancies. Traumatic or spontaneous rupture may also occur during pregnancy or in patients with cirrhosis and ascites.[37] These hernias are particularly prone to incarceration and strangulation. The hernial contents are usually the omentum and small or large intestine. Adhesions, which often develop between the omentum and the peritoneum, contribute to production of digestive symptoms and other complications.

The clinical diagnosis of an incarcerated umbilical hernia may be made on the occurrence of abdominal pain, vomiting, constipation, and local tenderness on pressure in the region of the umbilicus even if no obvious bulge is seen on the surface. Radiographs of the abdomen usually show evidence of intestinal obstruction and a tumorlike density of the hernia (Fig. 7–21).

In addition to supine, erect, and decubitus films of the abdomen, the coned-down lateral or cross-table views utilizing soft-tissue technique may be of value. The presence of gas-filled loops within the hernial sac indicates the likelihood of incomplete obstruction. If this is accompanied by fluid levels and distended intra-abdominal bowel loops, strangulation is probably complete. Contrast studies of the small and large intestine in the early stage provide confirmatory evidence, demonstrating narrowing of the bowel as it comes into relationship with the hernial ring and dilatation proximally. When the hernial content is primarily the omentum, a tumorlike density with stripes radiating from the opening of the sac may be seen (Fig. 7–22). Otherwise, the symptoms of an incarcerated omentum are quite similar to those of strangulated bowel obstruction.

VENTRAL HERNIA. The general term "ventral hernia" encompasses all protrusions of the viscera through the anterolateral abdominal wall except for herniations in the umbilical and groin regions.[37, 54]

MIDLINE. Midline ventral hernias emerge through the linea alba. The majority are located above the umbilicus and therefore are referred to as *epigastric hernias*. In

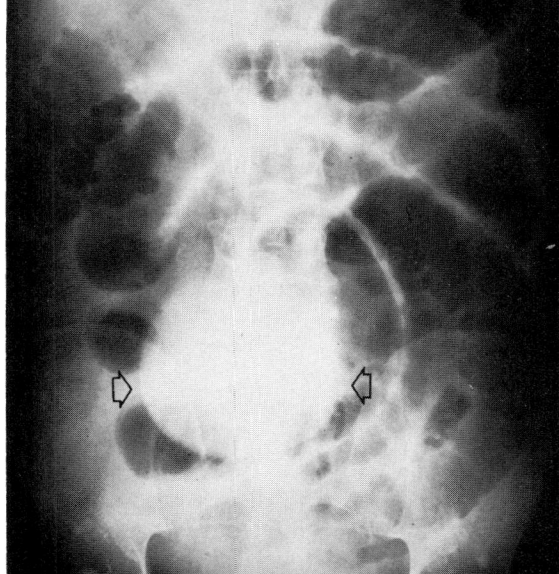

Figure 7–21. Strangulated umbilical hernia. Supine film of the abdomen demonstrates the tumorlike density of the hernia (arrows) and evidence of mechanical small bowel obstruction.

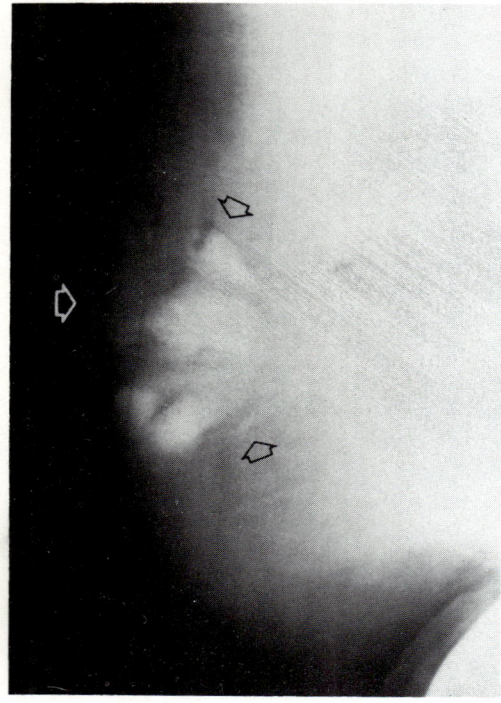

Figure 7–22. Strangulation of the omentum and small bowel in a small umbilical hernia. This coned-down lateral view of the anterior abdominal wall shows the soft tissue and fat densities of the congested loops and the omentum (arrows) radiating toward the small hernial orifice.

most instances, the hernial ring is a small, firm defect of less than 1.0 cm in diameter in the aponeurosis. The mushroom-like protrusion frequently consists of the omentum and preperitoneal fat, but the small and large bowel are occasionally involved. Incarceration of the herniated mass frequently occurs and may produce symptoms out of proportion to the objective manifestations. The localization of pain in the upper abdomen may simulate that of peptic ulcer disease except that it is aggravated by exertion.[54]

LATERAL. Lateral ventral hernias that appear through the semilunar line are also known as *spigelian hernias*.[22, 23, 37] The contents are usually the omentum and small bowel, and occasionally, the colon is included (Fig. 7–23).

The spigelian hernia occurs in every age group and with equal incidence in men and women. It may be bilateral and, at times, is associated with other ventral or inguinal hernias. Plain radiographs of the abdomen and barium studies of the gastrointestinal tract have been found most useful in establishing the preoperative diagnosis.[22, 23]

LUMBAR. Lumbar hernias emerge through two weak places in the loin. The lower of these, the inferior lumbar space, or Petit's triangle, lies just above the iliac crest between the external oblique and latissimus dorsi muscles. The larger superior lumbar space, or Grynfelt's triangle, is bounded above by the twelfth rib and inferior margin of the serratus posticus, inferolaterally by the internal oblique, and posteriorly by the erector spinae muscles.[37, 54] The lumbar hernias usually have a sac that consists of peritoneum or extraperitoneal tissue and that may contain fat, omentum, mesentery, small or large intestine, or kidneys (Fig. 7–24). The hernia usually presents as a bulging mass on coughing and rarely becomes incarcerated or strangulated.

INCISIONAL. Incisional hernias are traumatic hernias that may follow either accidental or surgical wounds of the abdominal wall.[1, 37, 54]

Incisional hernias usually contain the omentum and the small and large intestines.

HERNIAS — 305

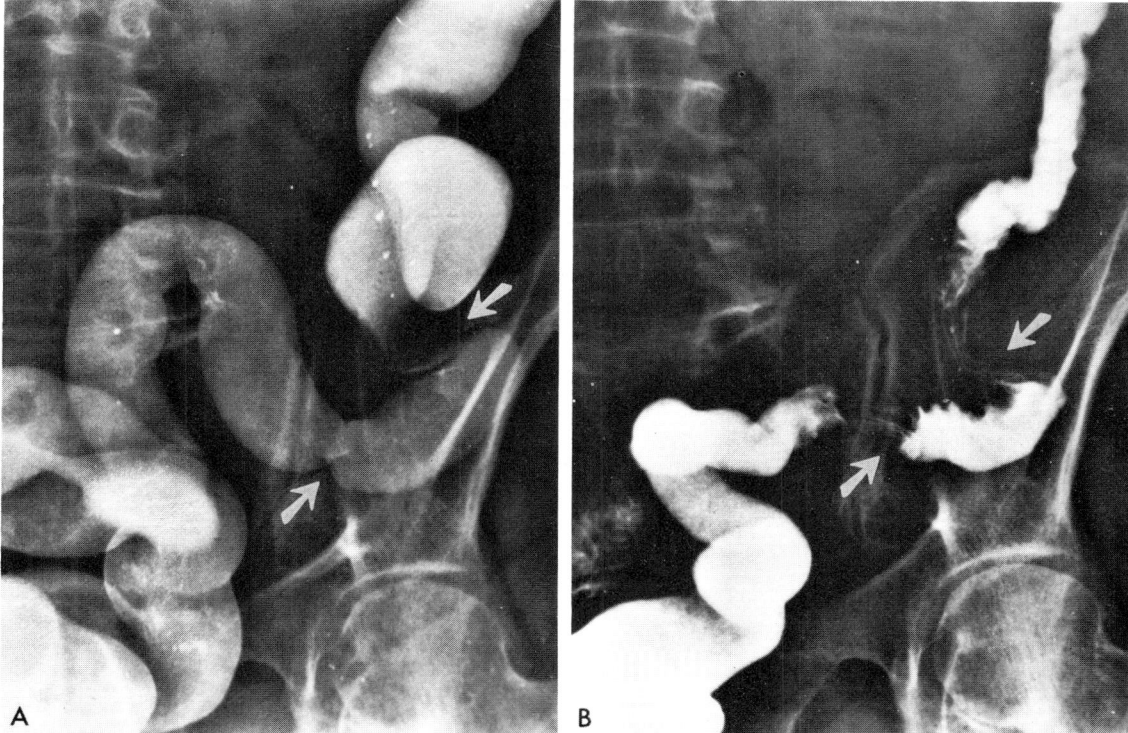

Figure 7–23. Spigelian hernia. *A* and *B*, The filled view and postevacuation film of a barium enema study reveal the herniation of a short segment of the sigmoid colon through the left semilunar line (arrows).

Symptoms and complications depend upon the size and rigidity of the aperture, as well as upon the existence of adhesions between the sac and its contents. Incarceration has been reported to occur in nearly one third of these hernias, but strangulation is seen in only 5 per cent.[37, 54] In general, the diagnosis is suspected on the basis of the

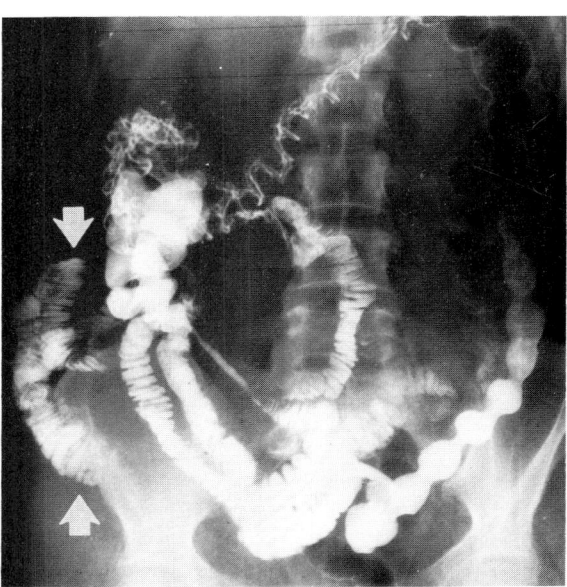

Figure 7–24. Lumbar hernia. The postevacuation radiograph of a barium enema study shows an ileal loop (arrows) herniating through the right inferior lumbar space or Petit's triangle.

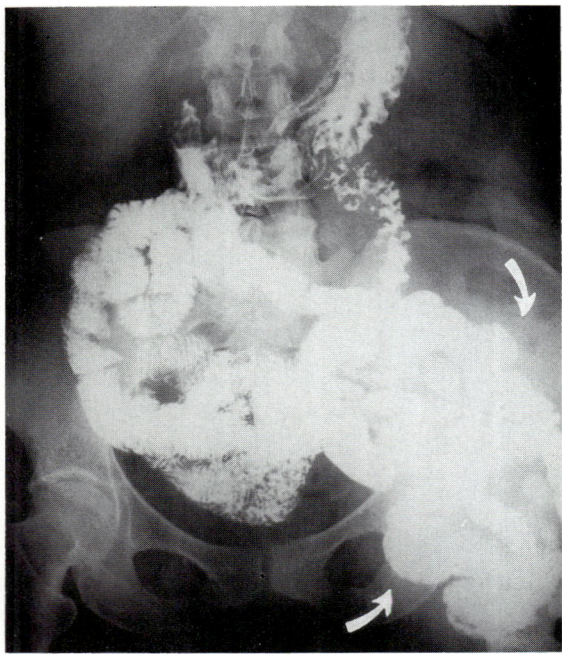

Figure 7–25. Large incisional hernia (arrows) following resection of the sigmoid colon for carcinoma.

clinical findings and is further confirmed by plain radiographs or barium studies of the gastrointestinal tract (Figs. 7–25 and 7–26).

INTERNAL ABDOMINAL HERNIAS

An internal hernia represents the protrusion of a viscus—essentially, a portion of the small intestine—through a normal peritoneal fossa or pathologic orifice within the confines of the adominalvity.[17] The majority of these hernias result from congenital

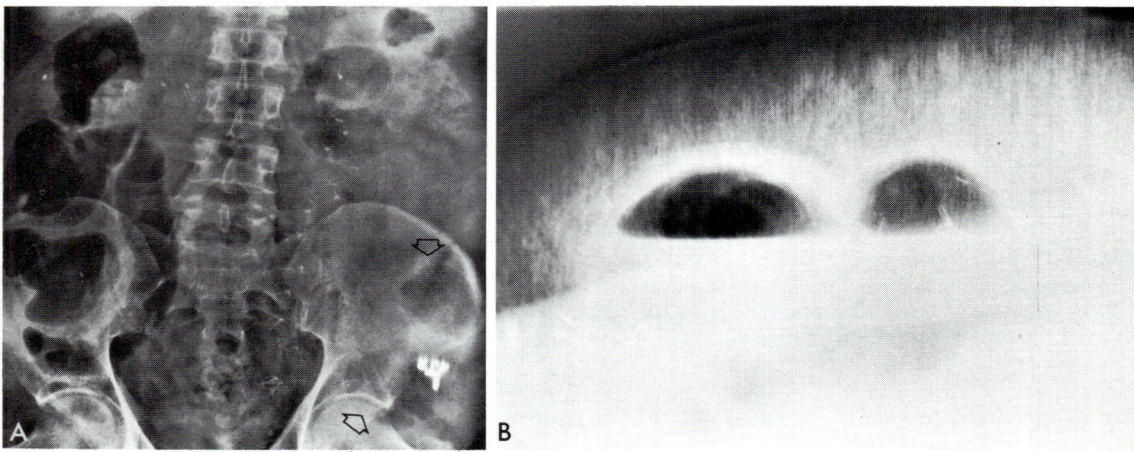

Figure 7–26. Incisional hernia with early strangulation. This patient had an infected Penrose drain site in the left lower abdomen after left hemicolectomy for diverticulitis. *A*, Supine film of the abdomen shows two gas-filled small bowel loops (arrows) over the left ilium. *B*, Cross-table lateral view with soft-tissue technique reveals air-fluid levels in small bowel loops projecting within the anterior abdominal wall. Note the thickened edematous wall of the herniated intestine.

anomalies of intestinal rotation and peritoneal attachment.[24, 34, 40, 51, 55] Acquired defects of the mesentery or peritoneum owing to abdominal surgery or trauma may also serve as the hernial ring, however.[20, 29, 32, 45, 53]

The autopsy incidence of internal hernia has been reported to be between 0.2 and 0.9 per cent.[24, 52] Many of these hernias are small and easily reducible, so that they may remain asymptomatic during life.[17, 31] In other cases, the patients usually present with a history of intermittent attacks of vague epigastric discomfort, colicky periumbilical pain, nausea, vomiting, and recurrent intestinal obstruction, especially after intake of a large meal.[24, 29, 31, 40, 52] In such patients radiologic diagnosis can be made if contrast studies are performed during symptomatic periods—prior to an often spontaneous reduction.[17, 31] The most important clinical manifestation is acute small bowel obstruction, however.

The radiologic features of various relatively common types of internal hernias are described and illustrated later in this chapter. Figure 7–27 shows the sites susceptible to occurrence and the relative incidence of internal hernias based on a collective review of 467 cases.[19] In general, the small bowel examination provides the most useful diagnostic hallmarks, which include (1) sacculation and crowding together of several small bowel loops due to encapsulation within the hernial sac, (2) segmental dilatation and prolonged stasis of barium in the herniated loops, and (3) abnormal location and disturbed arrangement of the small intestine.

Preoperative radiologic diagnosis of an internal hernia is important, because at laparotomy the hernia may not be easily recognizable once it has reduced spontaneously or following inadvertent traction. Furthermore, the usual exploratory laparotomy is often inadequate for evaluation of all significant peritoneal fossae and mesenteric defects that may serve as potential sites of herniation.[17, 31, 39]

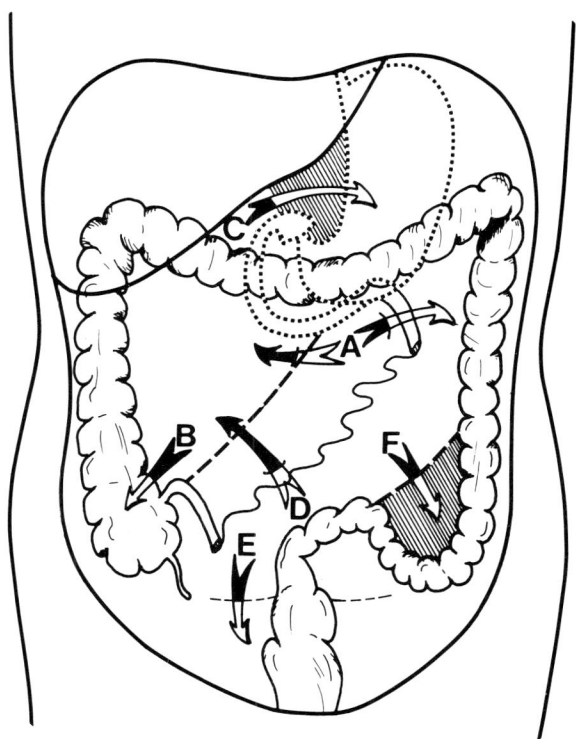

Figure 7–27. Location and relative incidence of internal hernias based on 467 cases. Paraduodenal hernias (A): 53 per cent; pericecal (B): 13 per cent; foramen of Winslow (C): 8 per cent; transmesenteric (D): 8 per cent; into pelvic structures (E): 7 per cent; and transmesosigmoid (F): 6 per cent. (*From* Ghahremani, G. G., and Meyers, M. A.: Internal abdominal hernias. Curr. Probl. Radiol., 5:1–30, 1975.)

Paraduodenal Hernias

Paraduodenal hernias are the most common type of intra-abdominal herniation and account for 53 per cent of reported cases.[15, 19, 24] These hernias are basically congenital in origin, representing entrapment of the small intestine beneath the mesentery of the colon during embryologic rotation of the midgut.[9, 54, 55]

Seventy-five per cent of paraduodenal hernias occur on the left side. The hernia frequently contains only a few jejunal loops and is spontaneously reducible. Since the afferent loop enters the sac from behind the point at which the duodenum emerges from its fixed retroperitoneal position, only the efferent loop of the intestine passes through the hernial orifice.

The right paraduodenal hernias account for the remaining 25 per cent of this group and involve the mesentericoparietal fossa of Waldeyer.[15, 24, 31] This peritoneal pocket in the jejunal mesentery has its orifice behind the superior mesenteric artery just inferior to the third portion of the duodenum. Because both afferent and efferent loops pass through the hernial orifice, the right paraduodenal hernias are usually more massive and fixed than those occurring on the left side.[17, 31]

The clinical manifestations of paraduodenal hernias range from intermittent, mild digestive complaints to acute intestinal obstruction with perhaps gangrene and peritonitis.[13, 15, 49] Recurrent postprandial epigastric pain, periumbilical cramps, and mild distention are frequently experienced prior to the onset of incarceration. It is during such symptomatic periods that contrast examinations of the gastrointestinal tract are most likely to provide the correct diagnosis.[17, 24, 30, 31, 34, 36, 39, 52] Once the hernia is spontaneously reduced, however, barium studies may be negative or show only a mild degree of dilatation, stasis, and mucosal edema of the involved small bowel loops.[17, 31]

In patients with a small left paraduodenal hernia (Fig. 7–28) a circumscribed mass of, usually, a few jejunal loops may be seen in the left upper quadrant immediately lateral to the ascending duodenum. The herniated loops may depress the distal transverse colon and indent the posterior wall of the stomach. Stasis of barium within the hernial contents and mild dilatation of the duodenum may be associated findings.

Large paraduodenal hernias can contain several or most of the small bowel loops. These form a circumscribed ovoid mass having its main axis lateral to the midline and its inferior border convex downward (Fig. 7–29). The encapsulation within the hernial sac prevents separation or displacement of the individual loops from the rest of the hernial contents during fluoroscopic manipulation. Stasis of the contrast material and dilatation of the herniated loops may also be evident. At the hernial orifice the efferent loop of the left paraduodenal hernia shows an abrupt change of caliber. In a right paraduodenal hernia, however, both the afferent and the efferent loops appear closely apposed and narrowed. Lateral films are particularly useful for detection of retroperitoneal displacement of the hernial content. On barium enema examination, the descending colon may be seen to be anterior, to the left, or posterior to a left paraduodenal hernia. The ascending colon always lies lateral to a right paraduodenal hernia, however, and the cecum is found in its normal position.[31]

The position of the major mesenteric vessels in the anterior margin of the neck of the paraduodenal hernial sac is important both embryologically and surgically. The inferior mesenteric vein and ascending left colic artery lie in the anteromedial free edge of the left paraduodenal hernia. The superior mesenteric artery and vein are located in the anteromedial free border of the right paraduodenal hernia.[12, 13, 46] Therefore, arteriographic visualization of these vessels, particularly of the position of their branches supplying the small bowel loops, can assist in radiologic diagnosis of paraduodenal hernias.[17, 30, 31] In a right paraduodenal hernia, the jejunal arteries that normally arise

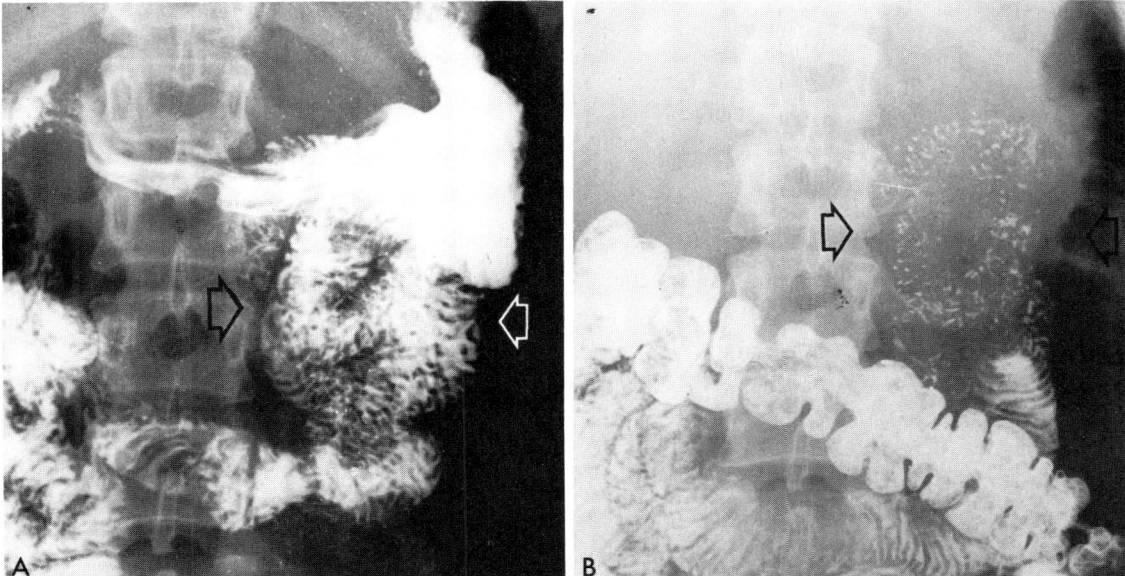

Figure 7-28. Small left paraduodenal hernia. *A,* This radiograph from a small bowel series shows a circumscribed ovoid mass of herniated jejunal loops immediately lateral to the ascending duodenum (arrows). *B,* Two-hour film demonstrates stasis of barium within these loops (arrows) and depression of the distal transverse colon. At surgery the hernial sac contained only a couple of feet of jejunum. This was readily reduced, and the peritoneal defect was repaired. (*From* Meyers, M. A.: Paraduodenal hernias. Radiologic and arteriographic diagnosis. Radiology 95:29-37, 1970.)

from the left side of the superior mesenteric artery are noted to reverse their direction and course behind the parent vessel to supply the herniated jejunal loops within the fossa of Waldeyer (Fig. 7-30). In a left paraduodenal hernia, the proximal jejunal arteries show an abrupt change of course along the medial border of the hernial orifice, where they are redirected posteriorly behind the inferior mesenteric vessels to accompany the herniated loops (see Fig. 7-29).

Foramen of Winslow Hernia

The protrusion of a viscus through the foramen of Winslow into the lesser omental sac accounts for 8 per cent of all internal hernias.[10, 19, 24]

Foramen of Winslow hernias contain the small intestine in 60 per cent of cases.[21, 24] The cecum, appendix, and ascending colon are involved in about 25 per cent; other viscera, such as the transverse colon, omentum, or gallbladder, are found occasionally.[17, 24]

This type of hernia usually affects middle-aged patients and presents as a sudden onset of crampy upper abdominal pain and progressive small bowel distention.[24]

The characteristic roentgen features of foramen-of-Winslow hernias follow:

1. Plain radiographs of the abdomen show evidence of mechanical small bowel obstruction as well as of the presence of gas-containing intestinal loops within the lesser sac medial and posterior to the stomach (Fig. 7-31).[10, 21, 24]

2. Upper gastrointestinal examination with contrast material demonstrates dis-

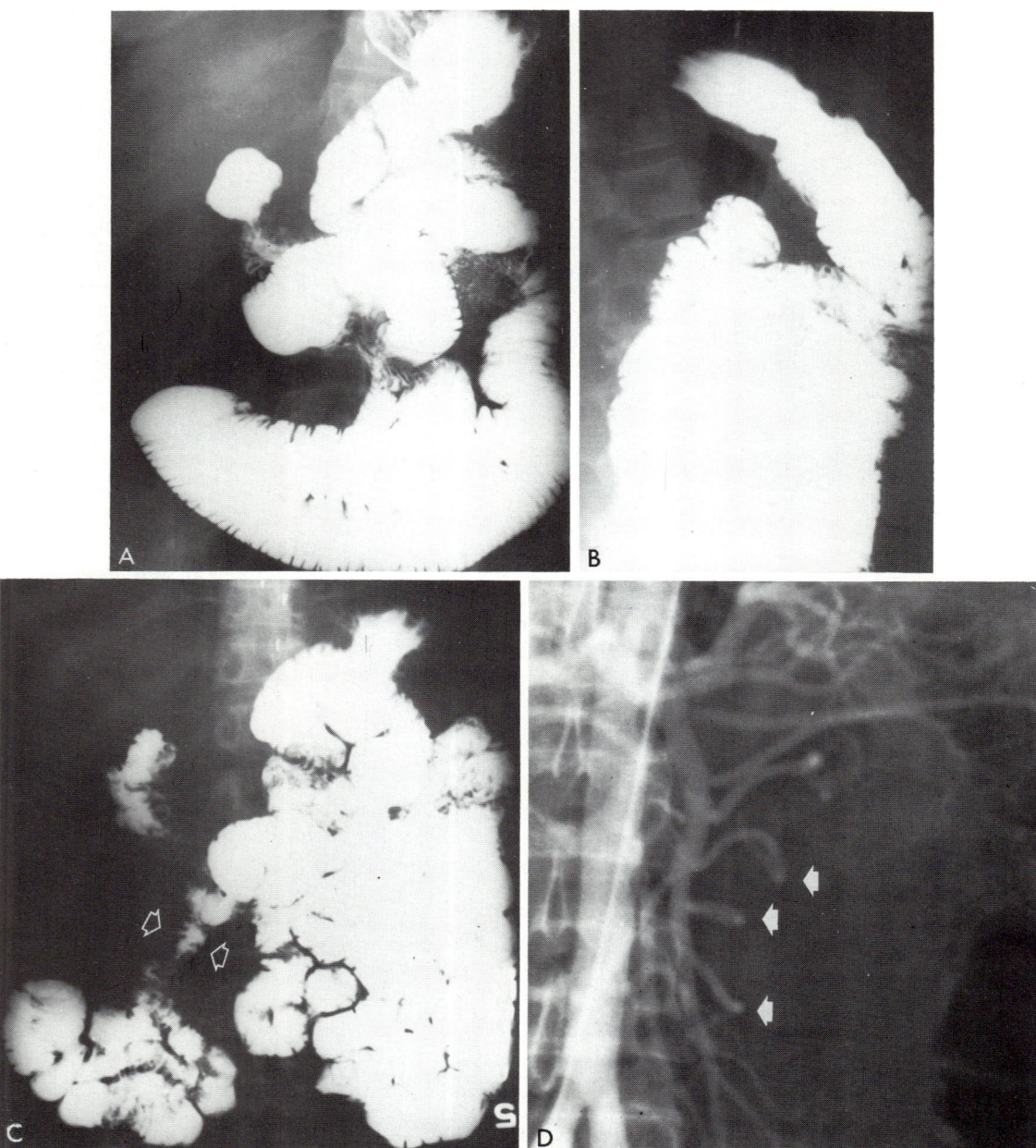

Figure 7–29. Large left paraduodenal hernia in a 42-year-old female with persistent postprandial pains despite multiple abdominal operations. *A,* Most of the small bowel loops are gathered in the left side of the abdomen, forming a circumscribed mass with a convex inferior margin. *B,* Lateral projection shows retroperitoneal displacement of the herniated intestine. *C,* A serial film demonstrates that the efferent loop (arrows) leads from the hernial sac to the normally situated distal ileum. *D,* Aortogram shows that the upper jejunal arteries are redirected medially just beyond their origins from the superior mesenteric artery (arrows). This characteristic reversal of their course indicates the posteromedial border of the hernial orifice, beyond which the intestinal loops herniate. (*From* Meyers, M. A.: Arteriographic diagnosis of internal (left paraduodenal) hernia. Radiology 92:1035–1037, 1969.)

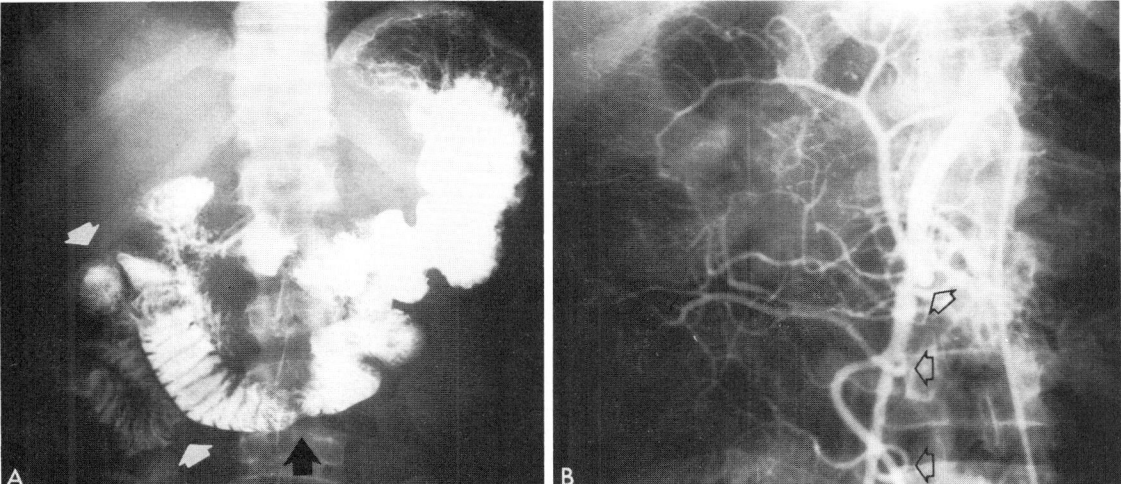

Figure 7–30. Right paraduodenal hernia. *A,* The right midabdomen is occupied by a circumscribed grouping of jejunal loops (white arrows) that have herniated into the ascending mesocolon and the right portion of the transverse mesocolon. The duodenum and ligamentum of Treitz are normally situated. The dilated afferent jejunal loop shows a localized constriction (black arrow) at the hernial orifice behind the superior mesenteric artery. *B,* Superior mesenteric arteriogram of another patient with a larger right paraduodenal hernia. Note that the jejunal branches originate from the left side, but abruptly change their direction (arrows) toward the right of the parent vessel to accompany the herniated jejunal loops.

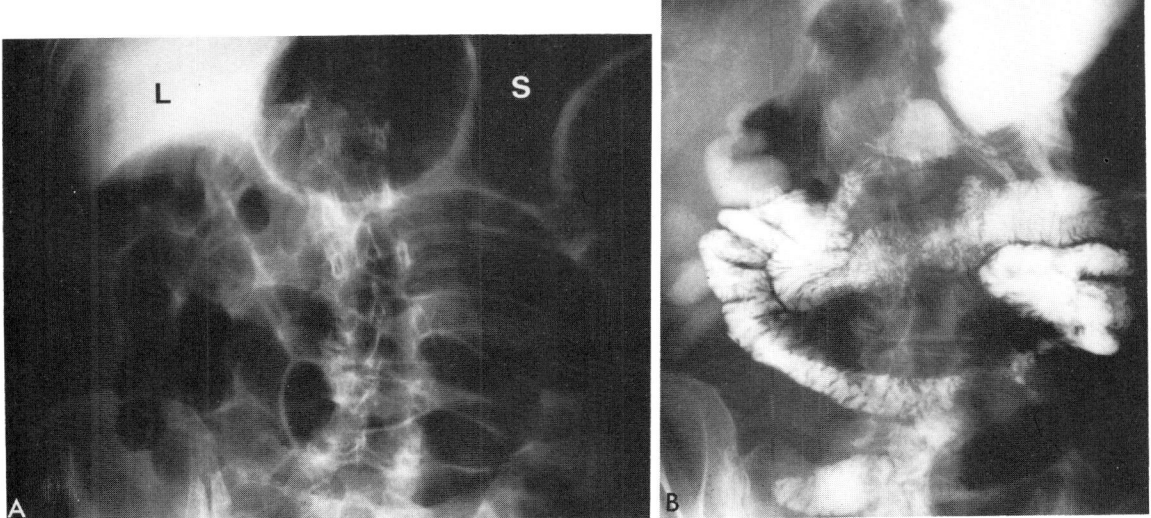

Figure 7–31. Cecal herniation through the foramen of Winslow. *A,* Supine abdominal film shows marked dilatation of the small bowel. An abnormal collection of gas is seen in the lesser peritoneal sac between the liver (L) and the stomach (S). *B,* Upper gastrointestinal series reveals displacement of the stomach and the first and second parts of the duodenum to the left. There is less gas in the small intestine and within the lesser sac owing to partial spontaneous reduction of the hernia. (*From* Henisz, A., Matesanz, J., and Westcott, J. L.: Cecal herniation through the foramen of Winslow. Radiology *112*:575–578, 1974.)

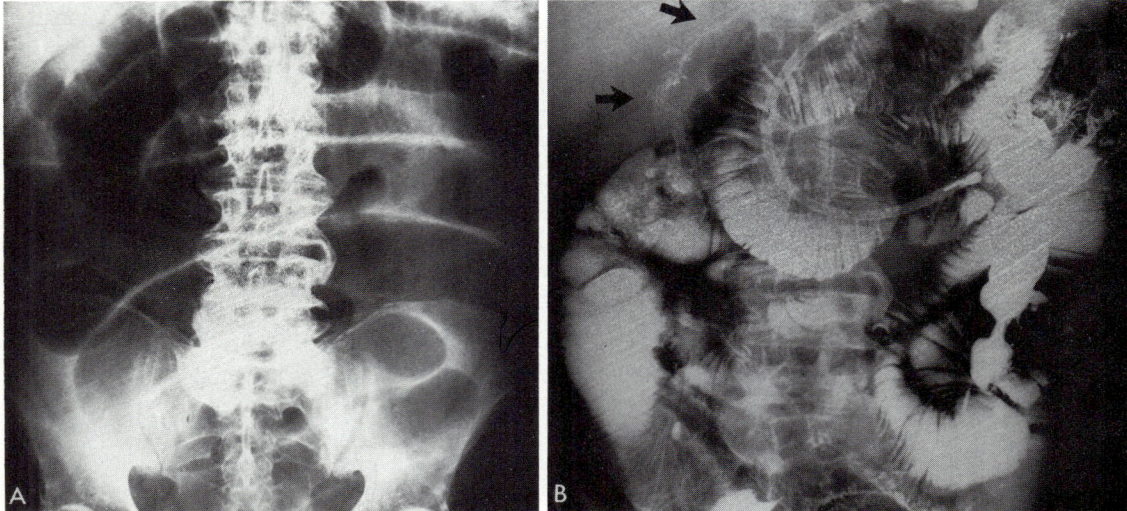

Figure 7–32. Foramen of Winslow hernia. *A,* Supine film of the abdomen reveals massive distention of the small bowel and absence of gas in the colon. *B,* A subsequent study with contrast material delineates the specific cause of the distal small bowel obstruction. The partially reduced and collapsed ileum and proximal colon (arrows) are seen to pass between the liver and duodenum in the direction of the foramen of Winslow.

placement of the stomach to the left and anteriorly by the mass of herniated loops. The first and second portions of the duodenum may also be deviated to the left side.[17, 21]

3. Small bowel series shows dilatation and hyperperistalsis of the more proximal small bowel loops owing to a mechanical obstruction at or near the location of the foramen of Winslow between the hilus of the liver and the duodenal bulb (Fig. 7–32).[17]

4. Barium enema examination may disclose a tapered narrowing or obstruction near the hepatic flexure if the cecum and ascending colon are among the herniated viscera.[10, 17, 21]

Pericecal Hernias

Four peritoneal fossae in the ileocecal region, as well as congenital and acquired defects in the mesentery of the cecum or appendix, may lead to development of a pericecal hernia.[34, 36, 43, 53, 55] The variety of other terms (ileocolic, retrocecal, ileocecal, paracecal) used to classify these hernias appear to have limited practical value in the radiologic differential diagnosis and surgical management.[17]

In the collective review of 467 internal hernias by Hansmann and Morton, 13 per cent involved the ileocecal region.[19] The clinical manifestations are usually intermittent episodes of right lower abdominal pain, tenderness, small bowel distention, nausea, and vomiting. Chronic incarceration may produce symptoms compatible with a periappendiceal abscess, Crohn's disease, or intestinal obstruction due to adhesions.[17, 36, 55]

In most cases, a portion of ileum passes through defects in the mesentery of the cecum to occupy the right paracolic gutter.[17, 36, 55] The correct diagnosis may be suggested on plain radiographs of the abdomen (Fig. 7–33). More useful are the delayed films of the small bowel series, or a barium enema examination in which reflux into the terminal ileum has been achieved. Careful fluoroscopic evaluation and radiographs in lateral and oblique projections are particularly valuable for the demonstration of the fixed position of herniated loops posterolateral to the cecum.[17]

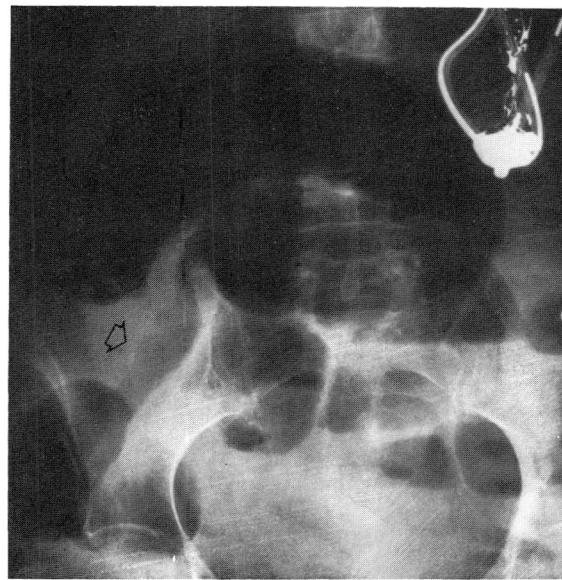

Figure 7–33. Pericecal hernia. The distal ileum protruding through a defect in the mesentery of the cecum is seen in the right lower abdomen, and there is gaseous distention of the proximal small intestine. The narrowed afferent segment of the herniated ileal loop (arrow) is identified. (*From* Ghahremani, G. G., and Meyers, M. A.: Internal abdominal hernias. Curr. Probl. Radiol. 5:1–30, 1975.)

Intersigmoid Hernias

The intersigmoid fossa is a peritoneal pouch formed between the two loops of the sigmoid colon and its mesentery. This pocket is found in 65 per cent of cadavers and serves as a potential site for an intersigmoid hernia.[7, 17, 55] This is usually a reducible hernia containing a few small bowel loops. Incarceration is surprisingly uncommon considering the high incidence of intersigmoid fossa among the general population.

The radiologic diagnosis of intersigmoid hernia is best made by retrograde filling of the small intestine during barium enema examination. Figure 7–34 shows the encapsulated ileal loops in a characteristic relationship to the sigmoid colon.

Two other similar, but rare, entities deserve a brief mention. These are (1) the *intramesosigmoid hernia,* which involves a defect of only one of the constituent mesenteric leaves, the separation of which forms the hernial sac,[7] and (2) the *transmesosigmoid hernia,* in which a usually large defect in both layers of the sigmoid mesentery allows herniation of the small bowel loops toward the left lower abdomen posterolateral to the sigmoid colon (Fig. 7–35).[7, 19, 36, 53]

It should be emphasized that radiologic differentiation of the three described types of hernia involving the mesosigmoid is often difficult and irrelevant in terms of their ultimate surgical management.[7, 34, 36, 53]

Transmesenteric Hernias

About 5 to 10 per cent of all internal hernias occur through defects in the mesentery of the small intestine.[19, 32, 53] An etiologic relationship to prenatal intestinal ischemic accidents seems probable, because such defects and associated herniation are frequently found adjacent to atretic intestinal segments in infants.[35] In fact, nearly 35 per cent of these hernias occur in the pediatric age group, in which they constitute the most common type of internal hernias.[35, 40] In adults, however, most of the mesenteric defects serving as the hernial ring are probably the result of previous surgery, abdominal trauma, or intraperitoneal inflammation.[32, 53]

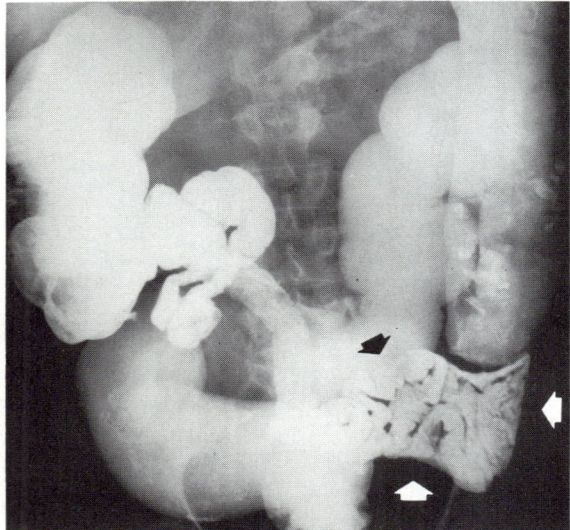

Figure 7–34. Intersigmoid hernia. Barium enema examination, with retrograde filling of the small bowel, shows the encapsulation of several ileal loops (arrows) within the intersigmoid fossa.

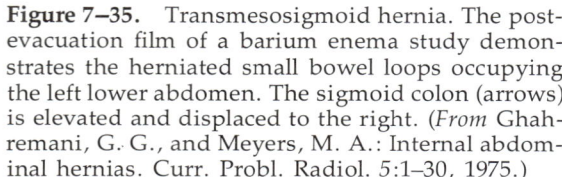

Figure 7–35. Transmesosigmoid hernia. The postevacuation film of a barium enema study demonstrates the herniated small bowel loops occupying the left lower abdomen. The sigmoid colon (arrows) is elevated and displaced to the right. (*From* Ghahremani, G. G., and Meyers, M. A.: Internal abdominal hernias. Curr. Probl. Radiol. 5:1–30, 1975.)

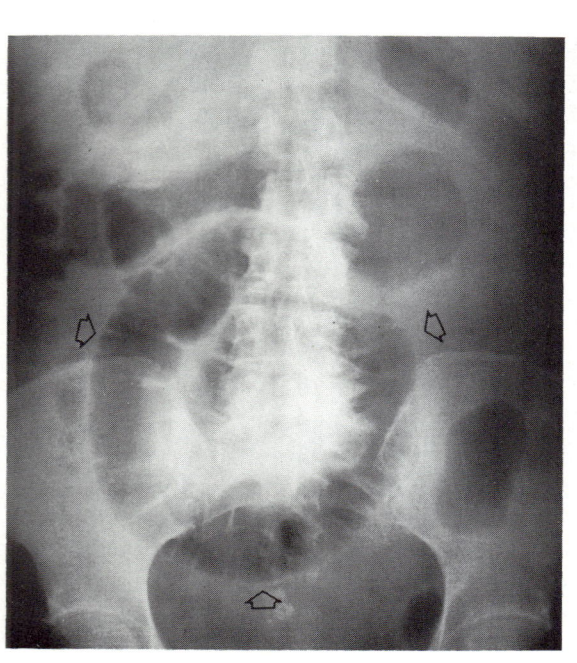

Figure 7–36. Herniation of a jejunal loop through a defect in the small bowel mesentery. Note the typical presentation of a distended closed loop (arrows) with approximation of its ends at the hernial orifice. (*From* Ghahremani, G. G., and Meyers, M. A.: Internal abdominal hernias. Curr. Probl. Radiol. 5:1–30, 1975.)

The mesenteric defects are often located close to the ligament of Treitz or the ileocecal valve.[17, 35, 43, 53] The usually small size of the defect and the absence of a limiting hernial sac accounts for a relatively high incidence of strangulation.[32, 35, 53] In such cases, the clinical presentation is severe periumbilical pain accompanied by small boel obstruction and hyperactive bowel sounds. A tender abdominal mass representing the Gordian knot of the herniated small intestine may occasionally be palpable.[40, 53]

Radiographs of the abdomen usually demonstrate mechanical small bowel obstruction and, occasionally, a single distended "closed loop" (Fig. 7–36). The small bowel series may further assist in the diagnosis by showing a constriction around the closely approximated afferent and efferent loops of the herniated intestine.[17, 43] These findings invariably signal a surgical emergency, although clinical and radiologic differentiation of the hernia from small bowel volvulus or entrapment beneath peritoneal adhesions may be impossible.[17] The early onset of strangulation and intestinal gangrene is a particular danger in cases of transmesenteric hernia.[32, 53] In fact, a mortality rate of about 50 per cent for surgically treated patients and 100 per cent for those without surgical treatment was found in a collective review of 95 patients.[32]

Retroanastomotic Hernias

These hernias are a well-recognized complication of gastrointestinal surgery.[20, 29, 33, 45]

The retroanastomotic hernias usually occur in patients who have undergone partial gastrectomy with gastrojejunostomy.[29, 33] It has been shown that patients who have antecolic gastrojejunostomies are particularly prone to this complication.[29] In both antecolic and retrocolic anastomosis, however, the superior border of the hernial ring is formed by the transverse mesocolon, the inferior border by the ligament of Treitz, and the anterior aspect by the gastrojejunostomy together with the afferent limb of the jejunum.[29]

The herniated loop is usually the efferent jejunal segment or, less commonly, an excessively long afferent limb that protrudes into the retroanastomotic space.[5, 17, 29] The herniation usually occurs in a right-to-left direction, so that the involved small bowel loops occupy the left upper quadrant of the abdomen (Fig. 7–37).

About half of these hernias manifest themselves within one month and another 25 per cent within one year after the operation.[45] The presenting symptoms are usually cramping abdominal pain and signs of a high small bowel obstruction. The herniated loops may sometimes be palpable as a tender mass in the left upper abdomen. In many instances, however, these nonspecific findings may be mistaken for stomal edema, dumping, or pancreatitis, and the correct diagnosis may be delayed until strangulation has developed.[5, 20, 29, 45] This contributes to the reported mortality rate of 32 per cent for surgically treated cases and almost 100 per cent for untreated patients.[29]

The correct diagnosis depends upon a careful fluoroscopic evaluation of the patient after the administration of contrast material. Prior knowledge of the type of surgical procedure performed is crucial in recognition of the radiologic findings, since the usual anatomic landmarks are absent or distorted. The examination discloses the fact that the obstruction is situated not at the gastric stoma but more distally in either of the anastomotic limbs. Gradual opacification of the partially obstructed efferent loop shows its abnormal position just lateral and posterior to the gastrojejunostomy (Fig. 7–37). Some degree of dilatation and stasis is usually associated. The diagnosis may be more difficult if the hernia involves the afferent limb.[5, 29] In such cases, the patency of the anastomosis and the efferent loop is easily demonstrated. Opacification of the afferent

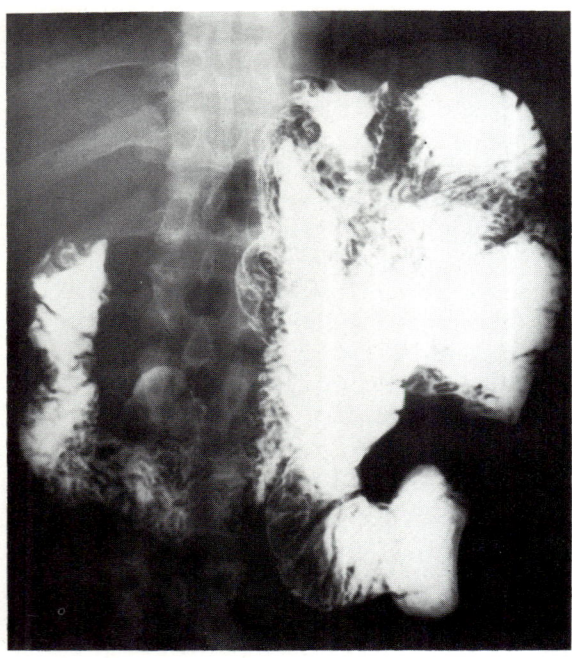

Figure 7–37. Retroanastomotic hernia in a patient with Billroth II gastrojejunostomy. The herniated efferent loop of jejunum forms a circumscribed mass in the left upper abdomen. The afferent loop with a duodenal diverticulum is also visualized.

limb itself may not occur or may be delayed, however. Clinically, these patients have rather constant pain and tenderness in the epigastrium, vomitus that does not contain bile, and usually, an elevated level of serum amylase.[29, 45]

An entity that must be differentiated from retroanastomotic hernia is the occasional herniation of both limbs of a gastrojejunostomy through the opening in the transverse mesocolon.[20] This is usually a complication of retrocolic anastomosis. In such cases, the upper gastrointestinal series shows a characteristic localized constriction and approximation of afferent and efferent loops a short distance below the site of anastomosis.[17, 20]

References

1. Akman, P. C.: A study of five hundred incisional hernias. J. Int. Coll. Surg. 37:125–142, 1962.
2. Avery, G. J., Berg, R. A., and Widmann, W. D.: The clinical value of pediatric herniography. Am. J. Dis. Child. 131:1255–1257, 1977.
3. Balison, J. R., Macgregor, A. M. C., and Woodward, E. R.: Postoperative diaphragmatic herniation following transthoracic fundoplication: a note of warning. Arch. Surg. 106:164–166, 1973.
4. Bell, J. W.: Chronically incarcerated hiatus hernia. Arch. Surg. 104:831–835, 1972.
5. Beranbaum, S. L., Lawrence, L., and Schwartz, S.: Roentgen exploration of the afferent loop. Radiology 91:932–941, 1968.
6. Berdon, W. E., Baker, D. H., and Amoury, R.: The rule of pulmonary hypoplasia in the prognosis of newborn infants with diaphragmatic hernia and eventration. Am. J. Roentgenol. 103:413–421, 1968.
7. Bertelsen, S., and Christiansen, J.: Internal hernia through mesenteric and mesocolic defects. A review of the literature and a report of two cases. Acta Chir. Scand. 133:426–428, 1967.
8. Bingham, J. A. W.: Herniation through congenital diaphragmatic defects. Br. J. Surg. 47:1–15, 1959.
9. Callander, C. L., Rusk, G. Y., and Nemir, A.: Mechanism, symptoms, and treatment of hernia into descending mesocolon (left duodenal hernia); plea for change in nomenclature. Surg. Gynecol. Obstet. 60:1052–1071, 1935.
10. Cimmino, C. V.: Lesser sac hernia via the foramen of Winslow. A case report. Radiology 60:57–59, 1953.
11. Ebert, P. A., Gaertner, R. A., and Zuidema, G. D.: Traumatic diaphragmatic hernia. Surg. Gynecol. Obstet. 125:59–65, 1967.
12. Efron, G., and Hyde, I.: Non-penetrating traumatic rupture of the diaphragm. Clin. Radiol. 18:394–398, 1967.

13. Filtzer, H., and Sedgewick, C. E.: Strangulated paraduodenal hernia. Report of a case. Surg. Clin. North Am. 53:371–374, 1973.
14. Fraser, R. G., and Paré, J. A. P.: Diagnosis of Diseases of the Chest. Vol. 2, Ed. 1. Philadelphia, W. B. Saunders Company, 1970, pp. 1224–1232.
15. Freund, H., and Berlatzky, Y.: Small paraduodenal hernias. Arch. Surg. 112:1180–1183, 1977.
16. Gerson, D. E., and Lewicki, A. M.: Intrathoracic stomach: when does it obstruct? Radiology 119:257–264, 1976.
17. Ghahremani, G. G., and Meyers, M. A.: Internal abdominal hernias. Curr. Probl. Radiol. 5:1–30, 1975.
18. Greenwood, R. D., Rosenthal, A., and Nadas, A. S.: Cardiovascular abnormalities associated with congenital diaphragmatic hernia. Pediatrics 57:92–97, 1976.
19. Hansmann, G. H., and Morton, S. A.: Intra-abdominal hernia. Report of a case and review of the literature. Arch. Surg. 39:973–986, 1939.
20. Hardy, J. D.: Problems associated with gastric surgery: review of 604 consecutive patients with annotation. Am. J. Surg. 108:699–716, 1964.
21. Henisz, A., Matesanz, J., and Westcott, J. L.: Cecal herniation through the foramen of Winslow. Radiology 112:575–578, 1974.
22. Holder, L. E., and Schneider, H. I.: Spigelian hernias: anatomy and roentgenographic manifestations. Radiology 112:309–313, 1974.
23. Hunter, T. B., Freundlich, I. M., and Zukoski, C. F.: Preoperative radiographic diagnosis of a spigelian hernia containing large and small bowel. Gastrointest. Radiol. 1:379–381, 1977.
24. Jones, T. W.: Paraduodenal hernia and hernias of the foramen of Winslow. In Nyhus, L. M., and Harkins, H. N. (eds.): Hernia. Philadelphia, J. B. Lippincott Company, 1964, pp. 577–601.
25. Keshishian, J. A., and Cox, P. A.: Diagnosis and management of strangulated diaphragmatic hernias. Surg. Gynecol. Obstet. 115:626–632, 1962.
26. Kozlowski, J. M., and Beal, J. M.: Obturator hernia. An elusive diagnosis. Arch. Surg. 112:1001–1002, 1977.
27. Lanuza, A.: The sign of the cane. A new radiological sign for the diagnosis of small Morgagni hernias. Radiology 101:293–296, 1971.
28. Liebeskind, A. L., Elkin, M., and Goldman, S. H.: Herniation of the bladder. Radiology 106:257–262, 1973.
29. Markowitz, A. M.: Retroanastomotic hernia. In Nyhus, L. M., and Harkins, H. N. (eds.): Hernia. Philadelphia, J. B. Lippincott Company, 1964, pp. 607–616.
30. Meyers, M. A.: Arteriographic diagnosis of internal (left paraduodenal) hernia. Radiology 92:1035–1037, 1969.
31. Meyers, M. A.: Paraduodenal hernias. Radiologic and arteriographic diagnosis. Radiology 95:29–37, 1970.
32. Mock, C. J., and Mock, H. E., Jr.: Strangulated internal hernia associated with trauma. Arch. Surg. 77:881–886, 1958.
33. Morton, C. B., Alrich, E. M., and Hill, L. D.: Internal hernia after gastrectomy. Ann. Surg. 141:759–764, 1955.
34. Mueller, E. C.: Congenital internal hernia. Am. J. Surg. 97:201–204, 1959.
35. Murphy, D. A.: Internal hernias in infancy and childhood. Surgery 55:311–315, 1964.
36. Nathan, H.: Internal hernia. J. Int. Coll. Surg. 34:563–571, 1960.
37. Nyhus, L. M., and Bombeck, C. T.: Hernias. In Sabiston, D. C., Jr.: Davis-Christopher Textbook of Surgery. The Biological Basis of Modern Surgical Practice. Philadelphia, W. B. Saunders Company, 1977, pp. 1335–1360.
38. Oh, K. S., Dorst, J. P., White, J. J., et al.: Positive-contrast peritoneography and herniography. Radiology 108:643–654, 1973.
39. Parsons, P. B.: Paraduodenal hernias. Am. J. Roentgenol. 69:563–589, 1953.
40. Pennell, T. C., and Shaffner, L. S.: Congenital internal hernia. Surg. Clin. North Am. 51:1355–1359, 1971.
41. Pollack, H. M., Popky, G. L., and Blumberg, M. L.: Hernias of the ureter. An anatomic-roentgenographic study. Radiology 117:275–281, 1975.
42. Reed, J. O., and Lang, E. F.: Diaphragmatic hernia in infancy. Am. J. Roentgenol. 82:437–449, 1959.
43. Rooney, J. A., Carroll, J. P., and Keeley, J. L.: Internal hernias due to defects in the meso-appendix and mesentery of small bowel, and probably Ivemark syndrome. Report of two cases. Ann. Surg. 157:254–258, 1963.
44. Rowe, M. I., Copelson, L. W., and Clatworthy, H. w., jr.: The patent processus vaginalis and the inguinal hernia. J. Pediatr. Surg. 4:102–107, 1969.
45. Sabesta, D. G., and Robson, M. C.: Petersen's retroanastomotic hernia. Am. J. Surg. 116:450–453, 1968.
46. Smith, L., and Lippert, K. M.: Peritoneo-pericardial diaphragmatic hernia. Ann. Surg. 148:798–804, 1958.
47. Sufian, S., and Matsumoto, T.: Intestinal obstruction. Am. J. Surg. 130:9–14, 1975.
48. Swischuk, L. E., and Stacy, T. M.: Herniography: radiologic investigation of inguinal hernia. Radiology 101:139–146, 1971.
49. Turner, F. W.: Gangrene and rupture of the stomach secondary to jejunal obstruction by an internal (paraduodenal) hernia: a case report. Can. J. Surg. 15:118–120, 1972.
50. Wallgast, G. F., and Hilts, J. M.: Littre's hernia, strangulation of Meckel's diverticulum in a femoral hernia and inguinal hernia. Am. Surg. 28:741–744, 1962.

51. Wang, C. A., and Welch, C. E.: Anomalies of intestinal rotation in adolescents and adults. Surgery 54:839–855, 1963.
52. Williams, A. J.; roentgen diagnosis of intra-abdominal hernia. An evaluation of the roentgen findings. Radiology 59:817–825, 1952.
53. Winterscheid, L. C.: Mesenteric hernia. In Nyhus, L. M., and Harkins, H. N. (eds.): Hernia, Philadelphia, J. B. Lippincott Company, 1964, pp. 602–605.
54. Zimmerman, L. M., and Anson, B. J.: Anatomy and Surgery of Hernia. Ed. 2. Baltimore, Williams & Wilkins Company, 1967.
55. Zimmerman, L. M., and Laufman, H.: Intra-abdominal hernias due to developmental and rotational anomalies. Ann. Surg. 138:82–91, 1953.

8

THE ESOPHAGUS

JOVITAS SKUCAS, M.D.
ROSCOE E. MILLER, M.D.

Part I

Disorders of Esophageal Motility

INTRODUCTION

The esophagus is a continuation of the hypopharynx and starts at the level of the cricopharyngeal muscle, at the level of the fifth and sixth cervical vertebrae. Narrow segments in the esophagus due to impressions of the aortic arch and left bronchus vary in extent among patients. The aortic arch impression, in particular, tends to be exaggerated in older people. At times, both of these impressions blend together to produce one smooth homogeneous narrowing in the midesophagus.

The heart, especially if enlarged, can produce an impression along the anterior margin of the lower third of the esophagus (Fig. 8–1). Fluoroscopy of this area in the lateral projection shows pulsations of the anterior wall of the esophagus synchronous with cardiac pulsations.

Air in the esophagus on routine chest films is not unusual; it can be seen even in the absence of disease.

The anatomy of the esophagus is best demonstrated with the patient in an upright position. With the patient thus positioned, however, gravity plays a large role in the progression of a bolus of food or barium, and if a motility disorder is suspected, the esophagus should also be studied with the patient recumbent. In the upright position, liquids travel through the esophagus faster than the primary peristaltic wave; the faster transit is the result of both gravity and the rapid contraction of the upper esophageal sphincter. The liquid bolus normally does not enter the stomach immediately, however, but is held up in the distal esophagus until the primary peristaltic wave reaches this area. At that time, the gastroesophageal junction opens and the bolus passes into

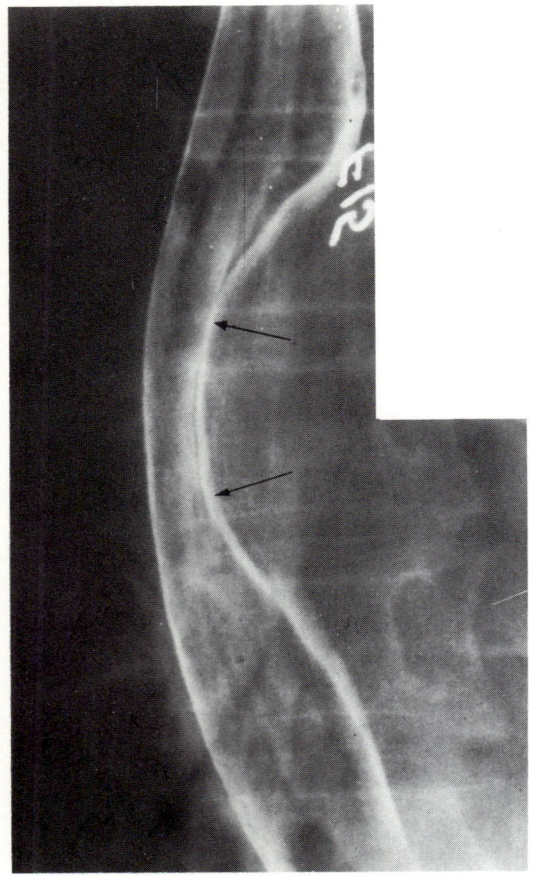

Figure 8–1. Esophageal displacement by an enlarged heart (arrows). (*From* Skucas, J.: The routine double-contrast examination of the esophagus. C.R.C. Crit. Rev. Diagn. Imaging *11*:121–143, 1978.)

the stomach. When the patient is in the recumbent position, a liquid, such as a barium sulfate suspension, normally travels at the speed of the primary peristaltic wave.

DISORDERS OF THE UPPER ESOPHAGEAL SPHINCTER

The upper esophageal sphincter is normally in a contracted state except during swallowing. Uncoordinated contractions, hypotonic contractions of the pharyngeal muscles, or failure of the cricopharyngeal muscle to relax may result in dysphagia and aspiration.

Some diseases involving the nervous system, such as poliomyelitis, multiple sclerosis, or a cerebrovascular accident, may result in dysphagia. After a high unilateral cervical vagotomy the cricopharyngeus may not relax.[18] Similar findings may be seen in cases of tumor involvement of the vagus nerve. If the involvement is sufficiently severe, aspiration can occur. Small amounts of aspirated material are best identified in a lateral projection (Fig. 8–2). Normally, contrast in the trachea induces vigorous coughing spasms. Intrabronchial impaction of barium sulfate is not a problem, since the barium compound does not dehydrate (Fig. 8–3).[9] In fact, there have been numerous studies advocating the use of barium sulfate as a bronchographic agent.[12,13] Of greater

THE ESOPHAGUS — 321

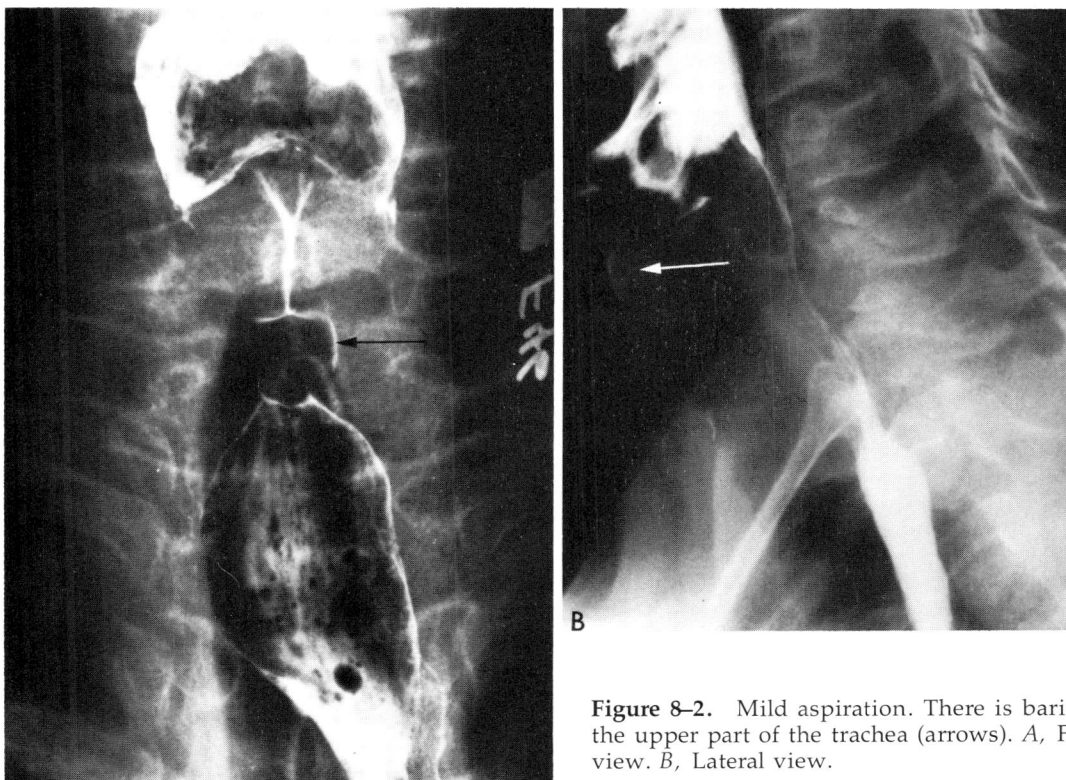

Figure 8–2. Mild aspiration. There is barium in the upper part of the trachea (arrows). *A,* Frontal view. *B,* Lateral view.

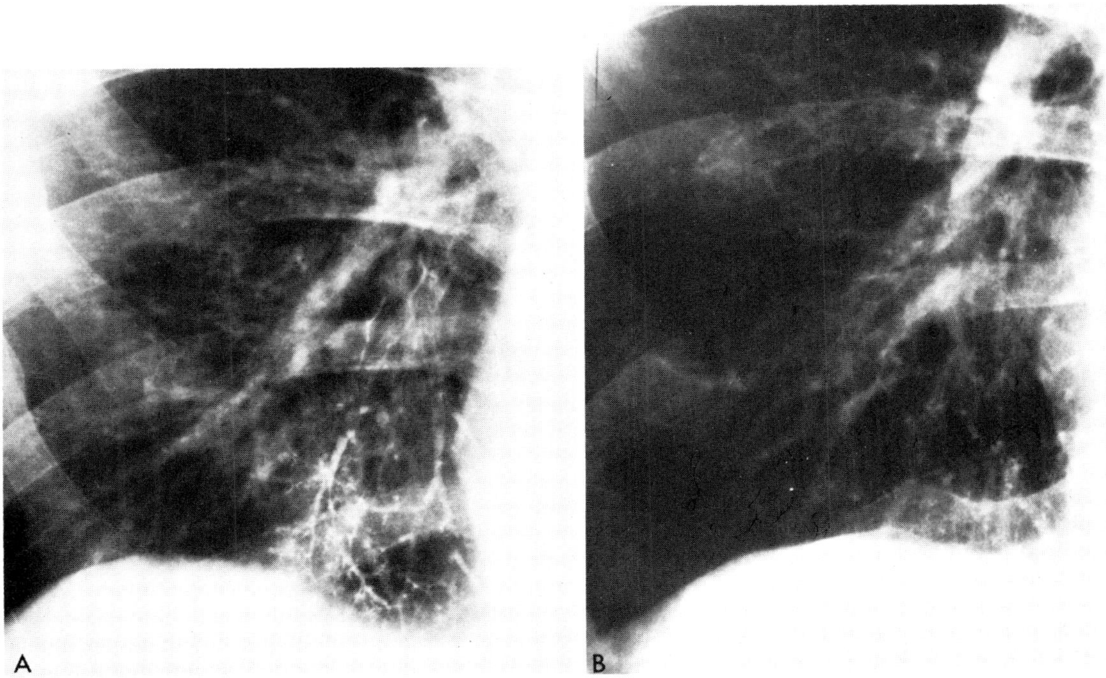

Figure 8–3. Aspiration. *A,* This radiograph was obtained immediately after a barium esophagogram and shows barium in the right lower lobe bronchi. *B,* Several hours later there has been almost complete clearing.

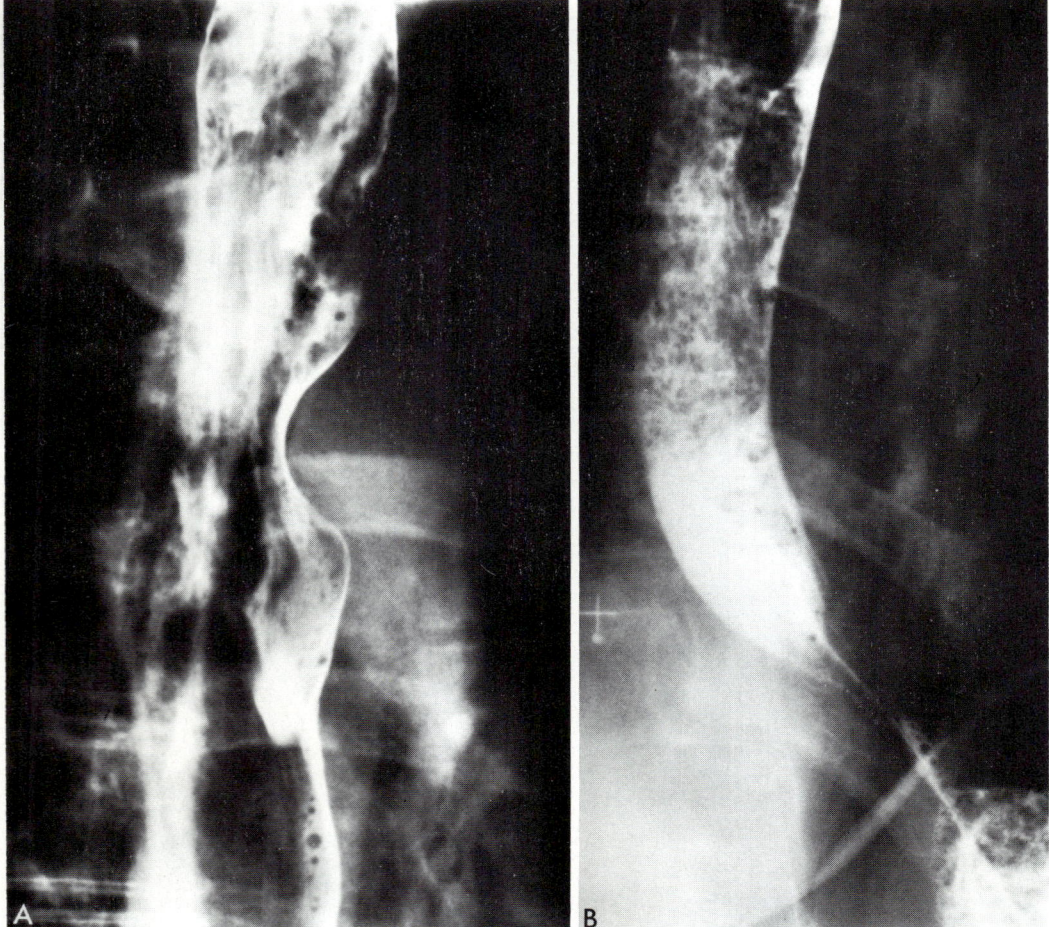

Figure 8–4. Myotonic dystrophy. Proximal (A) and distal (B) views of the esophagus in a 56-year-old woman show considerable dilatation, presence of secretions, and absent peristalsis. The esophageal contents emptied into the stomach mostly by gravity. There was no peristalsis even in the proximal part of the esophagus.

concern is the commonly associated recurrent aspiration of saliva and ingested liquids. This can lead to pulmonary atelectasis, bronchiectasis, pneumonia, or lung abscess.

Neuromuscular disorders may involve the pharyngoesophageal striated muscles only, both the striated and the smooth muscles, or only the smooth muscles of the esophagus. As an example, myotonic dystrophy can lead to dysphagia because of the involvement of the striated muscles or of both striated and smooth muscles (Fig. 8–4). The primary peristaltic wave is not initiated in 50 per cent of these patients.[19] The cricopharyngeal muscle seems relaxed in some myotonic patients, leading to regurgitation from the esophagus into the pharynx.

The pharyngeal muscles may be directly affected by diseases such as muscular dystrophy or dermatomyositis. The result is insufficient contraction of these muscles and stasis.

Abnormal function of the cricopharyngeal muscles is best evaluated in the lateral projection with the patient drinking a bolus of barium (Fig. 8–5). Although simple spot filming can be sufficient, a small-format camera at three to six frames per second, video tape, or cine recording is useful.

A myotomy may relieve obstruction at the cricopharyngeal level; the myotomy is helpful only if the other pharyngeal swallowing reflexes are intact, however. Thus, if the swallowing mechanism is also uncoordinated, aspiration can still occur in spite of a successful myotomy.[2, 3] Similarly, with significant tongue involvement, myotomy may be of little value.

Ideally, after a cricopharyngeal myotomy no residual narrowing should be seen. At times, however, varying degrees of failure of relaxation of the cricopharyngeal muscle persist.

After extensive pharyngeal and laryngeal surgery, dysphagia may be due to failure of the cricopharyngeal muscle to relax. Consequently, some surgeons advocate a cricopharyngeal myotomy when performing a laryngectomy to avoid subsequent dysphagia.[14]

ACHALASIA

Achalasia produces a functional obstruction of the distal esophagus, with dilatation proximally. The degree of dilatation varies with the duration and severity of the

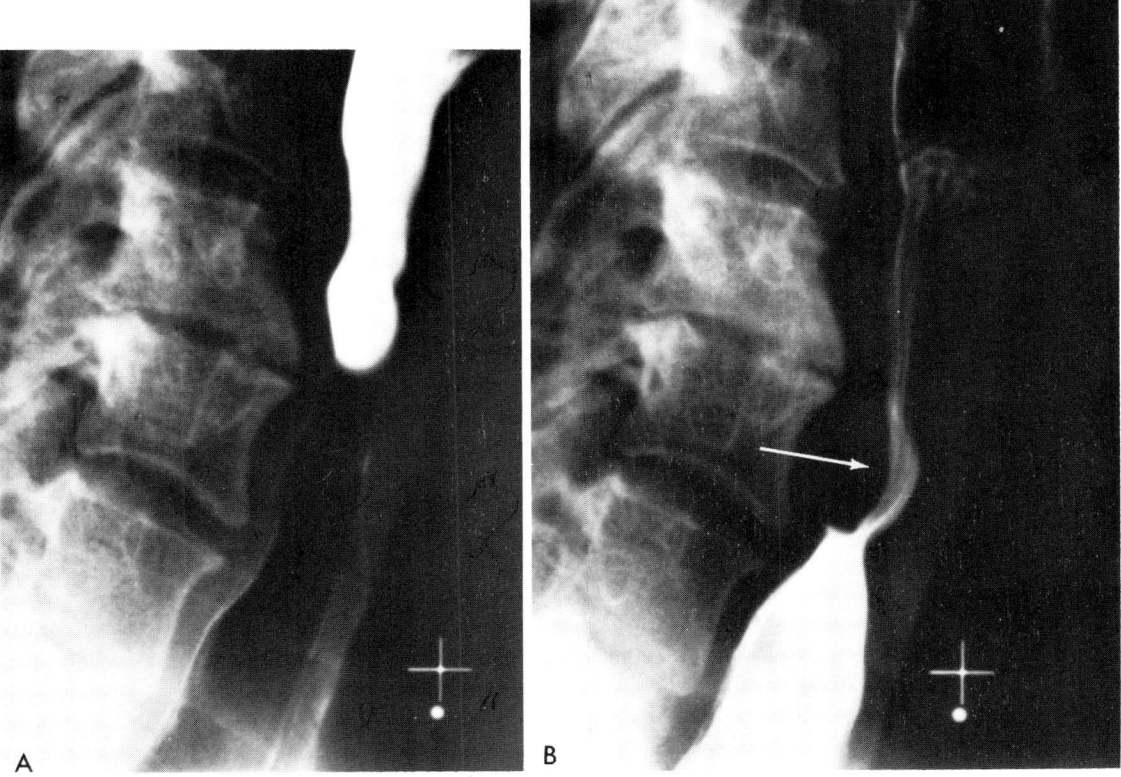

Figure 8–5. Prominent cricopharyngeal impression. A, The esophagus is distended by barium and air, and the cricopharyngeus muscle is relaxed. B, Immediately after the passage of the barium bolus there is a rather prominent contraction of the cricopharyngeus muscle (arrow).

disease. The disease involves the entire esophagus and is not limited to the gastroesophageal junction as was formerly thought.

Achalasia is generally a disease of adults; involvement in childhood is rare. Six cases of an infantile form, an autosomal recessive disorder, have been reported.[23]

Other names used in the past for achalasia include cardiospasm, megaesophagus, phrenospasm, esophageal dystonia, esophagectasia, and neuropathic dilatation.

In some South American countries, especially Brazil, a form of infection with *Trypanosoma cruzi* (Chagas' disease) may produce changes in the esophagus that are radiographically indistinguishable from achalasia. Occasionally, Chagas' disease is encountered also in the United States.

The diagnosis of achalasia usually can be readily made during esophagography (Fig. 8–6). There is considerable retained residue in a greatly dilated esophagus. At times, aspiration pneumonia occurs. There are weak, irregular, and ineffective contractions of the esophagus. Normal peristaltic waves are not seen. With the patient in a recumbent position, little barium enters the stomach. The distal segment of the esophagus dilates only intermittently, allowing the esophageal contents to spill into the stomach. In the upright position, usually a long column of barium is necessary to overcome the narrowed distal segment, and the esophagus still does not empty completely. The narrowed distal segment tends to change slightly, and considerable patience is required to show this segment even partially distended. The gastric air bubble can be either small or completely absent.

Radiographic aids can be used to help diagnose achalasia. Previously, methacholine (Mecholyl) was injected subcutaneously, producing extensive contractions

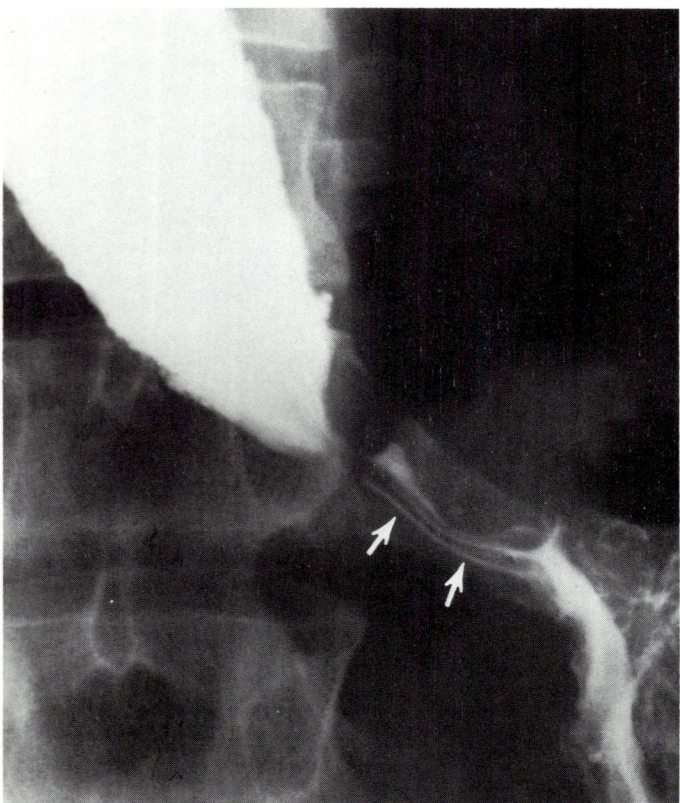

Figure 8–6. Achalasia. This 32-year-old man had progressive dysphagia. The esophagus is considerably dilated proximally, with a narrowed segment in the most distal portion (arrows). The esophageal folds in the narrowed region appear intact, and this area did distend slightly. No. peristalsis was seen.

throughout the esophagus. These contractions were still uncoordinated, did not result in significant esophageal emptying, and were associated with chest pain. A simpler test, which can be performed routinely, is to give the patient a dose of Seidlitz. The Seidlitz solutions, which consist of separate portions of tartaric acid and sodium bicarbonate, release carbon dioxide in the esophagus and result in marked distention. The rapid distention opens the narrowed lower segment, allowing adequate filling and subsequent emptying of the proximal esophagus.

There is an increased incidence of malignancy in long-standing achalasia. In one series, the time interval between the diagnosis of achalasia and subsequent carcinoma was 28 years.[24] Residual food in the dilated esophagus may hide a carcinoma, making diagnosis difficult.

A variant of the typically encountered achalasia is the so-called *vigorous achalasia*; in this condition there are powerful and uncoordinated spastic contractions throughout the esophagus. Radiologically, it can be difficult to differentiate vigorous achalasia from diffuse esophageal spasm, although there is dilatation of the esophagus in vigorous achalasia.[17]

The differential diagnosis of achalasia includes scleroderma, carcinoma, and numerous other inflammatory and neuromuscular diseases.

In scleroderma the distal segment is initially not narrowed. Later narrowing may occur because of the commonly associated reflux esophagitis. With a gaping esophageal junction there should be little confusion, but during the late stages after stricture development the differentiation can be difficult. Achalasia results in absent peristalsis throughout the esophagus, however; in cases of scleroderma the proximal one third has normal motility.

A tumor originating in the stomach or distal esophagus may invade the esophageal submucosa or muscle layers and mimic achalasia. Such secondary achalasia may even respond to the methacholine or Seidlitz test.[22] Rigidity of the esophagus or intraluminal polyps should be viewed with suspicion. Since the bulk of the tumor can be in the submucosa or muscle layers, even endoscopic biopsy may not initially reveal the malignancy.

Decreased peristalsis can also be seen with diabetes, chronic alcoholism, and such nervous system disease as parkinsonism. Myasthenia gravis produces feeble peristalsis in the striated upper portion of the esophagus; subsequent peristaltic waves can become weaker than the initial one. Lack of peristalsis can also be seen with reflux esophagitis and with the ingestion of corrosives.[20] The aperistalsis can be transient, or the inflammatory changes can progress to eventual stricture formation.

Treatment

The distal segment appears to be wider after therapeutic dilatation. The proximal portion still reveals abnormal contractions and dilatation; its diameter may decrease depending upon the effectiveness of the dilatation, however (Fig. 8–7).

Pneumatic dilatation of the esophagus in patients with achalasia can be associated with episodes of bradycardia. It has been suggested that premedication with atropine precede dilatation.[11]

In far-advanced disease there can be massive dilatation and elongation of the esophagus (Fig. 8–8). The most distal segment assumes a horizontal position, producing a 90 degree angulation at this level. Blind instrumentation of this segment can result in perforation; fluoroscopy, at times with varying amounts of a contrast medium, can aid in the successful passage into the stomach.

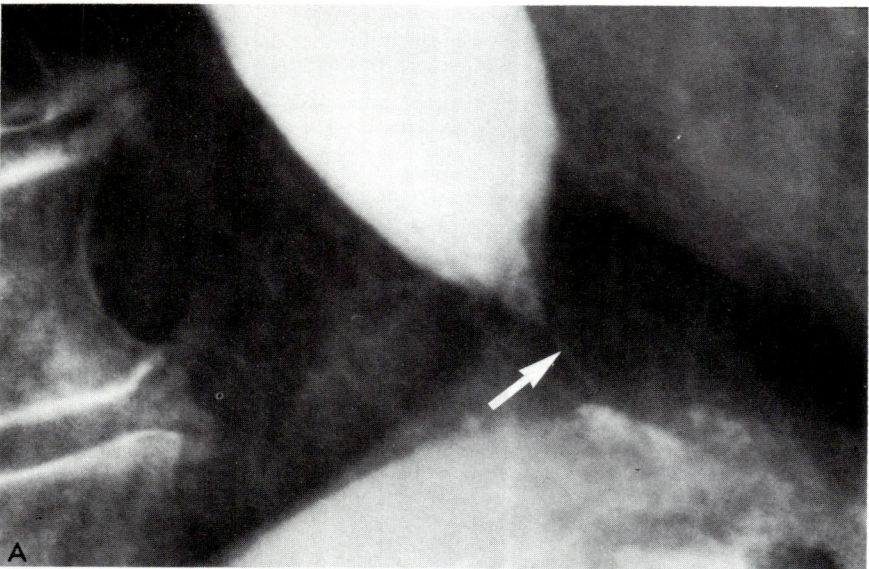

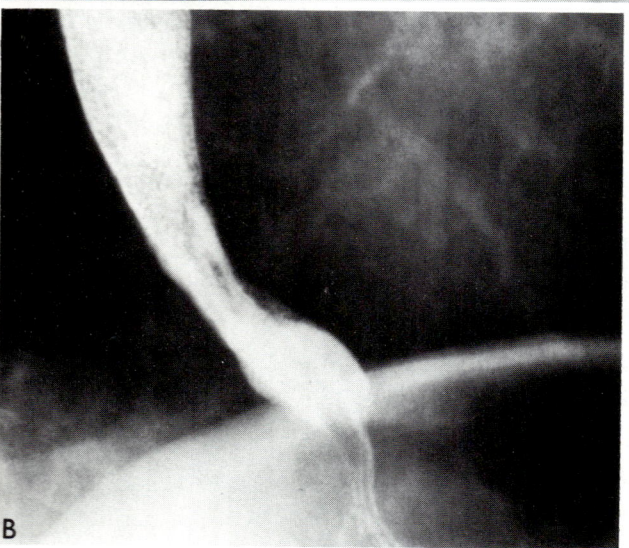

Figure 8–7. Achalasia. *A*, A 61-year-old man with long-standing achalasia has a dilated esophagus and a smoothly tapered distal section (arrow). There was no peristalsis present. *B*, After dilatation, the esophagus empties readily and is no longer as dilated, and the previously narrowed segment is considerably wider. No peristalsis was seen, however, the esophagus simply emptying passively by gravity.

Perforation following instrumentation can be limited to the wall of the esophagus, or it can extend into the mediastinum, pleural space, or occasionally even the peritoneal cavity. Small localized mucosal tears limited to the wall of the esophagus are not uncommon, are generally asymptomatic, and clear spontaneously with no therapy. Complete perforations, on the other hand, can rapidly lead to mediastinal widening and emphysema, or a pneumothorax, or both. Pneumoperitoneum can appear from a leak below the diaphragm.

The Heller esophagomyotomy, consisting of a longitudinal incision through the muscle of the distal esophagus, produces few postoperative radiologic signs. The previously narrowed segment may be wider (Fig. 8–9). There may be postoperative gastroesophageal reflux, unless an antireflux operation has also been performed. The dilated proximal esophagus may slowly decrease in caliber, usually during a period of weeks or months. The abnormal esophageal peristalsis remains unchanged, however. Some patients show little improvement after surgery (Fig. 8–10).

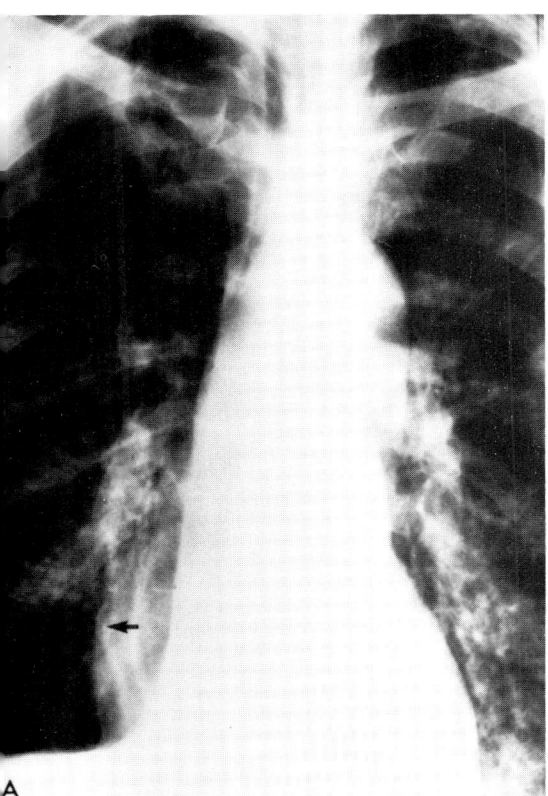
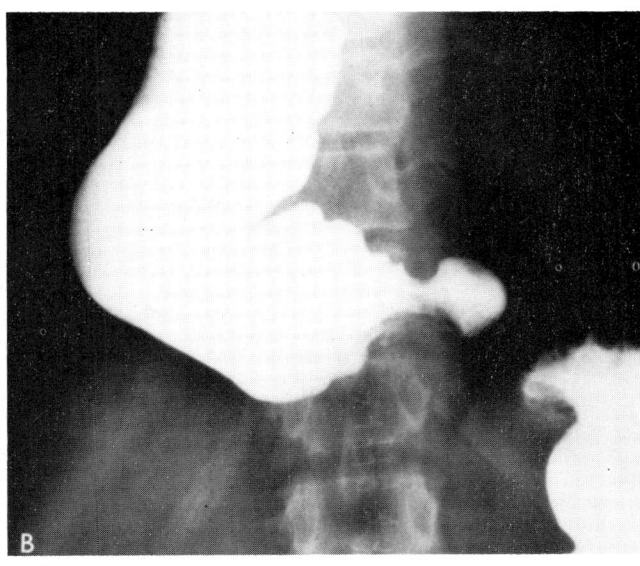

Figure 8–8. Far-advanced achalasia. *A,* A frontal chest film reveals a mottled appearance at the left base resulting from aspiration and a soft-tissue mass extending to the right of the mediastinum (arrow). *B,* An esophagogram shows the soft-tissue mass to be a greatly dilated esophagus. This 47-year-old man has already had a myotomy, with little improvement.

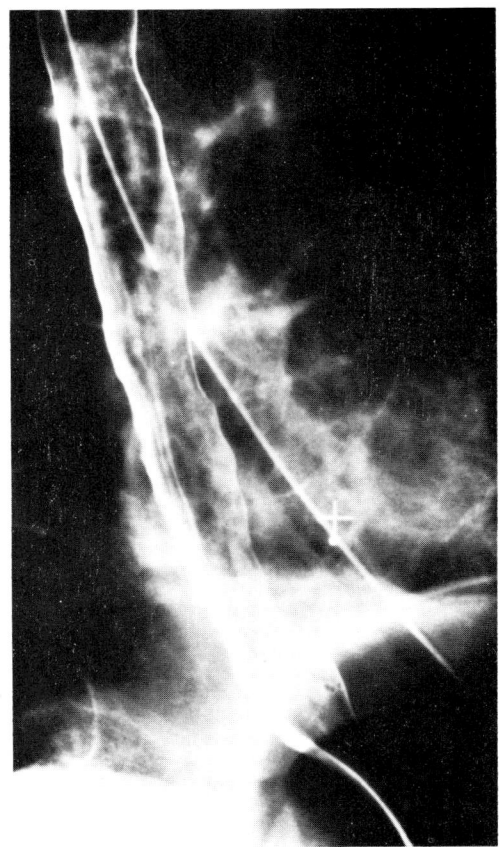

Figure 8–9. Post-Heller myotomy for achalasia. Same patient as shown in Fig. 8–7. Dysphagia recurred after dilatation, and the patient eventually underwent surgery. A postoperative esophagogram reveals a widely patent distal esophagus and a normal esophageal caliber. No peristalsis was present.

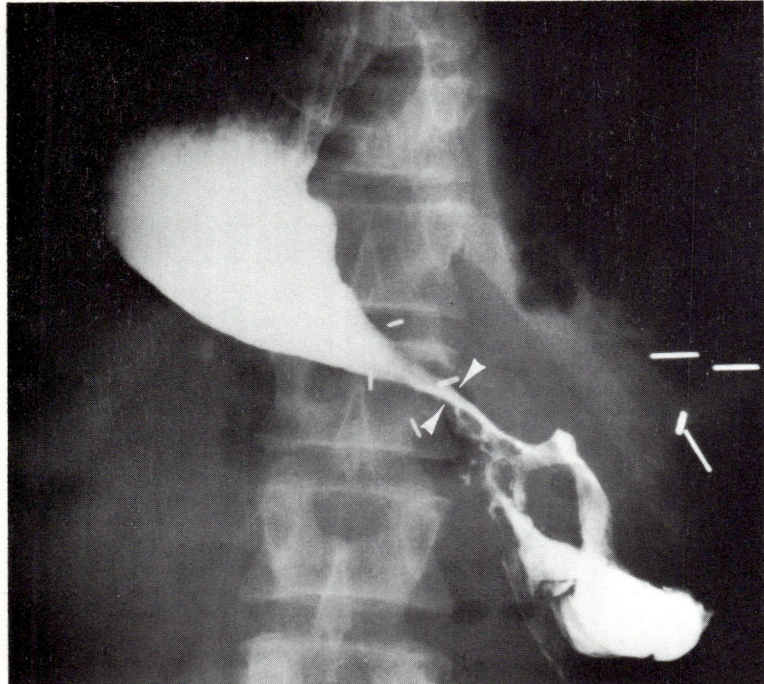

Figure 8–10. Megaesophagus due to achalasia. This 48-year-old man had undergone a Heller myotomy, partial gastrectomy, and more recently, an esophagojejunostomy. The anastomosis (arrowheads) is narrowed and the esophagus dilated.

DIFFUSE ESOPHAGEAL SPASM

In this disorder the esophagus contracts strongly but irregularly, producing no true peristaltic waves. Synonyms for this disorder include pseudodiverticulosis, tertiary esophagus, segmental spasms, primary disordered motor activity, functional diverticula, and corkscrew esophagus. The specific cause is not known. Dysphagia to both

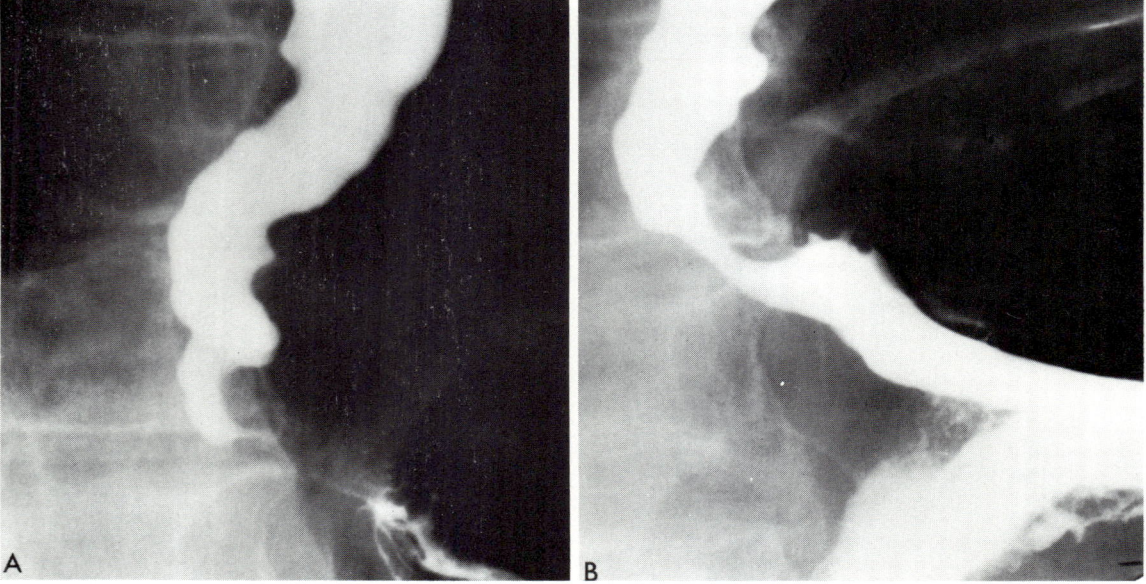

Figure 8–11. Diffuse esophageal spasm. A 70-year-old man had intermittent dysphagia and pain. An esophagogram reveals irregular and uncoordinated contractures in the lower esophagus. Although the distal portion of the esophagus is narrowed this segment did distend (A), and there is no proximal dilatation (B), distinguishing this entity from achalasia.

solids and liquids and associated weight loss may be present. The episodes of marked contraction may be associated with severe chest pain.[6, 8] The abnormality is usually limited to the lower two thirds of the esophagus (Fig. 8–11). There may be a considerable delay in the progression of barium, although the lower esophageal sphincter does relax. With long-standing disease there is considerable thickening of the esophageal wall, which can be identified between the intraluminal barium and the adjacent lung.[7, 10] Little or no dilatation is present. The marked irregular nonperistaltic contractions with intervening dilatations mimic diverticula. The outpouchings tend to appear at the same sites. Frequently, a small hiatus hernia is an associated finding.

The radiologic changes should be correlated with the patient's clinical status; at times, severe changes are seen radiologically although the patient is asymptomatic. Esophagoscopic findings are usually nonspecific.[6, 8]

Simple tertiary peristalsis, commonly called presbyesophagus or ripple esophagus, is not synonymous with diffuse esophageal spasm. Presbyesophagus is seen in older patients and usually is asymptomatic. The tertiary contractions are generally transient in nature, the esophageal wall is not thickened, and the spasm is not as striking (Fig. 8–12).

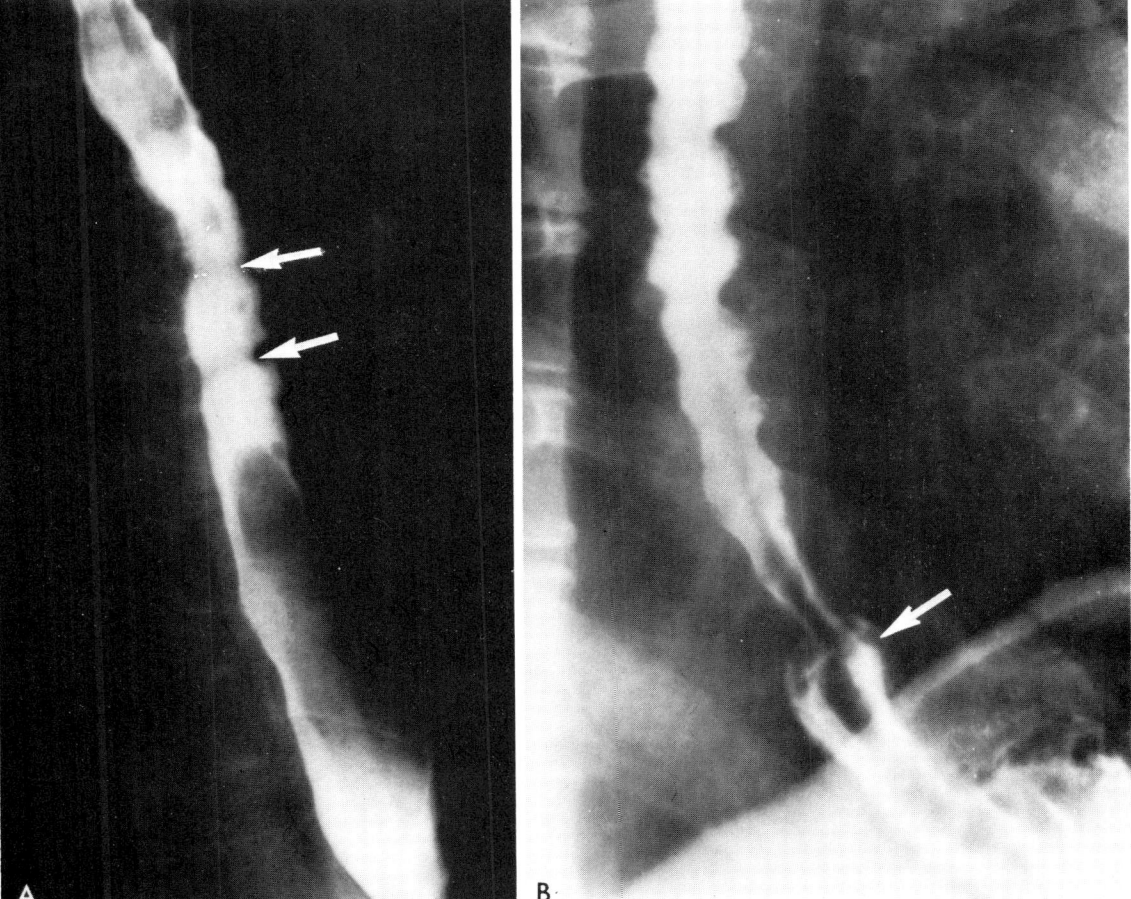

Figure 8–12. Presbyesophagus. Two different elderly patients exhibit intermittent tertiary contractions throughout the lower half of the esophagus. *A,* The tertiary contractions are mild (arrows), and peristalsis is present. *B,* More pronounced tertiary contractions are present, there is a hiatus hernia (arrow), and no peristalsis is seen in this more severely affected patient.

REFLUX ESOPHAGITIS

Reflux esophagitis may result from prior surgery in the gastroesophageal region or from systemic diseases such as scleroderma; it may be associated with a hiatus hernia or may be present without any other lesion. The reflux is best evaluated during fluoroscopy and recorded on cine or video tape.

Minimal pathologic changes of esophagitis limited to the mucosa produce no identifiable radiographic changes. The earliest radiologic change is hypoperistalsis.[20] At times the radiologist can simply take his time in obtaining numerous and different views of the esophagus without having the patient swallow any additional contrast agent. At least a portion of the study should be performed with the patient in the recumbent position, since gravity then plays no part and the hypoperistalsis is better visualized. The hypoperistalsis or even aperistalsis may be a transient phenomenon that eventually regresses, or it may lead to further complications. One may see nonperistaltic contractions or motor incoordination in the lower esophagus.

The endoscopic diagnosis of early esophagitis is also not foolproof, since there can be considerable discrepancy between the endoscopic diagnosis and the histologic findings of an accompany biopsy. The biopsy may not reveal significant inflammation of the mucosa, yet the endoscopist will describe a graphic picture of "diffuse inflammation."

The first anatomic change seen can be an irregularity of the lower esophageal folds (Fig. 8–13). At times, ulcers are present in the lower portion of the esophagus (Fig. 8–14). Although there may be considerable spasm present in the esophagus, this can usually be overcome by a large bolus of barium.

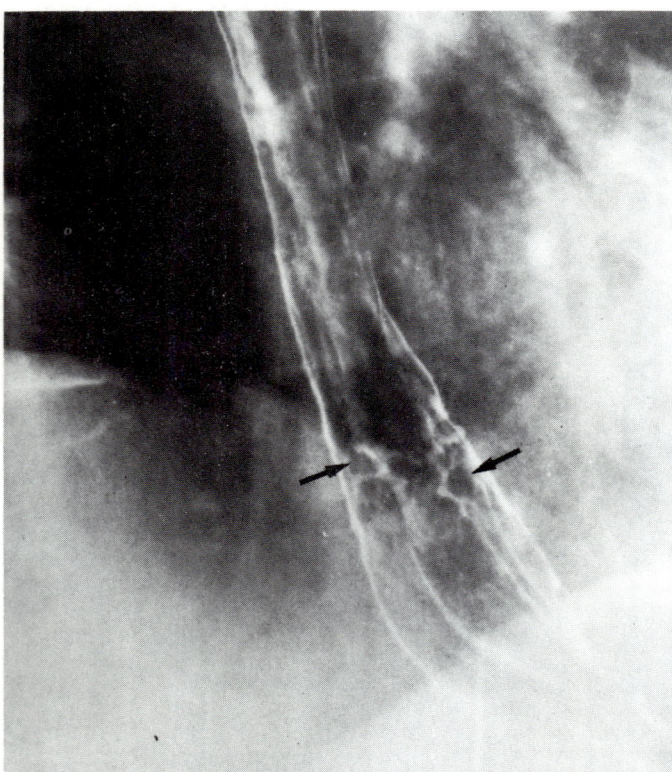

Figure 8–13. Reflux esophagitis. A small hiatus hernia is present. There are irregular folds and plaque-like defects throughout the gastroesophageal junction area (arrows). (*From* Skucas, J.: The routine double-contrast examination of the esophagus. C.R.C. Crit. Rev. Diagn. Imaging, *11*:121–143, 1978.)

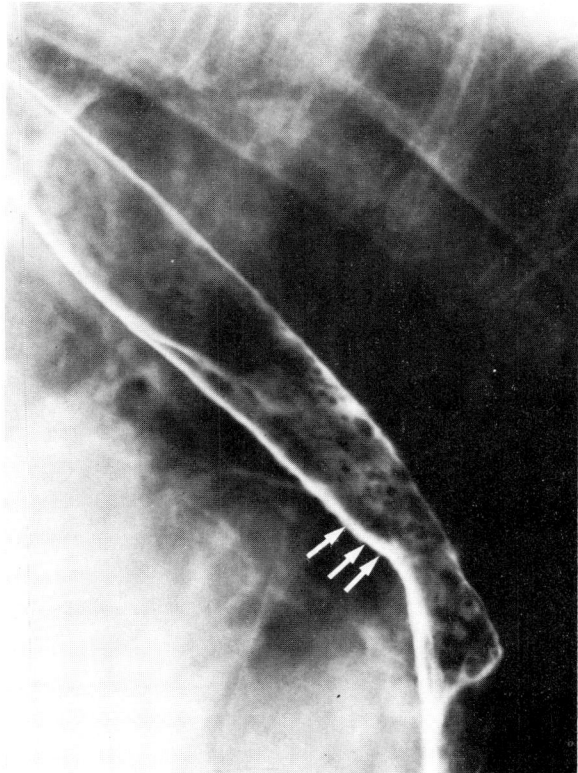

Figure 8–14. Reflux esophagitis with ulceration. Small irregular ulcers are present in the lower esophagus (arrows). (*From* Skucas, J.: The routine double-contrast examination of the esophagus. C.R.C. Crit. Rev. Diagn. Imaging, *11*:121–143, 1978.)

With further progression of the disease, there is fibrosis and narrowing of the esophageal lumen. The narrowing generally is smooth and symmetric, although occasionally a highly asymmetric stricture can be seen.

The patient's initial presentation may be the result of food impaction proximal to the stenotic segment. Occasionally the obstruction may be relieved through the use of glucagon, which acts as an antispasmodic agent.[5] The radiologic appearance of the esophagus after antireflux surgical procedures is discussed in the section on hiatus hernia (p. 361).

A nasogastric tube may result in reflux, followed by esophagitis and eventual ulcers or stricture. It is not unusual to see marked gastroesophageal reflux in the presence of a nasogastric tube. The onset of esophagitis can be insidious, a resultant severe stricture being the first clue to the extensive damage produced.

CONNECTIVE TISSUE DISORDERS

Several connective tissue disorders can involve the esophagus and produce dysphagia. Poor peristaltic activity is classically associated with scleroderma; occasionally, however, it is also associated with systemic lupus erythematosus or even with Raynaud's phenomenon without other disease being present.[21] In scleroderma, the disease is usually limited to the lower two thirds of the esophagus. Peristaltic activity is diminished and becomes totally absent in advanced disease, giving rise to an atonic, moderately dilated esophagus. Air may be seen in the esophagus on the chest film,

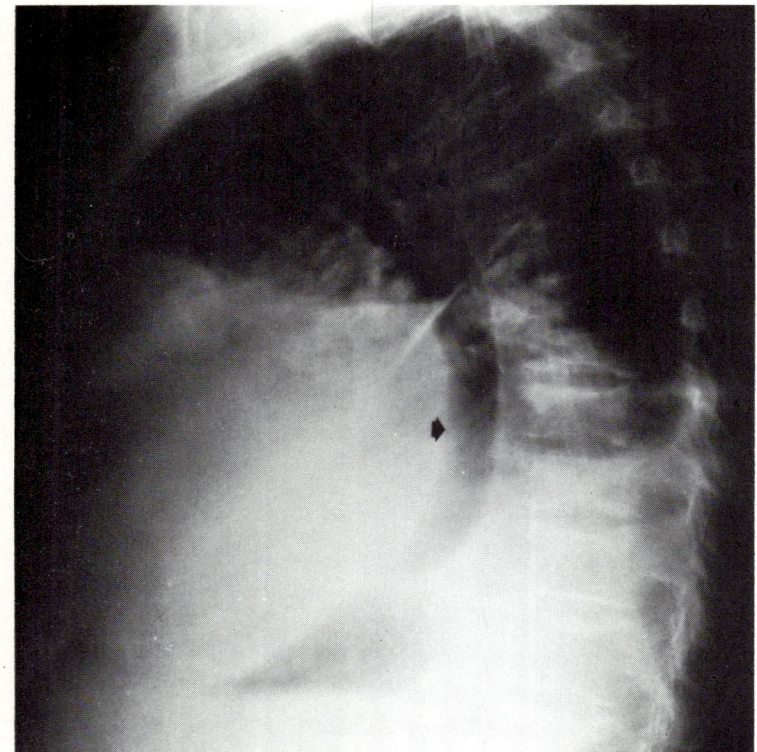

Figure 8–15. Scleroderma. An air-esophagogram is present (arrowhead). There is also extensive pulmonary disease.

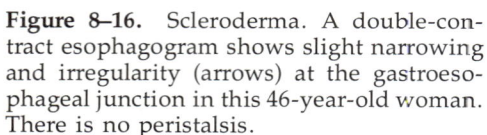

Figure 8–16. Scleroderma. A double-contract esophagogram shows slight narrowing and irregularity (arrows) at the gastroesophageal junction in this 46-year-old woman. There is no peristalsis.

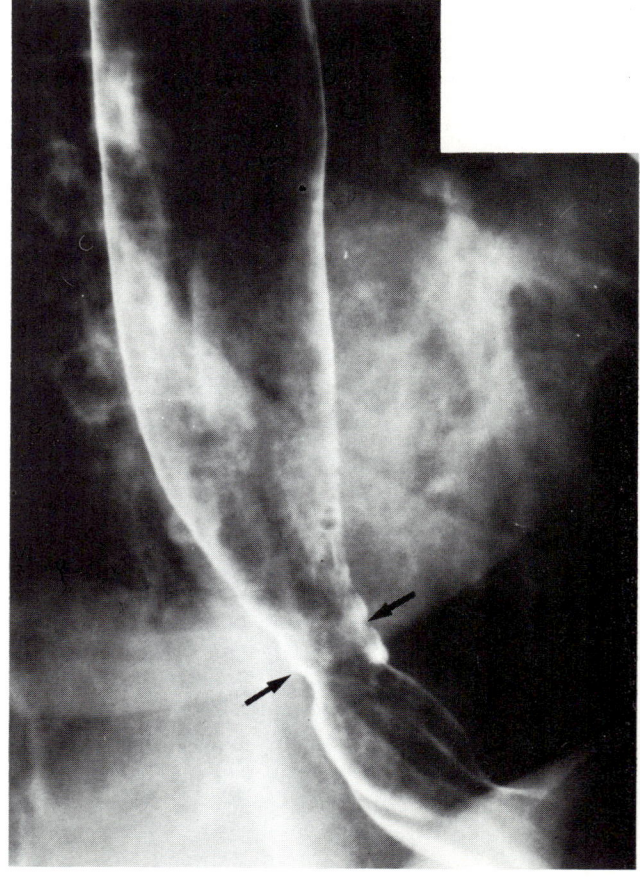

Figure 8–17. Scleroderma with stricture. There is a stricture at the gastroesophageal junction area (arrow). Considerable spasm is also present throughout this region. The distal two thirds of the esophagus lack peristalsis.

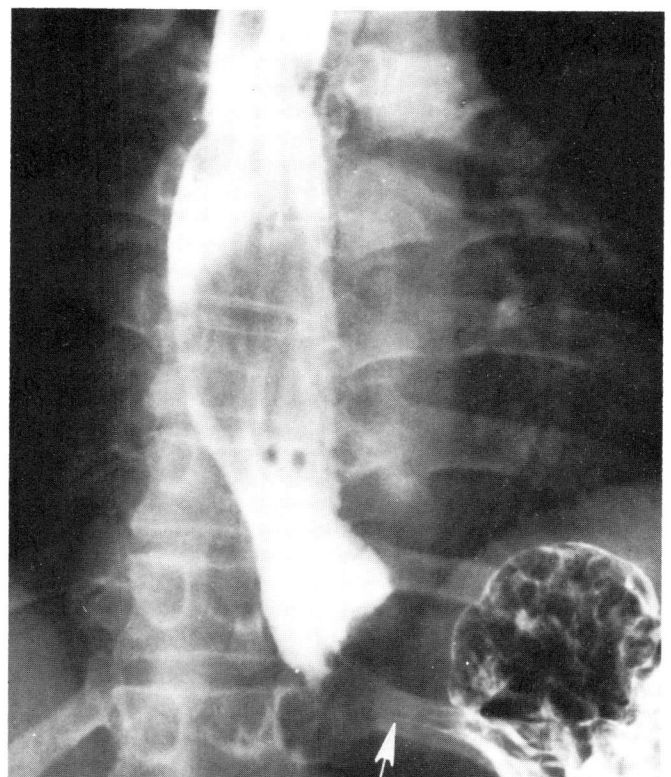

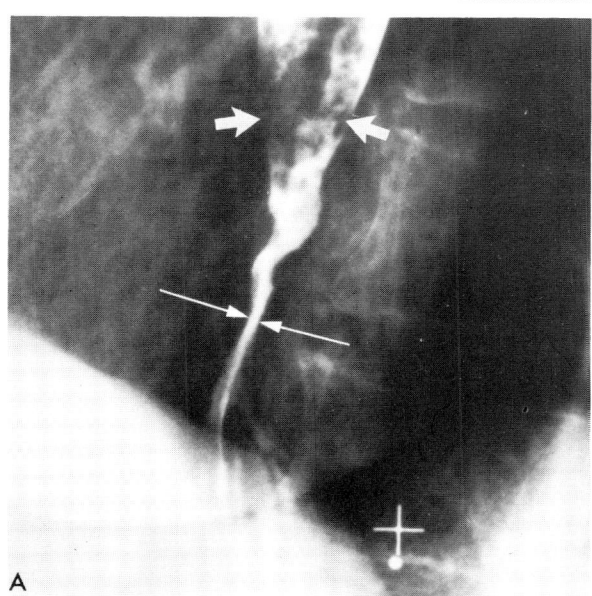

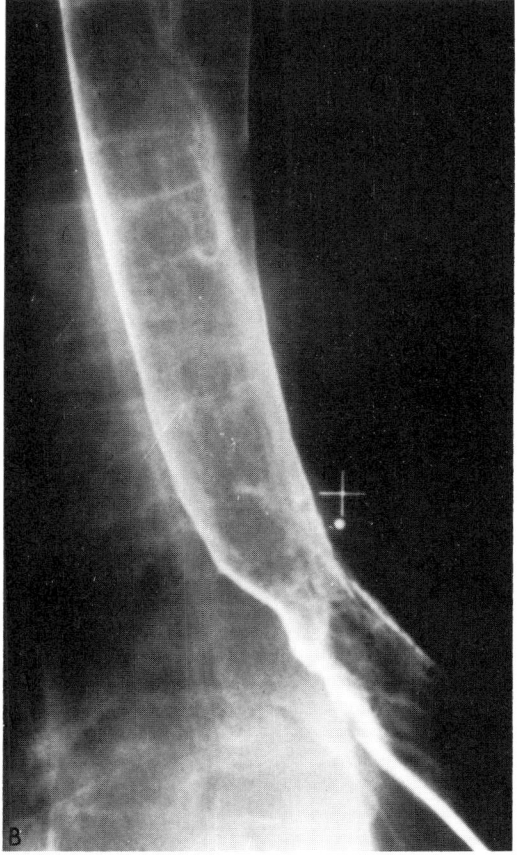

Figure 8–18. Scleroderma with esophageal obstruction. *A*, A 39-year-old woman with known scleroderma presented with acute dysphagia. There is a stricture in the distal esophagus (arrows), with an irregular intraluminal defect proximal to the stricture arrowheads. The defect was a piece of meat, which was subsequently removed by endoscopy. *B*, She subsequently underwent esophageal dilatation, and a follow-up esophagogram reveals an essentially normal lumen; no peristalsis was present, however.

especially on the lateral view (Fig. 8–15). In the upper third, peristalsis is usually normal.[16]

Initially, the diseased esophagogastric segment is patulous, and the esophagus empties rapidly in the erect position (in contradistinction to achalasia) (Fig. 8–16). In the recumbent position, however, barium may remain in the aperistaltic esophagus for a considerable period of time. Gastroesophageal reflux through the patulous junction is extremely common. The resultant reflux esophagitis may cause spasm, eventually leading to stricture (Fig. 8–17). Acute dysphagia may be a presenting symptom (Fig. 8–18*A*). The stricture may eventually require dilatation. Although after dilatation the lower esophagus can be patent, there still are no peristaltic waves present, and the esophagus simply empties by gravity (Fig. 8–18*B*).

Hiatus hernia is frequently seen in patients with esophageal scleroderma.

The radiologic appearance after surgery for stricture is outlined in the section on hiatus hernia (p. 361).

The changes secondary to dermatomyositis are similar to those of scleroderma, except that both the skeletal and smooth muscles are involved; thus, the changes can be seen throughout the entire esophagus rather than in just the lower two thirds.[15, 21] Occasionally, a patient with lupus erythematosus may have involvement of the pharynx.[4]

References

1. Banfield, W. J., and Hurwitz, A.: Esophageal stricture associated with nasogastric intubation. Arch. Intern. Med. *134*:1083–1086, 1974.
2. Bergman, A. B., and Lewicki, A. M.: Complete esophageal obstruction from cricopharyngeal achalasia. Radiology *123*:289–290, 1977.
3. Blakely, W. R., Garety, E. J., and Smith, D. E.: Section of the cricopharyngeus muscle for dysphagia. Arch. Surg. *96*:745–762, 1968.
4. Donner, M. W., and Siegel, C. I.: The evaluation of pharyngeal neuromuscular disorders by cinefluorography. Am. J. Roentgenol. *94*:299–307, 1965.
5. Ferrucci, J. T., Jr., and Long, J. A.: Radiologic treatment of esophageal food impaction using intravenous glucagon. Radiology *125*:25–28, 1977.
6. Gillies, M., Nicks, R., and Skyring, A.: Clinical, manometric, and pathological studies in diffuse esophageal spasm. Br. Med. J. *2*:527–530, 1967.
7. Gonzalez, G.: Diffuse esophageal spasm. Am. J. Roentgenol. *117*:251–258, 1973.
8. Henderson, R. D., Ho, C. S., and Davidson, J. W.: Primary disordered motor activity of the esophagus (diffuse spasm). Ann. Thorac. Surg. *18*:327–336, 1974.
9. House, A. J. S.: Barium sulfate as a bronchographic agent. *In* Miller, R. E., and Skucas, J. (eds.): Radiographic Contrast Agents. Baltimore, University Park Press, 1977, p. 403.
10. McNally, E. F., and Katz, I.: The roentgen diagnosis of diffuse esophageal spasm. Am. J. Roentgenol. *99*:218–222, 1967.
11. Markowiak, R., and Cohen, N. N.: Cardiovascular effects of pneumatic dilation of the cardioesophageal junction in achalasia. Gastrointest. Endosc. *19*:15–16, 1972.
12. Nelson, S. W., Cristoforidis, A. J., and Pratt, P. C.: Further experience with barium sulfate as a bronchographic contrast medium. Am. J. Roentgenol. *92*:595–614, 1964.
13. Nice, C. M., Waring, W. W., Killelea, D. E., et al.: Bronchography in infants and children; barium sulfate as a contrast agent. Am. J. Roentgenol. *91*:564–570, 1964.
14. Ogura, J. H., Saltzstein, S. L., and Spjut, H. J.: Experiences with conservation surgery in laryngeal and pharyngeal carcinoma. Laryngoscope *71*:258–276, 1967.
15. O'Hara, J. M., Szemes, G., and Lowman, R. M.: The esophageal lesions in dermatomyositis: a correlation of radiologic and pathologic findings. Radiology *89*:27–31, 1967.
16. Saladin, T. A., French, A. B., Zarafonetis, C. J. D., et al.: Esophageal motor abnormalities in scleroderma and related diseases. Am. J. Dig. Dis. *11*:522–535, 1966.
17. Sanderson, D. R., Ellis, F. H., Jr., Schlegel, J. F., et al.: Syndrome of vigorous achalasia: clinical and physiological observations. Dis. Chest *52*:508–517, 1967.
18. Seaman, W. B.: Functional disorders of the pharyngo-esophageal junction. Radiol. Clin. North Am. *7*:113–119, 1969.

19. Siegel, C. J., Hendrix, T. R., and Harvey, J. C.: The swallowing disorder in myotonia dystrophica. Gastroenterology 50:541–550, 1966.
20. Simeone, J. F., Burrell, M., Toffler, R., et al.: Aperistalsis and esophagitis. Radiology 123:9–14, 1977.
21. Stevens, M. B., Hookman, P., Siegel, C. I., et al.: Aperistalsis of the esophagus in patients with connective-tissue disorders and Raynaud's phenomenon. N. Engl. J. Med. 270:1218–1222, 1964.
22. Valdes-Dapena, A. M., and Stein, G. N.: Morphologic Pathology of the Alimentary Canal. Philadelphia, W. B. Saunders Company, 1970, pp. 16–20 and 92–105.
23. Westley, C. R., Herbst, J. J., Goldman, S., et al.: Infantile achalasia: inherited as an autosomal recessive disorder. J. Pediatr. 87:243–246, 1975.
24. Wychulis, A. R., Woolam, G. L., Anderson, H. A., et al.: Achalasia and carcinoma of the esophagus. J.A.M.A. 215:1638–1641, 1971.

Part II

Diverticula and Miscellaneous Conditions of the Esophagus

JOVITAS SKUCAS, M.D.
ROSCOE E. MILLER, M.D.

DIVERTICULA

Esophageal diverticula are saccular outpouchings from the esophageal lumen. Etiologically, diverticula can be subdivided into true (that is, containing all layers of the esophagus) or false, and pulsion, traction, or pulsion-traction diverticula. From a radiologic veiwpoint, classification by anatomic location is probably more useful. These diverticula occur characteristically at three separate locations: the pharyngoesophageal, midesophageal, and epiphrenic areas. Other locations are relatively rare, although occasionally one encounters generalized esophageal intramural diverticulosis. Rarely, an adjacent abscess ruptures into the esophagus; if the cavity persists, it may present with an appearance similar to that of a diverticulum.

Pharyngoesophageal Diverticula

True lateral pharyngeal diverticula are rare, although pseudodiverticular outpouchings of the lateral wall of the pharynx are not uncommon. These pseudodiverticula usually have no clinical significance (Fig. 8–19).

Pharyngoesophageal diverticula, known as Zenker's diverticula, are the most common type. These diverticula arise in the space bounded inferiorly by the transverse fibers and superiorly by the oblique fibers of the cricopharyngeal muscle and thus are pharyngeal in location. This space is a weak point known as Killian's dehiscence. The diverticula are probably acquired rather than congenital.

The radiologic appearance of a Zenker's diverticulum varies with its size. When small, there is an outpouching along the posterior wall of the cervical esophagus just above the cricopharyngeal muscle impression (Fig. 8–20). As the diverticulum becomes larger it may compress the adjacent esophagus. The larger diverticula generally extend laterally, and there is considerable stasis of secretions, food, and swallowed air. The

336 — THE ESOPHAGUS

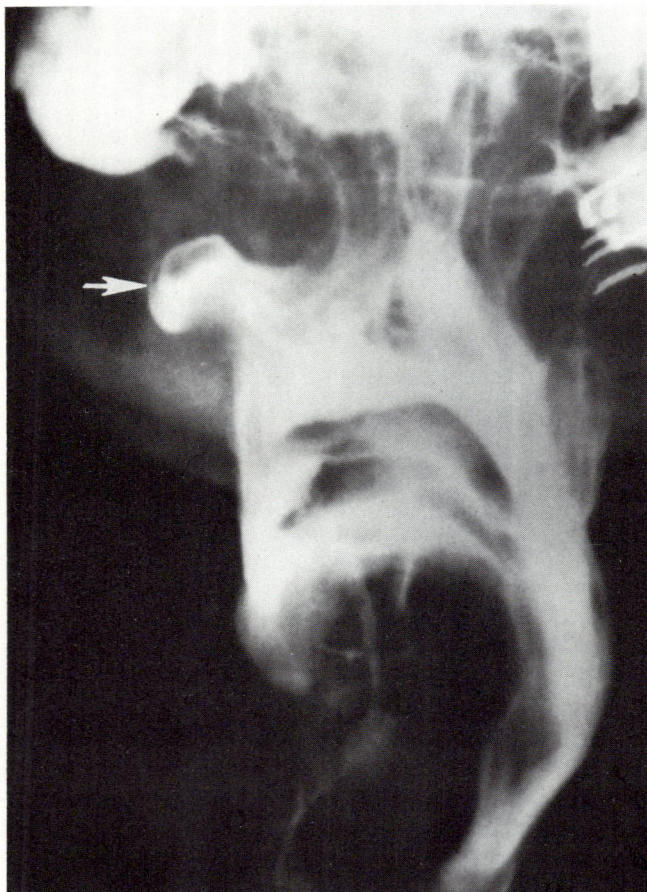

Figure 8–19. Pharyngeal pseudodiverticulum (arrow). These outpouchings usually are of no significance.

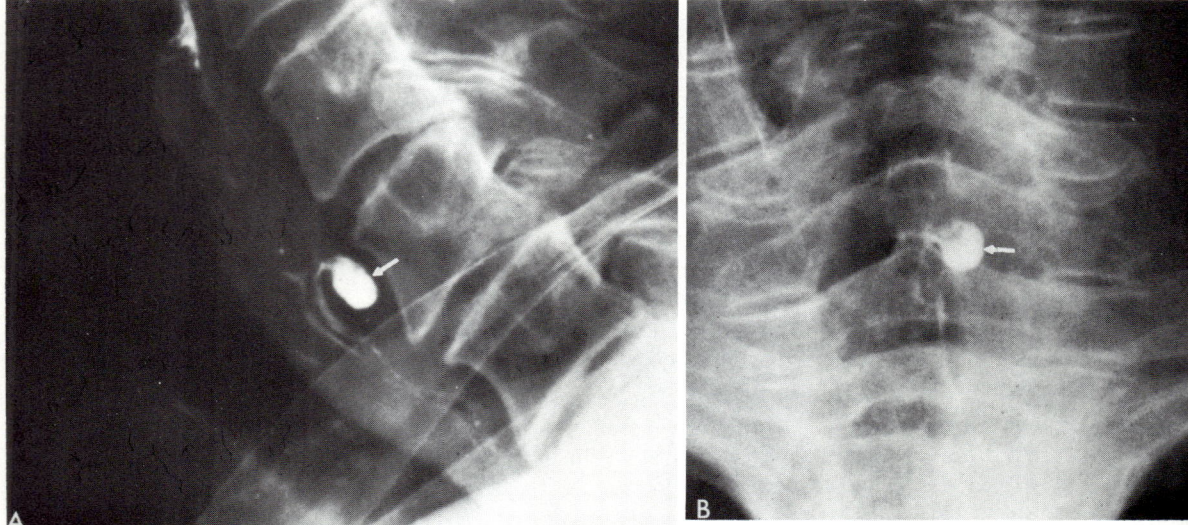

Figure 8–20. Zencker's diverticulum. *A,* Lateral view. *B,* Frontal view. There is a diverticulum extending posteriorly from the cervical esophagus (arrows), and the diverticulum displaces the adjacent esophagus. Even with a small diverticulum such as this there is considerable retention.

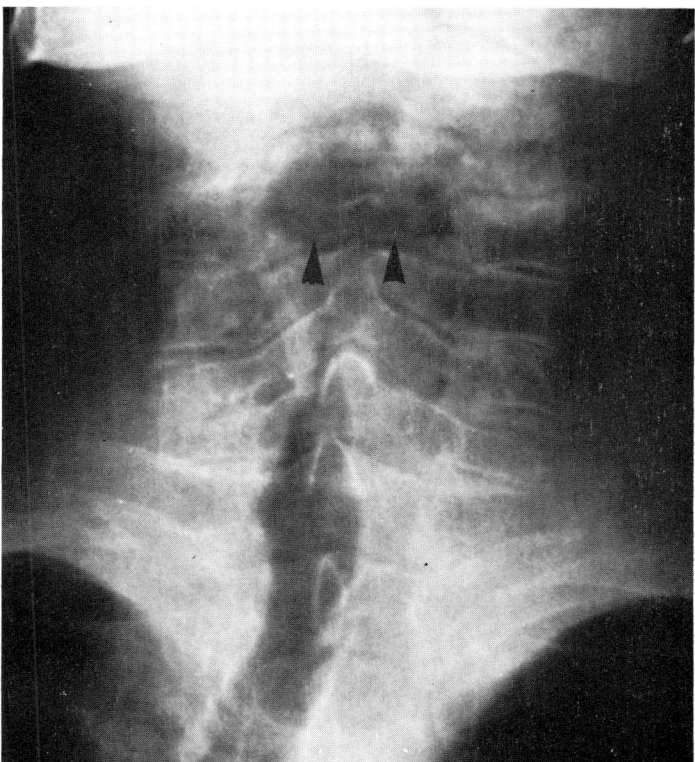

Figure 8–21. Large Zencker's diverticulum. An upright chest radiograph reveals an air-fluid level in the neck (arrowheads). A subsequent esophagogram showed that this represents a relatively large Zencker's diverticulum. The patient complained of regurgitation.

resultant air-fluid level can occasionally be seen on upright chest films (Fig. 8–21).

The neck of the diverticulum can be narrow. Invariably, in the upright position, contrast and secretions enter the diverticulum.

Small Zencker's diverticula are usually seen as incidental findings. With the larger diverticula, patients complain of regurgitation and dysphagia localized to the cervical esophagus. Chest films may reveal aspiration pneumonia due to the regurgitation. Occasionally, one finds ulcerations and perforations. Although unusual, malignant degeneration does occur in these diverticula.[22]

The postoperative diverticulectomy complications encountered, although rare, include localized infection and pharyngocutaneous fistula formation. Many surgeons perform a cricopharyngeal myotomy at the time of diverticulectomy.

Midthoracic Diverticula

Most midthoracic diverticula are asymptomatic and are simply incidental findings during esophagography. These diverticula are usually located in the carinal node region and extend anteriorly. The neck of the diverticulum can be either wide or narrow (Fig. 8–22). Occasionally, multiple diverticula are present. There is little stasis within these contractile diverticula, and filling and emptying can be observed during the passage of barium, since these traction diverticula contain all the esophageal muscle layers. Radiologically, there is no difficulty in differentiating these diverticula from ulcers.

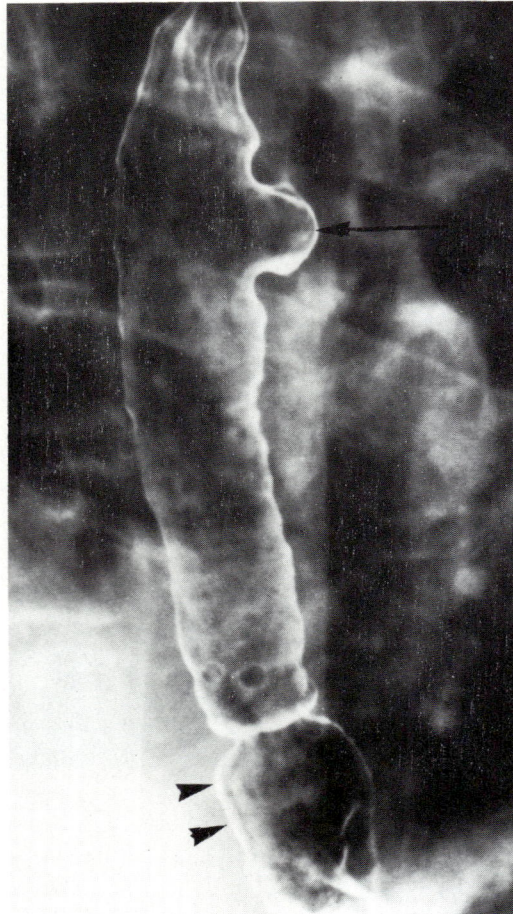

Figure 8–22. Midthoracic diverticulum. There is a diverticulum at the level of the carinal lymph nodes (arrow). The neck of the diverticulum is wide, and there was no stasis. The diverticulum was believed to be an incidental finding. The patient also has a hiatus hernia (arrowheads).

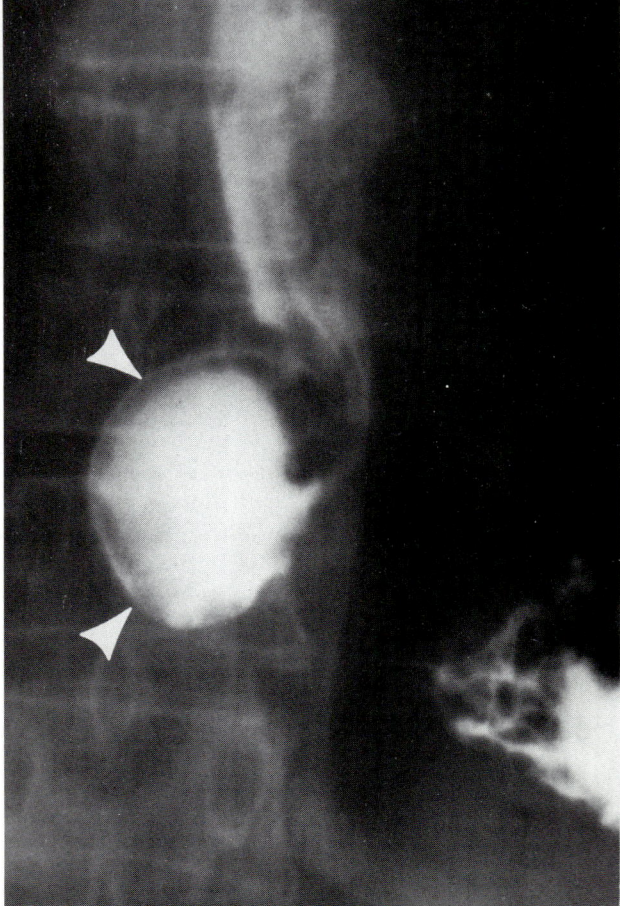

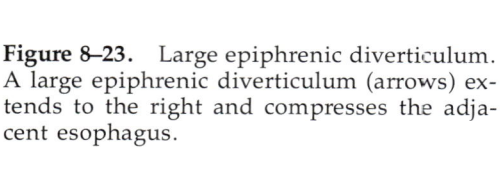

Figure 8–23. Large epiphrenic diverticulum. A large epiphrenic diverticulum (arrows) extends to the right and compresses the adjacent esophagus.

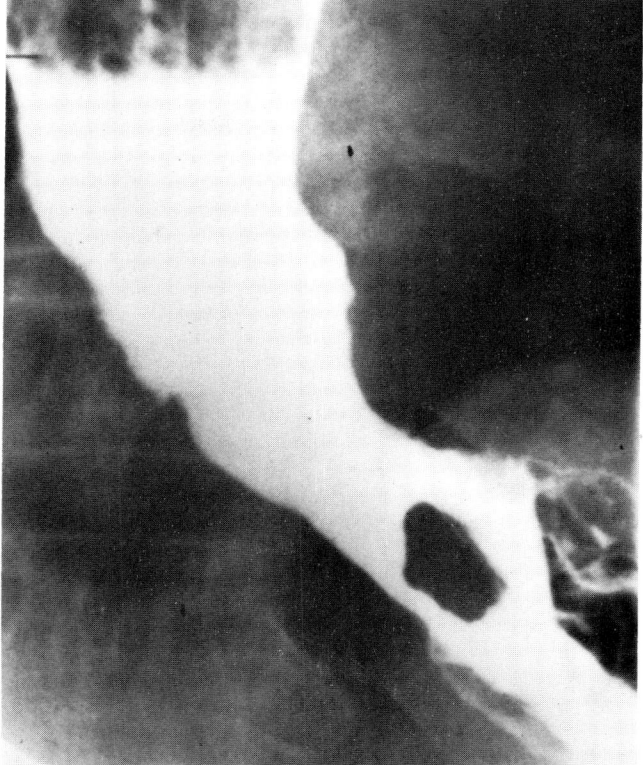

Figure 8–24. Postgastrodiverticular anastomosis. The patient had dysphagia seemingly due to an epiphrenic diverticulum and underwent surgery, which apparently consisted of an anastomosis between the diverticulum and the gastric fundus. The surgery was performed many years ago in Europe. The presence of a double esophageal lumen was confirmed by endoscopy.

Epiphrenic Diverticula

These diverticula are present in the distal 10 centimeters of the esophagus, usually extend to the right side, and are variable in size (Fig. 8–23). They empty slowly, and dysphagia due to esophageal compression may be present. There may be associated spasm of the esophagus. Familial occurrence of epiphrenic diverticula has been reported.[8]

Most of these diverticula are readily identified. They should be distinguished from the rare esophageal diverticulum located below the diaphragm, that is, the subphrenic diverticulum.[16]

After resection of an epiphrenic diverticulum, the esophagus appears normal. Occasionally, a surgical anastomosis may be made between the diverticulum and the stomach, leading to a double lumen (Fig. 8–24).

Intramural Diverticulosis

In this rare condition there are multiple small outpouchings scattered throughout the esophagus.[3, 10, 11] Often there is associated reflux esophagitis (Fig. 8–25).

Superficially these diverticula can be confused with multiple ulcerations throughout the esophagus. Although intramural diverticulosis has been described in association with moniliasis,[21, 24] the inflammatory process and ulcerations seen in cases of moniliasis may mimic diverticula and make the evaluation of true intramural divertic-

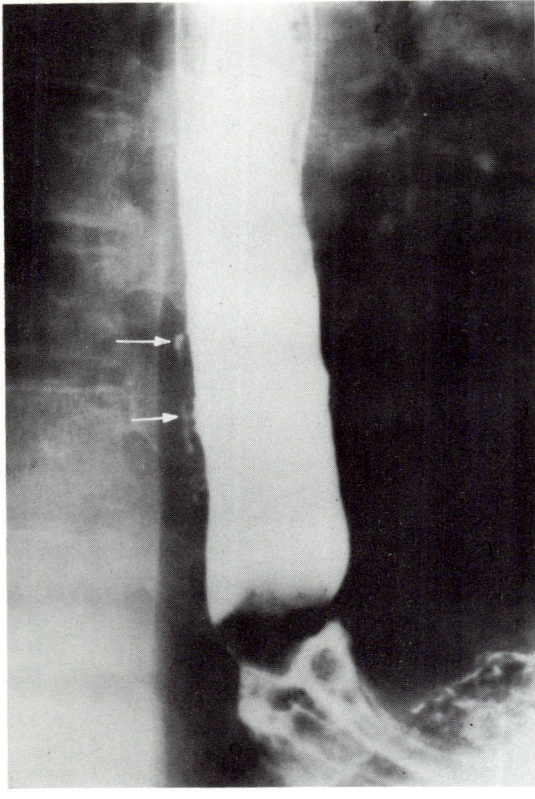

Figure 8–25. Intramural diverticulosis. There are numerous small outpouchings (arrows) in the lower part of the esophagus. These diverticula have relatively narrow necks and extend only into the wall of the esophagus. (Courtesy of J. Wandtke, M.D.)

ula difficult.[20] An association between the Paterson-Kelly (Plummer-Vinson) syndrome and intramural diverticulosis has been reported.[11]

The cause of these diverticula is not known. Uncoordinated esophageal motility and partial obstruction may be predisposing factors. Most of these diverticula are located in the proximal portion of the esophagus and appear to be associated with dysphagia or some other pathologic lesion.

Intraluminal Diverticulosis

An intraluminal esophageal diverticulum is rare. An esophagogram shows the diverticulum filled with barium and a thin radiolucent line separating the diverticulum from the esophageal lumen (Fig. 8–26). Rotation of the patient reveals the intraluminal location of the diverticulum.[17]

ESOPHAGEAL WEBS

The terms "Paterson-Kelly syndrome," "Plummer-Vinson syndrome," "sideropenic dysphagia," and "dysphagia with iron deficiency" have been used to describe anteriorly positioned webs in the upper esophagus. This syndrome is relatively infrequent in the United States. It may be associated with prior gastrectomy and secondary anemia. There is an increased incidence of carcinoma in these patients, the neoplasm

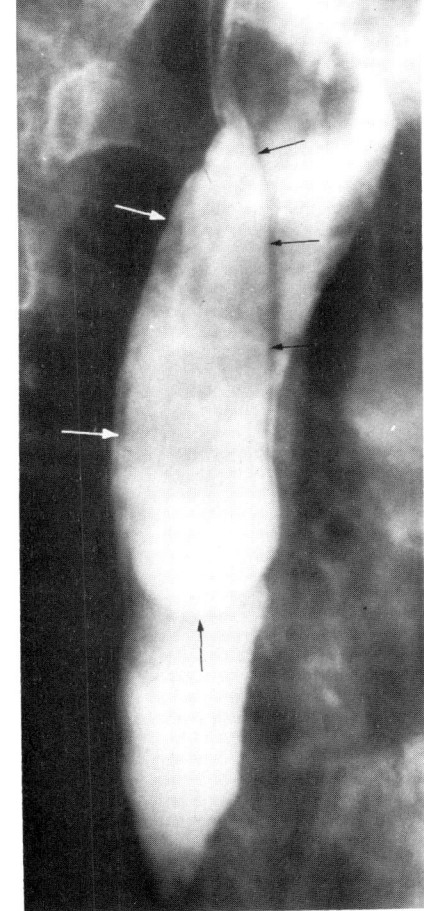

Figure 8–26. Intraluminal diverticulum. A large diverticulum (arrows) projects into the esophageal lumen. (*From* Schreiber, M. H., and Davis, M.: Intraluminal diverticulum of the esophagus. *129*:595–597, 1977.)

usually arising proximal to the web and involving either the oropharynx or the esophagus.

These webs are best seen in the lateral projection with the esophagus maximally distended by barium (Fig. 8–27). They usually project from the anterior wall and extend posteriorly to varying degrees. There may be a "jet phenomenon" with the barium being vigorously propelled through the narrowing produced by a web; technically excellent films should help differentiate this phenomenon from a long stricture.[18]

Webs similar to those seen in the Paterson-Kelly syndrome but not associated with any dysphagia or anemia are relatively common (Fig. 8–28). The full significance of these webs is still not known. Weblike defects may also result from prior surgery in the area (Fig. 8–29).

Lower esophageal rings are not uncommon even in asymptomatic patients. They are also best seen with the esophagus maximally distended with barium, and they are usually associated with a hiatal hernia. Dysphagia may be present if the diameter of the lumen is 13 mm or less. The significance of such a ring can be evaluated by having the patient swallow a barium tablet measuring 12.5 mm in diameter.[23] If the tablet is held up just proximal to the ring, even if the patient subsequently drinks water or

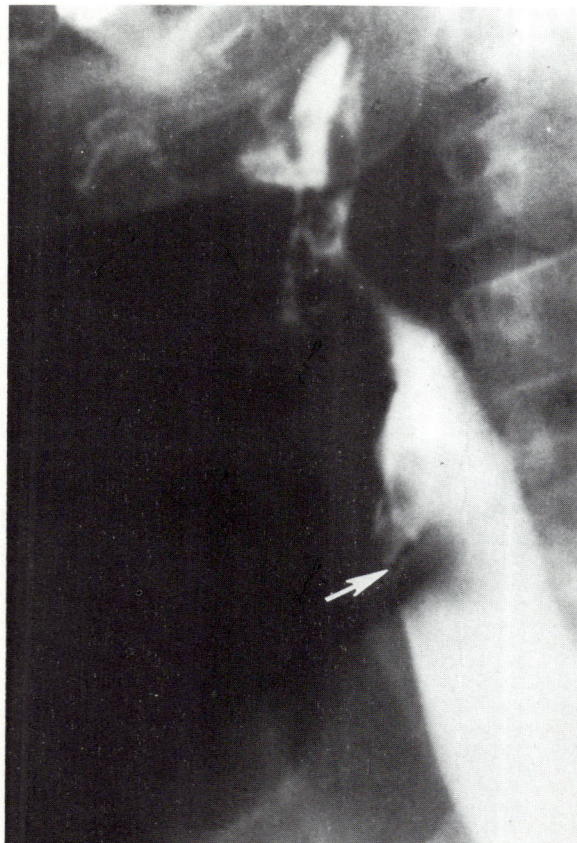

Figure 8–27. Probable Paterson-Kelly syndrome. This 45-year-old woman presented with dysphagia and subsequently was found to have iron-deficiency anemia. There is an anterior wall web (arrow) in the upper part of the esophagus.

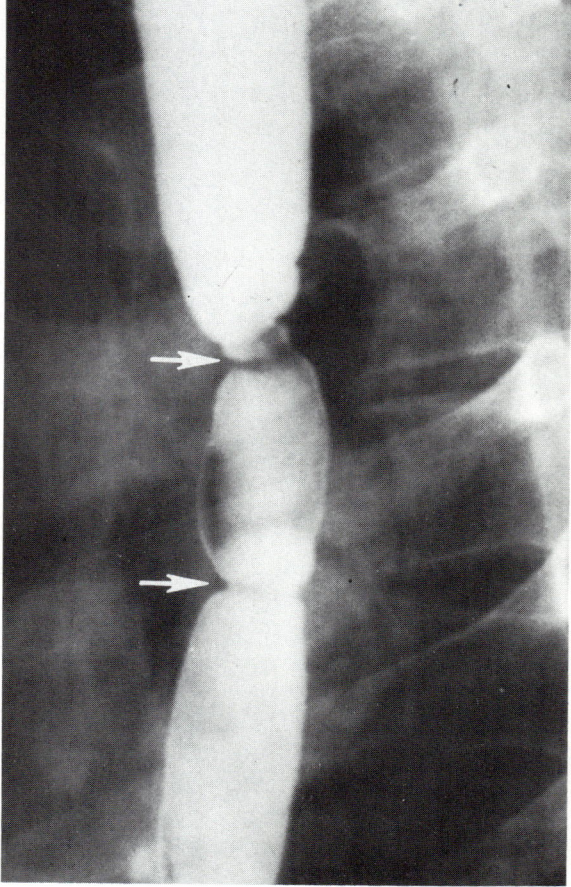

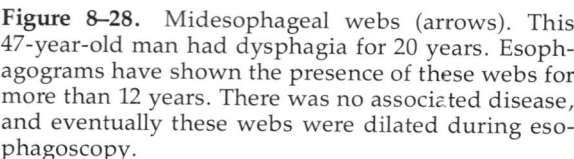

Figure 8–28. Midesophageal webs (arrows). This 47-year-old man had dysphagia for 20 years. Esophagograms have shown the presence of these webs for more than 12 years. There was no associated disease, and eventually these webs were dilated during esophagoscopy.

THE ESOPHAGUS — 343

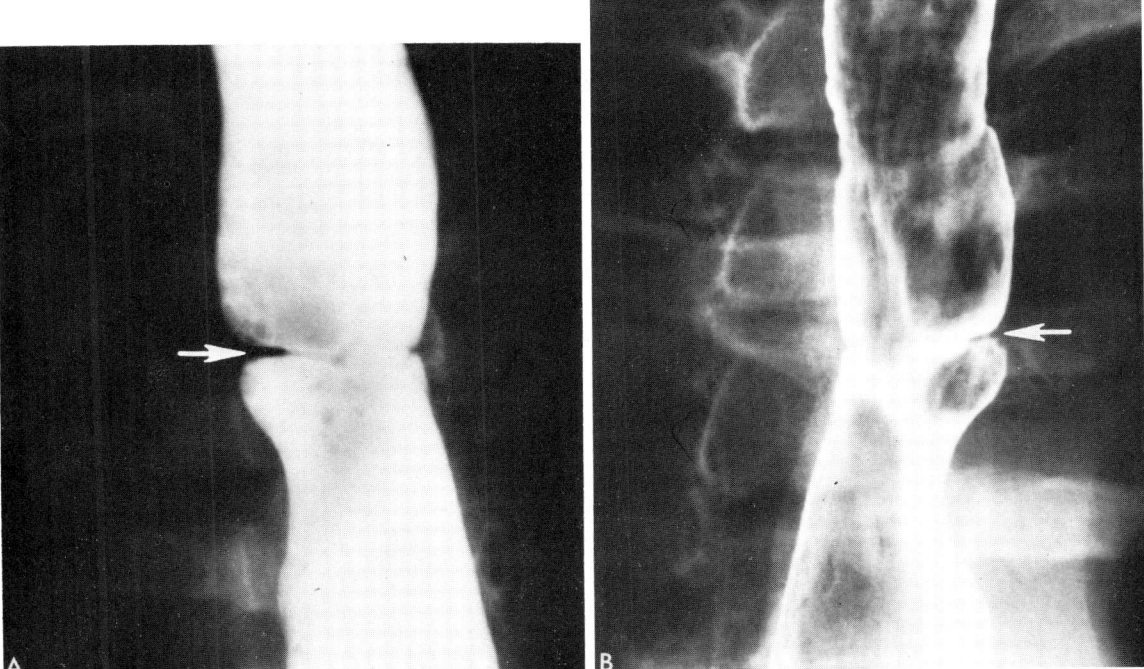

Figure 8–29. Midesophageal webs. This teenaged patient with dysphagia has a midesophageal web (arrows). As a baby she had had surgery for the repair of a tracheoesophageal fistula; the web seems to be secondary to the surgery. A, Full-column right posterior oblique view. B, Double-contrast left posterior oblique view.

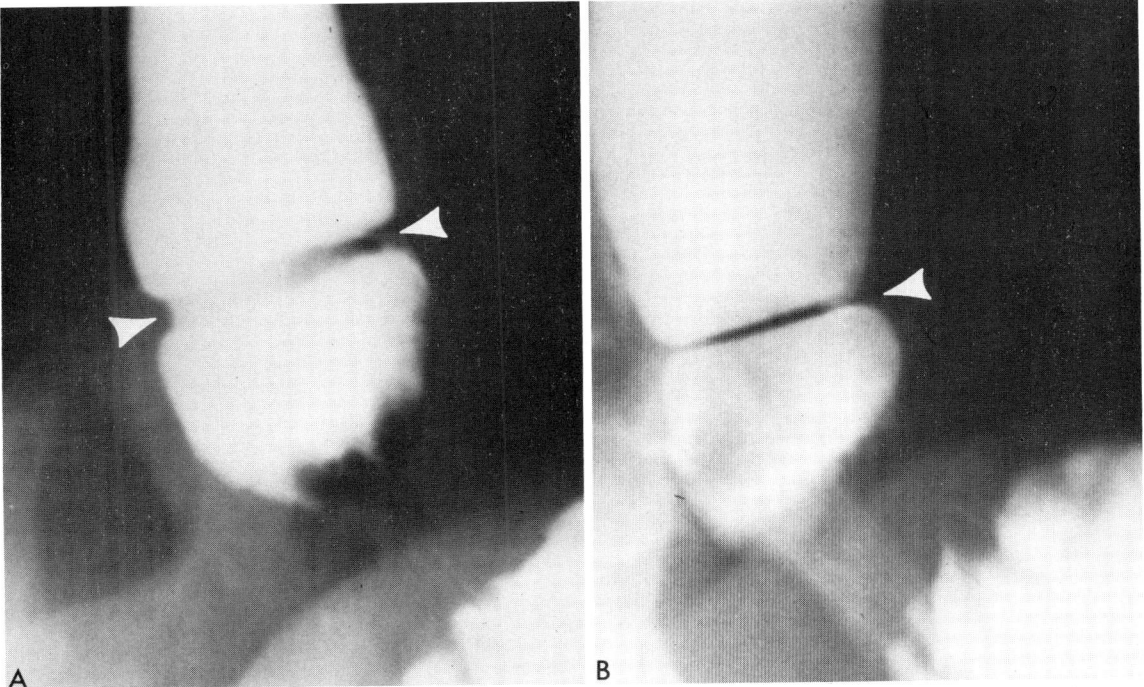

Figure 8–30. Lower esophageal rings and webs. A, Lower esophageal ring (Schatzki's ring) (arrowheads). The thin ring is mucosal in origin and marks the junction of the esophagogastric mucosa. B, Inferior esophageal sphincter (arrowhead). This ring varies in size at different times.

barium, the narrowing is probably significant. These rings can be either at the gastroesophageal mucosal junction or in the distal esophagus (Fig. 8–30).

Endoscopy may not reveal the smaller rings, since the mucosa throughout the area may be intact. If indicated, excision of these rings is performed during hiatal hernia repair. The postoperative radiologic appearance is discussed in the section on hiatus hernia (p. 361).

INFLAMMATORY AND INFECTIOUS DISEASES

The esophagus is relatively resistant to infection, with most infections occurring in debilitated or immunosuppressed patients. Tuberculosis and syphilis of the esophagus are rarely encountered today. Although there are occasional reports of opportun-

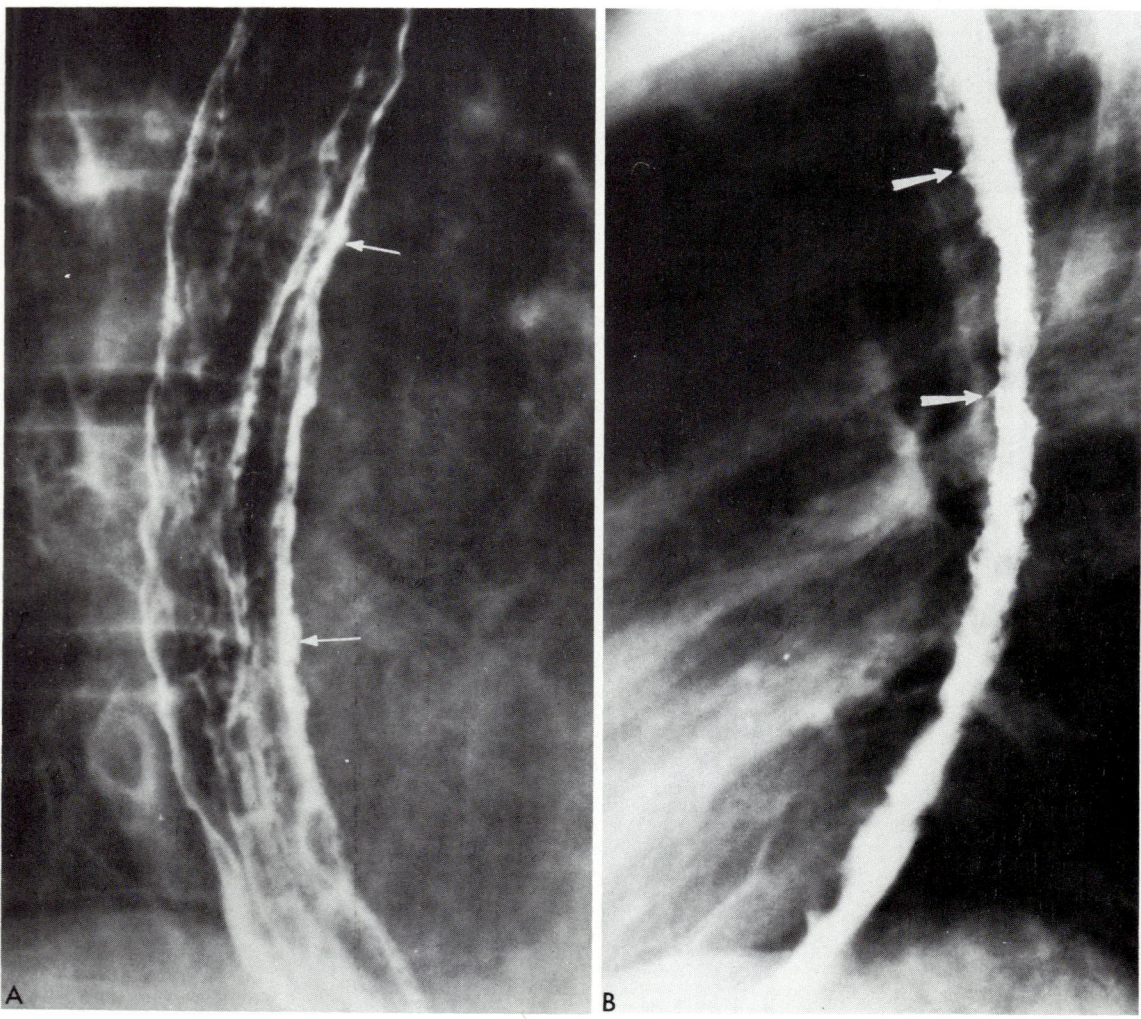

Figure 8–31. Esophageal moniliasis. Two different patients with proved esophageal moniliasis. The ulcerations throughout the esophagus are clearly evident (arrows). There was diffuse spasm throughout.

istic infection with such organisms as *Klebsiella*,[1] by far the most common organism is *Candida albicans (Monilia)*.

Moniliasis

Moniliasis of the esophagus is often, but not always, associated with infection of the mouth and oropharynx. The esophagus can reveal numerous intraluminal plaque-like defects and multiple ulcerations (Fig. 8–31). The ulcerations may be confused with intramural diverticulosis. Often there are diffuse spasms, and the patient complains of pain when drinking fluids or an effervescent solution.[2] Radiographically, the outline of the esophagus is usually diffuse and irregular.[13] The intraluminal plaque-like defects are known as "cobblestoning."[7] Rarely, a localized polypoid nodule occurs in cases of moniliasis of the esophagus, generally in association with an underlying malignancy.[9] An unusual complication is esophageal stricture.[15]

Herpes Infection

Herpes esophagitis is seen in severely debilitated or immunosuppressed patients. The esophagogram reveals plaque-like projections (Fig. 8–32). There may be numerous small ulcers.[14, 19] A double-contrast esophagogram aids in the diagnosis. The lesions do not change in size or shape with varying degrees of distention, which differentiates

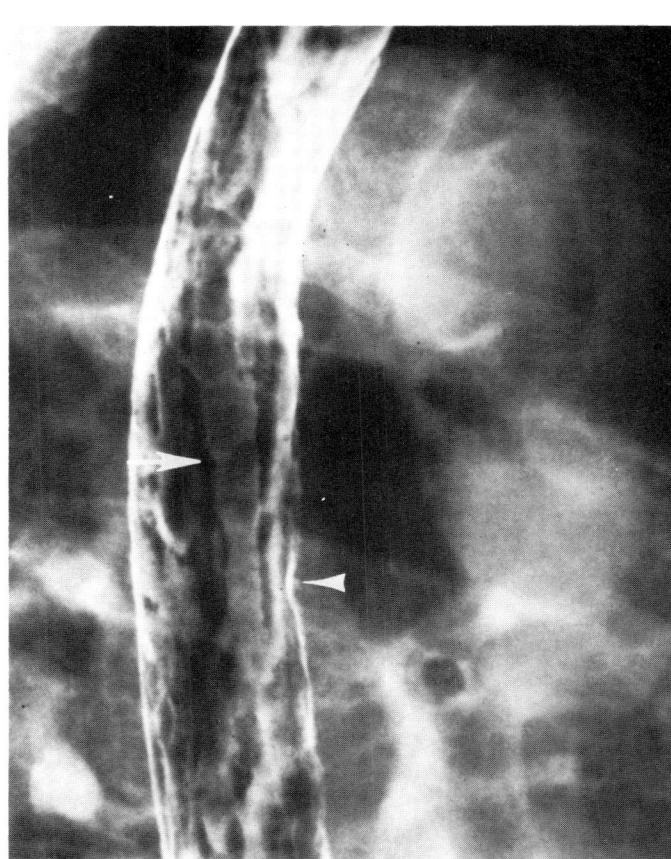

Figure 8–32. Herpes esophagitis. There are numerous linear, plaque-like defects scattered throughout the esophagus (arrow). Numerous ulcers are also present (arrowhead). (*From* Skucas, J., Schrank, W. W., Meyers, P. C., et al. Herpes esophagitis: a case studied by air contract esophagography. Am. J. Roentgenol. 128:497–499, 1977.)

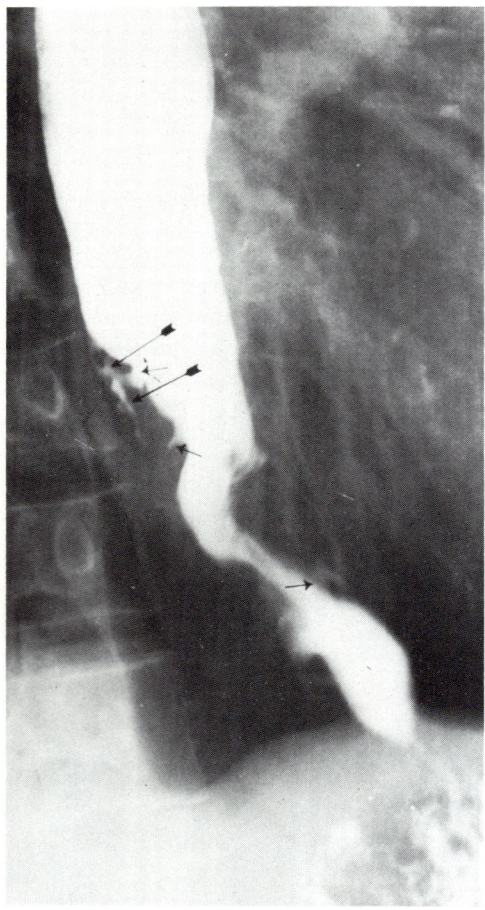

Figure 8–33. Crohn's disease of the esophagus. There are fistulous tracts (arrows) in the intramural portion of the distal esophagus. (*From* Cynn, W. S., Chon, H., Guregian, P. A., et al. Crohn's disease of the esophagus. Am. J. Roentgenol. *125*:359–364, 1975.)

them from varices. Generally, the lower two thirds of the esophagus is involved. These lesions closely resemble those of moniliasis, and differentiation between these two diseases can be difficult. Because of the common underlying associated diseases, moniliasis and herpes infection can coexist in the same patient. The differential diagnosis also includes acanthosis nigricans, which presents radiographically as a fine nodular pattern throughout the esophagus.[12]

Crohn's Disease

Crohn's disease involving the esophagus is unusual. In the few reported cases the esophagus appeared considerably strictured and the wall thickened. In the absence of disease involving other parts of the intestine, a diagnosis of Crohn's disease of the esophagus is highly unlikely. The diagnosis is difficult to confirm, since endoscopic biopsy may not produce adequate tissue or may be nonspecific.[6] Skip areas have not been seen in the esophagus. One report of two patients with Crohn's disease described multiple intramural fistulous tracts, with one patient acquiring an esophago-bronchial fistula (Fig. 8–33).[4] Associated mouth ulcerations have also been described.[5]

References

1. Athey, P., Goldstein, H. M., and Dodd, G. D.: Radiologic spectrum of opportunistic infections of the upper gastrointestinal tract. Am. J. Roentgenol. *129*:419–424, 1977.
2. Buckle, R. M., and Nichol, W. D.: Painful dysphagia due to monilial oesophagitis. Br. Med. J. *1*:821–822, 1964.
3. Culver, G. J., and Chaudhari, K. R.: Intramural esophageal diverticulosis. Am. J. Roentgenol. *99*:210–211, 1967.
4. Cynn, W. S., Chon, H., Gureghian, P. A., et al.: Crohn's disease of the esophagus. Am. J. Roentgenol. *125*:359–364, 1975.
5. Dyer, N. H., Cook, P. L., and Harper, R. A. K.: Esophageal stricture associated with Crohn's disease. Gut *10*:549–554, 1969.
6. Fröhlich, H., Huchzermeyer, H., and St. Stender, H.: Roentgenologic findings in regional esophagitis due to Crohn's disease. Fortschr. Geb. Roentgenstr. Nuklearmed. *125*:497–500, 1976.
7. Goldberg, H. I., and Dodds, W. J.: Cobblestone esophagus due to monilial infection. Am. J. Roentgenol. *104*:608–612, 1968.
8. Hird, W. E., and Hortenstine, C. B.: Familial esophageal epiphrenic diverticula. J.A.M.A. *171*:1924–1927, 1959.
9. Ho, C-S, Cullen, J. B., and Gray, R. R.: An unusual manifestation of esophageal moniliasis. Radiology *123*:287–288, 1977.
10. Hodes, P. J., Atkins, J. P., and Hodes, B. L.: Esophageal intramural diverticulosis. Am. J. Roentgenol. *96*:411–413, 1966.
11. Hüpscher, D. N.: Intramural diverticulosis of the esophagus. Radiol. Clin. Biol. *43*:144–154, 1974.
12. Itai, Y., Kogure, T., Okuyama, Y., et al.: Diffuse finely nodular lesions of the esophagus. Am. J. Roentgenol. *128*:563–566, 1977.
13. Lewicki, A. M., and Moore, J. P.: Esophageal moniliasis. A review of common and less frequent characteristics. Am. J. Roentgenol. *125*:218–225, 1975.
14. Meyers, C., Durkin, M. G., and Love, L.: Radiographic findings in herpetic esophagitis. Radiology *119*:21–22, 1976.
15. Ott, D. J., and Gelfand, D. W.: Esophageal stricture secondary to candidiasis. Gastrointest. Radiol. *2*:323–325, 1978.
16. Rettig, J.: Diverticulum of the abdominal portion of the esophagus. Gastroenterology *42*:781–783, 1962.
17. Schreiber, M. H., and Davis, M.: Intraluminal diverticulum of the esophagus. Am. J. Roentgenol. *129*:595–597, 1977.
18. Shauffer, I. A., Phillips, H. E., and Sequeira, J.: The jet phenomenon: a manifestation of esophageal web. Am. J. Roentgenol. *129*:747–748, 1977.
19. Skucas, J., Schrank, W. W., Meyers, P. C., et al.: Herpes esophagitis: a case studied by air contrast esophagography. Am. J. Roentgenol. *128*:497–499, 1977.
20. Smulewicz, J. J., and Dorfman, J.: Esophageal intramural diverticulosis: a re-evaluation. Radiology *101*:527–529, 1971.
21. Troupin, R. H.: Intramural esophageal diverticulosis and moniliasis. A possible association. Am. J. Roentgenol. *104*:613–616, 1968.
22. Turner, M. J.: Carcinoma as a complication of pharyngeal pouch. Br. J. Radiol. *36*:206–210, 1963.
23. Wolfe, B. S.: Use of a half inch barium tablet to detect minimal esophageal strictures. J. Mt. Sinai Hosp. *28*:80–82, 1961.
24. Zatzkin, H. R., Green, S., and LaVine, J. J.: Esophageal intramural diverticulosis. Radiology *90*:1193–1194, 1968.

Part III
Hiatus Hernia

JOVITAS SKUCAS, M.D.
ROSCOE E. MILLER, M.D.

Hiatus hernias can be classified into three types: paraesophageal hernia, sliding hernia, and a hernia associated with a congenitally short esophagus.

In a paraesophageal hernia the gastroesophageal junction is below the diaphragm, and a portion of the stomach herniates through the esophageal hiatus to lie alongside the esophagus. In a sliding hernia the gastroesophageal junction lies in the thorax. It is not unusual to see a mixed type of hernia. The short esophagus is a relatively rare congenital anomaly. Most patients with a congenitally short esophagus are children, and the gastroesophageal junction is in a fixed intrathoracic location.

The larger hernias can be readily identified on frontal or lateral chest radiographs (Fig. 8–34). The hernial sacs are usually well circumscribed, and an air-fluid level is present.

PARAESOPHAGEAL HIATUS HERNIA

Most paraesophageal hiatus hernias are not reducible and can thus be identified in both the upright and recumbent positions. An upper gastrointestinal examination should determine the location of the gastroesophageal junction, the size of the hernia, and the presence of ulcers or tumors within the hernia as well as other diseases in the stomach and duodenum. Frontal, lateral, and oblique views are necessary for full evaluation of the hernia.

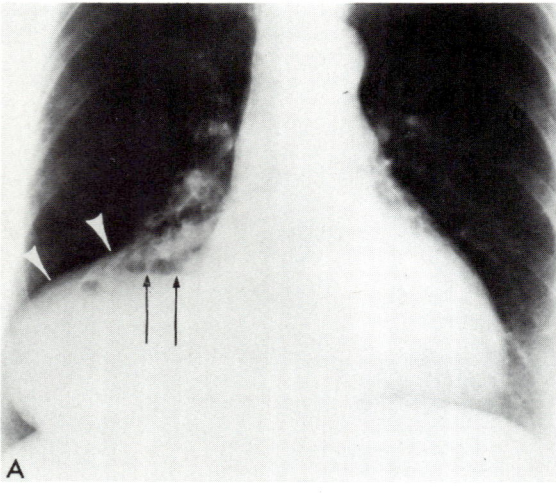
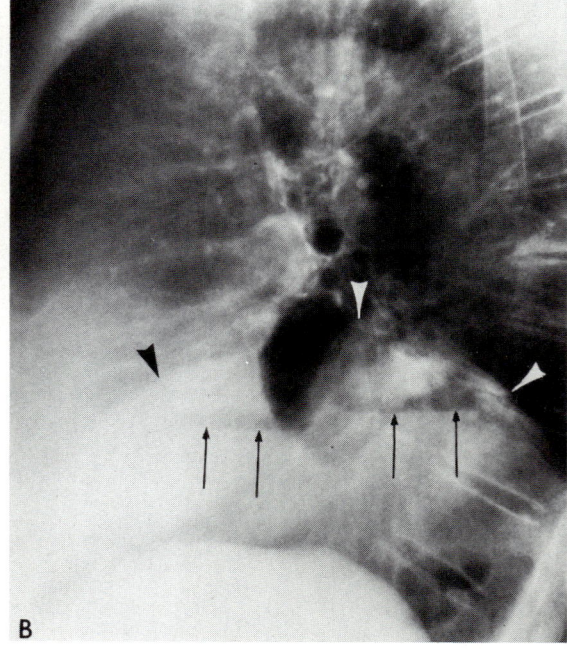

Figure 8–34. Hiatus hernia. The large hernia (arrowheads) is clearly seen on posteroanterior (A) and lateral chest (B) radiographs. The air-fluid level (arrows) in the hernia helps identify its true nature.

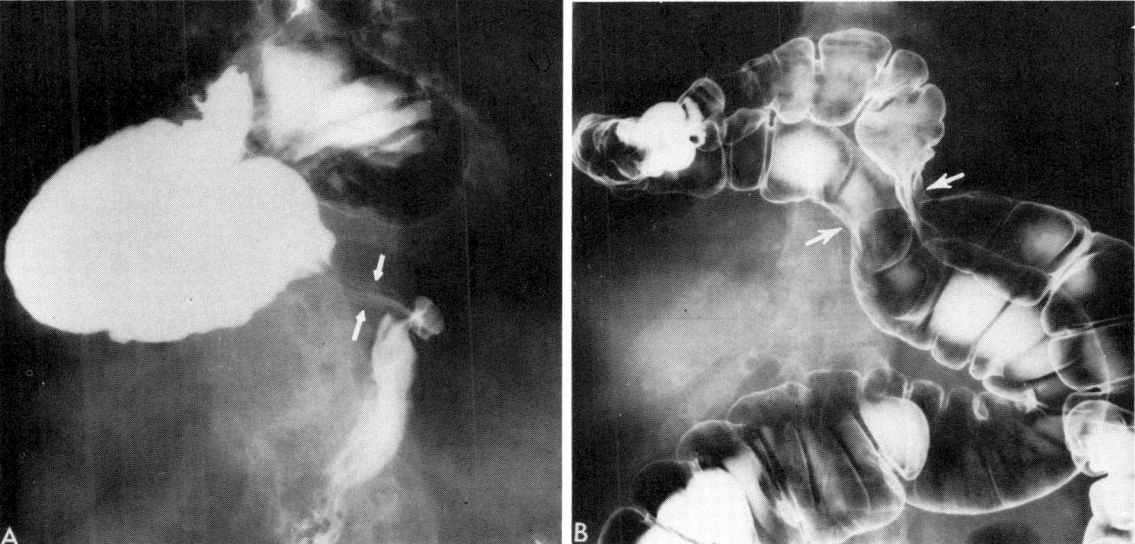

Figure 8–35. Large hiatus hernia. A, Almost the entire stomach is in the thorax. There is 180 degree gastric torsion, yet there is no obstruction. The antrum passes through the hiatus (arrows). B, A portion of the transverse colon was also in the chest. The narrowed diaphragmatic hiatus is clearly seen (arrows).

Complications encountered with large hernias include bleeding and obstruction. At times, there may be almost complete gastric herniation into the thorax (Fig. 8–35A). Transverse colon herniation through the hiatus may also be present (Fig. 8–35B). The fixed positions of the duodenum and the gastroesophageal junction serve as landmarks to identify organoaxial or mesenteroaxial torsion of the stomach during herniation into the thorax.[6] A 180-degree twist results in the so-called upside-down stomach.

A large hernia can be present without obstruction, although patients with this condition can present with sudden obstruction (Fig. 8–36). When the fundus is located inferiorly to the body of the stomach, ingested food and fluid tend to distend the fundus and compress the adjacent antrum at the hiatus. The passage of a nasogastric tube with decompression of the fundus may relieve the obstruction. A simple obstruction may be further complicated by volvulus of the stomach. At times both the fundus and the antrum are herniated into the thorax, the body of the stomach lying below the diaphragm (Fig. 8–37).

After the repair of a paraesophageal hernia there are no characteristic radiographic findings.

SLIDING HIATUS HERNIA

There is considerable controversy regarding the radiographic diagnosis of sliding hiatus hernia. Although the larger hernias are readily diagnosed, small sliding hiatus hernias can be difficult to demonstrate and their significance even more difficult to assess. Most of the smaller hernias are appreciated only in a recumbent position.

These hernias can vary from very small to very large (Fig. 8–38). They may be associated with gastroesophageal reflux, which is best demonstrated fluoroscopically or by cine or video tape.

When the hernia is reduced, a moon-shaped defect may be seen along the medial

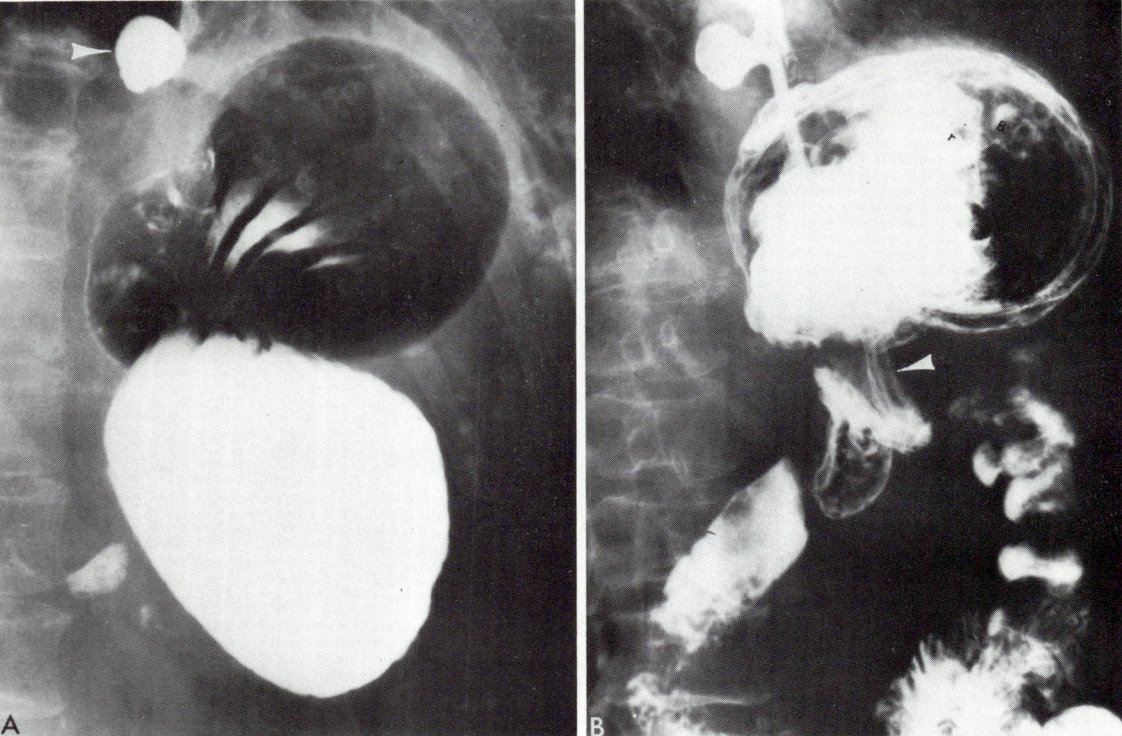

Figure 8–36. Gastric obstruction. *A,* An 80-year-old woman presented with acute gastric outlet obstruction. Most of her stomach is in the thorax. An incidental epiphrenic diverticulum is present (arrowhead). *B,* A nasogastric tube was passed, the stomach decompressed, and the obstruction spontaneously relieved. Partial gastric torsion is still present (arrowhead).

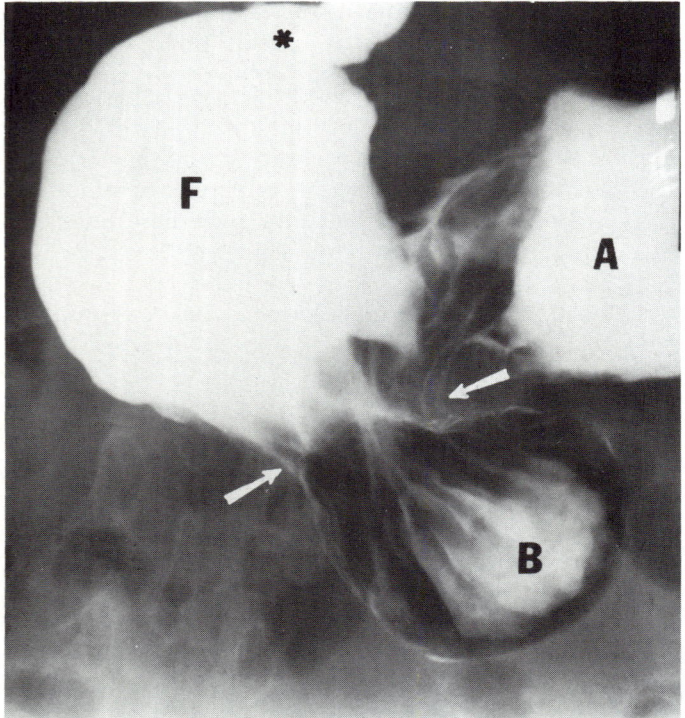

Figure 8–37. Compound hiatal hernia. The gastroesophageal junction (*) and fundus (F) are in the thorax, the body of the stomach (B) is in the abdomen below the esophageal hiatus (arrows), while the antrum (A) is lying alongside the fundus in the hernia. No obstruction was present.

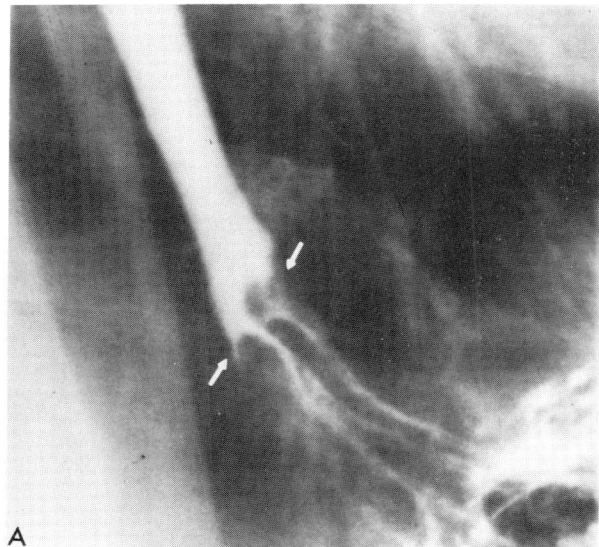
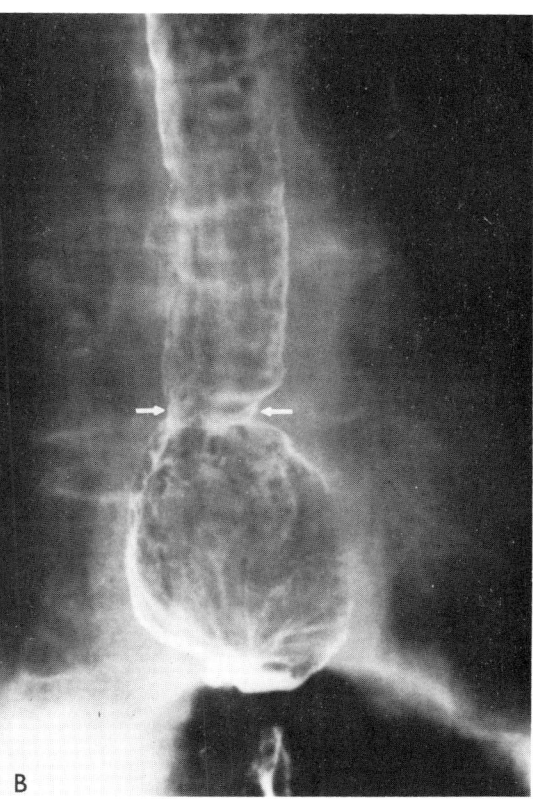

Figure 8–38. Sliding hiatus hernia. *A,* A small hiatus hernia is present. There are irregular folds at the gastroesophageal junction (arrows) indicating esophagitis. *B,* Another patient with a large sliding hiatus hernia. The hernia did not reduce completely even with the patient upright. The gastroesophageal junction is slightly narrowed (arrows). (*From* Skucas, J.: The routine double-contrast examination of the esophagus. C.R.C. Crit. Rev. Diagn. Imaging, *11*:121–143, 1978.)

aspect of the gastric fundus.[8] This pseudotumor may mimic a carcinoma, but the change in configuration of the pseudotumor during herniation aids in ready differentiation.

The complications of hiatus hernia and reflux include ulceration, esophagitis, and stricture. A common site of ulceration is at the esophageal hiatus (Fig. 8–39), but the ulcerations can be anywhere in the distal esophagus or in the hernia (Fig. 8–40). Large ulcers are not unusual.

Reflux esophagitis limited to the mucosa cannot be recognized with existing radiographic techniques. When there are small ulcerations extending into the submucosa, double-contrast esophagography can readily demonstrate these outpouchings (Fig. 8–41). The folds in the lower esophagus become thickened and irregular. The disease is generally limited to the lower esophagus, although it can extend proximally for varying lengths. There is gradual onset of dysphagia, and eventually a stricture develops. The strictures are usually sort, there is dilatation of the esophagus proximally, and there may be ulcers throughout the area (Fig. 8–42). Although most of these strictures are symmetric and do not present an irregular appearance, differentiating them from carcinoma can at times be difficult (Fig. 8–43). Endoscopic biopsy may likewise not yield a diagnosis. Numerous biopsy specimens from the area must be taken to exclude the diagnosis of neoplasm. If the endoscope cannot be advanced through a stricture, brush biopsy specimens may be helpful.

Although these strictures are generally short and limited to the lower esophagus, occasionally a long stricture is encountered.

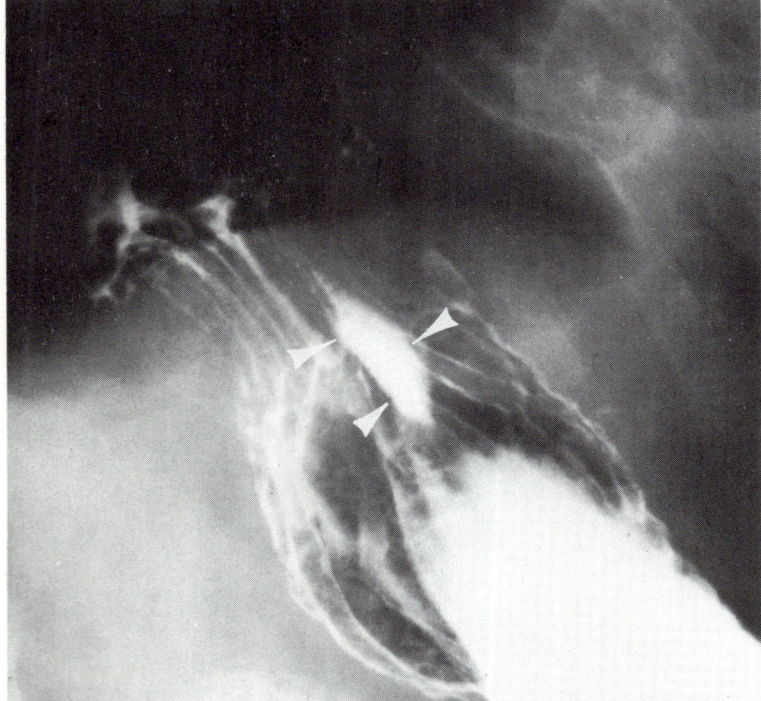

Figure 8–39. Hiatus hernia with ulcer. The ulcer is along the lesser curvature at the esophageal hiatus (arrowheads). This patient subsequently had a major upper gastrointestinal bleed from this ulcer.

Figure 8–40. Hiatus hernia with ulcer. The esophageal hiatus is wide. There is a deep, penetrating ulcer at the gastroesophageal junction (arrows). A mild stricture is also present. (*From* Skuras, J. and Schrank, W. W.: The routine air-contrast examination of the esophagus. Radiology *115*:482–484, 1975.)

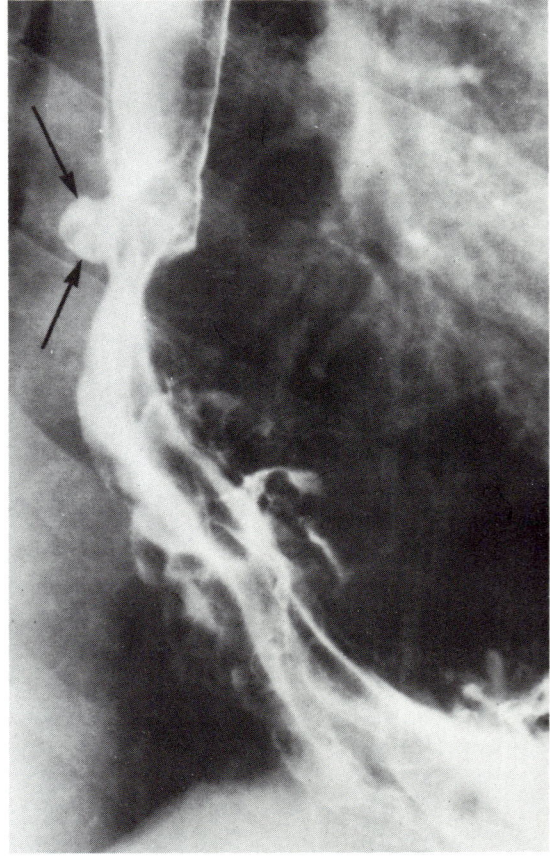

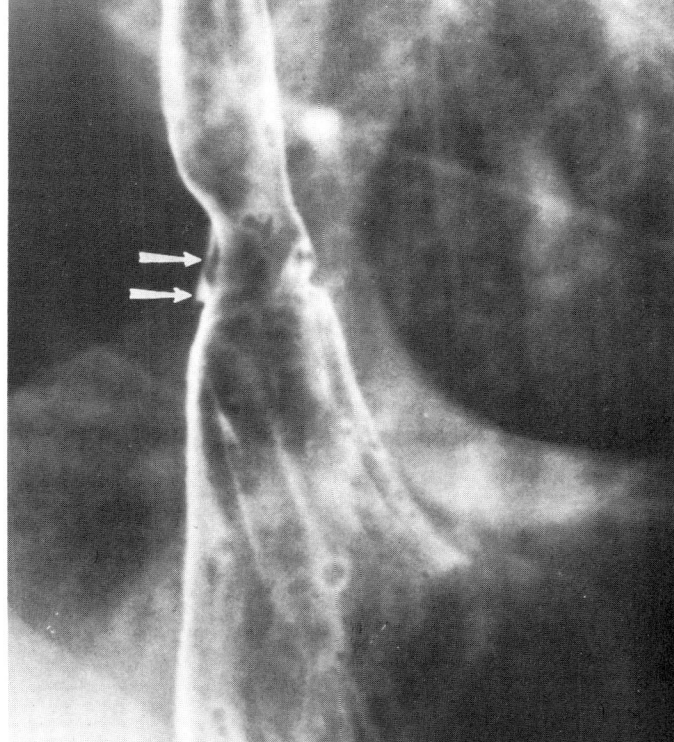

Figure 8–41. Hiatus hernia with ulcer. There is a linear longitudinal ulcer at the gastroesophageal junction (arrows). A rather wide hiatus is evident.

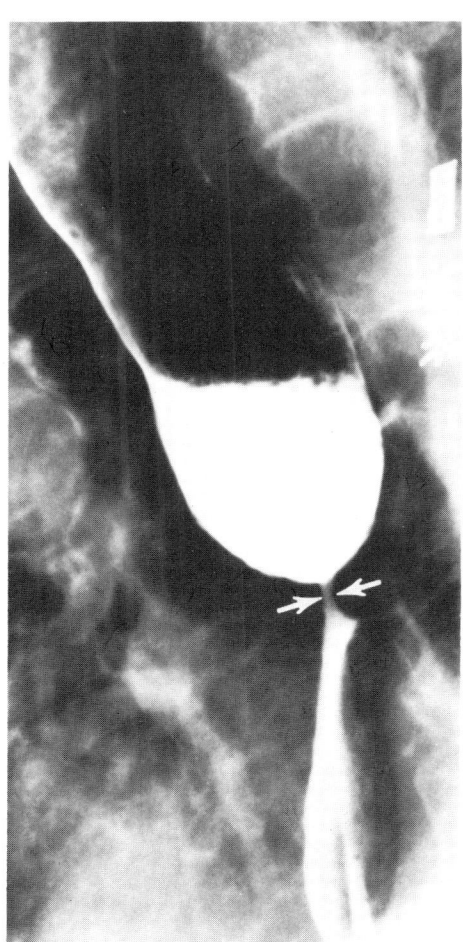

Figure 8–42. Hiatus hernia with stricture. A tight but symmetric stricture is present at the gastroesophageal junction (arrows). The patient had a long history of progressive dysphagia. As a result of the gradual onset, the esophagus proximal to the stricture has dilated considerably. (*From* Skucas, J.: The routine double-contrast examination of the esophagus. C.R.C. Crit. Rev. Diagn. Imaging, *11*:121–143, 1978.)

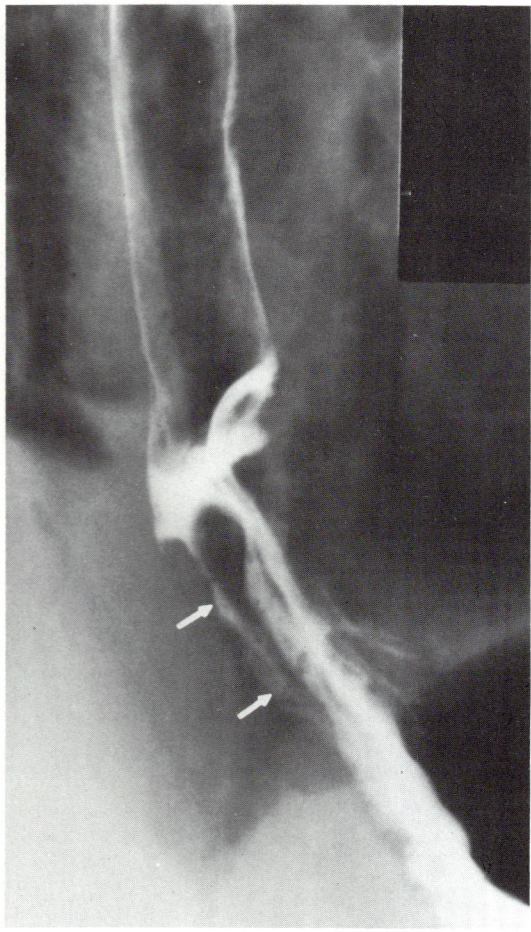

Figure 8–43. Reflux esophagitis mimicking carcinoma. This 54-year-old man had progressive dysphagia due to reflux esophagitis. There is a small hiatus hernia (arrows) with an irregular and asymmetric stricture at the gastroesophageal junction. This patient eventually underwent surgery because of his progressive symptoms. (*From* Skucas, J.: The routine double-contrast examination of the esophagus. C.R.C. Crit. Rev. Diagn. Imaging, 11:121–143, 1978.)

CONGENITALLY SHORT ESOPHAGUS

In this rare condition, seen almost exclusively in the pediatric age group, a portion of the stomach is fixed in an intrathoracic position. A similar appearance may be the result of gastroesophageal reflux with secondary inflammation and esophageal shortening. There may be associated splenic agenesis in some patients with a congenitally short esophagus.[14] A stricture can develop at the intrathoracic gastroesophageal junction (Fig. 8–44).

BARRETT'S ESOPHAGITIS

Occasionally the lower esophagus is lined by specialized columnar rather than squamous epithelium. Most investigators today believe that this condition is acquired, since most of these patients are in their fifties or sixties when first seen. Since the initial descriptions by Barrett,[1, 2] there has been considerable controversy about this condition. These columnar-lined esophageal segments are more common than previously was realized. Often the condition is associated with a hiatus hernia and reflux esophagitis. In one series, more than 80 per cent of the patients complained of dysphagia for solids for varying lengths of time.[13] Biopsy may reveal either the absence of parietal and chief cells or scattered gastric cells.[11] Although most of the resultant ulcers are in the columnar-lined portion of the esophagus, occasionally esophageal ulcers are found in the adjacent squamous epithelium.[13, 16] These ulcers, therefore, can occur anywhere throughout the esophagus (Fig. 8–45). The middle third of the esophagus is not an unusual location, the ulceration eventually progressing to a stricture (Fig. 8–46). Occasionally Barrett's esophagitis involves long segments of the esophagus, resulting in an extensive stricture and foreshortening (Fig. 8–47). The differentiation of this disease from a carcinoma can be difficult (Fig. 8–48); actually, there appears to be a higher incidence of carcinoma in the columnar-lined esophagus.[12]

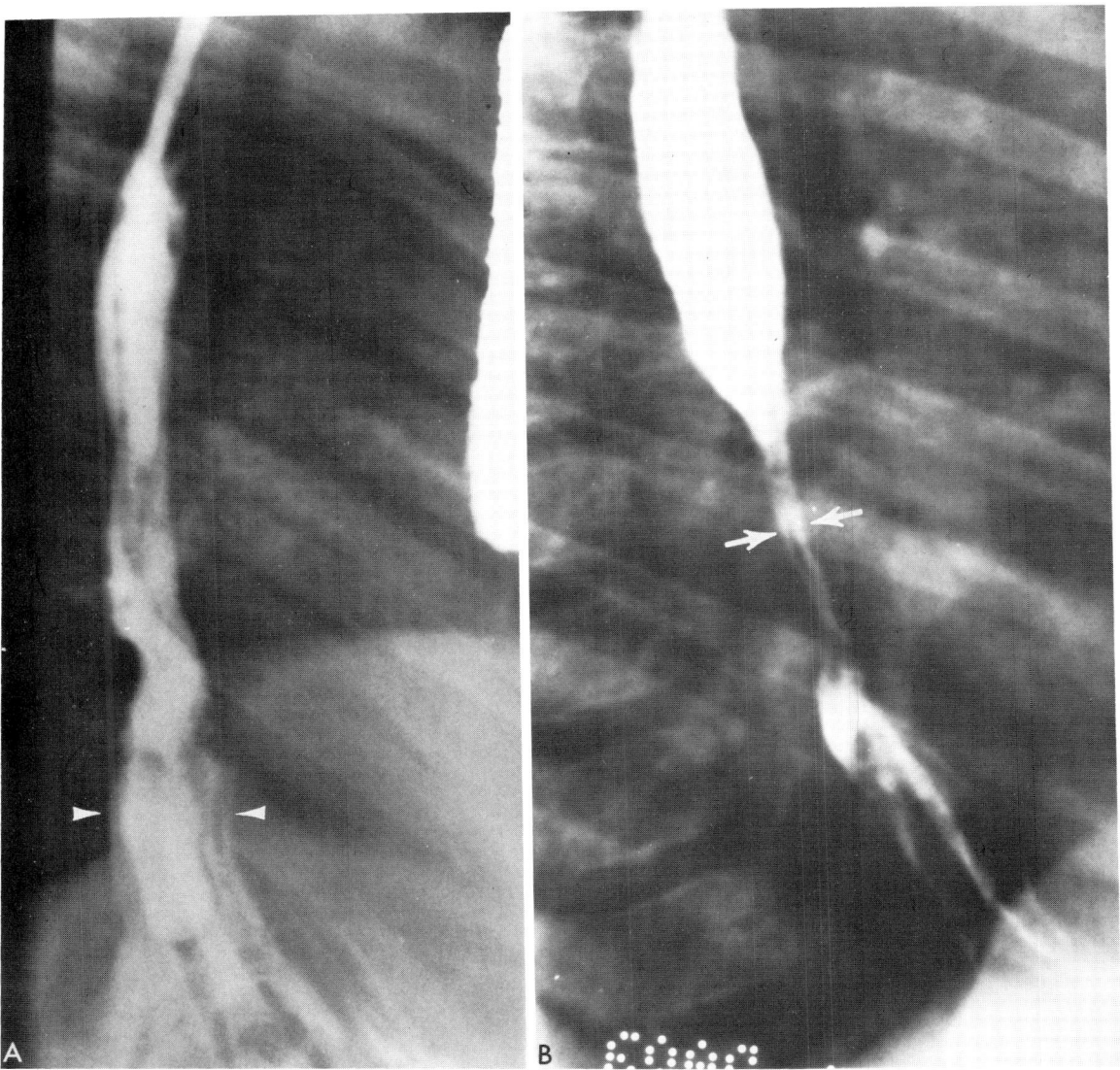

Figure 8–44. Congenital short esophagus. *A,* This 14-month-old baby has a hiatus hernia (arrowheads) and distortion at the gastroesophageal junction. *B,* Fourteen months later the hiatus hernia is still present, and there is also an esophageal stricture (arrows).

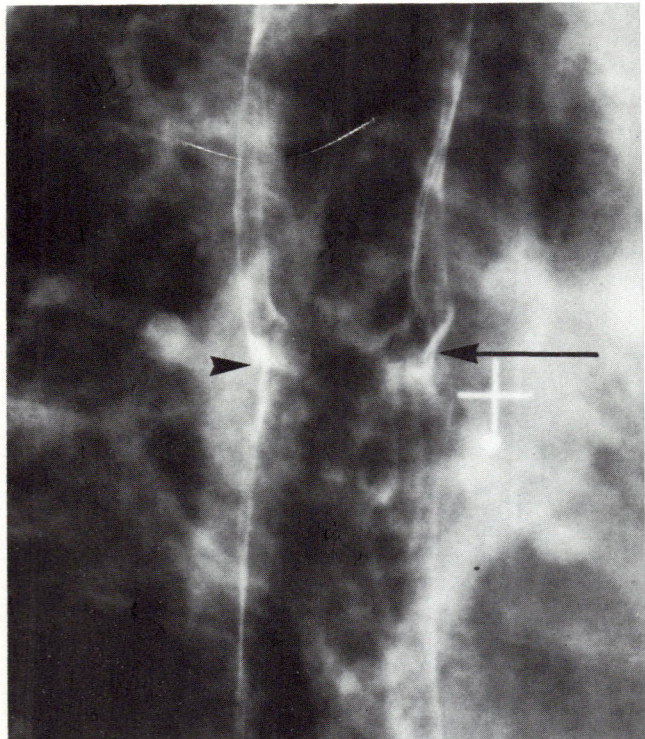

Figure 8–45. Barrett's esophagitis with ulcer. There is a mild stricture (arrow) and an ulcer (arrowhead) in the midesophagus in this 56-year-old man. The involved area was lined by columnar epithelium; superiorly and inferiorly the epithelium was squamous. (*From* Skucas, J.: The routine double-contrast examination of the esophagus. C.R.C. Crit. Rev. Diagn. Imaging, *11*:121–143, 1978.)

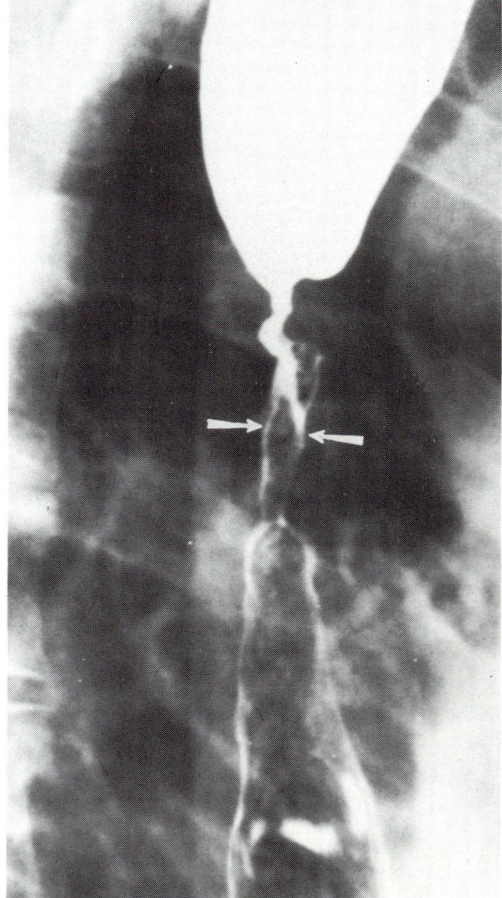

Figure 8–46. Barrett's esophagitis with stricture. This 49-year-old man had a two-month history of progressive dysphagia and 30-lb weight loss. There is an irregular long stricture in the midesophagus (arrows), with proximal esophageal dilatation. At esophagoscopy, the lesion appeared malignant, but subsequent resection revealed ectopic gastric mucosa.

Figure 8–47. Barrett's esophagitis with long stricture. A 52-year-old male with gradual onset of dysphagia. A stricture extends from the stomach and involves the lower half of the esophagus. The stricture has an undulating appearance, and the esophagus is foreshortened. Eventually the patient underwent resection of the involved area. (*From* Skucas, J.: The routine double-contrast examination of the esophagus. C.R.C. Crit. Rev. Diagn. Imaging 11:121–143, 1978.)

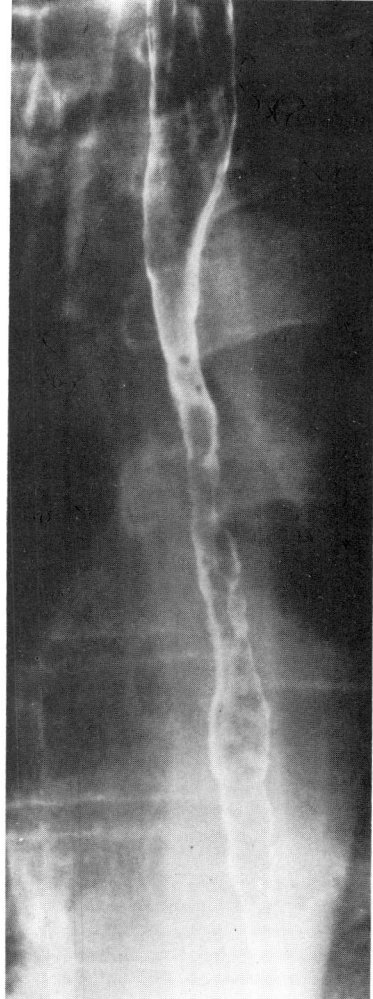

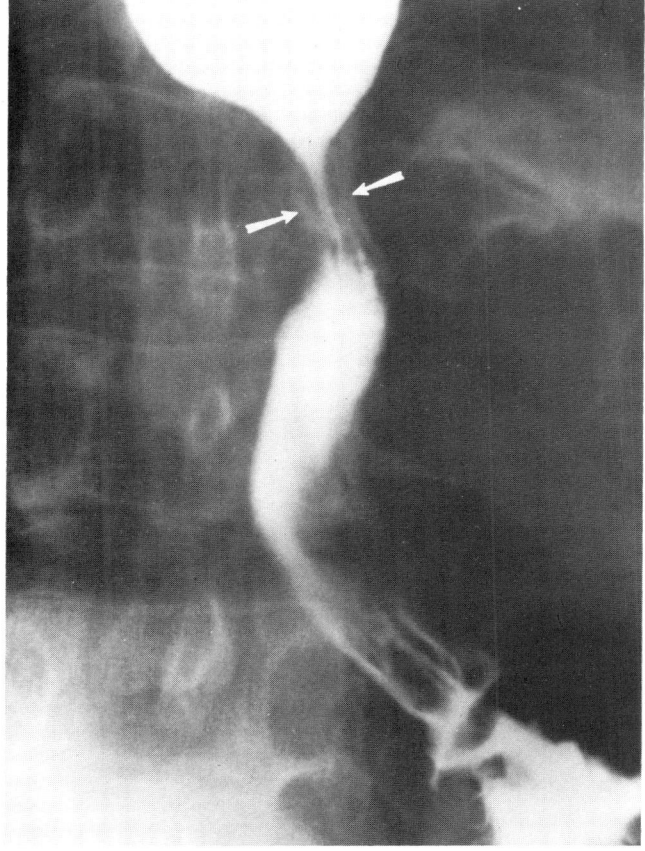

Figure 8–48. Esophageal carcinoma simulating a benign stricture. Squamous carcinoma in a 67-year-old male. The stricture is smooth and symmetric (arrows). There is also considerable dilatation in the proximal part of the esophagus.

Scintigraphy with ^{99m}Tc pertechnetate may be helpful in diagnosis.[3] There is an abnormal uptake of the radionuclide in the involved area. An antireflux procedure, such as fundoplication, can result in marked improvement.[10]

ESOPHAGOSCOPY AND ESOPHAGEAL DILATATION

Esophagoscopy and gastroscopy in a normal esophagus carry little risk. In the presence of inflammation, tumor, or undue tortuosity, however, the complication rate increases.

With suspected perforation, chest and abdominal radiographs may disclose pleural fluid, mediastinal gas, or pneumoperitoneum. Occasionally, however, pneumoperitoneum is seen even without perforation;[9] presumably the air dissects through tissue planes and eventually reaches the peritoneum. Perforation of the esophagus may result in subcutaneous emphysema. An esophagogram usually demonstrates a perforation

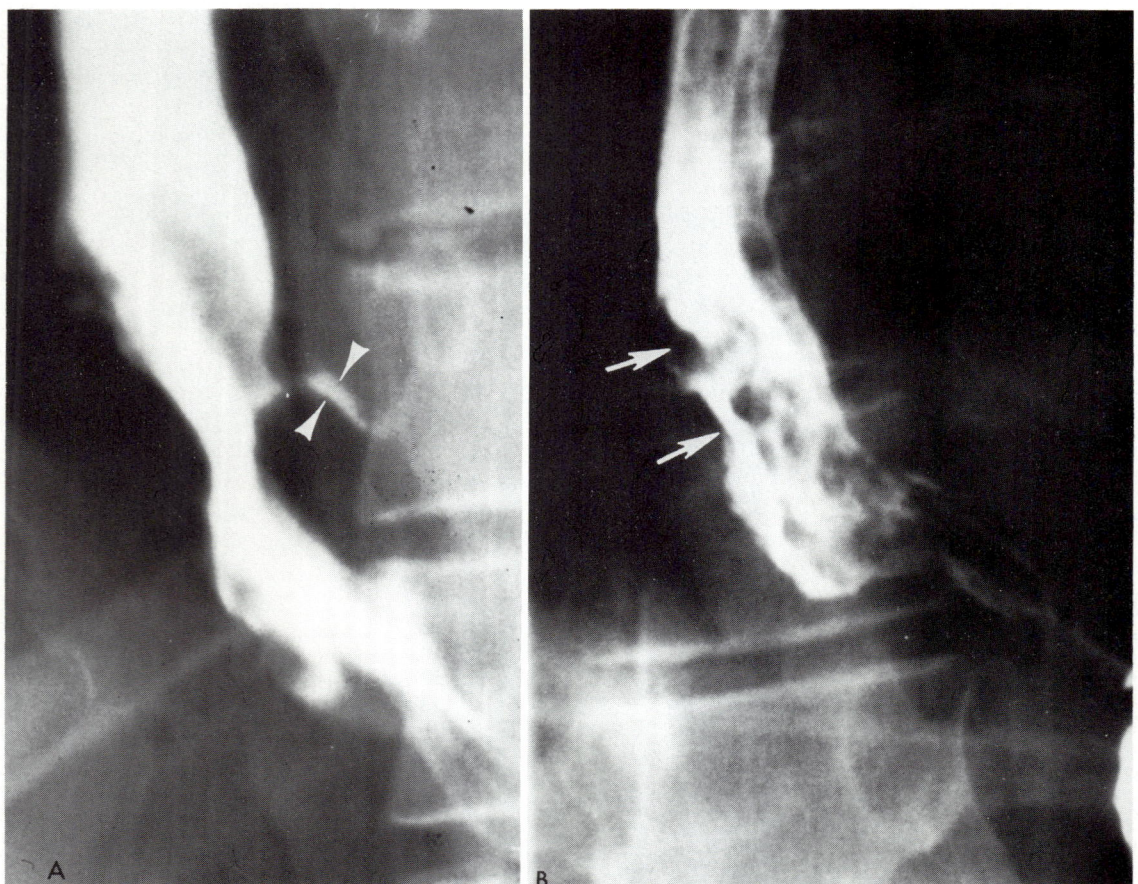

Figure 8–49. Esophageal perforation. This patient with dysphagia underwent endoscopy at another hospital. Only inflammatory changes were seen in the esophagus. A, Postendoscopy he had pain, and an esophagogram showed a localized perforation (arrowheads) and marked deformity throughout. He underwent surgery to repair the perforation. No tumor was appreciated at surgery. B, An esophagogram several days later again shows considerable distortion of the esophagus (arrows). His dysphagia progressed, surgery was again performed, and a carcinoma at the gastroesophageal junction was resected.

Figure 8–50. Prior esophageal perforation. A 71-year-old woman with long-standing achalasia who had undergone numerous prior surgical procedures, including an esophagojejunostomy, had a barium esophagogram performed shortly after esophageal perforation. Barium had extravasated into the mediastinal soft tissues. The current examination shows a dilated esophagus, indicated by the long air-fluid level (arrowheads), obstruction at the esophagojejunostomy site (large arrow), and residual barium in the soft tissues from the prior perforation (small arrows).

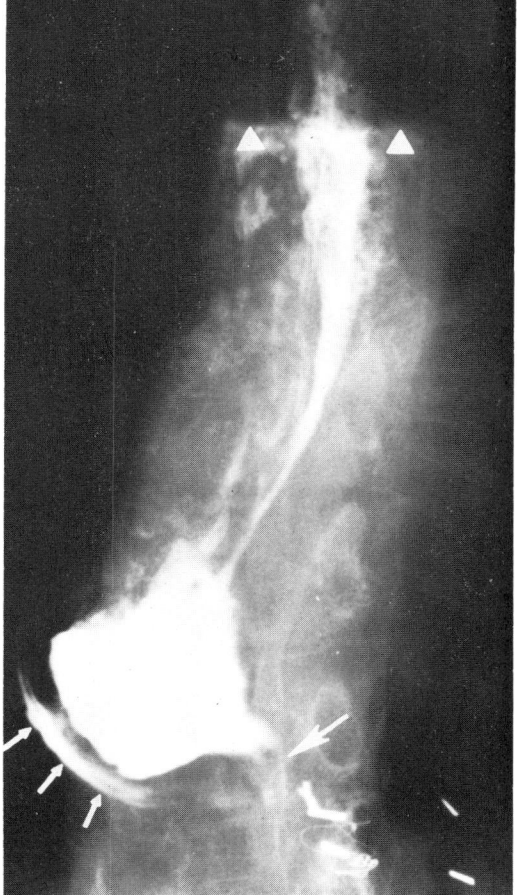

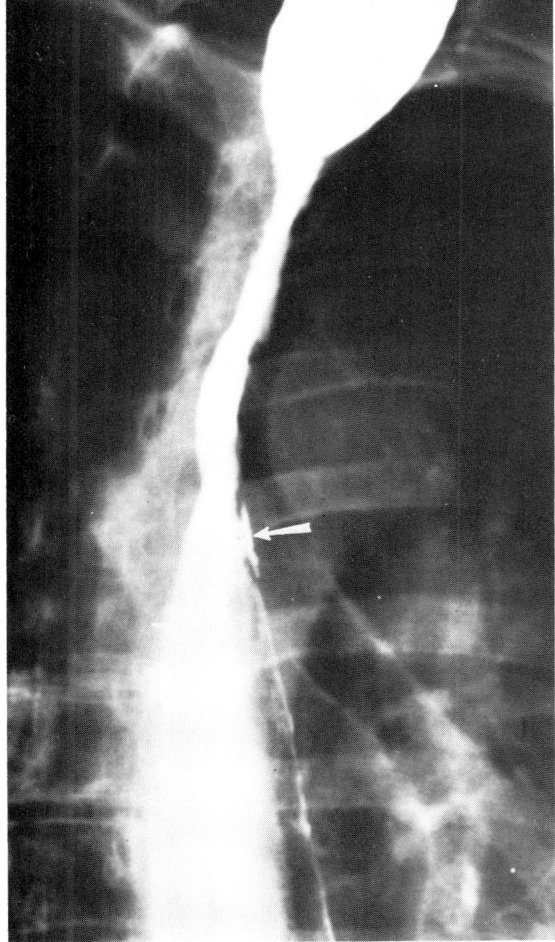

Figure 8–51. Intramural esophageal perforation. A 63-year-old woman with a midesophageal stricture underwent esophageal dilatation. An esophagogram taken after dilatation reveals intramural spread of contrast (arrow).

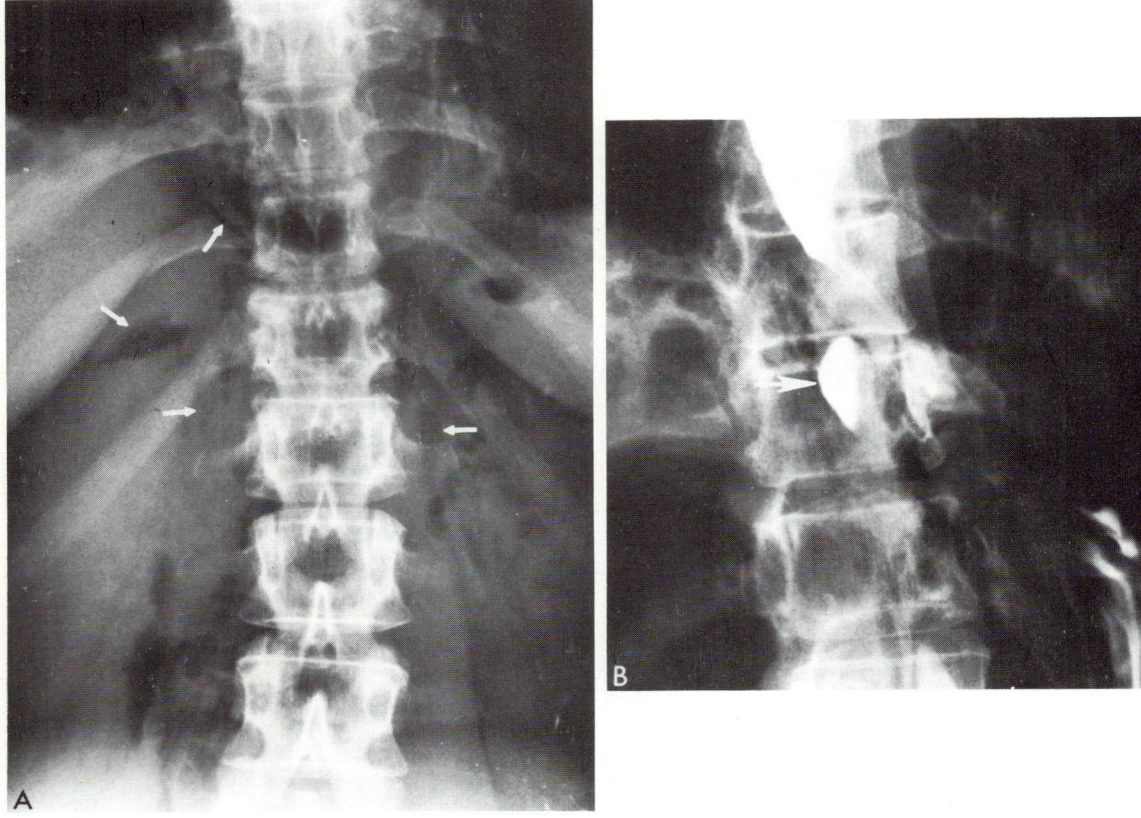

Figure 8–52. Transmural esophageal perforation. This 52-year-old woman had dilatation of a distal esophageal stricture resulting in perforation. A, Radiographs of the abdomen taken on admission reveal retroperitoneal gas (arrows). B, An emergency esophagogram locates the perforation in the distal esophagus (arrow).

Illustration and legend continued on the opposite page

(Fig. 8–49), although at times the initial examination may be normal. For study of a patient with suspected perforation, a water-soluble iodinated contrast medium should be used initially; if no obvious leak is seen, barium sulfate is employed for a more detailed study. At times a tube must be passed into the esophagus or stomach in order for an adequate study to be performed. If barium sulfate leaks into the surrounding tissues, residual barium may be evident for prolonged periods of time (Fig. 8–50).

During endoscopy, if the instrument is retroflexed in the stomach in order to better visualize the fundus and then is withdrawn, it can impact in the lower esophagus.[4]

After esophageal dilatation an esophagogram will demonstrate the resultant widening of the esophagus. There may be small intramural perforations, indicative of local trauma (Fig. 8–51). Most of these intramural, localized perforations are of little significance and heal spontaneously. On the other hand, if there has been transmural laceration of the esophagus, contrast leaks into either the mediastinum, the pleural space, or the abdomen, depending on the site of the perforation (Fig. 8–52).

Prior surgery on the esophagus can result in perforation, fistula formation, or stricture. At times the radiographic findings are bizarre (Fig. 8–53).

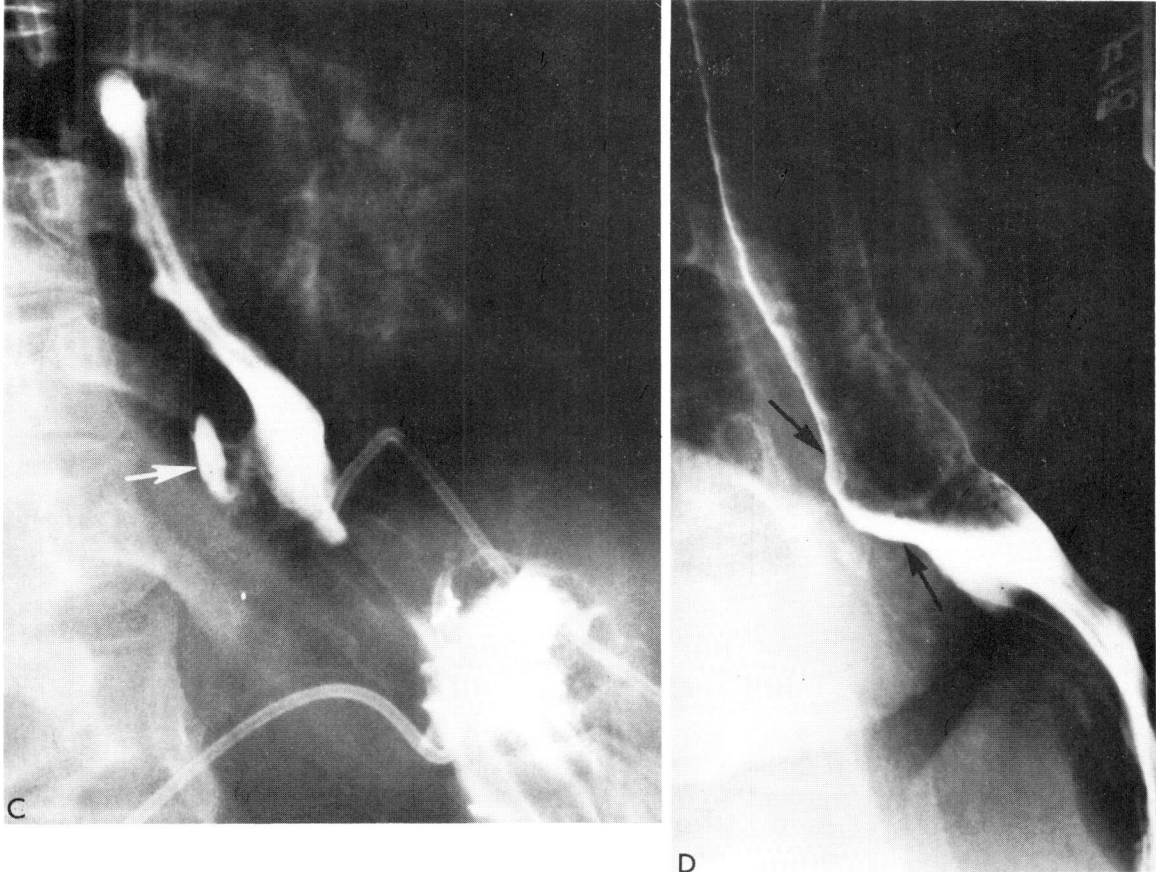

Figure 8–52 *Continued.* C, Nine days later, after surgical repair of the perforation, there is a well-defined outpouching at the site of perforation (arrow). D, A follow-up esophagogram taken five weeks later reveals only slight widening and distortion at the site of the previous perforation (arrows).

Esophageal obstruction due to an intramural hematoma from pneumatic dilatation has also been described.[7]

HIATUS HERNIA REPAIR

In the Belsey-Mark IV operation, the gastric fundus encircles the lower esophagus for approximately two thirds of its circumference. Surgery is performed through a left thoracotomy. A postoperative esophagogram shows a sharp angulation of the lower esophagus and a pseudotumor involving the cardia, with the lower esophagus passing through this mass (Fig. 8–54).

The Nissen fundoplication can be performed through either a thoracic or a transabdominal approach. The gastric fundus is wrapped around both sides of the esophagus and sutured together anteriorly (Fig. 8–55). The radiographic findings after a Nissen fundoplication are characteristic. There is a smoothly outlined and symmetric "mass" present at the cardia. This mass consists of the fundus wrapped around the

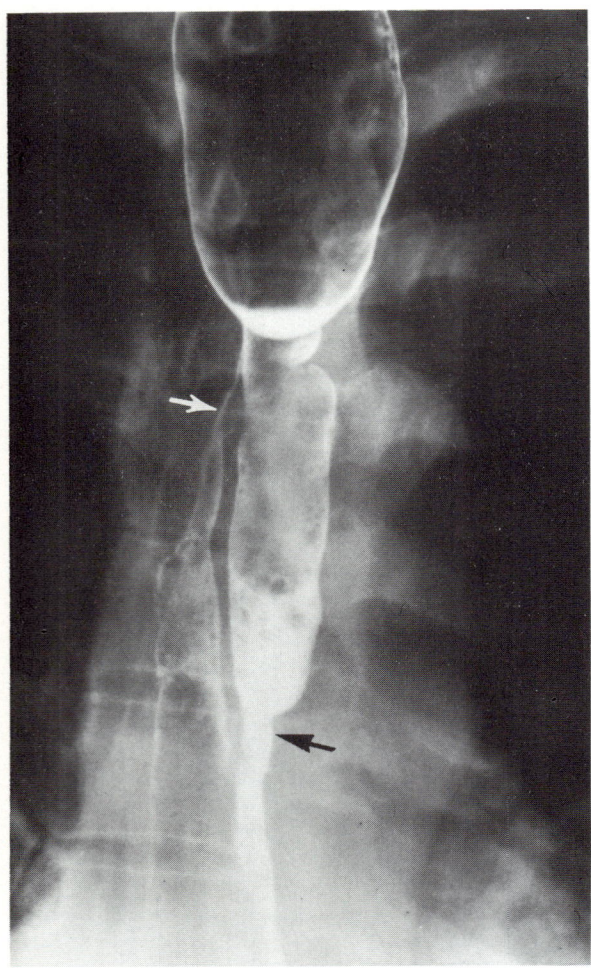

Figure 8–53. Double esophageal lumen. A 32-year-old woman who had ingested lye as a child and then undergone several corrective operations. She now has dysphagia, although she had been symptom-free for years. Both lumina are strictured (arrows). (*From* Skucas, J.: The routine double-contrast examination of the esophagus. C.R.C. Crit. Rev. Diagn. Imaging 11:121–143, 1978.)

esophagus; some barium or gas may be trapped in these folds. The esophagus can be seen tunneling through this mass (Fig. 8–56). The soft-tissue mass is more apparent immediately after surgery, owing to surrounding edema. Examinations performed months or years after fundoplication may reveal only a small defect (Fig. 8–57). Knowledge of the prior surgery and the typical radiographic appearance is essential to avoid confusing the soft-tissue mass with tumor. The well-preserved esophageal lumen and the well-defined gastroesophageal junction should allow ready differentiation, however.[15] Even if there is a recurrence of hiatal hernia after fundoplication, little or no reflux can be demonstrated radiographically.

The Hill procedure, also known as the posterior gastropexy, is performed through a transabdominal incision and consists of suturing the gastroesophageal junction to the median arcuate ligament. Usually the major radiologic postoperative feature is simply a smooth narrowing of the distal esophageal segment (Fig. 8–58), although some believe that the radiographic appearance of this operation is distinctive.

In the Thal fundal patch technique the serosa of the fundus is grafted over the strictured segment, resulting in some distortion of the gastric fundus.

Text continued on page 367.

THE ESOPHAGUS — 363

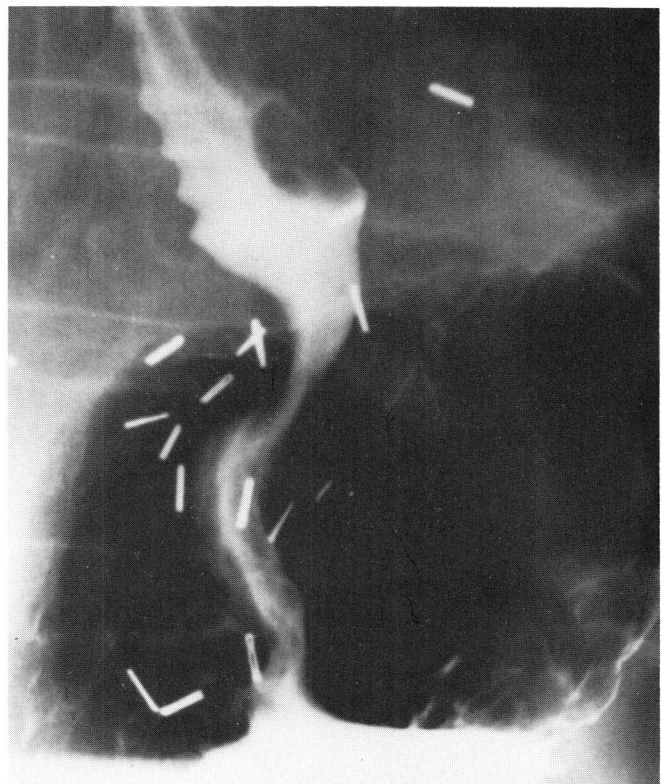

Figure 8–54. Post-Belsey operation. A 64-year-old man underwent repair of a hiatus hernia using the Belsey procedure. The distal esophagus is slightly narrowed and angulated.

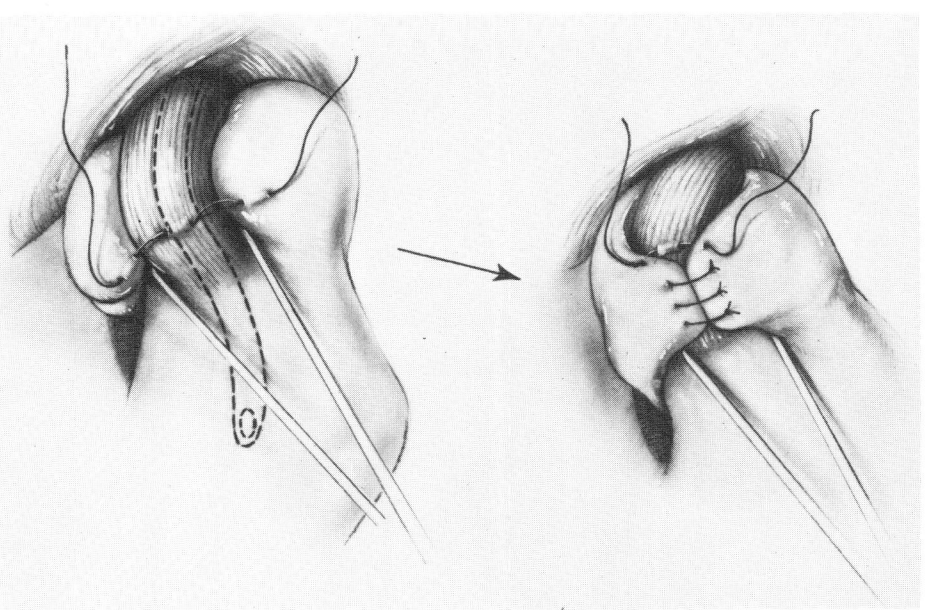

Figure 8–55. Diagram of the technique of Nissen fundoplication. A large-bore tube is in the esophagus to prevent excessive narrowing of the lumen. The hiatus hernia is reduced, and then the fundus is wrapped around the esophagus. (*From* Skucas, J., Mangla, J. C., Adams, J. T., et al.: An evaluation of the Nissen fundoplication. Radiology *118*:539–543, 1976.)

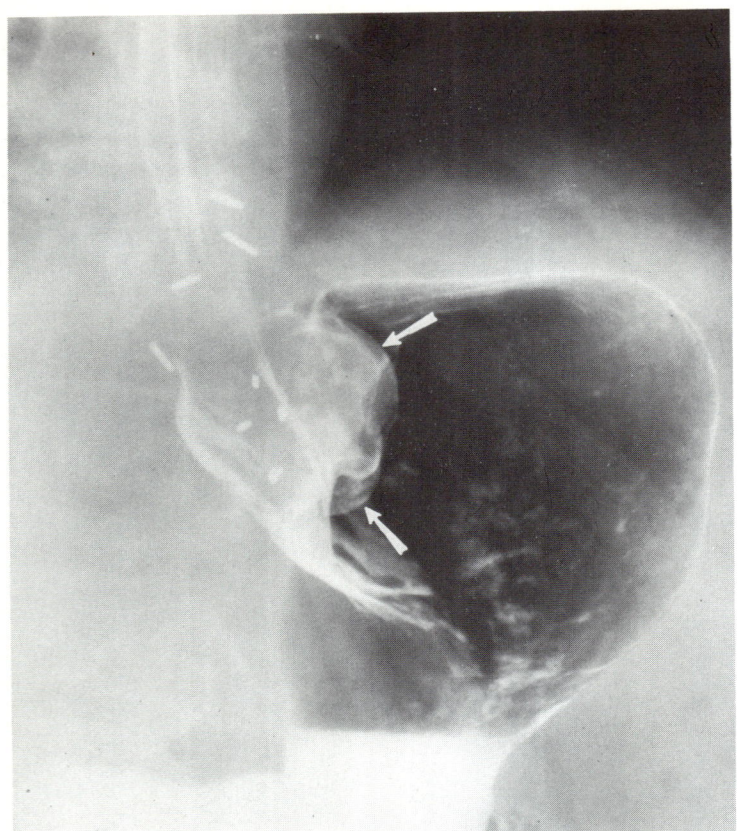

Figure 8–56. Post-Nissen fundoplication. An esophagogram performed 13 days after surgery shows the typical "pseudotumor" (arrows) and narrowed distal esophagus. (*From* Skucas, J., Mangla, J. C., Adams, J. T., et al: An evaluation of the Nissen fundoplication. Radiology *118*:539–543, 1976.)

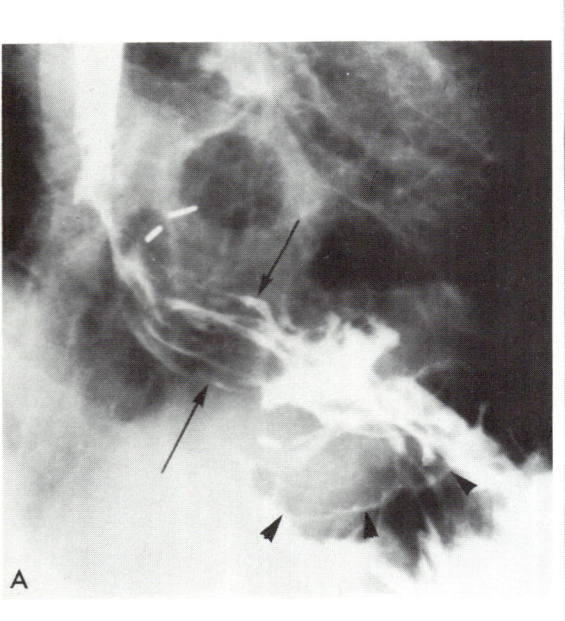
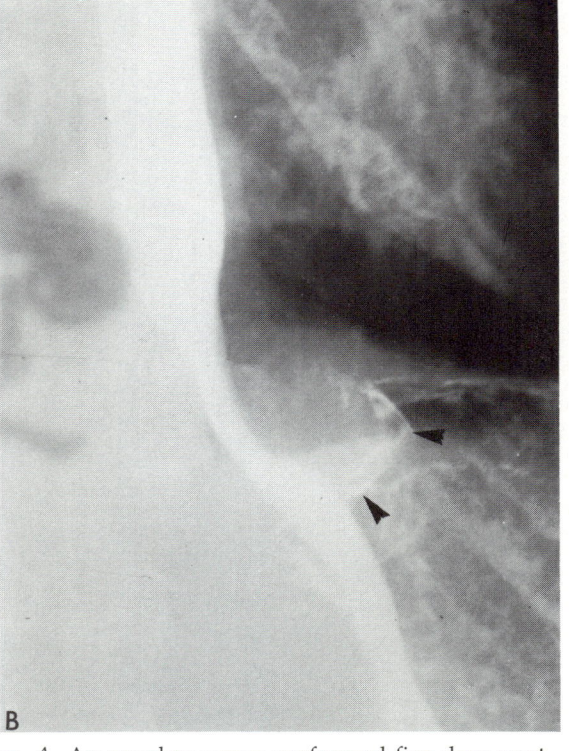

Figure 8–57. Pseudotumor of Nissen fundoplication. *A,* An esophagogram performed five days postfundoplication reveals a persistent hiatus hernia (arrows). There was no reflux. A prominent pseudotumor is also present (arrowheads). *B,* The same patient two years later. No hiatus hernia was evident, there was no reflux, and the patient was considerably improved. A residual pseudotumor, smaller than it was initially, persists (arrowheads). (*From* Skucas, J., Mangla, J. C., Adams, J. T. et al.: An evaluation of the Nissen fundoplication. Radiology, *118*:539–543, 1976.)

Figure 8–58. Post-Hill procedure. A 62-year-old woman after a Hill repair of a hiatal hernia. There is a smooth narrowing of the distal esophagus (arrows). No pseudotumor was present.

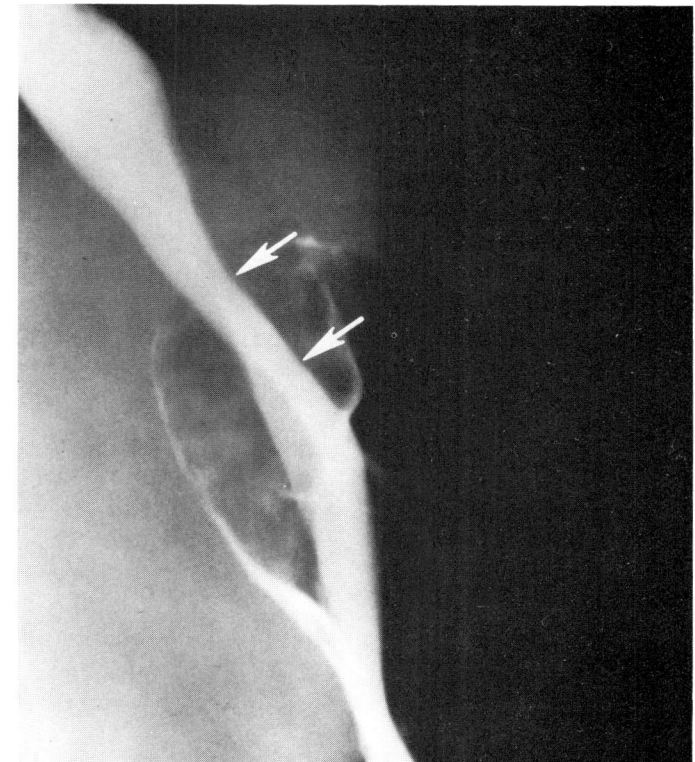

Figure 8–59. Empyema after hiatus hernia repair. This patient developed a left empyema after surgery. A chest tube was inserted (arrowhead) and gastric contents were aspirated. The chest tube has fortuitously been advanced through the gastropleural fistula into the stomach (straight arrow. An esophagogram outlines the fistula and the pleural extension of the empyema (curved arrows). Contrast is also draining through the chest tube.

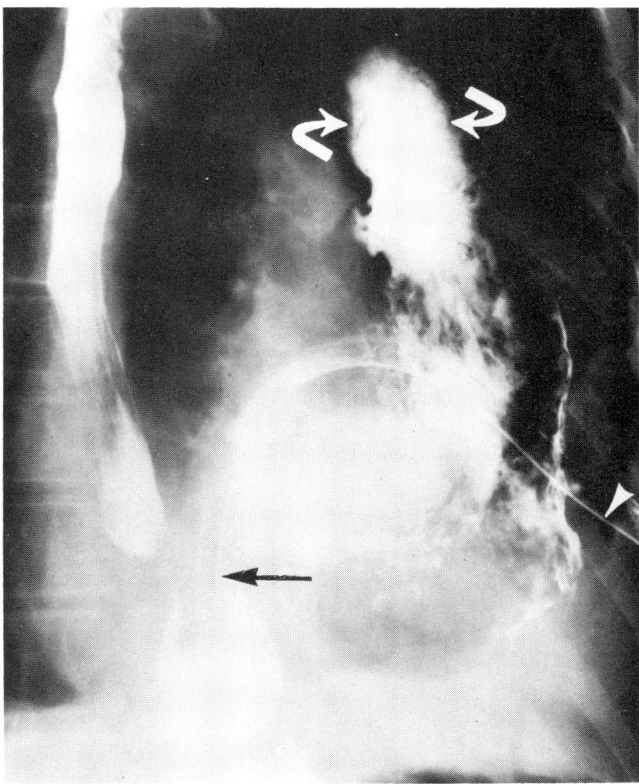

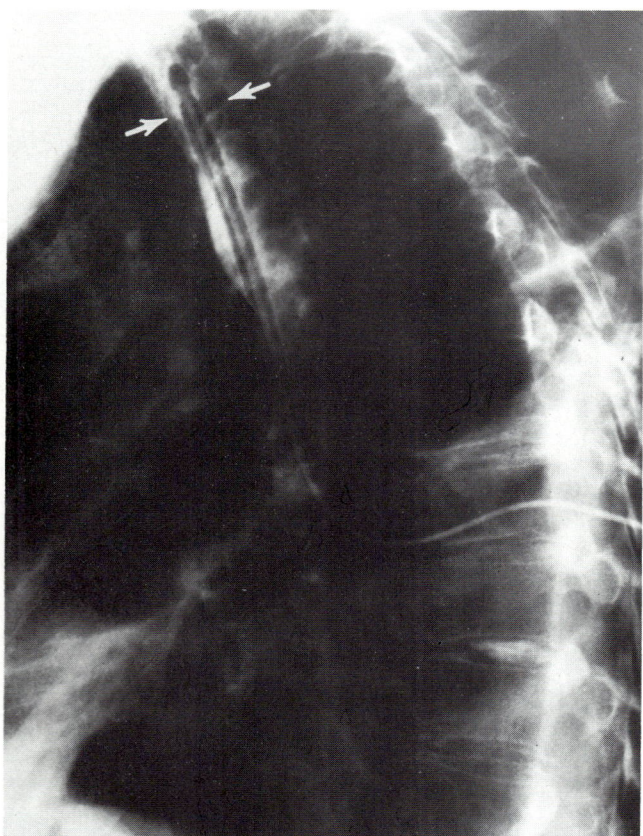

Figure 8–60. Esophagocutaneous fistula. A 60-year-old woman developed a cutaneous fistula after hiatus hernia surgery. A catheter was introduced into the fistula and contrast injected. The tip of the catheter is in the esophagus (arrows).

Figure 8–61. Subphrenic abscess after hiatus hernia repair. A 72-year-old woman underwent a Nissen fundoplication. Postoperatively she developed a left subphrenic abscess (arrowheads) communicating with the gastroesophageal region (arrow).

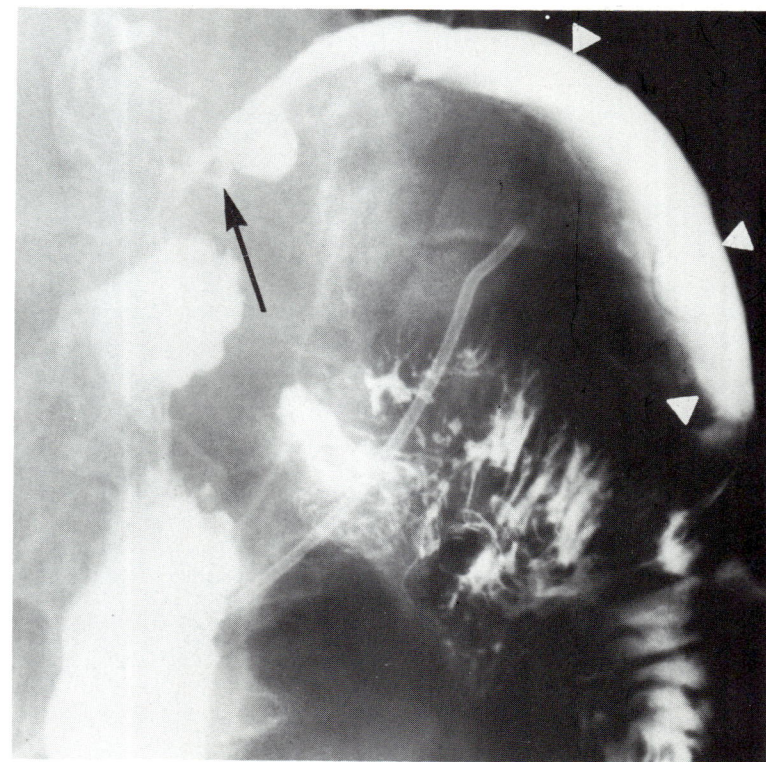

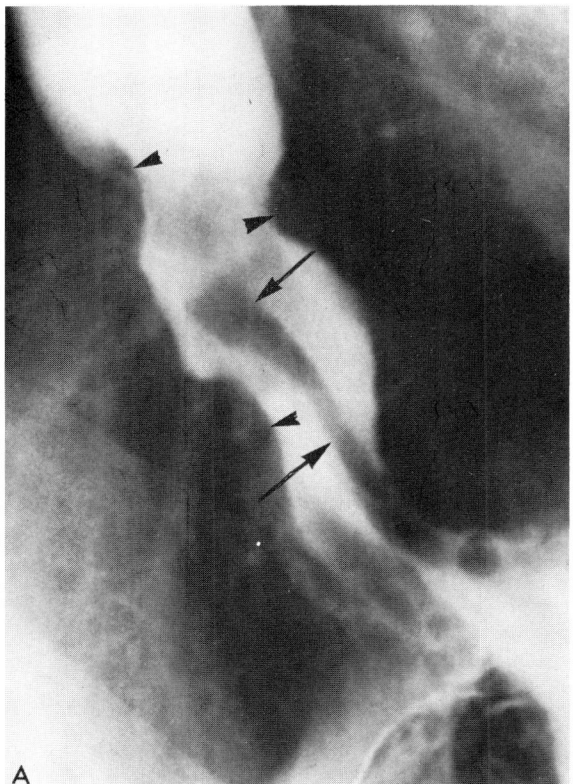
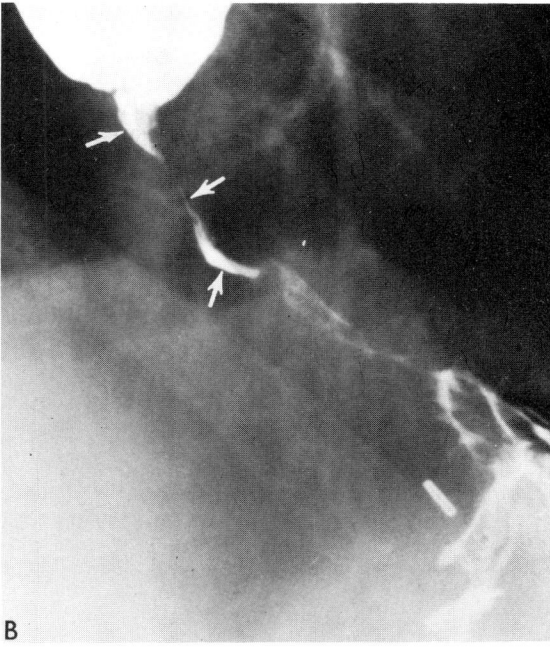

Figure 8–62. Carcinoma and hiatus hernia repair. *A*, This patient developed dysphagia, and an esophagogram revealed irregular asymmetric masses (arrowheads) and thickened folds (arrows) in the hiatus hernia, findings that are suspicious of an infiltrating lesion, but might also be due to inflammatory changes. The patient apparently underwent several other diagnostic tests, and eventually a hiatus hernia repair was performed. Apparently no tumor was discovered by the surgeon. *B*, The patient was referred to another hospital because of progressive dysphagia. An esophagogram taken five months after the initial study reveals a marked irregular stricture (arrows) with proximal dilatation. The stricture is due to extensive invasion by adenocarcinoma.

COMPLICATIONS OF HIATUS HERNIA REPAIR

Esophageal obstruction may occur after surgery. There may be postoperative abscess formation, causing a mottled appearance in either the mediastinum or the abdomen. Empyema may develop owing to a gastropleural fistula (Fig. 8–59). An esophagocutaneous fistula can develop (Fig. 8–60). If a leak occurs below the diaphragm, a left subphrenic abscess may result (Fig. 8–61).

The importance of a correct preoperative diagnosis is obvious. A carcinoma at the gastroesophageal region may result in progressive dysphagia and may mimic stenosis due to reflux esophagitis. Even during hiatus hernia repair, the surgeon may miss a carcinoma (Fig. 8–62).

References

1. Barrett, N. R.: Chronic peptic ulcer of the esophagus and "oesophagitis." Br. J. Surg. *38*:175–182, 1950.
2. Barrett, N. R.: The lower esophagus lined by columnar epithelium. Surgery *41*:881–894, 1957.
3. Berquist, T. H., Nolan, N. G., Stephens, D. H., et al.: Radioisotope scintigraphy in diagnosis of Barrett's esophagus. Am. J. Roentgenol. *123*:401–411, 1975.

4. Burke, E. L., and Roling, G. T.: Reflections on retroflexions. Gastrointest. Endosc. 17:99–100, 1971.
5. Feigin, D. S., James, A. E., Jr., Stitik, F. P., et al.: The radiological appearance of hiatal hernia repairs. Radiology 110:71–77, 1974.
6. Gerson, D. E., and Lewicki, A. M.: Intrathoracic stomach: when does it obstruct? Radiology 119:257–264, 1976.
7. Heceta, W. G., Wrobel, L. D., and Pate, J. W.: Esophageal obstruction due to intermuscular hematoma following pneumatic dilatation. Chest 69:115–117, 1976.
8. Kalokerinos, J.: The moon-shaped fundal defect of hiatus hernia: a new radiological sign. Aust. Radiol. 13:96–102, 1969.
9. Katz, D., Cano, R., and Antonelle, M.: Benign air dissection of the esophagus and stomach at fiberesophagoscopy. Gastrointest. Endosc. 19:72–74, 1974.
10. Mangla, J. C., Schenk, E. A., and Desbailets, L.: Pepsin secretion, pepsin, and gastrin in "Barrett's" esophagus. Gastroenterology 70:669–676, 1976.
11. Paull, A., Trier, J. S., Dalton, M. D., et al.: The histologic spectrum of Barrett's esophagus. N. Engl. J. Med. 295:476–480, 1976.
12. Poleynard, G. D., Marty, A. T., Birnbaum, W. B., et al.: Adenocarcinoma of the columnar-lined (Barrett) esophagus. Case report and review of the literature. Arch. Surg. 112:997–1000, 1977.
13. Robbins, A. H., Hermos, J. A., Schimmel, E. M., et al.: The columnar-lined esophagus—analysis of 26 cases. Radiology 123:1–7, 1977.
14. Shapiro, R. L.: Clinical Radiology of the Pediatric Abdomen and Gastrointestinal Tract. Baltimore, University Park Press, 1976, p. 28.
15. Skucas, J., Mangla, J. C., Adams, J. T., et al.: An evaluation of the Nissen fundoplication. Radiology 118:539–543, 1976.
16. Wolf, B. S., Marshak, R. H., and Som, M. L.: Peptic esophagitis and peptic ulceration of the esophagus. Am. J. Roentgenol. 79:741–759, 1958.

Part IV

Perforation of the Esophagus

DENIS J. O'CONNELL, M.R.C.P., F.R.C.R.

Perforation of the esophagus can no longer be considered an uncommon clinical entity. Its increasing incidence is directly related to the numerous endoscopic and therapeutic procedures now performed in many centers. Iatrogenic esophageal rupture is the most common cause of esophageal perforation, giving rise to 75 per cent of the cases in one series[3] and 50 per cent in another.[7] Several series have shown that mortality from esophageal perforation is related to delay in diagnosis, the site of perforation, and the presence of associated esophageal disease.[10] It is therefore important to be aware of the cases of esophageal rupture and to take rapid, appropriate steps to establish an early diagnosis of this potentially lethal condition. The causes of esophageal perforation are listed in Table 8–1.

Spontaneous perforation of the esophagus, first described by Boerhaave in 1924, is important to recognize because a delay in diagnosis is likely to have disastrous consequences. Although the clinical features have been well described, spontaneous esophageal rupture may mimic other acute thoracic and abdominal conditions. Accurate diagnosis is crucial, therefore, and in this regard, appropriate radiologic investigation has a significant role.

PATHOPHYSIOLOGY

Instrumental esophageal perforation tends to occur at the anatomic areas of esophageal narrowing, that is, the esophageal origin adjacent to C_6, the aortic arch, and the

TABLE 8–1. CAUSES OF ESOPHAGEAL PERFORATION

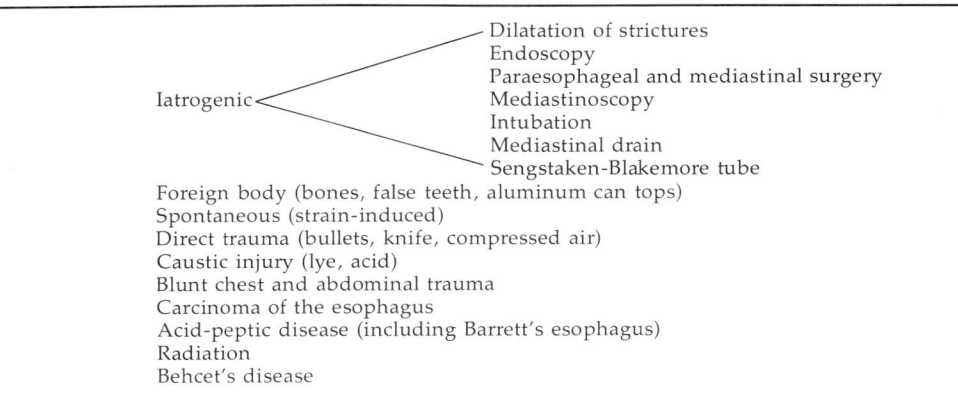

Iatrogenic
- Dilatation of strictures
- Endoscopy
- Paraesophageal and mediastinal surgery
- Mediastinoscopy
- Intubation
- Mediastinal drain
- Sengstaken-Blakemore tube

Foreign body (bones, false teeth, aluminum can tops)
Spontaneous (strain-induced)
Direct trauma (bullets, knife, compressed air)
Caustic injury (lye, acid)
Blunt chest and abdominal trauma
Carcinoma of the esophagus
Acid-peptic disease (including Barrett's esophagus)
Radiation
Behcet's disease

diaphragmatic hiatus. Passage of an endotracheal tube may cause perforation of the pyriform sinuses or cervical esophagus. Sharp foreign bodies (such as chicken bones) also tend to obstruct and perforate the cervical esophagus. Aluminum can tops ("pop-tops"), which have caused perforation of the cervical and thoracic esophagus in children, are relatively radiolucent and are difficult to appreciate even on the best-quality plain radiographs.[9]

Spontaneous, or strain-induced, esophageal rupture is reported with increasing frequency and constituted 35 per cent of the cases in a recent series of 33 esophageal perforations.[7] Although sudden vomiting is the usual cause, several reports have described spontaneous rupture after unusual physical straining, lifting, childbirth, defecation, and blunt abdominal trauma. The common denominator is a sudden violent increase in intra-abdominal pressure, which is transmitted to the relaxed lower esophagus. In the majority of cases, spontaneous rupture occurs in the left posterolateral aspect of the lower esophagus, and the tear is usually longitudinal and measures between 2 and 8 cm.[2] More than one tear may be present.[4] Rarely, spontaneous perforation may occur in the upper or middle third of the esophagus. Mackler[11] has shown that the lowest portion is the weakest part because of the lack of a supporting aorta, with only a thin layer of parietal pleura separating the left lower part of the esophagus from the left lung. The pressure needed to perforate the lower esophagus is approximately 5 pounds per square inch.

In children, the left lateral aspect of the esophagus is relatively well buttressed by the descending aorta, and higher pressures are needed to cause rupture. Neonatal spontaneous esophageal rupture has been described and usually occurs on the right side.[6]

Caustic strictures due to lye or acid ingestion may cause spontaneous perforation, but iatrogenic perforation following dilatation of a caustic stricture is much more common.

Most iatrogenic damage to the esophagus occurs during dilatation of strictures, hydrostatic dilatation for achalasia, removal of foreign bodies, and diagnostic esophagoscopy. More recently, however, iatrogenic esophageal rupture has been described in association with mediastinal drainage tubes, mediastinoscopy, fundoplication, vagotomy, and resection of pulmonary and mediastinal tumors. Emergency intubation may cause perforation of the hypopharynx or cervical esophagus. The esophageal obturator airway, extensively used by paramedical personnel during cardiopulmonary resuscitation, has also been associated with perforation of the cervical and distal esophagus.

CLINICAL FEATURES

Clinically, esophageal perforation can mimic a wide variety of acute abdominal and intrathoracic conditions, including perforated peptic ulcer, acute pancreatitis, mesenteric infarction, strangulated intrathoracic stomach, tension pneumothorax, aortic dissection, myocardial infarction, and pulmonary embolism. For this reason, the diagnosis of esophageal perforation, particularly the spontaneous variety, is not infrequently delayed. Although iatrogenic rupture is usually recognized during the procedure and surgical techniques have been considerably improved, the significant rates of mortality and morbidity associated with spontaneous, or strain-induced, esophageal rupture remain. A high index of suspicion and early radiologic investigation are of paramount importance in cases of possible esophageal rupture.

Although approximately 95 per cent of patients have low thoracic or epigastric pain [16] and 35 per cent also report back pain, pain may not be a significant feature of perforation of a previously diseased esophagus.[5] Clinical signs of esophageal perforation are inconstant,[10] and only about 50 per cent of patients with spontaneous esophageal rupture present with the classic triad of vomiting, low thoracic pain, and subcutaneous emphysema.[18] Dyspnea may be a prominent feature if a tension pneumothorax occurs. In one series, subcutaneous emphysema was detected in all patients with spontaneous rupture.[20] Abbott et al., however, stated that surgical emphysema may be undetectable clincally up to 24 hours after perforation, owing to the fact that most of the air leaking from the esophagus enters the pleural space.[20] According to one review of the literature, subcutaneous emphysema was palpable in only 60 per cent of cases.[15] A pleural effusion, usually left-sided, may be detectable clinically.

Neonatal spontaneous esophageal perforation presents differently, with cyanosis, tachycardia, and tachypnea, owing to a combination of a tension pneumomediastinum or tension hydropneumothorax. Although this condition is rare, it should be considered in the differential diagnosis of neonatal respiratory distress.

RADIOLOGIC EVALUATION

The radiologic examination of a patient with suspected esophageal perforation may be conveniently performed in two stages: the plain film examination and the contrast examination.

The most valuable diagnostic procedures are the upright chest radiograph[8, 10] and the contrast esophagogram.[16] Because the clinical picture of esophageal perforation is nonspecific, erect and supine abdominal radiographs are usually also obtained. These may help exclude the diagnosis of intestinal perforation and bowel infarction, but in the context of esophageal rupture they are of limited value, since subdiaphragmatic extension of free air from a perforated esophagus is rare.[10, 19]

Plain Film Examination

Many authors have emphasized the value of an early upright chest radiograph when this diagnosis is suspected. The earliest sign is the presence of linear collections of air in the fascial planes of the mediastinum. Free air may be seen outlining the border of the descending aorta and the aortic knob, or there may be small linear collections of air in the paratracheal regions (Fig. 8–63). As the volume of mediastinal gas increases, air may be seen in the fascial planes of the neck and supraclavicular regions (Figs. 8–64 to 8–67). Subdiaphragmatic extension of mediastinal emphysema

THE ESOPHAGUS — 371

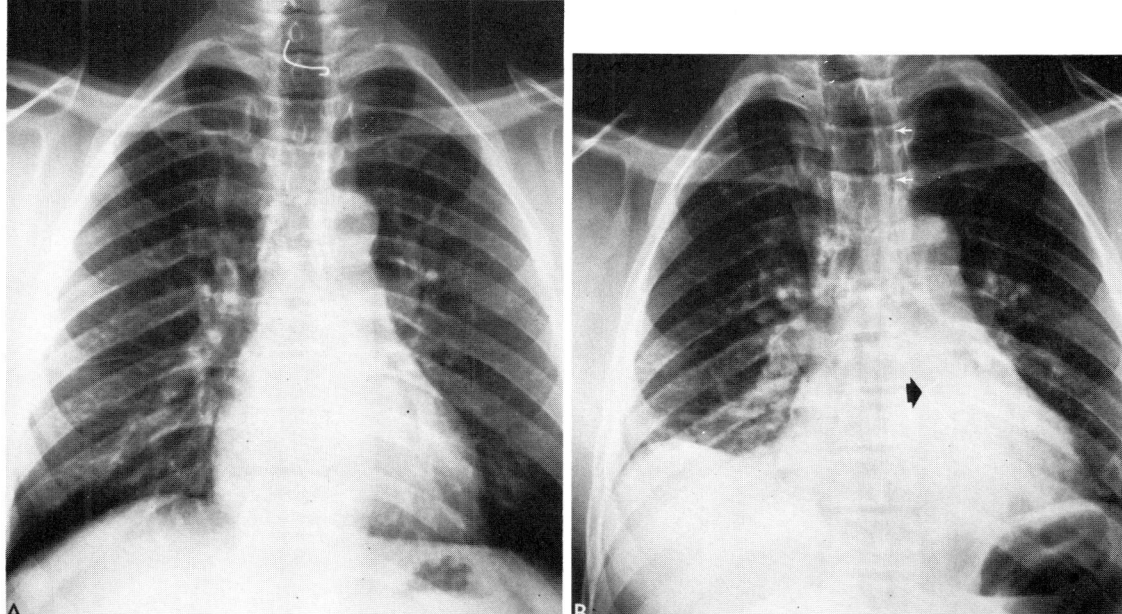

Figure 8–63. *A,* A 29-year-old male who swallowed dentures. The chest radiograph is normal. *B,* Twenty-four hours later, there is widening of the upper mediastinum. Note the linear collections of mediastinal air (white arrows) and the bilateral basal consolidation. The dentures are well to the left of the spine, and at surgery the esophagus was perforated.

is rare unless rupture of the subdiaphragmatic esophagus has occurred.[10, 14] If a radiograph is taken soon after the perforation and there is insufficient gas in the mediastinum to be appreciated, another radiograph should be taken after about two hours.

The diagnosis of subtle amounts of mediastinal emphysema depends on a sharp,

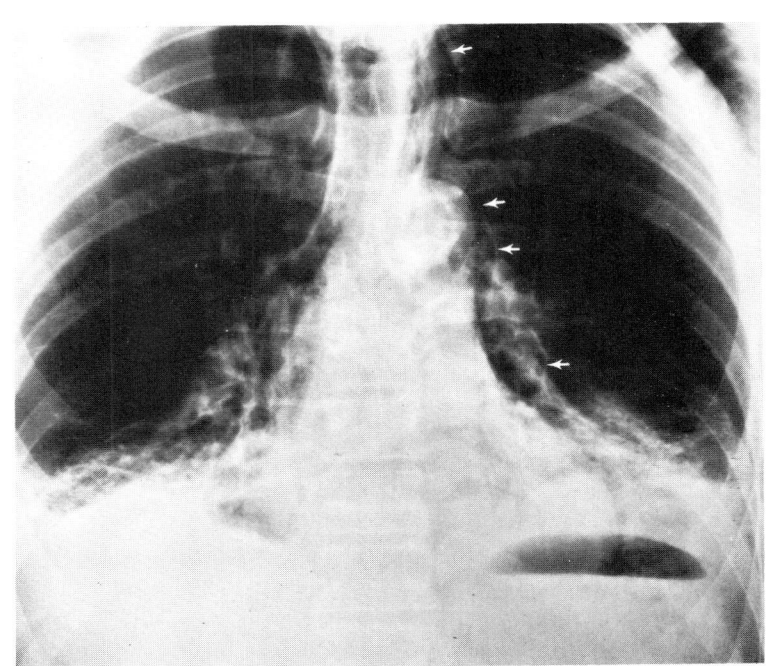

Figure 8–64. A 48-year-old female with spontaneous perforation one hour following laryngoscopy. There is extensive mediastinal emphysema (arrows) in the left paratracheal region and in the region of the aortic knob and left heart border. Surgical emphysema is present in the left axilla. There is bilateral basal consolidation and bilateral effusions. At surgery, a tear was found in the left lateral part of the lower esophagus.

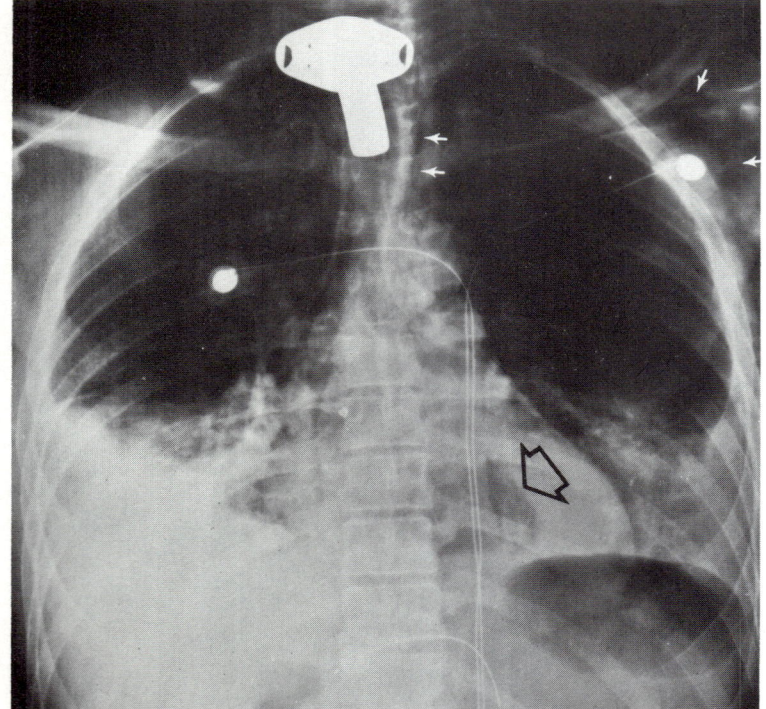

Figure 8–65. A 53-year-old female with spontaneous perforation three days after laryngectomy. There is mediastinal and surgical emphysema (white arrows). Note the large collection of air and fluid behind the heart (open arrow). There are bilateral effusions and infiltrates in both lower lobes.

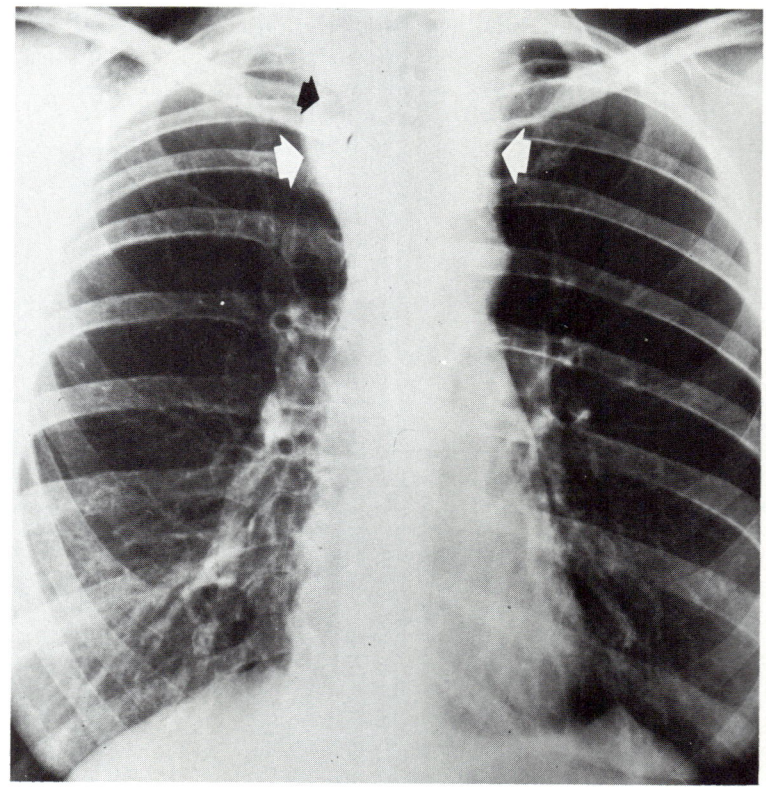

Figure 8–66. A 50-year-old male with dysphagia and fever 24 hours after esophagoscopy. The upper mediastinum is widened (white arrows). Note the abscess with the air-fluid level (black arrow) in the right paratracheal region. There is surgical emphysema in the right side of the neck. The esophagus was perforated just above the aortic arch.

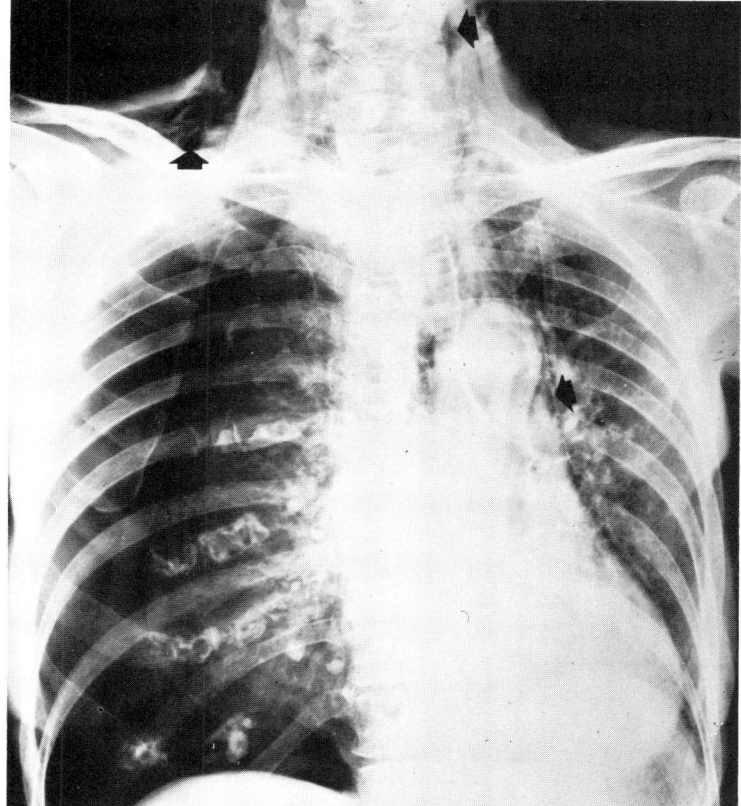

Figure 8–67. An 85-year-old female. Two hours after several unsuccessful attempts at esophagoscopy, she complained of dyspnea. There is a tension pneumothorax on the right, with displacement of mediastinal structures to the left. There is mediastinal emphysema, with air in the fascial planes of the neck and in the right supraclavicular region (arrows). The esophagus was perforated at the level of T_3.

properly exposed radiograph. Underexposure and lack of sharpness due to motion are the usual causes of missing the diagnosis in the early stages. It should be noted, however, that mediastinal emphysema may not be seen at any stage in as many as 40 per cent of cases.[13] Naclerio has described a V-shaped collection of air in the esophagodiaphragmatic recess, which represents early, localized mediastinal emphysema in the lower mediastinum.[12] This is a rare sign, however, and it is much more common for free air to diffuse throughout the mediastinum than to remain adjacent to an esophageal tear. An instrumental tear of the cervical esophagus results in characteristic vertical linear collections of air in the precervical soft tissues. There may also be a localized air-fluid collection with diffuse widening of the precervical soft tissues (Fig. 8–68). A plain lateral view of the neck is usually sufficient to establish the diagnosis, which can be confirmed by an esophagogram.

When the intrathoracic esophagus ruptures, fluid leaks from the perforated esophagus into the mediastinum. If the tear is in the mid- or lower esophagus, it is common to see the mediastinal fluid collection as a fusiform density, with an air-fluid level behind the heart (see Fig. 8–65). This sign is best appreciated on an overexposed or Bucky radiograph. The upper portion of the mediastinum widens to accommodate the increasing volume of mediastinal fluid. Mediastinal widening is best appreciated in the paratracheal regions. At this stage, the patient may have fever, cyanosis, hypotension, and tachycardia. These signs are probably due to increased mediastinal tension with subsequent compression of the major venous structures. In addition to medias-

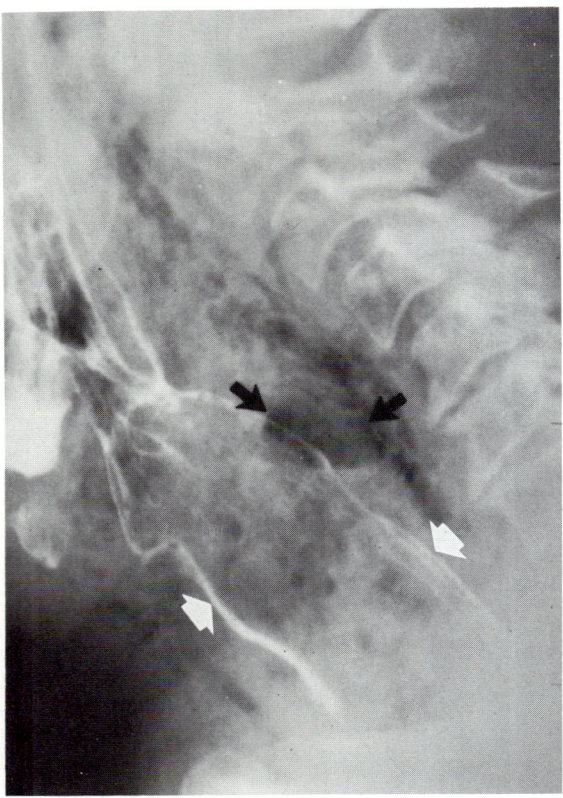

Figure 8–68. A 54-year-old female complained of neck pain and dysphagia following bronchoscopy. There is gas in the soft tissues and an abscess with an air-fluid level (black arrows). White arrows outline the barium-coated esophagus, displaced to one side and compressed by the large cervical abscess.

tinal widening, fluid collections in the upper mediastinum may cause anterior displacement of the trachea on the lateral chest radiograph.

A left pleural effusion with or without an associated pneumothorax occurs in 75 per cent of cases of perforation of the intrathoracic esophagus. The effusion occurs early if the pleura is torn with the esophagus, but there may be a delay of 24 to 48 hours before a sympathetic pleural effusion develops if pleural integrity is maintained. With spontaneous esophageal rupture, there is usually a tear in the adjacent parietal pleura, allowing gas and fluid to enter the left pleural space. This results in a hydropneumothorax, which may occasionally be under tension (see Fig. 8–67).

Pleural effusions are bilateral in approximately 7 per cent of cases,[2] but 5 per cent occur only on the right side. Several hours after the tear has occurred, it is common to find consolidation with or without collapse in the left lower lobe. The collapse consolidation is probably partly due to compression of the left lower lobe by the pleural fluid. In the first 24 hours after esophageal perforation, it is possible to demonstrate that the pleural fluid is free-flowing on a left lateral decubitus radiograph. This projection may often reveal subtle amounts of mediastinal air, which may not have been appreciable on the upright posteroanterior projection. A small pneumothorax may also be demonstrated along the mediastinal reflection of the parietal pleura. After 24 hours, it is inevitable that an empyema will be present if the pleura is torn. This should be suspected if there are loculated collections of pleural fluid or if the pleural fluid fails to move on the supine or lateral decubitus projections.

Contrast Examination

Whether or not the plain chest radiographic signs suggest esophageal perforation, when this diagnosis is suspected an esophagogram is indicated to confirm and localize the perforation (Figs. 8–69 to 8–71). Knowledge of the actual site of perforation, the volume of mediastinal fluid, and the presence of other esophageal disease, particularly obstruction, is important to the surgeon in making management decisions. With good technique it is often possible to demonstrate the site of the associated pleural tear, if there is one (Figs. 8–69 and 8–70).

There is some disagreement about the type of contrast medium to be used in suspected perforation of the esophagus. The majority of esophageal perforations are demonstrated by water-soluble Gastrografin, which diffuses through an esophageal tear and is absorbed from the mediastinum in a period of hours. Some authors, however, favor the use of barium because of its radiopacity. They justify the possible development of delayed adhesive mediastinitis by citing the superior definition produced by barium and reason that if a tear is demonstrated, the extravasated barium can be removed from the mediastinum at thoracotomy. Iodized oil (Lipiodol or Dionosil) should not be used because the high viscosity of this medium may fail to demonstrate small perforations.

A negative esophagogram does not necessarily exclude the diagnosis of esophageal rupture, although a false negative examination occurred in only one of 46 patients with esophageal rupture.[17]

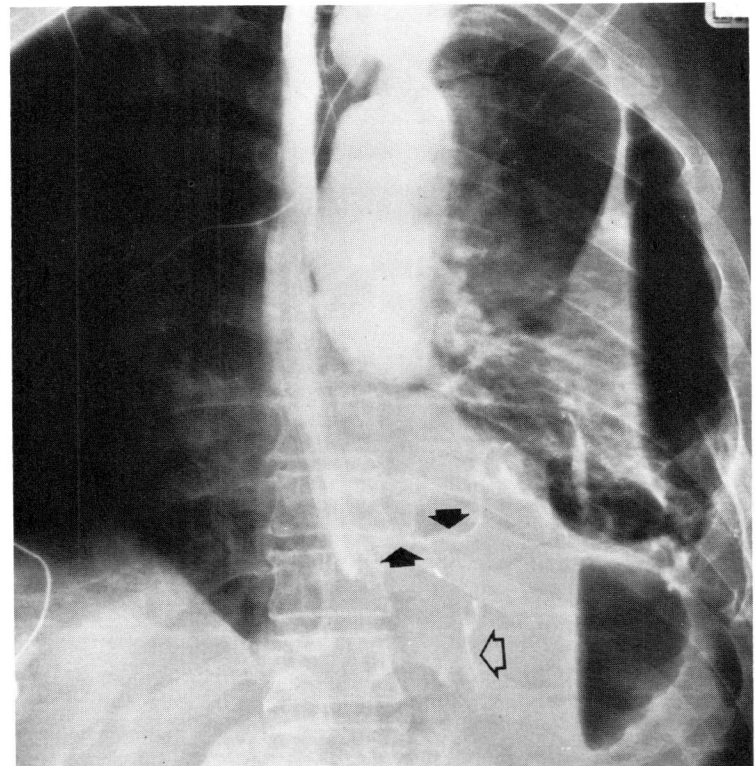

Figure 8–69. A 48-year-old male. Twenty-four hours after myotomy for achalasia he complained of chest pain. A Gastrografin esophagogram shows a leak from the lower esophagus (black arrows), with contrast tracking below the diaphragm (open arrow). This right lateral decubitus projection shows the large left hydropneumothorax. The left lower lobe is collapsed.

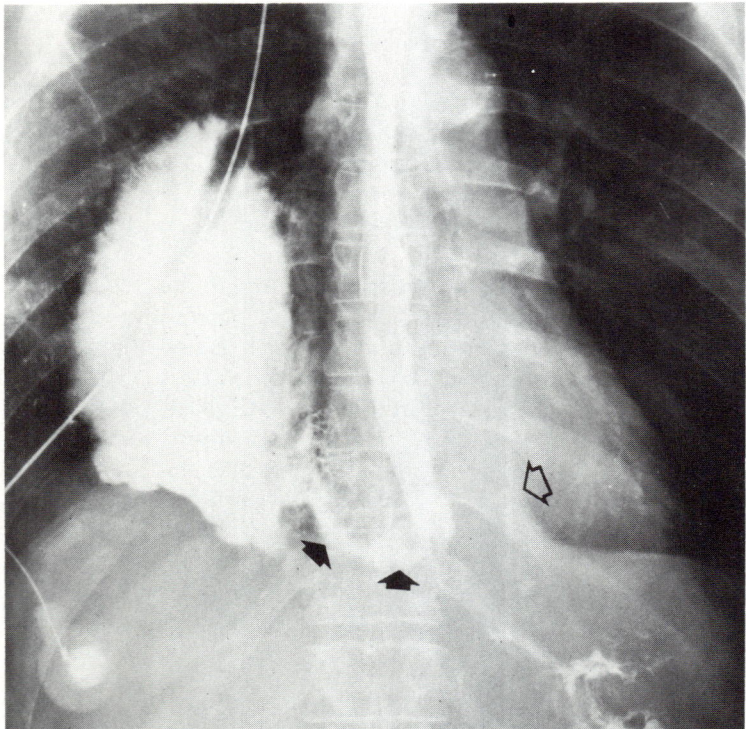

Figure 8–70. Spontaneous perforation in a 50-year-old female. This was not diagnosed until a right subphrenic abscess and right emphysema were drained. The esophageal and associated pleural tear are clearly demonstrated (black arrows), and contrast medium is pooling in the posterior part of the right pleural space. The left lower lobe is partly collapsed (open arrow).

The technique of examination for esophageal perforation is important. In the cervical region, anteroposterior and lateral views of the distended esophagus are adequate. If the patient is uncooperative, good spot films may be difficult to obtain, and the examination should be recorded on video tape or ciné. Supine and prone oblique projections of the intrathoracic esophagus should be taken. Some authors have advocated rocking the patient from side to side as he drinks the contrast medium,[14] but this is probably not necessary and may be difficult with an ill, uncooperative patient.

If adequate views of the distended esophagus are obtained, few, if any, perforations should be missed. Cross-table lateral decubitus views of the contrast-filled intrathoracic esophagus are of value if the routine views are negative (see Fig. 8–69). Some observers advocate passing a Ryle tube into the stomach and injecting contrast medium as the tube is withdrawn through the esophagus. This method has the advantage of giving good esophageal distention but necessitates passage of the tube across the site of the perforation, which may enlarge it.

The management of esophageal rupture depends on the site of the perforation. Perforations of the cervical esophagus require drainage of the precervical soft tissues, which usually results in spontaneous closure of the perforation. To confirm this, a repeat esophagogram may be performed. Rupture of the intrathoracic esophagus requires thoracotomy, closure of the defect, and drainage of the mediastinum. Serial chest radiographs should be obtained to confirm the resolution of the mediastinal and pleural fluid. Forty-eight hours after esophageal repair, another esophagogram should be taken to confirm the integrity of the repair. When a small leak is demonstrated, adequate drainage often results in its spontaneous closure.

After repair, the esophagogram may demonstrate plication defects at the anasto-

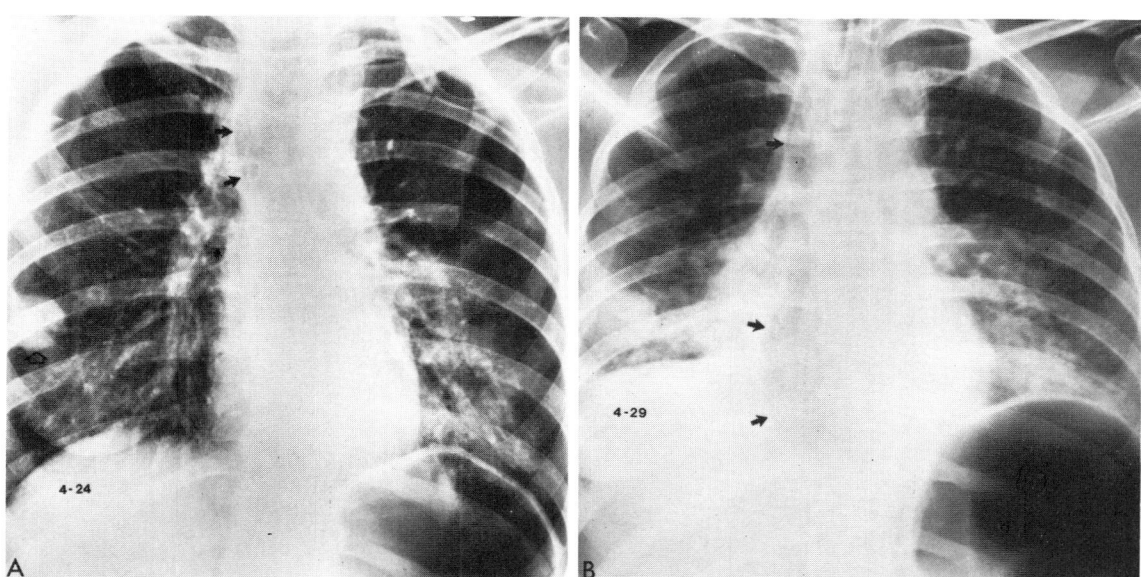
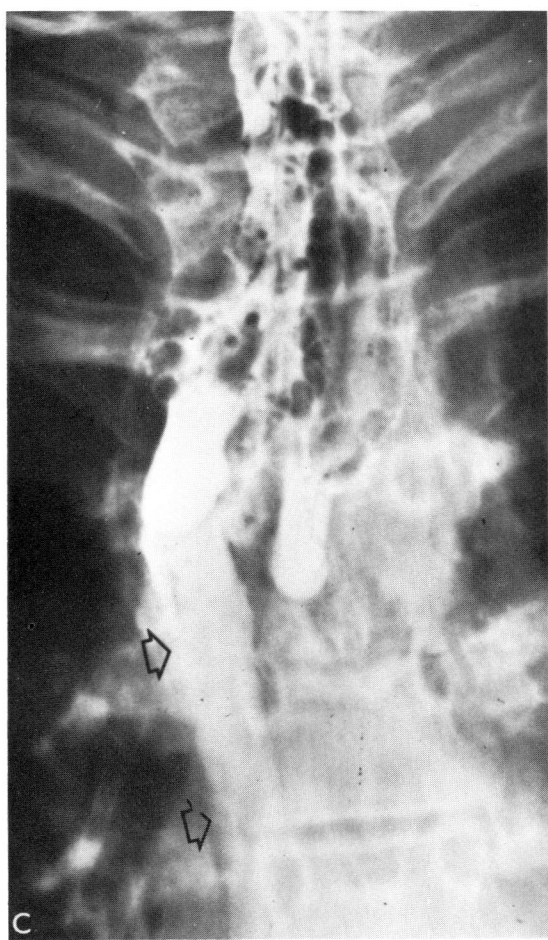

Figure 8–71. Hodgkin's disease and pulmonary involvement (open arrow), left lower lobe pneumonia, and documented esophageal candidiasis in a 29-year-old female. *A,* The mediastinum is wide owing to previous radiotherapy, but note the abnormal gas shadow in the right paratracheal region (black arrows). *B,* Five days later, there is a large fusiform collection of gas in the mediastinum (black arrows) and a right pleural effusion. *C,* Gastrografin swallow demonstrates extravasation into the mediastinal abscess (open arrow). At autopsy, a 2-cm by 2-cm defect due to spontaneous perforation was found in the upper esophagus.

motic site, which may give the mucosa a slightly nodular appearance. It is also common for a mild degree of stenosis to be demonstrated at the site of the repair. If there is a resolving mediastinal abscess, a smooth extrinsic defect resulting from pressure on the esophagus may also be present in the first few postoperative days.

References

1. Abbott, O. A., Mansour, K. A., Logan, W. D., Jr., et al.: Atraumatic so-called "spontaneous" rupture of the esophagus. A review of 47 personal cases with comments on a new method of surgical therapy. J. Thorac. Cardiovasc. Surg. 59:67–83, 1970.
2. Anderson, R. L.: Rupture of the esophagus. J. Thorac. Surg. 24:369–388, 1952.
3. Berry, B. E., and Ochsner, J. L.: Perforation of the esophagus. A 30 year review. J. Thorac. Cardiovasc. Surg. 65:1–7, 1973.
4. Christoforidis, A., and Nelson, S. W.: Spontaneous rupture of esophagus with emphasis on the roentgenologic diagnosis. Am. J. Roentgenol. 78:574–580, 1957.
5. Foster, J. H., Jolly, P. C., Sawyers, J. L., et al.: Esophageal perforation, diagnosis and treatment. Ann. Surg. 161:701–709, 1965.
6. Harell, G. S., Friedland, G. W., Daily, W. J., et al.: Neonatal Boerhaave's syndrome. Radiology 95:665–668, 1970.
7. Keighley, M. R. B., Girdwood, R. W., Wooler, G. H., et al.: Morbidity and mortality of esophageal perforation. Thorax 27:353–358, 1972.
8. Leading article: Management of esophageal perforation. Br. Med. J. 1:540, 1977.
9. Levick, R. K., and Robinson, A.: Case reports: the "invisible" can top. Br. J. Radiol. 50:594–596, 1977.
10. Loop, F. D., and Groves, L. K.: Esophageal perforations. Ann. Thorac. Surg. 10:571–587, 1970.
11. Mackler, S. A.: Spontaneous rupture of esophagus: experimental and clinical study. Surg. Gynecol. Obstet. 95:345–356, 1952.
12. Naclerio, E. A.: The "V sign" in diagnosis of spontaneous rupture of esophagus (early roentgen clue). Am. J. Surg. 93:291–298, 1957.
13. O'Connell, N. D.: Spontaneous rupture of the esophagus. Am. J. Roentgenol. 99:186–203, 1967.
14. Parkin, G. J. S.: The radiology of perforated esophagus. Clin. Radiol. 24:324–332, 1973.
15. Pate, J. W., Hughes, F. A., and Patton, J. B.: Spontaneous rupture of the esophagus. Am. Surg. 24:385–394, 1958.
16. Rosoff, L., and White, E. J.: Perforation of the esophagus. Am. J. Surg. 128:207–218, 1974.
17. Sawyers, J. L., Lane, C. E., Foster, J. H., et al.: Esophageal perforation. An increasing challenge. Ann. Thorac. Surg. 19:233–238, 1975.
18. Stephenson, H. E., Jr., McLeod, R. A., McCraw, J. B., et al.: Perforation of the esophagus. Am. J. Surg. 115:648–650, 1968.
19. Tesler, M. A., and Eisenberg, M. M.: Spontaneous esophageal rupture: collective review. Surg. Gynecol. Obstet. 117:1, 1963.
20. Triggiani, E., and Belsey, R.: Oesophageal trauma: incidence, diagnosis, and management. Thorax 32:241–249, 1977.

Part V
Corrosive Strictures of the Esophagus

HEBER MacMAHON, M.B.

INTRODUCTION

Corrosive esophagitis and stricture formation may result from ingestion of various caustic materials, such as lye, acid, detergents, and bleaches.[8] Most corrosive strictures result from either accidental ingestion by young children or attempted suicide by adults.

Sodium hydroxide (lye), one of the most frequently encountered corrosive agents, is apt to cause particularly severe injury. Sodium hydroxide is the active ingredient in many household drain cleaners, which, when ingested, rapidly produce liquefaction necrosis of the esophageal mucosa. Acids are less likely to cause severe esophageal injury, perhaps because they produce a coagulation necrosis of the mucosa, which tends to limit penetration. The major destructive effect of acids is seen in the antral region of the stomach, where they are retained by pyloric spasm. Household bleach occasionally causes severe strictures.[7] Clinitest tablets used to test urine for reducing substances have been ingested by children and adults and tend to produce a rather characteristic localized stricture of the upper midesophagus.[4]

Both acute and chronic esophagitis with stricture can result from certain tablet or capsule medications that have unrecognized corrosive properties. Hold-up of the medication is usually the result of some predisposing abnormality, such as an enlarged left atrium, an arteriosclerotic aorta, or a hiatal hernia. Implicated medications are slow potassium chloride tablets, tetracycline and doxycycline capsules, and quinidine and ferrous sulfate tablets.[17]

PATHOLOGY

The nature and extent of esophageal injury depend on the type of corrosive and its concentration and volume. The mildest cases show transient, superficial hyperemia and edema and heal without sequelae. A more severe burn may cause necrosis of all the layers of the esophagus and can extend to the periesophageal tissues with resultant mediastinitis or perforation. If the patient survives, a severe stricture inevitably results.

The temporal course in a typical case of lye ingestion can be divided into three phases.[10] The first stage is one of acute inflammation and necrosis during the first four days following ingestion. The mucosa is initially swollen and discolored. Ulceration develops within 24 hours, and microscopic examination shows necrosis of the esophageal wall to a variable depth, with thrombosis of submucosal vessels and intense inflammation of contiguous tissues.[12]

Ulceration and granulation characterize the second phase, which extends from the time when the mucosa sloughs at three to five days through the end of the second week. The esophageal wall is weakest at this time, and perforation may occur. The third phase is characterized by cicatrization and fibrosis, which become apparent after the second week. This results in narrowing of the lumen, sometimes with intraluminal adhesions. The mucosa and submucosa do not regenerate after a severe burn. Rigidity and aperistalsis or dysmotility may persist.

RADIOLOGIC FEATURES

Correct radiologic technique is important for optimal results. When a patient is seen in the acute phase following corrosive ingestion, a plain film of the chest should precede a contrast examination. This allows evaluation for aspiration, mediastinitis, and esophageal or gastric perforation. Aspiration is particularly likely in patients with pharyngeal burns, and a lateral soft tissue view of the neck may demonstrate severe edema of the pharyngeal tissues and supraglottic structures.[10] Respiratory distress may necessitate tracheotomy.[14] The patient with mediastinitis secondary to esophageal perforation is acutely ill. The chest radiograph may show mediastinal widening, pneumomediastinum, or pleural effusion. Lateral deviation of the paraspinal pleural reflection, thickening of the periesophageal soft tissue, and posterior indentation of the

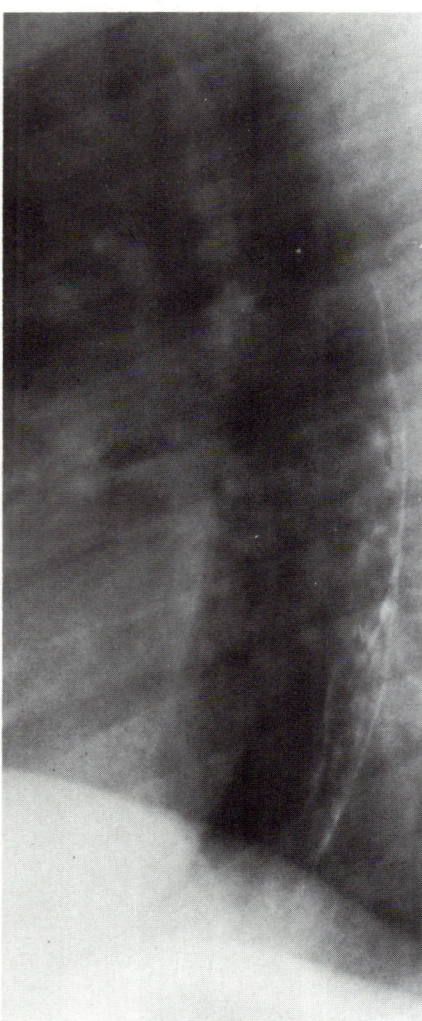

Figure 8–72. Lateral chest film shows dilated air-filled esophagus of a three-year-old child who had ingested lye (Liquid-plumr) 2 days earlier. There is intramural barium retention from an esophagogram performed the previous day. (*From* Martel, W.: Radiologic features of esophagogastritis secondary to extremely caustic agents. Radiology *103*:31–36, 1972. Reproduced by permission.)

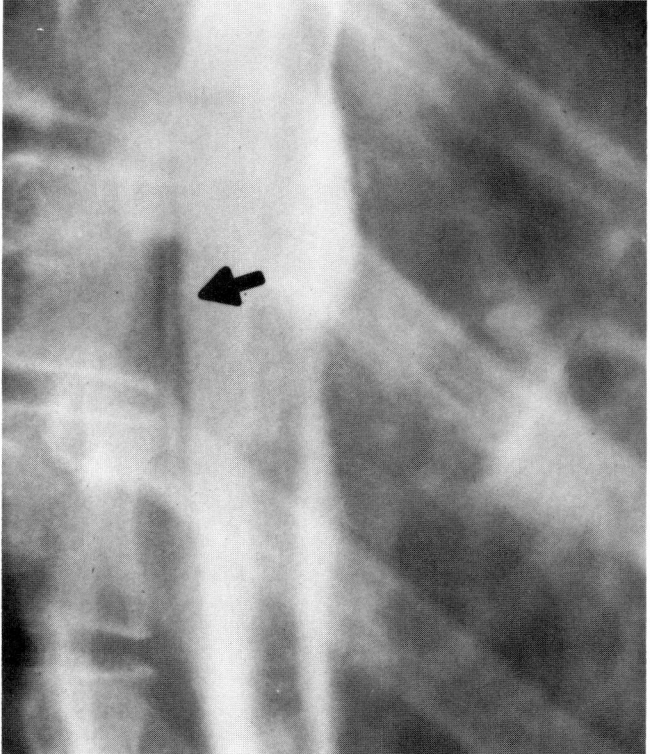

Figure 8–73. Esophagogram performed seven days after caustic ingestion shows the dissection of contrast material beneath partially sloughed mucosa (arrow). (*From* Martel, W.: Radiologic features of esophagogastritis secondary to extremely caustic agents. Radiology *103*:31–36, 1972. Reproduced by permission.)

trachea may be seen occasionally, however, in patients without radiologic evidence of perforation, presumably owing to chemical inflammation.[6] A dilated, atonic, air-filled esophagus is a frequent finding in the acute stage and may be visible on the chest film (Fig. 8–72). This has been attributed to damage to Auerbach's plexus.[15]

When there is a likelihood of perforation on the basis of the plain radiograph or on clinical grounds, the contrast examination should be started with water-soluble material (meglucamine diatrizoate or Gastrografin). This has the advantage of being quickly absorbed without adverse effects if it does enter the mediastinum. It provides less optimal mucosal coating than barium, however, and has an unpleasant taste. For the latter reason it may have to be instilled via a carefully positioned nasal tube in children. If the initial swallow shows no perforation, the study may be continued with barium. Video or ciné recording is useful for the documentation of motility disturbances.

The radiologic findings during the acute phase reflect the presence of edema, ulceration, and sloughing of the mucosa. They consist of blurring, scalloping, or straightening of the esophageal margins, and linear or plaque-like collections of contrast material may be seen in the esophageal wall. The latter finding indicates mucosal sloughing with intramural dissection, and these contrast collections may remain in the wall many hours after the examination (Figs. 8–72 and 8–73).[13] Dilation and atonicity of the esophagus are commonly present.[15] Diffuse, irregular ulceration may be visible throughout the esophagus after 24 hours (Fig. 8–74).

From the time that healing and fibrosis begin at two weeks, strictures become apparent. In many such cases, the initial esophagogram may have been normal (Fig. 8–75). Regular follow-up examinations are therefore indicated in all cases of corrosive

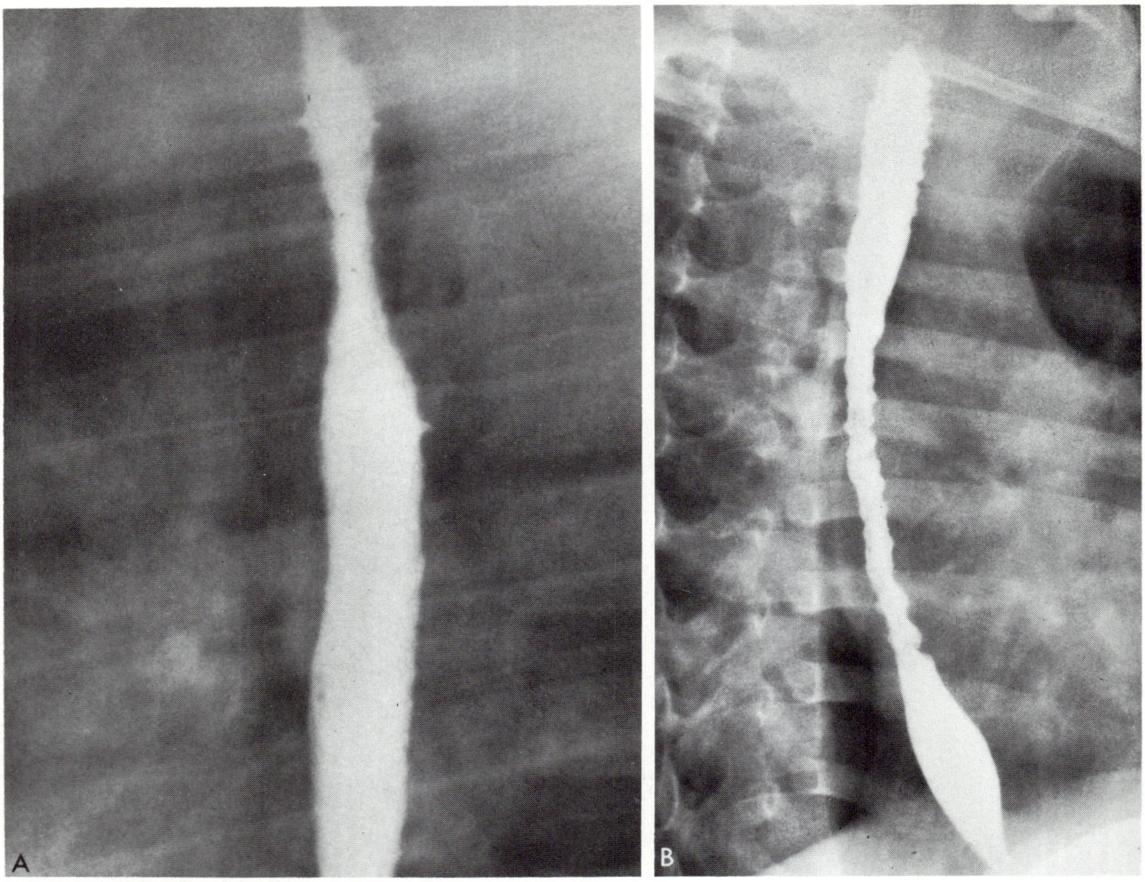

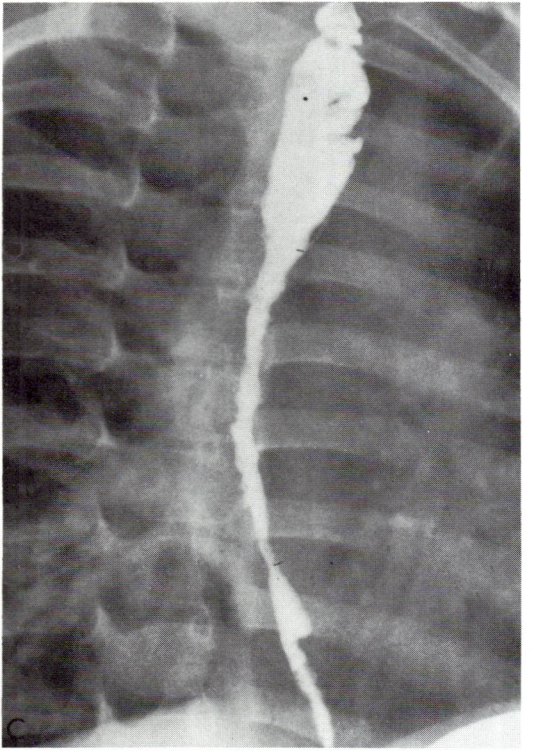

Figure 8–74. *A*, This three-year-old child swallowed an unknown quantity of lye. The initial examination shows diffuse esophageal ulceration. *B*, Two months later there is persistent ulceration, and luminal narrowing has become apparent. *C*, Six months after corrosive ingestion, there is extensive stricture formation, with persistent luminal irregularity. (Courtesy of W. H. McAlister, M.D.)

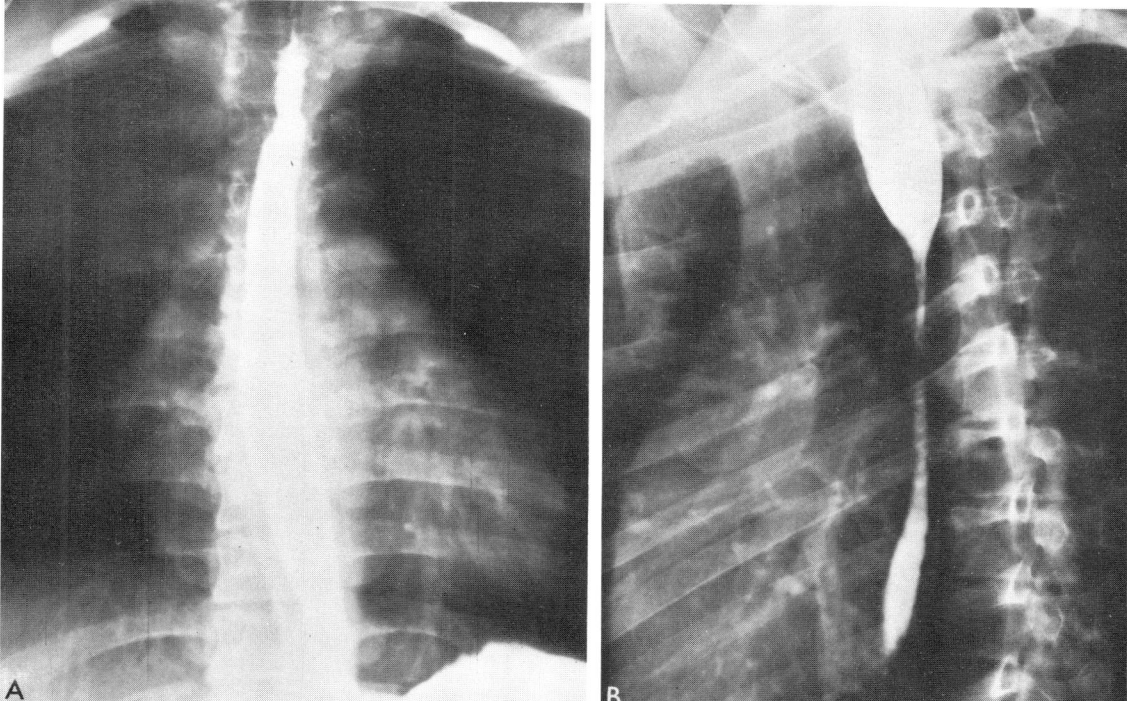

Figure 8–75. *A,* Initial esophagogram performed on a 21-year-old man who ingested a corrosive shows hypomotility but no evidence of ulceration or stricture. *B,* Examination six weeks later shows a typical corrosive stricture, with diffuse narrowing of the middle and distal esophagus. Note the smooth margins with gradual transition. (Courtesy of R. J. Stanley, M.D.)

ingestion, especially during the first six months. Stricture formation has been reported to occur in up to 50 per cent of untreated cases of corrosive ingestion, although when steroid and antibiotic therapy has been used, the incidence is considerably less.[1, 3]

Corrosive strictures may be localized, multiple, or continuous throughout the esophagus. Contrary to traditional teaching, the sites of strictures are not related to areas of anatomic narrowing but rather occur in random positions throughout the esophagus (Fig. 8–76). This is a reflection of segmental spasm, which occurs after caustic ingestion.[6] A constant feature, however, is sparing of the esophageal ampulla, also attributed to spasm.[16] One particular corrosive agent, the Clinitest tablet, invariably causes a localized stricture at the upper or midesophagus (Fig. 8–77).[4] Sodium hydroxide is the caustic ingredient.

In a typical corrosive stricture the margins are smooth and concentric, and mucosal folds are absent in the narrowed area. Occasionally, a caustic stricture may have an irregular outline and overhanging margins resembling a carcinoma. Thickening of the periesophageal tissues may be visible owing to surrounding fibrosis. Proximal dilatation and formation of wide-based diverticula within the strictured areas occur. Multiple outpouchings of the regenerated epithelium, probably due to intramural diverticulosis, are sometimes seen and have been attributed to chronically elevated intraluminal pressure (Fig. 8–78).[16]

Strictures are treated by bougienage insofar as possible, and repeated dilatation can produce impressive results (Fig. 8–79). In many cases of severe and extensive strictures, however, reconstructive surgery with bowel interposition must be performed. Use of inverted right colon with attached terminal ileum is favored by most

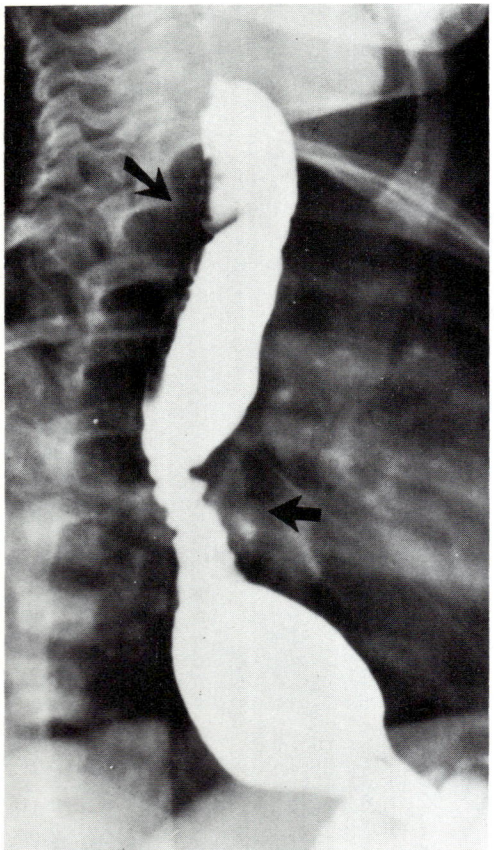

Figure 8–76. This two-year-old child swallowed lye one year ago; two areas of stricturing have occurred in the esophagus (arrows). In the area of the lower stricture, multiple tertiary contractions are apparent, indicating persistent dysmotility. A Nissen fundoplication has been performed for hiatus hernia and gastroesophageal reflux, which is a common complication of corrosive esophageal injury in children.

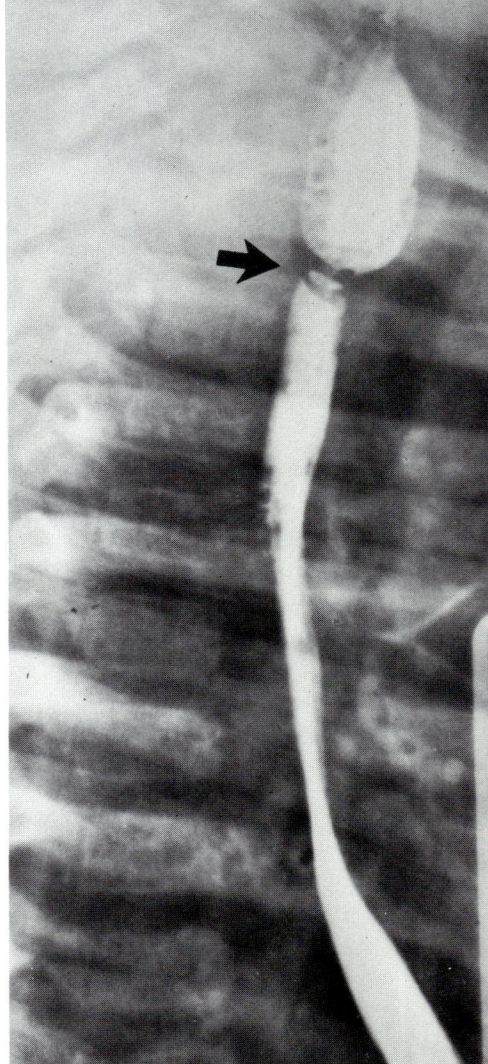

Figure 8–77. This infant had swallowed a Clinitest tablet two months previously. A localized ulcerated stricture of the upper esophagus resulted (arrow).

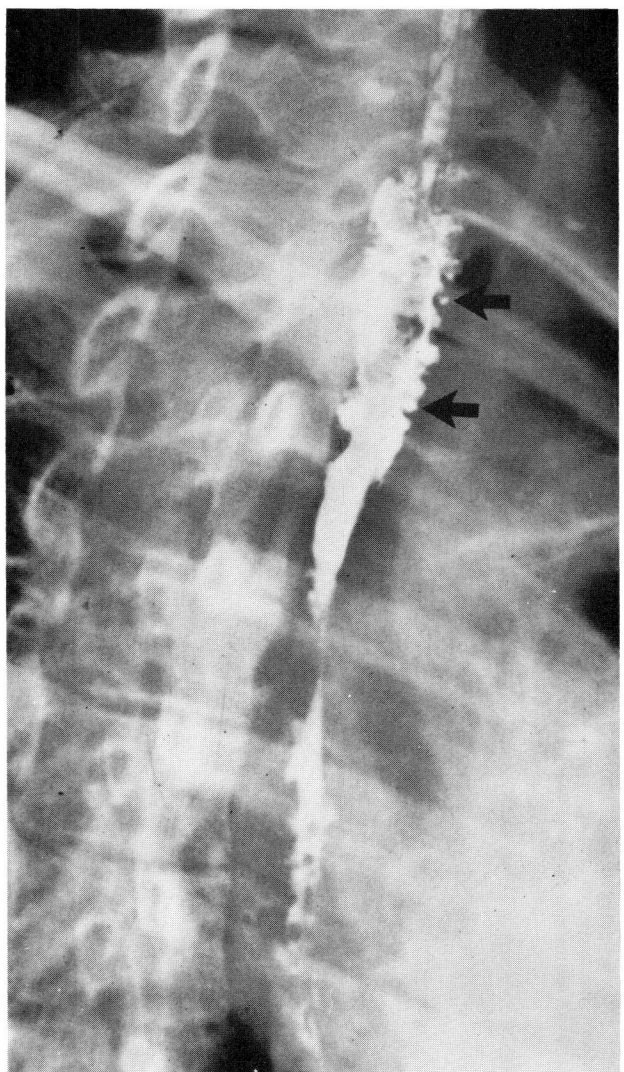

Figure 8–78. This 16-year-old female accidentally swallowed lye some months before this examination. The entire esophagus is severely strictured, and multiple small outpouchings of barium are apparent, probably owing to intramural diverticulosis (arrows). (Courtesy of R. J. Stanley, M.D.)

surgeons, although other colonic segments and gastric tube technique have also been successfully employed.[5, 9]

COMPLICATIONS

Apart from the stricture itself, long-term complications of corrosive ingestion include hiatus hernia, gastroesophageal reflux, mediastinal fibrosis, and carcinoma of the esophagus. In one follow-up study of 14 children after corrosive ingestion, four acquired hiatus hernias and two showed gastroesophageal reflux without hernia.[6] This was attributed to shortening of the esophagus secondary to fibrosis. Severe periesophageal fibrosis resulting in tracheal compression has also been described.

The incidence of esophageal carcinoma is significantly increased in patients with lye strictures.[11] The latent period in reported cases ranges from 16 to 42 years.[2] As a

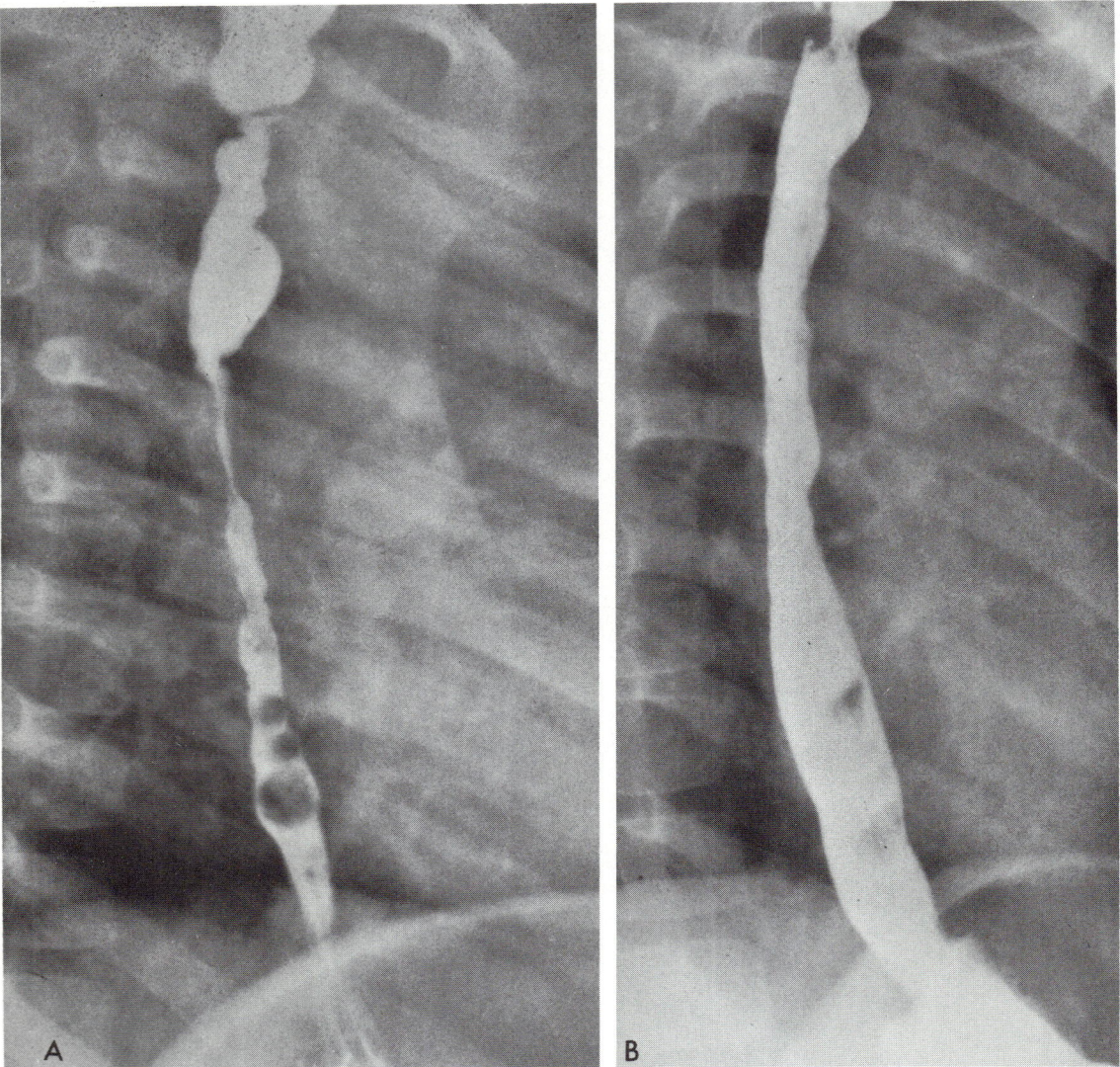

Figure 8–79. *A,* This esophagogram was performed about one year after lye ingestion by this child of two and one-half years. Severe strictures of the upper and middle esophagus are present. *B,* An examination five years later, following treatment by dilatation, shows a residual stricture at the thoracic inlet but only minimal residual narrowing in the middle esophagus. (Courtesy of W. H. McAlister, M.D.)

result, most of these patients are relatively young, compared with those in the general population with carcinoma. The tumor cell type in these cases is invariably epidermoid. Because these neoplasms arise in the area encased by fibrous tissue, local spread is inhibited and the prognosis is relatively favorable. Therefore, a change in symptoms or in the radiographic appearance of a long-established stricture should be viewed with suspicion and pursued with esophagoscopy. Unfortunately, negative biopsy findings are not conclusive, and surgical resection may have to be performed even in the absence of histologic proof of carcinoma.

References

1. Alford, B. R., and Harris, H. H.: Chemical burns of the mouth, pharynx and esophagus. Ann. Otol. Rhinol. Laryngol. 68:122–128, 1959.
2. Bigelow, N. H.: Carcinoma of the esophagus developing at the site of lye stricture. Cancer 6:1159–1164, 1953.
3. Borja, A. H., Randell, H. T., Jr., Thomas, T. C., et al.: Lye injuries of the esophagus: analysis of 90 cases of lye ingestion. J. Thorac. Cardiovasc. Surg. 57:533–538, 1969.
4. Burrington, J. D.: Clinitest burns of the esophagus. Ann. Thorac. Surg. 20:400–404, 1975.
5. Ein, S. H., Shandling, B., Simpson, J. S., et al.: A further look at the gastric tube as an esophageal replacement in infants and children. J. Pediatr. Surg. 8:859–868, 1973.
6. Franken, E. A., Jr.: Caustic damage of the gastrointestinal tract: roentgen features. Am. J. Roentgenol. 118:77–85, 1973.
7. French, R. J., Tabb, H. G., and Rutledge, L. J.: Esophageal stenosis produced by ingestion of bleach South. Med. J. 63:1140–1144, 1970.
8. Holinger, P. H.: Management of esophageal lesions caused by chemical burns. Ann. Otolaryngol. Rhinol. Laryngol. 77:819–829, 1968.
9. Hong, P. W., Seel, D. J., and Dietrick, R. B.: The use of colon in the surgical treatment of benign stricture of the esophagus. Ann. Surg. 160:202–209, 1964.
10. Johnson, E. E.: Study of corrosive esophagitis. Laryngoscope 73:1651–1696, 1963.
11. Lansing, P. B., Ferrante, W. A., and Ochsner, J. L.: Carcinoma of the esophagus at the site of lye stricture. Am. J. Surg. 118:108–111, 1969.
12. Leape, L. L., Ashcraft, K. W., Scarpelli, D. G., et al.: Hazard to health—liquid lye. N. Engl. J. Med. 284:578–581, 1971.
13. Martel, W.: Radiologic features of esophagogastritis secondary to extremely caustic agents. Radiology 103:31–36, 1972.
14. Middelkamp, J. N., Ferguson, T. B., Roper, C. L., et al.: The management and problems of caustic burns in children. J. Thorac. Cardiovasc. Surg. 57:341–347, 1969.
15. Simeone, J. F., Burrell, M., Toffler, R., et al.: Aperistalsis and esophagitis. Radiology 123:9–14, 1977.
16. Skene-Smith, H.: Caustic strictures of the esophagus. Br. J. Radiol. 48:646–648, 1975.
17. Teplick, J. G., et al.: Esophagitis caused by oral medication. Radiology 134:23–25, 1980.

Part VI

Tumors of the Esophagus

IGOR LAUFER, M.D.

INTRODUCTION

Benign tumors of the esophagus are rare.[1] Most patients presenting with esophageal symptoms resulting from tumor harbor an advanced carcinoma. In the vast majority of such patients, the radiologic findings are obvious and the diagnosis poses no difficulty. In these patients the barium swallow attains an accuracy of 90 per cent or more. An occasional patient with a small esophageal tumor may present with dysphagia, however. It has been found that 35 to 45 per cent of these small tumors have been missed on the initial radiologic study.[20, 29] The radiologic detection of small esophageal carcinomas presents a great challenge to radiologic technique and interpretative acumen.

Since the majority of patients with small tumors do not present with esophageal symptoms, it is important to consider those conditions that predispose to the development of esophageal carcinoma.[43] Among the conditions associated with a higher-than-normal incidence of esophageal carcinoma[43] are heavy smoking and drinking, celiac disease,[9] Bowen's disease, primary squamous carcinoma of the head and neck,[3]

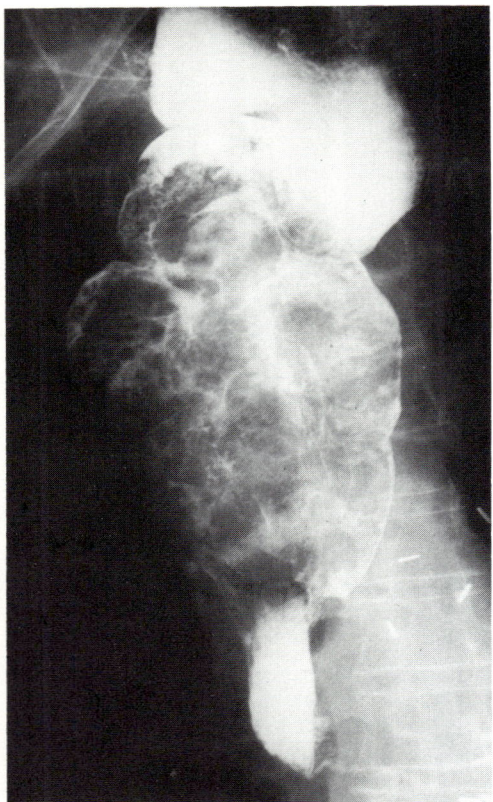

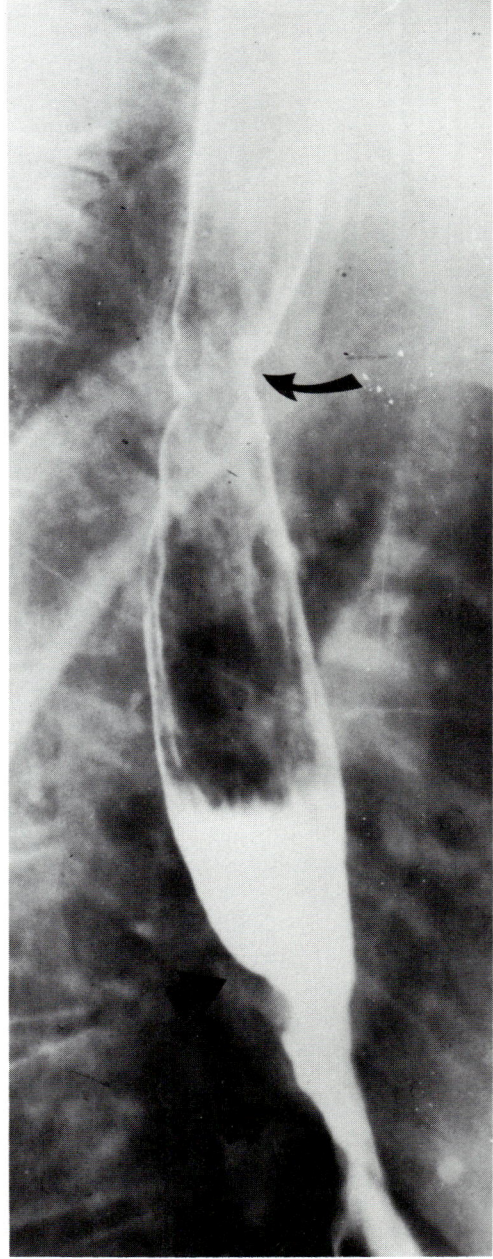

Figure 8–80. Malignant tumor in a patient with achalasia. There is a large bulky polypoid tumor occupying most of the thoracic esophagus. This proved to be a carcinosarcoma. There are numerous surgical clips from previous operations for relief of esophageal obstruction due to achalasia.

Figure 8–81. Adenocarcinoma in Barrett's esophagus. In the proximal third of the esophagus there are the typical findings of Barrett's esophagus, with slight narrowing and mucosal irregularity (curved arrow). In the distal esophagus there is a stricture with ulceration due to adenocarcinoma in the columnar-lined portion of the esophagus. (Courtesy of R. E. Koehler, M.D., St. Louis, Missouri.)

THE ESOPHAGUS — 389

achalasia (Fig. 8–80),[7] Barrett's esophagus (Fig. 8–81),[30] and tylosis (a rare dermatologic condition).[17] In the case of achalasia, retained food and secretions can obscure an esophageal tumor; thus, they should be removed by lavage prior to radiologic study if the presence of a complicating tumor is suspected. The middle third of the esophagus is the most common site (see Fig. 8–80). Patients with any of these predisposing conditions deserve regular and thorough screening examinations of the esophagus, even in the absence of esophageal symptoms (Fig. 8–82).[23]

DIAGNOSIS

Radiologic Techniques

The plain chest film may occasionally be helpful in the diagnosis of esophageal tumors. Widening of the retrotracheal stripe has been described as a sign of tumor

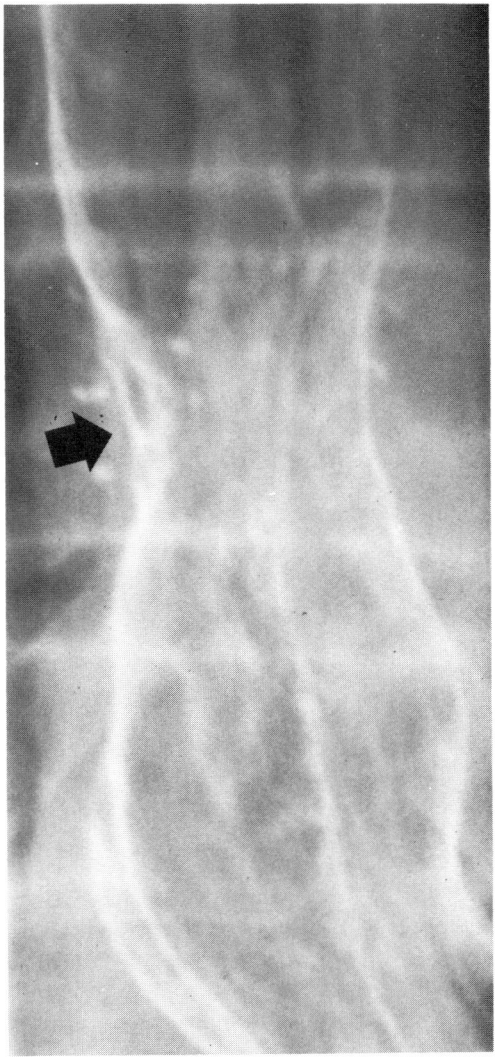

Figure 8–82. Asymptomatic squamous carcinoma. This upper gastrointestinal study was performed in a patient with a history of smoking and drinking. There were no symptoms referable to the esophagus. There is asymmetric flattening on the right lateral wall just above the gastroesophageal junction (arrow). This proved to be a squamous cell carcinoma. A few drops of residual Pantopaque from a previous myelogram are seen in the spinal canal.

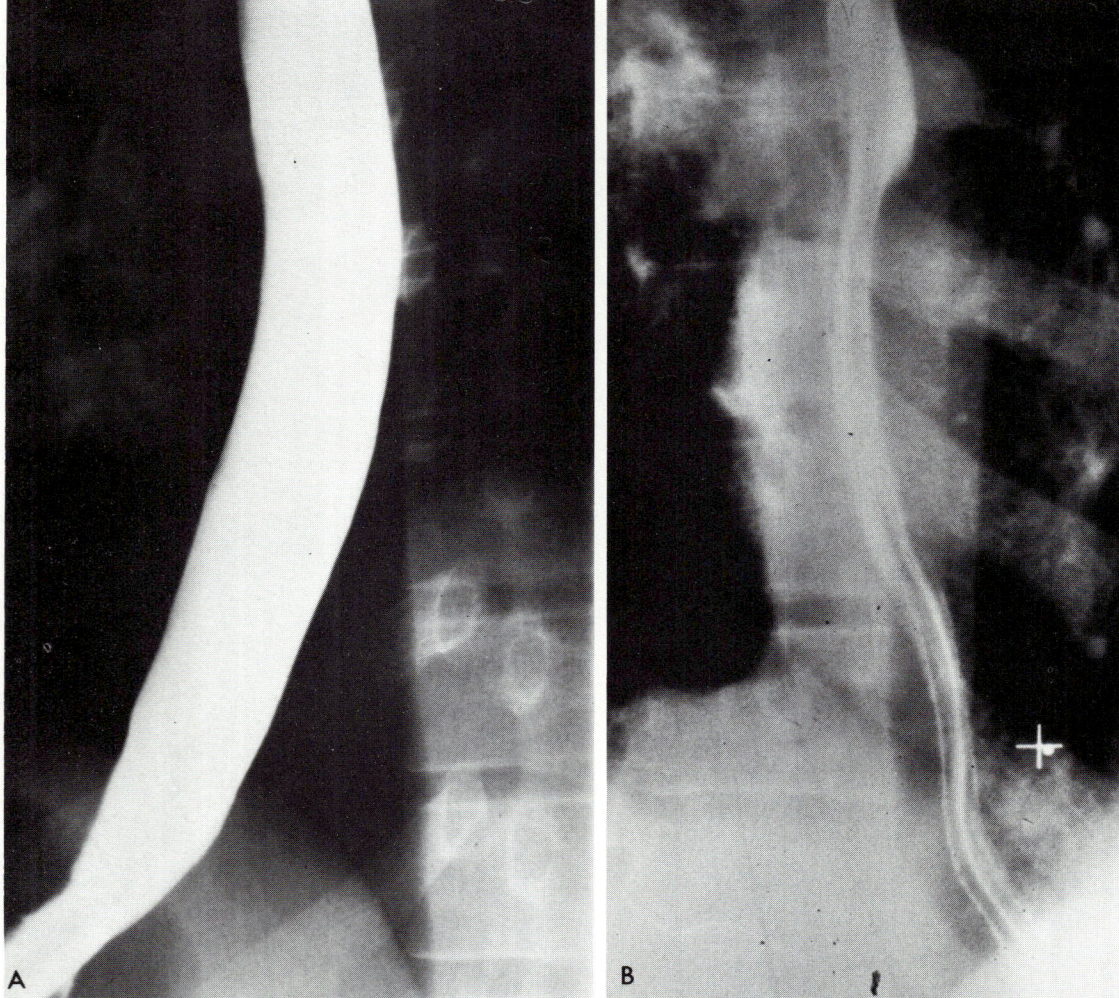

Figure 8–83. Components of a normal esophagram. *A,* Barium-filled view of the esophagus. *B,* The esophagus partially collapsed showing the normal longitudinal folds.

Illustration and legend continued on the opposite page

infiltration.[35] One may also see evidence of infiltrates due to aspiration in the lungs. Marked dilatation of the esophagus is usually not seen, since the obstruction is usually of much shorter duration than in patients with achalasia. In the majority of cases, a barium esophagogram is necessary to delineate the nature and extent of the lesion. A complete radiologic examination of the esophagus combines fluoroscopy, spot films, and, if needed, overhead radiographs. Fluroscopy is important in the assessment of peristaltic activity and for the detection of areas of slightly diminished distensibility. It is also important to observe the behavior of the lower esophagus and gastroesophageal junction.

Radiographs should be obtained to show the esophagus filled with barium (Fig. 8–83*A*). These views are particularly valuable for the demonstration of areas of limited

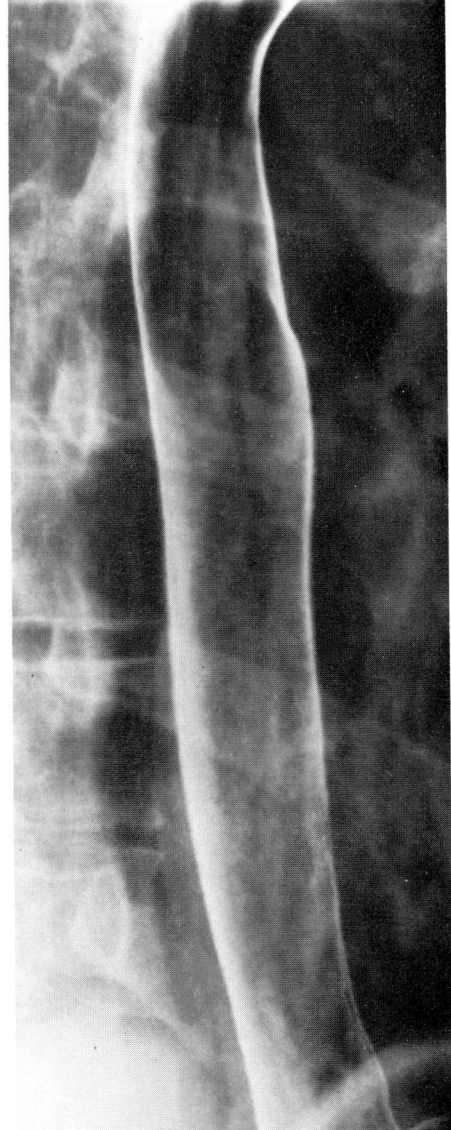

Figure 8–83 *Continued. C*, Double-contrast radiograph of a patient in the upright position.

distensibility and contour defects. Films should also be obtained with the esophagus collapsed to show the normal longitudinal folds (Fig. 8–83B). In some cases, it may be necessary to administer a barium paste in order to achieve adequate coating of the collapsed esophagus. In all patients with a suspicion of esophageal disease, double-contrast radiographs should also be obtained.[16, 22, 40, 41] These views are obtained with the patient upright, gulping a high-density barium suspension (Fig. 8–83C). If no abnormality has been seen during the fluoroscopic portion of the examination, overhead radiographs should be taken while the patient is drinking to distend the esophagus. If an abnormality is suspected in the pharynx or cervical esophagus, a dynamic form of imaging, such as cineradiography or video tape, is recommended. Rapid serial spot films exposed at the rate of three or four per second may also be used.

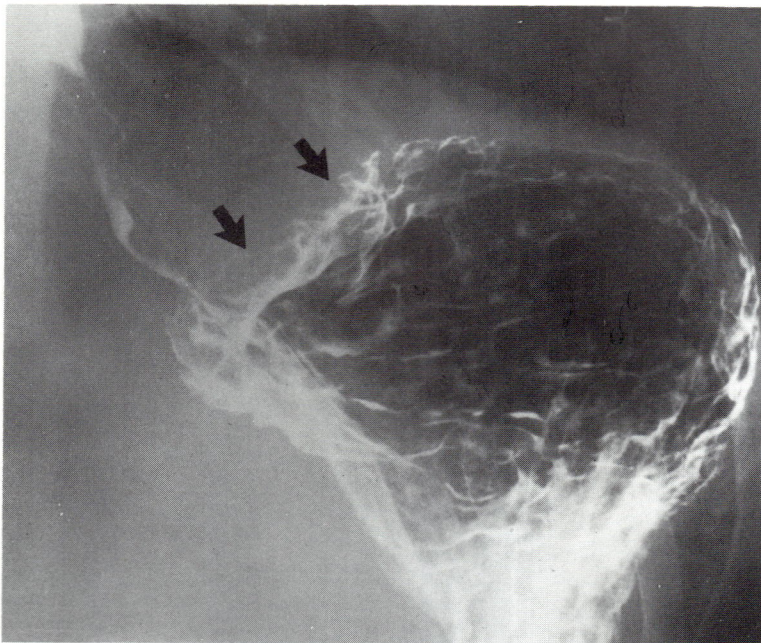

Figure 8–84. Dysphagia due to carcinoma of the fundus. This middle-aged man presented with dysphagia of recent onset. A double-contrast view of the fundus shows a mass lesion adjacent to the cardia (arrows). This proved to be a gastric carcinoma.

In any patient with esophageal symptoms, the examination must include the gastric fundus and cardia. Esophageal symptoms are frequently due to gastroesophageal reflux, and in addition, tumors or ulcers around the cardia frequently present with esophageal symptoms (Fig. 8–84). If an esophageal tumor has been found, the upper gastrointestinal tract should be surveyed for possible submucosal metastatic disease (Fig. 8–85).

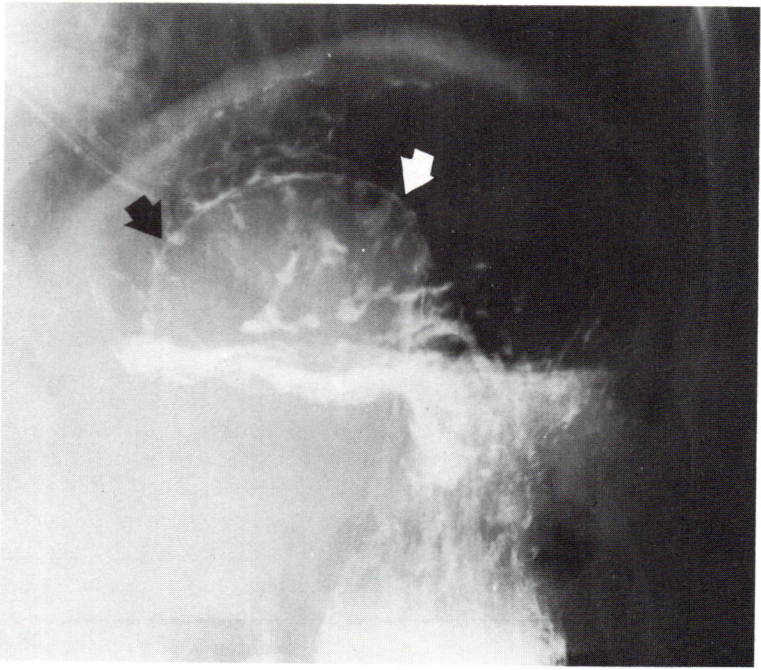

Figure 8–85. Gastric metastasis from esophageal carcinoma. There is a large submucosal mass (arrows) near the region of the gastric cardia. This was an incidental finding in this patient with esophageal carcinoma and represents a submucosal metastasis.

Benign Tumors

Most benign tumors in the esophagus are submucosal lesions, most commonly leiomyomas.[1] They usually show the characteristic features of a submucosal tumor—a smooth surface with a right angle between the tumor and the esophageal wall (Fig. 8–86A). When these tumors ulcerate, they may cause gastrointestinal bleeding (Fig. 8–86B). The differential diagnosis usually includes other types of connective tissue tumors, duplication cysts, and neurenteric cysts.

Benign epithelial tumors of the esophagus are particularly rare. Papillomas may be single or multiple and are usually found in older patients (Fig. 8–87).[21] Inflammatory and fibrovascular polyps are also found in the esophagus.[4, 26] These may have a typical pedunculated appearance. Pedunculated polyps due to lipomas have also been reported.[25]

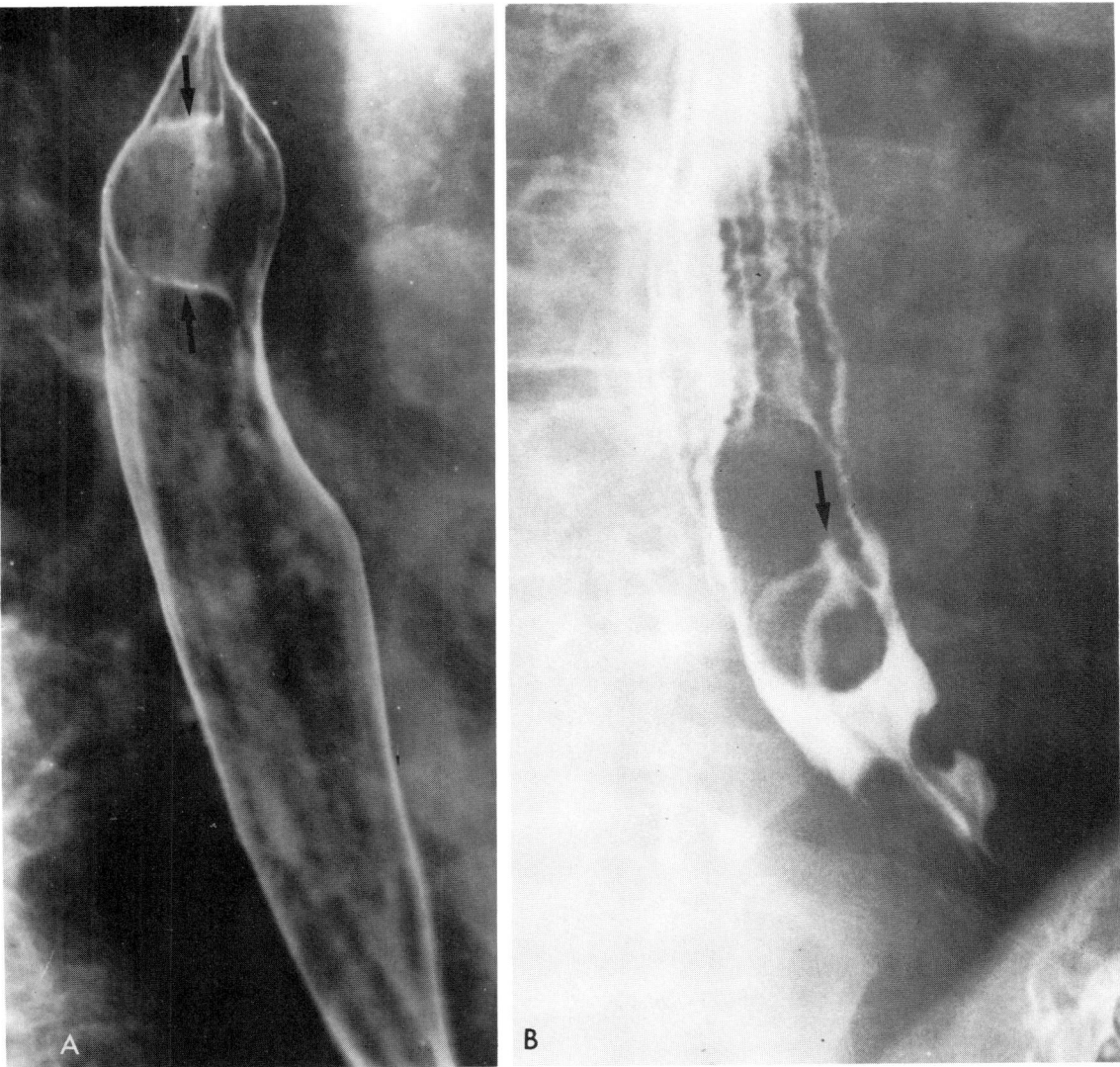

Figure 8–86. Benign submucosal tumors. *A,* Typical features of a submucosal tumor. There is a tumor in the proximal esophagus forming a right angle with the esophageal mucosa. The mucosal surface over the tumor is smooth. These are the typical features of a submucosal tumor, and this lesion was symptomatic. *B,* Ulcerated submucosal tumor. There is a smooth filling defect in the distal esophagus. There is a central ulcer (arrow). Such lesions frequently present with gastrointestinal bleeding.

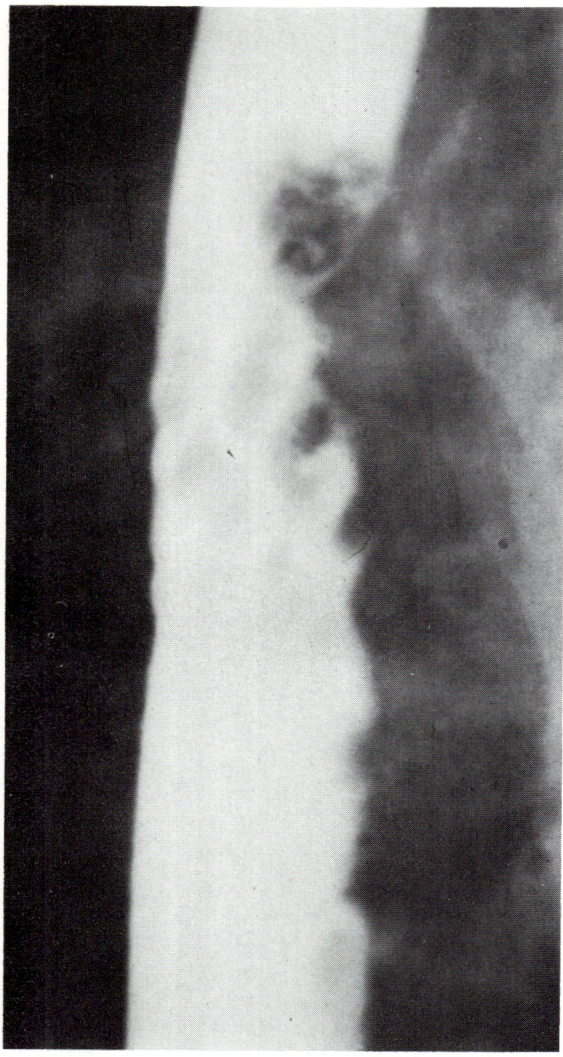

Figure 8–87. Esophageal papillomatosis. This close-up view of the midesophagus shows multiple small filling defects along the contour as well as *en face*. These filling defects were due to multiple esophageal papillomas.

Advanced Cancer

Carcinoma of the esophagus is a disease of the elderly with a marked male predominance. It is most commonly found at the distal end of the esophagus, diminishing in frequency at the proximal portions. The radiographic appearance of advanced esophageal cancer has four basic patterns: (1) Polypoid tumors are seen as intraluminal projections. In most cases, they are circumferential, but occasionally they involve the wall asymmetrically (Fig. 8–88A). (2) Infiltrative lesions result in an annular, constricted

Figure 8–88. Basic patterns of advanced esophageal cancer. *A*, Polypoid carcinoma. There is a lobulated polypoid carcinoma arising from the anterior wall of the esophagus. This tumor developed in a patient with nontropical sprue (*From* Laufer, I.: Double contrast radiology in the diagnosis of gastrointestinal cancer. *In* Glass, G. B. J. (ed.): Progress in Gastroenterology. Vol. 3. New York, Grune & Stratton, Inc., 1977.) *B*, Infiltrating carcinoma. This is a typical "apple-core" type of lesion characteristic of carcinoma throughout the gastrointestinal tract. *C*, Ulcerating carcinoma. The most prominent feature of this tumor is the ulcer (arrow) with relatively little mass effect. *D*, Varicoid carcinoma. This tumor of the midesophagus presents primarily as enlarged, tortuous folds, and the appearance may be suggestive of esophageal varices.

Illustrations on the opposite page

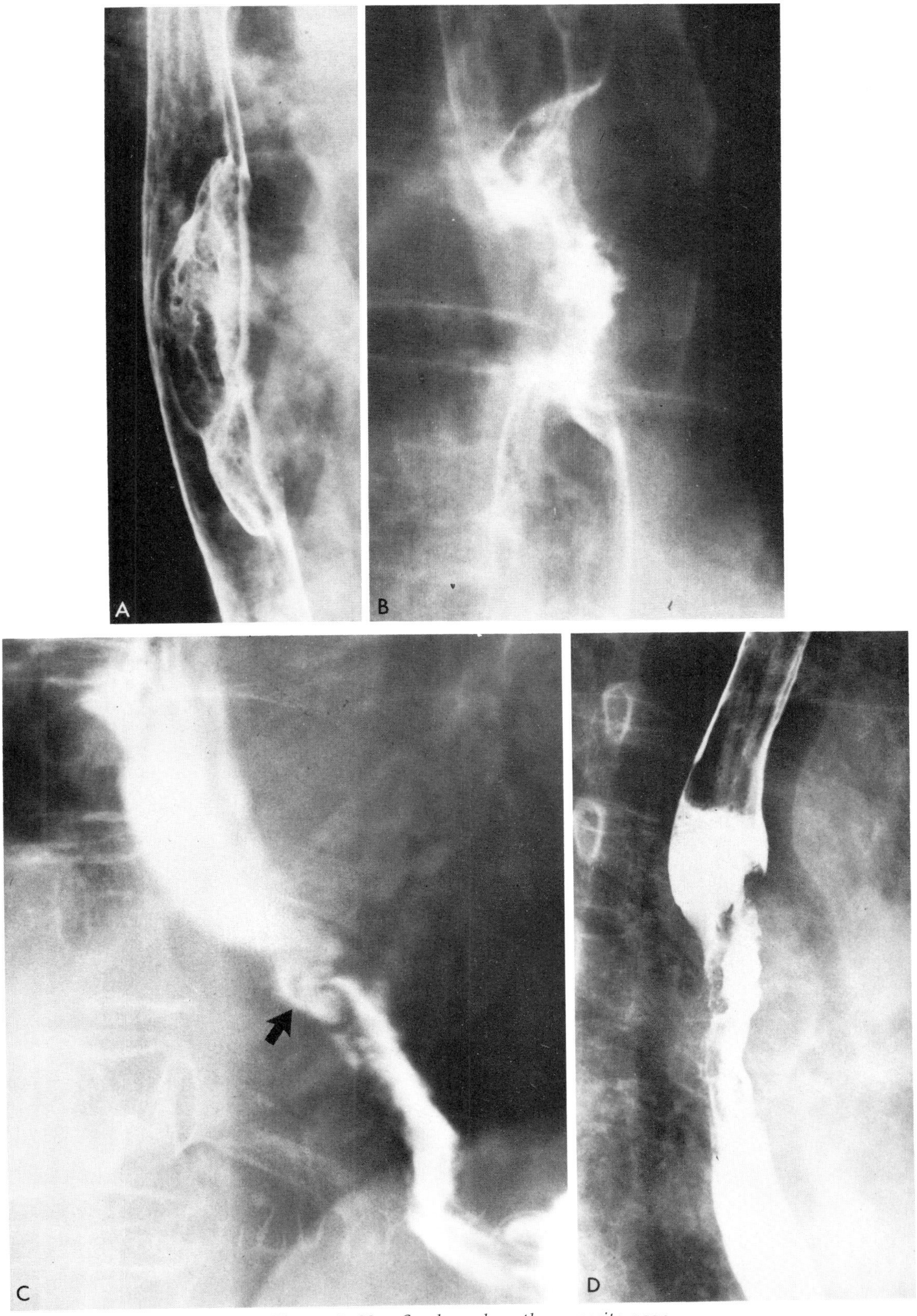

Figure 8–88. *See legend on the opposite page.*

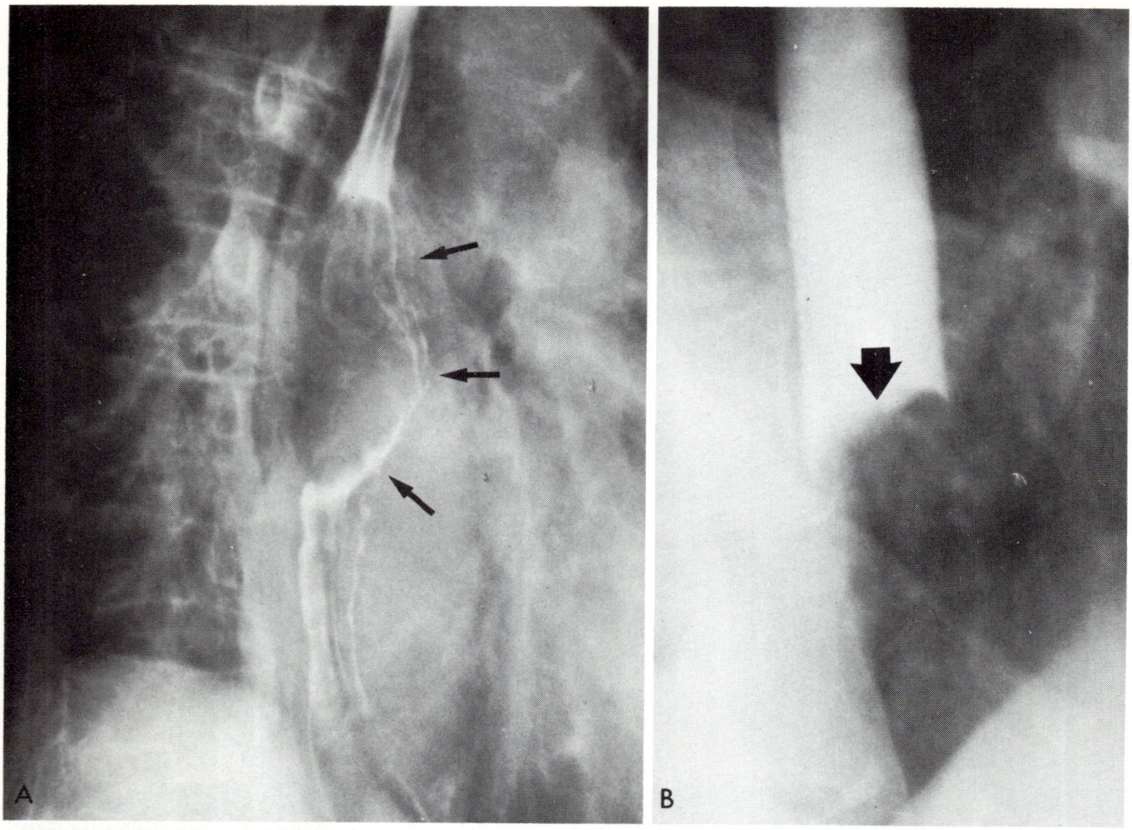

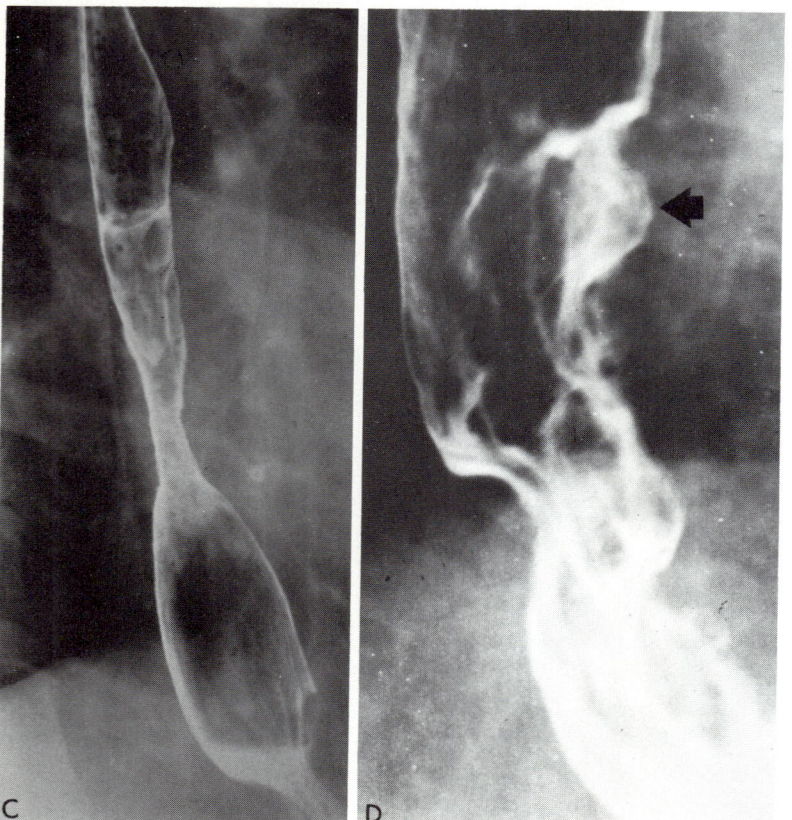

Figure 8–89. Differential diagnosis of advanced esophageal cancer. *A,* Carcinoma simulating an intramural lesion. This tumor in the midesophagus has a relatively smooth surface (arrows), and the mucosal folds appear to be intact. Nevertheless, it is a carcinoma. *B,* Foreign body in the esophagus. There is obstruction of the esophagus by a filling defect with a concave upper margin (arrow). This was due to an undigested piece of hot dog. *C,* Peptic stricture of the esophagus. There is a hiatus hernia, with narrowing of the esophagus extending from the gastroesophageal junction proximally. The stricture has smooth, tapering edges. *D,* Carcinoma of the cardia involving the distal esophagus. There is a mass lesion involving the left lateral wall of the esophagus with a mass and a large ulcer (arrow). This is due to adenocarcinoma originating in the stomach.

Illustration and legend continued on the opposite page

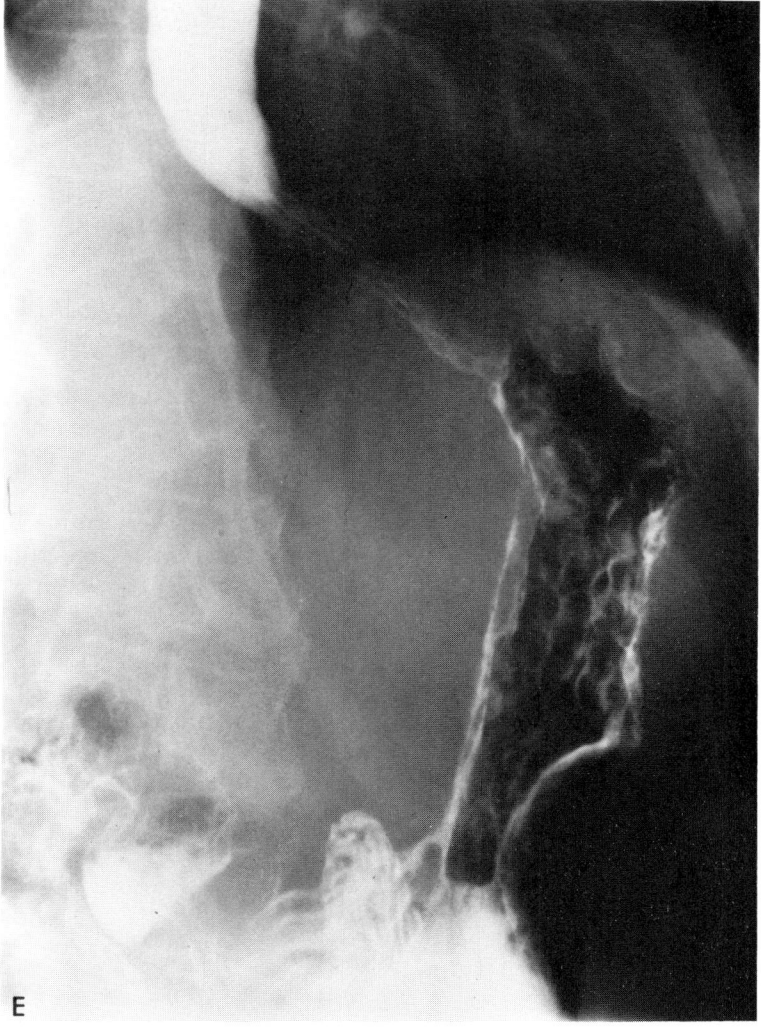

Figure 8–89 *Continued.* E, Submucosal spread of scirrhous gastric carcinoma that simulates achalasia. This middle-aged woman presented with dysphagia. There was impaired relaxation of the lower esophageal sphincter and no peristalsis in the body of the esophagus. There is obvious infiltration of the proximal half of the stomach, with involvement of the gastroesophageal junction. The radiologic and manometric abnormalities in the esophagus are due to the submucosal extension of the gastric tumor.

area, which is typical of carcinoma anywhere in the gastrointestinal tract (Fig. 8–88B). (3) The ulcerative type of carcinoma is uncommon. In this lesion, the most prominent feature is a flat mass with ulceration (Fig. 8–88C). (4) Varicoid carcinoma is the term applied to an esophageal carcinoma that presents primarily as enlarged, tortuous folds suggestive of esophageal varices (Fig. 8–88D).[24, 39] This type of carcinoma can be distinguished from varices by the stiffness of the wall and the unchanging appearance of the folds.

Several conditions must be considered in the differential diagnosis of esophageal carcinoma. Occasionally, a polypoid carcinoma has a very smooth surface and resembles a submucosal lesion (Fig. 8–89A). A smooth or irregular filling defect may also be seen in foreign body impaction within the esophagus (Fig. 8–89B). This may occur in patients with esophageal spasm or lower esophageal rings, in the absence of a fixed organic obstruction. The annular type of carcinoma must be distinguished from peptic stricture of the esophagus due to gastroesophageal reflux (Fig. 8–89C). Peptic strictures are almost always associated with a hiatus hernia and have smooth, tapering margins.

Malignant tumors involving the distal esophagus frequently arise in the gastric cardia or fundus and spread up the esophagus (Fig. 8–89D). Therefore, whenever the barium swallow shows a malignant lesion at or near the gastroesophageal junction, the stomach should also be examined to rule out a primary gastric tumor. In some patients, gastric carcinoma spreads submucosally along the esophagus and may produce a picture radiologically and manometrically indistinguishable from that of achalasia (Fig. 8–89E).

In many cases, a definitive histologic diagnosis cannot be made on the basis of the radiologic findings. In such cases, endoscopy, biopsy, and brushings are essential. These procedures are not infallible for the detection of malignancy in an esophageal lesion, however. If the radiologic findings are suggestive of malignancy and a lesion shows no evidence of regression over a short-term follow-up, operation may be necessary despite the negative results of the biopsies and cytologic tests.

Early Carcinoma

The early diagnosis of esophageal carcinoma represents a challenge in radiologic diagnosis. The findings in early tumors of the esophagus are very subtle, difficult to see fluoroscopically, and difficult to capture on film because of peristaltic activity within the esophagus. Early lesions may be encountered accidentally and rarely in asymptomatic patients (see Fig. 8–82), in the routine screening of patients with conditions predisposing to the development of esophageal carcinoma, or in the rare patients who present with symptoms resulting from a small lesion.[20]

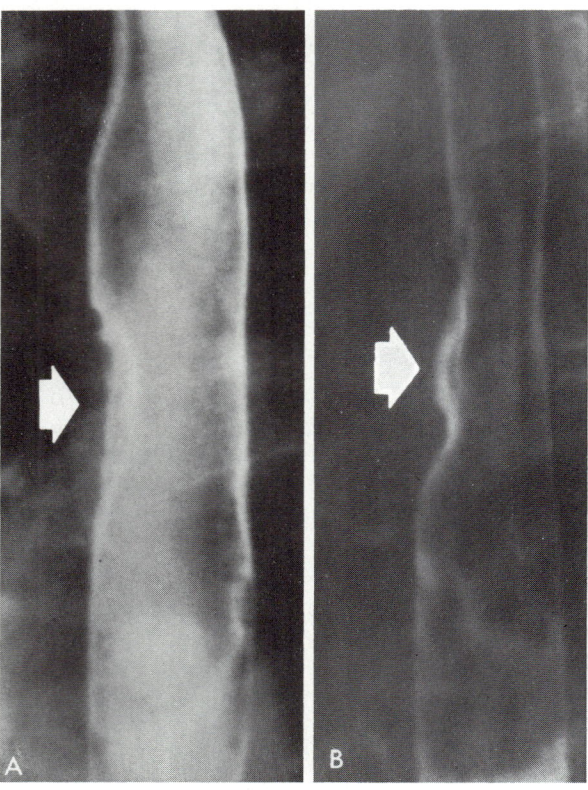

Figure 8–90. Early esophageal carcinoma. *A,* Plaque-like filling defect along the anterior wall of the esophagus due to a small esophageal carcinoma. *B,* Shallow ulceration in an early esophageal carcinoma.

Illustration and legend continued on the opposite page

THE ESOPHAGUS — 399

The most common manifestation of an early esophageal carcinoma is a plaque-like lesion. This may appear as a shallow filling defect or as an area of asymmetric stiffening of the esophageal wall (Fig. 8–90A). In many of these patients this is associated with a small central ulcer (Fig. 8–90B). As the tumors grow intraluminally, they may present as typical polypoid filling defects that may be seen in profile and *en face* (see Fig. 8–90C and D). Small lesions are best demonstrated on double-contrast radiographs.[16, 20]

In most cases, the changes due to an early esophageal carcinoma must be distinguished from the changes due to reflux esophagitis. The latter condition may also produce asymmetric stiffening of the esophageal wall (Fig. 8–91A) and be associated

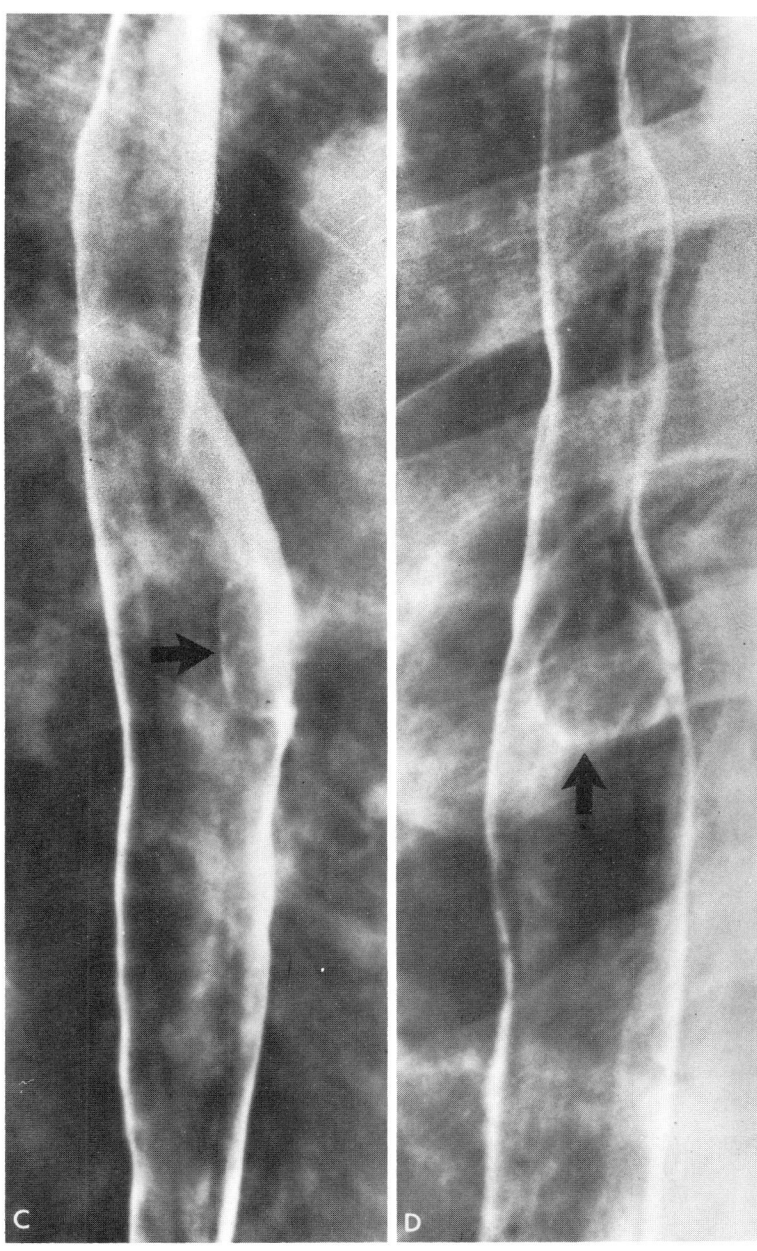

Figure 8–90 *Continued.* C and D, Early carcinoma presenting as a sessile polyp. The lesion is seen in profile (C) and *en face* (D). (A and B from Koehler, R. E., Moss, A. A., and Margulis, A. R.: Early radiographic manifestations of carcinoma of the esophagus. Radiology *119*:1–5, 1976. C from Goldstein, H. M., and Dodd, G. D.: Double-contrast esophagography. Gastrointest. Radiol. *1*:3–6, 1976. D courtesy of H. M. Goldstein, M.D., Houston, Texas.)

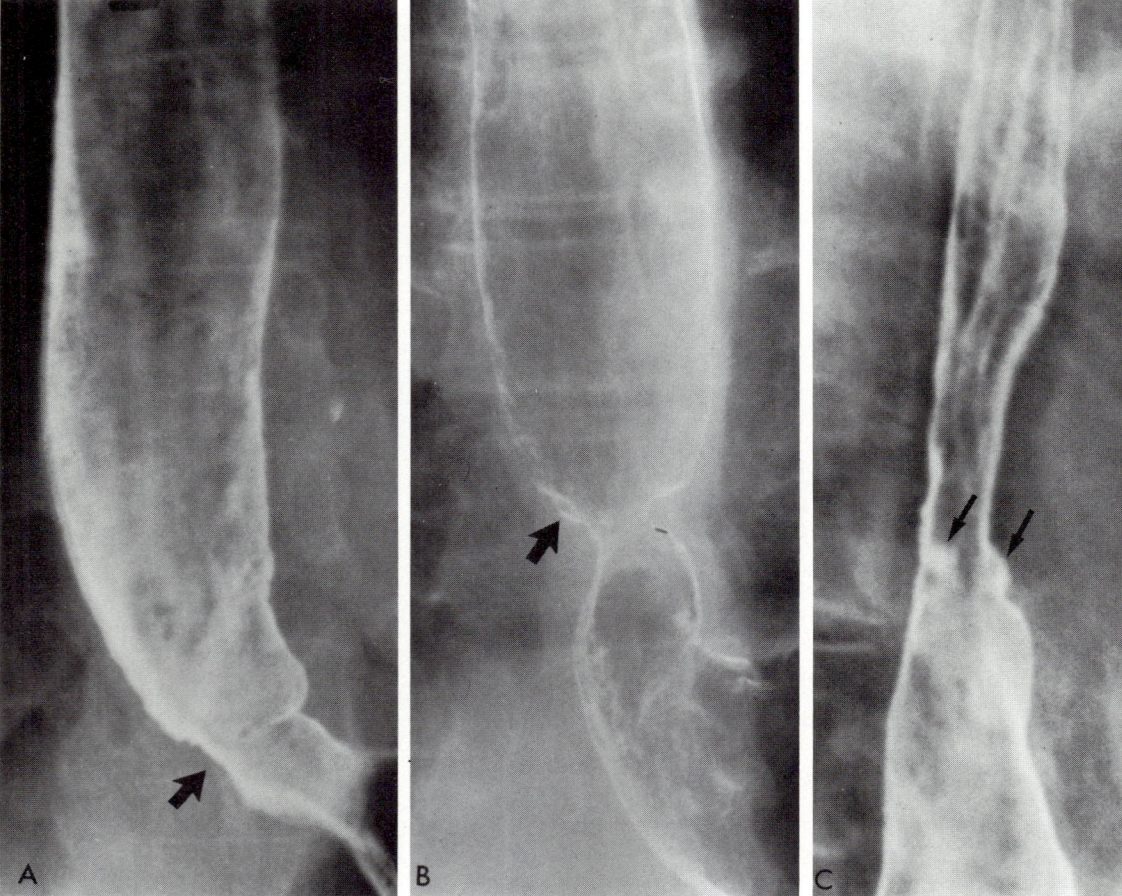

Figure 8–91. Differential diagnosis of early esophageal carcinoma. *A*, Reflux esophagitis. There is localized rigidity of the right wall (arrow) of the distal esophagus resulting from reflux esophagitis. *B*, Reflux esophagitis with stricture and ulceration. There is a hiatus hernia with reflux and narrowing at the esophagogastric anastomosis. A superficial ulcer is seen on the right lateral wall (arrow). This is associated with asymmetry and stiffening of the esophageal wall. *C*, Barrett's esophagus with narrowing, ulceration (arrows), and mucosal thickening (Courtesy of M. P. Banner, M.D., Philadelphia, Pennsylvania).

with superficial ulceration (Fig. 8–91*B*). Thickening of the esophageal folds may also give rise to mucosal nodularity. In the more proximal portion of the esophagus, changes simulating an early carcinoma may be produced by Barrett's esophagus, which may be associated with ulceration, nodularity, and rigidity (Fig. 8–91*C*).[36] In many of these cases, endoscopic biopsy and brushings for cytologic examination may be necessary to rule out carcinoma.

Other Malignant Tumors

Several other types of malignant tumors may involve the esophagus. Leiomyosarcoma may have the same features as benign leiomyoma, although it tends to be larger (Fig. 8–92*A*). There are several tumors that characteristically produce bulky, polypoid filling defects in the esophagus. Among these is the carcinosarcoma, which is a malignant tumor with combined epithelial and mesenchymal elements (see Fig. 8–80). These tumors have a much better prognosis than the usual squamous carcinoma.[19] Other tumors that produce a similar appearance include primary melanosarcoma (Fig. 8–92B)[38] and pseudosarcoma.[27] Lymphoma may also involve the esophagus, most often by direct extension from the stomach. The spectrum of radiologic findings includes an ulcerated mass, multiple submucosal nodules (Fig. 8–92C), and large folds simulating varices.[6]

Metastatic tumors may involve the esophagus in a variety of ways.[12] Bronchogenic carcinoma may invade the esophagus directly or secondarily from metastatic mediastinal lymph nodes. Mediastinal lymph nodes may also be involved by remote tumors (Fig. 8–93A). These enlarged lymph nodes invade the esophagus, resulting in an extrinsic ulcerated mass. There may also be serosal metastases to the esophagus. When these involve the gastroesophageal junction, a motility disturbance resembling achal-

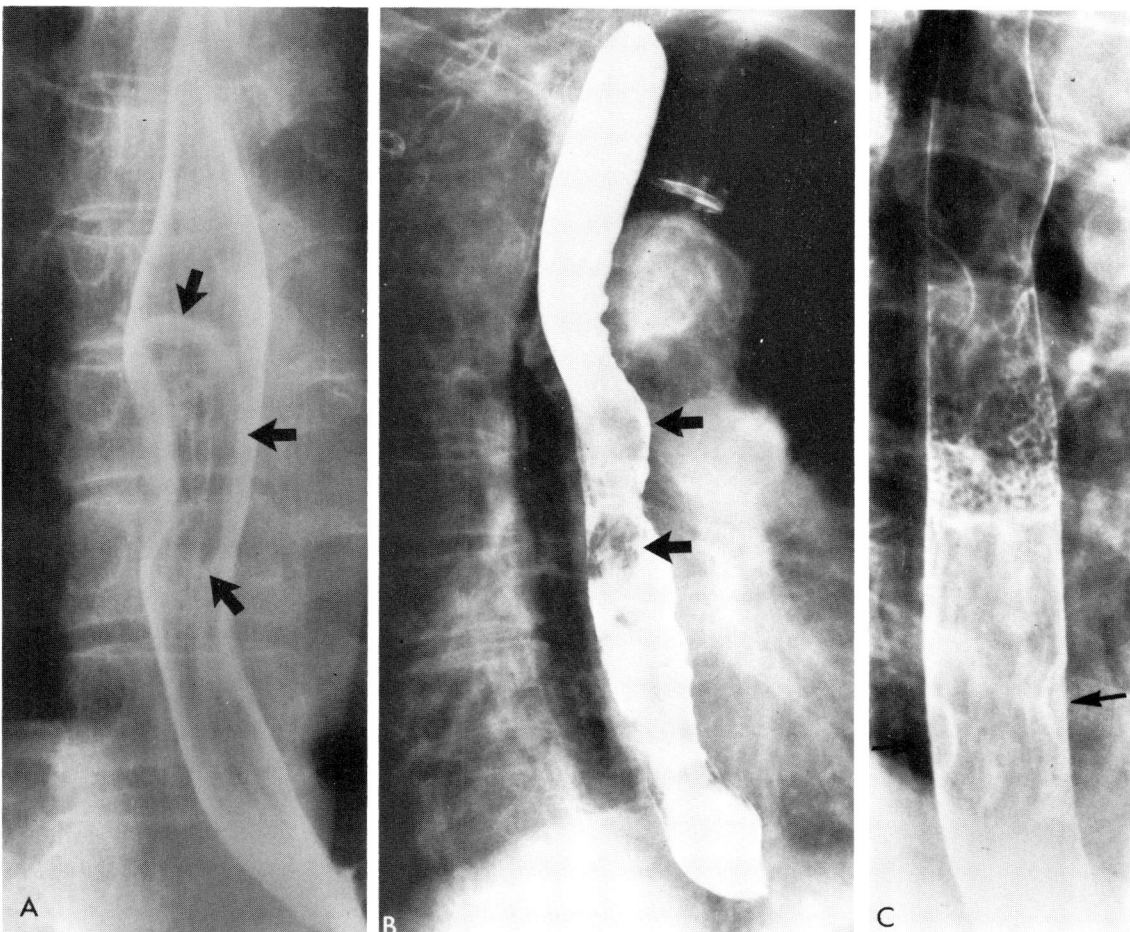

Figure 8–92. Other malignant tumors. A, Leiomyosarcoma. There is a large submucosal tumor in the midesophagus resulting from leiomyosarcoma. B, Melanosarcoma. There is a large polypoid tumor in the midesophagus owing to melanosarcoma. C, Lymphoma. There are multiple submucosal nodules in the esophagus owing to lymphoma. This patient also had lymphoma involving the colon. (A courtesy of A. Yamada, M.D., Tokyo, Japan. B courtesy of S. Antonmattei, M.D., Columbus, Ohio. C from Goldstein, H. M.: Esophagus. In Steckel, R. J., and Kagan, A. R. (eds.): Diagnosis and Staging of Cancer. A Radiologic Approach. Philadelphia, W. B. Saunders Company, 1976, pp. 110–128. By permission of Medical Communications, the University of Texas at Houston, M. D. Anderson Hospital and Tumor Institute.)

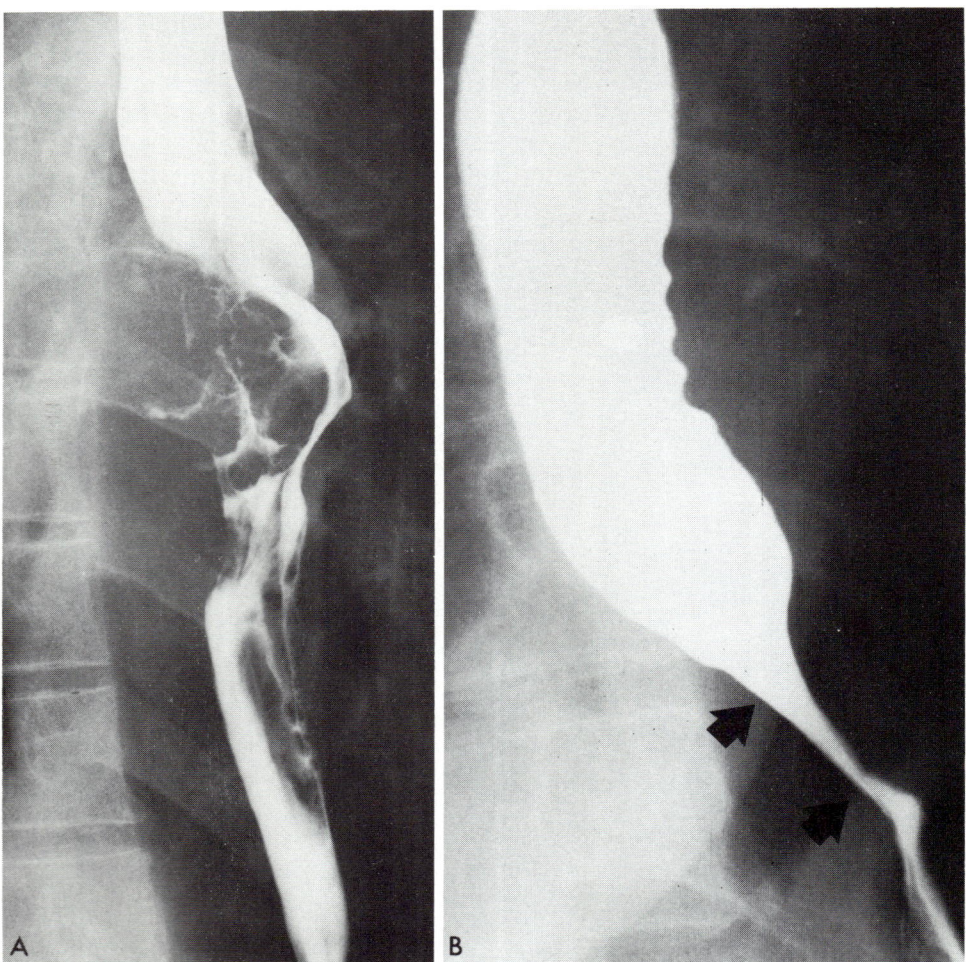

Figure 8–93. Metastatic disease involving the esophagus. *A,* Metastatic disease of subcarinal nodes invading the esophagus. There is an extrinsic, ulcerated mass involving the esophagus. This is due to metastatic disease from carcinoma of the cervix, involving the subcarinal nodes. *B,* Metastatic disease, simulating achalasia. There is tapered narrowing of the distal esophagus (arrow), and at fluoroscopy, there was absence of peristalsis and impaired relaxation of the lower esophageal sphincter. These findings were due to a submucosal metastatic deposit from ovarian carcinoma.

Illustration and legend continued on the opposite page

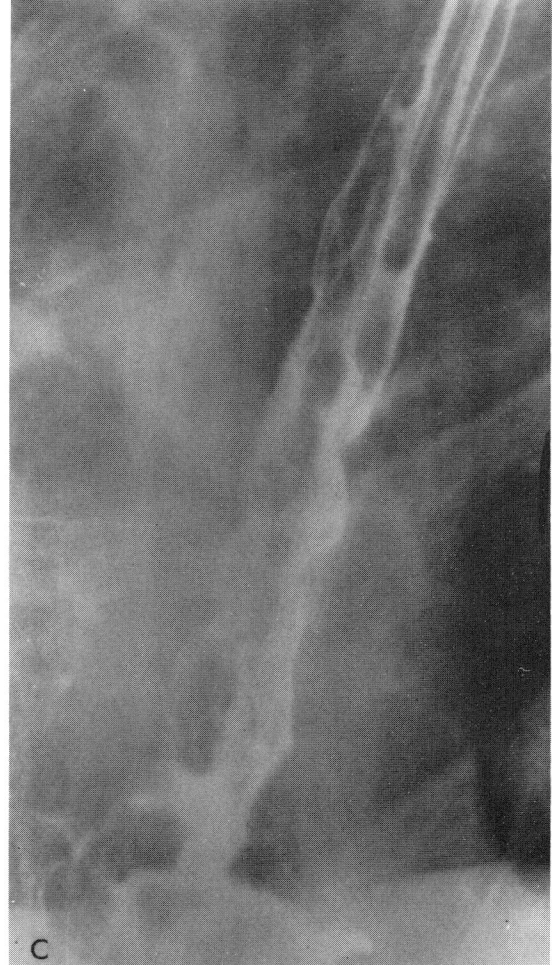

Figure 8–93 *Continued.* C, Extension of gastric carcinoma, simulating varices. There are thickened, tortuous folds in the distal esophagus, resembling esophageal varices. This finding is due to the mucosal extension of a gastric carcinoma along the esophagus.

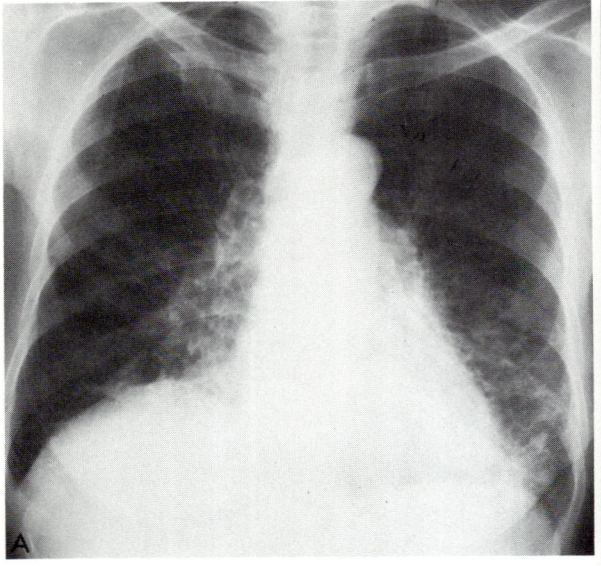
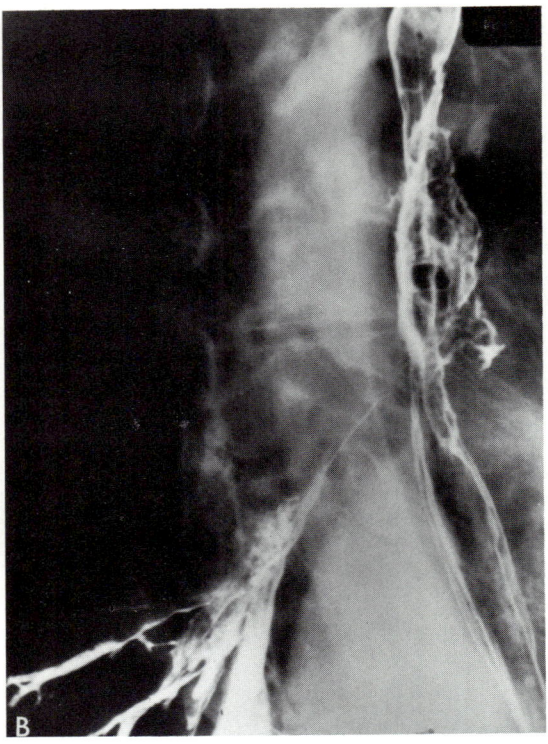

Figure 8–94. Complications of esophageal carcinoma. *A,* Aspiration. There are interstitial opacities in both lung fields, with cystic changes due to bronchiectasis secondary to repeated aspiration. *B,* Bronchoesophageal fistula. There is extensive tumor involving the midesophagus, with a bronchoesophageal fistula resulting in barium filling of the lower lobe bronchi.

asia may result (Fig. 8–93*B*). As mentioned previously, carcinoma of the stomach frequently extends along the esophagus. In most cases, the appearances are typical of a malignant lesion. Occasionally, however, a pattern of thickened, tortuous folds resembling varices may be seen (Fig. 8–93*C*). This is similar to the appearance of varicoid carcinoma.[24, 39]

COMPLICATIONS OF ESOPHAGEAL CARCINOMA. From a radiologic point of view, the major spontaneous complications of esophageal carcinoma are obstruction, aspiration (Fig. 8–94*A*), and tracheoesophageal or bronchoesophageal fistula (Fig. 8–94*B*). Aspiration is due to esophageal obstruction, whereas a fistula results from growth of the tumor into the adjacent airway. A fistula may also develop during the course of radiation therapy (Fig. 8–100*B* and *C*).

METHODS OF TREATMENT

Curative

Treatment of esophageal carcinoma may be either curative or palliative. Curative treatment is undertaken in patients without evidence of metastatic disease. In general, radiotherapy and surgery are the two treatment modalities that may be used. Surgical treatment with esophagogastric anastomosis is generally perferred for lesions of the distal esophagus, whereas radiation therapy is generally preferred for lesions of the cervical esophagus.[34] There is considerable variation in the therapeutic approach to the midesophagus, and either radiation therapy or surgery may be used. In many patients, radiotherapy has a dramatic effect on the primary tumor and results in virtually complete resolution (Fig. 8–95A and B). Nevertheless, most of these patients still succumb, because of either recurrent tumor or widespread metastatic disease. Radiation therapy may also be given preoperatively to reduce the size of the tumor.[32]

In most patients undergoing resection of a tumor, the stomach can be drawn up into the chest for an esophagogastric anastomosis (Fig. 8–96). In some patients this is not possible, however, and a loop of bowel must be interposed between the cervical esophagus and the stomach. Most commonly, this consists of a colonic interposition, using either the right colon with the terminal ileum anastomosed to the cervical esophagus, or the left colon. A barium enema and mesenteric angiography should be performed preoperatively to rule out unsuspected colonic or vascular diseases that might affect the interposed colon. Colonic interposition produces dramatic findings on the

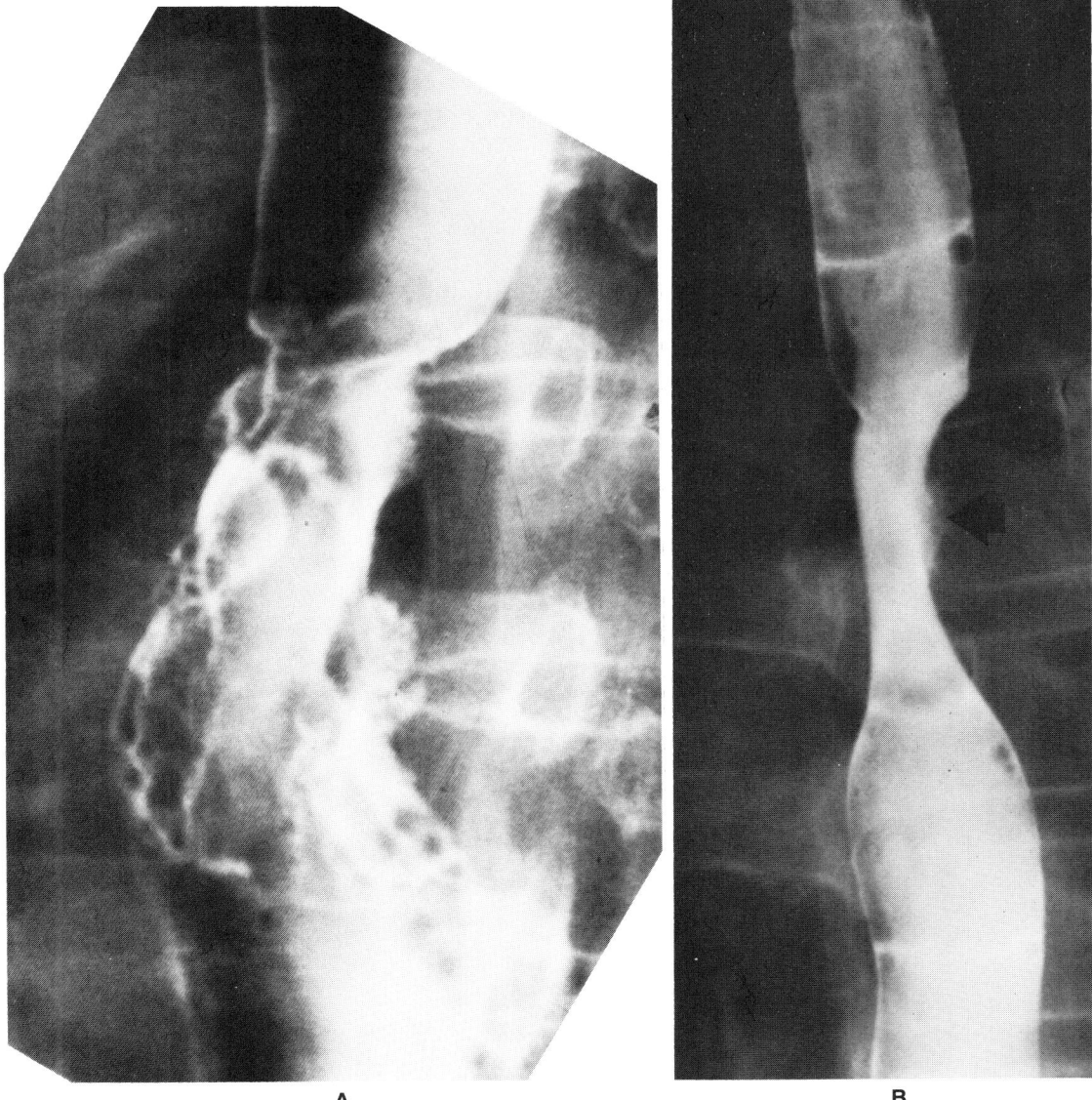

Figure 8–95. Good response to radiotherapy. *A*, Esophageal carcinoma with extensive ulceration. *B*, After radiotherapy the tumor has resolved almost completely, leaving only a stricture and an ulcer (arrow).

406 — THE ESOPHAGUS

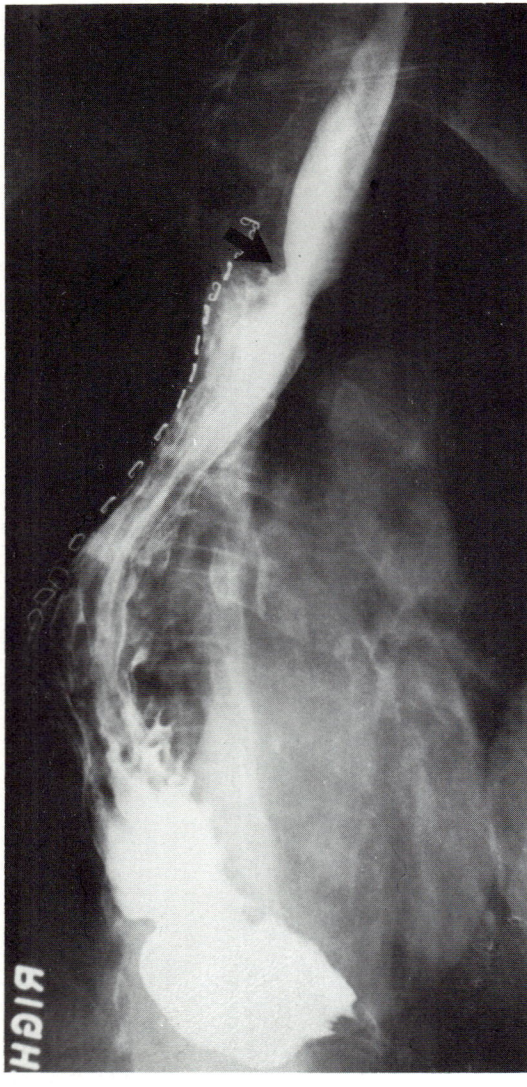

Figure 8–96. Normal appearance following esophagogastric anastomosis. This esophagogram was performed following esophagogastric resection and anastomosis. The stomach has been drawn up into the chest, and the anastomotic line is seen (arrow).

plain chest films, large air spaces being evident in the mediastinum that frequently contain fluid levels (Fig. 8–97A). On esophagography a tortuous, dilated colon is usually seen (Fig. 8–97B and C). This acts as a passive conduit for ingested materials. Occasionally, a loop of small bowel can be used for interposition.

Palliative

Palliative treatment is undertaken in patients who have evidence of disseminated disease or are otherwise unfit for curative treatment. Palliation is aimed at controlling symptoms due to obstruction or fistula.

Patients presenting with symptoms due to esophageal obstruction can be treated by radiation therapy at a dosage slightly lower than that used for curative treatment. In many patients some form of immediate relief of esophageal obstruction may be necessary, however, since the obstruction may initially be aggravated by the radiation therapy. Immediate relief can be obtained by some form of surgical bypass of the esophagus. Esophageal bougienage is an alternative to this form of treatment. In the presence of a tight stricture, this is started with the endoscopic passage of a wire

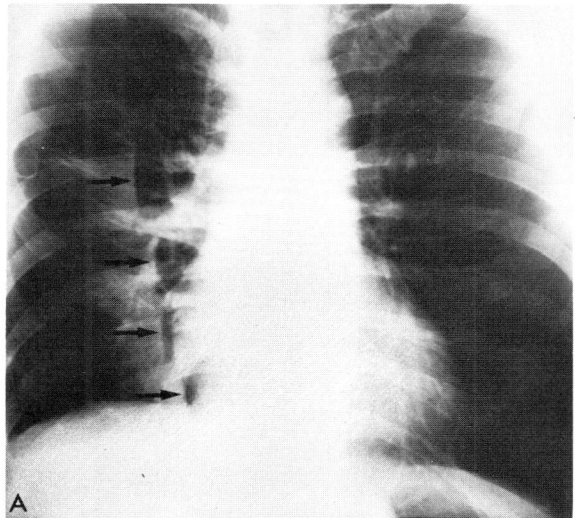

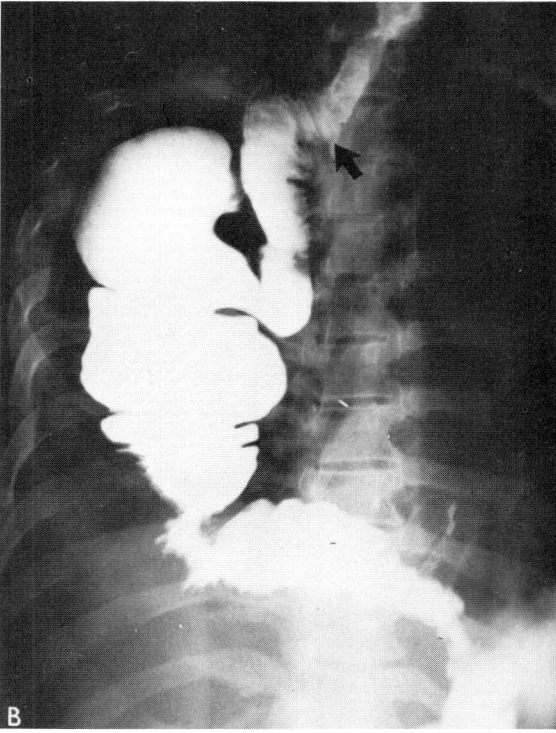

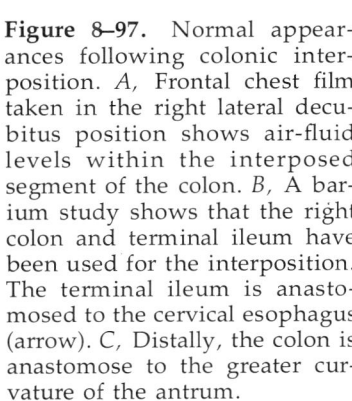

Figure 8–97. Normal appearances following colonic interposition. *A*, Frontal chest film taken in the right lateral decubitus position shows air-fluid levels within the interposed segment of the colon. *B*, A barium study shows that the right colon and terminal ileum have been used for the interposition. The terminal ileum is anastomosed to the cervical esophagus (arrow). *C*, Distally, the colon is anastomose to the greater curvature of the antrum.

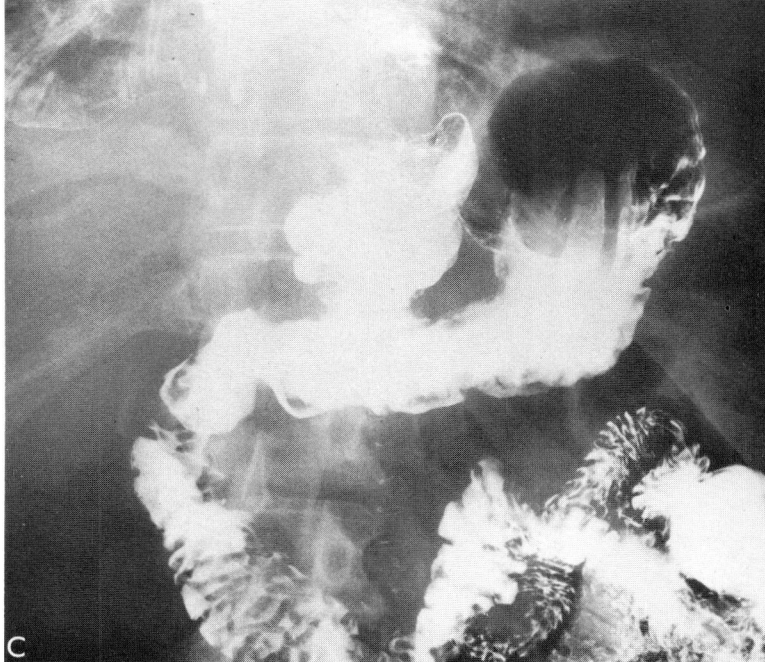

through the stricture and the passage of an olive dilator over the wire. Subsequent dilatations can be performed with Maloney or Hurst bougies.[2, 31]

Esophageal obstruction or fistula can also be palliated by esophageal bypass surgery. This may consist of a colonic interposition placed substernally or a reverse gastric "tube."[13] The gastric tube is fashioned from the greater curvature of the stomach. The antral end is brought up into the chest in a substernal location and anastomosed to the cervical esophagus. This operation represents relatively minor surgery, and the interposed gastric tube is well vascularized. This tends to minimize the incidence and severity of anastomotic leakage. This type of surgery can be recognized on plain films of the chest by the presence of the air-containing gastric tube in the retrosternal position (Fig. 8–98A). Abdominal films may show a crescentic arrangement of surgical staples along the greater curvature of the stomach.[11] A barium study outlines the gastric tube, the cervical anastomosis, and the residual portion of the stomach (Fig. 8–98B and C).

In some patients, palliation may be achieved by the passage of a firm tube to act as an esophageal prosthesis. As described by Celestin, this may be passed perorally while a gastrotomy is performed to pull the prosthesis into the stomach where it is anchored.[8] Alternatively, a prosthesis may be placed endoscopically following esoph-

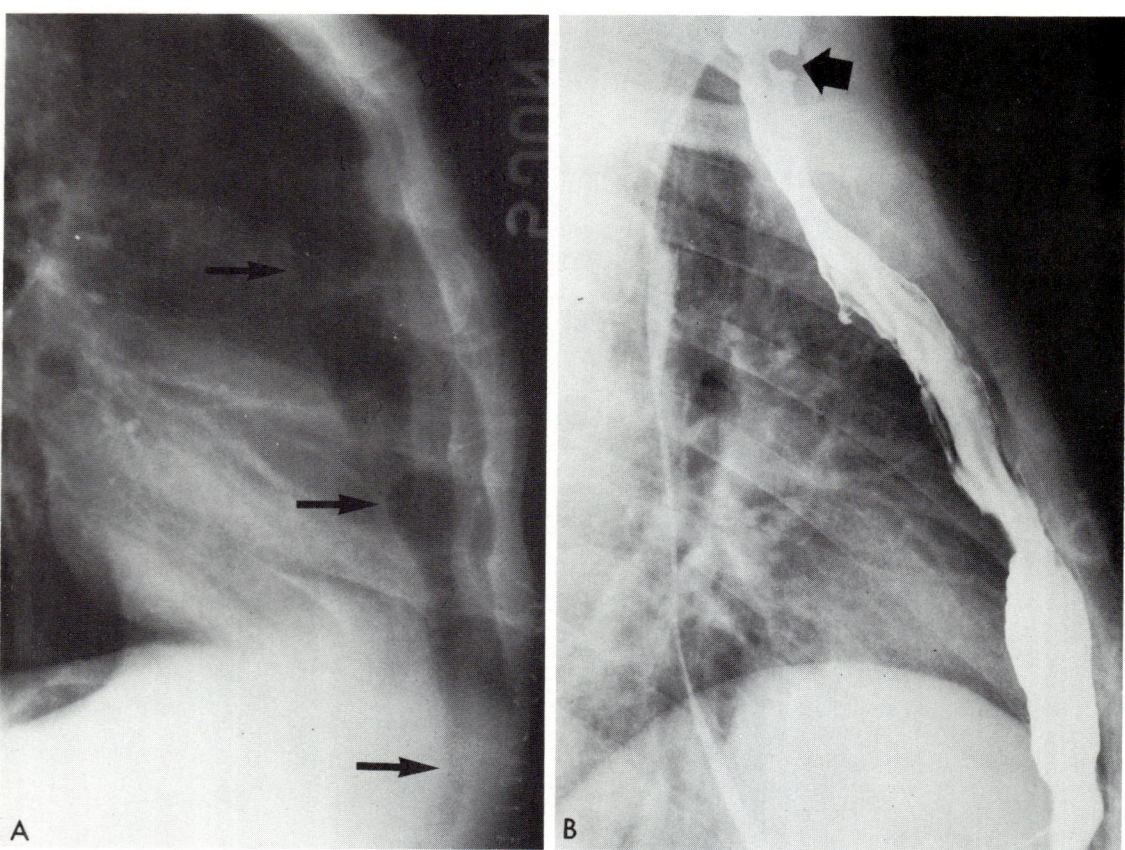

Figure 8–98. Reverse gastric tube. *A,* A lateral chest film shows the air shadows (arrows) in the retrosternal area within the gastric tube. *B,* A barium study shows the esophagogastric anastomosis (arrow), with barium outlining the gastric tube. Barium has also refluxed into the bypassed esophagus.

Illustration and legend continued on the opposite page

ageal dilatation.[31] The radiopaque tube can be recognized on a lateral chest film (Fig. 8–99A). A barium esophagogram performed after placement of the prosthesis should show the barium traversing the lumen of the prosthesis, with little or no passage between the prosthesis and the esophageal wall.[37] Effective palliation is not achieved if the barium passes around the tube and enters a fistula or site of perforation (Fig. 8–99B and C).

COMPLICATIONS OF TREATMENT

A multitude of complications may be encountered following treatment for esophageal tumors. These include complications of radiation therapy, general surgical complications, and the specific complications encountered with the various surgical procedures. These are summarized in Table 8–2.

Radiation Therapy

Radiotherapy may cause edema in the region of the esophageal tumor, which may result in a transient increase in the degree of esophageal obstruction. Radiation therapy

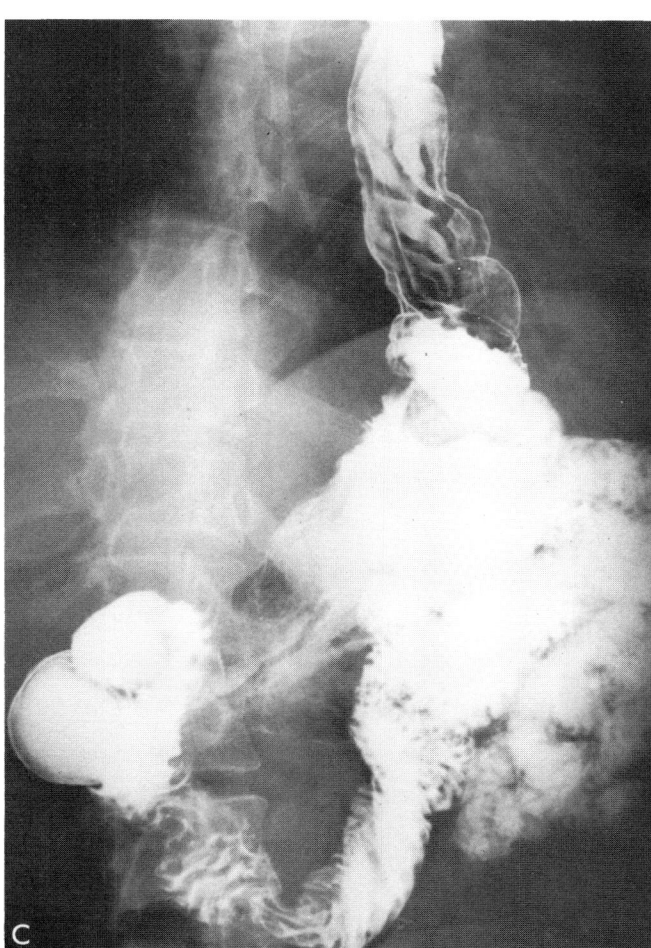

Figure 8–98 Continued. C, The gastric tube can be seen extending from the greater curvature of the stomach into the thoracic cavity. The gastric rugae within the tube are clearly delineated.

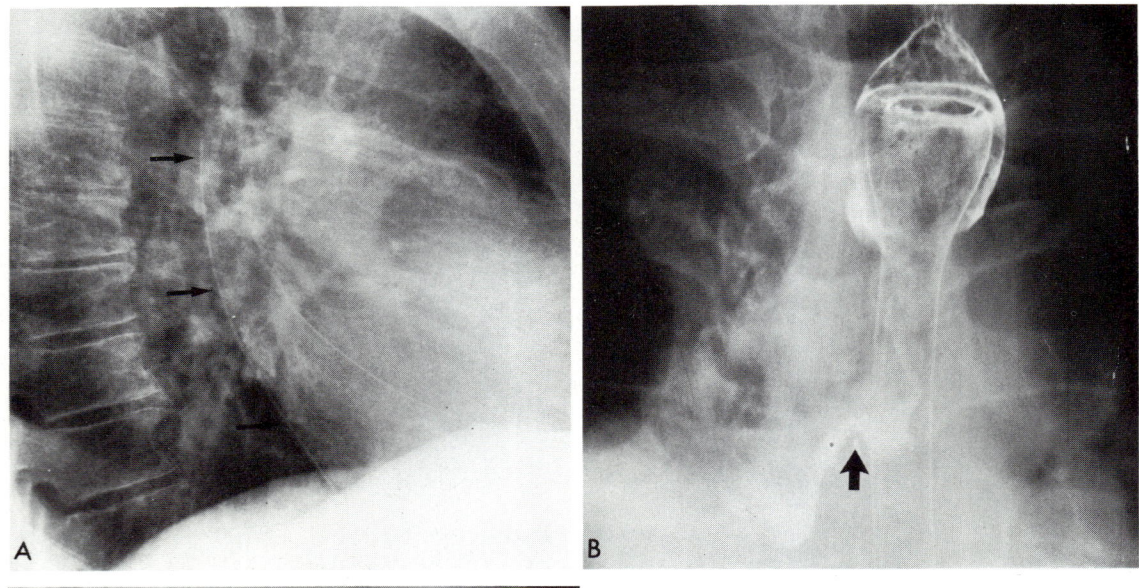
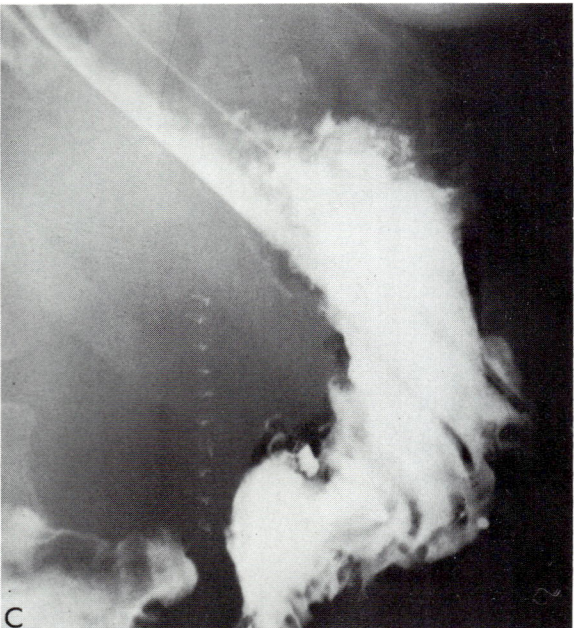

Figure 8–99. The Celestin tube. *A,* A lateral chest film shows the radiopaque Celestin tube in position within the esophagus (arrows). *B,* A barium esophagram outlines the Celestin tube. Some of the barium has passed around the tube and enters a site of esophageal perforation (arrow). *C,* The distal end of the tube is seen within the stomach.

TABLE 8-2. COMPLICATIONS OF TREATMENT FOR ESOPHAGEAL TUMORS

Radiation Therapy
    Obstruction
    Fistula
    Radiation stricture
    Extraintestinal damage—lungs, pericardium, spinal cord
General Surgical Complications (esophagogastric anastomosis and gastric tube)
    Hematoma, infection
    Anastomotic leak and sequelae
    Reflux and sequelae
Interposition
    Colonic disease—ischemia, diverticulitis
    Migration of abdominal colon
    Aspiration (damage to recurrent laryngeal nerve)
    Bile reflux esophagitis (jejunal interposition)
Celestin Tube
    Obstruction
    Perforation
    Migration
    Hemorrhage

may also cause necrosis of the tumor, which may result in a fistula to the airway (Fig. 8-100A and B) or in perforation and abscess (Fig. 8-100C). To a certain extent these complications may be avoided by the passage of a Celestin tube or by dilatation prior to institution of the radiation therapy. If the patient is fortunate enough to have a good response to this treatment, he still risks the development of a radiation-induced stricture (Fig. 8-101). This is rarely encountered, however, because of the small number of patients with a survival period long enough for this complication to arise.

General Surgical Complications

Patients undergoing esophageal resection with either direct anastomosis or interposition are subject to a series of complications.[5, 28] The most frequent and dreaded of these is leakage either at the esophagogastric anastomosis (Fig. 8-102) or at the proximal anastomosis in the case of an interposition. These leaks may be related to devascularization or ischemia of the anastomosed loop. Their development may be favored by the absence of a serosal lining in the esophagus.

Abnormalities on the chest film may give clues to the development of an anastomotic leak.[33] These abnormalities include widening of the mediastinum; mediastinal fluid level; mediastinal, cervical, or subcutaneous emphysema; pleural effusion; and hydropneumothorax. The precise findings depend on the length of time the leak has been present, its location, and whether it is confined to the mediastinum or has communicated with the pleural cavity. When an anastomotic leak is suspected, a contrast study is generally performed to define its location, size, and communications. Initially, a water-soluble contrast material, such as Gastrografin, should be used. If there is a leak and contrast material escapes into the mediastinum, it is not irritating and is reabsorbed. This contrast agent does not result in optimal radiographic detail, however. If the swallow of Gastrografin shows no leak the examination should be continued with barium. Barium has been shown to promote granuloma formation in the mediastinum.[18] If a leak is present, however, surgery is usually performed and the barium can be cleared.

Other possible general surgical complications include mediastinal hematoma and infection.

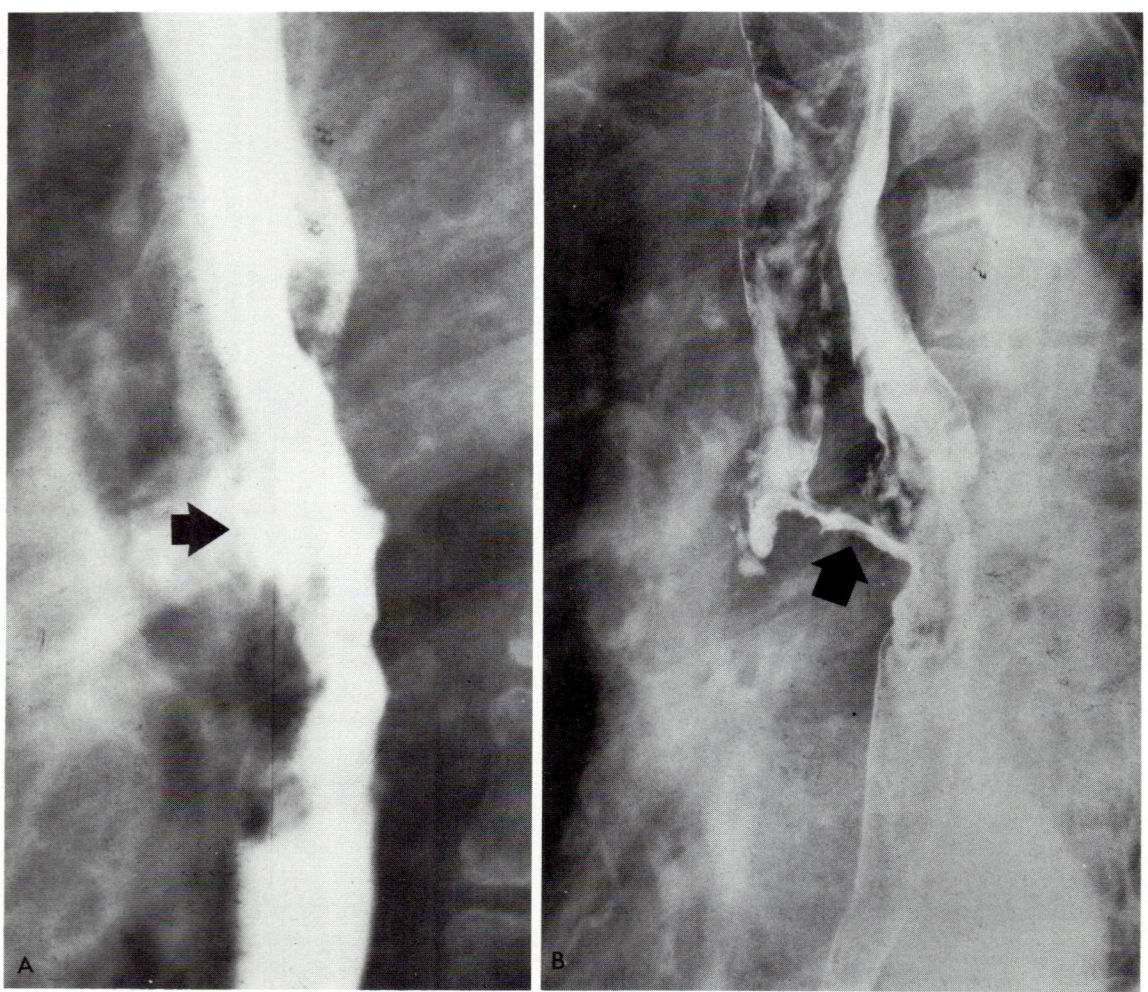

Figure 8–100. Complications of radiotherapy. *A* and *B*, Tracheoesophageal fistula. There is extensive tumor involving the midesophagus. One of the ulcerated areas (arrow) is immediately adjacent to the air shadow of the trachea *(A)*. Following radiation, a barium esophagogram *(B)* reveals a tracheoesophageal fistula (arrow), with barium filling the trachea.

Illustration and legend continued on the opposite page

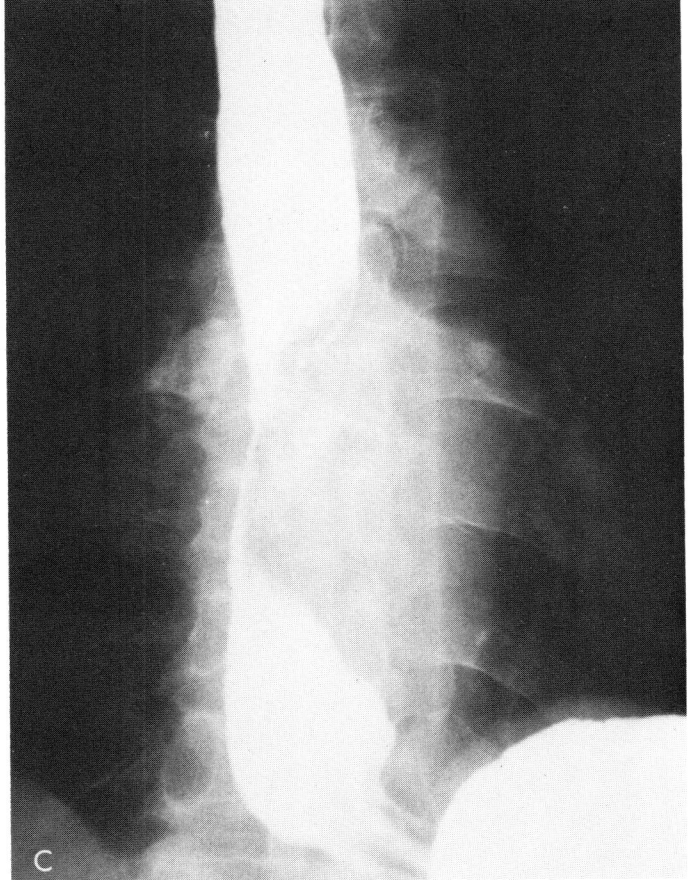

Figure 8–100 *Continued.* *C*, Esophageal perforation with abscess. This patient was irradiated for esophageal carcinoma and experienced an acute onset of dysphagia. A barium esophagogram shows an extrinsic mass compressing the esophagus. At operation, this was found to be an abscess due to perforation of the esophagus secondary to radiation therapy of the tumor. There was no residual tumor.

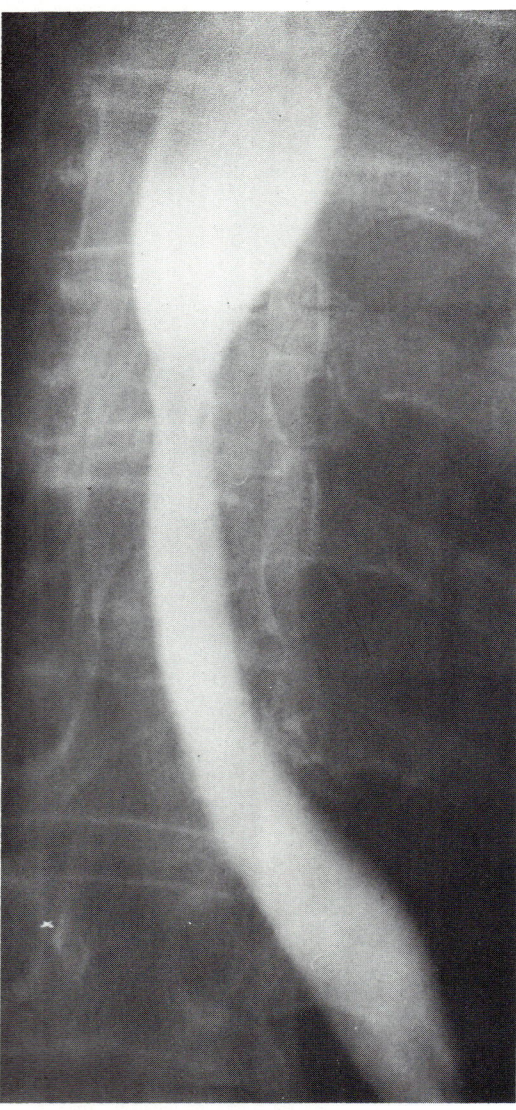

Figure 8–101. Radiation-induced stricture. This is a long stricture involving the distal half of the esophagus in a patient who was previously irradiated for esophageal carcinoma.

In the routine follow-up of a patient after esophageal resection, a Gastrografin-barium esophagogram is usually performed one week postoperatively, before the start of oral feeding. It is also advisable to obtain a barium esophagogram at two or three months to provide a record of the baseline appearance of the postsurgical anatomy should later complications develop.[42] Patients surviving an anastomotic leak may acquire a cutaneous fistula or a stricture at the anastomosis. Reflux of gastric contents may be a problem following esophageal resection. The resection removes the lower esophageal sphincter, allowing free reflux into the esophagus or interposed bowel. Many patients complain of some heartburn, but few survive long enough to acquire severe reflux esophagitis, ulceration, or stricture (Fig. 8–103).

The development of a radiologic abnormality at the anastomosis raises the possibility of recurrent carcinoma. In most cases the irregularity, nodularity, and narrowing make the diagnosis obvious (Fig. 8–104), but in some early cases, it may be necessary

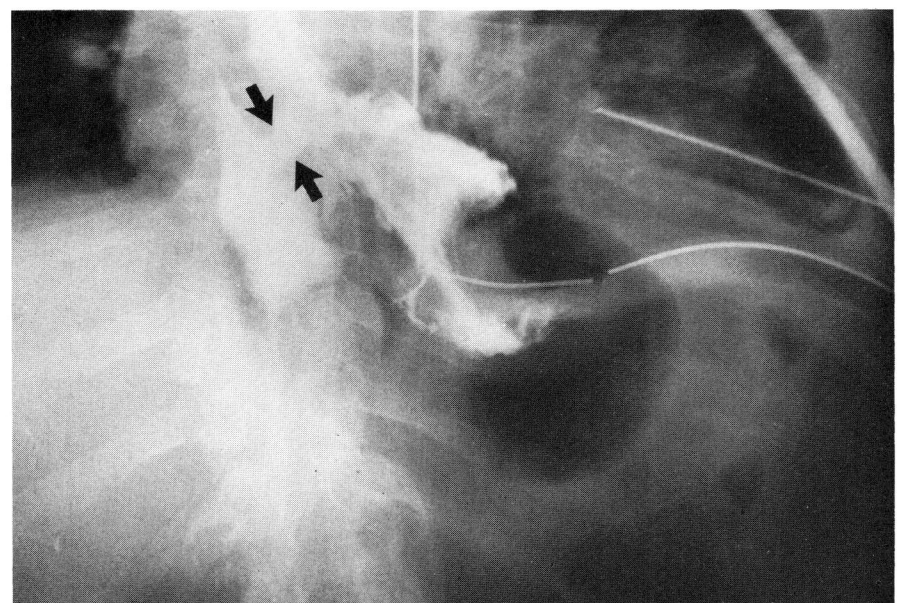

Figure 8–102. Anastomotic leak following the creation of an esophagogastric anastomosis. A Gastrografin esophagogram shows marked extravasation of contrast into a cavity from the right lateral aspect of the anastomotic site (arrows).

Figure 8–103. Anastomotic ulcer (arrow) following the creation of an esophagogastric anastomosis for benign esophageal tumor.

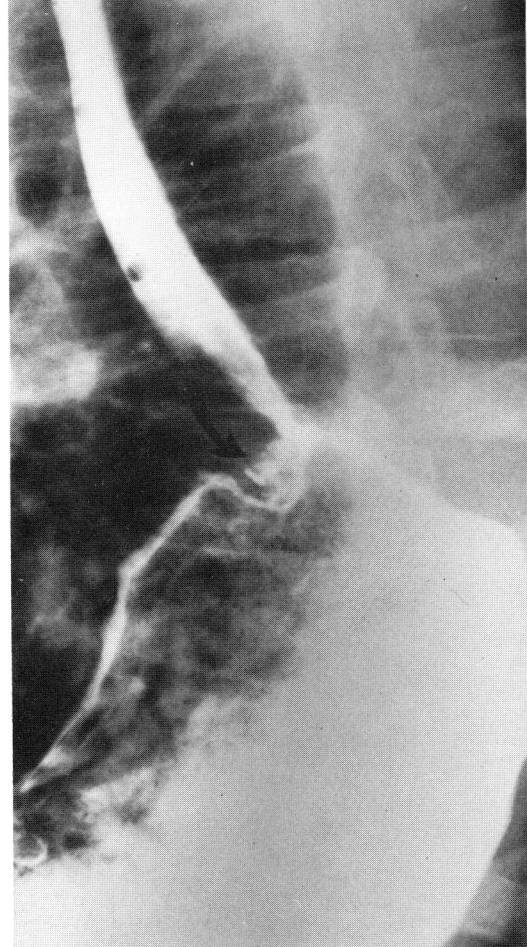

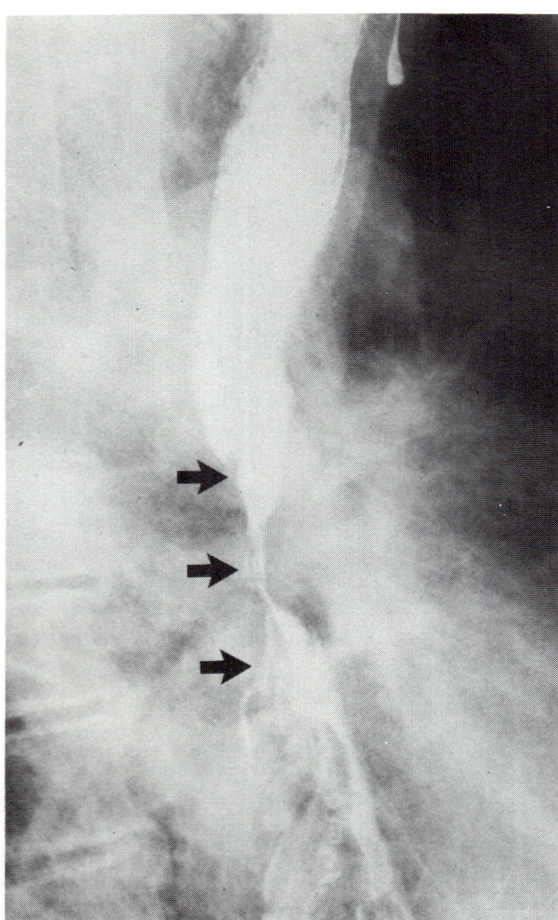

Figure 8–104. Recurrent carcinoma at the anastomosis. There has been an esophagogastric resection, with the creation of an esophagogastric anastomosis. There is an irregular narrowing at the anastomosis (arrows) resulting from recurrent carcinoma.

Figure 8–105. Slipped Celestin tube. This patient presented with dysphagia due to esophageal carcinoma. A Celestin tube had been inserted prior to radiation therapy. There was a good, direct response to radiation therapy, with shrinkage of the tumor. A barium study shows the barium-filled tube lying in the stomach. Because of the decrease in the size of the tumor, the Celestin tube was able to slip distally into the stomach. The tube was removed by laparotomy.

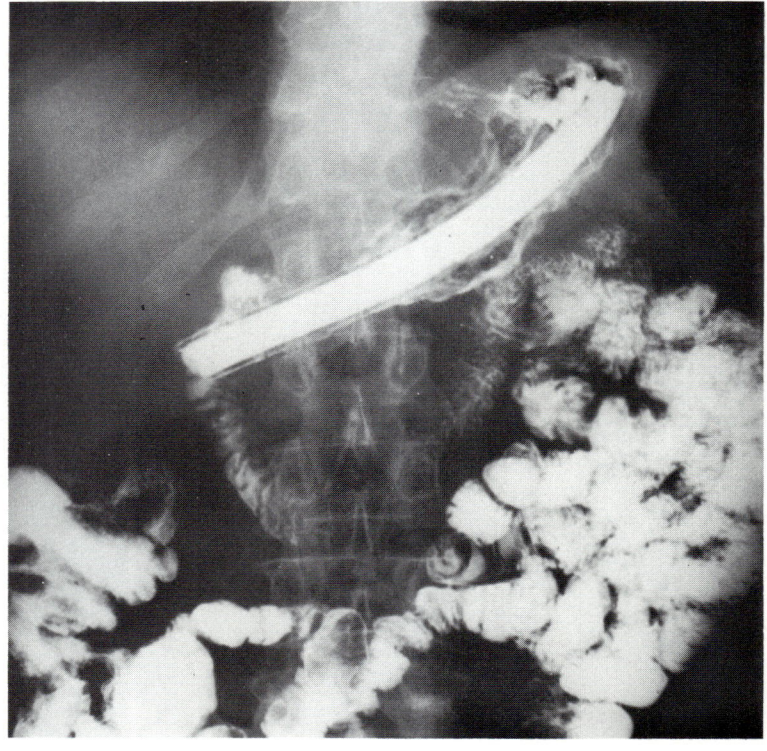

to resort to endoscopy and biopsy. If the tumor recurs submucosally, however, the biopsies and brushings may be unrevealing. In such cases, radiation therapy may be undertaken with a presumptive diagnosis of recurrent tumor.

Colonic Interposition

This operation carries with it the risk of general surgical complications, as well as a number of risks that are unique. The interposed colonic segment is subject to the usual colonic diseases, such as ischemia and diverticulitis. In addition, the portion of the colon that is left behind in the abdomen may migrate into the chest. This makes the intrathoracic portion redundant and elongated, and the resultant folding may cause a functional obstruction. In the formation of the cervical anastomosis, the recurrent laryngeal nerve may be damaged. This may give rise to postoperative aspiration.

Jejunal interposition is performed much less frequently. Although the small bowel has fewer intrinsic diseases, this operation is technically more difficult and is associated with reflux of bile into the esophagus, which may give rise to a severe esophagitis with ulceration and stricture.

Celestin Tube

Complications are rarely encountered with the insertion of a Celestin tube.[37] Occasionally obstruction, migration of the tube (Fig. 8–105), and hemorrhage occur, however.[10]

SUMMARY

Most patients with esophageal tumors present with advanced carcinoma of the esophagus. Radiologic diagnosis in these patients usually presents no difficulty. Occasionally, an opportunity arises to detect an early esophageal carcinoma. The radiologic findings in these patients may be very subtle and are best detected on double-contrast radiographs. Benign tumors and other malignant tumors rarely involve the esophagus. Surgery and radiation are the two primary modalities used for the treatment of esophageal carcinoma. Radiation may promote the development of perforation or tracheoesophageal fistula by causing necrosis of the tumor extending through the wall of the esophagus. Surgical procedures may be performed in the hope of achieving a cure or for the purpose of palliation. Palliative treatment usually consists of some form of bypass procedure—either a colonic interposition or a reverse gastric tube. The most feared complication of these procedures is the development of an anastomotic leak. Esophageal bougienage and placement of a Celestin tube can also be used for palliation.

References

1. Attah, E. B., and Hajdu, S. I.: Benign and malignant tumors of the esophagus at autopsy. J. Thorac. Cardiovasc. Surg. 55:396–404, 1968.
2. Boyce, H. W.: Cancer of the esophagus: the case for palliation. Hosp. Pract. 11:73–75, 1976.
3. Burdette, W. J., and Jesse, R.: Carcinoma of the cervical esophagus. J. Thorac. Cardiovasc. Surg. 63:41–52, 1972.
4. Burrell, M., and Toffler, R.: Fibrovascular polyp of the esophagus. Am. J. Dig. Dis. 18:714–718, 1973.
5. Calenoff, L., and Norfray, J.: The reconstructed esophagus. Am. J. Roentgenol. 125:864–876, 1975.
6. Carnovale, R. L., Goldstein, H. M., Zornoza, J. et al.: Radiologic manifestations of esophageal lymphoma. Am. J. Roentgenol. 128:751–754, 1977.
7. Carter, R., and Brewer, L.: Achalasia and esophageal carcinoma: studies in early diagnosis for improved surgical management. Am. J. Surg. 130:114–118, 1975.

8. Celestin, L. R.: Permanent intubation in inoperable cancer of the oesophagus and cardia. A new tube, Ann. R. Coll. Surg. Engl. 25:165–170, 1959.
9. Collins, S. M., Hamilton, J. D., Lewis, T. D., et al.: Small-bowel malabsoprtion and gastrointestinal malignancy. Radiology 126:603–609, 1978.
10. Duvoisin, G. E., Ellis, F. H., Jr., and Payne, W. S.: The value of palliative prosthesis in malignant lesions of the esophagus. Surg. Clin. North Am. 47:827–831, 1967.
11. Fetouh, S. A., Daffner, R. H., Postlethwait, R. W., et al.: Radiologic aspects of Beck gastric tube in esophageal reconstruction. Am. J. Roentgenol. 129:425–431, 1977.
12. Fisher, M. S.: Metastasis to the esophagus. Gastrointest. Radiol. 1:249–251, 1976.
13. Gavriliu, D.: Replacement of the esophagus by a reverse gastric tube. Curr. Probl. Surg. 12:36–64, 1975.
14. Gloyna, R. E., Zornoza, J., and Goldstein, H. M.: Primary ulcerative carcinoma of the esophagus. Am. J. Roentgenol. 129:559–600, 1977.
15. Goldstein, H. M.: Esophagus. In Steckel, R. J., and Kagan, A. R. (eds.): Diagnosis and Staging of Cancer. Philadelphia, W. B. Saunders and Company, 1976, pp. 110–128.
16. Goldstein, H. M., and Dodd, G. D.: Double-contrast esophagography. Gastrointest. Radiol. 1:3–6, 1976.
17. Harper, P. S., Harper, R. M. J., and Howel-Evans, A. W.: Carcinoma of the oesophagus with tylosis. Q. J. Med. 34:317–333, 1970.
18. James, A. E., Montali, R. J., Chaffee, V. et al.: Barium or Gastrografin: Which contrast media for diagnosis of esophageal tears? Gastroenterology 68:1103–1113, 1975.
19. Kenneweg, D. J., and Cimmino, C. V.: Carcinosarcoma of the esophagus. Am. J. Roentgenol. 101:482–484, 1967.
20. Koehler, R. E., Moss, A. A., and Margulis, A. R.: Early radiographic manifestations of carcinoma of the esophagus. Radiology 119:1–5, 1976.
21. Kostinanen, S., Teppo, L., and Virkkula, L.: Papilloma of the esophagus. Report of a case. Scand. J. Thorac. Cardiovasc. Surg. 7:95–97, 1973.
22. Laufer, I.: A simple method for routine double contrast study of the upper gastrointestinal tract. Radiology 117:513–518, 1975.
23. Laufer, I.: Double contrast radiology in the diagnosis of gastrointestinal cancer. In Glass, G. B. J. (ed.): Progress in Gastroenterology, Vol. 3. New York, Grune & Stratton, Inc., 1977, pp. 643–669.
24. Lawson, T. L., Dodds, W. J., and Sheft, D. J.: Carcinoma of the esophagus simulating varices. Am. J. Roentgenol. 107:83–85, 1969.
25. Liliequist, B., and Wiberg, A.: Pedunculated tumor of the esophagus. Two cases of lipoma. Acta Radiol. 15:383–392, 1974.
26. LiVolsi, V. A., and Perzin, K. H.: Inflammatory pseudotumors (inflammatory fibrous polyps) of the esophagus. A clinicopathologic study. Am. J. Dig. Dis. 20:475–481, 1975.
27. McCort, J. J.: Esophageal carcinosarcoma and pseudosarcoma. Radiology 102:519–524, 1972.
28. May, I. A., and Samson, P. C.: Esophageal reconstruction and replacements. Ann. Thorac. Surg. 7:249–277, 1969.
29. Moss, A. A., Koehler, R. E., and Margulis, A. R.: Initial accuracy of esophagograms in detection of small esophageal carcinoma. Am. J. Roentgenol. 127:909–913, 1976.
30. Naef, A., Savary, M., and Ozzello, L.: Columnar-lined lower esophagus—an acquired lesion with malignant predisposition. J. Thorac. Cardiovasc. Surg. 70:826–834, 1975.
31. Palmer, E. D.: Peroral prosthesis for the management of incurable esophageal carcinoma. Am. J. Gastroenterol. 59:487–498, 1973.
32. Parker, E. F., and Gregorie, H. B.: Carcinoma of the esophagus. Long-term results. J.A.M.A. 235:1016–1018, 1976.
33. Parkin, G. J. S.: The radiology of perforated oesophagus. Clin. Radiol. 24:324–332, 1973.
34. Pearson, J. G.: The value of radiotherapy in the management of esophageal cancer. Am. J. Roentgenol. 105:500–513, 1969.
35. Putman, C. E., Curtis, A. M., Westfried, M., et al.: Thickening of the posterior tracheal stripe: a sign of squamous cell carcinoma of the esophagus. Radiology 121:533–536, 1976.
36. Robbins, A. H., Hermos, J. A., Schimmel, E. M., et al.: The columnar-lined esophagus—analysis of 26 cases. Radiology 123:1–7, 1977.
37. Russell, E., Shapiro, R., and Wilson, G. L.: Radiologic aspects of Celestin tube intubation for incurable obstructive esophageal carcinoma. Radiology 102:531–532, 1972.
38. Saibil, E., Shapiro, R., and Wilson, G. L.: Radiologic aspects of Celestin tube intubation for incurable obstructive esophageal carcinoma. Radiology 102:531–532, 1972.
38. Saibil, E., and Palayew, M. J.: Primary malignant melanoma of the esophagus. Am. J. Gastroenterol. 61:63–67, 1974.
39. Silver, T. M., and Goldstein, H. M.: Varicoid carcinoma of the esophagus. Am. J. Dig. Dis. 19:56–58, 1974.
40. Skucas, J., and Schrank, W. W.: The routine air-contrast examination of the esophagus. Radiology 115:482–484, 1975.
41. Suzuki, H., Kobayashi, S., Endo, M., et al.: Diagnosis of early esophageal cancer. Surgery 71:99–103, 1971.
42. Tuszewski, F. K.: The radiologic appearance of the reconstructed esophagus. Acta Radiol. 12:193–216, 1972.
43. Wynder, E. L., and Mabuchi, K.: Cancer of the gastrointestinal tract: etiological and environmental factors. J.A.M.A. 226:1546–1548, 1973.

9

PEPTIC ULCER

ROBERT N. BERK, M.D.

During the past decade there has been a remarkable improvement in the radiologist's ability to detect gastric and duodenal ulcers and in his ability to differentiate reliably between benign and malignant gastric ulcer craters. Improved design of modern x-ray equipment has increased the quality of the fluoroscopic and radiographic images dramatically and has increased the ease and consistency with which they can be obtained. The introduction of effervescent powders, glucagon, and better barium preparations has made possible air-contrast radiographic studies of the gastric and duodenal mucosa in exquisite detail (Fig. 9–1).[2, 3, 9] Furthermore, Nelson, Wolf, and Marshak have simplified the task of differentiating between benign and malignant gastric ulcers by providing a clearer understanding of the anatomic basis for the radiographic features that are used to make the distinction.[8, 13, 15] Much of what follows is taken from the monumental work of these authors.

TECHNICAL CONSIDERATIONS

The ability to detect and classify ulcers of the stomach and duodenum on radiographic examination is distinctly impaired by the presence of blood clots and food residue in the crater, marked mucosal edema at the orifice of the ulcer, spasm of the adjacent gastric wall, excessive secretions in the stomach, and inability of the patient to cooperate. In these cases, a second examination performed one week after medical therapy often reveals an ulcer or discloses features that permit distinction between a benign ulcer and a carcinoma when these findings were not evident initially. While excessive secretions in the stomach of a patient who has fasted properly are a sign that a peptic ulcer may be present, they are also a forewarning that barium coating of the gastric wall and air-contrast studies will be inadequate for accurate evaluation of the stomach.

As in other radiographic procedures, the accuracy of the stomach examination depends on radiographic technique. Improperly exposed radiographs invariably lead to incorrect diagnoses. Premature flooding of the stomach with barium, failure to obtain both air contrast and compression views, an inadequate number of spot radiographs, and insufficient attention to any one of the three aspects of the examination (fluoros-

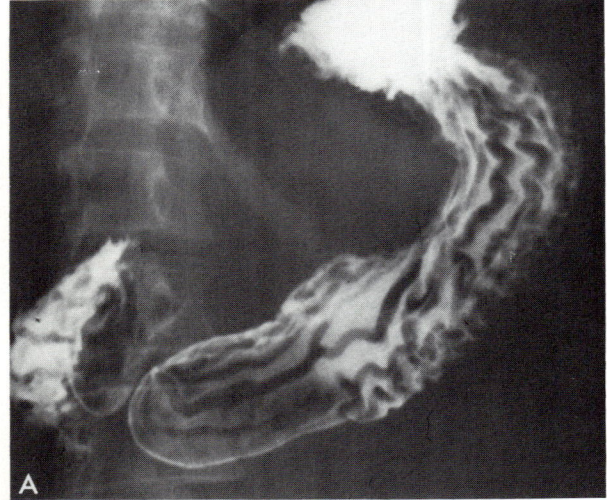

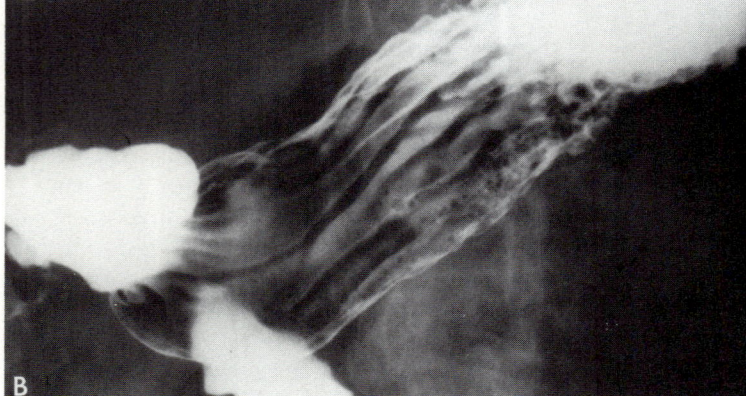

Figure 9–1. Normal supine air-contrast projections of the stomach. *A*, Left posterior oblique. *B*, Right posterior oblique.

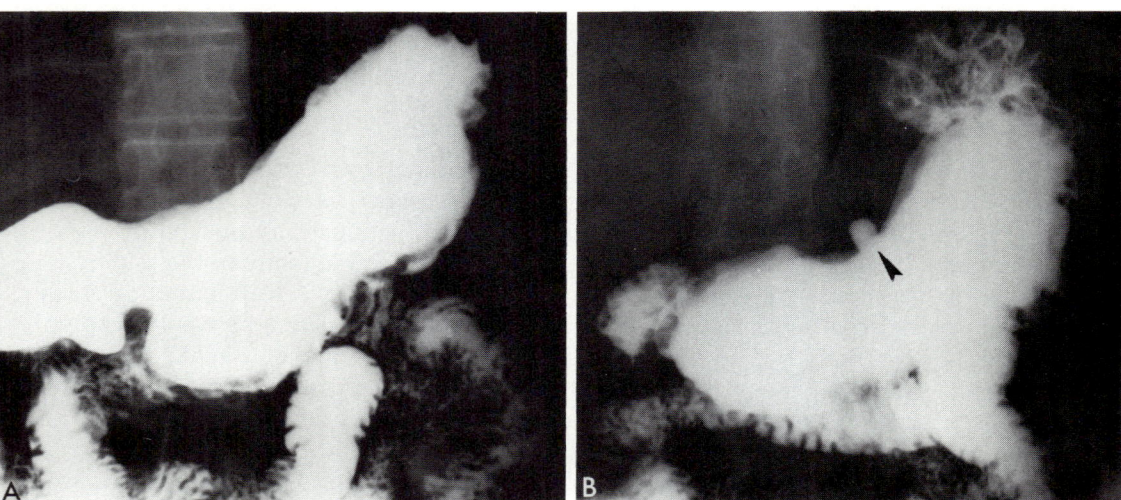

Figure 9–2. *A*, Prone view of the stomach in a patient whose stomach is high and transverse in position. *B*, Angling the radiographic tube 30 degrees toward the head elongates the lesser curvature and discloses a benign gastric ulcer (arrow) that is not visible in *A*.

copy, spot films, and radiographs) reduce the accuracy of the study. When the stomach is high and transverse in position, prone views made with the x-ray beam angled 30 degrees cephalad may disclose an ulcer in the lesser curvature that is not visible otherwise (Fig. 9–2).

Once a gastric ulcer is identified, every effort must be made to obtain spot-film radiographs of the lesion both in profile and *en face*, so that the criteria used to determine whether the lesion is benign or malignant can be evaluated optimally. Compression and air-contrast views are essential. Upright projections of the stomach when it is distended with barium can often demonstrate projection of lesser curvature ulcers beyond the gastric lumen when this feature is not apparent on radiographs made in other positions.

RADIOLOGIC FEATURES OF BENIGN GASTRIC ULCERS

According to Nelson, the presence of at least one radiographic sign indicating that the ulcer is benign is of great importance, but the presence of two or more is conclusive evidence of benignancy.[8] He lists the reliable signs that an ulcer is benign as follows: (1) penetration (projection of the ulcer crater beyond the normal contour of the stomach); (2) mucosal folds radiating into the orifice of the crater; (3) a single nodule in the base of the ulcer; (4) a smooth mound of edema surrounding a sharply defined crater; and (5) signs of undermining of the mucosa (Hampton's line, ulcer collar, "collar-button" shape, and crescent sign). Undermining is present when the base of an ulcer is wider than its orifice. The number, size, and location of ulcers cannot be used as criteria to distinguish benign from malignant ulcers.[8, 11–13, 15]

To evaluate these radiographic features in detail, it is convenient to divide them into those that can be seen optimally when the ulcer is viewed in profile and those that can be best identified when the ulcer is seen *en face*.[15] Because a benign ulcer is an erosion into and beyond the wall of the stomach, a benign ulcer crater projects beyond the normal gastric contour (penetration) (Fig. 9–3). This is in distinction to a malignant ulcer, in which the ulcer occurs in a tumor. In this case, the ulcer does not extend beyond the gastric wall because the tumor lies within the stomach. Another feature of a benign ulcer seen on profile projections of the crater is a small nodule in the base of the crater (Fig. 9–4). Nelson believes this is virtually diagnostic of a benign ulcer and is due to a blood clot in the base of the crater.[8] The clot is nearly always in the center of the crater, but it may be eccentric. The base of a malignant ulcer may be nodular, but the nodules are multiple and involve the orifice of the crater. A blood clot in the base of a malignant ulcer is rare, probably because gross bleeding is unusual. Carcinomas tend to ooze blood owing to multiple small bleeding points in the necrotic area (the ulcer), whereas erosion of a relatively large artery occurs in the base of a benign ulcer.

Once the gastric mucosa is destroyed in the formation of an ulcer, the submucosa is exposed to acid and pepsin. Because the submucosa is more susceptible to peptic digestion than the mucosa, the ulcer enlarges more rapidly in the submucosa and the mucosa becomes undermined. Consequently, the detection of undermining is evidence that acid is present and the ulcer is benign.[8] If there is no edema of the mucosa at the orifice of the ulcer, extension of the ulceration into the submucosa creates a lip of mucosa, which when viewed in profile radiographically produces a radiolucent 1-mm line across the orifice of the crater (Hampton's line) (Fig. 9–5A).[15] This is a rare finding, but it is pathognomonic of a benign ulcer. More frequently there is edema in the mucosa at the orifice, so that a radiolucent band (ulcer collar) rather than a Hampton line is created at the orifice of the ulcer (Fig. 9–5B and C). Marked edema of the mucosa at the

422 — PEPTIC ULCER

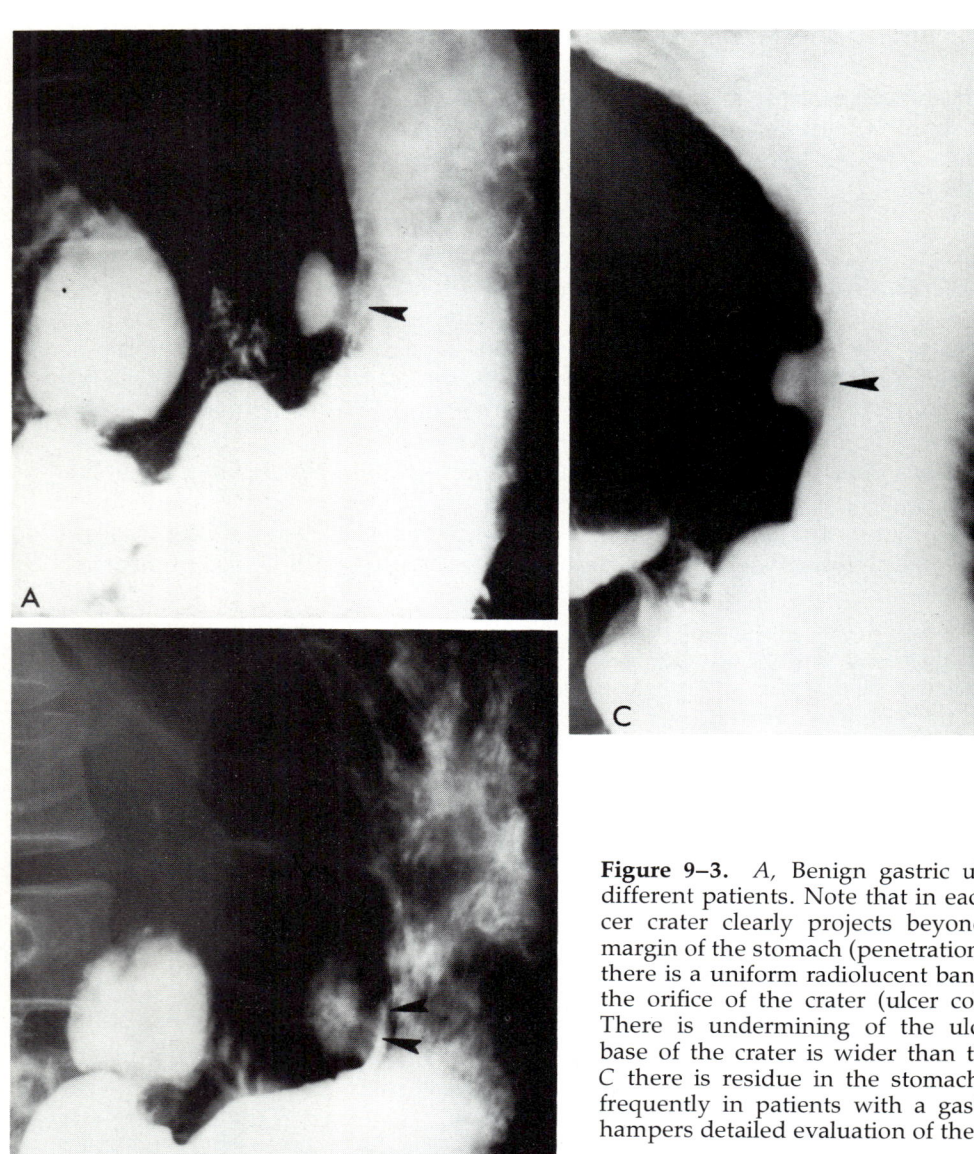

Figure 9–3. *A,* Benign gastric ulcers in three different patients. Note that in each case the ulcer crater clearly projects beyond the normal margin of the stomach (penetration), and in each there is a uniform radiolucent band of edema at the orifice of the crater (ulcer collar) (arrows). There is undermining of the ulcer in *A* (the base of the crater is wider than the orifice). In *C* there is residue in the stomach. This occurs frequently in patients with a gastric ulcer and hampers detailed evaluation of the crater.

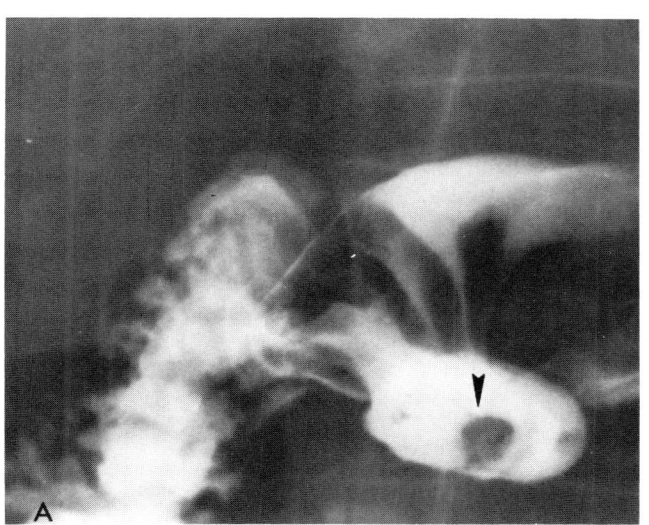
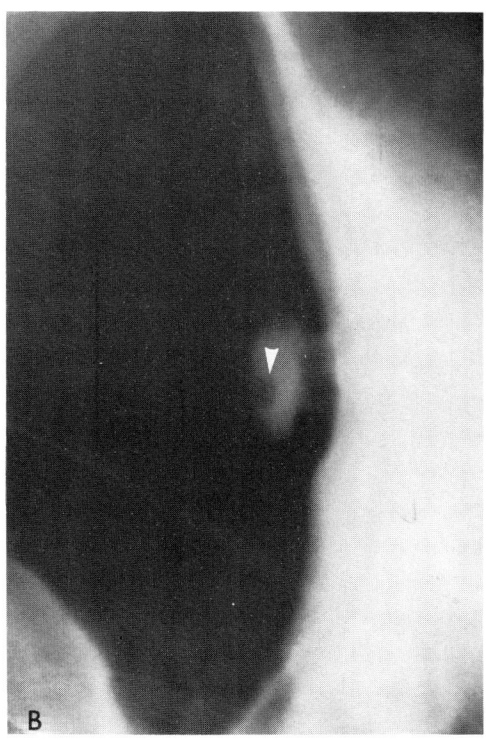

Figure 9–4. There is a small nodule in the base of both ulcer craters (arrow), which is a reliable sign of benignancy. *A,* The ulcer is along the greater curvature of the stomach. The crater projects beyond the normal lumen of the stomach, and there are distinct radiating folds to the orifice of the crater. *B,* In this lesser curvature ulcer penetration of the crater beyond the normal lumen of the stomach, undermining, and an ulcer collar are signs of benignancy.

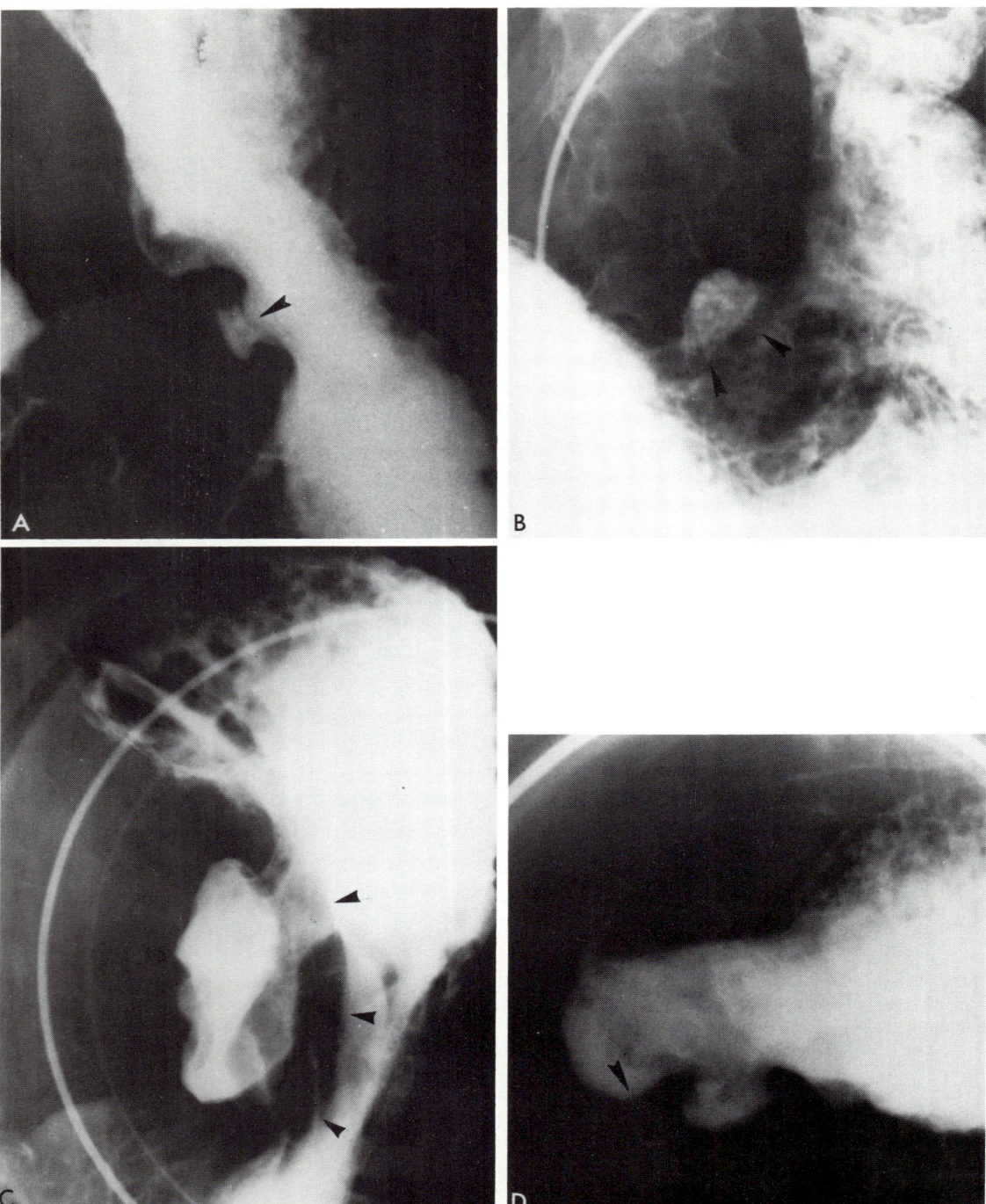

Figure 9–5. Profile characteristics of typical benign ulcers in four different patients. *A*, Benign ulcer along the lesser curvature of the stomach shows a 1-mm radiolucent line at the orifice of the crater (Hampton's line) (arrow). In *B* and *C* a uniform radiolucent band of edema is visible at the orifice of the crater (ulcer collar) (arrows). *D*, There is an ulcer in the greater curvature of the antrum showing an ulcer mound. Note that the tissue at the base of the crater is smooth. The ulcer is central, and there is an obtuse junction between the mound and the normal gastric wall (arrow).

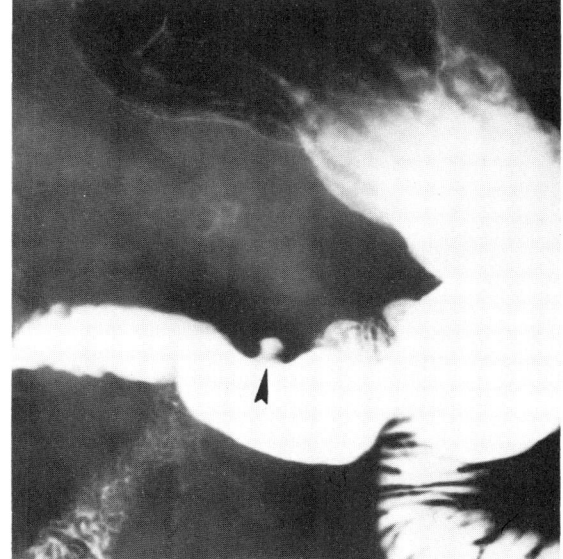

Figure 9–6. Benign ulcer crater along the lesser curvature of the stomach with a "collar-button" shape (arrow). The base of the ulcer is wider than the neck because peptic ulceration proceeds more rapidly in the submucosa than in the mucosa.

mouth of the crater, which is sometimes associated with spasm of the muscularis propria, creates a radiolucent mound of tissue that projects into the lumen on the radiograph (Fig. 9–5D). The benign nature of the ulcer mound is indicated by its smooth margin and gradual transition into the adjacent normal mucosa.

Undermining of the mucosa also tends to create an ulcer with a "collar-button" shape, in which the base of the crater is wider than the orifice (Fig. 9–6). If the mucosa at the mouth of an ulcer crater is enormously thickened by edema and inflammation, it may form a large mass of tissue that can prolapse into the ulcer, nearly occluding its lumen. In these cases, barium flows beneath the overhanging mass and assumes a crescent shape in the base of the ulcer (Fig. 9–7). This finding, termed the crescent sign by Nelson, is strong evidence that the ulcer is benign because it indicates that there is extensive undermining of the mucosa.[8]

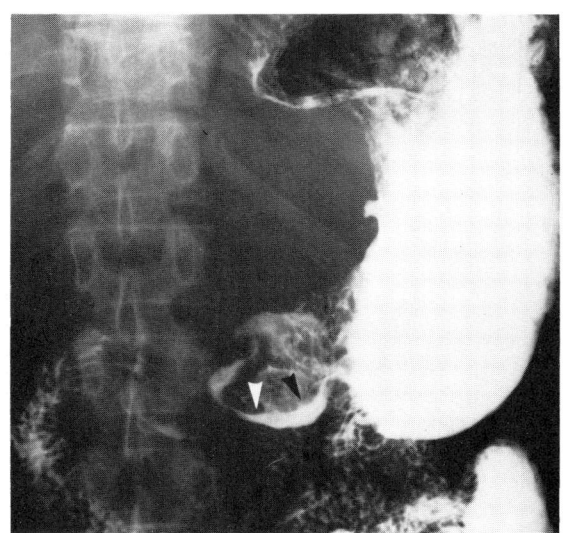

Figure 9–7. Benign ulcer in the antrum of the stomach demonstrating the crescent sign (arrows). The markedly edematous lips of the ulcer crater have prolapsed into the crater, so that only the base is filled with barium. Note also a second benign ulcer high on the lesser curvature.

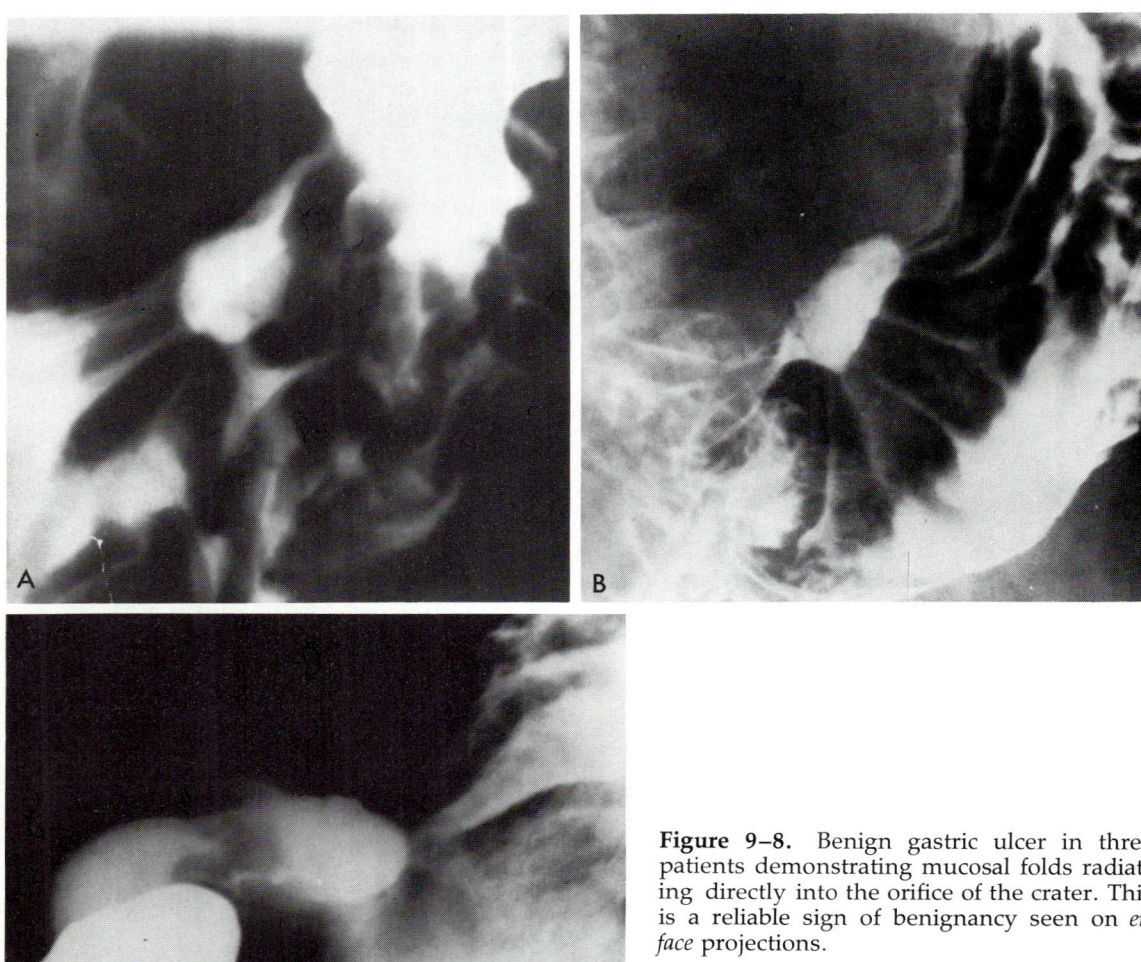

Figure 9–8. Benign gastric ulcer in three patients demonstrating mucosal folds radiating directly into the orifice of the crater. This is a reliable sign of benignancy seen on *en face* projections.

When the ulcer crater is viewed *en face*, the most reliable sign that the ulcer is benign is the presence of mucosal folds radiating directly into the orifice of the crater (Fig. 9–8).[15] This finding is of great diagnostic importance, because it indicates that the mucosa has not been destroyed or replaced by malignant tissue and that no tumor mass is present. Since most benign ulcers are at least as deep as they are broad, they have steep parallel walls, which produce a sharp margin when the crater is viewed *en face* (Fig. 9–9). When there is edema at the orifice of the crater, it produces a radiolucent mound that blends gradually into the adjacent normal mucosa (see Fig. 9 9). The ulcer is centrally located in the mound. Nodularity is absent in both the ulcer and the edematous tissue.

Figure 9–9. *En face* projection of a benign ulcer crater on the lesser curvature. The radiograph is made with the patient in the right posterior oblique projection. Notice that the crater is central in the edematous mass, and its margins are sharp. The edema blends gradually with the normal gastric wall.

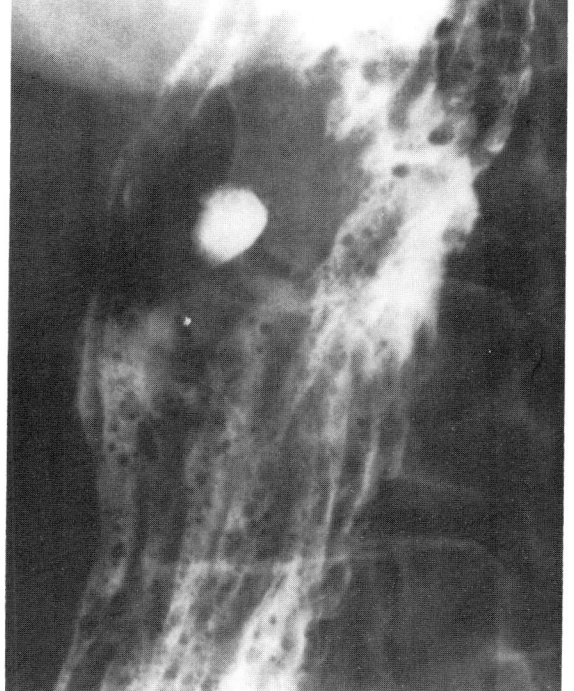

It is of interest to note that when upright projections demonstrate an air-fluid level in an ulcer, the crater is probably benign.[4] This sign indicates that most benign ulcers are deeper than they are wide. As a result, benign ulcers tend to trap air and fluid within the crater.

RADIOLOGIC FEATURES OF MALIGNANT GASTRIC ULCERS

The major radiographic features of a malignant ulcer are the presence of nodularity of the tissue surrounding the ulcer crater and in the orifice and floor of the crater, an abrupt transition of the mass at the orifice of the crater with the adjacent mucosa, and Carman's meniscus sign.[4, 13, 15] The crater fails to project beyond the normal gastric lumen; there are no radiating mucosal folds that reach the orifice of the ulcer; the crater is asymmetric in the tissue at its orifice; and the crater is usually wider than it is deep.

Figure 9–10 illustrates the abrupt transition of an ulcerating carcinoma into the normal adjacent gastric wall. This is typical of carcinomas throughout the gastrointestinal tract in which there is a well-demarcated edge of the tumor, rather than a gradual transition of an inflammatory process with normal adjacent mucosa. A carcinoma has a characteristic rolled edge. In many cases of malignant ulcers, nodularity of the crater and the adjacent tissue can be detected (Fig. 9–11). This finding is due to the presence of tumor excrescences, irregularities that are distinctly unusual in benign ulcers. In carcinomas, the nodularity can be seen in profile projections as well as *en face* views. In the latter, the crater is eccentric within a mass and radiating folds to the orifice of the crater are absent.

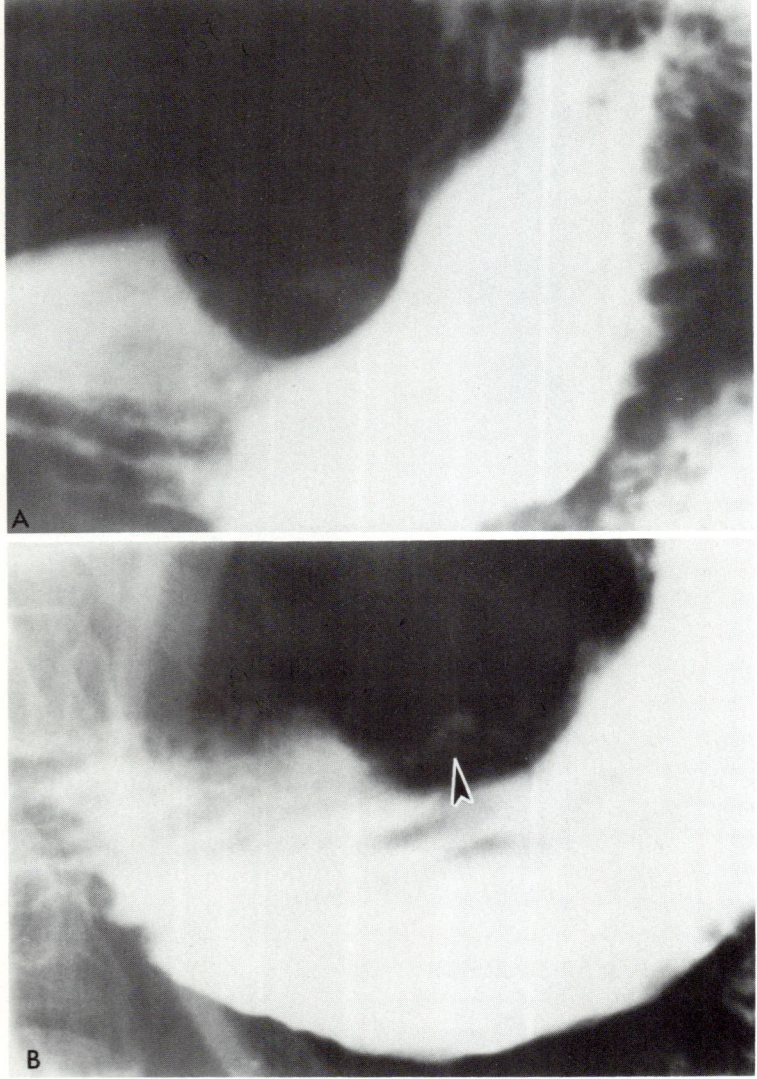

Figure 9–10. Malignant ulcer along the lesser curvature of the stomach at the incisura angularis. The irregular crater is visible in B (arrow). Note that the junction between the tumor and adjacent gastric wall is abrupt.

Carman's meniscus sign results from apposition of the two halves of the serpiginous rolled margin of the elevated tumor that forms the periphery of a gastric carcinoma. This occurs when the tumor straddles the lesser curvature (Figs. 9–12 and 9–13).[8] Barium caught within the tumor assumes a half-moon configuration (meniscus). The straight margin along the lesser curvature is the result of desmoplastic reaction in the center of the tumor. Nodularity in the periphery of the ulcerating carcinoma is characteristic.

It should be emphasized that while complete healing nearly always indicates that the ulcer was benign, on rare occasions a malignant ulcer completely resolves.[6, 8, 10] For this reason, follow-up examination after healing is indicated in all patients. Furthermore, a residual scar of a healed crater may be difficult to distinguish from incomplete healing (Fig. 9–14). A scar is usually pliable and fails to retain barium consistently. In cases in which differentiation is uncertain, follow-up examination shows that a scar persists without change.

PEPTIC ULCER — 429

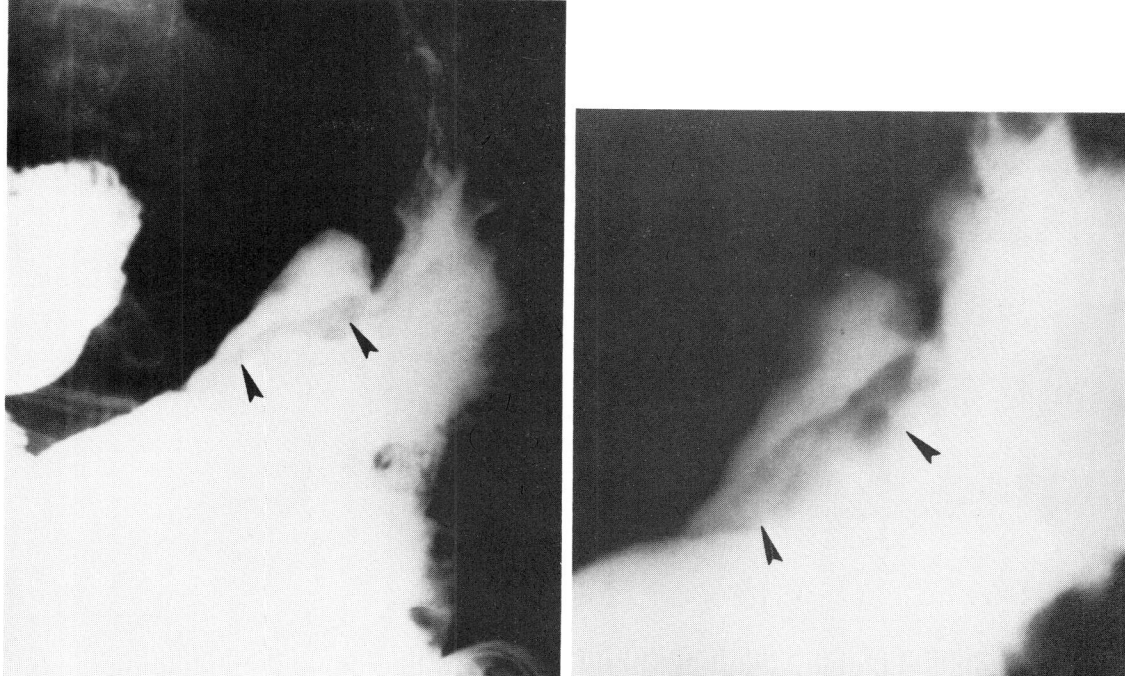

Figure 9–11. Malignant gastric ulcer along the lesser curvature of the stomach (arrows). Although the crater appears to project beyond the normal lumen of the stomach, the crater itself is asymmetric. There is prominent nodularity both within the crater and at its orifice. This is strong evidence that the crater is malignant.

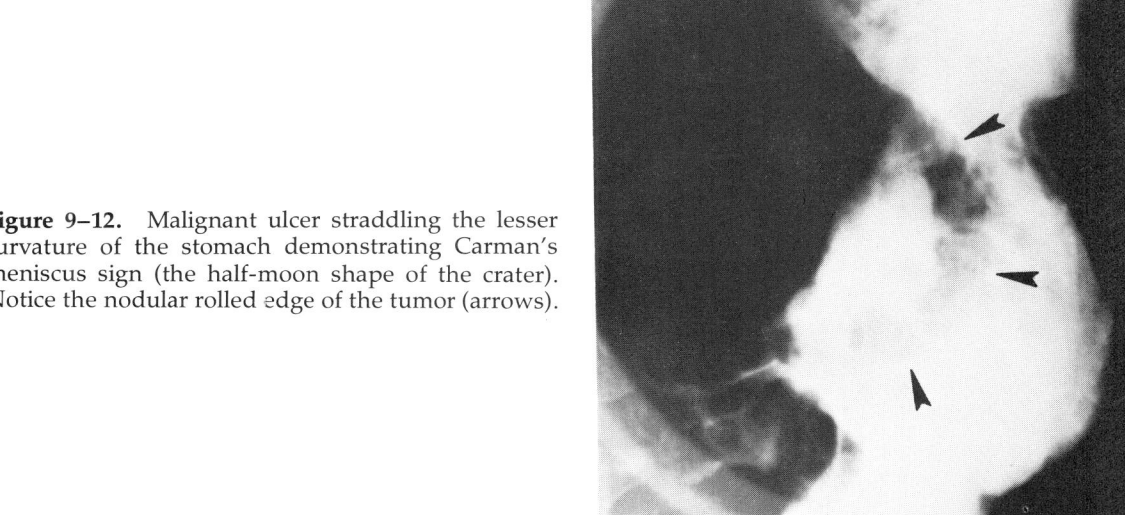

Figure 9–12. Malignant ulcer straddling the lesser curvature of the stomach demonstrating Carman's meniscus sign (the half-moon shape of the crater). Notice the nodular rolled edge of the tumor (arrows).

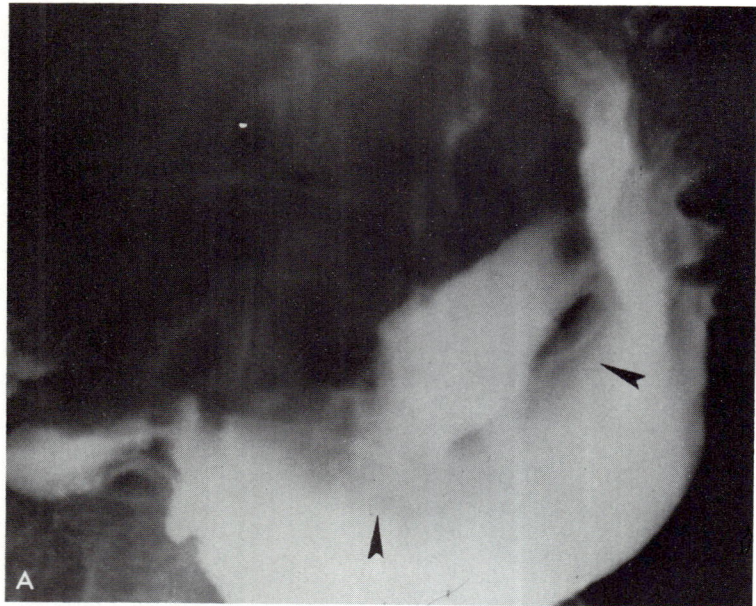
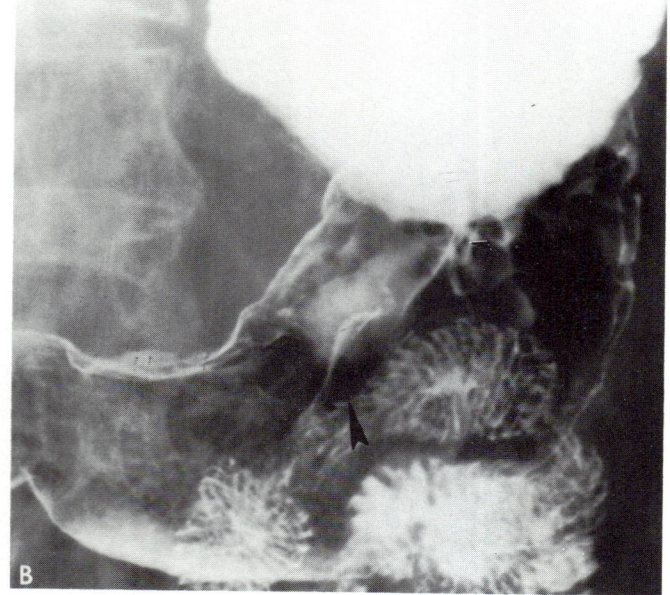

Figure 9–13. Large ulcerating carcinoma straddling the lesser curvature of the stomach demonstrating Carman's sign. The crater is filled with barium in *A*. The nodular rim of the carcinoma is apparent (arrowheads).

RADIOLOGIC FEATURES OF PREPYLORIC ULCERS

In a classic article in 1961, Wolf and Bryk described three types of ulcers that occur in the distal portion of the gastric antrum (the prepyloric region of the stomach).[14] The most common is a simple benign ulcer with a crater located on or near the lesser curvature (Fig. 9–15). The crater is less than 1 cm in diameter, there is often an ulcer collar or mound, and the mucosal pattern about the crater is intact. Motor activity of the antrum is normal, with no persistent spasm or deformity. The second type of prepyloric ulcer is also benign, but it is associated with antral deformity (Fig. 9–16). In these cases,

PEPTIC ULCER — 431

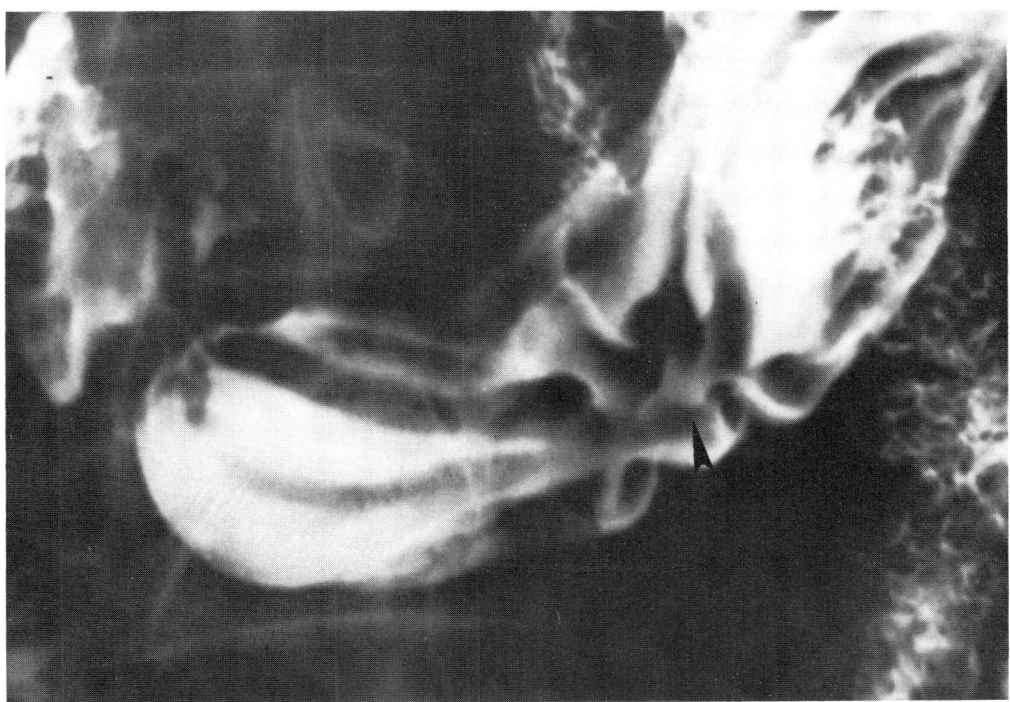

Figure 9–14. Scar from a healed benign gastric ulcer crater (arrow). The rugal folds radiate toward the original site of the ulcer.

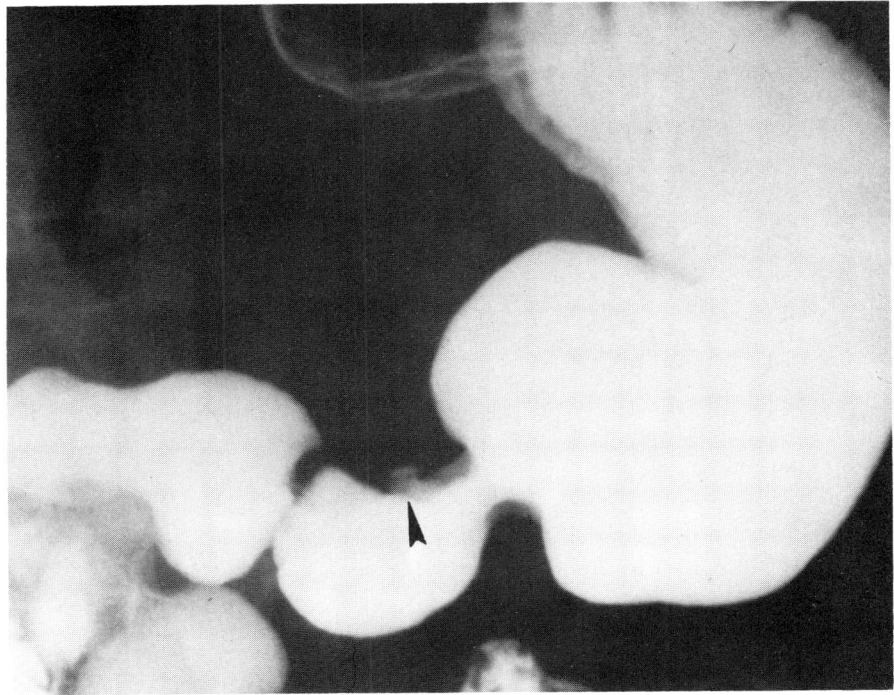

Figure 9–15. Benign ulcer of the gastric antrum (arrow). The ulcer projects beyond the lumen of the stomach and is not associated with narrowing of the antrum.

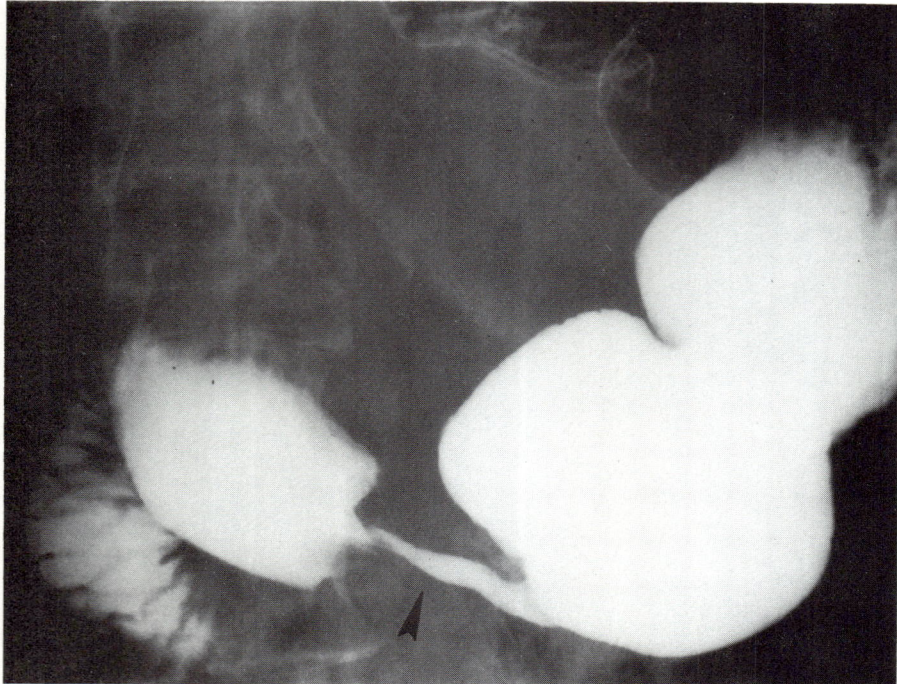

Figure 9–16. Benign gastric ulcer that completely encircles the gastric antrum (arrow). When the antrum is contracted, differentiation between benign and malignant ulcerating lesions is impossible.

the ulcer has penetrated through the muscularis propria and produced an intense desmoplastic response, which creates a persistent and often bizarre antral deformity. This type of penetrating calloused ulcer cannot be distinguished radiographically from the third type of prepyloric ulcer, an ulcerating carcinoma. In both situations there is a persistent antral narrowing.

RADIOLOGIC FEATURES OF DUODENAL ULCERS

No disease of the gastrointestinal tract is more often erroneously diagnosed radiographically than duodenal ulcer. This is regrettable because, in many cases, the correct diagnosis is subsequently overlooked, the patient suffers needless concern, or the patient's health record for insurance purposes is inappropriately tarnished. In order to make an accurate diagnosis of a duodenal ulcer, the quality of the radiographic examination must be such that an ulcer crater is demonstrated and confirmed by its persistence on a number of radiographs. This requires supine air-contrast and prone compression radiographs. Not every fleck of barium in the duodenal cap should be considered an ulcer. Indeed, most are collections of barium between mucosal folds. If the barium collection persists on multiple radiographs, however, the finding is not spurious and an accurate diagnosis of ulcer can be established (Fig. 9–17). Thickened mucosal folds radiating toward the crater are valuable confirmatory findings (Fig. 9–18). An active ulcer crater is particularly difficult to demonstrate in the presence of a deformed duodenal bulb (Fig. 9–19). Only a minority of patients with duodenal ulcer have deformity of the duodenal cap, spasm, or tenderness. Care should be taken not to confuse the pylorus viewed *en face* and superimposed on the duodenum with an ulcer crater (Fig. 9–20).

A large, penetrating duodenal ulcer may be associated with spasm and irritability that prevents filling of the crater with barium. In these cases, the administration of glucagon often relieves the spasm sufficiently to allow the crater to fill (Fig. 9–21). On occasion, the duodenal ulcer involves the entire duodenal bulb. In these cases, the ulcer is so large and so similar to the bulb in shape that it may be mistaken for the bulb itself (Figs. 9–22 and 9–23). This error can be avoided if the possibility is borne in mind, the irregular margins of the crater are recognized, and the presence of the crater without change in size or shape is detected on all of the radiographs. The normal duodenal bulb is pliable and changeable, whereas a giant ulcer crater is fixed and rigid.

Errors in diagnosis may also occur if a blood clot fills the ulcer so that the crater cannot fill with barium (Fig. 9–24). This is not infrequent in patients with a bleeding ulcer and can only be avoided by performing a second examination several days later when the clot has sloughed.

An important finding in some patients with a duodenal ulcer is the presence of a ring of barium that has the appearance of a small polyp or hypertrophied Brunner's glands (the ring sign) (Fig. 9–25). This may occur when barium empties out of an ulcer crater, depending on the patient's position. If the wall of the crater remains coated with barium, the barium creates a circular or ring density. When the shape of the ulcer is such that one wall is parallel to the x-ray beam and the other wall slopes, an incomplete ring may result (Fig. 9–26). The ring sign may also occur in association with gastric ulcers (Figs. 9–26 and 9–27).

Text continued on page 440.

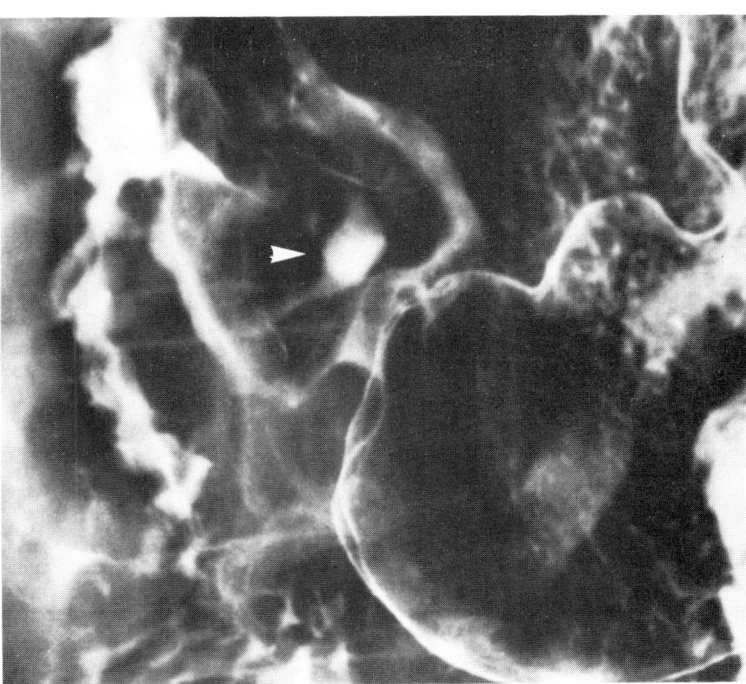

Figure 9–17. Supine air-contrast projection of the duodenal cap demonstrating a duodenal ulcer in the posterior wall (arrow).

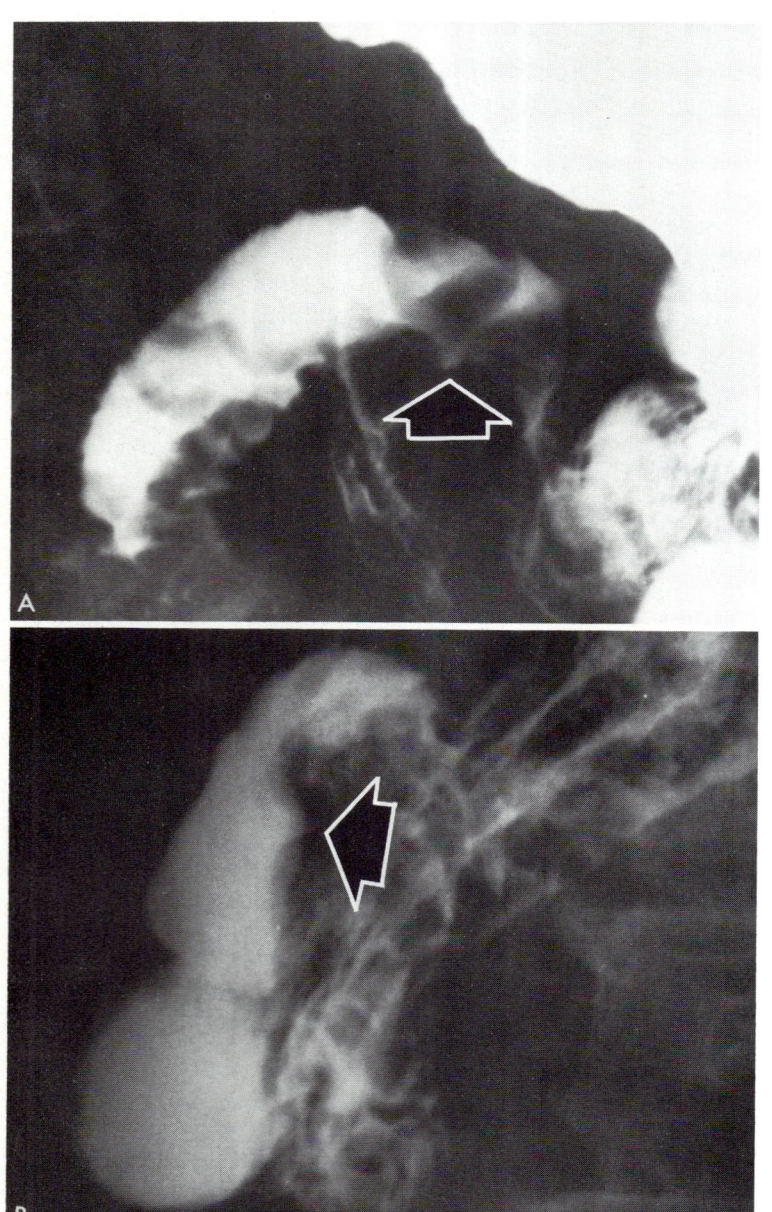

Figure 9–18. Small benign duodenal ulcer in the posterior wall with edematous radiating mucosal folds (arrow). The posterior position of the ulcer crater is visible when the patient is turned into the right posterior oblique projection.

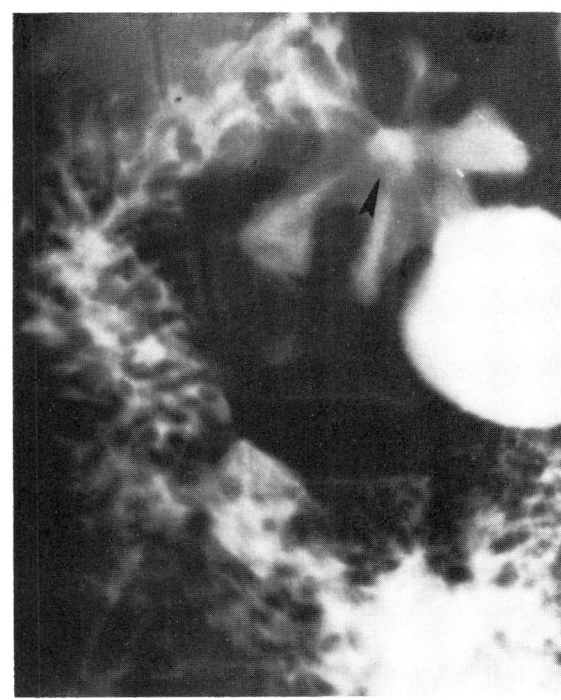

Figure 9–19. Duodenal ulcer in association with marked chronic deformity of a duodenal cap (arrow). Many active craters are missed in this circumstance, but the diagnosis of peptic ulcer disease is established.

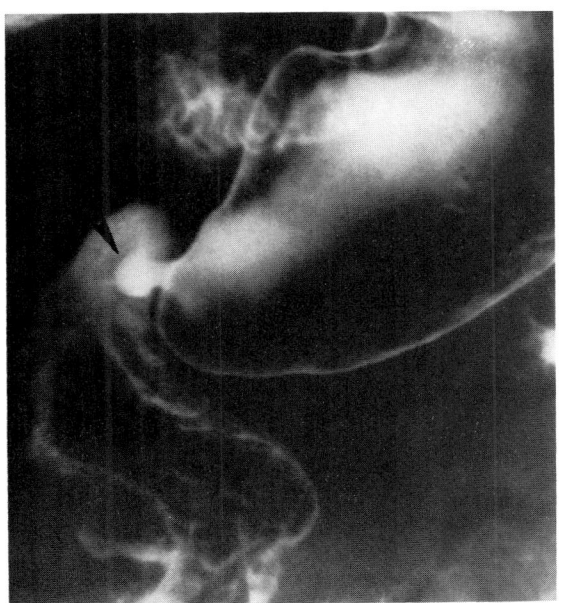

Figure 9–20. Superimposition of the pyloric canal in the duodenal cap may simulate a duodenal ulcer crater (arrow).

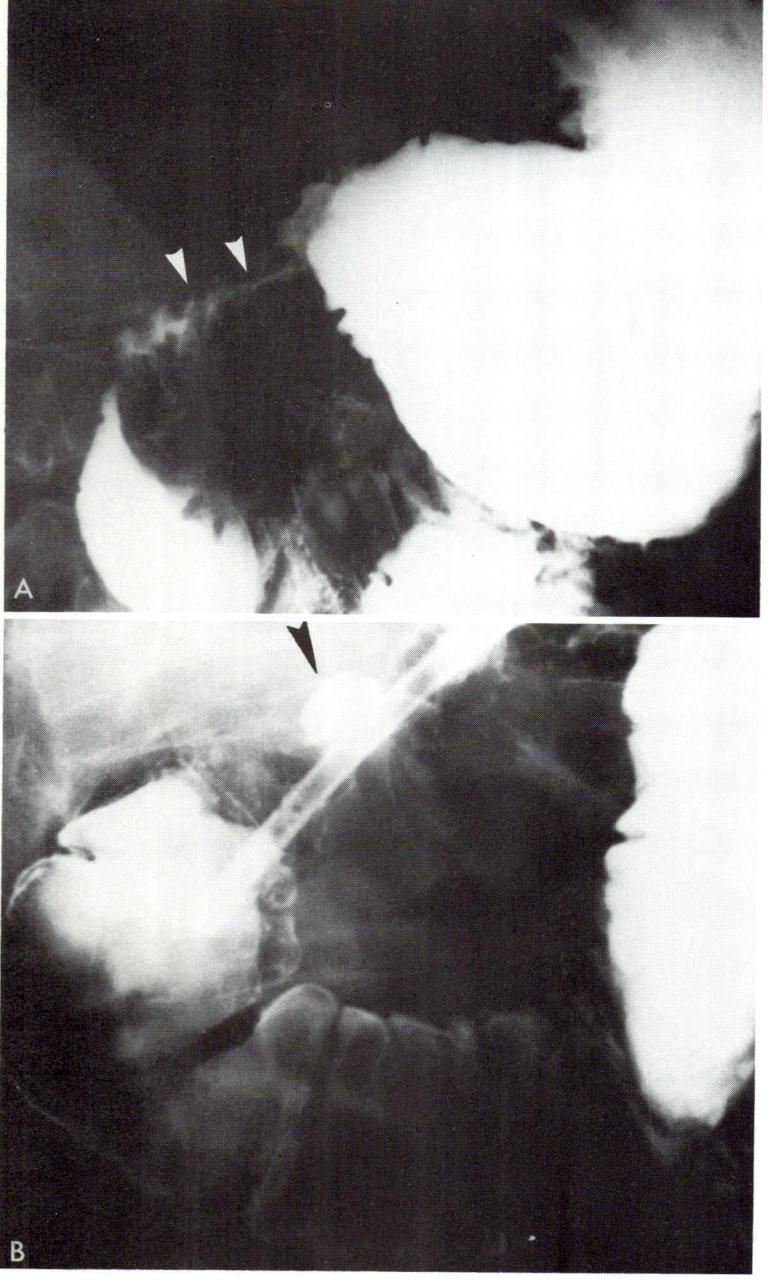

Figure 9–21. *A*, Marked spasm of the first portion of the duodenum is apparent with no evidence of an active ulcer crater (arrows). *B*, A large crater is visible following examination with glucagon and inflation of the duodenum with air via a nasogastric tube (arrow).

PEPTIC ULCER — 437

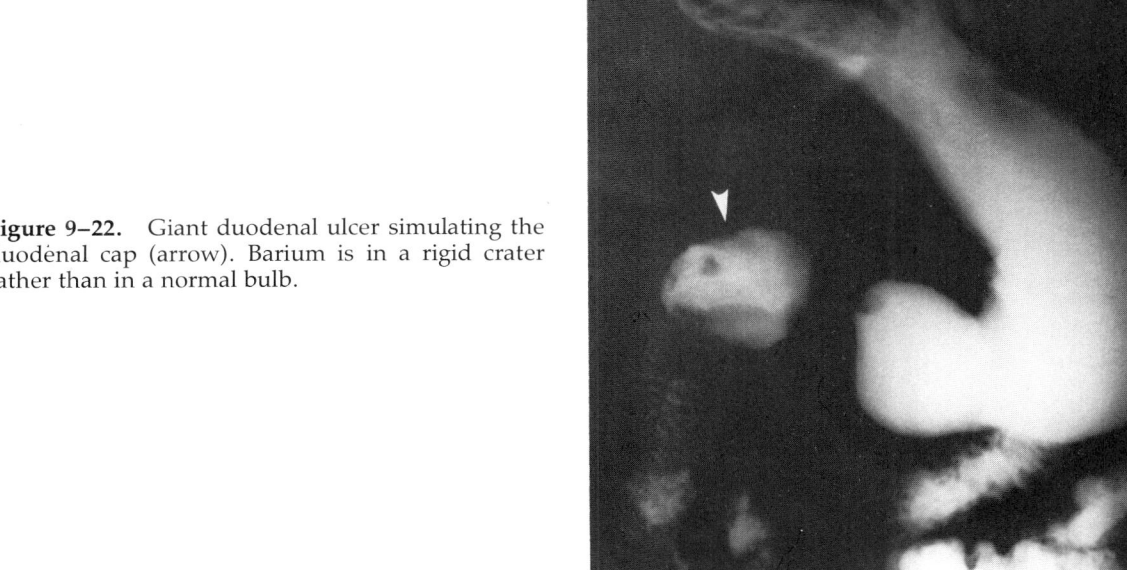

Figure 9–22. Giant duodenal ulcer simulating the duodenal cap (arrow). Barium is in a rigid crater rather than in a normal bulb.

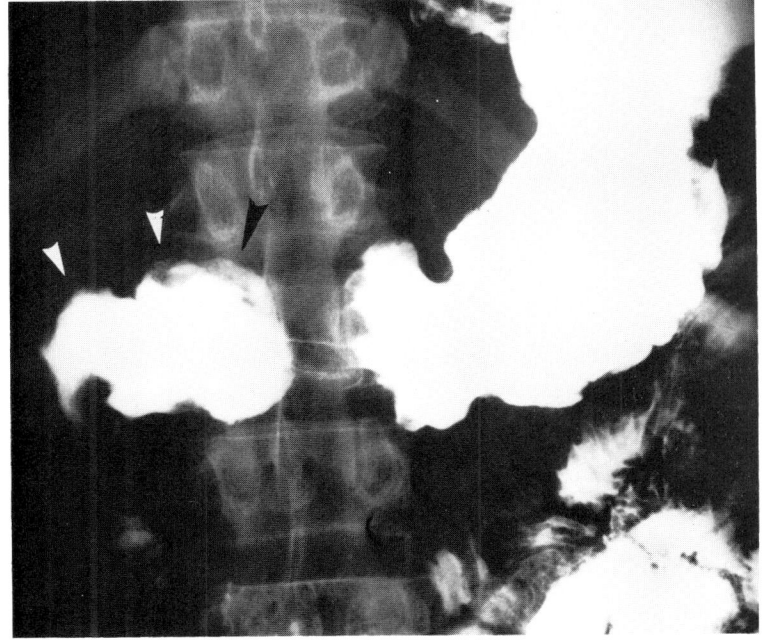

Figure 9–23. Giant duodenal ulcer simulating the duodenal cap (arrows). The marked marginal irregularity of the crater helps to differentiate the ulcer from the duodenal cap.

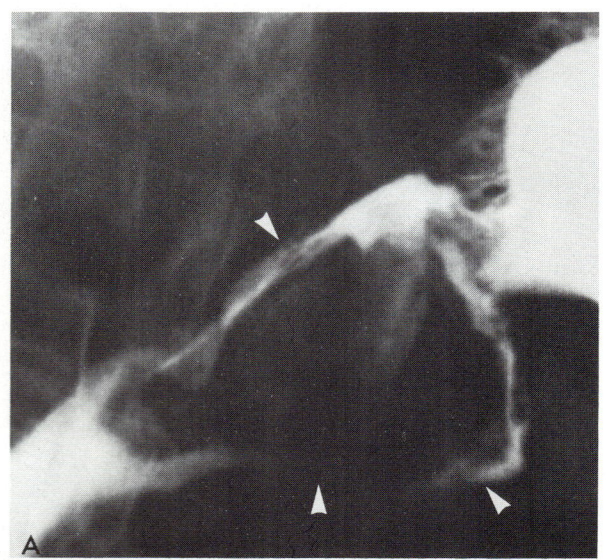
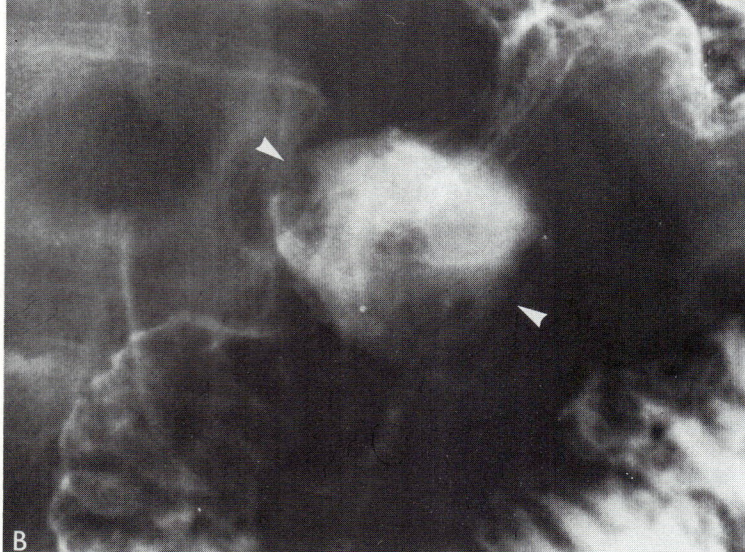

Figure 9–24. *A*, A mass is visible in the duodenal cap compatible with a benign tumor (arrows). *B*, Examination performed two days later shows a large duodenal ulcer (arrows). The initial study (*A*) failed to show the crater because it was filled with a blood clot that resembled a tumor. The clot had sloughed by the time the second examination was performed.

PEPTIC ULCER — 439

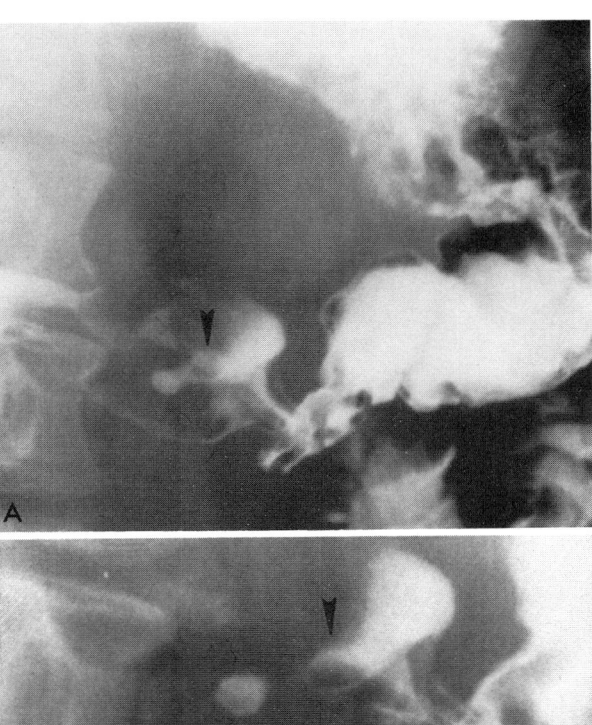

Figure 9–25. Supine left posterior oblique projections of the duodenal cap showing a duodenal ulcer filled with barium (*A* and *B*). A circular collection of barium is also visible (ring sign) (arrow). Supine right posterior projection (*C*) shows that this is an ulcer in the anterior wall of the duodenum in which only the walls of the crater are coated with barium. A second ulcer in the posterior wall is also visible (arrow).

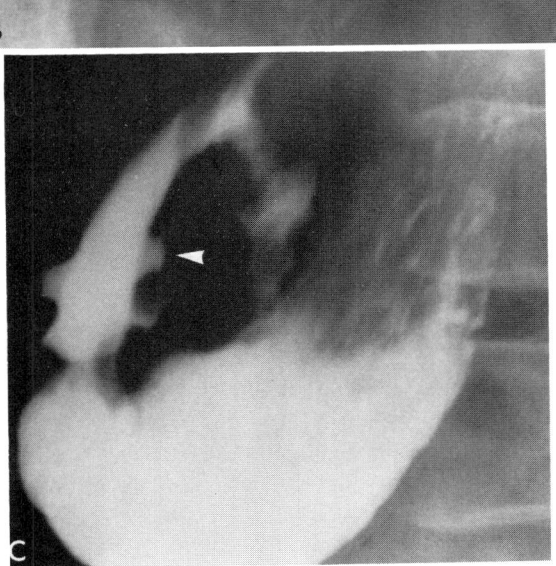

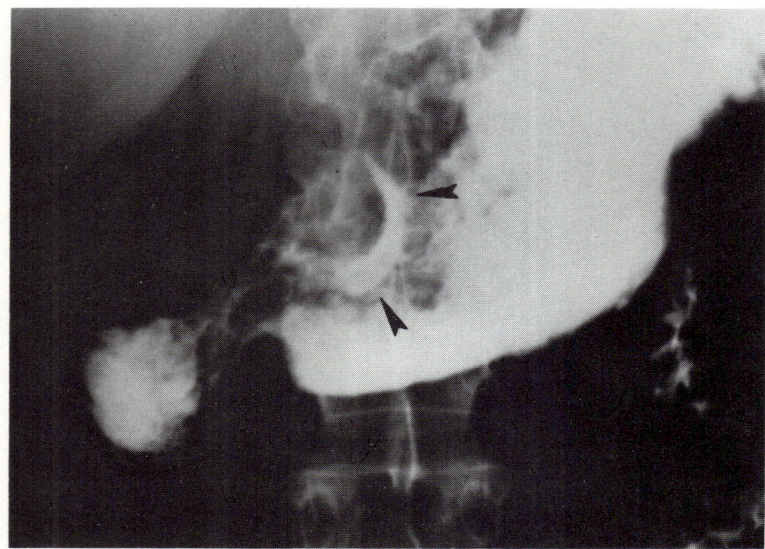

Figure 9–26. Incomplete ring sign (arrows) in a patient with a benign gastric ulcer of the lesser curvature penetrating into the lesser sac.

Postbulbar Duodenal Ulcers

Duodenal ulcers distal to the duodenal cap are unusual and frequently difficult to diagnose radiographically. Often the lesion is overlooked on initial gastrointestinal examinations, when insufficient attention is given to this portion of the duodenum. Detection of these ulcers is important because, like the bulbar variety, they may cause obstruction, pancreatitis, bleeding, and pain.

In some cases, the radiologic features are the same as those of bulbar ulcers in that an ulcer crater with edema of the adjacent mucosa can be demonstrated (Fig. 9–28). More often the finding is a ringlike narrowing in the duodenum with or without an ulcer crater (Fig. 9–29). In these cases particularly, the diagnosis is easily overlooked unless hypotonic duodenography is performed. The problem is similar to the one associated with the detection of a lower esophageal ring in that recognition of the abnormality requires full distention above and below the lesion. Even when this is achieved, the stricture may be hidden by superimposition of barium in the adjacent duodenal loops or in the distal portion of the stomach.

In a study of 12 cases reported by Bilboa et al., the strictures were eccentrically located in the second portion of the duodenum.[1] There was an abrupt transition to the normal duodenal caliber at both ends of the narrowed segment. The strictures varied from 2 to 15 mm in diameter and were 0.5 to 1 cm in length. Dilatation of the duodenum proximal to the stricture may be a helpful clue to the diagnosis (Fig. 9–29B).

Occasionally, large penetrating ulcers in the second portion of the duodenum cause jaundice and pancreatitis (Fig. 9–30). When pancreatitis is present, the duodenal loop is often widened and there may be effacement and spiculation of the duodenal mucosa (Fig. 9–31).

Figure 9–27. *A*, Supine left posterior oblique projection of the gastric antrum showing a circular radiolucency (the ring sign) owing to an incompletely filled benign ulcer in the anterior wall of the stomach (arrow). *B*, Prone projection in the same patient showing filling of the benign ulcer crater (arrow).

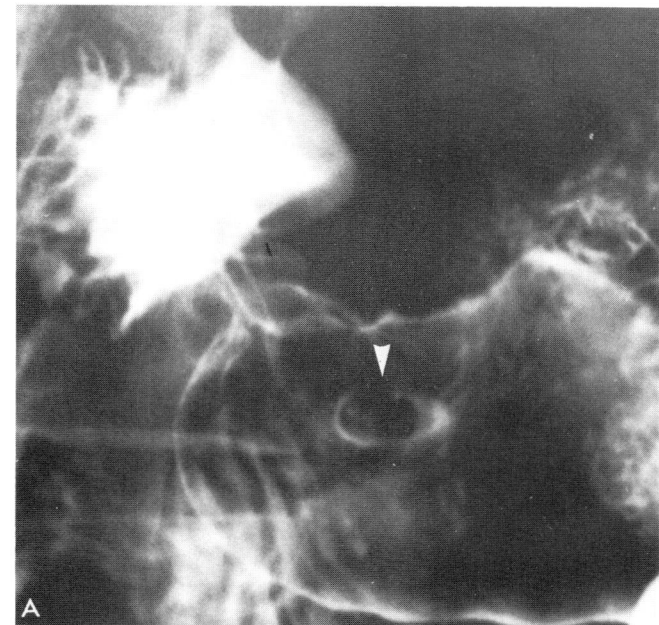
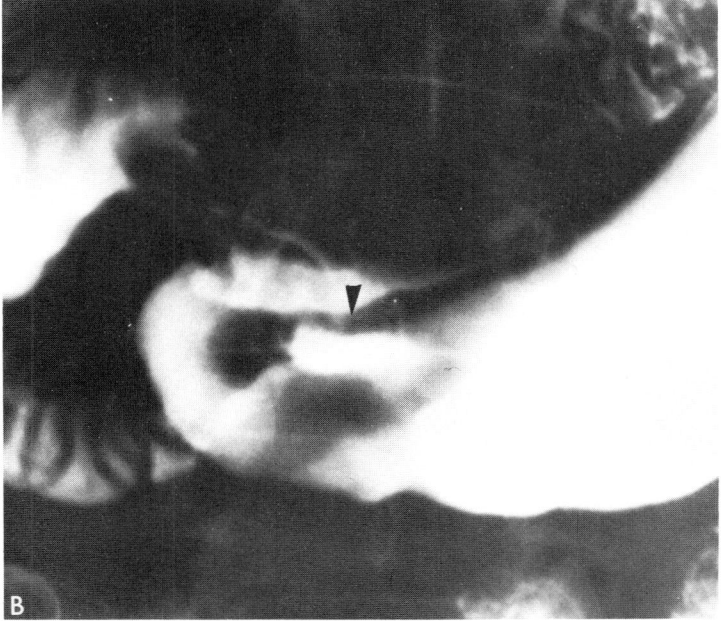

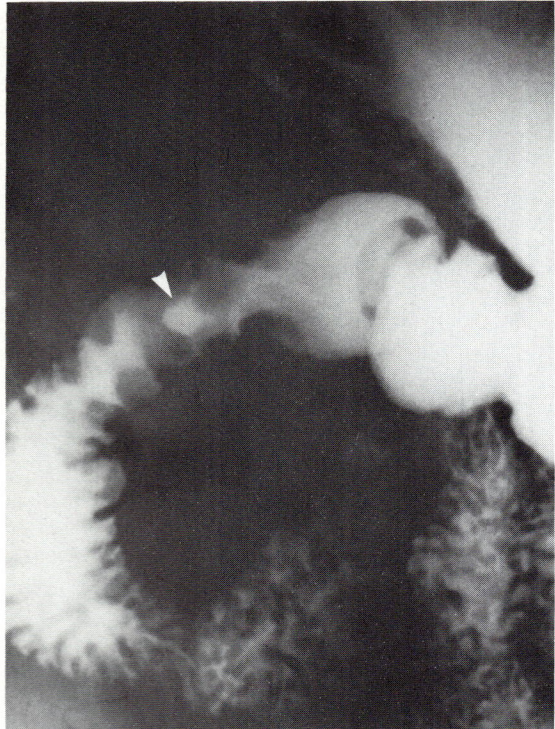

Figure 9-28. Benign duodenal ulcer in the second portion of the duodenum, with associated edema of the mucosal folds (arrow). The ulcer penetrated into the pancreas with subsequent pancreatitis, causing widening and effacement of the duodenal loop.

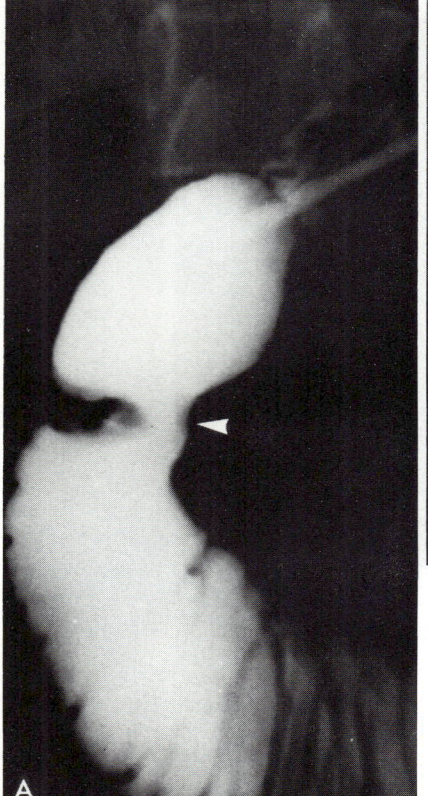
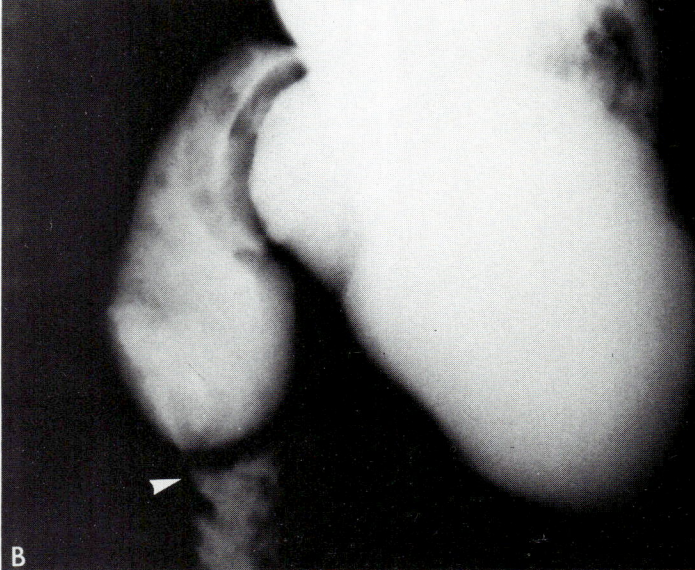

Figure 9-29. Diaphragm-like narrowing in the second portion of the duodenum (arrows) due to spasm associated with an active duodenal ulcer in two cases. There is obstructive dilatation of the duodenum proximal to the narrowing in *B*.

PEPTIC ULCER — 443

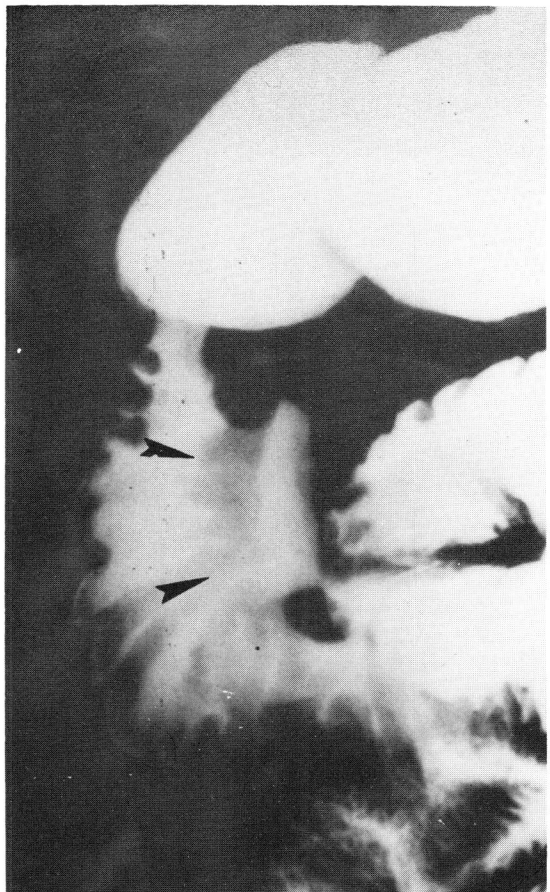

Figure 9–30. Large benign peptic ulcer in the second portion of the duodenum, with penetration, undermining and radiating mucosal folds, in a patient with abdominal pain and jaundice (arrows).

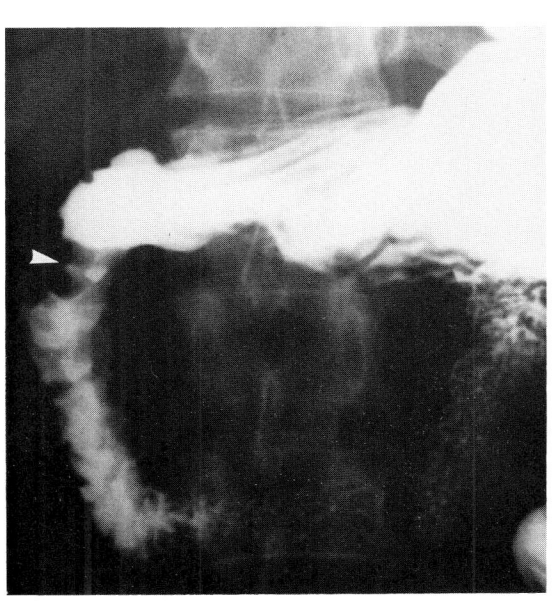

Figure 9–31. Active postbulbar duodenal ulcer with edema of the adjacent mucosal folds (arrow). There is widening of the duodenal loop owing to pancreatitis caused by penetration of the ulcer into the pancreas.

COMPLICATIONS OF THE PEPTIC ULCER THAT MAY REQUIRE SURGERY

Free perforation into the peritoneal space may occur in gastric or duodenal ulcers. In these cases the radiographic demonstration of free intraperitoneal air is conclusive evidence of the complication in the proper clinical setting (see Chapter 5).

As little as 1 ml of intraperitoneal air can be detected in patients with a perforated duodenal ulcer.[7] When large quantities of air are present, the falciform ligament or lateral umbilical ligaments may be identified (Fig. 9–32). Severe abdominal pain in most patients with a perforated duodenal ulcer almost always forces them to seek medical attention immediately. Consequently, the plain abdominal radiograph is usually made promptly after the perforation and before extensive peritonitis and paralytic ileus occur. As a result, free intraperitoneal air in the presence of extensive paralytic ileus is unusual in patients with a perforated duodenal ulcer.[5] In these cases, perforation of some other portion of the intestine, such as the colon, should be considered.

The perforation may be into the lesser sac or the pancreas, producing radiographic evidence of pancreatic enlargement (Fig. 9–33). It may be contained by tissues adjacent to the duodenal cap and result in the formation of an abscess (Fig. 9–34).

Massive upper gastrointestinal hemorrhage in a patient with documented peptic ulcer disease usually requires surgical intervention. When the site and origin of the massive, continuing bleeding are uncertain, angiographic localization is useful (see Chapter 14).

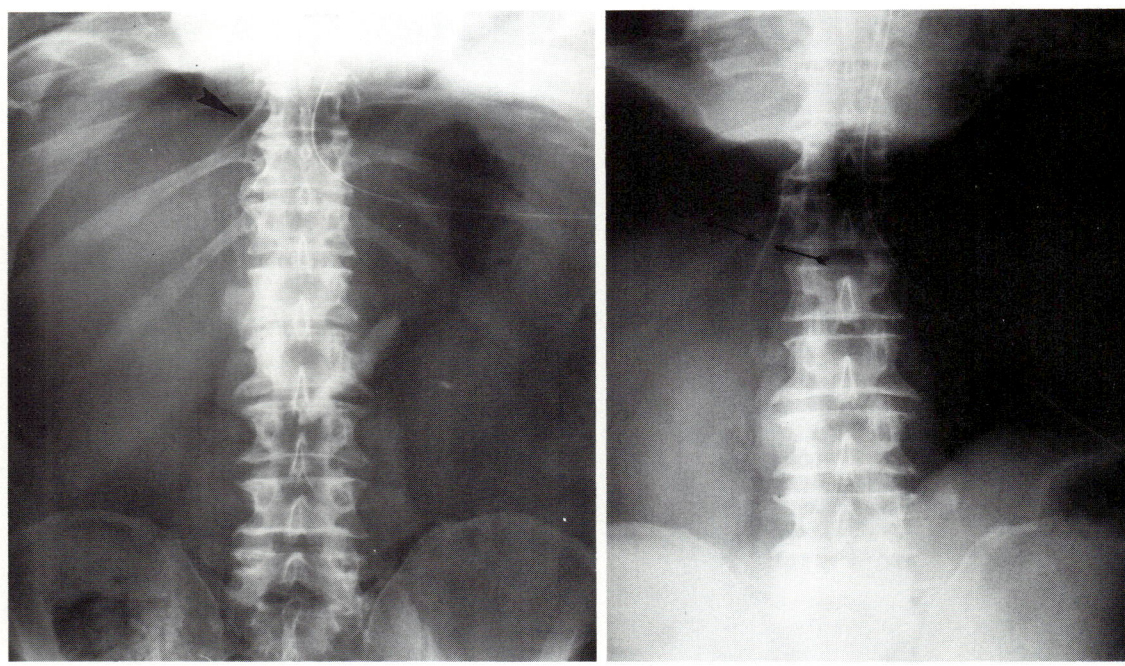

Figure 9–32. Supine (*A*) and upright (*B*) plain abdominal radiographs of a patient with a perforated gastric ulcer. There is a large amount of free intraperitoneal air. The falciform ligament is visible in both projections (arrows).

PEPTIC ULCER — 445

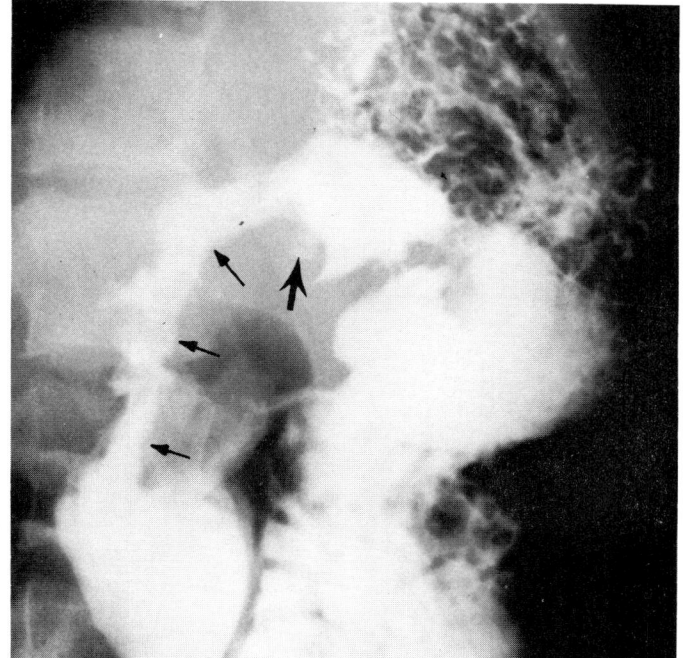

Figure 9–33. Perforation of a posterior-wall duodenal ulcer into the pancreas (large arrow), with compression and effacement of the duodenal loop due to pancreatitis (small arrows).

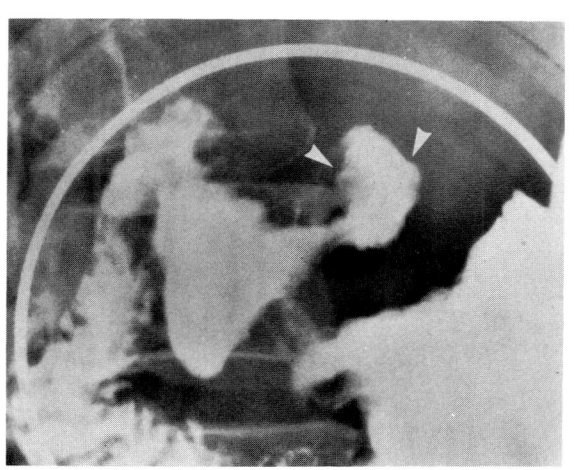

Figure 9–34. Localized perforation of a duodenal ulcer (arrows). Barium in the sealed-off perforation has the appearance of a deformed duodenal cap, but the collection was fixed and rigid on all projections.

446 — PEPTIC ULCER

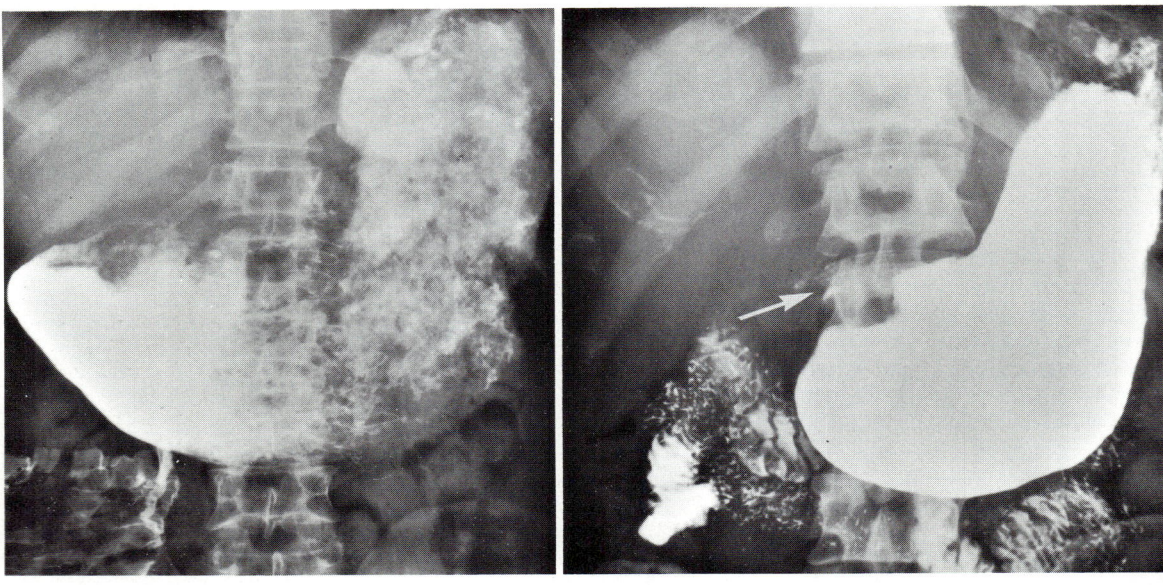

A **B**

Figure 9–35. Gastric outlet obstruction due to a duodenal ulcer. Initially, the stomach is dilated and contains a large amount of residue (*A*). After several days of nasogastric suction (*B*), a second examination shows marked deformity of the duodenal cap and a duodenal ulcer (arrow). The stomach is smaller, and residue is no longer present.

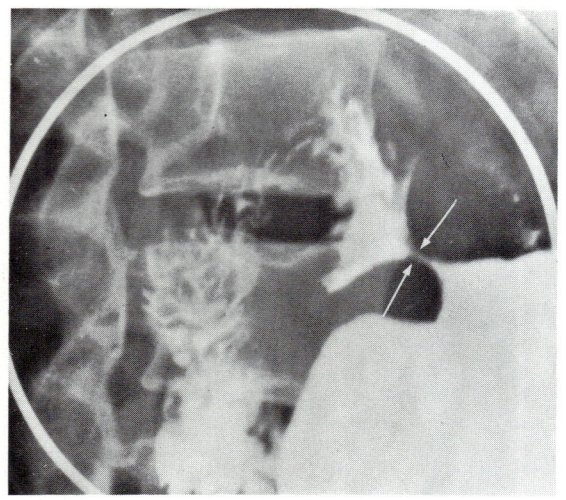

Figure 9–36. Gastric obstruction secondary to fibrosis caused by a recurrent pyloric ulcer. The pyloric canal is narrowed and elongated (arrows). No active ulcer crater is evident, and none was found at surgery.

References

1. Bilboa, M. K., Frische, L. H., Rösch, J., et al.: Postbulbar duodenal ulcer and ring stricture. Radiology *100*:27–37, 1971.
2. Gelfand, D. W., and Hachiya, J.: The double-contrast examination of the stomach using gas-producing granules and tablets. Radiology *93*:1381–1382, 1969.
3. Gelfand, D. W.: The Japanese-style double contrast examination of the stomach. Gastrointest. Radiol. *1*:7–19, 1976.
4. Harned, R. K., and Wolf, G. I.: Is an air-fluid level within a gastric ulcer a reliable roentgen sign of benignancy? Am. J. Gastroenterol. *67*:616–623, 1977.
5. Keefe, E. J., and Gagliardi, R. A.: Significance of ileus in perforated viscus. Am. J. Roentgenol. *117*:275–280, 1973.
6. Kirsh, I. E.: Radiological aspects of cancer after apparent healing. Veterans' Administration cooperative study on gastric ulcer. Gastroenterology *61*:606–622, 1971.
7. Miller, R. E., and Nelson, S. W.: The roentgenologic demonstration of tiny amounts of free intraperitoneal gas. Am. J. Roentgenol. *112*:574–578, 1971.
8. Nelson, S. W.: The discovery of gastric ulcers and the differential diagnosis between benignancy and malignancy. Radiol. Clin. North Am. *7*:5–15, 1969.
9. Obata, W. G.: A double-contrast technique for examination of the stomach using barium sulfate and simethicone. Am. J. Roentgenol. *115*:275–280, 1972.
10. Sakita, T., Aguro, Y., Takasu, S., et al.: Observations on the healing of ulcerations in early gastric cancer—the life cycle of the malignant ulcer. Gastroenterology *60*:835–844, 1971.
11. Sun, D. C. H., and Stempien, S. J.: Site and size of the ulcer as determinants of outcome. Veterans' Administration cooperative study on gastric ulcer. Gastroenterology. *61*:576–585, 1971.
12. Taxin, R. N., Livingston, P. A., and Seaman, W. B.: Multiple gastric ulcers: a radiographic sign of benignity? Radiology. *114*:23–27, 1975.
13. Wolf, B. S.: Observations on roentgen features of benign and malignant ulcers. Semin. Roentgenol. *6*:140–150, 1971.
14. Wolf, B. S., and Byrk, D.: Unequivocal benign gastric ulcers. Am. J. Roentgenol. *86*:1–15, 1961.
15. Wolf, B. S., and Marshak, R. H.: Profile features of benign gastric niches on roentgen examination. J. Mt. Sinai Hosp. N.Y. *24*:604–626, 1967.

10

THE STOMACH

ROBERT N. BERK, M.D.

Part I
Tumors

ADENOMATOUS POLYPS

There is an increased incidence of gastric polyps in patients with pernicious anemia, achlorhydria, atrophic gastritis, and carcinoma of the stomach. The relationship between polyps and carcinoma remains obscure, although most authorities now believe that like polyps of the colon, adenomatous polyps are the precursors of gastric carcinoma.[9] Of 138 patients with gastric polyps reported by Marshak and Feldman, 43 per cent had multiple polyps.[6] The polyps of one quarter of these were diffuse, the stomach being almost totally involved. The size of the lesions ranged from a few millimeters to 6 centimeters.

The large majority of polyps are small, smooth, unilobular, and sessile. A cluster of polyps is not infrequent (Fig. 10–1). The wall surrounding the polyp remains pliable and flexible, and no contour defect is present. The presence of a stalk and small size suggest that the polyp is benign. Sessile polyps larger than 2 cm are more likely to be malignant, although many are benign.[6] Despite the fact that bleeding occurs, the demonstration of an ulcer in a polyp is rare. When the polyp has a long stalk it may prolapse through the pylorus into the duodenum, either permanently or intermittently (Figs. 10–2 and 10–3).

The differential diagnosis includes carcinoid tumors, aberrant pancreatic tissue, inflammatory polyps; prominent rugal folds seen *en face*; retained food, medication, or blood clots; and gastric varices. Multiple gastric hamartomas occur in some patients with Peutz-Jeghers syndrome, and multiple adenomatous polyps may be a part of Gardner's syndrome.

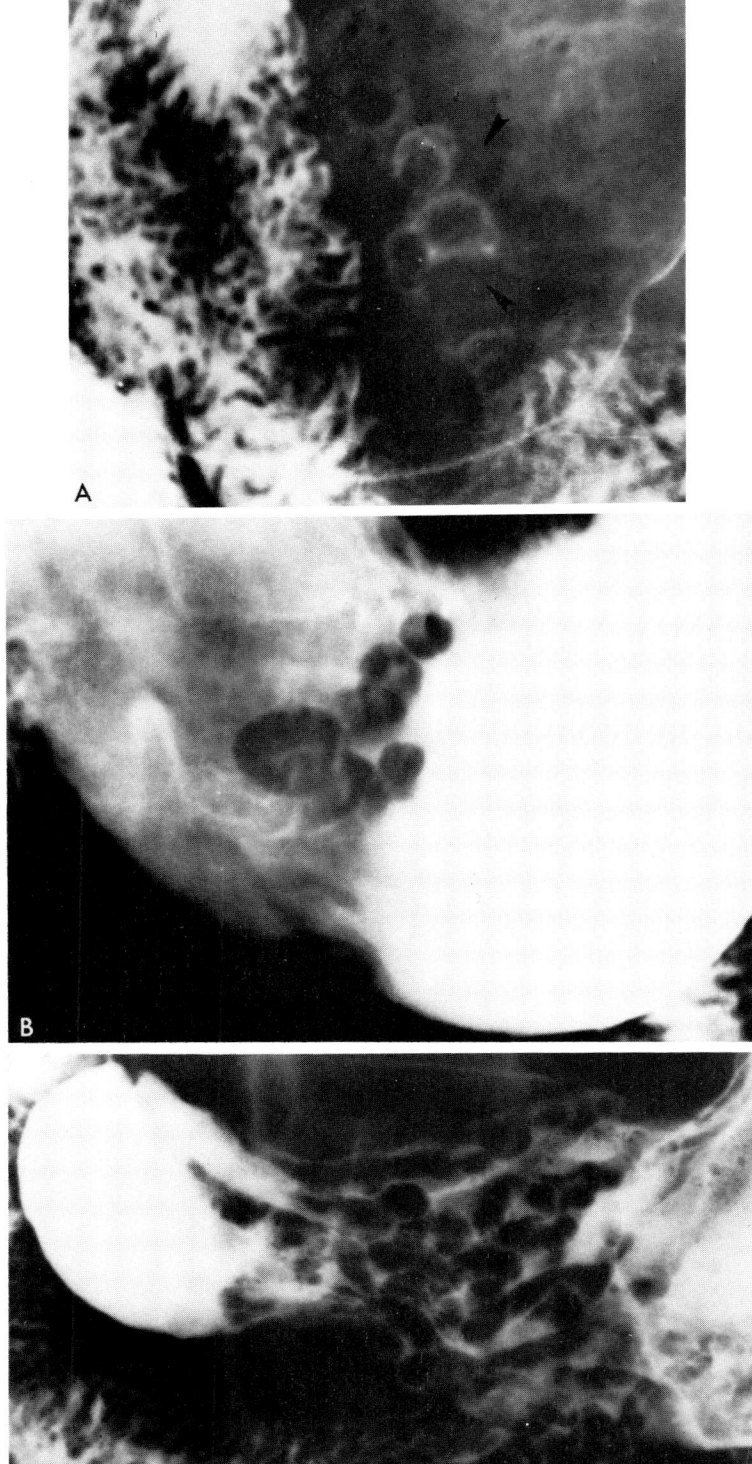

Figure 10–1. Multiple gastric polyps in three patients. *A*, Air-contrast supine projection (arrows). *B* and *C*, Prone compression views.

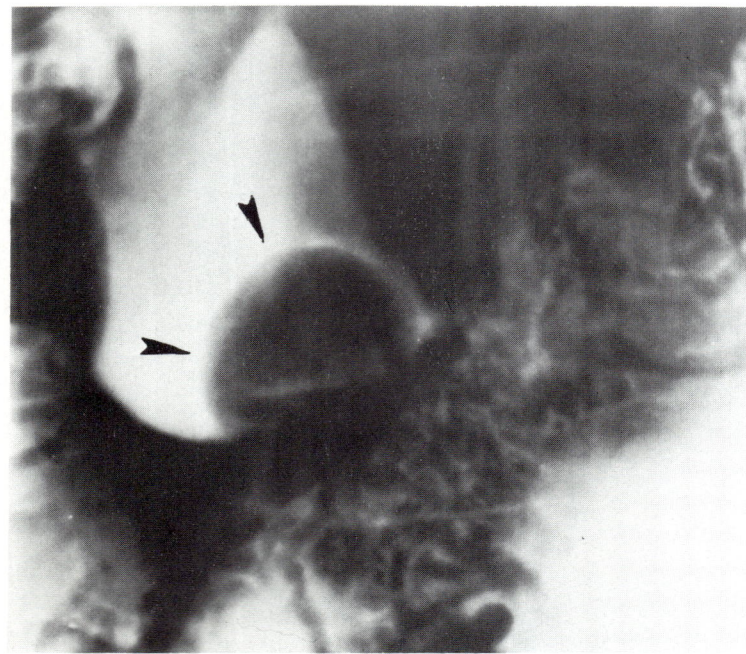

Figure 10–2. Gastric polyp projecting into the duodenal bulb (arrows). At surgery, a 2-cm gastric polyp on a 3-cm stock was impacted in the duodenum.

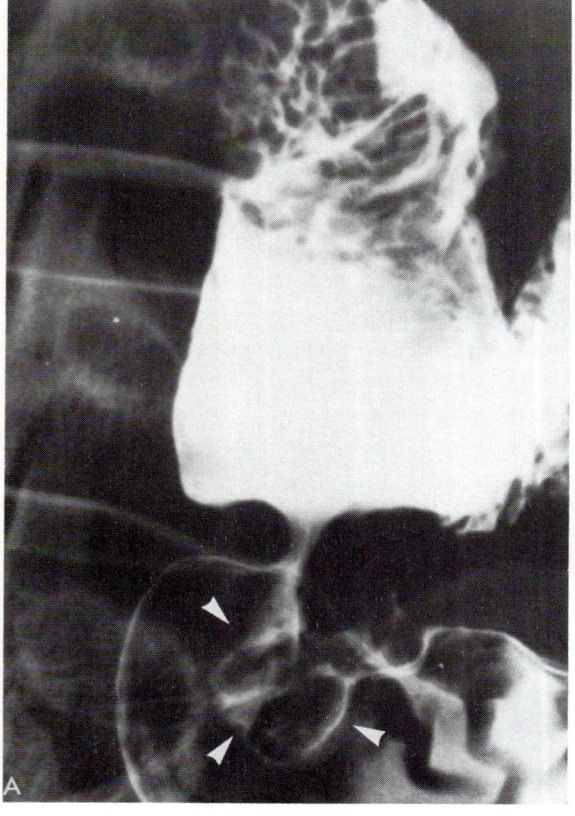
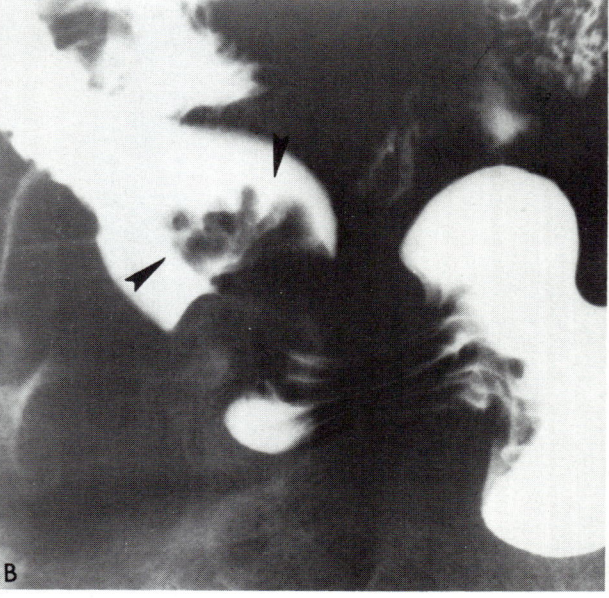

Figure 10–3. Cluster of gastric polyps that prolapse into the duodenal bulb (arrows). *A,* The polyps are visible in the gastric antrum. *B,* The polyps have prolapsed into the duodenum. At fluoroscopy, intermittent prolapse was evident.

BENIGN MESENCHYMAL TUMORS

Benign submucosal tumors of mesenchymal origin, such as leiomyomas, neurofibromas, and lipomas, are not rare and may cause bleeding, pain, or obstruction. Leiomyomas are the most common variety. The radiographic appearance of each of the tumors in this category is similar, so that differentiation between the various pathologic types is nearly always impossible (Figs. 10–4 and 10–5). Characteristically, these mural lesions have a smooth, sharply marginated surface that is usually quite distinct from the irregular, nodular surface of gastric carcinoma. Depending on the extent of the intraluminal growth, the angle formed by the tumor and the adjacent gastric wall may be obtuse or acute. Growth of the lesion (especially a leiomyoma) away from the lumen may produce a prominent exogastric mass that displaces adjacent structures away from the stomach. Ulcerations in the tumor are frequent (Fig. 10–6).

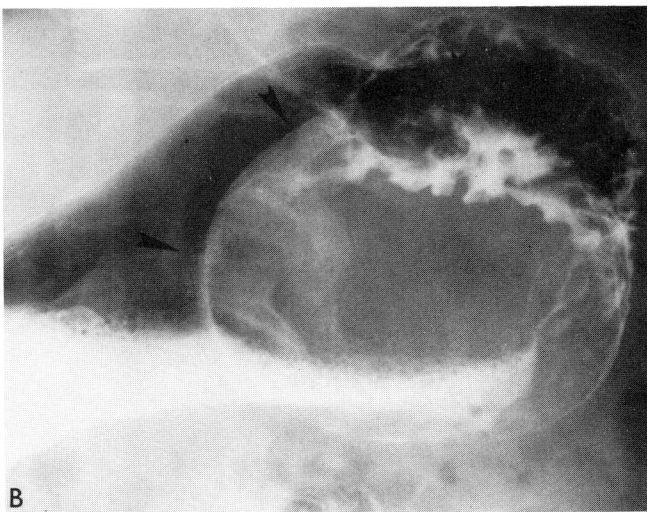

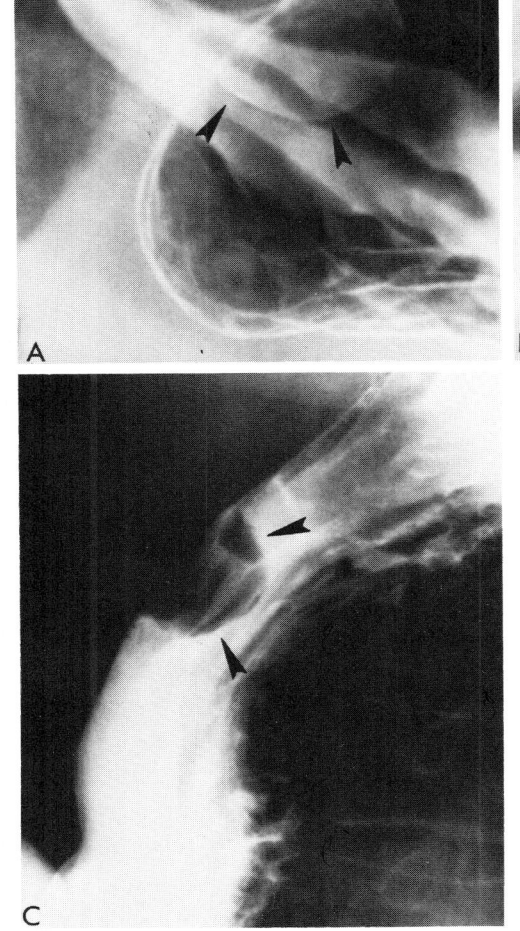

Figure 10–4. Gastric leiomyomas in three patients (arrows). *A*, Small leiomyoma in the fundus adjacent to the esophagogastric junction. *B*, Huge leiomyoma in the body of the stomach. *C*, Leiomyoma in the anterior wall of the stomach seen with the patient in the right posterior oblique projection. A smooth surface characteristic of a mural tumor is apparent in each case.

452 — THE STOMACH

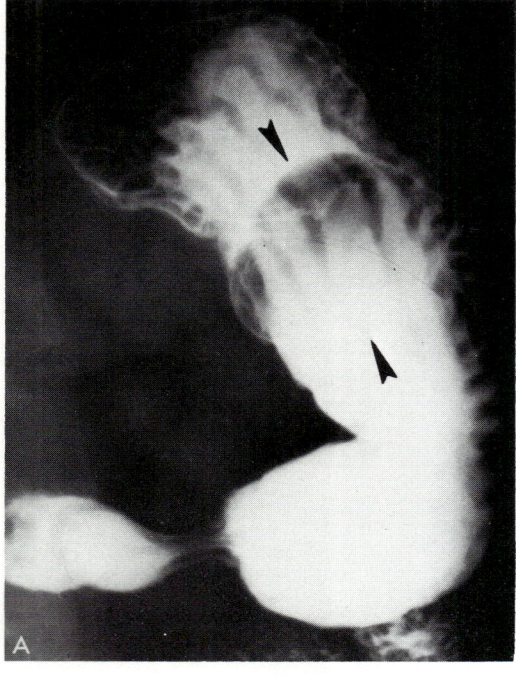
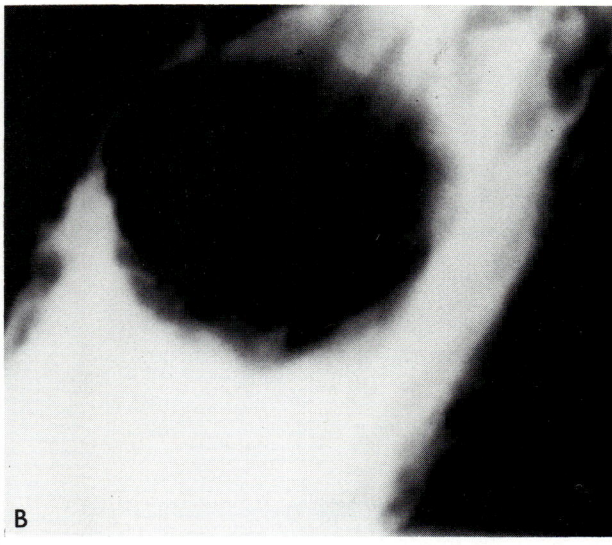

Figure 10–5. Large leiomyoma in the body of the stomach (arrows). The lesion is best seen on the radiograph made with compression B.

In the past decade a number of reports have appeared in the literature describing a bizarre smooth muscle tumor occurring predominantly in the stomach.[1] Stout classified the tumor as a leiomyoblastoma in an attempt to distinguish it from the benign leiomyoma and the highly malignant leiomyosarcoma.[10] The lesion has an unusual and characteristic histologic appearance consisting of rounded cells. There are no elongated, blunt-ended leiomyoblasts or myofibrils, which are seen in ordinary smooth muscle tumors. The rounded cells of the leiomyoblastoma are smooth muscle

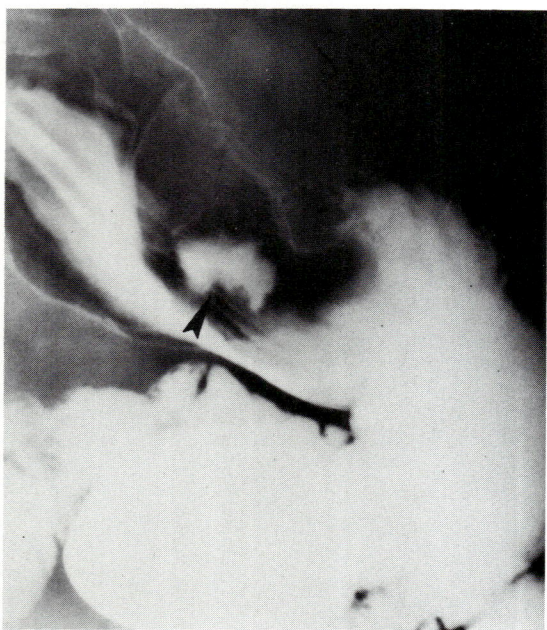

Figure 10–6. Neurolemmoma of the stomach. There is a large ulcer filled with barium in the tumor (arrow).

Figure 10–7. Large leiomyoblastoma of the stomach (arrows). *A*, Prone projection. *B*, Supine air-contrast projection. The smooth surface of the lesion is apparent and serves to differentiate the tumor from an adenocarcinoma.

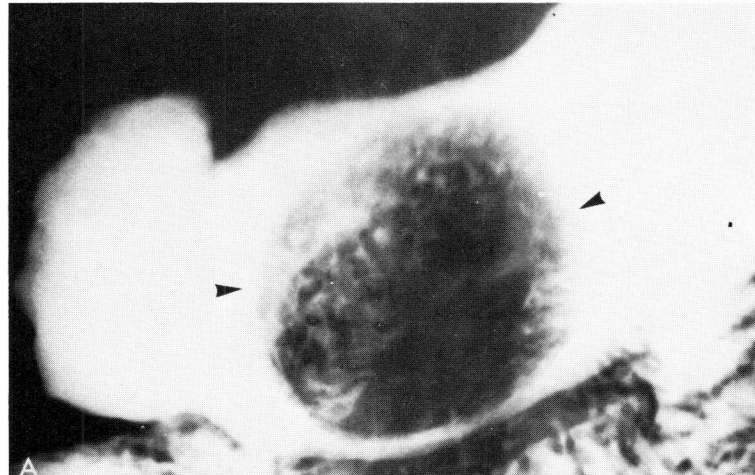
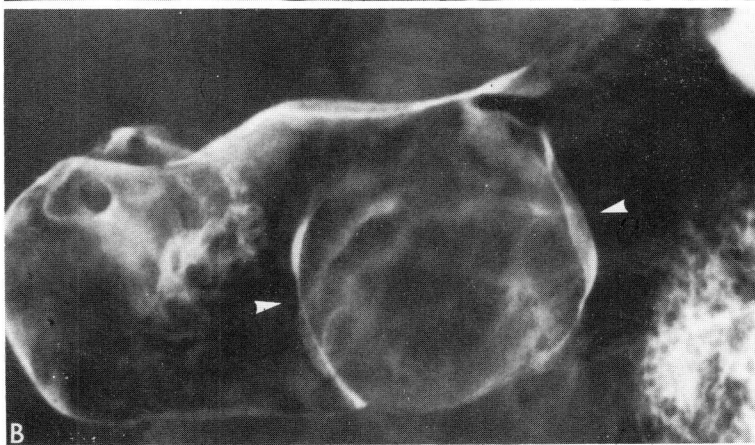

in origin, however, because occasional continuity between them and the more normal-appearing leiomyoblasts can be identified. Most cases are benign, but seven cases with distant metastases have been reported.[1]

Leiomyoblastomas are indistinguishable roentgenographically from other intramural lesions of the stomach (Fig. 10–7). As with leiomyomas, neuromas, glomus tumors, lipomas, and fibromas, the tumors produce a round, sharply marginated, smooth filling defect with a tendency to grow outward as well as into the gastric lumen. Ulceration is common, producing a central, sharply defined niche. Peristalsis is disturbed only if the tumor is large.

Gastric neurofibroma is a rare, benign tumor that may occur alone or in association with von Recklinghausen's multiple neurofibromatosis.[1] Up until 1962, only 29 cases had been reported in the literature, 5 of which were associated with cutaneous neurofibroma.[1] The incidence of malignant degeneration is 10 to 15 per cent whether or not the tumor is associated with multiple neurofibromatosis. The lesion presents the usual roentgenographic feature of a benign mural tumor (Fig. 10–8).

Lipomas of the stomach are submucosal tumors that have the same radiographic features as the other mesenchymal lesions (Fig. 10–9). When the tumor is large, however, a specific diagnosis may be possible if the relative radiolucency of the fat in the tumor can be detected. In some cases, the soft consistency of the lipoma may be evident because of a change in shape of the tumor.

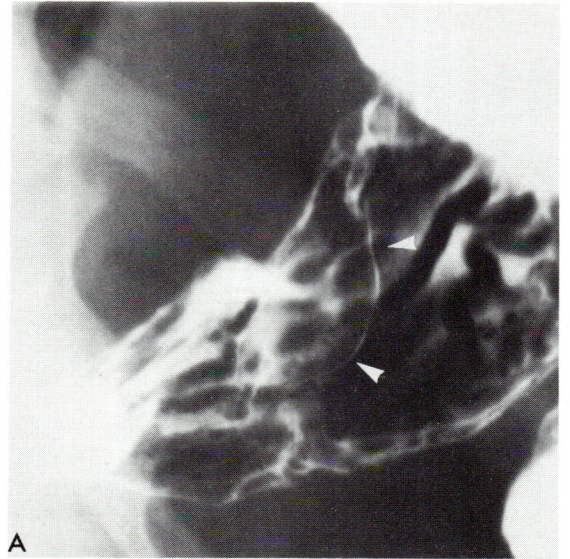

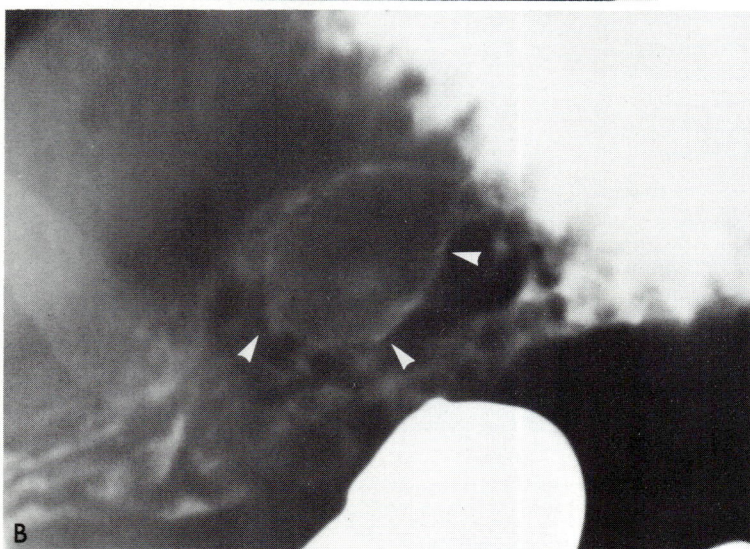

Figure 10–8. Neurofibroma of the stomach along the lesser curvature at the incisura angularis (arrows).

Figure 10–9. Large lipoma of the stomach at the incisura angularis (arrows). Relative radiolucency of the fat in the tumor is not apparent despite the large size of the mass.

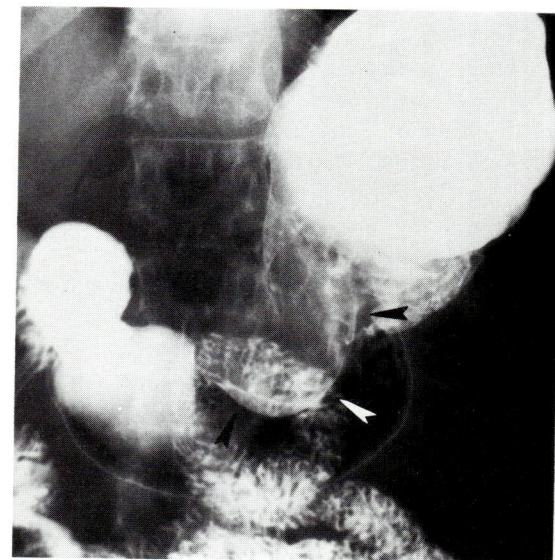

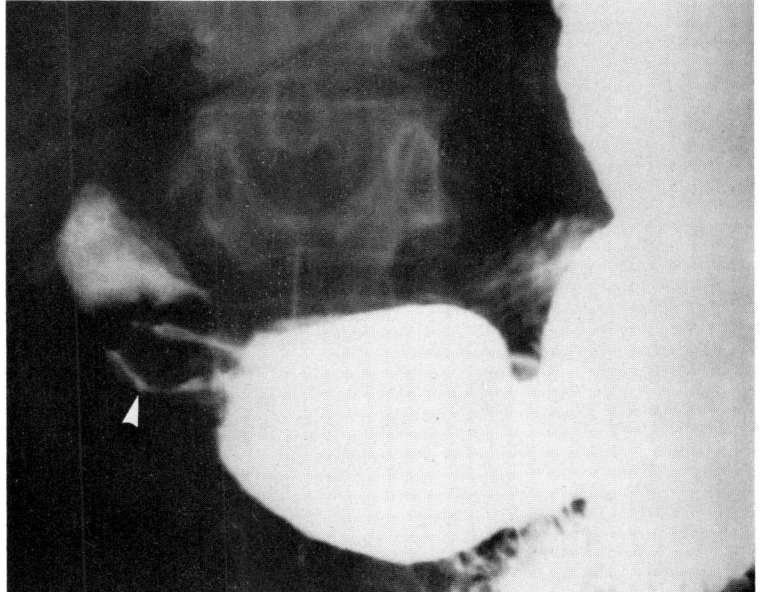

Figure 10–10. Relatively small adenocarcinoma of the stomach. There is an enlarged, irregular rugal fold visible in the gastric antrum (arrow). The patient refused treatment, and returned four years later with a huge infiltrating carcinoma in this location.

ADENOCARCINOMA OF THE STOMACH

Carcinoma of the stomach is rarely detected at an early stage, so that the tumor is usually large by the time the diagnosis is established. Early radiographic features include irregularly enlarged, beaded, or blunted rugal folds and localized areas of restricted distensibility (contour defect) (Figs. 10–10 to 10–13). Improved techniques for air-contrast examination of the gastric mucosa should lead to the detection of earlier lesions.[2] Like carcinoma in other portions of the gastrointestinal tract, three morphologic varieties occur.[11] The tumors may be infiltrating, polypoid, or ulcerat-

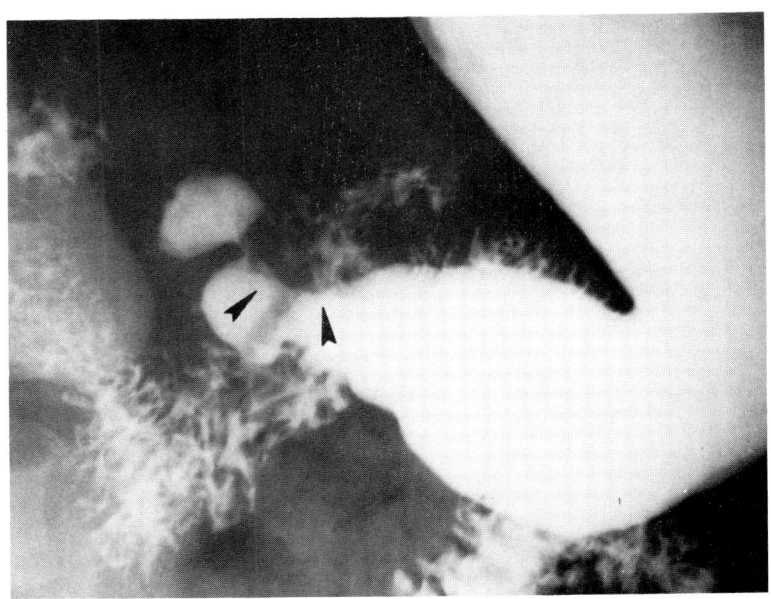

Figure 10–11. Relatively small adenocarcinoma of the stomach. There is asymmetry of the gastric antrum, with a contour defect along the lesser curvature (arrows). A prominent, irregular rugal fold is evident.

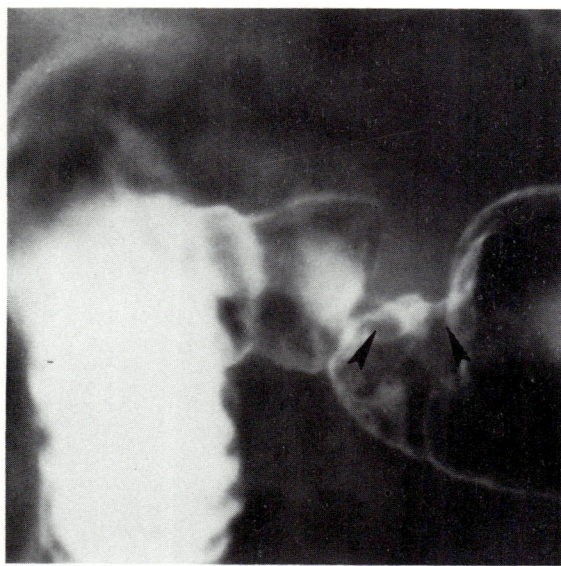

Figure 10–12. Relatively small adenocarcinoma of the gastric antrum adjacent to the pyloric canal. A prominent contour defect is apparent along the lesser curvature (arrows). Initial gastroscopic biopsies failed to show the tumor.

ing. Combinations of the three types are frequent. In nearly every case there is evidence of tumor nodularity, fixation, rigidity, and retraction as indications of the desmoplastic response associated with the tumor.

Rigidity, restricted distensibility, and imapired motility are the characteristic features of the infiltrating variety of adenocarcinoma. Submucosal extension of the tumor is often marked and may produce a "water-bottle," or linitis plastica, configuration (Figs. 10–14 and 10–15). When the tumor extends to the pylorus, the differential diagnosis includes stricture due to caustic ingestion, granulomatous diseases, such as syphilis and tuberculosis, and cicatrizing benign gastric ulcer.

Polypoid carcinomas nearly always have a lobulated surface that is distinct from

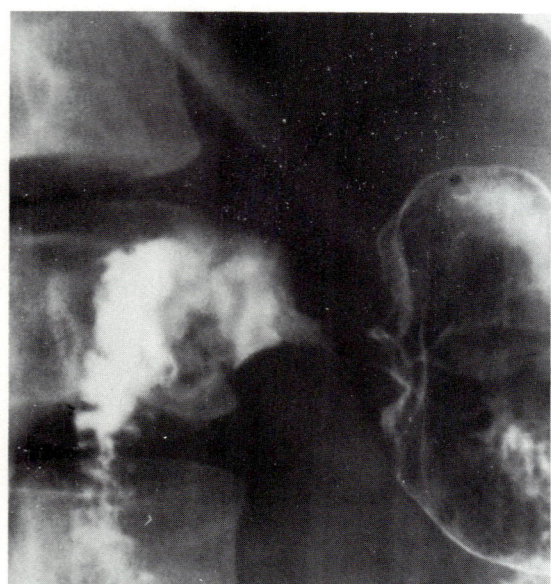

Figure 10–13 Adenocarcinoma of the gastric antrum extending across the pylorus. Extension into the duodenum is more common in cases of lymphoma.

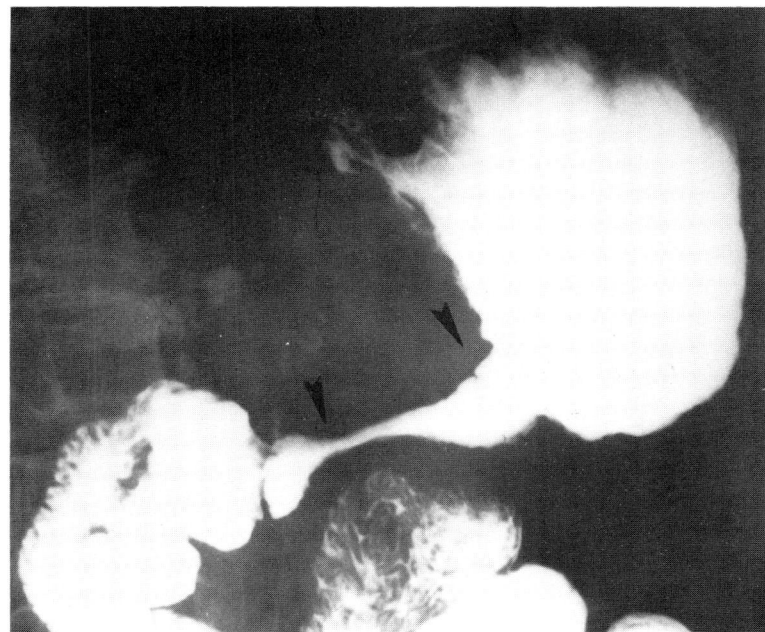
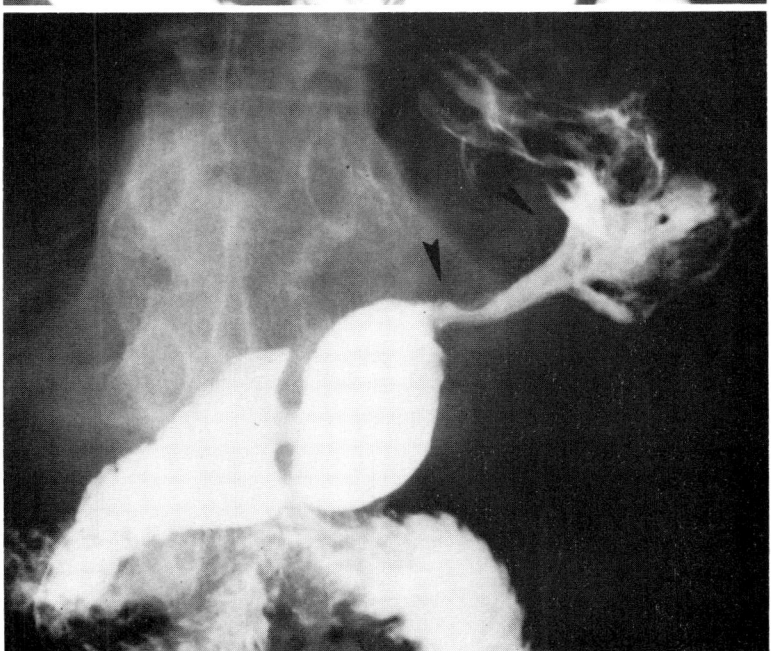

Figure 10–14. Infiltrating variety of gastric carcinoma in two patients. In each case there is segmental narrowing of the gastric lumen with abrupt margins (arrows). In both cases the antrum is spared.

the sharply marginated configuration of benign mural lesions (Figs. 10–16 and 10–17). The lesions are broad-based and have abrupt margins. The differentiation from bezoars is usually simple and is based on fixation of the tumor to the gastric wall.

Adenocarcinoma of the stomach of the ulcerating variety may present with radiologic features similar to those of benign gastric ulcers (Fig. 10–18). However, nodularity of the tissue surrounding the malignant ulcer crater, abrupt transition of the mass between the orifice of the crater and the adjacent mucosa, and failure of the

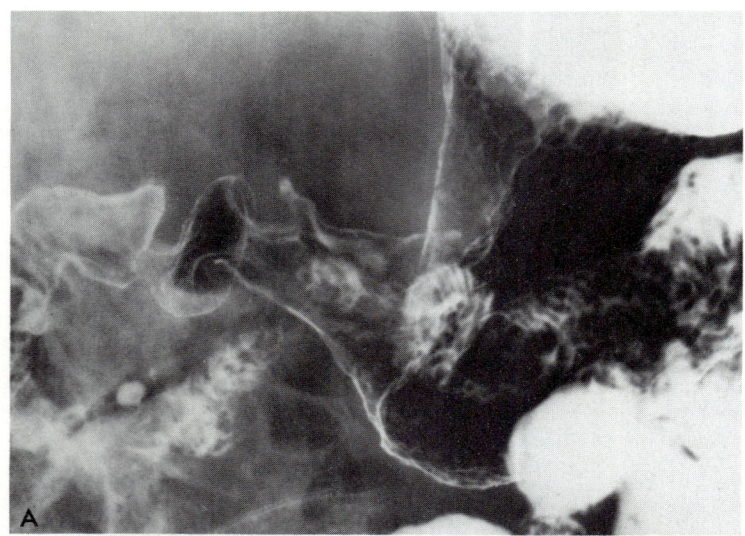
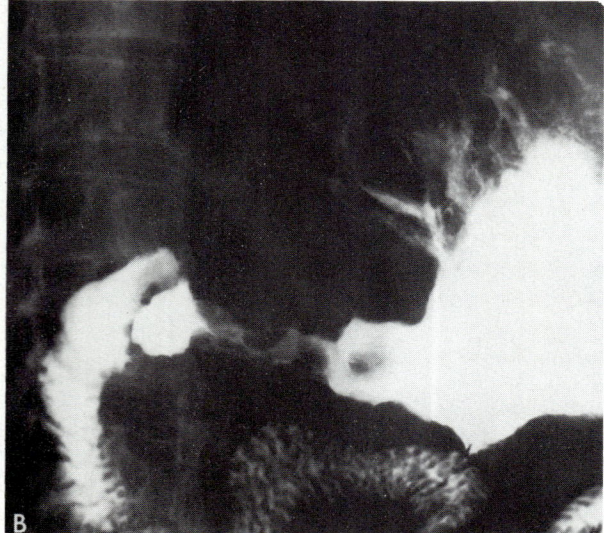

Figure 10–15. Infiltrating variety of gastric carcinoma in two patients. In both cases there is restricted distensibility of the gastric antrum. Nodularity of the lesion is apparent in *B*.

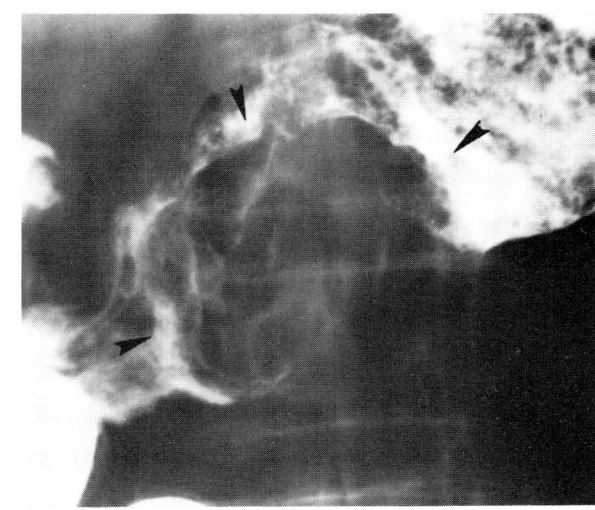

Figure 10–16. Polypoid variety of gastric carcinoma in two patients. In both cases the tumor mass is sessile on a broad base, and has an irregular nodular surface (arrows).

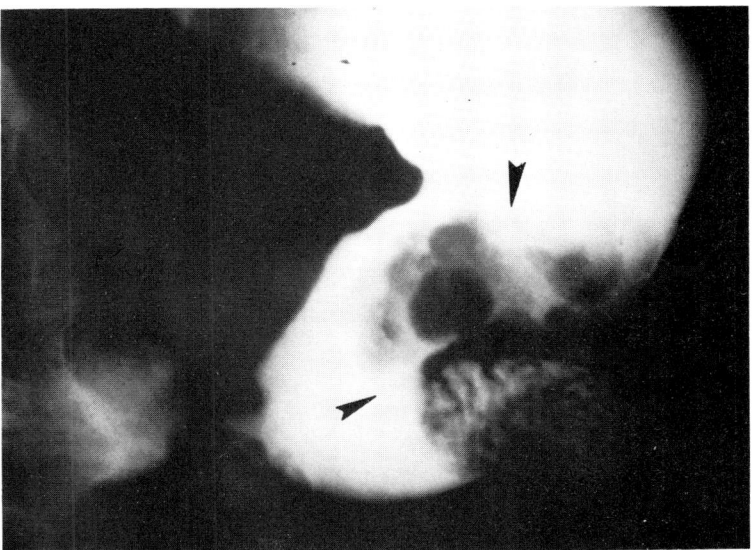

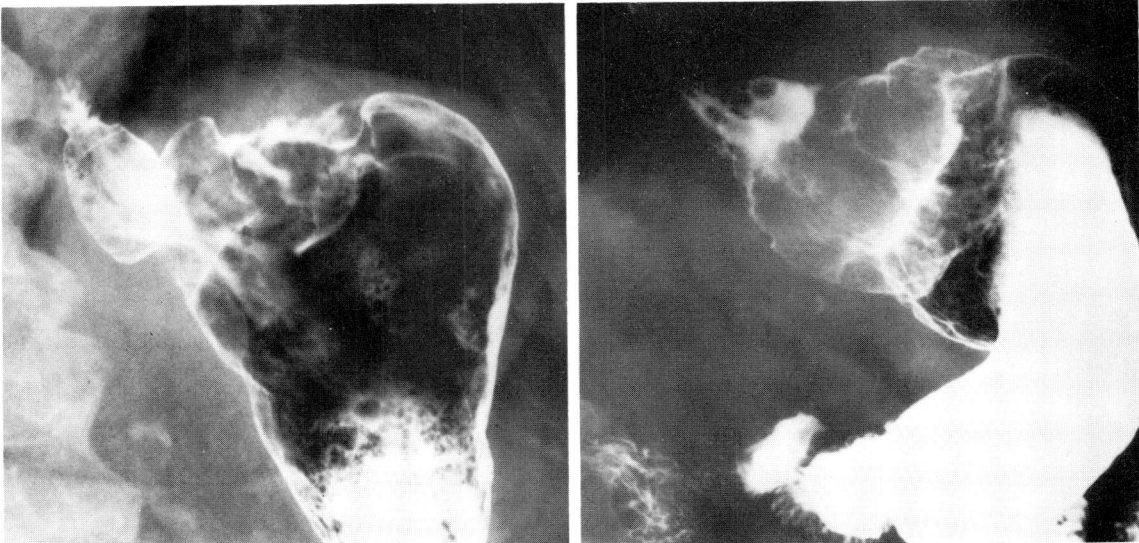

Figure 10–17. Polypoid variety of gastric carcinoma involving the gastric fundus in two patients. Distention of the fundus with gas is essential for the detection of smaller fundal tumors.

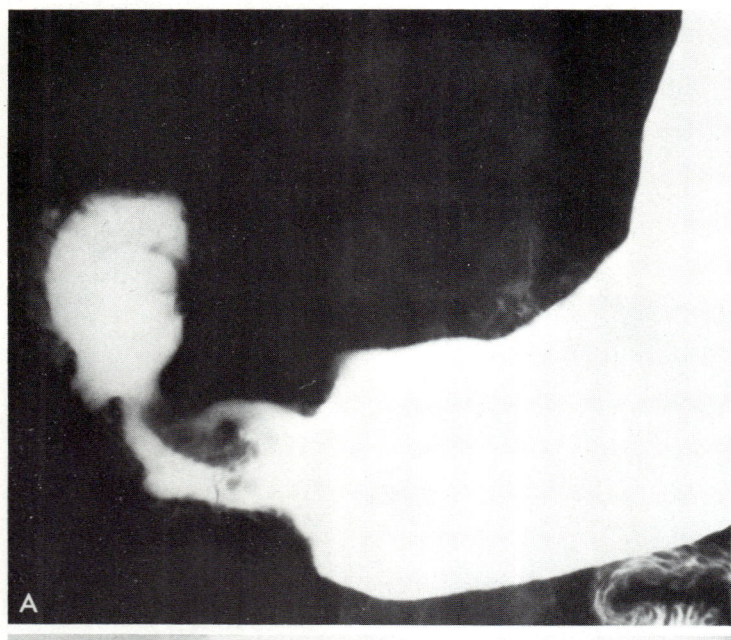
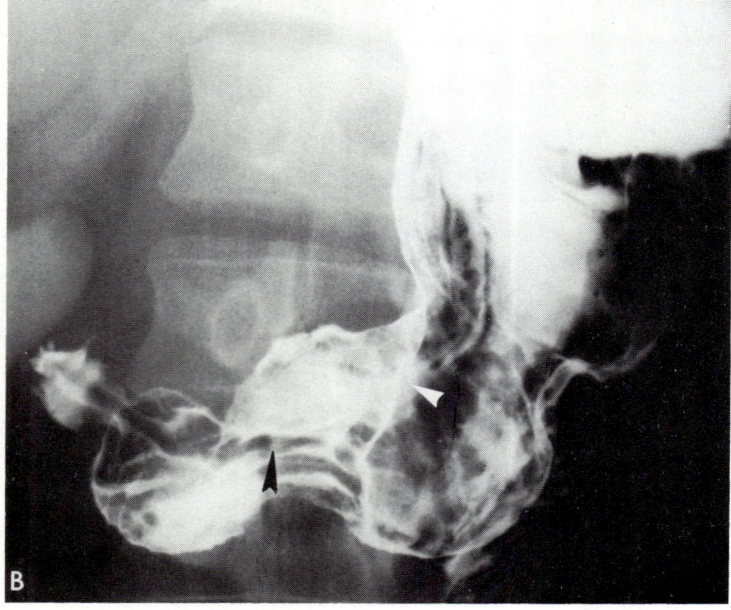

Figure 10–18. Ulcerating variety of gastric carcinoma involving the prepyloric area (*A*) and the lesser curvature at the incisura angularis (*B*) (arrows). In both cases typical malignant ulcers are evident.

THE STOMACH — 461

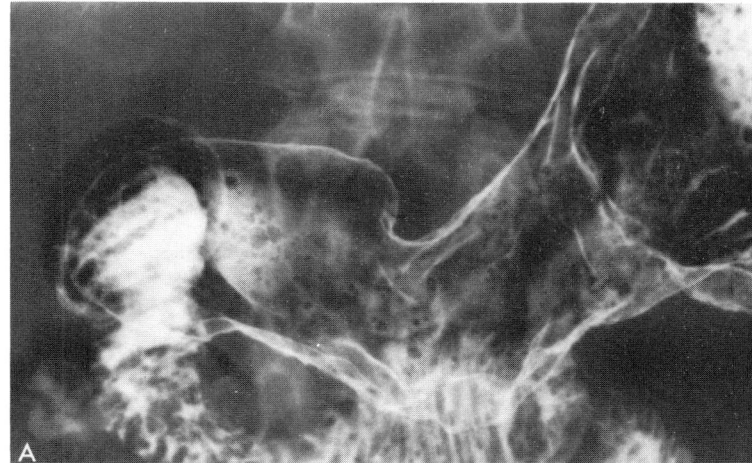
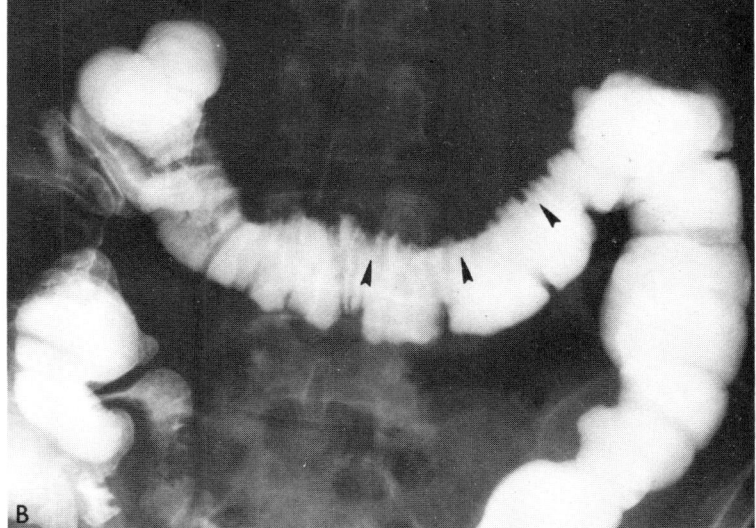

Figure 10–19. *A*, Supine air-contrast radiograph of the stomach showing restricted distensibility in the middle third. At fluoroscopy, motility was absent in this area. *B*, Barium enema examination in the same patient showing distortion of the haustra in the transverse colon (arrows) caused by direct extension of the gastric carcinoma down the gastrocolic omentum. Pleating of the margin of the colon is characteristic of metastatic disease and is due to the desmoplastic response produced by the tumor.

ulcer to penetrate beyond the normal lumen of the stomach are typical features that usually permit precise differentiation.

The proximity of the greater curvature of the stomach to the transverse colon is responsible for the frequent involvement of the colon via the gastrocolic omentum in cases of carcinoma of the stomach (Fig. 10–19). Pleating and retraction of the transverse colon are characteristic radiographic features that indicate involvement of the colon with metastatic disease.

LEIOMYOSARCOMA

Many cases of leiomyosarcoma of the stomach have the same radiographic appearance as benign leiomyomas. Differentiation in this situation depends on the number of mitoses seen histologically and is not possible radiographically. In other cases, however, the leiomyosarcoma presents as a huge, bizarre ulceration in which

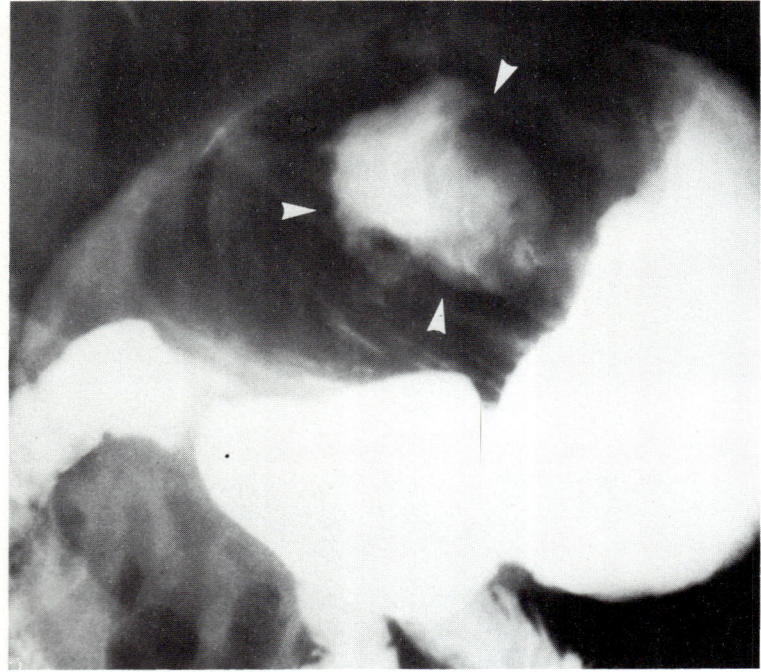

Figure 10–20. Cavitating leiomyosarcoma of the stomach. A large, irregular ulcer is visible in the gastric fundus (arrows). No tumor mass was evident radiographically or at gastroscopy. The tumor grew exophytically, with only a narrow attachment to the stomach.

the tumor mass itself may not be visible (Fig. 10–20). Exophytic growth often predominates, so that the origin of the tumor in the stomach may not be readily apparent.

GASTRIC LYMPHOMA

Menuck reported a retrospective analysis of 30 cases of gastric lymphoma and concluded that if careful attention is paid to the radiologic features, lymphoma can be distinguished from carcinoma in most cases.[7] He noted that gastric lymphoma usually presents as a much larger lesion than gastric carcinoma. The average size of the lymphomas was 11.9 cm; that of the gastric carcinomas was 5.6 cm. Both gastric carcinoma and lymphoma may involve the adjacent duodenum or esophagus, although extension to the duodenal bulb is more common in lymphoma (20 per cent) than in carcinoma (6 per cent). The most frequent primary radiographic finding in cases of gastric lymphoma is a diffuse infiltrating pattern consisting of enlarged, bizarre rugal folds without significant narrowing of the gastric lumen (Fig. 10–21). This was present in 56 per cent of the cases of gastric lymphoma but occurred in only 8 per cent of the cases of gastric carcinoma in Menuck's study.[7] Within the subgroups of lymphoma, Hodgkin's disease is quite different from lymphosarcoma and reticulum cell sarcoma in that the presenting lesion is much more comparable in size and radiographic appearance to gastric carcinoma.

Since most lymphomas do not evoke much of a desmoplastic response (Hodgkin's disease is the exception), they seldom produce significant narrowing of the lumen or loss of pliability even when the entire stomach is involved.[7] Furthermore, since a lymphoma has such extensive submucosal infiltration, the mucosa often is preserved and the submucosal infiltration is manifested as a nodular, bizarre rugal fold

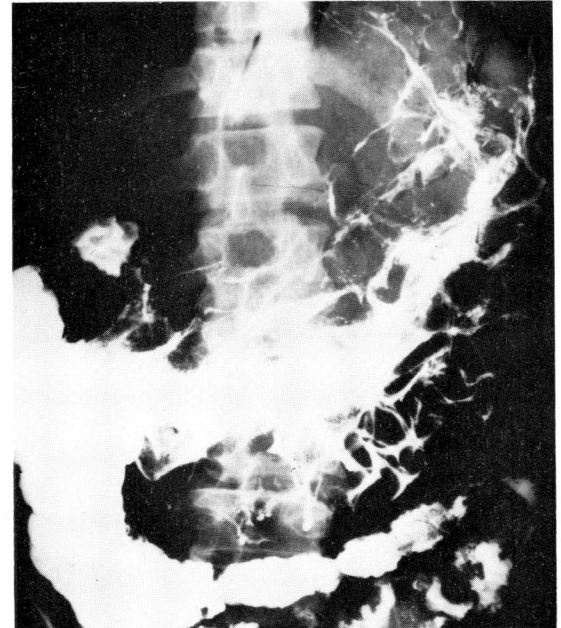

Figure 10–21. Typical lymphosarcoma of the stomach, with huge bizarre mucosal folds resulting from submucosal extension of the tumor. Barium is also present in the colon.

pattern (Fig. 10–21). This differs from the infiltrating gastric carcinoma, which usually has a pronounced desmoplastic response and extensive mucosal destruction, producing narrowing of the lumen, loss of pliability, and effacement and destruction of the gastric mucosal folds.

ADENOCARCINOMA OF THE DUODENUM (See also Chapter 11)

It is apparent from the large number of cases of adenocarcinoma of the duodenum now accumulated in the literature that the disease is not as rare as formerly thought. Up until 1961 over 601 cases were reported.[1] Although carcinoma of the small intestine accounts for only 3 per cent of all malignant gastrointestinal tumors, the incidence of carcinoma of the duodenum almost equals that of the jejunum and ileum combined.[3] The symptoms are nonspecific, and are usually similar to those of a peptic ulcer early in the disease. Later, there may be high intestinal obstruction, jaundice, hematemesis, and melena.

The tumors are grouped according to their relation to the ampulla of Vater. In the summary by Kleinerman et al. of 453 cases, 22 per cent were supra-ampullary, 60 per cent were periampullary, and 18 per cent were infra-ampullary.[5] The high incidence of the periampullary group is the result of the inclusion of some cases of carcinoma of the ampulla of Vater, usually considered to be distinct from duodenal carcinoma.

The radiographic features of adenocarcinoma of the duodenum are the same as those of carcinoma elsewhere in the gastrointestinal tract and can be classified as annular, infiltrating, or ulcerative (Fig. 10–22). Typical radiologic findings include effacement and thickening of the mucosal folds, rigidity, irregular polypoid filling defects, and dilatation. Because the lesion is unusual, inadequate attention is often

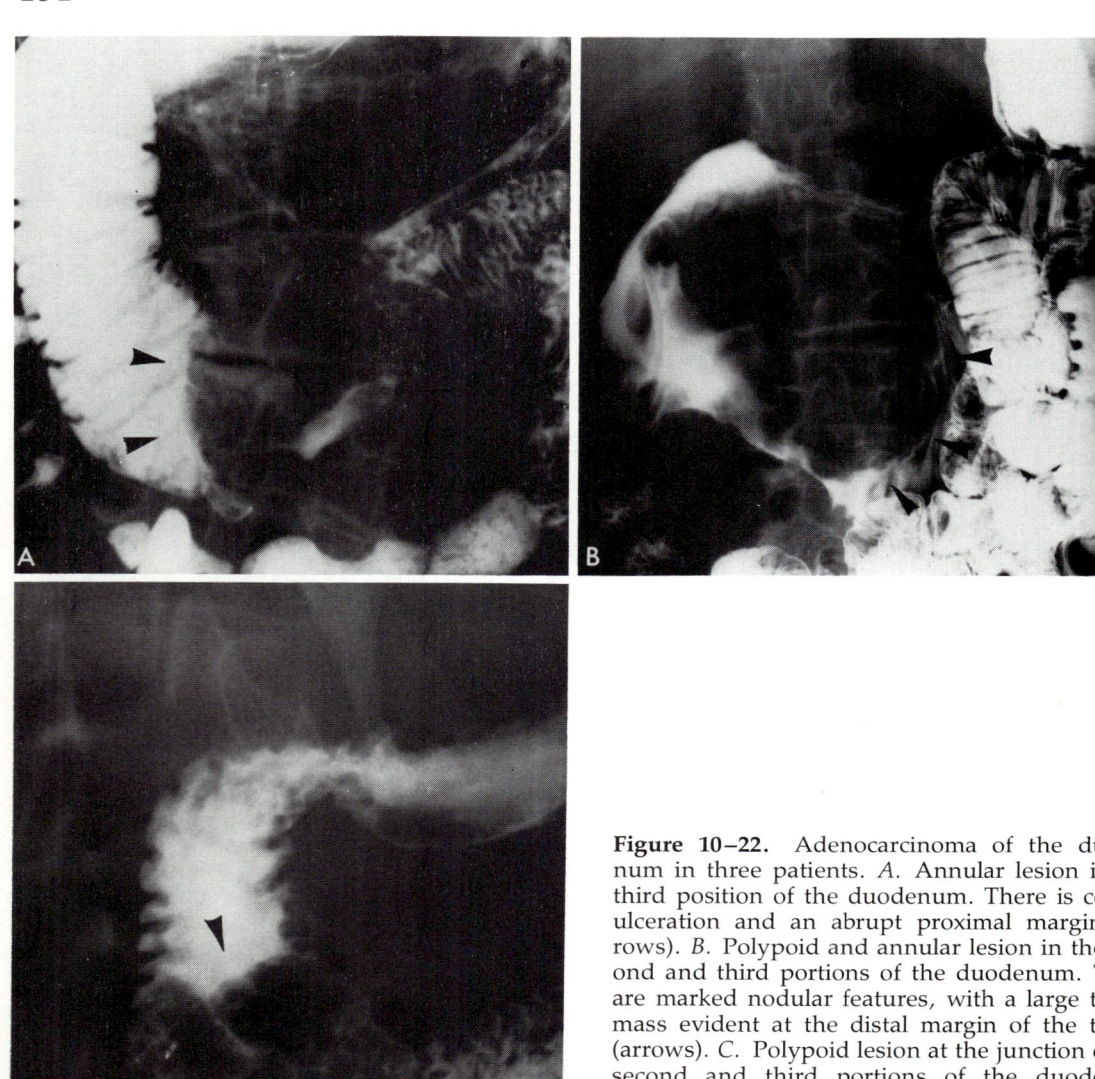

Figure 10–22. Adenocarcinoma of the duodenum in three patients. *A.* Annular lesion in the third position of the duodenum. There is central ulceration and an abrupt proximal margin (arrows). *B.* Polypoid and annular lesion in the second and third portions of the duodenum. There are marked nodular features, with a large tumor mass evident at the distal margin of the tumor (arrows). *C.* Polypoid lesion at the junction of the second and third portions of the duodenum (arrows).

given to the examination of the distal portion of the duodenum and the carcinoma may be overlooked.

Carcinoma confined to the duodenal cap is rare and presents several special problems in differential diagnosis (Fig. 10–23).[1] When the lesion is polypoid it may simulate Brunner's adenoma, an adenomatous polyp, or a carcinoid tumor. When the tumor is infiltrating, it simulates metastatic disease, contiguous involvement

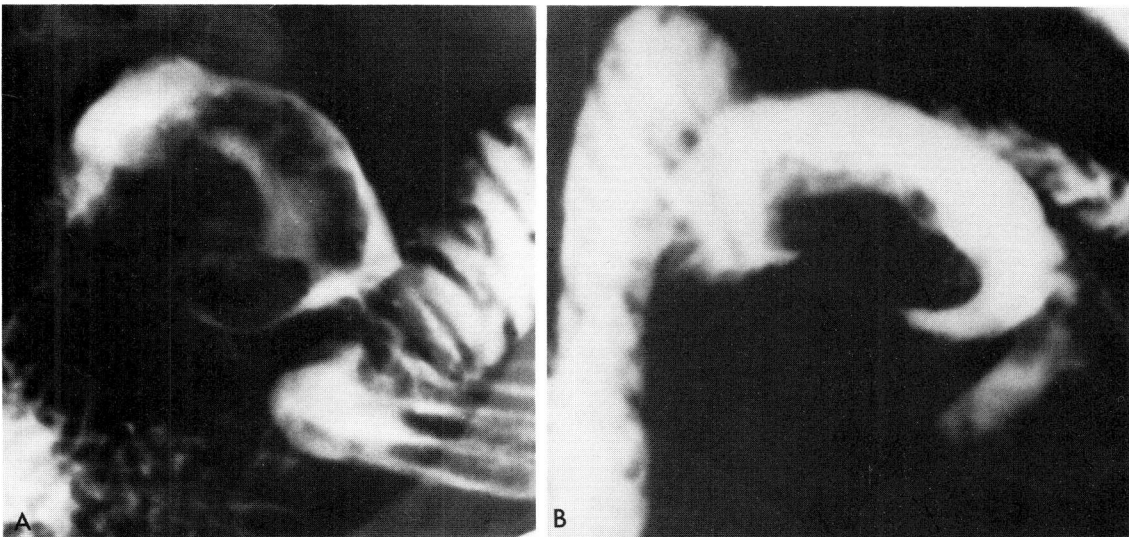

Figure 10–23. Adenocarcinoma of the duodenal bulb. The tumor is seen both *en face* (A) and in profile (B). At surgery, there was a polypoid adenocarcinoma of the duodenum confined to the first portion.

from carcinoma of the pancreas or gallbladder, annular pancreas, duodenal diverticula, or adhesions. Ulcerating carcinoma may simulate peptic ulcer, particularly in the postbulbar segment of the duodenum.

Carcinoma of the papilla of Vater typically produces an irregular polypoid mass

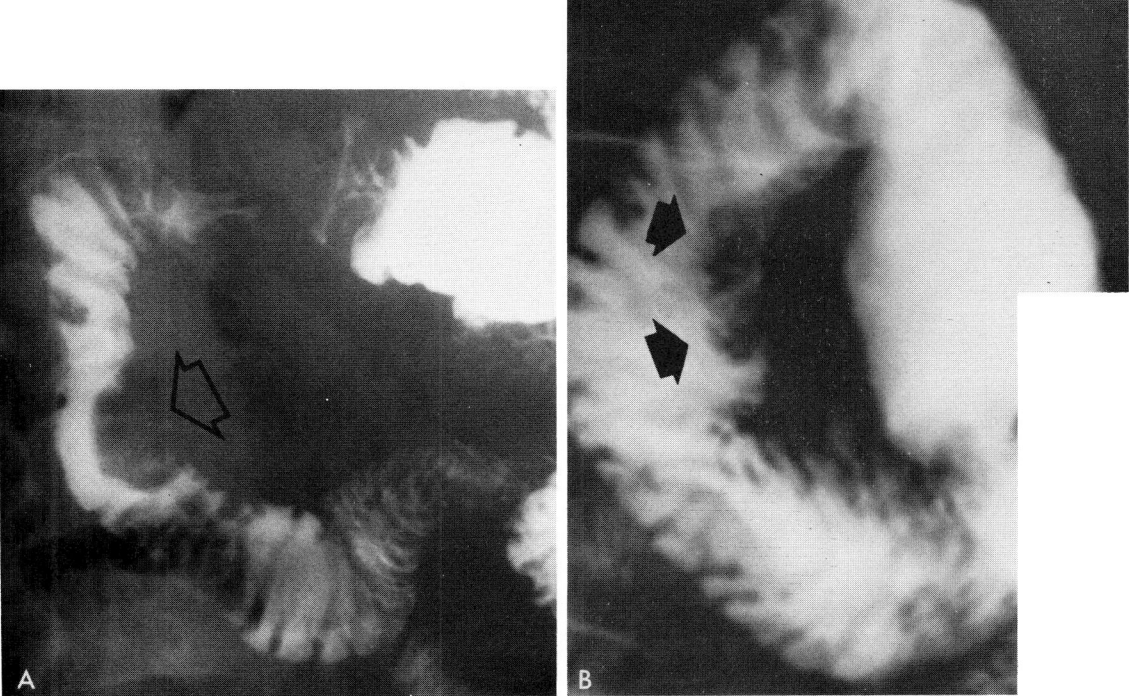

Figure 10–24. Adenocarcinoma of the papilla of Vater in two patients. In both cases, a polypoid mass with an irregular surface is evident at the papilla (arrows).

in the duodenal wall in the region of the papilla (Fig. 10–24). This differs from enlargement of the papilla of Vater due to edema associated with pancreatitis or an impacted gallstone, in which case the papilla is sharply marginated and smooth. When the papilla is edematous owing to pancreatitis (Poppel's sign), other effects of pancreatitis are apparent.

LYMPHOMA OF THE DUODENUM

The radiologic appearance of duodenal lymphoma is the same as that of lymphoma elsewhere in the small intestine. The tumor may be polypoid, annular, ulcerating, or aneurysmal (Fig. 10–25). Since concomitant desmoplastic reaction is unusual, obstruction is rarely marked.

METASTATIC DISEASE

Secondary neoplastic involvement of the stomach and duodenum is most commonly the result of direct extension from a contiguous tumor, such as carcinoma of the pancreas, or from a noncontiguous lesion, such as carcinoma of the transverse colon that spreads to the stomach or duodenum via the gastrocolic omentum. The radiographic changes produced by direct extension depend upon the site of the pri-

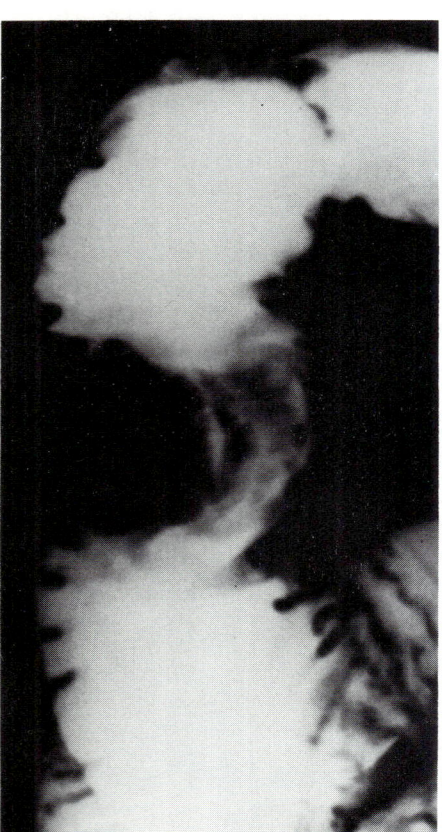

Figure 10–25. Lymphosarcoma of the duodenum. A polypoid mass is evident in the second portion of the duodenum.

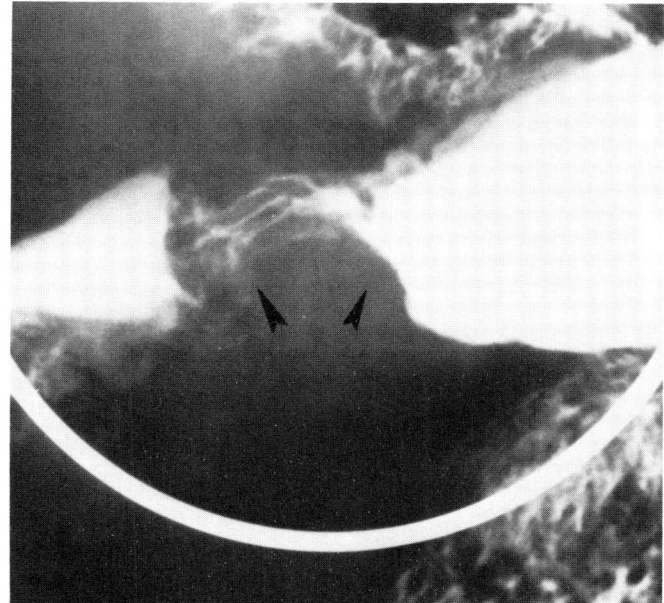

Figure 10–26. Carcinoma of the pancreas with direct extension to the stomach. A smooth tumor mass is visible along the greater curvature of the stomach owing to serosal involvement from the pancreatic tumor (arrows).

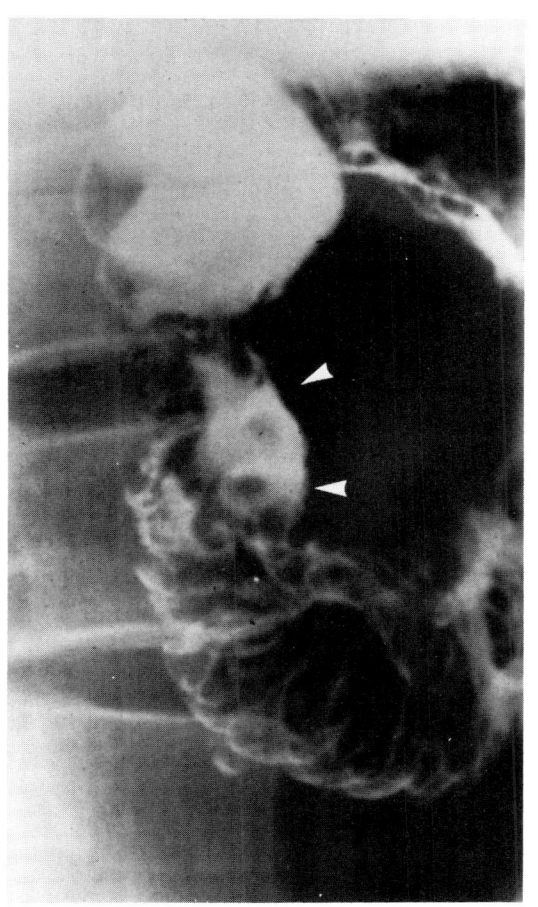

Figure 10–27. Carcinoma of the hepatic flexure of the colon with extension to lymph nodes adjacent to the duodenum. There is an ulcer of the second portion of the duodenum associated with narrowing due to metastatic carcinoma (arrows).

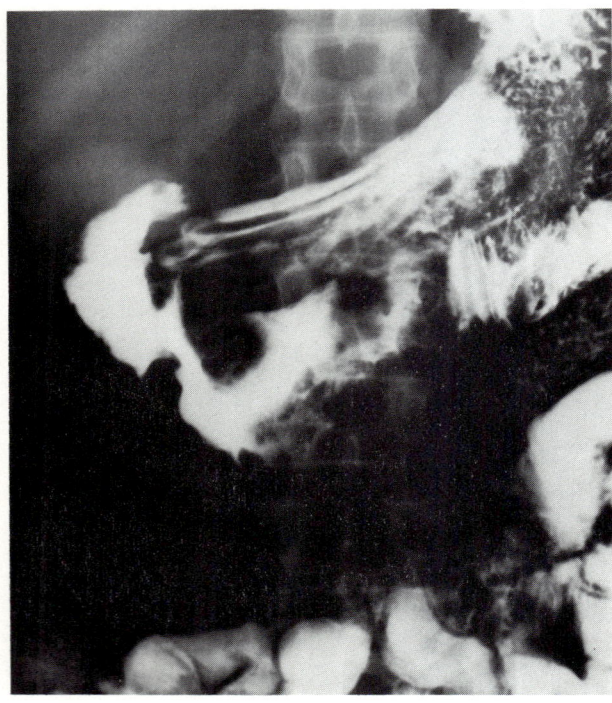

Figure 10–28. Huge retroperitoneal liposarcoma, with secondary involvement of the duodenum. A large extraluminal mass due to the primary retroperitoneal tumor is apparent.

mary tumor and the degree of gastric invasion. Keller et al. noted abnormal motility in the gastric antrum in association with gastric involvement by carcinoma of the pancreas. In their cases, fixation of the gastric wall by the adjacent carcinoma created abnormalities in distensibility, eccentric deformity, and asymmetric contractions, which they termed the struggling antrum.[4] The metastatic implant may produce a mass in the gastric wall with the radiographic features of a submucosal mural tumor (Fig. 10–26).

Metastatic involvement of the descending portion of the duodenum in cases of carcinoma of the hepatic flexure of the colon is not uncommon. The contiguity of the two structures and the intervening short fascial plan of the transverse mesocolon allow ready spread of the neoplastic process.[18] Extrinsic compression by enlarged nodes adjacent to the duodenum or actual extension of the tumor into the duodenal wall with ulceration may be detected (Fig. 10–27). Rarely, a tumor of the right renal pelvis can extend anteriorly to involve the descending duodenum.

Occasionally, a primary retroperitoneal tumor, such as lymphoma or liposarcoma, may involve the duodenum. In these cases there may be extensive distortion of the duodenal mucosa and irregular narrowing of the lumen. In most cases, however, the extraduodenal retroperitoneal mass is predominant (Fig. 10–28).

References

1. Berk, R. N., Scher, G. S., and Bode, D. F.: Unusual tumors of the gastrointestinal tract. Am. J. Roentgenol. 113:159–169, 1971.
2. Gelfand, D. W.: The Japanese-style double contrast examination of the stomach. Gastrointest. Radiol. 1:7–19, 1976.
3. Good, C. A.: Tumors of the small intestine. Am. J. Roentgenol. 89:685–705, 1962.

4. Keller, R. J., Khilnani, M. T., and Wolf, B. S.: The struggling antrum, a new sign of perigastric malignancy. Am. J. Roentgenol. *119*:300–307, 1973.
5. Kleinerman, J., Yardermian, K., and Tamaki, H. T.: Carcinoma of the duodenum. Ann. Intern. Med. *43*:451–465, 1950.
6. Marshak, R. H., and Feldman, F.: Gastric polyps. Am. J. Dig. Dis. *10*:909–935, 1965.
7. Menuck, L. S.: Gastric lymphoma, a radiologic diagnosis. Gastrointest. Radiol. *1*:157–163, 1976.
8. Meyers, M. A., and Whalen, J. P.: Roentgen significance of the duodenocolic relationships: an anatomic approach. Am. J. Roentgenol. *117*:263–274, 1973.
9. Monaco, A. P., Stanford, I. R., Castleman, B., et al.: Adenomatous polyps of the stomach. A clinical and pathological study of 153 cases. Cancer *15*:211–227, 1968.
10. Stout, P. F.: Bizarre smooth muscle tumors of stomach. Cancer *15*:400–409, 1962.
11. Templeton, F. E.: X-ray Examination of the Stomach. Chicago, University of Chicago Press, 1964, pp. 400–407.

Part II
Non-Neoplastic Diseases

ABERRANT PANCREATIC RESTS

Aberrant, heterotopic, or accessory pancreatic rests are islands of pancreatic tissue situated outside the normal confines of the pancreas. Most of these rests are located in the stomach and duodenum, but a substantial number are found elsewhere, such as in the jejunum, Meckel's diverticulum, gallbladder, liver, and spleen. Usually situated in the submucosa but sometimes extending into the muscle wall, the pancreatic rests appear as single, pale yellow or white, lobulated nodules that may easily be mistaken for neoplasms. The aberrant tissue consists of entoderm composed of

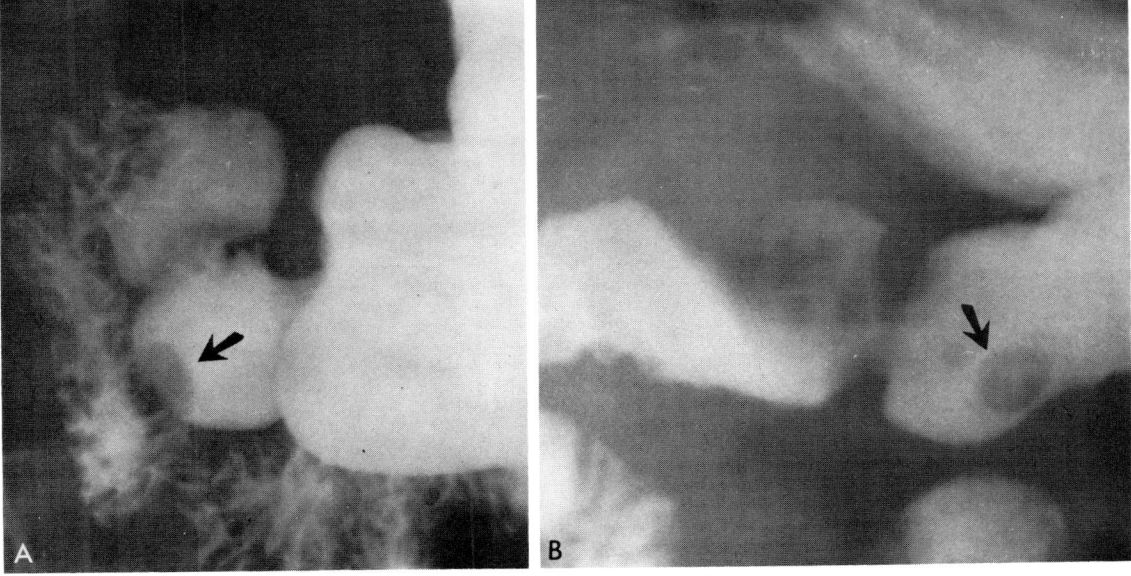

Figure 10–29. Typical aberrant pancreatic rest in the gastric antrum in two patients (arrows). Central umbilication is visible in *B*.

470 — THE STOMACH

all of the cell types normally found in the pancreas, often including islets of Langerhans. Pancreatitis with fat necrosis, islet cell tumors with hyperinsulinism, and pancreatic carcinoma with metastases may occur.

Pancreatic heterotopia is a congenital condition that can be encountered at any age. The lesions are usually discovered in the fourth and fifth decades of life, however; the diagnosis is infrequently made in childhood. This is not surprising in view of the fact that barium studies and abdominal surgery are more commonly performed in older patients. Most accessory pancreatic nodules in infants are in the range of 1 to 2 mm in diameter and are much smaller than those found in adults.[5] Consequently, the masses enlarge as the child grows to adulthood.

Most of the reports in the literature concerning the radiologic appearance of

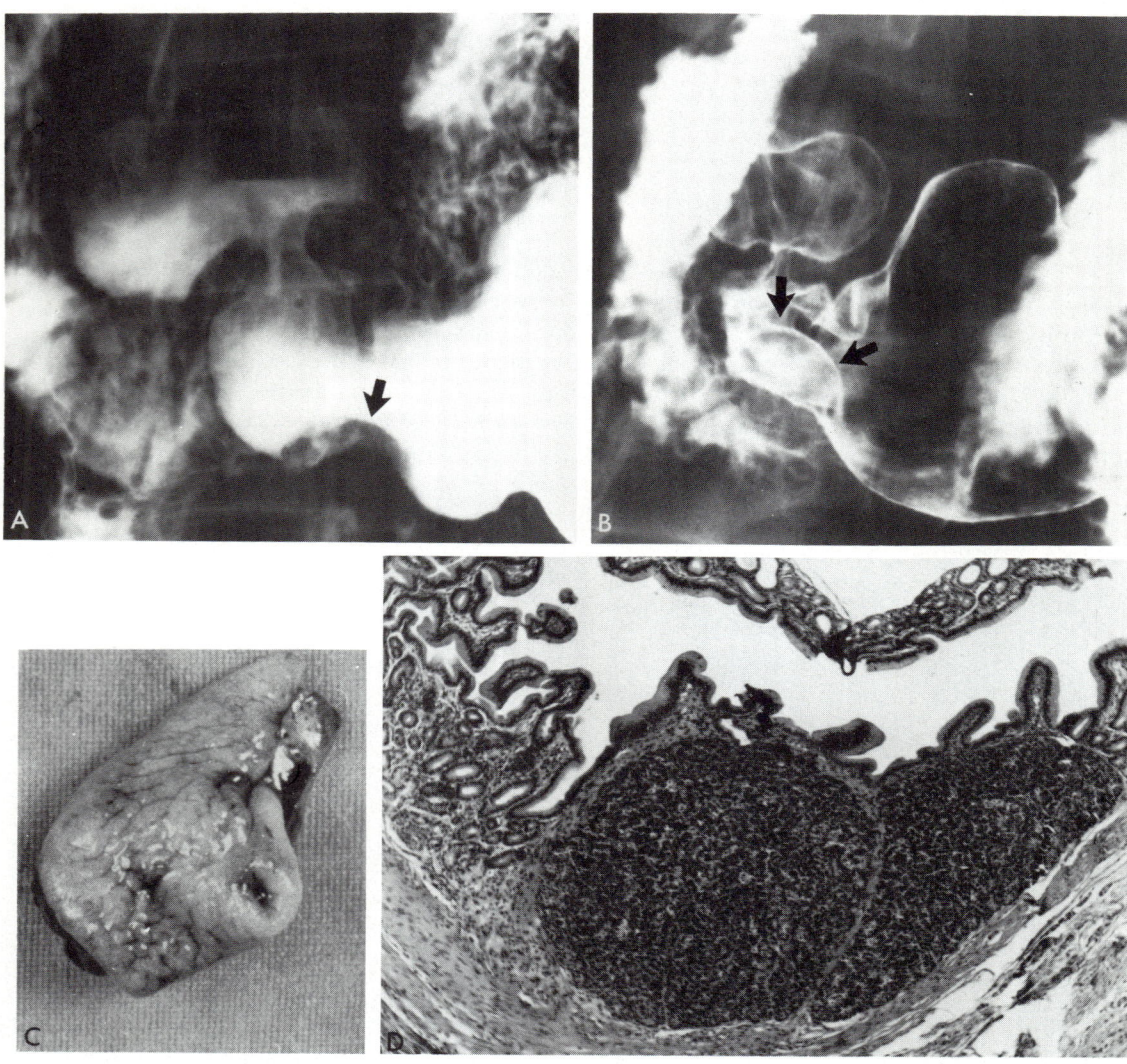

Figure 10–30. *A* and *B*, There is a smooth, broad-based intramural mass in the gastric antrum due to heterotopic pancreatic tissue (arrow). No central niche was visible in any projection. *C*, Photograph of the resected specimen showing a submucosal mass with a prominent central niche. *D*, Low-power photomicrograph showing a submucosal nodule composed of pancreatic cells arranged in a typical acinar pattern.

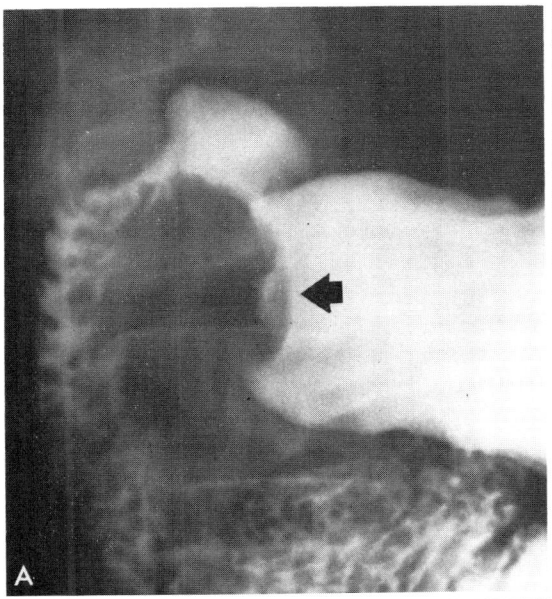
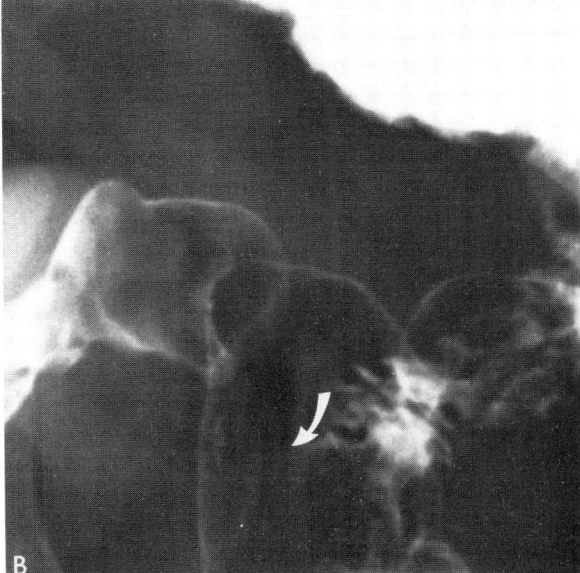
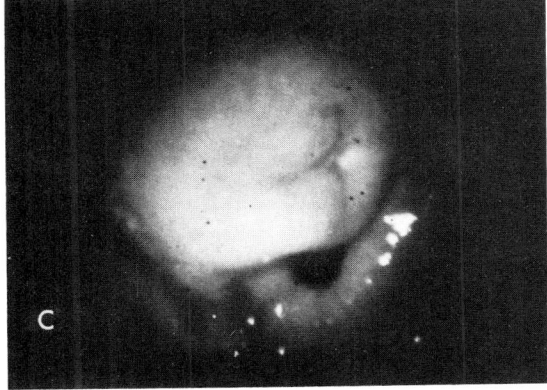

Figure 10–31. *A* and *B*, A smooth mural mass due to an aberrant pancreatic rest (arrow) is seen along the greater curvature of the stomach. A central niche is evident. *C*, Photograph of the pancreatic rest taken through the gastroscope.

aberrant pancreatic rests of the stomach describe a small usually round or oval mass that is sharply marginated and broad-based (Figs. 10–29 to 10–31). The mass is usually located along the greater curvature of the stomach, often in the prepyloric area, and always within 6 cm of the pyloric canal. The detection of a barium-filled niche or pit at the center of the lesion, representing a dimple leading to a ductal system, permits the specific diagnosis of heterotopic pancreatic tissue. The diameter of the orifice varies from 1 to 5 mm, and its depth varies from 5 to 10 mm.

In a review of 20 cases of pancreatic rests involving the stomach, Kilman and Berk confirmed that the typical finding is a smooth mass along the greater curvature or posterior wall of the stomach in the distal antrum or prepyloric area.[5] However, their study showed that heterotopic pancreatic tissue produces a broader spectrum of radiologic findings than previously supposed. In their series, more than twice as many pancreatic rests were found in the antrum than in the prepyloric area, and two of the antral lesions were more than 6 cm from the pyloric canal. Furthermore, the mass in 40 per cent of the cases appeared more sessile than broad-based and resembled a gastric polyp more than an intramural tumor. The mass was larger than 2 cm in almost half of the cases. More than half the lesions (55 per cent) did not have a

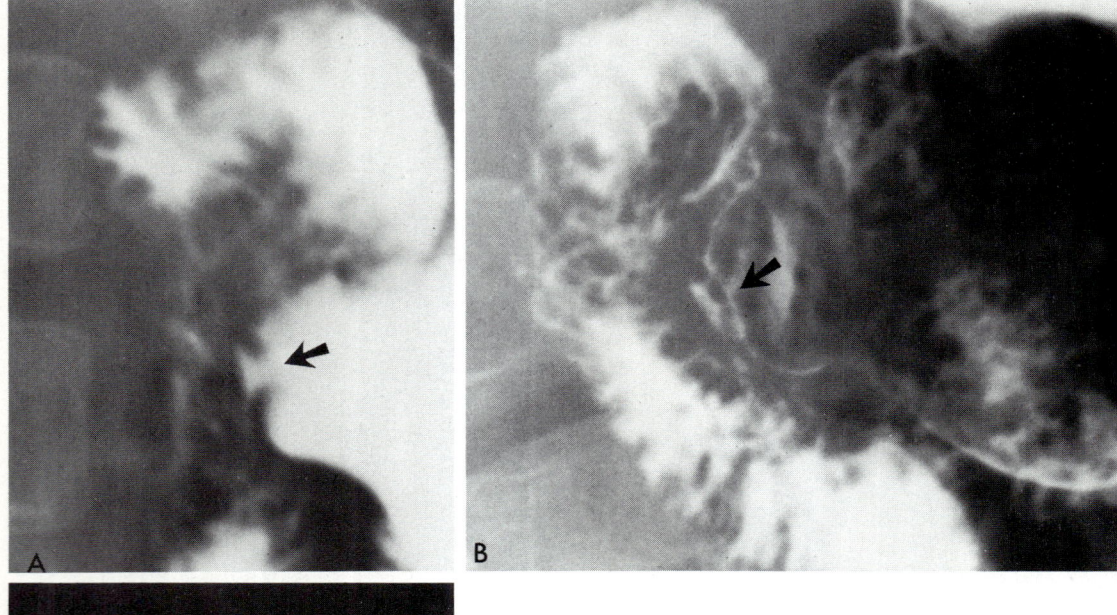
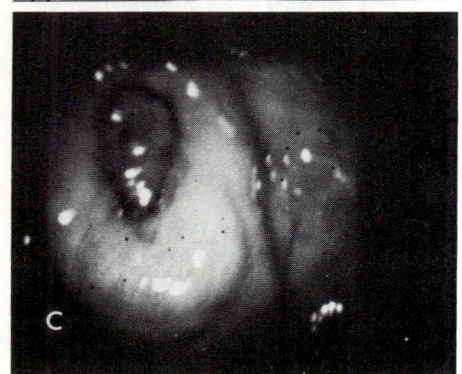

Figure 10–32. *A* and *B*. There is a persistent collection of barium along the greater curvature of the antrum due to an aberrant pancreatic rest with an unusually prominent central niche (arrow). *C*. Photograph made through the gastroscope showing the pancreatic rest.

central niche. Only 20 per cent of the cases had a small central umbilication, which could be considered typical. The umbilication in five of the cases was large in relation to the mass, resembling a healed gastric ulcer or an ulcerating intramural tumor. One patient had heterotopic pancreatic tissue with an unusually deep central umbilication that extended outside the gastric lumen (Fig. 10–32).

GASTRITIS

In the past, the diagnosis of gastritis was notoriously imprecise because of the poor correlation between radiographic and pathologic findings. Now, with improvements in gastroscopic techniques and the ability to perform a biopsy of the mucosa through the gastroscope, a more accurate diagnosis is possible.

It must be understood that the rugal folds seen radiographically include the lamina propria, the muscularis mucosa, and a variable portion of the submucosa, as well as the epithelium. Consequently, the folds often fail to reflect an abnormality even when gastritis is extensive. The thickness of the folds correlates well with the amount of acid secreted.[9] As a result, in many patients hypersecretion can be predicted when prominent rugal folds are detected.

Gastritis is usually classified according to whether the disease is acute or chronic. Acute gastritis may be bacterial (phlegmonous), corrosive, or erosive (acute hemorrhagic).[12] Chronic gastritis includes atrophic and hypertrophic gastritis (Ménétrier's disease) and granulomatous diseases such as Crohn's disease, syphilis, tuberculosis, and eosinophilic gastritis.

Erosive gastritis is a common cause of massive hematemesis and is usually seen in acutely ill patients, such as those with shock, uremia, sepsis, or trauma. Other predisposing factors include alcohol and a variety of drugs, such as acetylsalicylic acid, indomethacin, and steroids. The diagnosis is usually made gastroscopically, although bleeding can be detected angiographically. Because the ulcers are superficial, they are rarely detected by conventional barium studies of the stomach. Air-contrast techniques using effervescent powders and improved barium preparations allow more detailed evaluation of the gastric mucosa, however, so that even superficial erosions may be visible (Fig. 10–33).[6] The erosion may appear as flat, linear streaks, dots of barium, or targetlike lesions with a central collection of barium surrounded by a radiolucent halo.

Corrosive gastritis results from accidental or suicidal ingestions of acids or alkalis. Either may produce coagulation necrosis of the stomach, but acids are more likely to do so. Alkaline compounds are usually neutralized by the acid and food present in the stomach. Tissue necrosis may lead to perforation of the stomach, chronic scarring, or obstruction. In the acute stage, radiographic examination demonstrates mucosal edema, increased irritability, spasm, and exudate in the lumen (Fig. 10–34). The antrum of the stomach is often most extensively involved, and when healing is accompanied by extensive scarring, narrowing of the antrum may simulate carcinoma.

Acute gastritis resulting from alcohol ingestion or hyperacidity with or without an associated peptic ulcer can be suspected in patients with thickened rugal folds and excessive gastric secretions (Fig. 10–35). Rarely, similar findings are caused by an acute allergic reaction, such as in patients with hypersensitivity to penicillin. In

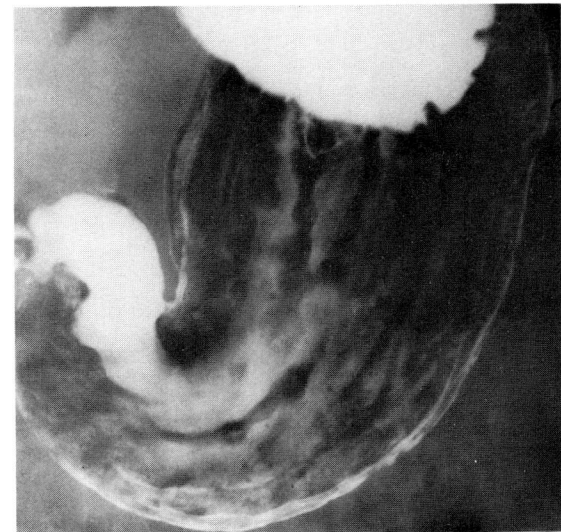

Figure 10–33. Supine air-contrast radiograph of the stomach showing multiple superficial ulcers caused by erosive gastritis.

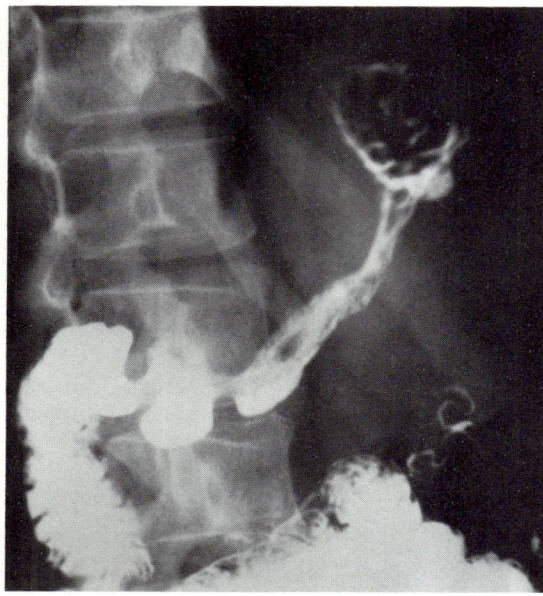

Figure 10–34. Upper gastrointestinal examination showing marked contraction of the stomach with edema of the mucosa due to acute corrosive gastritis. The patient had ingested lye one week earlier in a suicide attempt.

these cases, the response of the gastric mucosa is not unlike that of the skin and consists of urticaria, edema, and hemorrhage (Fig. 10–36).

Atrophic gastritis is a diffuse lesion of the stomach that most likely represents the endstage of chronic gastritis. It is seen regularly in patients with pernicious anemia, in whom both the mucosa and the muscularis are abnormally thin.[7] In these cases, the body and fundus of the stomach, where acid is secreted, are primarily

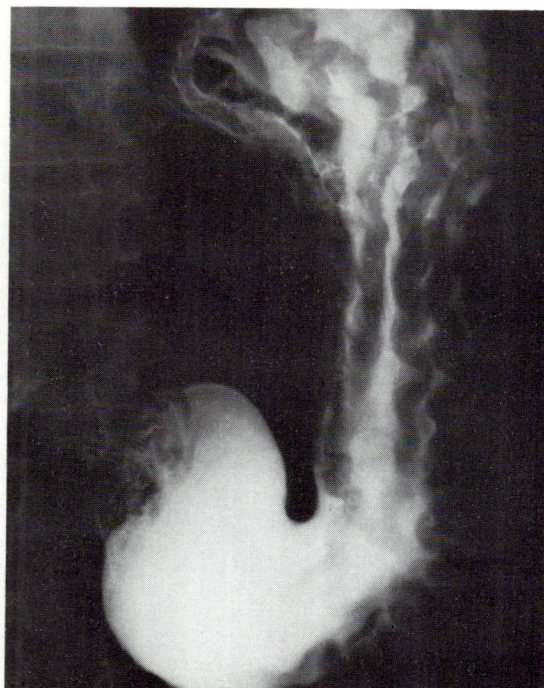

Figure 10–35. Upper gastrointestinal examination showing thickening of the rugal folds of the stomach resulting from alcoholic gastritis.

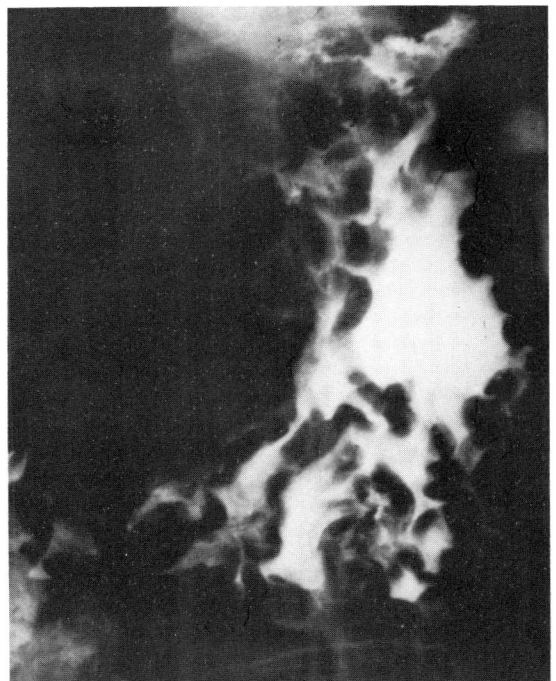

Figure 10–36. Upper gastrointestinal examination showing thickening of the gastric rugae due to an allergic reaction to penicillin. The patient had typical cutaneous manifestations of penicillin hypersensitivity. The stomach returned to normal as the cutaneous abnormalities subsided.

involved. The antrum is usually spared. Radiographically, the rugal folds are thin or absent, particularly in the fundus (bald fundus), and the stomach often assumes a tubular configuration (Fig. 10–37).

Another variety of acute gastritis is eosinophilic gastritis. Patients with this disease usually have a history of allergy, and nearly all have a marked peripheral eosin-

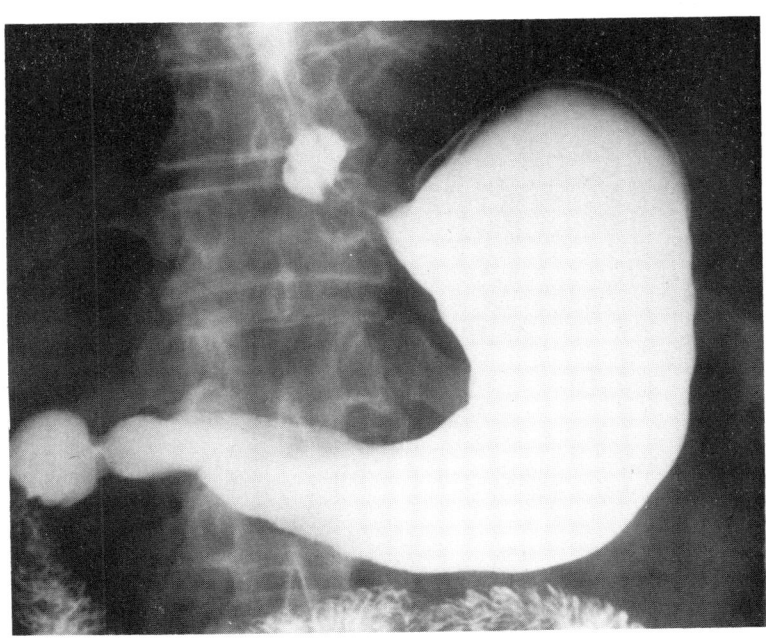

Figure 10–37. Upper gastrointestinal examination showing absence of rugal folds in the stomach, with a tubular configuration of the antrum in a patient with atrophic gastritis associated with pernicious anemia.

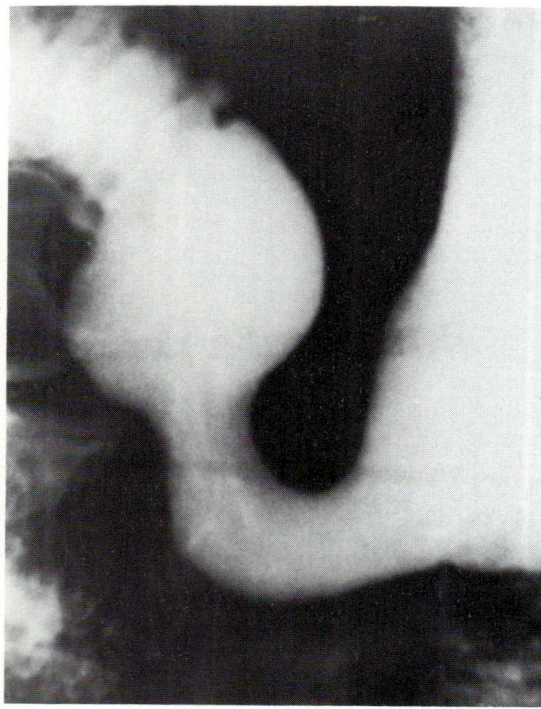

Figure 10–38. Upper gastrointestinal examination showing distortion of the antrum and pylorus due to eosinophilic gastritis.

ophilia. Infiltration of the distal portion of the stomach and proximal small intestine with eosinophils causes thickening of the rugal folds in the acute stage. The antrum is involved predominantly, so that when healing occurs the subsequent antral deformity may simulate antral carcinoma (Fig. 10–38).

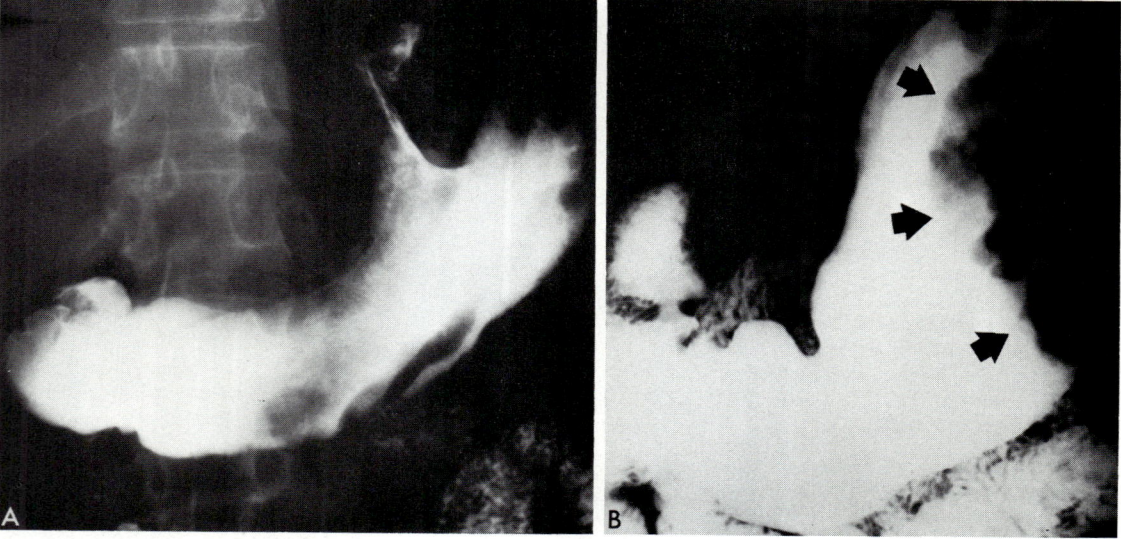

Figure 10–39. Ménétrier's disease in two patients. *A,* There are thickened rugal folds throughout the stomach. *B,* Localized enlarged rugal folds are present along the greater curvature in the proximal portion of the body of the stomach (arrows).

Ménétrier's disease is an uncommon form of gastritis of unknown origin, in which there is massive enlargement of the mucosal folds.[1] The disease is often localized, with a sharp demarcation existing between the abnormal and adjacent normal mucosa. Hypochlorhydria and protein-losing enteropathy are common but are not invariable.[11] Radiographic studies of the stomach show giant rugal folds either localized or spread throughout the stomach (Fig. 10–39). The antrum is usually, but not always, spared. Associated hypoproteinemia may cause thickening of the valvulae conniventes of the duodenum and jejunum.

ZOLLINGER-ELLISON SYNDROME

In 1955 Zollinger and Ellison described a syndrome characterized by markedly elevated rates of gastric acid secretion, severe recurrent peptic ulcers, and non-beta islet cell tumors of the pancreas.[13] The tumors that secrete gastrin, a potent stimulant of gastric acid secretion, are usually solitary, although multiple lesions are not uncommon. Sixty per cent are malignant, 30 per cent are adenomatous, and 10 per cent are hyperplastic. In one fourth of the cases the syndrome is associated with adenomas or hyperplasia in other endocrine glands (multiple endocrine adenoma syndrome).

The radiologic features of gastric hypersecretion are striking and suggest the diagnosis of the Zollinger-Ellison syndrome, even in the absence of a peptic ulcer.

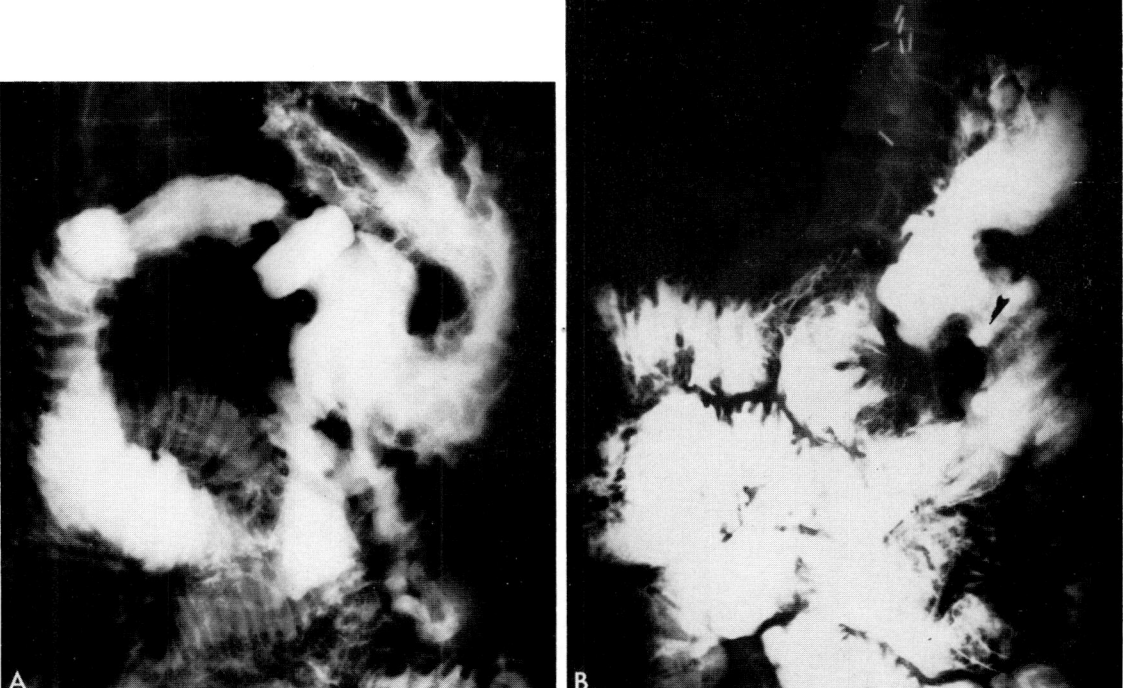

Figure 10–40. Zollinger-Ellison syndrome in two patients. *A*, Prominent rugal folds are present in the stomach and duodenum, and there are thickened valvulae conniventes in the jejunum indicative of chemical enteritis due to excessive acid secretion. The duodenal loop is dilated, and there are excessive secretions. *B*, The patient had a Billroth II hemigastrectomy. There is a marginal ulcer at the anastomosis (arrow) and edema of the mucosa of the stomach and small bowel.

These include fluid in the stomach despite an overnight fast, thickened rugal folds in the stomach and duodenum, dilatation of the second portion of the duodenum, edema and excessive fluid in the jejunum, and hypermotility (Fig. 10–40). The ulcers may be single or multiple, sometimes occur in unusual locations, are refractory to medical management, recur after surgical treatment, and are frequently large and penetrating. Two thirds are located in the first portion of the duodenum, and one quarter are in the jejunum distal to the ligament of Treitz.

GASTRIC DILATATION

Although acute dilatation of the stomach usually develops after surgery, it also occurs in association with a variety of acute and chronic infectious diseases, trauma, childbirth, and dietary indiscretion (Fig. 10–41). In these cases, prompt detection on plain abdominal radiographs is essential so that a nasogastric tube can be inserted to decompress the stomach. If gastric dilatation is not recognized early, pernicious vomiting, aspiration, and death from asphyxiation and cardiac arrest may occur. Rarely, perforation of the stomach may result.

When gastric dilatation appears following the application of a hip spica or body cast, it is known as the body-cast syndrome (Fig. 10–42).[3] Most authors attribute the dilatation to obstruction of the fourth portion of the duodenum resulting from compression by the superior mesenteric artery; yet, the point of obstruction is not routinely identified. Hyperextension and increased lumbar lordosis produced by the body cast associated with laxity of the abdominal musculature in asthenic patients cause displacement of the small intestine into the pelvis. This, in turn, produces traction on the mesentery and results in the duodenum's being compressed against

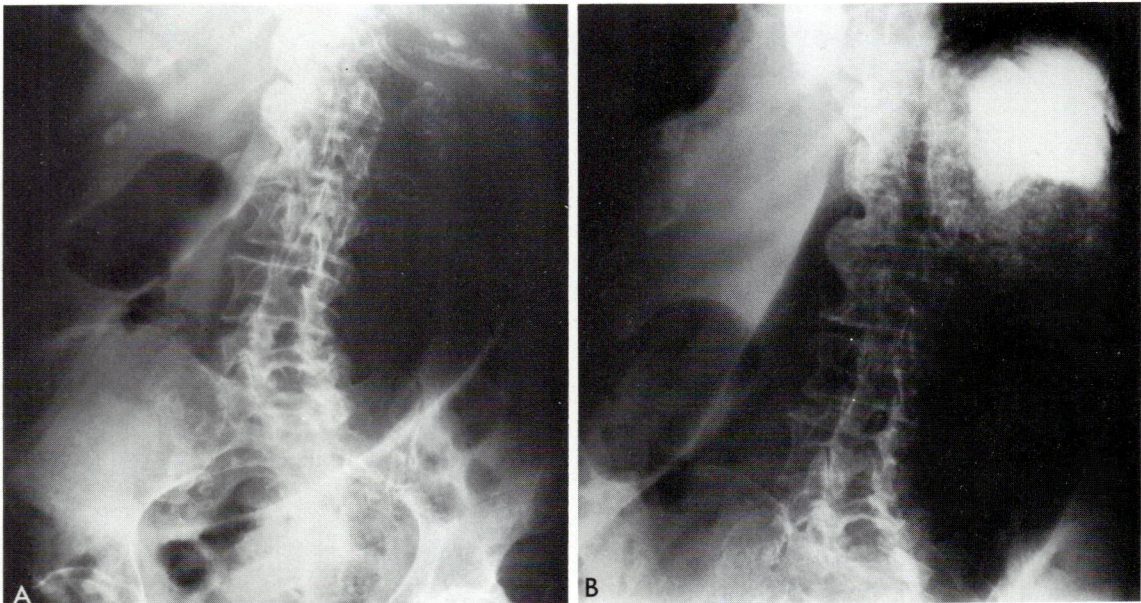

Figure 10–41. Acute gastric dilatation in a patient who had multiple fractures as a result of an auto accident. *A*, Supine projection showing the stomach filled with air. *B*, Supine projection after administration of barium identifies the stomach with certainty.

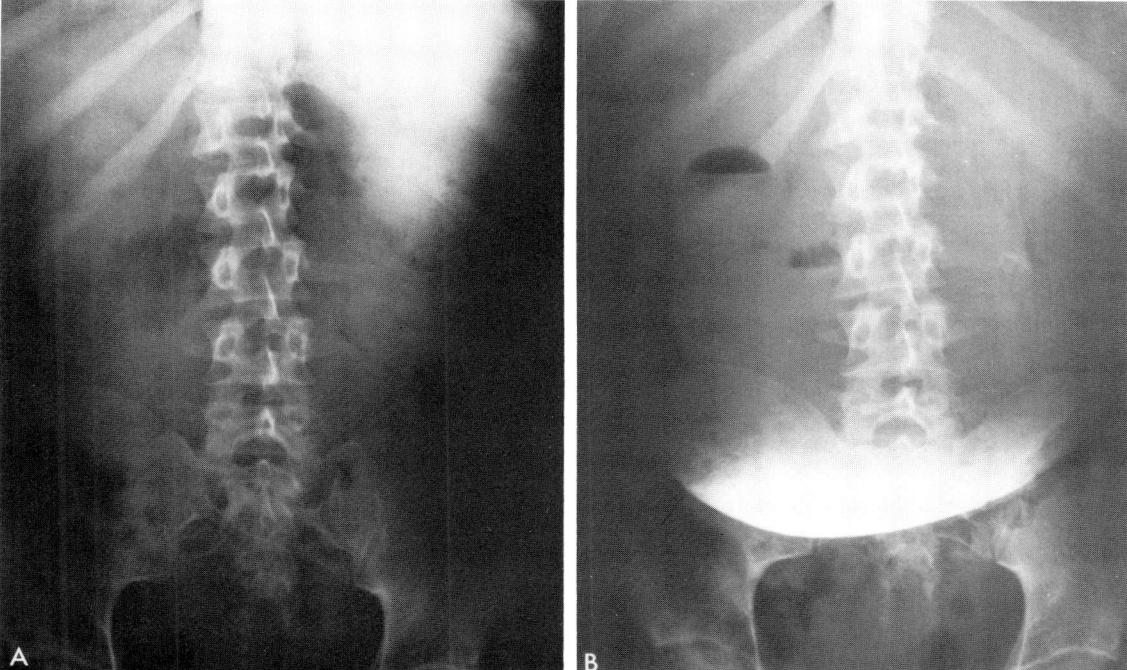

Figure 10–42. Acute gastric dilatation in a patient with the body-cast syndrome. *A*, Supine. *B*, Upright. The patient has been given a small amount of barium following removal of the body cast.

Figure 10–43. Diabetic gastropathy. Barium study shows a large amount of residue in the stomach despite an overnight fast. No organic lesion was present at the pylorus.

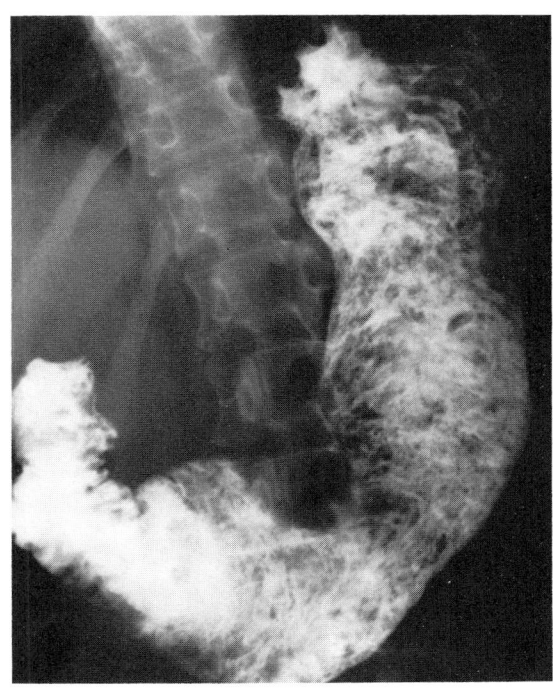

the spine by the superior mesenteric artery. Despite prompt removal of the cast, gastric dilatation may persist for some time.

Patients with diabetes mellitus may have impaired gastric emptying as a manifestation of visceral neuropathy. Radiographic examination of the stomach shows retention of food and secretions associated with diminution in peristalsis (Fig. 10–43). Pyloric obstruction can be excluded by failure to demonstrate an organic lesion at the pylorus.

MALLORY-WEISS SYNDROME

This syndrome of gastrointestinal hemorrhage is due to a nonperforating laceration of the gastroesophageal junction. Infrequently, the laceration is above or below the gastroesophageal junction. It is usually the result of forceful vomiting and is often associated with excessive alcoholic intake. Hematemesis is the usual presenting symptom; all degrees of severity of bleeding can occur.

Endoscopy is the most reliable method of diagnosis when active bleeding has diminished or ceased. Barium studies are usually unrevealing, although rarely a submucosal barium collection can be identified (Fig. 10–44).

During severe active bleeding, celiac arteriography discloses extravasation of the

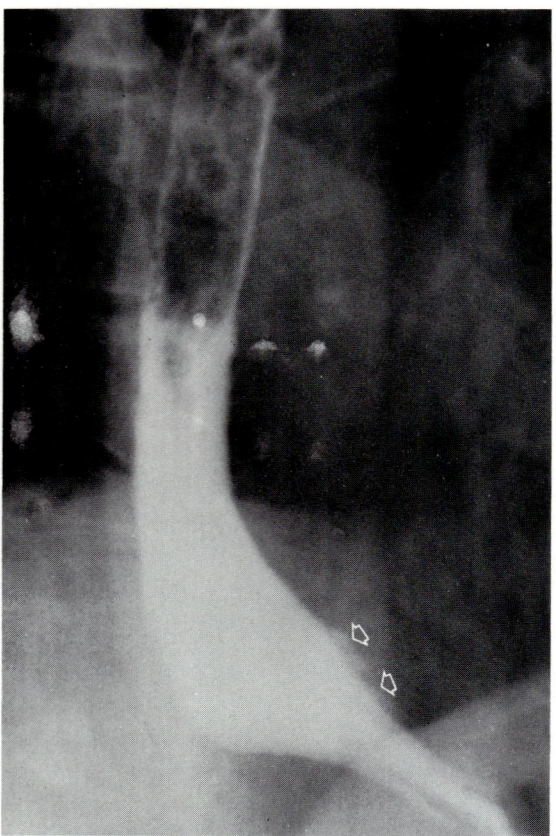

Figure 10–44. Mallory-Weiss syndrome. Esophagogram in a patient with hematemesis after a bout of vomiting reveals a collection of barium in the wall of the esophagus (arrows). Endoscopy confirmed the presence of a linear tear in the esophageal mucosa at the esophagogastric junction. (The tear is only rarely identified on barium studies.)

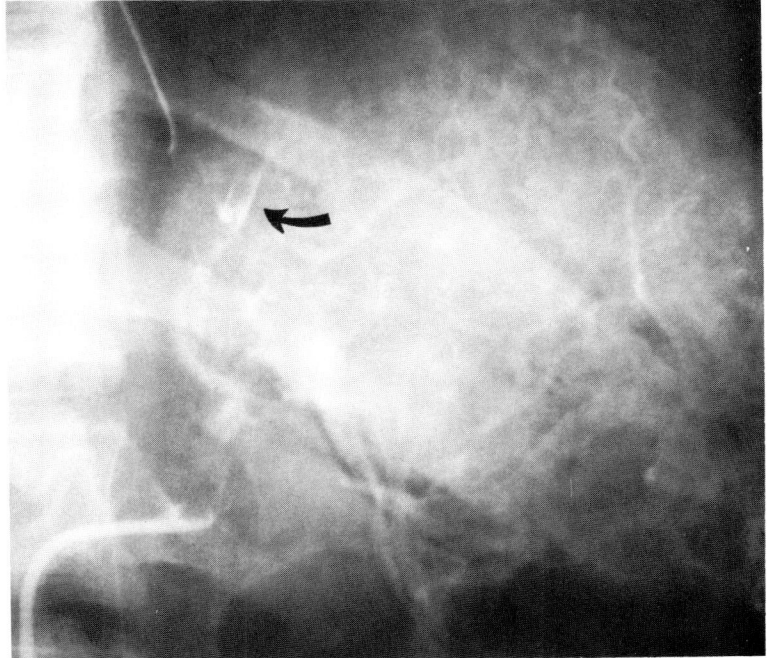

Figure 10–45. Angiogram in a patient with the Mallory-Weiss syndrome. Late phase of a selective splenic arteriogram shows extravasation of contrast material in the stomach in the vicinity of the esophagogastric junction (arrow).

contrast material into the lumen in the vicinity of the gastroesophageal junction (Figs. 10–45 and 10–46).

The bleeding stops spontaneously in most cases, but if it is persistent or recurrent intra-arterial infusion of vasopressin may be employed. Surgical intervention is only rarely necessary (see postemetic perforation of the esophagus [Boerhaave's syndrome], p. 368).[1]

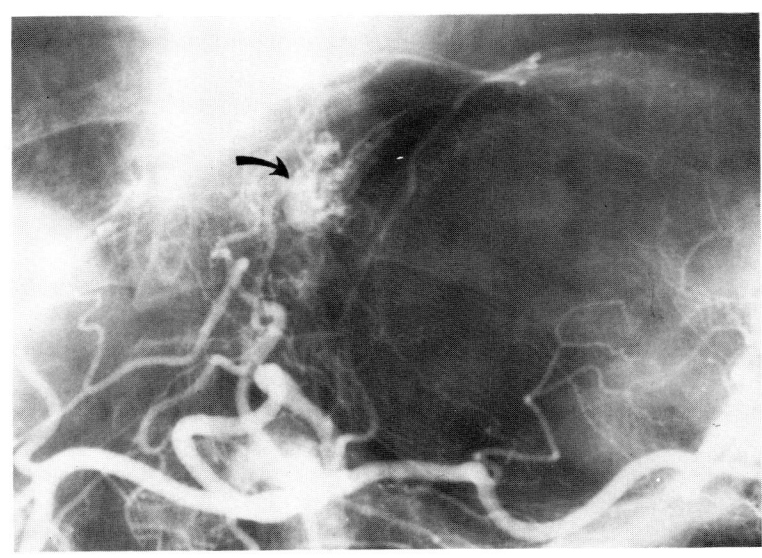

Figure 10–46. Celiac angiogram in a patient with the Mallory-Weiss syndrome. During the arterial phase, extravasation of contrast material (arrow) is evident near the esophagogastric junction.

VOLVULUS OF THE STOMACH

Twisting of the stomach on itself may occur in association with a hiatus hernia due to laxity of the ligamentous attachments of the stomach. The volvulus may be along the longitudinal axis of the stomach (organoaxial) or at right angles to this axis (mesenteroaxial).[10] The clinical and radiologic manifestations depend on whether there is an associated obstruction, ischemia or both. In the presence of an obstruction, symptoms are catastrophic and include retching with little or no vomitus. A nasogastric tube cannot be passed, and barium examination shows tapering of the distal esophagus with obstruction. In contrast, patients with a chronic volvulus have mild symptoms, consisting of bloating, eructation, and pyrosis. Plain abdominal radiographs may show air-fluid levels in the herniated portions of the stomach. The precise anatomic configuration of the stomach can usually be identified on barium studies (Fig. 10–47).

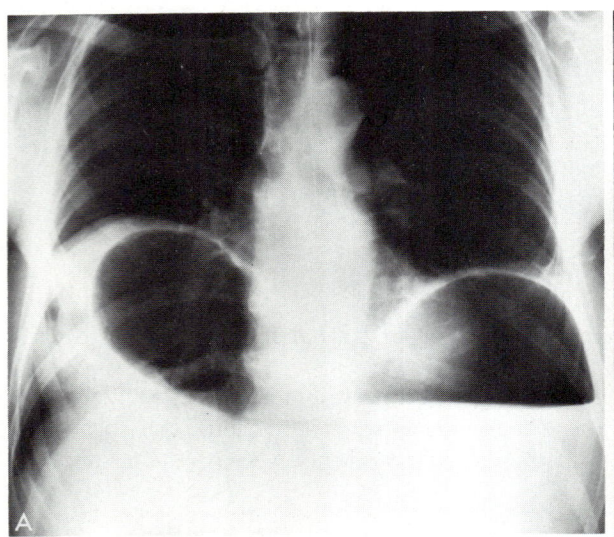
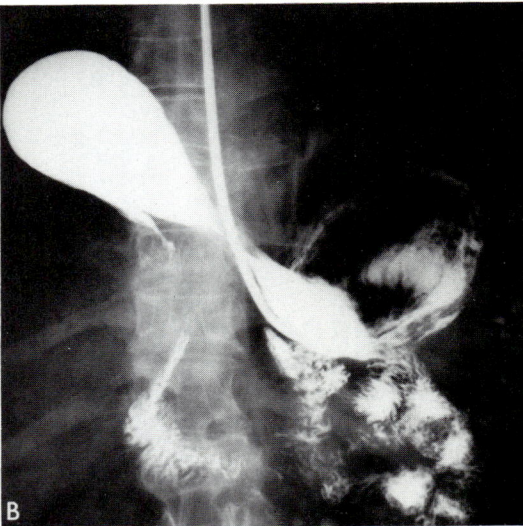
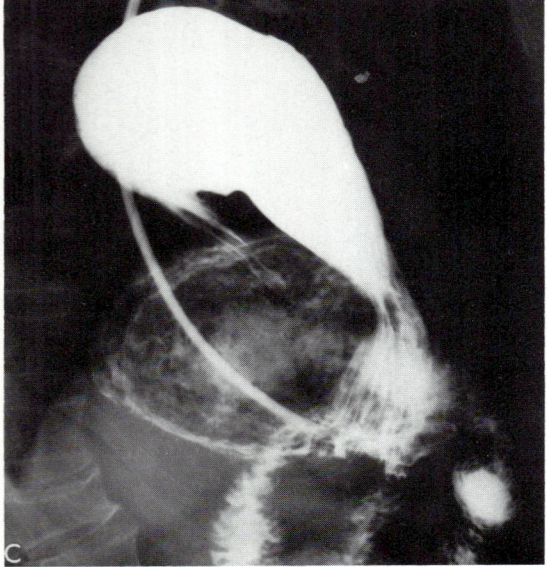

Figure 10–47. Mesenteroaxial volvulus associated with a hiatus hernia without obstruction or ischemia. *A,* Upright radiograph of the chest shows air-fluid levels in the fundus and antrum of the stomach. Frontal projection (*B*) and lateral view (*C*) show the gastric volvulus.

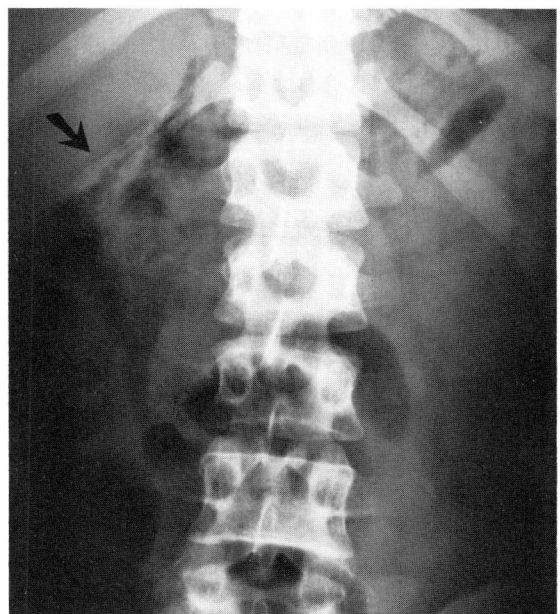

Figure 10–48. Plain abdominal radiograph shows free retroperitoneal air adjacent to the right kidney (arrow) in a patient with rupture of the duodenum due to a steering wheel injury.

DUODENAL RUPTURE (See also Chapter 11)

Because the duodenum is fixed retroperitoneally overlying the vertebral column, it is particularly susceptible to compression from blunt abdominal trauma.[4] Clinically combined injury of the pancreas and duodenum has a grave prognosis because of the deleterious effect of the pancreatitis on healing of the duodenal rupture.

Plain abdominal radiographs usually show retroperitoneal free air. This may appear as streaks or bubbles of gas around the kidney and along the right psoas margin (Fig. 10–48). The gas may dissect into the groin or mediastinum or enter the intraperitoneal space. Barium studies may disclose complete obstruction of the duodenum or an intramural mass due to a hematoma in the duodenal wall.

References

1. Baum, S., Nusbaum, M., et al.: Mallory-Weiss syndrome. Surgery 58:797, 1965.
2. Berensen, M. M., Sannella, J., and Freston, J. W.: Ménétrier's disease. Gastroenterology 70:257–263, 1976.
3. Berk, R. N., and Coulson, D. B.: The body cast syndrome. Radiology 94:303–305, 1970.
4. Eaton, S. R., and Ferrucci, J. T.: Radiology of the Pancreas and Duodenum. Philadelphia, W. B. Saunders Company, 1973, pp. 331–337.
5. Kilman, W. J.: The spectrum of radiographic features of aberrant pancreatic rests involving the stomach. Radiology 123:291–296, 1977.
6. Laufer, I., Hamilton, J., and Mullens, J. E.: Demonstration of superficial gastric erosions by double contrast radiography. Gastroenterology 68:387–391, 1975.
7. Laws, J. A., and Pitman, R. G.: The radiological features of pernicious anemia. Br. J. Radiol. 33:229–237, 1960.
8. Marshak, R. M., and Maklansky, D.: Diabetic gastropathy. Am. J. Dig. Dis. 9:366–369, 1964.
9. Moghadam, M., Gluckmann, R., and Eyler, W. R.: Radiologic assessment of gastric acid output. Radiology 89:888–892, 1967.
10. Raffin, S.: Diverticula, rupture and volvulus in gastrointestinal disease. In Sleisenger, M. H., and Fordtran, J. S. (eds.): Gastrointestinal Disease: Pathophysiology, Diagnosis, Management. Philadelphia, W. B. Saunders Company, 1973, pp. 608–616.

11. Reese, D. F.: Giant hypertrophy of the gastric mucosa (Ménétrier's disease). A correlation of the roentgenographic, pathologic and clinical findings. Am. J. Roentgenol. 88:619–626, 1962.
12. Seaman, W. B.: Non-neoplastic disease of the stomach. *In* Margulis, A. R., and Burhenne, H. J. (eds.): Alimentary Tract Roentgenology. St. Louis, The C. V. Mosby Company, 1973, pp. 589–648.
13. Zboralske, F. F., and Amberg, J. R.: Detection of Zollinger-Ellison syndrome, the radiologist's responsibility. Am. J. Roentgenol. *104:*529–543, 1968.

Part III
The Postoperative Stomach

TECHNIQUE OF EXAMINATION

The application of new air-contrast radiographic techniques to the postoperative stomach has been a major advance in the radiographic examination of the stomach after surgery. The traditional method, which depends on using a small amount of barium with appropriate compression and positioning, is difficult because of the rapid emptying of the gastric remnant and the inability to compress the remnant and the anastomosis owing to their position under the left rib cage. Consequently, the

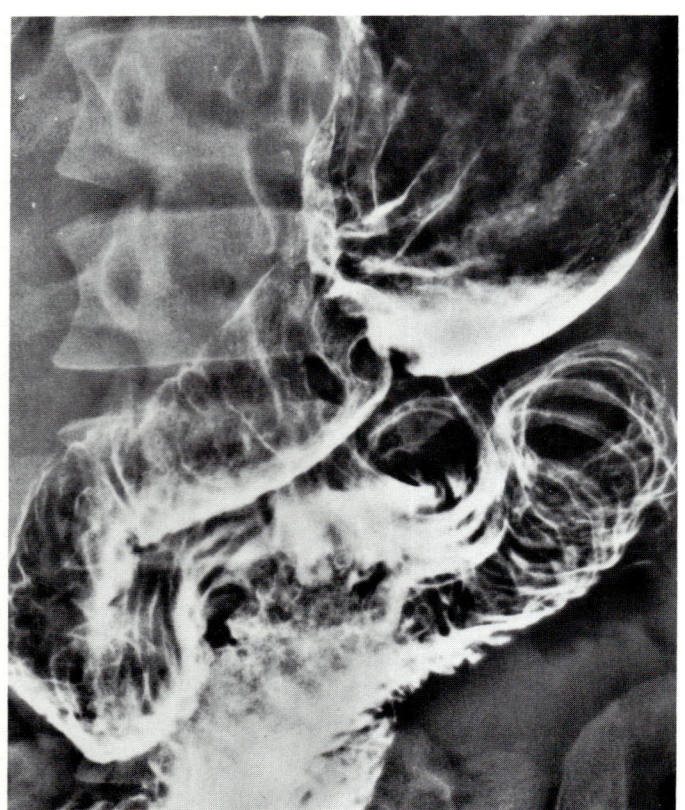

Figure 10–49. Radiographic examination of the stomach in a patient with a Billroth I hemigastrectomy using the air-contrast technique and hypotonia with glucagon. (Courtesy of R. P. Gold, M.D., and W. B. Seaman, M.D.)

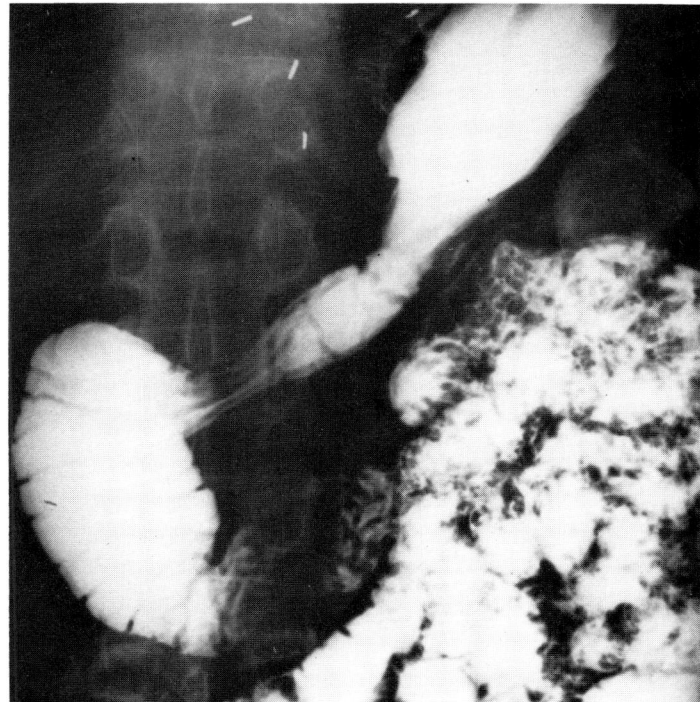

Figure 10–50. Conventional radiographic examination of the stomach in a patient with a Billroth I hemigastrectomy. Metallic clips are visible at the vagotomy site.

accuracy of the conventional examination is poor. The air-contrast technique is easier to perform, and the results are more reliable.[9]

The air-contrast procedure is performed by administering glucagon intravenously immediately before the examination to produce hypotonia of the stomach and small intestine. Double-contrast opacification of the stomach is accomplished by having the patient drink one of the improved barium preparations that coat the mucosa efficiently. This is followed by an effervescent powder and an antifoaming agent to provide gas in the stomach without bubbles. By properly positioning the patient and making serial radiographs, the gastric remnant and the afferent and efferent limbs of the anastomosis can be studied with great precision (Figs. 10–49 and 10–50). With the exception of suspected perforation or anastomotic rupture, there are no contraindications to the use of gastrointestinal hypotonia, distention, and barium coating of the mucosa.[9]

Burhenne emphasizes the importance of evaluating all of the basic components of gastric surgery when the postoperative patient is studied radiographically.[2] These include the extent of the gastric resection, the type of surgery, the size of the stoma, the rate of gastric emptying, the length of the afferent loop, and the direction of gastric emptying.

ANATOMY OF THE POSTOPERATIVE STOMACH

The most common types of surgical procedures involving the stomach include the Billroth I gastroduodenostomy, the Billroth II gastrojejunostomy, and pyloroplasty. In the first of these, a hemigastrectomy is performed and continuity is maintained between the stomach and duodenum by anastomosis of the stomach with the duodenum (Figs. 10–49 and 10–50). In the Billroth II procedure, the duodenal stump is closed and an anastomosis is made between the stomach and the jejunum (Fig. 10–51). The entire incised end of the stomach may be used for the anastomosis (the Pólya procedure), or only a portion of the lumen may be used for the anastomosis and the remainder closed (Hofmeister modification). The pyloroplasty is a technique used to widen the pyloric canal. The Whipple procedure consists of a hemigastrectomy with a gastrojejunostomy, a choledochojejunostomy, and a partial pancreatectomy (Fig. 10–52).

Several types of plication defects may be seen radiographically following Billroth I and II hemigastrectomies (Fig 10–53). These result from invagination of tissue adjacent to a suture line. The most striking of these is the Hofmeister defect, in which the plicated tissue at the margin of the gastrojejunostomy creates a bulky intraluminal mass often simulating a polypoid tumor.[8] Occasionally, a mass can be found in the duodenal stump owing to tissue inverted by the closure. Some plication defects can be distinguished from a tumor only by comparison with a baseline study performed in the postoperative period.

Following pyloroplasty pouchlike "pseudodiverticula" are characteristic (Fig. 10–54).[13] A large outpouching along the greater curvature aspect of the pylorus has been termed the beagle-ear sign by Burhenne.[4] An important finding after a pyloroplasty is that the pyloric canal can no longer be identified.

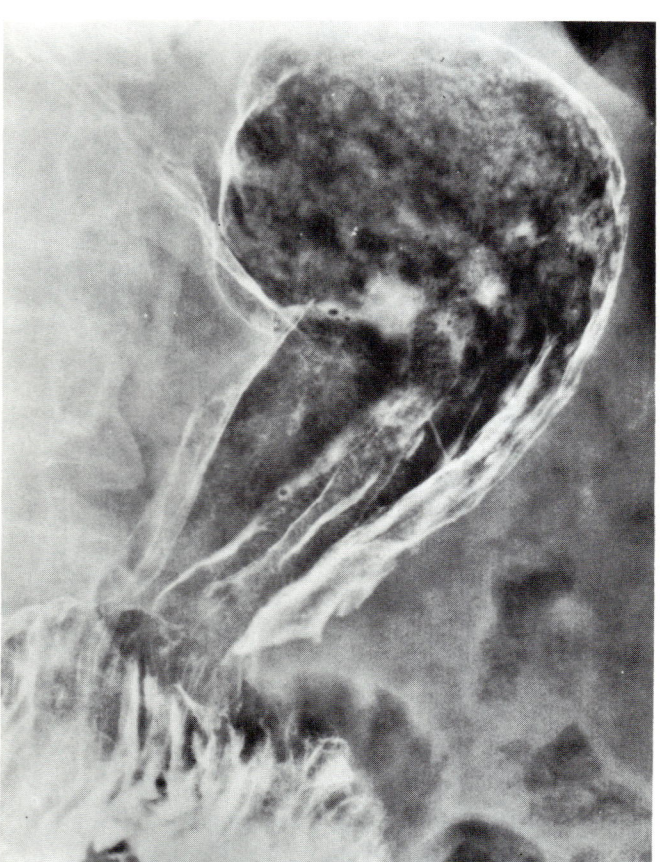

Figure 10–51. Radiographic examination of the stomach in a patient with a Billroth II hemigastrectomy using the air-contrast technique and hypotonia with glucagon. (Courtesy of R. P. Gold, M.D., and W. B. Seaman, M.D.)

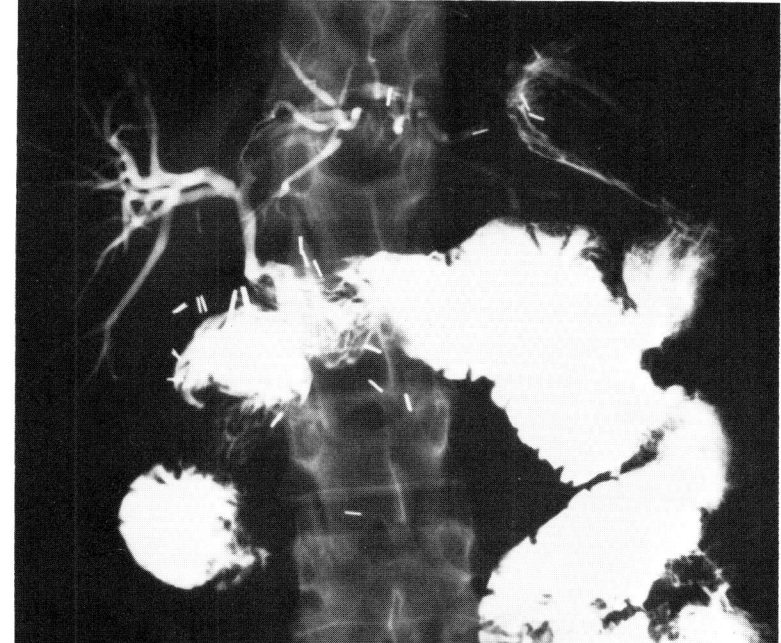

Figure 10–52. Radiographic examination of the stomach after a Whipple procedure. There is a Billroth II hemigastrectomy and a choledochojejunostomy. Barium is visible in the biliary tree.

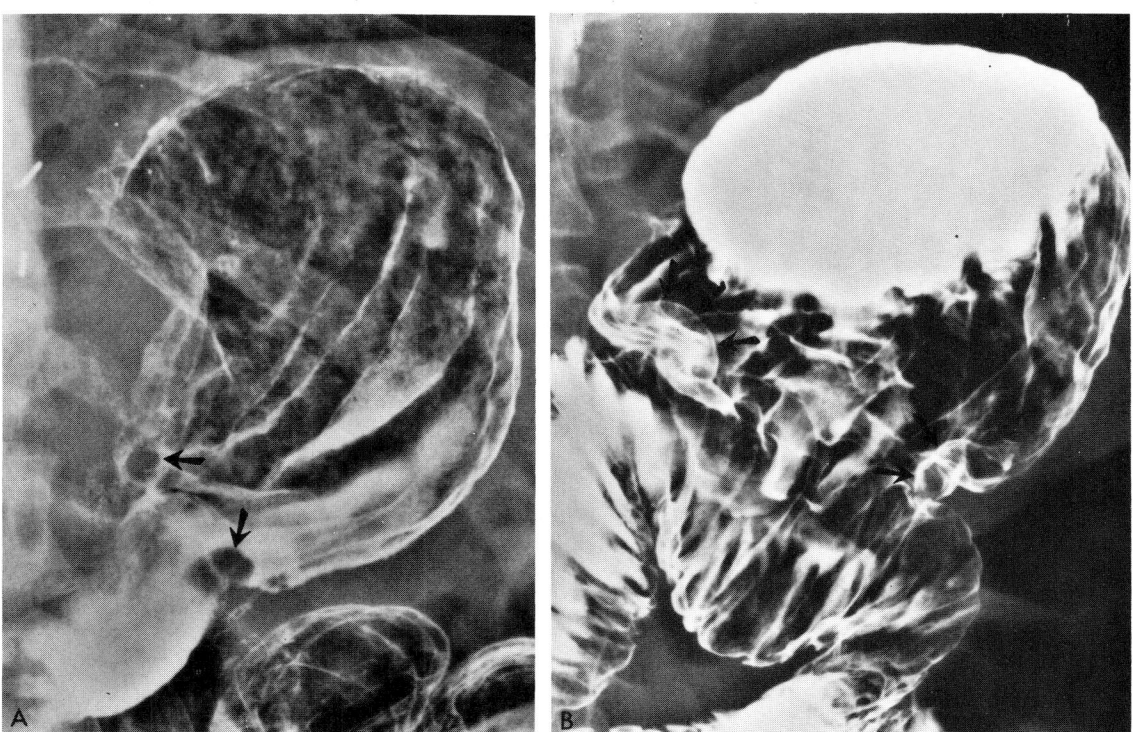

Figure 10–53. Nine examples of plication defects due to inversion of tissue at the suture line following gastric surgery. *A* and *B*, Plication defect in two patients following a Billroth II hemigastrectomy (Hofmeister modification) (arrows).

Illustration and legend continued on the following page.

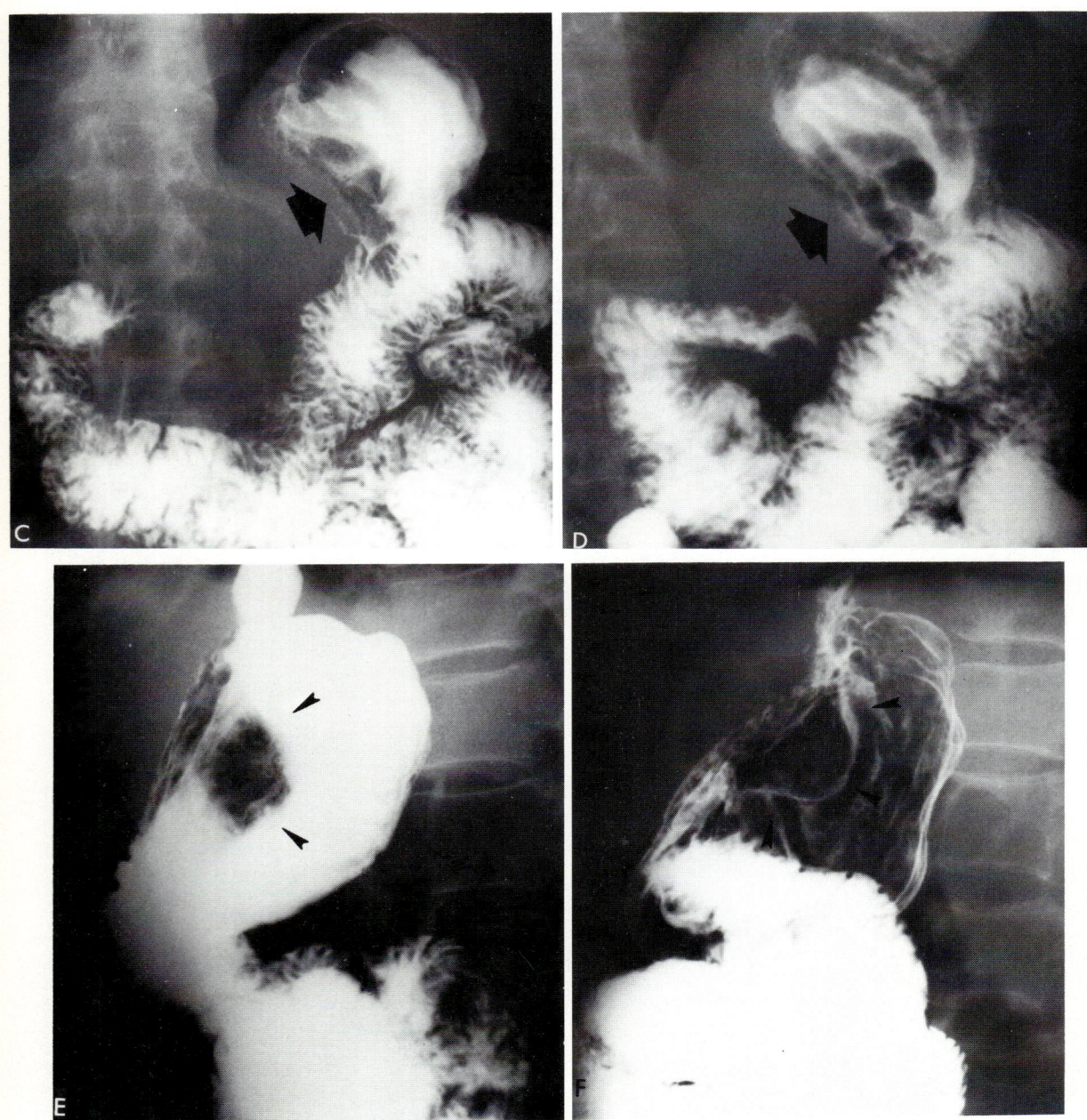

Figure 10–53. *Continued.* C to F, Large plication defects (arrows) producing a mass in the gastric wall in four additional patients with a Hofmeister type Billroth II hemigastrectomy. E and F are lateral projections.

Illustration and legend continued on the opposite page.

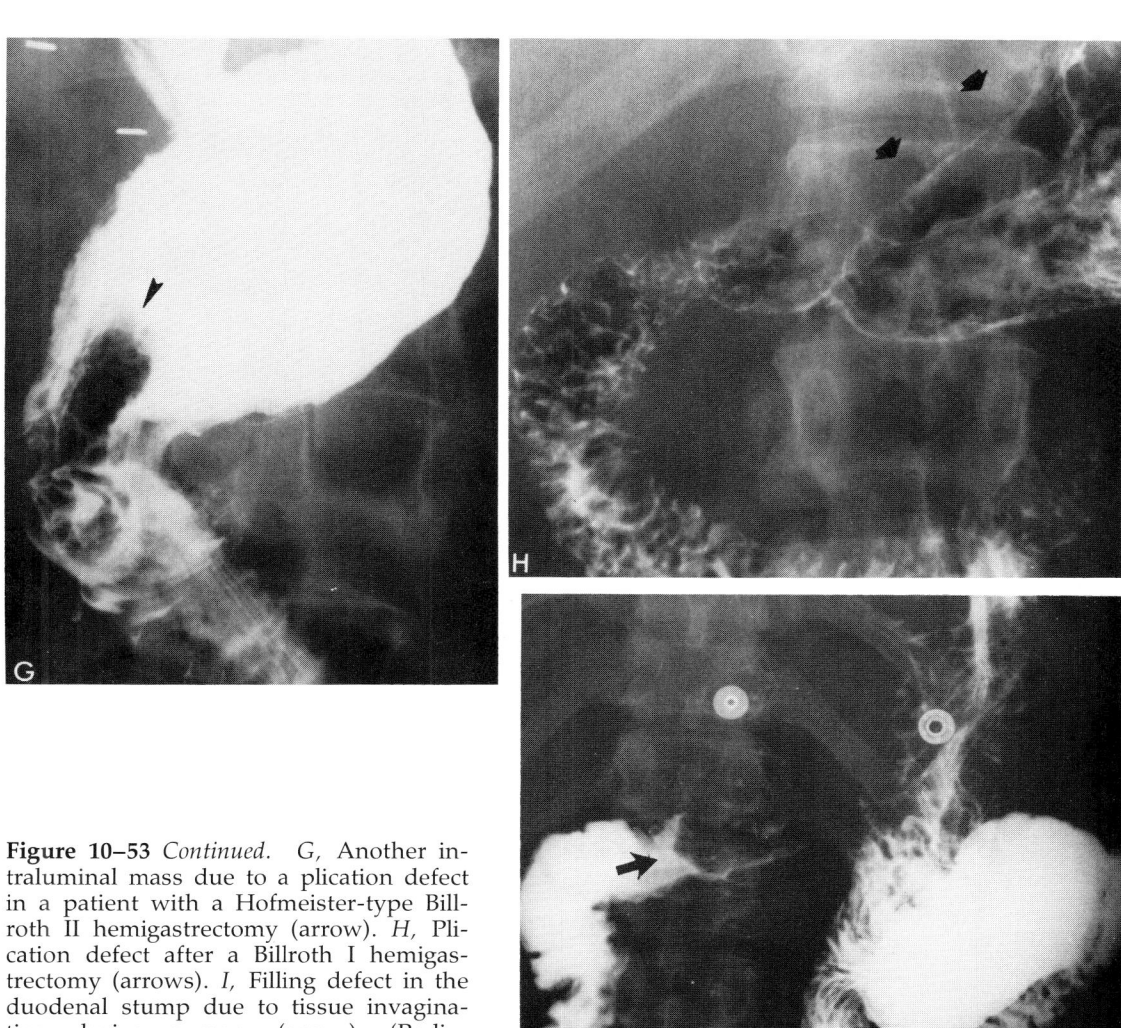

Figure 10–53 *Continued.* G, Another intraluminal mass due to a plication defect in a patient with a Hofmeister-type Billroth II hemigastrectomy (arrow). H, Plication defect after a Billroth I hemigastrectomy (arrows). I, Filling defect in the duodenal stump due to tissue invagination during surgery (arrow). (Radiographs *A* and *B* courtesy of R. P. Gold, M.D., and W. B. Seaman, M.D.)

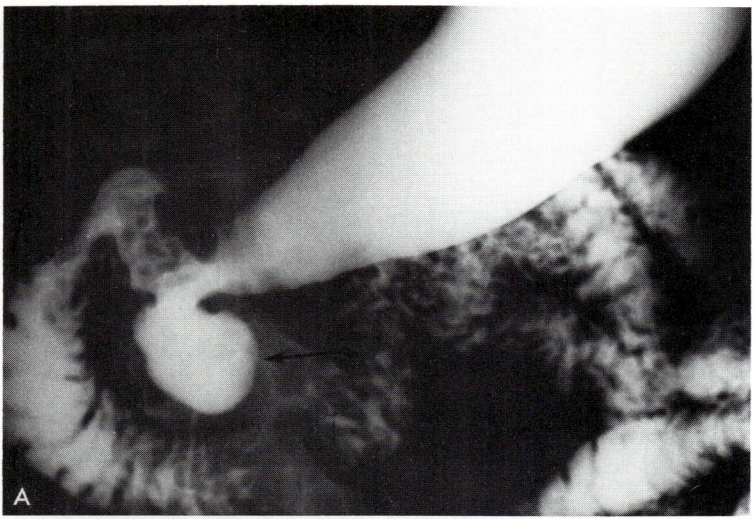

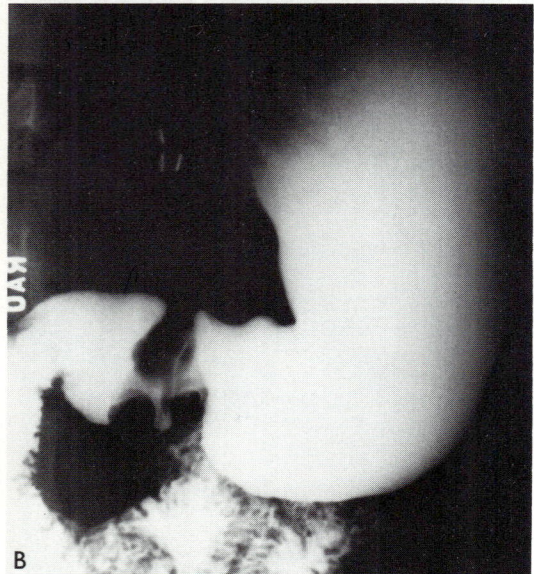

Figure 10–54. A and B, Postpyloroplasty changes in the stomach in two patients. In A, a prominent pseudodiverticulum is evident (the beagle-ear sign) (arrow).

Localized outpouches in the gastric wall simulating a gastric ulcer are often detected after removal of a gastrostomy tube (Fig. 10–55). Differentiation depends on detection of pliability in surgical defects; ulcers, by contrast are rigid.

Fundoplication procedures for the reduction of hiatus hernias create a large bulky mass in the gastric fundus on subsequent upper gastrointestinal examinations.[7] Unless the history of the surgery is known, the mass can easily be mistaken for a fundal carcinoma (Fig. 10–56).

POSTOPERATIVE COMPLICATIONS

Wound infection and intraperitoneal abscesses, general complications of abdominal surgery, are discussed elsewhere.

Figure 10–55. Localized outpouching of the greater curvature of the stomach ten years after the removal of a gastrostomy tube (arrow).

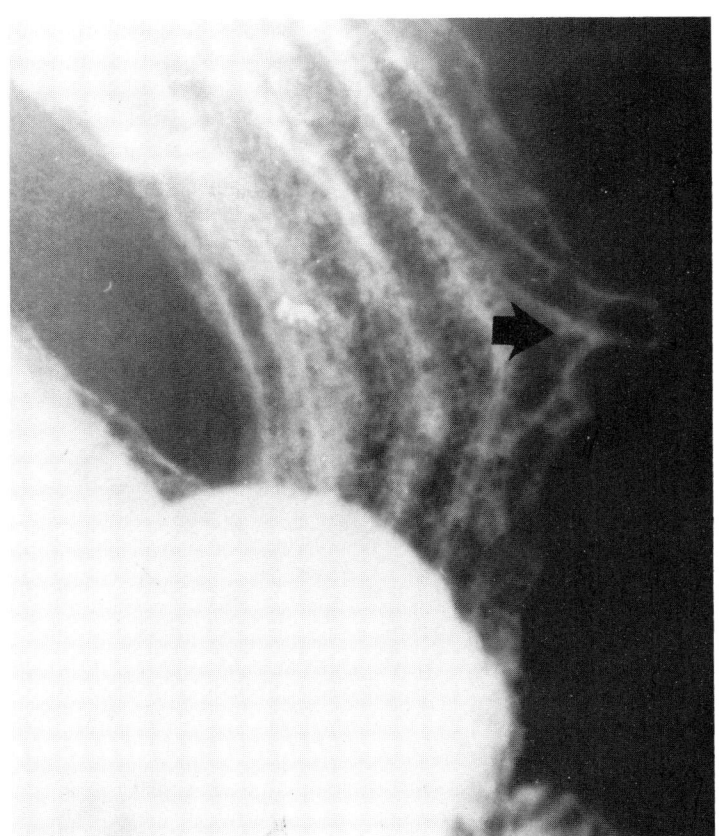

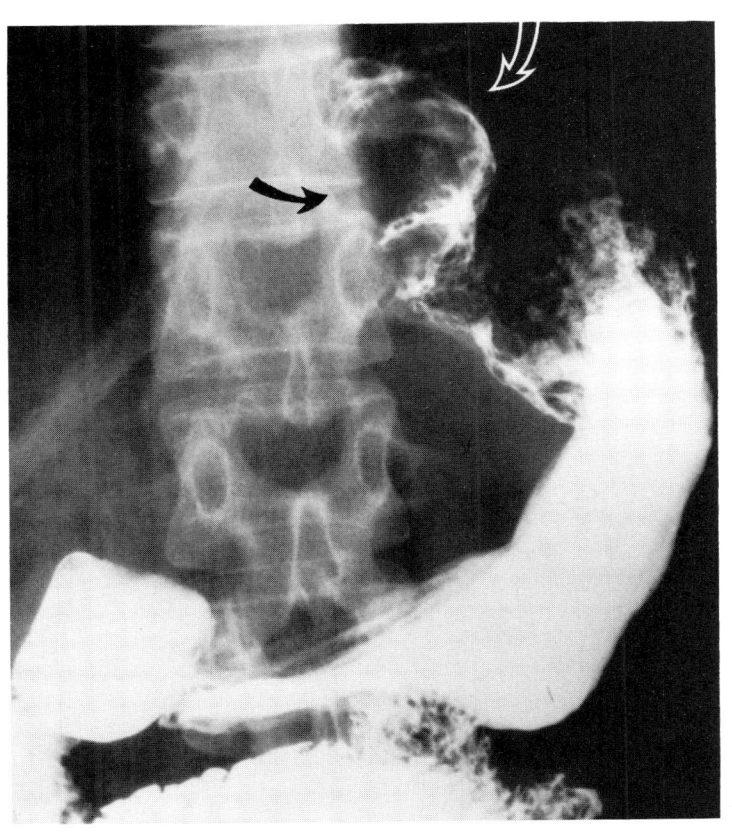

Figure 10–56. Large fundal mass created by a fundoplication procedure (arrow).

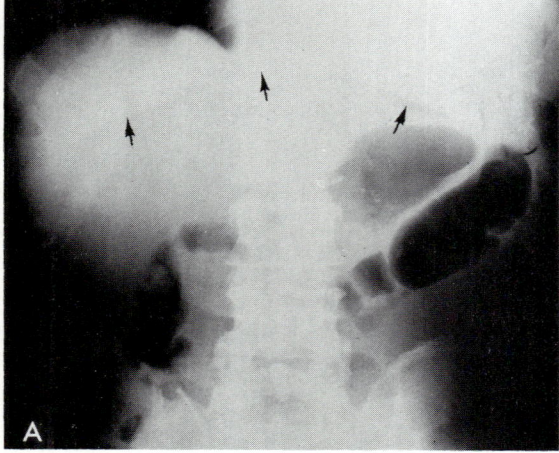
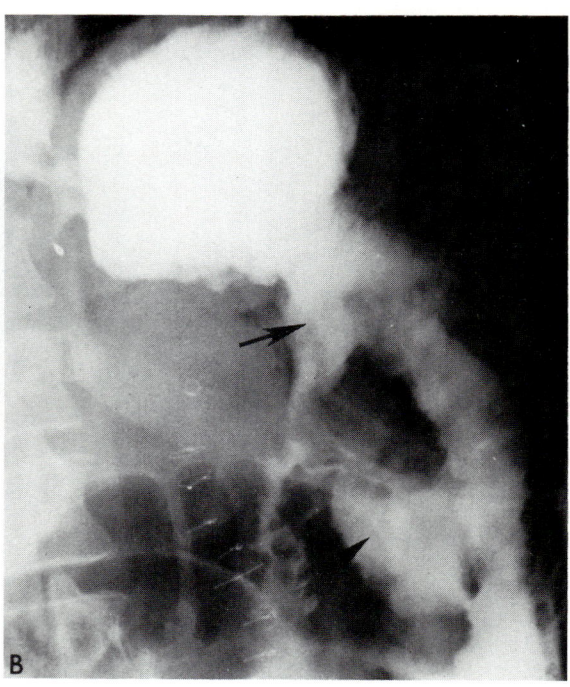

Figure 10–57. Leaking anastomosis one month after Billroth II hemigastrectomy. *A.* Supine plain abdominal radiograph shows free air in the lesser sac (arrows). *B.* Examination of the stomach with water-soluble contrast material discloses a leak from the anastomotic site (arrows).

A large anastomotic leak occurring after gastric surgery can be identified when extravasation of contrast material (the water-soluble media should be used) is identified either locally or in the peritoneal cavity (Fig. 10–57). Small leaks can lead to an abscess, which may create an air-containing mass adjacent to the gastric remnant (Fig. 10–58).

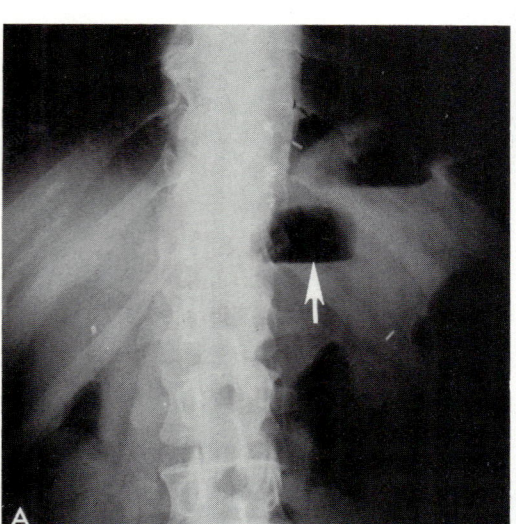
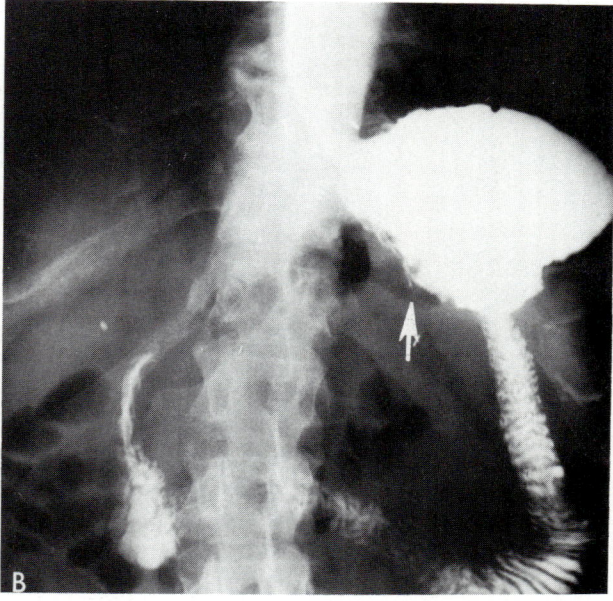

Figure 10–58. Abdominal abscess caused by a leak from the anastomosis following a Billroth II hemigastrectomy. *A*, Upright plain abdominal radiograph shows a collection of air and fluid (arrow) medial to the gastric remnant. *B*, Barium examination shows that the gas collection is extraluminal (arrow). At surgery, an abscess was found adjacent to the gastrojejunostomy with obstruction of the efferent loop.

Peptic ulceration at the anastomosis following gastric surgery (marginal or stomal ulcer) is much more common after surgery for duodenal ulcer than for gastric ulcer. The ulcer crater almost always occurs in the small bowel adjacent to the anastomosis. In patients with Billroth II procedures the ulcer occurs in the dependent portion of the efferent loop adjacent to the gastrojejunostomy. The cause of a marginal ulcer may be persistent acid secretion resulting from an incomplete vagotomy, the Zollinger-Ellison syndrome, or a retained gastric antrum.

Marginal ulcers may be difficult to demonstrate radiographically, if they are superficial or obscured by overlying loops of small bowel. Previous reports suggest that as many as 50 per cent of marginal ulcers are not recognized on upper gastrointestinal examination.[6] Improved radiographic techniques with double-contrast studies and hypotonia produced by glucagon will significantly reduce this figure.

The ulcer may be seen as a persistent collection of barium or a niche with adjacent mucosal edema (Figs. 10–59 to 10–62). Schatzki emphasized that rigidity, edema and irritability at the anastomosis are indicative of a marginal ulcer, even when the crater is not demonstrated.[10]

A marginal ulcer may penetrate the jejunal wall and erode into the adjacent portion of the colon, producing a jejunal-colic fistula (Fig. 10–63). This can cause pain, nausea, vomiting, and progressive weight loss from "bypass malabsorption." Radiographic diagnosis of this complication can be made on barium enema study, when there is filling of the gastric remnant or the jejunum *via* the colon. A barium meal may show the marginal ulcer and filling of the colon *via* the fistula.

Prolapse of gastric mucosa is a frequent finding following hemigastrectomy and is almost always asymptomatic (Fig. 10–64).[11] When viewed *en face* the prolapsed mucosa may simulate a tumor at the anastomosis, especially when the mucosa is superimposed on the gastric remnant.

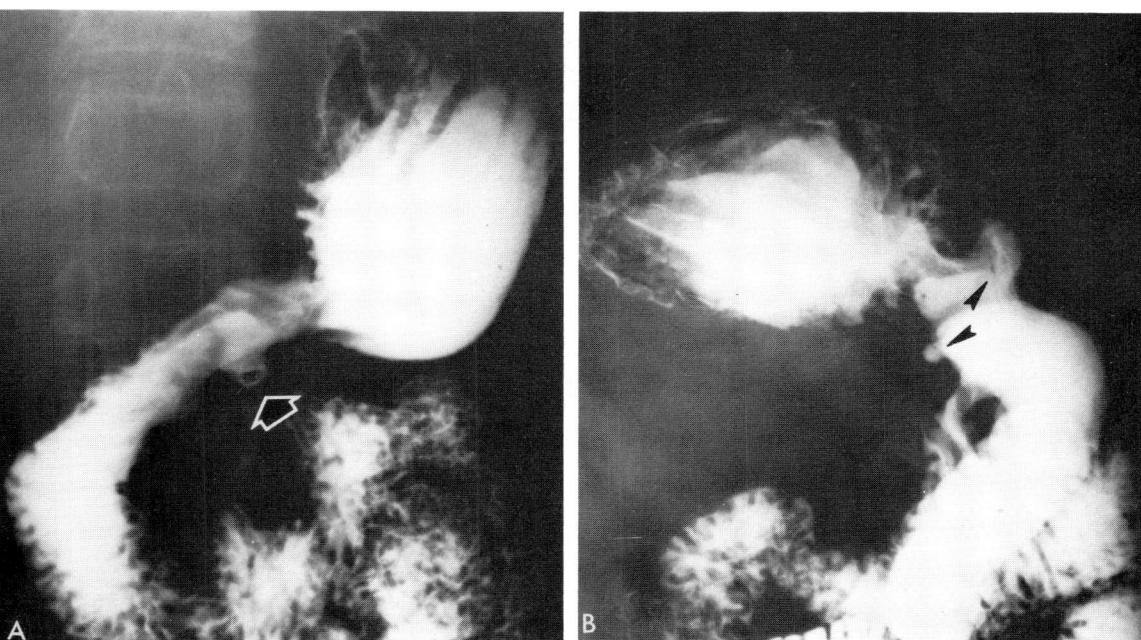

Figure 10–59. *A* and *B*, Marginal ulcers in two patients with Billroth I hemigastrectomies (arrows). Two ulcers are evident in *B*.

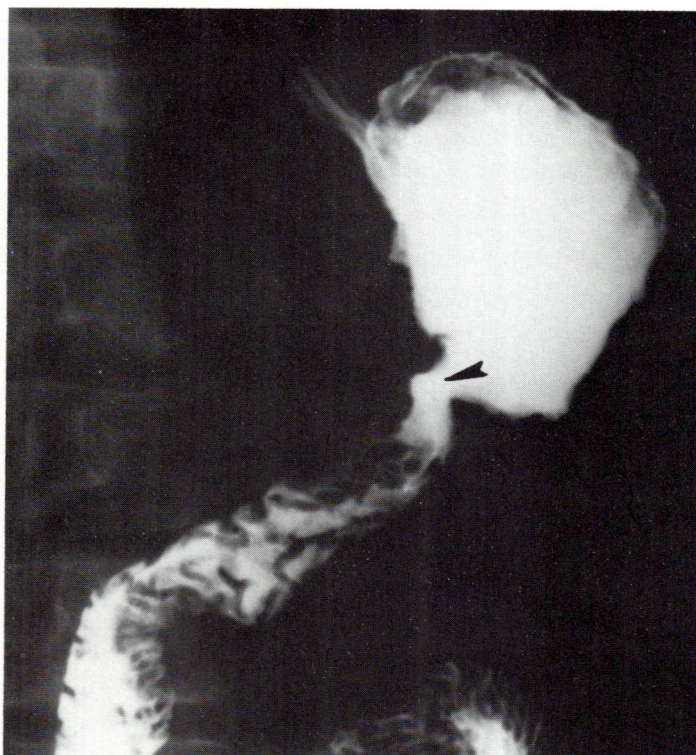

Figure 10–60. Marginal ulcer in another patient with a Billroth I hemigastrectomy (arrow).

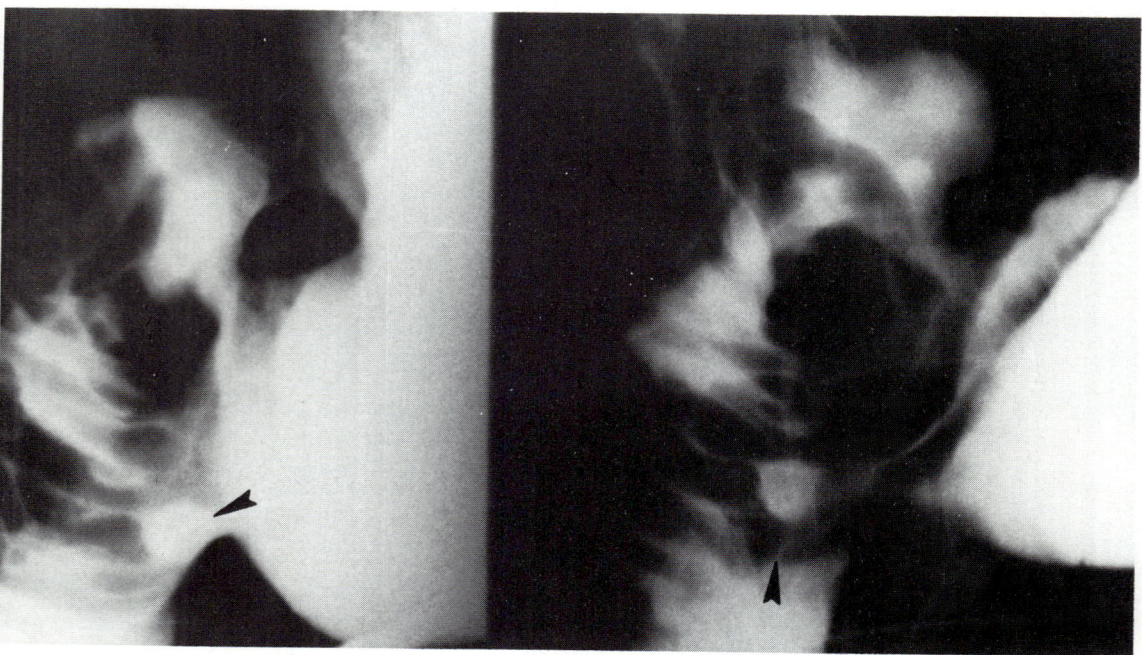

Figure 10–61. Marginal ulcer at the anastomosis after a Jabolay pyloroplasty (gastroduodenostomy) (arrows).

Figure 10–62. Two large marginal ulcers are visible in this patient following a Billroth I hemigastrectomy (arrows).

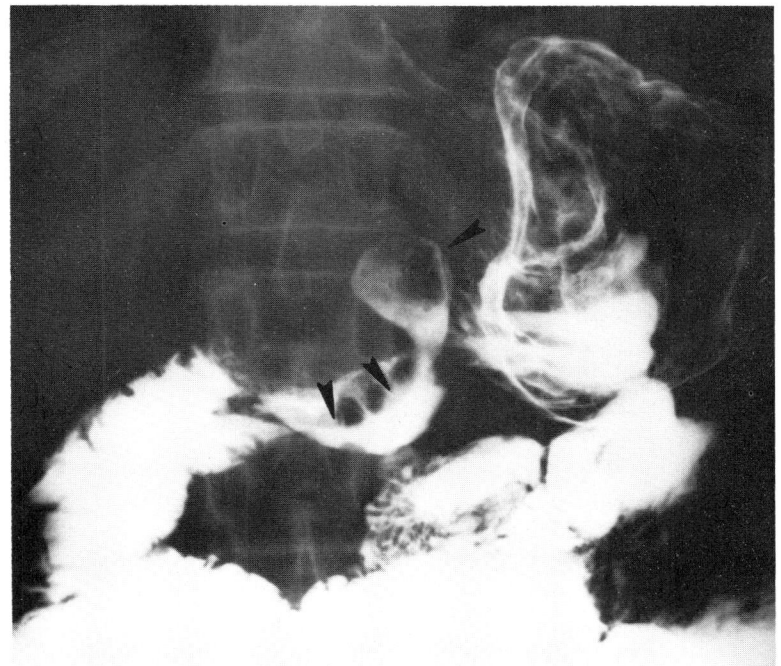

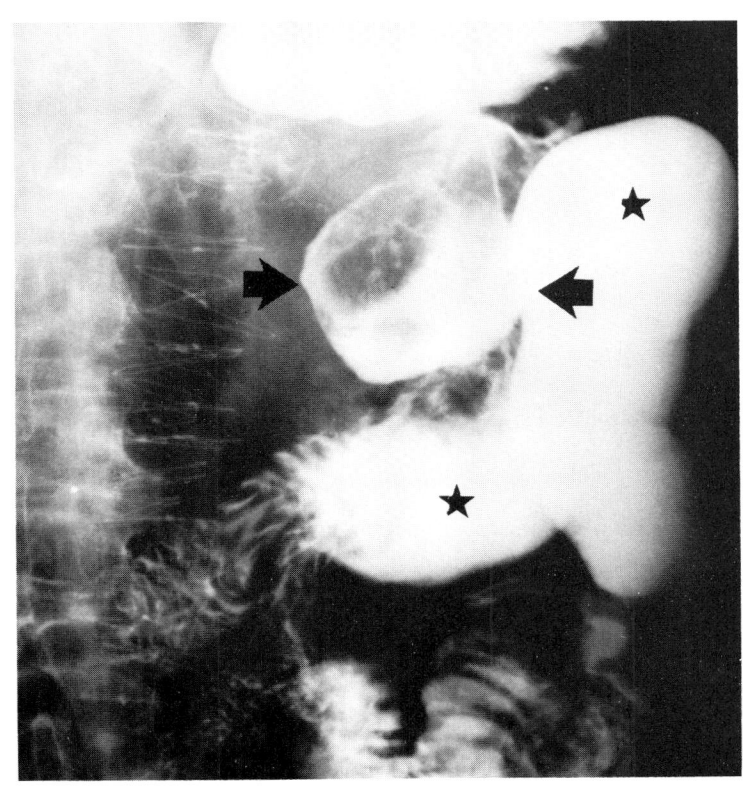

Figure 10–63. Upper gastrointestinal examination in a patient with a gastrojejunocolic fistula due to a marginal ulcer following a Billroth II hemigastrectomy. Barium is present in the gastric remnant and in the colon (stars). Barium also fills a huge marginal ulcer (arrows).

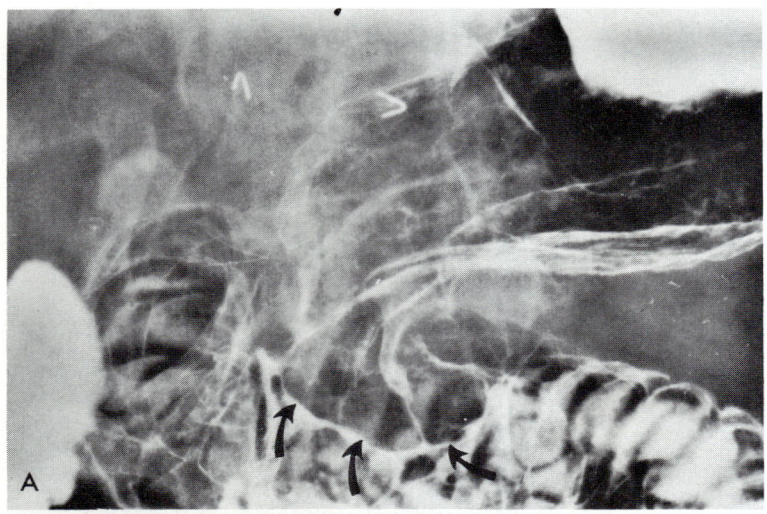

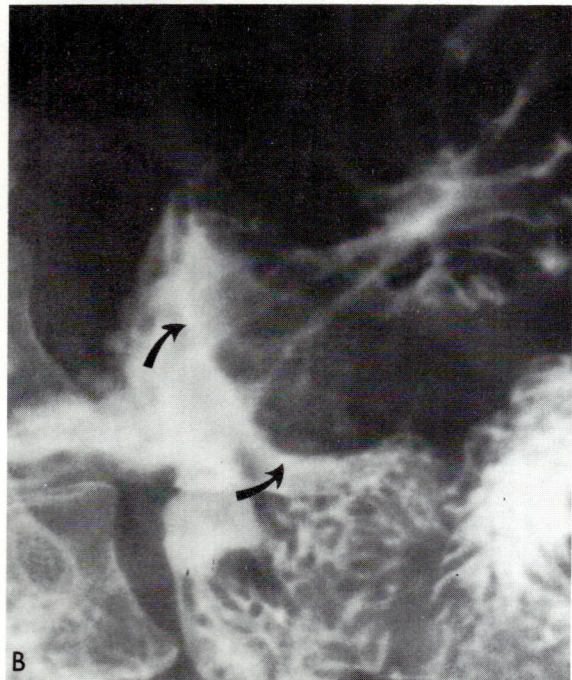

Figure 10–64. Three cases of prolapse of gastric mucosa into the small bowel following gastric surgery (arrows). A and B, Billroth II hemigastrectomy.

Illustration and legend continued on the opposite page.

Both retrograde and antegrade intussusception may occur. The jejunum invaginates into the gastric remnant in retrograde jejunogastric intussusception (Fig. 10–65). In other cases, the gastric pouch may intussuscept into the jejunum in a protograde fashion. Both varieties are usually intermittent.

Delayed gastric emptying and bezoar formation are among the most common postoperative complications following hemigastrectomy (Fig. 10–66).[12] Differentiation between retained food and a bezoar requires that the radiographic study be repeated after a 24-hour fast. The retained food will usually be passed, whereas a bezoar will persist on the subsequent examination.

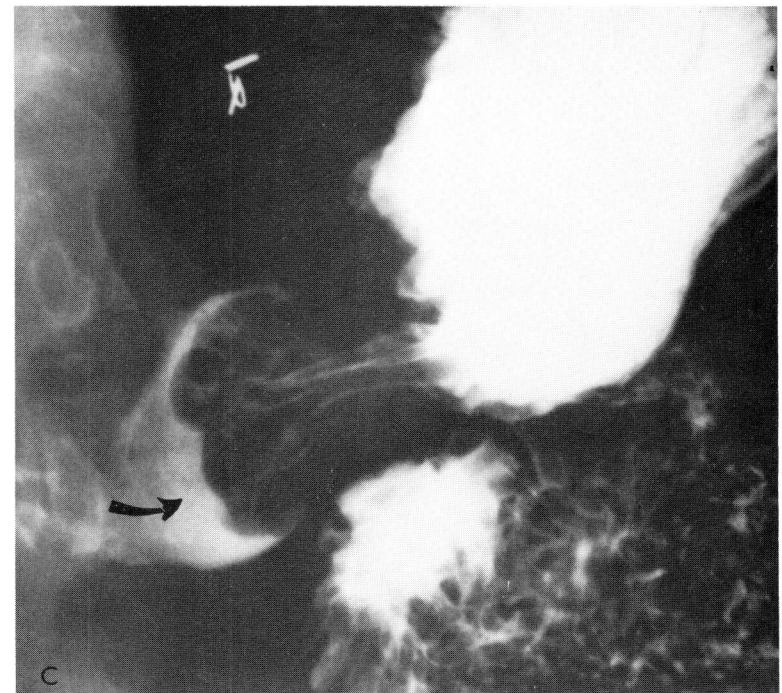

Figure 10–64. *Continued.* C, Billroth I hemigastrectomy. (Radiograph A courtesy of R. P. Gold, M.D., and W. B. Seaman, M.D.)

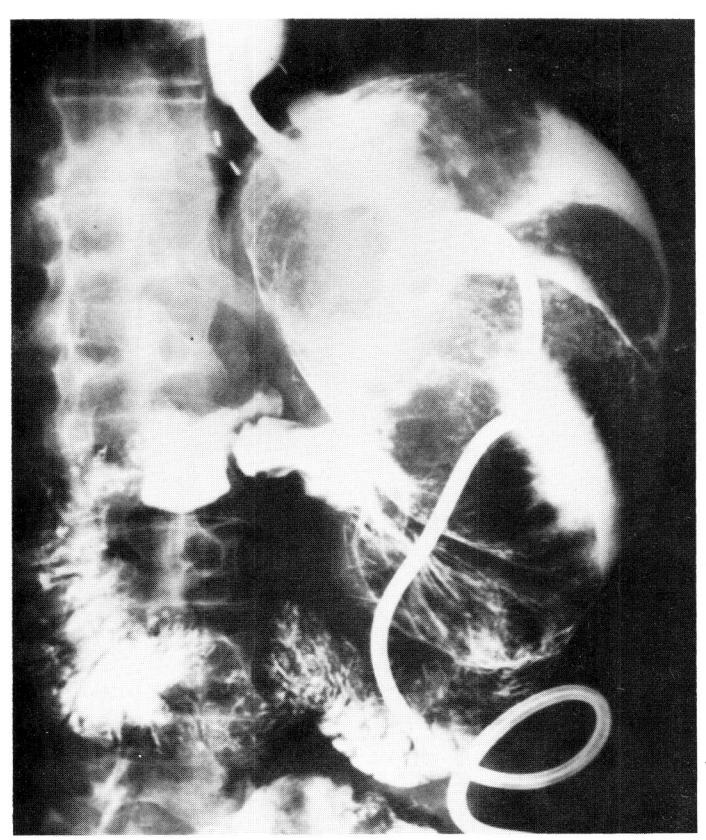

Figure 10–65. Retrograde jejunogastric intussusception in a patient with a gastrojejunostomy.

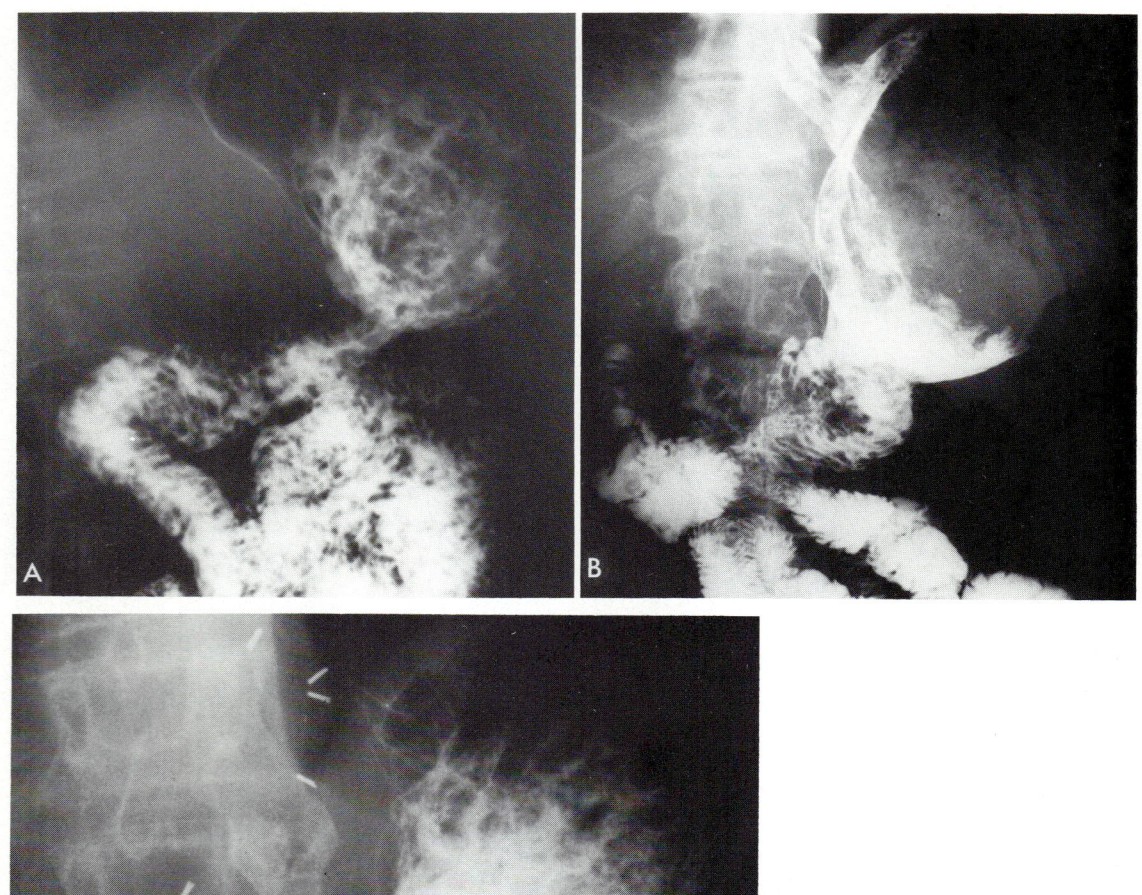

Figure 10–66. Gastric bezoars in three patients following hemigastrectomy.

The afferent loop syndrome occurs when there is stasis of food and secretions in the afferent loop.[4] This may be in association with obstruction of either the afferent or the efferent loop. When the syndrome is due to obstruction of the afferent loop, the loop dilates with bile and pancreatic juice. Radiologic examination may disclose the point of obstruction of either loop, nonfilling of the afferent loop, or cyclic filling and emptying of the afferent loop into the gastric remnant (Fig. 10–67).

Carter and Martel described two cases of contraction of the gastric antrum fol-

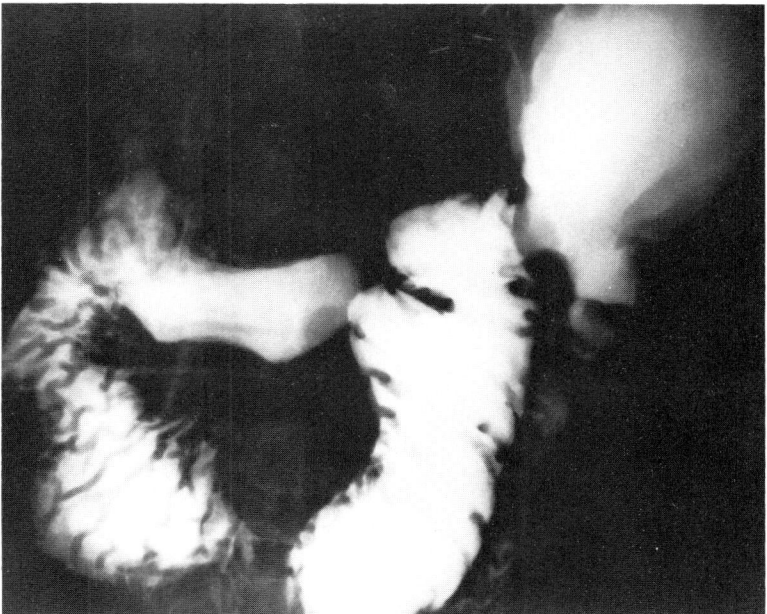

Figure 10–67. Afferent loop syndrome in a patient with a Billroth II hemigastrectomy. There is partial obstruction of the efferent loop resulting from adhesions. The afferent loop is dilated, and cyclic filling between the gastric remnant and the afferent loop was apparent at fluoroscopy.

lowing long-term gastroenterostomy.[5] The radiographic finding may be confused with scirrhous carcinoma of the stomach. In these cases the gastroenterostomy results in disuse of the antrum over many years, which leads to atrophy, contraction, and fibrosis (Fig. 10–68).

When a portion of the gastric antrum is left behind following gastric surgery, a source of gastrin remains.[3] Acid production continues, and recurrent marginal ulceration is frequent. The retained gastric antrum can be detected radiographically if there is sufficient filling of the afferent loop (Fig. 10–69). In these cases, reflux of barium from the duodenum into the antrum via the pylorus is apparent. Demonstra-

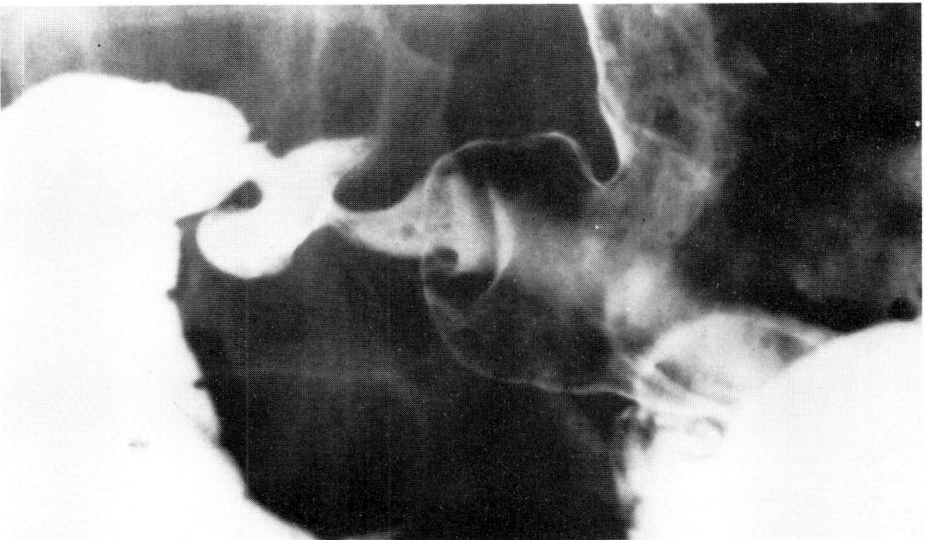

Figure 10–68. Contraction of the gastric antrum following long-term gastrojejunostomy.

tion of gastric mucosa is helpful in identifying the antrum. Care should be taken to distinguish filling of the duodenal stump or a duodenal diverticulum from a retained antrum.

Carcinoma of the gastric stump is generally defined as a carcinoma arising in the gastric remnant of a patient who has undergone a partial gastrectomy. These patients are primarily those who have had gastric surgery for benign lesions of the stomach or duodenum and whose surgery took place five years before the development of carcinoma. One hopes that none of these patients had an unsuspected gastric carcinoma at the time of gastric resection. Some authors also include in this group patients who have had gastric surgery for carcinoma of the stomach. In this circumstance, it is suggested that an interval of 10 or even 20 years should have elapsed to eliminate the possibility that the carcinoma is a recurrence of the primary tumor.[1]

In view of the increasing number of reports of this complication, carcinoma of the gastric stump should be recognized as a distinct clinical entity with characteristic clinical features and special diagnostic difficulties.[1] In one series, the duration of symptoms prior to diagnosis ranged from two months to two years, the average being nine months.[1] The radiologic diagnosis is difficult even if a high index of suspicion of carcinoma is maintained (Fig. 10–70). In some series, carcinoma was not demonstrated on radiographic examination in 17 to 70 per cent of the cases. Most postoperative patients have thick rugal folds in the gastric remnant, even though atrophic gastritis is a common finding histologically. Careful attention must be given to subtle localized thickening and irregularity of the gastric rugae and to evidence of rigidity and fixa-

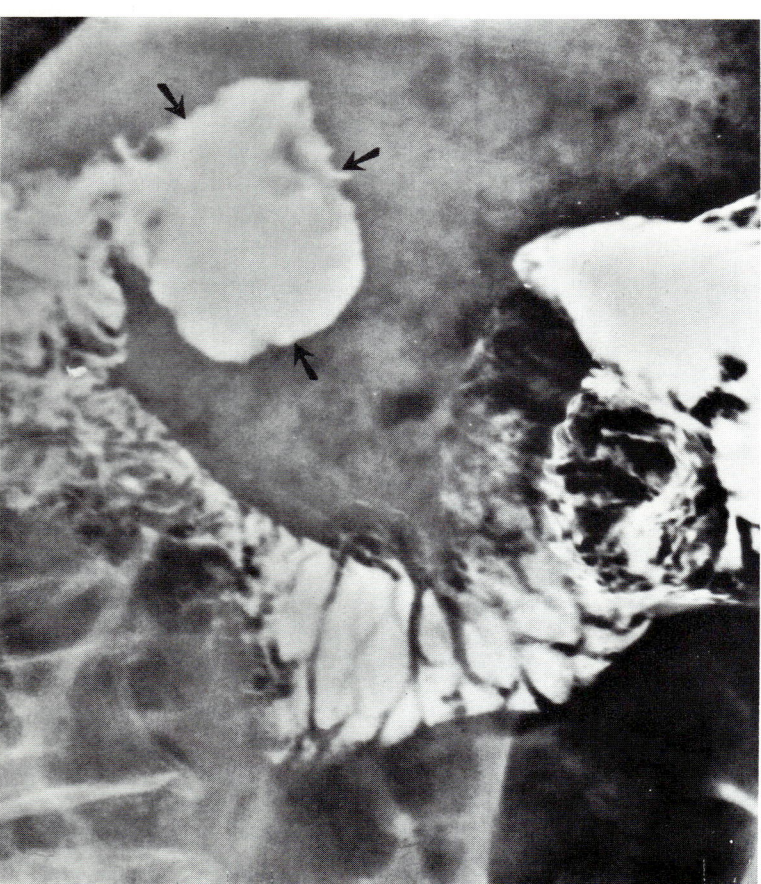

Figure 10–69. Barium in a retained gastric antrum (arrows) after a Billroth II hemigastrectomy. (Courtesy of R. P. Gold, M.D., and W. B. Seaman, M.D.)

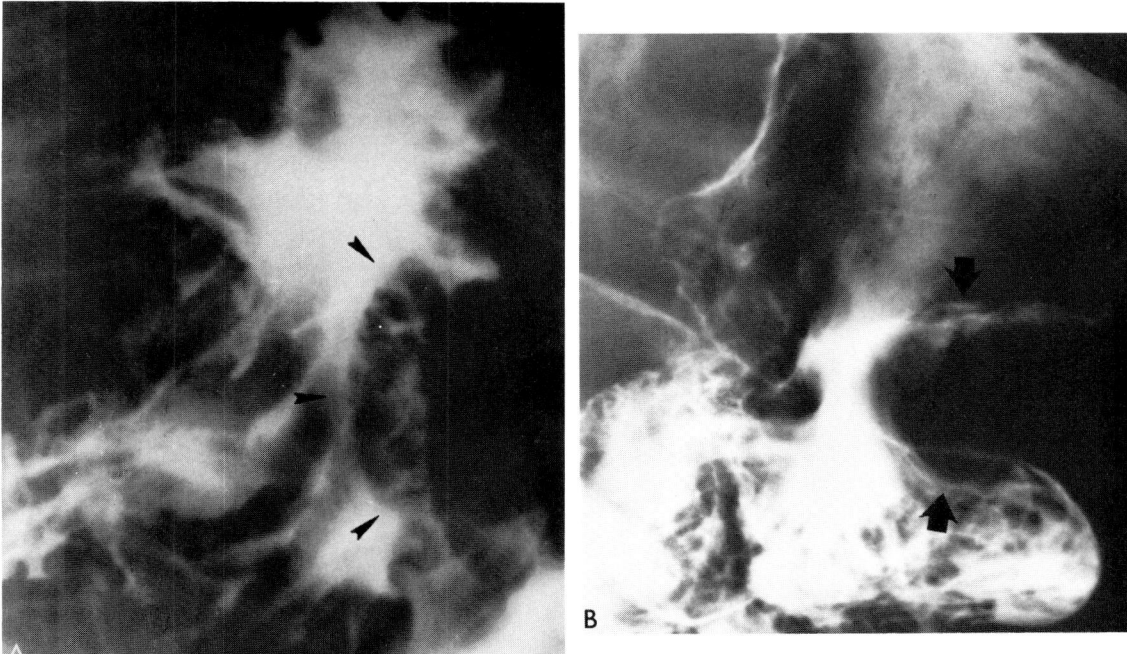

Figure 10–70. Carcinoma of the gastric remnant in two patients occurring ten years after the initial gastric resection. In both cases, a mass is visible in the gastric remnant at the anastomosis (arrows).

tion of the gastric wall. Multiple radiographs made with graded compression, gas distention, and adequate barium coating of the mucosa are essential. Comparison with previous postoperative radiographic studies is particularly important because it may demonstrate a change in the mucosal architecture in the gastric remnant, suggesting the occurrence of carcinoma. Knowledge that the tumor is almost always in the gastric remnant adjacent to the anastomosis is helpful in evaluating the radiographic findings.

References

1. Berk, R. N., Loeb, P. M., and Miao, Y. S.: Carcinoma of the gastric stump. J. Assoc. Can. Radiol 25:127–130, 1974.
2. Burhenne, H. J.: Roentgen anatomy and terminology of gastric surgery. Am. J. Roentgenol. 91:731–743, 1964.
3. Burhenne, H. J.: Retained gastric antrum. Am. J. Roentgenol. 101:459–465, 1967.
4. Burhenne, H. J.: Postoperative stomach. In Margulis, A., and Burhenne, H. J. (eds.): Philadelphia, W. B. Saunders Company, 1973, pp. 740–765.
5. Carter, T. L., and Martel, W.: Contraction of the gastric antrum following long term gastroenterostomy. Radiology 91:514–518, 1968.
6. Ellis, K.: Gastrojejunal ulcer. Radiology 71:187–193, 1958.
7. Ettinger, A., Paul, R. E., and Moean, J. M.: Gastric pseudotumor after fundoplication. Gastroenterology 61:299–303, 1971.
8. Fisher, M. S.: The Hofmeister defect, a normal change in the postoperative stomach. Am. J. Roentgenol. 84:1082–1083, 1960.
9. Gold, R., and Seaman, W. B.: The primary double contrast examination of the postoperative stomach. Radiology 124:297–306, 1977.
10. Schatzki, R.: The significance of rigidity of the jejunum in the diagnosis of postoperative jejunal ulcers. Am. J. Roentgenol. 103:330–340, 1968.
11. Seaman, W. B.: Prolapsed gastric mucosa through a gastrojejunostomy. Am. J. Roentgenol. 110:304–307, 1970.
12. Szemes, G., and Amberg, J. R.: Gastric bezoars after partial gastrectomy. Radiology 90:765–777, 1968.
13. Wilson, W. J., and Weintraub, H. D.: Postpyloroplasty antrum. Am. J. Roentgenol. 96:408–411, 1966.

11

DUODENUM

FRANCIS J. SCHOLZ, M.D.

BENIGN TUMORS

Primary benign tumors of the duodenum are rare (Figs. 11–1 and 11–2).[10, 18] Some variation in frequency is found from series to series because of the small numbers of tumors included in any one reported series. Adenomas are most common, especially when adenomas of Brunner's glands are included. Leiomyomas are probably second in frequency. After these two lesions the order of frequency is usually lipomas, pancreatic rests, hemangiomas, cysts, carcinoid tumors, gastric and biliary hamartomas, and other so-called rest tumors. Some of these tumors are not true neoplasms (cysts, pancreatic rests, hamartomas, and so forth) but must be included in the radiographic consideration of most duodenal tumors.

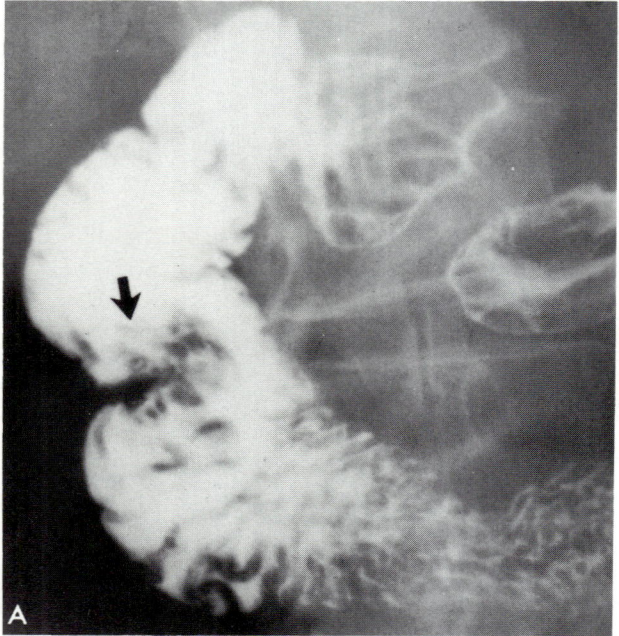

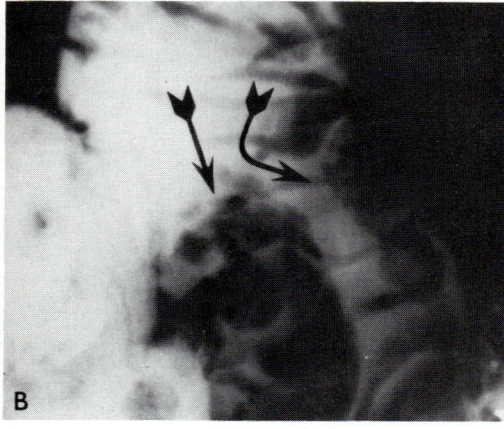

Figure 11–1. Sessile polyp. *A,* Lobulated sessile filling defect demonstrated in gastrointestinal series (arrow). *B,* Polyp confirmed on hypotonic examination (straight arrow). The differentiation of the papilla of Vater (curved arrow) from the adenoma allows for more precise surgical planning. The ampulla of Vater and biliary and pancreatic ducts were not involved, and excision of a portion of the duodenal wall removed the adenoma completely, leaving the ampullary mechanism intact.

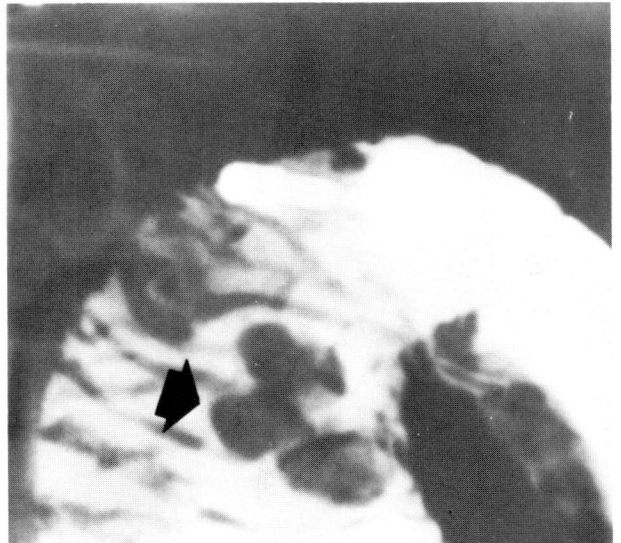

Figure 11–2. Lobulated benign adenoma demonstrated in the proximal descending duodenum (arrow) during hypotonic examination of the duodenum.

Adenomas

All benign tumors are either mucosal or extramucosal lesions. Adenomas are the only true mucosal tumors, and their radiographic appearance is identical to that of adenomas encountered anywhere in the gastrointestinal tract, namely, sessile or pedunculated filling defects. Sessile polyps may have a smooth or villous surface (see Fig. 11–1). Pedunculated polyps are seen less commonly in the duodenum and small bowel than in the colon.

Hyperplasia of Brunner's Glands

Brunner's glands are in the submucosa of the duodenum. They secrete an alkaline mucoid substance and are concentrated between the pylorus and the ampulla. Occasionally hypertrophy occurs, and these glands appear radiographically as smooth-surfaced nodules. True hyperplasia of Brunner's glands may be circumscribed with a few discrete, large submucosal filling defects (Fig. 11–3) or may become diffuse with innumerable tiny nodules. Hyperplastic Brunner's glands occur between the pylorus and the ampulla but occasionally have been seen in the more distal small bowel.

True neoplastic adenomas of Brunner's glands (Fig. 11–4) usually occur between the pylorus and the papilla of Vater and may be associated with adjacent hyperplastic Brunner's glands. Rarely, a pedunculated Brunner's gland adenoma has been found.[29] A malignant tumor has never been proven to originate from a Brunner's gland adenoma.

Lipomas

Lipomas are benign tumors arising from the submucosa (Fig. 11–5).[38] They are characterized radiographically as smooth, sharply defined, oval filling defects that change shape with peristalsis (as may congenital duplication cysts and choledochoceles). Rarely, a lipoma may ulcerate. Malignant lipomas of the duodenum are rare.

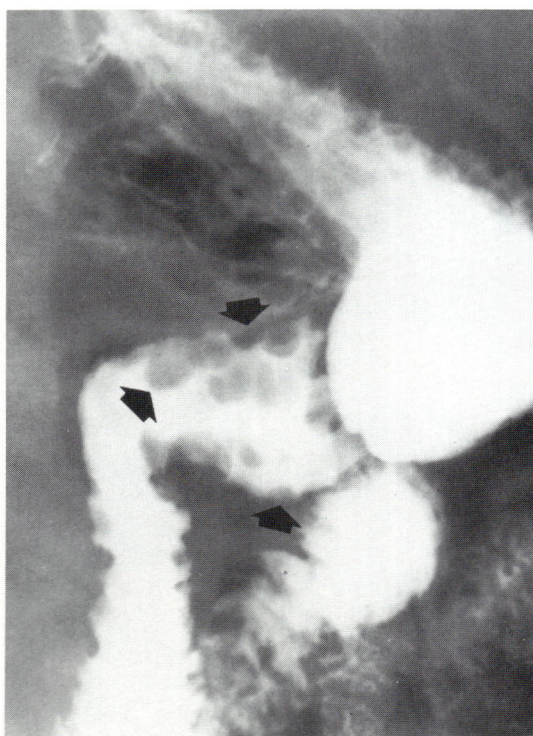

Figure 11–3. Multiple, sharply defined hypertrophied Brunner's glands (arrows) are seen in the duodenal bulb and the proximal descending limb of the duodenum.

Leiomyomas

Leiomyomas are tumors arising from smooth muscle in the duodenal wall. Primary duodenal carcinomas outnumber leiomyosarcomas in a ratio of 10 to 1.[17] Benign leiomyomas and malignant leiomyosarcomas share many characteristics and may not be clinically, radiographically, or even pathologically distinguishable. About one half are malignant. These tumors tend to be large, bulky, and sharply demarcated (Figs. 11–6 and 11–7). They may grow into the lumen or, more commonly, extraluminally, or

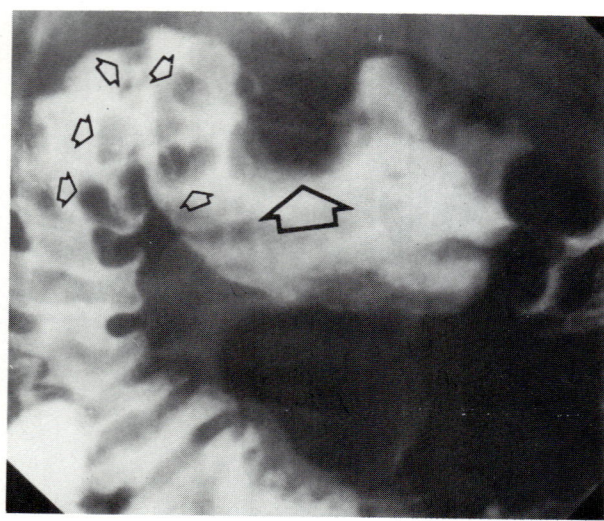

Figure 11–4. Adenoma of Brunner's gland. A large filling defect (large arrow) seen in the duodenal bulb subsequently proved to be a benign Brunner's gland adenoma of the duodenal bulb. Smaller nodular hyperplastic Brunner's glands are seen in the proximal postbulbar duodenum (small arrows).

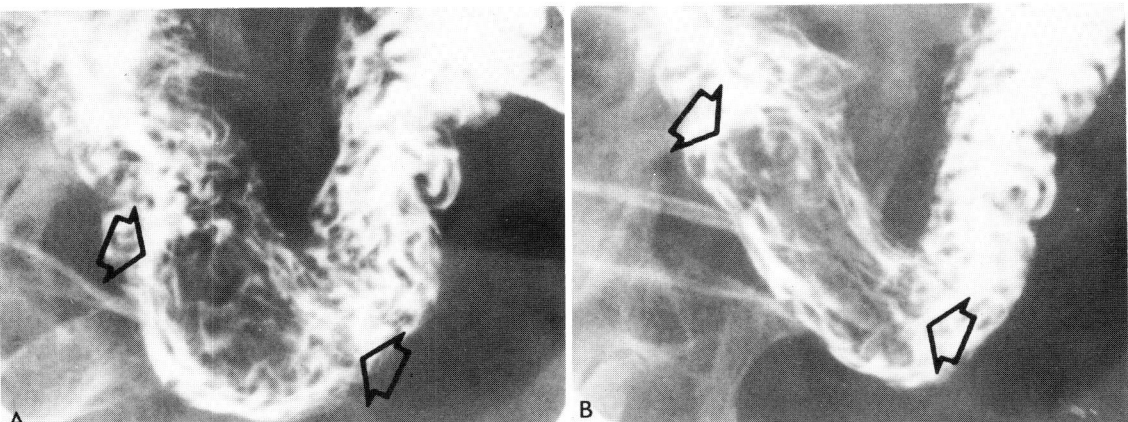

Figure 11–5. Lipoma. A persistent filling defect in the distal descending limb of the duodenum is seen to deform markedly with peristalsis. An oval defect (arrows, *A*) becomes markedly elongated (arrows, *B*). This is characteristic of soft lesions, such as lipomas, cysts, and choledochoceles.

they may grow in both directions with a dumbbell appearance. These tumors have a rich surface vascularity,[40] but with growth, the center of the tumor outgrows its blood supply and undergoes necrosis. The resultant large central necrotic ulcer cavity may extend a considerable distance from the duodenal lumen (Fig. 11–8).

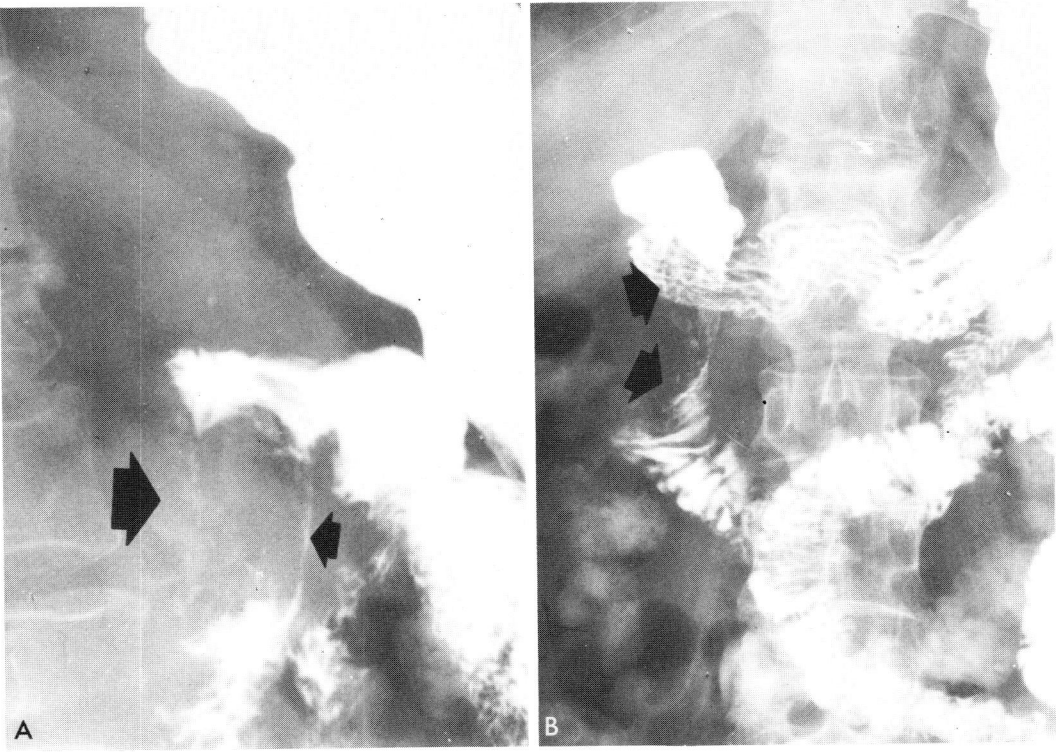

Figure 11–6. Leiomyoma. *A,* Large, oval filling defect demonstrated in the descending duodenum (arrows). At operation, a benign leiomyoma was removed. *B,* Tumor growth is primarily into the duodenal lumen, narrowing the lumen.

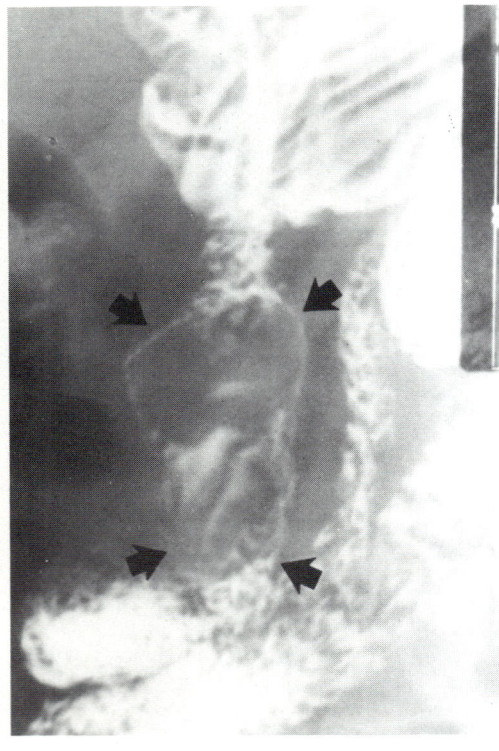

Figure 11–7. Leiomyoma. A large, bilobular filling defect in the distal descending limb of the duodenum. The barium is stretched around the leiomyoma, which protrudes into the duodenal lumen. This was found to be a benign leiomyoma at operation.

Pancreatic Rests

Pancreatic rests are non-neoplastic collections of normal pancreatic tissue in the submucosa of the duodenum, stomach, or jejunum. They are usually small (less than 2 cm in diameter), single, and asymptomatic. Radiographically, a typical submucosal filling defect is seen to have a smooth, dome-shaped appearance. A central dot of barium may be noted in the middle of the filling defect, representing barium in the duct

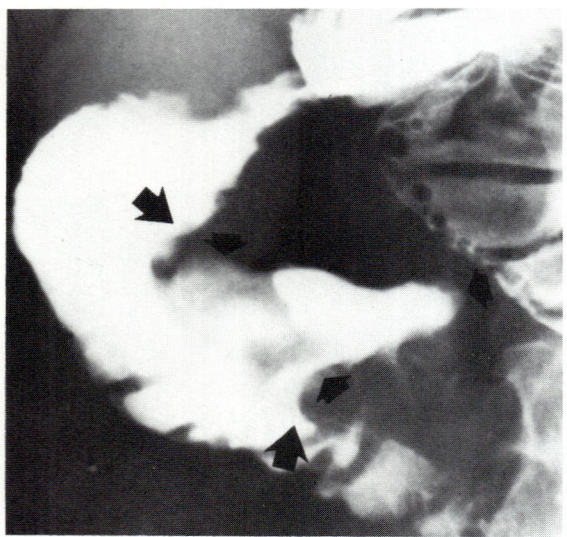

Figure 11–8. Leiomyosarcoma. The lesion (large arrows) arises from the medial wall of the descending portion of the duodenum. The mucosal folds on the opposite wall are intact. A large, irregular ulcer crater (delineated by three small arrows) arises from the center of the mass, and the crater extends a considerable distance from the duodenal lumen. The majority of growth of this leiomyosarcoma is extraluminal into the adjacent retroperitoneum, and only the tip of the tumor has grown into the duodenum.

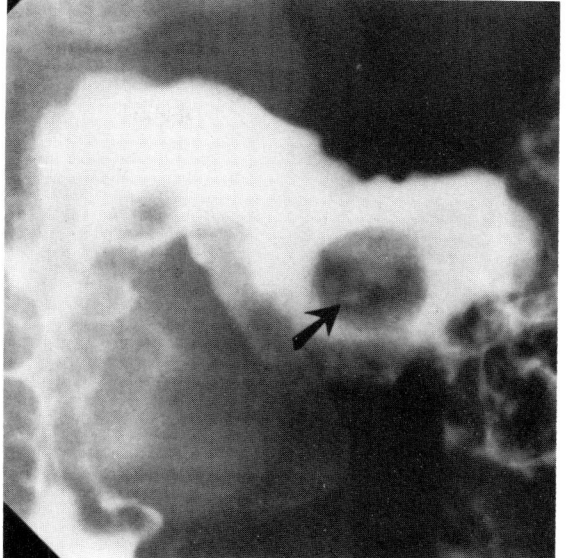

Figure 11–9. Ectopic pancreas. A round, sharply defined filling defect is noted in the duodenal bulb with an eccentric collection of barium. The collection of barium represents filling of the pancreatic duct that drains the ectopic pancreatic gland in the submucosa.

draining the ectopic pancreatic tissue (Fig. 11–9). Single pancreatic rests may not be distinguishable radiographically from ulcers or from small primary or metastatic tumors. Ulcers can usually be distinguished by obtaining a repeat examination to demonstrate ulcer healing. Other types of rests, such as ectopic gastric and biliary rests, may occur rarely in the duodenum.

Villous Tumors

The occurrence of villous tumors in the duodenum and small bowel is rare compared with their frequency in the colon. Fewer than 100 cases of duodenal villous tumors have been reported.[34, 39, 55] Between 25 and 50 per cent of villous tumors of the duodenum have some degree of malignancy, ranging from *in situ* to frankly invasive carcinoma. In one review, no malignancies were noted in patients younger than 50 years of age, and lesions less than 4 cm in diameter showed no evidence of invasion.[34] Electrolyte problems from the watery diarrhea seen in cases of villous tumors of the colon are not seen in cases of duodenal villous tumors because the entire length of small bowel is available for reabsorption of the fluid that "weeps" from these lesions. Radiographically, a typical appearance is noted: The barium is trapped in the interstices of the villous surface, giving a striated, reticulated, or "soap bubbly" appearance (Figs. 11–10 and 11–11). Villous tumors are more common in the proximal duodenum but occur throughout the length of the duodenum. Villous tumors arising from the papilla of Vater have been reported. Size and location are not reliable factors in excluding malignancy.[34, 39, 45]

MALIGNANT TUMORS

Malignant primary tumors of the duodenum are rare; metastatic tumors are encountered much more frequently. Any lesion or ulceration occurring distal to the duodenal bulb should be evaluated thoroughly for primary or secondary malignancy.

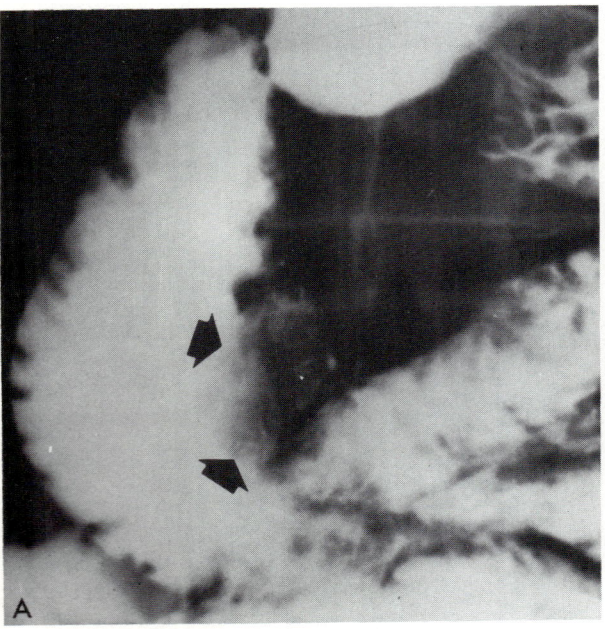
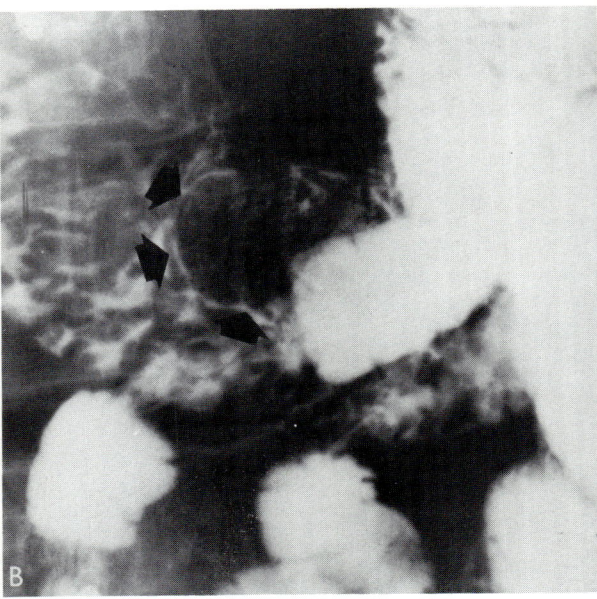
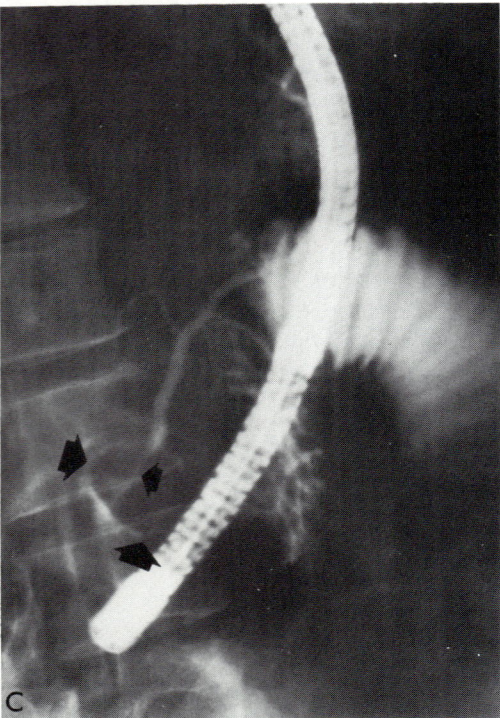

Figure 11–10. Villous adenoma. *A* and *B,* filling defect (arrows) is seen in the descending limb of the duodenum. It has a villous surface that fills with tiny collections of barium. This lacy or speckled appearance is characteristic of benign and malignant villous tumors. This was a benign villous adenoma arising from the papilla of Vater. *C,* The endoscopic pancreatogram shows that the tumor (two large arrows) is growing around and narrowing the ampullary portion (small arrow) of the pancreatic duct.

Carcinoma of the Duodenum (See also Chapter 12, Part VI and Figs. 12–63, 12–65, 12–74 to 76, 12–82)

Carcinoma of the duodenum is not common; it accounts for only 0.3 per cent of all malignant neoplasms of the gastrointestinal tract. Some of these lesions probably represent duodenal invasion from carcinoma arising in the pancreas, the common bile duct, or the gallbladder. "Periampullary cancer" is a term that includes tumors arising from the ampullary region of the duodenum or the closely adjacent pancreatic or common bile ducts and whose organ of origin cannot always be differentiated clinically, radiographically, or pathologically. Radiographically, early periampullary tumors may show only a prominent papilla if the growth of the tumor is still within the ampulla itself. Thus, jaundice and a prominent papilla require such additional diagnostic procedures as endoscopic retrograde cannulation and percutaneous transhepatic cholangiography. More advanced tumors show nodularity (Fig. 11–12), ulceration (Fig. 11–13), and finally, circumferential encasement of the duodenum (Fig. 11–14) like that seen in the apple-core lesion common in the colon. Carcinomas arising remotely from the ampullary region (*true* primary duodenal cancers) show characteristics identical to those of carcinomas in the remainder of the gastrointestinal tract. In one series, the correct diagnosis of duodenal carcinoma was made in 67 per cent of patients. In about 15 per cent of patients, other radiographic diagnoses—either benign stricture (9 per cent) or pancreatic carcinoma (6 per cent)—were made. In about 18 per cent of these patients, the duodenum was reported as normal.[50]

Morphologically, polypoid, infiltrating scirrhous (Fig. 11–15), or annular ulcerating forms may be seen.[5] Ulceration is common, and any ulceration seen distal to the duodenal bulb should be evaluated carefully for malignancy. Reports of duodenal carcinoma arising in patients with Gardner's syndrome or Peutz-Jeghers syndrome suggest a slightly higher incidence in individuals with these genetic disorders.[47, 55] Benign and malignant endocrine tumors occur in the duodenum, and these may not be demonstrated by the routine upper gastrointestinal barium series. These endocrine tumors are often small and are not apparent except by angiography or by surgical palpation. Both carcinoid and pancreatic islet cell tumors have been found in the duodenal wall.[21, 32, 54]

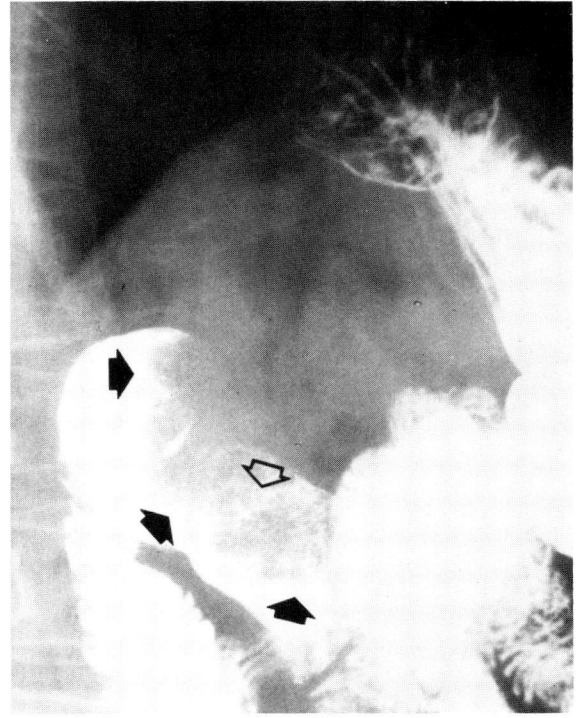

Figure 11–11. Villous adenoma. Solid arrows point to a large filling defect in the duodenal bulb. Multiple fine barium flecks are noted (open arrow), indicating barium trapped within the villous surface of tumor.

510 — DUODENUM

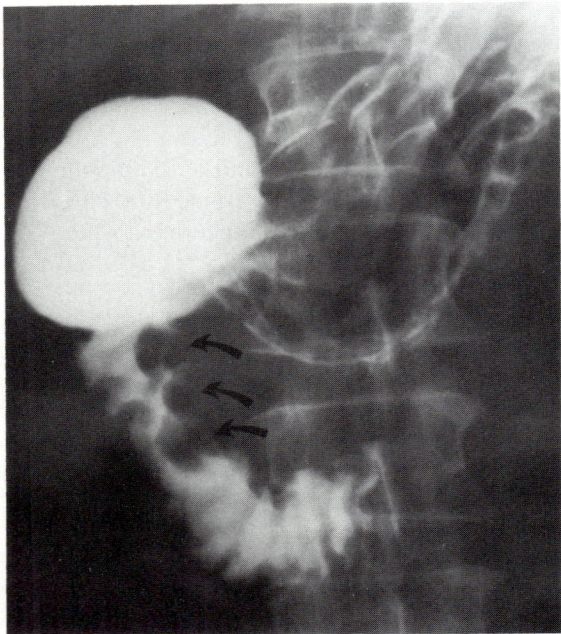

Figure 11–12. Carcinoma. Three arrows point to three distinct contiguous nodular filling defects. Mucosal destruction or ulceration is not evident. Any one of these could represent merely a prominent papilla, but three such defects must be considered ominous. Nodularity, rigidity, and ulceration are radiographic features that point a diagnosis of carcinoma of the ampulla of Vater.

Figure 11–13. Ulcerating carcinoma. A mass arises from the medial wall of the descending limb of the duodenum (solid arrows), and a large linear ulcer (open arrow) and several smaller linear ulcers are evident in the mass. The folds in the opposite wall are uninvolved.

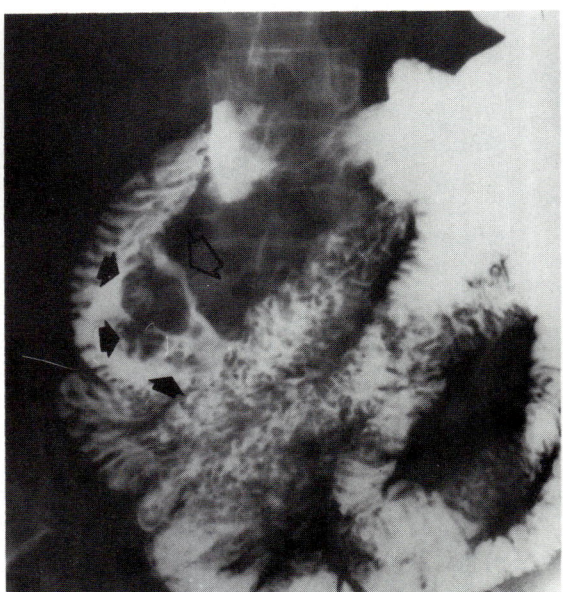

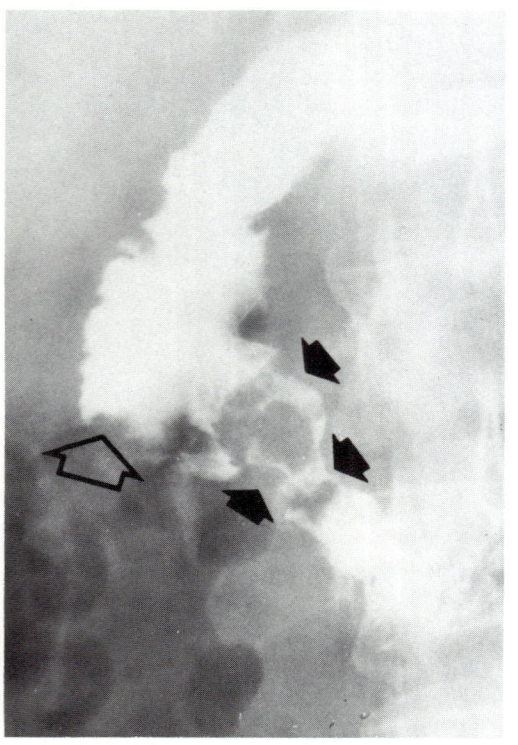

Figure 11–14. Ulcerating carcinoma. An abnormal narrowed segment of distal descending duodenum is noted with overhanging margins (open arrow) and numerous irregular linear ulcers (three solid arrows) extending through the ulcerated center of the tumor.

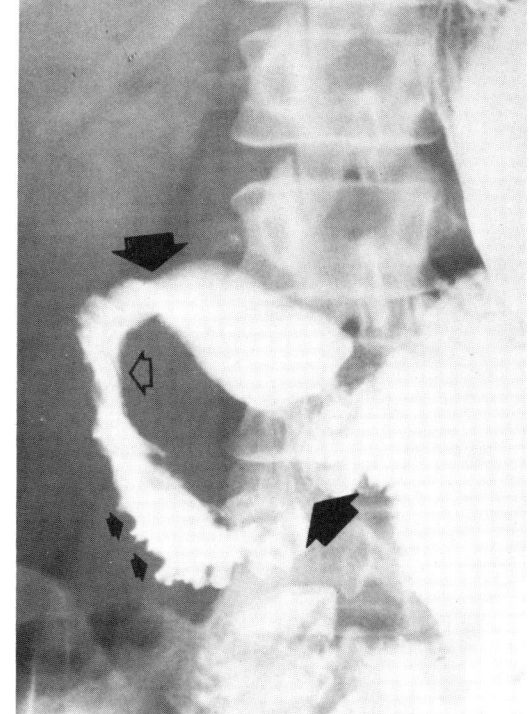

Figure 11–15. Scirrhous carcinoma. Incomplete distensibility of the duodenum between the duodenal bulb and the proximal ascending limb is apparent (large solid arrows). In the proximal duodenum the mucosal pattern is lost (open arrow), and in the distal duodenum irregular thickening of mucosal folds is present (small solid arrows). At operation, a majority of the duodenum was infiltrated with scirrhous tumor.

Lymphomas of the Duodenum

Involvement of the duodenum by lymphoma is rare. The duodenum may be involved secondarily owing to invasion by retroperitoneal lymphoma or may be involved primarily as part of diffuse gastrointestinal lymphoma (Fig. 11–16). Lymphoma is rarely confined to the duodenum.[3] All cell types have been seen. Radiographically, lymphoma has numerous and varying characteristics. It may be finely nodular, grossly polypoid, infiltrative (with mucosal fold changes, such as fold thickening, flattening, constriction, or aneurysmal dilatation of the segment, all with or without mucosal ulceration), excavative (with mucosal ulceration extending into adjacent lymphomatous masses), or extrinsic mesenteric (with extrinsic mass effect). Lymphoma may mimic other, more common, duodenal deformities, such as those due to hyperplasia of Brunner's glands, pancreatitis, Crohn's disease, and peptic ulceration. Because the disease usually is not limited to the duodenum, evaluation of the rest of the gastrointestinal tract prevents confusion of lymphoma with benign processes.

Metastatic Disease

The duodenum is often involved by metastatic disease, more commonly by invasion from contiguous organs than by hematogenous or lymphatic spread from distant sites. The entire length of the duodenum is contiguous to the pancreas, and pancreatic carcinoma (Figs. 11–17 and 11–18) is the most frequent invading neoplasm. Carcinoma of the gallbladder (Fig. 11–19), colon (Fig. 11–20), or kidneys may involve the duodenum by contiguity. The duodenal bulb and immediate postbulbar portion may be deformed or even invaded by metastatic nodes in the liver hilum. The changes of

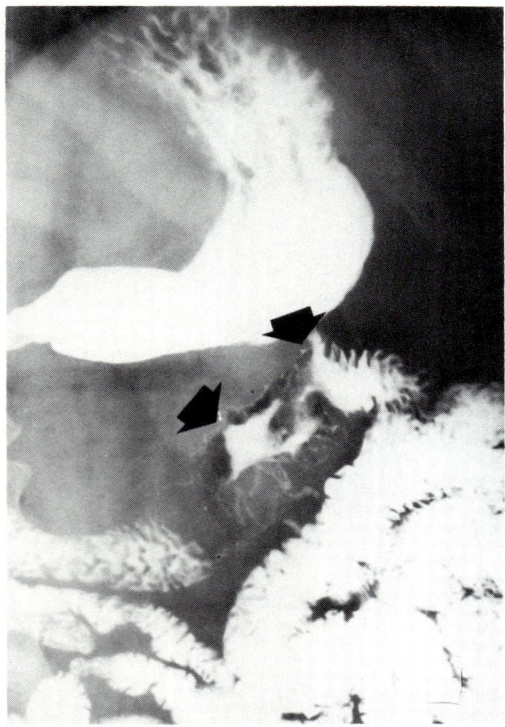

Figure 11–16. Lymphoma. An abnormal ulcerated segment (arrows) is visible in the distal duodenum at the ligament of Treitz. The entire circumference of this segment is involved, but the lumen appears to be dilated rather than constricted. Aneurysmal dilatation is one characteristic of lymphoma of the gastrointestinal tract that, when seen, helps to differentiate it from carcinoma. When carcinoma involves the entire circumference, it almost always narrows the lumen.

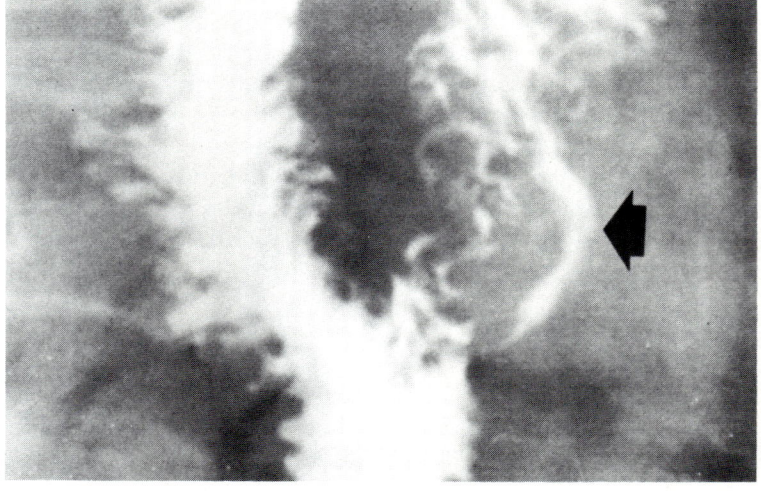

Figure 11–17. Metastasis. The arrow points to linear ulcer in the proximal ascending portion of the duodenum. Carcinoma of the pancreas has invaded this portion of the duodenum.

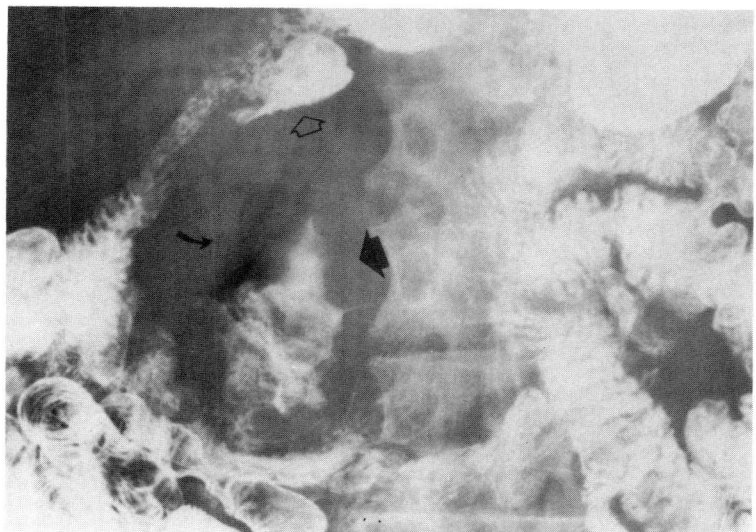

Figure 11-18. Carcinoma of the pancreas invading the duodenum. The duodenal sweep is widened. Deformity is evident in a diverticulum arising from the proximal descending duodenum (open arrow). Invasion of a diverticulum arising from the descending limb of the duodenum has occurred, and air is demonstrated within the necrotic center of the tumor (curved arrow). Amorphous barium passes into the necrotic tumor (solid straight arrow) from the perforated duodenal diverticulum. (*From* Kessler, R. M., and Scholz, F. J.: Carcinoma of the pancreas. Contemp. Surg. 6:74, 1975.)

metastatic disease in the duodenum are typical of metastatic invasion anywhere in the gastrointestinal tract and include fixation of mucosal folds, spiculation, nodularity, and ulceration. Annular constricting and obstructing lesions indistinguishable from primary duodenal carcinoma may be encountered. Attempted resections of primary tumors in contiguous organs may lead to duodenal perforations (see Fig. 11-20) resulting from involvement of the duodenum.

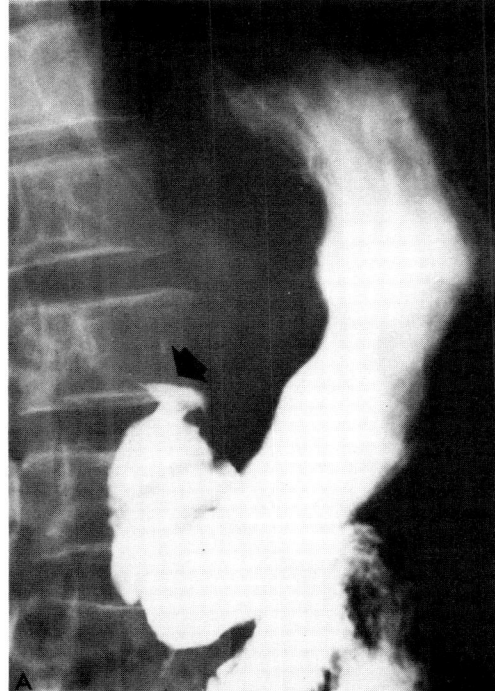
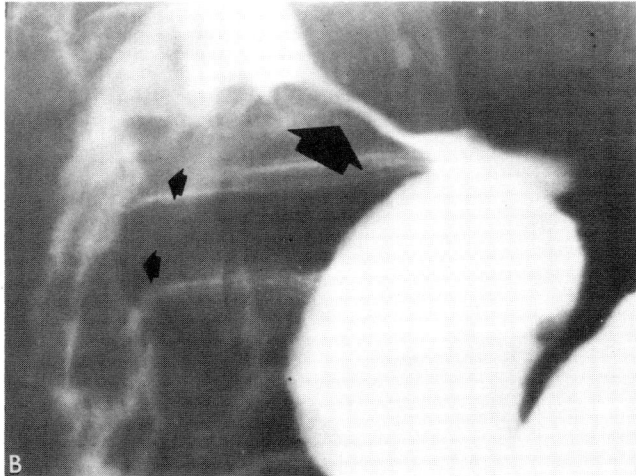

Figure 11-19. Encasement of the midportion and the apex of the duodenal bulb (large arrow, *A* and *B*) and distortion of the mucosal pattern in the proximal descending limb of the duodenum (small arrows, *B*). At operation, carcinoma of the gallbladder was found invading the descending portion of the duodenum and encasing the duodenal bulb.

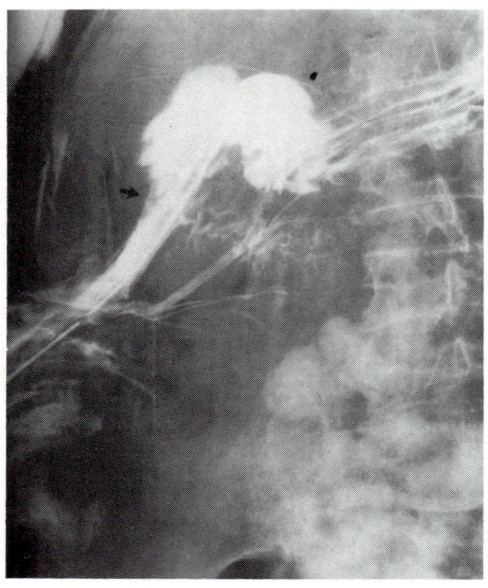

Figure 11–20. Carcinoma of hepatic flexure of the colon with enteric drainage from an incision after resection. A swallow of water-soluble contrast material demonstrates the contrast material passing from the descending limb of the duodenum into a drainage tube that has been placed in the draining wound (arrow).

PSEUDOTUMORS

Many lesions of the duodenum fit the literal meaning of the word "tumor," that is, a swelling, but not its current meaning, neoplasia. Such pseudotumors include cysts, edematous papillae of Vater (from common duct calculi, pancreatitis, or duodenitis), choledochoceles, flexure and intussusception pseudopolyps, and surgical scars.

Cysts of the Duodenum

The majority of duodenal cysts are enteric or duplication cysts. These are submucosal cysts lined with enteric mucosa that probably begin embryologically during the sixth to tenth fetal week. At this stage, the entire hollow enteric canal undergoes rapid growth, and the core fills with rapidly proliferating cells that obliterate the entire intestinal lumen. By the tenth week, numerous discontinuous vacuoles form in the gastrointestinal tract and eventually coalesce to form one continuous gastrointestinal lumen. Two parallel, longitudinal vacuoles in the descending duodenum are the last to coalesce. If a vacuole fails to coalesce into the enteric lumen, it remains a blind cyst that may gradually enlarge as lining cells are shed into the lumen of the cyst. A true enteric duplication cyst contains clear, colorless fluid. Such lesions can occur throughout the gastrointestinal tract, and approximately 5 per cent occur in the duodenum.[25]

In the duodenum, enteric duplication cysts are usually in the descending limb along the concave (pancreatic) surface and are either contiguous to or near the papilla of Vater. Approximately 13 per cent contain ectopic gastric mucosa.[51] Although probably of congenital origin and usually diagnosed within the first decade, duplication cysts have been seen in elderly patients; they are rarely multiple.[7]

There are two forms of duodenal duplications: cystic and tubular. Cystic lesions, as discussed previously, are usually entirely within the wall of the duodenum. The rare communicating tubular duodenal duplication usually communicates with the gastrointestinal tract, and the tubular duplication may extend through the diaphragm into the chest. Commonly, this type of duplication contains ectopic gastric mucosa. The tubular form probably has an embryologic origin distinctly different from that of the cystic form.

Radiographically, duplication cysts are pliable, submucosal, oval filling defects in the descending portion of the duodenum (Fig. 11–21). Pliability may be noted on fluoroscopy with manual palpation or peristaltic activity. Duplication cysts rarely may communicate with the lumen of the gastrointestinal tract or the biliary tree. With biliary communication, confusion with choledochal cysts and choledochoceles may occur.

Edema of the Papilla

The papilla of Vater is a normal papillary eminence, or "tumor," occurring in most persons. Its size is usually less than 1 cm in diameter. However, Poppel et al. state that "increase in size alone up to 3 cm in length, 1.2 cm in width, and 1.2 cm in profile may still be possibly within the normal in the absence of any other abnormality."[43] It has, therefore, become mandatory to demonstrate additional abnormalities or to obtain clinical or laboratory confirmation before an abnormality is postulated.

With adjacent inflammatory processes, such as pancreatitis (Fig. 11–22), impaction or passage of a common bile duct calculus (Fig. 11–23), and duodenitis, the papilla may

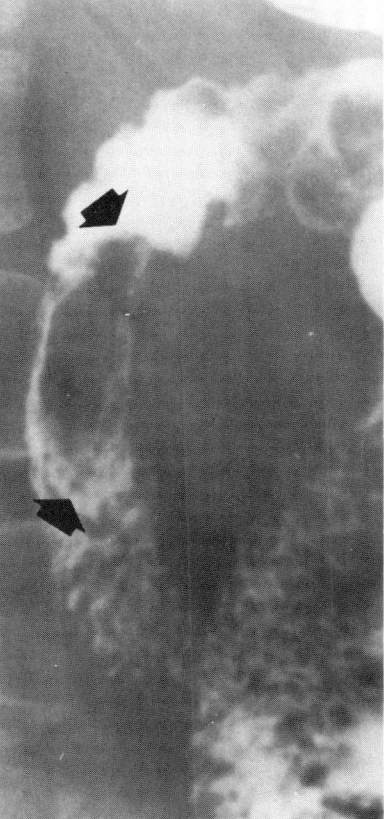

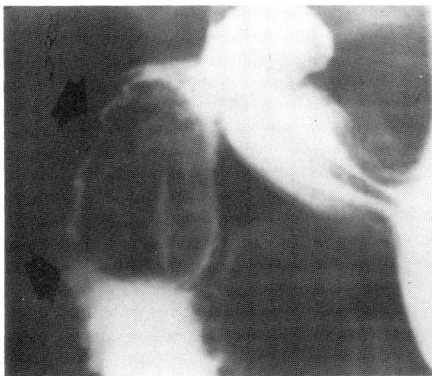

Figure 11–21. Duplication cyst. A smoothly marginated filling defect is evident in the proximal duodenum (arrows). This changed shape with peristalsis from a more round (B) to a more elongated oval (A). Pliability in a filling defect is characteristic of cysts, lipomas, and choledochoceles.

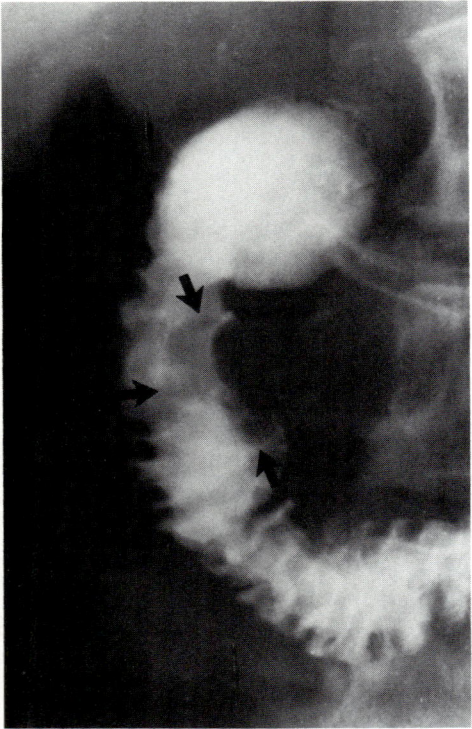

Figure 11–22. Edematous papilla of Vater. A large filling defect is seen in the medial posterior wall of the descending limb of the duodenum. Thickened mucosal folds appear in the adjacent duodenum. An edematous papilla is the diagnosis. An edematous papilla may be seen with pancreatitis, common bile duct calculi, or duodenitis. It may not be distinguishable radiographically from ampullary carcinoma, and correlation with the patient's clinical findings are required. Endoscopy may be necessary.

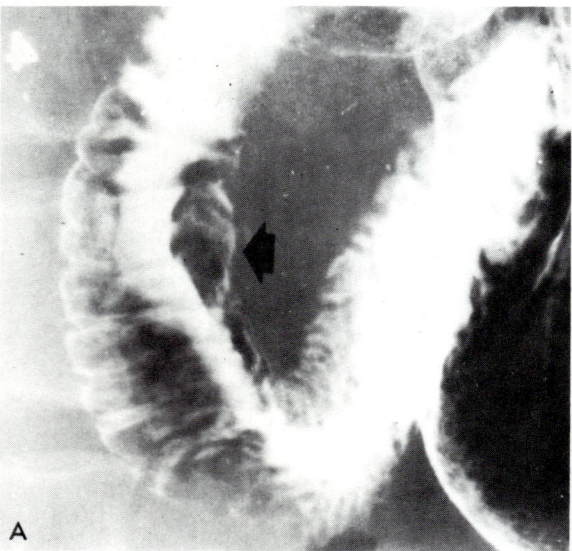

Figure 11–23. Calculus in common bile duct. A, Abdominal pain and abnormal liver function prompted a gastrointestinal series that shows persistent prominence of the papilla of Vater (arrow). B, Endoscopic cannulation demonstrates edema of the papilla of Vater (small arrows). The distal common duct is normal in diameter, but a large oval calculus is found in the midportion of the common bile duct (large arrow), and the biliary tree proximal to this is dilated. Edema of the papilla need not always occur with impaction of calculi in the distal common duct. Edema may persist after passage of the calculi, and in this patient, a smaller stone had most likely passed recently into the duodenum.

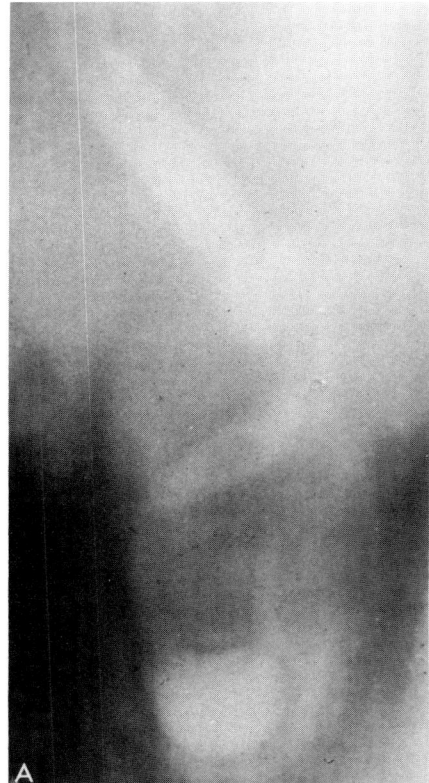
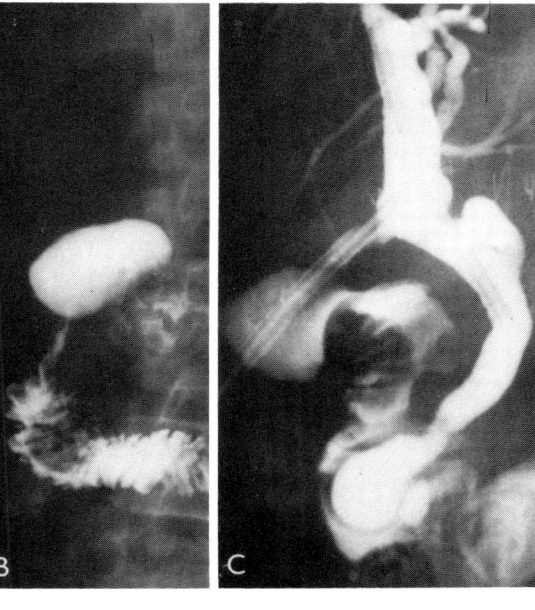

Figure 11–24. Choledochocele. *A,* Intravenous cholangiogram. Tomography shows cystic dilatation of the terminal common bile duct. *B,* Upper gastrointestinal series. A sharply defined filling defect is seen in the mid-descending limb of the duodenum. Fluoroscopy showed evidence of changeability during peristalsis. *C,* T-tube cholangiogram. Cystic dilatation of the terminal common bile duct, which is projecting into the duodenal lumen, is seen. Contrast material in the duodenum demonstrates the intraluminal position of the choledochocele and confirms it to be the filling defect noted on the gastrointestinal series. The lumen of the choledochocele is separated from the lumen of the duodenum by a membrane composed of two layers of mucosa—one layer of enteric mucosa lining the choledochocele and one layer of duodenal mucosa covering the choledochocele. (*From* Scholz, F. J., Carrera, G. F., and Larson, C. R.: The choledochocele: correlation of radiological, clinical and pathological findings. Radiology *118:*25–28, 1976.)

become edematous and markedly increased in size. In such instances, abnormal clinical or laboratory findings (for example, jaundice or elevated level of serum amylase) combined with the radiographically prominent papilla alert the clinician to investigate further the ampullary axis (biliary tree, pancreas, and duodenum). Endoscopic retrograde cholangiopancreatography, ultrasonography, computerized axial tomography, and intravenous or percutaneous cholangiography usually aid in establishing a correct diagnosis. A prominent papilla alone, with no abnormal laboratory or clinical findings, can be observed closely for a suitable clinical period.

Choledochocele

The choledochocele (Fig. 11–24) is a rare lesion of uncertain origin that is believed by some to be a congenital diverticulum of the ampulla of Vater, by others to be an enterogenous cyst of the duodenum communicating with the biliary and pancreatic ducts, and by still others to be an acquired dilatation of the terminal common bile duct secondary to inflammatory stenosis of the papilla of Vater. No matter what its origin, it can be defined clinically, surgically, and radiographically as a cystic dilatation of the terminal common bile duct projecting wholly or partly into the duodenal lumen.[48] It does not fill during the upper gastrointestinal series but does appear similar to a cyst projecting into and occasionally even occluding the duodenal lumen. It is opacified during cholangiography, whether intravenous, operative, retrograde, or percutaneous. Most patients present with recurring abdominal pain. Occasionally, jaundice, cholangitis, pancreatitis, and gastrointestinal bleeding occur. Choledocholithiasis or calculi in the choledochocele have been reported to occur in 31 per cent of patients.[48] The pancreatic duct usually drains either directly into the choledochocele or into the ampulla, which then drains into the choledochocele. Because of these varying relationships, surgical reports of these lesions stress that the ducts should have probes placed in them before surgical excision is attempted. The choledochocele is lined by enteric mucosa.

Duodenotomy Pseudotumors

During biliary or pancreatic operation, the duodenum may be opened for sphincterotomy or for evaluation of the ampulla. The incision is usually on the lateral aspect of the descending duodenum. Closure of this opening produces a variety of inversion defects that may subsequently mimic disease. Two types of appearances have been described in the lateral wall of the duodenum: one, a polypoid masslike defect (Fig. 11–25), and the other, a convex, tapered indentation (Fig. 11–26); bizarre configurations also may be seen, however. A history of pancreatic or duodenal operations in a patient with a deformity or mass in the descending limb of the duodenum should alert one to the possibility of a pseudotumor.[33]

Intussusception Pseudotumors

The duodenal bulb is bounded by two tubular structures, the tubular duodenum and the tubular pylorus. Because each has a smaller diameter than the bulb itself, each can prolapse or intussuscept into it. Invagination of the pylorus or antrum into the

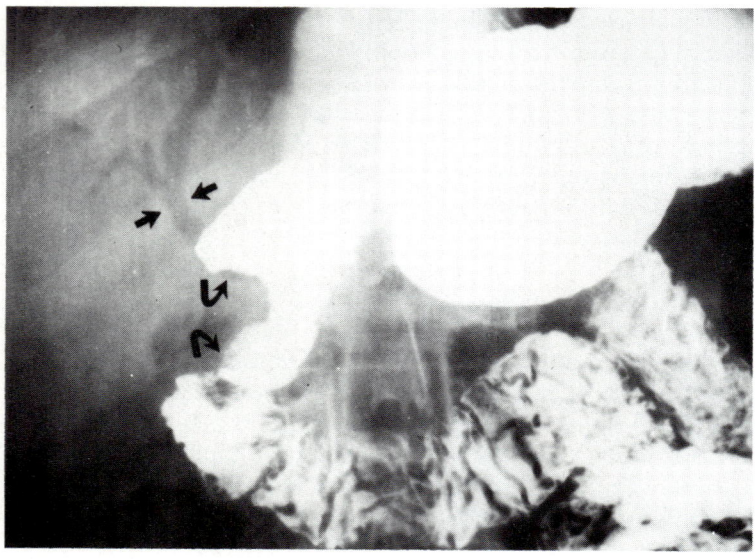

Figure 11–25. Postoperative pseudotumor. A large duodenotomy defect (curved arrows) is demonstrated in the descending duodenum. Air is demonstrated in the biliary tree (straight arrows).

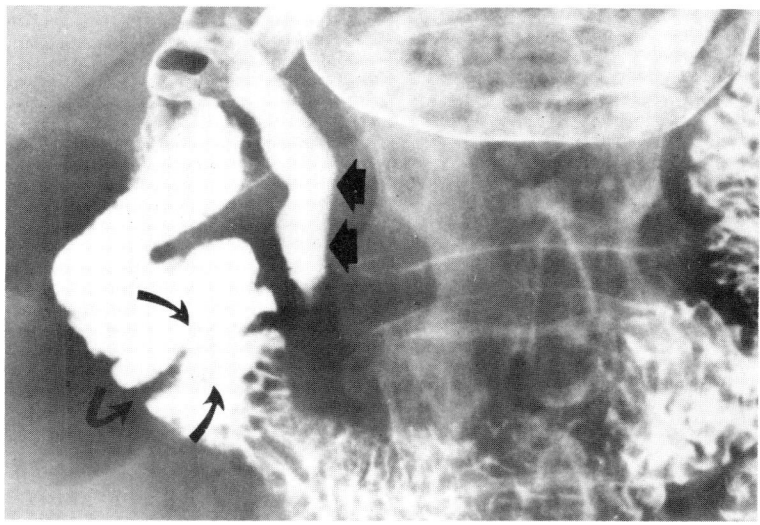

Figure 11–26. Postoperative pseudotumor. Curved arrows point to a filling defect in the descending duodenum opposite the region of the papilla. This represents the inverted site of closure of the duodenotomy. Because of sphincteroplasty, barium refluxes into the common bile duct (paired large arrows).

duodenal bulb may simulate a mass, but it is usually transient and inconstant, and careful fluoroscopy shows normal peripyloric anatomy (Fig. 11–27). Rarely, the bulb may telescope transiently over its tubular postbulbar portion, giving a pseudotumor appearance, but again, careful fluoroscopy clarifies this appearance. Persistent or nonreducible invagination may be seen in adult hypertrophic pyloric stenosis and is one diagnostic component of this entity. Occasionally, a gastric polyp intussuscepts into the duodenal bulb.

Flexure Pseudotumors

Whenever a tubular structure bends to a 90° or sharper angle, the wall of the tube along the concave aspect of the bend tends to be noticeably less distensible than the convex wall. This is true in the duodenum as well as in the small bowel and colon. Incomplete distensibility may cause a noticeable bunching up of the mucosa and give

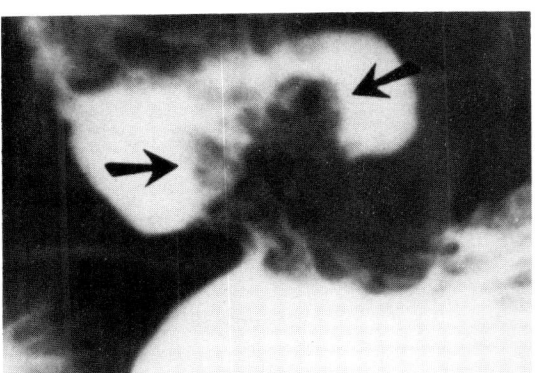 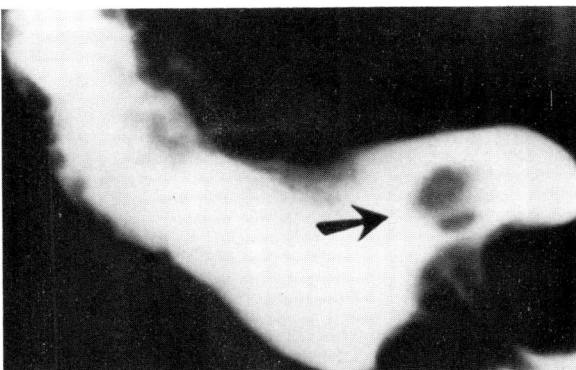

Figure 11–27. Pseudotumor. A mass noted in the base of the duodenal bulb is seen to change with peristalsis (arrows). The majority of the defect was believed to be due to invagination of the pylorus into the base of the duodenal bulb. A small filling defect persisted, however. At endoscopy, a small submucosal "bump" was noted that was consistent with a pancreatic rest, solitary Brunner's gland, or a submucosal process, such as leiomyoma or carcinoid tumor. Follow-up study for several years showed no change.

the appearance of a filling defect.[8] In the duodenum, this occurs classically at the junction of the apex of the bulb and the tubular proximal descending limb (Fig. 11–28). An abrupt flexure anywhere in the duodenum, however, may resemble such a filling defect (Fig. 11–29). If a radiograph can be obtained with the flexure in profile, the acute bend can be shown (see Fig. 11–29). Often, barium trapped in the bunched, nondistensible folds mimics an ulcer. Changeability during rotation and peristalsis usually permits exclusion of the diagnosis of neoplasm or other disease.

Obstruction

Many lesions already discussed may occasionally or frequently cause obstructive symptoms. The following entities are almost always associated with obstructive symptoms, and patients present with recurring nausea and vomiting.

Annular Pancreas

With incomplete rotation and fusion of the dorsal and ventral pancreatic buds that normally arise from opposite walls of the descending duodenum, a collar of remnant pancreatic tissue surrounds the descending limb of the duodenum. This collar usually narrows the postbulbar portion of the duodenum, and patients are usually neonates with high intestinal obstruction. Not all such collars are tight enough to cause an immediate neonatal problem, however, and symptoms may arise in adults. Pancreatitis in the adult may precipitate obstructive symptoms when the edematous pancreatic collar further narrows the duodenal lumen (Figs. 11–30 and 11–31).

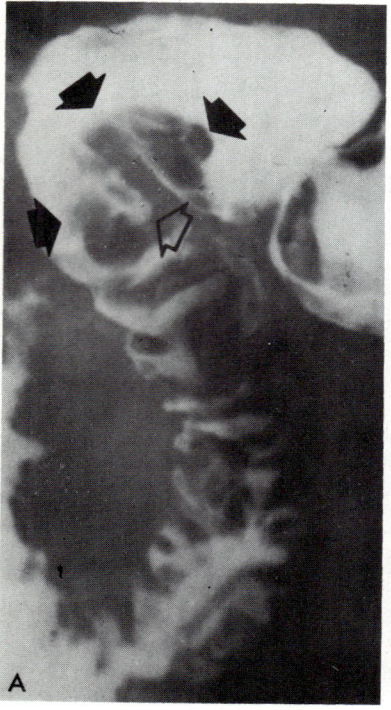
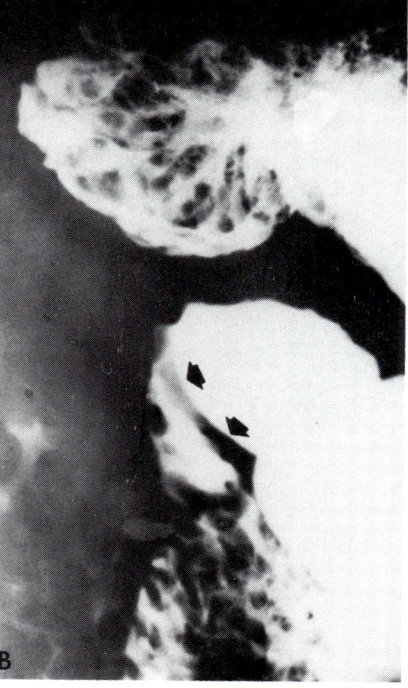

Figure 11–28. Pseudotumor. *A,* A polypoid filling defect is seen in the apex of the bulb and the proximal descending limb of the duodenum (three solid arrows). The collection of barium in the center (open arrow) suggests an ulcer crater. This is a classic flexure pseudotumor or flexure pseudoulcer with a mass simulated at the bend of the duodenum. *B,* With an increase in obliquity, this lesion disappears and is replaced by an abrupt fold (two arrows). Rotation during fluoroscopy confirmed that the pseudotumor was due to an abrupt fold or bend in the duodenum.

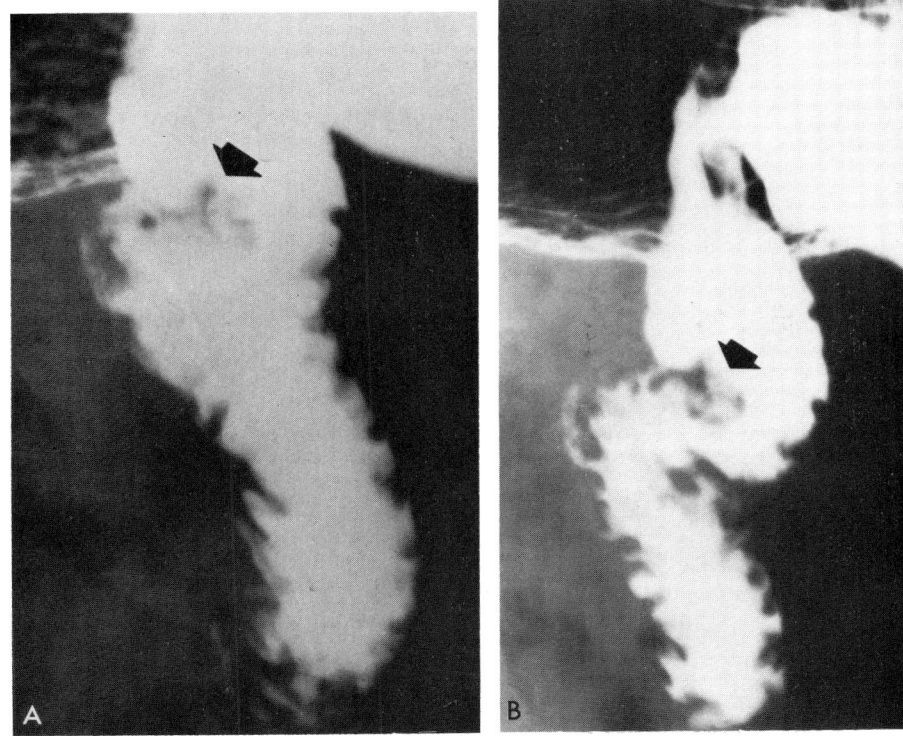
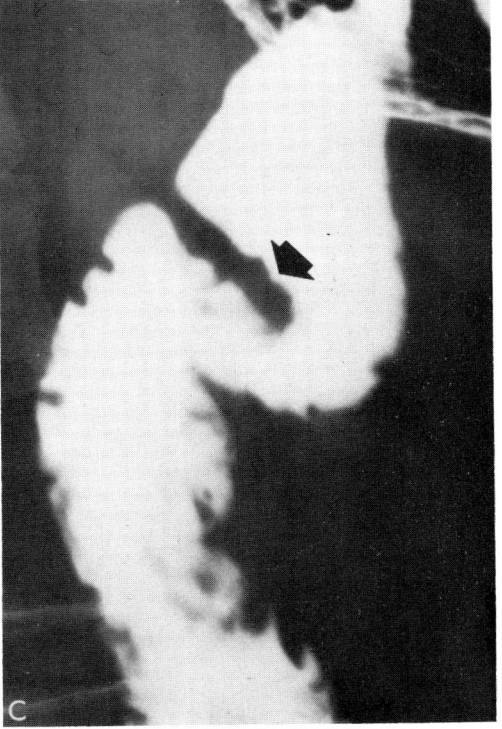

Figure 11–29. Pseudotumor. *A,* At fluoroscopy, a poorly defined filling defect (arrow) is seen in the proximal descending limb of the duodenum. *B,* With gradual rotation of the patient, this becomes more distinct (arrow). *C,* Finally, with more complete rotation, this is confirmed to be a flexure pseudotumor due to an abrupt bend (arrow) in the duodenum.

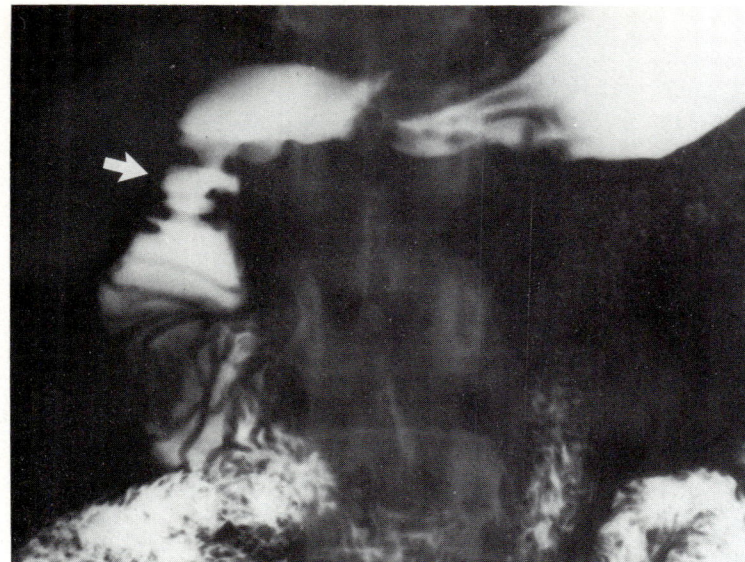

Figure 11-30. Annular narrowing and incomplete distensibility in the proximal descending duodenum (arrow). The presence of annular pancreas was confirmed at surgery.

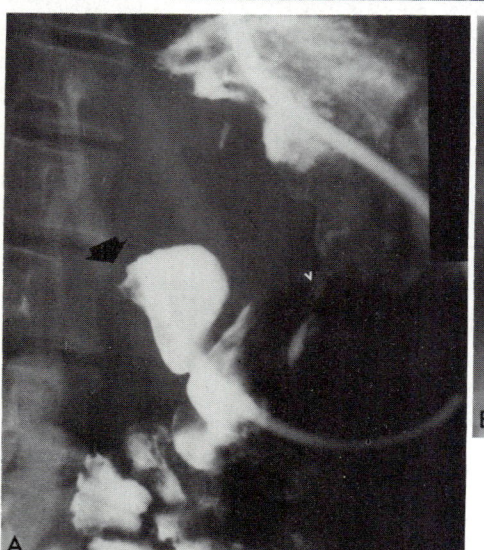

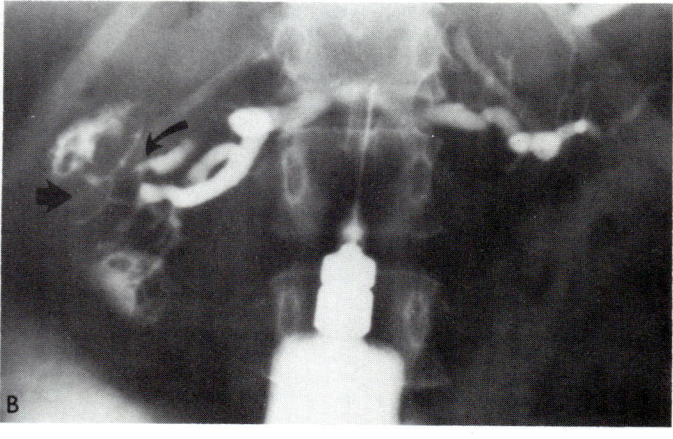

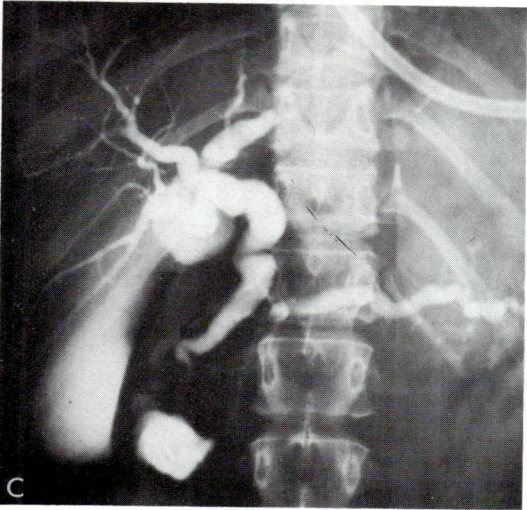

Figure 11-31. Annular pancreas. This patient as an infant had duodenal obstruction from an annular pancreas, which required gastrojejunostomy. As a young adult, the patient experienced pain and was re-examined. *A*, Complete obstruction was noted at the apex of the duodenal bulb (arrow) with drainage of the stomach via a gastrojejunostomy. At operation, chronic pancreatitis was found, and a distal pancreaticojejunostomy was performed, resulting in clinical improvement. *B*, Operative pancreatography demonstrates opacification of the pancreatic ducts (arrow) within the annular pancreas itself. The pancreatic duct drained into the duodenum via the main and accessory ducts giving rise to two separate puddles of contrast material in the duodenum, presumably above and below the constricted duodenal segment. Minimal filling of the common bile duct (curved arrow) is subsequently well opacified. *C*, Separate operative cholangiography demonstrates relationship of common duct (curved arrow), pancreatic duct, and annular pancreas.

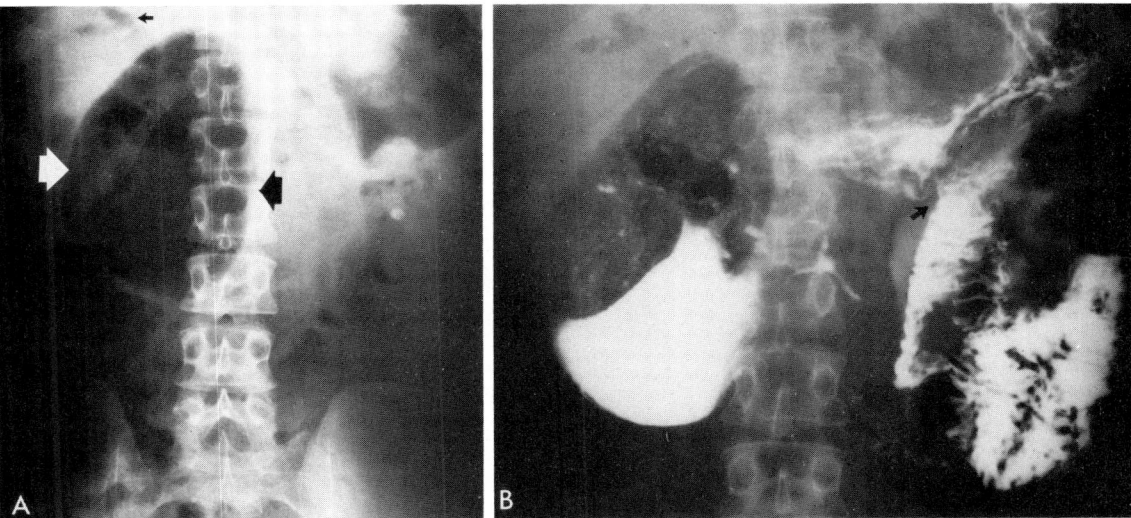

Figure 11–32. Duodenal atresia—late complications. This patient with trisomy required a gastrojejunostomy after birth because of duodenal atresia. Attacks of cholangitis, nausea, and vomiting occurred when the patient was a young adult. *A*, A film of the abdomen shows a large air-filled oval structure (large arrows) in the right upper quadrant and air in the intrahepatic bile ducts (small arrow). *B*, A gastrointestinal series shows a well-functioning gastrojejunostomy (arrow), but barium also drains via the antrum into the oval structure. This was found at operation to be a chronically dilated duodenum. Duodenojejunostomy relieved all symptoms. Multiple anomalies of the bile ducts were also noted.

Postbulbar ring strictures may be caused by processes other than annular pancreas. In the case of postbulbar ulcers, healing may cause circumferential fibrotic scarring. It may be very difficult or impossible radiographically, surgically, or pathologically to differentiate stricture due to postbulbar ulcer from annular pancreas.

Most strictures probably represent postbulbar ulcer scarring. Duodenal atresia occurs and is corrected in the newborn, but complications may arise years later, especially after gastrojejunostomy (Fig. 11–32). Other causes for duodenal stenoses include peritoneal colohepatic bands (Ladd's bands), seen in incomplete rotation or nonrotation of the colon,[25] and the rare preduodenal portal vein, in which the portal vein crosses in front of, rather than behind, the duodenum.[6, 22]

Intraluminal Duodenal Diverticulum

The intraluminal duodenal diverticulum is a rare entity with a characteristic radiographic appearance (Fig. 11–33).[35, 44, 58] An increased incidence in Down's syndrome is reported.[14, 46] Its origin is probably related to the period of vacuole coalescence in early embryologic life (see Cysts of the Duodenum, p. 514). If a transverse portion of the wall between the two major duodenal vacuoles fails to disappear, a duodenal diaphragm remains.[44] If this is complete, the neonate will have complete duodenal obstruction requiring immediate surgical correction. If the diaphragm is incomplete and an opening permitting passage of food is present, however, the patient presents later in life with the entity known as the intraluminal duodenal diverticulum. Gradual peristaltic pressure on the intact portion of the diaphragm causes progressive invagination, until the diaphragm has the typical windsock or comet-shaped appearance. The site of attachment is always in the descending limb, usually at, or just above or below, the papilla of Vater. It is lined on both sides by duodenal mucosa. Symptoms usually do not

524 — DUODENUM

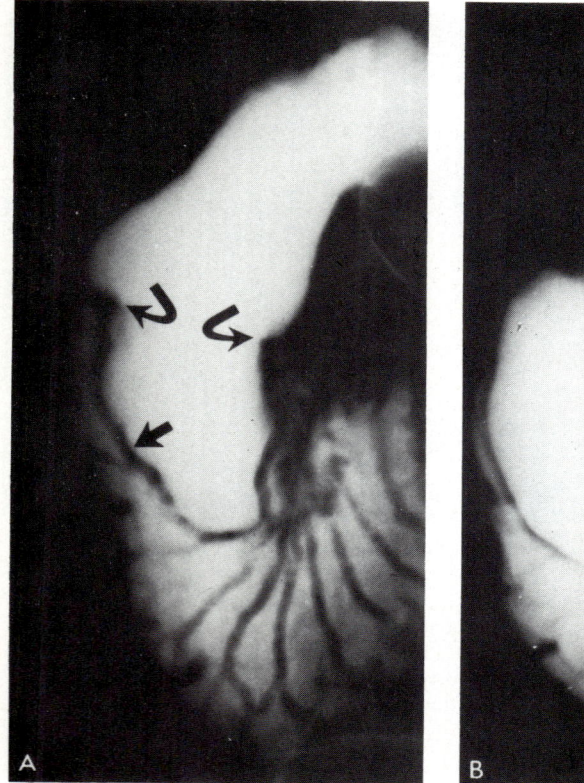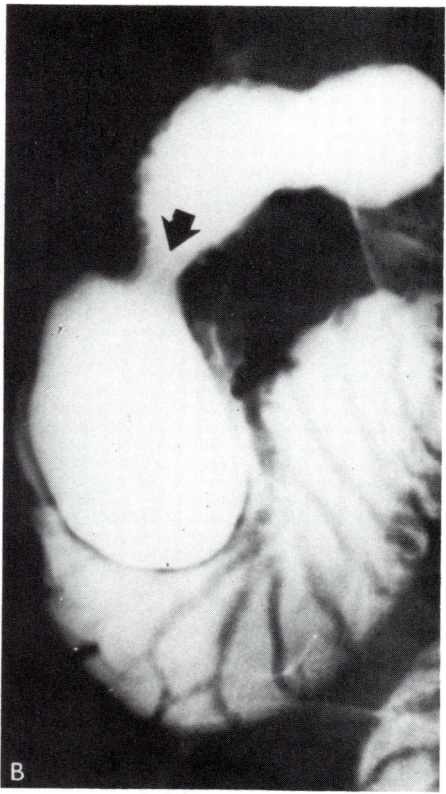

Figure 11–33. The typical appearance of an intraluminal duodenal diverticulum can be noted. *A,* The straight arrow shows the thin membrane of the diverticulum, which is lined on the inside and covered on the outside by duodenal mucosa. Dilatation of the duodenum is evident proximal to the attachment (curved arrows) of the membranous diaphragm to the duodenal wall. *B,* A peristaltic wave demonstrates the pliability of the diverticulum and the ballooning of its fundus that occurs as each peristaltic wave squeezes it from its orifice (arrow) to its fundus.

occur until adulthood, when the diverticulum has attained considerable size. The pain, nausea, and vomiting may be due not only to degrees of duodenal obstruction but also to peristaltic pressure pulling or stretching the intraluminal diverticulum. The fundus of the diverticulum may stretch to the ligament of Treitz because of chronic peristaltic traction. Ingested foreign bodies, such as fruit pits, may be trapped within the intraluminal duodenal diverticulum.

Superior Mesenteric Artery Syndrome

Considerable controversy exists about the superior mesenteric artery syndrome. Most clinicians agree that such a syndrome exists but disagree about its origin, severity, frequency, and treatment. Some believe that a superior mesenteric artery syndrome is secondary to obstruction of the duodenum from the acute angle formed by the superior mesenteric artery and the aorta and that certain factors precipitate obstruction of the duodenum at this point. The classic syndrome (Figs. 11–34 and 11–35) consists of nausea and vomiting in association with most or all of the following radiographic features: duodenal dilatation; intermittent reversal of peristaltic activity in the duodenum, producing a churning to-and-fro activity; delay of transit through the gastro-

DUODENUM — 525

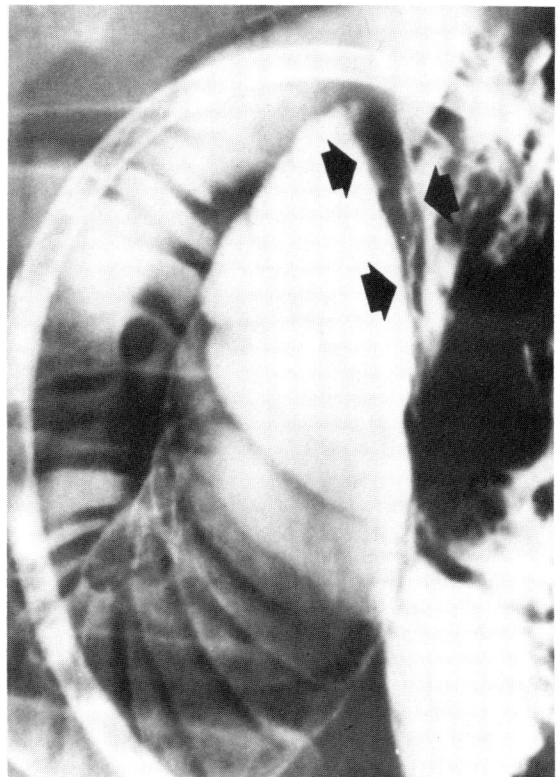

Figure 11–34. Superior mesenteric artery impression. The arrows point to a tubular impression seen on hypotonic duodenography (induced ileus). The insufflation of air into the hypotonic duodenum shows transient trapping of air in the duodenum proximal to the tubular impression, and a nondistended duodenum can be seen behind the single arrow. This patient was not operated on because symptoms were not believed to be related to the superior mesenteric artery impression.

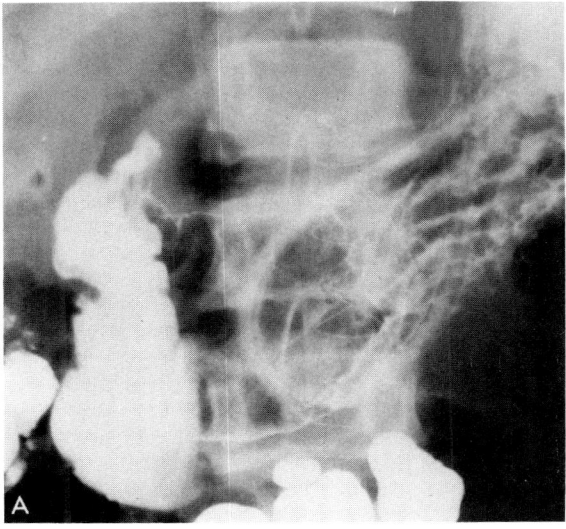

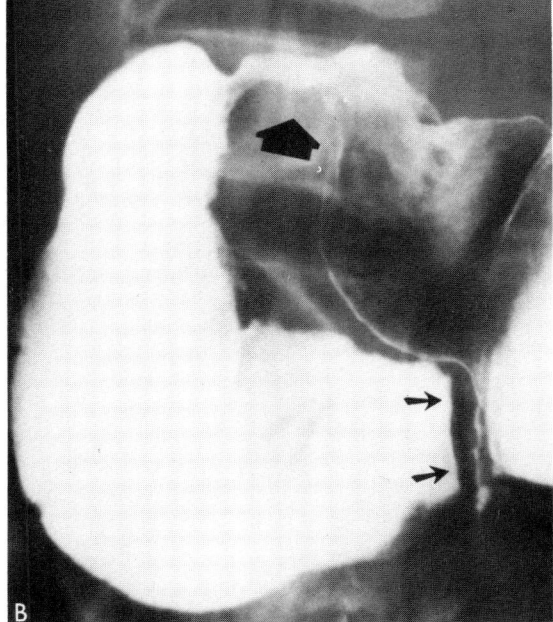

Figure 11–35. Superior mesenteric artery syndrome. *A,* Barium persists in a dilated descending duodenum, abruptly terminating where the duodenum crosses the spine. *B,* Gastroduodenal Crohn's disease with loss of pyloric anatomic landmarks is apparent. The antrum and the duodenal bulb are narrowed, and the pyloric canal is widened (large arrow). A tubular impression (small arrows) on the ascending portion of the duodenum represents a superior mesenteric artery impression. Persistent vomiting gradually improved only after release of the duodenum from the ligament of Treitz. The patient's symptoms had not responded to previous gastrojejunostomy. (Courtesy of Edward B. Singleton, M.D., St. Luke's Episcopal Hospital, Houston, Texas.)

duodenal region for several hours; abrupt obstruction, with an oblique cutoff in the distal duodenum with normal caliber of the duodenum distal to the superior mesenteric artery impression; and more prompt passage of barium in the knee-chest position. The syndrome has been seen in children and adults, and several predisposing events appear to precipitate the acute syndrome. Application of body casts,[27] acute weight loss, forced supine immobility,[26] severe trauma, operation, and severe burns[52] have been noted as precipitating events. Chronic syndrome without known predisposing factors is unusual.[42]

Some investigators, however, question whether obstruction plays a primary etiologic role in the syndrome—or any role at all. They believe that the syndrome is a reflection of a temporary or permanent generalized neuromuscular disorder that is most manifest in the duodenum with relative duodenal atony and dilatation. Dilatation of the duodenum is seen in both symptomatic and asymptomatic patients with progressive systemic sclerosis,[24] systemic lupus erythematosus, Ehlers-Danlos syndrome,[2] pancreatitis,[49] diabetes, regional enteritis, and idiopathic megaduodenum,[1] and after vagotomy. In each of these entities, all of the radiographic features of the superior mesenteric artery syndrome have been noted, but the common feature is a neuromuscular disorder, a "paralytic ileus" of the duodenum.

The truth may lie between these two extremes. Most likely the ileus does play some role in precipitating or accentuating obstructive symptoms related to the crossing point of the duodenum and superior mesenteric artery. In many instances, conservative treatment (for example, nasogastric suction or the removal of a body cast) provides relief. If the ileus does not respond to conservative therapy, duodenojejunostomy may be required. Even though opinions concerning its origin and treatment vary, the

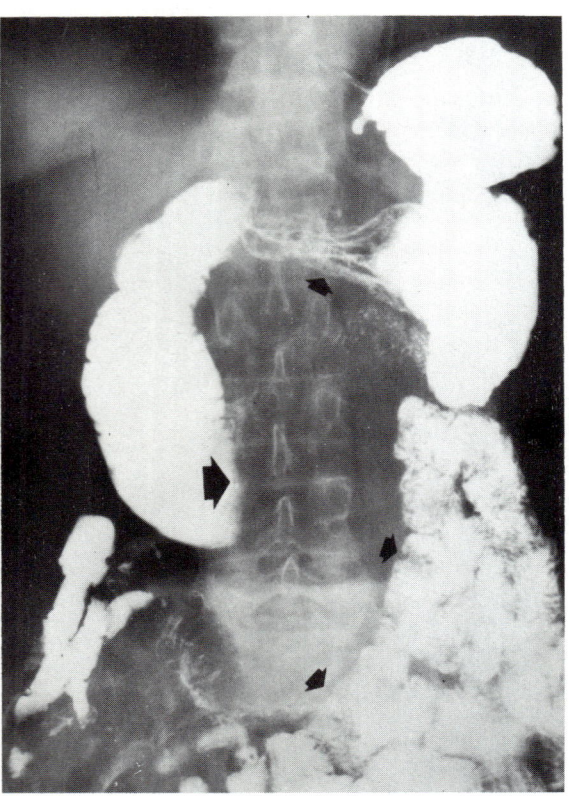

Figure 11–36. Aortic aneurysm. Symptoms of intermittent upper abdominal obstruction led to a gastrointestinal series that showed a dilated duodenum changing abruptly (large arrow) to a more normal duodenal caliber. The patient has a large, pulsatile abdominal mass, and associated pressure on the antrum of the stomach (upper small arrow) and on the small bowel (lower small arrows) is apparent.

superior mesenteric artery syndrome with persistent vomiting has occasionally been fatal when not diagnosed early. With early diagnosis, operative and nonoperative therapy have both been effective.

Aneurysms

Aortic aneurysms may cause obstruction of the duodenum. Aneurysmal enlargement of the aorta encroaches on the angle formed by the superior mesenteric artery and aorta. The radiographic changes in the duodenum may be identical to those of the superior mesenteric artery syndrome. Usually, however, aneurysms large enough to cause enteric obstructive symptoms also cause typical mass effects on the stomach and small and large bowel and are clinically apparent as a pulsatile abdominal mass (Fig. 11–36).

TRAUMA

Blunt and penetrating injuries to the abdomen often involve the duodenum. The most common penetrating injury occurs during an abdominal operation. Because the duodenum straddles the epigastrium, any upper abdominal operation may affect the duodenum. Similarly, blunt abdominal trauma often results in duodenal hematomas.

Hematoma

Hematomas of the gastrointestinal tract from blunt abdominal trauma occur most commonly in the duodenum, usually in the region where the duodenum crosses the spine. A blunt force can compress the fixed retroperitoneal duodenum against the spine or posterior abdominal wall musculature. The hematoma forms between the serosa and the muscularis and usually compresses the lumen eccentrically. The lumen becomes crescent-shaped in cross section, and barium in this distorted lumen fills the crescentically stretched mucosal folds giving a coiled-spring appearance (Fig. 11–37).[21] With resolution or diffusion of the organized hematoma, the masslike effect diminishes. The mucosal folds in resolving hematomas are edematous. The appearance of diffuse edema has been likened to a picket fence or stack of coins (Figs. 11–38 and 11–39), which may also be seen in spontaneous diffuse hemorrhage resulting from anticoagulation or bleeding diatheses.[56] An organized hematoma, with its coiled-spring appearance, is not seen with such spontaneous hemorrhages.

Often, duodenal hematomas are associated with retroperitoneal hematomas and pancreatic and liver trauma, and sorting one element from another may be difficult radiographically. The coiled-spring appearance of the duodenal hematoma and the "stack of coins" or "picket fence" appearance of resolving hematomas should alert the physician to the likelihood of a duodenal hematoma and stimulate a search for associated intra-abdominal trauma.

Aortoenteric and Paraprosthetic-Enteric Fistulas

The ascending portion of the duodenum is associated intimately with both the superior mesenteric artery anteriorly and the aorta posteriorly. The intimate aortoduo-

528 — DUODENUM

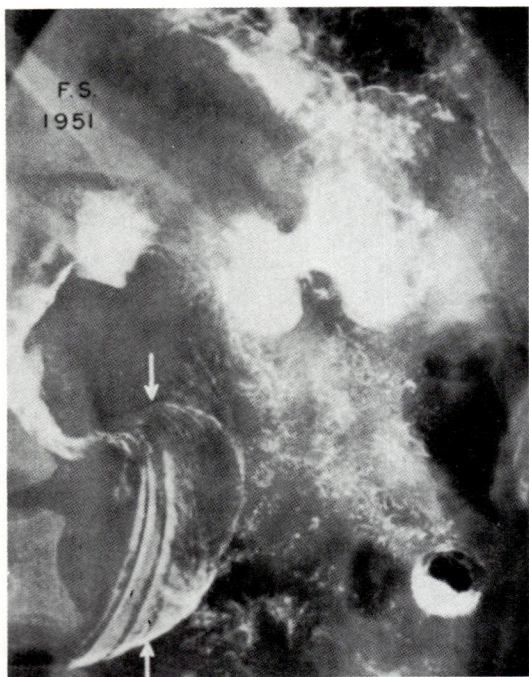

Figure 11–37. An upper gastrointestinal radiograph showing the "coiled spring sign" (arrow) indicative of post-trauma duodenal hematoma. (*From* Felson, B., and Levin, E. J.: Intramural hematoma of the duodenum. A diagnostic roentgen sign. Radiology *68:*823–829, 1954.)

Figure 11–38. Duodenal hematoma. A "picket fence" appearance is seen in the ascending portion of the distal duodenum (between arrows). Deformity of the adjacent portion of the jejunum is present. Intramural hematoma was diagnosed and treated conservatively in this patient who suffered blunt trauma to the midepigastrium. The follow-up examination showed a normal duodenum.

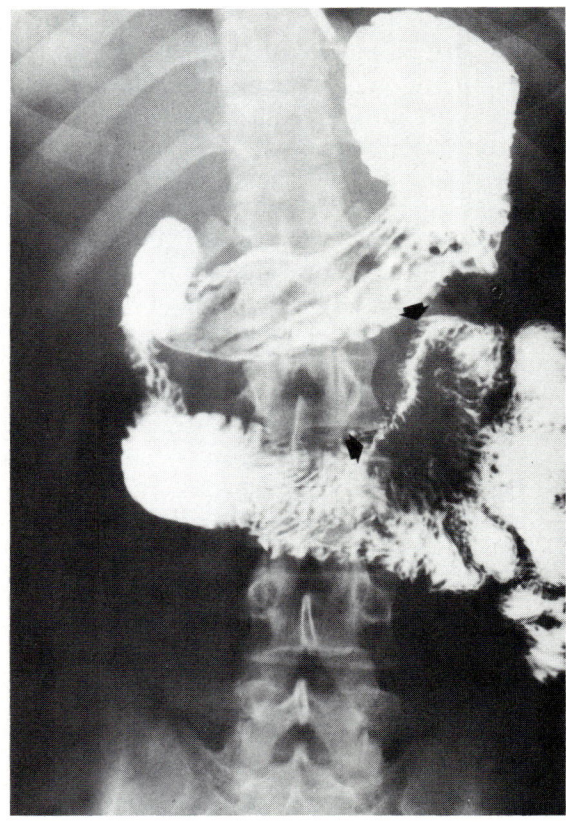

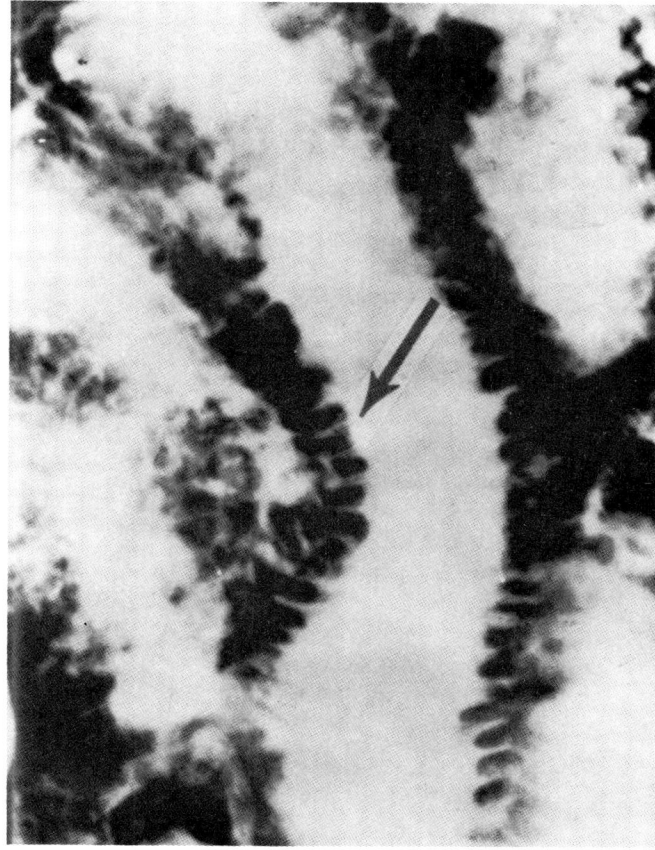

Figure 11–39. Spontaneous hemorrhage into the duodenum in a patient receiving anticoagulant therapy. The spiculated "stack of coins" appearance is characteristic of the fold thickening (arrow) seen in hemorrhage resulting from anticoagulant therapy and bleeding diatheses and occasionally seen in resolving traumatic hematomas. (*From* Fullen, W. D., Selle, J. G., Whitely, D. H., et al.: Intramural duodenal hematoma. Ann. Surg. *179:*549–556, 1974.)

denal relationship also plays a role in the formation of fistulas between the duodenum and the aorta (aortoenteric fistula) or aortic bed (paraprosthetic-enteric fistula). Paraprosthetic communication with the jejunum, ileum, and sigmoid colon has been reported.[15, 19]

Patients with aortoenteric fistulas usually present with acute upper and lower gastrointestinal hemorrhage, although the hemorrhage may be intermittent for several days or weeks. Patients whose fistulas communicate only with the duodenum and the adjacent periprosthetic tissue plane without communication with the aortic lumen usually present with chronic sepsis for weeks, months, and occasionally, years. Rarely, spontaneous fistulas occur without previous aortic operation, especially in instances of aortic aneurysm. More commonly, duodenal aortic and duodenal paraprosthetic fistulas occur after aortic resection and graft procedures,[15, 19] renal artery bypass grafts,[30] and aortofemoral bypass grafts,[15, 19] in which sepsis develops in the groin wound (Fig. 11–40).

The radiographic diagnosis may be made by aortography in patients with active bleeding. In patients without gastrointestinal bleeding, a gastrointestinal series may show a fistula between the duodenum and the periaortic tissues in paraprosthetic-enteric fistulas. Pressure on the duodenum from an acute hematoma or a chronic abscess may be the only demonstrable abnormality and, when minimal, may not be distinguishable from postoperative distortion. If a skin fistula is present, cutaneous fistulography may permit the diagnosis of a paraprosthetic-enteric fistula. Even in the absence of conclusive radiographic studies, however, the clinical diagnosis of aortoen-

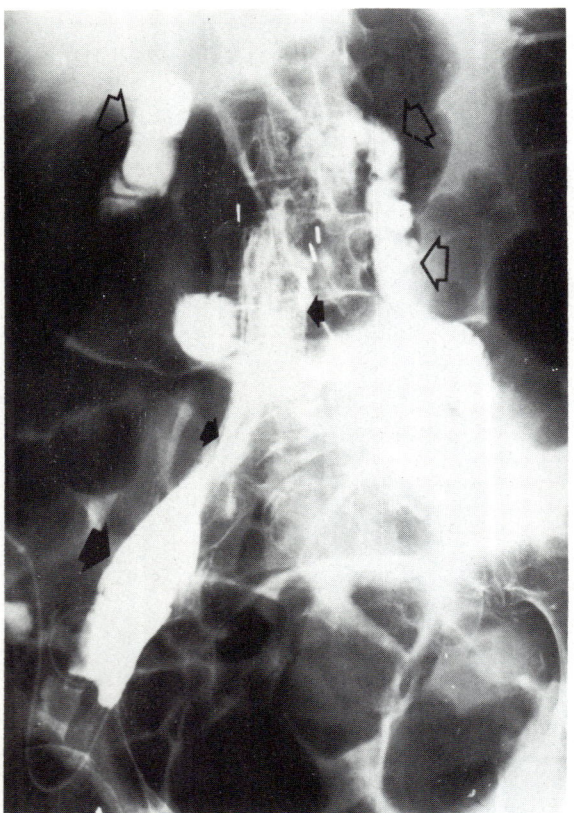

Figure 11–40. Aortic graft—duodenal fistula. A fistula developed from the right groin. Several years earlier, the patient had had an aortoiliac bypass graft. Injection of a Foley catheter inserted into the right groin tract (large solid arrow) demonstrated contrast material tracking along and outlining the cloth pattern of the graft (small solid arrows). Contrast material passed from the aortic graft bed into the ascending duodenum delineating the duodenum and the small bowel (open arrows). (Courtesy of Stefan Schatzki, Mount Auburn Hospital, Cambridge, Massachusetts.)

teric or paraprosthetic-enteric fistula must be considered in every instance of abdominal aortic reconstruction with late hemorrhagic or septic complications.[19] The duodenum is the most common site of involvement, and attention should be focused on the distal portion of the duodenum.

Ampullary Disconnection

A rare complication of Billroth I or Billroth II procedures is ampullary disconnection, also termed ampullary transection or avulsion of the ampulla of Vater (Figs. 11–41 and 11–42).[11, 12, 16, 53] With dissection of the proximal descending limb of the duodenum before stump closure in a Billroth II procedure or duodenal mobilization for anastomosis in a Billroth I procedure, the ampulla may be transected or avulsed forcibly from its insertion into the duodenal wall. About one fourth of such disconnections are not recognized and are not repaired during the initial surgical procedure. The diagnosis is made postoperatively when bile begins to drain from the incision. Fistulography shows contrast filling the biliary and pancreatic ducts without filling the duodenum. Lack of duodenal filling is the key finding in differentiating disconnection from a breakdown in the anastomosis (Billroth I) or duodenal stump closure (Billroth II). Rarely, ampullary disconnection may be seen after blunt abdominal trauma.[4] Peritonitis usually develops, and radiographic evaluation is not required in such instances.

Figure 11–41. Ampullary disconnection. Fistulogram shows simultaneous injection of both pancreatic and common bile ducts but not of the duodenum, pathognomonic of disconnection of the ampulla. Variation in the shape of the terminal portion (arrow) more clearly seen on fluoroscopy as rhythmic contractions confirms the integrity of the sphincter of Oddi. (*From* Corlette, M. B.: Disconnection of the ampulla of Vater. Surg. Gynecol. Obstet. *141:*915–918, 1975. Reproduced by permission of Surgery, Gynecology & Obstetrics.)

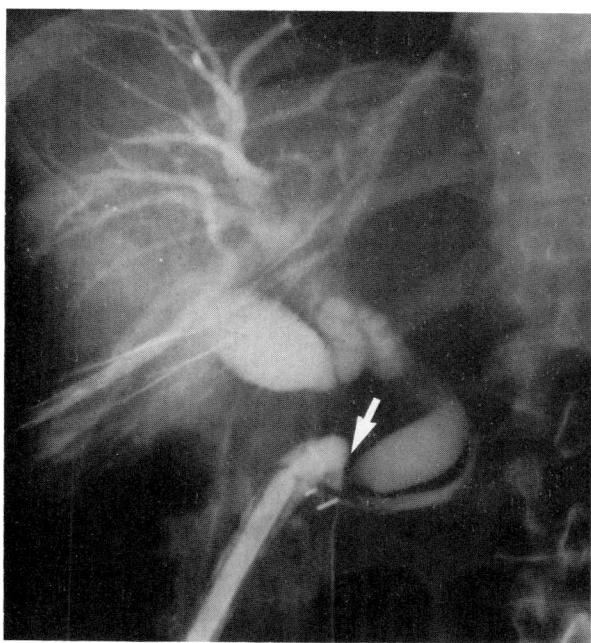

Stump Leak

One cause of subhepatic and subphrenic collections and enteric-cutaneous drainage after Billroth II procedures is a leak from the closed end or stump of the duodenum (Fig. 11–43). If proper regional drainage can be maintained to prevent the formation of a sterile or infected abscess, such stump leaks may heal spontaneously. It is important to obtain a radiograph before the administration of any contrast agent. The only clue to such a leak may be filling of the lumen of a sump drainage tube. With oral administra-

Figure 11–42. Ampullary disconnection. After surgical reimplantation of the ampulla into a Roux-en-Y jejunostomy, a control T-tube cholangiogram shows dye entering the Roux-en-Y limb. Passage of dye into the limb occurred at physiologic pressure. Fluoroscopy again confirmed the functional integrity of the sphincter. (*From* Corlette, M. B.: Disconnection of the ampulla of Vater. Surg. Gynecol. Obstet. *141:*915–918, 1975. Reproduced by permission of Surgery, Gynecology & Obstetrics.)

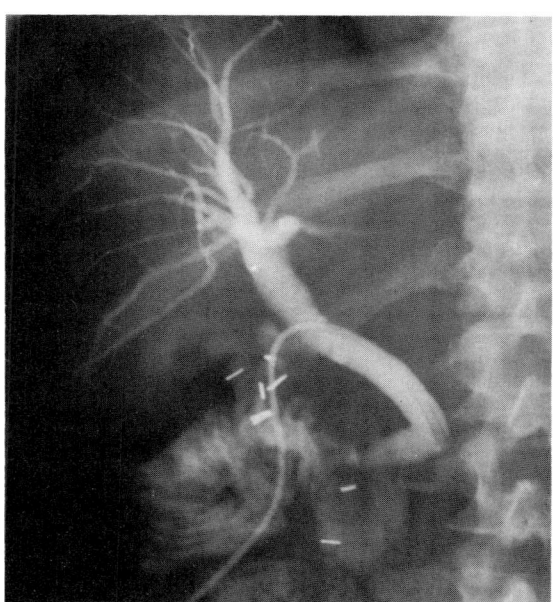

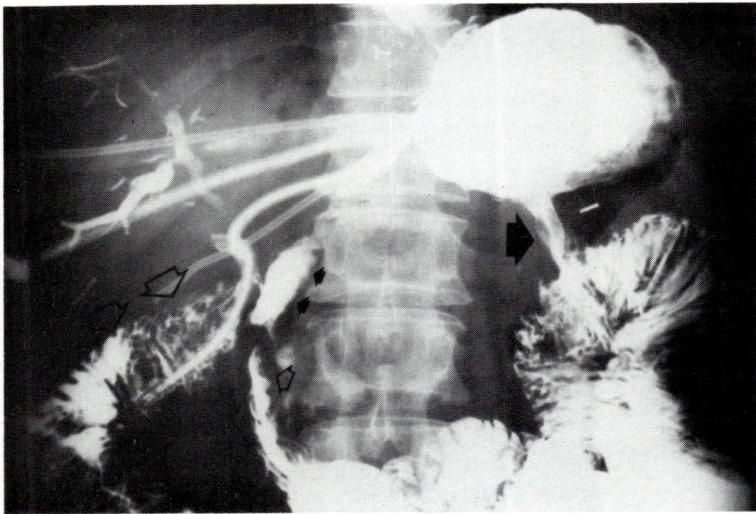

Figure 11–43. Stump leak. Persisting drainage from a wound in the right upper abdominal quadrant after a hepaticojejunostomy and gastroenterostomy for chronic pancreatitis. The large solid arrow shows functioning gastrojejunal anastomosis. Two open arrows point to barium in the jejunal limb, one limb of the T tube being filled with barium. Barium has refluxed into the intrahepatic ducts. The small open arrow points to the closed stump of the duodenum with a small trickle of barium in the subhepatic space (two small solid arrows). This eventually closed spontaneously.

tion of water-soluble contrast agents, the resulting contrast in the tube of the lumen may be faint, and only comparison with the preliminary radiograph will confirm that an enteric sump tube–cutaneous communication exists.

MISCELLANEOUS CONDITIONS

Crohn's Disease of the Duodenum

Crohn's disease of the duodenum is relatively uncommon and occurs in about 1 or 2 per cent of all patients with Crohn's disease.[36] The duodenal involvement may precede or follow the diagnosis of Crohn's disease elsewhere in the gastrointestinal tract. Occasionally, the duodenum may be the only site of involvement. Concurrent involvement of the gastric antrum and duodenal bulb is more common than is isolated involvement of either the stomach or the duodenum. Involvement of the antrum, pylorus, and duodenal bulb often leads to obliteration of the normal pyloric canal. In these instances, the antrum is narrowed, the pylorus is widened, and the duodenal bulb is narrowed, yielding a uniform tubular appearance that has been called a pseudo-post-Billroth I appearance (Fig. 11–44).[41] The radiographic findings in the duodenum include thickened folds, ulceration, pseudodiverticula, and short- or long-segment strictures (string sign). Involvement in or about the papilla of Vater may lead either to a patulous, incompetent sphincter of Oddi or to a fistula with reflux of barium into the common bile duct or pancreatic duct. Hepatic abscess and pancreatitis are reported complications.[37, 59] A duodenocolic fistula between the descending portion of the duodenum and the proximal transverse colon may cause a short bowel or blind loop syndrome or both. The colon, the duodenum, or both may be the diseased organ from which the fistula originates.

Duodenal Diverticular Disease

Diverticula occur frequently in the duodenum. The majority are acquired diverticula, consisting of only a mucosal layer herniated through the muscular wall of the duodenum. Rarely, an acquired diverticulum contains all layers of the duodenal wall and is secondary to traction from an adjacent inflammatory process. Congenital duodenal diverticula, which might be more properly classified as communicating duodenal duplication cysts or as tubular duodenal duplications, are rare.

Usually a single acquired diverticulum, the perivatarian diverticulum, is seen in the mid-descending duodenum in the ampullary window. Diverticula may be multiple and may occur anywhere in the duodenum, sometimes attaining considerable size (Fig. 11–45). The perivatarian diverticulum occurs in 3 per cent of patients.[41] The ampullary window is the channel through which the common ampulla or the separate pancreatic and biliary ducts normally pass. It is the weakest part of the duodenal wall and a frequent site of diverticulum formation (Figs. 11–46 and 11–47). This diverticulum usually arises parallel to the ampulla. With progressive enlargement of the diverticulum, the portion of the duodenal mucosa containing the ampulla itself sometimes herniates and the diverticulum contains the ampulla (see Fig. 11–47). The ampullary and other duodenal diverticula rarely undergo ulceration or perforation.[9, 28] The preoperative radiographic diagnosis of a perforated duodenal diverticulum is rarely made. The gastrointestinal series may show no abnormality because the neck of the diverticulum has become sealed or may show extravasation of contrast material into the adjacent retroperitoneum but without evidence of the preexisting diverticulum. Free

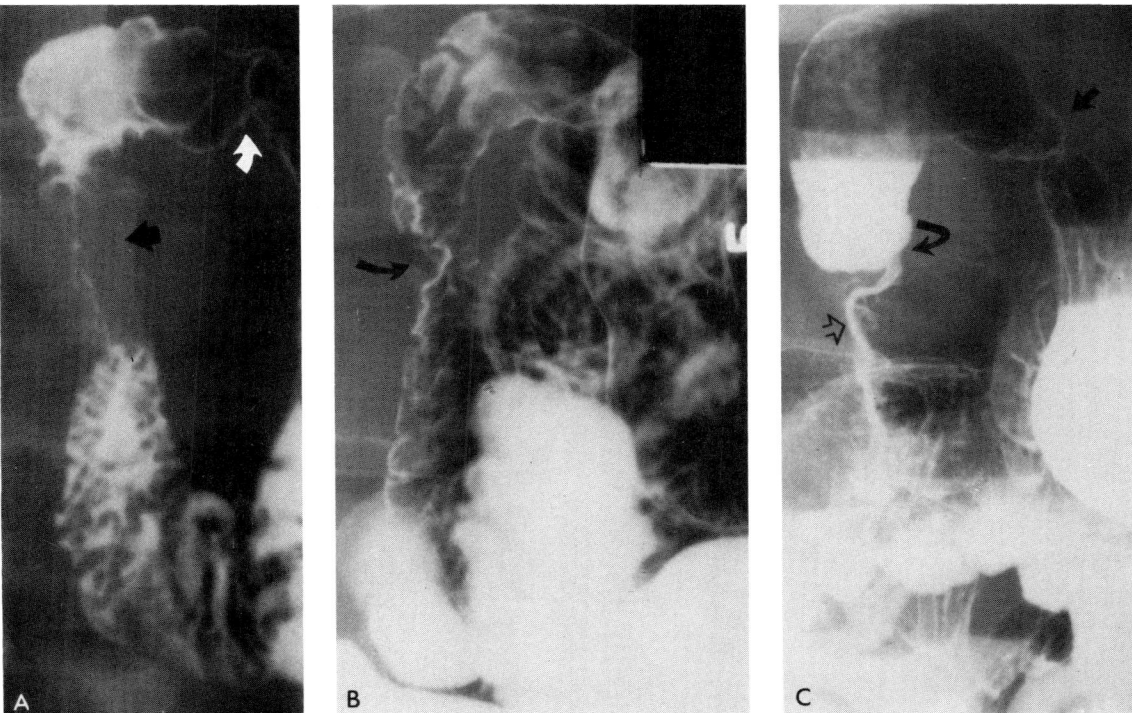

Figure 11–44. Crohn's disease. *A,* Incomplete distensibility (black arrow) of the descending limb of the duodenum and of the base of the duodenal bulb (white arrow) suggests the presence of Crohn's disease in this patient with known ileocecal Crohn's disease. *B,* After 0.5 mg of glucagon was administered intravenously, distensibility was somewhat better, but focal narrowing and nodularity persisted (curved arrow). *C,* The upright radiograph demonstrates a focal stenotic ring (curved arrow) with obstruction and an air barium level above. A thin stream of barium drained slowly through this narrowing (open arrow). The narrowed base of the duodenal bulb is visible again (straight black arrow). After endoscopy and a biopsy that confirmed the diagnosis of Crohn's disease, symptomatic improvement occurred with steroid therapy (Fig. 11–35).

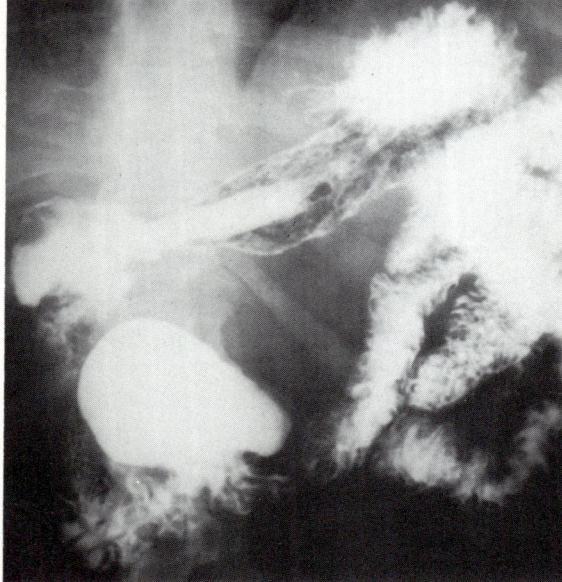

Figure 11–45. A giant duodenal diverticulum may be seen in asymptomatic patients. A massive diverticulum is visible in the proximal ascending limb of the duodenum.

intraperitoneal air is usually not evident because the duodenum, except for the bulb, is a retroperitoneal organ. Recognition of retroperitoneal air on a radiograph should suggest, among other diagnoses, perforation of the duodenum.[57] When ulceration occurs without perforation (Fig. 11–48), only rarely is a preoperative diagnosis made. With

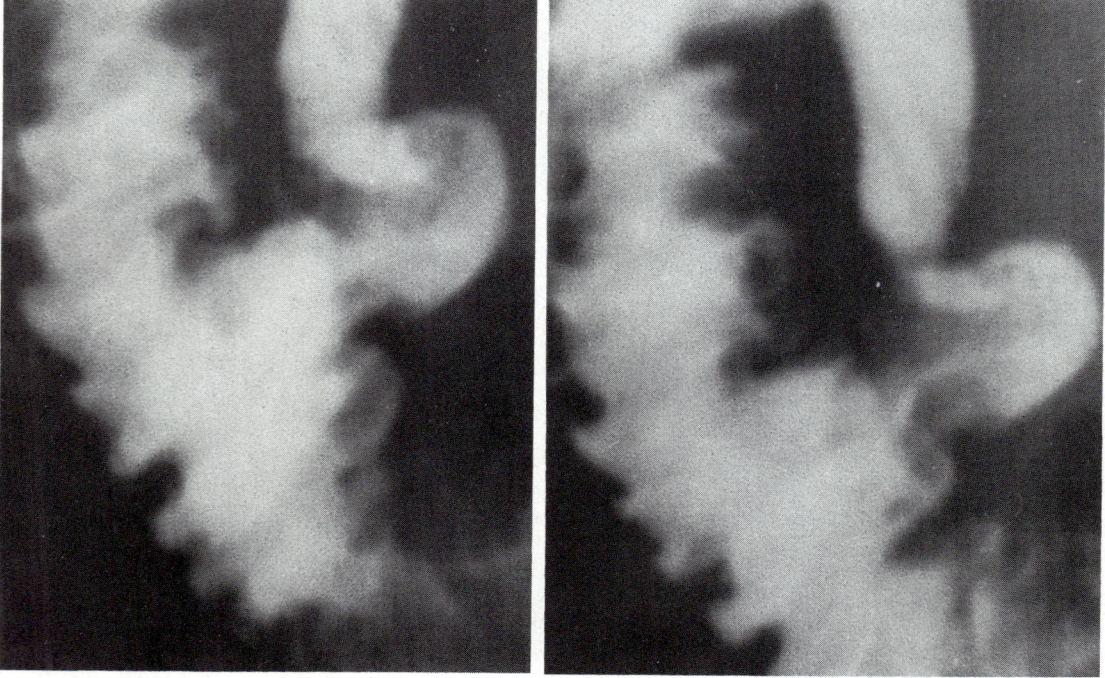

Figure 11–46. The distal common bile duct is seen draining into a diverticulum arising from the window (fenestra) in the duodenum through which the ampulla normally passes.

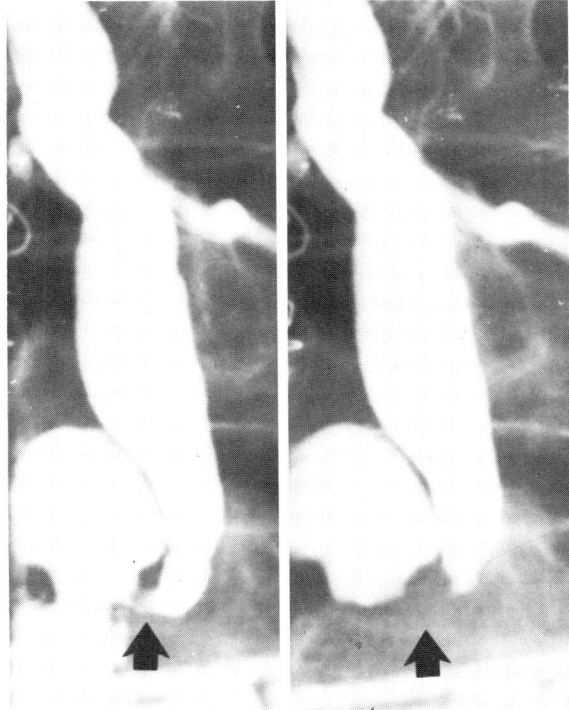

Figure 11-47. The common bile duct is seen entering the inferior wall of the diverticulum arising from the ampullary window. An intact sphincter has herniated through the hiatus and can be seen relaxed (left) and contracted (right.)

acute bleeding, angiography confirms active bleeding with contrast extravasation but only occasionally indicates its origin from a duodenal diverticulum.[23] Endoscopy usually does not disclose the location of the ulcer within the diverticulum unless blood is noted draining from the orifice of the diverticulum. Rarely, barium fills and delineates a crater within a diverticulum (see Fig. 11-18). Duodenal diverticula may be deformed from adjacent inflammatory or neoplastic pancreatic diseases (see Fig. 11-18).

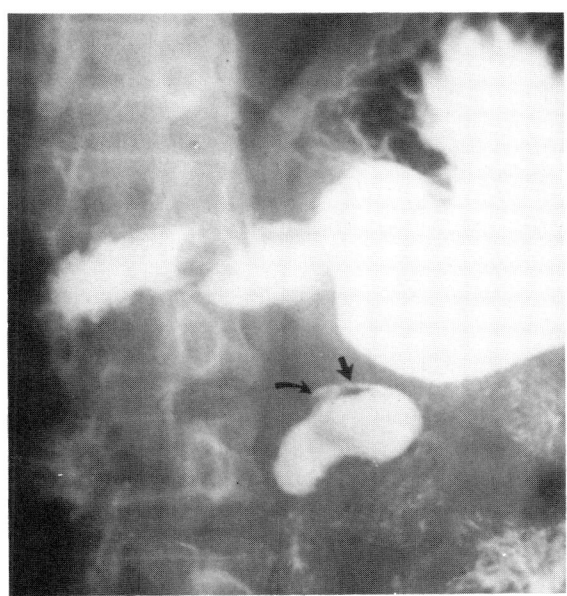

Figure 11-48. Bleeding ulceration in duodenal diverticulum. A diverticulum in the ascending limb of the duodenum had been noted on previous examinations of this patient with recurrent gastrointestinal bleeding. The presence of an ulcer (curved arrow) and a mucosal sinus tract (straight arrow) seen on upper gastrointestinal series was confirmed at operation to be the source of gastrointestinal blood loss. Fortunately, ulcers rarely occur in duodenal diverticula. Ulceration may occur in duodenal diverticula from stasis of gastric secretions within the diverticula or from acid produced from heterotopic gastric mucosa that may occur in congenital duodenal diverticula.

Considerable uncertainty exists about the clinical significance of insertion of the common bile duct and pancreatic ducts into a duodenal diverticulum. Disagreement exists about whether this anomaly plays any significant role in clinical disease, choledocholithiasis, cholangitis, or pancreatitis.[13, 41]

References

1. Anderson, F. H.: Megaduodenum. A case report and literature review. Am. J. Gastroenterol. 62:509–515, 1974.
2. Bain, N. H.: Ehlers-Danlos syndrome. Case report. Am. J. Gastroenterol. 67:167–170, 1977.
3. Balikian, J. P., Nassar, N. T.; Shamma'a, M. H., et al.: Primary lymphomas of the small intestine including the duodenum. A roentgen analysis of twenty-nine cases. Am. J. Roentgenol. 107:131–141, 1969.
4. Balsano, N. A., and Reynolds, B. M.: Rupture of the common duct and ampulla of Vater due to blunt trauma. Ann. Surg. 178:200–203, 1973.
5. Bosse, G., and Neely, J. A.: Roentgenologic findings in primary malignant tumors of the duodenum. Report of 27 cases. Am. J. Roentgenol. 107:111–118, 1969.
6. Braun, P., Collin, P. P., and Ducharme, J. C.: Preduodenal portal vein: a significant entity? Report of two cases and review of the literature. Can. J. Surg. 17:316–319, 322, 1974.
7. Broker, H. M., and Hay, L. J.: Case report of 2 spherical duplications of second portion of duodenum in 54-year-old patient. Surgery 37:996–1001, 1955.
8. Burrell, M., and Toffler, R.: Flexural pseudolesions of the duodenum. Radiology 120:313–315, 1976.
9. Cavanagh, J. E.: Enteroliths and perforation of duodenal diverticula. Arch. Surg. 100:614–618, 1970.
10. Chavez, C. M., Conn, J. H., and Fain, W. R.: Primary tumors of the duodenum. South. Med. J. 63:1001–1004, 1970.
11. Clemmesen, T., and Baden, H.: Accidental transection of the ampulla of Vater at surgery for duodenal ulcer. Acta Chir. Scand. 136:497–502, 1970.
12. Corlette, M. B.: Disconnection of the ampulla of Vater. Surg. Gynecol. Obstet. 141:915–918, 1975.
13. Costopoulos, L. B., and Miller, J. D. R.: Insertion of the common bile duct and pancreatic duct into duodenal dive-ticula. Radiology 89:256–262, 1967.
14. Curtis, G. T., Simpson, W., and Lowdon, A. G.: Intraluminal diverticulum of the duodenum in a mongol. Clin. Radiol. 16:289–291, 1965.
15. Dalinka, M. K., Gohel, V. K., Schaffer, B., et al.: Gastrointestinal complications of aortic bypass surgery. Clin. Radiol. 27:255–258, 1975.
16. Danese, C. A., Margolese, R., Dreiling, D. A., et al.: Disconnection of the papilla of Vater. A complication of gastric surgery. Am. J. Gastroenterol. 53:446–459, 1970.
17. Dodds, J. J., and Beahrs, O. H.: Leiomyosarcoma of the duodenum. Am. J. Surg. 105:245–249, 1963.
18. Ebert, R. E., Parkhurst, G. F., Melendy, O. A., et al.: Primary tumors of duodenum. Surg. Gynecol. Obstet. 97:135–139, 1953.
19. Elliott, J. P., Jr., Smith, R. F., and Szilagyi, D. E.: Aortoenteric and paraprosthetic-enteric fistulas. Arch. Surg. 108:479–490, 1974.
20. Evans, W. E., Armstrong, R. G., Schulte, W., et al.: Ulcerogenic tumor of the duodenum. Am. J. Surg. 124:596–599, 1972.
21. Felson, B., and Levin, E. J.: Intramural hematoma of the duodenum. A diagnostic roentgen sign. Radiology 68:823–829, 1954.
22. Friedland, G. W., Mason, R., and Poole, G. J.: Ladd's bands in older children, adolescents, and adults. Radiology 95:363–368, 1970.
23. Ghahremani, G. G., and Hietala, S. O.: Arteriography of a bleeding duodenal diverticulum. Am. J. Dig. Dis. 22:445–448, 1977.
24. Gondos, B.: Duodenal compression defect and the "superior mesenteric artery syndrome." Radiology 123:575–580, 1977.
25. Gross, R. E.: The Surgery of Infancy and Childhood; Its Principles and Techniques. Philadelphia, W. B. Saunders Company, 1953, p. 245.
26. Hall, L. W.: The cast syndrome incognito. Am. J. Surg. 127:371–376, 1974.
27. Hughes, J. P., McEntire, J. E., and Setze, T.: Cast syndrome. Duodenal dilation or obstruction in a patient in a body cast, with review of the literature. Arch. Surg. 108:230–232, 1974.
28. Juler, G. L., List, J. W., Stemmer, E. A., et al.: Perforating duodenal diverticulitis. Arch. Surg. 99:572–578, 1969.
29. Kaplan, E. L., Dyson, W. L., and Fitts, W. T., Jr.: Hyperplasia of Brunner's glands of the duodenum. Surg. Gynecol. Obstet. 126:371–375, 1968.
30. Keeffe, E. B., Krippaehne, W. W., Rösch, J., et al.: Aortoduodenal fistula: complication of renal artery bypass graft. Gastroenterology 67:1240–1244, 1974.

31. Kessler, R. M., and Scholz, F. J.: Carcinoma of the pancreas. Contemp. Surg. 6:74, 1975.
32. Kibbey, W. E., Sirinek, K. R., Pace, W. G., et al.: Primary duodenal tumors. A diagnostic and therapeutic dilemma. Arch. Surg. 111:377–380, 1976.
33. Kim, S. K., and Proto, A. V.: Duodenotomy defect. Br. J. Radiol. 48:811–813, 1975.
34. Kutin, N. D., Ranson, J. H., Gouge, T. H., et al.: Villous tumors of the duodenum. Ann. Surg. 181:164–168, 1975.
35. Laudan, J. C., and Norton, G. I.: Intraluminal duodenal diverticulum. Am. J. Roentgenol. 90:756–760, 1963.
36. Legge, D. A., Carlson, H. C., and Judd, E. S.: Roentgenologic features of regional enteritis of the upper gastrointestinal tract. Am. J. Roentgenol. 110:355–360, 1970.
37. Legge, D. A., Carlson, H. C., and Hoffman, H. N.: A roentgenologic sign of regional enteritis of the duodenum. Radiology 100:37–39, 1971.
38. Lukash, W. M., Osborne, D. P., Brown, L. T., et al.: Lipoma of duodenum. Report of a case. Am. J. Gastroenterol. 49:494–498, 1968.
39. Meltzer, A. D., Ostrum, B. I., and Isard, H. J.: Villous tumors of the stomach and duodenum; report of three cases. Radiology 87:511–513, 1966.
40. Meyers, M. A., and King, M. C.: Leiomyosarcoma of the duodenum. Angiographic findings and report of a case. Clin. Radiol. 22:257–260, 1971.
41. Nelson, J. A., and Burhenne, H. J.: Anomalous biliary and pancreatic duct insertion into duodenal diverticula. Radiology 120:49–52, 1976.
42. Nugent, F. W., Braasch, J. W., and Epstein, H.: Diagnosis and surgical treatment of arteriomesenteric obstruction of the duodenum. J.A.M.A. 196:1091–1093, 1966.
43. Poppel, M. H., Jacobson, H. G., and Smith, R. W.: The Roentgen Aspects of the Papilla and Ampulla of Vater. Springfield, Illinois, Charles C Thomas, Publisher, 1953.
44. Pratt, A., Jr.: Current concepts of the obstructing duodenal diaphragm. Radiology 100:637–643, 1971.
45. Ring, E. J., Ferrucci, J. T., Jr., Eaton, S. B., Jr., et al.: Villous adenomas of the duodenum. Radiology 104:45–48, 1972.
46. Sampliner, J., Kollins, S. A., and Hermann, R. E.: Intraluminal duodenal diverticulum associated with trisomy. Am. J. Roentgenol. 127:677–679, 1976.
47. Schnur, P. L., David, E., Brown, P. W., Jr., et al.: Adenocarcinoma of the duodenum and the Gardner syndrome. J.A.M.A. 223:1229–1232, 1973.
48. Scholz, F. J., Carrera, G. F., and Larsen, C. R.: The choledochocele: correlation of radiological, clinical and pathological findings. Radiology 118:25–28, 1976.
49. Simon, M., and Lerner, M. A.: Duodenal compression by the mesenteric root in acute pancreatitis and inflammatory conditions of the bowel. Radiology 79:75–81, 1962.
50. Spira, I. A., Ghazi, A., and Wolff, W. I.: Primary adenocarcinoma of the duodenum. Cancer 39:1721–1726, 1977.
51. Thompson, N. W., and Labow, S. S.: Duplication of the duodenum in the adult. Arch. Surg. 94:301–306, 1967.
52. Wallace, R. G., and Howard, W. B.: Acute superior mesenteric artery syndrome in the severely burned patient. Radiology 94:307–310, 1970.
53. Warren, K. W.: Pancreatic considerations in gastric surgery. J.A.M.A. 154:803–810, 1954.
54. Warren, K. W., McDonald, W. M., and Logan, J. H.: Periampullary and duodenal carcinoid tumours. Gut 5:448–453, 1964.
55. Warren, K. W., Kune, G. A., and Poulantzas, J. K.: Peutz-Jeghers syndrome with carcinoma of the duodenum and jejunum. Lahey Clin. Found. Bull. 14:97–102, 1965.
56. Wiot, J. F., Weinstein, A. S., and Felson, B.: Duodenal hematoma induced by coumarin. Am. J. Roentgenol. 86:70–75, 1961.
57. Wolfe, R. D., and Pearl, M. J.: Acute perforation of duodenal diverticulum with roentgenographic demonstration of localized retroperitoneal emphysema. Radiology 104:301–302, 1972.
58. Yang, T. S., Greenspan, A., Farber, M., et al.: Intraluminal duodenal diverticulum. Arch. Surg. 109:113–115, 1974.
59. Zarnow, H., Grant, T. H., Spellberg, M., et al.: Unusual complications of regional enteritis. Duodeno-biliary fistula and hepatic abscess. J.A.M.A. 235:1880–1881, 1976.

12

THE SMALL INTESTINE

Part I

Small Bowel Obstruction

STEVEN H. OMINSKY, M.D.

ALEXANDER R. MARGULIS, M.D.

PLAIN FILM EXAMINATION

Supine and upright abdominal views and an upright posteroanterior chest view are necessary for the evaluation of a patient with suspected small bowel obstruction. A horizontal beam film is necessary to detect air-fluid levels. If an upright abdominal view is impossible to obtain because of the patient's condition, a lateral decubitus view of the abdomen with the patient's left side down should be taken. An upright posteroanterior chest film is necessary to rule out the possibility of conditions that may cause an ileus, such as lower lobe pneumonia, congestive heart failure, or scleroderma, and also to determine whether there is free air under the diaphragm.

Simple Mechanical Obstruction

A mechanical obstruction results in the distention of small bowel loops because of the increased amount of gas or fluid that accumulates proximal to the site of obstruction. The small bowel and colon distal to the obstruction are either normal in size or partially collapsed. Small bowel loops wider than 3 cm in diameter are considered distended.

GAS-DISTENDED SMALL BOWEL LOOPS. Since the colon may normally be larger than 3 cm in diameter, it is important to differentiate a dilated small bowel from a normal or dilated large bowel. The location of gas-filled loops is extremely important in making this distinction. When the small bowel is obstructed, the loops

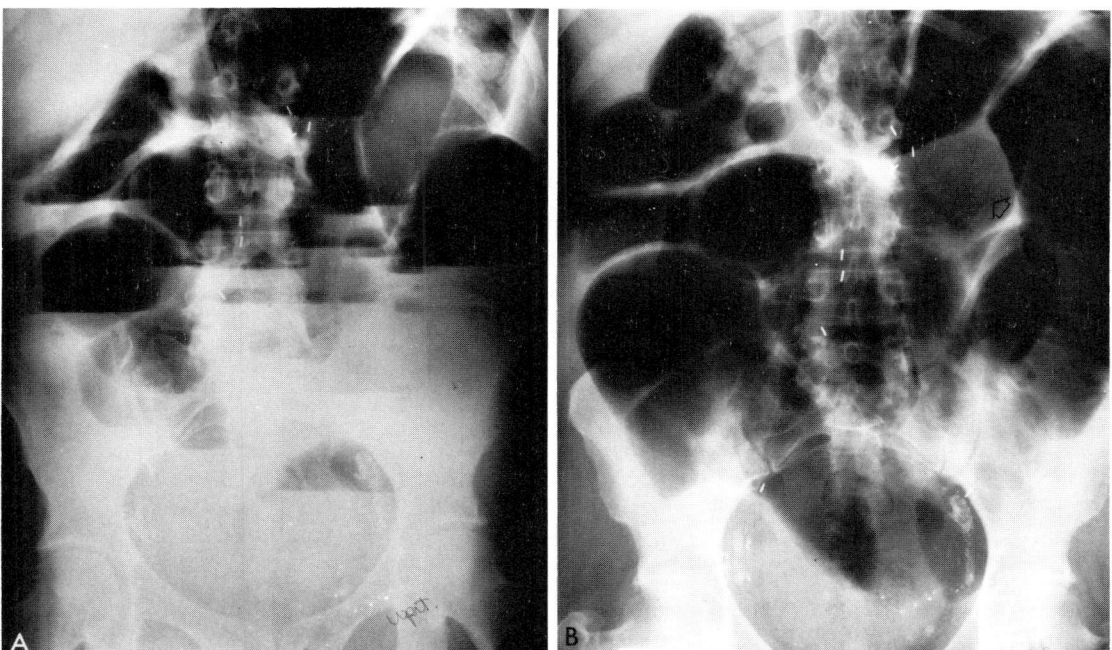

Figure 12–1. Upright (*A*) and supine (*B*) views of a patient with a low small bowel obstruction secondary to adhesions. Note the valvulae conniventes extending across the diameter of the bowel (*B*, arrow).

are seen in the midportion of the abdomen (Fig. 12–1): If many loops are dilated and gas-filled, there may be an oblique orientation from the right lower quadrant to the left upper quadrant along the axis of the small bowel mesentery. The large bowel lies along the peripheral portions of the abdomen, with the ascending and descending portions of the colon positioned laterally and the transverse colon positioned along the superior portion of the abdomen (Fig. 12–2). If the transverse colon or sigmoid colon has a long mesentery, these segments may be located in the central portion of the supine or upright abdominal film. Knowledge of the configuration as well as of the location of dilated loops is necessary for the differentiation of the small from the large bowel. The valvulae conniventes in the small bowel extend across its entire diameter (see Fig. 12–1*B*), whereas the large bowel haustra usually do not extend across the diameter of the colon. In addition, the haustra indent the walls of the colon, and when distended the colon wall has a slightly irregular contour (see Fig. 12–2*B*). Conversely, the small bowel has parallel walls without indentation by the valvulae. Sometimes distinction is difficult.

Generally, the more numerous the dilated loops, the more distal is the level of obstruction. The diameter of the dilated small bowel loops probably depends on the chronicity and completeness of the obstruction, the widest loops being seen in long-standing cases of partial obstruction.[2]

FLUID-DISTENDED SMALL BOWEL LOOPS. Most gas in the bowel seen on the x-ray is secondary to air swallowing. If a patient fails to swallow much air, the obstructed bowel contains little or no gas but is dilated with fluid because of the failure of fluid transport beyond the obstruction. When a small amount of gas is present in the distended bowel, it may be seen on the upright view trapped between the valvulae in the superior portion of the small intestinal loop. This collection of trapped gas densities has a linear configuration and has been called the string-of-beads sign. It is a reliable indicator of a mechanical small bowel obstruction. When slightly more gas

540 — THE SMALL INTESTINE

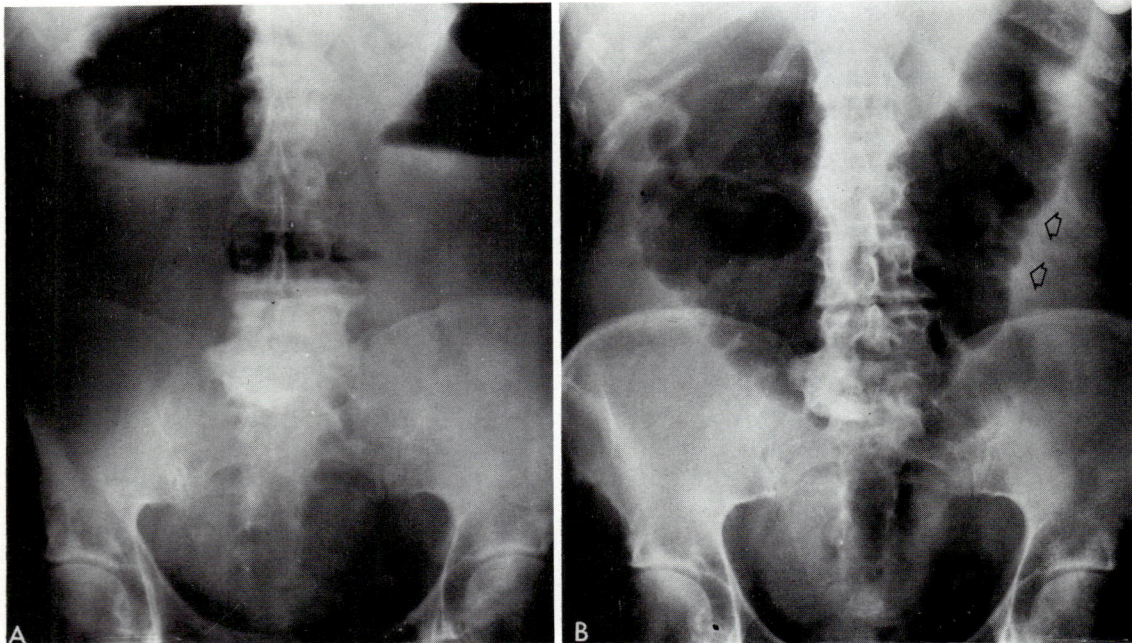

Figure 12–2. Upright (*A*) and supine (*B*) views of a patient with an obstructing splenic flexure carcinoma. Note the indented wall of the colon resulting from the haustra (arrows).

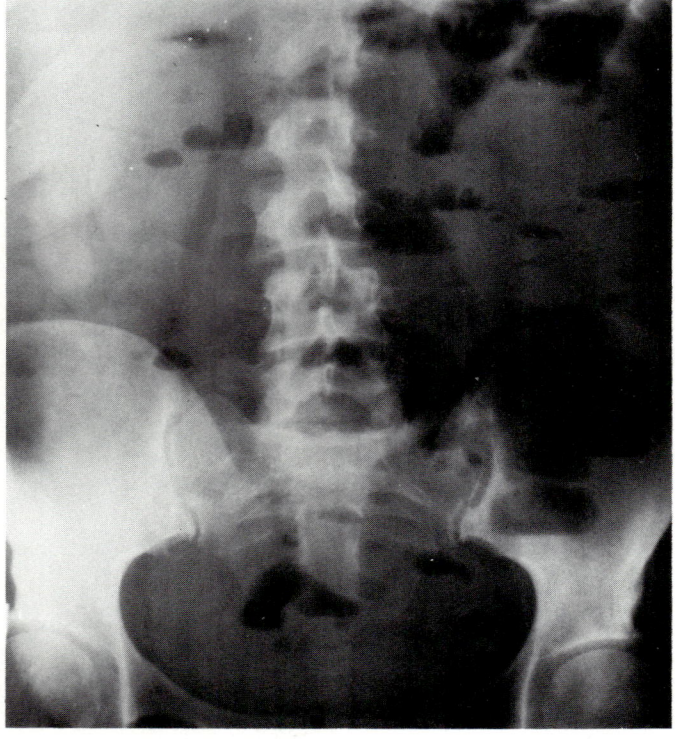

Figure 12–3. Upright view of a patient with small bowel obstruction and multiple small air-fluid levels.

is present, multiple small air-fluid levels are seen on the upright film (Fig. 12–3). Since there is usually a small amount of fluid in the small bowel of the normal person, occasional air-fluid levels are not abnormal. However, the presence of more than two air-fluid levels in dilated loops of small intestine indicates an abnormal production or retention of fluid. This may be due to dynamic or adynamic causes. An increased production of fluid can be seen in gastroenteritis, and multiple air-fluid levels may be evident on the upright films of patients with this condition. Gastroenteritis should be differentiated from obstruction or ileus clinically.

Diagnosis is most difficult when obstructed loops contain no gas because the patient is not swallowing air or has nasogastric suction. In this case, the gasless abdomen film may show sausage-shaped loops of bowel of soft tissue density outlined by serosal fat and measuring more than 3 cm in diameter. Visualization of these loops requires good film technique and close inspection.

METEORISM. When large amounts of gas are swallowed, distended gas-filled small bowel or small and large bowel loops may be seen. This occurs normally in infants and edentulous adults who eat by sucking and is called meteorism or aerophagy. It is also seen in patients with painful conditions, such as fractures or ureteral calculi, or following uncomplicated surgery. In the postoperative period, meteorism is commonly mistaken for adynamic ileus.[7] Since meteorism is caused by increased air swallowing and not by abnormal fluid transport, an increased amount of fluid with air-fluid levels is not present. This absence of air-fluid levels distinguishes meteorism from small bowel obstruction.

Strangulation Obstruction

Strangulation develops when the circulation to the obstructed intestine is impaired. This condition can eventually produce gangrene, perforation, and peritonitis. Unfortunately, strangulation obstruction is more difficult to diagnose than simple obstruction, its diagnosis being dependent upon the recognition of subtle findings.

This condition usually occurs as a result of volvulus of the small bowel about adhesive bands. It may also be found in cases of external or internal herniation of the bowel.

FIXATION OF BOWEL LOOP. When upright and supine views are compared, a gas- or fluid-filled loop may show an unchanged position. In this case, the presence of a closed loop obstruction, with the bowel fixed at two points by adhesion or hernia, should be suspected.[4] Supine films taken at five-minute intervals also help to demonstrate a complicated obstruction. If there is a minimal change in the position of gas and fluid within the bowel loops and no change in the position of the loops, a complication such as strangulation, perforation, or volvulus may be present.[1]

PSEUDOTUMOR SIGN. In cases of closed loop obstruction, the fluid-filled small bowel loop may have the configuration of a mass and produces extrinsic pressure defects in adjacent structures, such as the bladder and colon (Fig. 12–4). This mass is fixed and can be differentiated from the nonfixed fluid-filled small bowel loops of simple obstruction, which do not indent adjacent structures.

ABSENCE OF VALVULAE CONNIVENTES. Ischemia of a bowel loop results in edema and submucosal hemorrhage. The valvulae become effaced, and the bowel has a nodular contour (Fig. 12–5). This effacement of the valvulae can also be seen in cases of ischemia due to thromboembolic disease and in cases of acute bowel inflammation. The combination of fixed bowel loops and effacement is strongly suggestive of a strangulated obstruction.[4]

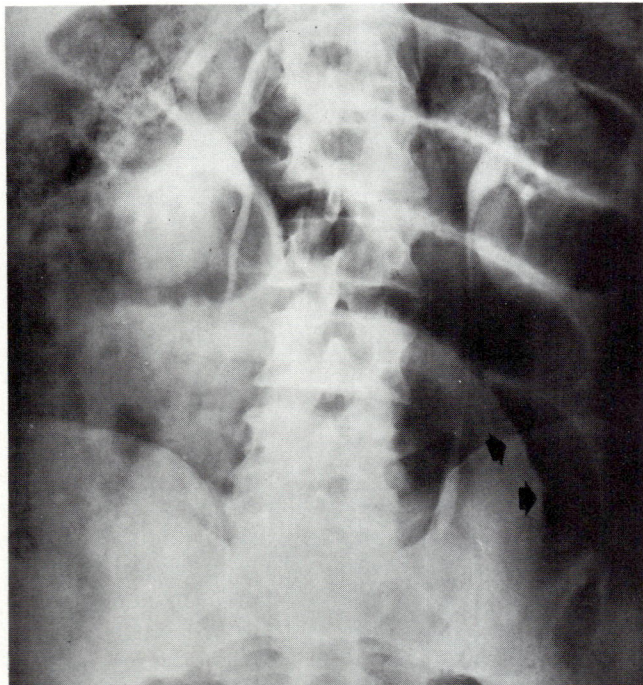

Figure 12–4. Pseudotumor in a case of closed loop obstruction. Note the mass that is producing an extrinsic defect in the adjacent dilated small bowel (arrows).

Figure 12–5. Sigmoid volvulus and intestinal knot with strangulation of ileal loops. The small bowel has a nodular contour (arrows).

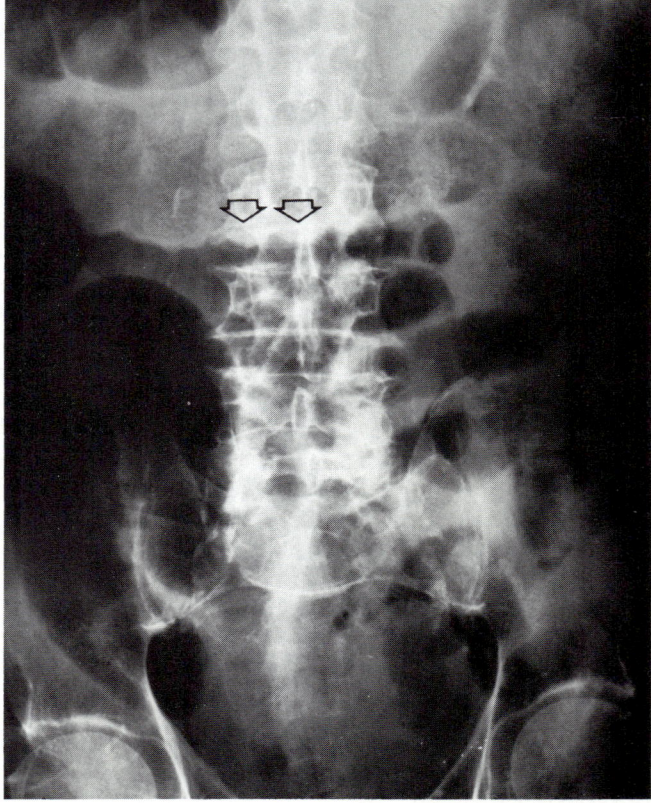

ABSENCE OF BOWEL GAS. A gasless abdomen can be seen in cases of low strangulating obstruction. The most common cause of a gasless abdomen, however, is acute pancreatitis. Other causes include nasogastric suction, mesenteric infarction, esophageal or pyloric obstruction, and simple mechanical obstruction accompanied by repeated vomiting.

Adynamic Ileus and Pseudo-obstruction

Mechanical small bowel obstruction must be differentiated from adynamic ileus, which can also cause bowel distention. Adynamic ileus occurs after abdominal surgery and anesthesia. Spine fractures, retroperitoneal hemorrhage, and distention of other organs, such as the bladder and ureter, may also result in an adynamic ileus. The plain film findings in patients with adynamic ileus are distention of the small and large bowel and frequently of the stomach as well. A low colonic obstruction with an incompetent ileocecal valve may also result in colon and small bowel distention, and a barium enema may sometimes be necessary to distinguish adynamic ileus from a low colonic obstruction. Air-fluid levels at different heights or at the same level may be seen in cases of both adynamic ileus and mechanical obstruction and are of no value in distinguishing the two.

A patient may have clinical and radiologic evidence of a small bowel obstruction although true obstruction is not present. This intestinal pseudo-obstruction occurs in patients with generalized disease that alters intestinal motor function.[8] Diseases such as pancreatitis (Fig. 12–6), renal failure, lower lobe pneumonia, scleroderma, myx-

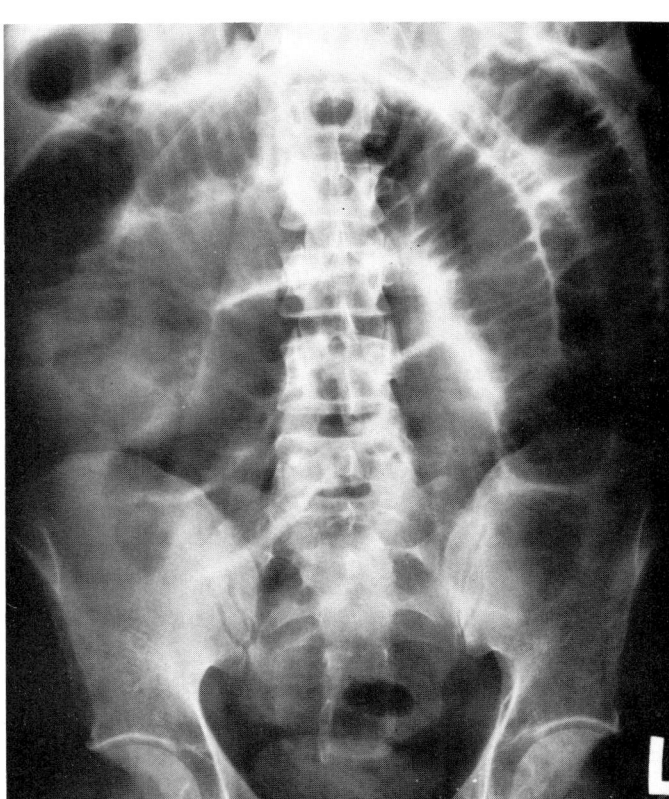

Figure 12–6. Acute pancreatitis and marked small bowel ileus.

544 — THE SMALL INTESTINE

edema, and systemic amyloidosis can interfere with intestinal motor transport and produce a pseudo-obstruction. In these diseases a barium study is necessary to distinguish pseudo-obstruction from actual obstruction. Postoperative hypokalemia, vagotomy, and postoperative narcotic analgesia may also interfere with intestinal transport and mimic a mechanical obstruction.

Small Bowel Obstruction After Pelvic Surgery

A common occurrence on the second to fifth day after pelvic surgery is the onset of vomiting and abdominal distention. The supine and upright films show findings typical of mechanical obstruction. These patients have local paralysis of the pelvic small intestine owing to manipulation at surgery, or local inflammation with a resulting block in intestinal transport. The clinical picture improves spontaneously or with the aid of intubation after several days. Surgery is not necessary, but in questionable cases barium can be given to rule out actual obstruction.

CONTRAST EXAMINATIONS

Barium Enema and Retrograde Small Bowel Study

As mentioned previously, a barium enema may be necessary to differentiate a low colonic obstruction from a paralytic ileus. A barium enema is also necessary

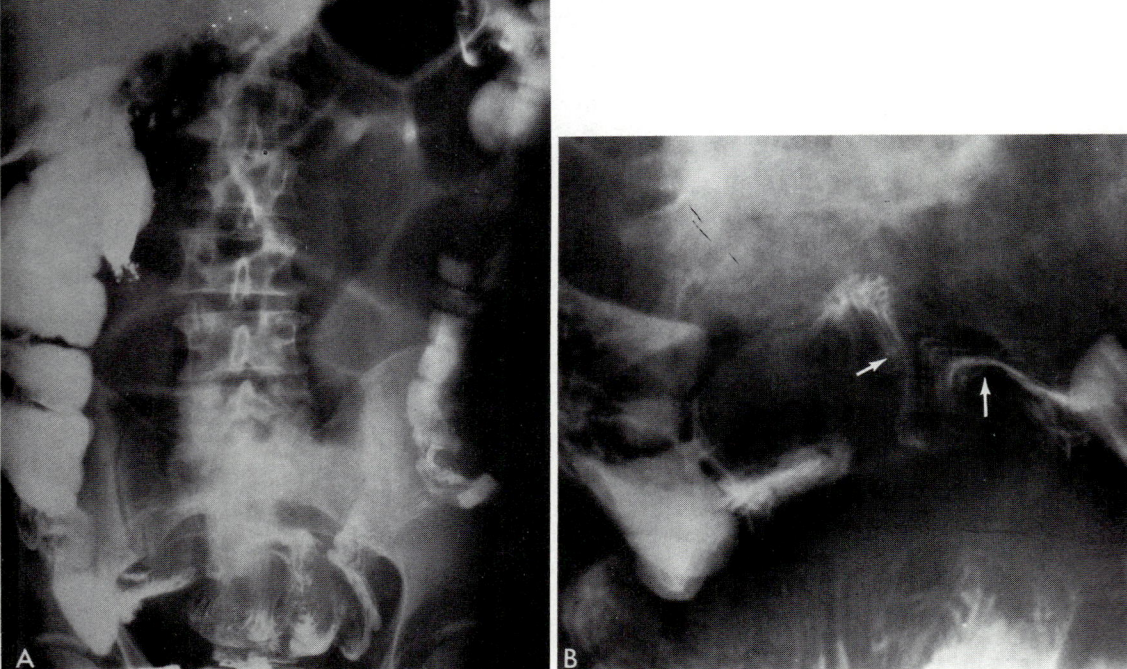

Figure 12–7. *A,* Barium enema study of a patient with a gas-filled dilated small bowel. *B,* Spot film shows marked angulation of the distal small bowel with the preservation of mucosal folds (arrows). An adhesion was found in the distal ileum at surgery.

THE SMALL INTESTINE — 545

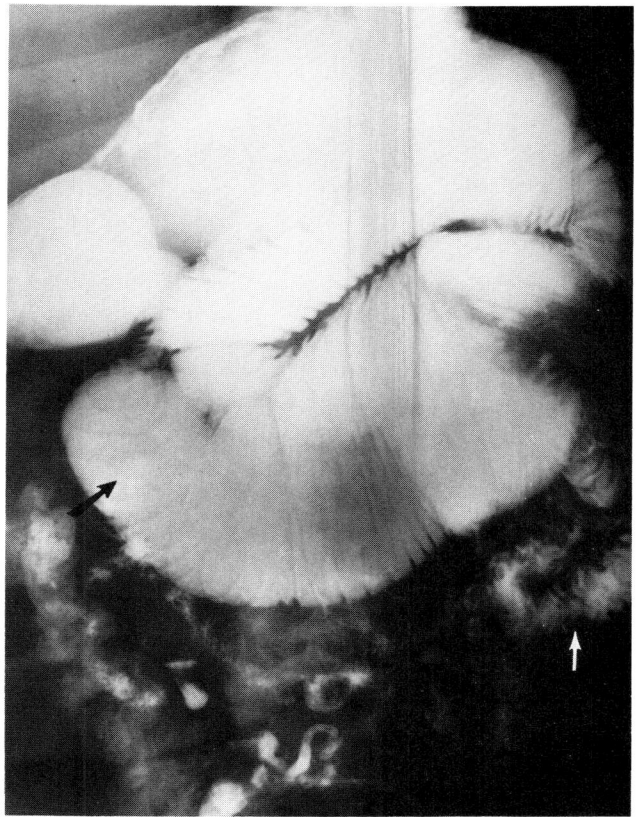

Figure 12–8. Oral barium examination showing partial high small bowel obstruction. Note the marked difference in the caliber of the bowel proximal (black arrow) from the bowel distal (white arrow) to the obstruction.

when plain films show distended bowel loops and a colonic obstruction cannot be differentiated from a low small bowel obstruction. If peroral barium is given in this situation and a colonic obstruction is present, the barium may inspissate in the colon proximal to the obstruction. A barium enema study is also an excellent way to examine the distal small bowel.[5] If an obstruction is present in the ileum, the type of obstruction may be delineated by barium reflux into the ileum (Fig. 12–7). One drawback to this method of studying the distal bowel is that in a small percentage of cases the ileocecal valve remains competent even after the administration of glucagon. A subsequent peroral study can be initiated, however, without fear of barium inspissation in the colon.

Peroral Barium Examination

When an obstruction is localized to the upper or middle portion of the small intestine by the plain film examination or when a mechanical obstruction must be differentiated from a localized ileus, barium should be administered, either orally or via a nasogastric tube. The barium does not convert a partial small bowel obstruction to a complete obstruction, since the increased intestinal fluid proximal to an obstruction prevents the barium from inspissating. Barium provides excellent visualization of the site of obstruction (Fig. 12–8) and may also demonstrate the cause of obstruction (that is, adhesions, a tumor, an extrinsic mass, or a twist).[6] One disadvantage of an antegrade study is that barium may move slowly when a complete obstruction is present. If a rapid diagnosis is critical for the surgeon, barium can be instilled via a nasogastric tube advanced to the ligament of Treitz (Fig. 12–9). Enteroclysis can be performed by adding large volumes (up to 600 ml) of water to large volumes (up to 600 ml) of barium by infusion. Because of the slow transport of oral barium to a distal small bowel obstruction and the resulting delay in diagnosis, a barium enema with retrograde small bowel filling is the procedure of choice for the examination of a low small bowel obstruction.

Water-Soluble Iodine-Containing Contrast Agents

An antegrade or retrograde examination with water-soluble iodine-containing contrast is indicated when a perforation in the gastrointestinal tract is suspected. If leakage from a bowel anastomosis is suspected or if a stab wound or other trauma with possible perforation has occurred, a water-soluble contrast examination should be performed. There are, however, several disadvantages in using water-soluble iodine-containing contrast instead of barium to study a small bowel obstruction. Since water-soluble contrast media are hyperosmolar solutions and act as saline cathartics, they can cause dehydration. This complication is a problem in infants[3] and in elderly persons with tenuous fluid balances; these patients must be carefully monitored for potential hypovolemia. The dilution that occurs in the intestine with these hyperosmolar contrast agents makes it difficult to identify the exact site of a bowel obstruction. In addition, partial obstructions may be missed because of rapid transit time.

TYPES OF BOWEL OBSTRUCTION

Extrinsic Obstruction

The most common cause of small bowel obstruction in adults is an adhesion from prior surgery. In these patients the barium study shows marked angulation and kinking of the obstructed bowel segment, but the mucosal folds are preserved (see Fig. 12–7B). Another finding is a club-shaped, dilated bowel just proximal to the site of obstruction that abruptly becomes partially collapsed just distal to the obstruction (Fig. 12–10). The mucosal folds are preserved (see Fig. 12–8). This pattern is seen when the obstruction is due to a single adhesive band compressing the bowel. External hernias are the second most common cause of small bowel obstruction in adults. There is compression of the small intestine as it passes through the hernia neck, but again the mucosal folds are preserved. When serosal metastases compress and obstruct the small intestine, there is usually marked irregularity and destruction of the small bowel mucosal folds (Fig. 12–11).

Intrinsic Obstruction

Strictures may result from a primary carcinoma of the small bowel with a mass effect and mucosal destruction indistinguishable from that of serosal metastases invading and destroying the mucosa. The diagnosis of strictures secondary to a chronic inflammatory disease, such as Crohn's disease, is indicated by the clinical history and by the presence of inflammatory changes elsewhere in the small bowel. Radia-

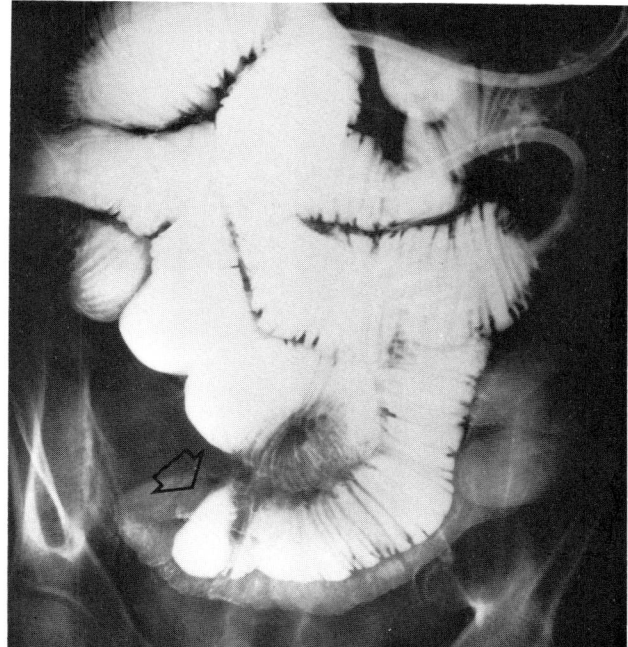

Figure 12–9. Small bowel barium examination via a tube demonstrates a jejunal obstruction (arrow) secondary to an adhesion.

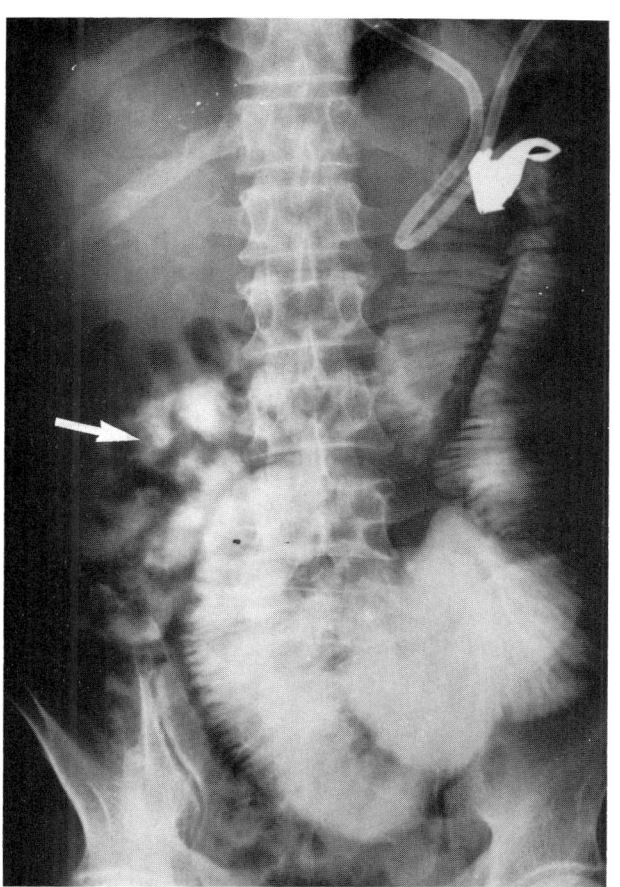

Figure 12–10. One-hour film of a patient who had undergone a partial gastrectomy one week earlier. The contrast is a water-soluble agent. There is a partial obstruction in the distal jejunum. Partially collapsed loops of the proximal ileum (arrow) are filling with contrast, which has passed the site of obstruction.

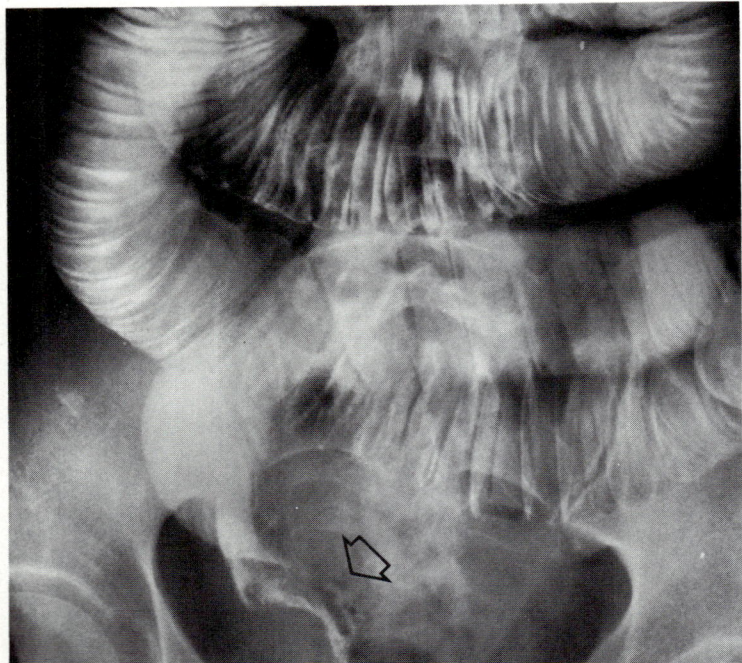

Figure 12–11. A peroral barium study of a patient with small bowel obstruction secondary to lung carcinoma and serosal metastasis. Note the irregular configuration of the small bowel and the mucosal destruction at the site of obstruction (arrow).

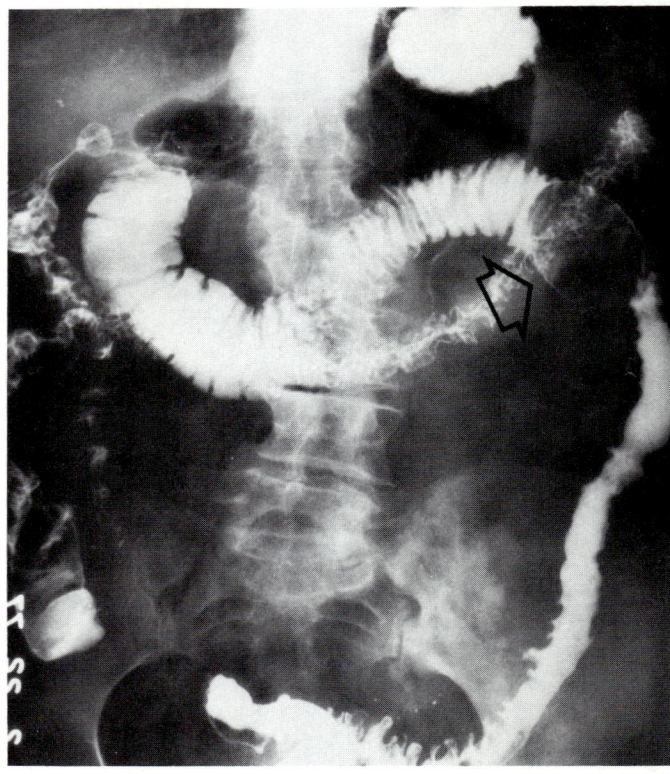

Figure 12–12. Gallstone obstruction. A patient with a gallstone ileus and impacted stone at the level of the ligament of Treitz (arrow). A duodenocolic fistula is present, with barium in the colon.

THE SMALL INTESTINE — 549

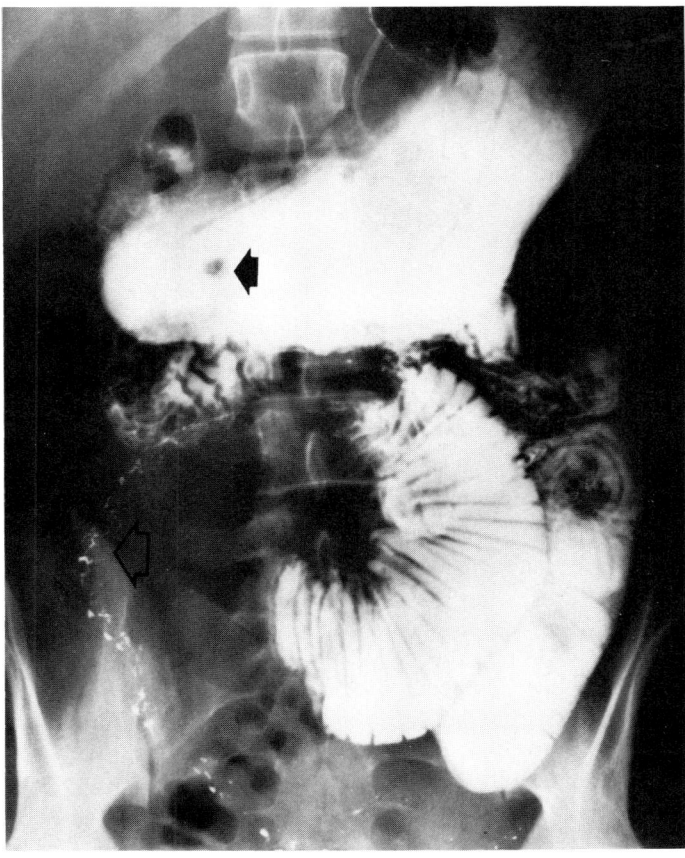

Figure 12–13. Intussusception. A patient with Peutz-Jehgers syndrome and a long intussusception (large arrow) with a stringlike appearance. Note the polyp in the stomach (small arrow).

tion strictures usually have a smooth, tapered configuration, and again, the clinical history is extremely important in their diagnosis.

Obturation of Intestinal Lumen

Large polypoid tumors, bezoars, and large gallstones that obstruct the small bowel lumen are easily identified and outlined during the barium examination (Fig. 12–12). Intussusception may also obstruct the small bowel lumen. In adults, polypoid tumors usually lead the intussusceptum. In Peutz-Jehgers syndrome, mechanical small bowel obstruction secondary to intussusception is frequently the presenting clinical problem. When an antegrade barium examination is performed in cases of intussusception, barium in the lumen of the narrowed intussusceptum has a narrow stringlike appearance (Fig. 12–13), unlike the typical coiled-spring appearance of barium between the intussusceptum and intussuscipiens in a retrograde examination.

References

1. Bryk, D.: Functional evaluation of small bowel obstruction by successive abdominal roentgenograms. Am. J. Roentgenol. *116*:262–275, 1972.

2. Bryk, D.: A radiological evaluation of small bowel activity in the acute abdomen. C.R.C. Crit. Rev. Diagn. Imaging 9:99–128, 1977.
3. Harris, P. D., Neuhauser, E. B. D., and Gerth, R.: The osmotic effect of water soluble contrast media on circulating plasma volume. Am. J. Roentgenol. 91:694–698, 1964.
4. Levin, B.: Mechanical small bowel obstruction. Semin. Roentgenol. 8:281–297, 1973.
5. Miller, R. E.: Complete reflux small bowel examination. Radiology 84:457–463, 1965.
6. Nelson, S. W., and Christoforidis, A. J.: The use of barium sulfate suspensions in the diagnosis of acute disease of the small intestine. Am. J. Roentgenol. 104:505–519, 1968.
7. Schwartz, S. S.: The differential diagnosis of intestinal obstruction. Semin. Roentgenol. 8:323–338, 1973.
8. Seaman, W. B.: Motor dysfunction of the gastrointestinal tract. Am. J. Roentgenol. 116:235–244, 1972.

Part II

Regional Enteritis

(See also Inflammatory Bowel Disease, Chapter 13, Part II)

STEVEN H. OMINSKY, M.D.
ALEXANDER R. MARGULIS, M.D.

Regional enteritis, or Crohn's disease, is an inflammatory disease of unknown etiology that can occur in any portion of the alimentary tract. Although originally described by Crohn as a disease limited to the terminal ileum,[3] it soon became apparent that the condition can affect any portion of the small bowel as well as the colon. Although the terminal ileum remains the most common site of involvement, Crohn's disease has been detected from the esophagus to the rectum. In addition, anal disease with fissures, ulcers, fistulas, and perianal abscesses frequently coexists with colon disease and less often with small bowel disease. Anal lesions may predate the onset of large or small bowel disease. The colon may be involved, with no evidence of small bowel disease. When colon and small bowel disease coexist, the latter may be a direct extension of colonic involvement or may be separated by a normal segment of bowel. Involvement of the upper intestinal tract is being recognized with greater frequency. The incidence of involvement of the duodenum may be as high as 15 per cent;[14] it occasionally precedes the onset of disease elsewhere in the intestinal tract. Stomach involvement is also being detected with greater frequency, especially with the increased use of endoscopy and double-contrast radiographic techniques. Although the location of bowel involvement may vary, the pathologic features of Crohn's disease are constant.

PATHOLOGY

Since the radiographic appearance of Crohn's disease is a direct reflection of the macroscopic pathologic changes, an appreciation of the macroscopic appearance is essential in the understanding and interpretation of the radiographic findings. Grossly, the involved bowel appears thickened owing to fibrosis and edema. Lymphangiectasia and fibrosis characteristically involve the entire bowel wall, including the submucosa, intermuscular septa, and subserosa, so that the process is both transmural and cicatrizing.[19] The changes are typically segmental, with evidence of normal intervening bowel—"skip" lesions. Because Crohn's disease is a transmural disease with serosal involvement, loops of bowel can become adherent to one another or to pelvic organs. The mesentery adjacent to the involved bowel is thickened and contains enlarged lymph nodes.

The earliest mucosal changes are tiny aphthoid ulcers, often present in seemingly uninvolved mucosa.[13] These are tiny ulcerations with a white base and slightly elevated margins on a background of normal mucosa. Histologically, they are minute foci of ulceration over lymph follicles. Larger ulcers may have a discontinuous linear or serpiginous appearance. A cobblestone appearance may be present owing to linear ulcerations and intervening edematous mucosa and submucosa. Fissures, if present, may penetrate the bowel wall and produce fistulas or local serosal adhesions.

Microscopically, there is transmural inflammatory change, the submucosa being more involved than the mucosa. Although ulceration coexists, there is little glandular disorganization, even in areas adjacent to the ulcers.[17] Lymphoid aggregates in the submucosal-mucosal junction and within the submucosa and sarcoidlike noncaseating granulomas in the submucosa and serosa are characteristic of Crohn's disease. The granulomas in Crohn's disease tend to develop in and around lymphatics and appear to be responsible for the lymphatic blockade and subsequent lymphangiectasis seen in Crohn's disease. Submural fibrosis, if extensive, is responsible for areas of stenosis.

RADIOLOGIC FINDINGS

The submucosal and, to a lesser extent, mucosal inflammatory changes are the cause of the early radiologic findings. The terminal ileum is the most common site of involvement in the small bowel, and spasm of this segment recognized fluoroscopically may be the earliest manifestation of Crohn's disease. The valvulae conniventes, which are normally thin and parallel, become slightly thickened and distorted and may be associated with spasm and irritability. When inflammatory change is more extensive, the mucosal folds may be irregularly thickened, resulting in marked distortion, and the contour of the intervening mucosa may be blunted.

The earliest ulcerations—aphthoid ulcers—can be seen radiologically if a double-contrast examination is used. There is a pinpoint central collection of barium and a round radiolucent halo surrounding the barium. This results in a target or bullseye configuration.[9] The aphthoid ulcers are easiest to see in the colon after the administration of a double-contrast barium enema, but they may also be seen in the lower small bowel during the double-contrast enema or a double-contrast small bowel examination. The double-contrast gastrointestinal series may also reveal these ulcerations in the stomach or the duodenum. When they increase in size, the ulcers may assume a linear configuration both parallel and perpendicular to the long axis of the intestine (Fig. 12–14). The "cobblestones" seen occasionally on gross inspection, resulting from transverse and longitudinal ulcerations adjacent to edematous mucosa, appear radiologically as a symmetric, evenly spaced series of filling defects involving the total diameter of the bowel lumen. With more advanced disease, the symmetric appearance of cobblestoning gives way to an asymmetric network of barium-filled ulcerations, and the appearance becomes more reticulated.[11]

The transverse ulcerations may have various configurations radiologically. One that is frequently seen is the narrow-based linear fissure extending at right angles from the bowel lumen. Since the bowel wall at the ulcer site is usually thickened, the fissure-ulcer extending into the thickening bowel wall can be long. Longitudinal ulcer tracts running parallel to the axis of the bowel lumen but located in the subserosa are characteristic of Crohn's disease. These ulcer tracts are most common in the sigmoid colon. If diverticula of the colon are also present, distinction between Crohn's disease and diverticulitis can be difficult.

Because of the thickening of the bowel wall, the barium-filled lumen becomes narrower in caliber. Early in the course of the disease the radiographic narrowing may be primarily due to spasm; it is a transient phenomenon. As the disease progresses, however, the narrowing becomes fixed. The normal pliability of the bowel is lost, and the bowel becomes straightened and rigid (Fig. 12–15). Loops of bowel are separated from one another because of increased bowel wall thickness, and frequently the bowel appears to be draped around a mass. Although this mass effect may be due to perforation and abscess, more often it is secondary to induration of the mesentery and enlargement of the lymph nodes adjacent to the affected bowel loop. If the fibrosis in the bowel wall is asymmetric, pseudodiverticula are produced as the skip areas of cicatrization, often along one side of the bowel, intermittently retract the bowel lumen. More advanced fibrosis circumferentially involving the bowel lumen leads to marked luminal narrowing and stenotic bowel segments. The involved bowel segments are fixed in position, and their position does not vary when serial small bowel films are obtained.

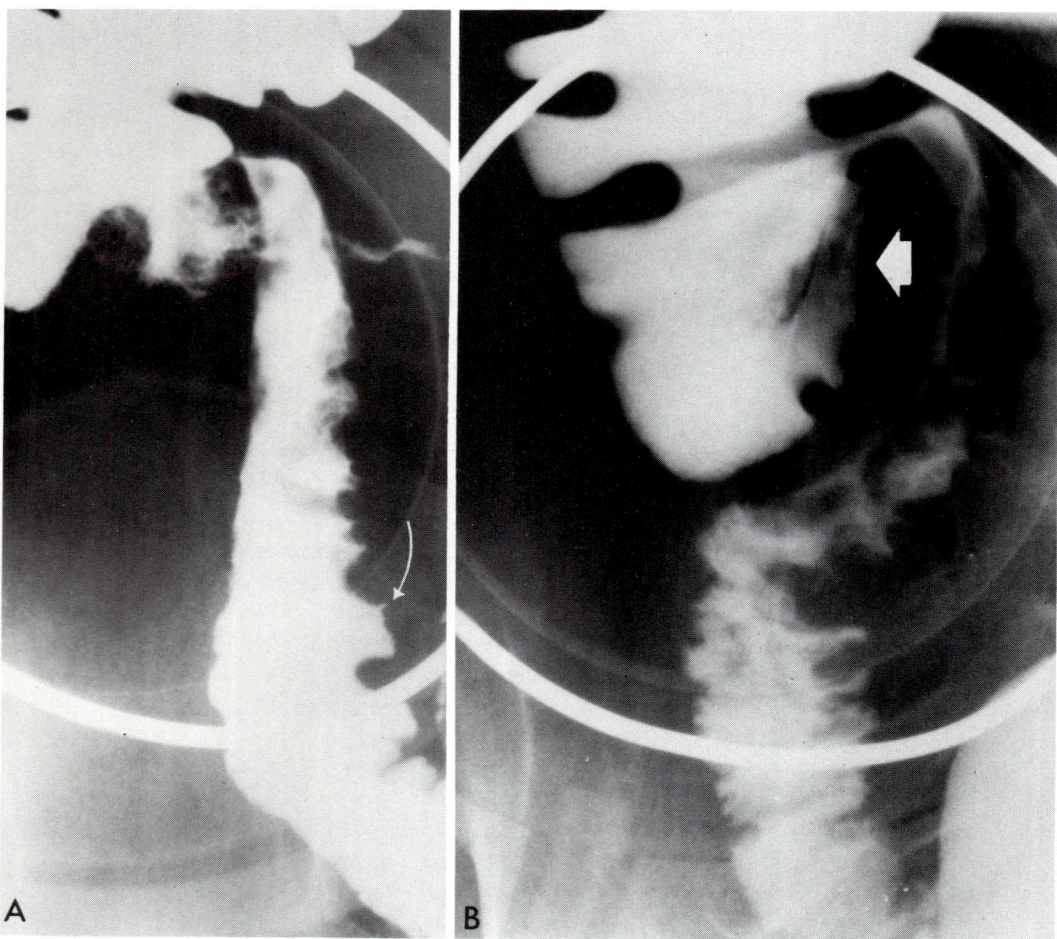

Figure 12–14. *A,* Spot film of the terminal ileum from a small bowel series of a 20-year-old female with Crohn's disease. There is straightening of the lateral wall of the terminal ileum and an irregular nodular contour to the medial wall. A small ulcer is present on the medial wall (arrow). *B,* Retrograde filling of the terminal ileum during a barium enema in the same patient. There are longitudinal and transverse ulcers and a deformity at the medial base of the cecum (arrow).

Illustration and legend continued on the opposite page.

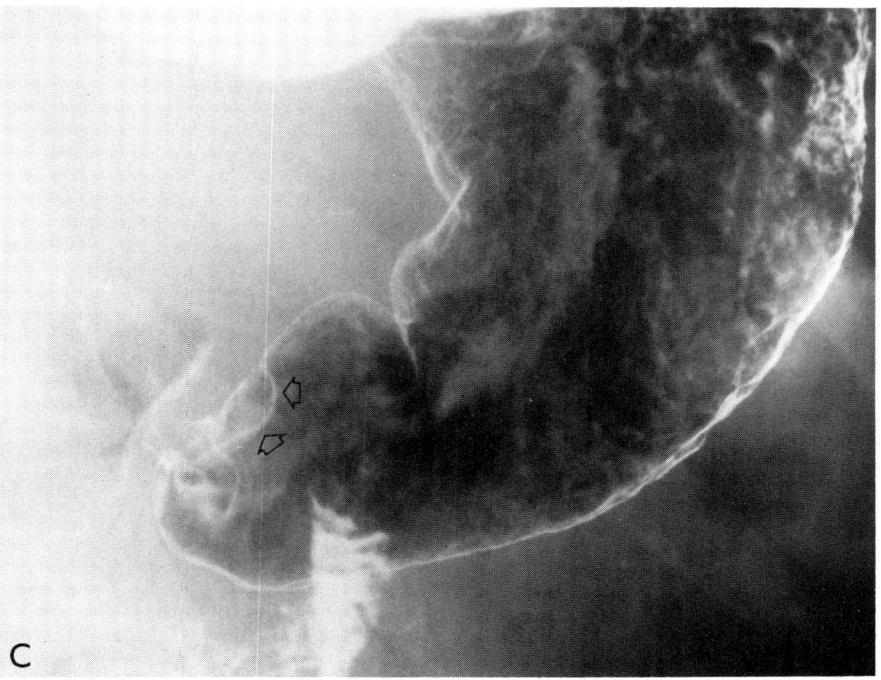

Figure 12–14 *Continued.* C, Double-contrast examination of the stomach of the same patient. Localized thickened folds simulate a mass in the antrum (arrows). Endoscopy demonstrated erythematous antral folds with superficial erosions. The antrum is the most common site of involvement in the stomach of the patient with Crohn's disease.

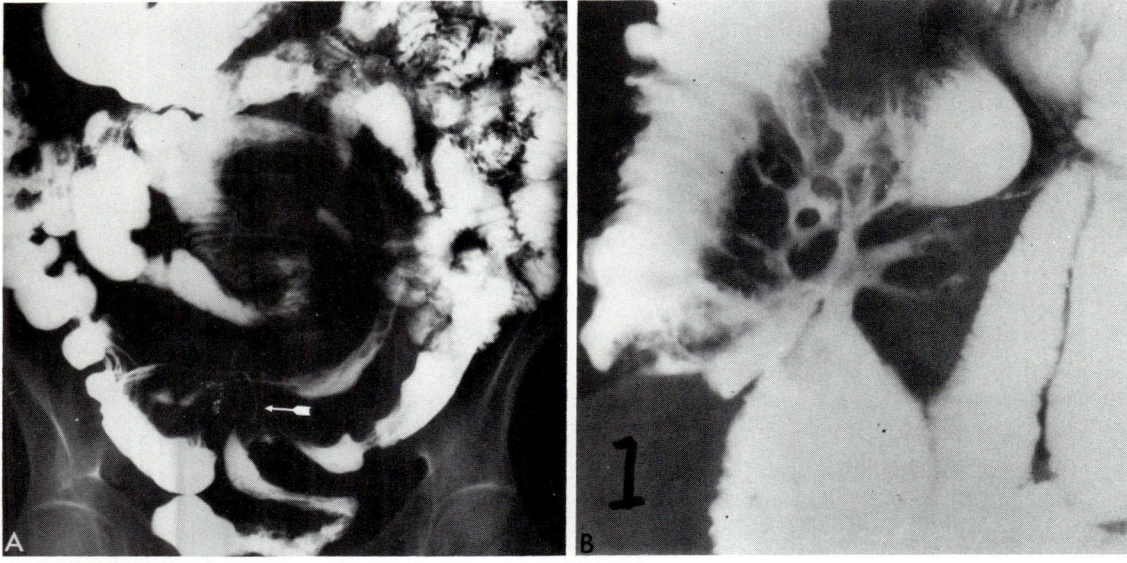

Figure 12–15. Fistula formation in Crohn's disease. *A*, Small bowel examination of a patient with Crohn's disease. There is a long segment of stenosis in the distal ileum and separation of the bowel loops. There is an ileosigmoid fistula (arrow). *B*, Patient with an eight-year history of regional enteritis. Upper gastrointestinal series demonstrates multiple fistulous tracts from the terminal ileum to the ascending colon.

Illustration and legend continued on the opposite page.

COMPLICATIONS OF REGIONAL ENTERITIS

Intestinal Complications

PARTIAL OBSTRUCTION. Stenosis leading to partial bowel obstruction is responsible for the distressing symptom of crampy abdominal pain. Radiologically the stenotic segment may vary in length from 1- to 2-cm areas to much larger segments of rigid narrowing. The margins of the stenotic segments are usually tapered and do not have the overhanging edges seen in malignant obstructions. Even though stricture formation and partial small bowel obstruction are common, complete obstruction is unusual even in severe disease and is rarely a surgical emergency.[11] It is important not to confuse the transient narrowing of spastic irritable bowel (string sign) with the fixed narrowing secondary to extensive fibrosis. In the latter case, there is dilatation of the bowel just proximal to the partial obstruction (Fig. 12–16). Frequently there are multiple areas of stenotic bowel separated by uninvolved or minimally involved bowel loops. Enteroliths may become lodged in the bowel just proximal to the obstruction.

FISTULAS AND ABSCESSES. If a fissure-ulcer continues through the bowel wall and extends extramurally, it may remain localized in the intraperitoneal space and form an abscess, or it may continue to penetrate into adjacent viscera to become a fistula.[20] Fistulas may extend from one loop of bowel to another (see Fig. 12–15) or from the bowel to the vagina, bladder, or abdominal wall. Multiple fistulas often arise proximal to a stricture or from a mesenteric abscess. Occasionally, overlapping bowel that is matted together by adhesions prevents the visualization of fistulas on the barium examination. Rectal filling prior to filling of the proximal colon may be the only finding

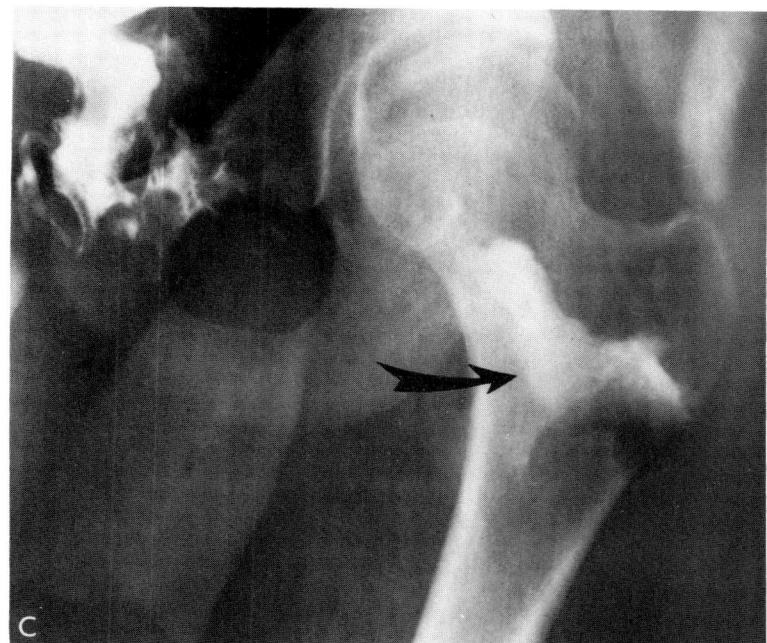

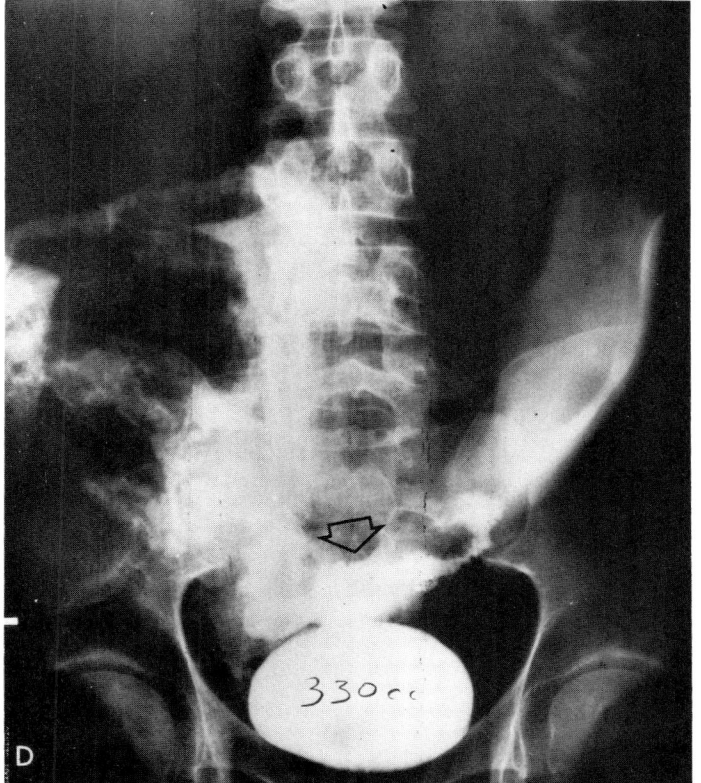

Figure 12–15. *Continued. C,* Crohn's disease of the colon and a perirectal fistula leading to a left buttock abscess (arrow). *D,* Regional enteritis and bladder fistula. Retrograde cystogram demonstrates communication with the small bowel (arrow) and free intraperitoneal contrast extravasation.

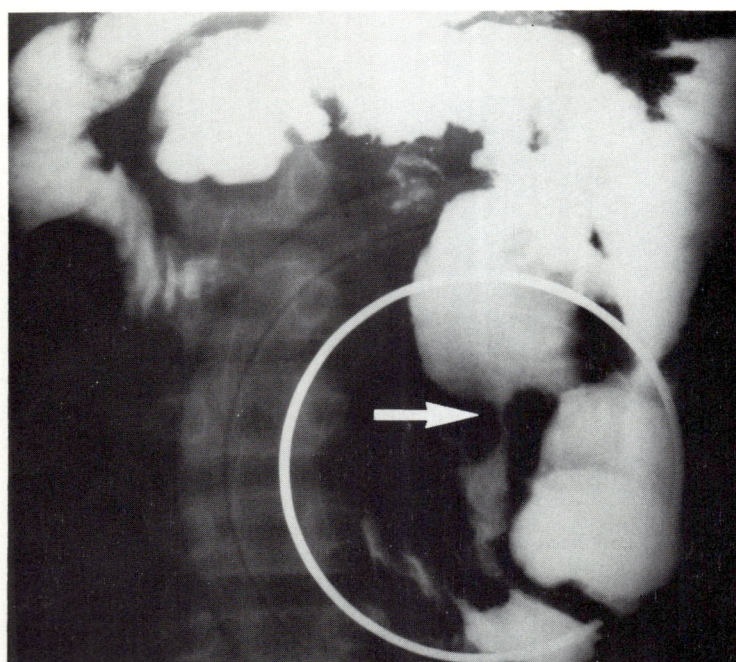

Figure 12–16. Crohn's disease and partial obstruction. There are several dilated loops of small bowel proximal to a stricture (arrow).

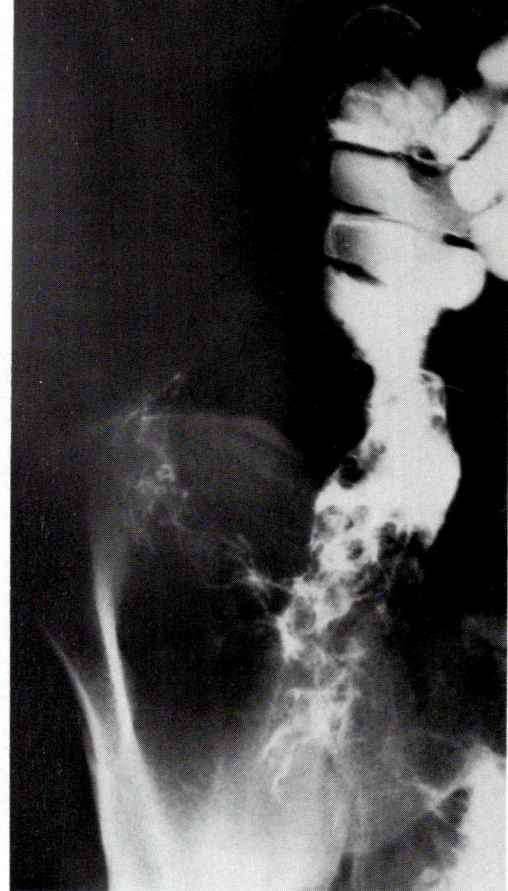

Figure 12–17. Crohn's disease and abscess of the right flank. Upper gastrointestinal series shows displacement of the right colon and a fistula dissecting into the right flank.

in the case of an enterosigmoid fistula on a small bowel examination. Multiple fistulas are a sign of advanced active disease.

Abscesses (Figs. 12–17 and 12–18) are usually located in the pelvis and present as soft tissue areas that displace or deform adjacent strictures. Small gas bubbles or larger air collections with air-fluid levels on horizontal beam films may be present. The proximity of the ileum to the psoas muscle may result in the occurrence of psoas abscess in Crohn's disease.[8] On the plain film there may be bulging of the psoas muscle, lumbar scoliosis, or linear gas densities within the psoas abscess that continue across the hip joint toward the lesser trochanter. Septic hip arthritis may also result as an extension of the psoas abscess.[10] Extraperitoneal extension of a pelvic abscess may result in osteomyelitis of the iliac bone. The focal destructive process in the iliac bone simulates primary or metastatic bone disease; however, a small bowel series can demonstrate the fistulas and inflammatory bowel changes of Crohn's disease.[5]

POSTOPERATIVE RECURRENCE. Recurrent disease after surgery has the same radiologic manifestations as the original disease. Contour irregularities, edema, ulcerations, fistulas, and stenosis all occur after surgery (Fig. 12–19). Recurrence is most commonly seen at the site of the new terminal ileum and may extend into the colon (Fig. 12–20). Recurrent disease appears more frequently in those patients who had active disease, fistula, and abscess prior to surgery than in those with the chronic changes of stenosis without fistula.

MALABSORPTION. Patients with extensive Crohn's disease may have malabsorption for a variety of reasons. The enterohepatic circulation, which is dependent on intact terminal ileal mucosa for recirculation, may be interrupted and result in de-

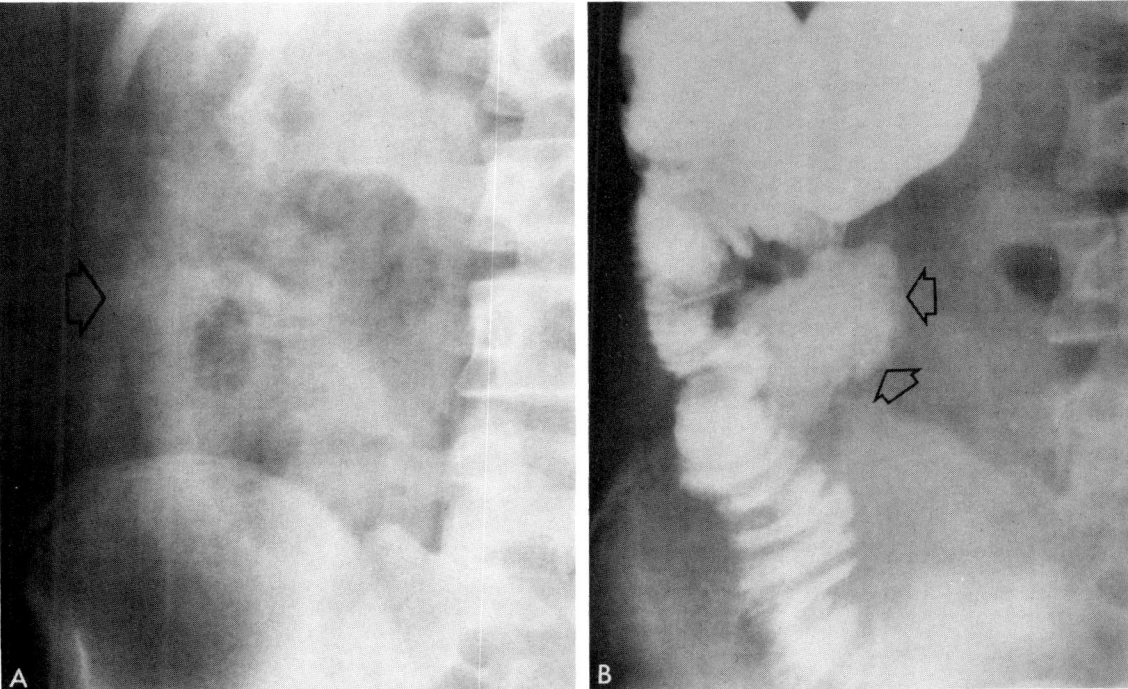

Figure 12–18. Right flank abscess secondary to perforation at ileocolostomy site in a patient with regional enteritis. *A,* Plain film of the right upper quadrant shows loss of the flank stripe (arrow). *B,* Barium enema of the same area shows a large collection of barium (arrows) in the abscess cavity adjacent to the ileocolostomy site.

creased levels of bile salts and fat malabsorption. Blind loops, secondary to areas of stricture and intervening areas of bowel dilatation or to surgery and bypass of bowel segments, result in bacterial overgrowth and deconjugation of bile salts. Lymphatic obstruction secondary to perilymphatic granulomas as well as repeated surgical resection leading to a short bowel syndrome is a potential cause of malabsorption.

RARE INTESTINAL COMPLICATIONS. When perforation of the bowel occurs in Crohn's disease, the perforation is usually rapidly sealed off. As a result, perforation with free air under the hemidiaphragms is extremely rare, but it can occur.[12, 15] Another rare manifestation of Crohn's disease is massive gastrointestinal hemorrhage. Angiography may be helpful in locating the source of bleeding.[16] Although hemorrhagic episodes tend to recur, bleeding often subsides spontaneously and the patient remains well for variable lengths of time.[2] Toxic megacolon may occur in cases of Crohn's disease but is less common and more benign than the toxic megacolon associated with ulcerative colitis. Toxic dilatation limited to the ileum has also been reported.[6]

Patients with long-standing regional enteritis have an increased risk of acquiring adenocarcinoma compared with the general population.[7] Diagnosis is frequently difficult, since the tumor may develop in a surgically bypassed loop of bowel or the radiologic findings may simulate recurring inflammatory disease. Adenocarcinoma is rarely diagnosed preoperatively. These patients usually acquire partial small bowel

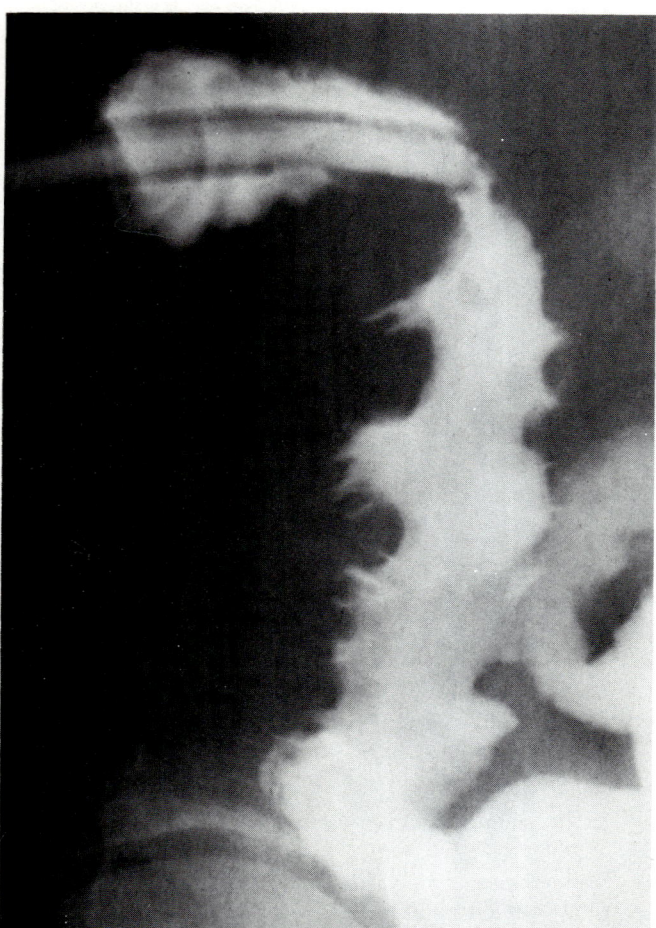

Figure 12–19. Recurrent Crohn's disease. Retrograde filling of the ileum through the ileostomy stoma in a patient with recurrent Crohn's disease. There are multiple ulcerations associated with marked mucosal edema in the ileum just proximal to the ileostomy.

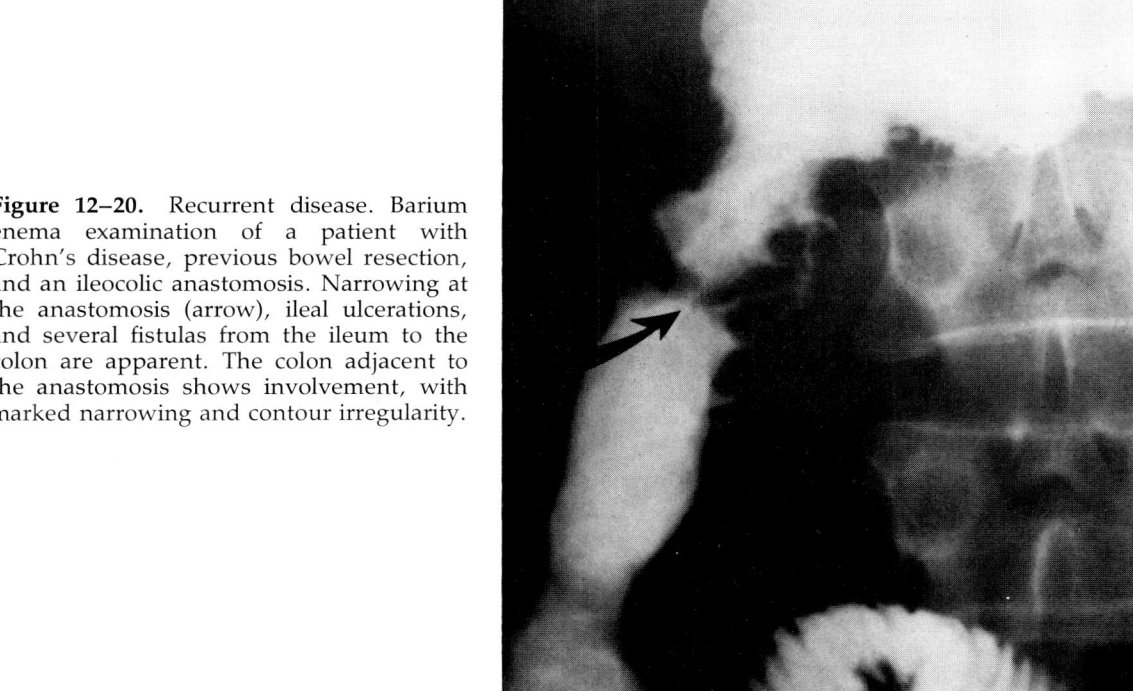

Figure 12–20. Recurrent disease. Barium enema examination of a patient with Crohn's disease, previous bowel resection, and an ileocolic anastomosis. Narrowing at the anastomosis (arrow), ileal ulcerations, and several fistulas from the ileum to the colon are apparent. The colon adjacent to the anastomosis shows involvement, with marked narrowing and contour irregularity.

obstruction after long periods of inflammatory disease quiescence. Carcinoma should be considered in the differential diagnosis when patients with Crohn's disease of long standing have a new partial obstruction.

Extraintestinal Complications

Patients with Crohn's disease have an increased incidence of gallstones. This may be due to the decreased bile salt pool resulting from failure of resorption in the diseased terminal ileum. Other hepatobiliary abnormalities reported in Crohn's disease include fatty degeneration of the liver, pericholangitis, and sclerosing cholangitis. Endoscopic retrograde cholangiography or percutaneous transhepatic cholangiography of patients with sclerosing cholangitis demonstrates intrahepatic ductal stenosis, ectasia, decreased arborization, and obstruction. Extrahepatic radiographic abnormalities include ductal stenosis, ductal diverticula, and mural irregularities.[18]

Patients with long-standing Crohn's disease have an increased incidence of nonopaque uric acid and radiopaque oxalate renal calculi. Oxalate calculi are caused by excessive absorption of dietary oxalate in the presence of nonabsorbed fatty acids. Scout films for small bowel series should always be checked to determine whether radiopaque oxalate renal calculi are present. Other urinary tract complications associated with Crohn's disease are fistulas and abscesses involving the bladder, kidneys, or ureters; hydronephrosis; and obstruction of the ureter secondary to retroperitoneal fibrosis or abscess. Radiographically, unilateral dilatation of a ureter, usually to the level of the pelvic brim, may be seen. The right ureter, being closest to the terminal

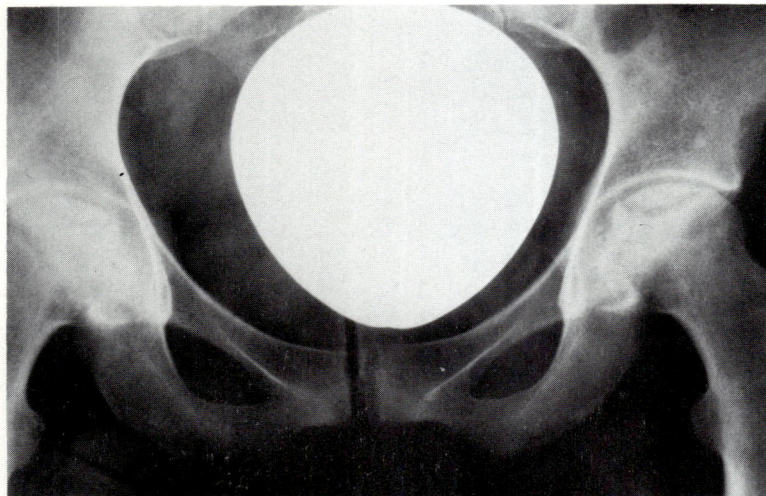

Figure 12–21. Aseptic necrosis. Pelvis film of a patient with Crohn's disease who has had steroid therapy demonstrates bilateral aseptic necrosis of the femoral heads.

ileum, is much more frequently involved.[1] Bladder deformities may be secondary to pelvic abscesses, adjacent fibrosis, or enlarged adjacent lymph nodes.

In addition to osteomyelitis of the iliac bone and septic arthritis of the hip, the bone and joint complications of Crohn's disease include aseptic necrosis secondary to steroid therapy (Fig. 12–21), growth failure in children, sacroiliitis, and polysynovitis predominantly affecting large joints.

DIFFERENTIAL DIAGNOSIS

Acute inflammatory disease secondary to appendicitis or pelvic inflammatory disease may produce radiographic changes that are identical to those of acute regional enteritis and may be differentiated only at surgery. Usually, however, patients with Crohn's disease have a clinical history suggesting a more chronic inflammatory process. Intestinal tuberculosis may also have radiographic findings that are indistinguishable from Crohn's disease. Both diseases are characterized by contour irregularities, thickened mucosal folds, and large ulcerations. A helpful diagnostic finding is that major involvement in ileocecal tuberculosis is usually on the cecal side of the valve. A wide gaping of the valve associated with narrowing of the immediately adjacent ileum and circumferential, rather than eccentric, bowel involvement may also be helpful in distinguishing tuberculosis from Crohn's disease.

Crohn's disease of the colon may also at times be indistinguishable radiologically from ulcerative colitis. Deep ulcers, asymmetric involvement, skip areas, abscesses of rectal diseases, and particularly, terminal ileal disease are features that help to distinguish Crohn's colitis from ulcerative colitis.

In children and young adults, multiple small filling defects in the terminal ileum, secondary to lymphoid hyperplasia, may simulate the cobblestone pattern of Crohn's disease. The bowel shows no wall thickening or rigidity but instead demonstrates a normal pliability.[4] Lymphoid hyperplasia due to lymphatic obstruction has also been seen in cases of Crohn's disease, but other evidence of inflammatory change is always present.

Lymphosarcoma with thickened mucosal folds, ulcerative fistulas, and intraluminal nodules may simulate Crohn's disease. The ulcerations in lymphosarcoma are usually larger and more irregular, without the linear configuration often seen in Crohn's disease. Stenosis is uncommon. The nodules may be larger and more irregular in shape than the cobblestone nodular defects of Crohn's disease. Clinically there is often evidence of widespread lymphatic disease.

Radiation enteritis is differentiated from Crohn's disease by the clinical history. Henoch-Schönlein purpura can result in edematous mucosal folds and may mimic Crohn's disease if the onset of hematuria, typical rash, and arthralgia is delayed. Patients with bleeding diatheses may also have thickened small bowel folds secondary to intramural hemorrhage. Again, the clinical history is essential in the diagnosis.

Other conditions that sometimes mimic Crohn's enteritis radiographically include strongyloidiasis, vascular infarction, severe Giardia infestation, eosinophilic gastroenteritis, and diffuse metastatic involvement of the mesentery.

References

1. Bagby, R. J., Clements, J. L., Jr., Patrick, J. W., et al.: Genitourinary complications of granulomatous bowel disease. Am. J. Roentgenol. *117*:297–306, 1973.
2. Corona, F. E., and Dyck, W. P.: Massive gastrointestinal hemorrhage as the sole clinical manifestation of regional enteritis. Am. J. Dig. Dis. *18*:1001–1004, 1973.
3. Crohn, B. B., Ginzburg, L., and Oppenheimer, G. D.: Regional ileitis; a pathological and clinical entity. J.A.M.A. *99*:1323–1328, 1932.
4. Franken, E. A., Jr., Smith, J. A., and Fitzgerald, J. R.: Regional enteritis in children: clinical and roentgen features. C.R.C. Crit. Rev. Diagn. Imaging *10*:163–185, 1977.
5. Ghahremani, G. G.: Osteomyelitis of the ilium in patients with Crohn's disease. Am. J. Roentgenol. *118*:364–370, 1973.
6. Greene, L., Kresch, L., and Held, B.: Acute toxic dilatation limited to the ileum in Crohn's disease. Am. J. Dig. Dis. *17*:439–446, 1972.
7. Hoffman, J. P., Taft, D. A., Wheelis, R. F., et al.: Adenocarcinoma in regional enteritis of the small intestine. Arch. Surg. *112*:606–611, 1977.
8. Kyle, J.: Psoas abscess in Crohn's disease. Gastroenterology *61*:149–155, 1971.
9. Laufer, I., and Costopoulos, L.: Early lesions of Crohn's disease. Am. J. Roentgenol. *130*:307–311, 1978.
10. London, D., and Fitton, J. M.: Acute septic arthritis complicating Crohn's disease. Br. J. Surg., *57*:536–537, 1970.
11. Marshak, R. H., and Lindner, A. E.: Radiology of the Small Intestine. Philadelphia, W. B. Saunders Company, 1970, p. 167.
12. Mogadam, M., and Priest, R. J.: Necrotizing enteritis in Crohn's disease of the small bowel. Gastroenterology *56*:337–341, 1969.
13. Morson, B. C.: The early histological lesion of Crohn's disease. Proc. R. Soc. Med. *65*:71–72, 1972.
14. Moss, A. A.: Inflammatory bowel disease: update 1978. *In* Margulis, A. R., and Gooding, C. A. (eds.): Diagnostic Radiology 1978. San Francisco, University of California at San Francisco Extended Programs in Medical Education, 1978, pp. 383–400.
15. Nasr, K., Morowitz, D. A., Anderson, J. G. D., et al.: Free perforation in regional enteritis. Gut *10*:106–108, 1969.
16. Podolny, G. A.: Crohn's disease presenting with massive lower gastrointestinal hemorrhage. Am. J. Roentgenol. *130*:368–370, 1978.
17. Price, A. B., and Morson, B. C.: Inflammatory bowel disease: the surgical pathology of Crohn's disease and ulcerative colitis. Hum. Pathol. *6*:7–29, 1975.
18. Rohrmann, C. A., Jr., Ansel, H. J., Freeny, P. C., et al.: Cholangiographic abnormalities in patients with inflammatory bowel disease. Diagn. Radiol. *127*:635–641, 1978.
19. Sommers, S. C.: Ulcerative and granulomatous colitis. Am. J. Roentgenol. *130*:817–823, 1978.
20. Steinberg, D. M., Cooke, W. T., and Alexander-Williams, J.: Abscess and fistulae in Crohn's disease. Gut *14*:865–869, 1973.
21. Yentis, L.: Henoch-Schönlein purpura mimicking acute appendicitis and Crohn's disease. Br. J. Radiol. *46*:555–556, 1973.

Part III
Malabsorption Syndromes

STEVEN H. OMINSKY, M.D.
ALEXANDER R. MARGULIS, M.D.

Malabsorption can be defined as any disorder in which the intestinal absorption of nutrients is impaired. Physiologically, normal absorption in the intestine is extremely complex, and many diseases can result in the impaired absorption of fat, carbohydrates, proteins, vitamins, electrolytes, minerals, and water.

There are almost as many classifications of malabsorption diseases as there are causes. This discussion is confined to malabsorption disorders that have abnormalities demonstrable in the small bowel roentgen examination. For purposes of simplification, six types of disorders are discussed (Table 12–1): (1) abnormalities resulting in decreased effective bowel length; (2) abnormalities resulting in bacterial overgrowth; (3) abnormalities that decrease digestive activity; (4) intrinsic small bowel mucosal or submucosal abnormalities; (5) abnormalities with lymphatic obstruction; and (6) infections. The first two types are usually related to surgical intervention and, as such, are of special interest to the surgeon. The other disorders include diseases treated by the

TABLE 12–1. MALABSORPTION DISORDERS WITH SMALL INTESTINE RADIOGRAPHIC ABNORMALITIES

Causes of Malabsorption Related to Surgical Intervention
  Decrease in Effective Bowel Length
    Partial or total gastrectomy
    Short bowel syndrome
    Bypass surgery for morbid obesity
    Fistula
  Bacterial Overgrowth
    Blind loops
    Afferent loop syndrome

Other Causes of Malabsorption with Radiographic Manifestations
  Bacterial Overgrowth
    Scleroderma
    Small bowel diverticula
    Idiopathic pseudo-obstruction
  Decreased Digestive Activity
    Pancreatic insufficiency
    Bile acid insufficiency
  Intrinsic Mucosal and Submucosal Abnormalities
    Celiac sprue
    Whipple's disease
    Amyloidosis
    Eosinophilic gastroenteritis
    Crohn's disease
    Radiation enteritis
  Abnormalities of Lymphatic Obstruction
    Congenital lymphangiectasia
    Lymphoma

Other Causes of Lymphatic Obstruction
  Infections
    Giardiasis
    Strongyloides stercoralis
    Tropical sprue

surgeon, such as bile duct obstruction, Crohn's disease, lymphoma, and pancreatic insufficiency. This classification omits causes of malabsorption in which diagnosis depends exclusively on biopsy, blood chemistry, or drug history and in which radiologic examination plays no diagnostic role.

CAUSES OF MALABSORPTION RELATED TO SURGICAL INTERVENTION

Decrease in Effective Bowel Length

PARTIAL OR TOTAL GASTRECTOMY. Malabsorption can occur following complete or partial gastrectomy, resulting in an increased fat content of the stool, decreased vitamin B_{12} absorption,[4] iron deficiency anemia,[14] or decreased serum calcium levels.[10] Altered reservoir function of the gastric remnant plays an important role in malabsorption, since rapid gastric emptying leads to the dilution of pancreatic proteolytic and lipolytic enzymes and of bile salts.[25] Malabsorption and caloric loss are often further complicated by decreased food intake secondary to early satiety or "fear of dumping" syndrome. Truncal or selective vagotomy also may result in diarrhea and steatorrhea, although the reason for this has not yet been established.

The radiographic appearance of the small bowel in patients with partial gastric resection is usually normal. Mild dilatation of the proximal small bowel is frequently seen after a vagotomy. Dilution of barium may occur, especially in patients with diarrhea. Occasionally, cases of latent celiac sprue become active after gastric surgery, presumably because of contact with increased concentrations of gluten.[12] Radiographically, the patients in whom this occurs may have the small bowel dilatation and hypersecretion seen in patients with typical adult celiac sprue. Vagotomy may also unmask asymptomatic adult celiac disease (Fig. 12–22).[19] Altered calcium metabolism may result in osteoporosis or osteomalacia or both. The abdominal film may demonstrate wedging and biconcave vertebral bodies, rib fractures, accentuated bony trabeculae, or lucent pseudofracture lines in the pubic rami.[5]

SHORT BOWEL SYNDROME. A short bowel syndrome may result from repeated resections of the small bowel necessitated by trauma, infarction, recurrent tumor, or inflammatory bowel disease. If the patient can be supported by intravenous hyperalimentation, the remaining portions of the jejunum may undergo hypertrophy, dilatation, and elongation. The upper gastrointestinal examination can demonstrate this dilatation and mucosal fold thickening and determine the length of the remaining small bowel (Fig. 12–23). Patients with massive resections also may have gastric hypersecretion[8] and an increased risk of acquiring a peptic ulcer.

Limited resections of terminal ileum, such as may be performed in patients with Crohn's disease, also may result in malabsorption, since this segment of bowel absorbs vitamin B_{12} and is also responsible for the active absorption of bile salts back into the enterohepatic circulation. Patients with resection of 2 or more feet of terminal ileum require life-long vitamin B_{12} replacement.[25] Because of the cathartic action of bile salts on the colon, malabsorption and watery diarrhea occur in patients with ileal resection.

BYPASS SURGERY FOR MORBID OBESITY. When malabsorption is deliberately produced by bypass surgery for morbid obesity, complications may result. In one study, obstruction was the most common complication.[20] Unlike the usual postsurgical intestinal obstruction, most of these cases were due not to adhesions but to intussusception (Fig. 12–24),[8] incarcerated hernia, and volvulus.[22] These patients also have a higher than normal incidence of acute cholecystitis and renal oxalate stones (see also Part IX, pp. 637–645).

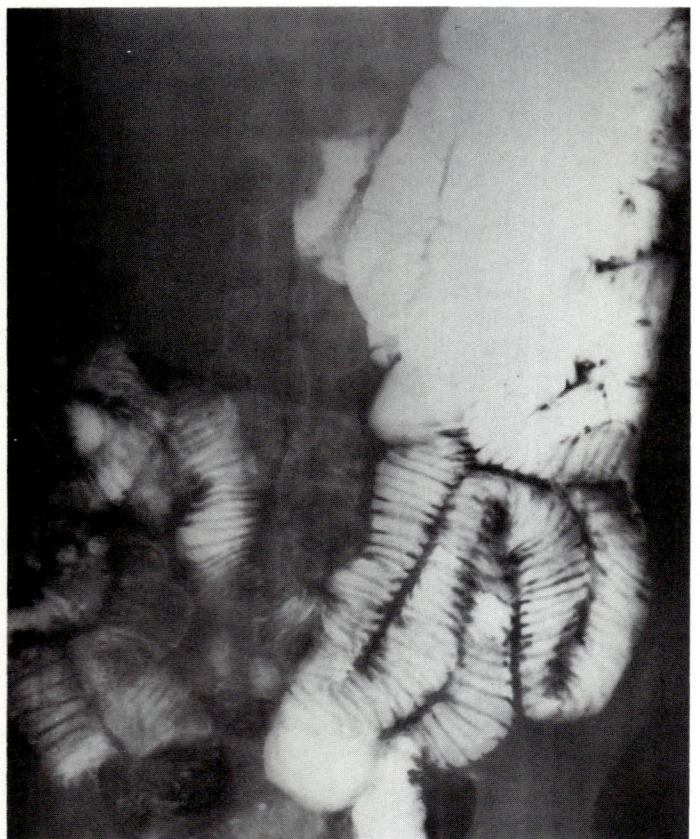

Figure 12–22. Celiac disease after vagotomy. This patient had an esophagectomy with esophagogastrostomy and vagotomy for esophogeal carcinoma. Two months after surgery the patient acquired marked steatorrhea. A small bowel biopsy demonstrated broad flat intestinal villi and infiltration of the lamina propria by lymphocytes, plasma cells, and eosinophils. A film from the small bowel examination shows dilatation of the middle and distal jejunum. The steatorrhea ceased after a gluten-free diet was instituted. (*From* Moss, A. A.: Postvagotomy unmasking of nontropical sprue. Gastrointest. Radiol. *1:*173–175, 1976. Reproduced by permission.)

Figure 12–23. Short bowel syndrome. This patient had a superior mesenteric artery infarction during abdominal surgery, and a small bowel resection with a duodenocolic anastomosis was performed. Three months after surgery an upper gastrointestinal series showed marked dilatation and fold thickening in the remaining duodenum.

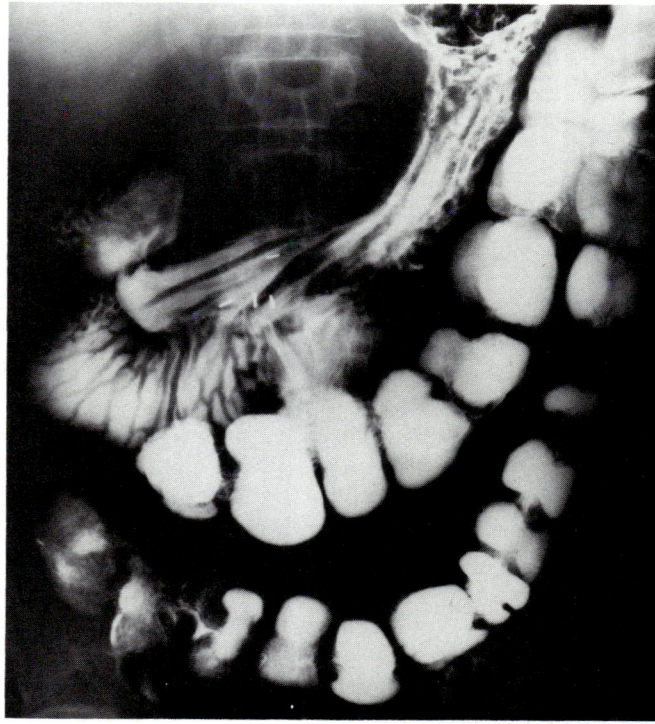

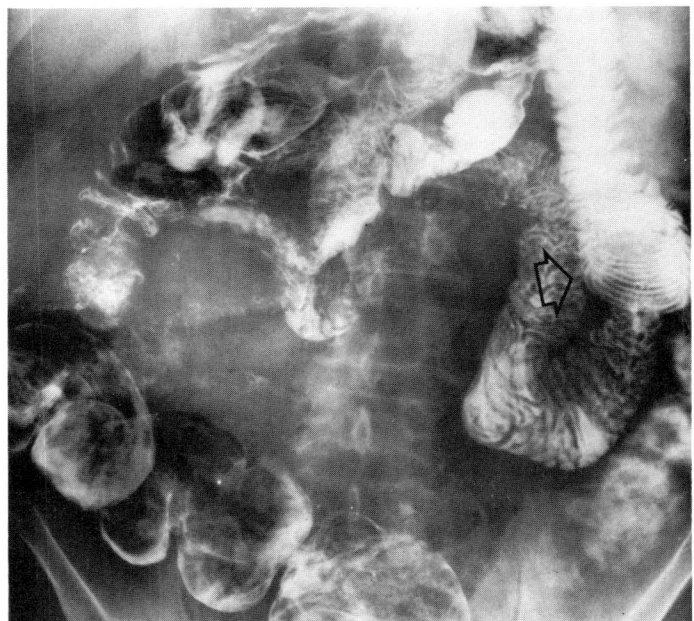

Figure 12-24. In a patient with bypass surgery for weight reduction there is partial obstruction due to a jejunojejunal intussusception (arrow).

FISTULA. When fistulas create a bypass of large portions of the small bowel or of vital portions, such as the terminal ileum, malabsorption occurs. Since the main portion of the intestinal stream is diverted, such a fistula can be demonstrated with a barium small bowel examination. A surgically created fistula of this type occurs when a gastroileostomy is inadvertently performed instead of a gastrojejunostomy. This results in rapid weight loss, hunger after meals, and passage of undigested food. Survival is unlikely unless the gastroileostomy is eliminated. An upper gastrointestinal examination provides an immediate diagnosis of the presence of a gastroileostomy.

Gastrojejunocolic fistula, a sequela of marginal ulceration, also results in rapid weight loss and a high mortality rate if not recognized early. Barium enema is usually more effective than an upper gastrointestinal series in diagnosing this complication (Fig. 12–25). Gastrocolic fistula with malabsorption may also occur as a result of carcinoma of the stomach or the colon.

Bacterial Overgrowth

Bacterial overgrowth decreases conjugated bile salts and increases the free bile acids in the lumen of the upper small intestine, resulting in decreased lipid solubilization, with malabsorption and consequent steatorrhea.[17] Bacteria also take up vitamin B_{12}, both unbound and bound to intrinsic factor, causing a B_{12} deficiency. Bacterial overgrowth can occur when there is hypomotility and stasis of the contents of the small intestine or from contamination of the upper small bowel by colonic contents. This may be due to a fistula or to resection of the lower small intestine and the ileocecal valve. The barium small bowel examination is ideally suited to the detection of fistulas and stasis.

BLIND LOOPS. A true blind loop is a segment of small intestine into which contents pass but cannot exit at a normal rate.[25] Strictures of the small bowel with intervening areas of dilatation can be found during the stenotic phase of regional enteritis or in cases of radiation enteritis. These strictures result in a blind loop

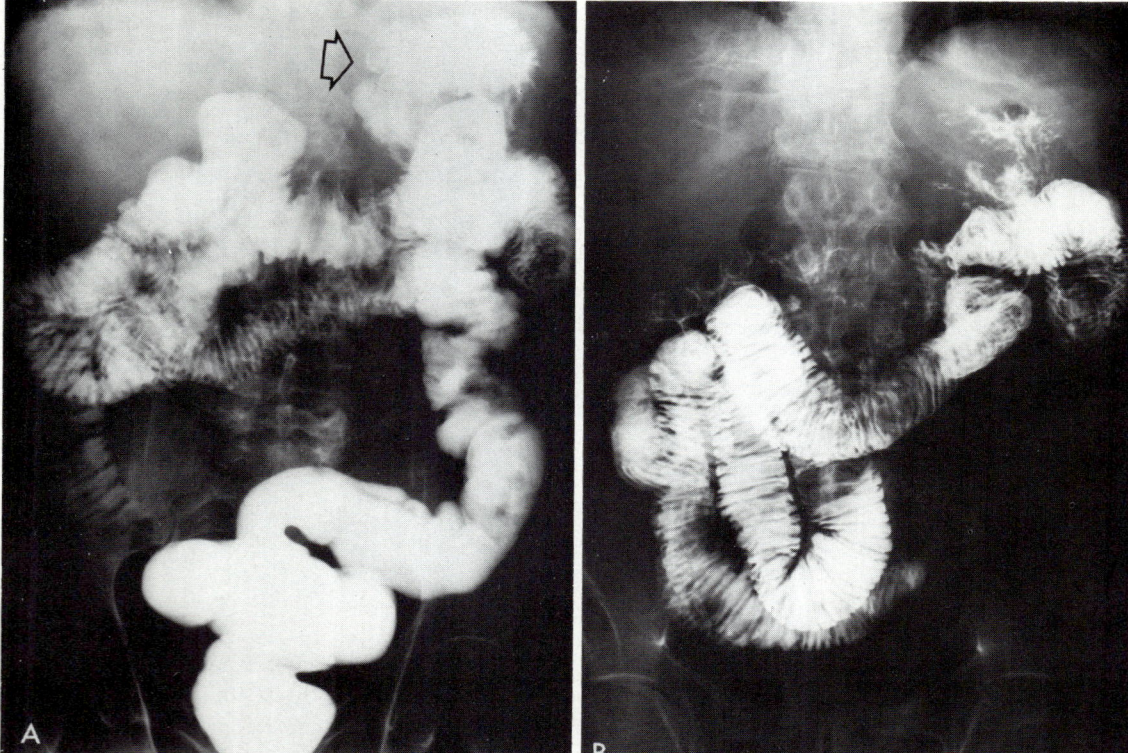

Figure 12–25. *A,* Barium enema examination in a patient who had Billroth II surgery for peptic ulcer disease. The patient experienced diarrhea, weight loss, and anemia. There is a gastrojejunocolic fistula secondary to a marginal ulcer, with reflux of barium into the stomach (arrow) and the jejunum. *B,* Postevacuation film of the same patient with a large amount of residual barium in the jejunum.

syndrome, with stasis and bacterial overgrowth. Blind loops may result from congenital small bowel duplications. Surgically created blind loops are frequently associated with side-to-side intestinal anastomosis, especially when a partially defunctionalized ileal loop has been excluded from the mainstream by an ileotransverse colostomy or an ileosigmoidostomy. A side-to-side anastomosis may also result in a recirculation phenomenon and bacterial overgrowth.

AFFERENT LOOP SYNDROME. The blind loop syndrome can occur following a gastrojejunostomy if there is stasis in the afferent loop; this is known as the afferent loop syndrome. Afferent loop filling in the upper gastrointestinal series is not abnormal, but preferential filling, distention, and stasis of the afferent loop are. If the afferent loop is already distended and filled with food contents, the barium may not enter the loop or may just outline the retained food (Fig. 12–26).

OTHER CAUSES OF MALABSORPTION WITH RADIOGRAPHIC MANIFESTATIONS

Bacterial Overgrowth

SCLERODERMA. Scleroderma involving the small intestine produces hypomotility and bowel stasis, resulting in bacterial overgrowth and malabsorption.[15] This complication usually occurs in cases of advanced disease. The radiologic findings are characterized by hypomotility and areas of dilatation, especially in the descending portion of the duodenum, without evidence of organic obstruction (Fig. 12–27). Another finding is pseudosacculations of the small intestine and colon, which resemble diverticula but have wide necks. This is the result of asymmetric bowel wall fibrosis. Bowel wall fibrosis may also cause thinning of the valvulae conniventes. Pneumatosis intestinalis may be present as well. Scleroderma with dilatation may superficially resemble the dilatation of sprue, but the two can be differentiated because the hypersecretion and dilution of barium that occurs in sprue does not occur in scleroderma. Patients with sprue also usually have normal bowel motility.

SMALL BOWEL DIVERTICULA. Multiple small bowel diverticula may also result in stasis and bacterial overgrowth. A plain film of the abdomen may show multiple large bubble-shaped gas densities, especially in the left upper quadrant. These gas collections may simulate colon gas if they are small and oriented in a linear configura-

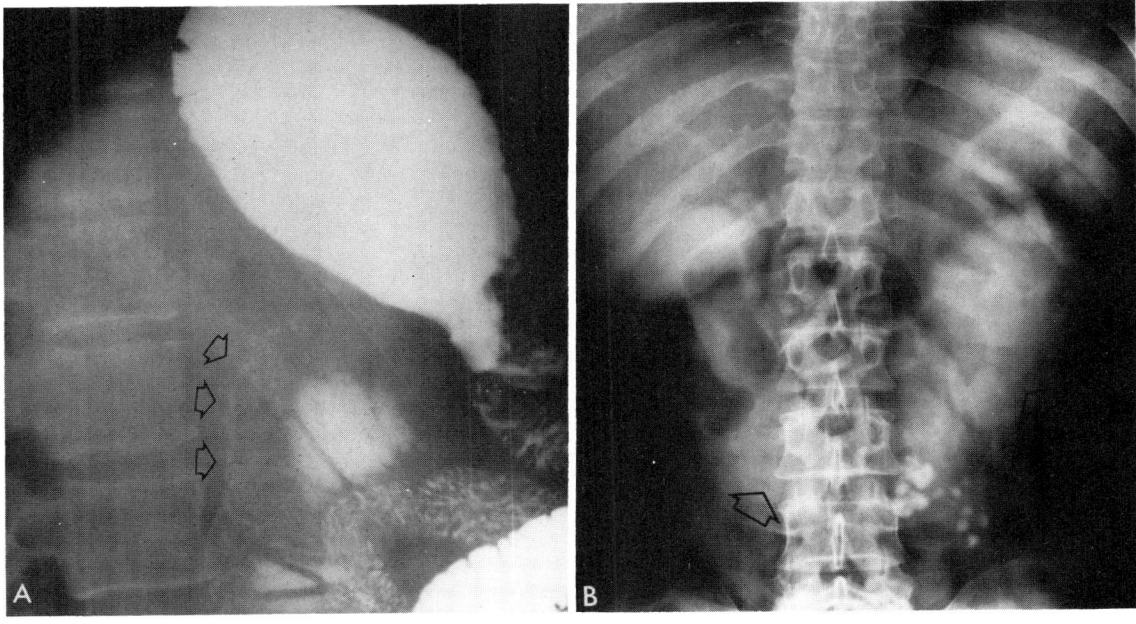

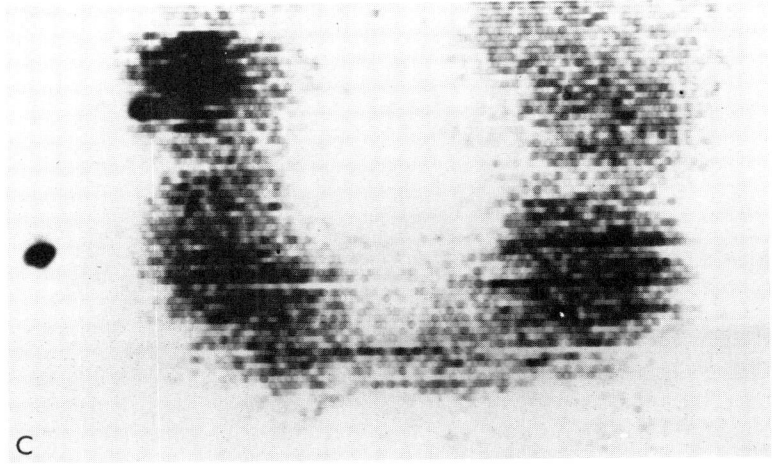

Figure 12–26. *A*, Billroth II anastomosis and malabsorption. A lateral view from an upper gastrointestinal series shows a small amount of contrast outlining a dilated bowel loop (arrows). *B*, A film of the same patient after an intravenous cholangiogram shows marked dilatation of the afferent loop (arrows). *C*, Four-hour ^{131}I rose Bengal scan of the same patient shows the marked dilatation of the afferent loop.

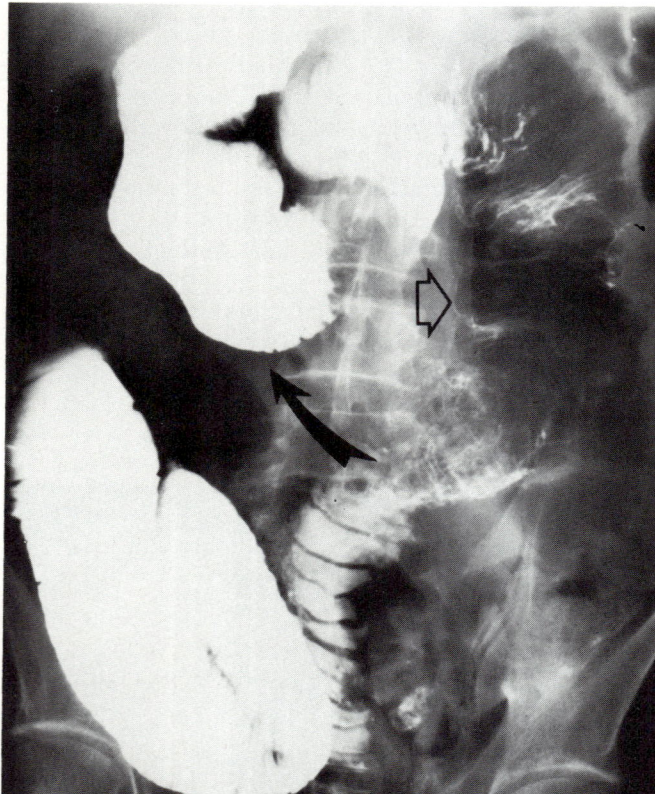

Figure 12–27. Upper gastrointestinal series of a patient with scleroderma and malabsorption. Note the dilatation of the descending duodenum (long arrow) and the proximal jejunum (open arrow) as well as, to a lesser degree, dilatation of the small bowel in the right lower quadrant.

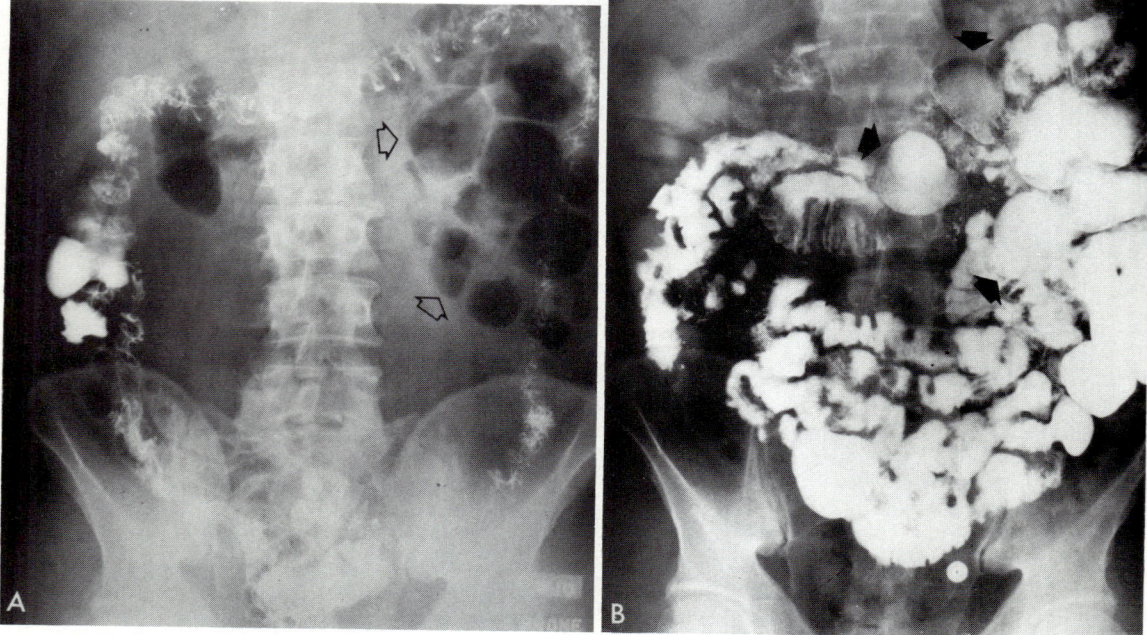

Figure 12–28. Jejunal diverticula. *A*, Postevacuation film, after a barium enema, demonstrates unusual round collections of gas in the left upper quadrant (arrows), which have thin walls where they coalesce. *B*, Small bowel examination confirms the presence of multiple large jejunal diverticula (arrows) in this patient with malabsorption.

tion. If they are large, they may coalesce with intervening walls that are thinner than haustra (Fig. 12–28A). A small bowel series confirms the presence of the diverticula (Fig. 12–28B). Diverticula must be differentiated from the pseudosacculations of scleroderma, which have wide necks, in contrast to the narrowed necks of true diverticula.

IDIOPATHIC PSEUDO-OBSTRUCTION. Small bowel and colon dilatation with hypomotility may also occur in cases of pseudo-obstruction,[24] which is characterized by intermittent bouts of marked intestinal ileus. Plain film findings include bowel dilatation simulating a large or small bowel obstruction; however, a small bowel series merely shows dilatation and delayed transit without focal obstruction. Stasis leads to bacterial overgrowth and malabsorption in some patients.

Decreased Digestive Activity

PANCREATIC INSUFFICIENCY. Patients with chronic pancreatitis, cystic fibrosis, or pancreatic carcinoma may have malabsorption secondary to pancreatic acinar loss or pancreatic duct obstruction. The absence of pancreatic lipase results in steatorrhea. Radiographically, the small bowel is usually normal; occasionally, however, patients with severe chronic pancreatitis demonstrate increased secretions and dilution of barium in the small bowel, without the dilatation seen in sprue (Fig. 12–29).

BILE ACID INSUFFICIENCY. Malabsorption of fat because of insufficient bile salts can occur in primary liver disease or in bile duct obstruction. Small bowel radiographic examination is usually normal as in pancreatic insufficiency. However, an occasional patient with steatorrhea may show small bowel dilatation and hypersecretion.

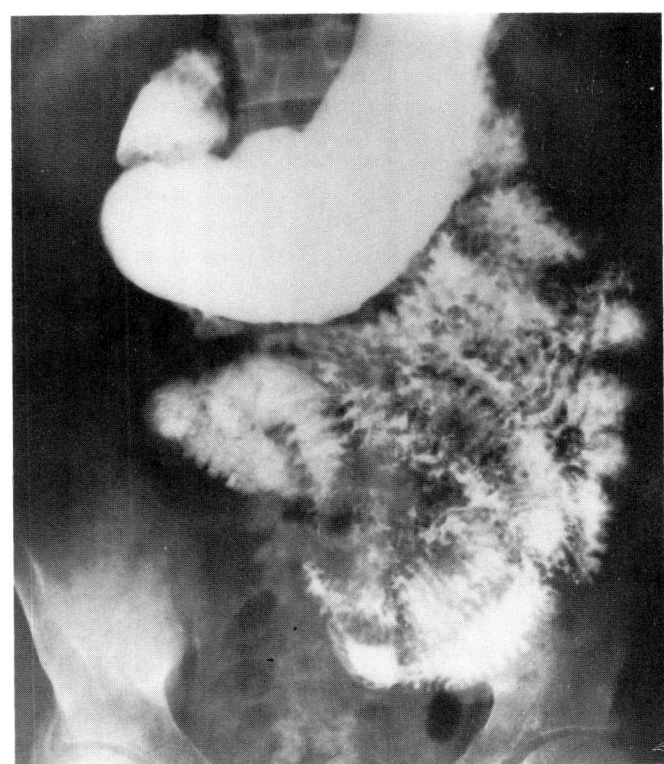

Figure 12–29. Malabsorption from pancreatic insufficiency. This 25-year-old patient had severe diabetes, pancreatic insufficiency, and malabsorption. A small bowel series shows increased secretions, dilution of the barium, and thickened small bowel folds. At autopsy, there was marked pancreatic fibrosis, and sections of the small intestine were normal.

Intrinsic Mucosal and Submucosal Abnormalities

CELIAC DISEASE. Adult and childhood celiac disease affect the small bowel mucosa, resulting in flattened or absent villi, cuboidal instead of elongated absorptive cells, and infiltration of the lamina propria with lymphocytes and plasma cells. The jejunum is affected more than the ileum.

Dilatation and hypersecretion are the radiologic hallmarks of celiac disease. Dilatation is most commonly seen in the midjejunum (Fig. 12–30), but it may be generalized in the small intestine. The extent of bowel dilatation appears to be related to the severity of the disease; it is most pronounced in advanced cases.[18] The amount of dilatation in one loop may vary during the course of the small bowel series. Prolonged transit time may occur in some cases with markedly dilated loops. Peristalsis may become disordered and transient. Nonobstructive intussusceptions may occur.

Patients with celiac disease also have an excessive amount of fluid in the small bowel. The term "hypersecretion" has been applied, although the origin of the increased fluid is unclear. The increased fluid produces air-fluid levels on the upright plain film and also dilutes the barium as it passes through the small intestine (Fig. 12–31A). Modern barium suspensions, with micropulverized barium, do not show the fragmentation and clumping that was associated with increased fluid in the small intestine when coarser barium was routinely used. Normal-sized or thinned folds without irregularity are seen. The complications of small intestinal lymphoma[11] and,

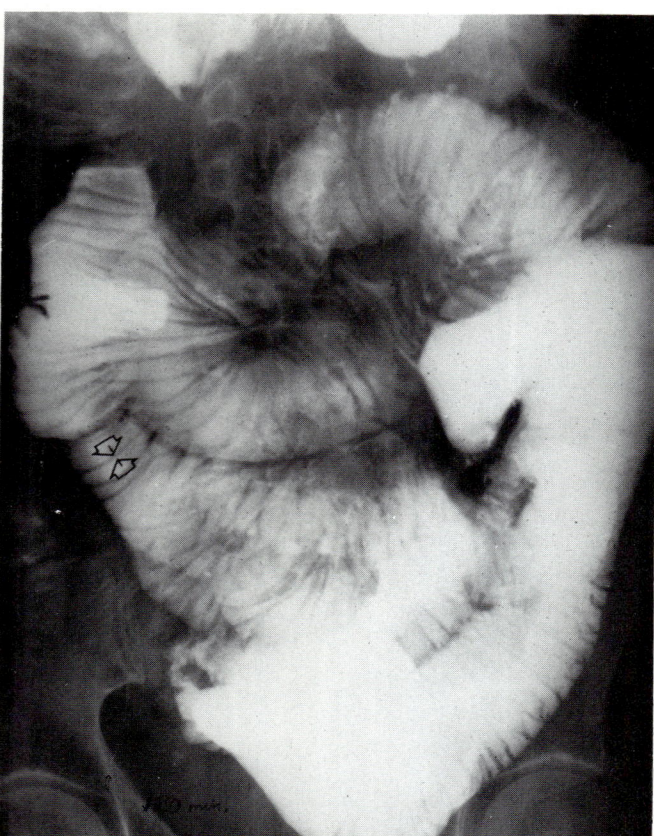

Figure 12–30. Celiac disease. Two-hour small bowel film of a patient with celiac disease. The bowel is dilated, and the barium is partially diluted secondary to hypersecretion. The mucosal folds are slightly thinned (arrows).

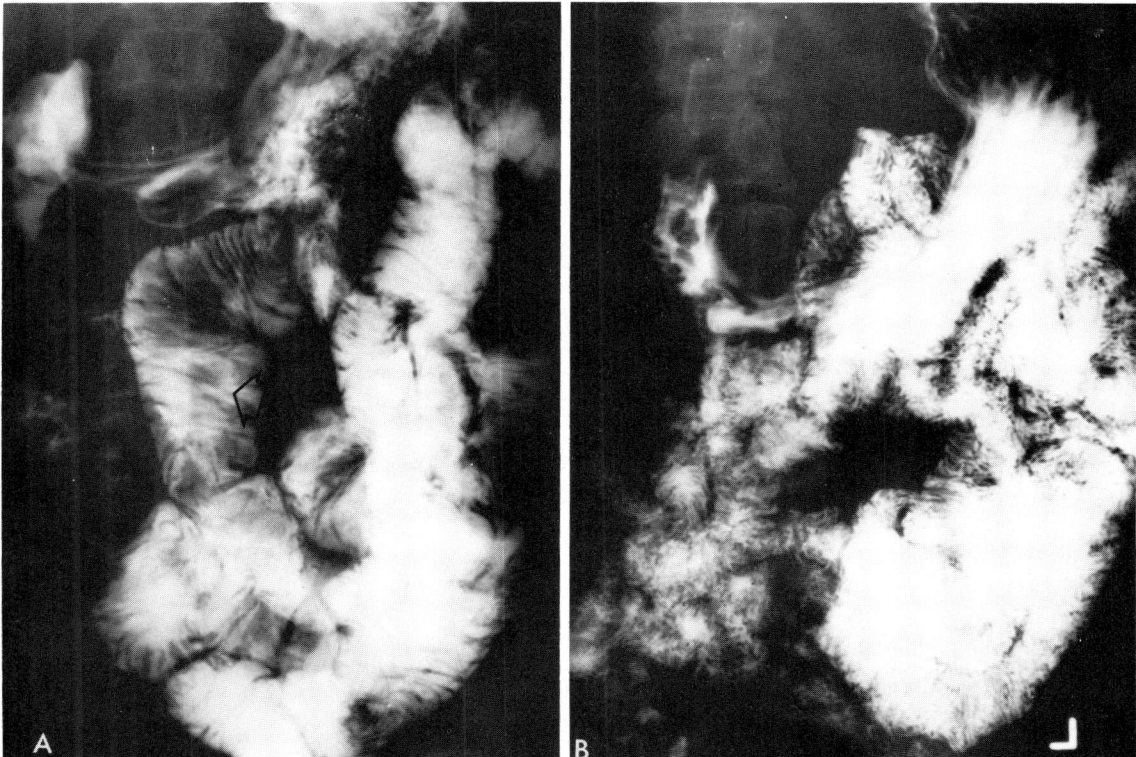

Figure 12–31. *A,* Patient with celiac disease and jejunal dilatation (arrow). *B,* The same patient after a gluten-free diet. The jejunum has returned to a normal caliber.

less commonly, small bowel carcinoma[3] can occur in patients with celiac disease. If lymphoma develops in patients with celiac disease, the mucosal folds become thickened and nodular, and extraluminal extrinsic mass defects may be present. A less common complication of celiac disease is ulceration with hemorrhage or perforation.[1] Osteomalacia with bone fractures secondary to the impaired absorption of vitamin D and calcium is another complication.

WHIPPLE'S DISEASE. Whipple's disease is a systemic condition caused by an organism that has the ultrastructural morphologic state of a bacterium.[26] Its clinical signs and symptoms are abdominal distention, diarrhea, and steatorrhea, and occasionally lymphadenopathy, fever, and arthritis. Intestinal biopsy shows thickening and edema of the lamina propria and infiltration of the lamina with PAS-positive macrophages. Some lymphatic dilatation may also be present. Unlike that in celiac disease, the epithelium in Whipple's disease is only slightly affected, resulting in some attenuation in the height of the epithelial cells. The PAS-positive granules seen in the macrophages are thought to be remnants of the cell wall of phagocytized bacilli. After antibiotic therapy the PAS-positive macrophages disappear, and the mucosa reverts to normal.

Thickened and sometimes nodular mucosal folds are seen on the barium small bowel examination (Fig. 12–32). There may be marked irregularity, with a serpiginous and redundant configuration of the thickened valvulae as they cross the small bowel lumen. The duodenum and jejunum are primarily affected. The ileum is usually normal, and there is little or no bowel dilatation or increase in bowel secretions. The bowel remains pliable.

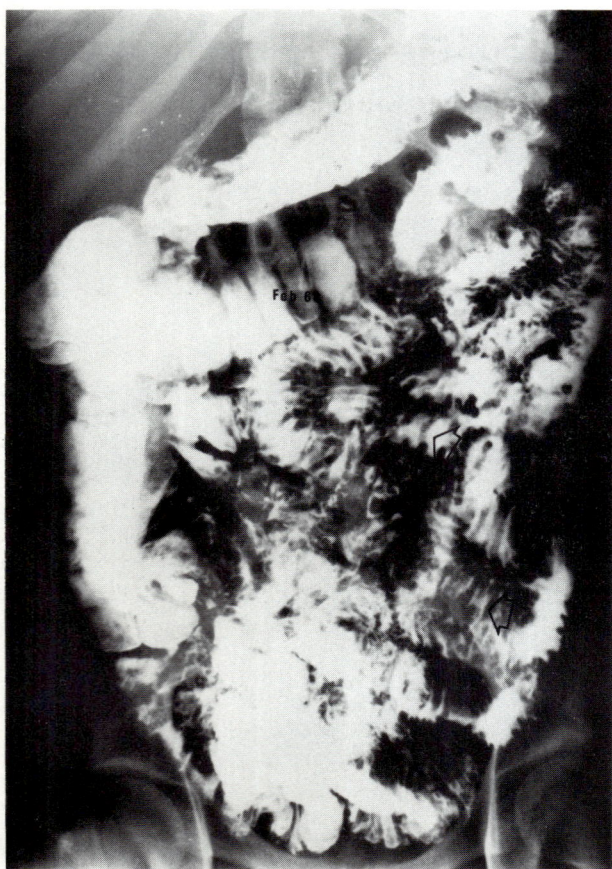

Figure 12–32. Whipple's disease. This adult male presented with crampy abdominal pain; diarrhea; weight loss; steatorrhea; and inguinal, axillary, and cervical adenopathy. PAS-positive macrophages were present in small bowel biopsy tissue. The small bowel folds are thickened and serpiginous (arrows).

AMYLOIDOSIS. The small intestine is often involved by systemic amyloidosis.[23] Patients may have cramping abdominal pain, protein-losing enteropathy, and malabsorption. The bowel is affected in primary amyloidosis when the latter is associated with paraprotein disease, most commonly multiple myeloma. Secondary amyloidosis due to chronic infections or chronic joint and bone disease rarely involves the small bowel.[13] There is perivascular deposition of amyloid accompanied by the eventual narrowing of blood vessels and amyloid deposition in the lamina propria. Gradually, the muscular wall of the bowel may be replaced by amyloid.

The principal radiographic finding in cases of amyloid disease of the small intestine is thickening of the mucosal folds or valvulae conniventes. This thickening is uniform, with no localized nodularity (Fig. 12–33). There is no dilatation of the bowel and no hypersecretion. The distribution is uniform throughout the small intestine, and the ileal mucosal folds may resemble the jejunum—an appearance that has been termed jejunization. This distribution helps to differentiate amyloidosis of the small intestine from Whipple's disease. The absence of secretions and dilatation helps differentiate it from celiac disease. Decreased motor activity occurs in advanced cases secondary to muscle fiber replacement and the involvement of the autonomic innervation.

EOSINOPHILIC GASTROENTERITIS. These patients usually have a history of allergy and present with intermittent nausea, vomiting, and crampy abdominal pain, often connected with specific food intolerances. They may have diarrhea and malabsorption.

Almost all of the patients have eosinophilia. Small bowel biopsy reveals marked infiltration of eosinophils in the lamina propria. The disease affects the stomach and small intestine. In the case of gastric involvement the antrum is usually affected, with resultant thickening and rigidity. Narrowing in the antrum may simulate a carcinoma. A cobblestone appearance, with multiple polypoid defects, may be present. The small bowel changes are mainly due to submucosal edema, which causes widened and blunted mucosal folds or complete fold effacement.[2] Irregular luminal narrowing and spasm may also occur. Radiographically, the disease is occasionally limited to the small intestine, without antral involvement.

CROHN'S DISEASE AND RADIATION ENTERITIS. Both of these conditions can cause malabsorption. Although primarily diseases of the bowel wall, they both may also result in fistulas, lymphatic obstruction, and strictures with blind loops, thus initiating malabsorption in a number of ways. These diseases are discussed in detail elsewhere.

Abnormalities of Lymphatic Obstruction

After the absorption of fatty acids and monoglycerides into the small intestine, mucosal cell re-esterification and the formation of chylomicrons occur. These chylomicrons move from the mucosal cell into the intestinal lymphatic system. Lymphatic obstruction with lipid retention in dilated lymphatics results in steatorrhea. Hypopro-

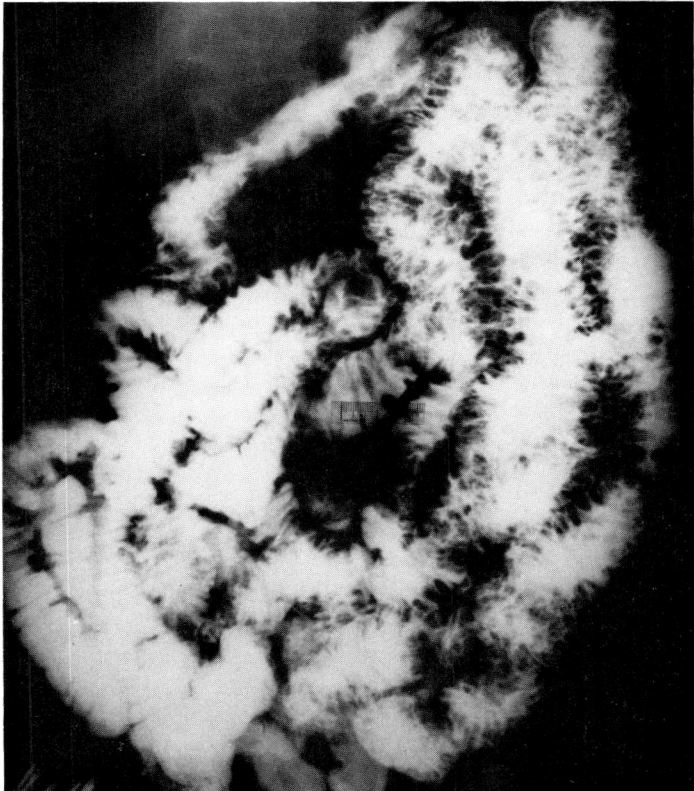

Figure 12–33. Amyloidosis. This film of a patient with multiple myeloma and small bowel amyloidosis shows marked thickening of mucosal folds in the duodenum, jejunum, and ileum. There is no hypersecretion.

teinemia also occurs, as a result of the exudation of protein into the lumen of the intestine through the dilated and engorged lacteals.

CONGENITAL LYMPHANGIECTASIA. Patients with congenital lymphangiectasia acquire edema early in life. Fever, intermittent diarrhea, steatorrhea, and generalized anasarca may be present. The cause of this disorder is unknown, but in patients with a family history of the condition it may represent a congenital malformation of the lymphatic system. The bowel is edematous, and biopsy of the small intestine shows dilatation of the lymphatics in the small intestinal mucosa and submucosa.

Radiographically, there is marked thickening of the mucosal folds. The folds are usually regular without a nodular appearance, but they may be redundant and excessive.[18] There is some hypersecretion but no dilatation of the bowel loops (Fig. 12–34). The hypersecretion helps differentiate lymphangiectasia from the thickened folds of amyloidosis. In lymphangiectasia the fold thickening is usually greater than that seen in other cases of hypoproteinemia, such as cirrhosis or nephrosis.

LYMPHOMA. Lymphoma of the small bowel is described in detail in another section (p. 611). Although localized primary lymphoma and systemic lymphoma with small bowel involvement may occasionally result in malabsorption, patients with primary diffuse intestinal lymphoma have a high incidence of malabsorption. These

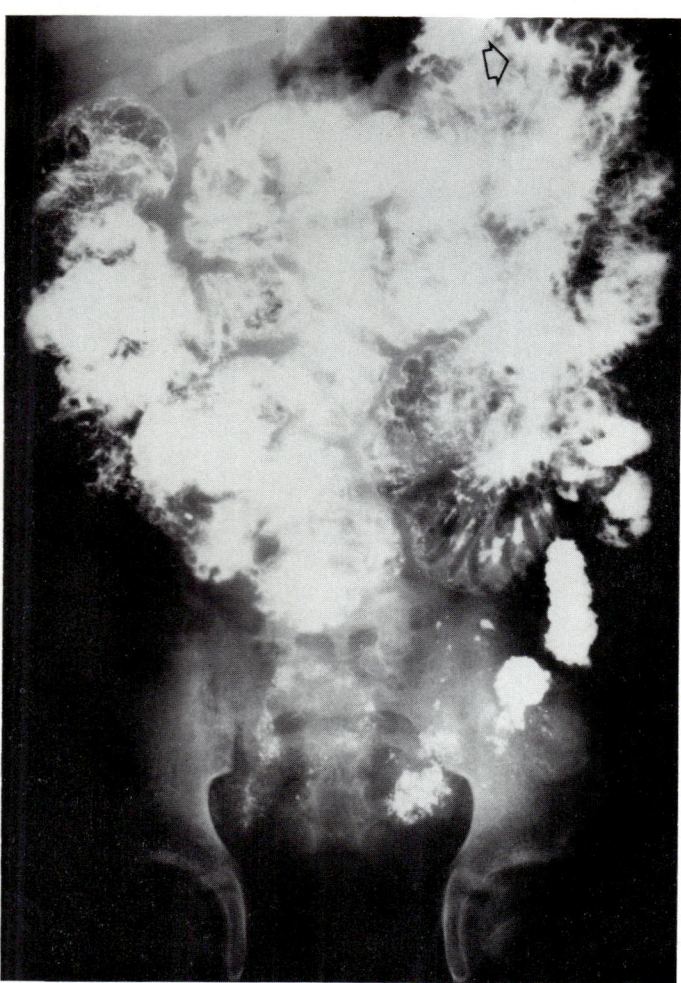

Figure 12–34. Congenital lymphangiectasia. There is dilution of the barium and thickened, nodular small bowel folds (arrow) in this young female.

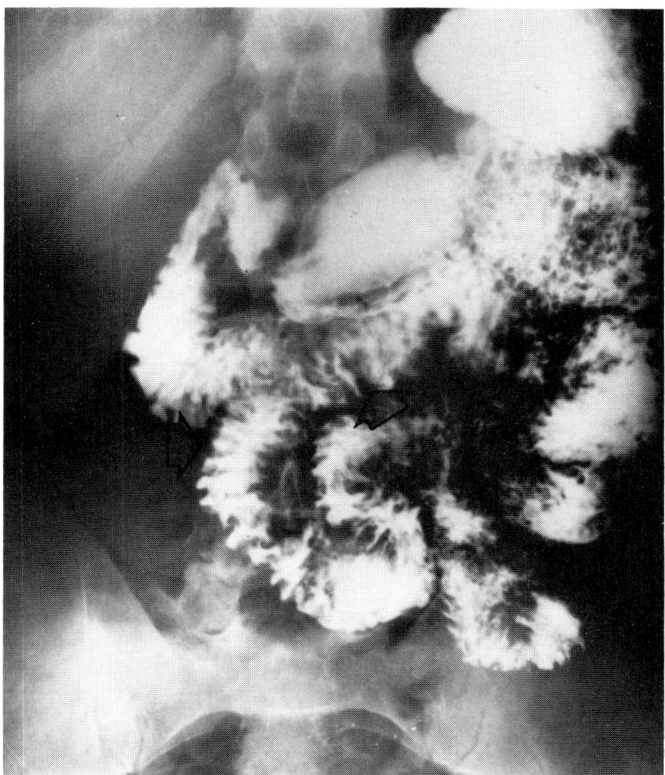

Figure 12–35. A patient with giardiasis and thickened irregular folds (arrows) in the duodenum and proximal jejunum.

patients frequently are adolescents from the Middle East or the Mediterranean basin. They have weight loss, diarrhea, and steatorrhea, but unlike patients with celiac disease they have more abdominal pain and anorexia. Radiologic findings show diffuse coarse, thickened folds, which tend to affect the distal jejunum and ileal segments. Occasionally, small intraluminal masses are seen. Bowel dilatation and hypersecretion may also be present. The distribution in the distal small bowel and the thickened folds help differentiate primary diffuse lymphoma from celiac disease.

OTHER CAUSES OF LYMPHATIC OBSTRUCTION. Desmoplastic changes in the small bowel mesentery from tuberculosis, radiation, or metastatic malignant carcinoid syndrome produce lymphatic obstruction and may cause steatorrhea. Dilated lymphatics in patients with retroperitoneal fibrosis and constructive pericarditis have also been described.

Infections

GIARDIASIS. Patients with *Giardia lamblia* infection are usually asymptomatic. With heavy infestations, diarrhea and steatorrhea may occur. The latter is more common in children and may clinically resemble celiac disease. Patients with hypogammaglobulinemia have an increased incidence of giardiasis. A small bowel biopsy may show acute and chronic inflammatory epithelial changes.

The radiographic features of giardiasis include thickening of the mucosal folds primarily affecting the duodenum and the proximal jejunum (Fig. 12–35). Luminal narrowing may be present, and there is frequently spasm of the affected loops, with rapid transit time through these loops. Increased secretions may occur. When patients have dysgammaglobulinemia, lymphoid hyperplasia may also be seen as multiple small filling defects, primarily in the proximal small bowel[21] but also in the terminal ileum and right colon in some cases.

STRONGYLOIDES STERCORALIS. Patients with Strongyloides infection may be asymptomatic, but diarrhea, nausea, vomiting, and malabsorption can occur. Penetration of the skin by the filiform larvae can result in infection of the lungs with pneumonia and pulmonary edema. Ingested larvae take up residence in the proximal small intestine. Radiographically, as in the case of giardiasis, there are nonspecific inflammatory changes—edema and thickening of the duodenal and proximal jejunal mucosal folds. Severe cases may show ulceration or stricture. In chronic cases, tubelike, rigid jejunal loops are characteristic. Colon ulcerations and mucosal edema indistinguishable from ulcerative colitis may be present on a barium enema examination.[6]

TROPICAL SPRUE. Although its cause has not been identified, tropical sprue is thought to result from an infectious agent because of its epidemic occurrence. Recurring diarrhea and malabsorption lead to steatorrhea, xylose malabsorption, and vitamin B_{12} malabsorption. The radiologic findings are similar to those of nontropical sprue (celiac disease), but the small bowel folds can be thick and edematous in tropical sprue.

References

1. Blau, J. S., Stolzenberg, J., and Toffler, R. B.: Small bowel ulcerations: an unusual complication of celiac disease. J. Can. Assoc. Radiol. 25:77–78, 1974.
2. Burhenne, H. J., and Carbone, J. V.: Eosinophilic gastroenteritis. Am. J. Roentgenol. 96:332–338, 1966.
3. Collins, S. M., Hamilton, J. D., Lewis, T. D., et al.: Small bowel malabsorption and gastrointestinal malignancy. Radiology 126:603–609, 1978.
4. Cueto, J., Urdaneta, L. F., Belin, R. P., et al.: Vitamin B_{12} and iron deficiency after partial gastrectomy. Arch. Surg. 91:995–997, 1965.
5. Deller, D. J., and Begley, M. D.: Bone changes after partial gastrectomy: Calcium metabolism and the bones after partial gastrectomy. I. Clinical features and radiology of the bones. Aust. Ann. Med. 12:282–294, 1963.
6. Drasin, G. F., Moss, J. P., and Cheng, S. H.: Strongyloides stercoralis colitis: findings in four cases. Radiology 126:619–621, 1978.
7. Fikri, E., and Cassella, R. R.: Jejunoileal bypass for massive obesity: results and complications. Ann. Surg. 179:460–464, 1974.
8. Frederick, P. L., Sizer, J. S., and Osborne, M. P.: Relation of massive bowel resection to gastric secretion. N. Engl. J. Med. 222:509, 1965.
9. Gregory, J. G., Starlcoff, E. B., Miyai, K., et al.: Urologic complications of ileal bypass for morbid obesity. J. Urol. 113:521–524, 1975.
10. Hall, G. H., and Neale, G.: Bone rarefaction after partial gastrectomy. Ann. Intern. Med. 59:455–463, 1963.
11. Harris, O. D., Cooke, W. T., Thompson, H., et al.: Malignancy in adult celiac disease and idiopathic steatorrhea. Am. J. Med. 42:899–912, 1967.
12. Hedberg, C. A., Melnyk, C. S., and Johnson, C. F.: Gluten enteropathy appearing after gastric surgery. Gastroenterology 50:796–804, 1966.
13. Herskovic, T., Bartholomew, L. G., and Green, P. A.: Amyloidosis and malabsorption syndrome. Arch. Intern. Med. 114:629–633, 1964.
14. Hines, J. D., Hoffbrand, A. V., and Mollin, D. L.: The hematologic complications following partial gastrectomy. A study of 292 patients. Am. J. Med. 43:555–569, 1967.
15. Kahn, I. J., Jeffries, G. H., and Sleisenger, M. H.: Malabsorption in intestinal scleroderma. N. Engl. J. Med. 274:1339–1344, 1966.
16. Kiefer, E. D.: Postgastrectomy syndrome. Am. J. Gastroenterol. 35:352–360, 1961.
17. Kim, Y. S., Spritz, M., Blum, M., et al.: The role of altered bile acid metabolism in the steatorrhea of experimental blind loop. J. Clin. Invest. 45:956–962, 1966.
18. Marshak, R. H., and Lindner, A. E.: Radiology of the Small Intestine. Philadelphia, W. B. Saunders Company, 1970, p. 13.
19. Moss, A. A.: Postvagotomy unmasking of nontropical sprue. Gastrointest. Radiol. 1:173–175, 1976.
20. Moss, A. A., Goldberg, H. D., and Koehler, R. E.: Radiographic evaluation of complications after jejunoileal bypass surgery. Am. J. Roentgenol. 127:737–741, 1976.

21. Olmstead, W. W., and Reagin, D. E.: Pathophysiology of enlargement of the small bowel fold. Am. J. Roentgenol. *127*:423–428, 1976.
22. Payne, J. H., de Wind, L., Schwab, C. E., et al.: Surgical treatment of morbid obesity: sixteen years of experience. Arch. Surg. *106*:432–437, 1973.
23. Pear, B.: Radiographic studies of amyloidosis. Crit. Rev. Radiol. Sci. *3*:425–452, 1972.
24. Pearson, A. J., Braechwa-Ajdukiewicz, A., and McCarthy, C. F.: Intestinal pseudo-obstruction with bacterial overgrowth in the small intestine. Am J. Dig. Dis. *14*:200–205, 1969.
25. Sleisenger, M. H., and Brandborg, L. L.: Malabsorption. Major Problems of Internal Medicine. Vol. 13. Philadelphia, W. B. Saunders Company, 1977, p. 206.
26. Trier, J. S.: Whipple's disease. *In* Sleisenger, M. H., and Fordtran, J. S. (eds.): Gastrointestinal Diseases. Philadelphia, W. B. Saunders Company, 1973, p. 538.

Part IV

Appendicitis

STEVEN H. OMINSKY, M.D.
ALEXANDER R. MARGULIS, M.D.

Physicians usually make the diagnosis of appendicitis on the basis of the patient's medical history and physical examination. Typically, laboratory and x-ray examinations play a secondary role. Unfortunately, appendicitis frequently has an atypical presentation, especially in young children and in the elderly. When the clinical presentation is confusing, radiology can play an important role not only in suggesting the diagnosis of appendicitis but also in excluding the diagnoses of other conditions. When the appendix is perforated, the radiographic examination is often essential in the preoperative evaluation of the location and extent of the abscess process.

ACUTE APPENDICITIS

Plain Film Examination

The plain films of patients with suspected acute appendicitis should include supine and upright or left lateral decubitus abdominal films as well as an upright chest film. The findings on plain abdominal radiographs are positive in 60 to 70 per cent of cases of acute appendicitis; the incidence of positive findings is 90 to 95 per cent when the appendix is perforated.[13] Although several findings are pathognomonic, other findings indicate only the presence of a nonspecific inflammatory process in the right lower quadrant.

PATHOGNOMONIC FINDINGS

APPENDICOLITH. An appendicolith is a concretion with sufficient calcium to be opaque on the plain film. It is the most important plain film finding. In the presence of appropriate symptoms, an appendicolith is diagnostic of acute appendicitis and should be regarded as an absolute indication for surgical intervention.

Appendicoliths are usually oval or round, with well-defined or laminated margins. Seventy-seven per cent are less than 2 cm in diameter.[5] There may be multiple appendicoliths in some cases; these are usually faceted and linear in configuration. The typical location of an appendicolith is lateral to the right sacroiliac joint and overlying the midportion of the right iliac bone (Fig. 12–36). Because of malrotation or nonrotation of the colon an appendicolith may be in the right upper or left upper quadrant; the diagnosis of appendicolith is still possible, however, if the abnormal location of the cecum is known from a previous barium enema examination.

Appendicoliths may be confused with gallstones, bone islands, mesenteric nodes, or phleboliths on the plain film. Gallstones are usually located in the right upper quadrant and are adjacent to the hepatic flexure, which is usually identified because of the presence of stool or gas. Low-lying gallbladders are usually adjacent to the hepatic flexure rather than to the cecum. A bone island does not shift in position when the upright and supine views are compared. Mesenteric nodes, on the other hand, are unusually mobile, upright views differing greatly from supine views. Mesenteric nodes also have a characteristic punctate, granular calcification and irregular margins. Phleboliths have a typical round, smooth appearance and are fixed in position overlying the lower pelvis. They are usually multiple and bilateral.

In addition to being the most accurate sign of acute appendicitis, appendicoliths are associated with a higher incidence of perforation and gangrene.[10] It is important that the surgeon be aware of the presence of an appendicolith, since if not removed during surgery for perforation, it may act as a nidus for infection or fistula formation.

GAS IN THE APPENDIX. Gas may occasionally be seen in the normal appendix, especially when the appendix is located more cephalad than the cecum, as in the case of malrotation or of retrocecal appendix. In the proper clinical setting, a gas-filled appendix that is distended, or has an air-fluid level on the upright view, or is fixed in position on upright and supine views is almost certainly acutely inflamed. Appendiceal gas is uncommon, occurring in less than 1 per cent of cases of appendicitis. Care must be taken not to confuse an edematous, narrowed, terminal ileal bowel segment with a distended gas-filled appendix.

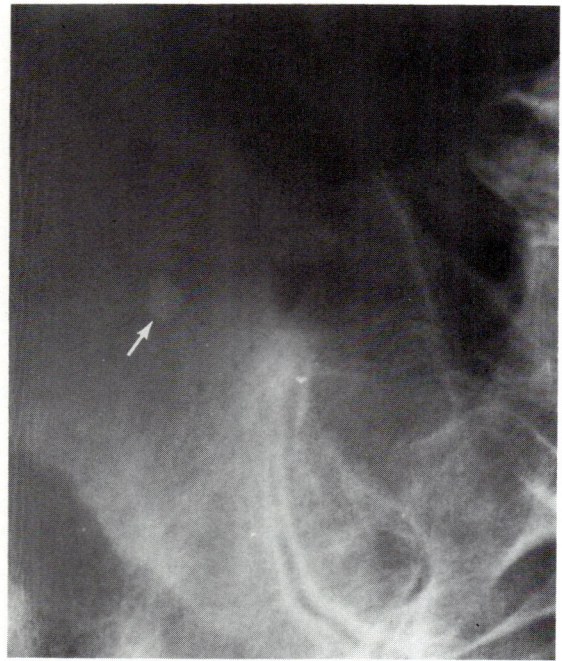

Figure 12–36. Appendicolith (arrow) with a typical oval shape and a laminated margin.

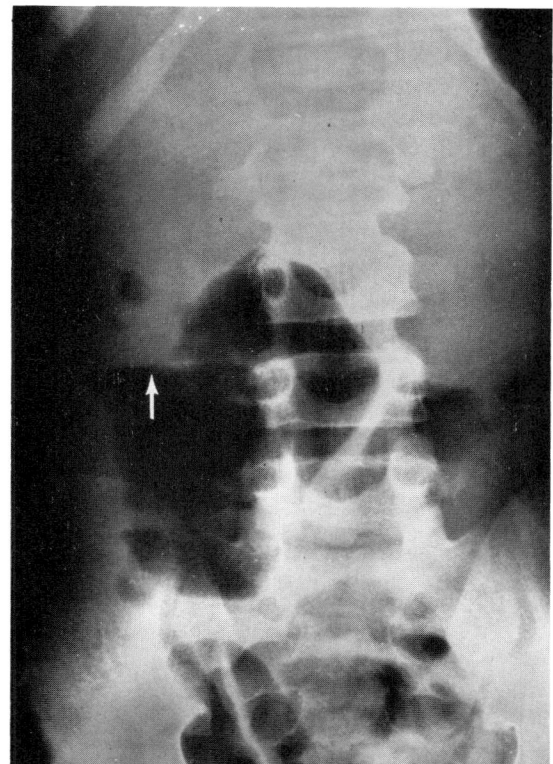

Figure 12–37. Air-fluid level (arrow) in the cecum. Note the medial displacement of the lateral well of the ascending colon in a patient with appendicitis and perforation.

SUGGESTIVE FINDINGS. The following findings are caused by an inflammatory process in the region of the appendix. Although such findings are nonspecific for appendicitis, they do suggest an inflammatory process in the area of the appendix, and in many clinical settings, appendicitis is the most likely diagnosis.

CECUM. The most important finding in the cecum is an air-fluid level confined to the cecum on the upright view (Fig. 12–37) or to the ascending colon on the lateral decubitus view. When fluid levels are distributed throughout the colon or the colon and small intestine, other diagnoses, such as acute gastroenteritis and distal colon obstruction, should be considered. The cecum is frequently dilated and the haustra are thickened secondary to submucosal edema. If the cecum is filled with gas, an inflamed appendiceal mass may produce an extrinsic contour defect at the base of the cecum. If the cecum is dilated and filled with fluid, it simulates a right lower quadrant mass.

TERMINAL ILEUM. An air-fluid level in the terminal ileum, alone or in conjunction with a cecal air-fluid level, is a significant finding. The terminal ileum may be dilated or decreased in caliber because of edematous, thickened walls. When there is a fluid exudate adjacent to an edematous appendix and omentum, an ill-defined increased density is present in the right lower quadrant. The combination of cecal and terminal ileal dilatation, air-fluid levels, and right lower quadrant haze is called appendiceal ileus and is highly suggestive of acute appendicitis.[12]

SUPPORTING SIGNS. The following signs help in diagnosis if found in conjunction with the signs just mentioned.

PSOAS MUSCLE. When the psoas muscle is in contact with an adjacent inflammatory process, contraction secondary to irritation produces lumbar scoliosis (Fig. 12–38). This sign is helpful in diagnosing young adults and especially young children and

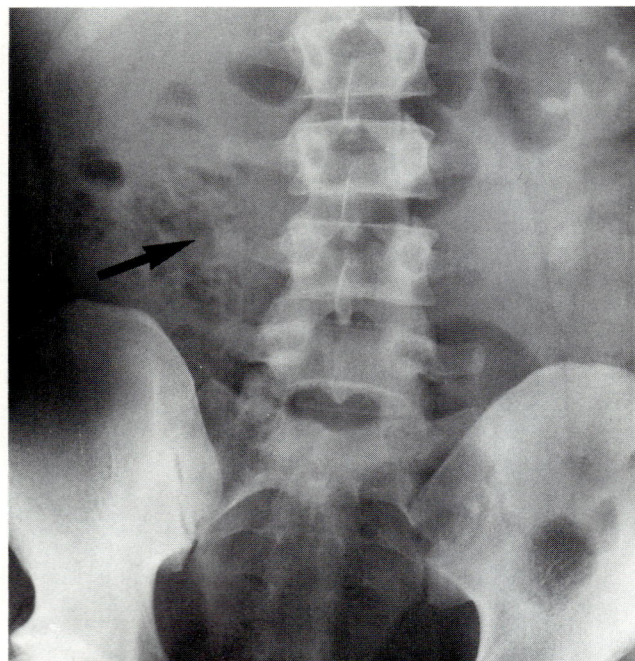

Figure 12–38. Periappendiceal abscess. There is scoliosis, obliteration of the right psoas margin, and a collection of gas bubbles (arrow) above the right iliac crest. (Courtesy of Arthur Gronner, M.D., Oakland, California.)

infants, in whom the examination may be difficult and the history atypical.[14] Edema extending into the fat adjacent to the muscle obliterates the psoas margin on the plain film. Unfortunately, the visualization of psoas muscle margins is variable in normal people and depends on positioning of the patient and the amount of fat adjacent to the psoas muscle. This obliteration is more significant when limited to the lower half of the right psoas muscle.

FLANK STRIPE. The flank stripe is the extraperitoneal fat between the parietal peritoneum and the fascia transversalis. Inflammatory processes adjacent to the lateral peritoneum transude fluid into the extraperitoneal fat, and by changing the fat to fluid density they obliterate the lucent flank stripe. This sign may indicate an inflamed laterally positioned or retrocecal appendix. In infants, the obliteration of the flank stripe is seen in association with a focal thickening of the lateral abdominal wall and is a helpful localizing sign.

Barium Enema

When the clinical signs and the plain films are not diagnostic of appendicitis or when other conditions, such as Crohn's disease, cecal diverticulitis, and cecal carcinoma with perforation, must be ruled out, a barium enema is indicated. This is a safe procedure even in cases of perforation or gangrene, since barium does not usually fill the occluded lumen of the inflamed appendix and the free spilling of barium from a perforated appendix is prevented. If barium does enter a partially occluded appendiceal lumen and then leaves by way of a perforation, the barium is contained by the periappendiceal abscess cavity. Soter has performed barium enemas without complication in more than 800 patients with suspected appendicitis,[11] and Schey has used barium enemas without complication when the diagnosis of appendicitis was difficult

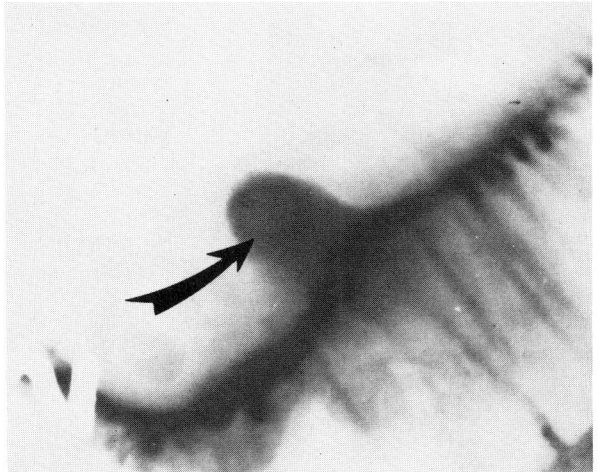

Figure 12–39. Barium enema with indentation of the base of the cecum in a patient with acute appendicitis. Note the appendicolith (arrow).

in children.[9] Since preliminary cleansing preparations are unnecessary, the barium enema can be performed without delay.

CECAL ABNORMALITIES. An extrinsic defect at the base of the cecum is the most important sign of cecal abnormality (Fig. 12–39). The defect is usually located at the medial wall below the ileocecal valve. The preservation of the mucosal folds distinguishes the extrinsic mass from an abnormality of mucosal origin, such as a cecal carcinoma. A characteristic configuration is a biconcave defect, the so-called reverse-3 sign, that is due to a small amount of filling of the proximal portion of the appendix (Fig. 12–40). Extrinsic filling defects may also be seen on the lateral wall of the terminal ileum.

APPENDIX. In addition to a cecal extrinsic mass there is nonfilling of the appendix. (In approximately 15 per cent of cases the normal appendix will not fill with

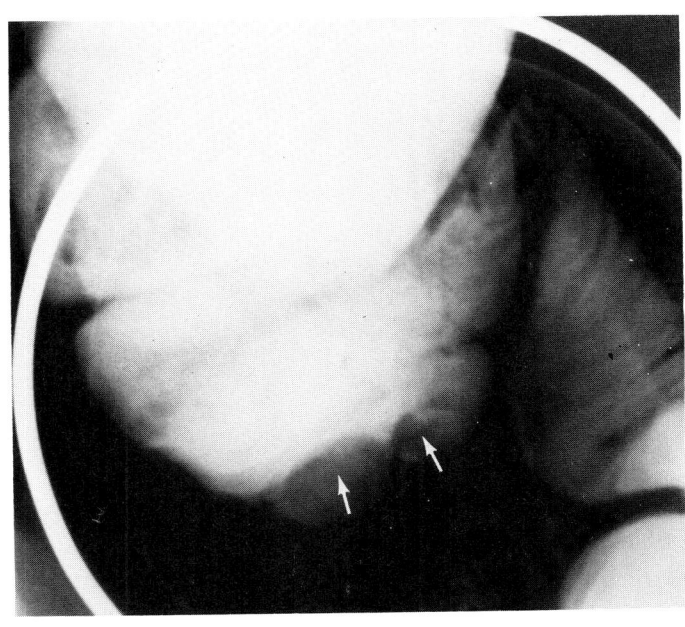

Figure 12–40. Barium enema and biconcave defect (figure 3 sign) on the base of the cecum (arrows) in a patient with acute appendicitis. (*From* Joffe, N.: Radiology of acute appendicitis and its complications. CRC Crit. Rev. Radiol. Nucl. Med. 7:150, 1975. Reproduced by permission.)

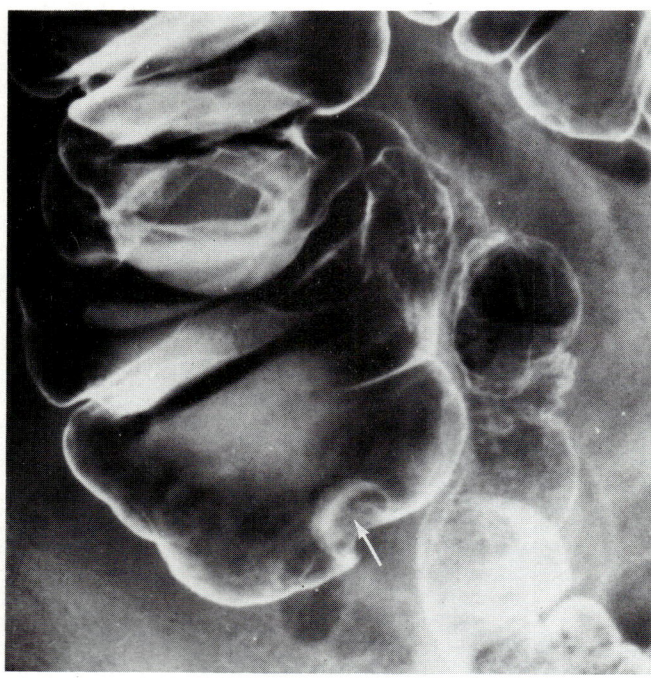

Figure 12–41. Postappendectomy stump defect (arrow) at the base of the cecum. This should not be confused with a tumor.

barium, so that nonfilling of the appendix alone is not diagnostic. Complete filling of the appendix must be obtained, since obstruction and inflammation may be limited to the middle or distal appendix. The distal tip of the appendix should be rounded and slightly bulbous. Any irregular or squared-off configuration of the distal appendix should be considered abnormal. Other diseases and abnormalities, such as an appendiceal carcinoma, intussusception, mucocele, or metastatic implant, may result in nonfilling of the appendix and an extrinsic cecal defect. These abnormalities, however, do not cause inflammatory signs and symptoms clinically. A history of appendectomy explains the nonfilling of the appendix and a cecal defect from an inverted or deformed stump (Fig. 12–41).

COMPLICATIONS OF APPENDICITIS

Although the radiologic findings in cases of acute appendicitis can be significant, the contribution of the radiologist in assessing complications of appendicitis is usually vital. The newer diagnostic imaging modalities, such as gray-scale ultrasonography and computerized tomography, as well as nuclear medicine and standard radiographic techniques, are unquestionably the important preoperative procedures for locating abscesses and fistulas.

Perforation and Pneumoperitoneum

Since perforation of the appendix usually occurs distal to the obstructed lumen, free air is rarely seen under the diaphragm on the erect abdominal view or outlining the liver margin on the decubitus view. It occurs in approximately 1 per cent of cases of appendicitis, and when present, is a small collection. Localized extraluminal gas bubbles may be the result of perforation, but they are usually secondary to the bacterial production of gas and indicate the presence of an abscess. Linear gas in the wall of the cecum in a patient with an appendiceal abscess most likely represents dissection by gas produced by bacteria.[3]

Diffuse Peritonitis

When perforation is not localized to the periappendiceal area, the resulting diffuse peritonitis produces a generalized adynamic ileus. This is seen on the plain film as a dilatation of both the large and the small bowels, with air-fluid levels appearing on the upright or decubitus view. Little change in the configuration of the bowel loops occurs when films are taken at short intervals.[1] If the ileus affects predominantly the large or the small bowel, then the diagnosis of mechanical large or small bowel obstruction may be difficult to exclude. A mechanical small bowel obstruction may also be a complication of perforated appendicitis when an inflammatory mass obstructs a small bowel loop (Fig. 12–42). Mechanical small bowel obstructions usually are the result of adhesions, however, and are most common postoperatively.

Free Fluid

The outporing of exudate associated with peritonitis separates small bowel loops and displaces the ascending colon medially away from the lateral abdominal wall (see

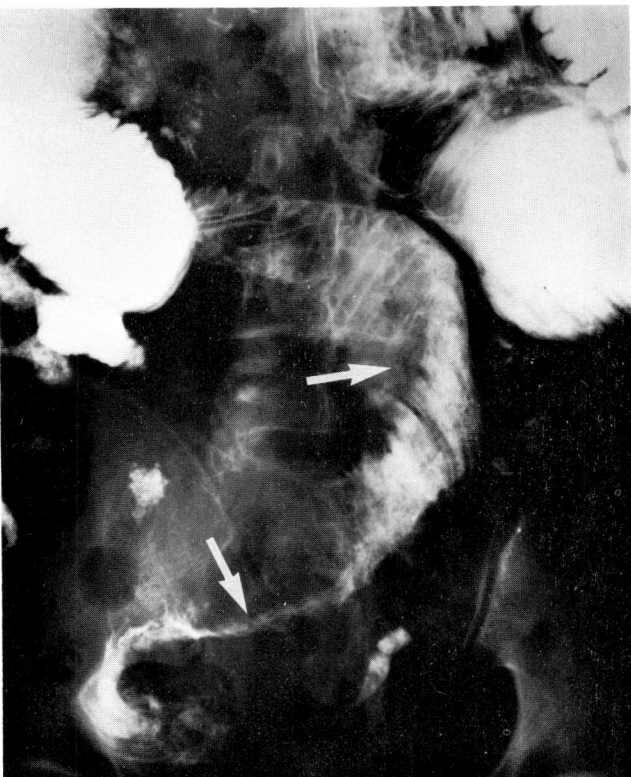

Figure 12–42. Periappendiceal abscess resulting in a small bowel obstruction. A loop of small bowel is draped around a large right lower quadrant mass (arrows).

Fig. 12–37). Fluid tends to gravitate to the pelvis, and a soft tissue mass overlying the pelvis superior to the bladder may be seen on plain films. Ultrasound is very accurate in diagnosing the presence of free intra-abdominal fluid.

Abscess

PERIAPPENDICEAL ABSCESS. When confined to the periappendiceal area, an abscess produces an extrinsic defect on the air- or barium-filled cecum. The defect is larger than the defect seen with simple acute appendicitis. Extrinsic defects of the lateral wall of the terminal ileum and medial displacement of the terminal ileum also occur (Fig. 12–43). Multiple small, lucent gas densities may sometimes be seen in the area of the mass. Barium may enter an abscess cavity (Fig. 12–44), but this is not serious, since the abscess is sealed off from the remainder of the abdomen.

Ultrasound or CT studies usually demonstrate the periappendiceal abscess and its size and extent.

REMOTE ABSCESS. Spread of infection may proceed via gravity to the dependent pelvis. Plain abdominal films may show gas collections, which do not shift position with upright and supine views. In addition, gas may outline the psoas muscle or kidney. A pelvic abscess can result in an extrinsic defect on the right superior portion of the bladder (Fig. 12–45) or may compress the rectum, sigmoid, or pelvic small bowel. In addition to a bladder defect, an intravenous pyelogram may show a partially dilated or medially deviated right ureter.[2] In children, urinary tract symptoms and right-sided hydronephrosis demonstrated by excretory urography may be due to inflammatory obstruction from appendicitis (Fig. 12–46).[8]

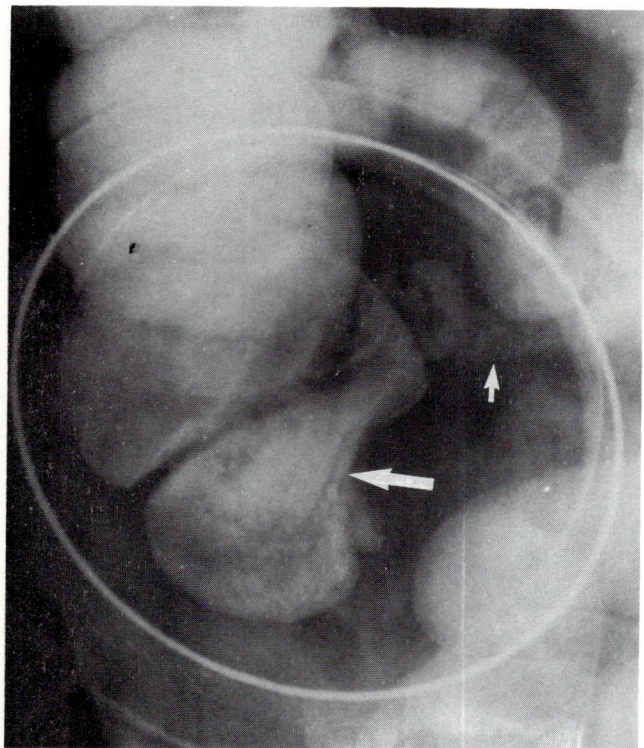

Figure 12–43. Periappendiceal abscess. An inflammatory mass is producing a pressure defect on the cecum (large arrow) and elevating the terminal ileum (small arrow).

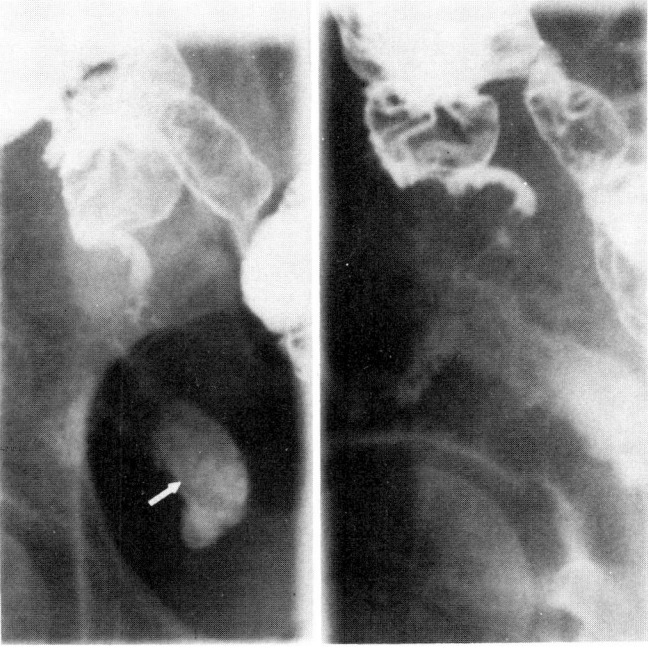

Figure 12–44. Periappendiceal abscess. Barium enema examination in a patient with suspected perforating cecal carcinoma. There is filling of the proximal portion of the appendix with a sharp distal margin and leak of barium in a large abscess cavity (arrow). (*From* Joffe, N.: Radiology of acute appendicitis and its complications. CRC Crit. Rev. Radiol. Nucl. Med. 7:142, 1975. Reproduced by permission.)

Spread may proceed along the right paracolic gutter to the anterior and then posterior subhepatic space and to the right subphrenic space. A subphrenic abscess can produce a right pleural effusion (Fig. 12–47). Subphrenic and subhepatic abscesses are best evaluated by ultrasound (Fig. 12–48). Fluid collections are echo-free and conduct sound well. Abscesses are frequently elliptic in shape and have well-defined margins, although they are less sharp than those of a fluid-filled viscus. In the subhepatic space, care must be taken to identify the gallbladder and not confuse it with a subhepatic

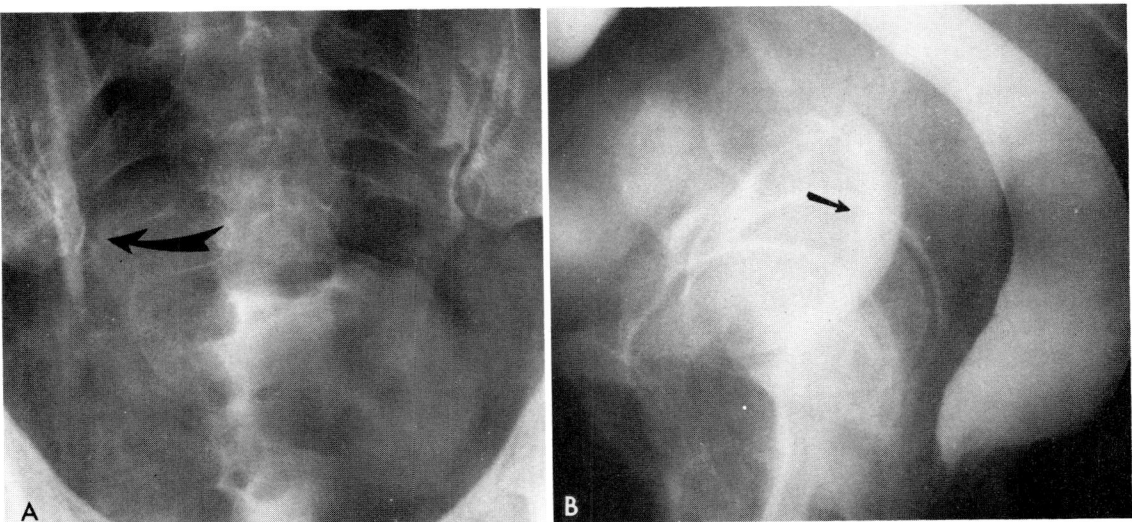

Figure 12–45. Pelvic abscess. Compression on the right side (*A*) and anterior portion of the bladder (arrow, *B*) by a large pelvic abscess secondary to appendiceal perforation. There is also slight dilatation of the right lower ureter (arrow).

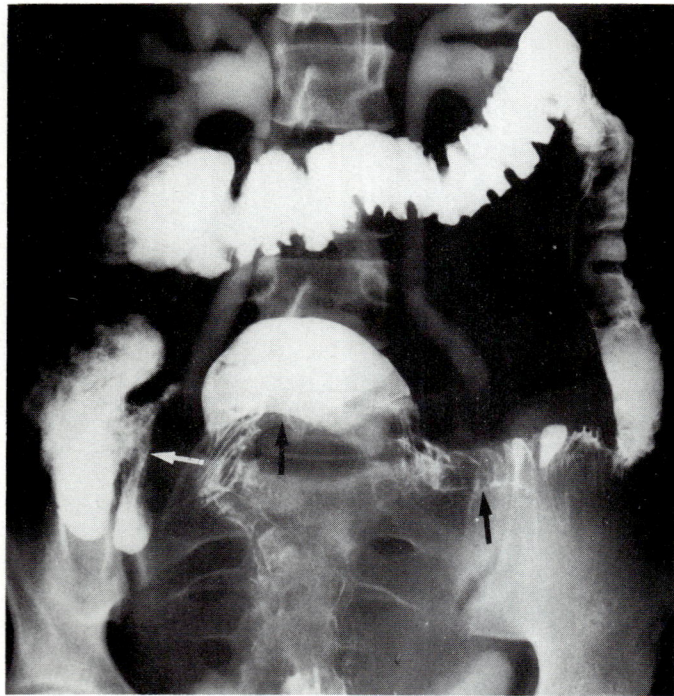

Figure 12–46. Periappendiceal and pelvic abscess in a 15-year-old girl. The large pelvic inflammatory mass is compressing the cecum (white arrow), elevating and compressing the sigmoid (black arrows) and compressing both lower ureters, causing dilatation of both upper urinary tracts.

abscess.[4] The extent of abscess involvement in the retroperitoneum is best evaluated with computerized tomography or ultrasound.

Gallium-67 localizes in inflammatory as well as in tumor tissue. In contrast to tumor scanning, scanning for a site of infection can be performed as easily as six hours after the

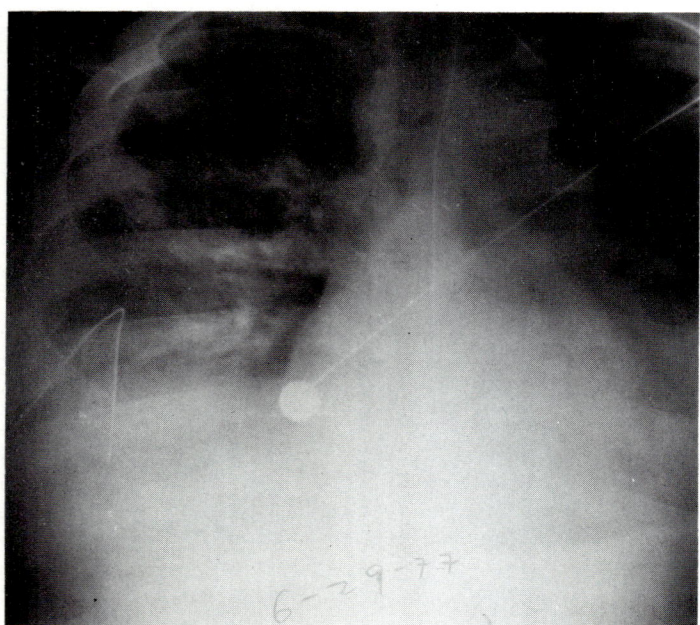

Figure 12–47. Right-sided empyema in a patient with appendiceal perforation and intra-abdominal abscess. (Courtesy of Arthur Gronner, M.D., Oakland, California.)

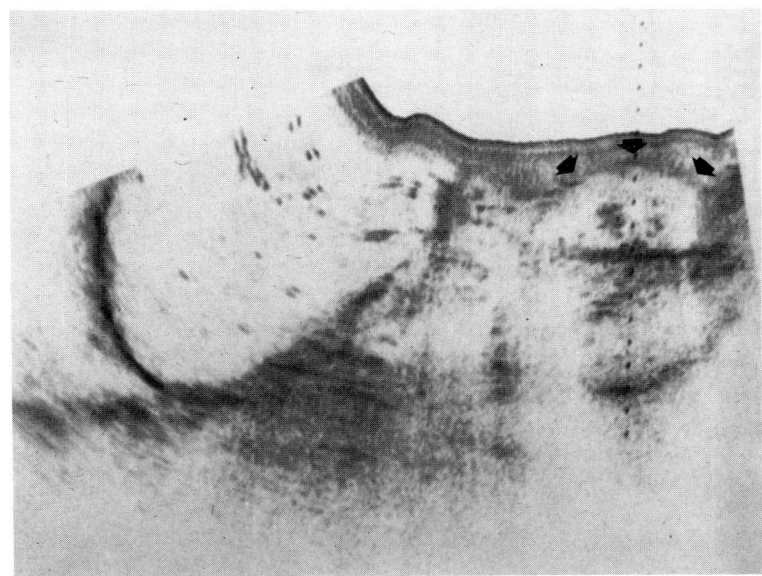

Figure 12–48. Periappendiceal abscess. Sagittal ultrasonal scan showing sonolucent mass (arrows) with central area of echoes.

injection of isotope,[6] although 24-hour scans are preferable. Gallium scanning is useful when a patient presents with a fever of unknown origin resulting from an indolent inflammatory process (Fig. 12–49). It is also useful when multiple abscess sites must be localized prior to surgery.

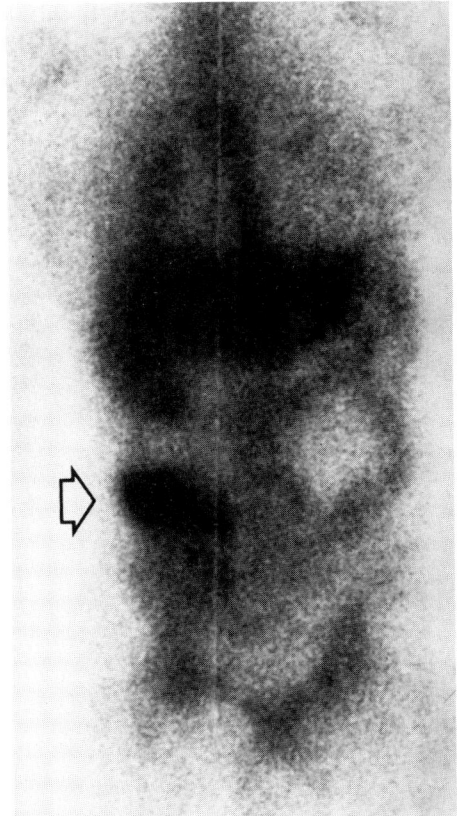

Figure 12–49. Appendiceal abscess: gallium scan. A 24-hour ^{67}gallium scan in an immunosuppressed renal transplant patient with a fever of unknown origin. There is a localized collection of isotope in the right lower quadrant (arrow).

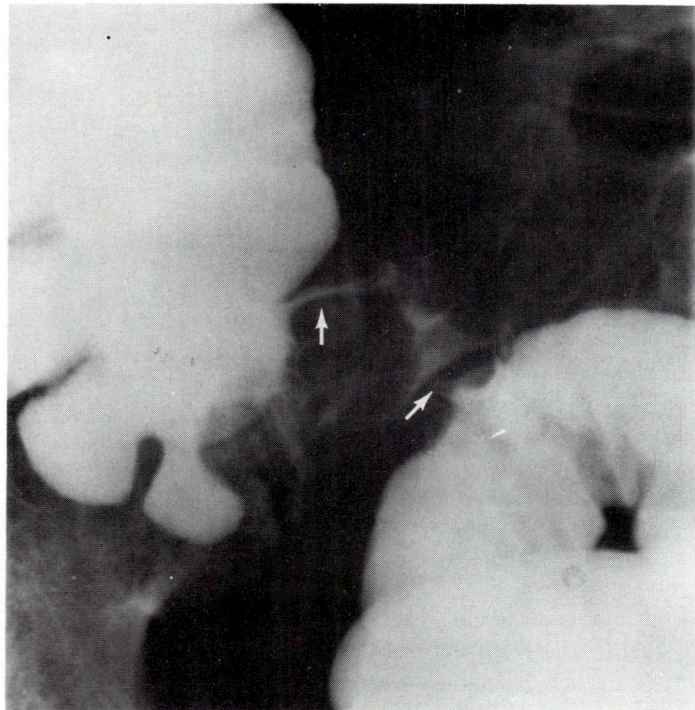

Figure 12–50. Cecal-sigmoid fistula (arrows) in a patient with rectal bleeding. The distal end of the ruptured appendix has embedded in the sigmoid at the site of the fistulous opening. (*From* Joffe, N.: Some unusual roentgenologic findings associated with acute perforative appendicitis. Radiology *110*:301, 1974. Reproduced by permission.)

Figure 12–51. Postoperative bleeding. Barium enema five days after appendectomy in a 15-year-old male with rectal bleeding. Note the narrowing of the cecum and the nodularity of the walls (arrows) secondary to submucosal hemorrhage. A bleeding appendiceal artery was found at surgery.

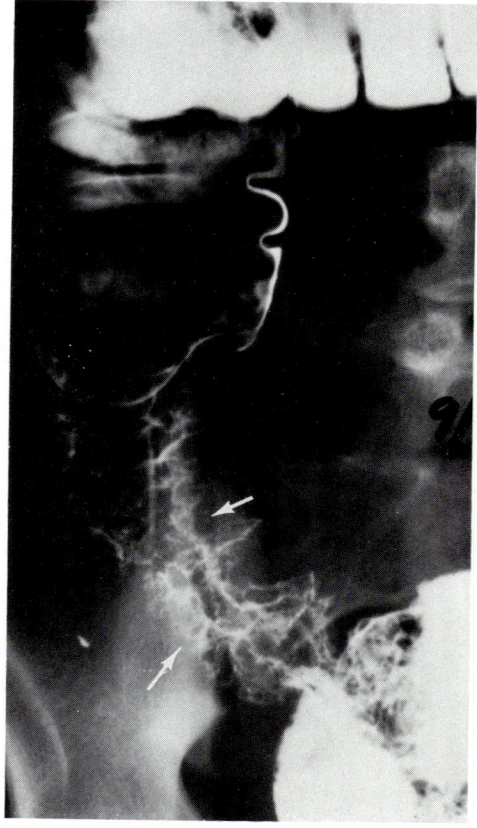

Appendiceal Fistula

Fistulization from the appendix most frequently occurs to the bladder. This is best demonstrated on a barium enema study. The cecum and terminal ileum are the most common bowel sites, but fistulization to the duodenum, jejunum, ascending colon, and sigmoid can occur. Preoperative demonstrations of these fistulas are dependent on barium studies (Fig. 12–50).

Complications of Surgery

Abscesses developing postoperatively produce the same plain film, barium, CT, and ultrasound findings as preoperative appendiceal abscesses. Adhesions following surgery can result in partial or complete small bowel obstruction. Plain films show dilated small bowel loops and little or no gas in the colon. Barium studies show an abrupt change in the caliber of the bowel, with preservation of the mucosal folds. Frequently there is an acute angulation of the bowel at the site of the obstruction.

Postoperative bleeding at the surgical site produces a mass effect and luminal narrowing. A barium enema may show spasm and luminal narrowing at the bleeding site. Nodularity of the cecal bowel wall may occur secondary to submucosal hemorrhage (Fig. 12–51).

References

1. Bryk, D.: Functional evaluation of small bowel obstruction by successive abdominal roentgenograms. Am. J. Roentgenol. 116:262–275, 1972.
2. Chiu, C. L., and Gambach, R. R.: Radiographic ureteral changes with appendicitis. J. Can. Assoc. Radiol. 25:154–160, 1974.
3. DiDonato, L. R.: Pneumatosis coli secondary to acute appendicitis. Radiology 120:90, 1976.
4. Doust, B., and Doust, V.: Ultrasonic diagnosis of abdominal abscesses. Am. J. Dig. Dis. 21:569–576, 1972.
5. Felson, B., and Bernhard, C. M.: Roentgenologic diagnosis of appendiceal calculi. Radiology 49:178–191, 1947.
6. Hopkins, C. B., Kan, M., and Mende, C. W.: Early ^{67}Ga scintography for the localization of abdominal abscesses. J. Nucl. Med. 16:990–992, 1975.
7. Joffe, N.: Radiology of acute appendicitis and its complications. C.R.C. Crit. Rev. Clin. Radiol. Nucl. Med. 7:97–160, 1975.
8. Moncada, R., Raffensberger, J., Wasserman, D., et al.: Hydronephrosis secondary to acute appendicitis in children. Pediatr. Radiol. 2:121–124, 1974.
9. Schey, W. L.: Use of barium in the diagnosis of appendicitis in children. Am. J. Roentgenol. 118:95–103, 1973.
10. Shaw, R. E.: Appendix calculi and acute appendicitis. Br. J. Surg. 52:451–459, 1965.
11. Soter, C. S.: The use of barium in the diagnosis of acute appendicitis, a new radiologic sign. Clin. Radiol. 19:410–415, 1968.
12. Soter, C. S.: The contribution of the radiologist to the diagnosis of acute appendicitis. Semin. Radiol. 8:375–388, 1973.
13. Soteropoulous, C., and Gilmore, J. H.: Roentgen diagnosis of acute appendicitis. Radiology 71:246–256, 1958.
14. Wilkinson, R. H., Bartlett, R. H., and Eraklis, A. J.: Diagnosis of appendicitis in infancy. Am. J. Dis. Child. 118:687–690, 1969.

Part V
Radiation Enteritis

STEVEN H. OMINSKY, M.D.
ALEXANDER R. MARGULIS, M.D.

ACUTE SMALL BOWEL INJURY

Individuals receiving lethal doses of whole-body irradiation rapidly acquire severe diarrhea and intestinal hemorrhage. This is due to the cessation of the production of new cells in the intestinal generative zone within the crypts of the intestinal epithelium[10] and subsequent damage to active transport processes. Following therapeutic irradiation, the basic abnormalities, although the same, are less extensive and are self-limiting. Intestinal epithelium shows decreased mitoses in the intestinal crypt cells and decreased height in crypts and villi. Patients with pelvic irradiation frequently have diarrhea, tenesmus, or constipation at the end of treatment or a few weeks after treatment. These symptoms are usually secondary to acute proctitis, and the mucosa of the rectum appears engorged and edematous and may bleed easily with the manipulation of the proctoscope.[1] A barium enema shows edematous changes in the rectum and sigmoid colon as well as rectal or sigmoid spasm. Occasionally, nausea and vomiting are also associated with the diarrhea of acute irradiation injury. A small bowel series may reveal dilated, atonic small bowel loops.[9] This adynamic ileus responds to conservative therapy.

CHRONIC SMALL BOWEL INJURY

Pathology

Progressive vasculitis, rather than the alteration of the epithelial proliferative kinetics, is the cause of chronic intestinal injury.[2] Endarteritis with luminal narrowing results in progressive tissue hypoxia. Fibrosis with thick strands of hyalinized connective tissue replaces and thickens the muscular and submucosal layers of the affected bowel. Tissue hypoxia can lead to gangrene, perforation, abscess, and peritonitis. If fibrosis predominates, then partial or complete bowel obstruction may result. Patients with pre-existing vascular disease secondary to hypertension or diabetes have an increased risk of experiencing small bowel complications from irradiation.[8] Thin patients and those with previous abdominal surgery resulting in the fixation of small bowel loops in the pelvis also have an increased risk of complications from pelvic irradiation. If a patient scheduled for pelvic irradiation has had previous abdominal surgery and adhesions are suspected, a small bowel study can be extremely helpful in determining whether loops of small bowel are fixed in the pelvis. If fixed loops are demonstrated, the course of therapy can be modified.

At surgery, the walls of the small intestine damaged by irradiation are thickened, stiff, and inelastic.[5] The loops may be matted together. The serosal surface is opaque, white, and indurated. Fibrosis also affects the bowel mesentery, which is shortened and also thicker and stiffer than normal. The mucosa typically shows atrophy or shallow ulceration; rarely, it shows complete denudation.

Radiologic Findings

The radiologic changes in radiation enteritis are a direct result of the pathologic changes. The submucosa is primarily involved, being thickened owing to edema and fibrosis; this results in the marked thickening and straightening of the mucosal folds, as opposed to the serpiginous thickening of mucosal folds secondary to infiltrative lesions, as in Whipple's disease and amyloidosis, which primarily affect the mucosa rather than the submucosa. The bowel contour may have a spiked configuration owing to the compression of the bowel lumen between thickened folds. If the submucosa is greatly thickened, complete effacement of the mucosal folds results (Fig. 12–52). The contour of the bowel may be irregular and may even have a nodular configuration. The thickening of the bowel wall also results in the separation of adjacent small bowel loops. The thickened loops show diminished or absent peristalsis at fluoroscopy. Because of fibrosis and shortening of the small bowel mesentery, sharp angulation of bowel loops may occur (Fig. 12–53). There may be localized tethering of one wall of a bowel loop.

Submucosal thickening can be seen, owing to the infiltration of blood, inflammatory cells, edema, or recurrent tumor. The findings of small bowel submucosal thickening can also be seen in Crohn's disease, bleeding disorders, acute thromboembolic disease, and metastasis. A clinical history is necessary to make a diagnosis of radiation enteritis and to exclude the diagnosis of other diseases with similar radiologic findings. If the bowel has a nodular appearance, the differentiation between recurrent tumor and radiation enteritis can be difficult without biopsy. The use of angiography has been advocated to differentiate radiation change from recurrent tumor when differential diagnosis is impossible with a conventional barium study.[3] In adenocarcinoma, the arteries supplying the tumor may be dilated with large numbers of tiny tumor vessels, whereas in radiation enteritis the lesions are relatively avascular.

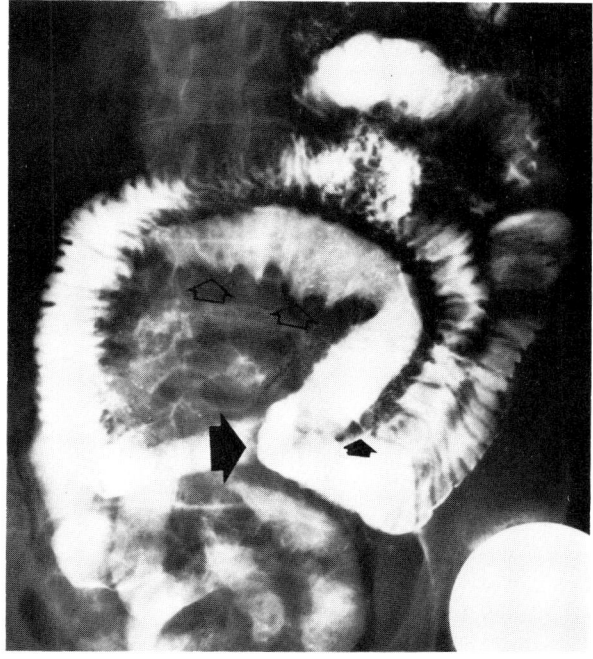

Figure 12–52. Small bowel series in a patient with pelvic irradiation. Note the separation of the bowel loops and the acute angulation of the bowel (large solid arrow). Also note the effacement and irregular contour of the bowel (open arrows). A small fistula is present (small solid arrow).

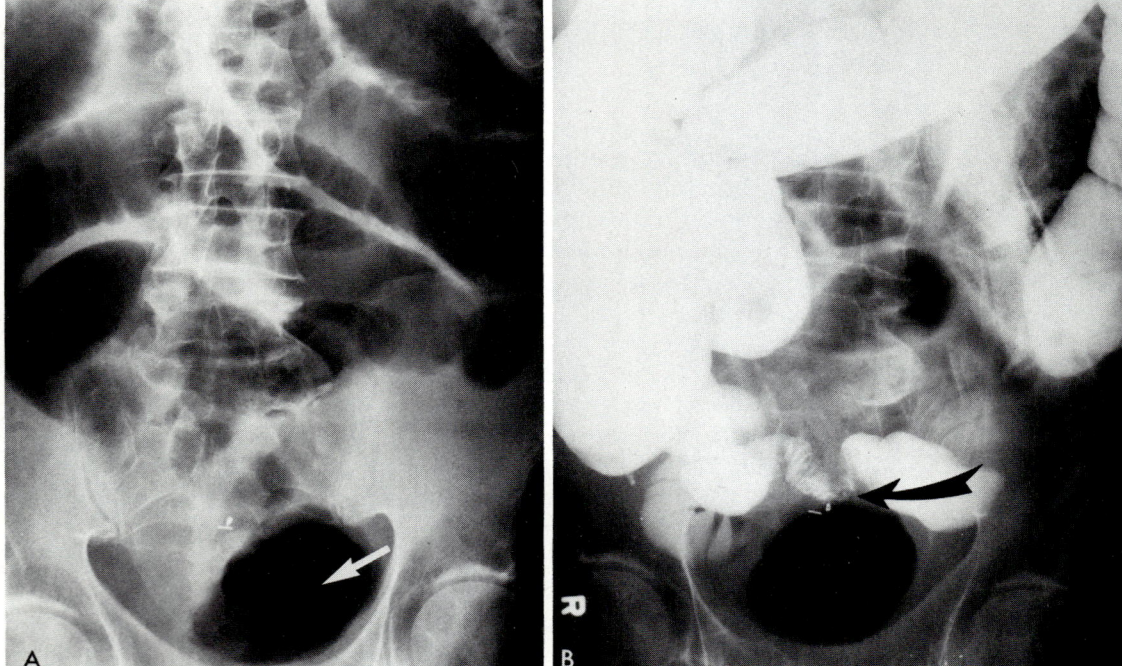

Figure 12–53. Pelvic irradiation and small bowel obstruction (A). There are dilated small bowel loops and air in the bladder (arrow) secondary to an enterovesical fistula. B, Retrograde enema in the same patient via a descending colon colostomy. The ileal folds are thickened and angulated at the site of partial obstruction (arrow), and a small amount of barium has passed to the dilated small bowel just proximal to the obstructed site.

COMPLICATIONS OF CHRONIC SMALL BOWEL RADIATION INJURY

Stricture and Obstruction

When progressive fibrosis narrows the intestinal lumen, partial or complete small bowel obstruction occurs, with dilatation of the small bowel loops and small bowel air-fluid levels appearing on the plain films (see Fig. 12–53A). Low small bowel obstructions can be delineated with a barium enema (see Fig. 12–53B) and high strictures with a barium small bowel series. Strictures are usually short, measuring from 0.5 to 4 cm in length, and they may be multiple.[7] A smooth, tapering configuration is more common than nodular, irregular narrowing. When adhesions are present from previous surgery the combination of an adhesion with a partially narrowed lumen secondary to fibrosis may result in complete small bowel obstruction.

Ulceration and Hemorrhage

Although superficial ulcerations are found on gross inspection of irradiated small bowel, ulcers large enough to be seen on a small bowel series are rare. Deep ulcer tracts seen on a small bowel series have been described and are thought to be secondary to incipient fistulas.[6] Mesenteric angiography may show the site or sites of hemorrhage when acute bleeding occurs.

Fistulas

Small intestinal fistulas secondary to irradiation are a grave complication with a high mortality rate.[5] Barium studies can demonstrate the fistulas when the bowel loops are separated, as is frequently the case. Adhesions and fibrosis of the mesentery may result in matting together of the small bowel loops, however. Individual loops of bowel may not be recognized, and fistulas in these loops as well as other irradiation changes may be missed. Fistulas to the bladder due to pelvic irradiation are not uncommon and result in pneumaturia. Plain films reveal air in the bladder (see Fig. 12–53A).

Perforation and Abscess

Ischemia from radiation endarteritis can lead to gangrene, perforation, and abscess formation. Free air in the abdomen can be demonstrated under the hemidiaphragms on the upright chest film or adjacent to the lateral aspect of the liver on the left-side-down lateral decubitus view of the abdomen. When free air is present, water-soluble contrast agents may be useful in locating the site of perforation. Abscesses displace bowel loops on the plain film or the barium study. Collections of bubbles without a bowel configuration localized to an area of the abdomen should also raise the suspicion of an abscess. Computed tomography and ultrasound are excellent methods for locating and evaluating abdominal abscesses.

Anastomosis Breakdown

The extent of vascular compromise in the small intestine may be difficult to detect at surgery, and for this reason bypass surgery is advocated rather than local excision and anastomosis. Irradiated tissue heals poorly. Primary resection and anastomosis of small intestine has an increased risk of leakage and sepsis. Ileus or mechanical obstruction secondary to abscess formation results in dilated bowel on the postoperative plain film. Water-soluble contrast may be helpful in documenting the breakdown of an anastomosis but is usually not necessary.

Malabsorption

Patients with extensive small bowel changes, especially of the ileum, may present with steatorrhea, decreased calcium levels, and tetany as well as abnormalities due to B_{12} avitaminosis.[12] Differentiation must be made from sprue, which produces dilatation of the bowel and increased secretions but no submucosal abnormalities. Malabsorption may also be secondary to progressive bowel resections, leading to a short bowel syndrome. Blind loop syndrome or stricture formation may also be the cause of malabsorption.

GASTROINTESTINAL TRACT CHANGES

Esophagus

Radiation changes in the esophagus can result in altered esophageal motility. Primary peristaltic waves seen with a barium study may be interrupted at the site of

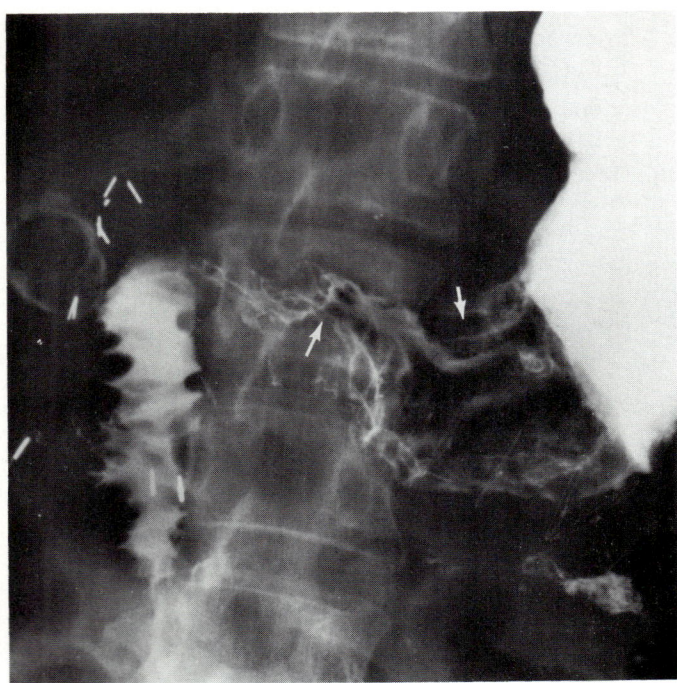

Figure 12–54. Postirradiation gastritis and duodenitis. Upper gastrointestinal series in a patient with irradiation to the head of the pancreas. Gastric folds and duodenal folds are thickened, and there is narrowing of the antrum (arrows). Gastric involvement is sharply limited to the irradiated lower third of the stomach.

irradiation, with nonperistaltic tertiary contractions continuing distally from the site of irradiation.[4] Esophageal stricture with smooth, tapering margins and no localized irregularity and, less commonly, frank ulceration at the site of irradiation can also occur.

Stomach

Radiation to the stomach can result in ulcers that are radiologically indistinguishable from typical benign gastric ulcers. Unlike typical ulcer patients, patients with radiation ulcers have unrelenting pain, unrelievable by antacids. These ulcers heal slowly, if at all. Reduced motility and emptying as well as spasm may be seen in the irradiated stomach,[11] and there may be fixed narrowing of the pyloroantral region of the stomach. Marked prominence of the mucosal folds (Fig. 12–54) is frequently seen, and superficial mucosal ulcerations or effacement of the mucosa have also been described.[11]

Colon

The changes in the colon are similar to those in the small intestine. Submucosal disease results in thickened folds and spasm (Fig. 12–55). Stenoses and strictures are usually smooth and tapering (Fig. 12–56), but occasionally the underlying fibrosis has an irregular component, and narrowing may be irregular on the barium enema examination. This is more common in the anterior rectal wall, and biopsy may be necessary to

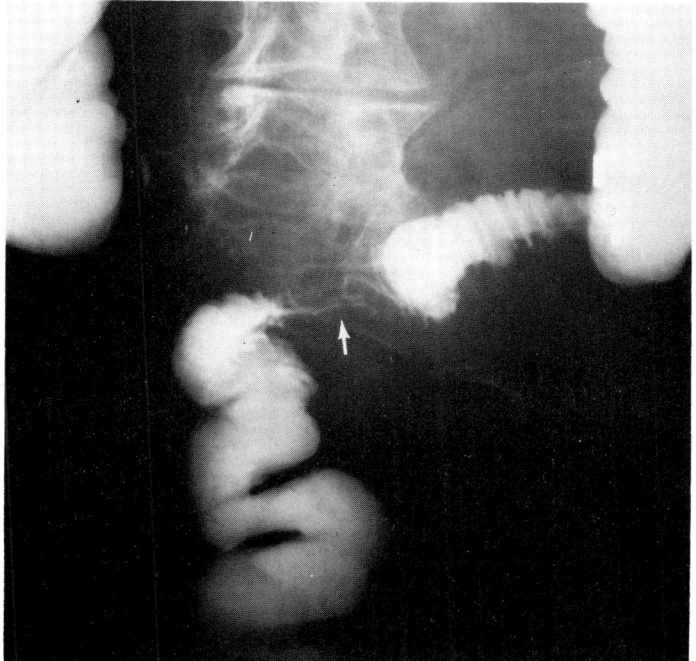

Figure 12–55. Postirradiation sigmoiditis. Barium enema in a patient with pelvic irradiation. Note the thickened rectosigmoid mucosa and associated sigmoid spasm (arrow).

rule out the possibility of recurrent tumor. Ulceration can also occur, and the anterior rectal wall is a common site. Breakdown and fistula from the anterior rectal wall can result in a rectovaginal fistula, which is best demonstrated in the lateral rectal view during the barium enema examination.

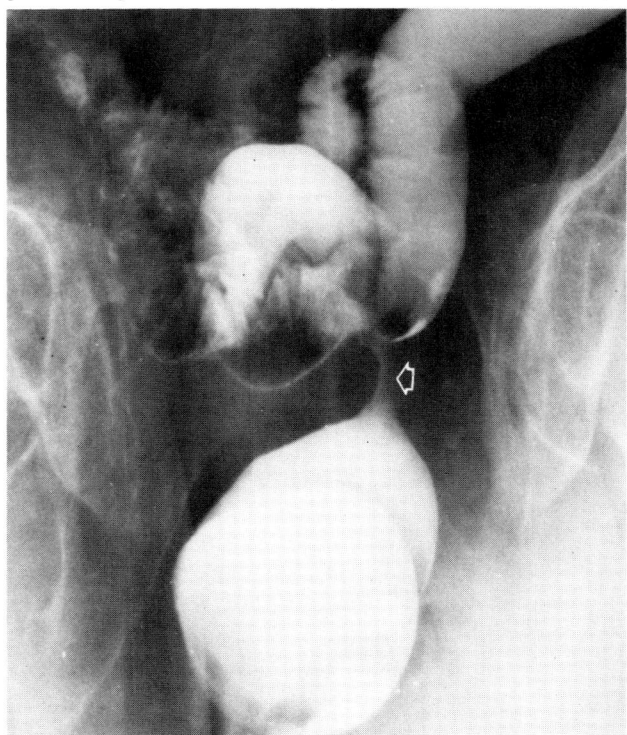

Figure 12–56. Postirradiation stricture. Barium enema examination in a patient with irradiation for cancer of the cervix. There is a rectosigmoid stricture with a smooth, gradually tapering configuration (arrow).

References

1. Ashbaugh, D. G., and Owens, J. C.: Intestinal complications following irradiation for gynecologic cancer. Arch. Surg. *87*:100–107, 1963.
2. De Cosse, J. J.: Radiation injury to the intestinal tract. *In* Sabiston, D. C., Jr. (ed.): Davis-Christopher Textbook of Surgery. Ed. 11. Philadelphia, W. B. Saunders Company, 1977, p. 1060.
3. Dencker, H., Holmdahl, K. H., Lunderquist, A., et al.: Mesenteric angiography in patients with radiation therapy to the bowel after pelvic irradiation. Am. J. Radiol. *114*:476–481, 1972.
4. Goldstein, H. M., Rogers, L. F., Fletcher, G. H., et al.: Radiological manifestations of radiation-induced injury to the normal upper gastrointestinal tract. Radiology *117*:135–140, 1975.
5. Graham, J. B., and Villalba, R. J.: Damage to the small intestine by radiotherapy. Surg. Gynecol. Obstet. *116*:665–668, 1963.
6. Halls, J. M.: Radiation damage to the small intestine. Clin. Radiol. *16*:173–176, 1965.
7. Joelsson, I., Räf, L., and Söderberg, G.: Stenosis of the small bowel as a complication in radiation therapy of carcinoma of the uterine cervix. Acta Radiol. *10*:593–603, 1971.
8. Maruyama, Y., Van Nagell, J. R., Jr., Utley, J., et al.: Radiation and small bowel complications in cervical carcinoma therapy. Radiology *112*:699–703, 1974.
9. Mason, G. R., Dietrich, P., Friedland, G. W., et al.: The radiological findings in radiation-induced enteritis and colitis: a review of 30 cases. Clin. Radiol. *21*:232–247, 1970.
10. Quastler, H.: The nature of intestinal radiation death. Radiat. Res. *4*:303–320, 1956.
11. Roswit, B., Malsky, S. J., and Reid, C. B.: Severe radiation injuries of the stomach, small intestine, colon and rectum. Am. J. Roentgenol. *114*:460–475, 1972.
12. Wellwood, J. M., and Jackson, B. T.: The intestinal complications of radiotherapy. Br. J. Surg. *60*:814–818, 1973.

Part VI

Tumors

H. C. CARLSON, M.D.

INTRODUCTION

(See also Chapter 11, The Duodenum)

The incidence of neoplasms in the small intestine is relatively low compared with other portions of the gastrointestinal tract, such as the stomach and colon. Neoplasms of the small intestine constitute only about 2 per cent of all gastrointestinal neoplasms (and are frequently an unexpected surgical or autopsy finding). Nevertheless, if the radiologic examination is undertaken with interest, effort, and discipline, small bowel tumors will be detected more frequently.[3, 5, 6, 15, 20]

INCIDENCE

If all neoplasms of the small intestine are considered, there are about an equal number of benign and malignant lesions. About two thirds of benign lesions are found at autopsy and one third at surgery; the reverse is true of malignant lesions. If carcinoid tumors are excluded, almost 90 per cent of malignant tumors of the small intestine are found at surgery. This undoubtedly reflects the high incidence of obstruction and hemorrhage associated with these lesions, which often leads to surgical exploration of the abdomen. Of all tumors found in the small intestine at the time of operation, about two thirds are malignant.[5, 13]

INVESTIGATIVE MODALITIES

Contrast Examination

A moderate number of patients with small bowel neoplasms present with high-grade and even complete obstruction of the small intestine. In these cases, only plain abdominal films are necessary or desirable to make the diagnosis. Contrast examination will only delay the inevitable surgical management of the lesion. However, most lesions do not present in this dramatic way, and contrast examination of the small bowel should be made, using a nonflocculating barium suspension. Soluble contrast medium should almost never be used, since it is extremely hypertonic and becomes so dilute that it allows only the distinction between complete and incomplete obstruction.

After at least 12 ounces of barium suspension have been ingested, a substantial portion of duodenum and jejunum should be opacified and examined fluoroscopically and with palpation. Then the patient can be given an additional 6 ounces of barium, returning in about 15 minutes for further examination. Thereafter, 20 to 30 minutes may elapse between films and fluoroscopy until the entire small intestine and the cecum have been thoroughly opacified and studied. Spot films can be exposed to record abnormalities. Careful fluoroscopy is paramount for the successful examination of the small intestine.

Angiography

Selective arteriography is most useful when the patient is actively bleeding and after a gastric or esophageal source is excluded by prompt endoscopy. Extravasation of contrast medium into the lumen of the small intestine during angiography constitutes irrefutable evidence of the site of hemorrhage. However, the examination often does not delineate the nature of the lesion. Nevertheless, the site of bleeding and the identification of the artery supplying the bleeding site are critical information, especially if surgical management must be undertaken. The selective catheter can be used to administer vasopressive substances or even embolic material in order to control a hemorrhage. Vasopressive substances can also be administered systemically, and re-examination through the selective catheter can be carried out in order to determine whether the hemorrhage has been controlled.

Angiography can be used in patients with chronic gastrointestinal blood loss, in whom conventional studies have not revealed any pathologic abnormality. This is particularly true in vascular malformations of the small intestine and in smooth muscle tumors of the small intestine. Approximately two thirds of the lesions are largely extraluminal and do not produce luminal abnormalities on barium examination.[22]

Computerized Tomography and Ultrasound

Currently, the usefulness of these modalities in the detection and identification of small bowel neoplasms seems quite limited. At present, their chief value is in the detection of associated mesenteric and retroperitoneal lymph node metastases. These studies can also determine whether palpable abdominal masses are cystic, solid, or vascular.

SYMPTOMS AND SIGNS

Only about one fifth of all patients with benign neoplasms of the small intestine develop clinical manifestations, whereas about 90 per cent of patients with malignant lesions have related symptoms and signs.

In the case of benign lesions, the usual symptoms are pain, melena, and weakness. The most common signs are weight loss, anemia, and the presence of a palpable abdominal mass. Pain is usually caused by obstruction of the small intestine, which is almost always due to intussusception. Obstruction directly caused by a benign mass in or adjacent to the small intestinal lumen, without intussusception, is extremely uncommon. Intussusception is usually transient and is one of the major roentgenologic signs that allow the detection of an intraluminal pedunculated mass which otherwise may elude visualization. Anemia and melena are usually associated with ulceration, which, however, is uncommon in benign lesions.

Malignant small intestinal neoplasms tend to cause obstruction by infiltration of the entire circumference of the bowel wall. Pain is usually due to obstruction but may also be caused by nerve invasion. A pedunculated intraluminal malignant mass can also result in intussusception. Malignant lesions very frequently undergo necrosis and ulceration and consequently are often associated with hemorrhage and weight loss.

A palpable mass may occur in either benign or malignant lesions. In benign lesions it is usually due to a large tumor mass but occasionally results from a relatively fixed segment of intussusception. In malignant tumors, the mass may represent either the tumor itself or metastases to mesenteric or retroperitoneal nodes.[3, 5, 13]

ROENTGENOLOGIC SIGNS

The plain film of the abdomen is usually negative but may reveal small intestinal obstruction or evidence of bowel perforation. Barium study of the small intestine is far more informative. During the examination, there may be mild and often transient dilatation of a segment of small intestine associated with an adjacent area of narrowing. Marked narrowing readily detects and localizes the lesion, but if the narrowing is slight, even mildly distended, barium-filled bowel proximal to the narrowing is significant.

The presence of intussusception, which is usually transient, is also a convincing sign in the adult of possible intraluminal lead mass. If the transient intussusception is already established, the barium will disclose only slight dilatation proximal to a marked narrowing of the lumen and elongated linear mucosal patterns through the intussuscepted segment. If the intussusception occurs after barium coating of the segment, the invaginated portion with all of its reflections will be visible as the characteristic "packed coil-spring" appearance. Only after the intussusception has reduced itself can the presence or absence of an intraluminal mass be determined.[4]

Lack of mobility and pliability of segments of the small intestine is an important sign of involvement with a disease process. This can be most efficiently and convincingly demonstrated by fluoroscopy and by vigorous palpation of the intestinal loops. Fixation of a loop with respect to other intra-abdominal organs and rigidity of segments of the small intestine are most important in recognizing segments of diseased bowel. Increased focal thickness of small intestinal folds is another very important sign of neoplasm. Even more significant is localized absence of normal mucosal pattern, usually indicating an area of necrosis and ulceration. These changes are almost always accompanied by some rigidity of the segment.

PATHOLOGIC TYPES

Leiomyoma and Leiomyosarcoma

INCIDENCE AND DISTRIBUTION. Leiomyoma is by far the most common benign tumor of the small intestine, constituting about one third of all such lesions. About one half are found at operation and one half at autopsy. Leiomyosarcomas are much less common, only about one sixth of smooth muscle tumors being malignant.

Both the benign and the malignant forms occur considerably more frequently in the duodenum than in the jejunum and ileum.[5, 13, 22]

GROSS PATHOLOGY. Leiomyomas and sarcomas arise from the smooth muscle elements of the bowel wall and form rather cellular masses that most commonly have a spherical form. Lobulation is frequent, and some tumors even have a flat or spiral configuration.

The size of these neoplasms varies greatly, with a medium diameter of about 5 cm. Only about one of five projects chiefly into the lumen, and rarely may develop a pedicle. Discovery of smooth muscle tumors by barium examination is often difficult, especially when the masses project mainly from the serosal surface and do not deform the intestinal lumen.

The surface of the tumor is often highly vascular and may bleed massively if mucosal ulceration occurs. Necrosis is rather common in the large growths. This necrotic material may liquefy and empty into the intestinal lumen through a rather small mucosal ulceration, resulting in a gas- and fluid-filled cavity.[22, 25]

SYMPTOMS AND SIGNS. Clinical manifestations occur in only about one fourth of cases of benign smooth muscle tumors, the rest being discovered at autopsy or incidentally at the time of surgery. Almost all malignant smooth muscle tumors develop symptoms and signs.

About one half of symptomatic patients with leiomyoma have pain, probably due to intermittent partial obstruction or to tumor necrosis. About one half have intermittent, often massive, hemorrhage, and about one fifth have a palpable mass.

In patients with leiomyosarcoma, blood loss, pain, and palpable mass alone or in combination occur in about two thirds of cases. Obstruction is relatively uncommon, occurring in only about one fourth of cases. About half of these are due to intussusception.

X-RAY AND BARIUM STUDIES. If the tumor mass is pedunculated, it may be seen directly as a round filling defect within the lumen, or it may cause intussusception. A mass with a demonstrable deep, pitlike ulcer crater is highly suggestive of smooth muscle tumor. The same is true if a relatively large cavity communicating with the intestinal lumen can be demonstrated. However, sarcomatous lesions of non-smooth muscle character can produce a similar picture, and not all leiomyosarcomas ulcerate. Distinction between benign and malignant smooth muscle neoplasms by roentgenographic means is usually impossible (Figs. 12–57 to 12–60).[1, 5, 13]

ANGIOGRAPHY. Because of their high degree of vascularity, smooth muscle tumors can be readily demonstrated in the small vessel phase during angiography. If the mass is homogeneously vascular and is spherical or lobulated, a histologic diagnosis can be strongly suggested (Fig. 12–61). This is particularly true if there is also a history of unexplained, intermittent interstitial hemorrhage and normal barium examinations. The presence of malignancy cannot be excluded, however.

If the lesion is actively bleeding, extravasation of contrast agent into the interstitial lumen further documents the source of hemorrhage.[2, 10, 18, 26]

600 — THE SMALL INTESTINE

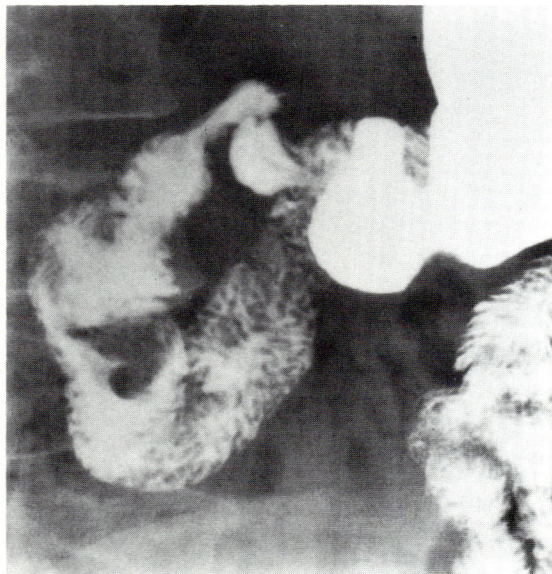

Figure 12–57. Lobulated, localized leiomyosarcoma on a broad pedicle in the second portion of the duodenum.

Figure 12–58. Leiomyosarcoma in the jejunum. The patient is a 58-year-old male with a mostly exophytic, lobulated, cavitating (arrows) tumor. One lobule of the mass fixes and deforms the bowel just caudal to the cavity.

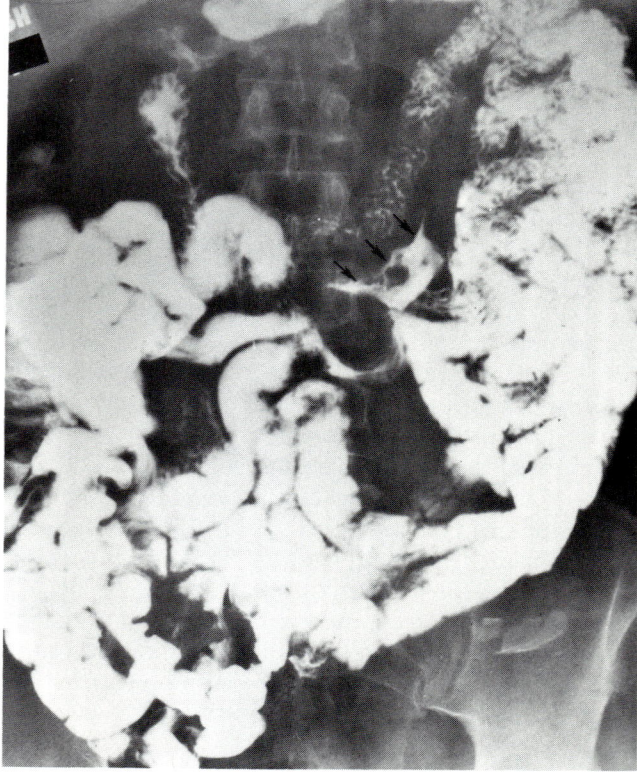

THE SMALL INTESTINE — 601

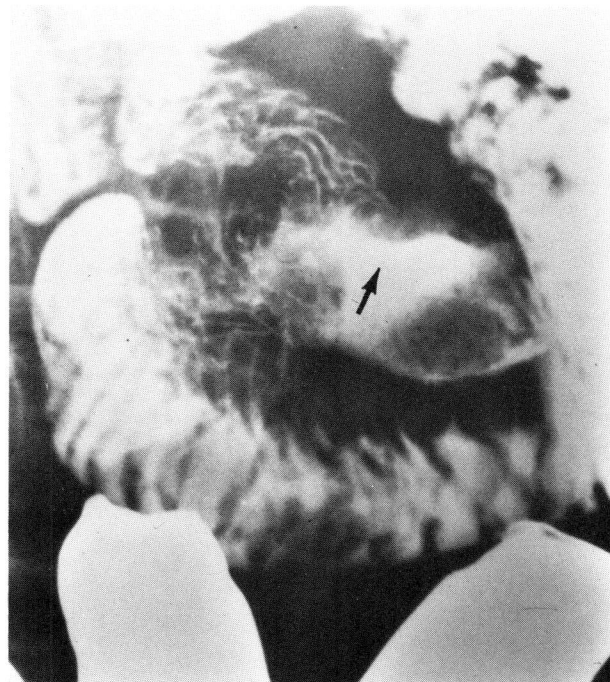

Figure 12–59. Cavitating leiomyosarcoma communicating with the jejunal lumen. The barium collection (arrow) is within the cavitating lesion. The solid portions are producing the filling defects.

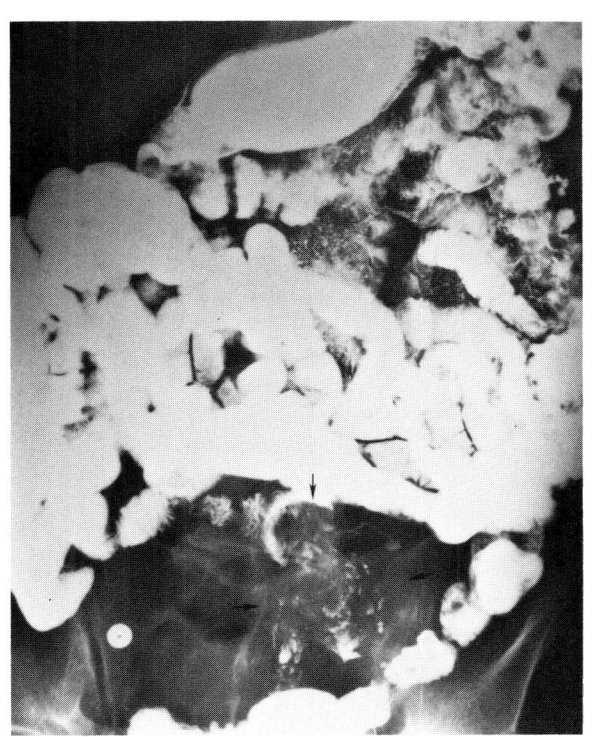

Figure 12–60. A 20-cm lobulated leiomyosarcoma with one lobule projecting into the ileal lumen (vertical arrow) and a large cavitating mass communicating with the lumen (horizontal arrows). The mass was not palpable on physical examination, and the patient had fever of undetermined origin.

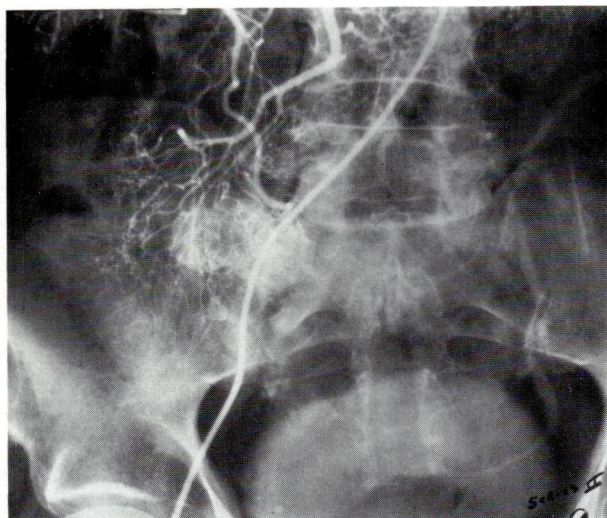

Figure 12–61. Angiogram showing vascular blush of lobulated leiomyosarcoma of the ileum in a patient with several episodes of large-volume lower intestinal hemorrhages. Earlier barium studies had been negative.

Benign Glandular Tumors (Polyps)

Benign tumors composed chiefly of glandular elements can be found in all segments of the small intestine but are much more common in the duodenum. These are one half as common as smooth muscle tumors.[5, 13]

PATHOLOGY. These lesions usually occur as pedunculated masses but are occasionally rather sessile. About two thirds of them are hamartomas, containing glands, smooth muscle, vessels, and connective tissue. They occur primarily in Peutz-Jeghers syndrome. The remaining third are true adenomatous growths, ectopic gastric tissue, and hyperplastic collections of Brunner's glands in the duodenum. The only type having significant malignant potential is the true adenoma, a very rare lesion.[5]

SYMPTOMS AND SIGNS. Those patients with multiple or diffuse hamartomatous polyps may have the characteristic mucosal and skin pigmentation of Peutz-Jeghers syndrome. Patients with Gardner's syndrome occasionally have adenomatous lesions in the small bowel, although these are much more common in the colon.

All of the glandular masses can ulcerate or become necrotic and cause intestinal hemorrhage. More commonly, however, intussusception occurs, resulting in transient obstruction and pain.

RADIOGRAPHIC DIAGNOSIS. Masses less than 1 cm in diameter usually elude detection on the barium examination. Larger lesions may appear as a filling defect attached to the mucosa by a broad or narrow pedicle. Often, only the finding of intussusception suggests the presence of the mass. It is impossible to predict the histologic composition from the x-ray appearance alone (Figs. 12–62 and 12–63).

GASTROINTESTINAL POLYPOSIS. All three segments of the gastrointestinal tract—stomach, small intestine, and colon—may be afflicted with polyposis, alone or in combination. Regardless of their histologic character, these masses may ulcerate and bleed or cause obstruction due to intussusception. Surgical excision of an offending small bowel polyp is the definitive treatment.

PEUTZ-JEGHERS SYNDROME. In this syndrome, small, localized deposits of melanin in the mucous membrane of the oral cavity or the skin of the lips, eyes, nose, and digits are associated with multiple hamartomatous polyps in the small intestine (Fig. 12–64). The small intestinal polyps are almost always multiple, usually diffuse,

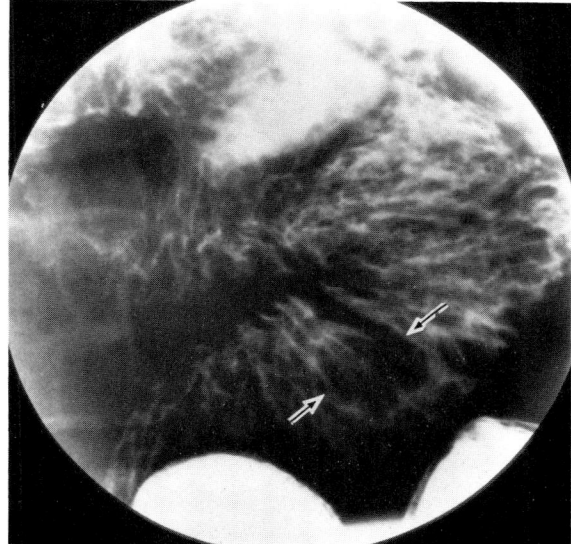

Figure 12–62. Pedunculated adenomatous polyp (arrows) in the jejunum.

and have almost no malignant potential. About half the cases have associated polyps in the stomach or colon. In the colon they may be a mixture of hamartomas and adenomas; the latter have a distinct malignant potential. If there are many adenomatous lesions present in the colon, prophylactic resection may be considered. There is

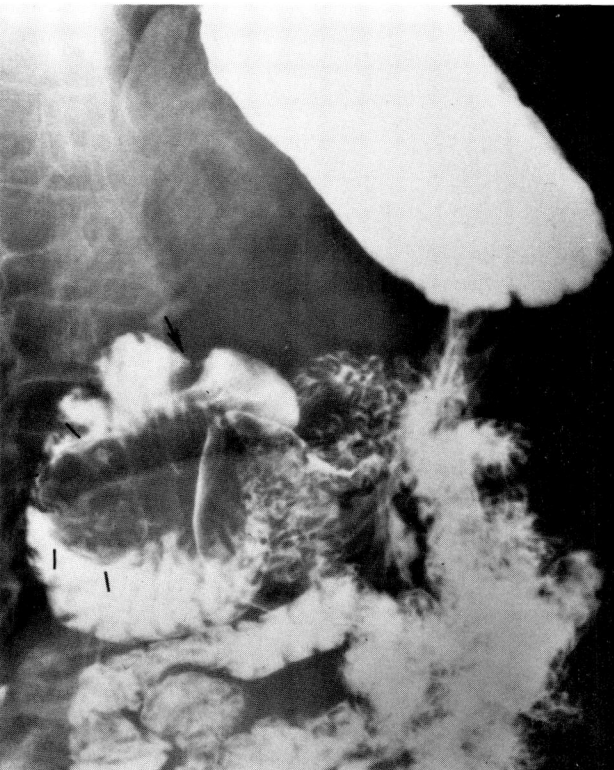

Figure 12–63. Large Brunner's gland hamartoma on a stalk (arrow) arising in the duodenal bulb.

604 — THE SMALL INTESTINE

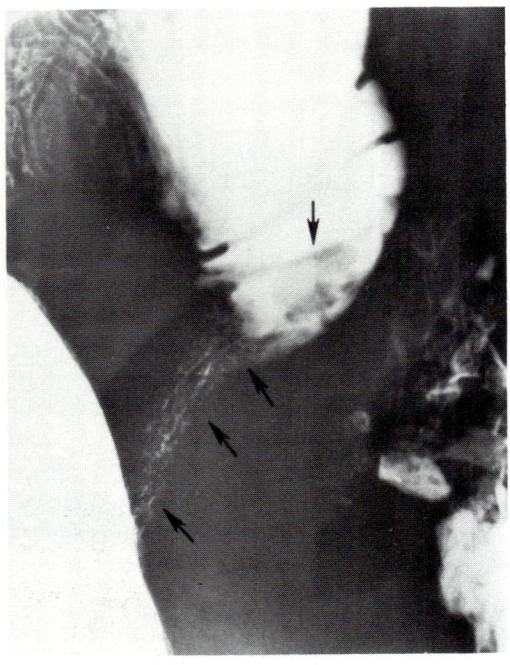

Figure 12–64. Peutz-Jeghers syndrome with an intraluminal jejunal hamartoma (vertical arrow) just proximal to an established intussusception caused by similar distal polyps. Only the central channel of the intussusception is opacified (oblique arrows).

an apparent increased incidence of carcinoma of the duodenum in these patients.[12, 19]

GARDNER'S SYNDROME. In this association of osteomas, skin tumors, and multiple polyps in the colon, there is a high rate of carcinoma of the colon. Prophylactic resection of the colon is often indicated. Multiple adenomatous polyps in the small intestine and even the stomach are sometimes associated. These may require local surgical excision (Figs. 12–65 and 12–66).[14, 21]

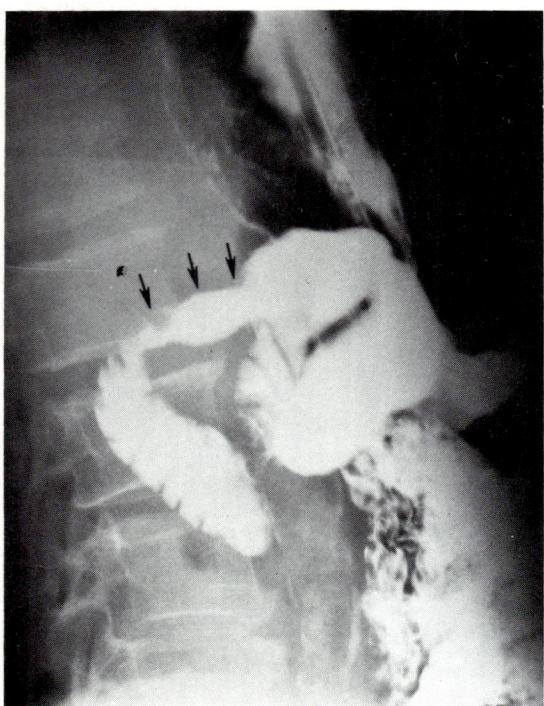

Figure 12–65. Inoperable, annular, ulcerating adenocarcinoma of the second part of the duodenum (arrows). Subtotal colectomy and ileorectostomy had been performed 24 years before for multiple colonic polyps.

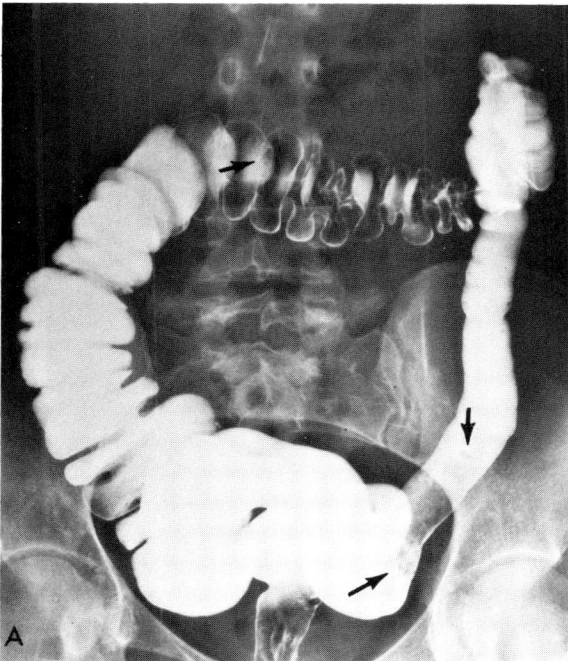 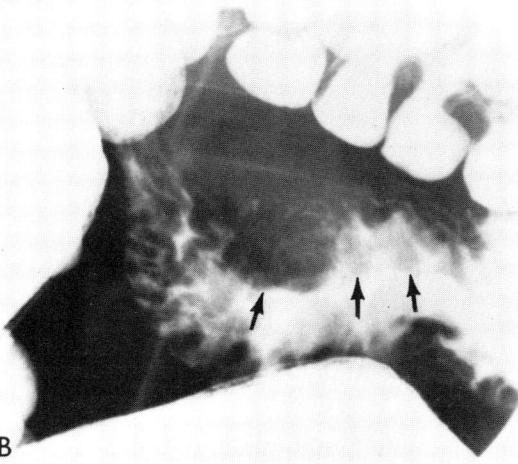

Figure 12–66. *A*, Gardner's syndrome with multiple colonic polyps (arrows). Total colectomy was done. *B*, Same patient with a cluster of adenomatous polyps (arrows) in the duodenum which were locally excised.

Lipoma

Lipomas may occur in any portion of the small intestine but are discovered most frequently in the duodenum and terminal ileum.[5, 13]

PATHOLOGY. The lipoma arises in the submucosa and may protrude into the lumen, covered by mucosa. It consists of fat-filled cells with a fibrous framework. The surface is very smooth and the mass soft and pliable. It is relatively hypovascular.

SYMPTOMS AND SIGNS. Only about one fourth of all lipomas are found at surgery, and only about one sixth develop clinical manifestations. They may cause intussusception and lead to pain from transient obstruction. About one third of the symptomatic lesions ulcerate and bleed.[23]

RADIOGRAPHIC DIAGNOSIS. Because the duodenum and terminal ileum are relatively fixed and more thoroughly examined with compression, lipomas are discovered in these segments more often than in other segments of the small intestine. The tumors are soft, easily deformed, and frequently overlooked. In the mobile portions of the small bowel, usually intussusception first calls attention to the tumor's presence. If the mass is unusually large it may be readily seen as a smooth filling defect. Lipomas may attain a diameter of 6 cm but are usually quite small (Figs. 12–67 and 12–68).[5, 13]

Hemangioma

Although not infrequent, hemangiomas are rarely diagnosed preoperatively. They occur chiefly in the jejunum and ileum; 15 per cent are incidental findings at

THE SMALL INTESTINE

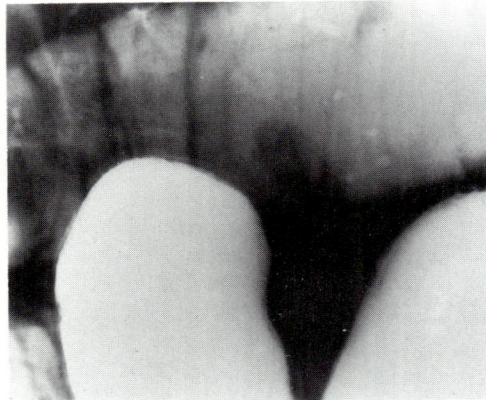

Figure 12–67. Small lipoma of jejunum. Symptoms of intermittent bowel obstruction were present.

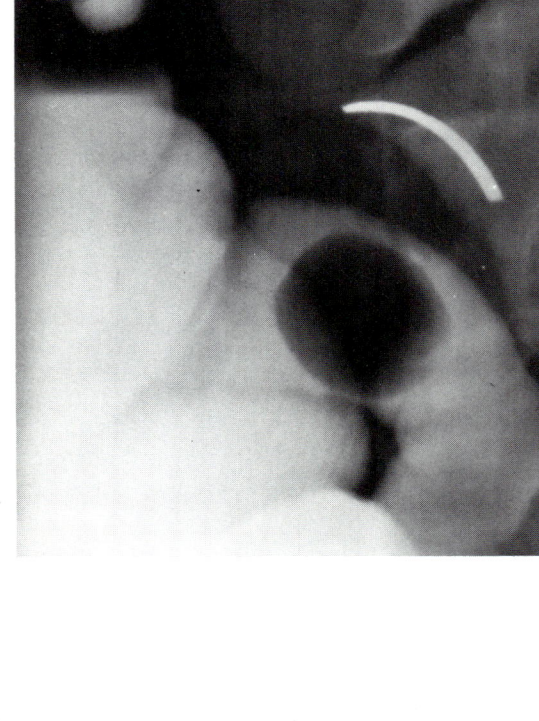

Figure 12–68. Very smooth, pliable lipoma in the terminal ileum seen during barium enema.

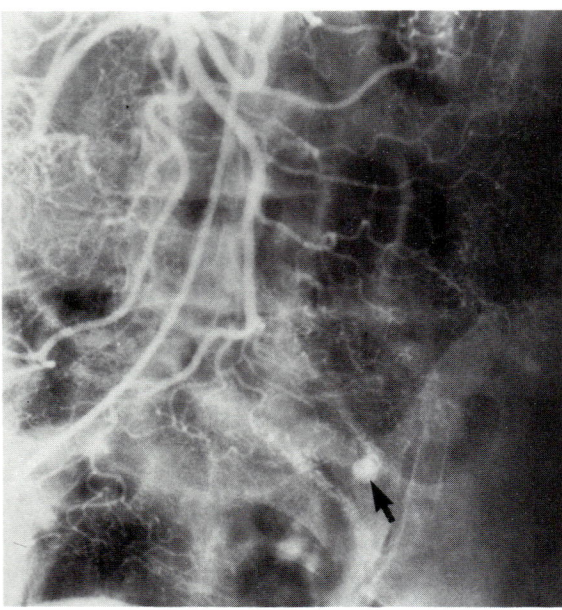

Figure 12–69. Capillary hemangioma (arrow) in the distal ileum of a 72-year-old male. Unexplained anemia was found on routine physical examination. A barium examination of the entire gut was normal. Hemangioma of the liver was revealed on an angiogram.

autopsy. Clinical manifestations (chiefly hemörrhage) occur in only one sixth of cases.

The lesions are small and soft and may permeate the entire bowel wall thickness, but usually do not deform the lumen and are rarely found during barium examination. In fact, they are often overlooked at surgical exploration. In patients with unexplained intestinal bleeding, preoperative diagnosis can often be made angiographically (Fig. 12–69). If hemangiomas are found in other portions of the body, especially the skin, intestinal bleeding should suggest the possibility of intestinal hemangioma. Vascular abnormalities in the small intestine, either small nodular hemangiomas or spider telangiectasias, may also be associated with Rendu-Osler-Weber syndrome.[5, 11, 13]

Miscellaneous Tumors

Almost all tissues in the intestine can form neoplasms, and neurofibromas, fibromas, and lymphangiomas as well as ectopic pancreatic tissue are occasionally found (Fig. 12–70). Most of these are asymptomatic unless ulceration or intussusception occurs.

Malignant Tumors in General

If carcinoids are excluded, nearly all malignant small bowel tumors cause profound clinical manifestations. Because of this, nine tenths of them are found at operation rather than at autopsy. They should be detected roentgenologically in about that same proportion, if the examination is carried out with interest and care.[3, 5, 13]

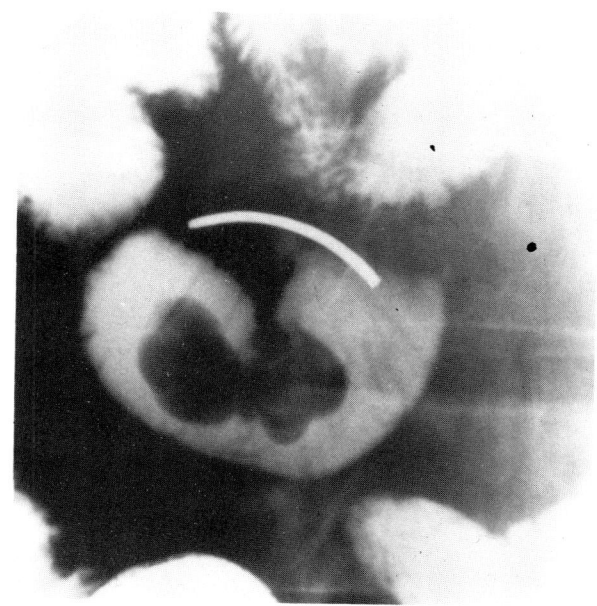

Figure 12–70. Lobulated lymphangioma of the jejunum in a 65-year-old male. The form and consistency also suggest hemangioma and lipoma.

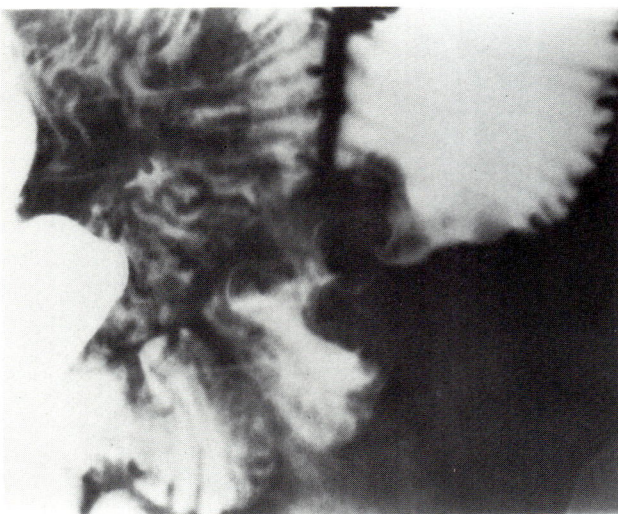

Figure 12–71. Short, annular, localized adenocarcinoma of the jejunum. The patient had been evaluated previously for blood loss but had never had a small bowel examination.

Adenocarcinoma

Primary adenocarcinomas of the small intestine occur chiefly in the duodenum and jejunum and are relatively uncommon in the ileum. They are most common in the duodenum.

PATHOLOGY. By far the most common gross form is an infiltrative, annular, constricting process. Much less commonly, the growth may form a sessile polypoid mass, or rarely, one suspended from a pedicle. The annular lesion may be very short and may resemble a fibrotic stricture. Invasion of the normal tissues of the bowel results in a rather active fibrotic process that causes narrowing of the lumen. Gross ulceration of the narrowed segment may or may not be present, but extensive necrosis and cavitation are uncommon.

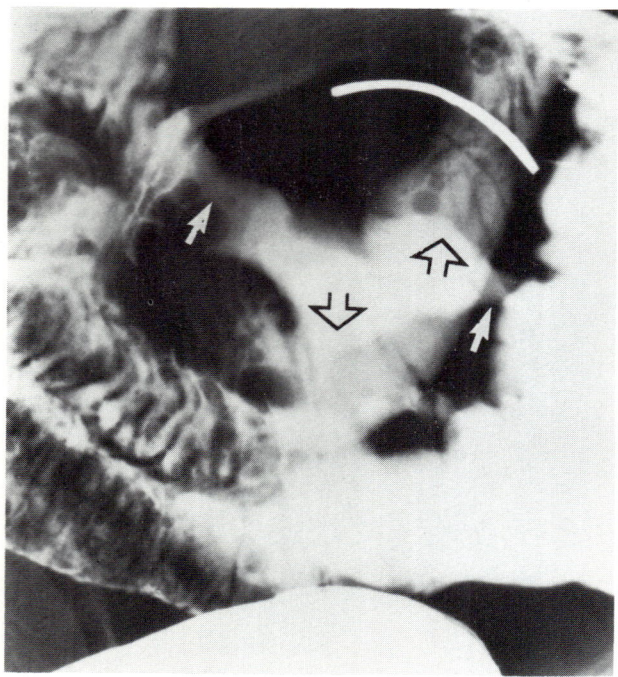

Figure 12–72. Annular (black and white arrows) ulcerating (open arrows) primary adenocarcinoma of the ileum. The patient had been anemic for several months and had had multiple x-rays of the stomach and colon but no previous small bowel examination.

THE SMALL INTESTINE — 609

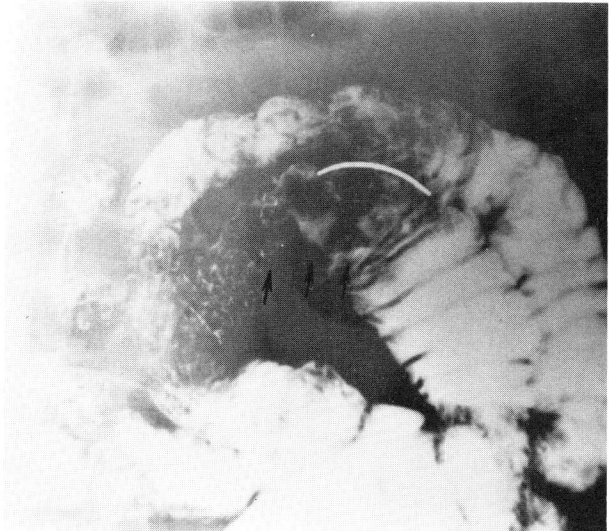

Figure 12–73. Partially obstructing, nodular necrotic primary adenocarcinoma of the jejunum. The form is somewhat suggestive of lymephoma.

SYMPTOMS AND SIGNS. About nine tenths of all patients exhibit clinical manifestations. Of these, about two thirds have pain or evidence of obstruction, approximately one half experience blood loss, and about one third have a palpable mass.

RADIOGRAPHIC DIAGNOSIS. The roentgenologic findings reflect the gross pathologic findings. The most common appearance is an annular, partially obstructing process in the duodenum or jejunum. The obstruction is almost always caused by direct narrowing of the lumen rather than by intussusception. The transition zone between the distensible and constricted segments is usually very abrupt but may be quite smooth owing to the infiltrative character of the neoplasm. Somewhat polypoid excrescences may protrude into the distensible lumen, however, and this readily identifies the lesion as malignant.[5, 13]

Infrequently, the adenocarcinoma appears as a sessile polypoid mass, a pedunculated polyp, or a plaque-like ulcerated mass. In general, any ulcerated mass in the small intestine should be considered a malignant neoplasm (Figs. 12–71 to 12–76).

Radiographic distinction from a solitary metastatic lesion is often impossible.

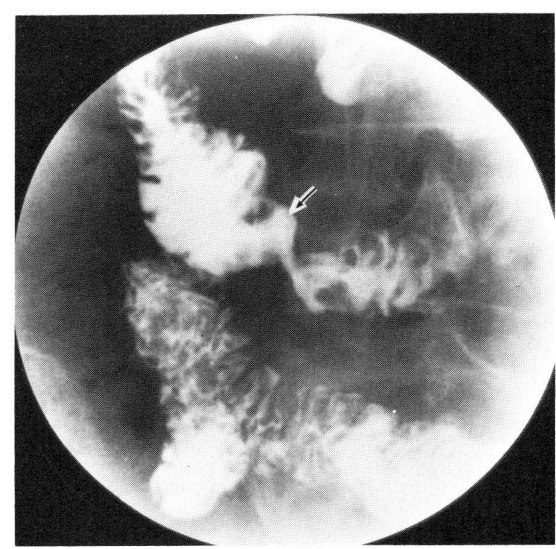

Figure 12–74. Localized adenocarcinoma of the third portion of the duodenum with ulceration (arrow) and marked narrowing.

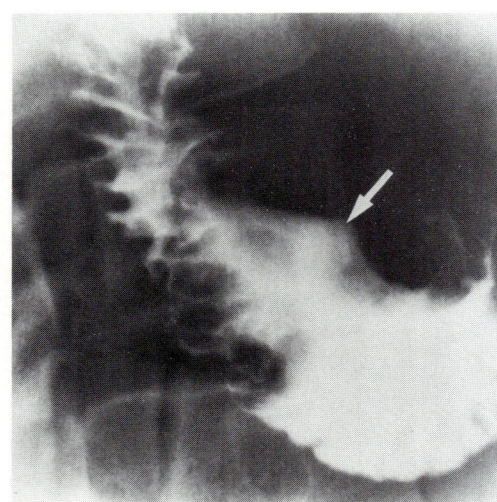

Figure 12–75. Primary carcinoma of the third portion of the duodenum with extensive ulceration (arrow) but little narrowing. The appearance is somewhat suggestive of lymphoma.

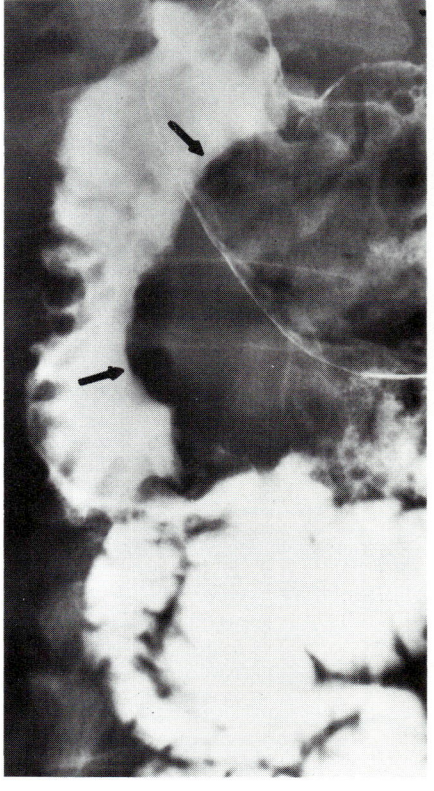

Figure 12–76. Villous adenoma of the second portion of the duodenum (arrows) with adenocarcinoma arising near the papilla. The bile duct was dilated on CT examination, but the patient had no history of jaundice and serum bilirubin level was normal.

Malignant Lymphoma

Primary malignant lymphoma of the small bowel is about two thirds as common as primary adenocarcinoma. However, there may be involvement of the small bowel as part of widespread, multisystem lymphoma. The primary variety occurs almost exclusively in the jejunum and ileum and rarely in the duodenum. If the duodenum is involved, it is usually as a part of more extensive retroperitoneal node disease.[5, 13]

PATHOLOGY. Malignant lymphoma is a very cellular growth which excites very little tissue reaction. It infiltrates the mucosa and muscularis rather extensively and only infrequently narrows the lumen. As the cellular growth becomes larger and more extensive, necrosis often occurs in the mass and the overlying mucosa, and this may result in widening of the intestinal lumen or in cavitation.

The gross form can be quite variable, and single, fairly large polyps as well as annular lesions may occur. Occasionally, the mucosa is extensively involved with innumerable small polypoid nodules which are often also found in the colon and rectum. If multiple lesions are found, multisystem lymphoma or some other form of metastatic disease should be strongly considered, since only about 3 per cent of cases of primary small bowel lymphoma have multiple sites of origin.[5, 13]

SYMPTOMS AND SIGNS. Pain and other obstructive symptoms are very common but are less severe than in adenocarcinoma. High-grade obstruction is rare. A palpable mass is found in about two thirds of patients, and evidence of blood loss in about half that number.

RADIOGRAPHIC DIAGNOSIS. The most characteristic roentgenologic finding is a rather long lesion involving the entire circumference of the bowel wall with extensive ulceration of the surface of the lumen. This surface may have a rather smooth, nodular appearance. There is often evidence of a mass in the adjacent mesentery. These findings are highly suggestive of lymphoma. Diffuse lymphomatous involvement may appear as thickened folds, diffuse nodulation, or multiple masses, often in combination. However, when there is a sessile mass, an annular constricting lesion, submucosal infiltration alone, or diffuse nodularity, other possibilities must be considered.[5, 7, 13, 16]

Associated splenomegaly is strongly suggestive of advanced-stage lymphoma.

The various histologic varieties of malignant lymphoma cannot be distinguished radiographically (Figs. 12–77 to 12–86).

Text continued on page 616.

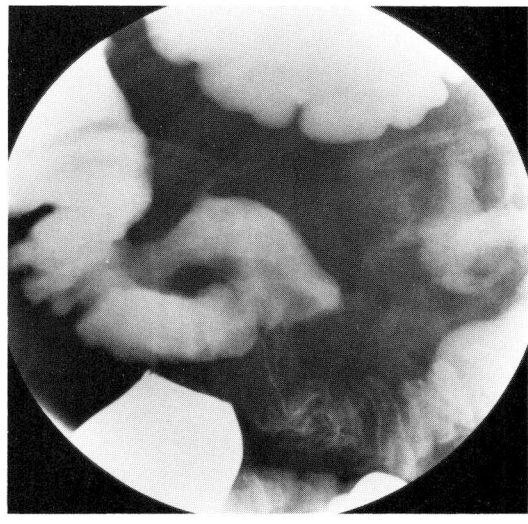

Figure 12–77. Ulcerated malignant lymphoma of the terminal ileum with "aneurysmal dilatation." Ultrasound showed extensive retroperitoneal node enlargement.

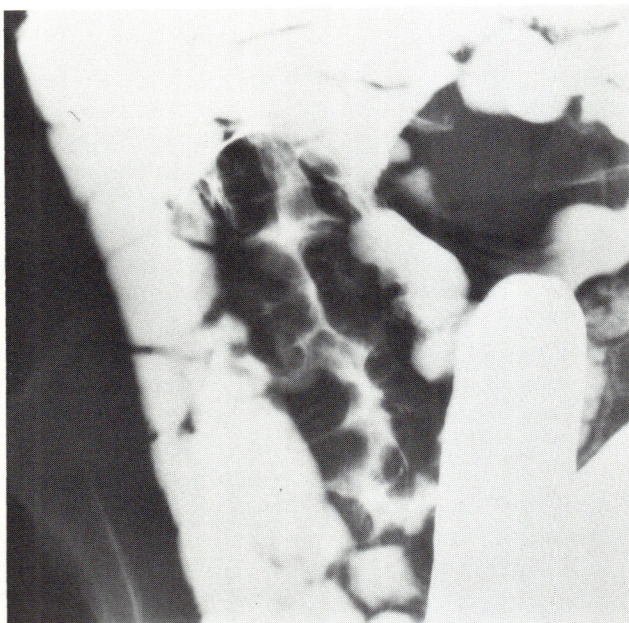

Figure 12–78. Nodular submucosal malignant lymphoma in the terminal ileum, producing a thumbprinting appearance.

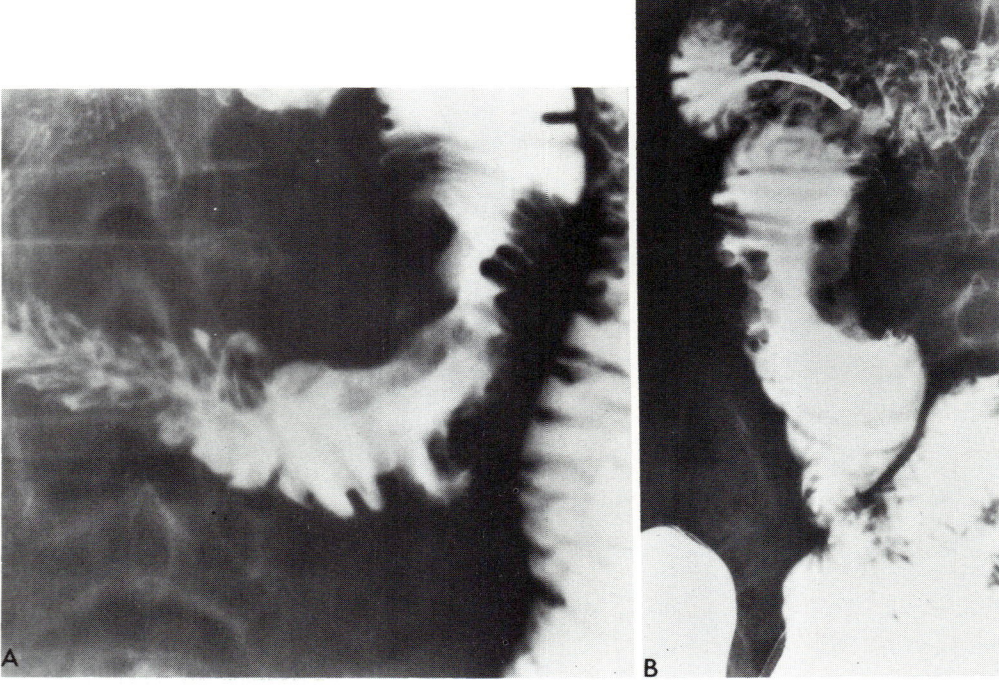

Figure 12–79. *A* and *B*, Multiple sites of infiltrating, extensively ulcerating, malignant lymphoma in the jejunum.

THE SMALL INTESTINE — 613

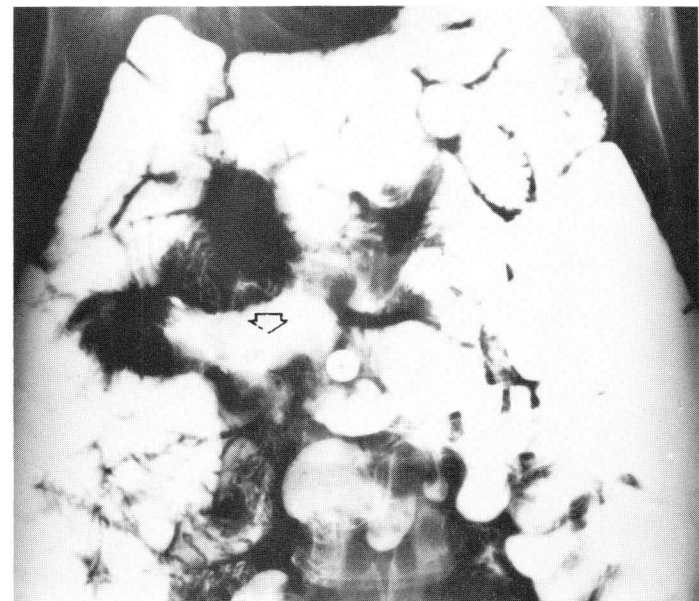

Figure 12–80. Malignant lymphoma demonstrating a cavitating (arrow) mass in the mesentery communicating with the lumen of the jejunum. The appearance is similar to cavitating smooth muscle tumors.

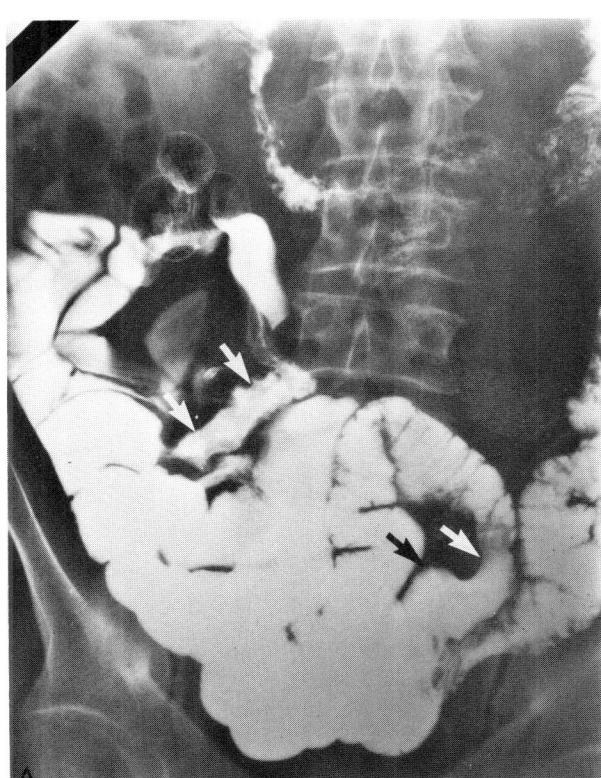

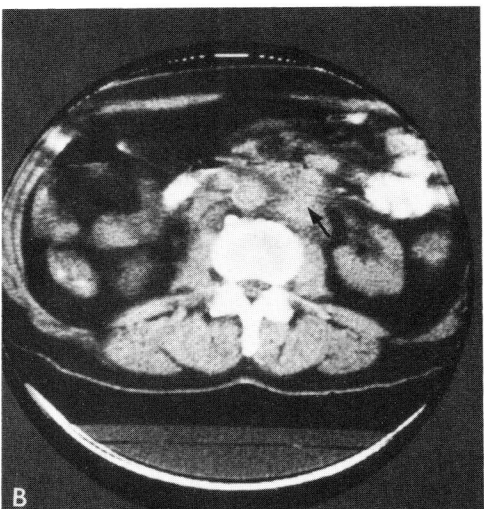

Figure 12–81. *A*, Multiple sites of malignant lymphoma (arrows) demonstrating infiltration and extensive ulceration, resulting in widening of the intestinal lumen. *B*, CT scan showed large retroperitoneal nodes (arrow).

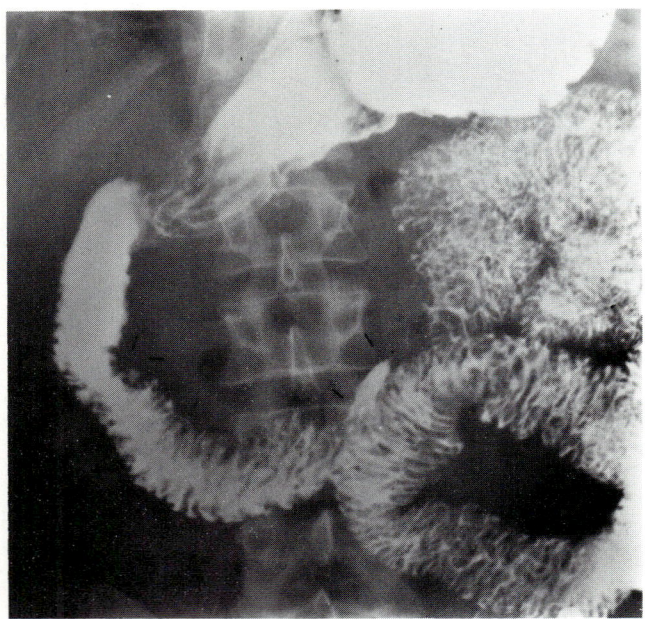

Figure 12–82. Two lymphomatous masses in the duodenum with intact mucosa over the proximal one (left arrows) and broad ulceration of the distal (right arrows). Lymphangiogram showed extensive retroperitoneal node involvement.

Figure 12–83. Malignant lymphoma causing narrowing (arrow) and marked jejunal obstruction.

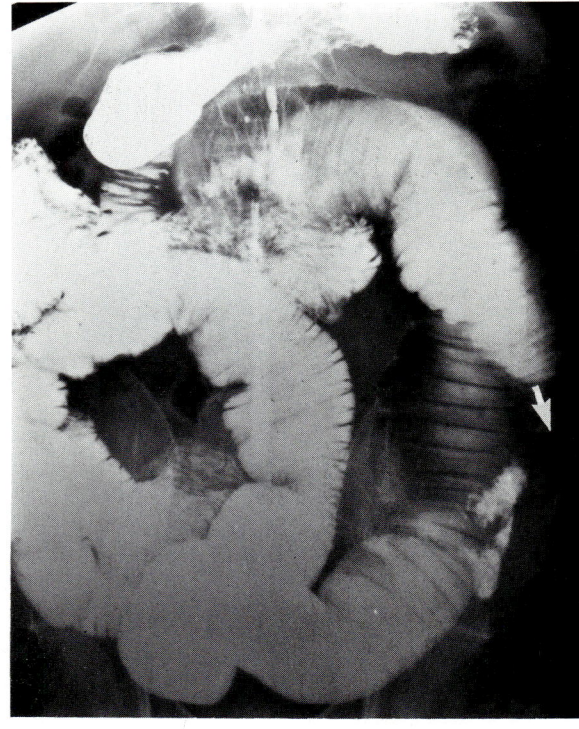

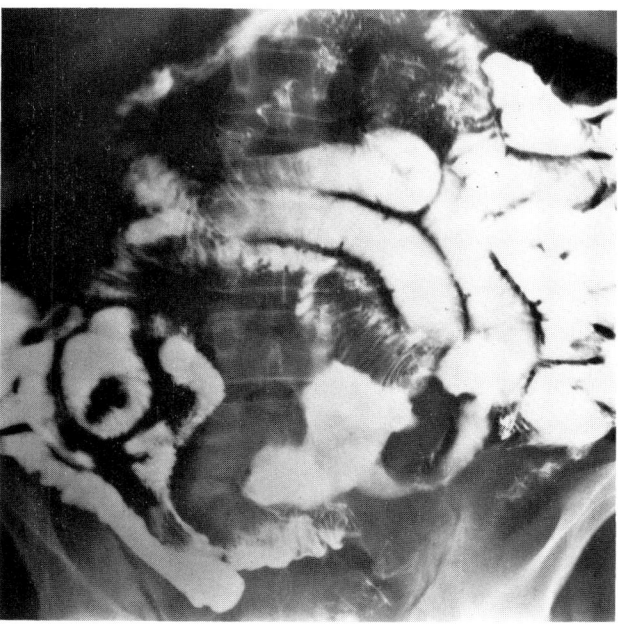

Figure 12–84. In a patient suffering from chronic blood loss there are multiple sites of malignant lymphoma in the jejunum and ileum showing intussusception, intramural infiltration, annular narrowing, and a large cavitating communicating mass. The spleen and retroperitoneal nodes were also involved.

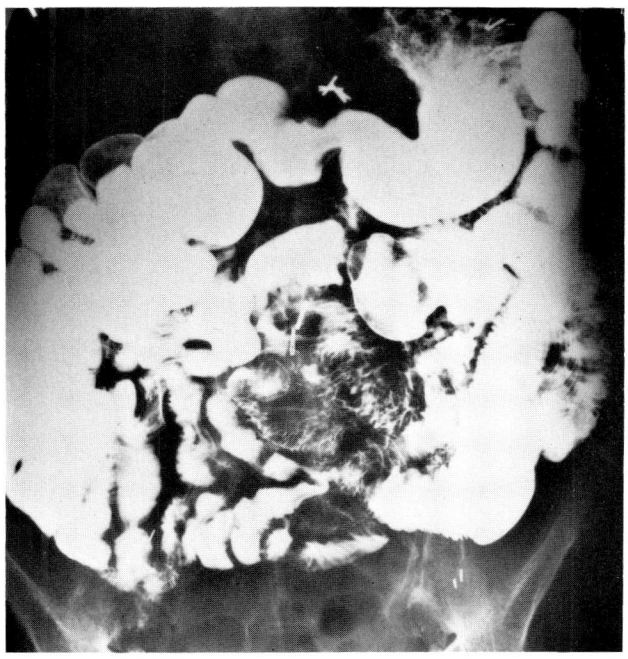

Figure 12–85. Malignant lymphoma (Hodgkin's disease) showing polypoid masses, infiltration, and fixation of the bowel.

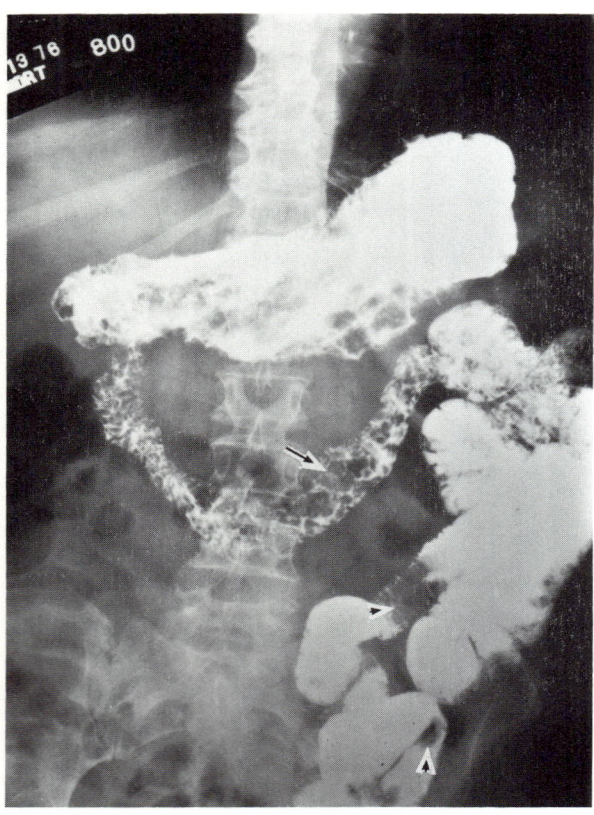

Figure 12–86. Diffuse involvement of the small intestine with multiple lymphomatous masses (arrows). The stomach and colon were also involved as well as the retroperitoneal nodes, which are invading the duodenum (larger arrow).

Metastatic Tumors

Most secondary small bowel neoplasms are associated with disseminated peritoneal disease. In a significant number of cases, however, single or multiple metastases involve the small bowel alone, without evidence of diffuse peritoneal involvement or direct extension. Symptoms and signs are quite like those of a primary neoplasm. The radiographic appearance of metastatic masses is extremely variable.

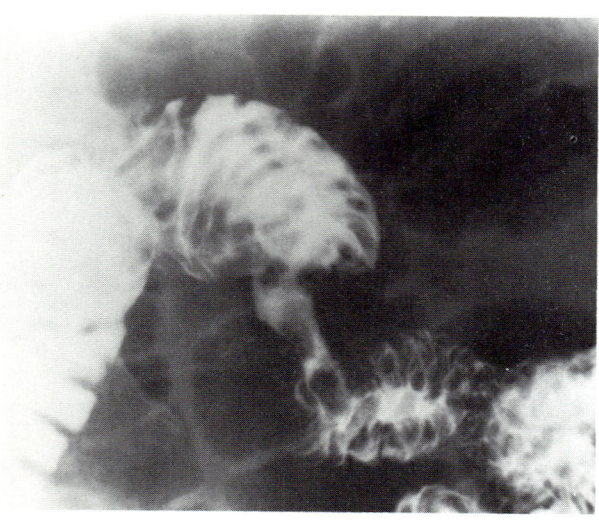

Figure 12–87. Short, annular, partially obstructive metastasis to the midjejunum from carcinoma of the pancreas. The appearance is very much like that of primary carcinoma.

THE SMALL INTESTINE — 617

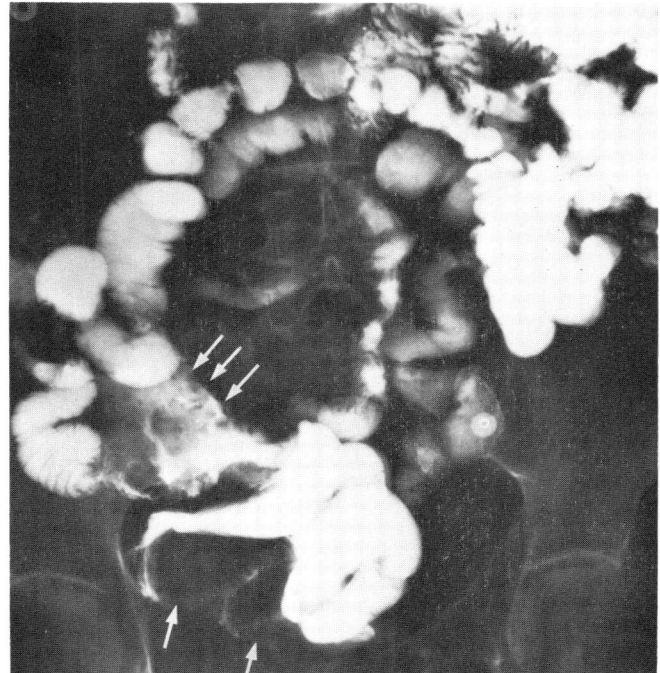

Figure 12–88. Metastatic squamous cell carcinoma from the urinary bladder causing multiple extramucosal masses (lower arrows) and an ulcerating mass (upper arrows) in the ileum.

Although they are usually multiple, solitary lesions are not rare and usually cannot be distinguished radiographically from a primary neoplasm. Metastases can appear as a polyp, as intramural infiltration with the formation of an extramucosal mass, as an annular constriction, or as necrosis with widening of the lumen or formation of a

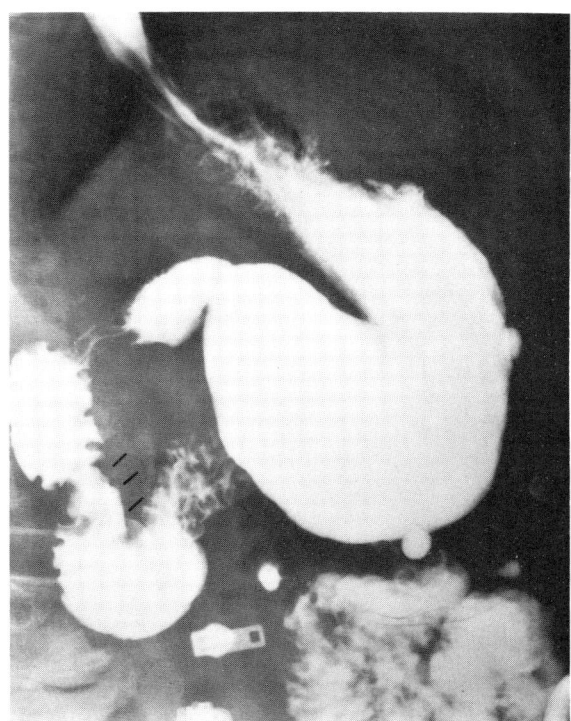

Figure 12–89. Extension of carcinoma of the pancreas to the duodenum, causing an annular ulcerating lesion (arrows) resembling primary carcinoma.

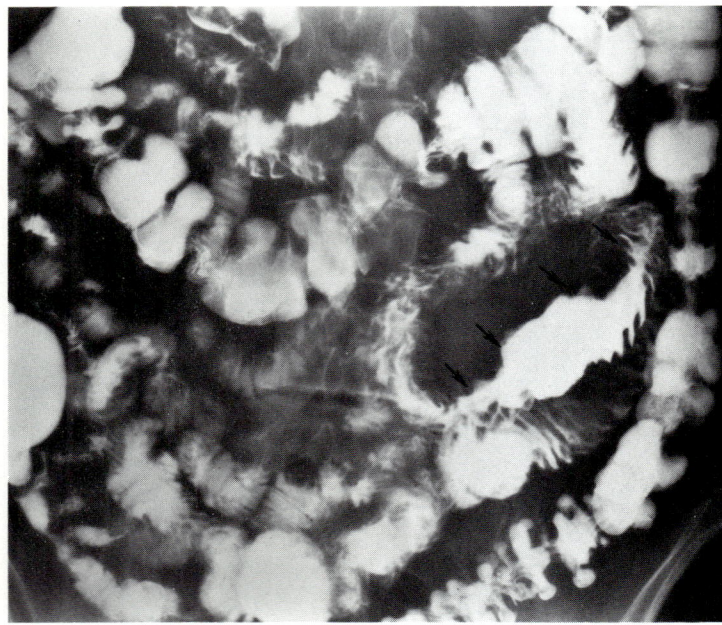

Figure 12–90. Metastatic melanosarcoma in the jejunum, with infiltration and extensive necrosis resulting in widening of the lumen (arrows), an appearance very suggestive of lymphosarcoma.

communicating cavity. Very cellular lesions, such as melanosarcoma, are very much prone to extensive necrosis. Multiple lesions of varied form in the small intestine in a patient with known primary malignant neoplasm should make metastases a paramount consideration. Malignant lymphoma can result in almost identical lesions (Figs. 12–87 to 12–90).[5, 8, 24, 27]

POSTOPERATIVE COMPLICATIONS

Obstruction

After abdominal surgery of any sort, pain and abdominal distention often raise the question of possible mechanical small bowel obstruction. Most often, the clinical picture is due to disorganization of the propulsive motor activity of the small intestine. The plain films usually confirm this by showing relatively moderate gaseous distention of both the small and the large intestine. Likewise, if there is high-grade mechanical obstruction of the small intestine, plain films are diagnostic in about three out of four cases. If the plain film findings are not clear, contrast medium either by mouth or by tube is simple and highly diagnostic. Barium suspension can be used instead of water-soluble contrast unless there has been recent colon surgery.

Hemorrhage

Severe postoperative hemorrhage is investigated by gastric aspiration, gastroscopy, and, if necessary, by angiography. If there has been recent resective small bowel surgery, angiography is especially useful in identifying bleeding from the anastomotic site(s) (Fig. 12–91).

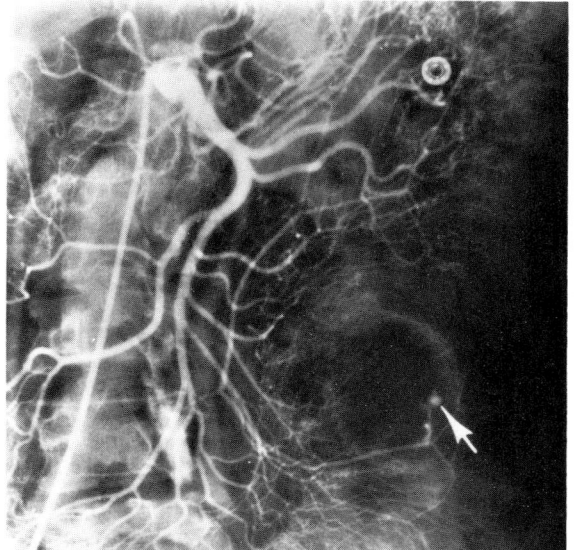

Figure 12–91. Massive postoperative hemorrhage following segmental resection of the jejunum for ulcerated lipoma. Arteriogram showed extravasation of contrast (arrow) near line of surgical staples. The briskly bleeding artery was surgically ligated.

SUMMARY

1. Small intestinal neoplasms are not common, but malignant lesions should be detected in 80 to 90 per cent of cases by careful radiologic studies.

2. Careful, frequent fluoroscopy and manual compression are fundamental in the examination of the small bowel.

3. Angiography is most useful during active bleeding. However, it will often demonstrate vascular and smooth muscle tumors even in the absence of active hemorrhage. These lesions are often very difficult to demonstrate by barium examination.

4. Although benign neoplasms are more common than malignant ones, about two thirds of all tumors removed surgically are malignant.

5. Any mass in the small intestine in a patient with appropriate symptoms has a rather significant likelihood of being malignant. If there is radiographic evidence of ulceration, the mass is almost certainly malignant.

6. If there are multiple lesions in the small intestine that form masses and exhibit ulceration and narrowing of the lumen, they probably represent either multisystem lymphoma or metastatic malignant neoplasm.

References

1. Baker, H. L., Jr., and Good, C. A.: Smooth-muscle tumors of the alimentary tract: their roentgen manifestations. Am. J. Roentgenol. *74:*246–255, 1955.
2. Burrows, F. G. O., Dodds, W. N., and Thompson, H.: Diagnosis of a leiomyoma of the small intestine by selective angiography. Br. J. Surg. *64:*145–146, 1977.
3. Broders, A. C., Jr., Hightower, N. C., Jr., Hunt, W. H., III, et al.: Primary neoplasms of the small bowel: analysis of one hundred two cases. Arch. Surg. *79:*753–760, 1959.
4. Carlson, H. C.: Small intestinal intussusception: an easily misunderstood sign. Am. J. Roentgenol. *15*(2):338–339, 1970.
5. Carlson, H. C., and Good, C. A.: Neoplasms of the small bowel. *In* Margulis, H. R., and Burhenne, H. J. (eds.): Alimentary Tract Roentgenology. Vol. 2. St. Louis, The C. V. Mosby Company, 1973, pp. 865–902.

6. Cooley, R. N.: The diagnostic accuracy of radiologic studies of the biliary tract, small intestine and colon. Am. J. Med. Sci. 246:610–638, 1963.
7. Cupps, R. E., Hodgson, J. R., Dockerty, M. B., et al.: Primary lymphoma in the small intestine: problems of roentgenologic diagnosis. Radiology 92:1354–1362, 1969.
8. De Castro, C. A., Dockerty, M. B., and Mayo, C. W.: Metastatic tumors of the small intestines. Surg. Gynecol. Obstet. 105:159–165, 1957.
9. Farmer, R. G., and Hawk, W. A.: Metastatic tumors of the small bowel. Gastroenterology 47:496–504, 1964.
10. Forbes, W. St. C., Nolan, D. J., Fletcher, E. W. L., et al.: Small bowel melena: 2 cases diagnosed by angiography. Br. J. Surg. 65:168–170, 1978.
11. Gentry, R. W., Dockerty, M. B., and Clagett, O. T.: Collective review: vascular malformations and vascular tumors of gastrointestinal tract. Int. Abstr. Surg. 88:281–323, 1949.
12. Godard, J. E., Dodds, W. J., Phillips, J. C., et al.: Peutz-Jeghers syndrome: clinical and roentgenographic features. Am. J. Roentgenol. 113(2):316–324, 1971.
13. Good, C. A.: Tumors of the small intestine: Caldwell Lecture, 1962. Am. J. Roentgenol. 89:685–705, 1963.
14. Grosberg, S. J.: Gardner's syndrome and villous adenoma of jejunum. Am. Surg. 41:177–178, 1975.
15. Keats, R. E., and Sakai, H. Q.: An evaluation of the sources of error in the roentgenologic diagnosis of neoplasms of the small intestine. Gastroenterology 29:554, 1955.
16. Marshak, R. H., Wolf, B. S., and Eliasoph, J.: The roentgen findings in lymphosarcoma of the small intestine. Am. J. Roentgenol. 86:682–692, 1961.
17. Moertel, C. G., Hill, J. R., and Adson, M. A.: Management of multiple polyposis of the large bowel. Cancer 28:160–164, July, 1971.
18. Ramer, M., Mitty, H. A., and Baron, M. G.: Angiography in leiomyomatous neoplasms of the small bowel. Am. J. Roentgenol. 113(2):263–268, 1971.
19. Reid, J. D.: Intestinal carcinoma in the Peutz-Jeghers syndrome. J.A.M.A. 229(7):833–834, 1974.
20. River L., Silverstein, J., and Tope, J. W.: Collective review: benign neoplasms of small intestine; a critical comprehensive review with reports of 20 new cases. Int. Abstr. Surg. 102:1–38, 1956.
21. Ross, J. E., and Mara, J. E.: Small bowel polyps and carcinoma in multiple intestinal polyposis. Arch. Surg. 108:736–738, 1974.
22. Skandalakis, J. E., Gray, S. W., Shepard, D., et al.: Smooth Muscle Tumors of the Alimentary Tract: Leiomyomas and Leiomyosarcomas—A Review of 2,525 Cases. Springfield, Illinois, Charles C Thomas, Publisher, 1962.
23. Smith, F. R., and Mayo C. W.: Submucous lipomas of the small intestine. Am. J. Surg. 80:922–928, 1950.
24. Smith, S. J., Carlson, H. C., and Gisvold, J. J.: Secondary neoplasms of the small bowel. Radiology 125(1):29–33, 1977.
25. Starr, G. F., and Dockerty, M. B.: Leiomyomas and leiomyosarcomas of the small intestine. Cancer 8:101–111, 1955.
26. Stothert, J. C., Riaz, M. A., Joyce, P. F., et al.: Preoperative angiographic diagnosis of small bowel leiomyomas. Arch. Surg. 113:643, 1978.
27. Watanabe, H., Enjoji, M., Yao, T., et al.: Accompanying gastro-enteric lesions in familial adenomatosis coli. Acta Pathol. Jap. 27(6):823–839, 1977.
28. Zboralski, F. F., and Bessolo, R. J.: Metastatic carcinoma to the mesentery and gut. Radiology 88:302, 1967.

Part VII

Carcinoid Tumors and the Carcinoid Syndrome

H. C. CARLSON, M.D.

INTRODUCTION

As the name implies, carcinoid is a tumor that histologically appears to be a cancer but clinically usually does not behave like cancer. Long symptomatic periods, occasionally lasting more than 20 years, may elapse before the diagnosis is made.

INCIDENCE AND LOCATION

Almost all gastrointestinal carcinoid tumors of clinical importance are located in the small intestine. They occur rather infrequently in the duodenum, where they are found as a small polypoid lesion on x-ray examination, and they also occur in the rectum, where they are seen as small submucosal nodules at proctoscopy. Appendiceal carcinoids, although relatively common, never metastasize.

Of lesions in the small intestine, about 2 per cent are found in the duodenum, about 7 per cent in the jejunum, and about 90 per cent in the ileum. In the ileum, about two thirds are located in the lower third of the organ, the majority in the distal 2 feet.

They are the most common tumors found in the small intestine, but the majority do not cause symptoms and are incidental findings at surgery or autopsy.

Of the symptomatic tumors in the small intestine, carcinoid is slightly less common than adenocarcinoma. Most symptomatic carcinoids are in the ileum.[3, 6, 8]

PATHOLOGY

These neoplasms arise from the chromaffin cells at the base of the crypts of Lieberkühn and have an affinity for silver stain. They are almost always rather small, about 75 per cent being less than 1.5 cm in diameter. The primary tumor is rarely symptomatic, although it can cause intussusception, and very rarely, ulceration and bleeding. Metastases occur much more frequently if the primary carcinoid is 2 cm or more in diameter.

Multicentricity is a striking feature of carcinoid, and almost one third of cases have more than one primary mass. In addition, about one fourth of all carcinoid tumors are associated with an unrelated malignancy at another site, including the intestines, lung, and breast.

Invasive carcinoids that infiltrate the muscularis, peritoneum, and mesentery can cause an intense fibrous reaction which is responsible for a buckling deformity which can cause mechanical bowel obstruction. Less common mechanisms of obstruction are narrowing of the lumen by invasion, intussusception, and volvulus.

Metastases to lymph nodes can produce huge masses in the mesentery, from which spread to the liver occurs. In cases of symptomatic carcinoid, about 90 per cent have regional lymph node metastasis, and almost 40 per cent hepatic deposits. The tumor rarely extends beyond the abdominal cavity, although metastases to the pleura and bone marrow have been reported.[6, 8]

CLINICAL COURSE

Almost all patients with symptomatic carcinoid experience abdominal pain. In about half, it is the characteristic pain of mechanical intestinal obstruction, while in the rest it is vague and nonspecific. Ultimately, about half the patients develop diarrhea and experience weight loss, and a minority experience flushing or constipation.

Abnormal physical findings are infrequent, but there may be a palpable abdominal mass, usually on the right, a distended abdomen, and least often, hepatomegaly. Signs and symptoms of bleeding are rare. Symptoms persist for an average of four years before diagnosis is made.

A few patients present with an acute abdomen, which results from massive

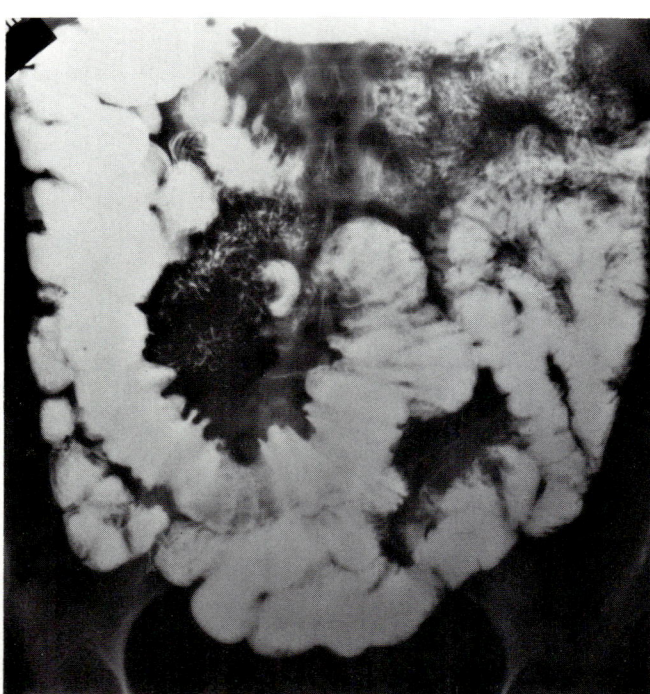

Figure 12–92. Malignant carcinoid of the ileum, with mesenteric extension and kinking of the lumen (arrow) causing obstruction. Metastasis is present in lymph nodes, but none was demonstrated in the liver.

mesenteric lymph nodes causing volvulus or constriction of the superior mesenteric vessels sufficient to produce massive small bowel infarction.[8, 10]

RADIOGRAPHIC DIAGNOSIS

Since almost all significant intestinal carcinoids are associated with abdominal pain and about half with symptoms of bowel obstruction, x-ray examination of the small bowel and colon are almost always requested by the clinician.

The findings of partial mechanical obstruction due to buckling of the ileal lumen from a fibrosing peritoneal and mesenteric pathologic process should strongly suggest this diagnosis (Fig. 12–92). If combined with the demonstration of an intraluminal mass in a patient with a long history of abdominal pain and diarrhea, the diagnosis can be strongly suspected (Fig. 12–93). A combination of suggestive roentgenologic findings should be followed by the determination of 24-hour urinary excretion of 5-hydroxyindoleacetic acid (5-HIAA), the degradation product of serotonin produced by the tumor.[1, 2, 3, 7]

Any pathologic process that infiltrates the intestinal wall and induces a fibrotic response by the peritoneum and mesentery resembles carcinoid (Fig. 12–94). Peritoneal carcinomatosis, an inflammatory process resulting from bowel perforation or sometimes from regional enteritis can produce a fibrotic mesenteric response and resemble carcinoid change. Lymphoma frequently enters into the radiographic differential diagnosis.

Unfortunately, most cases of symptomatic carcinoid already have extensive metastases to the mesentery, liver, and peritoneum. Ultrasound, computed tomography, and angiography may be helpful in detecting hepatic and mesenteric masses (Fig. 12–95). If a localized hepatic metastasis can be demonstrated, resection of the liver and mesenteric mass may prove remarkably palliative. Even if the metastatic process

Figure 12–93. Multiple carcinoid nodules in the terminal ileum (arrows), with an invasive carcinoid proximal to this site. Mesenteric nodes were metastatically involved.

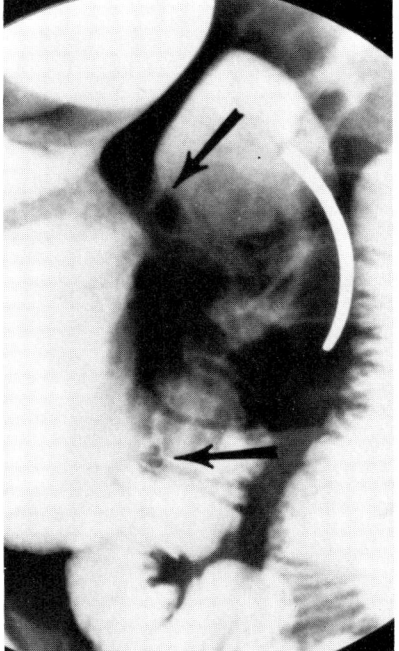

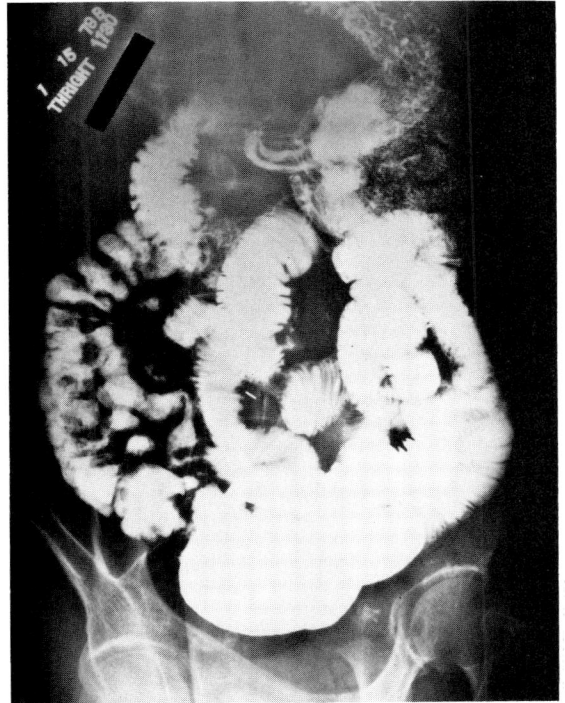

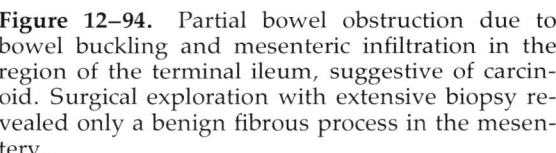

Figure 12–94. Partial bowel obstruction due to bowel buckling and mesenteric infiltration in the region of the terminal ileum, suggestive of carcinoid. Surgical exploration with extensive biopsy revealed only a benign fibrous process in the mesentery.

Figure 12–95. CT scan shows multiple metastatic masses in the liver from a carcinoid mass in the lumen of a partially obstructed small intestine. The patient had flushing, tachycardia, and elevated 5-HIAA in the urine but only slight, intermittent abdominal pain. No therapy was given.

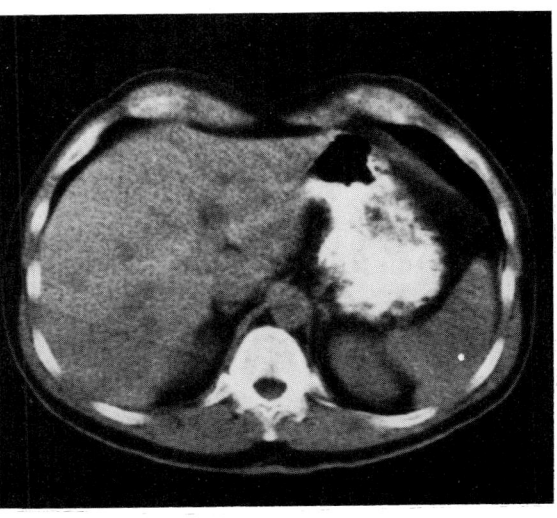

is diffuse, significant control of the malignant process can be accomplished by chemotherapy in a substantial proportion of cases. In all of these cases, the diagnosis can be made confidently if the urinary 5-HIAA is elevated.

CLINICAL COURSE

In spite of extensive metastases, in over 90 per cent of symptomatic cases the surgical removal of as much tumor tissue as possible can result in remarkable relief of symptoms and long survival. Even simply bypassing an obstructing lesion can produce symptomatic relief and long survival. Of course, if symptoms are not severe, treatment may be withheld until such time as the risks of chemotherapy or surgery are justified by the discomfort, disability, or life-threatening character of the situation.[8]

SURVIVAL

Usually, surgical exploration or liver biopsy is necessary for a histologic diagnosis unless excess 5-HIAA can be demonstrated in the urine. Somewhat more than half of these explored cases are considered resectable, even though almost all have peritoneal or nodal metastases. The five-year survival of this group is almost 70 per cent. Patients considered inoperable have an encouraging five-year survival rate (40 per cent) even with hepatic masses (20 per cent). The mean survival time between diagnosis and death from metastasis is eight years.

CARCINOID SYNDROME

In a small group of patients with intestinal carcinoid tumor, the clinical course is characterized by periodic flushing of the skin, diarrhea, tachycardia, and occasionally, wheezing. These patients all have extensive metastases, usually to the liver and the mesenteric nodes. The tumor produces 5-hydroxytryptamine (serotonin), a pressor agent that is normally deactivated by the liver and lungs to inert 5 hydroxyindoleacetic acid which is then excreted by the kidneys. When the hepatic deposits produce quantities of 5-HIAA greater than the deactivating capacity of the lung, the systemic effects of the syndrome occur. Serotonin also has a direct fibrotic effect on the valves and endothelium of the right heart, causing valve dysfunction. The left heart valves are not affected, presumably because much of the serotonin has been deactivated by the lung.[3, 12]

The most common symptom in carcinoid syndrome is flushing, followed closely by diarrhea. The diarrhea probably results from the direct entry of serotonin into the mesenteric circulation and its effect on the small intestinal smooth muscle.

A surprising number of patients with carcinoid syndrome die of extensive small bowel infarction. This is due to mechanical compression of the mesenteric vessels by the extensive tumor mass and to vasoconstrictive effect of serotonin.[4, 5, 8–11] In addition, elastic fiber proliferation in and around the mesenteric vessels occurs in a large proportion of patients with malignant carcinoid tumor and extensive metastases. This may be the dominant mechanism of mesenteric vascular narrowing in extensive carcinoid tumor and may account for the relatively frequent occurrence of ileal necrosis.[4, 5, 8–11]

SUMMARY

1. Carcinoid tumor is one of the most common symptom-producing tumors of the small intestine. It is by far the most common tumor involving the ileum.
2. With an understanding of the pathologic nature and clinical course of intestinal carcinoid, the radiologic diagnosis should be made more frequently and precisely than in the past.
3. Even though most patients with symptomatic intestinal carcinoid have extensive metastases, the detection and identification of the lesions can result in effective palliative therapy. Modern radiologic methods, such as computed tomography, angiography, and ultrasound, can make substantial contributions to the management of patients, including those with carcinoid syndrome.

References

1. Bancks, N. H., Goldstein, H. M., and Dodd, G. D.: The roentgenologic spectrum of small intestine carcinoid tumors. Am. J. Roentgenol. 123(2):274–280, 1975.
2. Boijsen, E., Kaude, J., and Tylen, U.: Radiologic diagnosis of ileal carcinoid tumors. Acta Radiol. Diagn. 15:65–82, 1974.
3. Carlson, H. C., and Good, C. A.: Neoplasms of the small bowel. In Margulis, H. R., and Burhenne, H. J. (eds.): Alimentary Tract Roentgenology. Vol. 2. St. Louis, The C. V. Mosby Company, 1973, pp. 865–902.
4. Chapuis, P., and Weedon, D.: Ischaemic ileal necrosis and carcinoid tumor. Aust. N. Z. J. Surg. 46(1):63–64, 1976.
5. Claps, R. J., Lande, A., Lilienfeld, R., et al.: Angiographic demonstration of an ileal carcinoid. Radiology 103:87–88, 1972.
6. MacDonald, R. A.: A study of 356 carcinoids of the gastrointestinal tract: report of four new cases of the carcinoid syndrome. Am. J. Med. 21:867, 1956.
7. Miller, E. R., and Herrmann, W. W.: Argentaffin tumors of the small bowel: a roentgen sign of malignant change. Radiology 39:214, 1942.
8. Moertel, C. G., Sauer, W. G., Dockerty, M. B., et al.: Life history of the carcinoid tumor of the small intestine. Cancer 14:901–912, 1961.
9. Murray-Lyon, I. M., Rake, M. O., Marshall, A. K., et al.: Malignant carcinoid tumor with gangrene of small intestine. Br. Med. J. 4:770–771, 1973.
10. Qizilbash, A. H.: Carcinoid tumors, vascular elastosis, and ischemic disease of the small intestine. Dis. Colon Rectum 20(7):554–560, 1977.
11. Shimkin, P. M., DeVita, V. T., and Doppman, J. L.: Arteriography of an ileal carcinoid tumor. J. Can. Assoc. Radiol. 22:259–260, 1971.
12. Tilson, M. D.: Carcinoid syndrome. Surg. Clin. North Am. 54(2):409–423, 1974.

Part VIII
Meckel's Diverticulum

J. GEORGE TEPLICK, M.D.
M. E. HASKIN, M.D.

Meckel's diverticulum is an uncommon remnant of the fetal omphalomesenteric duct (vitelline duct), which extends from the umbilicus to the distal ileum. Failure of closure of the intestinal end of this duct results in an ileal diverticulum, from which a fibrous remnant of the obliterated duct frequently extends to the umbilicus.

The diverticulum may have a broad or narrow base from the ileum and is always on the antimesenteric surface, from 40 to 95 cm proximal to the ileocecal valve. It is usually from 2 to 4 cm in diameter but occasionally can be huge. It lies in the middle or lower abdomen, preponderantly, but not always, on the right side (Fig. 12–96). The incidence of Meckel's diverticulum in the general population is from 0.3 to 2.0 per cent.[14]

The diverticulum contains all layers of the small intestine and has contractile activities similar to those of a normal small intestinal loop. Ectopic gastric mucosa in varying amounts is found in 15 to 50 per cent of cases.[8, 15] Often the gastric mucosa extends into the adjacent ileal mucosa. Rarely, ectopic pancreatic tissue is also present.

The overwhelming majority of Meckel's diverticula are asymptomatic and are an incidental finding at surgery or autopsy. A nondiseased diverticulum is only rarely discovered on contrast studies of the gastrointestinal tract (Fig. 12–97). A number of disease processes are specifically related to Meckel's diverticulum.[3, 14] These include:

1. Peptic ulceration in ectopic gastric mucosa.
2. Inflammation with or without ulceration. Complications of perforation, abscess, and peritonitis may also occur.
3. Intussusception in which the diverticulum is the lead point.
4. Internal herniation or volvulus from entrapment of an ileal loop around the fibrous remnant of the omphalomesenteric duct.
5. Calculus (enterolith) formation within the diverticulum.

The most common (50 per cent) clinical manifestation of a diseased Meckel diverticulum is gastrointestinal bleeding caused by peptic ulceration in the ectopic gastric mucosa. As in a gastric or duodenal ulcer, the bleeding may be episodic, severe,

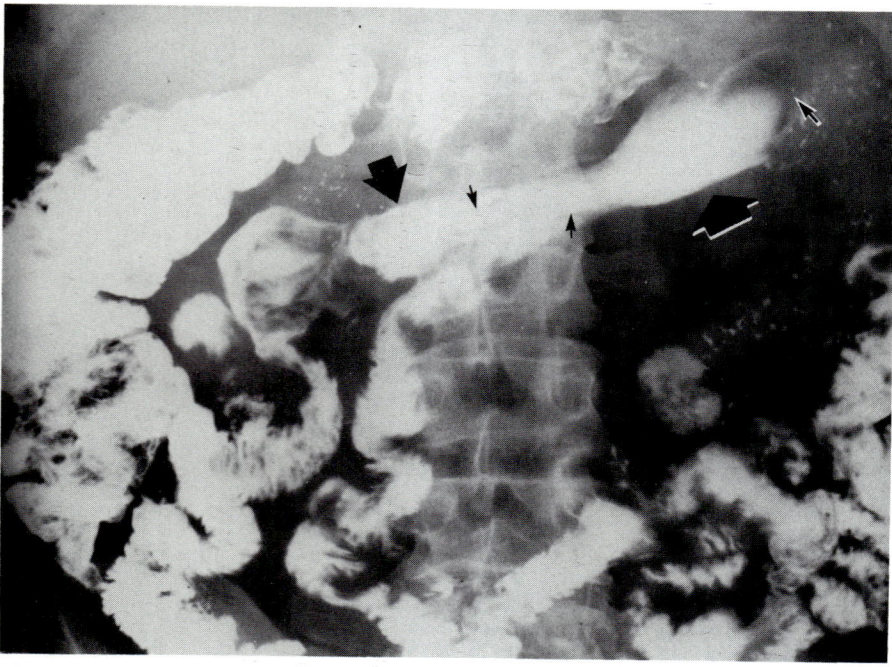

Figure 12–96. Bleeding Meckel's diverticulum. A small bowel study demonstrates a long diverticulum (large arrows) arising from the ileum on the right and extending into the left upper abdomen. Note the air (small black arrow) in the distal part of the sac. Linear gastric-like mucosa is present (small arrows).

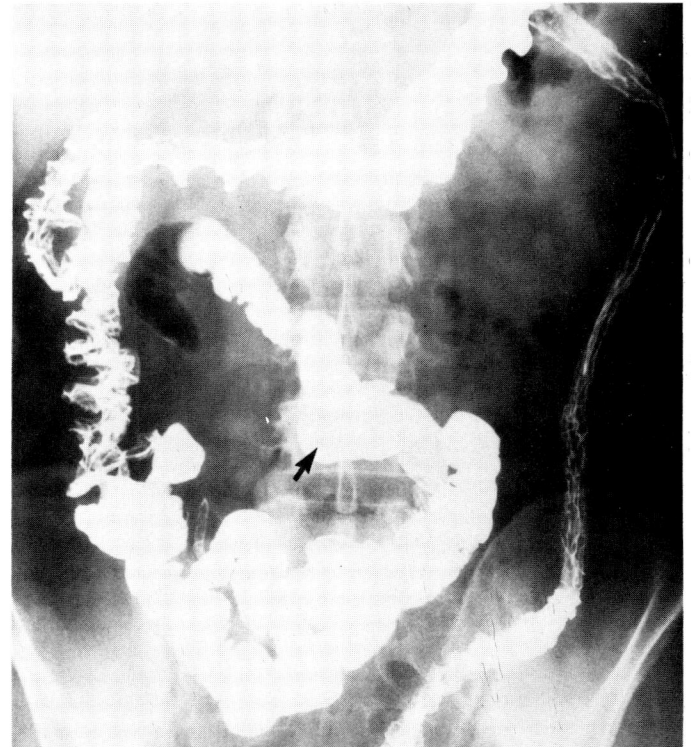

Figure 12–97. Asymptomatic Meckel's diverticulum in a 35-year-old man. On the postevacuation barium enema films, the diverticulum was transiently filled (arrow); a later small bowel study failed to demonstrate the diverticulum. The diverticulum was identified at surgery performed one year later for gallstones.

or mild. It most often occurs in children and young adults. The bleeding is generally manifested by *red* blood via rectum; tarry stools alone are uncommon.

Abdominal pain, often vague and of varying degrees of severity, may sometimes accompany the bleeding. Abdominal pain or discomfort may be the only symptom of an ulcerated or inflamed Meckel diverticulum.

Acute Meckel's diverticulitis may cause severe abdominal pain, tenderness, fever, and leukocytosis. It can closely mimic acute appendicitis, although the tenderness or inflammatory mass is more medial than in appendicitis. The acute diverticulitis, if untreated, may lead to perforation, abscess, and even a generalized peritonitis.

Clinical symptoms of acute intestinal obstruction can result from volvulus of a small bowel loop around the vitelline duct remnant or from intussusception of the diverticulum (Fig. 12–105). Obstruction represents about 25 per cent of the clinical disorders from Meckel's diverticula.

RADIOLOGIC DIAGNOSIS

The radiologic modalities employed for detection of a symptomatic Meckel diverticulum are: (1) abdominal films and barium contrast studies of the gastrointestinal tract; (2) radionuclide study with ^{99m}Tc pertechnetate; and (3) angiography.

Contrast studies of the gastrointestinal tract generally fail to demonstrate Meckel's diverticulum.[3, 10, 17] Owing to its contractility, the diverticulum usually cannot be identified or distinguished from other small bowel segments. Occasionally, on a barium enema study there may be sufficient reflux into the small bowel to permit its opacification and recognition (Fig. 12–97). An inflamed or ulcerated Meckel diverticulum frequently has decreased contractibility and may remain filled after the surrounding small bowel has emptied, enabling identification (Figs. 12–98 to 12–102). Rarely, a bleeding diverticulum may be identified by a filling defect of a clot (Fig. 12–100) or of noncalcified enteroliths.

Occasionally, a persistent collection of gas may accumulate within an inflamed Meckel diverticulum (Fig. 12–103); a small bowel study may reveal barium entering or filling the air-containing sac (see Figs. 12–96 and 12–103). The configuration, the presence of gastric-like folds, and normal adjacent small bowel distinguish it from a communicating abscess. A distended inflamed diverticulum may appear as a mass separating the small bowel loops (Fig. 12–104).

Volvulus or intussusception will appear as a nonspecific small bowel obstruction. Contrast studies will demonstrate the site of obstruction or intussusception (Fig. 12–105), but the diverticulum itself will not be identified.

The development of calculi (enteroliths) within Meckel's diverticulum is rare[5, 6] and is probably due to stasis from a narrow neck or associated chronic diverticular inflammation or both (Fig. 12–106). Single or multiple calculi are present; the latter are usually faceted. About 25 per cent are sufficiently calcified to be identified on a plain abdomen film[6] and must be differentiated from colonic enterolith, appendolith, ureteral calculus, gallstone in the gastrointestinal tract, node, or stone in a bladder diverticulum. The small bowel contrast study will usually demonstrate barium within the calculus-containing sac (Fig. 12–106).

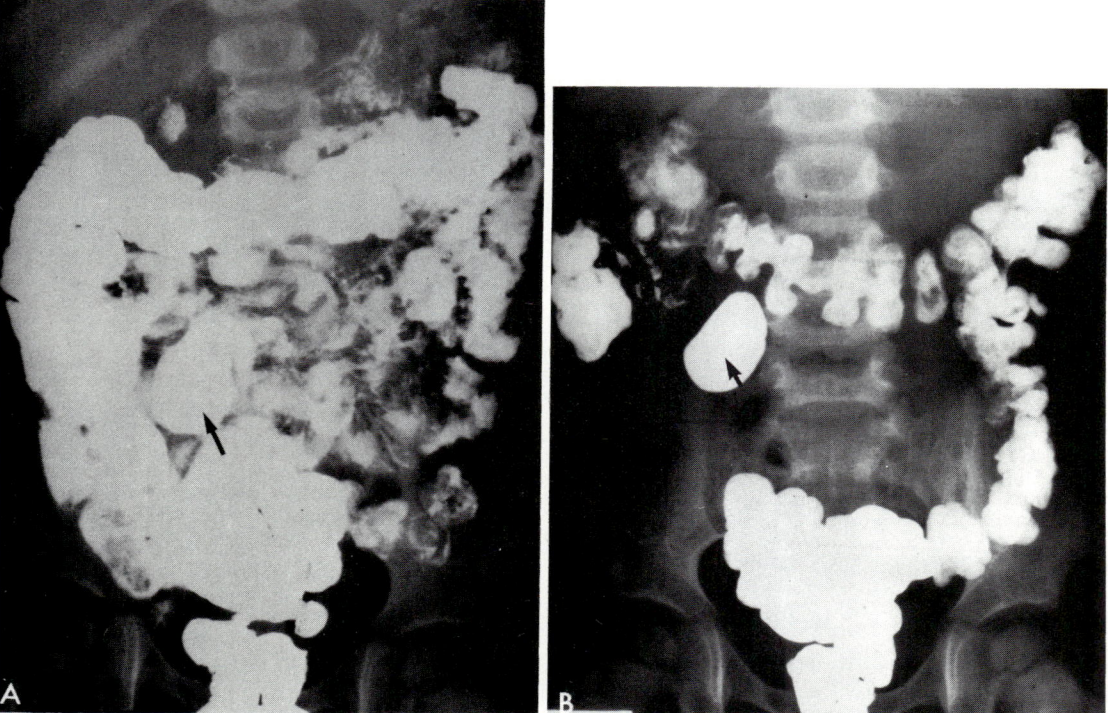

Figure 12–98. Bleeding diverticulum in a three-year-old boy. Crampy abdominal pain and red blood in stools led to an upper gastrointestinal study. The collection of barium in the Meckel's diverticulum was best seen on the 90-minute (A) and 24-hour (B) films (arrows).

THE SMALL INTESTINE — 629

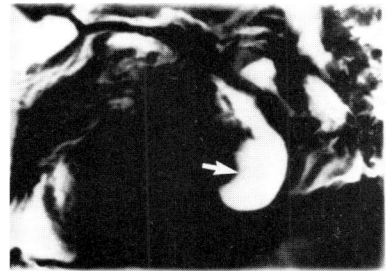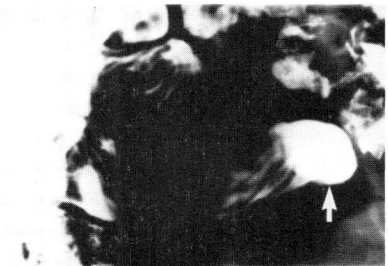

Figure 12–99. Bleeding Meckel's diverticulum in a six-year-old boy. The diverticulum in the right lower quadrant is readily identified (arrows).

Overall, the recognition of Meckel's diverticulum on barium studies is infrequent to rare. Meguid[10] emphasizes the pitifully poor yield of the barium studies, reporting no identification in 29 patients later proved to have Meckel's diverticulum.

In 11 symptomatic cases, Dalinka[3] reported identification of the diverticulum in two, both on small bowel studies. None was identified in eight asymptomatic patients.

Radionuclide diagnosis of Meckel's diverticulum can often be made, utilizing intravenously administered sodium technetium^{99m} pertechnetate.[1, 7-9, 11, 13, 15] Both normal and ectopic gastric mucosa selectively secrete the TcO$_4$ ion, probably by the same cellular mechanism that secretes the chloride ion. Only about 16 to 25 per cent of

Text continued on page 633.

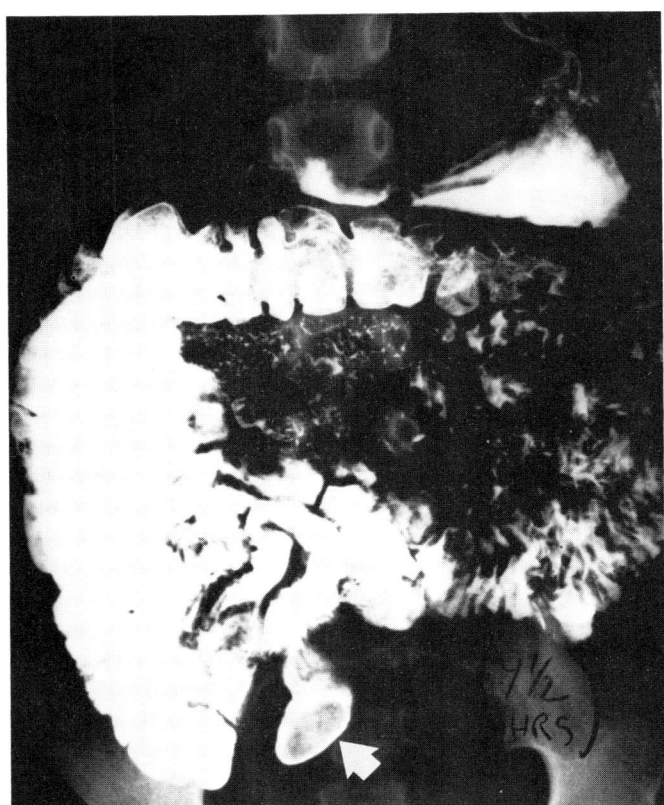

Figure 12–100. Clot in bleeding Meckel's diverticulum. The barium-filled diverticulum (arrow) in the right lower quadrant contains a lucent defect due to a clot.

630 — THE SMALL INTESTINE

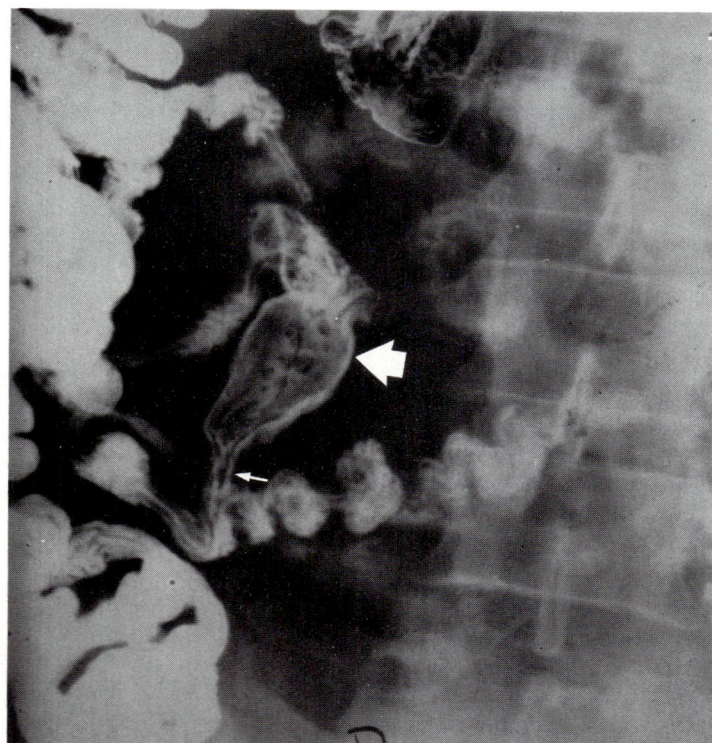

Figure 12–101. Young adult with bleeding Meckel's diverticulum. The neck (small arrow) and the diverticulum sac containing gastric-like mucosa (large arrow) are clearly identified in the right midabdomen.

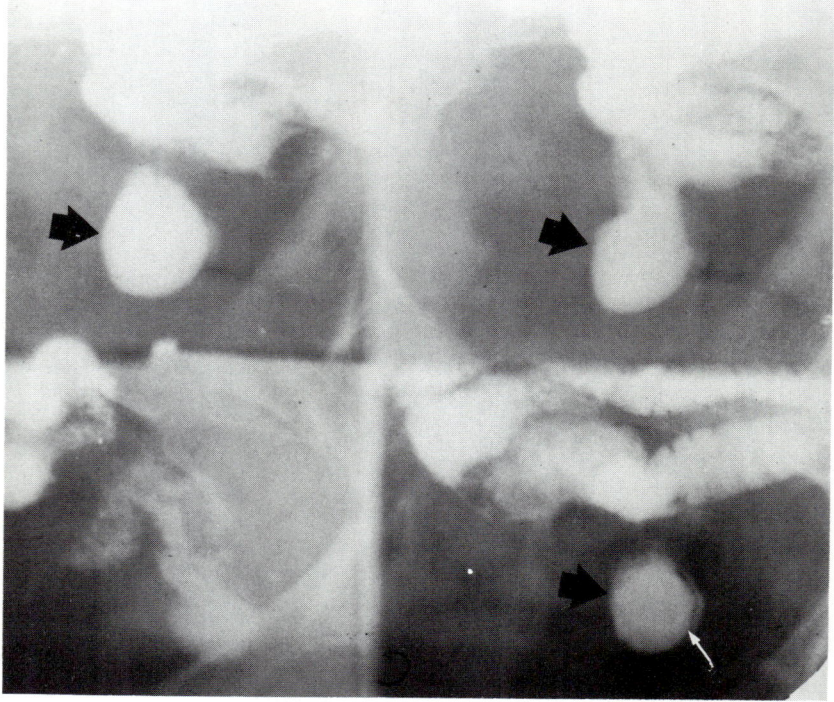

Figure 12–102. Bleeding Meckel's diverticulum in young adult. The diverticulum (black arrow) is seen on the right side of the pelvis and contains gastriclike mucosa (white arrow).

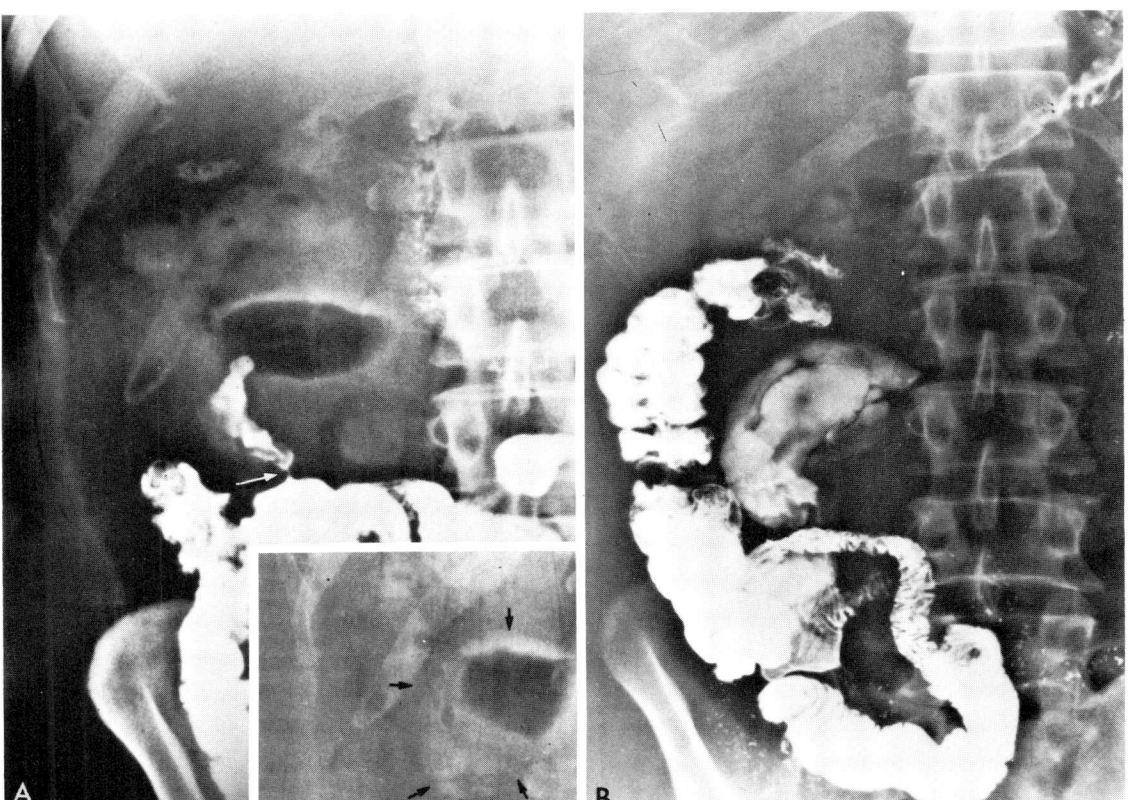

Figure 12–103. Bleeding Meckel's diverticulum in a 55-year-old man. *A,* Inset of portion of the plain film shows a gas collection beneath the right twelfth rib. After barium ingestion, a narrow tract (white arrow) is seen extending from a distal ileal loop into the gas collection. Note the gastric-type folds in the barium-filled portion of the diverticulum. *B,* Later, entire Meckel's diverticulum is filled with barium.

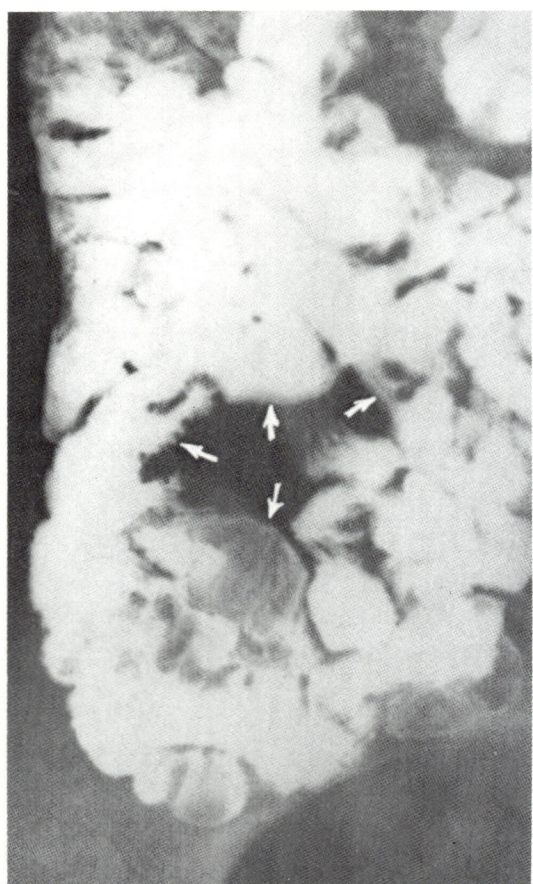

Figure 12–104. Inflamed bleeding Meckel's diverticulum in a child. The separation of the small bowel loops in the right lower quadrant (arrows) was due to a distended inflamed Meckel's diverticulum, which did not fill with barium. (*From* White, A. F., Oh, K. S., et al.: Radiologic manifestations of Meckel's diverticulum. Am. J. Roentgenol. *118:*86–94, 1973. Reproduced by permission.)

Figure 12–105. Intussusception of Meckel's diverticulum. Barium enema shows intussusception (arrows) into the ascending colon. At surgery, a Meckel's diverticulum was found to be the lead point. (*From* White, A. F., Oh, K. S., et al.: Radiologic manifestations of Meckel's diverticulum. Am. J. Roentgenol. *118:*86–94, 1973. Reproduced by permission.)

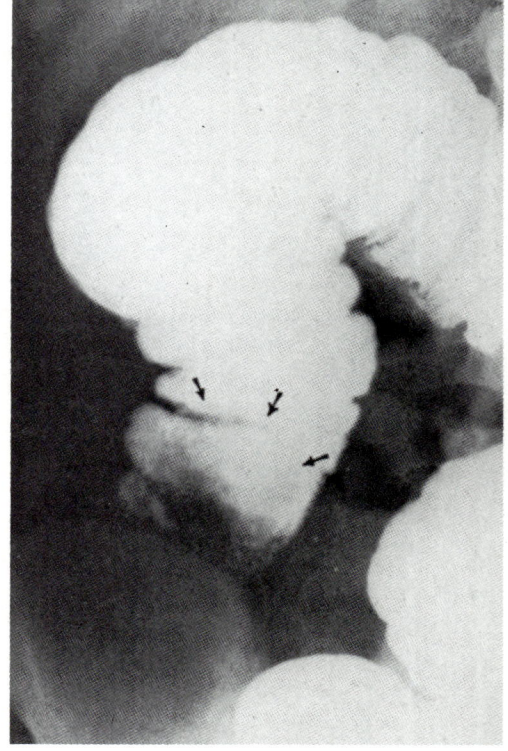

THE SMALL INTESTINE — 633

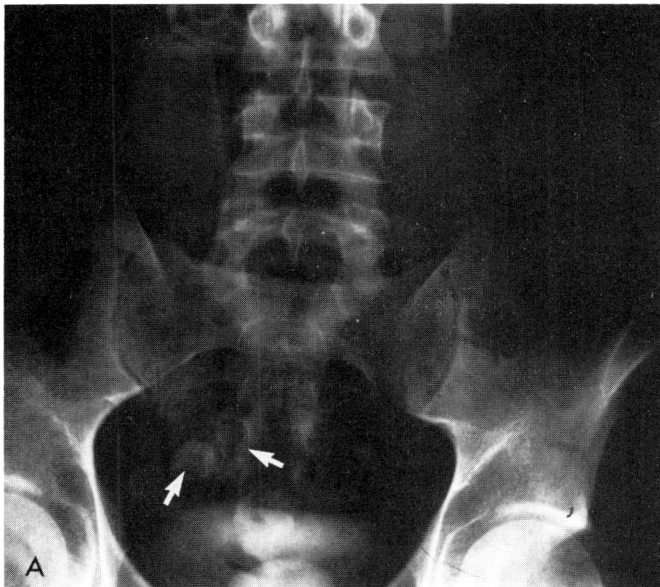

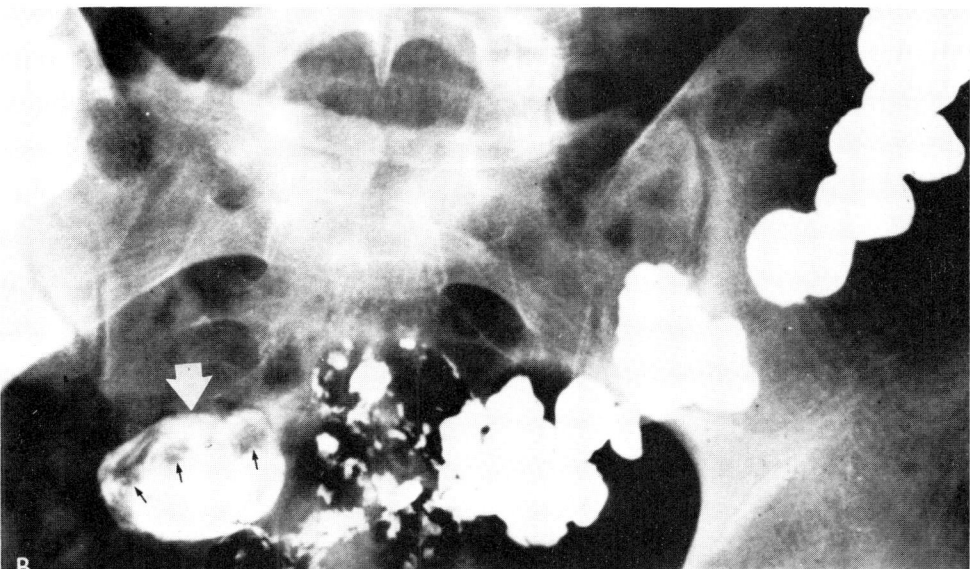

Figure 12–106. Enteroliths in Meckel's diverticulum. *A,* The faceted calculi (arrow) in the right lower quadrant are outside the urinary tract. *B,* A 24-hour film after an upper gastrointestinal study shows barium in the diverticulum (white arrow), which can be identified as completely separate from the barium-filled colon. The calculi are seen as filling defects (black arrows).

Meckel's diverticula contain sufficient ectopic gastric mucosa to produce a positive scan,[14, 15] but almost every bleeding diverticulum contains adequate ectopic mucosa for scan identification.[15] The dose of the isotope is 75 to 100 mcg per kg. Premedication with oral potassium perchlorate is often employed in order to block thyroid uptake. Scanning is generally performed at 30 to 45 minutes, 4 hours, and occasionally at 24 hours (Fig. 12–107).

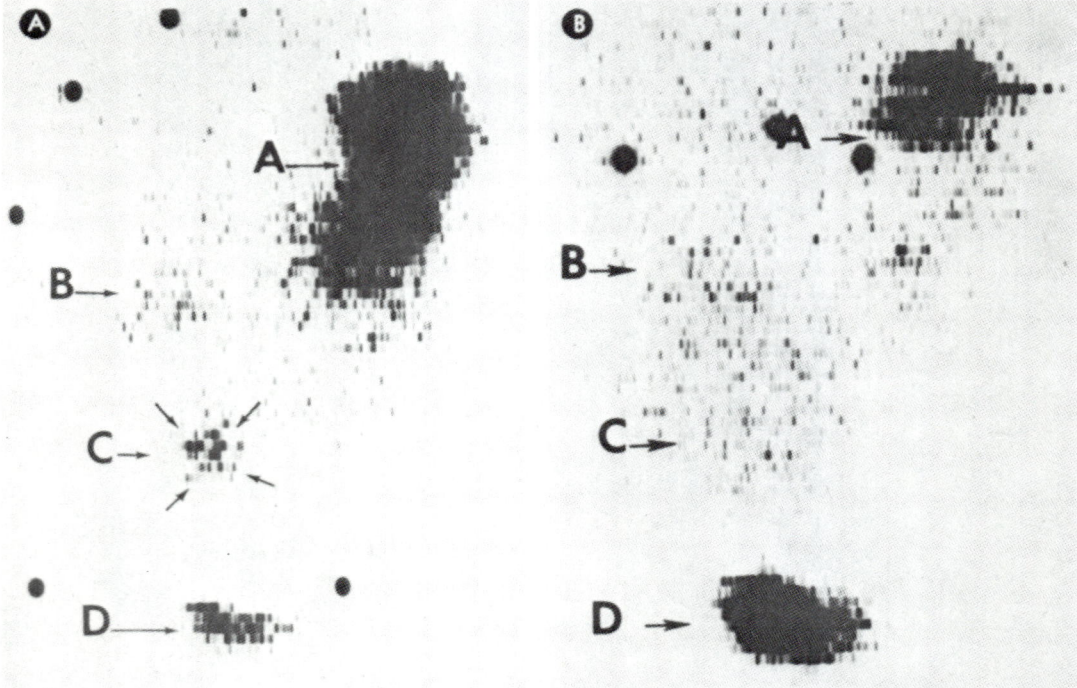
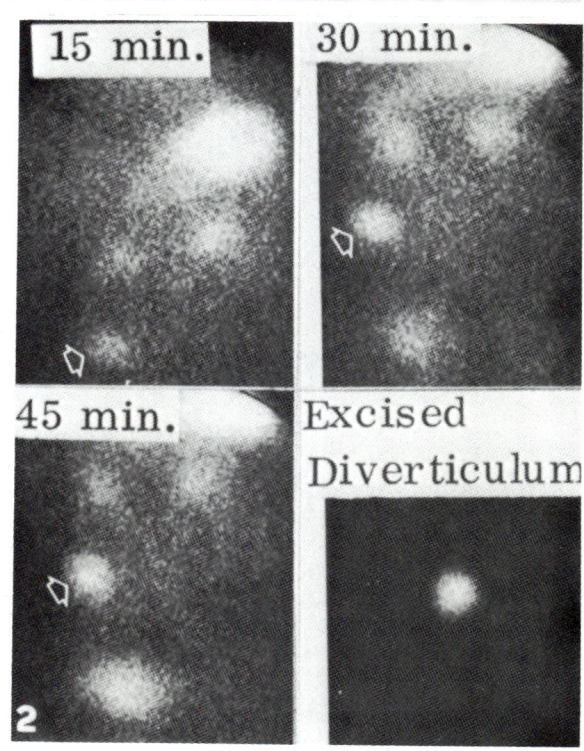

Figure 12–107. Positive technetium scans in two children with bleeding Meckel's diverticulum. A and B, In this child with rectal bleeding, the barium studies of the small bowel and colon were negative. The preoperative scan (A) shows uptake by the diverticulum at area C (arrows). On the scan made after surgical removal of the diverticulum (B), uptake at area C is no longer seen. Uptake in the stomach (A→) and duodenum (B→) and excreted technetium in the bladder (D→) are normally seen in a technetium pertechnetate scan. C, In an eight-month-old infant with rectal bleeding, the scan shows uptake of the diverticulum in the right midabdomen, beginning at 15 minutes and intensifying at 45 minutes (arrows). (A and B are from White, A: F., Oh, K. S., et al.: Radiologic manifestations of Meckel's diverticulum. Am. J. Roentgenol. 118:86–94, 1973. C is from Rosenthall, L., Henry, J. N., et al.: Radiopertechnetate imaging of Meckel's diverticulum. Radiology 105:371–373, 1972. Reproduced by permission.)

THE SMALL INTESTINE — 635

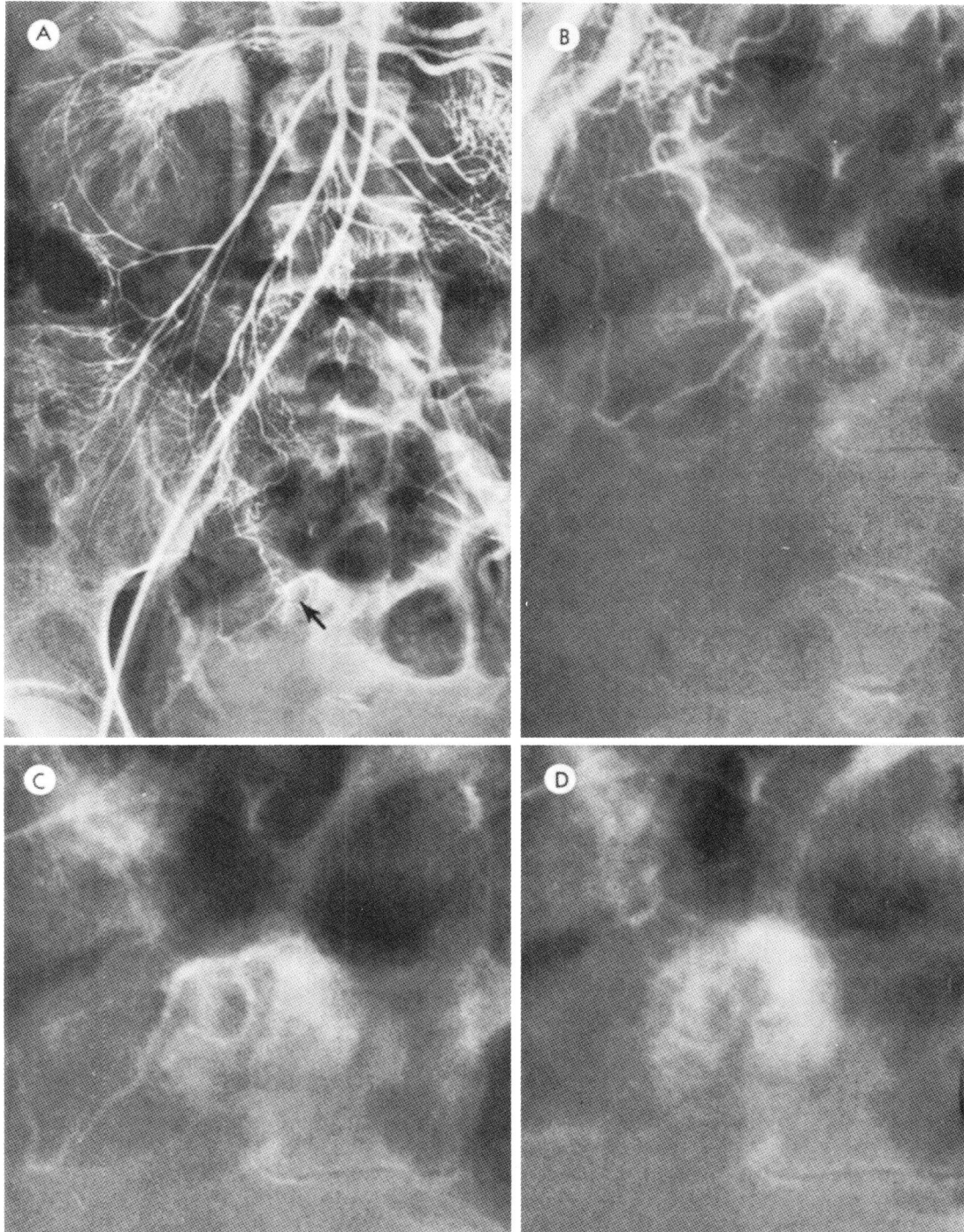

Figure 12–108. Bleeding Meckel's diverticulum; mesenteric arteriogram. *A,* An irregular vessel is seen in the ileal area (arrow). *B,* Close-up view of vessel. *C* and *D,* Later films show irregular "stain" around this vessel owing to extravasation and gastric mucosa vascularity. (*From* White, A. F., Oh, K. S., et al.: Radiologic manifestations of Meckel's diverticulum. Am. J. Roentgenol. *118:*86–94, 1973. Reproduced by permission.)

The technetium nucleotide study is a convenient noninvasive method for establishing a preoperative diagnosis of bleeding Meckel's diverticulum, since the bleeding develops in ulcerated ectopic gastric mucosa in virtually every case. Leonidas and Germann[8] had only one preoperative false negative scan in thirteen cases of bleeding Meckel's diverticula. Others have had comparable success.[1, 8, 9, 11, 15, 17]

Bequist[1] found no false positive results in 100 cases in which a search was made for Meckel's diverticulum by radioisotope scanning. However, others report false positive scans in a variety of conditions, including telangiectatic lesions of the small bowel, peptic ulceration of the small bowel, aneurysm of abdominal vessels, partial intestinal obstruction, and duplication cysts containing gastric mucosa.[9, 12, 16]

Mesenteric and celiac arteriography can be used to locate the site of bleeding if the rate of bleeding is at least 0.5 cc per minute (Fig. 12–108).[2, 4, 11] Even when Meckel's diverticulum is identified by the technetium scan in a severely bleeding patient, mesenteric arteriography is often performed to confirm that the bleeding is arising from the diverticulum.

If the bleeding rate is insufficient to demonstrate extravasation of contrast during arteriography, a focal deep capillary stain may sometimes mark the site of Meckel's diverticulum. This stain is probably in hypervascular ectopic gastric mucosa.[4] In a patient with persistent severe gastrointestinal bleeding of undetermined cause, immediate mesenteric arteriography is the most prudent procedure for identifying the site of bleeding and making the decision for therapy.

If the bleeding is mild and not life-threatening, investigation should begin with contrast studies of the upper gastrointestinal tract. Although these very rarely demonstrate the diverticulum, they serve to rule out the more common causes of gastrointestinal bleeding. Negative studies, particularly in children and young adults, should be followed by a technetium pertechnetate scan, which will prove positive in almost every case.

References

1. Bequist, T. H., Nolan, N. G., and Stephen, D. H.: Specificity of ^{99M}Tc in scintographic cases of Meckel's diverticulum. J. Nucl. Med. *16:*515, 1975.
2. Bree, R. L., and Reuter, S. R.: Angiographic demonstration of bleeding Meckel's diverticulum. Radiology *108:*287–288, 1973.
3. Dalinka, M. K., and Wunder, J. F.: Meckel's diverticulum and its complications, with emphasis on roentgen demonstration. Radiology *106:*295–298, 1973.
4. Farris, H. C., and Whitley, J. E.: Angiographic demonstration of Meckel's diverticulum. Radiology *108:*285–286, 1973.
5. Gershater, R.: Enterolith causing bleeding in a patient with Meckel's diverticulum. Radiology *120:*327–328, 1976.
6. Hirschy, J. C., Thorpe, J. J., and Cortese, A. F.: Meckel's stones. Radiology *119:*19–20, 1976.
7. Ho, J. E., and Kunieczny, K. M.: Sodium pertechnetate Tc 99 M scan: an aid in evaluation of gastrointestinal bleeding. Pediatrics *56:*34–40, 1975.
8. Leonidas, J. C., and Germann, D. R.: Technetium-99M pertechnetate imaging in diagnosis of Meckel's diverticulum. Arch. Dis. Child. *49:*21–26, 1974.
9. Martin, G. I., Kutner, F. R., and Moser, L.: Diagnosis of Meckel's diverticulum by radioisotope scanning. Pediatrics *57:*11–12, 1976.
10. Meguid, M. M., Wilkinson, R. H., et al.: Futility of barium sulfate in diagnosis of bleeding Meckel's diverticulum. Arch. Surg. *108:*361–362, 1974.
11. Muroff, L. R., Casarella, W. J., and Johnson, P. M.: Preoperative diagnosis of Meckel's diverticulum. J.A.M.A. *229:*1900–1902, 1974.
12. Rodgers, B. M., and Youssef, S.: False positive scan for Meckel's diverticulum. J. Pediatr. *87:*239–240, 1975.
13. Rosenthall, L., Henry, J. N., et al.: Radiopertechnetate imaging of Meckel's diverticulum. Radiology *105:*371–373, 1972.

14. Sabiston, D. C. (ed.): Davis-Christopher Textbook of Surgery. Ed. 11. Philadelphia, W. B. Saunders Company, 1977, p. 1042.
15. Schusseim, A., and Levy, L. M.: Pre-operative diagnosis of bleeding Meckel's diverticulum. J. Pediatr. 82:45, 1973.
16. Siddiqui, A., Ryo, U. Y., and Pinsky, S. M.: A-V malformation simulating Meckel's diverticulum on ^{99m}Tc-pertechnetate abdominal scintigraphy. Radiology 122:173–174, 1977.
17. White, A. F., Oh, K. S., et al.: Radiologic manifestations of Meckel's diverticulum. Am. J. Roentgenol. 118:86–94, 1973.

Part IX

Radiology after Intestinal Bypass Surgery for Morbid Obesity

MATHIS P. FRICK, M.D.
EUGENE GEDGAUDAS, M.D.

INTRODUCTION

Intestinal bypass procedures have become established in recent years as a method of treating morbid exogenous obesity.[2, 7, 8, 13–16, 20, 29, 46, 48–50, 52, 54, 55, 57, 58, 70] In gastric bypass, a small proximal gastric pouch and a narrow gastrojejunostomy (approximately 0.8 to 1.2 cm in diameter) limit food intake. About 80 to 90 per cent of the distal stomach is bypassed.[15, 36, 70] Jejunoileal bypass (JIB), as described by Payne and DeWind[48, 49] and others,[10, 24, 46, 54] reduces the absorptive surface of the small bowel. Many complications after intestinal bypass[5, 21–24, 30, 34, 35, 38, 44] are diagnosed by radiologic means. Knowledge of typical normal and abnormal postoperative radiographic findings is essen-

TYPICAL RADIOGRAPHIC FINDINGS FOLLOWING INTESTINAL BYPASS

Stomach

Gastric bypass resembles a Billroth II procedure.[15, 36, 37] Several features should be evaluated radiographically, including the width and appearance of the gastrojejunostomy, the size and rate of emptying of the proximal gastric pouch, and the diameter and mucosal pattern of the jejunum. Initially, the stoma should be studied with a small amount of barium. Extreme left anterior oblique or left lateral projections demonstrate the stoma to best advantage (Fig. 12–109A). The afferent loop usually can be identified, but nonfilling is not necessarily pathologic. Incomplete filling of the distal gastric pouch may rarely mimic extravasation.[15]

Small Bowel

Following JIB, several features should be evaluated radiographically, including the type of anastomosis, transit time, appearance of mucosa, approximate length and

638 — THE SMALL INTESTINE

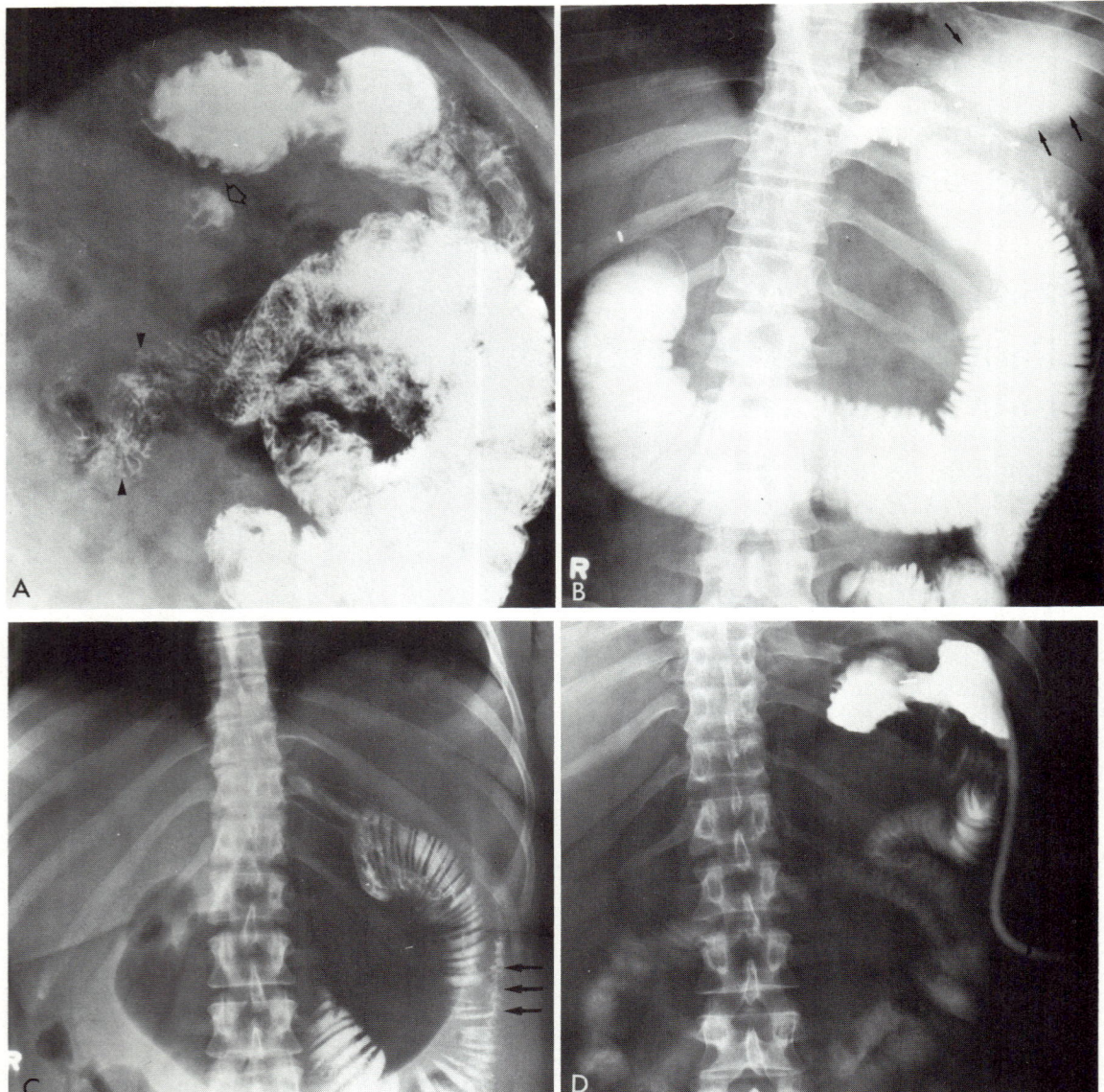

Figure 12–109. Gastric bypass. *A*, Left anterior oblique position demonstrates the proximal gastric pouch and gastrojejunostomy. Note partial filling of the afferent loop (closed arrows) and distal gastric pouch (open arrow). *B*, Partial obstruction at gastrojejunostomy, similar to that shown in C. Leaky anastomosis in distal gastric pouch causes extravasation of contrast into the left subphrenic space (arrows). *C*, Partial obstruction at gastrojejunostomy. There is preferential filling of distended afferent loop and poor filling of efferent loop (arrows). Note the air-distended distal gastric pouch. *D*, Leakage at site of gastrojejunostomy. Fistulogram shows communication of left subphrenic abscess cavity with gastric pouch and efferent loop.

degree of dilatation of functioning small bowel, distribution of air-fluid levels, and presence and extent of reflux into the bypassed segment.

Accurate assessment of transit time requires serial radiographs at five-minute intervals after barium ingestion. The patient's size may prohibit spot filming. However, the anastomosis is usually well demonstrated on overhead radiographs (Fig.

12–110A) Barium should be followed beyond the stoma of the bypassed segment, which may empty into the cecum or into the transverse or left colon, depending on the surgical procedure.

Normal transit times from pylorus to cecum are shortened to five to ten minutes (Fig. 12–110A). The functioning small bowel segment increases in length and caliber following JIB in the majority of patients (Fig. 12–110A).[3, 43, 50, 67] Postoperative mucosal hypertrophy is seen in about 85 per cent of cases (Fig. 12–110A).[3, 18] Those changes limited to the terminal ileum have been termed jejunization.[3, 67] If the radiographic appearance of the distal ileum approaches that of the colon, this is called colonization.[3, 67]

Air-fluid levels are expected postoperatively in large or small bowel or both in approximately 90 per cent of patients[3, 67] and should not be misdiagnosed as bowel obstruction (Fig. 12–111). Increased air-fluid levels in the small bowel alone are rare.[67]

A small amount of reflux into the bypassed small bowel segment after Payne's procedure is common and not significant (see Fig. 12–110B).[3, 72]

Colon

Dilatation of the colon to a diameter of more than 7 cm is seen in half of patients following JIB (Fig. 12–111).[4, 24, 43] Megacolon is considered a normal postoperative finding[67]; however, differentiation from neurogenic or toxic megacolon is necessary. Unlike toxic megacolon, the margins of megacolon after JIB are regular and not

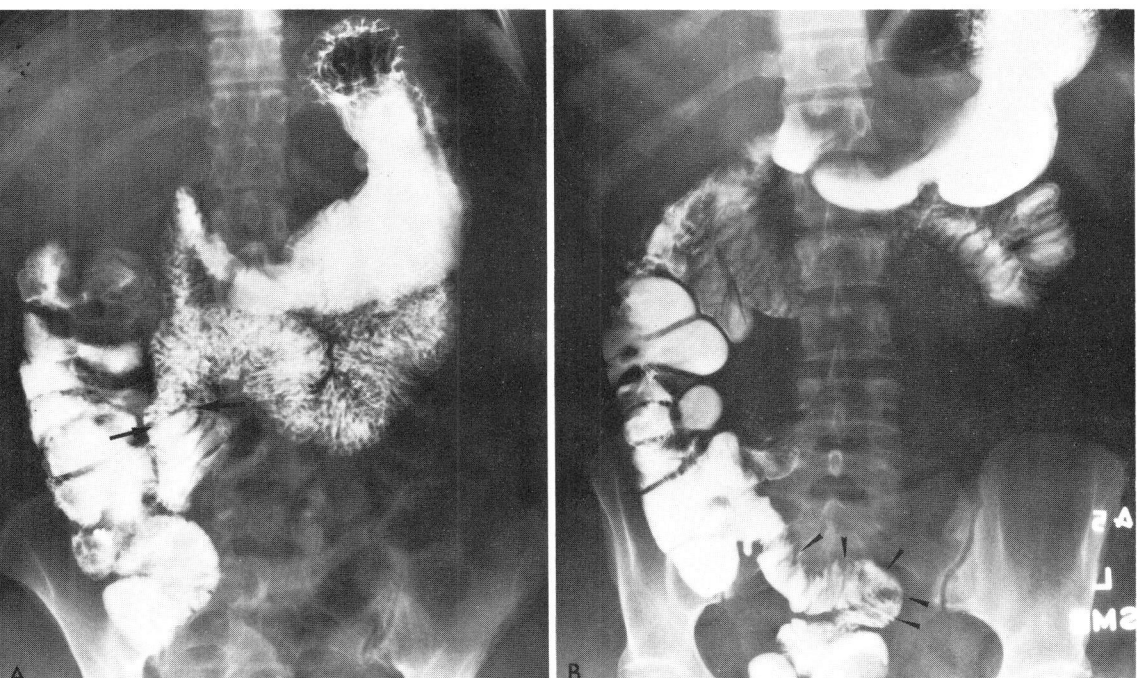

Figure 12–110. *A,* Jejunoileal bypass (Scott procedure) with end-to-end jejunoileostomy (arrow). Normal transit time (~ten minutes). Note dilatation and mucosal hypertrophy of jejunum. (Incidentally a benign gastric ulcer is seen.) *B,* There is moderate reflux through ileocecostomy into bypassed ileum (arrows).

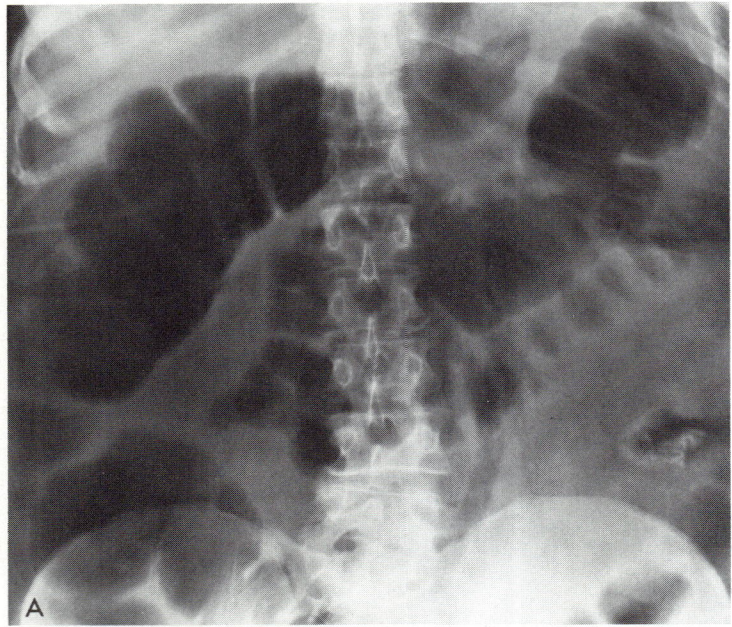
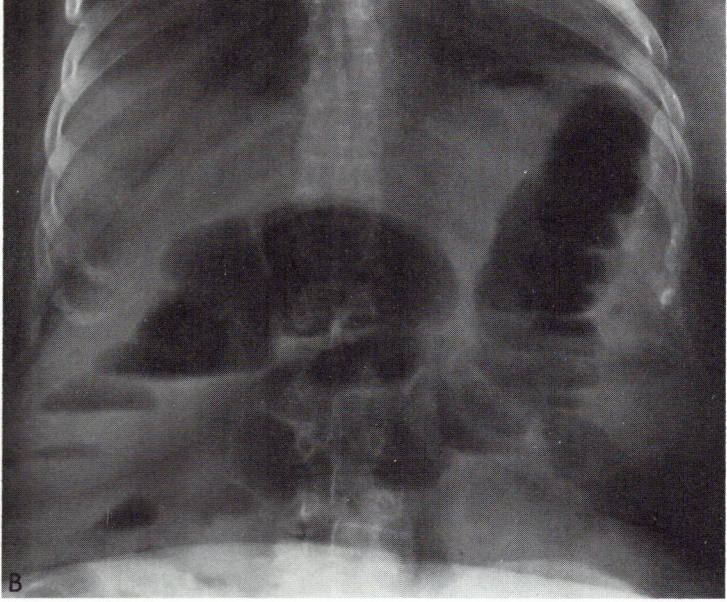

Figure 12–111. Flat (*A*) and upright (*B*) abdominal radiograph after jejunoileal bypass. Multiple air-fluid levels are seen in small bowel and colon. There is colonic distention (megacolon) but not obstruction.

ulcerated. Recognition of this "pseudo-obstruction" avoids unnecessary re-exploration.[4, 43, 45, 67]

Gallbladder

An oral cholecystogram after JIB may fail to visualize a normal gallbladder, since the surface area for absorption of contrast is reduced.[67, 71] Therefore, following JIB all patients should take the biliary agent for two consecutive days prior to imaging.

RADIOGRAPHIC EVALUATION OF POSTOPERATIVE COMPLICATIONS

Early Complications after Gastric Bypass and Jejunoileal Bypass

A major complication after gastric bypass or JIB in the early postoperative period is leakage at the site of the anastomosis (see Fig. 12–109D). Radiographic examinations usually require the use of a water-soluble contrast agent.

Obstruction at the anastomosis causes distention of the proximal gastric pouch or afferent loop after gastric bypass (see Fig. 12–109B and C) or marked distention of pre-anastomotic loops after JIB (see Fig. 12–114).

Late Complications after Gastric Bypass

Late complications after gastric bypass are similar to those after Billroth II procedures and include esophagitis, gastritis, and stomal ulceration. A major complication is an ulcer at the gastrojejunostomy, a finding reported in 1 to 2 per cent of patients.[15, 37] An old scarred ulcer may obstruct the gastroenterostomy and enlarge the proximal gastric pouch with or without bezoar formation.[15]

Failure to lose weight may be caused by enlargement of the proximal gastric pouch or dilatation of the gastrojejunostomy. Stomal widening results in faster emptying of the proximal gastric pouch and marked increase in the size of the jejunum, which then assumes gastric reservoir function.[37]

Late Complications after Jejunoileal Bypass

The most common late postoperative complication after JIB is bowel obstruction, occurring in about 3 to 10 per cent of patients.[8, 43] Barium enema examinations with small bowel reflux usually exclude obstruction of functioning or bypassed bowel segments (Fig. 12–112B).

Obstruction of the functioning segment may be due to narrowing or volvulus at the anastomotic site, incarceration of an external or internal hernia (through a mesenteric defect), and very rarely, adhesions.[43] Radiographically, there is marked distention of pre-anastomotic small bowel loops (Fig. 12–113).

Obstruction of the bypassed segment is usually caused by intussusception of the bypassed ileal segment into the colon—a complication occurring in 0.5 to 4.0 per cent of patients.[63] A "pseudotumor" or a separation of surgical clips is the most common presentation on abdominal plain radiographs.[63]

"Bypass enteropathy"[19] or "bypass enteritis"[47] is characterized by increased diarrhea, diffuse abdominal tenderness, and fever. The presumed etiology is overgrowth of enteric bacteria in the bypassed bowel. Treatment is conservative.[19, 47] Plain radiographs of the abdomen exhibit distended loops in the bypassed segment with air-fluid levels. There may be associated pneumatosis intestinalis. Pneumatosis[23, 31, 35, 47, 61, 69]—with or without pneumoperitoneum—is not a specific radiographic finding of "bypass enteritis" and may be encountered in asymptomatic patients after JIB (Fig. 12–114).[23] Pneumatosis may involve the bypassed ileum,[31] the functioning small bowel,[69] or the colon.[23]

Ultimate failure to lose weight may be caused by reflux into long segments of

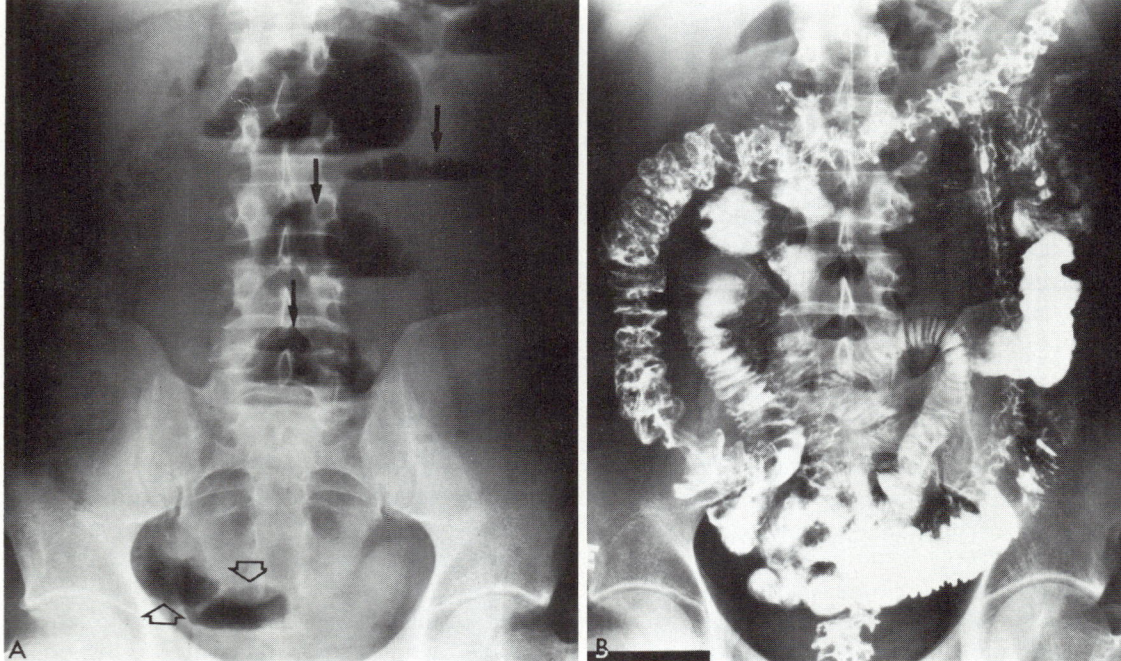

Figure 12–112. *A,* Multiple air-fluid levels in functioning (closed arrows) and bypassed small bowel (open arrows). *B,* Barium enema with reflux into functioning and bypassed segments. No obstruction is present.

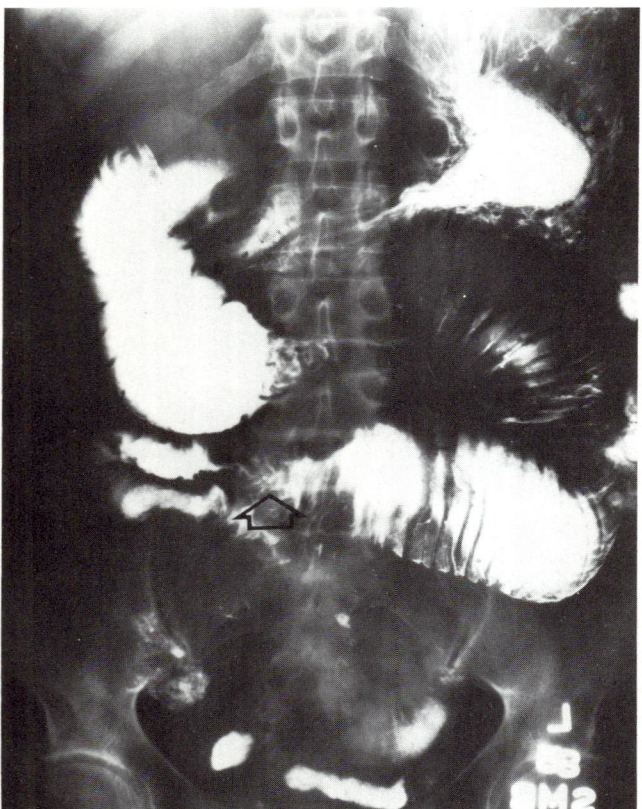

Figure 12–113. Adhesions (open arrow) causing partial obstruction of the functioning small bowel segment.

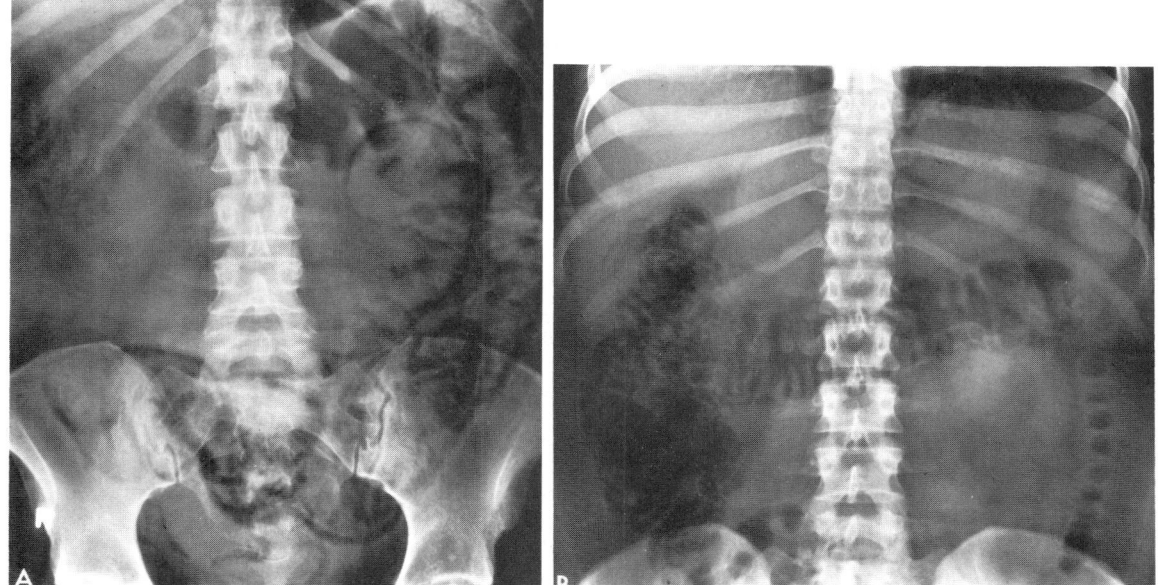

Figure 12–114. A and B, Pneumatosis intestinalis in two patients after jejunoileal bypass. (Courtesy of Samuel E. Feinberg, M.D.)

bypassed small bowel, particularly in association with slow emptying of these segments (Fig. 12–115).[3, 72]

Other intra-abdominal complications after JIB include an increased incidence of cholelithiasis,[71] cholecystitis,[2, 25, 50, 71] and various forms of liver failure.[1, 8]

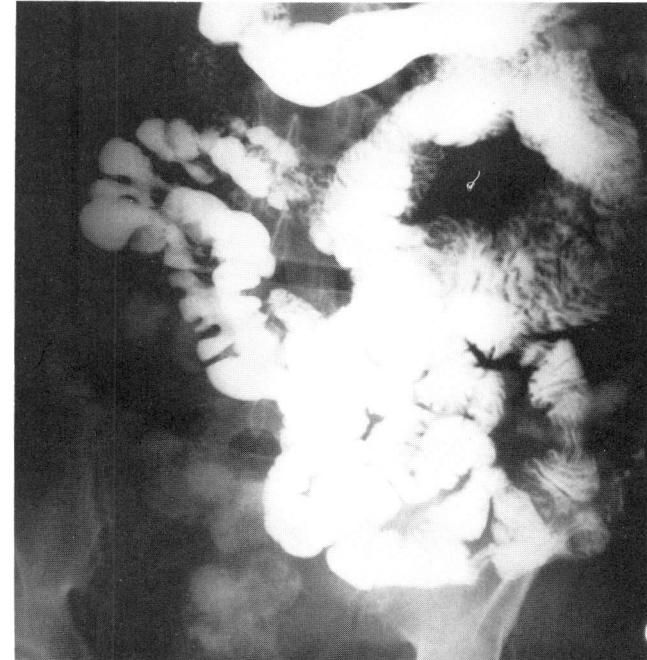

Figure 12–115. Massive reflux into bypassed segment may account for the patient's failure to lose weight.

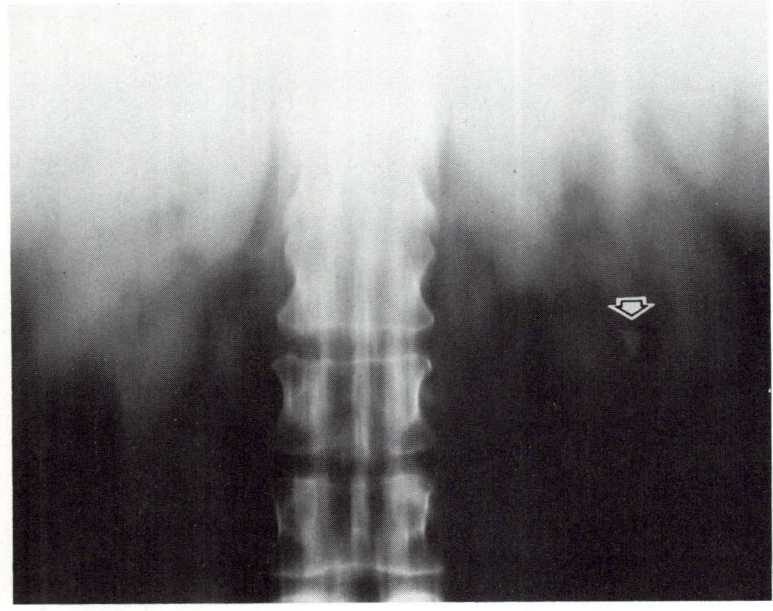

Figure 12–116. Calcium oxalate stone in left renal collecting system (arrow) after jejunoileal bypass.

Urinary tract stones, apparently due to increased urinary excretion of oxalate, develop in 3 to 30 per cent of patients after JIB (Fig. 12–116).[17, 26, 41, 45, 66, 72]

Arthritis is a complication of JIB in 25 to 30 per cent of patients.[40, 59, 68] It may involve sacroiliac joints symmetrically, similar to arthritis associated with ulcerative colitis or Crohn's disease.[9, 28, 42, 53]

References

1. Andreassy, M. R. J., Haff, R. C., and Lobritz, R. W.: Liver failure after jejunoileal shunt. Arch. Surg. 110:332, 1975.
2. Baber, J. C., Hayden, W. F., and Thompson, B. W.: Intestinal bypass operations for obesity. Am. J. Surg. 126:769–772, 1973.
3. Balthazar, E. J., and Goldfine, S.: Jejunileal bypass. Roentgenographic observations. Am. J. Roentgenol. 125:138–142, 1975.
4. Barry, R. E., Benfield, J. E., and Bray, G. A.: Colonic pseudo-obstruction: a new complication of jejunoileal bypass. Clin. Res. 23:391A, 1975.
5. Bondar, G. F., and Pisesky, W.: Complications of small intestinal short-circuiting for obesity. Arch. Surg. 94:707–716, 1967.
6. Booth, C. C.: The metabolic effects of intestinal resection in man. Postgrad. Med. J. 37:725–739, 1961.
7. Braasch, J. W.: The surgical treatment of obesity: a study in applied physiology. Surg. Clin. North Am. 51:667–673, 1971.
8. Bray, G. A.: Intestinal bypass operation as a treatment for obesity. Ann. Intern. Med. 85:97, 1976.
9. Brewerton, D. A., Caffrey, M., and Nicholls, A.: HL-A 27 and arthropathies associated with ulcerative colitis and psoriasis. Lancet 1:956–958, 1974.
10. Brill, A. B., Sandstead, H. H., and Price, R.: Changes in body composition after jejunoileal bypass in morbidly obese patients. Am. J. Surg. 123:49–56, 1972.
11. Brown, R. G., O'Leary, J. P., and Woodward, E. R.: Hepatic effects of jejunoileal bypass for morbid obesity. Am. J. Surg. 127:53–58, 1974.
12. Buchanan, R., and Wilkins, R.: Arthritis after jejunoileostomy. Arthritis Rheum. 15:644–645, 1972.
13. Buchwald, H., Varco, B. L., Moore, R. B., et al.: Intestinal bypass procedures: partial ileal bypass for hyperlipidemia and jejunoileal bypass for obesity. Curr. Probl. Surg. 1–51, 1975.
14. Buchwald, H., Schwartz, M. Z., and Varco, R. L.: Surgical treatment of obesity. Adv. Surg. 235, 1975.
15. Cohen, W. N., Mason, E. E., and Blommers, T.: Gastric bypass for morbid obesity. Radiology 122:609–612, 1977.

16. DeMuth, W. E., and Rottenstein, H. S.: Death associated with hypocalcemia after small bowel short circuiting. N. Engl. J. Med. 270:1239–1240, 1964.
17. Dickstein, S. S., and Frame, B.: Urinary tract calculi after intestinal shunt operations for the treatment of obesity. Surg. Gynecol. Obstet. 136:257–260, 1973.
18. Dowling, R. H., and Booth, C. C.: Functional compensation after small bowel resection in man: demonstration by direct measurement. Lancet 2:146–147, 1966.
19. Drenick, F. J., Ament, M. F., Finegold, S. M., et al.: Bypass enteropathy: intestinal and systemic manifestations following small-bowel bypass. J.A.M.A. 236:269, 1976.
20. Drenick, E. J., Simmons, F., and Murphy, J. F.: Effect on hepatic morphology of treatment of obesity by fasting, reducing diets and small bowel bypass. N. Engl. J. Med. 282:829–834, 1970.
21. Editorial: Complications of intestinal bypass for obesity. J.A.M.A. 200:158, 1967.
22. Editorial: Obesity, small-bowel bypass and liver disease. N. Engl. J. Med. 282:870, 1970.
23. Feinberg, S. B., Schwartz, M. Z., Clifford, S., et al.: Significance of pneumatosis cystoides intestinalis after jejunoileal bypass. Am. J. Surg. 133:149–152, 1977.
24. Fikri, E., and Cassella, R. R.: Jejunoileal bypass for massive obesity: results and complications in fifty-two patients. Ann. Surg. 179:460–464, 1974.
25. Gazet, J-C., Pilkington, T. R. E., Kalucy, R. S., et al.: Treatment of gross obesity by jejunal bypass. Br. Med. J. 4:311–314, 1974.
26. Gregory, J. G., Starkloff, E. B., Miyai, K., et al.: Urologic complications of ileal bypass operation for morbid obesity. J. Urol. 113:521–524, 1975.
27. Harmon, J. W., Aliapoulos, M., and Braasch, J. W.: The excluded small-bowel segment. A source of complications after small-bowel bypass. Arch. Surg. 111:953–954, 1976.
28. Haslock, I., and Wright, V.: The arthritis associated with intestinal disease. Bull. Rheum. Dis. 24:750, 1973.
29. Hirsch, J.: Jejunoileal shunt for obesity. N. Engl. J. Med. 290:962–963, 1974.
30. Holzbach, R. T., Wieland, R. G., and Lieber, C. S.: Hepatic lipid in morbid obesity. Assessment at and subsequent to jejunoileal bypass. N. Engl. J. Med. 290:296–299, 1974.
31. Ikard, R. W.: Pneumatosis cystoides intestinalis following intestinal bypass. Am. Surg. 43:467–470, 1977.
32. Jewell, W. R., Hermreck, A. S., and Hardin, C. A.: Complications of jejunoileal bypass for morbid obesity. Arch. Surg. 110:1039–1042, 1975.
33. Kaufmann, W.: Intussusception—a late complication of small bowel bypass for obesity. J.A.M.A. 202:1147, 1967.
34. Lewis, L. A., Turnbull, R. B., and Page, I. H.: Effects of jejunocolic shunt on obesity, serum lipoproteins, lipids, and electrolytes. Arch. Intern. Med. 117:4–16, 1966.
35. Martyak, S. N., and Curtis, L. E.: Pneumatosis intestinalis. A complication of jejunoileal bypass. J.A.M.A. 235:1038–1039, 1976.
36. Mason, E. E., and Ito, C.: Gastric bypass. Ann. Surg. 170:329–339, 1969.
37. Mason, E. E., Printen, K. J., and Hartford, C. E.: Optimizing results of gastric bypass. Ann. Surg. 182:405–414, 1975.
38. Mason, E. E., and Printen, K. J.: Metabolic considerations in reconstitution of the small intestine after jejunoileal bypass. Surg. Gynecol. Obstet. 142:177–183, 1976.
39. McGill, D. B., Humpherys, S. R., and Baggenstoss, A. H.: Cirrhosis and death after jejunoileal shunt. Gastroenterology 63:872–877, 1972.
40. Mir-Madjlessi, S. H., Mackenzie, A. H., and Winkelmann, E. I.: Articular complications in obese patients after jejunocolic bypass. Cleveland Clin. Quart. 41:119, 1974.
41. Mobley, J. E., and Hardison, W.: Nephrolithiasis following intestinal bypass for obesity. Urology 3:639–641, 1974.
42. Morris, R. I., Metzger, A. L., and Bluestone, R. M.: Use of HLA-A-W27 in arthropathies of inflammatory bowel disease. N. Engl. J. Med. 290:1117–1119, 1974.
43. Moss, A. A., Goldberg, H. I., and Koeler, R. E.: Radiographic evaluation of complications after jejunoileal bypass surgery. Am. J. Roentgenol. 127:737–741, 1976.
44. Moxley, R. T., Pozefsky, T., and Lockwood, D. H.: Protein nutrition and liver disease after jejunoileal bypass for morbid obesity. N. Engl. J. Med., 290:921–926, 1974.
45. O'Leary, J. P., Thomas, W. C., and Woodward, E. R.: Urinary tract stone after small bowel bypass for morbid obesity. Am. J. Surg. 127:142–147, 1974.
46. Pace, W. G., Large, J. W., and Thomford, N. R.: A modification of the jejunoileal bypass. Am. Surg. 128:631–632, 1974.
47. Passard, E., Drenick, E., and Wilson, S. F.: Bypass enteritis. A new complication of jejunoileal bypass for obesity. Am. Surg. 131:169, 1976.
48. Payne, J. H., DeWind, L. T., and Commond, R. R.: Metabolic observations in patients with jejunocolic shunts. Am. J. Surg. 106:273–289, 1963.
49. Payne, J. H., and DeWind, L. T.: Surgical treatment of obesity. Am. J. Surg. 118:141–147, 1969.
50. Payne, J. H., DeWind, L. T., Schwab, C. E., et al.: Surgical treatment of morbid obesity: sixteen years of experience. Arch. Surg. 106:432–437, 1973.
51. Quaade, F., Juhl, E., Feldt-Rasmussen, K., et al.: Blind-loop reflux in relation to weight loss in obese patients treated with jejunoileal anastomosis. Scand. J. Gastroenterol. 6:537–541, 1971.

52. Randolph, J. G., Weintraub, W. H., and Rigg, A.: Jejunoileal bypass for morbid obesity in adolescents. J. Pediatr. Surg. 9:341–345, 1974.
53. Rose, E., Espinoza, L. R., and Osterland, O. K.: Intestinal bypass arthritis: association with circulating immune complexes and HLA B27. J. Rheumatol. 4:129–134, 1977.
54. Salmon, P. A.: The results of small intestinal bypass operation for the treatment of obesity. Surg. Gynecol. Obstet. 132:965–979, 1971.
55. Schwartz, M., Varco, R., and Buchwald, H.: Preoperative preparation, operative technique, and postoperative care of patients undergoing jejunoileal bypass for massive exogenous obesity. J. Surg. Res. 14:147–150, 1973.
56. Scott, H. W., Law, D. H., Sandstead, H. H., et al.: Jejunoileal shunt in surgical treatment of morbid obesity. Ann. Surg. 171:770–782, 1970.
57. Scott, H. W., and Law, D. H., IV: Clinical appraisal of jejunoileal shunt in patients with morbid obesity. Am. J. Surg. 117:246–253, 1969.
58. Scott, H. W., Sandstead, H. H., Brill, A. B., et al.: Experience with new technique of intestinal bypass in treatment of morbid obesity. Ann. Surg. 174:560–572, 1971.
59. Shagrin, J. W., Frame, B., and Dunca, H.: Polyarthritis in obese patients with intestinal bypass. Ann. Intern. Med. 75:377–380, 1971.
60. Shibata, H. R., MacKenzie, J. R., and Long, R. C.: Metabolic effects of controlled jejunocolic bypass. Arch. Surg. 95:413–428, 1967.
61. Sicard, G. A., Vaughan, R., and Wise, L.: Pneumatosis cystoides intestinalis: an unusual complication of jejunoileal bypass. Surgery 79:480–484, 1976.
62. Solow, C., Silberfarb, P. M., and Swift, K.: Psychosocial effects of intestinal bypass surgery for severe obesity. N. Engl. J. Med. 290:300–304, 1974.
63. Starkloff, G. B., Shively, R. A., and Gregory, J. G.: Jejunal intussusception following small bowel bypass for morbid obesity. Ann. Surg. 185:386–390, 1977.
64. Starkloff, G. B., Donovan, J. P., Ramach, K. R., et al.: Metabolic intestinal surgery. Arch. Surg. 110:652–657, 1975.
65. Tanga, M. R., Waddel, W. G., and Wellington, J. I.: Jejunal intussusception: a complication of small bowel bypass for intractable obesity. Can. J. Surg. 13:168–169, 1970.
66. Vainder, M., and Kelly, J.: Renal tubular dysfunction secondary to jejunoileal bypass. J.A.M.A. 235:1257–1258, 1976.
67. Wade, D. H., Richards, V., and Burhenne, H. J.: Radiographic changes after small bowel bypass for morbid obesity. Radiol. Clin. North Am. 14:493–498, 1976.
68. Wands, J. R., Lamont, J. T., and Mann, R.: Arthritis associated with intestinal bypass procedure for morbid obesity. N. Engl. J. Med. 294:121–124, 1976.
69. Wandtke, J., Skucas, J., Spataro, R., et al.: Pneumatosis intestinalis as a complication of jejunoileal bypass. Am. J. Roentgenol. 129:601–604, 1977.
70. Weismann, R. E.: Surgical palliation of massive and severe obesity. Am. J. Surg. 125:437–446, 1973.
71. Wise, L. W., and Stein, T.: Biliary and urinary calculi. Pathogenesis following small bowel bypass for obesity. Arch. Surg. 110:1043–1047, 1975.
72. Woodward, E., Payne, J. H., Salmon, P. A., et al.: Morbid obesity. Arch. Surg. 110:1440–1445, 1975.

13

THE LARGE BOWEL

Part I

Non-Neoplastic Lesions

CHARLES M. NICE, JR., M.D., Ph.D.
FRANCIS A. PUYAU, M.D.

STANDARD IMAGING STUDIES

Roentgen examination of the colon and rectum is complementary to digital examination of the rectum and sigmoidoscopic and colonoscopic examination. Therefore, correlation of the examination findings is of the utmost importance.

Considerable information may sometimes be gathered from the plain roentgenogram. The thick haustral pattern of the colon may often be distinguished from the thinner valvulae conniventes of the small intestine. The gas in the colon may suggest the presence of an obstruction. At times, intraluminal masses may be outlined. The lumen widened by the toxic dilatation of ulcerative colitis and the lumen narrowed by vascular insufficiency may be distinctive enough to be recognized on plain roentgenograms.

The barium enema examination should utilize a controlled barium suspension with high kilovoltage technique. Very high weight-to-volume concentrations of barium coupled with low kilovoltage technique can cause marked gradations in contrast in filming the gastrointestinal tract. Although such levels of contrast are desirable in certain radiographic techniques, such as arteriography, small intraluminal filling defects can be overlooked in examination of the colon. Optimal demonstration of intraluminal filling defects can be achieved with a suspension of 300 gm of barium in 2500 ml of water and filming at 125 to 150 kvp.

Because of the complex shape of the colon, no single view allows adequate definition of all parts, and therefore when totally filled the abdomen should be filmed in multiple projections (Fig. 13–1*A* to *C*). The rectosigmoid junction is frequently obscured

Text continued on page 651

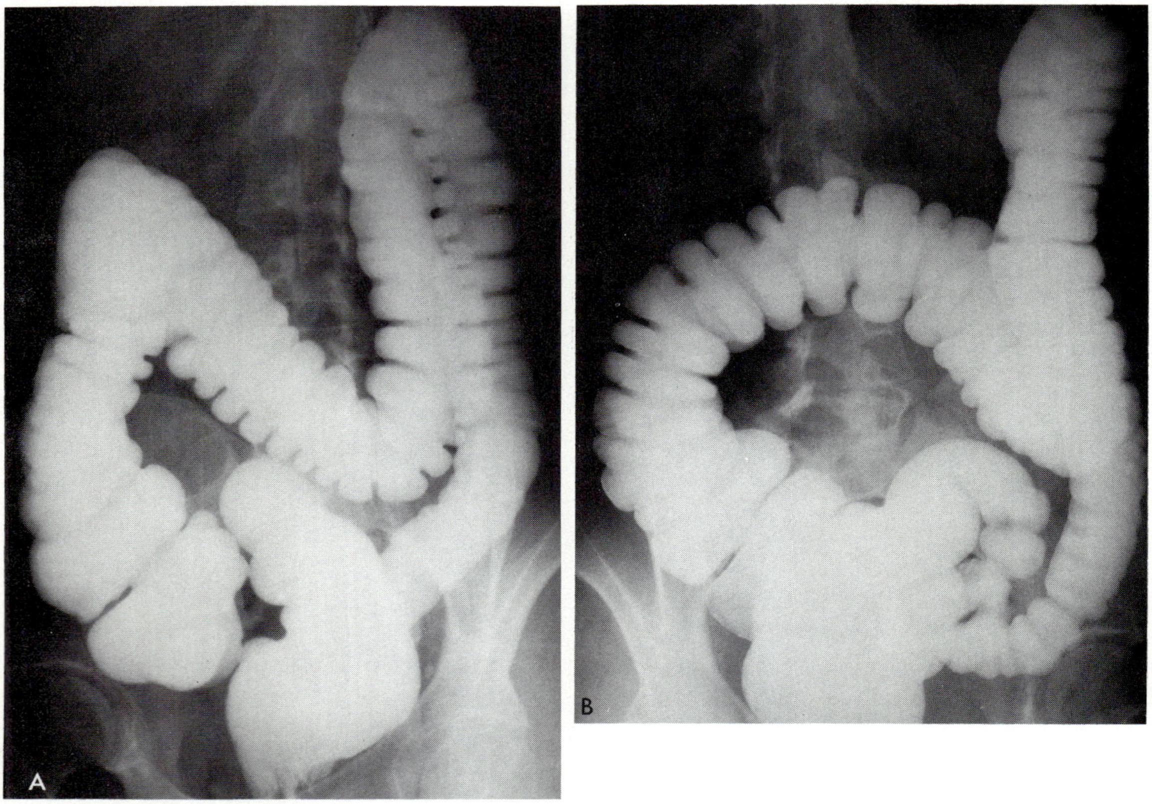

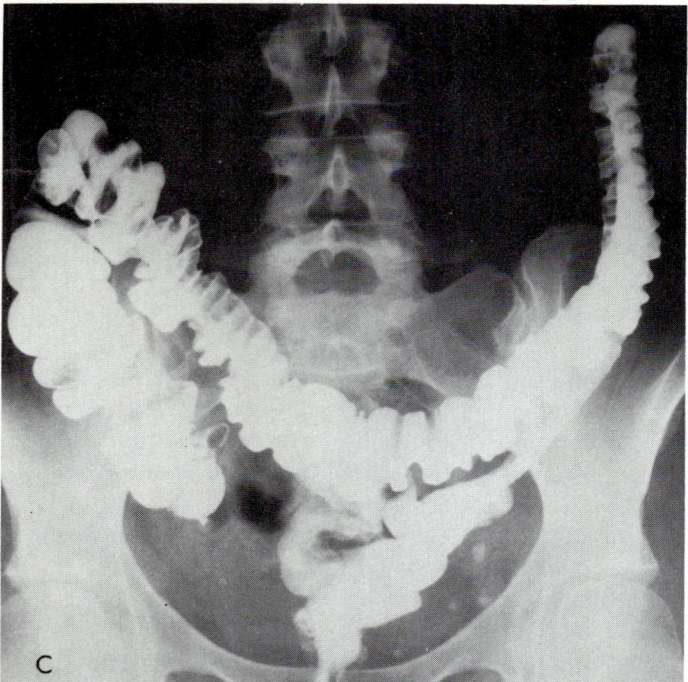

Figure 13–1. Normal colon. *A,* Right posterior oblique filled colon. *B,* Left posterior oblique filled colon. *C,* Post-evacuation.

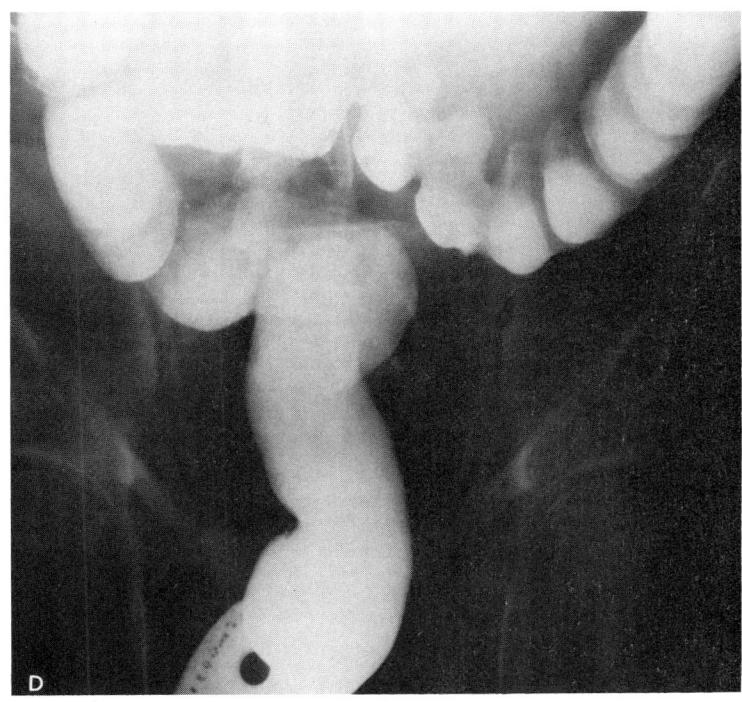

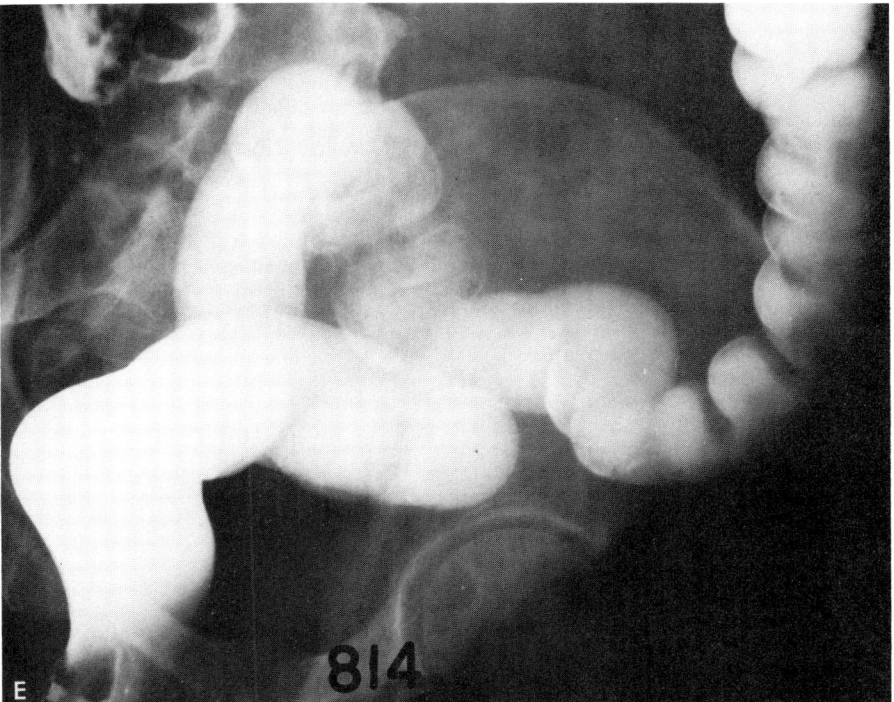

Figure 13–1 Continued. D, Angled view of rectosigmoid. E, Oblique view of rectosigmoid.

Illustration and legend continued on the following page

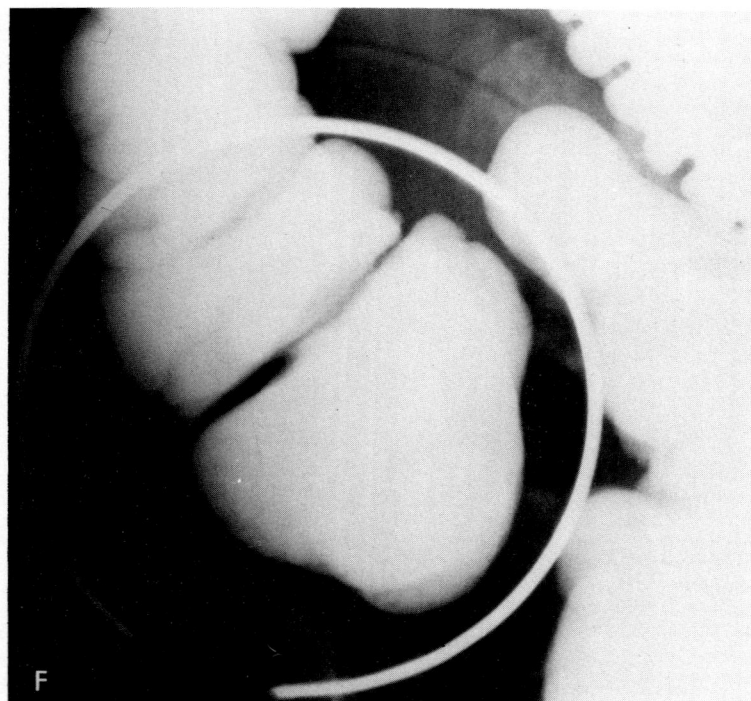

Figure 13–1 *Continued.* F, Spot film of cecum with compression.

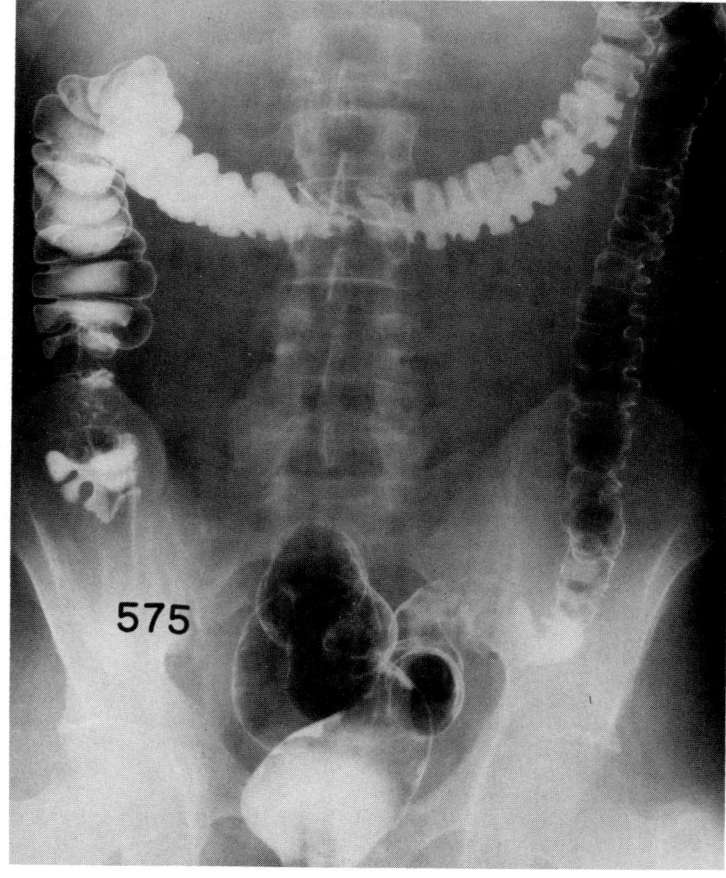

Figure 13–2. Anteroposterior view of double-contrast examination. The transverse colon does not show much air-filling, although the rest of the colon shows good double contrast. Normally, multiple roentgenograms are taken, including oblique, upright, and lateral decubitus views of the double-contrast study.

by overlapping loops and is best demonstrated by angled (Fig. 13–1D) or oblique (Fig. 13–1E) views. Spot filming during fluoroscopic filming with compression allows special definition of individual segments, such as the cecum (Fig. 13–1F). A postevacuation study permits better evaluation of the detail of the mucosal pattern than a study of the totally filled colon (see Fig. 13–1C).

Air-contrast technique (Fig. 13–2) is used when there is still unexplained blood in the stool, following routine barium enema, or to corroborate the presence of a suspected intraluminal lesion. There are an increasing number of advocates of air-contrast study as the first examination. There is no question that with careful preparation, careful selection of barium suspension, and optimal roentgen technique, the air-contrast colon study gives more information than the routine barium enema. However, the latter is still quite useful as a first study, since most lesions, even relatively small polyps, can be demonstrated with good technique. At times the two studies definitely have complementary value. On rare occasions, under difficult conditions, it may be advisable to outline the colon by taking delayed films after a barium meal (Fig. 13–3).

Many observers stress the importance of the type of barium used; however, most manufacturers do not list the additives in their barium products. Miller[49] tested many barium suspensions and concluded that equal parts of Intropaque and Unibaryt C at a density of 6.0 give the best visualization of the colonic mucosa. From time to time, a special variation of colonic examination, such as the water–double-contrast barium enema, is suggested.[58]

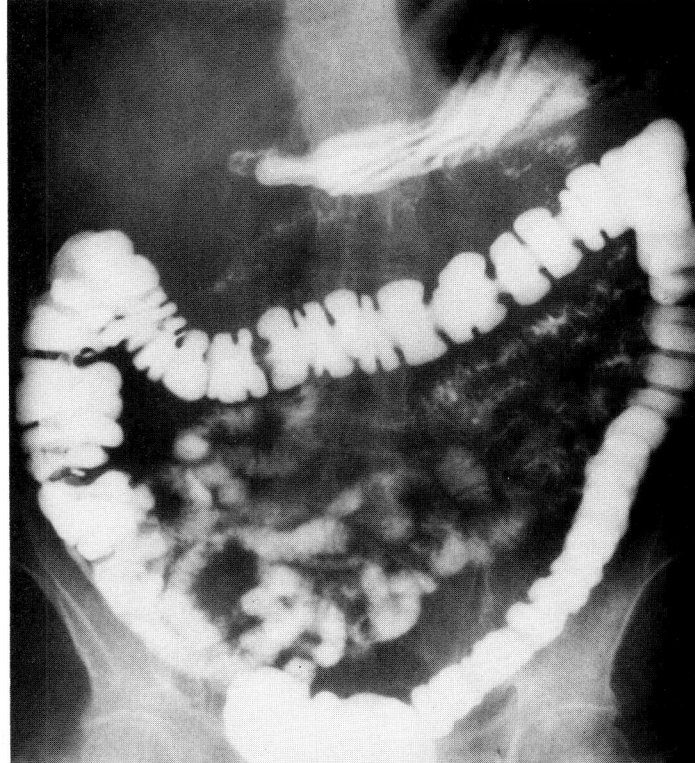

Figure 13–3. Colon opacification by antegrade barium after oral ingestion for upper gastrointestinal tract study.

OTHER IMAGING STUDIES

The ultrasound scan may occasionally be of considerable value in studying disease processes adjacent to the colon. If a mass is shown displacing the sigmoid colon in the female pelvis, ultrasound scanning helps determine whether it is solid or cystic. Ultrasound may also demonstrate a mass originating in the pancreas, kidney, spleen, gallbladder, or liver that has been shown to displace the colon.

Computed tomography may also be useful in the study of masses or abscesses involving the abdomen and pelvis. In studying the upper abdominal structures, dilute contrast may be given by mouth to outline the stomach and duodenum, and intravenous contrast may be given to label the kidneys. When the lower abdomen and pelvis are studied, dilute barium suspension or water-soluble contrast may be given by rectum, and intravenous contrast may be used to opacify the ureters and bladder.

Isotope studies, such as the radioactive gallium scan, may be used to visualize abscesses in the abdomen and pelvis. The liver scan with technetium sulphur colloid may be used to demonstrate metastases from colonic carcinoma.

PREPARATION

Many methods of preparation of the colon have been described in the literature. Certain basic principles should be emphasized. Of paramount importance are a nonresidue diet for 48 hours, ample fluid intake, a laxative the night before the examination, and a suppository or cleansing enema on the morning of the examination. It is important that a cleansing enema should reach the ascending colon.

No preparation is given to infants with possible Hirschsprung disease or to patients with an acute abdomen, suspected perforation, or severe obstruction. If fecal material is still obscuring detail in a routine study, the patient may be allowed to evacuate the barium, and a second barium enema may be given. Air-contrast may be used immediately following a barium enema or may be scheduled for the next day if too much of the ileum has been filled with barium.

ROENTGEN ANATOMY

The relationships between the colon and other structures are useful in analyzing masses in the abdomen.[71] The cecum is usually in the right lower quadrant over the midportion of the iliac bone but may extend deep into the right side of the pelvis. The ascending and descending portions of the colon are not suspended on a mesentery, and the posterior wall of each is retroperitoneal. Therefore, a mass lesion behind either the ascending or the descending colon is retroperitoneal, usually a renal mass or a retroperitoneal tumor. An enlarged liver or gallbladder or a mass in the upper pole of the right kidney may depress the hepatic flexure or proximal transverse colon in the right upper quadrant. Although masses in the pancreatic head will enlarge the duodenal loop, a mass in the body of the pancreas may occur between the stomach and the transverse colon.[31] A mass in the tail of the pancreas may be behind the body of the stomach, but may also lie between the stomach and the splenic flexure, or be nestled within the two loops of the splenic flexure. An enlarged spleen may depress the splenic flexure of the colon. In the pelvic region, intraperitoneal masses may displace the sigmoid colon posteriorly, while retroperitoneal masses may displace the rectum or

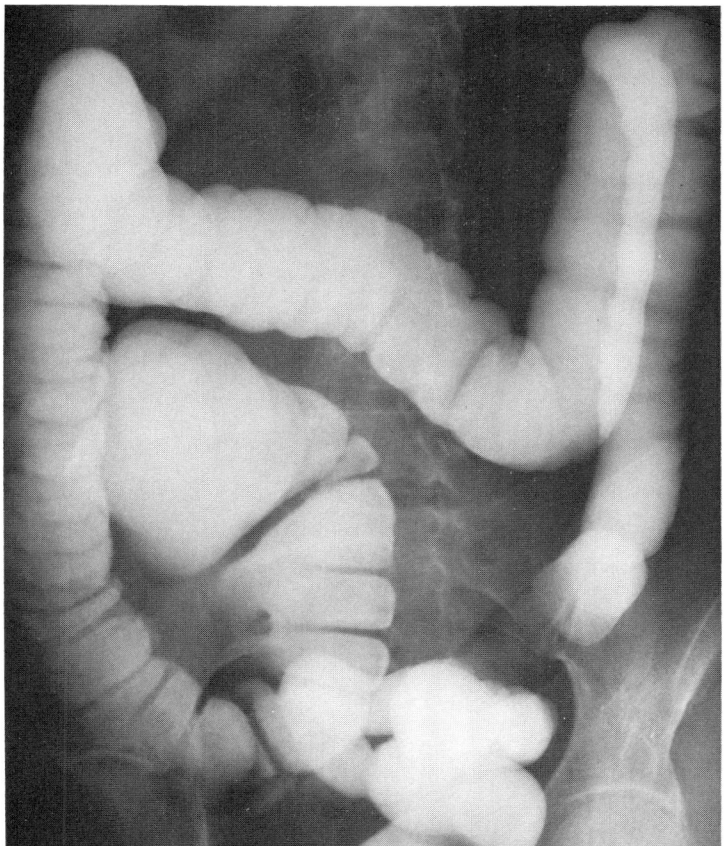

Figure 13–4. Redundant or mobile cecum. The cecal tip lies directly under the transverse colon.

sigmoid colon anteriorly. Absence of the left kidney may allow the splenic flexure or the tail of the pancreas to shift and lie in the renal fossa.

Several normal variations of the colon may be seen. The inverted cecum is a mild form of nonrotation. The mobile cecum is on a mesentery and deviates medially (Fig. 13–4). The cecal bascule (Fig. 13–5) is a condition in which the cecum is reflected straight upward anterior to the ascending colon. Partial or near duplication of the colon (Fig. 13–6) is a rare anomaly. The congenital diaphragm (Fig. 13–7) and atresia of the colon (Fig. 13–8) are very rare anomalies which may be associated with obstruction early in life.

THE POSTOPERATIVE COLON

One of the most elementary surgical procedures on the colon is the colostomy (Fig. 13–9). The barium enema examination may be used to examine the remaining colon proximal or distal to the colostomy. Great care must be used, since there is danger of perforation near the colostomy site, especially if any type of inflated device is used inside the stoma (Fig. 13–10).

Following any type of colonic resection, the barium enema may be used to study the anastomotic site and uncover any new or recurrent disease process. It is important,

Text continued on page 658

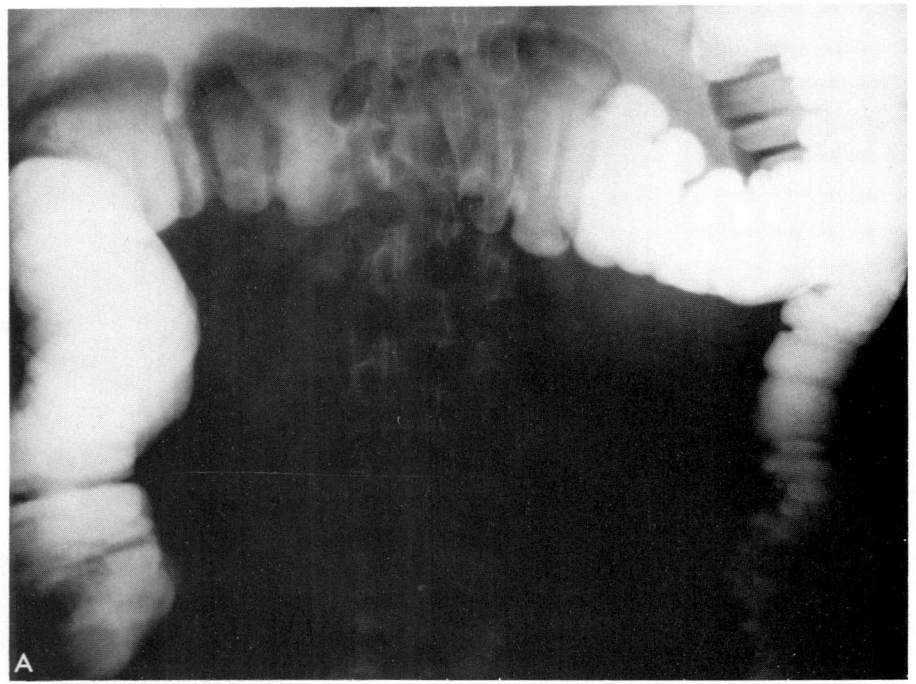
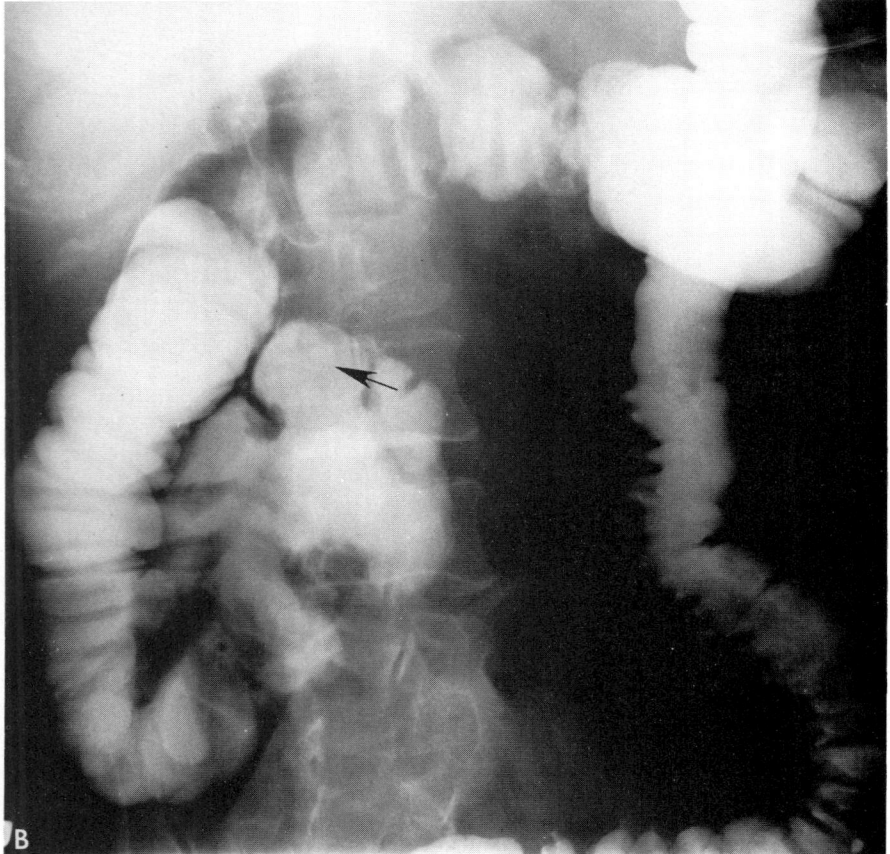

Figure 13–5. Cecal bascule. *A,* In the anteroposterior view, the cecum is lying directly in front of the ascending colon and cannot be well outlined or evaluated. *B,* In the left posterior oblique view, the cecum (arrow) can be seen adjacent to the ascending colon.

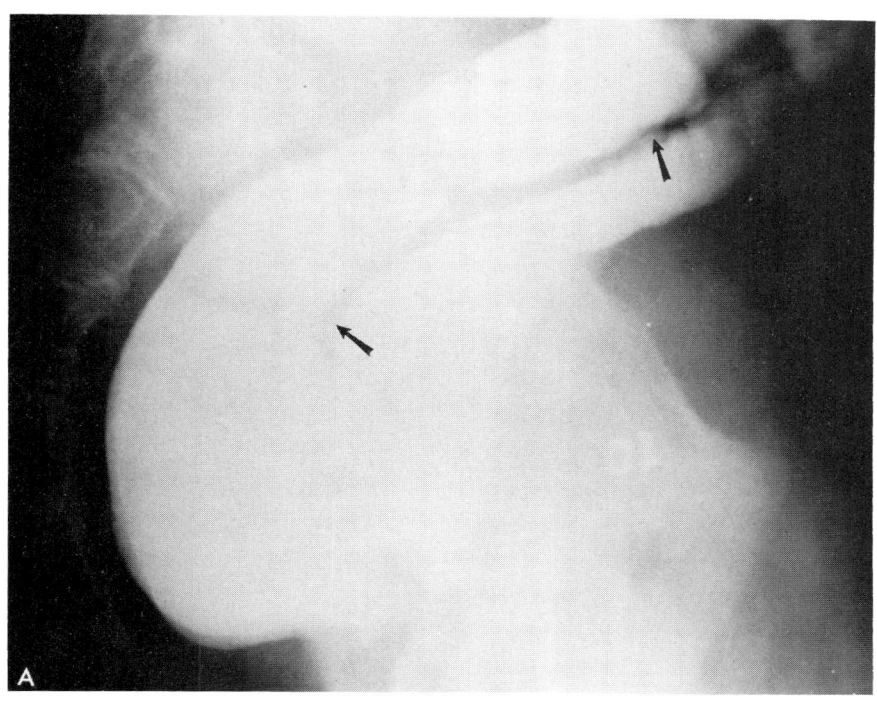

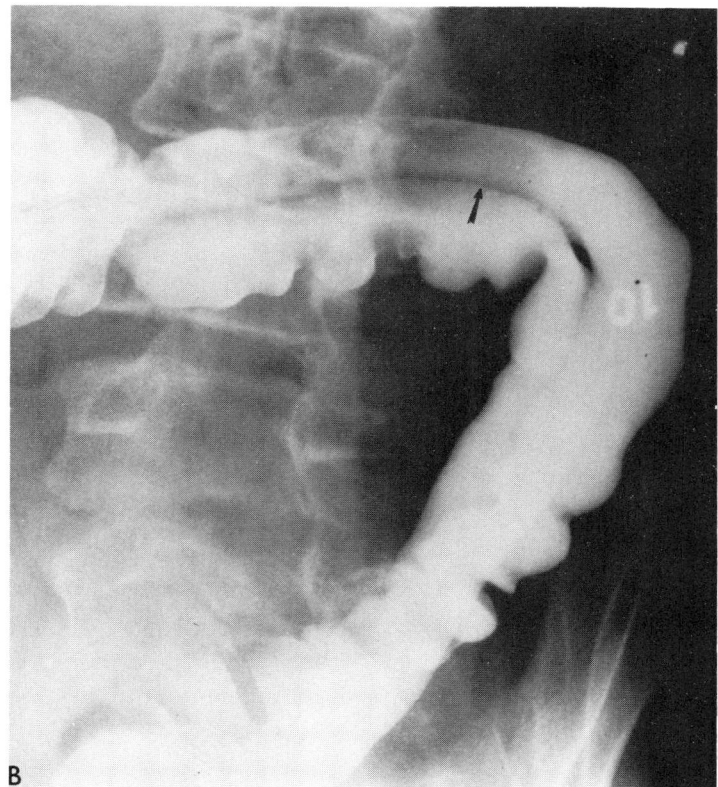

Figure 13–6. Duplication of the colon. The two lumina of the sigmoid (*A*) and the left colon, including a portion of the transverse colon (*B*), are clearly seen. The septum (arrows) separating the two channels is also visualized.

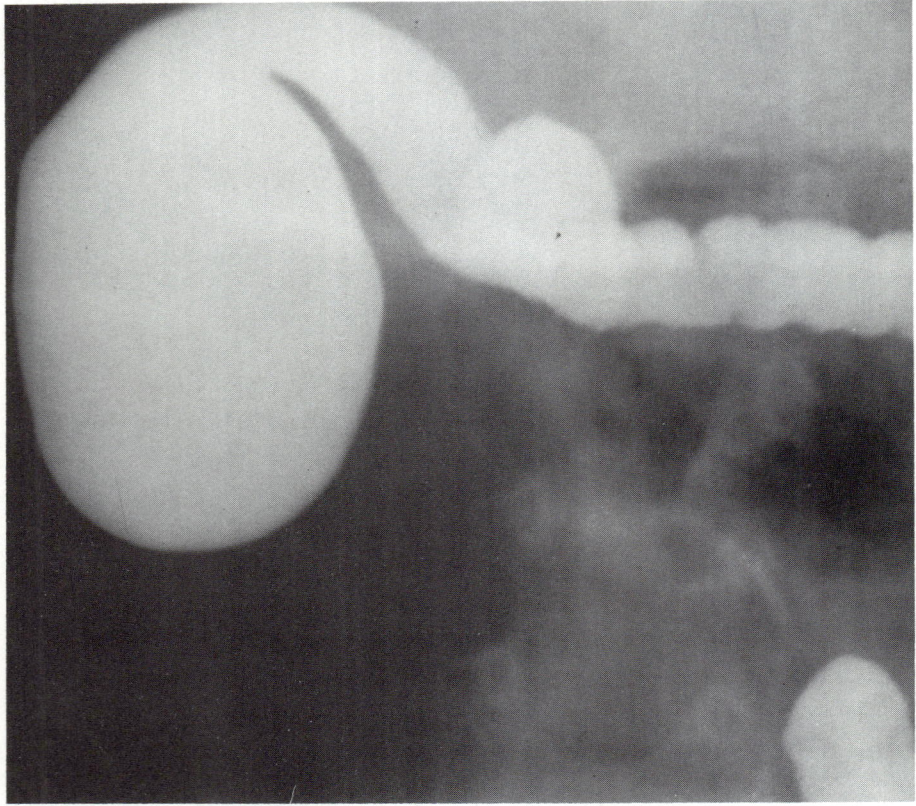

Figure 13–7. Congenital diaphragm in the ascending colon. The retrograde barium stops just above the level of the ileocecal valve at the site of the congenital diaphragm. Note the gaseous distention of the small bowel.

THE LARGE BOWEL — 657

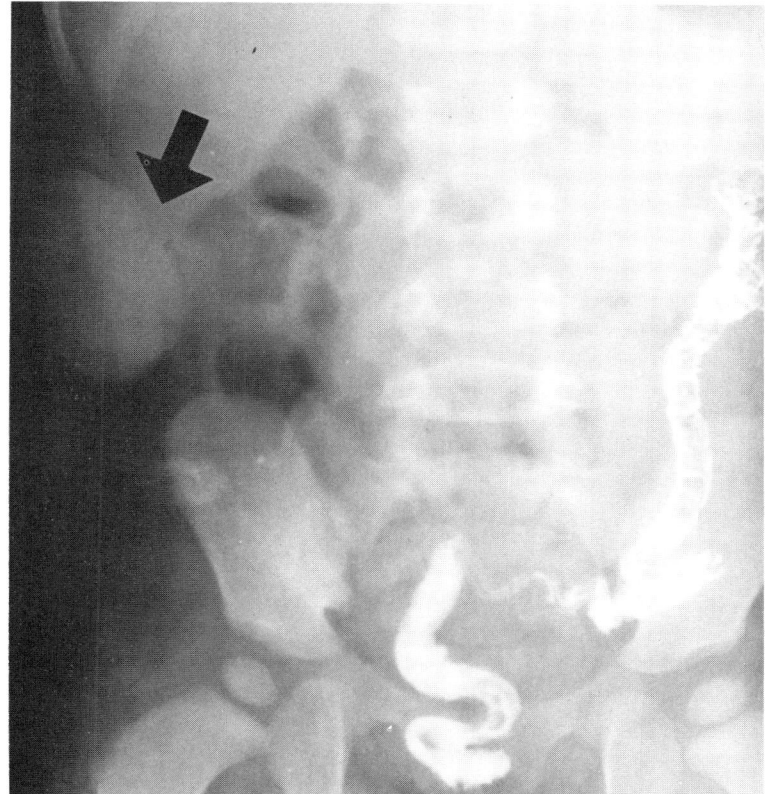

Figure 13–8. Atresia of the transverse colon. The arrow points to an ascending colostomy. The retrograde flow of barium is obstructed near the level of the splenic flexure. There was atresia between the hepatic and the splenic flexures of the colon.

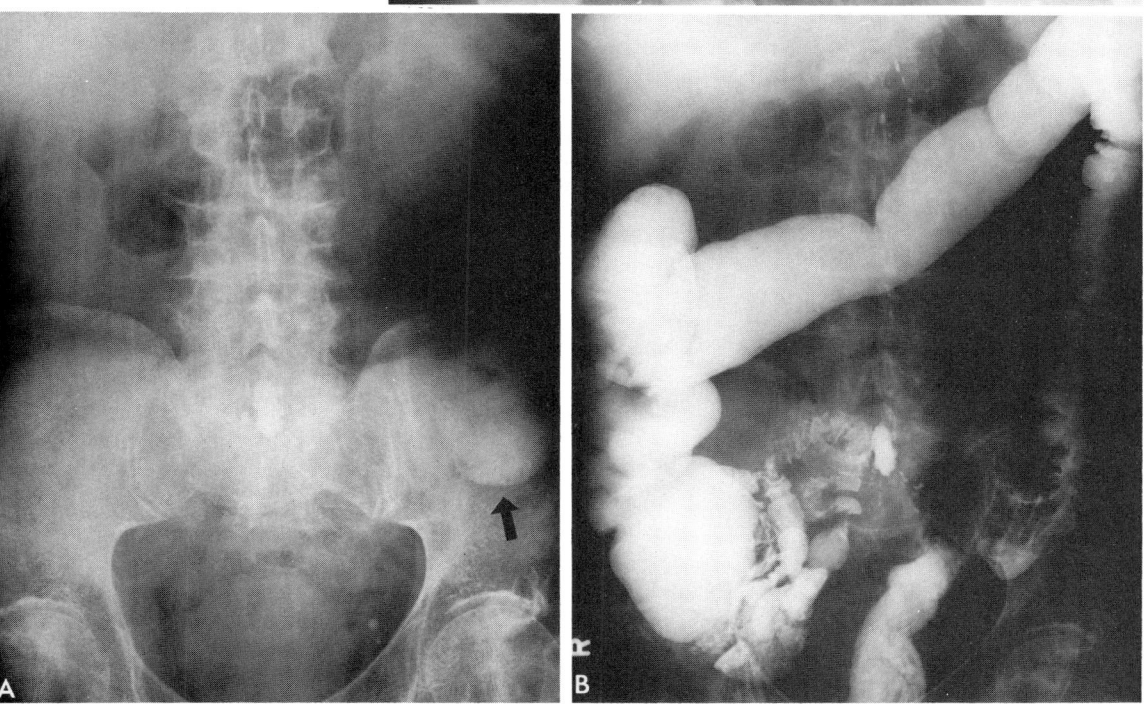

Figure 13–9. Double-barreled colostomy. *A,* The colostomy produces a soft-tissue shadow on abdominal film (arrow). *B,* The colon and terminal ileum were filled by barium injection through one barrel of the colostomy. The filling of the sigmoid was obtained by rectal instillation of barium.

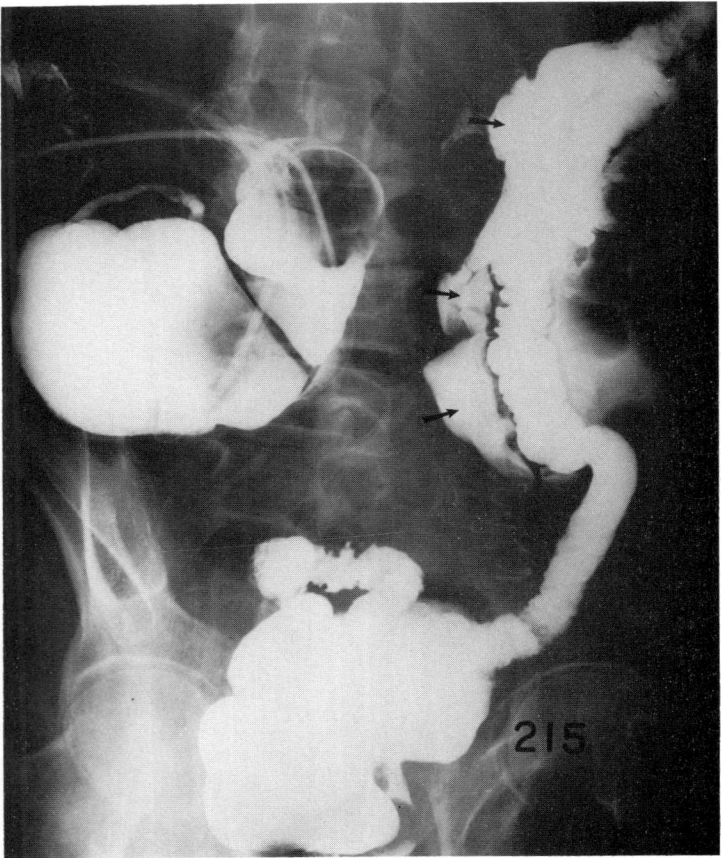

Figure 13–10. Extravasation of barium (arrows) around the upper descending colon at a colostomy site. This resulted from a barium enema, but the stoma had been obstructed by an inflated balloon, allowing perforation at the colostomy site and extravasation.

therefore, to know in advance whether the patient has had an ileotransverse colostomy (Fig. 13–11), an ileosigmoidostomy (Fig. 13–12), or some form of colocolostomy (Figs. 13–13 and 13–14). In each there is shortening of the total length of the colon depending on the length of the segment removed. An examination two to four weeks after surgery may serve as a baseline for later comparison. If the anastomosis changes and becomes asymmetric or narrowed, the possibility of recurrent tumor should be considered (Fig. 13–15). Sometimes a narrowing that has developed at the anastomosis is only a benign stricture.

BLUNT TRAUMA

In patients exposed to blunt trauma, the colon may be injured by a direct blow, by shearing forces generated by compression between the anterior abdominal wall and the lumbar spine or pelvis, or by shearing associated with the use of lap-type seat belts.[79] Bowel laceration may lead to peritonitis. Injury to blood vessels may produce hemorrhage, intramural hematoma, or pseudoaneurysms of vessels. The latter may be shown on arteriography. Intramural hematoma may cause a localized indentation or constriction.

Ischemia of the bowel wall following blunt trauma may heal completely, may cause bowel necrosis and peritonitis, or may produce a late focal stenosis. With traumatic

Text continued on page 663

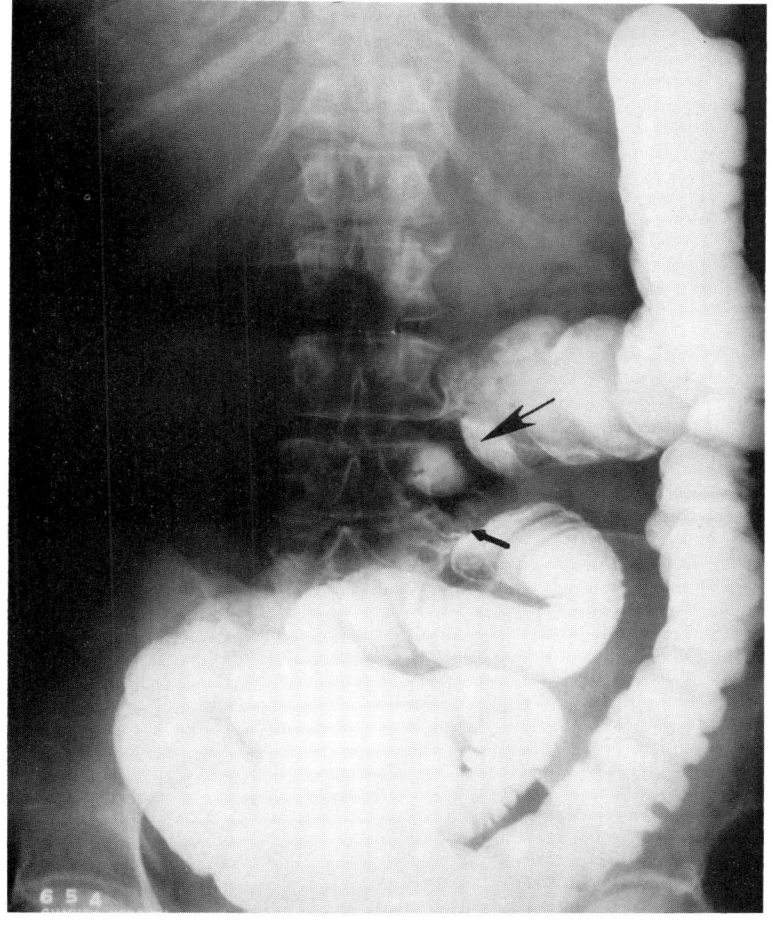

Figure 13–11. Ileotransverse colostomy. The ileum (small arrow) is anastomosed to the midtransverse colon (large arrow). The rest of the right colon has been resected.

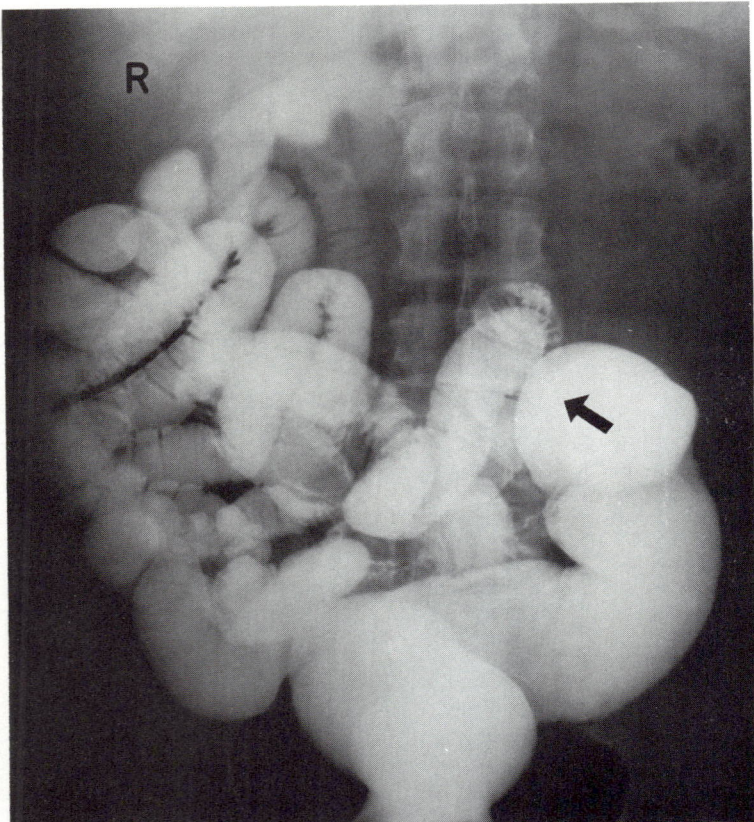

Figure 13–12. Ileosigmoidostomy. The small bowel is anastomosed to the sigmoid (arrow).

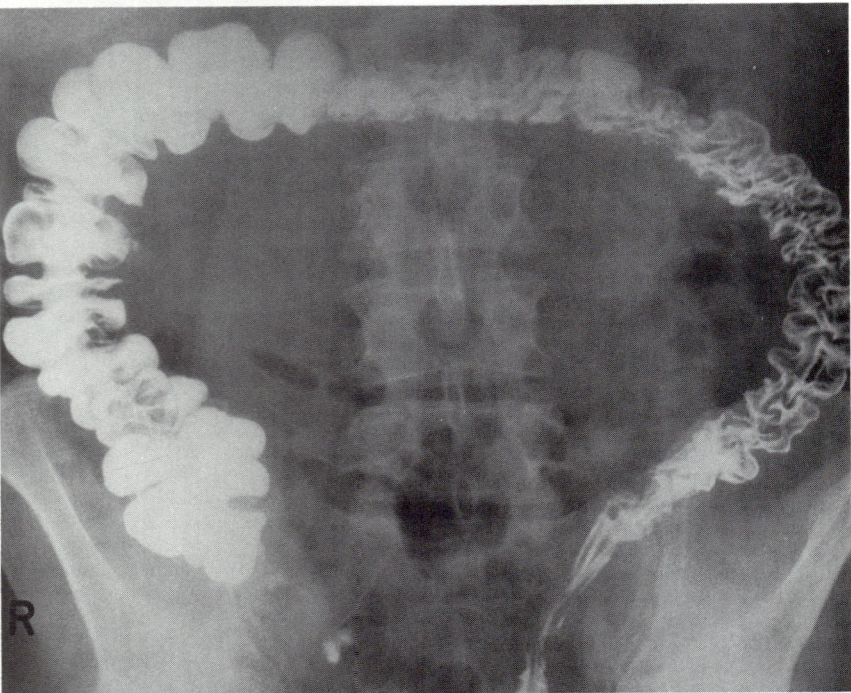

Figure 13–13. Appearance of the colon after partial resection of the left colon. Note the straight sigmoid and the marked shortening of the sigmoid, most of which has been resected.

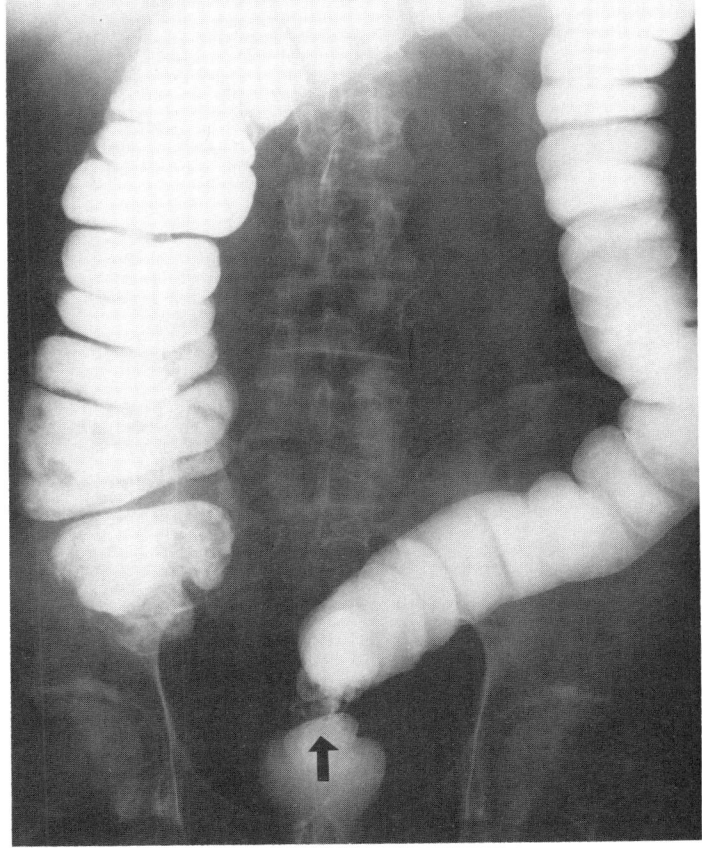

Figure 13–14. Postoperative appearance of anastomoses (arrow) following resection of most of the sigmoid. There has been a low anastomosis to the rectum. Because the irregularity of the anastomosis can be confused with recurrent tumor, baseline examinations shortly after surgery are helpful for evaluating possible recurrences at the anastomotic site on later examinations.

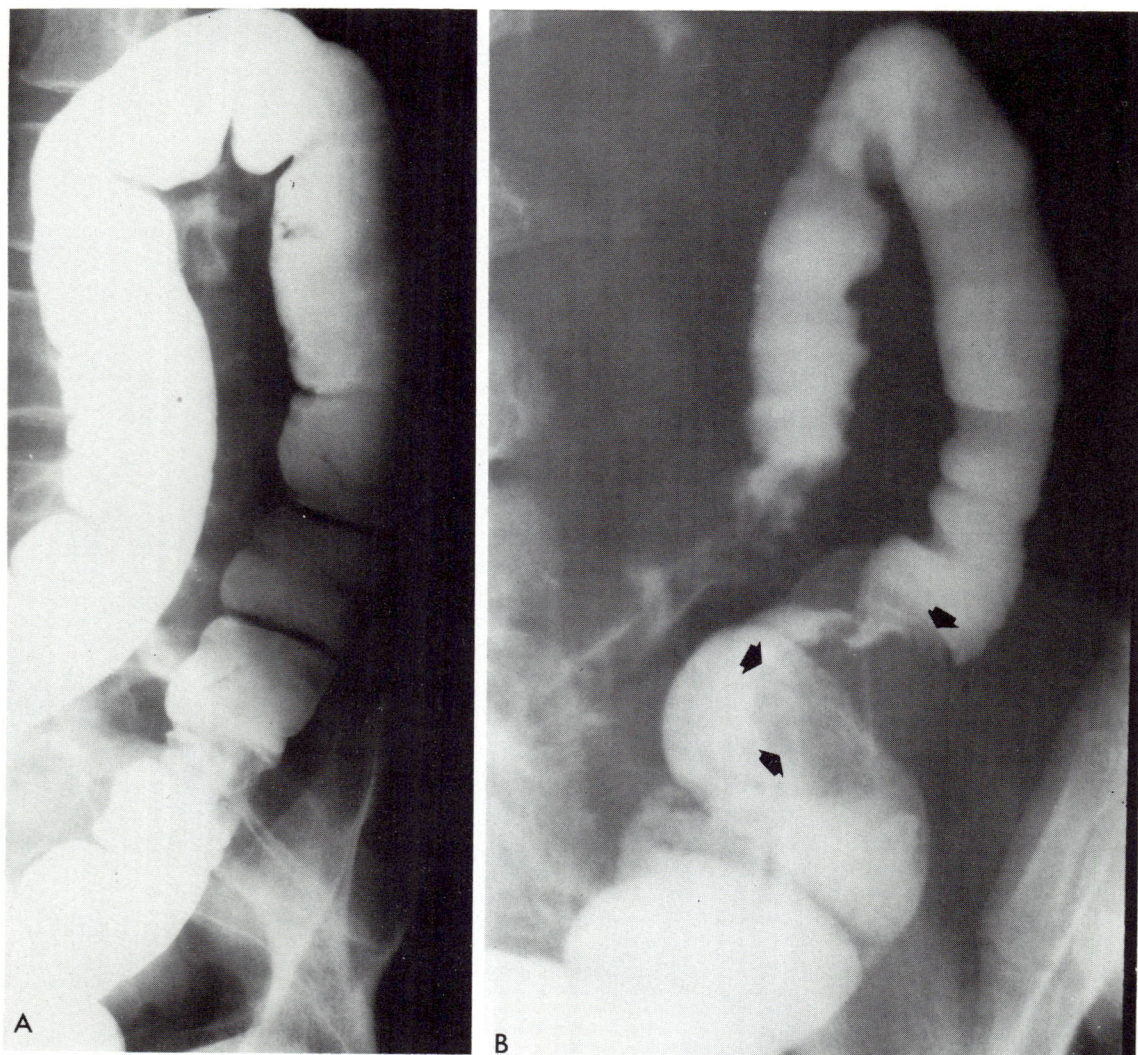

Figure 13–15. Recurrent tumor and edema at anastomotic site. *A*, The anastomosis (arrow) is fairly normal in appearance. The bowel irregularity is usually a normal anastomotic finding. *B*, A year later, there is a large filling defect (arrows) due to a recurrent tumor at the anastomotic site.

rupture of the diaphragm, the colon may be entrapped in the chest and become obstructed (Fig. 13–16).

PERITONITIS

Peritonitis may produce an adynamic dilatation of the colon as well as of the small bowel. Peritonitis can arise from a hematogenous infection or from perforation of a hollow viscus within the abdomen. However, generalized peritonitis or a localized peritonitis with abscess formation may also result from colonic perforation following previous surgery, sigmoidoscopic examination (Fig. 13–17),[33] barium enema, or rupture of a diverticulum in a region involved by diverticulitis (Fig. 13–18).

VOLVULUS

Volvulus implies twisting of a loop of bowel. In the colon, sigmoid volvulus is most common, followed by cecal volvulus, and the rare volvulus of the transverse[24, 54] or descending colon.

In the sigmoid volvulus, the plain roentgenogram may show two large symmetric gas-filled loops in the central abdomen within a slender opaque line between the loops

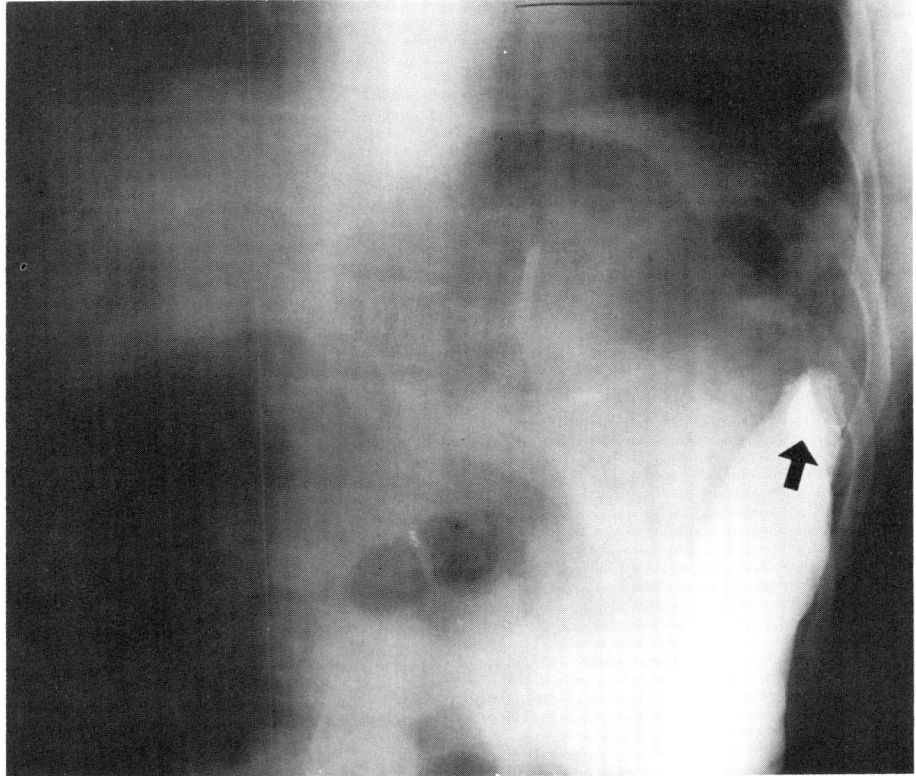

Figure 13–16. The tapering obstruction (arrow) of the upper descending colon is secondary to entrapment of a post-traumatic diaphragmatic hernia of the colon.

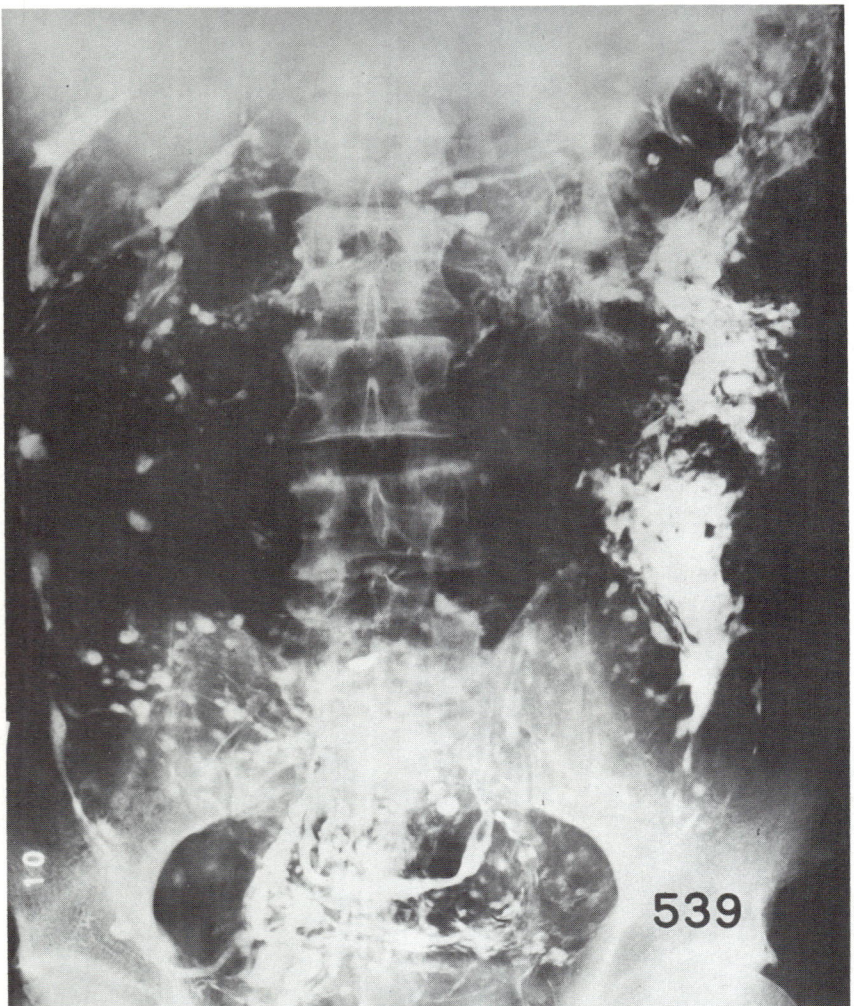

Figure 13–17. Barium scattered throughout the peritoneum after perforation of the sigmoid by sigmoidoscopy. A severe peritonitis developed.

pointing into the pelvis (Fig. 13–19). Sigmoid volvulus may be reduced by proctoscopic examination, insertion of a rectal tube, or administration of a saline or barium enema. Cecal volvulus accounts for about 15 per cent of cases of volvulus and occurs when the ascending colon is on an anomalous mesentery. With twisting, the cecum distends and may be found in the central abdomen or even in the left upper quadrant. It can frequently be recognized on the plain roentgenogram as a huge bean-shaped distended loop of bowel. The ileocecal valve may be seen on the right; the small bowel is obstructed, and an air-fluid level is seen in the cecum. In any type of volvulus the barium enema shows a tapering or "beak" at the site of the twisting (Fig. 13–20). Obstruction similar to cecal volvulus occurs with the "cecal bascule," in which the cecum is folded anterior to the ascending colon.[6] A rare type of severe obstruction is produced by the intestinal knot syndrome, which consists of sigmoid volvulus with a loop of ileum wrapped around the twisted area. Because both colon and small bowel are obstructed, the entire abdomen seems filled with distended loops.[55]

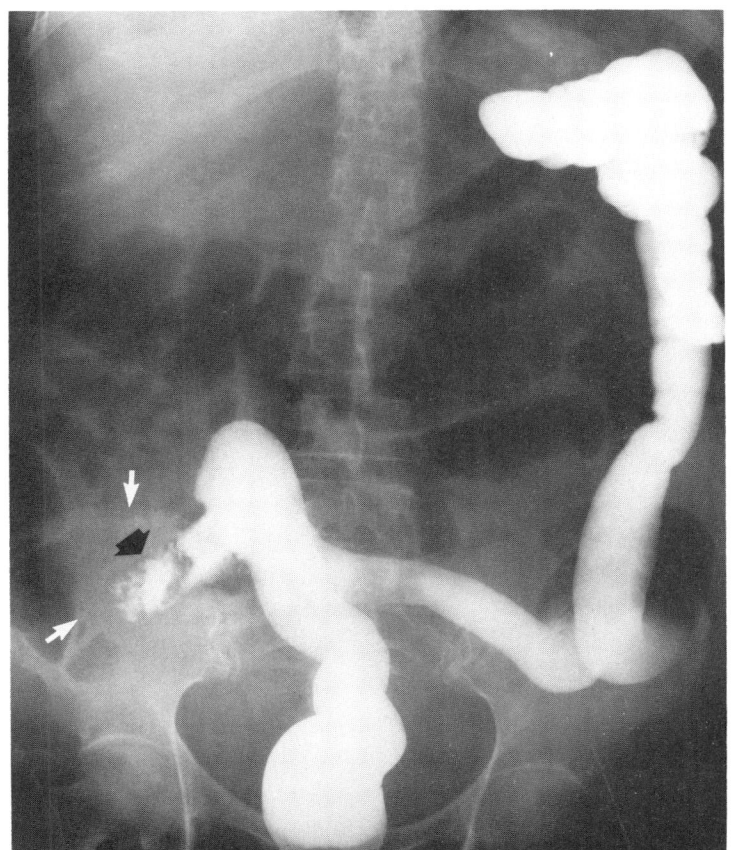

Figure 13–18. Perforated sigmoid diverticulitis. The soft-tissue mass (white arrows) and the extravasated barium (black arrow) are part of an abscess from diverticulitis of the sigmoid.

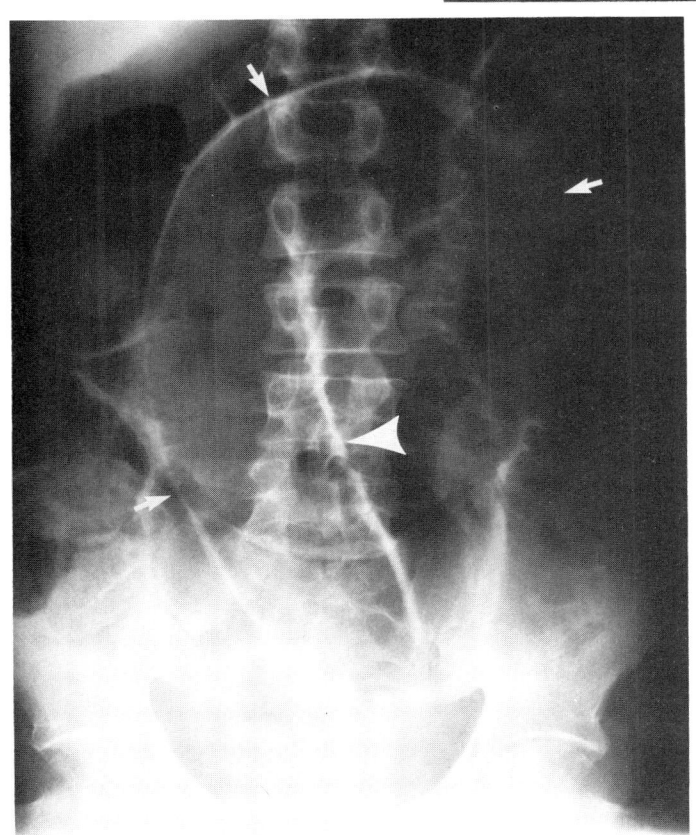

Figure 13–19. Sigmoid volvulus; plain film. The large oval-shaped, gas-filled density (white arrows), with the central opaque line extending down to the pelvic area (arrowhead), is typical of sigmoid volvulus. The point of volvulus is at the lower end of the white line, which represents the walls of the adjacent volvulated loops.

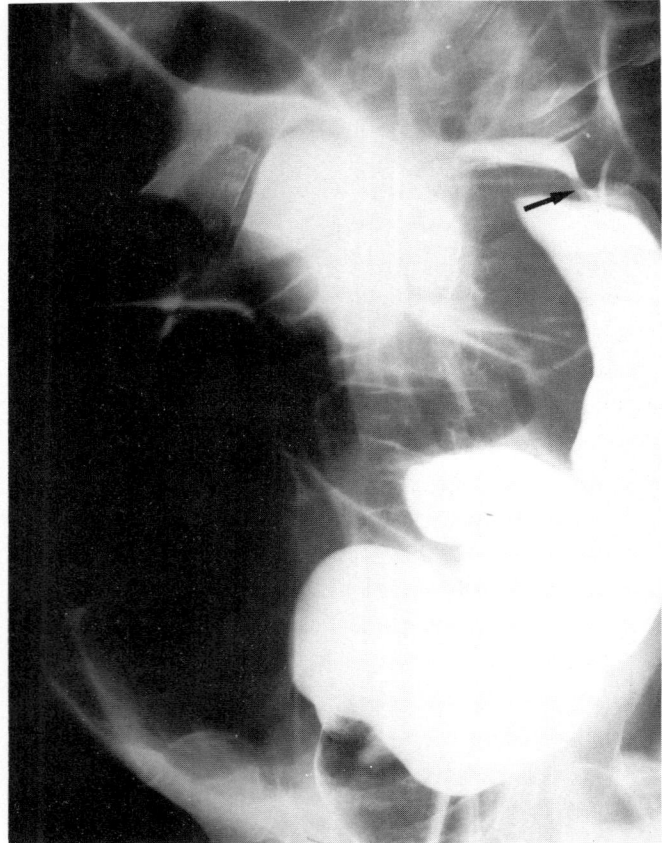

Figure 13–20. Volvulus of the descending colon. The barium enema shows a twisted narrowing (arrows) at the point of volvulus with a little barium extending proximal to the greatly dilated volvulated area. This type of volvulus is quite unusual.

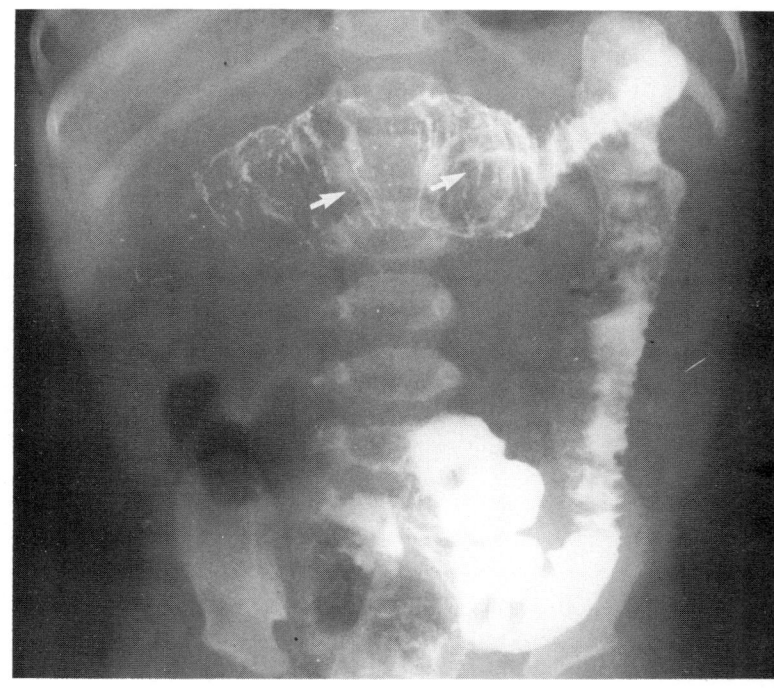

Figure 13–21. Ileocolic intussusception. The barium enema is characteristic, the intussuscepted area having a dilated, somewhat coiled-spring appearance (arrows). No barium could penetrate the intussuscepted area, which consisted of ileum. Often these intussusceptions can be reduced by the pressure of the barium enema.

INTUSSUSCEPTION

In the first year or two of life, spontaneous ileocolic intussusception may occur; this may be reduced by barium enema during the first 24 hours if no signs of sepsis have appeared. In later childhood and adulthood, ileoileal, ileocolic, and colocolic forms of intussusception are associated with a tumor or some other localized abnormality (such as Meckel's diverticulum) which initiates the process.[25] The intussusception invaginates the intussuscipens, resulting in a "coil-spring" pattern when barium is administered (Fig. 13–21).

FECAL IMPACTION

Considerable fecal material is usually found in infants and young children with Hirschsprung disease, and it may become impacted in the sigmoid. There is also an idiopathic or psychogenic megacolon that occurs in childhood and adult life, in which the colon is dilated to the anal sphincter (Fig. 13–22). Occasionally, depressed or dehydrated patients develop a hard mass of fecal material in the rectum, or rectosigmoid, leading to considerable retention of feces in the proximal dilated colon. An impaction may simulate an intraluminal mass (Fig. 13–23) and, if large enough, cause a complete obstruction to retrograde barium flow (Fig. 13–24). The radiographic appearance of the impaction and the intact colonic or rectal wall will usually distinguish it from a neoplastic mass.

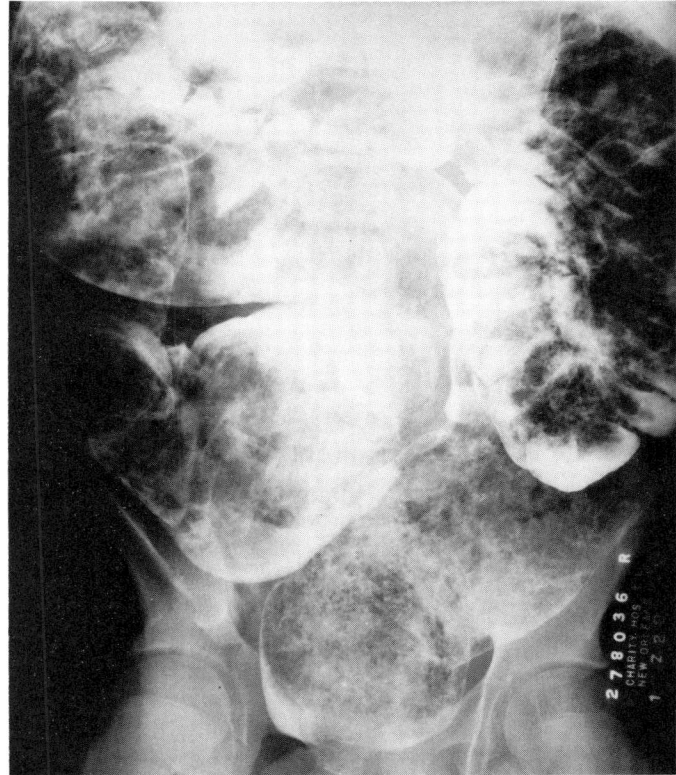

Figure 13–22. Idiopathic megacolon. The entire colon is greatly dilated and filled with fecal material throughout. Note that the dilatation and fecal collections extend down to the lower rectum, in contrast to most cases of Hirschsprung's megacolon.

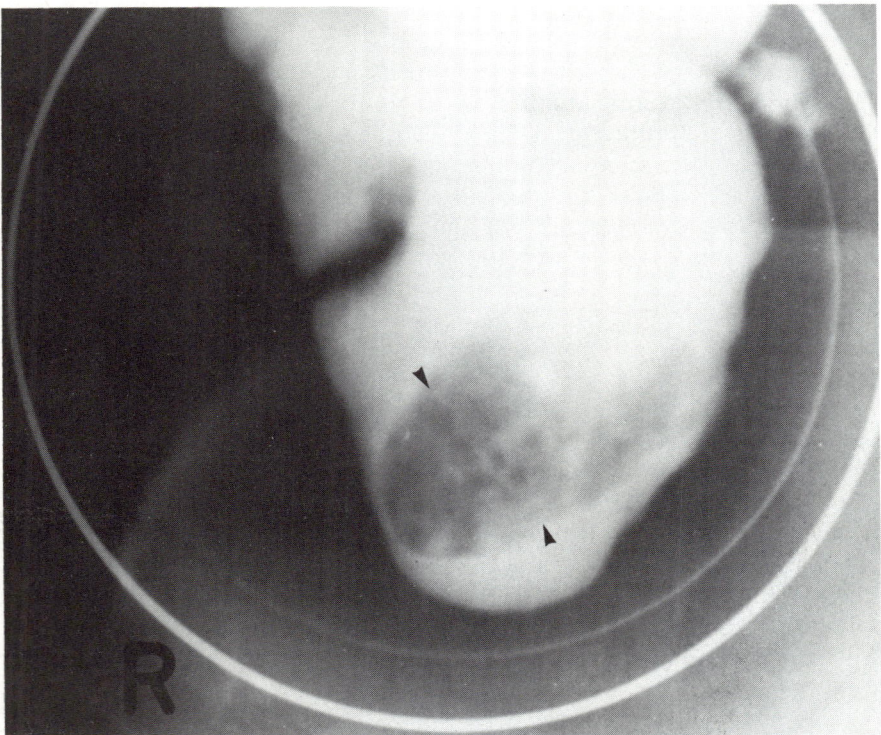

Figure 13–23. Fecalith in the cecum appears as a large filling defect (arrows). The mottled appearance within the defect is fairly characteristic of impacted feces, although occasionally a villous adenoma can give the same appearance. However, note that the walls of the cecum appear to be intact, which favors an interluminal fecal collection rather than a wall tumor.

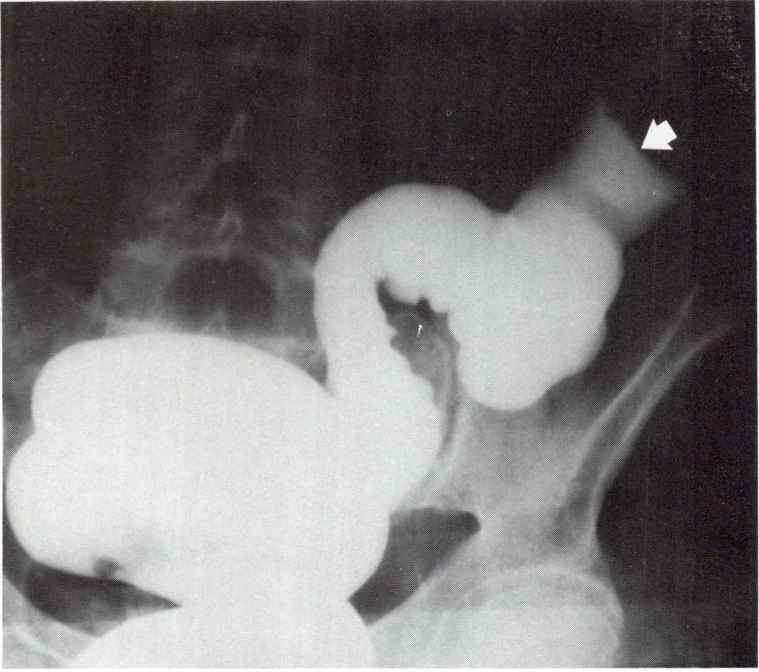

Figure 13–24. Fecal impaction in descending colon. The obstruction (arrow) at the descending colon was due to a large fecal impaction simulating a tumor. Most fecal impactions occur in the rectum and sigmoid.

DIVERTICULOSIS AND DIVERTICULITIS

Diverticula are small round or pear-shaped protrusions of mucosa through the muscular layer of the colon, which are covered only by serosa. The absence of a muscular layer is responsible for their slow and inadequate emptying. The circular muscle of the colon is often thickened in a segment that contains numerous diverticula.

The number of diverticula may vary from a single pouch to several hundred. Diverticula are most frequent and numerous in the sigmoid, with progressively decreasing incidence in the descending, transverse, and right colon. Their number and frequency increase with age; diverticula are rare before age 35.

Even without superimposed diverticulitis, diverticular bleeding occasionally occurs, most often in the right colon. When the bleeding is severe, arteriography may show extravasation of contrast material into the diverticulum or the adjacent colon.

Diverticulitis is most common in the sigmoid. Initially, the inflammatory changes are limited to the mucosa of the pouch, and radiographic changes may be absent or show only focal irritability and spasm. With involvement of the serosa and surrounding tissues, an inflammatory pericolonic soft-tissue mass (Fig. 13–25) or frank abscess (Fig. 13–26) becomes apparent. Ulceration may lead to internal fistulous tracts, sometimes parallel to the colon or extending into the pericolonic collection (Figs. 13–27 and 13–28). Fistulas to adjacent organs can occur, usually to the bladder but also to the ileum or the female genital organs (Figs. 13–29 and 13–30). In uncertain cases, ultrasound may confirm the presence of a pericolonic collection.

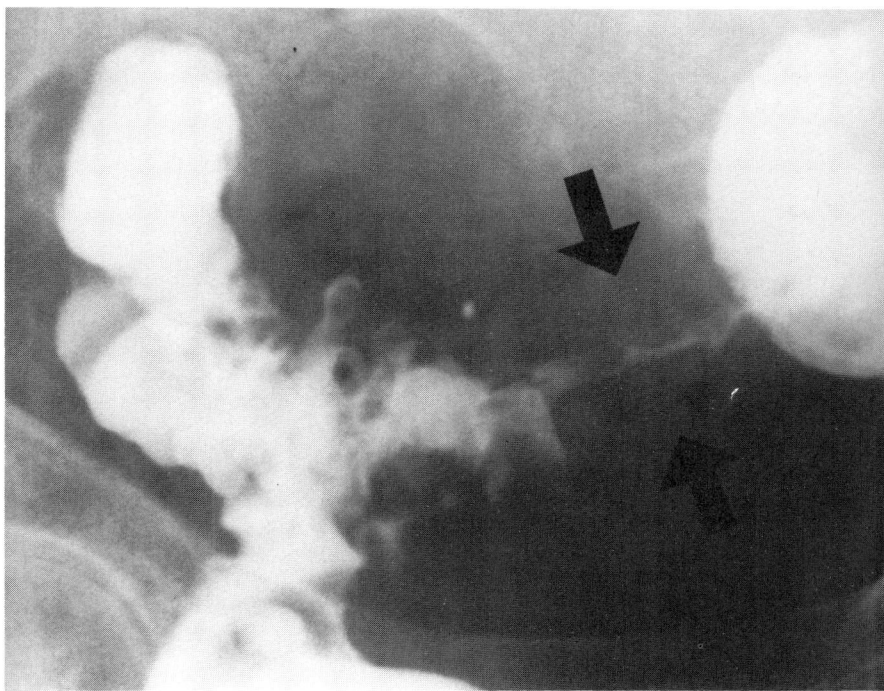

Figure 13–25. Diverticulitis. The sigmoid is narrowed and somewhat irregular and surrounded by a large soft-tissue mass (arrows). Although there are no significant shelving (or shoulder) defects, the appearance nevertheless is quite similar to that of a large carcinoma. The soft-tissue mass of the space was a pericolonic inflammatory mass.

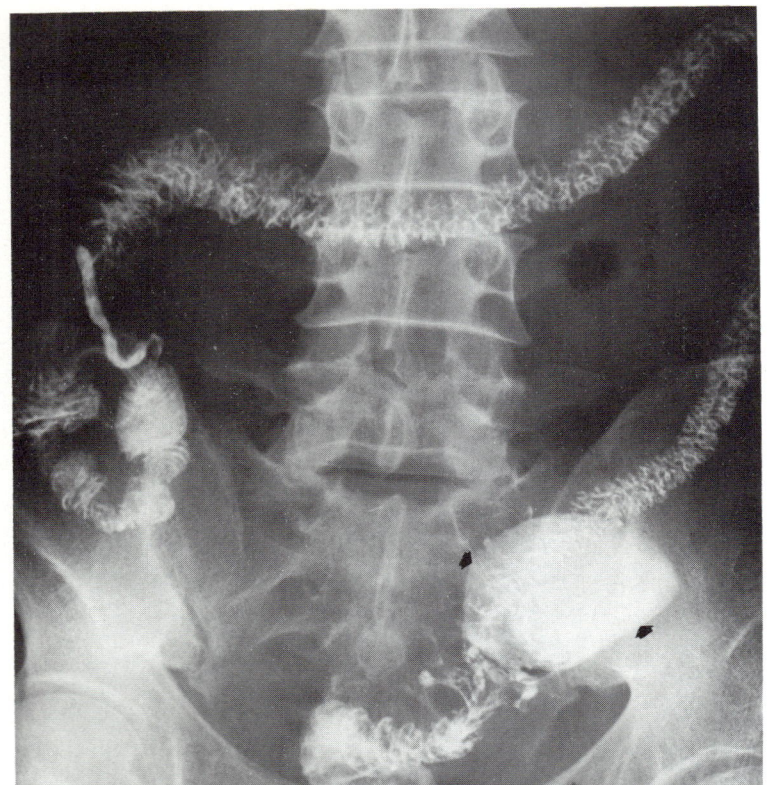

Figure 13-26. Diverticular abscess. The diverticula in the sigmoid and the mild irregularity are associated with a large collection of barium (arrows) in an abscess cavity due to perforation of one of the inflamed diverticula.

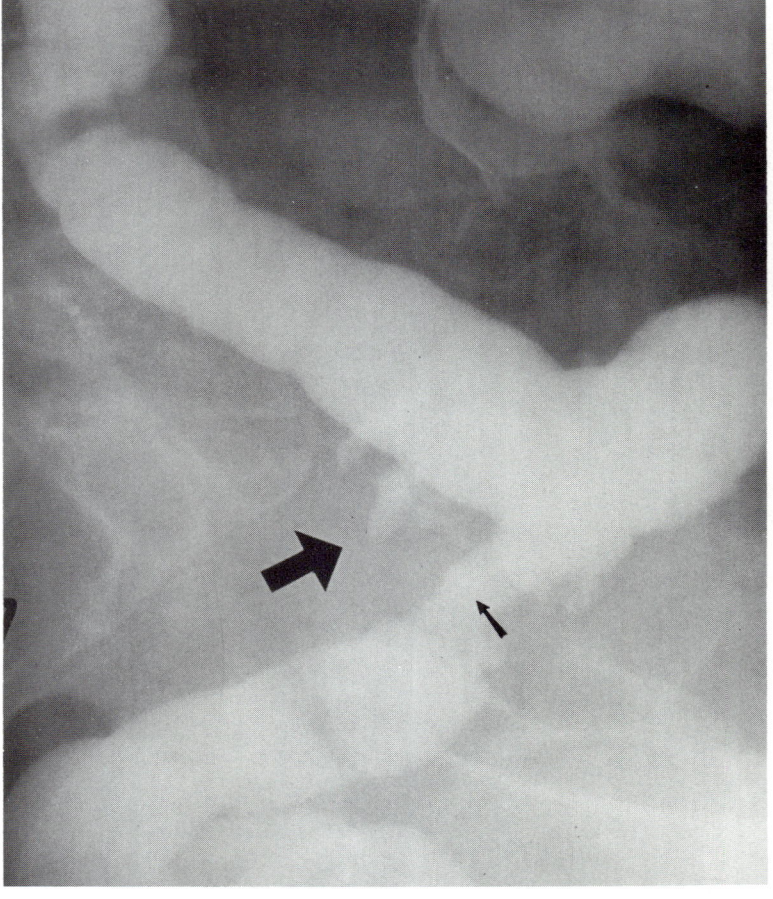

Figure 13-27. Sigmoid diverticulitis with internal fistula. The irregular, narrowed sigmoid (small arrow) is the site of the diverticulitis. Tracks of barium extend from this inflamed area posteriorly (large arrow).

THE LARGE BOWEL — 671

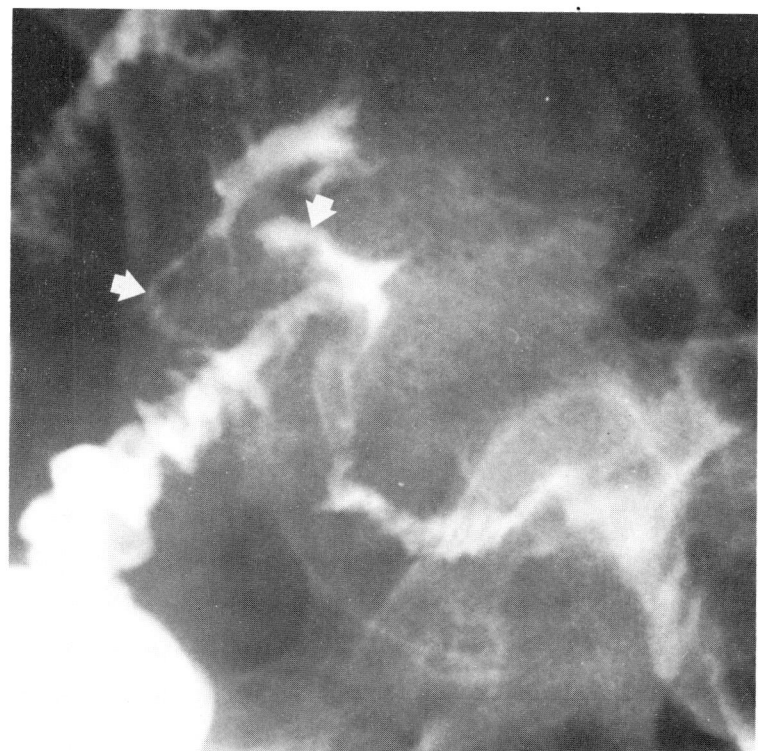

Figure 13–28. The sigmoid is narrowed and irregular owing to diverticulitis. Multiple fistulous tracks extend from the inflamed area (arrows).

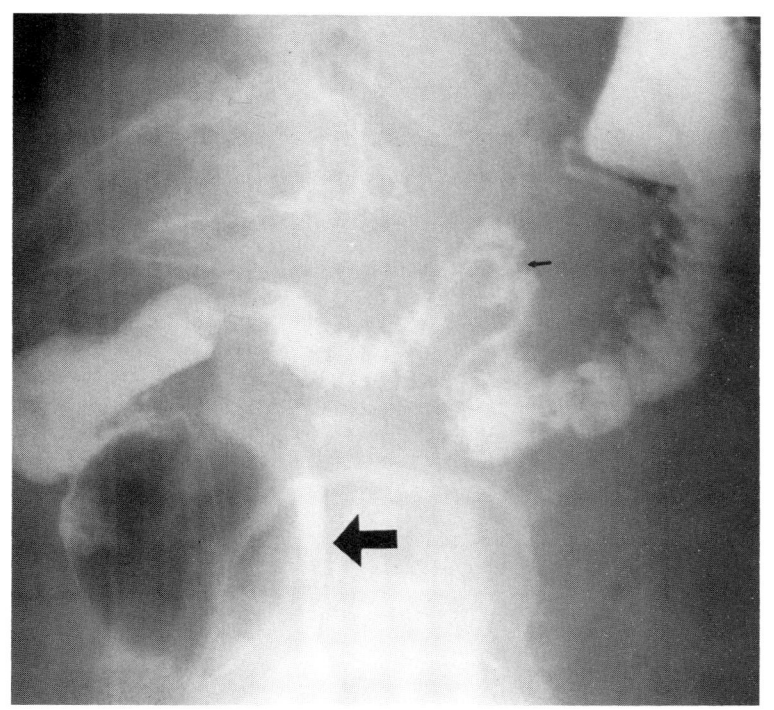

Figure 13–29. Sigmoid diverticulitis with fistula to the vagina. The area of diverticulitis (small arrow) has fistulized into the vagina (large arrow). The sinus tract is not completely demonstrated on this study.

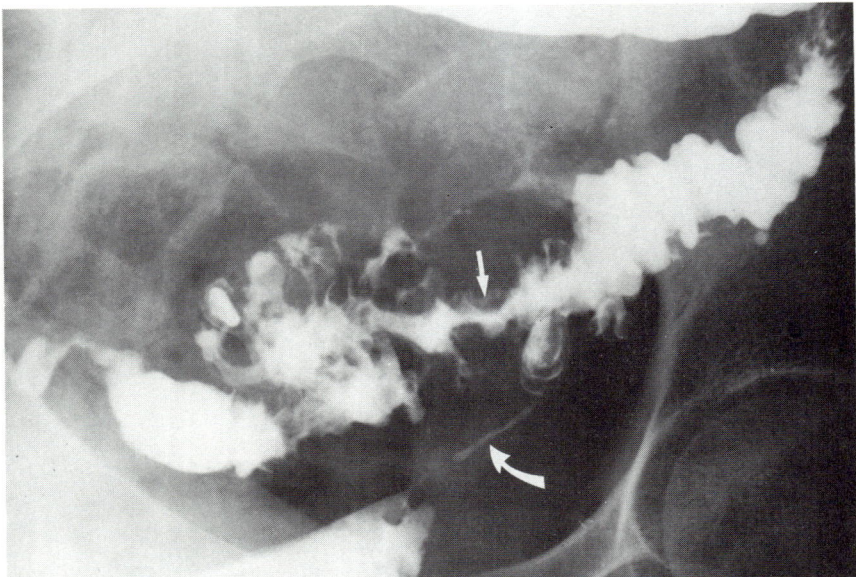

Figure 13–30. Sigmoid diverticulitis with fistulization into the uterus. From the irregular area of diverticulitis (small arrow), there is a fistulous tract (large arrow) extending into the uterus.

Sometimes radiographic differentiation from carcinoma or focal Crohn's disease is difficult or impossible. Rarely, carcinoma may fortuitously coexist with diverticulitis (Fig. 13–31).

In suspected acute diverticulitis, barium enema study should be performed cautiously in order to avoid perforation.

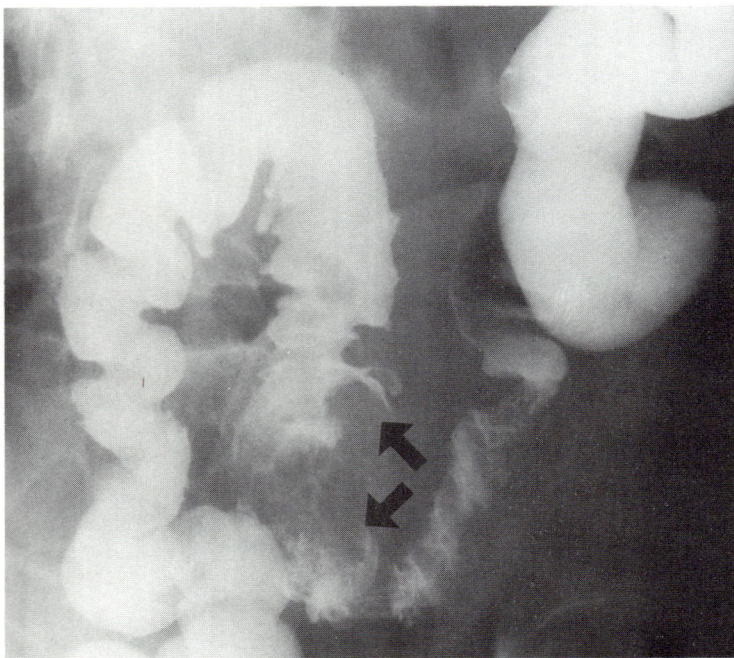

Figure 13–31. Diverticulitis with associated carcinoma. The large defect (arrows) in the area of the diverticulitis is a carcinoma. The relation is fortuitous, since diverticulitis does not predispose to carcinoma.

INFLAMMATORY DISEASES

Ulcerative and granulomatous colitis are discussed in Part II of this chapter (pp. 688 to 721.)

Pseudomembranous or staphylococcal *enterocolitis* is an infrequent complication of antibiotic therapy or may occur proximal to an obstructing lesion. Symptoms may vary from mild diarrhea, fever, and vomiting to shock.

The pseudomembrane may be seen on sigmoidoscopy. On barium enema the haustral pattern is distorted, and the normal mucosal pattern is replaced by a grossly irregular pattern. Ulcerations and defects from edema and pseudomembranes are frequent. Radiographically, the appearance simulates acute ulcerative or infectious colitis (Fig. 13–32).

Lymphogranuloma venereum primarily involves the rectum and often the sigmoid colon and is more common in women. There is a narrowing due to spasm and ulceration, leading eventually to fibrous stricture. Blind internal sinus tracts are common, and fistulas to skin or vagina may occur (Fig. 13–33).

Ileocecal tuberculosis produces nonspecific inflammatory changes involving the terminal ileum and the cecum. Amebiasis may involve the cecum but usually spares the terminal ileum. Crohn's disease may involve the terminal ileum and cecum, and occasionally ulcerative colitis is accompanied by backwash ileitis, so all three conditions have to be considered when there is inflammatory change on both sides of the

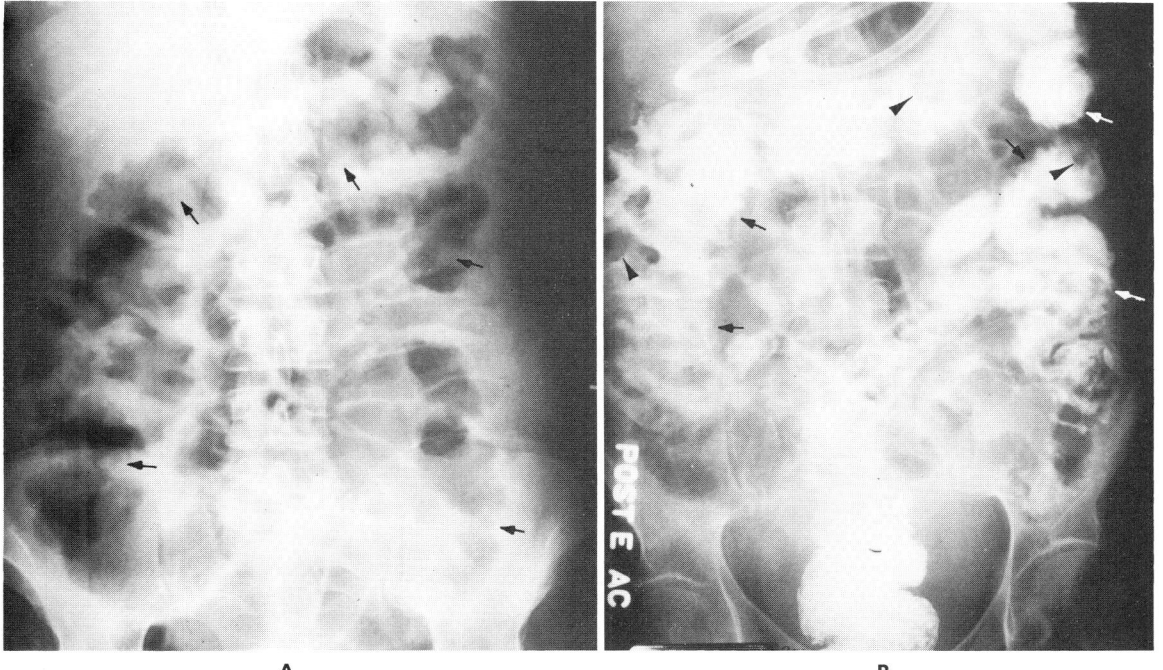

Figure 13–32. *A*, A 47-year-old woman receiving clindamycin developed pain, diarrhea, abdominal distention, and rectal bleeding. An abdominal film reveals an ileus, with distention of both small and large bowel. Throughout the colon, irregularities and large defects are seen (*arrows*).

B, Barium enema discloses diffuse defects (*arrowheads*) and ulcer-like irregular projections (*arrows*) throughout the colon. The large defects were due to pseudomembranous plaques, producing a somewhat distinctive appearance. However, differentiation from acute ulcerative colitis with pseudopolyps or from acute bacterial colitis with extensive wall edema cannot be made solely from the radiographic appearance.

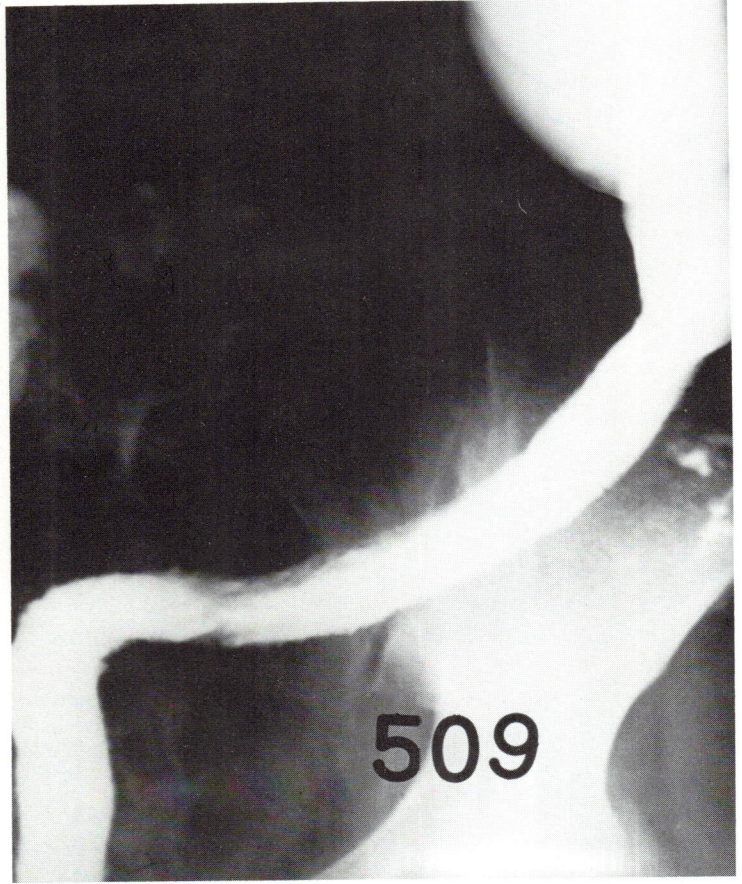

Figure 13–33. Lymphogranuloma venereum. There is marked narrowing of the rectum and sigmoid associated with irregular walls, some of which are the result of ulcerations. The marked stenosis of the rectum and sigmoid is fairly characteristic of lymphogranuloma venereum. Frequently, the ulcerations extend into the soft tissues, producing internal small blind fistulas.

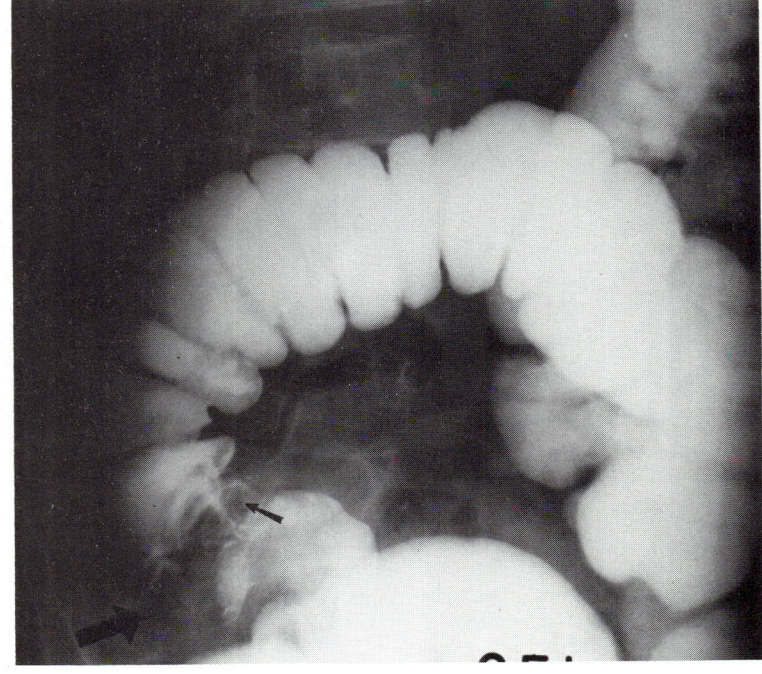

Figure 13–34. Actinomycosis of the cecum. There is irregularity of the cecum with some defects (arrows). This is not a specific finding and could be due to a neoplasm or to a chronic inflammatory lesion. Actinomycosis in the intestinal tract has a tendency to localize in the cecum and occasionally may cause fistulization to the skin or internal organs.

ileocecal valve. With tuberculosis there may be evidence of calcification in the intestinal lesions or active tuberculosis in the chest, whereas in Crohn's disease there may be skip areas in the small bowel or colon. Rarely, histoplasmosis[14] or anisakiasis[62] may involve the ileocecal region and simulate tuberculosis. Anisakiasis is a parasitic infestation associated with eating raw, pickled, or slightly salted fish. Occasionally, actinomycosis may involve the cecum (Fig. 13–34).

Amebiasis may occur as an acute general colonic inflammation with multiple tiny mucosal ulcers seen along the margin of the entire colon down to and including the rectum.[10] This picture may simulate that of chronic ulcerative colitis. The granulomatous form of amebiasis may cause narrowing of the cecum and may involve the right colon, simulating Crohn's disease. Usually the terminal ileum is spared in amebic infection (Fig. 13–35). Occasionally, amebiasis may produce a "thumbprinting" pattern, simulating ischemic colitis.

Ascariasis is an infestation of roundworms which usually is found in the small intestine. However, sometimes large masses of worms may extend into the ascending colon (Fig. 13–36) and may even cause partial obstruction.

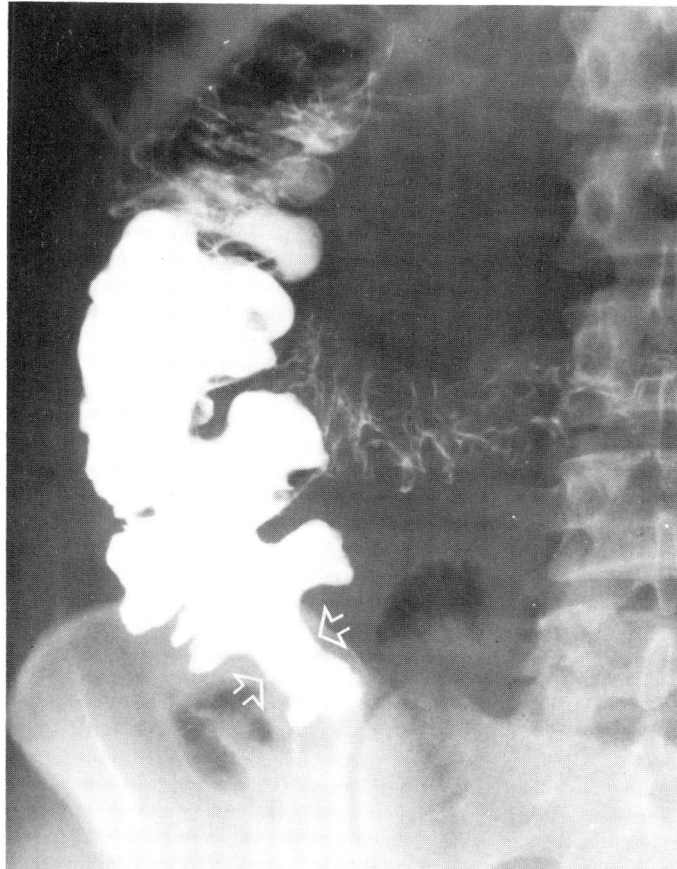

Figure 13–35. Amebiasis of the cecum. The cecum is smoothly and markedly narrowed (arrows), a characteristic result of chronic amebiasis of the cecum. The cecum is a favored area, but any portion of the colon can be involved by chronic amebiasis.

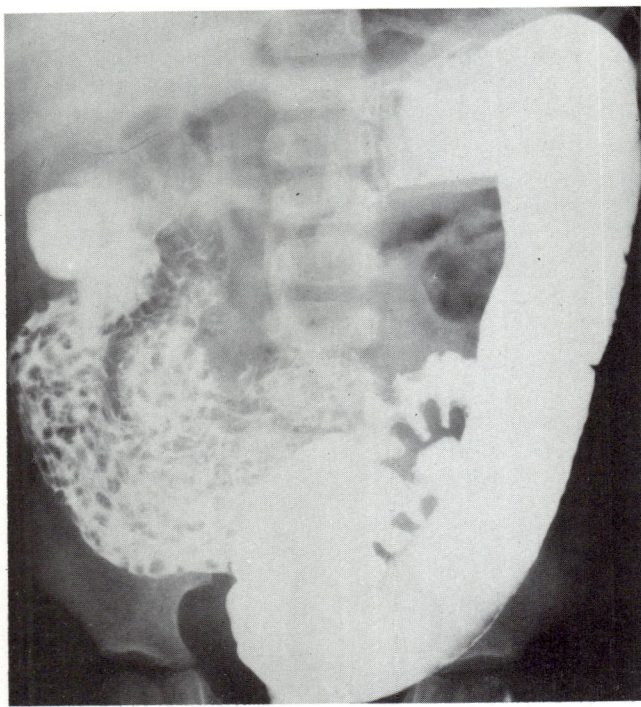

Figure 13–36. Massive ascariasis of the terminal ileum and ascending colon. The defects in the terminal ileum and ascending colon are due to huge numbers of worms. Occasionally, these can cause a mechanical obstruction.

VASCULAR LESIONS

Vascular lesions involving the colon may be due to acute or gradual occlusion of a major artery, occlusion of multiple small arteries, or venous thrombosis. With occlusion of the superior mesenteric artery, plain roentgenograms may show gaseous distention of the small bowel and the right colon up to the splenic flexure. At other times a nonspecific ileus pattern is seen. With venous occlusion, there may be a thickened bowel wall with a narrow gas-filled lumen. With both arterial and venous obstruction, the bowel tends to fill with fluid, and so-called strangulation obstruction occurs.

Localized ischemic colitis may occur in nonspecific small-vessel sclerosis, in cardiac disease, in collagen diseases, such as polyarteritis, and after surgery.[48] On barium enema the mucosa may be edematous with patchy ulceration, and multiple marginal indentations referred to as thumbprinting may be seen (Fig. 13–37). These findings may resolve, or the colon may gradually show a relative constriction or stenosis over a period of several weeks or months (Fig. 13–38). Very rarely, thromboangiitis obliterans[63] may involve mesenteric vessels and cause circumferential narrowing of the colon.

With increasing use of arteriography, *vascular ectasias or small arteriovenous malformations* have been seen, frequently in the region of the cecum.[7, 19, 22, 69] These often cause life-threatening blood loss. On superior mesenteric arteriography, a small branch of the ileocolic artery may be seen entering a small vascular malformation, with early venous filling (Fig. 13–39).

RADIATION INJURY

Radiation injury following large-dosage therapy of lesions of the cervix or other pelvic tumors may decrease vascular supply and cause nonspecific inflammatory

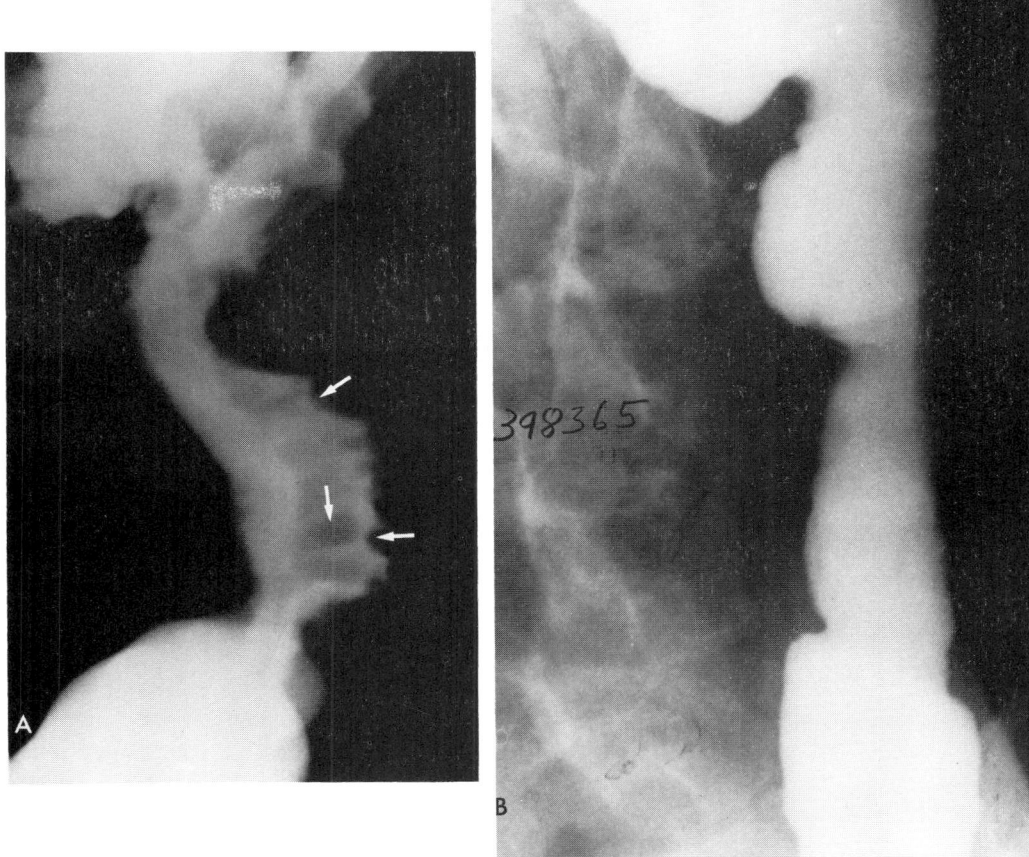

Figure 13–37. Ischemia of the colon. *A*, There are typical thumbprinting changes (arrows) in the upper descending colon. These are associated with some areas of narrowing due to spasm. The narrowing and thumbprinting are fairly characteristic findings of ischemia. *B*, One week later, there has been marked improvement in the appearance of this involved portion of the colon, which has returned to almost normal. (Courtesy of Christopher Merritt, M.D., New Orleans.)

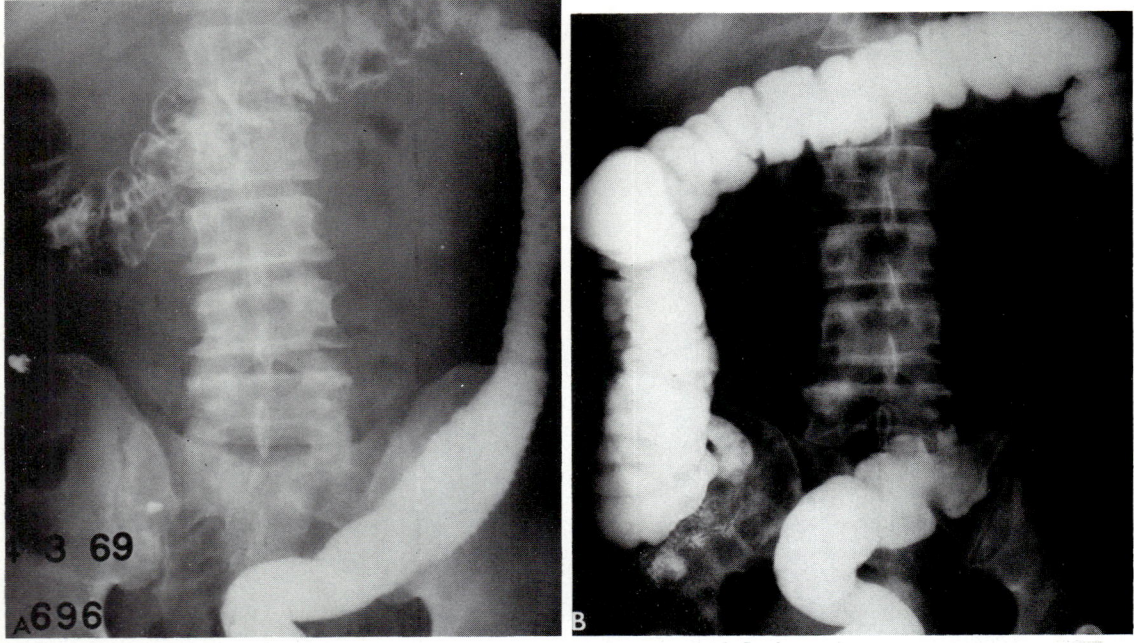

Figure 13–38. Ischemic colon and late stricture. *A*, The descending colon and sigmoid show some irritability and evidence of scalloping and thumbprinting due to acute ischemia. *B*, Four months later, there is a long stricture of the descending colon. (Courtesy of W. V. Weldon, M.D., Birmingham, Alabama.)

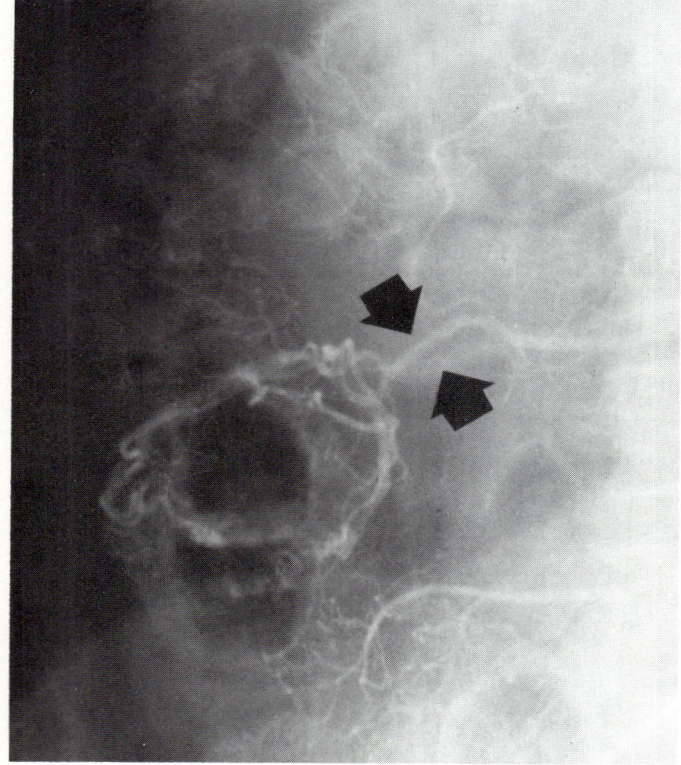

Figure 13–39. Arteriovenous malformation of the cecum; arteriogram. The ileocolic artery (upper arrow) is supplying a tortuous collection of vessels representing the malformation in the cecum. Early venous filling is seen (lower arrow).

THE LARGE BOWEL — 679

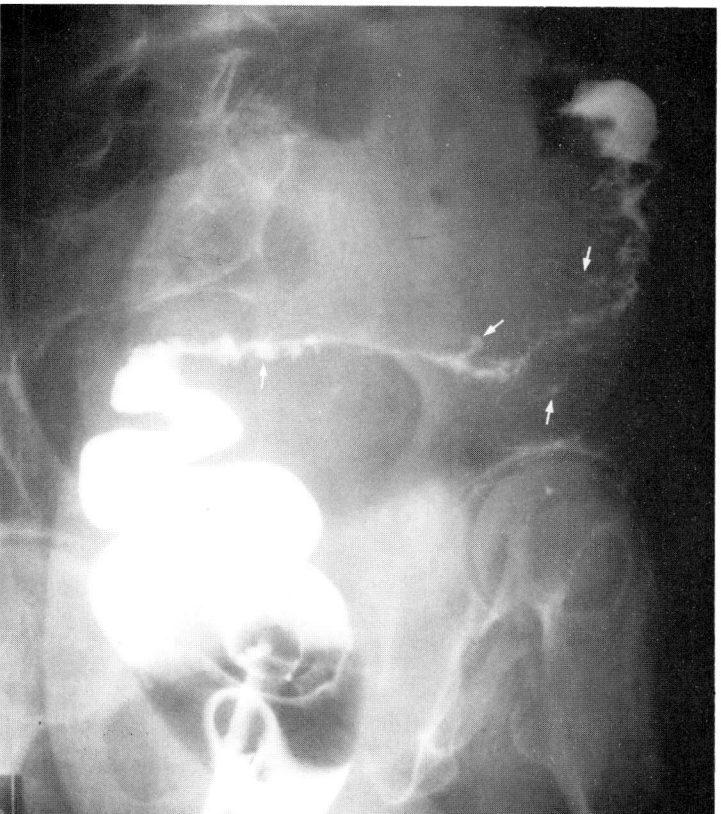

Figure 13–40. Late radiation injury. The sigmoid is markedly narrowed and irregular, with multiple ulcerations and small fistulous tracks (arrows). These are permanent changes and can cause obstruction or fistulous connection to adjacent structures.

mucosal change in the rectum and sigmoid colon. Severe injury can lead to stenosis (Fig. 13–40). Rectovaginal fistulas can result from radiation necrosis of a bowel wall.

MISCELLANEOUS BENIGN LESIONS

Pneumatosis cystoides intestinalis is characterized by multiple gas-containing cysts in the subserosal area (Fig. 13–41) and may somewhat simulate the thumbprinting of ischemic colitis or vaguely resemble multiple polyposis. The air lucencies, however, will be seen to extend beyond the barium margin, a distinctive finding. This condition may be relatively benign and disappear spontaneously. However, there are severe inflammatory or necrotizing forms of enterocolitis that may be complicated by gas in the bowel wall. In children, the intramural gas may sometimes extend into the portal veins, usually an ominous finding. Similar findings are occasionally seen in small bowel necrosis from ischemia. Pneumatosis may occasionally be seen in patients with carcinoma, scleroderma, cystic fibrosis, or leukemia treated by steroids.

Endometriosis and uterine endometrial cells may implant any place in the peritoneal cavity. The rectum and sigmoid are the most commonly involved parts of the gastrointestinal tract. Partial obstruction may be associated with cramping pain, diarrhea, or constipation. Symptoms may be exaggerated during menstruation. Barium enema reveals a partially constricting lesion (Fig. 13–42) that may be relatively short or long and tends to remain extramucosal.

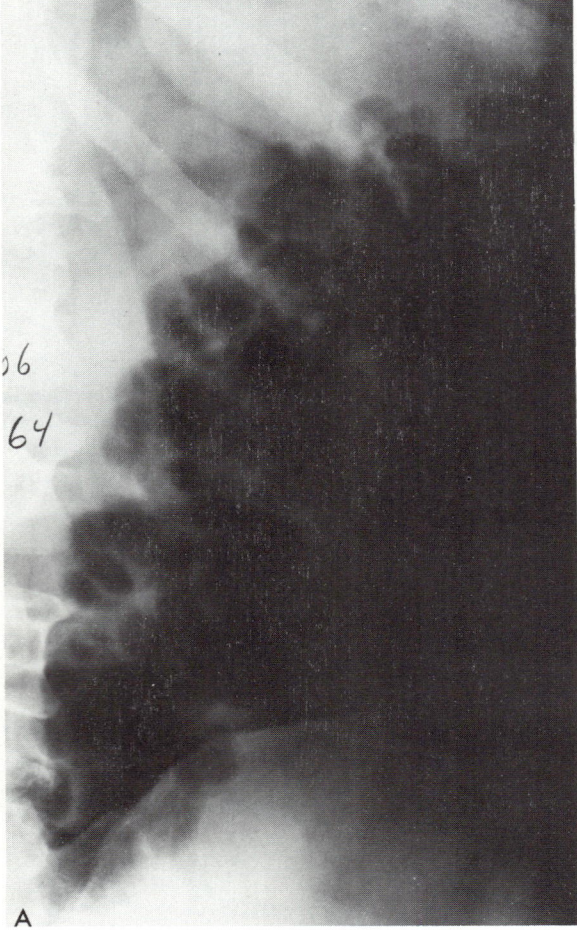
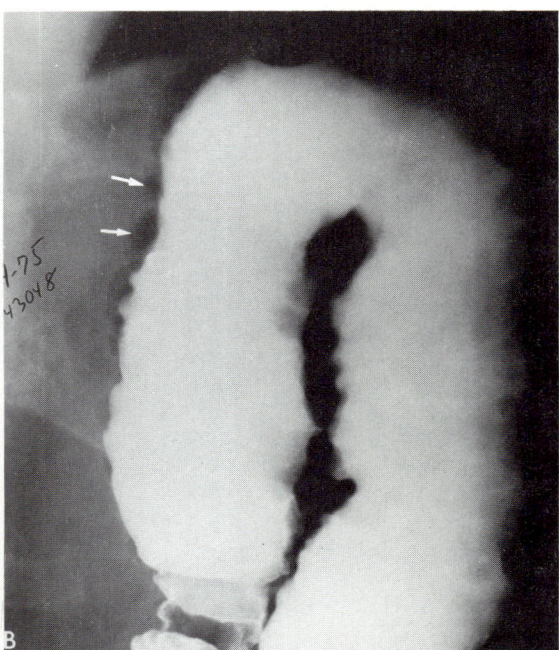

Figure 13–41. Pneumatosis cystoides intestinalis. *A,* A plain film demonstrates multiple rounded collections of gas throughout the distal transverse colon. These are cystlike collections of gas within the wall of the colon. *B,* In another patient, the barium enema shows multiple irregularities of the contour of the distal transverse and descending colon, similar to thumbprinting. However, the defects that are due to intramural gas collections can be seen extending as gas shadows beyond the barium (arrows), a characteristic finding of this type of pneumatosis.

The *lipoma* is the second most common benign tumor of the colon but far less frequent than adenoma. The lipoma is quite radiolucent (Fig. 13–43), is submucosal, and may show some evidence of pliability.[72] The use of a water enema has been suggested when lipoma is suspected, since fat is more radiolucent than water and this lesion will appear as a lucent defect in the water-filled bowel. Enlargement of the ileocecal valve by fatty infiltration or true lipoma may simulate a carcinoma (Fig. 13–44).[4]

Carcinoid tumors of the cecum and right side of the colon are quite rare and sometimes highly malignant. The carcinoid syndrome of skin flushing, asthmatic attacks, diarrhea, and right-heart endocardial fibroelastosis may be present when there are hepatic metastases. The latter interfere with tryptophan metabolism, so that elevated levels of bradykinins and serotonin occur. Rectal carcinoids are not usually associated with the carcinoid syndrome. About one third are over 2 cm in diameter and malignant. Carcinoid may also involve other parts of the colon (Fig. 13–45).

Colitis cystica profunda is a benign process, usually involving the rectum or rectosigmoid and appearing as one or several polypoid masses (Fig. 13–46). It is usually seen in younger adults. Microscopically, there are small cystic mucous lakes lined with normal epithelium beneath the mucosa. Rectal bleeding, mucorrhea, and diarrhea may occur. The lesion is benign but may be mistaken for carcinoma.[52]

Text continued on page 684

THE LARGE BOWEL — 681

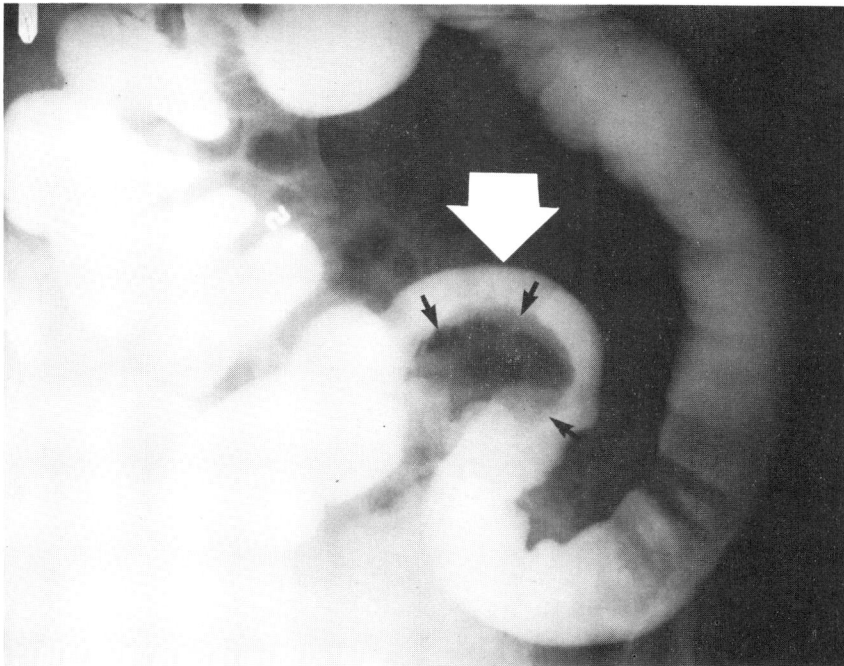

Figure 13–42. Endometriosis of the sigmoid colon. A loop of sigmoid (large arrow) shows a large scalloped defect involving the inferior wall (arrow). This appearance is characteristic of an intramural lesion.

Figure 13–43. Lipoma of the colon. The smooth defect in the descending colon (arrow) was a submucosal lipoma extending into the lumen. Radiographically, it may be difficult to distinguish a lipoma from a large polyp. Sometimes a plain water enema is employed to demonstrate the lucency of the lipoma relative to water.

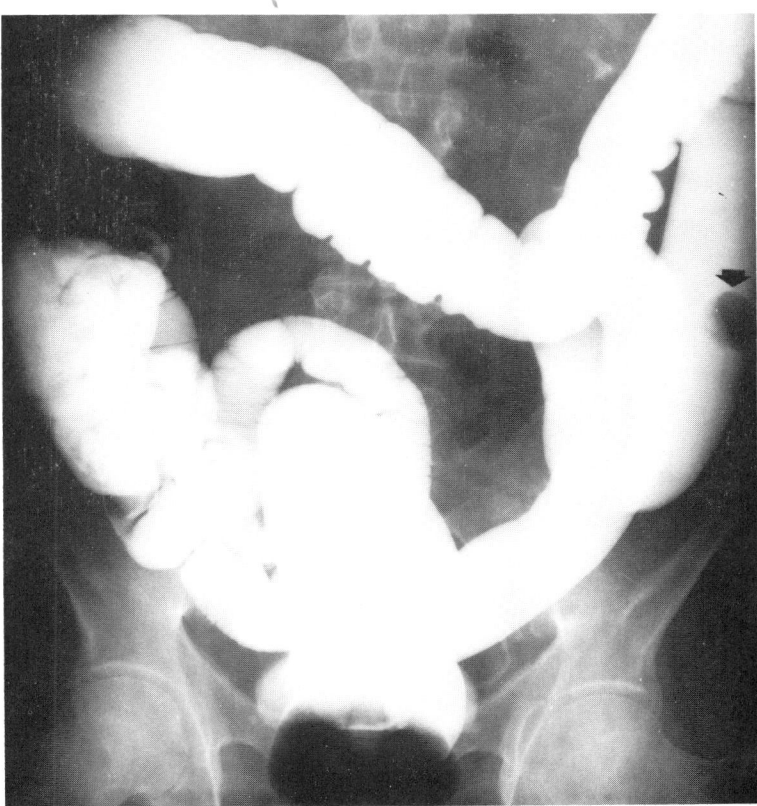

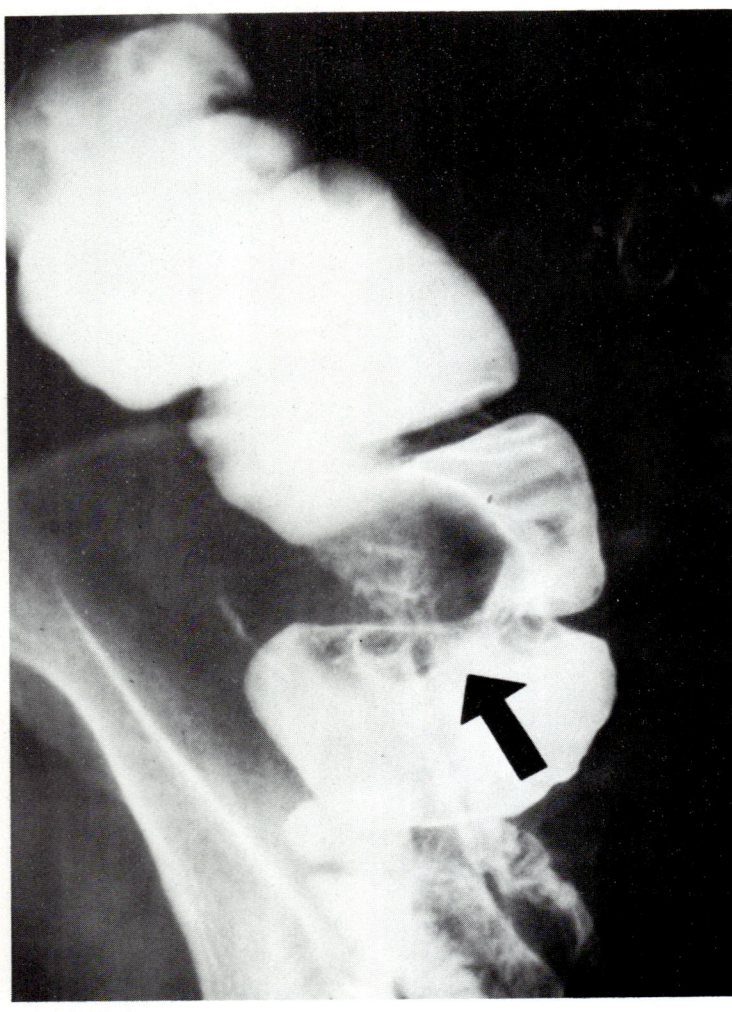

Figure 13–44. Lipoma of the ileocecal valve. The large smooth defect (arrow) is a lipoma of the ileocecal valve. Lipomatous infiltration is a common cause of enlargement of the ileocecal valve.

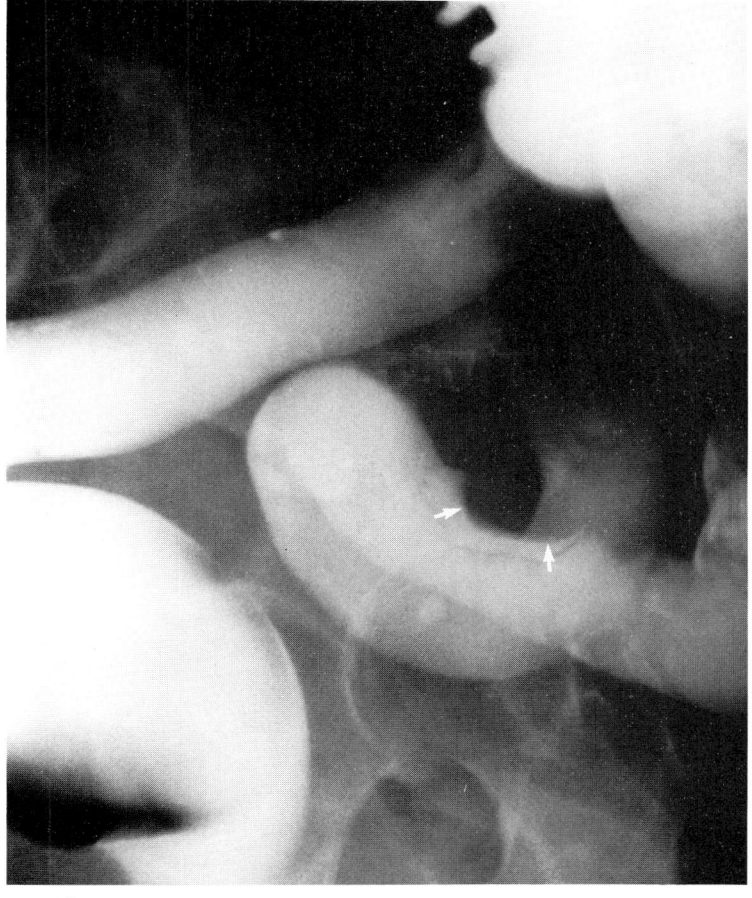

Figure 13–45. Carcinoid of the sigmoid colon. The defect on the superior wall of the sigmoid (white arrows) proved to be a carcinoid. Submucosal lesions, such as carcinoid, lipoma, neurofibroma, or endometriosis, may have similar radiographic appearances.

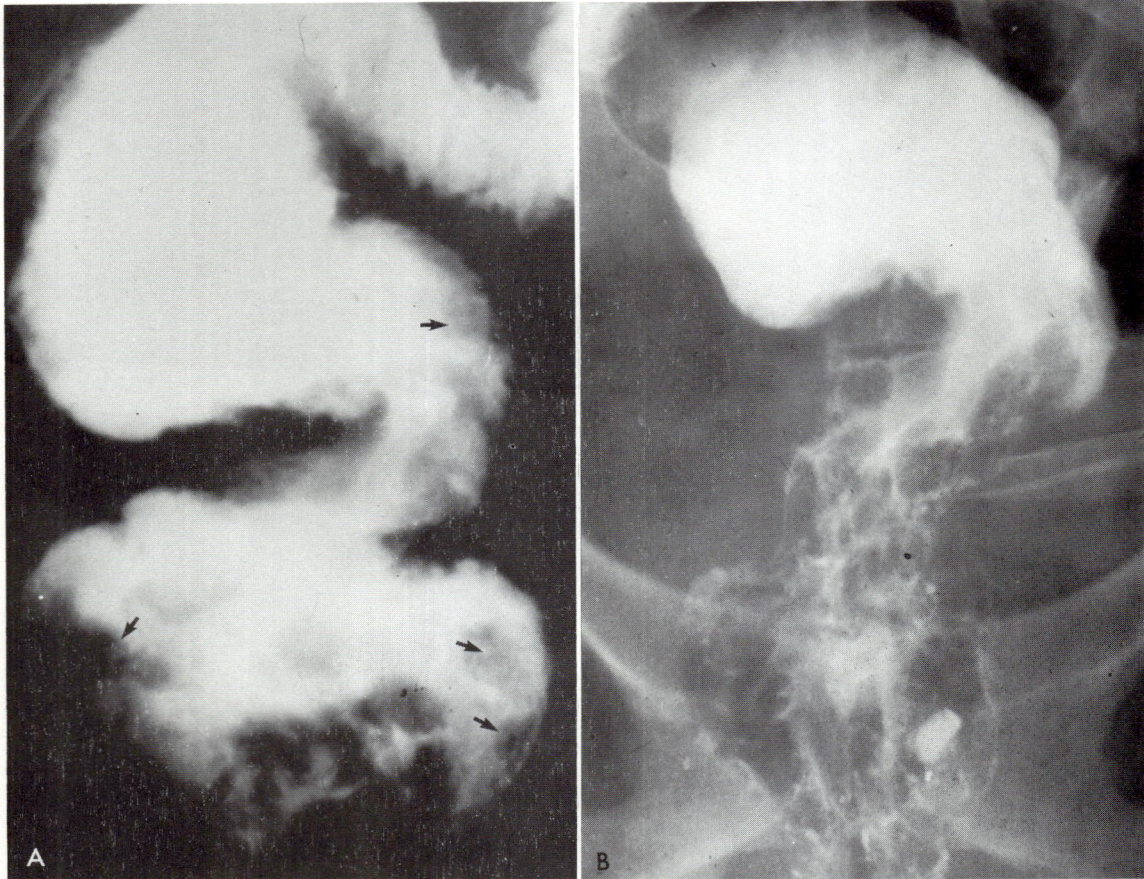

Figure 13-46. Colitis cystica profunda. *A,* There are multiple nodular defects throughout the rectum and rectosigmoid area (arrows). *B,* The postevacuation film shows to better advantage the multiple defects. Radiographically, it may be impossible to distinguish this lesion from a nodular carcinoma. (Courtesy Dr. Arthur Clemett, New York.)

A *hemangioma*[23] may sometimes be suspected when phleboliths are seen adjacent and parallel to the barium column. The lesion is quite pliable and submucosal, so that there is very little or no filling defect or wall irregularity. On the postevacuation film the distortion of the mucosal pattern produced by the extramural hemangioma may sometimes be seen. However, hemangiomas are rarely detected on routine barium enema studies. The increasing use of double-contrast studies has enhanced detection of small mucosal and submucosal lesions of all varieties.

Cathartic colon[76] may be difficult to differentiate from the quiescent phase of long-standing, ulcerative colitis. The clinical history helps in evaluating the radiologic findings. In cathartic colon there may be loss or alteration of the haustral pattern, unusually variable or fleeting contractions, and inconstant narrowing, more pronounced on the right side. The ileocecal valve may be gaping, and the terminal ileum may show similar changes. In severe cases the left side of the colon may also be involved (Fig. 13-47). The flexures are usually in normal position. The sigmoid and rectum are normally distensible.

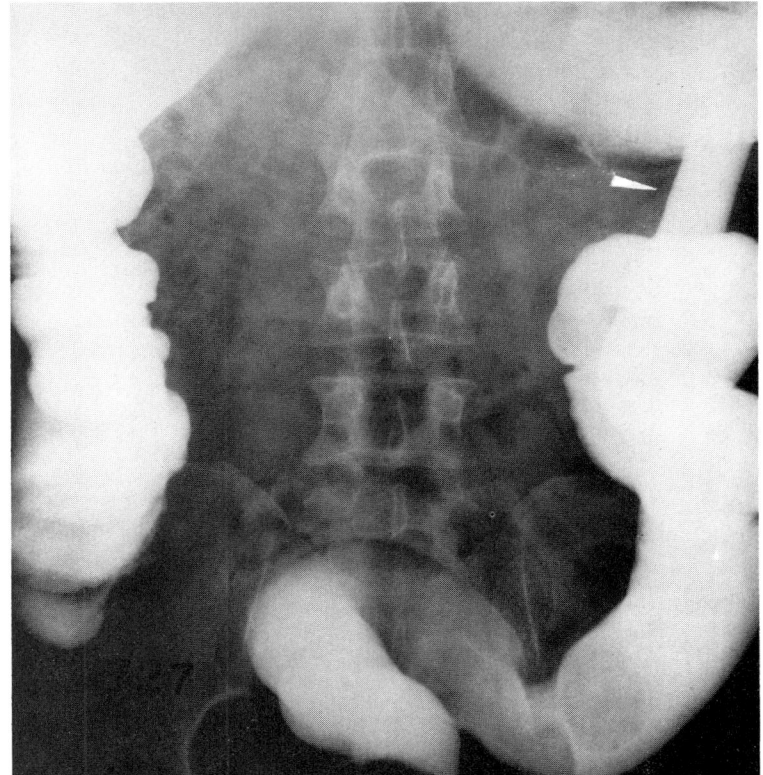

Figure 13–47. Cathartic colon. Normal haustral markings are lacking. Areas of tubular narrowing (arrowhead) and spasm are characteristic.

UNUSUAL LESIONS

1. *Intestinal ganglioneuromatosis* is often associated with medullary thyroid carcinoma and pheochromocytoma. Barium enema demonstrates a distinctive triad of (a) an abnormal haustral pattern in the filled colon, (b) thickened mucosal folds on postevacuation films, and (c) colonic diverticula.[1]

2. *Urticaria* of the colon may produce raised plaques of focal submucosal edema visible on barium enema examination.[5]

3. *Angioneurotic edema* of the colon produces blisterlike, rounded, edematous mucosal imprints in a localized segment on barium enema studies.[30]

4. An *appendix epiploica* may calcify and rarely may become detached and freely mobile in the peritoneal cavity.[8] Torsion, thrombosis, or gangrene involving an appendix epiploica may produce indentation or stenosis of the colon.[32]

5. *Malakoplakia*, usually seen in the urinary tract, may present as a polypoid mass in the cecum.[68]

6. *Pseudotumors* of the colon due to adhesions or fibrous bands appear as intraluminal or intramural masses.[34]

7. *Schistosomiasis* has been reported to produce calcification in the left colon as well as rectosigmoid polyposis and protein-losing enteropathy.[37]

8. A solitary or nonspecific *benign ulcer* of the colon may be demonstrated on barium enema in children or adults.[42]

9. A *rectal stone* may be seen in patients with unusually heavy intake of substances such as milk of magnesia.[38, 72]

10. Patients with *herpes zoster* may show small polygonal mucosal blebs or small ulcerations involving a short segment of the colon.[46]

11. *Extramedullary plasmacytoma* may rarely present as a polypoid mass in the colon.[51]

12. *Behçet's disease*, initially described as a syndrome consisting of oral ulcers, genital ulcers, and ocular inflammation, may also involve multiple other systems. The patients may present with arthritis, a variety of dermatologic lesions, thrombophlebitis, central nervous system involvement, and an unusual colitis. Discrete, peptic-type ulcers, with normal intervening mucosa and normal overall configuration of the colon, are seen on radiography and endoscopy.[71]

13. *Chagas disease*, a relatively common condition in Central and Latin America, causes a generalized degeneration of autonomic ganglia and usually presents as megaesophagus or megacolon.[74]

References

1. Anderson, T. E., Spackman, T. J., and Schwartz, S. S.: Roentgen findings in intestinal ganglioneuromatosis. Radiology *101*:93–96, 1971.
2. Asch, T., Milikow, E., and Gump, F.: Giant gas cyst of the sigmoid. Radiology *96*:409–410, 1970.
3. Berk, R. N.: Barium enema examination in acute appendicitis. J.A.M.A. *236*:394–396, 1976.
4. Berk, R. N., Davis, G. B., and Cholhassey, E. B.: Lipomatosis of the ileocecal valve. Am. J. Roentgenol. *119*:323–328, 1973.
5. Berk, R. N., and Millman, S. J.: Urticaria of the colon. Radiology *99*:539–540, 1971.
6. Bobroff, L. M., Messinger, N. H., Subbarao, K., et al.: The cecal bascule. Am. J. Roentgenol. *115*:249–252, 1972.
7. Boley, S. J., Sprayregen, S., Sammartano, R. J., et al.: The pathophysiologic basis for the angiographic signs of vascular ectasias of the colon. Radiology *125*:615–621, 1977.
8. Borg, S. A., Whitehouse, G. H., and Griffiths, G. J.: A mobile calcified amputated appendix epiploica. Am. J. Roentgenol. *127*:349–350, 1976.
9. Bryk, D.: Ulcerative colitis proximal to an obstructing surgical colonic stricture. Radiology *91*:786–787, 1968.
10. Cardoso, J. M., Kimura, K., Stoopen, M., et al.: Radiology of invasive amebiasis of the colon. Am. J. Roentgenol. *128*:935–941, 1977.
11. Cohen, L. E., Smith, C. J., Pister, J. D., et al.: Clindamycin (Cleocin) colitis. Am. J. Roentgenol. *121*:301–304, 1974.
12. Cohen, W. N.: Roentgenographic evaluation of the rectal valves of Houston in the normal and in ulcerative colitis. Am. J. Roentgenol. *114*:580–583, 1968.
13. Damron, J. R., Lieber, A., and Simmons, T.: Rectal diverticula. Radiology *115*:599–601, 1975.
14. Dietz, M. W.: Ileocecal histoplasmosis. Radiology *91*:285–289, 1968.
15. Dysart, D. N., and Stewart, H. R.: Special angled roentgenography for lesions of the rectosigmoid. Am. J. Roentgenol. *96*:285–291, 1966.
16. Farman, J., Rabinowitz, J. G., and Meyer, M. A.: Roentgenology of infectious colitis. Am. J. Roentgenol. *119*:375–381, 1973.
17. Federman, J., Goldstein, M. E., and Weingarten, B.: Malignant lymphoma of over fifteen years' duration masquerading as ulcerative colitis. Am. J. Roentgenol. *89*:771–778, 1963.
18. Felson, B., and Wiot, J. F.: Some interesting right lower quadrant entities. Radiol. Clin. North Am. *7*:83–95, 1969.
19. Foster, J. H., Morgan, C. V., Therlkell, J. B., et al.: Vascular malformation of the appendiceal stump. J.A.M.A. *215*:636–638, 1971.
20. Franken, E. A., Bixler, D., Fitzgeral, J. F., et al.: Juvenile polyposis of the colon. Eur. Soc. Paediatr. Radiol. *18*:499–504, 1974.
21. Gardiner, G. A.: "Backwash ileitis" with pseudopolyposis. Am. J. Roentgenol. *129*:506–507, 1977.
22. Gennant, H. K., and Ranninger, K.: Vascular dysplasias of the ascending colon: report of two cases and review of the literature. Am. J. Roentgenol. *115*:349–354, 1972.
23. Ghahremani, G. G., Kangarloo. H., Volberg, F., et al.: Diffuse cavernous hemangioma of the colon in the Klippel-Trenaunay syndrome. Radiology *118*:673–678, 1976.
24. Gibson, J. Y.: Volvulus of the transverse colon. South. Med. J. *65*:1150–1151, 1972.
25. Gorske, K.: Intussusception of the proximal appendix into the colon. Radiology *91*:791, 1968.
26. Govoni, A. F., Burdman, D., Teicher, I., et al.: Enterogenous cyst of the colon presenting as a retroperitoneal tumor in an adult. Am. J. Roentgenol. *123*:320–329, 1975.

27. Govoni, A. F., and Smulewicz, J. J.: Large diverticulum of the anal canal. Am. J. Roentgenol. 121:344–347, 1974.
28. Gundersen, A. L., and Kreiter, R. L.: Cecal lithiasis secondary to cecal stenosis. J.A.M.A. 205:210–212, 1968.
29. Holloway, W. J.: Clindamycin-associated colitis. South. Med. J. 68:1469–1470, 1975.
30. Johnson, T. H., Jr., and Caldwell, K. W.: Angioneurotic edema of the colon. Radiology 99:61–63, 1971.
31. Kent, K. H.: Extrinsic lesions affecting the transverse colon. Am. J. Roentgenol. 89:779–786, 1963.
32. Kirsh, D., and Drosd, R. E.: Roentgen change in disease of the appendices epiploicae. Am. J. Roentgenol. 81:640–649, 1959.
33. Kiser, J. L., Spratt, J. S., Jr., and Johnson, C. A.: Colon perforations occurring during sigmoidoscopic examinations and barium enemas. Missouri Med. 65:969–974, 1968.
34. Kyaw, M. M., and Koehler, P. R.: Pseudotumors of colon due to adhesions. Radiology 103:597–599, 1972.
35. Kyaw, M. M., Gallagher, T., and Haines, J. O.: Cloacogenic carcinoma of the anorectal junction: roentgenologic diagnosis. Am. J. Roentgenol. 115:384–391, 1972.
36. Laufer, I., Mullens, J. E., and Hamilton, J.: Correlation of endoscopy and double-contrast radiography in the early stages of ulcerative and granulomatous colitis. Radiology 118:1–5, 1976.
37. Lehman, S., Jr., Farid, Z., Bassily, S., et al.: Colonic calcification and polyposis in schistosomiasis. Radiology 98:379–380, 1971.
38. Lieber, A., and Alavi, S. M.: Rectal stone, report of a case. Am. J. Digest. Dis. 15:287–290, 1970.
39. Lim, M. S.: Gas-filled appendix: lack of diagnostic specificity. Am. J. Roentgenol. 128:209–210, 1977.
40. McDonald, J. B., and Middleton, P. J.: Tuberculosis of the colon simulating carcinoma. Radiology 118:293–294, 1976.
41. McKechnie, J. C., Bynum, T. E., Bentlif, P. S., et al.: Ulcerative proctitis. South. Med. J. 67:1052–1056, 1974.
42. Magilner, A. D.: Solitary benign ulcer of the colon in childhood. Radiology 105:113–114, 1972.
43. Mainzer, F., and Minagi, H.: Giant sigmoid diverticulum. Am. J. Roentgenol. 113:352–354, 1971.
44. Margulis, A. R.: Radiology of ulcerating colitis. Radiology 105:251–263, 1972.
45. Margulis, A. R.: Goldberg, H. I., Lawson, T. L., et al.: The overlapping spectrum of ulcerative and granulomatous colitis: a roentgenographic-pathologic study. Am. J. Roentgenol. 113:325–334, 1971.
46. Menuck, L. S., Brahme, F., Amberg, J., et al.: Colonic changes of herpes zoster. Am. J. Roentgenol. 127:273–276, 1976.
47. Messinger, N. H., Bobroff, L. M., and Beneventano, T. C.: Lymphosarcoma of the colon. Am. J. Roentgenol. 117:281–286, 1973.
48. Meyers, M. A.: Griffiths' point: critical anastomosis at the splenic flexure. Am. J. Roentgenol. 126:77–94, 1976.
49. Miller, R. E., and Skucas, J.: Radiographic Contrast Agents. Baltimore, University Park Press, 1977.
50. Miller, W. T., DePoto, D. W., Scholl, H. W., et al.: Evanescent colitis in the young adult: a new entity. Radiology 100:71–78, 1971.
51. Miller, W. A.: Extramedullary plasmacytoma of the colon. J. Can. Assoc. Radiol. 21:33–34, 1970.
52. Mulder, H., and teVelde, J.: Colitis cystica profunda. Radiol. Clin. Biol. 43:529–539, 1974.
53. Nelson, J. A., Margulis, A. R., Goldberg, H. E., et al.: Ulcerative and granulomatous colitis. Am. J. Roentgenol. 119:369–374, 1973.
54. Newton, N. A., and Reines, H. D.: Transverse colon volvulus: case reports and review. Am. J. Roentgenol. 128:69–72, 1977.
55. North, L. B., and Weens, H. S.: The intestinal knot syndrome. Am. J. Roentgenol. 92:1042–1047, 1964.
56. Pear, B. L., and Wolff, J. N.: Epidermoid cyst of the cecum. J.A.M.A. 207:1516–1517, 1969.
57. Peterson, R. B., Meseroll, W. P., Shrago, G. G., et al.: Radiographic features of colitis associated with the hemolytic-uremic syndrome. Radiology 118:667–671, 1976.
58. Pochaczevsky, R.: The water double contrast barium enema study. Am. J. Roentgenol. 121:326–333, 1974.
59. Press, H. C., Jr., and Davis, T. W.: Ingested foreign bodies simulating polyposis: report of six cases. Am. J. Roentgenol. 127:1040–1042, 1976.
60. Rabinowitz, J. G., Farman, J., Dallemand, S., et al.: Giant sigmoid diverticulum. Am. J. Roentgenol. 121:338–343, 1974.
61. Raskin, M. M., Viamonte, M., and Viamonte, M., Jr.: Primary linitis plastica carcinoma of the colon. Radiology 113:17–22, 1974.
62. Richman, R. H., and Lewicki, A. M.: Right ileocolitis secondary to anisakiasis. Am. J. Roentgenol. 119:329–331, 1973.
63. Sachs, I. L., Klima, T., and Frankel, N. B.: Thromboangiitis obliterans of the transverse colon. J.A.M.A. 238:336–337, 1977.
64. Sacks, B. A., Joffe, N., and Antonioli, D. A.: Metastatic melanoma presenting clinically as multiple colonic polyps. Am. J. Roentgenol. 129:511–513, 1977.
65. Sannella, N. A.: Inguinal hernia and colon carcinoma: presentation of a series and analysis. Surgery 73:434–437, 1973.
66. Seaman, W. B.: Unusual roentgen manifestations of large bowel cancer. Semin. Roentgenol. 11:89–99, 1976.

67. Soter, C. S.: The contribution of the radiologist to the diagnosis of acute appendicitis. Semin. Roentgenol. 8:375–388, 1973.
68. Spjut, H. J., and Navarrete, A.: Pathology of the colon. In Margulis, A. R., and Burhenne, H. J. (eds.): Alimentary Tract Roentgenology. St. Louis, The C. V. Mosby Company, 1973.
69. Sprayregen, S., and Boley, S. J.: Vascular ectasias of the right colon. J.A.M.A. 239:962–964, 1978.
70. Stanley, P., Fry, I. K., Dawson, A. M., et al.: Radiological signs of ulcerative colitis and Crohn's disease of the colon. Clin. Radiol. 22:434–442, 1971.
71. Stanley, R. J., Tedesco, F. J., Melson, G. L., et al.: The colitis of Behçet's disease: a clinical-radiographic correlation. Radiology 114:603–604, 1975.
72. Thompson, R. J., and Barry, W. F., Jr.: Rectal calculus. Radiology 96:411–412, 1970.
73. Thompson, W. M., Kelvin, F. M., and Rice, R. P.: Inflammation and necrosis of the transverse colon secondary to pancreatitis. Am. J. Roentgenol. 128:943–948, 1977.
74. Todd, I. P., Porter, N. H., Morson, B. C., et al.: Chagas disease of the colon and rectum. Gut 10:1009–1014, 1969.
75. Tully, T. E., and Feinberg, S. B.: A reappearance of antibiotic-induced pseudomembranous enterocolitis. Radiology 110:563–567, 1974.
76. Urso, F. P., Urso, M. J., and Lee, C. H.: The cathartic colon: pathological findings and radiological/pathological correlation. Radiology 116:557–559, 1975.
77. Weinrib, M., and Sheehy, T. W.: Colitis associated with clindamycin therapy. South. Med. J. 68:1471–1474, 1975.
78. Wener, L.: The angle prone projection: its value in diagnosis of low-lying lesions. Am. J. Roentgenol. 110:393–398, 1970.
79. Westcott, J. L., and Smith, J. R. V.: Mesentery and colon injuries secondary to blunt trauma. Radiology 114:597–600, 1975.
80. Whalen, J. P.: Anatomy of the colon: guide to intraabdominal pathology. Am. J. Roentgenol. 125:3–20, 1975.
81. Wolf, B. S.: Lipoma of the colon. J.A.M.A. 235:2225–2227, 1976.
82. Youker, J. E., Dodds, W. T., and Welin, S.: Colonic polyps. In Margulis, A. R., and Burhenne, H. J. (eds.): Alimentary Tract Roentgenology. St. Louis, The C. V. Mosby Company, 1973.

Part II
Inflammatory Bowel Disease

RICHARD GARDINER, M.D.

Inflammatory bowel diseases, such as ulcerative colitis and Crohn's disease, are reported to be difficult to detect and differentiate, especially in their early stages when objective findings may be subtle.[3, 13, 17] With the advent of colonic endoscopy much has been learned of the mucosal changes that take place in these conditions. Excellent correlation can now be made between the endoscopic evaluation of the mucosal surface and the findings on high-quality double-contrast radiologic studies.

METHOD OF EXAMINATION

The available evidence indicates that double-contrast examination of the colon is the most effective method for the radiologic evaluation of inflammatory bowel diseases and bowel neoplasia.[9–11, 14] The exquisite detail of the gut's surface anatomy that is obtained with double-contrast examinations provides demonstration of subtle pathologic changes. Early or subtle surface changes are often difficult or impossible to detect on full-column barium enema studies. Frequently, the full extent of involvement cannot be assessed on full-column study even when an excellent postevacuation film is obtained.

Patient comfort and diagnostic accuracy both may be improved if parenteral glucagon is used to induce bowel hypotonia during the double-contrast study.[15] A detailed description of patient preparation and materials and methods for performing double-contrast examinations is available in the literature.[5]

ULCERATIVE COLITIS

Radiologic Appearance

PLAIN FILM   Air-filled colonic segments on plain films of the abdomen in patients with ulcerative colitis may show: (1) loss of normal haustral pattern; (2) a scalloped or wavy appearance of the contour of the bowel and, occasionally, deep, toothlike projections; and (3) numerous broad-based, polypoid projections extending into the lumen from the bowel wall.[16] These plain film findings are infrequent except in advanced cases.

When toxic dilatation of the colon (megacolon) is clinically suspected, radiologic examination should be limited to plain noncontrast film studies. It is dangerous to administer an enema to a patient with toxic dilatation of the colon, since this may lead to perforation of the thinned colonic mucosa.[21] It has been suggested that an objective diagnosis of megacolon complicating ulcerative colitis may be established by either of the following criteria: (1) an abnormal gas-filled transverse colon that exceeds 6 cm in diameter and presents as the most distended segment of colon; and (2) a subserosal radiolucent line paralleling the colon.[16] Multiple polypoid defects in the gas-filled distended transverse colon are virtually diagnostic (Fig. 13–48).

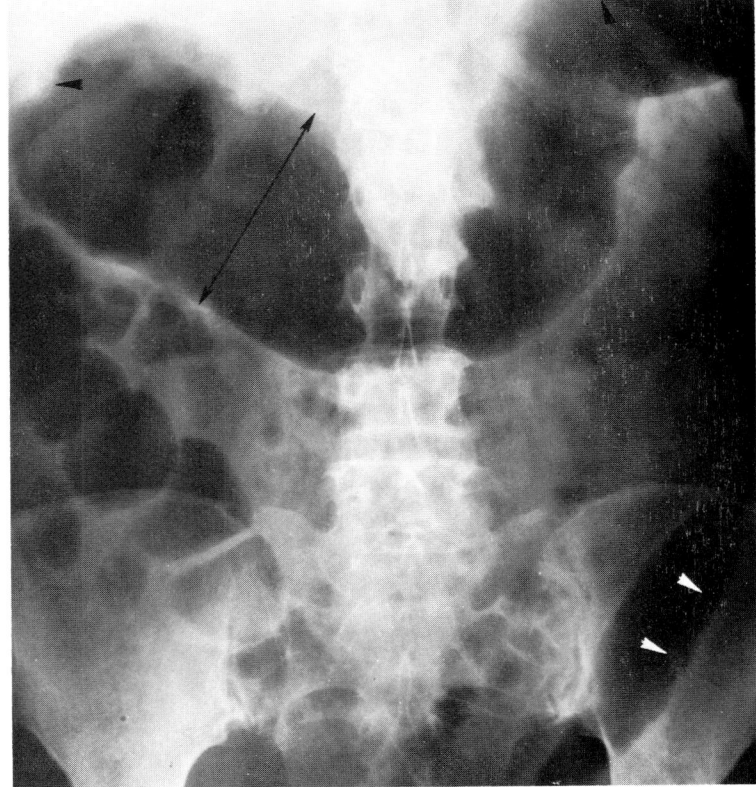

Figure 13–48. Acute megacolon in ulcerative colitis. The transverse colon is greater than 6 cm in diameter (double-headed arrow), and the transverse and sigmoid portions of the colon contain multiple polypoid projections into the bowel lumen (arrowheads).

BARIUM ENEMA. In patients whose clinical condition permits, the double-contrast, enema is an excellent method for determining the presence and extent of ulcerative colitis. Involvement in ulcerative colitis may be confined to the rectum (Fig. 13–49), which is invariably involved, or may extend continuously orad to include any segment up to the entire large bowel in continuity with a short segment of terminal ileum. The latter is termed backwash ileitis.[26] Involvement in the diseased segment of large bowel is diffuse, symmetric, continuous, and total. Instead of the normal smooth appearance, the mucosa is irregular and granular, often with shallow ulcerations and inflammatory pseudopolyps. Periproctitis may cause an increase in the presacral space and a narrowing of the rectosigmoid colon lumen (see Fig. 13–49; Figs. 13–50 to 13–53).[24] When present, backwash ileitis is usually associated with an incompetent ileocecal valve and total large bowel involvement. The involved terminal ileum is flaccid and has an appearance similar to that of the diseased large bowel.

Text continued on page 694

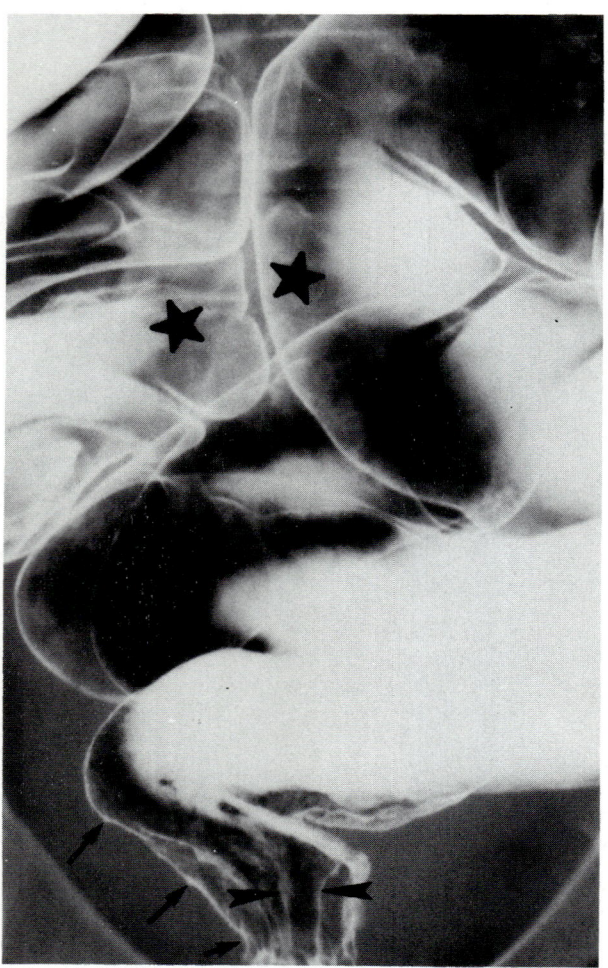

Figure 13–49. Ulcerative proctitis. Double-contrast study. The rectal mucosal folds are thickened (arrowheads) and irregular (arrows). The sigmoid and cecal colonic mucosa (asterisks) and the rest of the colon are normal.

Figure 13–50. Ulcerative colitis of the rectum and sigmoid. Double-contrast study. Frontal (A) and lateral (B) views of the rectosigmoid show fine mucosal ulcerations involving the entire sigmoid colon and rectum. Shallow ulcerations and mucosal granularity extend orad from the rectum with total, continuous, symmetric, and diffuse involvement of the diseased segment.

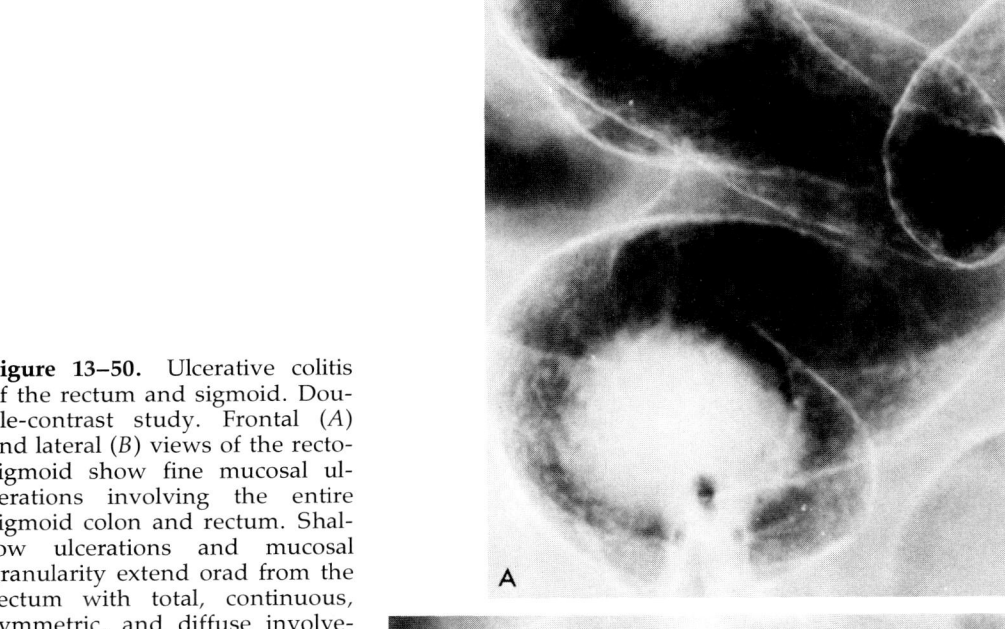
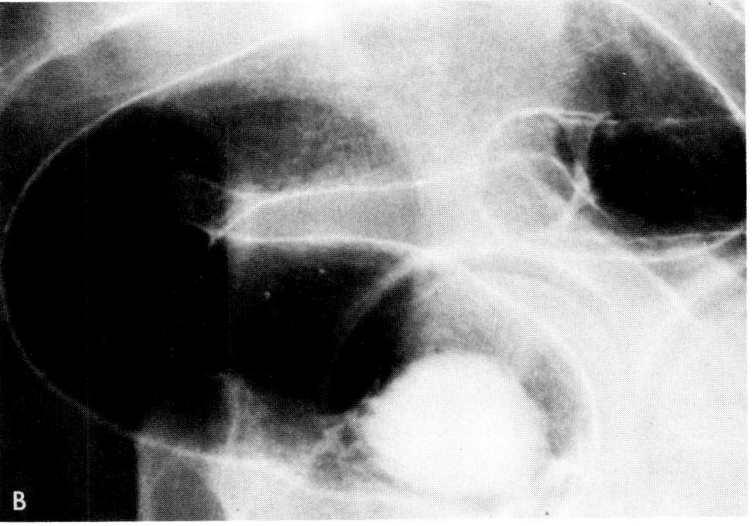

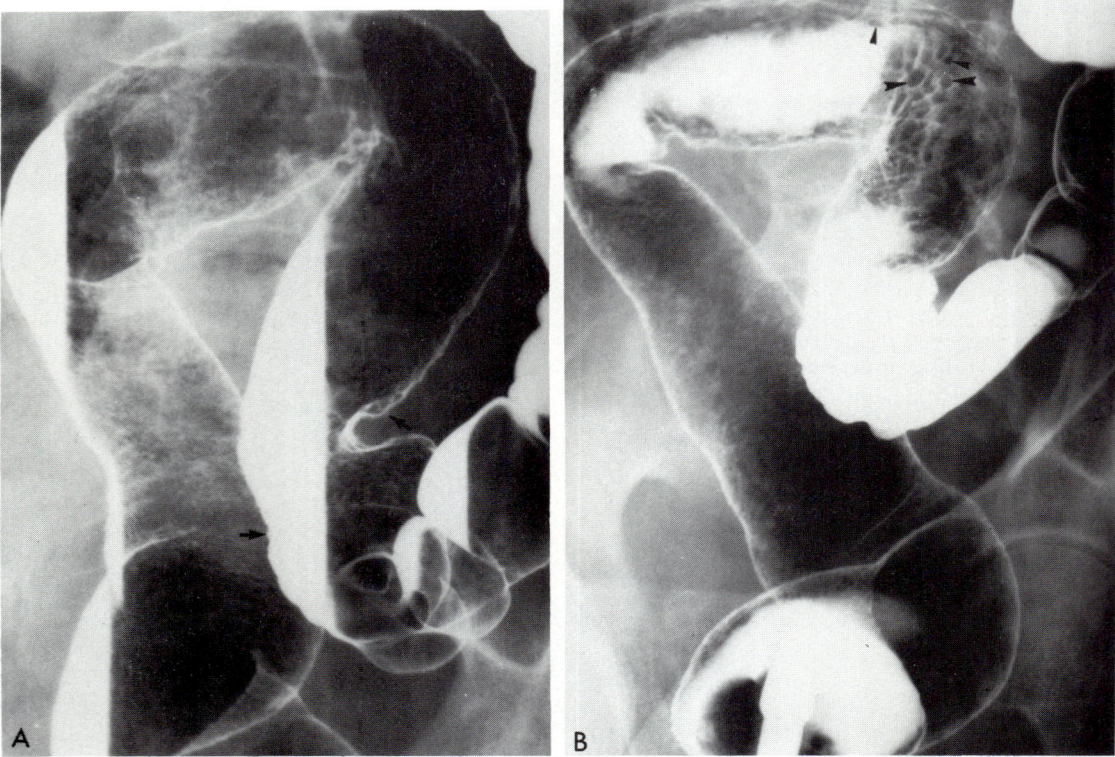

Figure 13–51. Ulcerative colitis of rectum and sigmoid. Double-contrast study. *A*, The bowel has a fine, granular appearance on the *en face* view; small ulcerations (arrows) can be seen in the profile view. *B*, Polypoid projections (arrowheads) in the sigmoid colon represent inflammatory polyps.

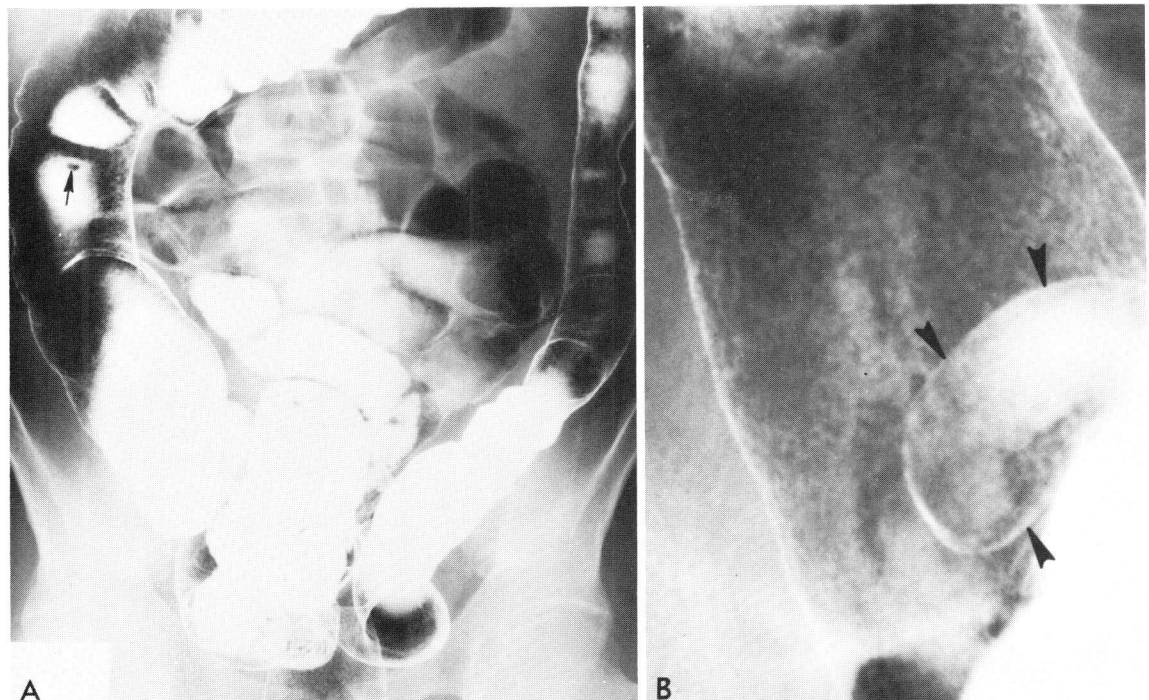

Figure 13–52. Chronic ulcerative colitis of entire colon. Double-contrast study. *A,* Pancolitis is evident, with symmetrical, diffuse mucosal granularity involving the entire large bowel from the cecum to the anus. An inflammatory polyp is present in the proximal colon (arrow). No normal mucosa is present. *B,* The ileocecal valve is patulous, and the terminal ileum (arrowheads) is widened and devoid of the normal mucosal folds, indicating backwash ileitis.

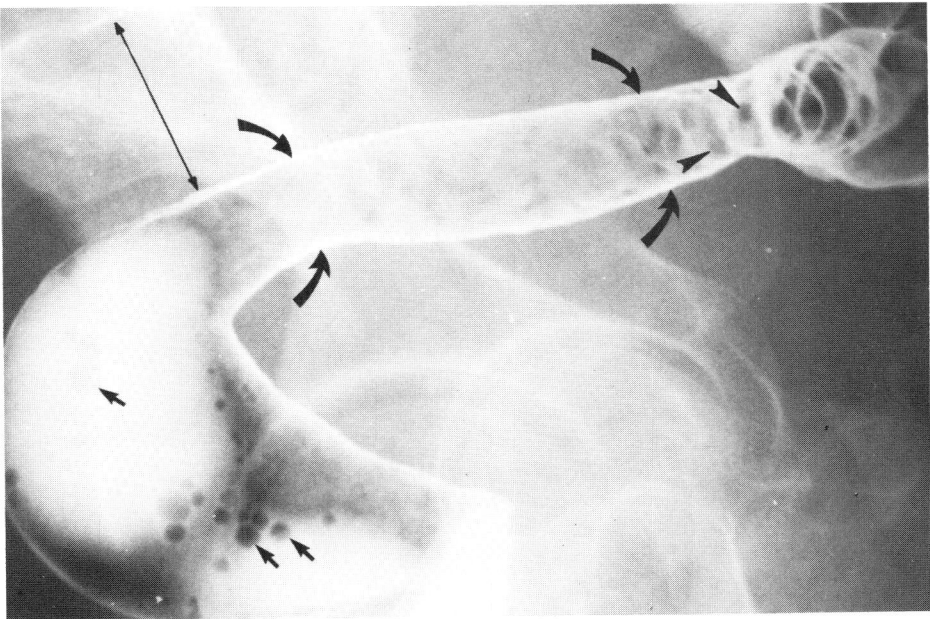

Figure 13–53. Chronic ulcerative colitis. Double-contrast study. Periproctitis has increased the presacral space (double-headed arrow). The sigmoid colon (curved arrows) is narrowed. The small lucencies (arrows) in the rectum are gas bubbles. Several round lucencies in the distal sigmoid colon represent postinflammatory polyps (arrowheads).

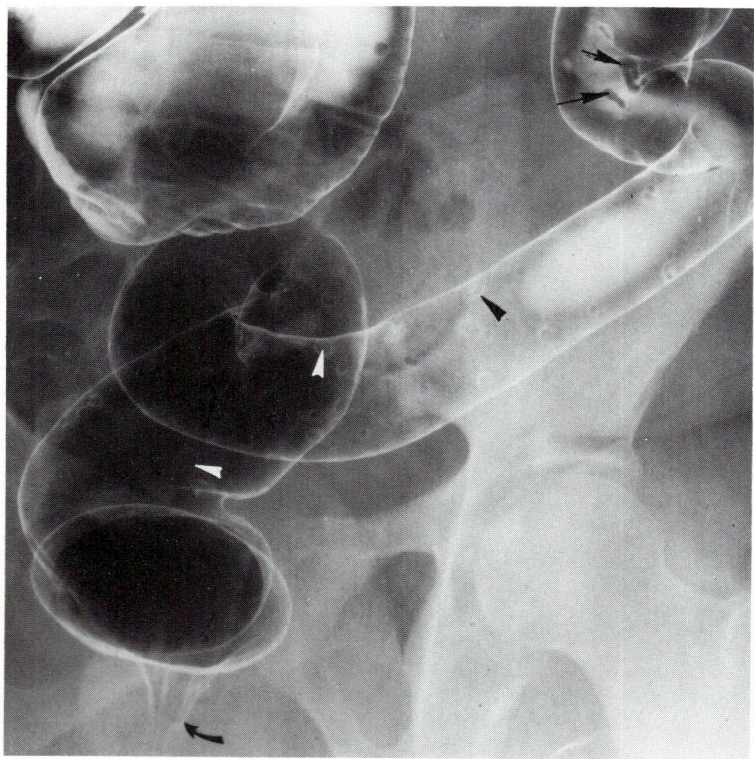

Figure 13–54. Inactive ulcerative colitis. Double-contrast study. The background mucosa is normal, with no evidence of ulceration or granularity, and the anal folds (curved arrow) are not edematous. However, as sequelae of the acute phase of the disease, multiple postinflammatory polyps (arrowheads), some with a filiform shape (arrows), are present throughout the sigmoid colon.

Polypoid Changes and Carcinoma

Several kinds of "polyps" are found in patients with ulcerative colitis. Adenomatous and hyperplastic (metaplastic) polyps may be found in any large bowel. Patients with ulcerative colitis and extensive confluent ulceration may also develop pseudopolyps, which can be detected on barium enema examinations. Although three histologic types of pseudopolyps have been described,[12] they are usually indistinguishable from one another or from adenomatous or hyperplastic polyps on radiologic examination. Polyps on a background of granular, inflamed mucosa, with or without ulceration, are called inflammatory polyps (see Figs. 13–51, 13–52, 13–56, and 13–59). Polyps on the smooth mucosa of quiescent inflammatory bowel disease are called postinflammatory polyps (Figs. 13–53 and 13–54). Inflammatory and postinflammatory polyps may assume an elongated, filiform shape (Fig. 13–54)[28] and may sometimes be connected to the bowel wall in two places forming "mucosal bridges" (see Fig. 13–76).[6] The uniform small size of the submucosal defects of nodular lymphoid hyperplasia helps to distinguish this presumably nonspecific response to inflammatory bowel disease[19] from other polypoid changes (Fig. 13–55).

There is an increased incidence of colorectal cancer in patients with ulcerative colitis, especially when large bowel involvement is total and long-standing (Figs. 13–56 and 13–57; see Fig. 13–93).[18] Unfortunately, colorectal carcinoma complicating chronic ulcerative colitis may be a relatively flat growth,[8, 18] making radiologic or endoscopic detection difficult.[2] There is some indication that colonic dysplasia (precarci-

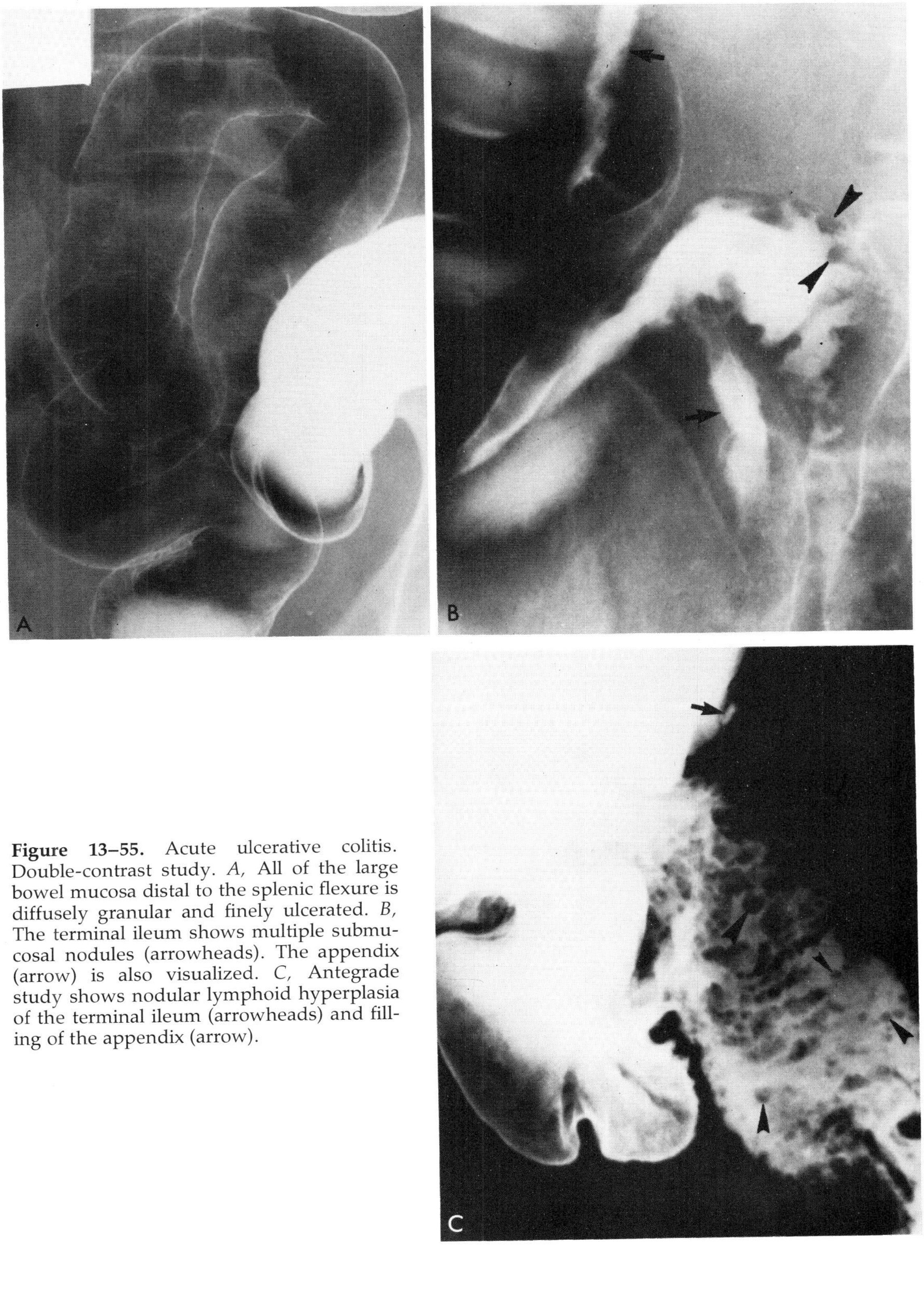

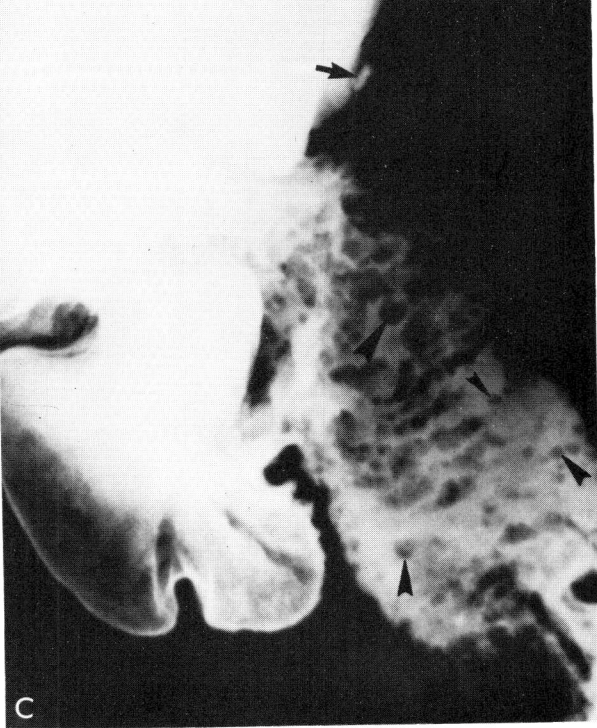

Figure 13–55. Acute ulcerative colitis. Double-contrast study. *A*, All of the large bowel mucosa distal to the splenic flexure is diffusely granular and finely ulcerated. *B*, The terminal ileum shows multiple submucosal nodules (arrowheads). The appendix (arrow) is also visualized. *C*, Antegrade study shows nodular lymphoid hyperplasia of the terminal ileum (arrowheads) and filling of the appendix (arrow).

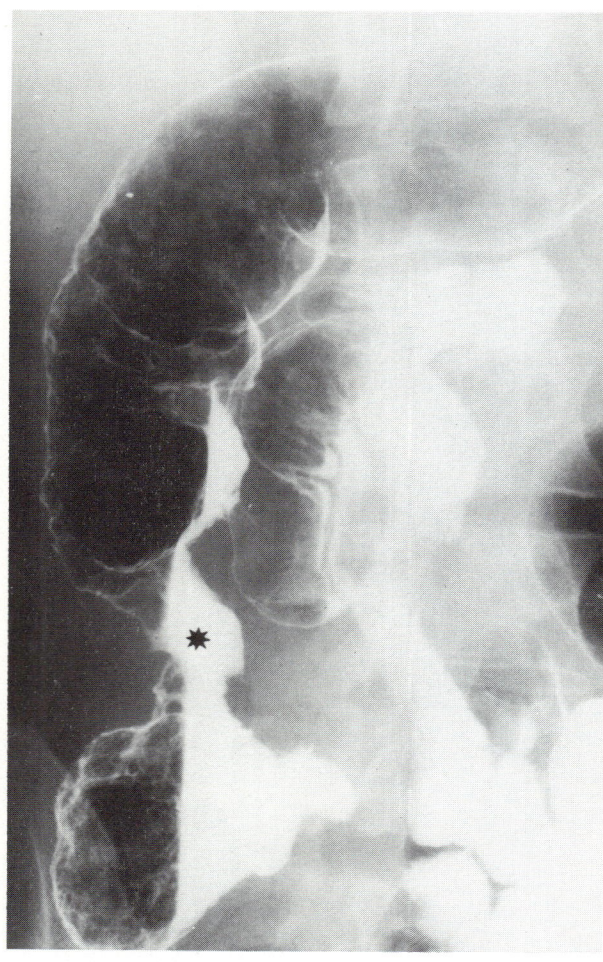

Figure 13–56. Carcinoma complicating ulcerative colitis. A 28-year-old man had a nontender right lower quadrant mass, anemia, and occult blood in his stool. Twenty years earlier he had been hospitalized for colitis. Since then he had been asymptomatic. Double-contrast enema examination shows an encircling carcinoma (asterisk) of the proximal ascending colon. The surface of the colon surrounding the carcinoma is irregular and contains multiple inflammatory polyps and several adenomatous polyps.

noma) may be detectable by double-contrast enema examination in patients with chronic ulcerative colitis.[4] If true, then periodic examinations may provide a satisfactory monitor for the development of malignancy.

Unlike Crohn's disease, ulcerative colitis is rarely complicated by inflammatory masses and fistulas. A small percentage of cases of ulcerative colitis are associated with sclerosing cholangitis or with spondylitis, especially sacroiliitis.

Post-Therapy Changes

It is essential that the radiologist obtain an accurate and complete clinical history for evaluating the follow-up radiologic examinations (Fig. 13–58). Since medical therapy may alter the appearance of the bowel, knowledge of the treatment administered may enable the radiologist to evaluate the radiographic images more accurately. For example, the absence of rectal involvement in a patient with otherwise typical findings for ulcerative colitis might be puzzling and confusing unless the radiologist learns that the patient has received corticosteroid enemas, which can locally reverse the mucosal changes of ulcerative colitis (Fig. 13–59). Similarly, partial bowel resection may necessitate technical modifications of the barium study.

Text continued on page 701

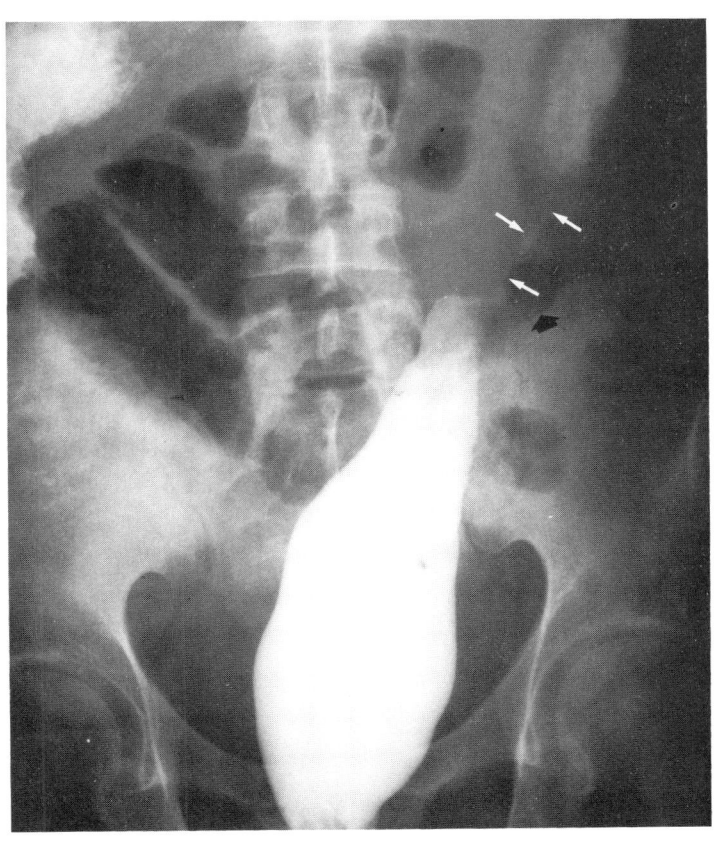

Figure 13–57. Stricture-like carcinoma complicating chronic ulcerative colitis. The long stricture-like narrowing (white arrows) in the sigmoid was an encircling carcinoma. The portions of the colon opacified by barium show the characteristic mucosal loss and postinflammatory polyps of chronic ulcerative colitis (disregard the black arrow).

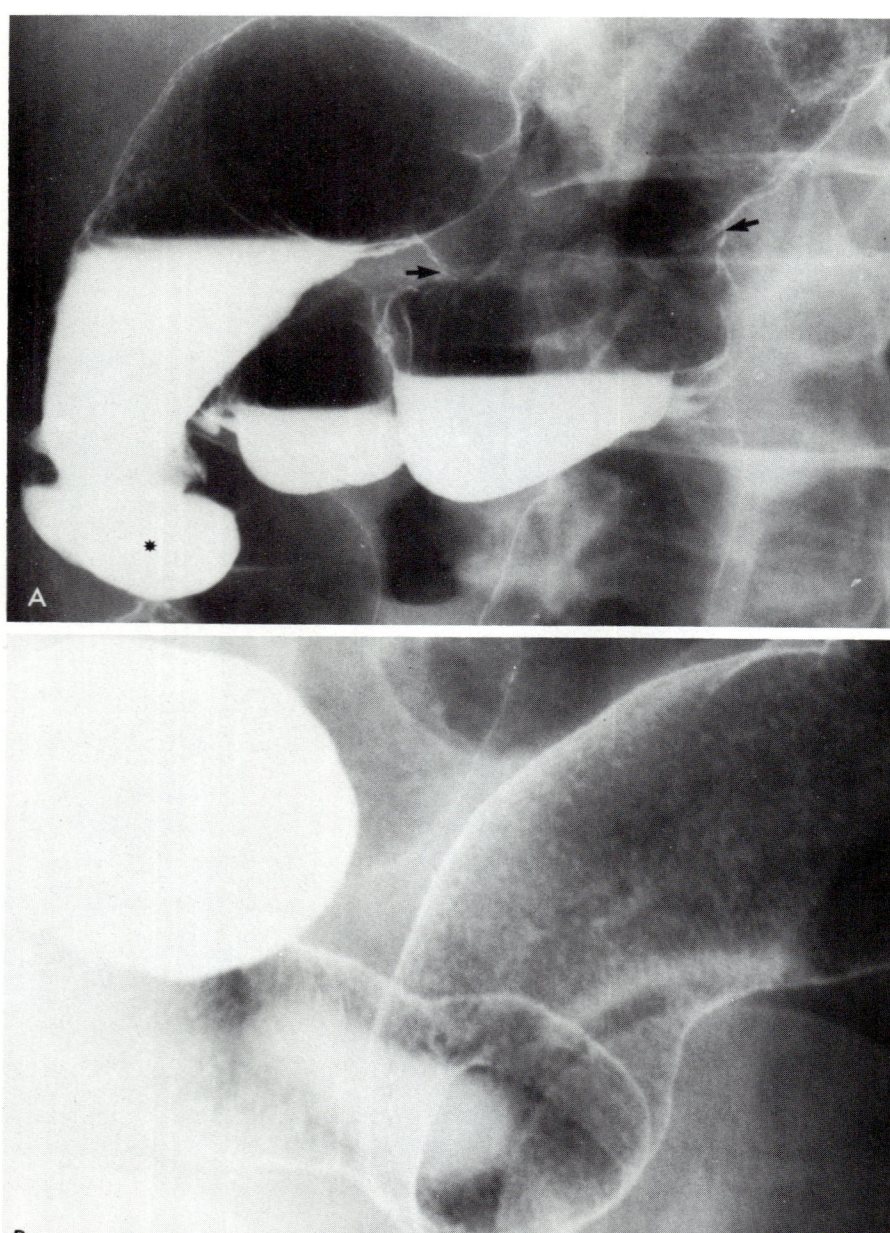

Figure 13–58. Recurrent carcinoma of colon in unrecognized ulcerative colitis. A 38-year-old man with bowel problems since early youth had a right hemicolectomy for carcinoma of the cecum performed ten months previously. A small bowel resection for tumor recurrence had been performed one month prior to this examination. *A*, An ileotransverse side-to-side anastomosis (between arrows) separates the finely granular large bowel mucosa from the normal small bowel mucosa. The most proximal portion of the large bowel is indicated by the asterisk. *B*, Fine mucosal granularity also involves the sigmoid.

Figure 13–58 *Continued.* C, Extrinsic impression (arrowheads) on the anterior surface of the rectum indicates tumor implants in the cul-de-sac. Until this examination, ulcerative colitis had not been suspected.

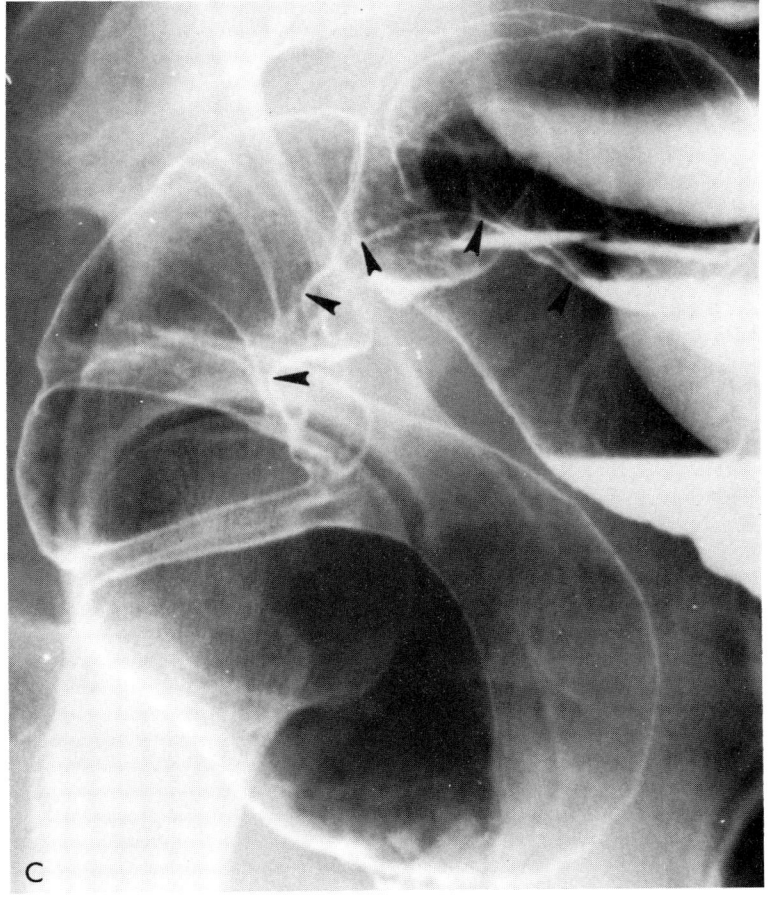

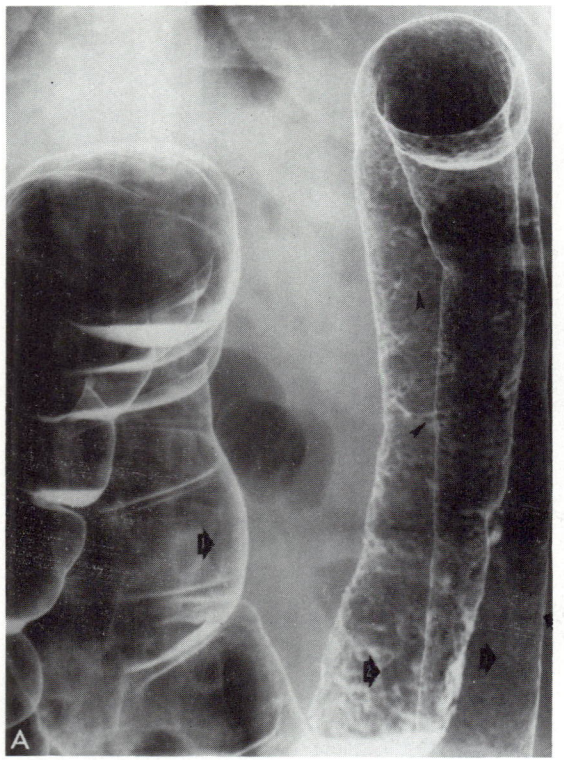 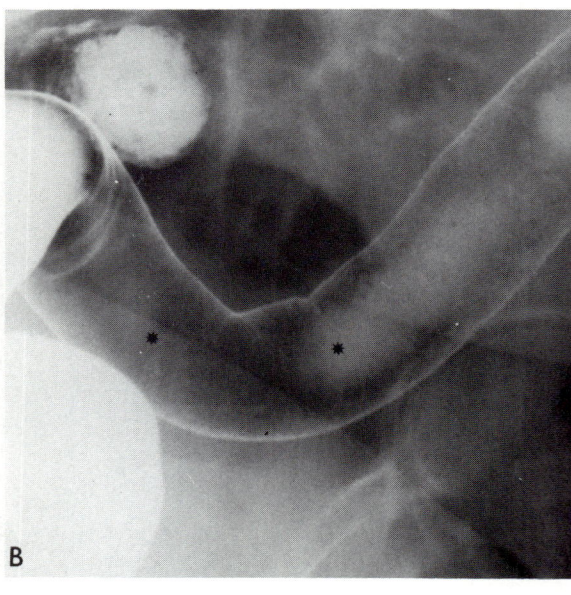

Figure 13–59. Chronic ulcerative colitis. Improvement of distal colon and rectum from corticosteroid enemas. *A*, The proximal colon (arrow #1) is normal. An abrupt transition is present in the distal transverse colon, with severe mucosal irregularity and inflammatory polyposis (arrowheads) in the distal transverse colon (arrow #2.) The degree of mucosal involvement progressively diminishes from a severely involved splenic flexure with a coarse pattern to moderately granular mucosa involving the descending colon (arrow #3) and finely granular mucosa in the proximal sigmoid colon. *B*, The fine granularity in the proximal sigmoid colon gradually fades (between the asterisks) into a normal mucosal appearance in the distal sigmoid colon and the rectum.

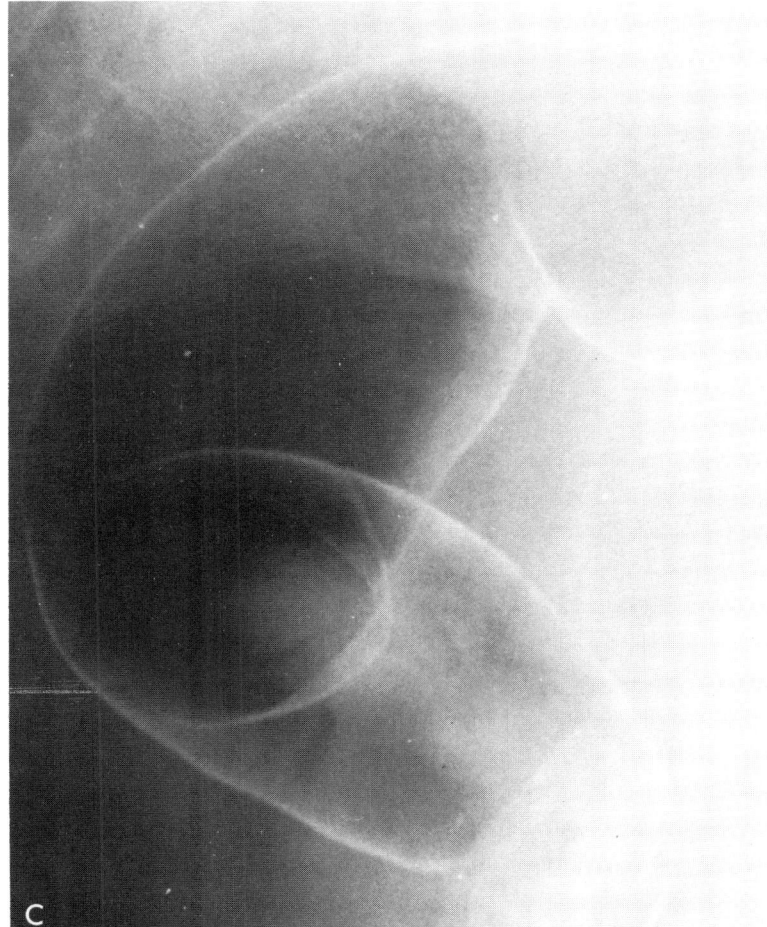

Figure 13–59 *Continued.* C, A lateral view of the rectum shows the mucosa to be normal. Mucosal healing from corticosteroid enemas is most marked in the rectum and decreases cephalad.

CROHN'S DISEASE

Radiologic Appearance

Barium studies are almost always necessary to evaluate patients for Crohn's disease, but plain film examination may occasionally be helpful and should be made prior to barium administration.[22] Though toxic dilatation of the colon is very uncommon in Crohn's disease[17] its occurrence contraindicates barium enema examination. If the plain film shows fixed, separated loops of small bowel, indicating bowel wall thickening, and if the wall appears irregular, the findings suggest Crohn's disease and barium studies are indicated.

One of the hallmarks of Crohn's disease on double-contrast studies is discrete, mucous membrane ulcers, either on an edematous or on an otherwise normal background.[9, 11, 25] These ulcers are different from those found in ulcerative colitis and are called aphthous, aphthoid, or aphthic. They are of varying sizes and shapes, may penetrate deeply into the submucosa, and may be asymmetrically present in several scattered segments of bowel with intervening normal mucosa. Edema immediately adjacent to an aphthous ulcer may appear as a dark ring ("halo") surrounding the barium-filled ulcer. Short, transverse lines that represent "transverse grooves between swollen mucosal folds" may be a finding unique to Crohn's disease.[25] Bowel wall thickening may cause luminal narrowing with segmental strictures, and if involvement is asymmetric, may produce pseudodiverticula. When luminal narrowing due to bowel wall thickening and spasm is associated with diffuse ulcerations the bowel may have the appearance of a piece of frayed string. This is the "string sign" of Crohn's disease. Sinus tracts, fistulas, and pericolonic inflammatory masses are common in Crohn's disease and very rare in ulcerative colitis (Figs. 13–60 to 13–63; see Figs. 13–68 and 13–72).[23, 26] Inflammatory polyps and "mucosal bridges"[6] may also develop (see Fig. 13–76).

Segmental Crohn's disease, especially if limited to the sigmoid, may be difficult to distinguish from diverticulitis.

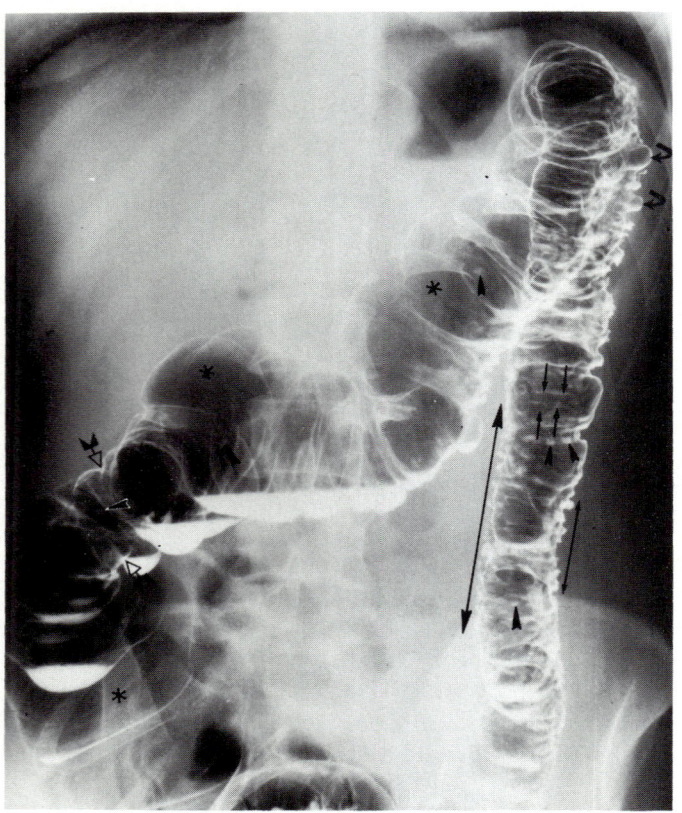

Figure 13–60. Crohn's disease. Typical findings on double-contrast enema. The findings include multiple aphthoid ulcers *en face* (arrowheads), deep and undermining ulcers (double-headed arrows), areas of normal background mucosa (asterisks), transverse lines (arrows), asymmetric, pseudodiverticula (curved arrows), and a short segment of narrowed bowel (open-headed arrows). Skip areas and asymmetric involvement are commonly found in Crohn's disease, in contrast to the continuous and total circumferential involvement in ulcerative colitis.

Figure 13–61. Crohn's disease. Sinus tract. A short sinus tract (white arrow) extends from the medial wall of the mid-descending colon. Transverse lines (arrows) are present in the descending colon. The large bowel proximally and distally is normal (asterisks).

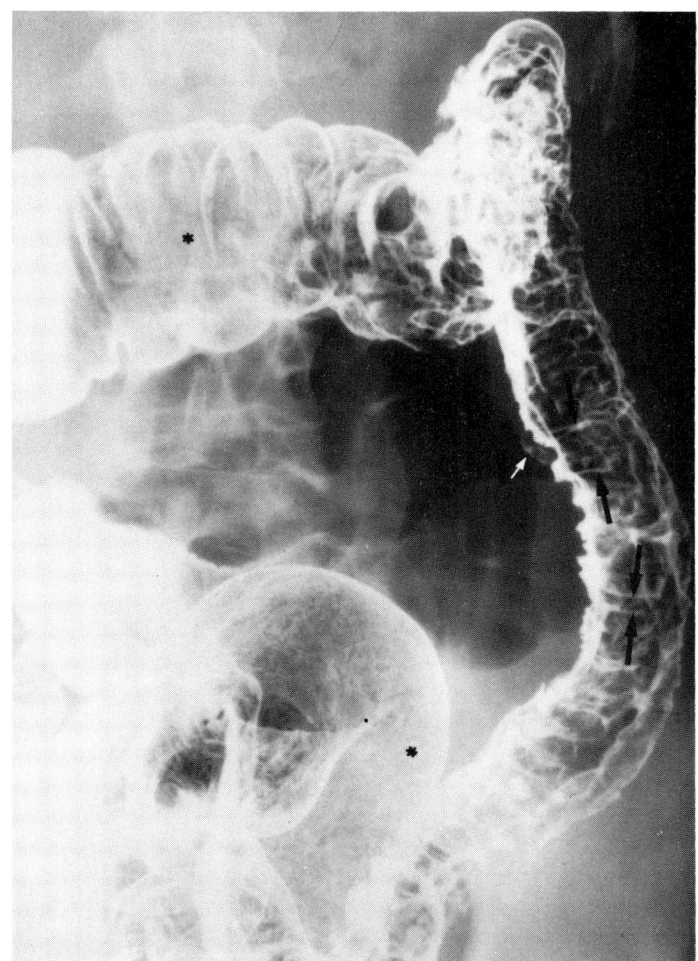

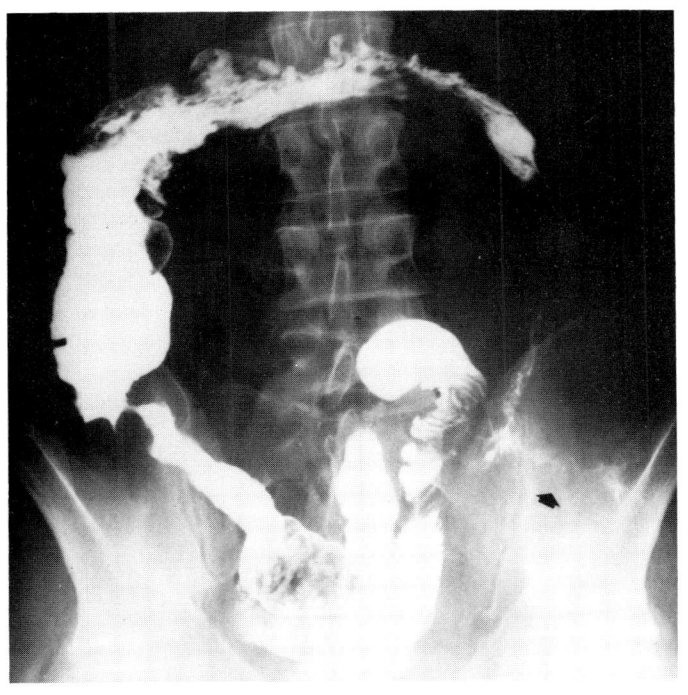

Figure 13–62. Crohn's disease. Colonic-cutaneous fistula. The entire colon and terminal ileum are involved with advanced Crohn's disease. A fistulous tract (arrow) extends from the lower descending colon to the skin.

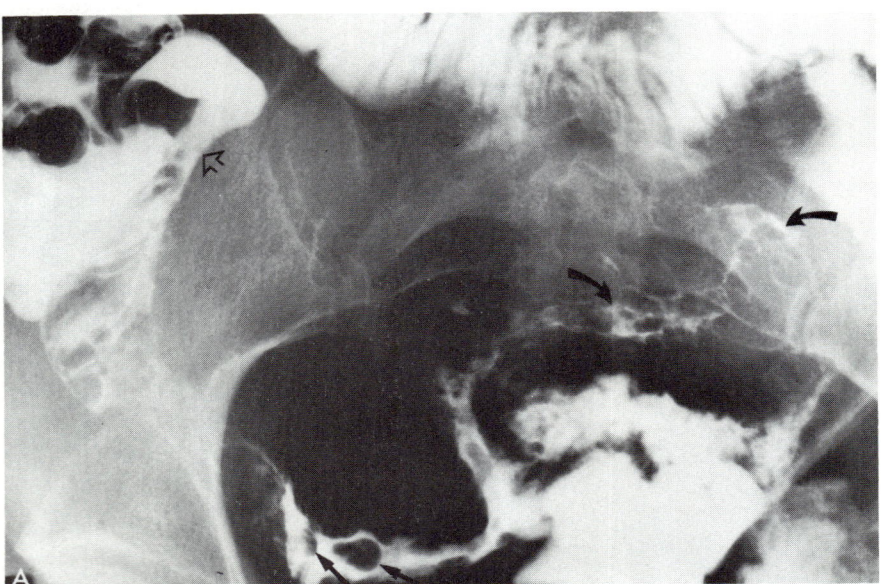
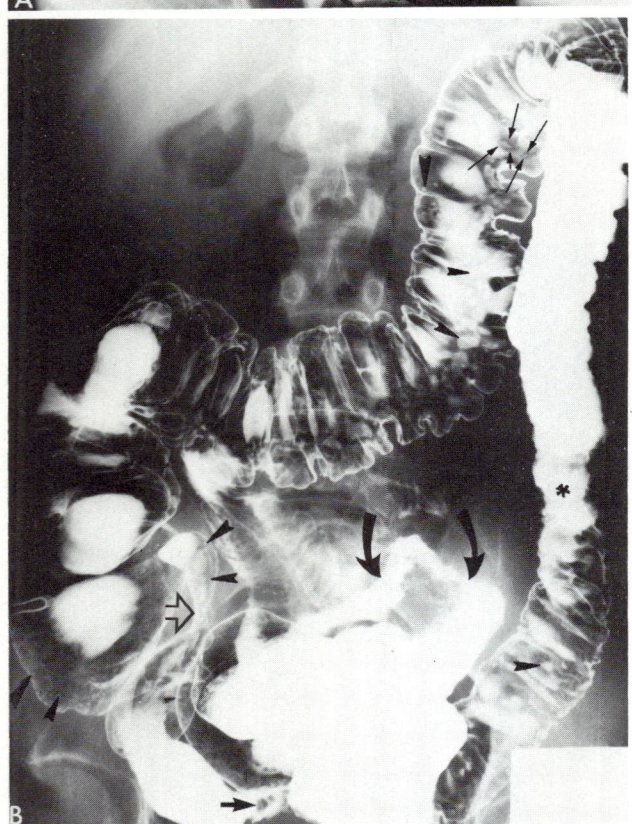

Figure 13–63. Granulomatous enterocolitis (Crohn's disease). A, Antegrade study shows an ulcerated (cruved arrows) and narrowed (open arrow) terminal ileum with submucosal nodules (arrows). B, Double-contrast enema confirms the ileal findings (curved arrows, arrow, and open arrow) and also uncovers segmentally located aphthous ulcers (arrowheads) in the terminal ileum, the cecum, the transverse colon, and at the descending sigmoid colon junction. Rings of edema ("halos") (small arrows) surround several of the large discrete (aphthous) ulcers in the distal transverse colon. The lumen of the mid-descending colon is narrowed (asterisk).

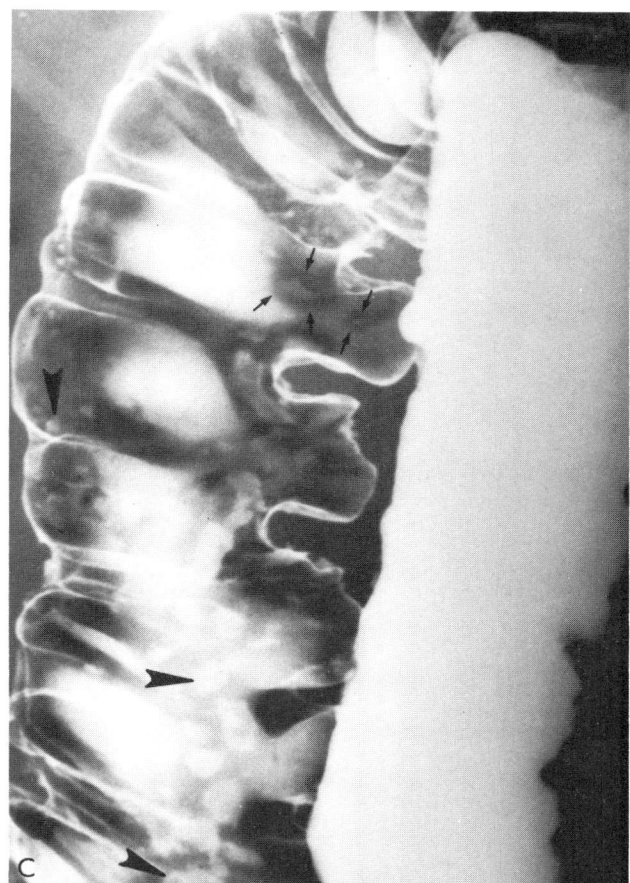

Figure 13-63 *Continued.* C, A close-up view of the distal transverse colon shows the aphthous ulcers (arrowheads) with the surrounding rings of edema (arrows).

Extent and Spread of Disease

In the vast majority of cases, Crohn's disease is confined to the ileum or large bowel or both. Rarely, other portions of the alimentary tract are primarily involved.[26] Colon involvement is most often right-sided and segmental. Spread to adjacent or noncontiguous portions of the enterocolonic tract may occur, usually slowly and over a period of years, in contrast to the rapid contiguous spread in some cases of ulcerative colitis.[26]

The complications include sinus tracts, mesenteric and pericolonic inflammatory masses, and fistulas to other bowel loops, the duodenum, the bladder, the vagina, a ureter, or the skin. Stenotic strictures leading to obstruction are not rare. Arthritis, especially a sacroiliitis, is sometimes associated, although it occurs more frequently in patients with ulcerative colitis.

Contrast studies will enable determination of the extent of alimentary tract involvement (Figs. 13–63 to 13–68).

Text continued on page 711.

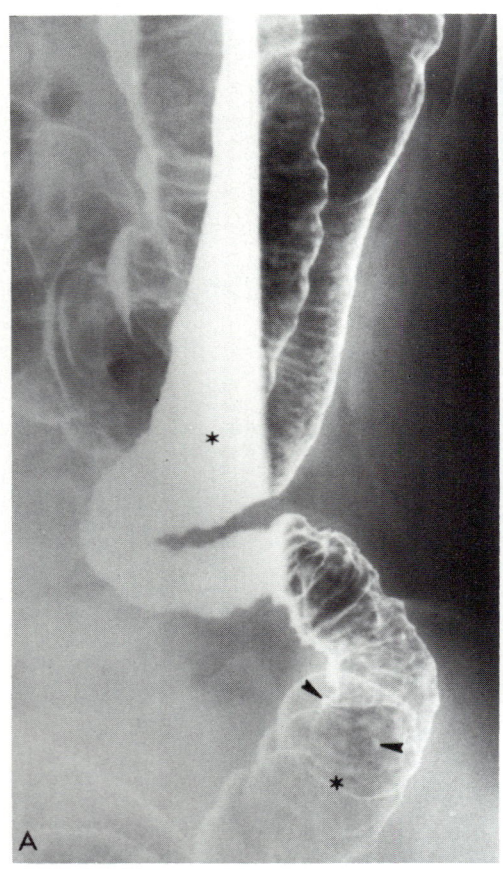
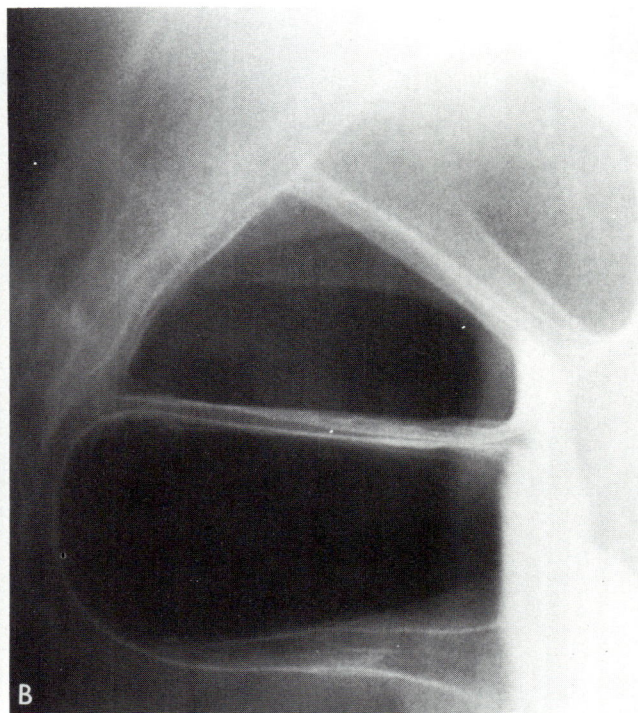

Figure 13–64. Progressive Crohn's disease of colon. *A* and *B*, Aphthous ulcers (arrowheads) are present in a short segment (between asterisks) at the descending–sigmoid junction, associated with luminal narrowing. The rectum (*B*) is normal.

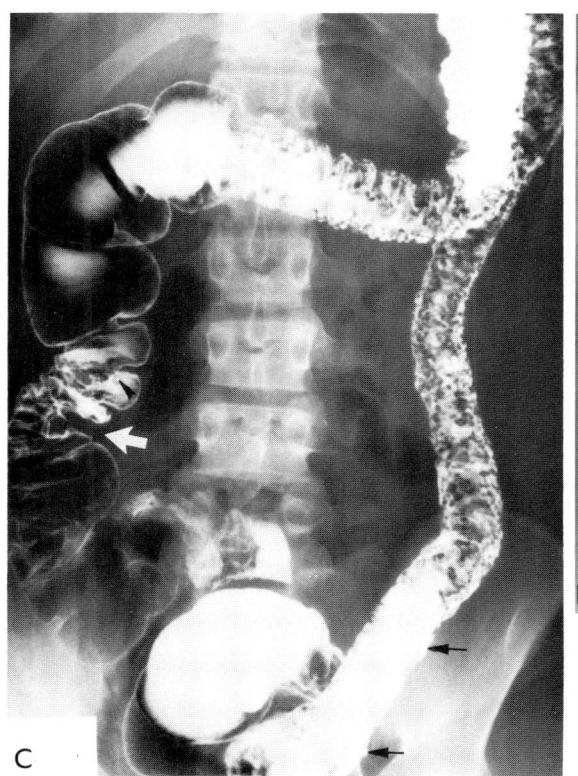
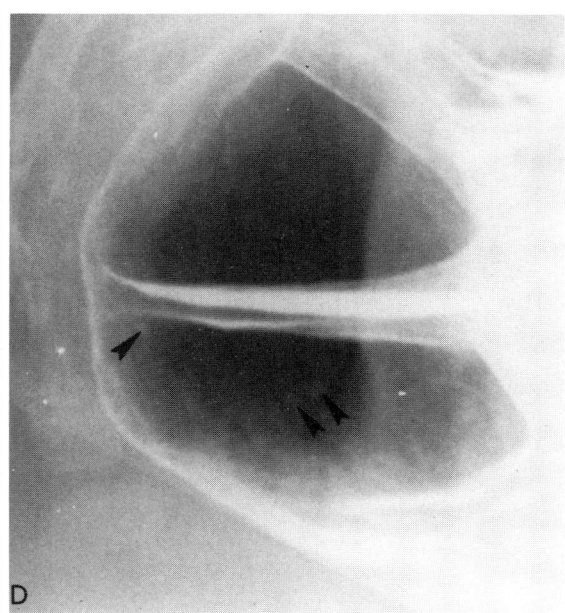

Figure 13–64 *Continued.* C and D, A double-contrast study five months later shows continuous involvement from the midtransverse colon to the distal sigmoid with deep undermined ulcers (thin arrows). The hepatic flexure is spared, but in the mid-ascending colon there is segmental narrowing (thick arrow) and aphthous ulceration (arrowhead). In the rectum (D), aphthoid ulcers (arrowheads) are now present.

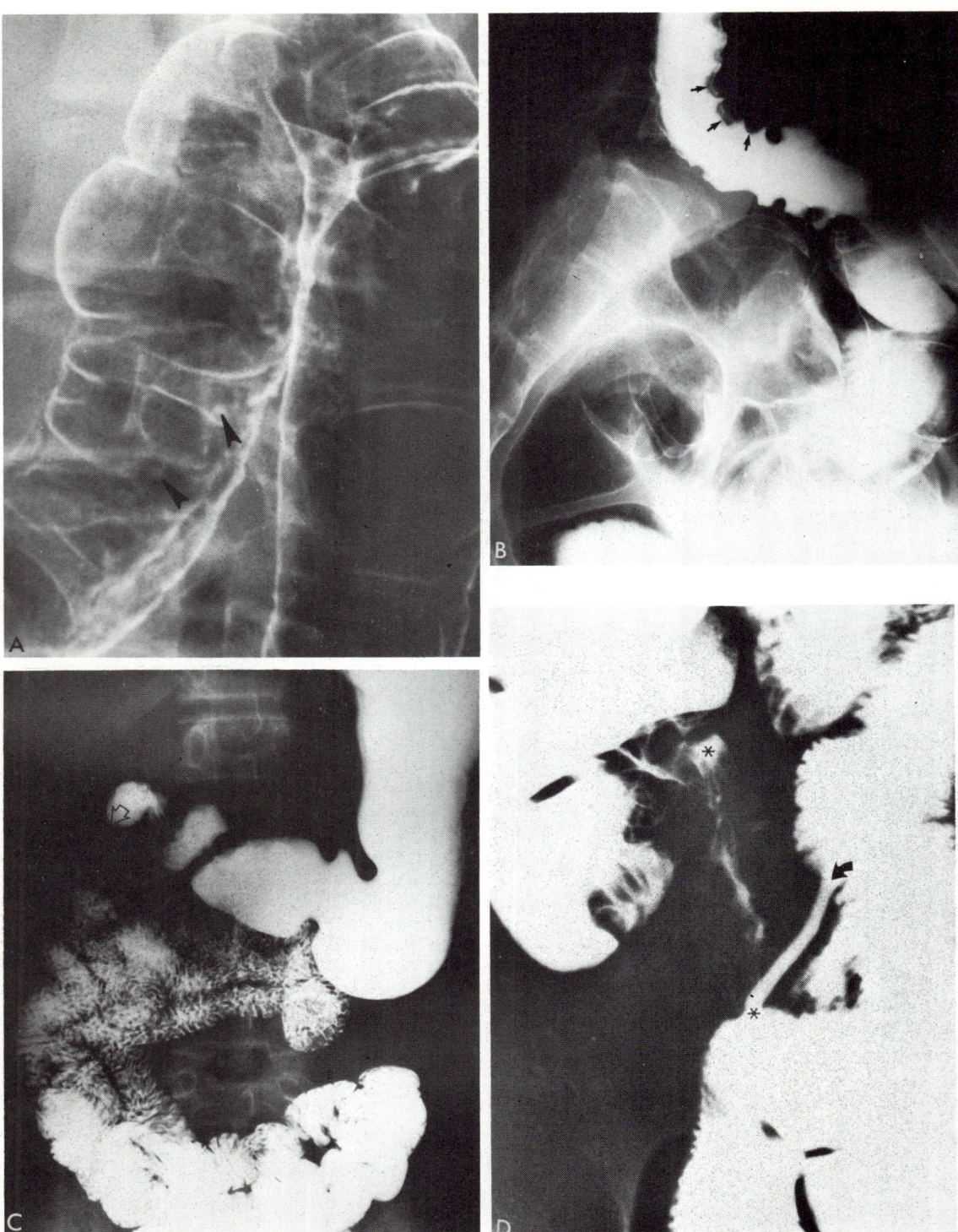

Figure 13–65. Crohn's disease in young woman, previously mislabeled as ulcerative colitis. *A,* Aphthoid ulcers (arrowheads) are present on a normal mucosal background with asymmetric involvement at the distal transverse colon. *B,* Thickened and distorted haustral folds (arrows) are present in the proximal sigmoid colon. *C,* The descending duodenum (open arrow) is narrowed owing to spasm and involvement with Crohn's disease. *D,* The terminal ileum (between the asterisks) shows luminal narrowing produced by bowel wall thickening and spasm, with associated ulceration. This is the "string sign" of Crohn's disease. A segment of the barium filled appendix is seen between the curved arrow and the asterisk.

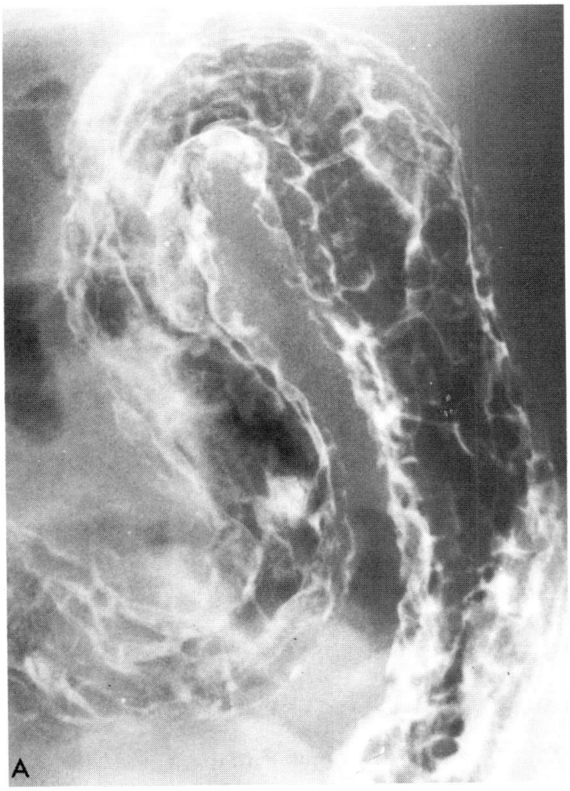

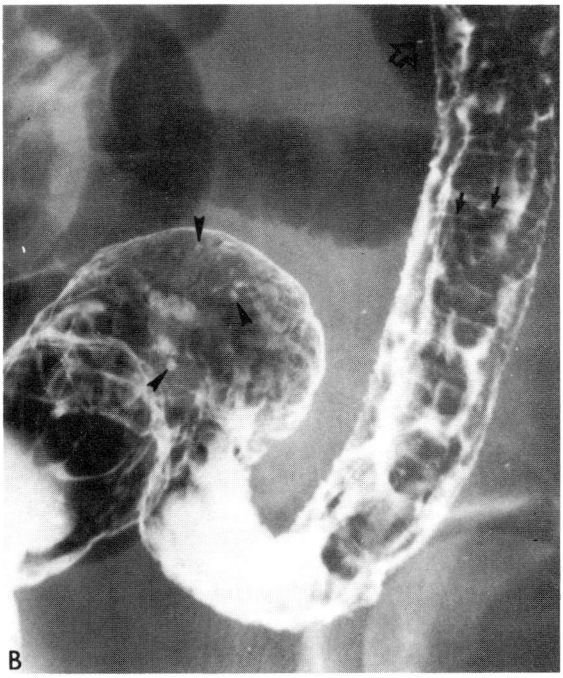

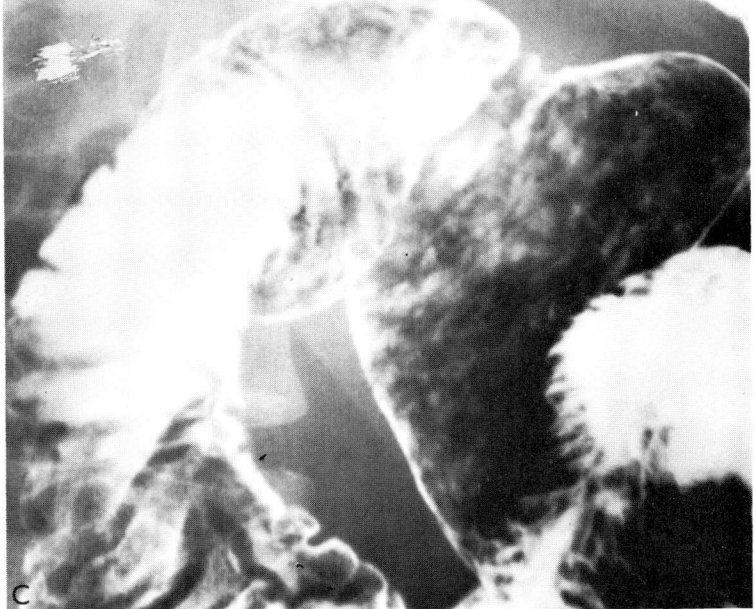

Figure 13–66. Crohn's disease of colon and stomach. *A*, Deep, linear, longitudinal and transverse ulcers and fissures are present in the distal transverse and proximal descending portions of the colon, producing a cobblestone pattern. *B*, Aphthous ulcers (arrowheads) are located in the sigmoid colon, and transverse grooves (arrows) are in the distal descending colon. A short sinus tract (open arrow) is located in the distal descending colon. *C*, An erosive gastritis involves the antrum.

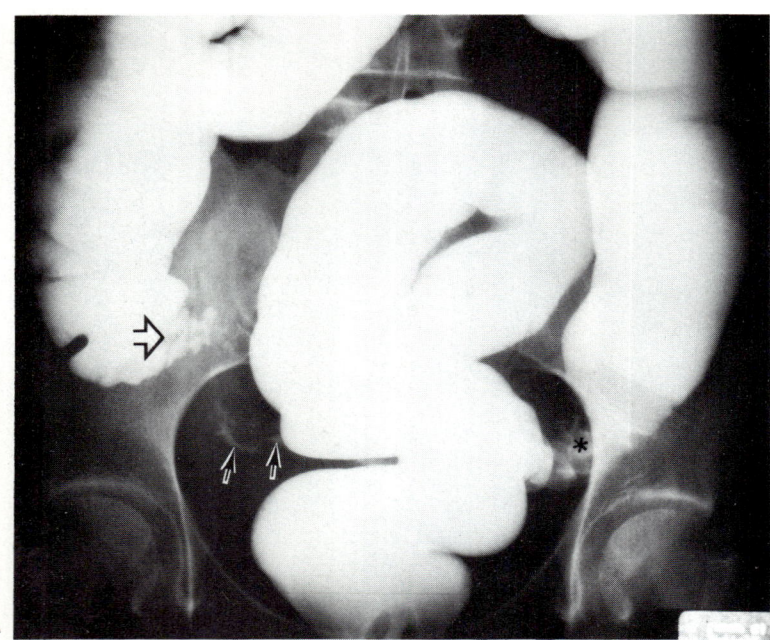
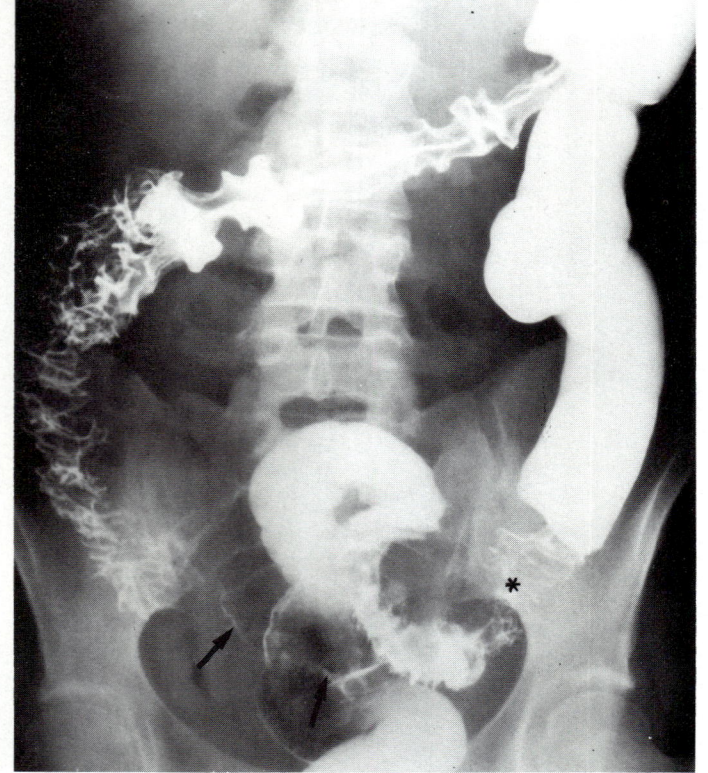

Figure 13–67. Crohn's disease of terminal ileum secondarily involving the sigmoid by contiguity. *A,* On the filled-colon film the narrowed terminal ileum (arrows) produces a string sign, and spasm is present in both the cecal tip (open arrow) and the sigmoid colon (asterisk). *B,* The postevacuation view again shows the string sign in the terminal ileum (arrows) and confirms the distortion of a segment of sigmoid colon (asterisk) with apparently intact mucosa. Abdominal exploration revealed Crohn's disease of the ileum adherent to the sigmoid, with an ileosigmoid colon fistula.

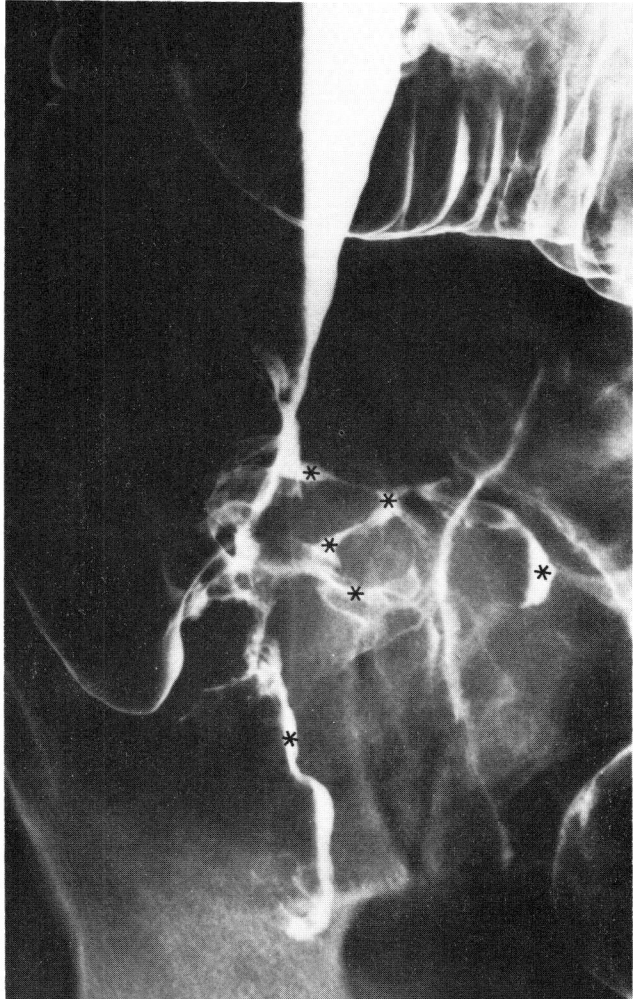

Figure 13–68. Multiple fistulas in Crohn's disease. Multiple ileoileal and ileocolic fistulas (asterisks) are present without evidence of primary involvement of the large bowel.

Types of Examination

Both antegrade and retrograde studies of the alimentary tract are useful in evaluating for Crohn's disease, and the studies are frequently complementary (see Figs. 13–63 and 13–65; Figs. 13–69 and 13–70). If a retrograde double-contrast study is possible, it usually demonstrates the nature and extent of disease in the colon and terminal ileum better than an antegrade study. Antegrade study of the small bowel, either with ingested barium suspension or with barium suspension injected through a long intestinal tube (enteroclysis) can be extremely helpful in evaluating the extent of small bowel involvement. Enteroclysis also permits double-contrast studies of the small bowel to be performed.[7] Contrast examination of the esophagus, stomach, and duodenum for Crohn's disease should be made. Double-contrast studies of the upper alimentary tract may reveal minimal mucosal changes of Crohn's disease that would escape detection on routine contrast studies (Figs. 13–71 and 13–72).[5]

Text continued on page 717

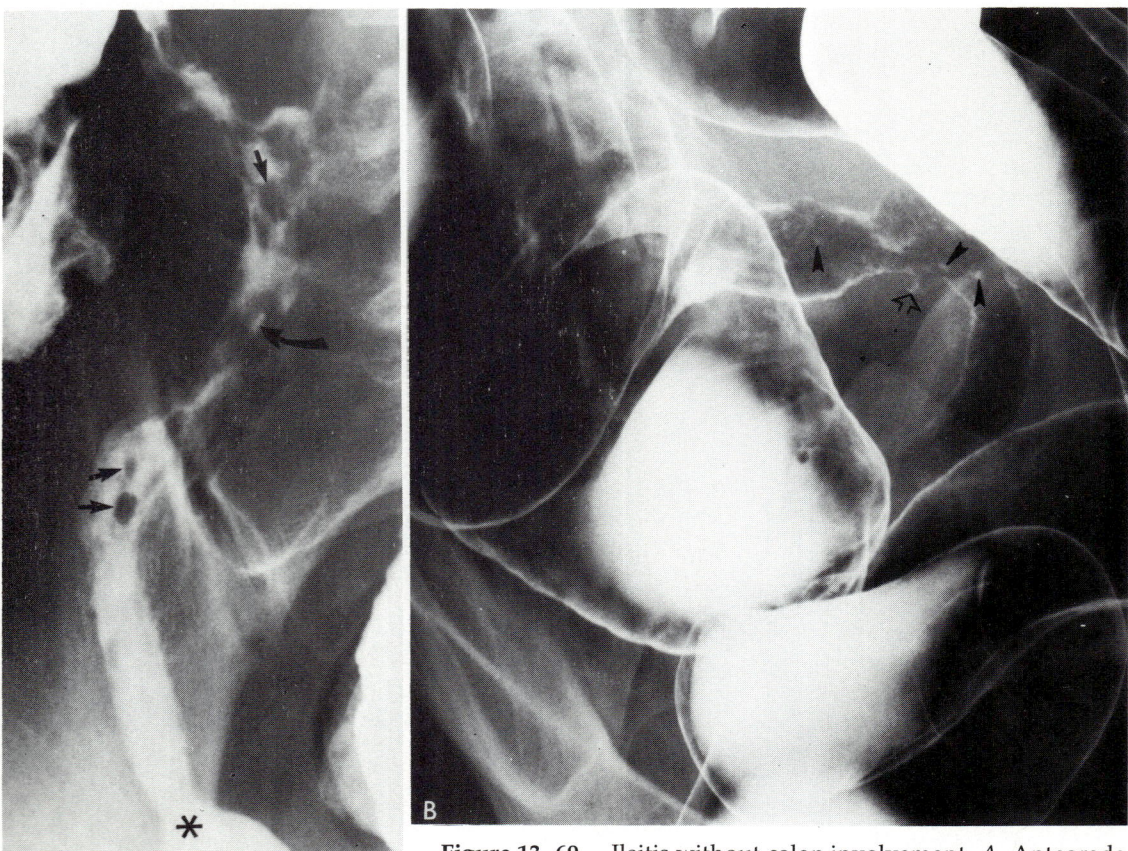

Figure 13–69. Ileitis without colon involvement. *A*, Antegrade study suggests luminal narrowing of the terminal ileum (distal to the asterisk), with an indistinct scalloped mucosal border, questionable ulceration (curved arrow), and nodularity (arrows). The cecum seems abnormal. *B*, On the double-contrast enema examination, the caliber of the small bowel is shown to be normal, but distinct aphthous ulcers (arrowheads) are present adjacent to a probable short sinus tract (open arrow). The colon is entirely normal. Double-contrast study is more accurate in determining minimal mucosal disease than a full-column study.

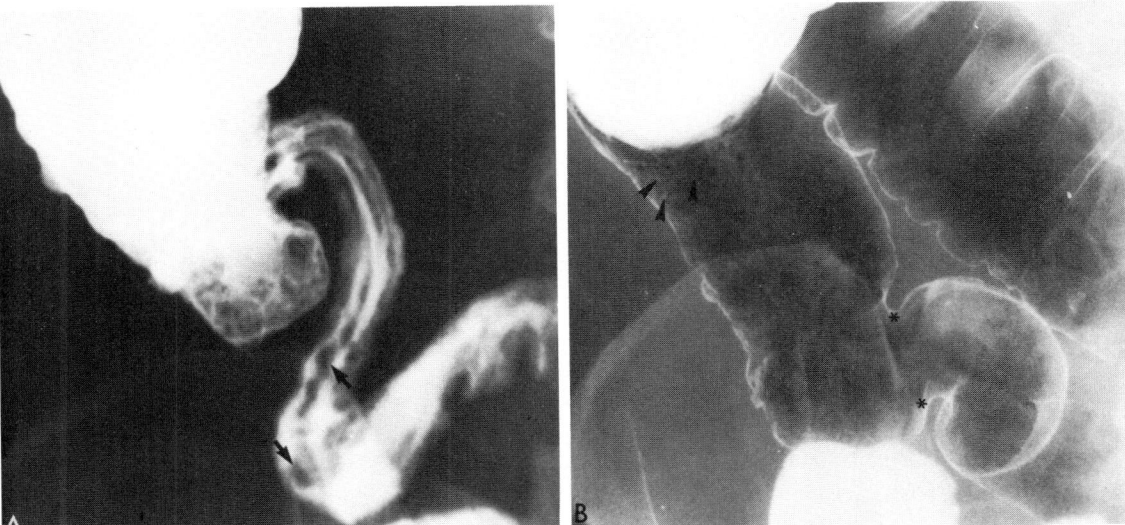

Figure 13–70. Suspicious ileal disease clarified by double-contrast study. *A,* Antegrade study of the terminal ileum appears abnormal, with longitudinal folds and a nodular (arrows) cobblestoned pattern proximally. *B,* Double-contrast enema demonstrates aphthous ulcers (arrowheads) in the proximal colon, with a normal large bowel distally. The ileocecal valve is patulous (between asterisks), and the small intestine is normal. Colonoscopy with biopsy confirmed that Crohn's disease was confined to the colon, and the ileum was spared.

714 — THE LARGE BOWEL

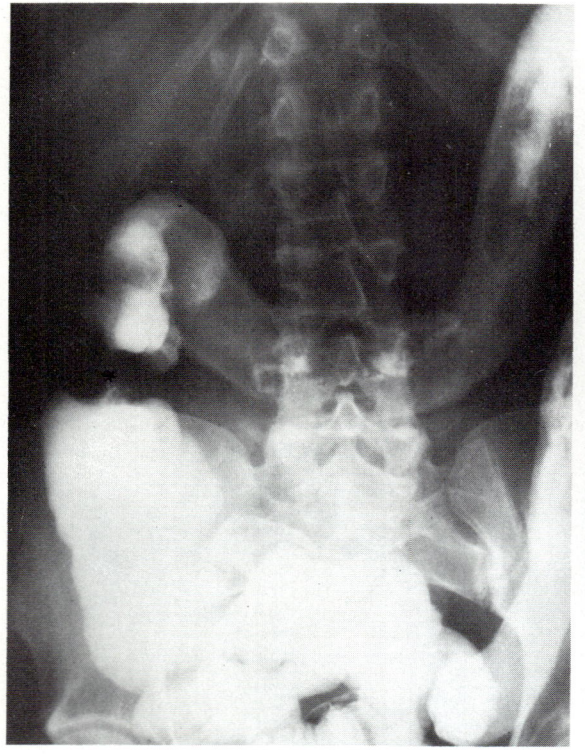

A

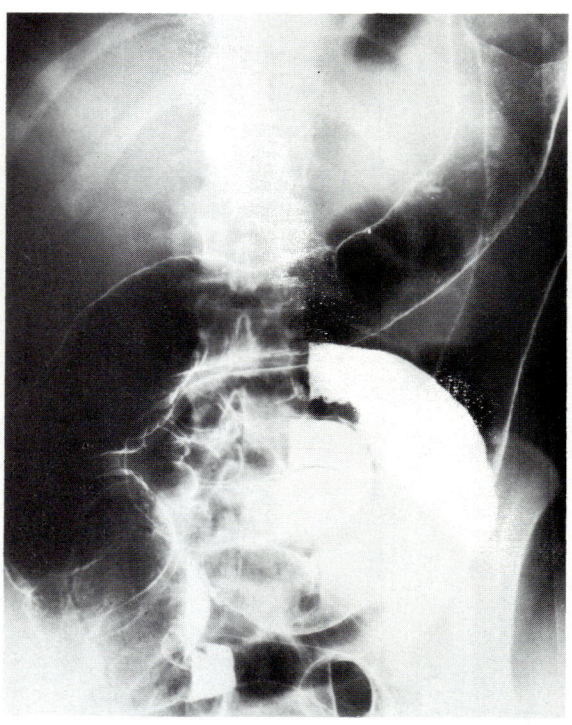

B

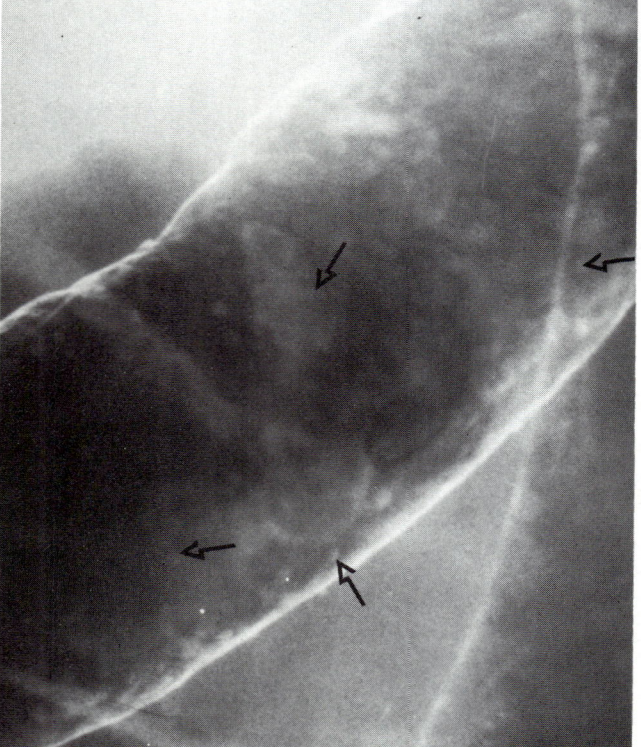

C

Figure 13–71. Ulcerative colitis versus Crohn's disease; clarification by double-contrast study. *A,* A full-column barium enema (performed 19 months earlier) was interpreted as ulcerative colitis because of effaced mucosal folds and absent haustra. The narrowing (asterisk) in the ascending colon was due to spasm. *B,* However, double-contrast enema shows aphthous ulcers involving the colon from the cecum to the mid-descending colon with a skip area in the rectum. The terminal ileum is normal. *C,* A close-up view of the distal transverse colon shows multiple aphthous ulcers (open arrowheads). The correct diagnosis of Crohn's disease was made by this double-contrast examination.

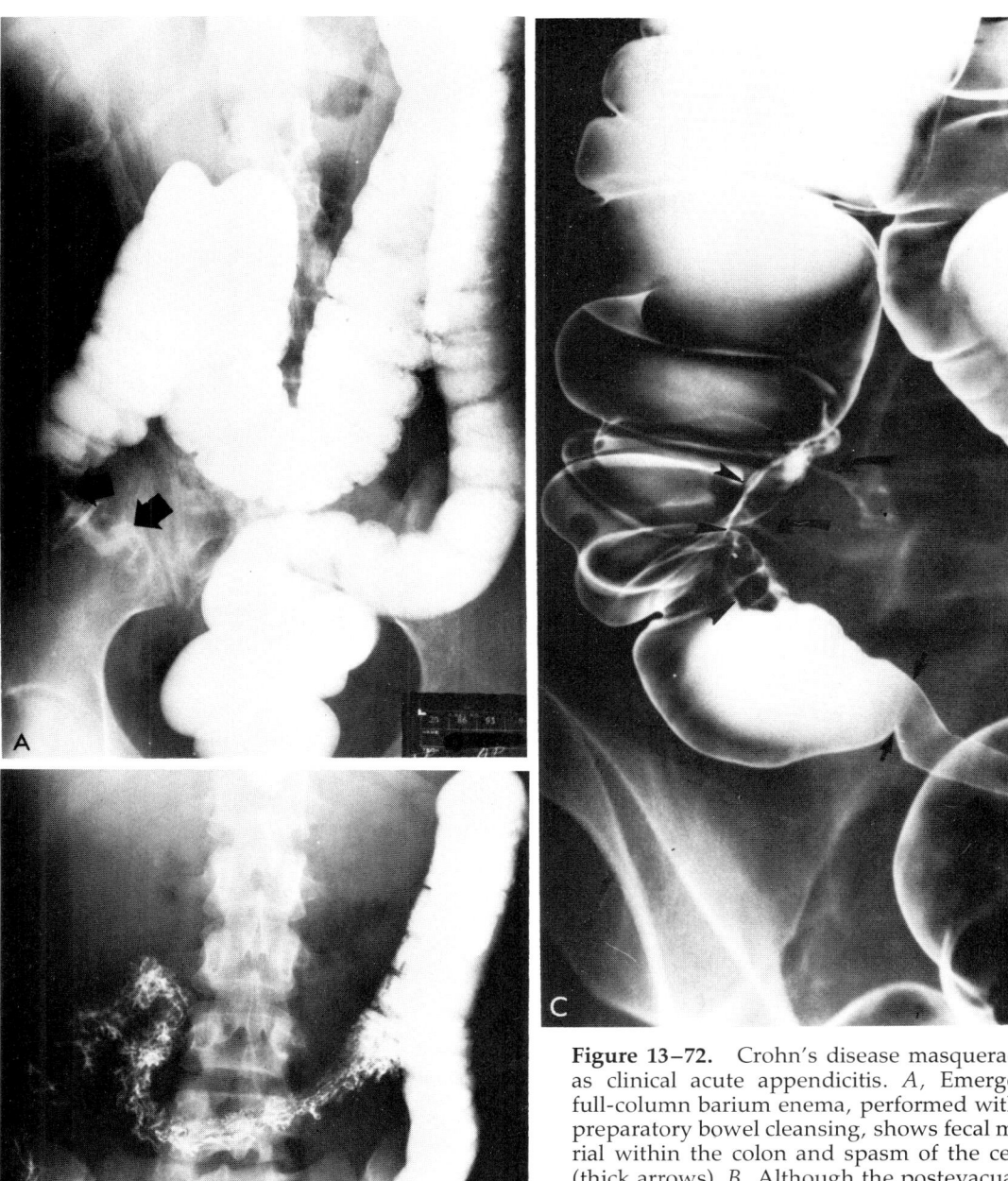

Figure 13–72. Crohn's disease masquerading as clinical acute appendicitis. *A,* Emergency full-column barium enema, performed without preparatory bowel cleansing, shows fecal material within the colon and spasm of the cecum (thick arrows). *B,* Although the postevacuation view shows the appendix to fill completely to its tip (asterisk), irregularity of the luminal surface near the base of the appendix (arrows) causes suspicion of appendiceal abnormality. *C,* Double-contrast enema examination performed after a single 2-liter cleansing enema shows the appendix to be completely normal both at its base (arrows) and at its tip (asterisk). However, two short tracts (curved arrows) of barium are present at the medial wall of the proximal large bowel in the region of the ileocecal valve, with adjacent extrinsic colon impression (arrowheads). The large bowel is otherwise normal. A disgnosis was made of Crohn's disease extending to the colon from adjacent diseased small bowel. Double-contrast enema, after bowel cleansing, should be done if acute appendicitis is suspected clinically.

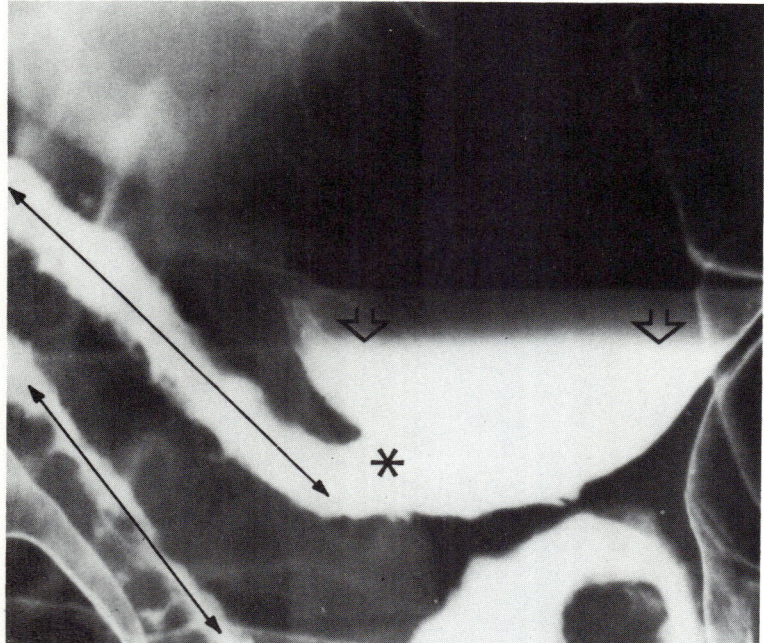

Figure 13–73. Recurrent ileal disease after ileocolic resection. The anastomotic site (asterisk) is in the midtransverse colon. Recurrent ulceration is seen in the small bowel (double-headed arrows), but the colon appears free from recurrence.

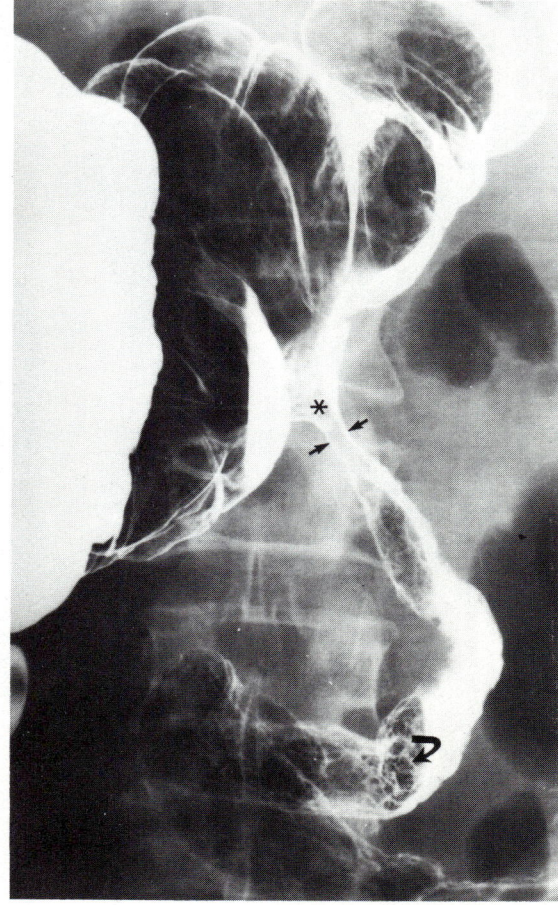

Figure 13–74. Recurrence in ileum 23 years after ileotransverse colostomy for Crohn's disease. The colon is normal. The terminal ileum, just proximal to the anastomosis (asterisk) is narrowed (arrows), and although the ileum has a nodular appearance (curved arrow), no ulcerations are identified.

Post-Therapy Changes

After either resective or bypass surgery has been performed, radiologic examination can help detect recurrences or complications (Figs. 13–73 to 13–78).

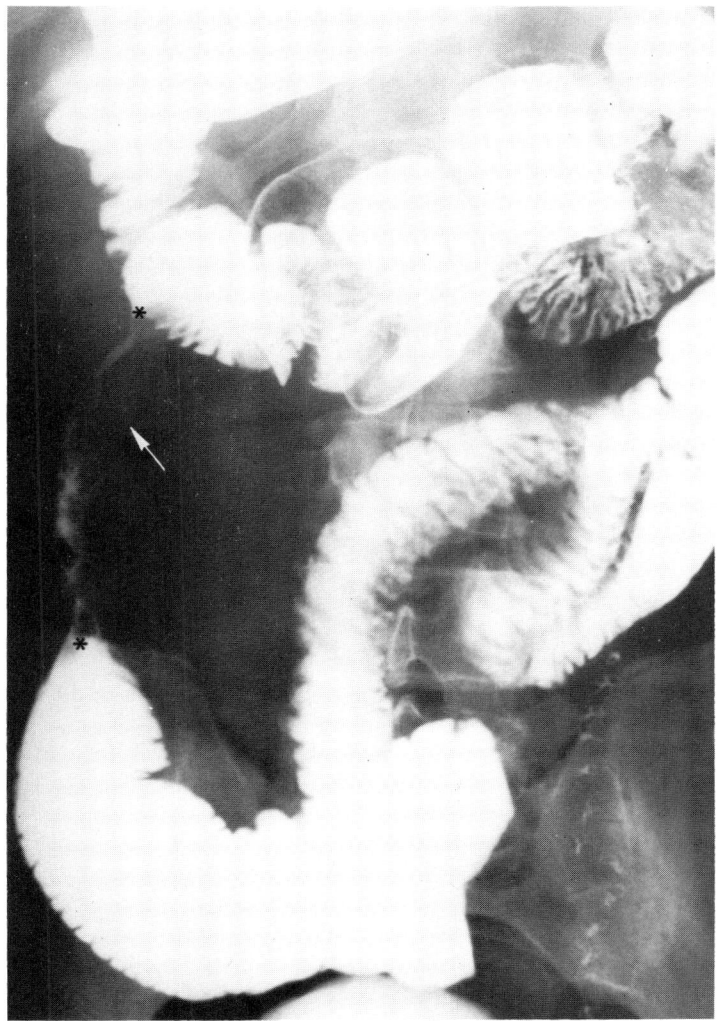

Figure 13–75. Ileal recurrence 17 years after ileocolic resection for Crohn's disease. Antegrade small bowel study shows that the small bowel is dilated proximal to a nodular, narrowed preanastomotic segment (between asterisks). A short sinus tract (arrow) extends inferomedially from the small bowel, indicating small bowel recurrence.

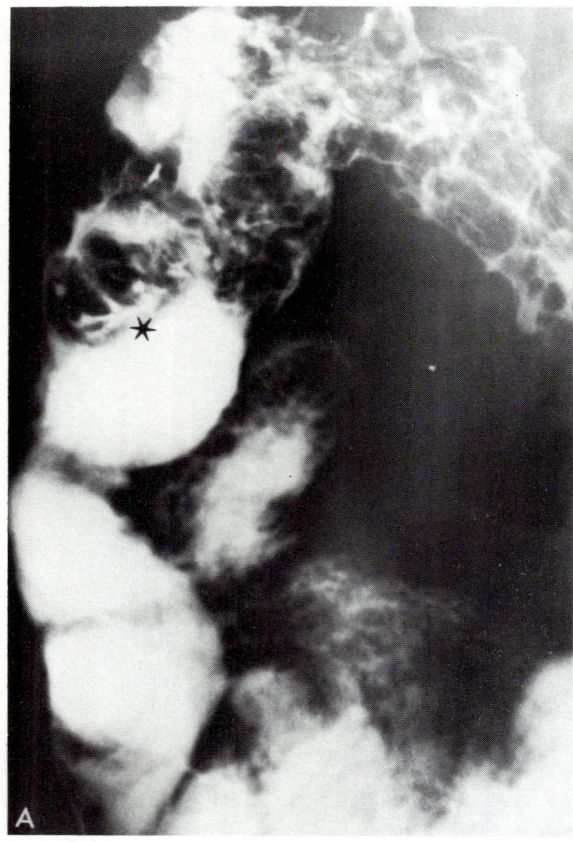
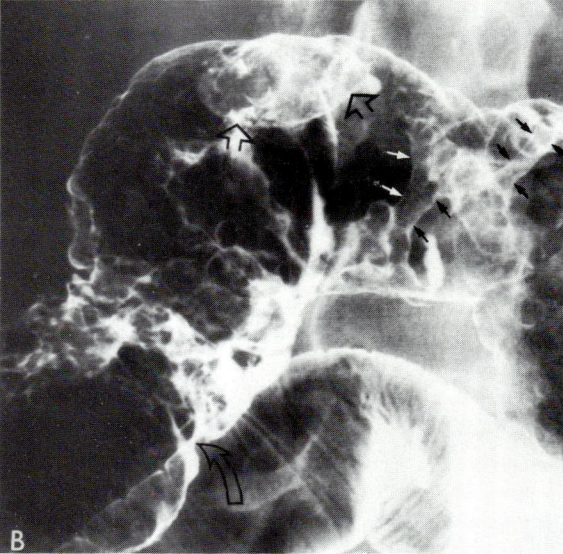

Figure 13–76. Recurrent colonic disease in 27-year-old woman after several ileocolic resections. *A*, Antegrade study of the terminal ileum and proximal colon raises the question of colonic abnormality. The anastomosis (asterisk) is identified. *B*, Double-contrast enema shows the terminal ileum to be normal. An abrupt transition is clearly identified at the ileocolic anastomotic site (curved arrow). Inflammatory polyps, some quite large (open arrows), and mucosal bridges (short arrows) are located in the proximal colon.

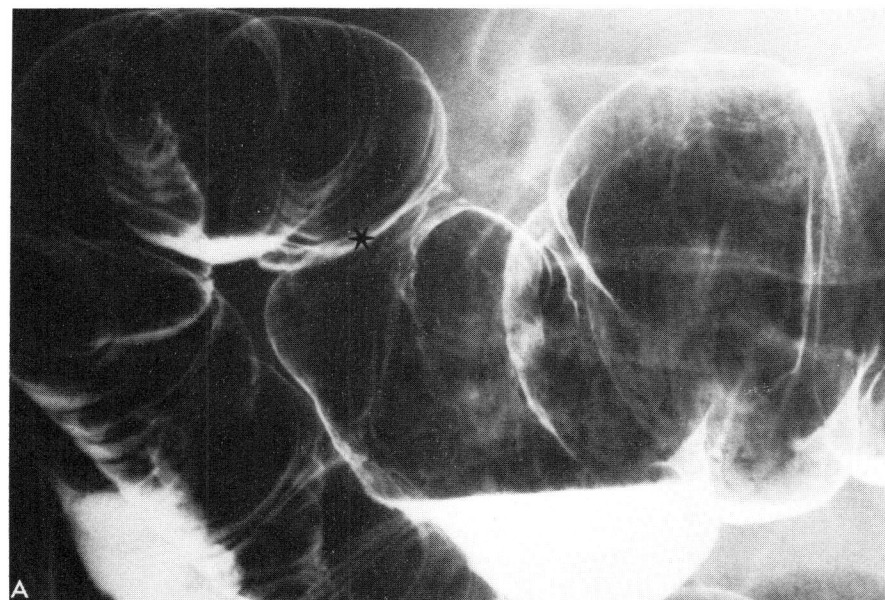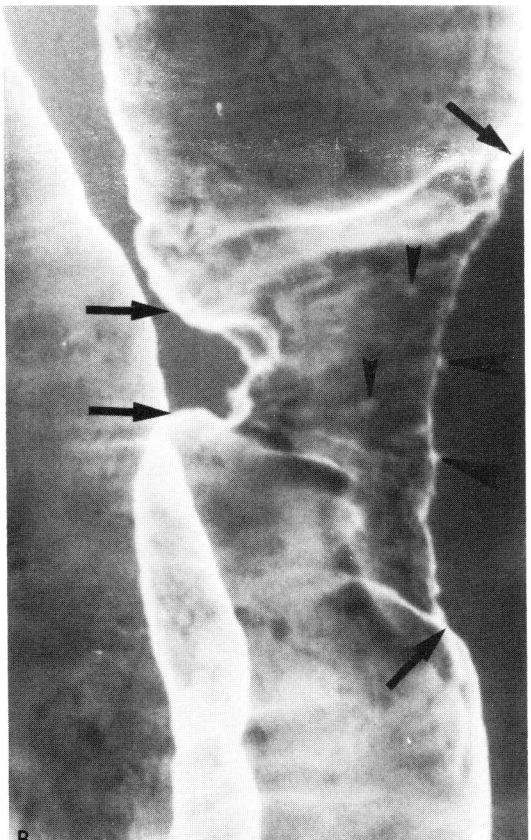

Figure 13–77. Recurrent Crohn's disease 12 years after right hemicolectomy for cecal disease. *A,* Double-contrast enema shows the terminal ileum and adjacent colon at the anastomotic site (asterisk) to be normal. *B,* A short, asymmetric stricture (between the arrows) is located in the proximal descending colon, with multiple aphthous ulcers (arrowheads) seen both *en face* and in profile.

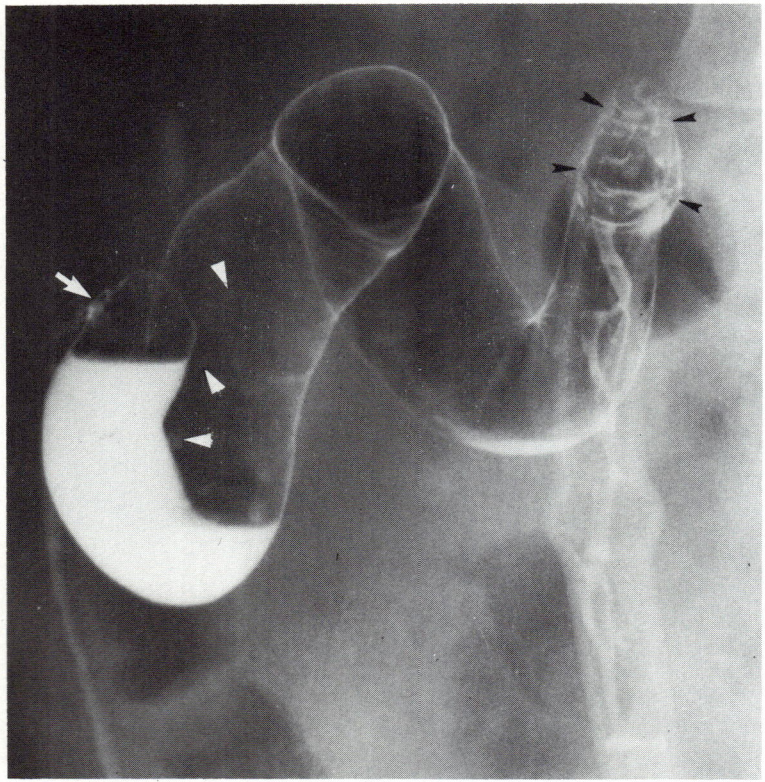

Figure 13–78. Recurrent Crohn's disease after multiple bowel resections and colostomies in a 23-year-old woman. Double-contrast examination of an excluded bowel segment with two stomas shows a catheter tip in the proximal stoma (black arrowheads) and a balloon externally occluding the distal stoma (arrow) during the examination. Aphthoid ulcers (white arrowheads) are present in this segment of colon.

SUMMARY

In ulcerative colitis, the disease process extends continuously orad from the rectum with the diseased mucosa symmetrically and diffusely involved with granularity, shallow ulcerations, or both. It should be possible to identify an abrupt transition zone between the abnormal bowel distally and the normal bowel proximally. The terminal ileum is usually spared, but backwash ileitis may be present in patients whose entire large bowel is involved. Polypoid projections into the lumen may represent pseudopolyps, inflammatory polyps, postinflammatory polyps, hyperplastic (metaplastic) polyps, adenomatous polyps, or carcinoma. Both colonic dysplasia (precarcinoma) and carcinoma may often be difficult to detect.

In Crohn's disease, the terminal ileum and large bowel are most frequently affected, but any part of the alimentary tract may be involved. The involvement is asymmetric and may be discontinuous, including several segments of abnormal bowel with intervening normal mucosa. Asymmetric bowel wall involvement may produce pseudodiverticula, and discontinuous involvement may lead to segmental strictures. The ulcers of Crohn's disease are typically discrete mucous membrane (aphthous) ulcers, which may be deep, located on a normal or edematous mucosal background. The presence of transverse grooves, sinus tracts, or fistulas strongly indicates Crohn's disease over ulcerative colitis.

With proper patient preparation and meticulous double-contrast technique, the early, accurate detection and differentiation of ulcerative colitis and Crohn's disease usually can be made. However, in far advanced disease without small bowel involvement, radiographic and even clinical differentiation may be difficult or impossible. From radiographic features alone, it may be impossible to distinguish diffuse ulcerative or Crohn's colitis from other infectious colitides, including pseudomembranous colitis. Segmental lesions, such as ischemic colitis, diverticulitis, amebiasis, schistosomiasis, or even tuberculosis, can simulate segmental Crohn's disease radiographically.

References

1. Brahme, F., and Fork, F-T.: Dynamic aspects of colonic Crohn's disease. Radiologe 15:463–468, 1975.
2. Crowson, T. D., Ferrante, W. F., and Gathright, J. B., Jr.: Colonoscopy: inefficacy for early carcinoma detection in patients with ulcerative colitis. J.A.M.A. 236:2651–2652, 1976.
3. Ferrucci, J. T., Jr.: Case records of the Massachussetts General Hospital. N. Engl. J. Med. 286:147–153, 1972.
4. Frank, P. H., Riddell, R. H., Feczko, P. J., et al.: Radiological detection of colonic dysplasia (precarcinoma) in chronic ulcerative colitis. Gastrointest. Radiol. 3:209–219, 1978.
5. Gardiner, R.: Details of the current materials and methods for performing double contrast examinations of the alimentary tract. (Unpublished observations; may be obtained by writing directly to the author.)
6. Hammerman, A. M., Shatz, B. A., and Susman, N.: Radiographic characteristics of colonic "mucosal bridges": sequelae of inflammatory bowel disease. Radiology 127:611–614, 1978.
7. Herlinger, H.: A modified technique for the double-contrast small bowel enema. Gastrointest. Radiol. 3:201–207, 1978.
8. James, E. M., and Carlson, H. C.: Chronic ulcerative colitis and colon cancer: Can radiographic appearance predict survival patterns? Am. J. Roentgenol. 130:825–830, 1978.
9. Kelvin, F. M., Oddson, T. A., Rice, R. P., et al.: Double contrast barium enema in Crohn's disease and ulcerative colitis. Am. J. Roentgenol. 131:207–213, 1978.
10. Laufer, I.: The double-contrast enema: myths and misconceptions. Gastrointest. Radiol. 1:19–31, 1976.
11. Laufer, I., Mullens, J. E., and Hamilton, J.: Correlation of endoscopy and double-contrast radiography in the early stages of ulcerative and granulomatous colitis. Radiology 118:1–5, 1976.
12. Lumb, G., and Protheroe, R. H. B.: Ulcerative colitis: a pathologic study of 152 surgical specimens. Gastroenterology 34:381–407, 1958.
13. Margulis, A. R., Goldberg, H. I., Lawson, T. L., et al.: The overlapping spectrum of ulcerative and granulomatous colitis: a roentgenographic-pathologic study. Am. J. Roentgenol. 113:325–334, 1971.
14. Miller, R. E.: The barium enema in the high-risk carcinoma patient. Radiology 123:813–814, 1977.
15. Miller, R. E., Chernish, S. M., and Brunelle, R. L.: Gastrointestinal radiography with glucagon. Gastrointest. Radiol. 4:1–10, 1979.
16. Neschis, M., Siegelman, S. S., and Parker, J. G.: Diagnosis in management of the megacolon of ulcerative colitis. Gastroenterology 55:251–259, 1968.
17. Price, A. B.: Difficulties in the differential diagnosis of ulcerative colitis and Crohn's disease. In Yardley, J. H., Morson, B. C., and Abell, M. R. (eds.): The Gastrointestinal Tract. Baltimore, The Williams & Wilkins Company, 1977, pp. 1–14.
18. Riddell, R. H.: The precarcinomatous lesion of ulcerative colitis. In Yardley, J. H., Morson, B. C., and Abell, M. R. (eds.): The Gastrointestinal Tract. Baltimore, The Williams & Wilkins Company, 1977, pp. 109–123.
19. Selke, A. C., Jr., Jona, J. Z., and Belin, R. P.: Massive enlargement of the ileocecal valve due to lymphoid hyperplasia. Am. J. Roentgenol. 127:518–520, 1976.
20. Shimkin, P. M.: Radiology of acute appendicitis. Am. J. Roentgenol. 130:1001–1004, 1978.
21. Simon, M., Shapiro, J. H., Parker, J. G., et al.: The diagnosis and treatment of dilatation of the colon in severe ulcerative colitis: a diagnostic roentgen sign. Am. J. Roentgenol. 87:655–669, 1962.
22. Simpson, S. A., and Lewin, J. R.: Plain roentgenography in diagnosis of chronic ulcerative colitis and terminal ileitis. Am. J. Roentgenol. 84:306–315, 1960.
23. Stanley, P., Fry, I. K., Dawson, A. M., et al.: Radiological signs of ulcerative colitis and Crohn's disease of the colon. Clin. Radiol. 22:434–442, 1971.
24. Teplick, S. K., Stark, T., Clark, R. E., et al.: The retrorectal space. Clin. Radiol. 29:177–184, 1978.
25. Welin, S., and Welin, G.: A pathognomonic roentgenologic sign of regional ileitis (Crohn's disease). Dis. Colon Rectum 16:473–478, 1973.
26. Williams, G. T., and Morson, B. C.: The pathology of inflammatory bowel disease. Curr. Concepts Gastroenterol. 4(4):5–12, 1978.
27. Yardley, J. H., and Donowitz, M.: Colo-rectal biopsy in inflammatory bowel disease. In Yardley, J. H., Morson, B. C., and Abell, M. R. (eds.): The Gastrointestinal Tract. Baltimore, The Williams & Wilkins Company, 1977, pp. 50–94.
28. Zegel, H. G., and Laufer, I.: Filiform polyposis. Radiology 127:615–619, 1978.

Part III
Precancerous and Malignant Lesions

RICHARD GARDINER, M.D.

According to predictions made in 1979, colorectal and lung carcinoma will be the most frequently encountered internal malignancies in the United States.[18] Three quarters of the large bowel cancers will be discovered in patients between 50 and 80 years of age; the sex incidence will be about equal. In all likelihood, colorectal carcinoma develops from pre-existing lesions, rather than arising *de novo*.[15] Owing to its slow growth rate and tendency to metastasize late, as opposed to lung cancer, large bowel cancer can be detected at an earlier stage, so that the rate of cure can be significantly improved. Radiologic examination currently offers the safest, easiest, fastest, and cheapest method of accurately assessing the entire large bowel for carcinoma, even in its early stages. Clinical examination, fecal occult blood testing, and internal direct inspection with proctosigmoidoscopy or colonoscopy or both are complementary examination methods. This chapter will focus on both colorectal carcinoma and its precursors.

Several colonic polyposis syndromes strongly predispose to the development of colorectal carcinoma. Although the adenomatous polyp accounts for three quarters of all large bowel neoplasms, fewer than one polyp in twenty undergoes malignant transformation.[15] Isolated adenomatous polyps and the polyposis syndromes will be discussed in Part IV. On the other hand, villous adenomas and tubulovillous adenomas (which have histologic features of both villous adenomas and adenomatous polyps) have incidences of malignant degeneration reaching 50 per cent.[1, 15, 16, 20] Both these important premalignant lesions and colorectal carcinoma will be discussed in detail.

Since the risk of developing colorectal carcinoma may exceed 60 per cent in patients with long-standing ulcerative colitis, especially if the colitis involves the entire colon,[5] several examples of malignancy developing on a background of ulcerative colitis will be shown. Crohn's disease is a much less frequent malignant precursor. Examples of the postoperative appearance of the large bowel will be discussed and shown, since surgical resection is the mainstay for the treatment of colonic malignancy. Normal postoperative anatomy, several complications of surgery, and metachronous tumors will be illustrated.

RADIOGRAPHIC EXAMINATION TECHNIQUES

The barium enema is the major primary study for detecting large bowel neoplasms. The full-column barium enema may fail to disclose at least 10 per cent of colonic carcinomas and an even higher percentage of smaller, noncancerous polypoid lesions.[13, 16] However, there is much evidence indicating that the double-contrast enema is quite sensitive for identifying these tumors.[7, 8, 11, 13, 16, 21]

Effective bowel cleansing is essential for either type of examination and is achieved through diet modification, laxatives, and full-colon (2- to 3-liter) lukewarm cleansings.[9, 12] A poorly prepared bowel containing either residual liquid or particulate matter can prevent satisfactory mucosal coating, produce factitious tumorlike findings (Fig. 13–79), or obscure an existing tumor.

A barium sulfate suspension, specifically prepared for the type of examination to be performed, is used. A suspension that readily coats the bowel is used for the

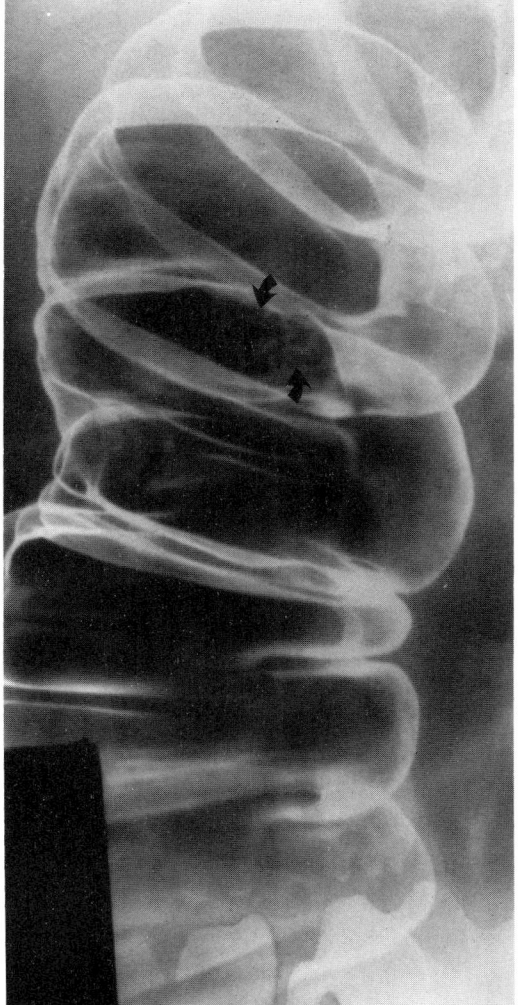

Figure 13–79. Feces mimicking villous adenoma. An otherwise clean colon contains a bubbly-appearing filling defect (arrows) in the ascending colon which has the typical appearance of a villous adenoma but, in fact, represents retained feces.

double-contrast enema. Approximately 2 to 3 liters of air are then gradually instilled, the patient is rotated, and the table is tilted to ensure that the entire large bowel is coated with barium suspension and distended with air. For the full-column enema the suspension should be sufficiently dilute and the kilovoltage sufficiently high to permit proper penetration of the column of barium.[3]

Both types of examinations include radiographs and spot films taken with graded compression of all portions of the large bowel from the anus to the appendix and also the ileum, if small bowel reflux occurs. The postevacuation view may add crucial information to the full-column barium enema (Fig. 13–80), but it is not helpful with the double-contrast technique. Patient discomfort is usually relieved by the prompt hypotonic effect on the bowel of 0.5 mg of intravenous glucagon.[10]

Occasionally, when the barium enema examination does not display tumors to the best advantage, or when the patient is unable to hold the enema solution, an antegrade study of the bowel is necessary (Fig. 13–81). In these examinations the barium suspension is administered per mouth. When the suspension has reached the area of interest, the glucagon is given parenterally and the air is inflated per rectum.

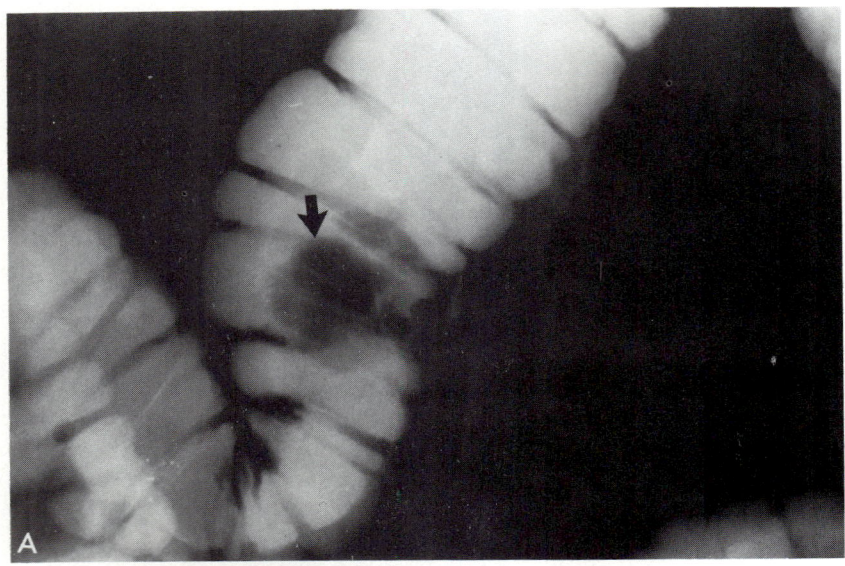
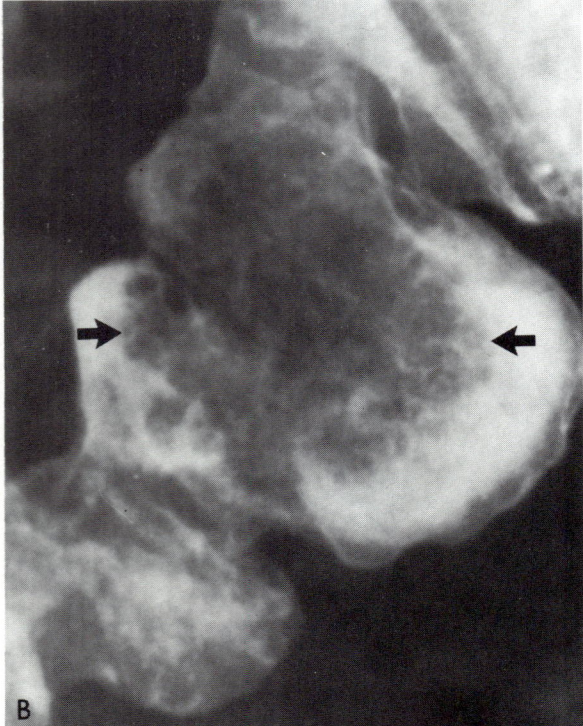

Figure 13–80. Transverse colon benign villous adenoma on filled and postevacuation views. *A,* A 3-cm polypoid villous adenoma (arrow) displaces the barium suspension in the transverse colon. *B,* Barium suspension trapped in the fronds of the tumor (arrows) on this postevacuation view permits identification of the characteristic network appearance of the tumor's surface.

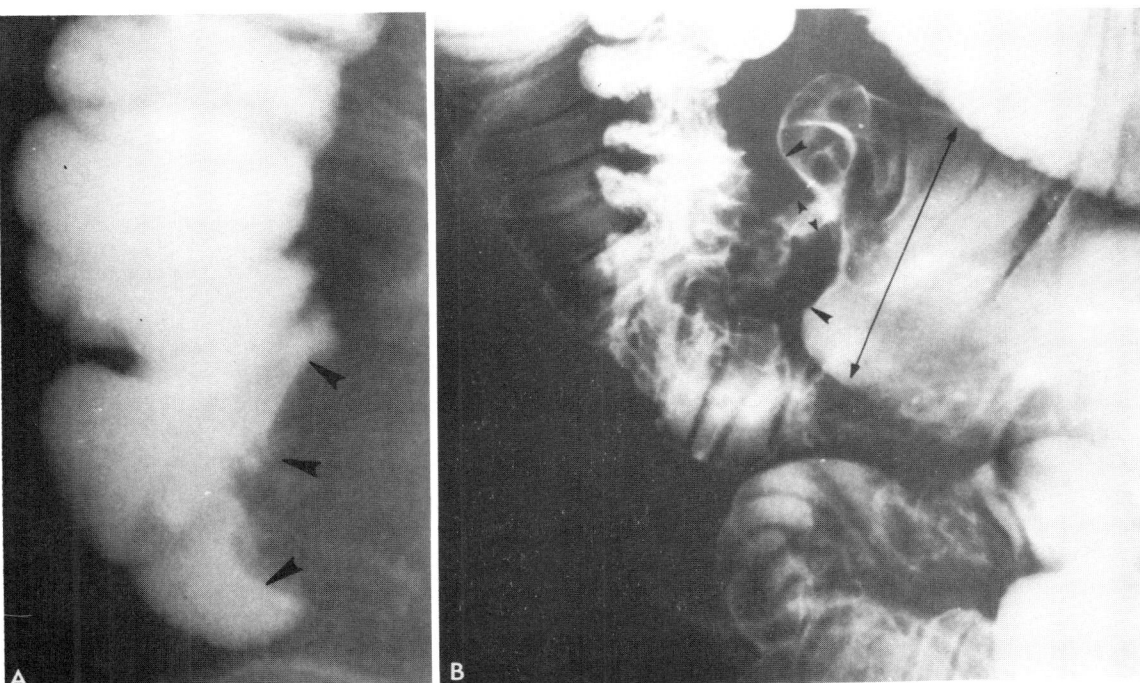

Figure 13–81. Obstructing ileocecal valve carcinoma. *A,* Barium enema shows what appears to be extrinsic impression on the medial portion of the cecum and proximal ascending colon (large arrowheads). *B,* An antegrade study demonstrates an encircling carcinoma of the ileocecal valve (small arrowheads) with shouldering at the proximal edge of the tumor (medium arrowheads). The small intestine is dilated (two-headed arrow) proximal to the tumor.

VILLOUS ADENOMA

Both tubulovillous adenomas and villous adenomas have strong tendencies to undergo malignant transformation. Combined, they represent one fourth of colorectal neoplasms but produce approximately two thirds of colorectal carcinomas. Most patients coming to medical attention because of these tumors have either rectal bleeding or diarrhea. Occasionally, villous adenomas produce copious mucous diarrhea with excessive secretion of potassium, which leads to significant hypokalemia. The vast majority of villous adenomas are located in the rectum or the sigmoid and, although they are usually sessile, they may be pedunculated.[1, 20] Typically, the lesions are soft, with a cauliflower-like appearance.

Radiographically, the usual villous adenoma appears as a polypoid, sessile lesion, frequently indistinguishable from other polypoid lesions. After the secretions have been washed from the interstices of a villous adenoma, the barium suspension may insinuate itself in and among the deeply creviced folds of the tumor and produce a reticulated, bubbly, cobblestone, mosaic pattern. This appearance is especially notable on the postevacuation view of a full-column barium enema (see Fig. 13–80).[20] The double-contrast enema may also show the gross warty appearance of these large tumors (Fig. 13–82).

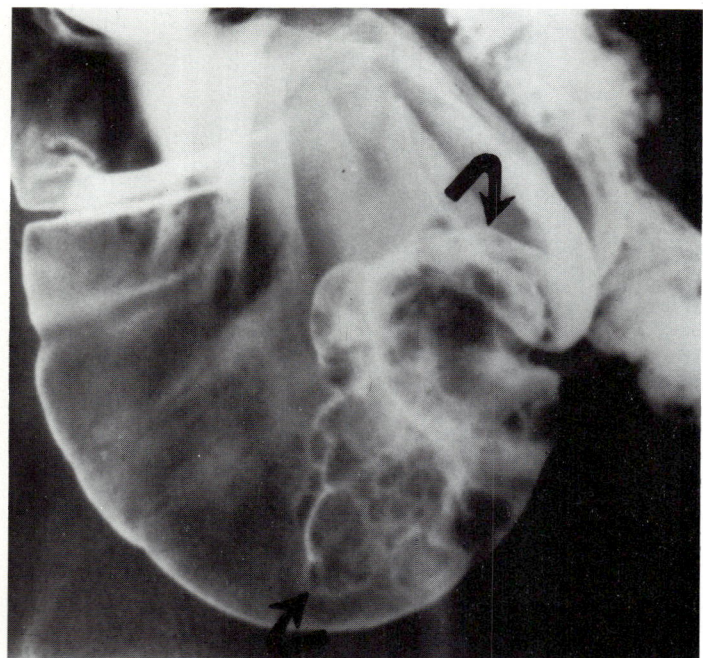

Figure 13–82. Cecal villous adenoma with malignant transformation. This 5-cm cecal pole villous adenoma (curved arrows) has a typical bubbly appearance, with barium suspension entrapped in its interstices. Foci of adenocarcinoma were present in the tumor.

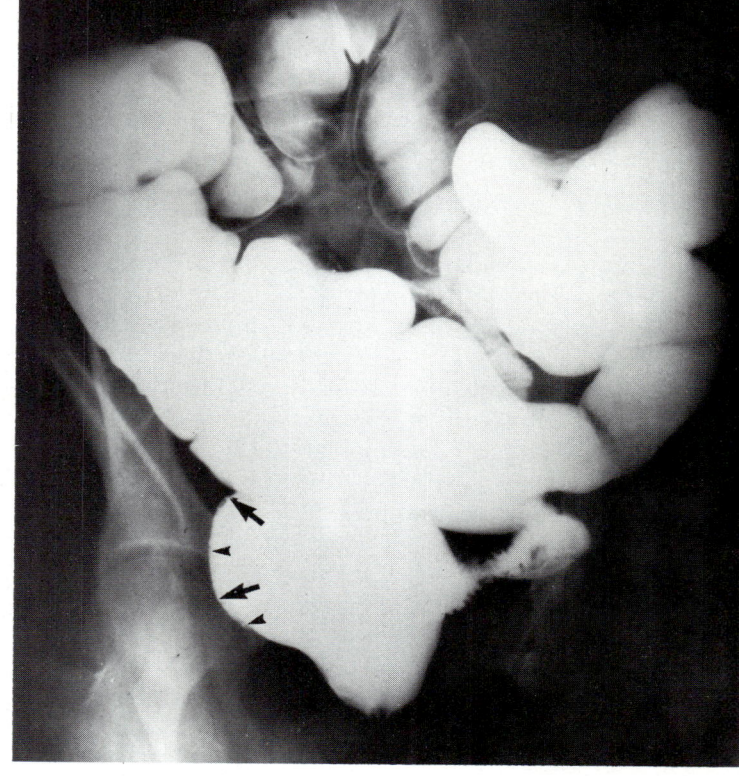

Figure 13–83. Rectal villous adenoma. A villous adenoma arises from the right lateral wall of the rectum producing a subtle, serrated profile.

Since villous adenomas may produce plateaulike growth that is just barely raised from the bowel surface,[15] the full-column barium enema may display these relatively flat tumors only in the profile view (Fig. 13–83). Therefore, the entire circumference of the colon is viewed in profile to help detect low, flat lesions. The double-contrast enema examination permits detection of very small villous adenomas, even those located in the large-caliber cecum (Fig. 13–84). Retained feces that have adhered to the bowel wall can very closely resemble villous tumors (see Fig. 13–79). In some instances it may not be possible to distinguish whether a particular abnormality represents retained adherent feces or a true tumor. In these cases, after further bowel cleansing, either radiologic reexamination or colonoscopy may be necessary.

Enlargement or change in the shape of a villous adenoma often heralds malignant degeneration (Fig. 13–85). Also, a large, sessile, coarsely patterned villous adenoma should raise strong suspicion of malignant degeneration (Figs. 13–86 and 13–87). Large bowel villous adenomas not infrequently coexist with colorectal carcinoma (Fig. 13–88).[1, 15]

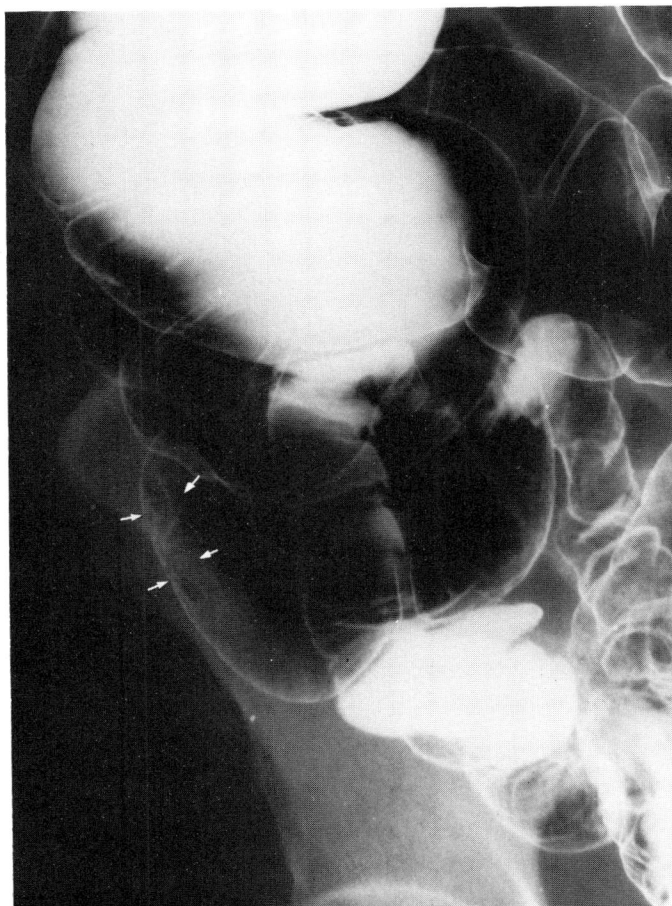

Figure 13–84. Cecal villous adenoma. A benign villous adenoma of the cecum, 3 mm in height and 2 cm in diameter, (arrows) has a typical warty appearance.

728 — THE LARGE BOWEL

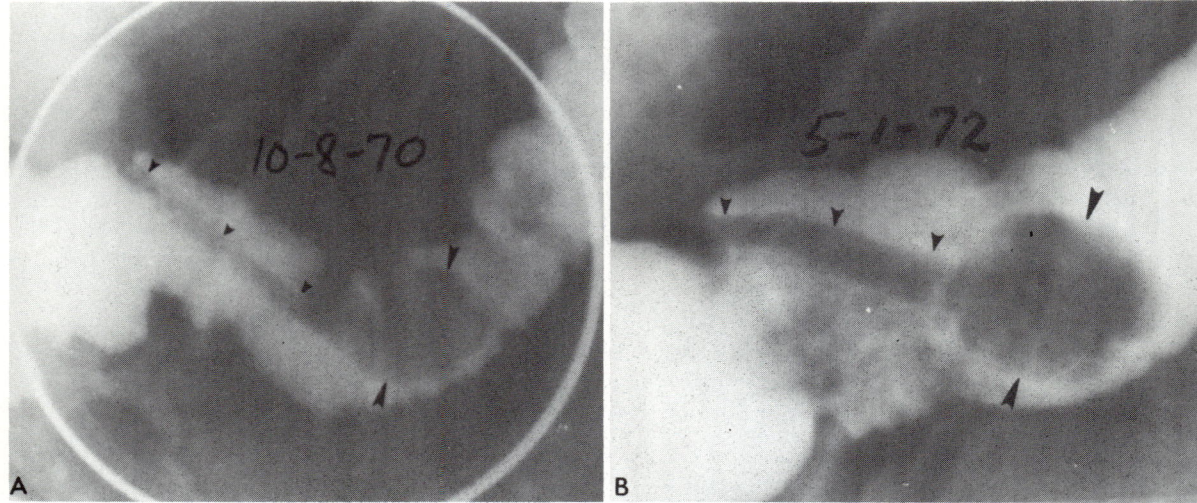

Figure 13–85. Sigmoid colon carcinoma *in situ* developing in a tubulovillous adenoma. Malignant transformation of a tubulovillous adenoma is indicated in serial examinations by a change in the tumor's shape and size. The pedicle (arrowheads) shortens and widens as its head (large arrowheads) enlarges. *A,* On the initial examination the stalk is 50 mm in length and 4 mm wide, and the smooth head is 20 mm in diameter. *B,* Nineteen months later the stalk has shortened and thickened (35 mm long and 8 mm wide), and the now irregular head of the polyp has increased to 25 mm in diameter. Carcinoma *in situ* had arisen in the villous adenoma portion of this intermediate polyp.

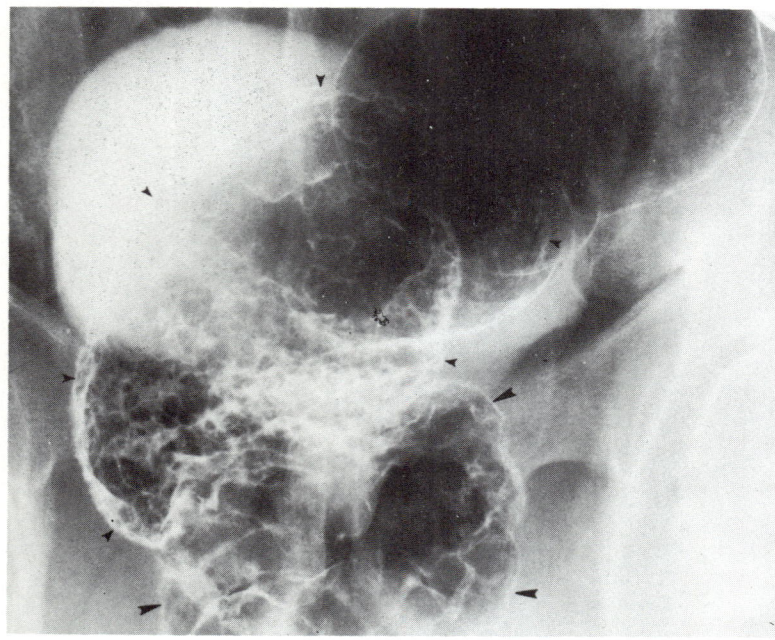

Figure 13–86. Rectal carcinoma in a villous adenoma. Carcinoma has developed in an intermittently prolapsing rectal villous adenoma. The tumor has a delicate, reticulated pattern proximally (small arrowheads) and a coarse, nodular pattern distally (large arrowheads).

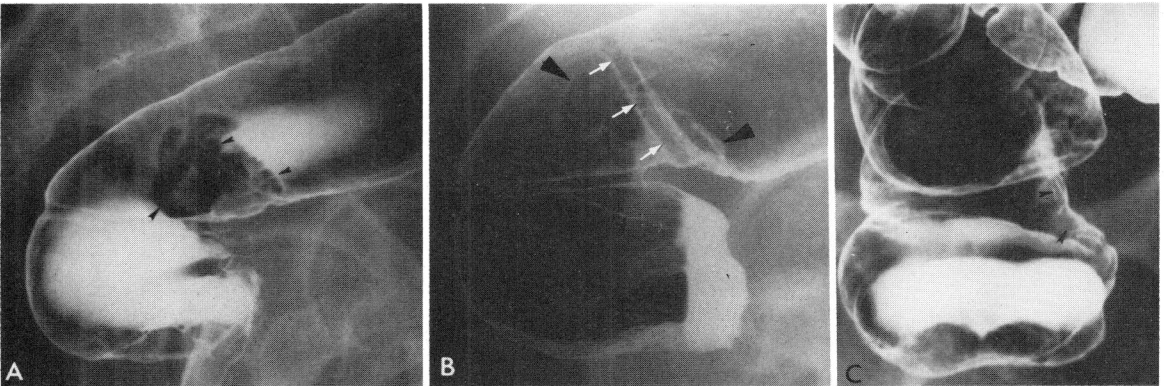

Figure 13–87. Rectal carcinoma in a tubulovillous adenoma. A sessile tubulovillous adenoma has developed invasive carcinoma in its villous adenoma component. Only a small portion of the tumor contains the histologic features of an adenomatous polyp, while villous adenoma comprises the bulk of the tumor. The tumor (arrowheads) is on the left wall of the colon, and a rectal fold (arrows) is on the right lateral wall. *A*, The tumor is located in a shallow puddle of contrast material in this left lateral view with a vertical x-ray beam. The barium suspension abuts the tumor, indicating its proximal and distal extent. *B*, The prone horizontal beam view simultaneously shows the tumor and an overlying rectal fold. Both structures are coated with barium and outlined with air. Neither structure affects the other, indicating that they are on opposite rectal walls and that the tumor is not circumferential. *C*, The prone view with a vertical beam confirms that the tumor is located on the left wall of the rectum. The radiologic appearance does not reveal that a tubulovillous adenoma was the underlying lesion of this adenocarcinoma.

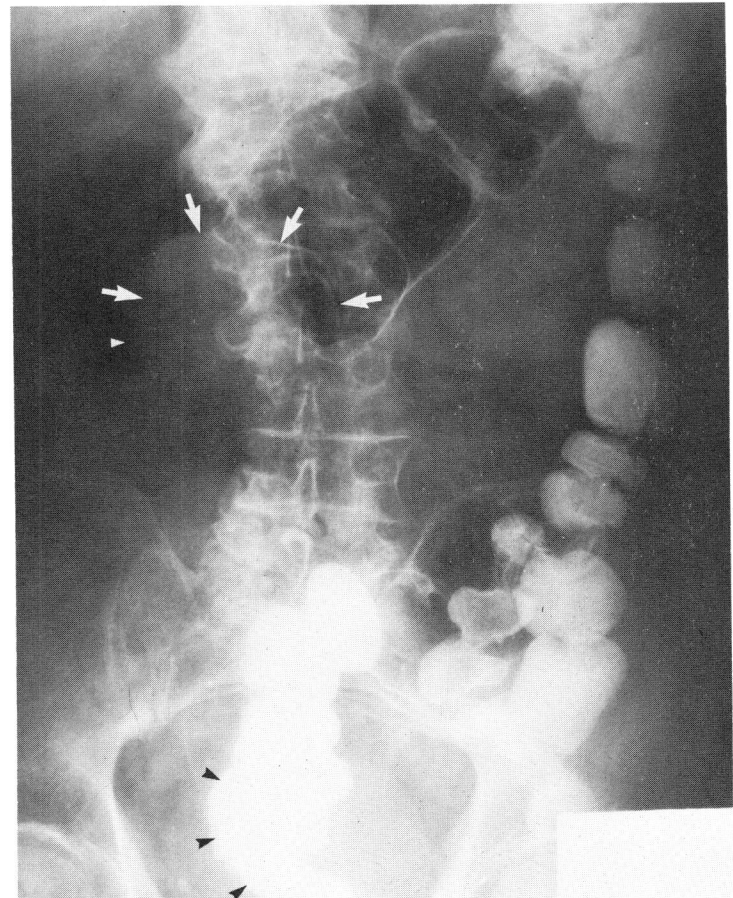

Figure 13–88. Rectal villous adenoma and obstructing transverse colon carcinoma. A dilute barium suspension enema, performed as an emergency to evaluate for bowel obstruction, outlines the distal portion of the transverse colon carcinoma. Gas in the proximal transverse colon outlines the proximal portion of this obstructing tumor (arrows). A benign villous adenoma with a typical bubbly appearance is synchronously present in the rectum (arrowheads).

COLORECTAL CARCINOMA

Clinical Features

Statistics indicate that carcinomas involving the right side of the colon usually are polypoid, fungating, nonobstructing lesions, and carcinomas of the more distal portions of the large bowel usually are encircling, obstructing lesions.[22] However, the appearance of colorectal carcinoma depends more upon the stage of growth than upon the location of the tumor. Since the circumference of the colon is greater proximally than distally and its contents are liquid, right-sided colon tumors take longer to encircle the bowel and cause obstruction than left-sided tumors. Therefore, the symptoms of right-sided lesions usually are abdominal pain, anemia, or abdominal mass, whereas the symptoms of left colon carcinomas most often include obstruction, change of bowel habits, or bleeding in addition to abdominal pain.[22] Since the stool is more formed and solid in the rectum, rectal carcinomas produce bleeding, diminished caliber of stool, change in bowel habits, either a sense of incomplete evacuation or tenesmus, and rectal mass.[22] Barium enema x-ray examination and proctosigmoidoscopy are complementary methods of examining the rectum and sigmoid,[6, 11, 19, 21] where more than one half of colorectal carcinomas are located.[1, 14, 16]

Radiologic Features

Except in cases of ulcerative colitis, in which colorectal carcinoma develops from areas of epithelial dysplasia, large bowel carcinoma arises in benign neoplasms[1, 15] that

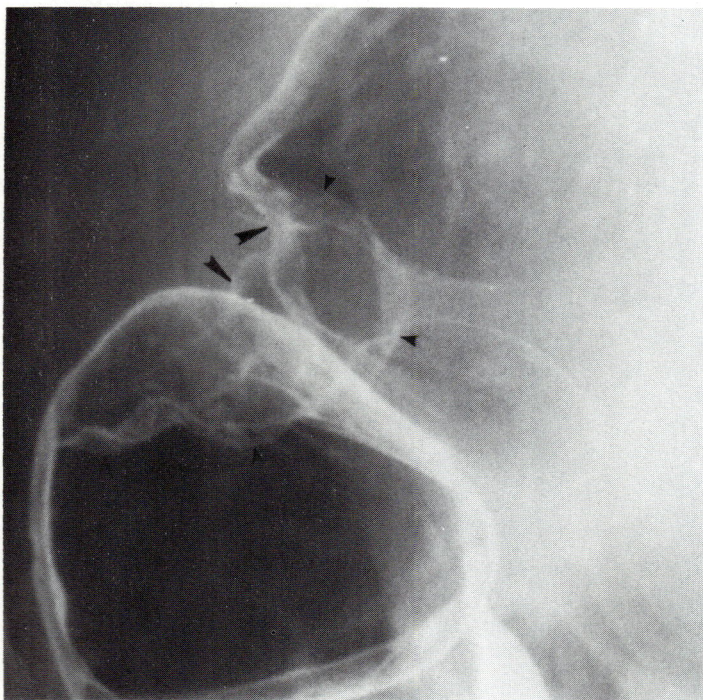

Figure 13–89. Rectal carcinoma. Irregularity of the posterior aspect of the rectum (large arrowheads) indicates invasion of the bowel wall by a polypoid carcinoma (small arrowheads).

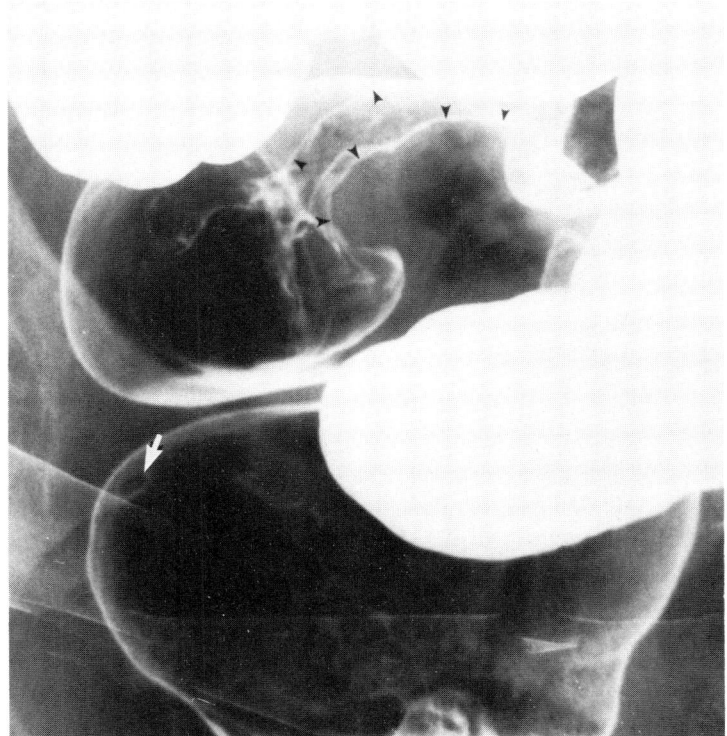

Figure 13–90. Sigmoid colon carcinoma and adenomatous polyp. An encircling carcinoma of the distal sigmoid (arrowheads) is seen through the air-distended, barium-coated rectum. An adenomatous polyp, 6 mm in diameter and 2 mm in height (arrow), is present in the rectum, distal to the carcinoma.

have already produced a growth protruding into the bowel lumen. The radiographic detection of both benign neoplasms and colorectal carcinoma therefore depends upon the ability to observe a mass encroaching into the bowel. The smaller the neoplasm, the less likely it is to be malignant, but even small tumors may harbor cancer.[15] Tumors have about a 1 per cent incidence of containing carcinoma if they are less than 1 cm in diameter; a 10 per cent chance if they are 1 to 2 cm in diameter, and an almost 50 per cent likelihood if they are over 2 cm in diameter.[15] Full-column barium enemas are unlikely to detect very small tumors,[13] and double-contrast enemas also may miss a small mass if not performed and interpreted expertly.

The smallest colorectal carcinomas appear on barium enema examinations as smooth protrusions into the bowel lumen. As they grow, they may develop either an irregular surface[9] or, if they have deeply invaded the bowel wall, an irregular base at their point of attachment to the bowel (Fig. 13–89). Some carcinomas enlarge, producing growth predominantly into the lumen with relatively little lateral extension of the base. This growth pattern yields a bubbly protruded tumor. Other tumors grow both into the lumen and along the bowel wall, both circumferentially and longitudinally, producing a sharply marginated encircling tumor. The sharply demarcated edge between the tumor and the normal bowel mucosa is referred to as the shoulder of the tumor. These tumors produce the usual appearance of advanced colorectal carcinomas (Figs. 13–90 to 13–92). Rarely, the tumors grow predominantly submucosally in the bowel wall, with little or no luminal protrusion. This is the unusual infiltrative type of colorectal carcinoma, which may be difficult to detect either radiologically or endoscopically. It can appear as a smooth, gradually tapered luminal narrowing that resembles a

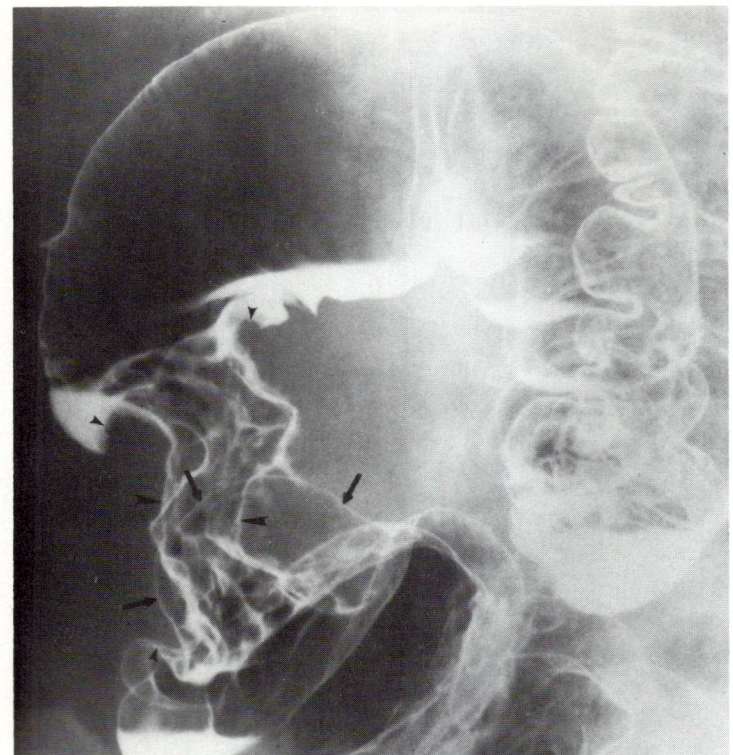

Figure 13–91. Ascending colon carcinoma. An ascending colon carcinoma encircles the bowel, producing luminal narrowing (large arrowheads). The tumor's shoulders (small arrowheads) and surface details are accurately depicted. Part of the lesion is visible through the air-distended colon (arrows), proximal to the lesion.

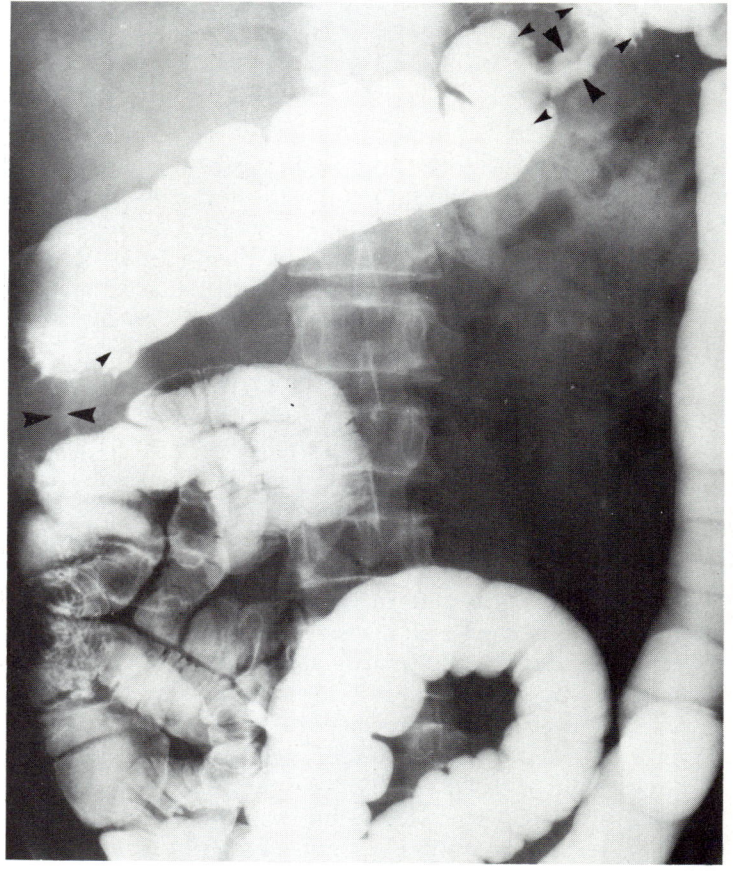

Figure 13–92. Synchronous ascending and transverse colon carcinomas. Encircling carcinomas (large arrowheads) are located in the distal ascending and transverse portion of the colon. The shelflike edges of the two synchronous tumors (small arrowheads) are discernible.

stricture rather than a tumor. Sometimes these shoulderless tumors extend longitudinally for many centimeters, and it is difficult to evaluate their true extent. Although usually of the typically encircling type (Figs. 13–93 and 13–94), scirrhouse carcinomas arising in patients with ulcerative colitis may have this infiltrative appearance and be mistaken for benign strictures (see Fig. 13–58).[2,6] Benign strictures are, however, rare in ulcerative colitis.

The typical encircling protruded colorectal carcinoma rarely extends longtudinally for more than 6 cm, because by the time it has grown that far along the bowel, it usually also has extended sufficiently around and into the bowel lumen to produce bowel obstruction (Fig. 13–95; see Figs. 13–81 and 13–88). Though large bowel tumors usually obstruct by encirclement with luminal narrowing, they occasionally produce intussusception with resultant obstruction. The tumor, which leads the intussusceptum, may be identified after hydrostatic reduction of the intussusception by the barium enema (Fig. 13–96). Bulky or pedunculated rectal tumors may prolapse through the rectum (see Fig. 13–86).

Colorectal carcinoma may ulcerate or even on occasion perforate the bowel wall. When perforation occurs, a track of contrast material may be seen extending from the expected confines of the bowel lumen. However, when the site of perforation has sealed off, which is the usual case, the diagnosis must be made by indirect signs, such as bowel displacement or even bowel obstruction produced by a pericolonic abscess (Fig. 13–97). If a perforation does not become confined to the pericolonic tissues, fistula formation can develop to other segments of the bowel (Fig. 13–98) or to other organs. These fistulas can be radiologically evaluated after the administration of contrast material by rectal infusion, by oral ingestion, or by fistula injection through the noncolonic site of the fistula, such as the skin, bladder, or vagina.

Text continued on page 738

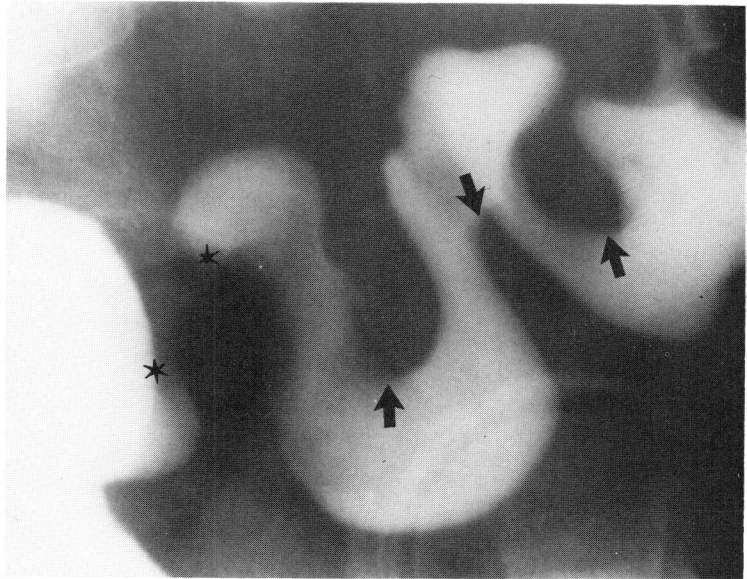

Figure 13–93. Sigmoid colon carcinoma with serosal implants in chronic ulcerative colitis. Twenty years after the onset of ulcerative colitis, an encircling carcinoma narrows the bowel lumen (between asterisks). Multiple serosal implants (arrows) angulate and indent the bowel.

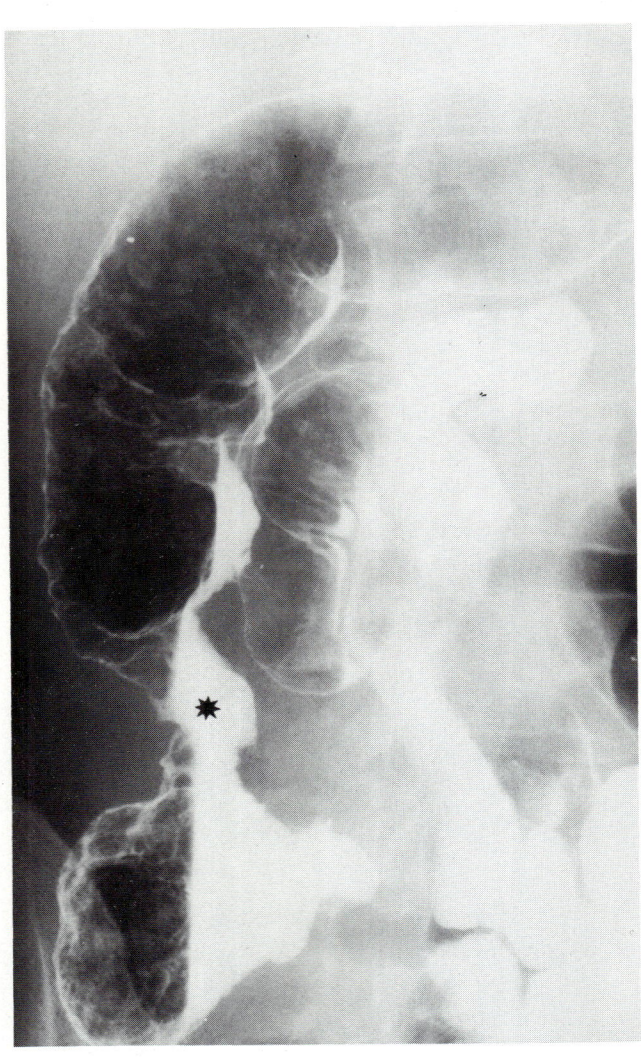

Figure 13–94. Ascending colon carcinoma in ulcerative colitis. An encircling carcinoma (asterisk) is located in the proximal ascending colon. The bowel surface surrounding the abruptly marginated tumor is irregular and contains multiple inflammatory polyps and several adenomatous polyps.

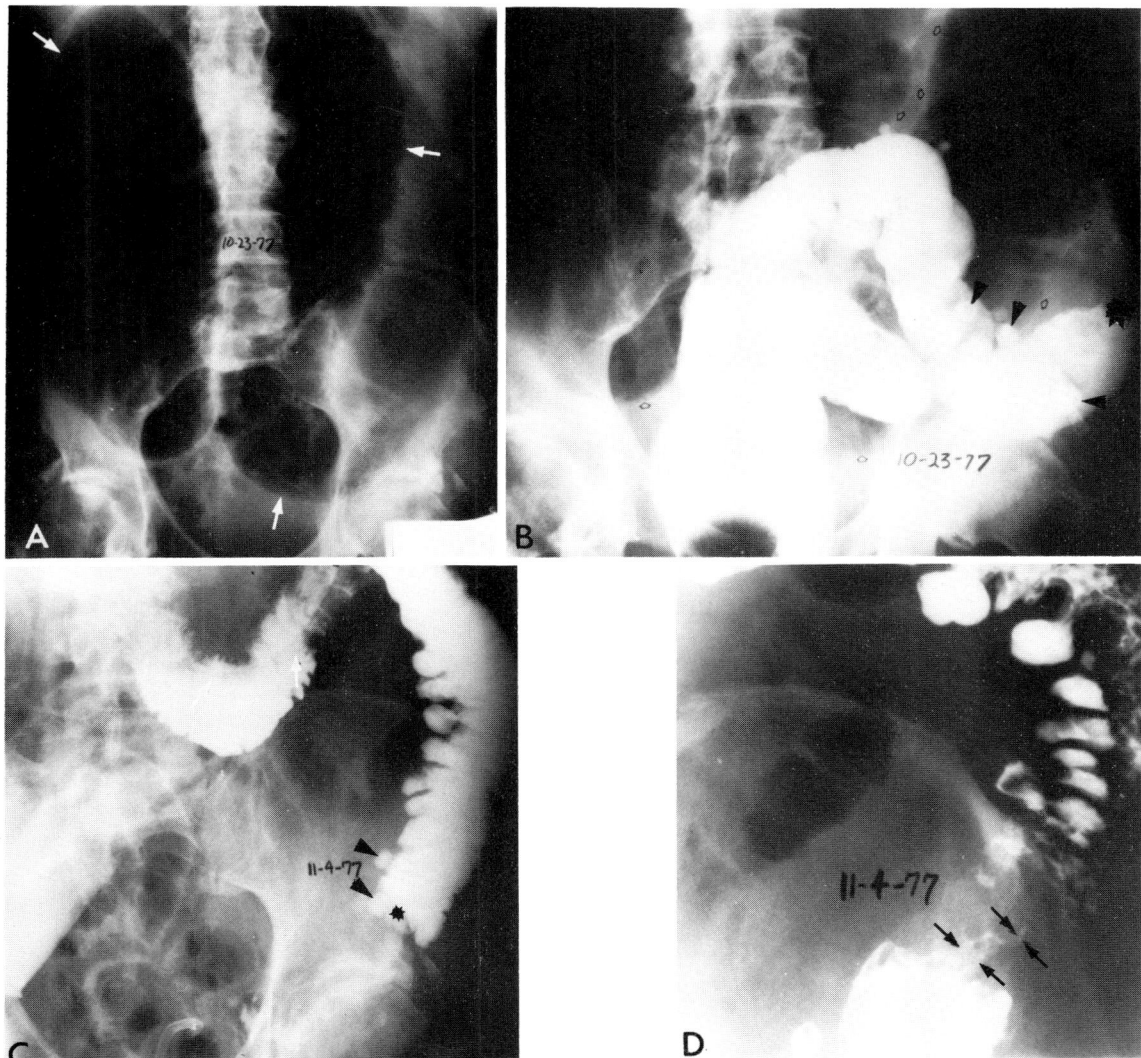

Figure 13–95. Obstructing sigmoid colon carcinoma simulating diverticulitis. *A,* Plain film of the abdomen shows dilated colon (white and open arrows) proximal to a distal colonic obstruction. *B,* Barium enema on the same day shows complete retrograde obstruction (asterisk) near the junction of the descending and the sigmoid colon. Multiple diverticula (large arrowheads) are present distal to the obstruction. Proximal colonic distention persists (open arrows). At surgery, the distinction between diverticulitis and carcinoma could not be made, so a diverting transverse colostomy was performed. *C,* Two weeks later, an antegrade study was performed through a catheter (white arrows) placed in the distal limb of the transverse colostomy. Diverticula are identified (large arrowheads) proximal to the obstruction. An apparently complete antegrade obstruction was initially encountered (asterisk). *D,* However, a delayed film shows that the obstruction was not complete and that luminal narrowing (small arrows) was produced by an encircling carcinoma.

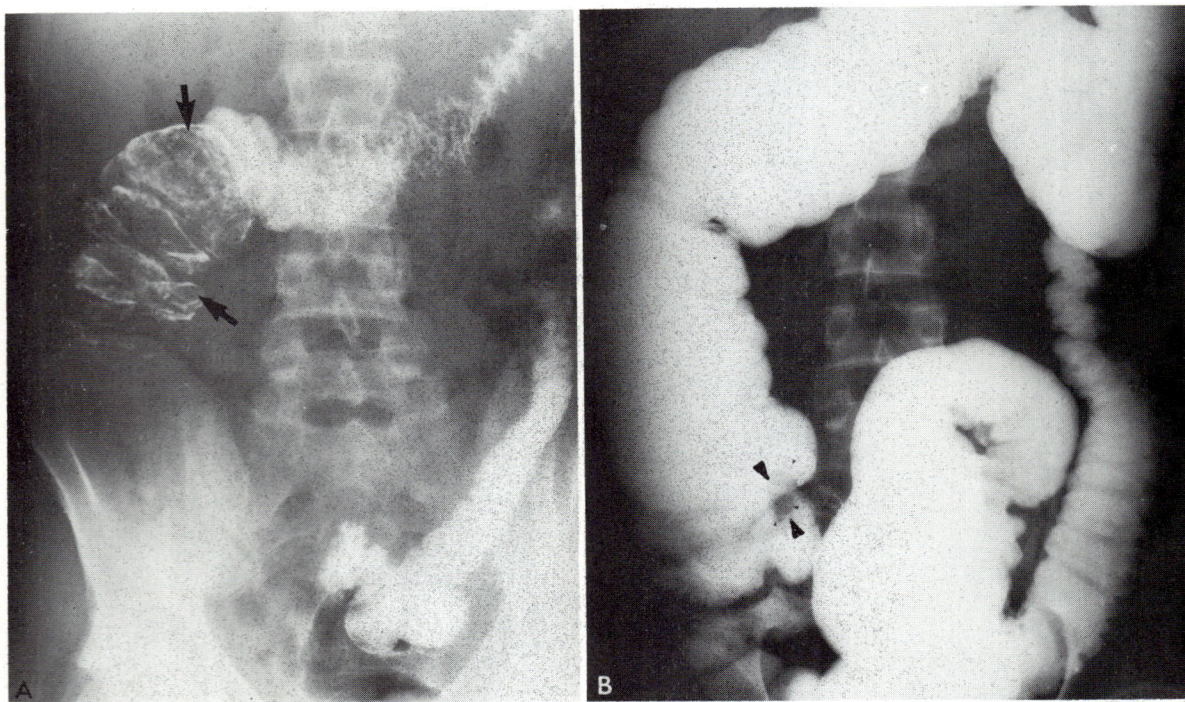

Figure 13–96. Intussuscepting obstructing ileocecal valve carcinoma. *A,* An intussusception is present (large arrows) near the hepatic flexure. *B,* After hydrostatic reduction of the intussusception by the enema, the lead point is shown to be a carcinoma (arrowheads) adjacent to the ileocecal valve.

Figure 13–97. Perforating sigmoid colon carcinoma simulating diverticulitis. *A,* An ulcerated carcinoma (small arrowheads) has perforated the sigmoid colon. An extrinsic mass resulting from the perforation impresses upon the sigmoid colon (large arrowheads) proximal to the tumor. This resembles diverticulitis with perisigmoid abscess. *B,* A spot film shows the ulcerated tumor (arrowheads) to better advantage.

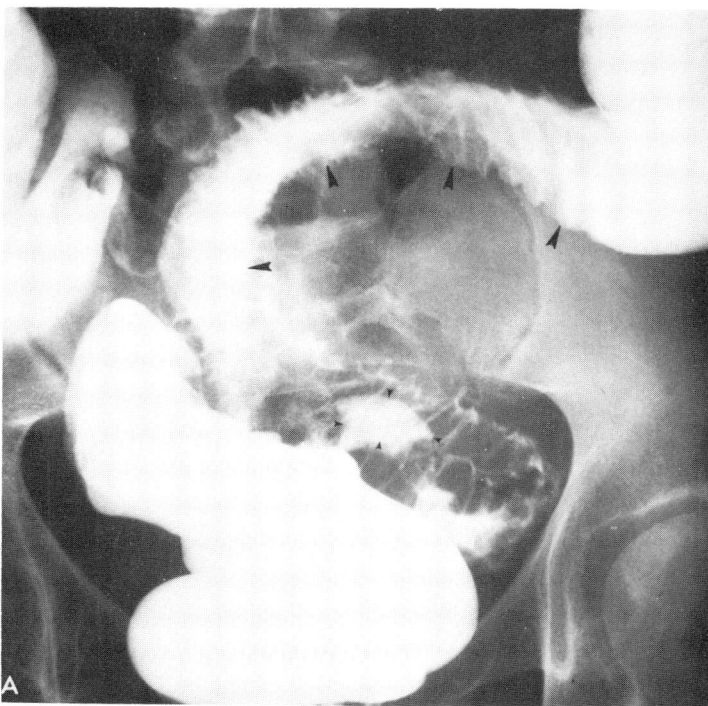
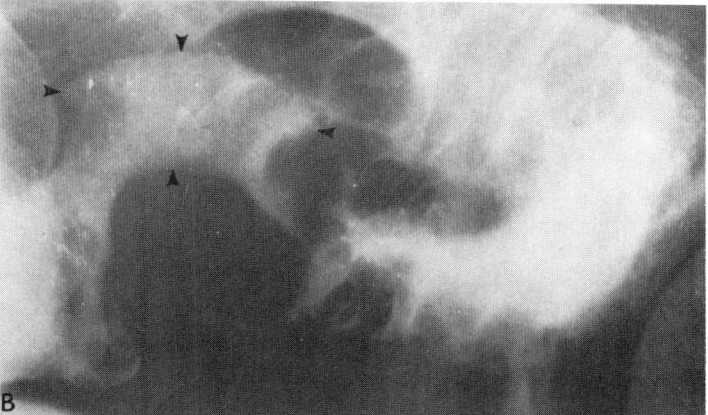

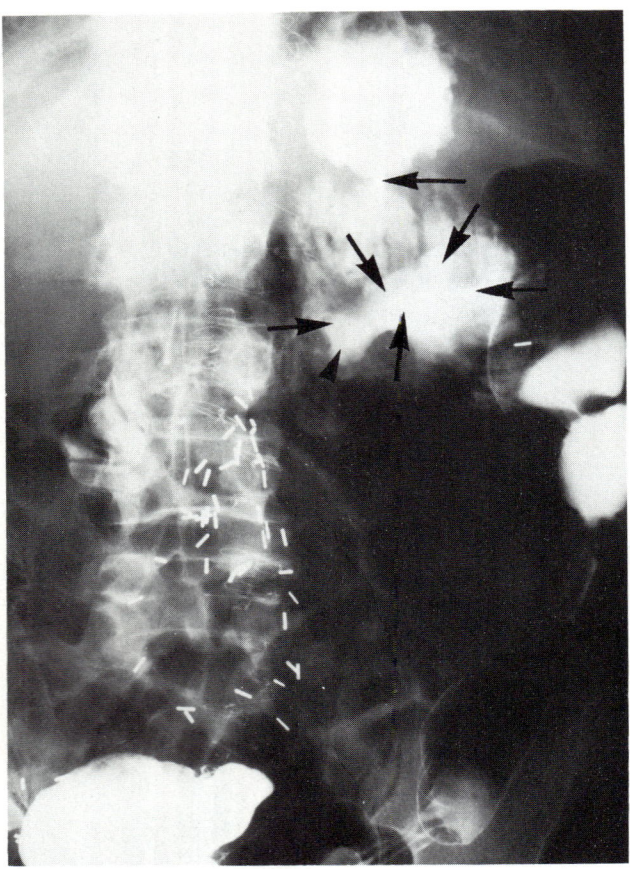

Figure 13–98. Transverse colon carcinoma with jejunocolic fistula. Several years after right hemicolectomy for carcinoma of the proximal colon and antrectomy and gastrojejunostomy for peptic ulcer disease, a large ulcerated (arrows) carcinoma is found in the transverse colon. There is fistulization to the jejunum and entrance of contrast material into the gastric pouch through the gastrojejunostomy (top arrow). The combination of surgery and tumor perforation produces the equivalent of a gastrojejunocolic fistula.

Occasionally, large bowel carcinoma can be detected by the appearance of calcification within the tumor, especially if the carcinoma is of the mucoid type. Involved lymph nodes may also calcify with mucoid carcinoma. The liver and lungs are the most common distant metastatic sites for colorectal carcinoma, and intraperitoneal spread is not uncommon (Fig. 13–99).

RADIOLOGIC DIFFERENTIAL DIAGNOSIS. Many conditions may simulate colorectal carcinoma, and colorectal carcinoma may masquerade as other diseases (Table 13–1). Whenever the diagnosis is uncertain, colonoscopic evaluation is indicated. In some instances, however, definitive distinction can be made only after surgical intervention.

Diverticular disease is the condition that most often produces diagnostic difficulty, and colorectal carcinoma not infrequently resembles diverticulitis. Diverticulitis develops a pericolonic inflammatory process that produces bowel wall edema. The mucosal folds swell, and the outline of the bowel lumen becomes irregular. The inflammatory distortion may be sufficient to cause partial or complete bowel obstruction. However, in diverticulitis there is no intraluminal tumor, and the inflammatory process may involve a longer segment of bowel (greater than 6 cm) than is usual for large bowel cancer (see Figs. 13–95 and 13–97).

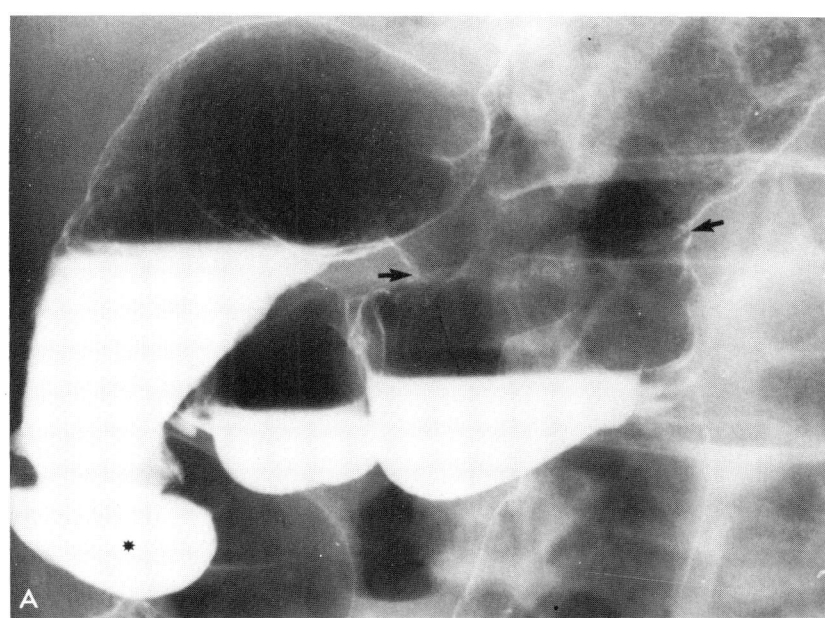
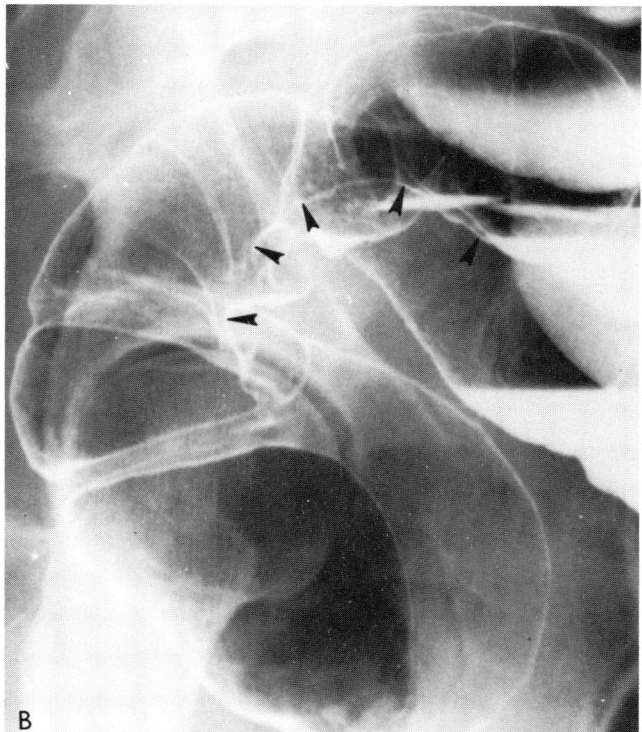

Figure 13–99. Cul-de-sac tumor after right hemicolectomy for cecal carcinoma in ulcerative colitis. *A,* An ileotransverse side-to-side anastomosis (between arrows) separates the finely granular colon mucosa, involved with ulcerative colitis, from the normal small bowel. The most proximal portion of the colon is indicated by the asterisk. *B,* Smooth, extrinsic impression (arrowheads) on the anterior surface of the rectum indicates tumor implants in the cul-de-sac.

TABLE 13–1. DIFFERNTIAL DIAGNOSIS OF COLORECTAL CARCINOMA

Inflammation
 Diverticulitis
 Ulcerative colitis
 Crohn's disease
 Amebiasis
 Lymphogranuloma venereum
 Tuberculosis
 Actinomycosis
 Radiation injury
 Ischemia
 Appendicitis

Tumors
 Benign
 Lymphoma
 Carcinoid
 Metastases

Miscellaneous
 Spasm
 Adhesions & Bands
 Endometriosis
 Postoperative
 Hemorrhoids
 Feces or Gas

Spasm may temporarily mimic carcinoma, but it can usually be distinguished by its transience. If it is persistent, intravenous glucagon almost always obliterates it. Also, close inspection of the radiographs usually reveals that intraluminal mass with tumor shoulders is absent and that the mucosa is intact with wavy, not jagged or shaggy, contours (Fig. 13–100).

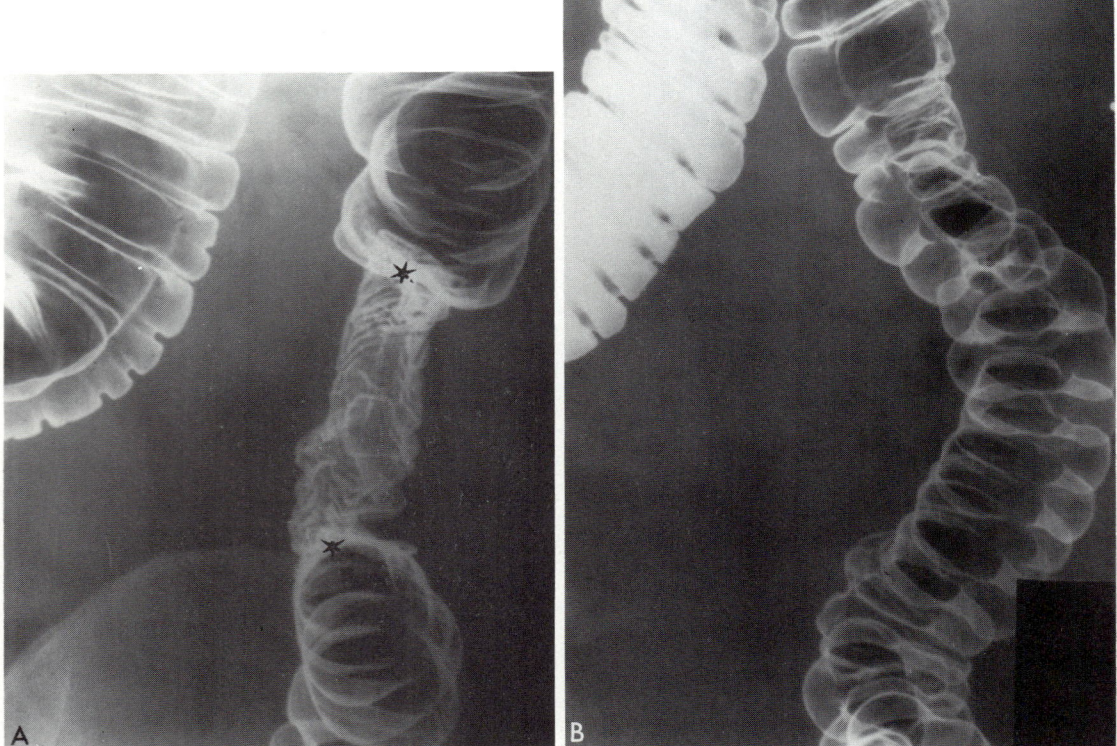

Figure 13–100. Large bowel spasm mimicking carcinoma. *A*, A short segment (between asterisks) in the descending colon is narrowed with a wavy irregular surface. Although the transition to normal-appearing bowel is abrupt both proximally and distally, there are no tumor shoulders as in Figure 13–91*B*. Moments later, without the use of hypotonic agents, the bowel is normal, indicating that the narrowing was due to transient spasm.

Lymphoma is a very rare large bowel neoplasm that is submucosal in origin, in contradistinction to the mucosally arising carcinoma. Most often it appears as many nodular lesions of various sizes. However, on rare occasions it appears as an annular constricting lesion, radiographically indistinguishable from carcinoma. Sometimes it manifests as a bulky, ulcerating mass suggesting carcinoma but involving a longer segment than is usually involved with carcinoma.

Rather than appearing as a distinct mass, rectal carcinomas that are located just proximal to the anus may mimic hemorrhoids (Fig. 13–101). With increased intraluminal pressure or with gravitational drainage of blood, hemorrhoids may change in size whereas tumors retain their size. However, direct visual inspection is recommended for all questionable lesions.

POSTOPERATIVE FEATURES. The postoperative radiologic examination is tailored to the specific needs of each patient. When the x-ray examination is performed in the immediate postoperative period to evaluate for anastomotic integrity and patency, prior bowel cleansing is unnecessary. Water-soluble contrast is used for these examinations, which are confined to the segments of bowel adjacent to the anastomosis. Bowel cleansing is necessary after the immediate postoperative period, and even defunctionalized segments of bowel that are to be studied are cleansed of residual mucus and other material to permit optimal examination. Because the rectal sphincter enables the patient to retain the enema, it is almost always easier to perform examinations through the rectum. However, patients whose examination must be performed through a colostomy can still be afforded the benefits of a double-contrast examination (Fig. 13–102).[4] Parenteral glucagon is used for colostomy enemas to eliminate bowel spasm, thereby reducing pain and helping the patient to retain the enema.

Complications of surgery, tumor recurrences, and metachronous lesions can be detected by the radiologic examination of patients with previous resections for

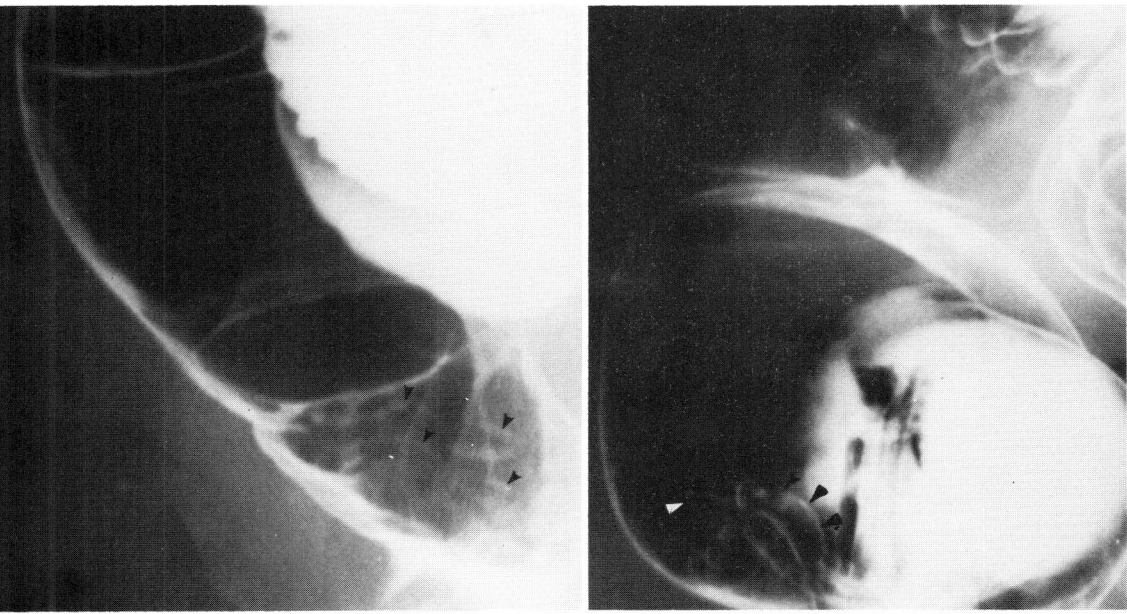

Figure 13–101. Rectal carcinoma simulating hemorrhoids. The distal portion of the rectum contains a few short, subtle, wavy folds, produced by the irregular surface of a small carcinoma (arrowheads) that resembles hemorrhoids.

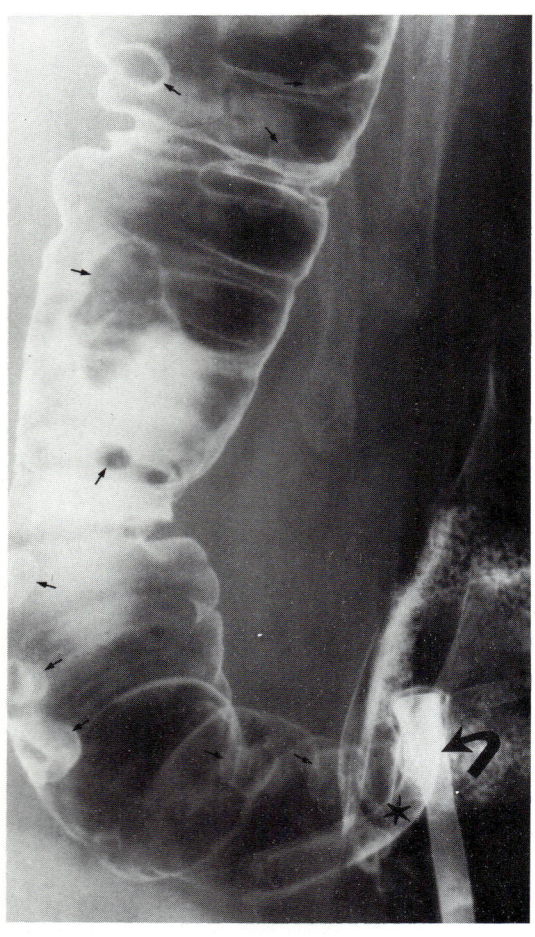

Figure 13–102. Colostomy enema with multiple neoplasms. Eleven years after sigmoid colon resection for carcinoma, a barium enema performed through a catheter (curved arrow) placed in a descending colon colostomy (asterisk) shows multiple, varying-sized polypoid neoplasms (arrows). A large metachronous adenocarcinoma was present in the cecum.

colorectal carcinoma. A satisfactory anastomosis connects the correct bowel segments, maintains the bowel lumen, and does not leak (Fig 13–103; see Fig. 13–99). The luminal surface of the bowel is often so smooth and regular in end-to-end colonocolonic anastomoses that the site of anastomosis is hard to locate, but it may be identified by subtle disruption of the regular haustral pattern (Fig. 13–104). If the anastomosis is between the ileum and the colon, the demarcation between the small bowel and the colon is usually evidenced by the abrupt change both in mucosal folds and in bowel caliber, even in end-to-end anastomoses (Figs. 13–105 and 13–106). Sometimes, postoperative deformity from distorted bowel or suture defects may mimic tumor, and endoscopic evaluation is necessary to exclude the presence of recurrent tumor (Figs. 13–107 and 13–108).

Anastomotic dehiscence in the immediate postoperative period following low anterior resection is often asymptomatic, so radiologic study is necessary for accurate assessment of the integrity of the anastomosis.[17] Anastomotic dehiscence is diagnosed by identifying water-soluble contrast material projecting outside the bowel lumen (Fig. 13–109). Late bowel stenosis can be identified by the barium enema as a smoothly tapered, narrowed segment at the anastomotic site (Fig. 13–110). Serial radiologic examinations are helpful in assessing the progress or regression of both perforations and stenoses.

Recurrent tumor at an anastomotic site is not unusual and may be difficult to distinguish from postoperative deformity (see Figs. 13–107, 13–108, and 13–110A) unless prior postoperative studies are available for comparison. Changes in the appearance of an anastomotic site after the immediate postoperative period are unlikely to be caused by a benign condition, and malignancy should be suspected when any change occurs. New second malignancies occur with sufficient frequency to justify regular follow-up studies (see Figs. 13–98 and 13–102).[1, 15]

Text continued on page 748

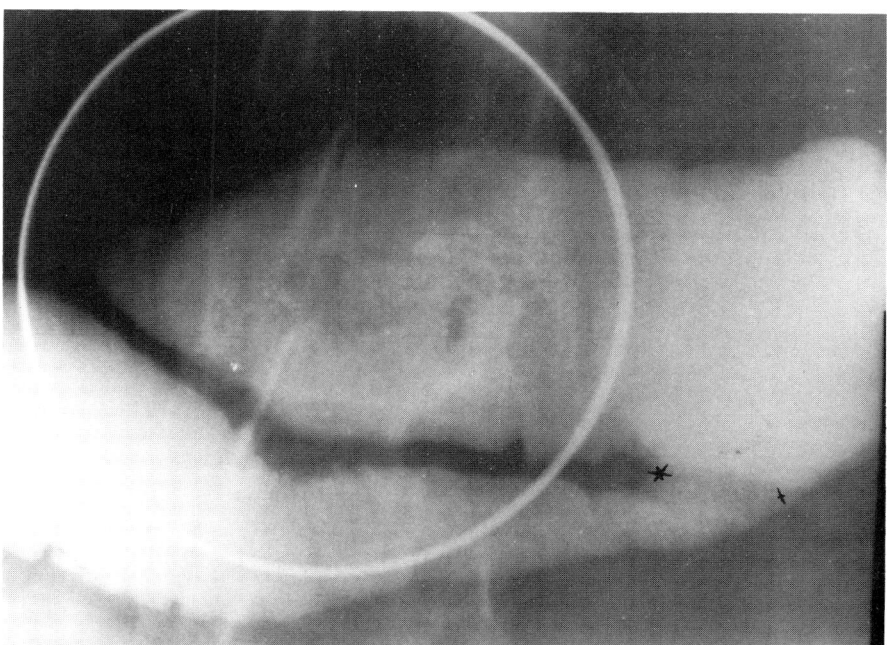

Figure 13–103. End-to-side ileotransverse anastomosis. An end-to-side ileotransverse anastomosis (between asterisks) is patent with no evidence of recurrence or stenosis.

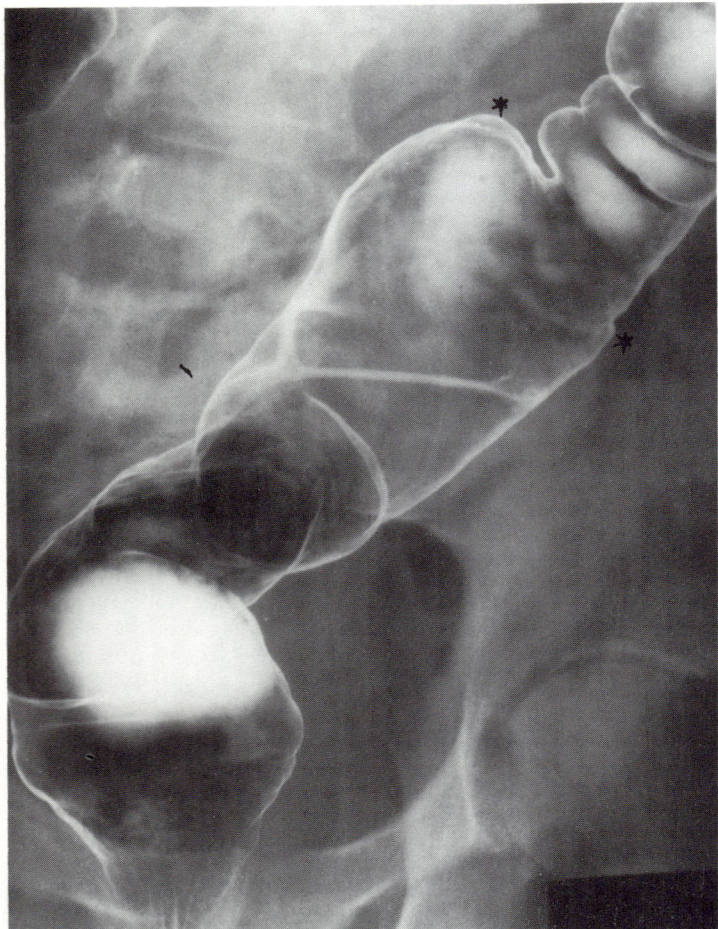

Figure 13–104. End-to-end sigmoid anastomosis. Eight years after partial sigmoid resection, the anastomosis (between asterisks) appears normal. The anastomosis is identified by the change in the haustral appearance on the superior surface and the slight bowel wall irregularity on the inferior surface.

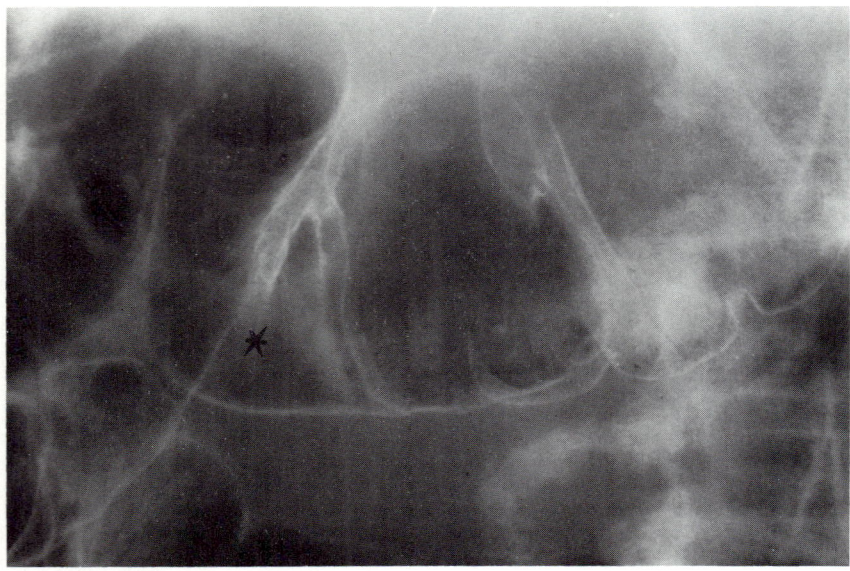

Figure 13–105. End-to-end ileotransverse anastomosis. Following right hemicolectomy for carcinoma of the ascending colon, an end-to-end ileotransverse anastomosis is seen (asterisk) to be normal.

THE LARGE BOWEL — 745

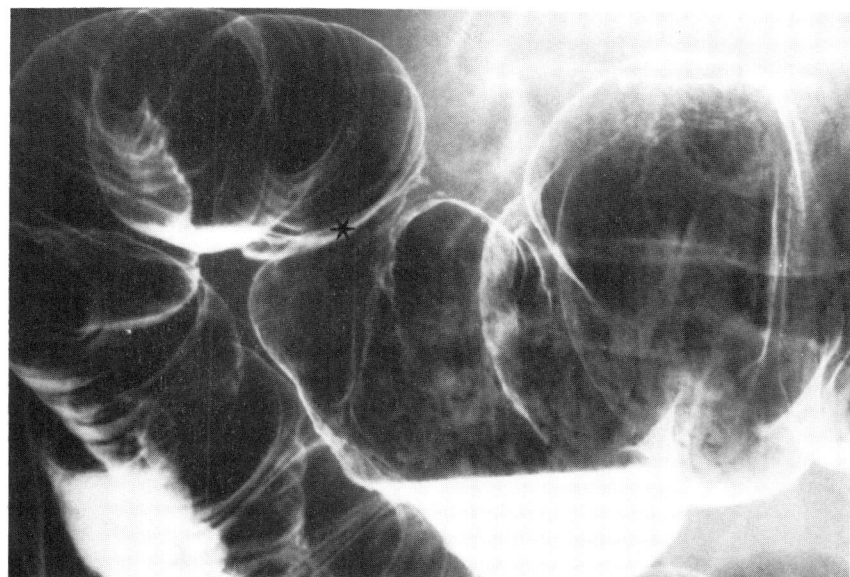

Figure 13–106. End-to-end ileotransverse anastomosis. The end-to-end anastomosis (asterisk), performed for Crohn's disease, has a normal appearance.

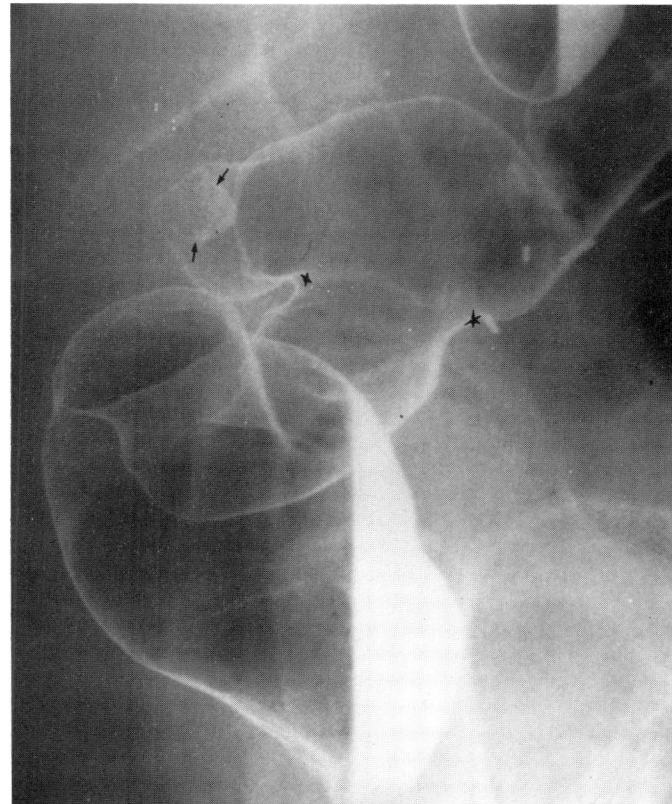

Figure 13–107. Side-to-end sigmoid anastomosis with postoperative deformity. A patent, normal-appearing anastomosis (between asterisks) is present following partial sigmoid resection. Postsurgical deformity (arrows) is seen at the stump closure.

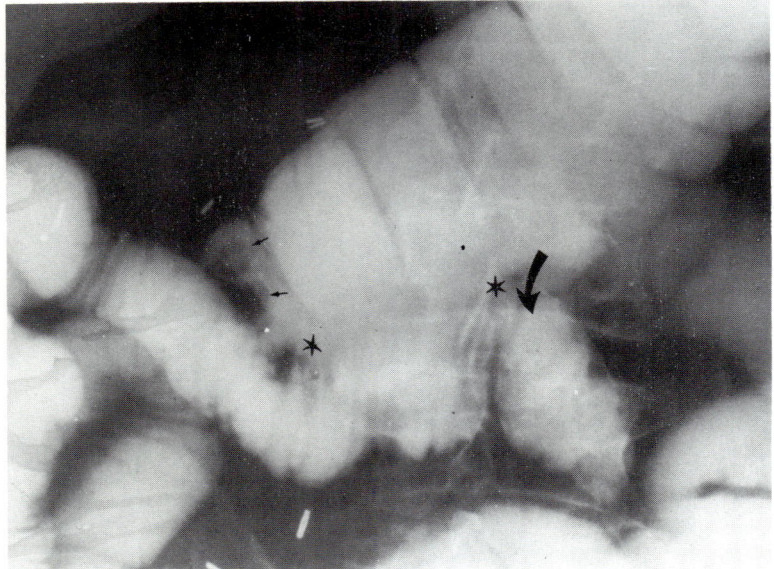

Figure 13–108. Side-to-side ileotransverse anastomosis with postoperative deformity. A side-to-side anastomosis has been constructed with a wide-open stoma (between asterisks). Postoperative deformity, which is present at the most proximal end of the remaining colon, is produced by mucosal enfolding (arrows), not by tumor recurrence. The ileum distal to the anastomosis (curved arrow) is normal.

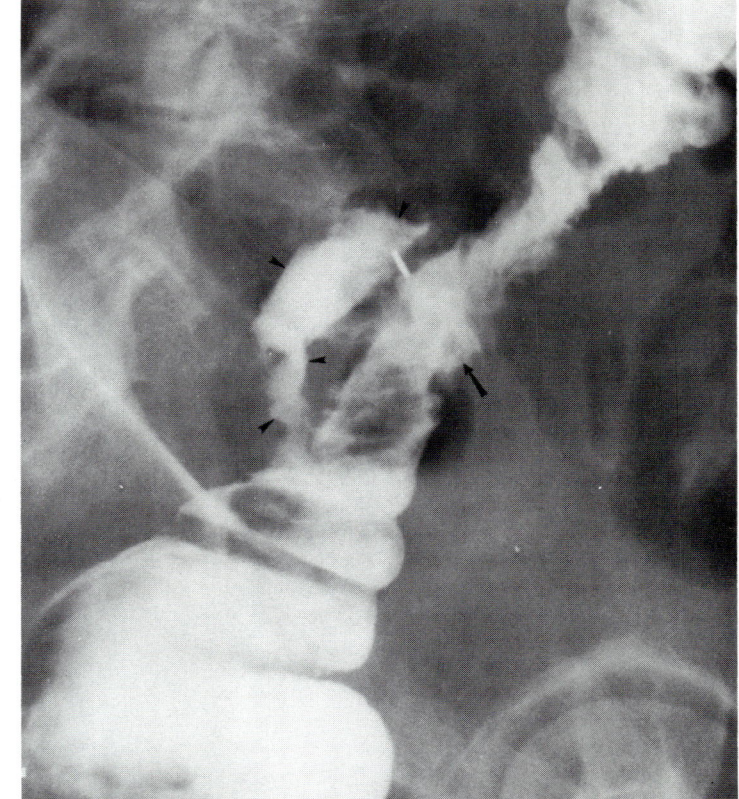

Figure 13–109. Low rectal anastomotic perforation. Nine days after low anterior bowel resection for rectal carcinoma, a limited full-column enema performed with water-soluble contrast and without bowel cleansing shows a collection of contrast material (arrowheads) outside of the bowel lumen. This indicates perforation adjacent to the narrowed bowel segment at the anastomotic site (arrow).

THE LARGE BOWEL — 747

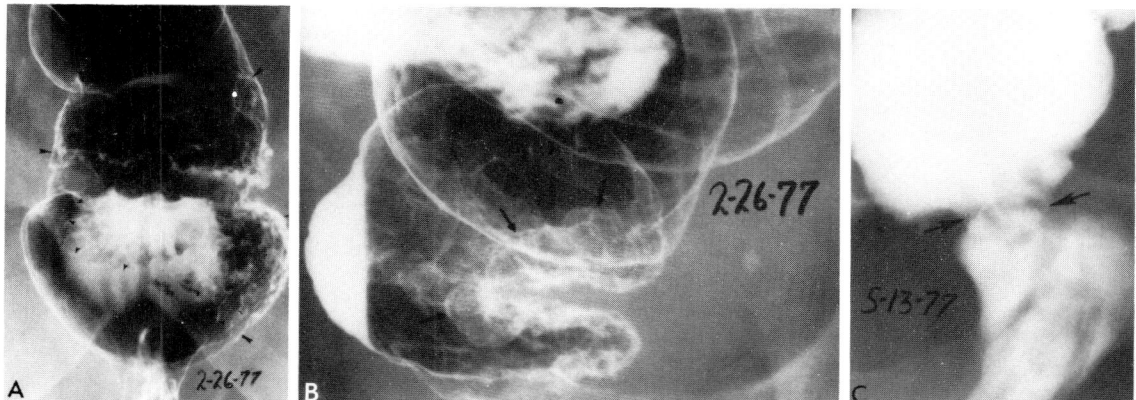

Figure 13–110. Rectal villous adenoma and narrowed rectosigmoid anastomosis. *A,* A large benign villous adenoma (large arrowheads) is present in the rectum. The distal rectum is spared (small arrowheads). *B,* A view from the same examination, but with insufficient distention, gives the false impression that the distal rectum is entirely involved. The nodular pattern to the left lateral wall of the rectum (small arrows) raises the question of carcinoma developing in the villous adenoma. *C,* Barium enema performed ten weeks postoperatively shows that the end-to-end rectosigmoid anastomosis (large arrows) is narrowed but without perforation or obstruction.

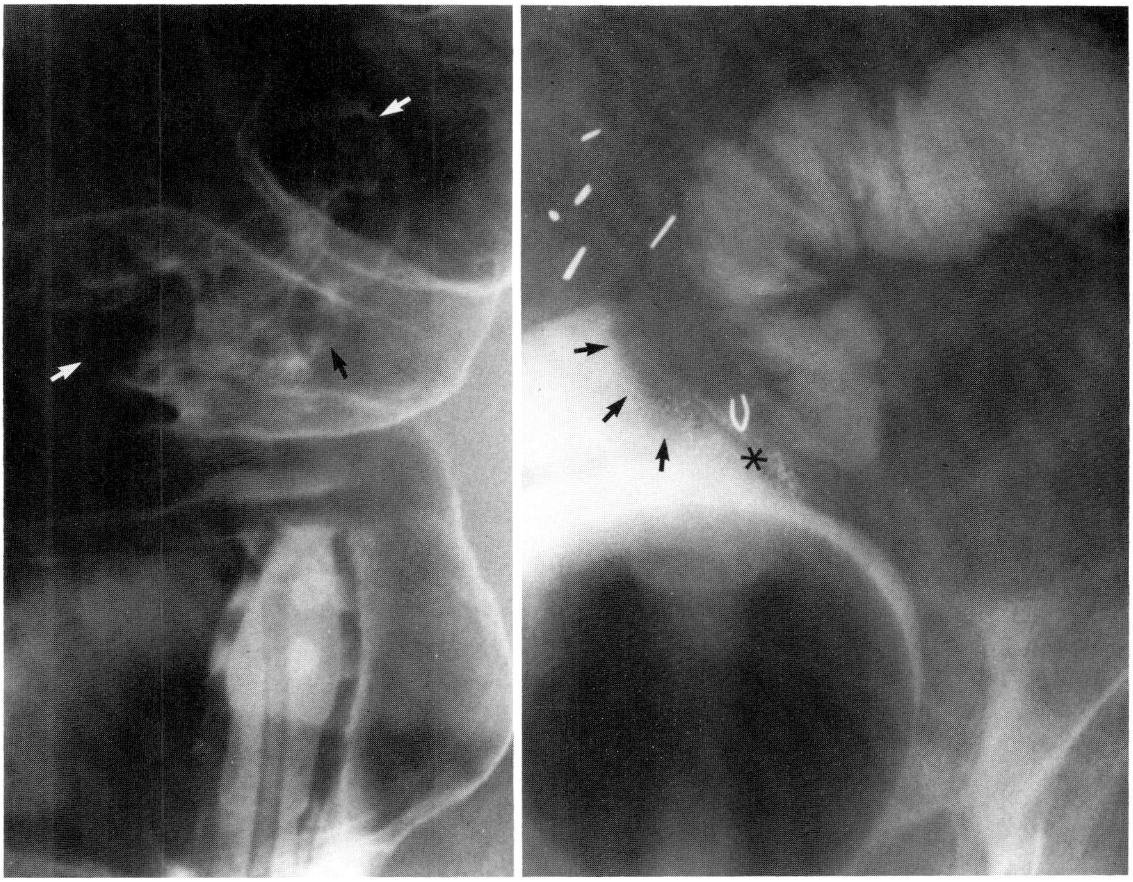

Figure 13–110A. Recurrent rectal adenocarcinoma after surgical resection. *Left,* A bulky tumor (arrows) protrudes into the rectal lumen. *Right,* The end-to-end anastomosis is identified (asterisk), and tumor has recurred (arrows) in the distal segment.

References

1. Enterline, H. T.: Polyps and cancer of the large bowel. *In* Morson, B. C.: Pathology of the Gastro-Intestinal Tract. Berlin, Springer-Verlag, 1976, pp. 97–141.
2. Fennessy, J. J., Sparberg, M. B., and Kirsner, J. B.: Radiological findings in carcinoma of the colon complicating chronic ulcerative colitis. Gut 9:383–397, 1968.
3. Figiel, S. J.: Colon examination technique. *In* Detection of Colon Lesions, First Standardization Conference, 1969. Chicago, American College of Radiology, 1973, pp. 132–145.
4. Goldstein, H. M., and Miller, M. H.: Air contrast examination in patients with colostomies. Am. J. Roentgenol. *127*:607–610, 1976.
5. Greenstein, A. J., Sachar, D. B., Smith, H., et al.: Cancer in universal and left-sided ulcerative colitis: factors determining risk. Gastroenterology 77:290–294, 1979.
6. Hodgson, J. R., and Sauer, W. G.: The roentgenologic features of carcinoma in chronic ulcerative colitis. Am. J. Roentgenol. *86*:91–96, 1961.
7. Laufer, I.: The double-contrast enema: myths and misconceptions. Gastrointest. Radiol. *1*:19–31, 1976.
8. Laufer, I.: Double contrast radiology in the diagnosis of gastrointestinal cancer. *In* Glass, G. B. J.: Progress in Gastroenterology, Vol. 3. New York, Grune & Stratton, 1977, pp. 643–669.
9. Levin, B., and Gardiner, R.: Early detection and diagnosis of large bowel cancer. *In* Enker, W. E.: Carcinoma of the Colon and Rectum. Chicago, Year Book Medical Publishers, Inc., 1978, pp. 3–17.
10. Miller, R. E., Chernish, S. M., and Brunelle, R. L.: Gastrointestinal radiography with glucagon. Gastrointest. Radiol. 4:1–10, 1979.
11. Miller, R. E.: Examination of the colon. Curr. Probl. Radiol. *5*(2):1–40, 1975.
12. Miller, R. E.: The clean colon. Gastroenterology *70*:289–290, 1976.
13. Miller, R. E.: The barium enema in the high-risk carcinoma patient. Radiology *123*:813–814, 1977.
14. Morgenstern, L., and Lee, S. E.: Spatial distribution of colonic carcinoma. Arch. Surg. *113*:1142–1143, 1978.
15. Morson, B. C.: Genesis of colorectal cancer. Clin. Gastroenterol. *5*:505–525, 1976.
16. Ott, D. J., and Gelfand, D. W.: Colorectal tumors: pathology and detection. Am. J. Roentgenol. *131*:691–695, 1978.
17. Sharefkin, J., Joffe, N., Silen, W., et al.: Anastomotic dehiscence after low anterior resection of the rectum. Am. J. Surg. *135*:519–523, 1978.
18. Silverberg, E.: Cancer statistics, 1979. CA *29*:6–21, 1979.
19. Stevenson, G. W., Gardiner, R., Somers, S., et al.: Radiology of the rectum: a challenge. Audiovisual Refresher Course. Chicago, The Radiological Society of North America, 1978.
20. Turek, R. E., Davis, W. C., Wilson, W. J., et al.: The roentgenographic diagnosis of villous tumors of the colon. Am. J. Roentgenol. *113*:349–351, 1971.
21. Welin, S., and Welin, G.: The Double Contrast Examination of the Colon: Experiences with the Welin Modification. Stuttgart, Georg Thieme Publishers, 1976.
22. Wooley, P. V., III: Clinical manifestations of cancer of the colon and rectum. Semin. Oncol. *3*:373–376, 1976.

Part IV

Colonic Polyposis and Associated Syndromes

GEORGE N. STEIN, M.D.
GERALD M. KLEIN, M.D.

GARDNER'S SYNDROME

In the early 1950's, Gardner and his coworkers wrote a series of articles describing a syndrome manifested by the triad of colonic polyposis, soft tissue tumors, and bony tumors (osteomas) (Fig. 13–111).[17] This syndrome was noted to be familial and inherited as a mendelian dominant trait. These patients often have cosmetic deformities secondary to bony or soft tissue tumors.

Figure 13–111. Gardner's syndrome. *A* and *B*, Anteroposterior film from a double-contrast enema demonstrating multiple tiny polyps distributed throughout the colon. *C*, Mandibular osteomas (arrows). *D*, Lateral view of the skull demonstrating multiple osteoma. (*From* Youker, J. E., Dodds, W. J., et al.: Colonic polyps. *In* Margulis, A. R., and Burhenne, H. J. (eds.): Alimentary Tract Roentgenology. Ed. 2. St. Louis, The C. V. Mosby Company, 1973. Reproduced by permission.)

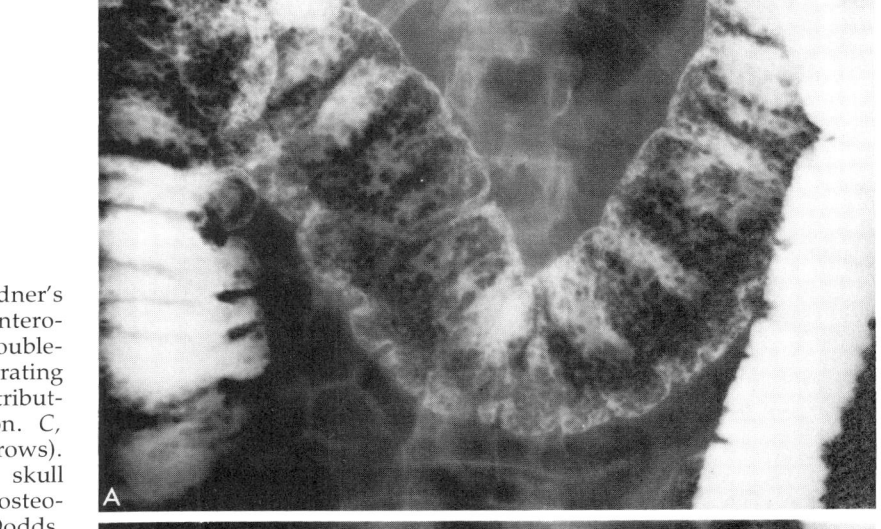
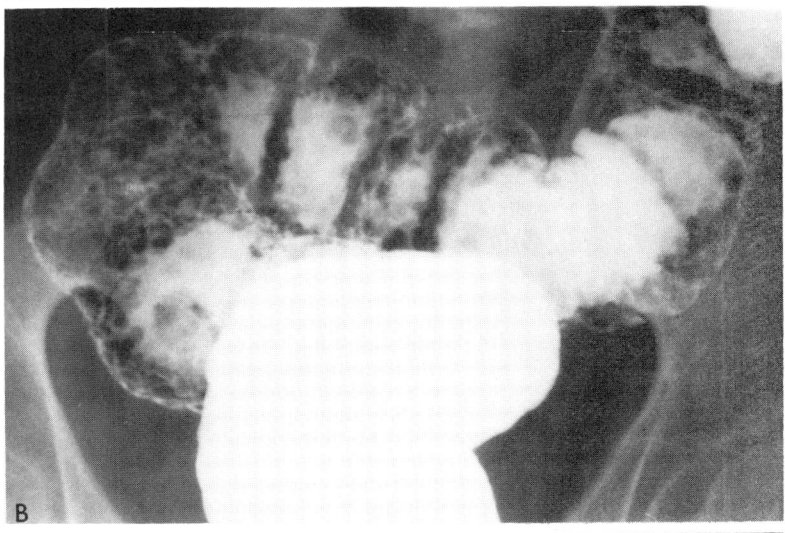
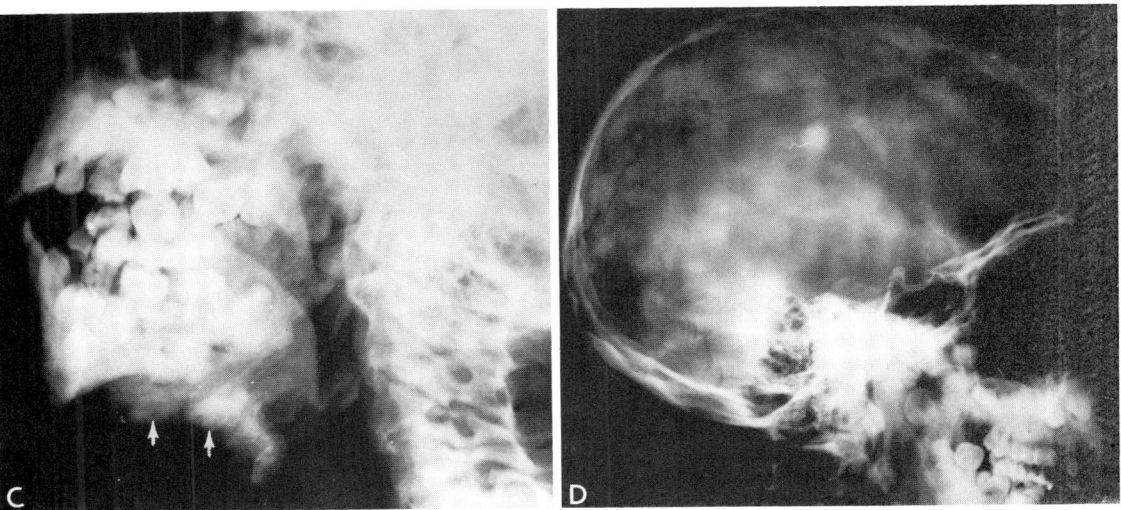

The osteomas may vary in size from slight localized cortical thickening to large protuberant masses. Almost any bone may be involved, although localized cortical thickening of the long tubular bones is most common (Fig. 13–112). Large osteomas of the mandibular angle are characteristic;[8] osteomas of the skull are also common. Dental abnormalities, including compound odontoma, multiple impacted supernumerary and permanent teeth, and carious teeth, have also been noted.[15] The soft tissue lesions consist of sebaceous cysts that appear most commonly on the face, back, and extremities. Benign tumors, such as fibromas, lipomas, leiomyomas, and neurofibromas, also occur,[11] and occasionally malignant soft tissue tumors, such as fibrosarcoma, are noted. These patients also exhibit a tendency toward fibrous tissue overgrowth, resulting in keloid formation and excessive scarring at sites of injury. Desmoid tumors have also been associated with the syndrome.[34]

Intestinal polyps occur almost exclusively in the colon (rarely in the small bowel or stomach), generally appearing in adolescence; they increase in size and number during succeeding years. Eventually the entire colon may become covered by polyps (see Fig. 13–111A and B). Diagnosis may be made by proctosigmoidoscopy or barium enema or both. Histologically, the polyps are adenomas and there is a high incidence (virtually 100 per cent) of colonic carcinoma if the colon is not removed. The polyps usually become clinically apparent when the patient enters the third decade, and malignant changes develop about 15 years later, with death resulting when the patient is in his early forties. Because of the almost inevitable development of malignancy in these patients, prophylactic colectomy is the recognized treatment of choice. Whether to perform an ileostomy and remove the rectum or to perform an ileorectal anastomosis

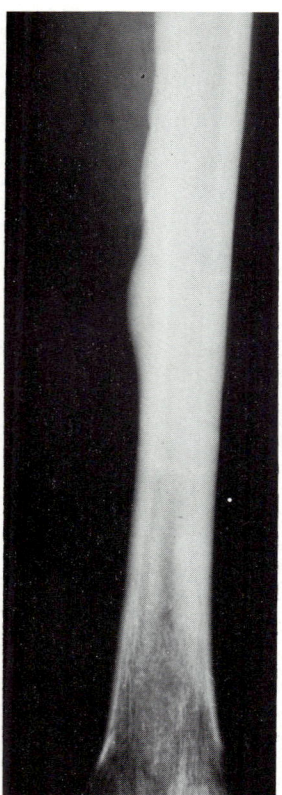

Figure 13–112. Gardner's syndrome. Localized cortical thickening of the femur. (*From* Youker, J. E., Dodds, W. J., et al.: Colonic polyps. *In* Margulis, A. R., and Burhenne, H. J. (eds.): Alimentary Tract Roentgenology. Ed. 2, St. Louis, The C. V. Mosby Company, 1973. Reproduced by permission.)

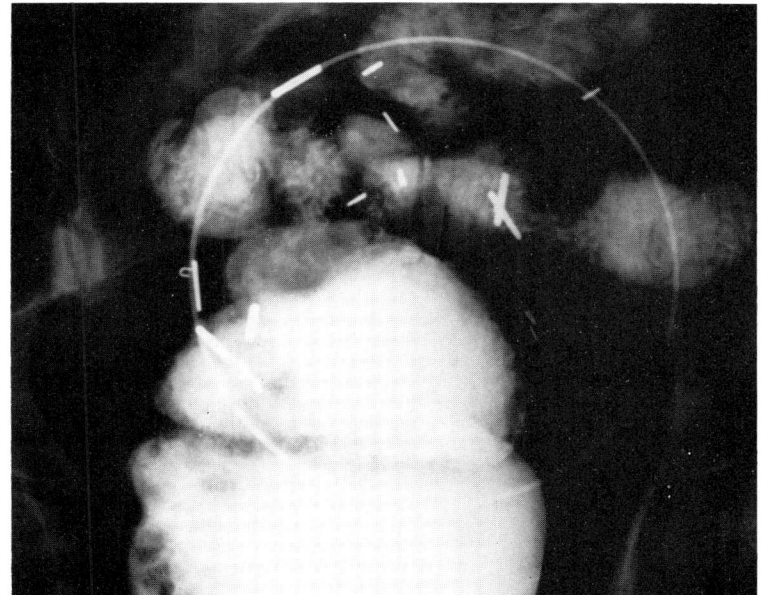

Figure 13–113. Gardner's syndrome. Barium enema demonstrating an ileorectal anastomosis.

(Fig. 13–113) is still debated. Retention of the rectum may be associated with an increase in the number of polyps in this area and the eventual development of carcinoma in the retained segment. If the rectum is not removed, close follow-up of this area by interval proctoscopy must be performed and rectal polyps fulgurated. Moertal and his coworkers believe that ileorectal anastomosis can be attempted in patients who do not have significant polypoid disease of the rectum, that is, patients with 20 or fewer polyps in the rectum; however, if rectal involvement is more severe than this, total colectomy and ileostomy should be performed because of the high incidence of carcinoma development in the retained rectal segment and the poor prognosis of these patients.[27]

POLYPS OF THE COLON AND RECTUM

Polyp is a clinical term referring to a localized lesion protruding into the intestinal lumen. It is a description of the gross morphologic condition and not a histologic diagnosis. Histologically, benign adenomatous lesions of the colon can be divided into two main groups—adenomatous polyps and villous adenomas. Villous adenomas are much less frequent (making up approximately 3 per cent of all tumors in the colon but up to 15 per cent of all the tumors in the rectosigmoid region);[38] villous tumors are considered much more likely to be malignant and invasive, however.[40] The incidence of polyps in the colon increases with age. Blatt found that in a series of 446 colons examined in consecutive autopsies, 38.6 per cent of those cadavers of patients older than 30 had polyps.[5] Of these approximately half were less than 5 mm, 34 per cent were 6 to 10 mm, and 13 per cent were from 11 to 20 mm. Others have found the incidence in the asymptomatic population to vary from 5.4 to to 19 per cent.[13, 31] The frequency with which polyps are demonstrated by barium enema is directly proportional to the degree of the radiologist's interest and care. Ideally, the barium enema should be able to detect lesions in the 3- to 5-mm size range, since malignancy in polyps smaller than 5 mm is exceedingly rare and is uncommon in polyps in the 5-mm range. The use of the new sophisticated double-contrast barium enema has considerably increased the detection of very small polyps and other mucosal lesions.[14, 35] The endoscopist, of course, can detect still smaller lesions. In Blatt's series, no polyp smaller than 1.1 cm was malignant.[5] One must recognize, however, that it is almost impossible to determine accurately the benignancy or malignancy of a polypoid tumor based solely on its roentgen configuration (Fig. 13–114).

Marshak believes that one can make a good guess about histology on the basis of size, shape, the presence of a pedicle, and the presence of a contour defect of the bowel wall at the site of attachment of the polyp.[24] He thinks that circular lesions smaller than 1 cm are benign but that irregularly shaped lesions are suspicious for malignancy. Lesions on a pedicle may be watched if the head of the lesion measures less than 1.5 cm and repeat examinations are done at regular intervals for evidence of change in size or shortening of the pedicle, findings that suggest malignancy. An irregular bowel wall contour defect indicates malignancy regardless of polyp size. These lesions show evidence of bowel wall invasion and should not be removed by colonoscopy but rather by segmental bowel resection.

Almost all polypoid tumors 3 cm or larger are carcinomas.[1] Those between 2 and 3 cm are malignant in two thirds of cases. Probably the critical size for the removal of a polypoid lesion, in balancing the risk of morbidity of polypectomy by colotomy against the risk of carcinoma, is 1 cm. Colonoscopic polypectomy has become an accepted mode of treatment for polyps. It is Ottenjann's belief that polyps up to 2 cm can be removed with reasonable safety by this method.[30] Wolff and Shinya have removed polyps as large as 5 cm colonoscopically without significant complication except for one episode of bleeding requiring transfusion.[43] Other complications have been reported, however, and will be discussed later.

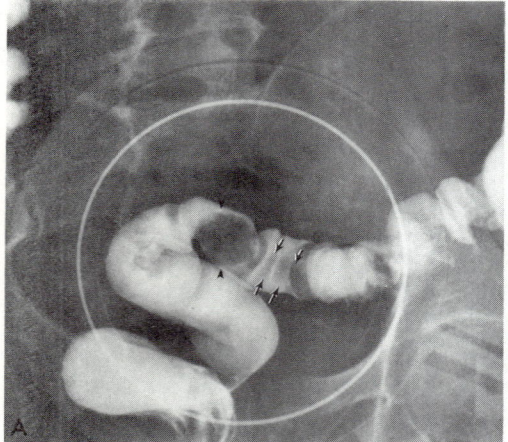 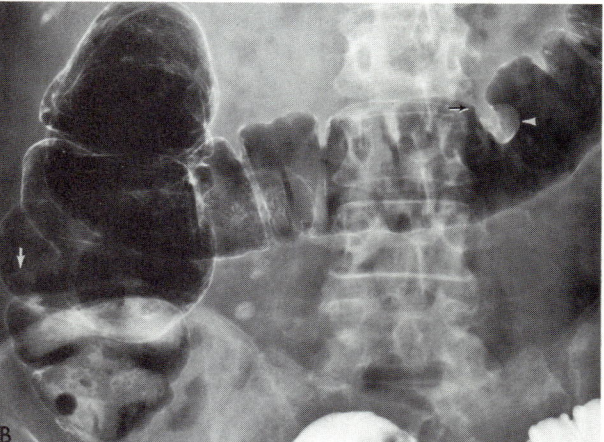

Figure 13–114. Multiple polyps, benign and malignant. *A*, Oblique film of the barium-filled sigmoid showing a 25-mm polyp (arrowheads) with a faintly discernible pedicle (arrows). *B*, Posteroanterior view of the colon after double-contrast enema showing a small barium-coated lesion on the lateral aspect of the cecum (white arrow), seen on multiple films, and a second lesion in the transverse colon (arrowhead) on a short pedicle (black arrow). All of these lesions were thought to represent benign polyps: the cecal lesion because of its small size and smooth appearance, the sigmoid lesion because of its long pedicle, and the transverse colon lesion because of its size and pedicle (even though the pedicle was a short one). Histologically, however, the transverse colon lesion was found to be carcinoma with malignant infiltration into the adjacent bowel wall but without lymph node involvement. (Courtesy of The American College of Radiology. *From* Stein, G. N., and Finkelstein, A. K.: Atlas of Tumor Radiology: The Duodenum, Small Intestine and Colon. Chicago, Year Book Medical Publishers, 1973. Reproduced by permission.)

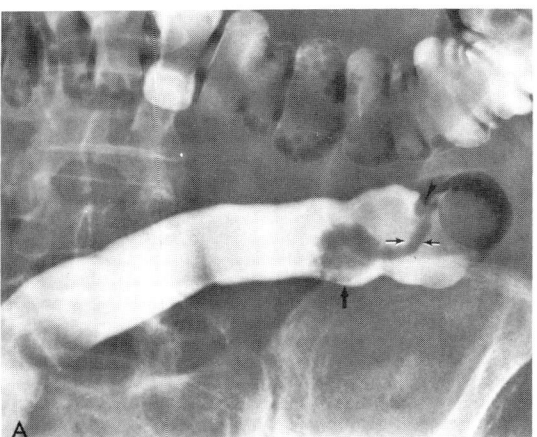 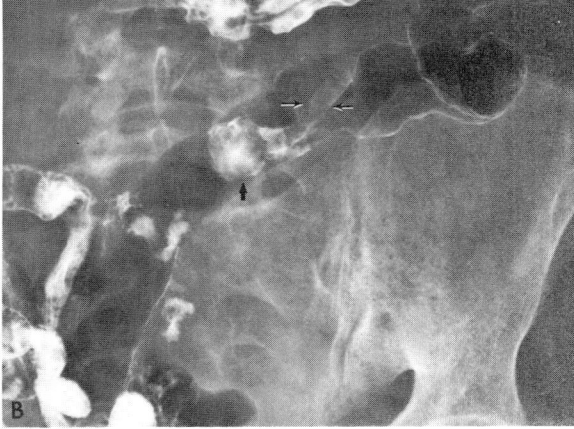

Figure 13–115. Pedunculated polyp. *A,* Double-contrast enema with barium in the sigmoid colon outlining a rounded radiolucent mass (large arrow). Note the long linear radiolucent stalk attaching it to the wall (small arrows) and the smooth indentation of the wall of the sigmoid at the site of attachment (arrowhead). *B,* Barium coating the polyp (large arrow) and stalk (small arrows), with air filling the sigmoid colon. (Courtesy of The American College of Radiology. *From* Stein, G. N., and Finkelstein, A. K.: Atlas of Tumor Radiology: The Duodenum, Small Intestine and Colon. Chicago, Year Book Medical Publishers, 1973. Reproduced by permission.)

According to some clinical reports, up to 75 per cent of all polyps are located in the rectosigmoid area.[30] Blatt's study reveals far different localization, with only 32 per cent in the sigmoid, 26.6 per cent in the cecum, and the rest fairly evenly distributed in the remainder of the colon.[5] This distribution varies somewhat from that of colonic cancers, which are more prevalent at both ends of the colon.[1] The incidence of colonic malignancy is much higher in those patients with multiple polyps than in those with one polyp (see Fig. 13–14).[6, 31] Multiple polyps are common, the reported incidence varying from 27 to 42 per cent.[5, 13, 19]

Grossly, polyps can be divided into several types: They can be either sessile or pedunculated. When pedunculated (Fig. 13–115), the stalk acts as a barrier between the carcinoma that may develop in the polyp and the adjacent normal bowel wall; the stalk must be involved in the malignant process for the tumor to be termed invasive. Histologically, 90 per cent of all colorectal polyps are benign adenomas.[16] Radiographically, these appear as flat radiolucent defects in the barium column if sessile (Fig. 13–116) and seen in profile, and as relatively round defects if shown *en face;* occasionally, a pedunculated polyp is seen *en face* and presents the "bull's eye" sign owing to barium coating the head and the stalk (Fig. 13–117).

Villous tumors make up 1 to 3 per cent of all colorectal polyps.[16, 42] Their surfaces are usually nodular and interspersed with deep clefts (Fig. 13–118). The vast majority occur in the rectum and sigmoid. Barium enema shows a polypoid lesion without evidence of infiltration of the wall or ulceration and with a characteristic surface appearance—described as variable collections of barium between the fronds of the tumor, giving the appearance of a fine-to-coarse network of barium streaks within the mass.[42] These lesions change shape and appearance with the filling and emptying of the colon. As in the case of polypoid tumors, one cannot tell which of these tumors is benign or malignant by radiographs alone (Figs. 13–119 and 13–120), although the majority are benign.

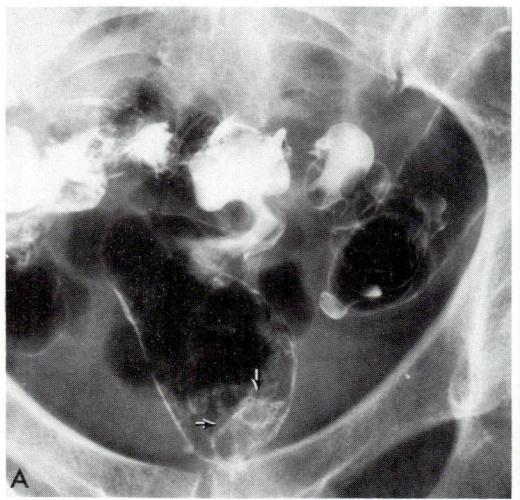
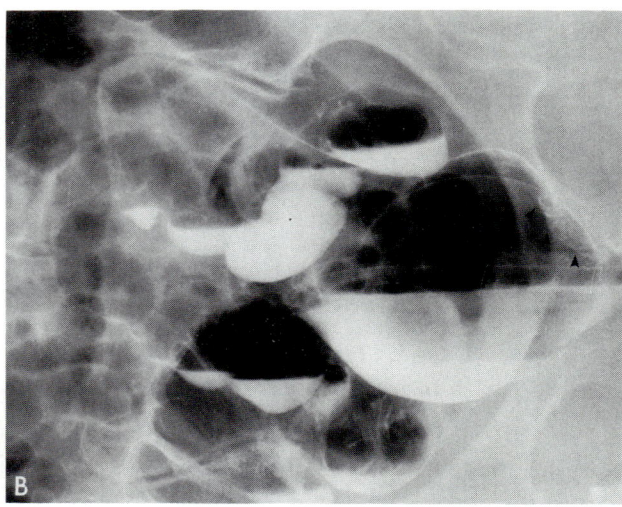
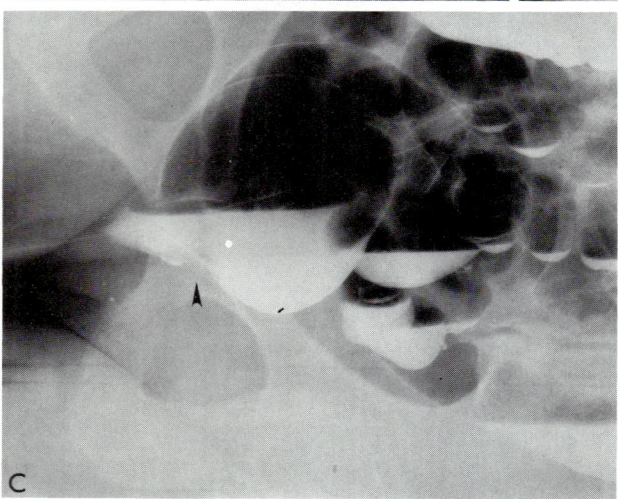

Figure 13–116. Sessile polyp of the rectum. *A*, Anteroposterior film of the rectosigmoid region from a double-contrast enema, showing a barium-coated flat irregular lesion on the left side of the rectum (arrows). Histologically, this was a benign adenomatous polyp. *B*, Decubitus film from a double-contrast enema with the right side down shows the lesion (arrowhead) coated with barium and surrounded by air. *C*, Decubitus film with the left side down shows the lesion as a filling defect surrounded by barium (arrowhead).

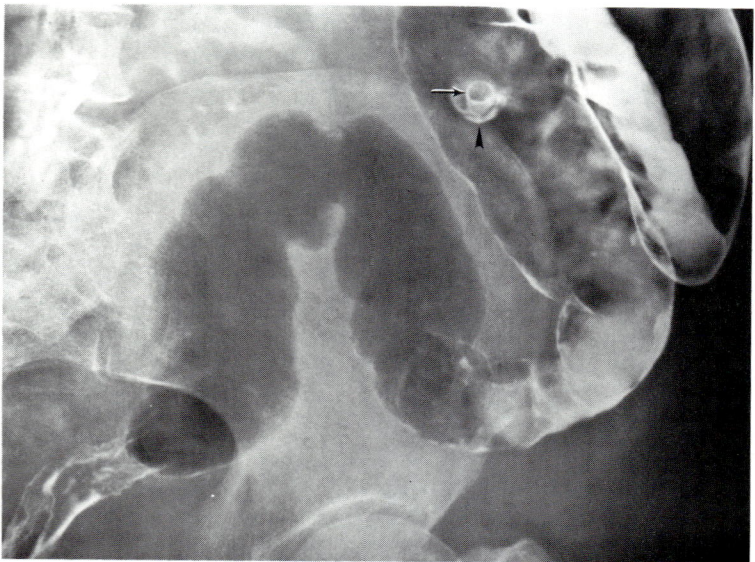

Figure 13–117. Pedunculated polyp. Left posterior oblique film from a double-contrast enema shows a barium covered filling defect in the sigmoid colon measuring 15 mm (arrowhead). Within its outlines and slightly off center there is a second ring of barium measuring 7 mm (arrow). The second smaller ring represents barium coating the pedicle of the polyp, while the larger coated structure is the head of the polyp. This picture, often seen when a pedunculated polyp is viewed on end, is referred to as the bull's eye sign. (Courtesy of The American College of Radiology. *From* Stein, G. N., and Finkelstein, A. K.: Atlas of Tumor Radiology: The Duodenum, Small Intestine and Colon. Chicago, Year Book Medical Publishers, 1973. Reproduced by permission.)

Figure 13–118. Benign villous tumor. Lateral view of the rectum from a double-contrast enema showing a barium-coated lesion with a slightly nodular surface (arrowheads) arising from the posterior rectal wall. Note the streaks of barium within the lesion representing barium trapped within the deep clefts of the lesion, a characteristic appearance of villous tumor. (Courtesy of The American College of Radiology. *From* Stein, G. N., and Finkelstein, A. K.: Atlas of Tumor Radiology: The Duodenum, Small Intestine and Colon. Chicago, Year Book Medical Publishers, 1973. Reproduced by permission.)

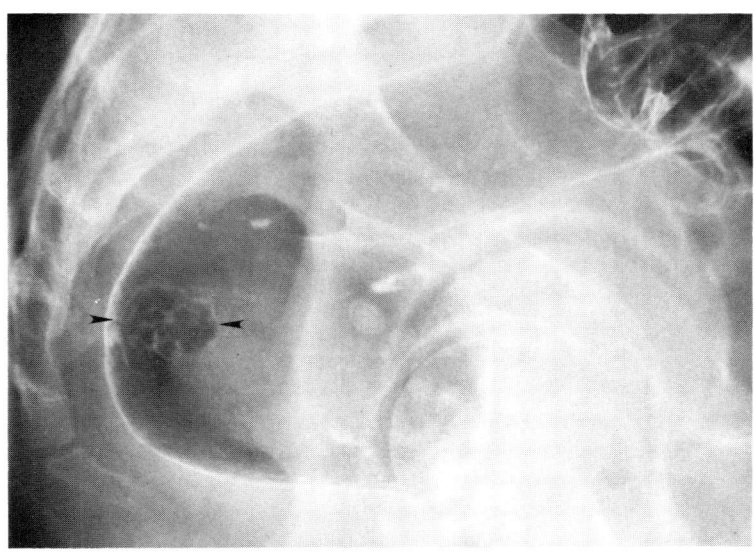

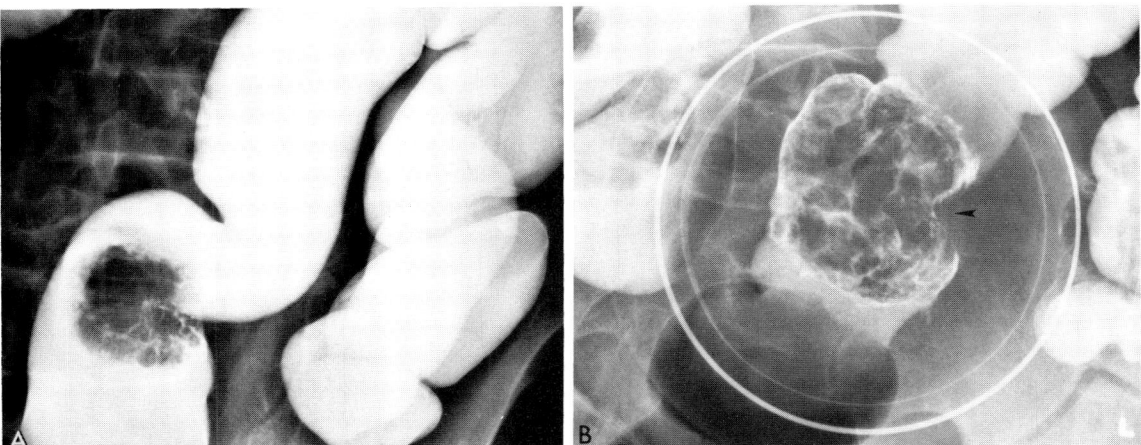

Figure 13–119. Malignant villous tumor. *A,* Posteroanterior film of the barium-filled sigmoid colon showing an irregularly rounded lesion measuring 4 cm in diameter. Its marginal outline is irregular, indicating its nodularity, and a lacy pattern is seen inferiorly on its surface, representing barium caught in surface crevices. *B,* Double-contrast film of the sigmoid region with compression showing better the lacy appearance of the tumor. Note also the indentation of the bowel wall at the site of attachment of the tumor (arrowhead), suggesting invasion of the bowel wall at this site. (Courtesy of The American College of Radiology. *From* Stein, G. N., and Finkelstein, A. K.: Atlas of Tumor Radiology: The Duodenum, Small Intestine and Colon. Chicago, Year Book Medical Publishers, 1973.)

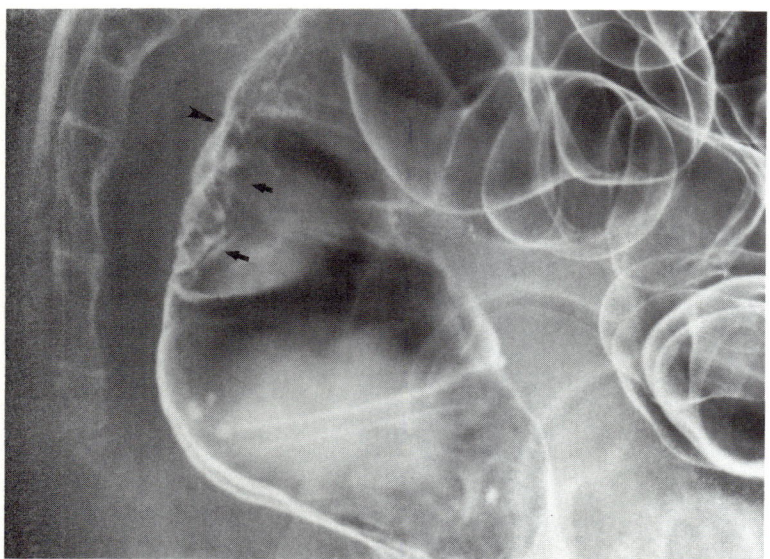

Figure 13–120. Malignant villous tumor. Double-contrast enema film of the rectum in the lateral projection shows an irregular flat lesion of the posterior rectal wall (arrows), again exhibiting a lacy surface appearance. There is some dimpling of the upper posterior rectal wall (arrowhead), suggesting malignancy. (Courtesy of The American College of Radiology. *From* Stein, G. N., and Finkelstein, A. K.: Atlas of Tumor Radiology: The Duodenum, Small Intestine and Colon. Chicago, Year Book Medical Publishers, 1973. Reproduced by permission.)

Another group are the benign adenomas containing invasive carcinoma. Enterline and his associates believe these occur in up to 3 per cent of all adenomatous polyps, whereas others believe that these lesions represent carcinoma that arises from normal colonic mucosa that happens to cover a benign polyp.[14, 37] The larger the polyp, the more likely it is to be malignant (Fig. 13–121).

Finally, there are small carcinomas that radiographically resemble or mimic polyps but histologically contain no benign component. Investigators have noted an increased incidence of carcinoma in the colons of patients who have or have had polyps (Figs. 13–122 and 13–123). Some claim that carcinoma arises directly from adenomatous polyps, although others disclaim this. In truth, there is little conclusive evidence to support the theory of direct origin of carcinoma from adenomatous polyps.[1, 37] There is strong evidence that this occurs in villous tumors, however (Fig. 13–124); these make up approximately 3 per cent of all colonic polyps and exhibit invasive carcinoma in from 8 to 30 per cent of cases.[20, 43]

What is the treatment of a polyp? Before colonoscopic polypectomy came into use, treatment depended upon the physician's opinion about the risk of malignancy versus the risk of surgical removal of the polyp. It was believed that polyps larger than 1 cm should be removed if clinically feasible. Those smaller than 1 cm could be examined with reasonable safety at six month intervals for a time, to determine if any growth occurred (see Fig. 13–121), and if a doubling time of 6 to 12 months was noted, malignancy would be strongly suspected. No growth over several years indicated probable benignancy. Of course, the complications of colotomy are well known, the major ones being an anastomotic leak and infection (Figs. 13–125 to 13–127). With the advent of colonoscopic polypectomy, lesions that previously would have been watched or resected by colotomy are now being removed via the colonoscope. Williams performs colonoscopy on patients with polyps measuring 6 to 7 mm that have been demonstrated by barium enema.[41] Colonoscopy is performed because of the potential for growth of the polyp and the possibility of finding other adenomas that had not been identified by barium enema. All visualized polyps are removed. The follow-up consists of annual sigmoidoscopy and clinical examination, an air-contrast barium enema being per-

Text continued on page 761

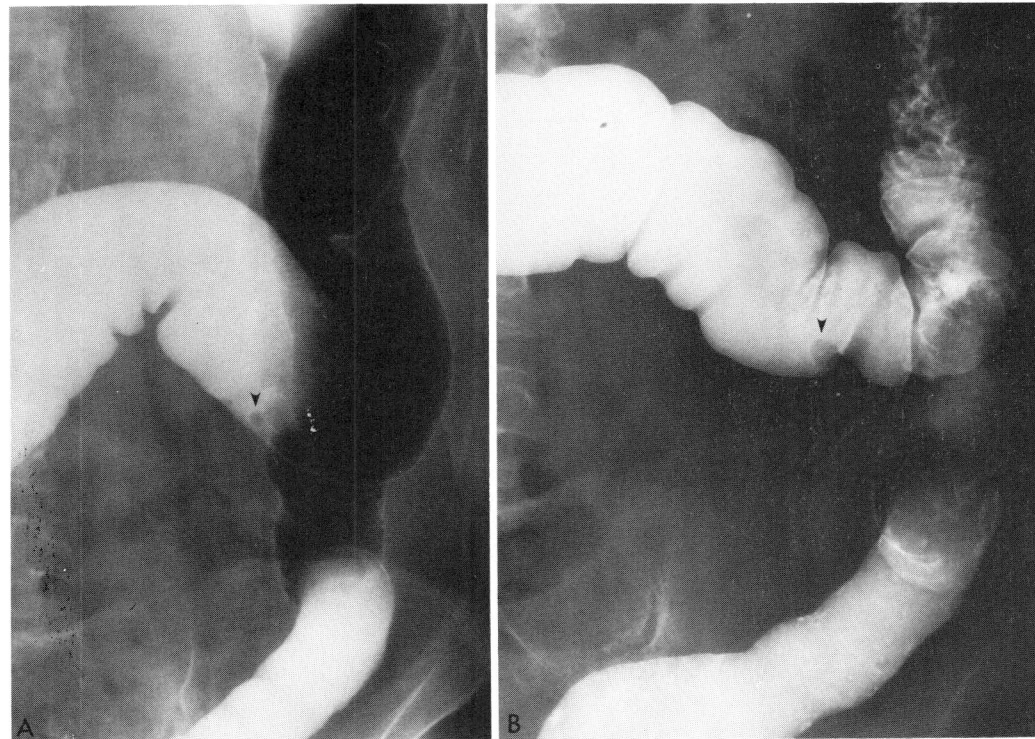

Figure 13–121. Enlarging adenomatous polyp. *A*, Film from a double-contrast enema of the distal transverse and descending colon showing a small round lucency (arrowhead) near the inferior aspect of the distal transverse colon. *B*, Frontal view of the distal transverse and descending colon from a double-contrast enema performed four years after the original study reveals a significant increase in the size of the lesion in the distal transverse colon (arrowhead). The lesion is now more than three times larger than on the previous study. Histologically, this is a benign adenoma. Although the change in size was worrisome, the long interval required for this change in size indicates that the lesion is very slow growing.

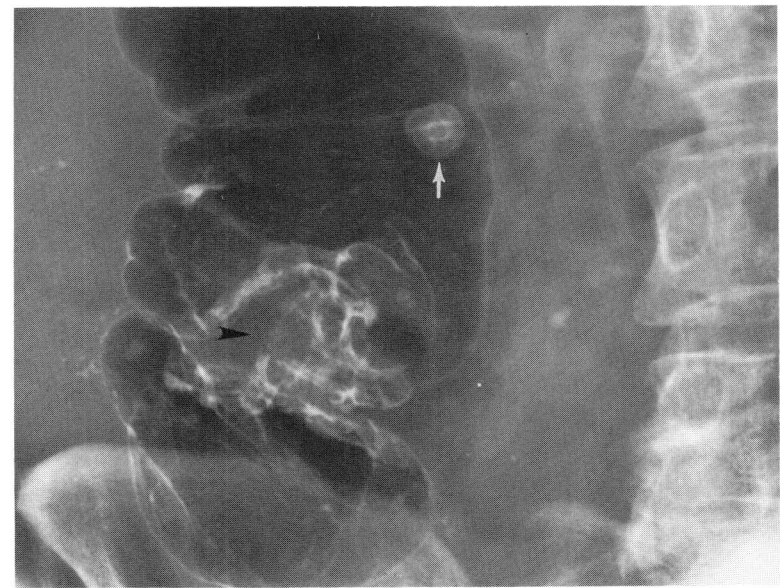

Figure 13–122. Carcinoma of the cecum adjacent to a benign pedunculated polyp. Posteroanterior view of the ascending colon from a double-contrast enema: Note the annular constricting lesion of the cecum (arrowhead) with overhanging edges and mucosal destruction, typical of carcinoma. A barium-coated lucency in the ascending colon measuring 12 mm (arrow) is seen near the carcinoma. This lesion exhibits the "bull's eye" sign, indicating that is is a pedunculated polyp. (Courtesy of The American College of Radiology. *From* Stein, G. N., and Finkelstein, A. K.: Atlas of Tumor Radiology: The Duodenum, Small Intestine and Colon. Chicago, Year Book Medical Publishers, 1973. Reproduced by permission.)

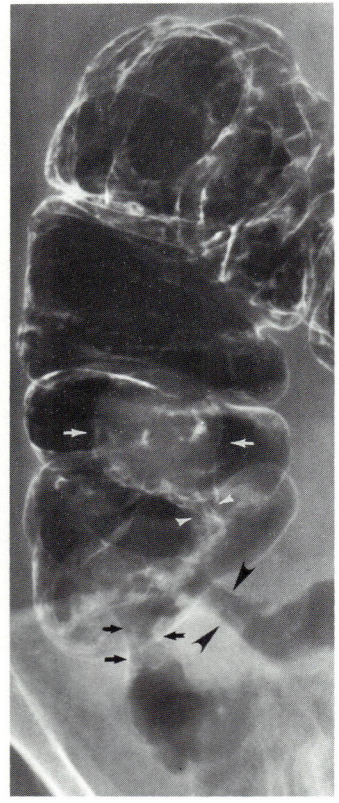

Figure 13–123. Cecal carcinoma with adjacent adenomatous polyp. A posteroanterior view of the ascending colon from a double-contrast enema: Note the smooth, round 3.5 cm barium-coated soft tissue density (white arrows) within the proximal ascending colon, attached by a short pedicle (white arrowheads). Note the air-filled terminal ileum (black arrowheads) and also the marked distortion and narrowing of the cecum below the ileocecal junction (black arrows) secondary to an infiltrating carcinoma. Histologically, the polyp was found to be benign in spite of its size. (Courtesy of The American College of Radiology. *From* Stein, G. N., and Finkelstein, A. K.: Atlas of Tumor Radiology: The Duodenum, Small Intestine and Colon. Chicago, Year Book Medical Publishers, 1973. Reproduced by permission.)

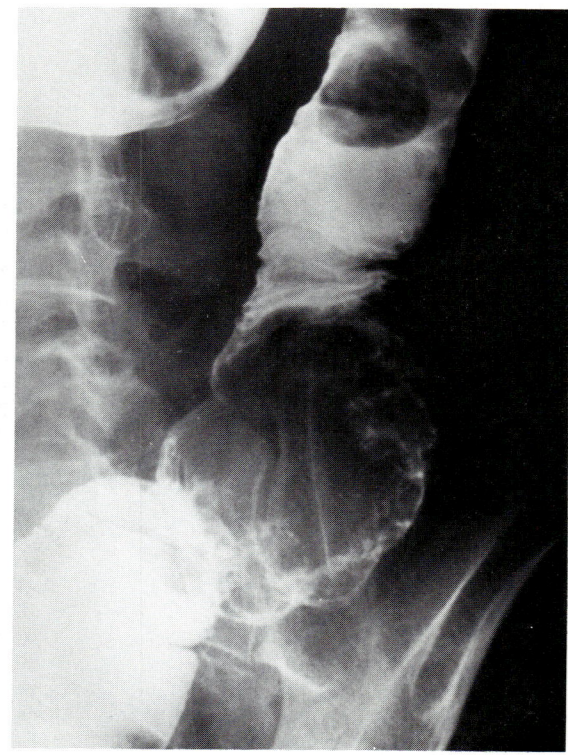

Figure 13–124. Villous adenocarcinoma. Barium-filled sigmoid colon showing a large intraluminal tumor that exhibits a lacy architecture in its periphery. The lesion is expanding the bowel lumen but shows no signs of wall invasion. Only its size speaks for malignancy. The multiple filling defects proximal and distal to the lesion represent residue.

THE LARGE BOWEL — 759

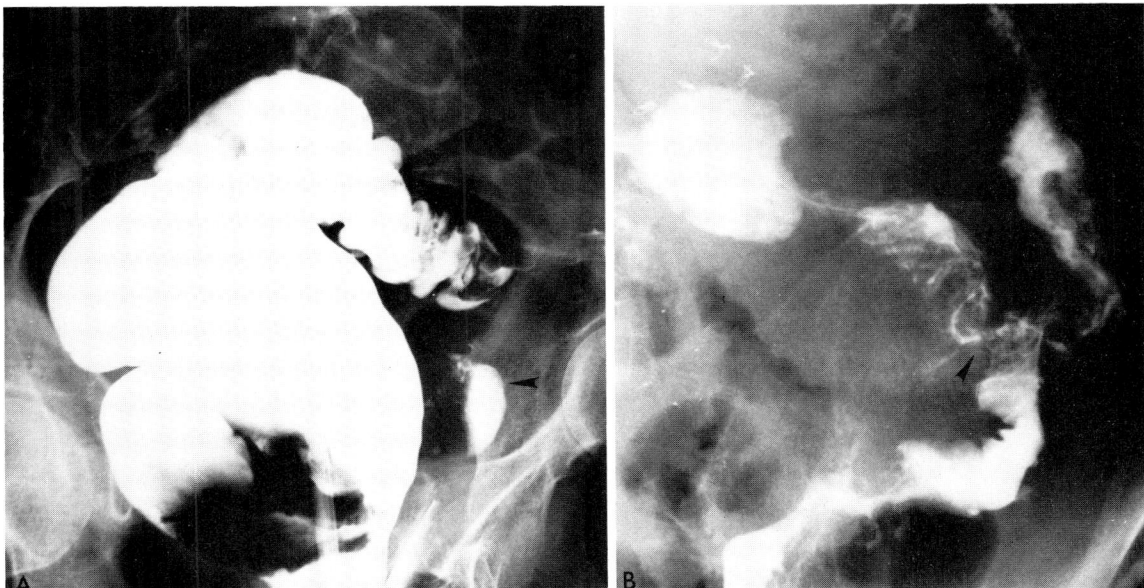

Figure 13–125. Postoperative fistulas. *A,* Oblique film of the barium-filled sigmoid colon showing a fistulous tract from the sigmoid colon into a confined pelvic abscess (arrowhead). *B,* Anteroposterior film of the barium-filled descending colon reveals a fistula (arrowhead) between the colon and the small intestine. (*A,* Courtesy of the Philadelphia General Hospital and the Mutter Museum of the Philadelphia College of Physicians.)

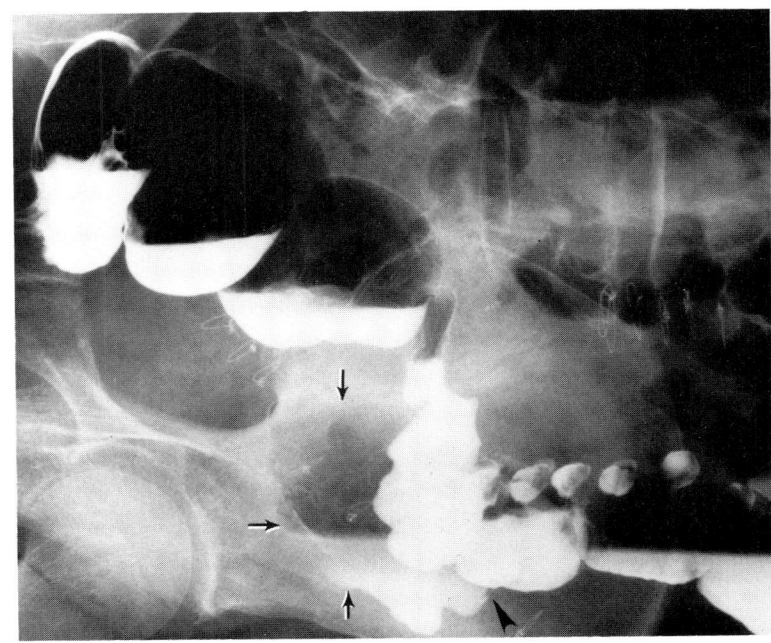

Figure 13–126. Postoperative abscess and fistula. Left-side-down decubitus film of the double-contrast enema following segmental colonic resection shows extraluminal barium adjacent to the descending colon. The barium is located in a paracolic abscess (arrows) that is communicating with the bowel by a fistulous tract (arrowhead).

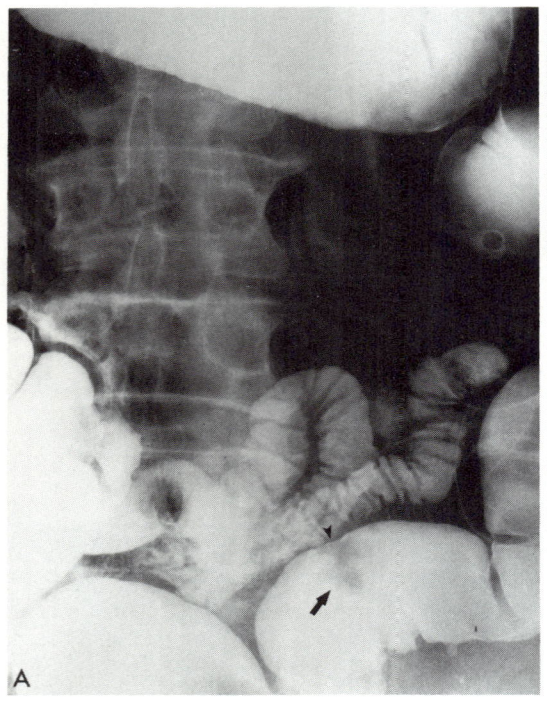
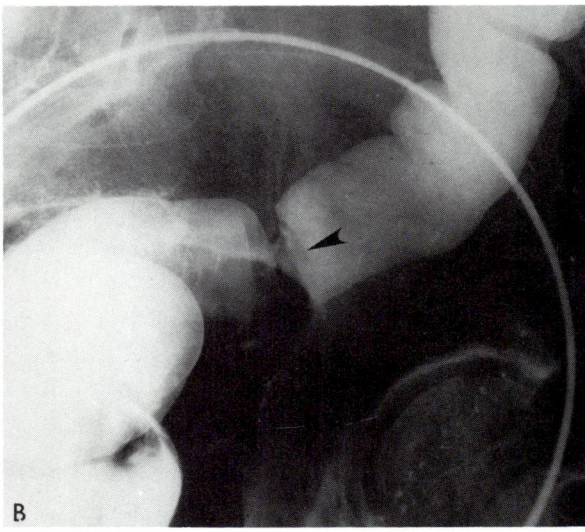

Figure 13–127. Postoperative anastomotic stricture. *A*, Anteroposterior barium-filled film of the sigmoid colon reveals an irregularly shaped filling defect (arrow) in the barium column, associated with some dimpling of the bowel wall at the sight of attachment (arrowhead). This was resected and found to be a sessile adenocarcinoma. *B*, Oblique film of the barium-filled sigmoid colon 16 months later shows no evidence of tumor recurrence, but there is a stricture (arrowhead) at the site of the anastomosis.

formed every three to five years for the detection of new polyps. Some authors recommend local bowel resection following colonoscopic removal of a polyp with malignant change.[22] Williams thinks this is not necessary if the carcinoma is of a low or average grade of malignancy; this opinion is based on the work of Carden and Morsen.[7]

Potential complications of colonoscopic polypectomy include bleeding and perforation.[4] Berci et al., in a series of 3850 colonoscopies and 901 polypectomies, reported a total perforation rate of 0.25 per cent. Seven of ten were thought to be related to the manipulation of the instrument rather than to the polypectomy. Cauterization of a polyp at its base or pedicle may result in coagulation necrosis of the colonic wall and produce perforation. The bleeding rate was 0.82 per cent, and the morbidity rate was 0.43 per cent. These results compare favorably with the reported morbidity rate of 20 per cent after laparotomy, colotomy, and polypectomy.[23] Mural perforation may cause an abscess (see Fig. 13–126); other complications have been reported less frequently. According to Meyers, clinical signs of perforation may be immediate or delayed, and the x-ray examination may be crucial for the diagnosis.[26] The presence of intra- or extraperitoneal air or both and the location of the air can help in localizing the site of perforation. Free perforation is about four times more common than a confined perforation.[9] Extraperitoneal rupture usually follows a more benign course than intraperitoneal rupture, and may not be discovered for several days. Meyers recommends routine abdominal films for the detection of possible perforation after all diagnostic and therapeutic colonoscopies. If perforation does occur, considerable free air is seen because the colon is usually distended with air for easier passage of the colonoscope. Meyers' study details where free air may be present following the perforation and how this free air aids in localizing the site of perforation. Free intraperitoneal air is indicated on a supine film by visualization of the falciform ligament, demonstration of both sides of the bowel wall, and increased radiolucency in the abdomen. Since most procedures are performed on the left side of the colon, free intraperitoneal air usually indicates a perforation in the region of the sigmoid colon or at the site of an anterior polypectomy. Extraperitoneal air most commonly arises from a perforation of the rectum or the posterior wall of the descending colon. Acute diverticular perforation usually gives rise to extraperitoneal air because most diverticula—75 per cent according to a study by Meyers[26]—face the extraperitoneal tissues. These perforations only occasionally give rise to intraperitoneal air. Perforation of the sigmoid or transverse colon into the mesentery also results in extraperitoneal gas. Anatomic studies have shown the extraperitoneal space to be divided into three compartments by fascial planes: anterior pararenal, perirenal, and posterior pararenal spaces.

Meyers and Ghahremani state that rectal perforation is indicated by gas ascending the posterior pararenal spaces bilaterally, with lucent areas paralleling the lateral borders of the psoas muscles; superiorly it sometimes extends as high as the upper renal pole and adrenal gland, the medial border of the spleen and liver, the medial crus of the diaphragm, and the immediate subphrenic tissues. Extension into the flank fat stripes, anterior abdominal walls, scrotum, and mediastinum may occur. Extraperitoneal (posterior) perforation of the sigmoid, descending, or ascending colon results in a unilateral collection of gas within the anterior pararenal space, shown by a collection of mottled lucent areas with a generally vertical axis. These characteristics extend medially over the psoas muscle to approach the spine, but do not usually infiltrate the flank stripe. Perforation of the sigmoid colon at a site between the leaves of the mesacolon may give rise to extraperitoneal gas within the anterior pararenal space bilaterally. Both intra- and extraperitoneal gas may be seen depending upon the site and size of the colonic perforation (Fig. 13–128).[25]

These patterns of gas distribution are extremely helpful in determining the site of perforation, since this may not always be demonstrated on emergency water-soluble contrast enema.

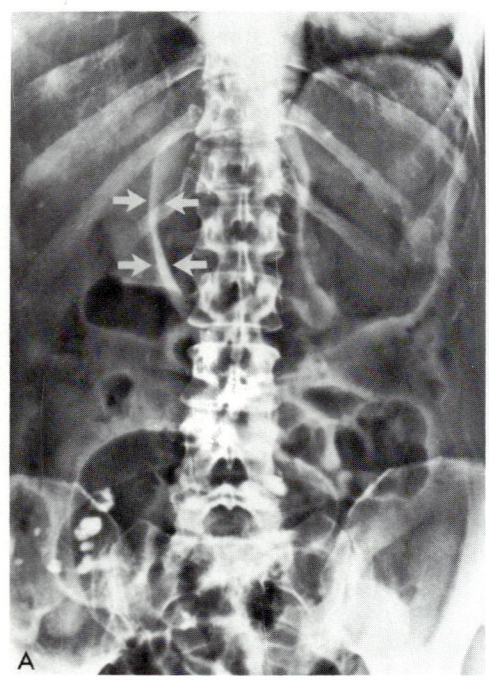
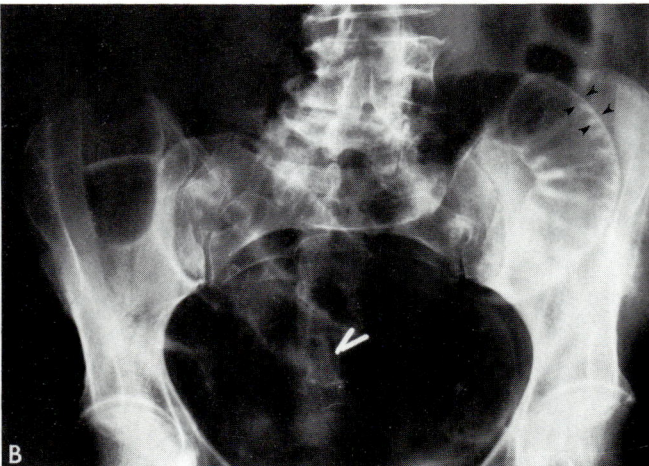

Figure 13–128. Endoscopic perforation: two cases. *A* and *B*, Sigmoid perforation. *A*, Gross free intraperitoneal air outlining the falciform ligament (arrows). *B*, Free intraperitoneal air allowing visualization of both sides of the bowel wall (arrowheads).

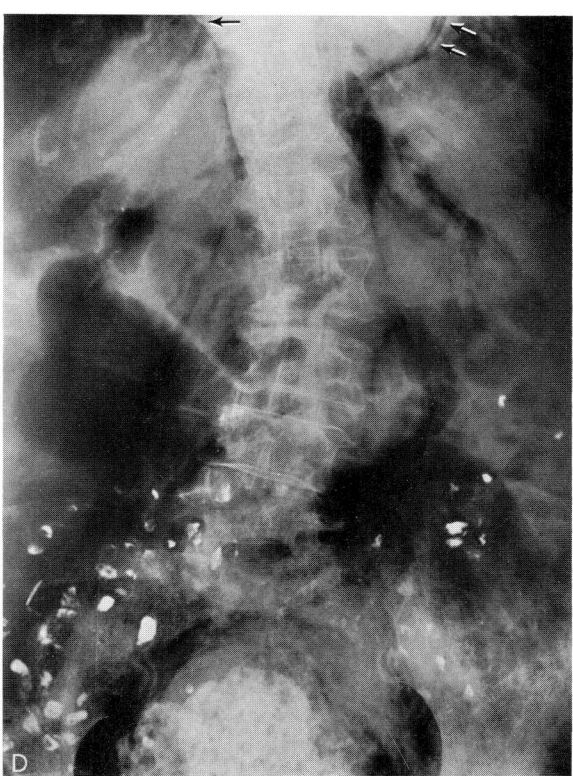

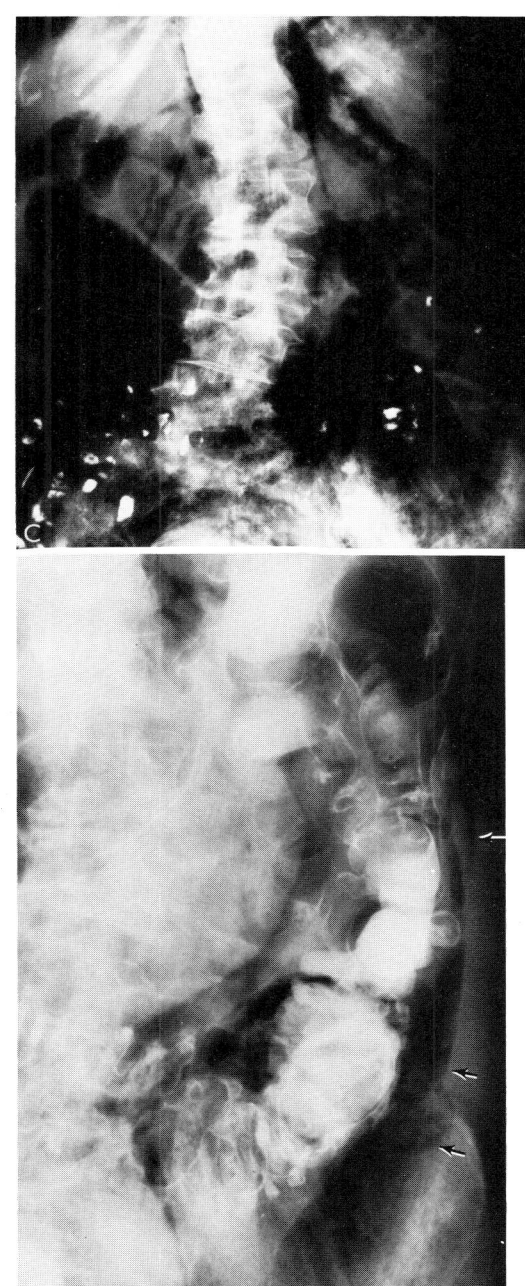

Figure 13–128 *Continued.* C to E, Rectal perforation. C, Supine film of the abdomen showing extraperitoneal free air in the pararenal areas and outlining the lateral margins of both psoas muscles. The upper poles of the kidneys, medial border of the spleen, and immediate subphrenic tissues are also seen. *D,* Note the extension of the air from the abdomen into the pericardial sac (arrows). *E,* Supine film of the left colon from a double-contrast enema showing free extraperitoneal air in the paracolic region (arrows) but no evidence of contrast extravasation. (*A* and *B* from Meyers, M. A., and Ghahremani, G. G.: Colon complications of fiberoptic endoscopy. II. Colonoscopy. Radiology *115:*301–307, 1975. Reproduced by permission.)

Juvenile Polyps

Juvenile gastrointestinal polyposis syndromes comprise a group of conditions varying from single or multiple polyps in the colon to multiple lesions throughout the entire gastrointestinal tract. Although this type of polyp is occasionally seen in adults, it is most frequent in children and adolescents. The generalized form is believed to be familial, with a dominant genotype and a variable age-dependent expression.[32] Interestingly, in succeeding generations, this disorder is seen to manifest itself at earlier ages. Grossly, the polyps appear smooth and round; histologically, they exhibit an epithelial component surrounded by abundant connective tissue stroma that often displays a primitive mesenchymal appearance.[28] The epithelial element is arranged in tubules associated with possible overproduction or retention of mucus in cystic spaces. Surface epithelial cells may be absent in these polyps, especially those arising in the rectum, owing to infection or ulceration. These polyps are also called retention or inflammatory polyps.

Most of these polyps, approximately 75 per cent, develop as isolated colonic lesions in childhood. Even when multiple, there are rarely more than several.[33] They may be present at birth or become evident later. These polyps may produce acute or chronic blood loss from the gastrointestinal tract or recurrent bouts of intussusception. Rarer

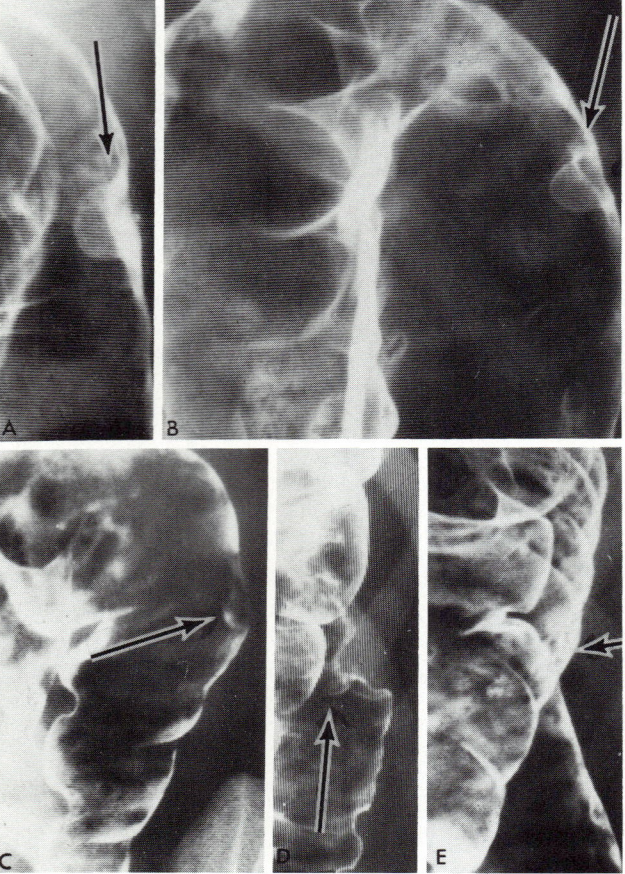

Figure 13–129. Regression in size of a polyp in a five-year-old child from 9 mm to 4 mm during a four and a half year period. *A*, December 21, 1953. *B*, August 8, 1955. *C*, January 31, 1956. *D*, August 16, 1957. *E*, February 10, 1958. (*From* Welin, S., Youker, J., and Spratt, J. S.: The rates and patterns of growth of 375 tumors of the large intestine and rectum observed serially by double contrast enema study (Malmö technique). Am. J. Roentgenol. 90:673–678, 1963. Reproduced by permission.)

symptoms include abdominal pain and diarrhea. Barium enema examination demonstrates round, pedunculated polyps or radiolucent defects, seen most commonly in the rectum or sigmoid colon. Because the lesions are totally benign and have a tendency toward regression or autoamputation (Fig. 13–129), operative treatment should be reserved for those cases in which serious symptoms are present. When surgery is required, treatment should be conservative in order to preserve maximal gastrointestinal surface area and function.

Hyperplastic Polyps

These are small, sessile, smooth-surfaced, and usually multiple mucosal excrescences. Most are smaller than 5 mm, and they rarely exceed 1 cm. They probably result from a non-neoplastic proliferation of the upper crypt and surface epithelial cells of the colon.[18] These lesions are common, with reported incidences of from 25 to 80 per cent of all people.[2, 3, 28, 29] They are not premalignant and have no proven relationship to adenomatous polyps. This is not meant to imply that all small polyps in this size range are hyperplastic polyps, however. Minute true adenomatous polyps do occur and make up approximately 10 per cent of all small polyps in the size range of 3 to 5 mm.[18] The remaining 90 per cent are hyperplastic polyps. The uniform structure, small size, and common occurrence of these polyps in all adult age groups indicate that they are limited in growth potential. Some may actually undergo spontaneous regression.[3] They are usually asymptomatic and discovered on routine examinations of the colon.

FAMILIAL POLYPOSIS

Familial polyposis is an uncommon entity in which there is a pathologic proliferation of epithelial lining cells resulting in the formation of colonic polyps. These may be villous, sessile, or pedunculated and often cover the entire colon from the ileocecal valve to the anus. The rectum and the left colon are more frequently involved (Figs. 13–130 and 13–131), and involvement of the stomach and small bowel occurs in less than 5 per cent of all cases.[44] The disease is transmitted as a mendelian dominant trait without regard to sex and with a high penetrance. Generally the polyps become clinically apparent at approximately age 20. Malignant changes develop about 15 years later, and unless treated the patients die from cancer in their early forties. Clinically, symptoms usually occur in the third and fourth decades of life, the average age at the onset of symptoms being approximately 30. Since a high percentage of asymptomatic patients already have a carcinoma at the time of the first barium enema and others acquire malignancy within two years of discovery of this syndrome,[39] polyps should be looked for in relatives of those known to have the disease; annual barium enema and colonoscopic examinations should be performed on patients older than 20 even before symptoms become apparent. Multiple carcinomas also occur.

The most common presenting symptom is rectal bleeding, occurring in more than 75 per cent of the patients. It may be severe enough to cause anemia. Diarrhea is noted in over 50 per cent of patients, and other symptoms occur less frequently. Since colon carcinoma invariably develops in these patients, the need for early diagnosis is extremely important. With total colectomy the threat of carcinoma is removed. Debate persists, however, regarding whether total colectomy and ileostomy should be performed. Moertel believes that the rectum should be removed in those patients with multiple polyps in the rectum at the time of surgery, because of the high incidence of

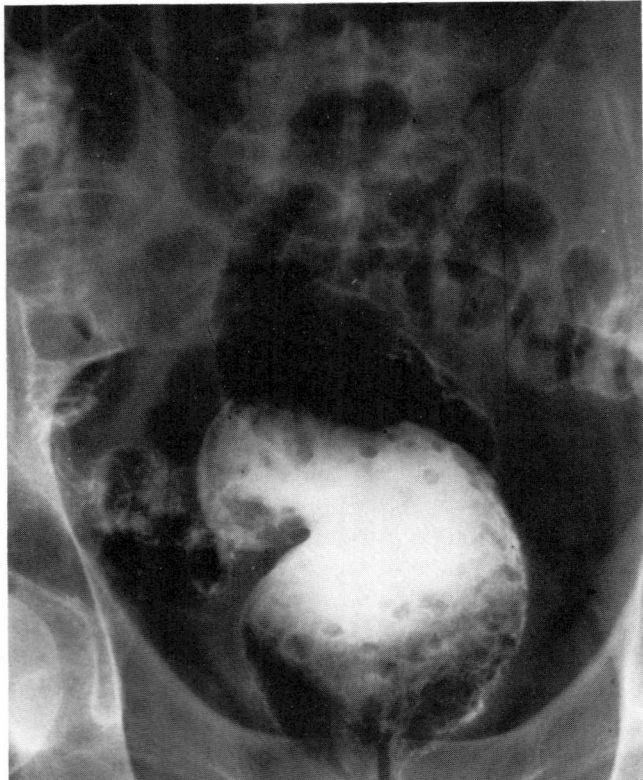

Figure 13–130. Familial polyposis. Anteroposterior film of the barium-filled rectum showing multiple small filling defects representing polyps. (Courtesy of The Philadelphia General Hospital and the Mutter Museum of the Philadelphia College of Physicians.)

Figure 13–131. Familial polyposis. Posteranterior view of a barium-filled colon showing multiple filling defects throughout the colon but especially on the left side. These defects are multiple polyps. (Courtesy of the Philadelphia General Hospital and the Mutter Museum of the Philadelphia College of Physicians.)

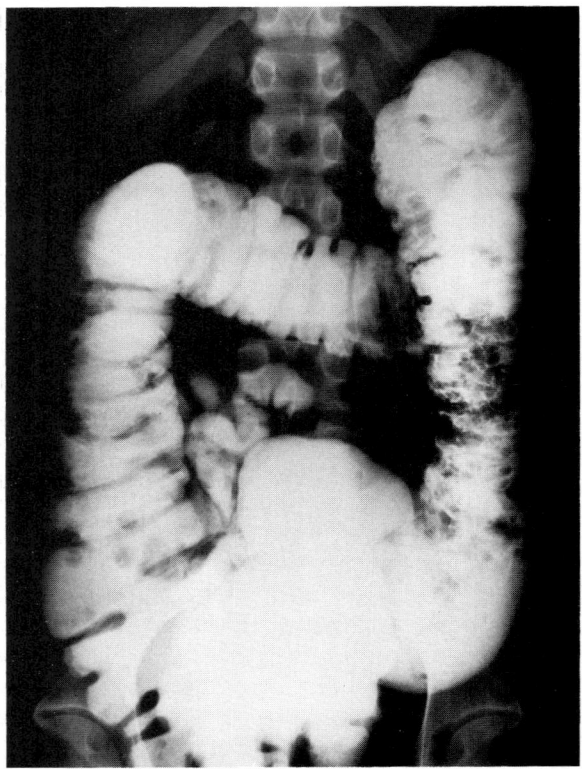

rectal carcinoma despite adequate follow-up.[27] Others think that in reliable patients the rectum can be retained if there are frequent proctosigmoidoscopic examinations. Some believe that polyps in the retained rectum may actually decrease in size following ileorectal anastomosis, but the mechanism for this is not fully understood.[10, 21] If polyps are noted on follow-up, they can be excised or fulgurated. With fulguration there is the risk of rectal stricture and perforation.

Differential diagnosis of familial polyposis includes nonfamilial multiple polyps, pseudopolyposis in ulcerative colitis, juvenile polyposis, Peutz-Jeghers syndrome, Gardner's syndrome, and Cronkhite-Canada syndrome. Juvenile polyposis and Gardner's syndrome have been discussed previously (see p. 748 and p. 764). Nonfamilial multiple polyps (Figs. 13–132 and 13–133) appear later in life than the familial type; these polyps are fewer in number and tend to be located in the rectum and sigmoid. With this type there is no family history of polyposis.

Pseudopolyposis (Figs. 13–134 and 13–135) seen in chronic inflammatory diseases of the colon, such as ulcerative colitis, may also look similar; these lesions represent inflammatory masses made up of hyperplastic mucosal remnants. Other roentgen changes of ulcerative colitis are usually evident, including absence or irregularity of the haustral markings, luminal narrowing, shortening of the colon, and mucosal ulceration, which should distinguish this from familial polyposis. It must be stressed, however, that differential diagnosis on the basis of the appearance of the polyps alone is impossible.

Peutz-Jeghers syndrome (Figs. 13–136 and 13–137) rarely offers a problem, since the polyps, which are really hamartomas, involve the small bowel in 95 per cent of these patients. These lesions are benign and have no malignant potential. The colonic lesions may be difficult to distinguish from adenomatous polyps,[28] since they are also proliferative mucosal lesions. There is colorectal involvement in approximately 30 per

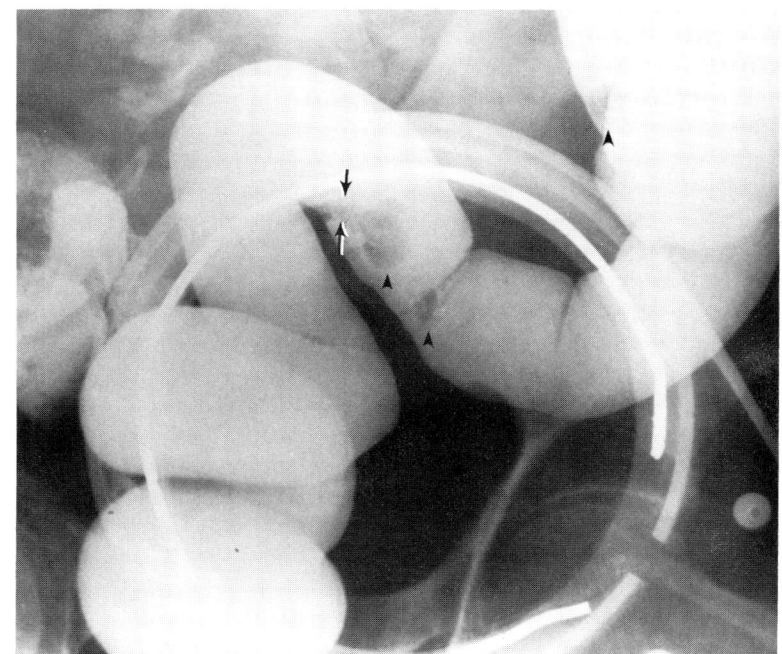

Figure 13–132. Nonfamilial multiple polyps. Oblique film of the barium-filled rectosigmoid with compression, showing three round smooth filling defects in the barium column (arrowheads). The largest lesion is attached by a stalk (arrows). The remaining results of the barium enema was negative; there was no family history of polyps.

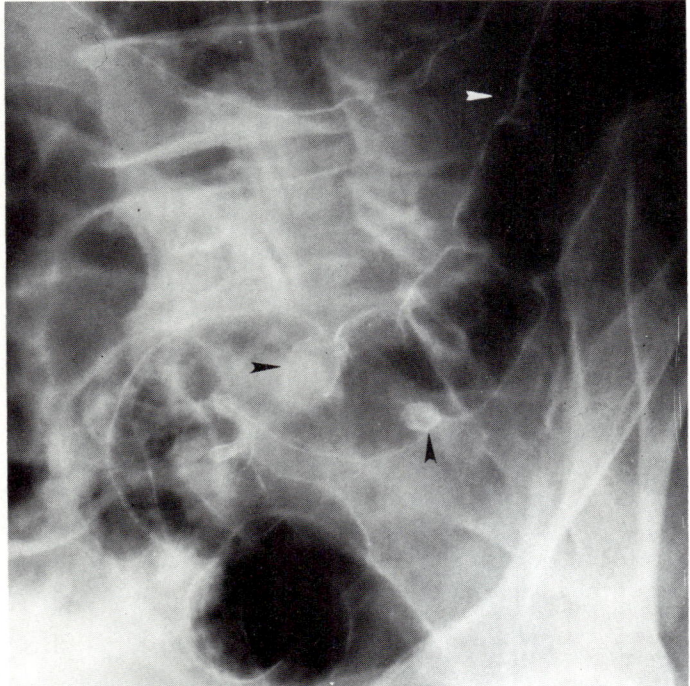

Figure 13–133. Nonfamilial multiple polyps. Oblique film of the sigmoid colon from a double-contrast enema showing defects on the left side of the colon (arrowheads). There was no family history of colonic polyps.

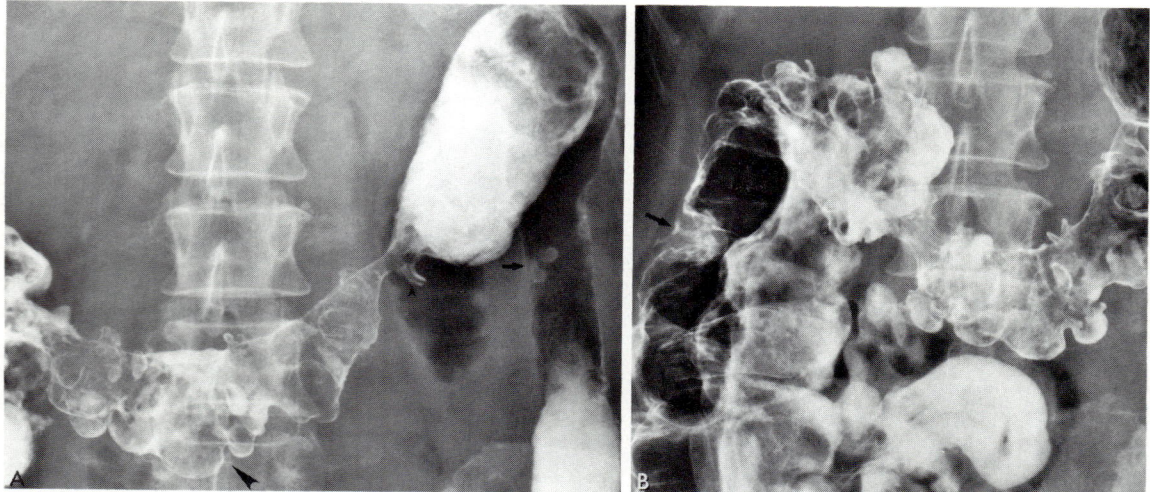

Figure 13–134. Inflammatory polyps in granulomatous colitis. *A,* Posteranterior view of the transverse and descending colon from a double-contrast enema. Note the generalized loss of haustrations and the peculiar sacculations (large arrowhead) on the inferior aspect of the transverse colon. A small projection of barium on the inferior aspect of the transverse colon (small arrowhead) represents a fistula. Several small barium-coated lucencies in the descending colon are pseudopolyps (arrow). *B,* Posteroanterior view of the right colon from a double-contrast enema shows a 2-cm sessile polyp (arrow) with ulceration arising from the ascending colon. The previously described changes in the transverse colon are again seen. Histologically, the large polyp is a benign inflammatory polyp. (Courtesy of The American College of Radiology. *From* Stein, G. N., and Finkelstein, A. K.: Atlas of Tumor Radiology: The Duodenum, Small Intestine and Colon. Chicago, Year Book Medical Publishers, 1973. Reproduced by permission.)

Figure 13–135. Diffuse inflammatory polyposis and chronic ulcerative colitis. Posteroanterior view of the colon from a double-contrast enema showing slight narrowing of the colon with areas of mild marginal fuzziness secondary to ulcerative colitis. Note the multiple small barium-coated filling defects throughout the colon secondary to inflammatory polyps. The small collections of barium in the rectum represent acute ulcerations, indicating reactivation of the disease (arrowheads). These polyps are readily differentiated from familial polyposis by the other changes of ulcerative colitis seen in this patient. (Courtesy of The American College of Radiology. *From* Stein, G. N., and Finkelstein, A. K.: Atlas of Tumor Radiology: The Duodenum, Small Intestine and Colon. Chicago, Year Book Medical Publishers, 1973. Reproduced by permission.)

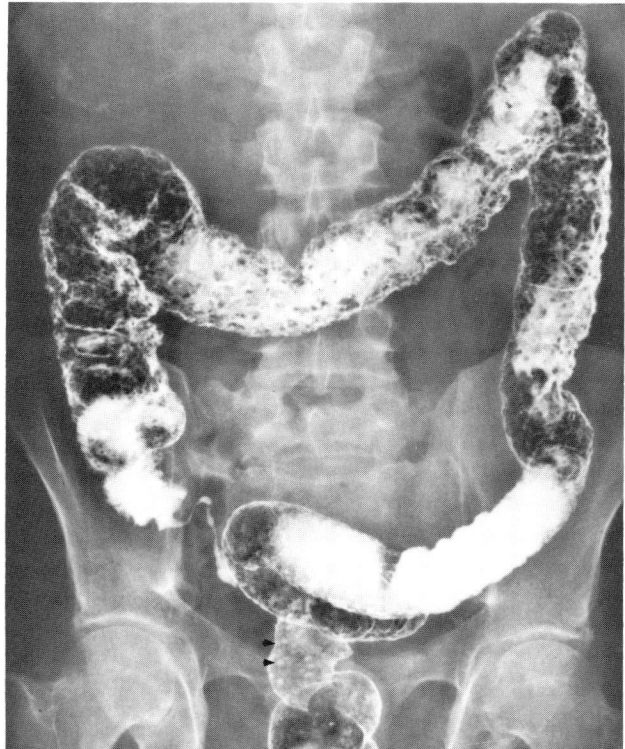

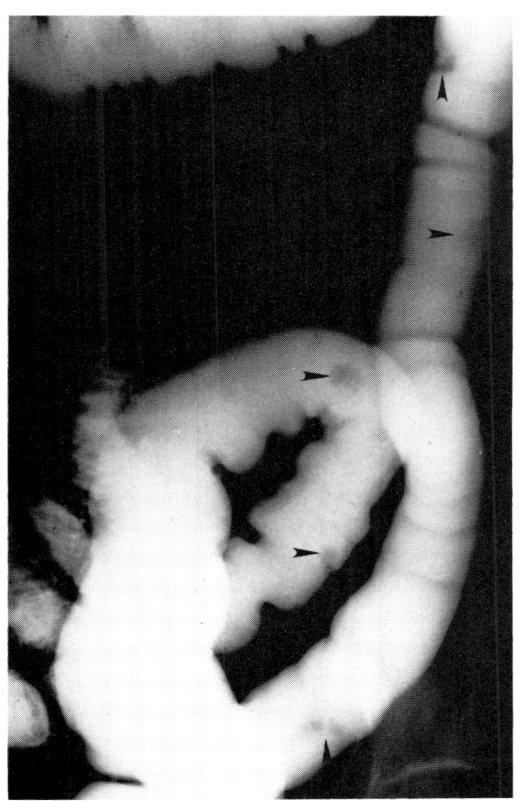

Figure 13–136. Peutz-Jeghers syndrome. Posteroanterior film of the barium-filled left colon demonstrates several small sessile filling defects (arrowheads) in the barium column. (Courtesy of The Philadelphia General Hospital and the Mutter Museum of the Philadelphia College of Physicians.)

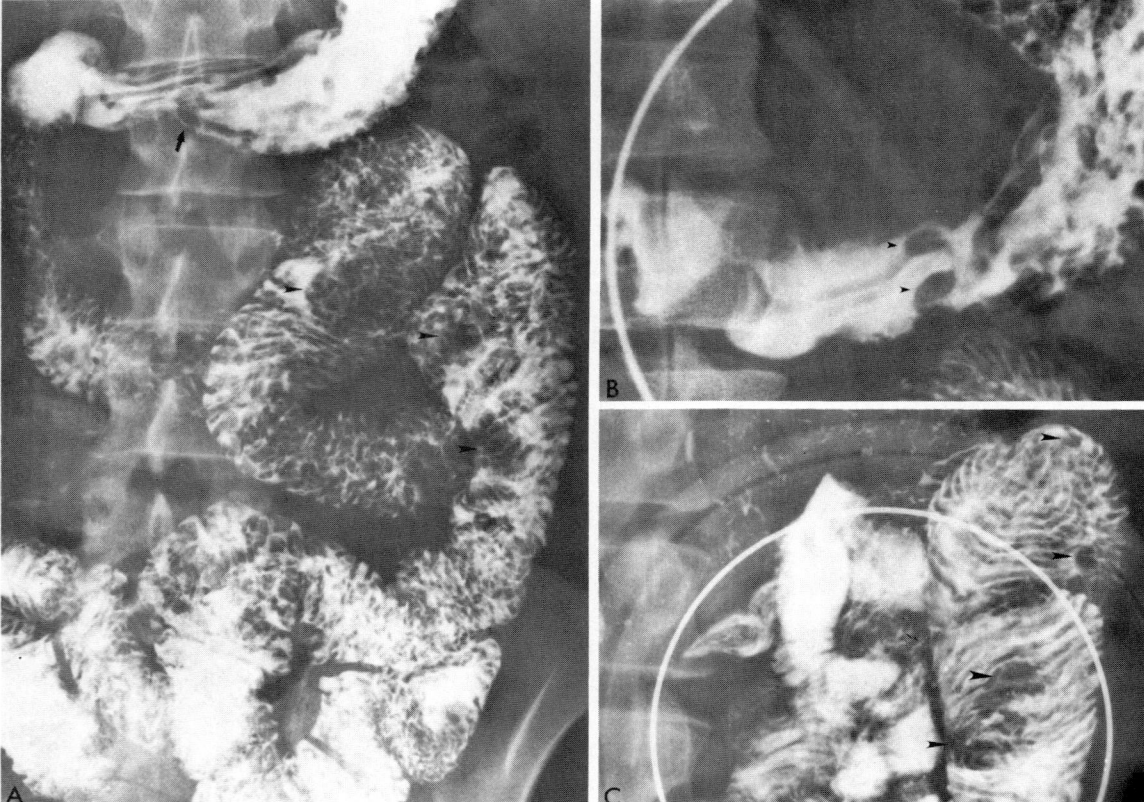

Figure 13–137. Peutz-Jeghers syndrome. *A,* Posteroanterior view of the distal stomach and proximal small bowel showing multiple lucent filling defects in the proximal small bowel (arrowheads) as well as one in the gastric antrum (arrow). *B,* Oblique view of the stomach with compression shows two oval polyps (arrowheads) identified in the antrum. *C,* Posteroanterior view of the proximal small bowel with compression enhances the appearance of the multiple polyps (arrowheads). (Courtesy of The American College of Radiology. *From* Stein, G. N., and Finkelstein, A. K.: Atlas of Tumor Radiology: The Duodenum, Small Intestine and Colon. Chicago, Year Book Medical Publishers, 1973. Reproduced by permission.)

cent of cases. The lesions are usually pedunculated and number from two to a dozen or more. Diffuse carpeting of the colon, such as is present in familial polyposis, has not yet been reported.

In the rare Cronkhite-Canada syndrome, gastric and diffuse colonic polyps are associated with ectodermal changes. Small bowel polyps are also present in about half the cases. The lesions are histologically similar to juvenile polyps.[1,2]

Other conditions that may simulate multiple polyposis causing multiple filling defects on barium enema examination include retained fecal material, nodular lymphoid hyperplasia, pneumatosis intestinales (Fig. 13–138), neurofibromatosis, and lymphosarcoma (Fig. 13–139). None of these lesions is actually associated with polyps.

Figure 13–138. Pneumatosis intestinalis. Posteroanterior film of the barium-filled left side of the colon showing multiple smooth marginal irregularities involving the rectosigmoid and sigmoid regions. These irregularities are associated with multiple marginal lucencies (arrowheads) secondary to air-filled cysts within the wall of the colon. Note the air-filled cyst in the proximal sigmoid colon (arrow), which radiographically resembles a polyp.

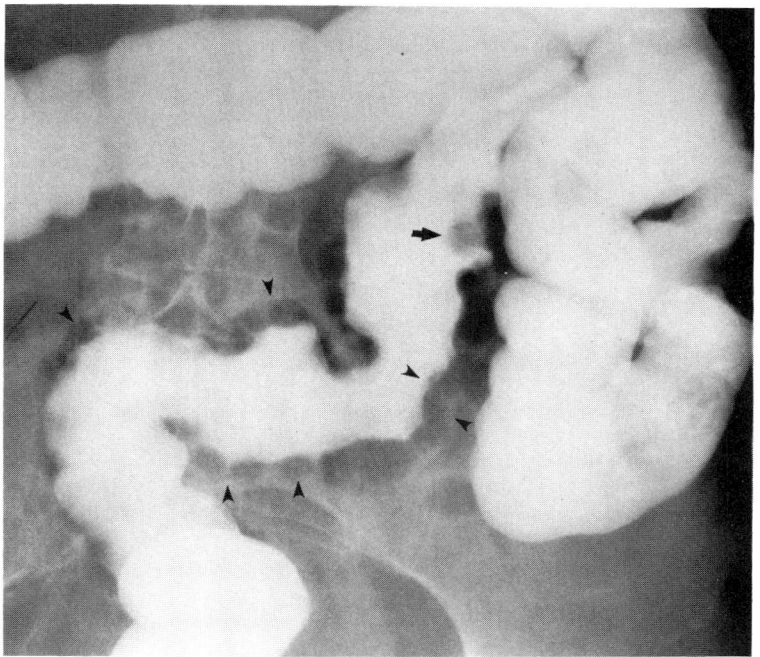

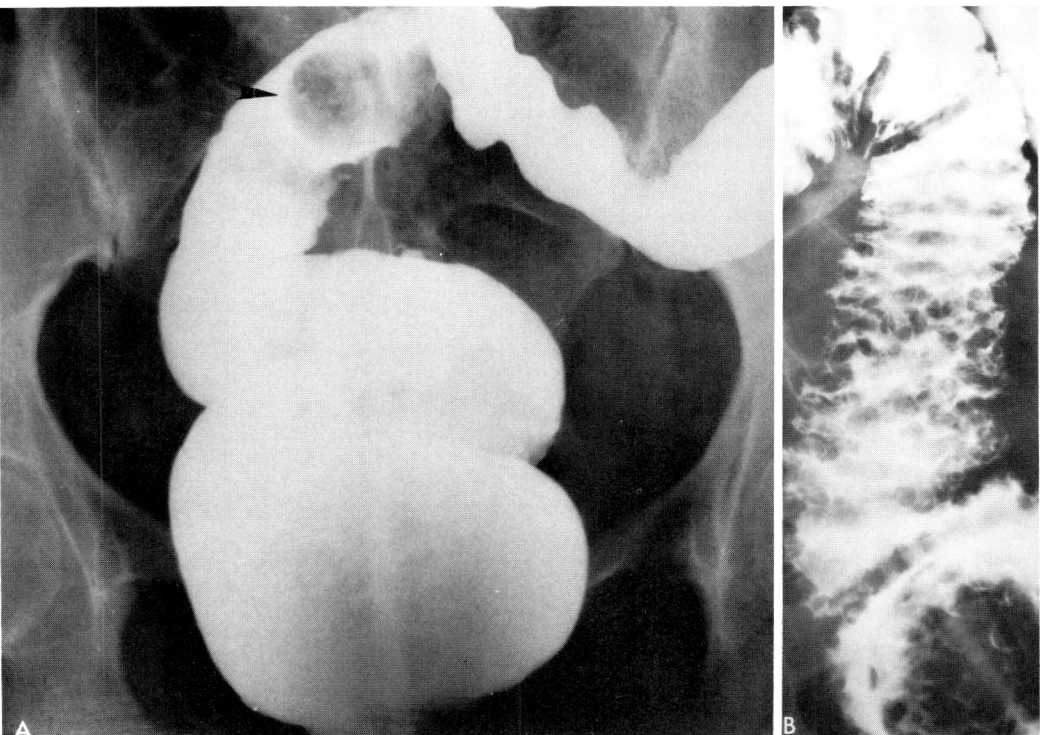

Figure 13–139. *A,* A film of the barium-filled rectosigmoid reveals one round filling defect in the sigmoid colon (arrowhead). Other lesions were present in the colon in this patient with proven neurofibromatosis. *B,* Film of the barium-filled rectosigmoid reveals multiple nodular radiolucencies, relatively uniform in size. Slight irregularity of the luminal outline is also noted. Biopsy revealed extensive lymphosarcoma. (*B,* Courtesy of The American College of Radiology. *From* Stein, G. N., and Finkelstein, A. K.: Atlas of Tumor Radiology: The Duodenum, Small Intestine and Colon. Chicago, Year Book Medical Publishers, 1973. Reproduced by permission.)

References

1. Ackerman, L. V., and Spratt, J. S.: Do adenomatous polyps become cancer? Editorial. Gastroenterology 44:905–908, 1963.
2. Arthur, J. F.: The significance of small mucosal polyps of the rectum. Proc. R. Soc. Med. 55:703–704, 1962.
3. Arthur, J. F.: Structure and significance of metaplastic nodules in the rectal mucosa. J. Clin Pathol. 21:735–743, 1968.
4. Berci, G., Panish, J. F., Schapiro, M., et al.: Complications of colonoscopy and polypectomy: Report of Southern California Society for Gastrointestinal Endoscopy. Gastroenterology 67:584–585, 1974.
5. Blatt, L. J.: Polyps of the colon and rectum: incidence and distribution. Dis. Colon Rectum 4:277–282, 1961.
6. Bockus, H. L., Tachdjian, V., Ferguson, L. K., et al.: Adenomatous polyp of the colon and rectum; its relation to carcinoma. Gastroenterology 41:225–232, 1961.
7. Carden, A. B. G., and Morson, B. C.: Recurrence after local excision of malignant polyps of rectum. Proc. R. Soc. Med. 57:559–561, 1964.
8. Chang, C. H., Piatt, E. D., Thomas, K. E., et al.: Bone abnormalities in Gardner's syndrome. Am. J. Roentgenol. 103:645–652, 1968.
9. Colcher, H.: Prevention and treatment of complications of diagnostic coloscopy and of polypectomy. Presenting at the Annual Meeting of the American Society of Gastrointestinal Endoscopy, San Francisco, Calif., 1974.
10. Cole, J. W., McKalen, A., and Powell, J.: The role of ileal contents in the spontaneous regression of rectal adenomas. Dis. Colon Rectum 4:413–418, 1961.
11. Coli, R. D., Moore, J. P., La Marche, P. H., Gardner's syndrome: a revisit to a previously described family. J. Dig. Dis. 15:551–568, 1970.
12. Diner, W. C.: Cronkhite-Canada syndrome. Radiology 105:715–716, 1972.
13. Enquist, I. F.: The incidence and significance of polyps of the colon and rectum. Surgery 42:681–688, 1957.
14. Enterline, H. T., Evans, G. W., Mercado-Lugo, R., et al.: Malignant potential of adenomas of the colon and rectum. J.A.M.A. 179:322–330, 1962.
15. Fader, M., Kline, S. M., Spatz, S. S., et al.: Gardner's syndrome (intestinal polyposis, osteomas, sebaceous cysts) and a new dental discovery. Oral Surg. 15:153–172, 1962.
16. Finkelstein, A. K., Stein, G. N., and Roy, R. H.: Colonic polyps: a radiologist's viewpoint. Radiol. Clin. North Am. 1:175–194, 1963.
17. Gardner, E. J., and Richards, R. C.: Multiple cutaneous and subcutaneous lesions occurring simultaneously with hereditary polyposis and osteomatosis. Amer. J. Hum. Genet. 5:139–147, 1953.
18. Goldman, H., Ming, S., and Hickok, D. F.: Nature and significance of hyperplastic polyps of the human colon. Arch. Pathol. 89:349–354, 1970.
19. Helwig, E. B.: The evaluation of adenomas of the large intestine and their relation to carcinoma. Surg. Gynecol. Obstet. 84:36–49, 1947.
20. Hines, M. D., Hanley, P. H., Ray, J. E., et al.: Villous tumors of the colon and rectum. Dis. Colon Rectum 1:128, 1958.
21. Hubbard, T. B.: Familial polyposis of the colon. The fate of the retained rectum after colectomy in children. Am. Surg. 23:577–586, 1957.
22. Jackson, B. R.: Adenomas of the colon: the rationale for resection as the treatment of choice. Dis. Colon Rectum 13:47–58, 1970.
23. Kleinfield, G., and Gump., F. E.: Complications of colotomy and polypectomy. Surg. Gynecol. Obstet. 111:726, 1960.
24. Marshak, R. H., Lindner, A. E., and Maklansky, D.: Adenomatous polyps of the colon—a rational approach. J.A.M.A. 235:2856, 1976.
25. Meyers, M. A., and Ghahremani, G. G.: Complications of fiberoptic endoscopy. II. Colonoscopy. Radiology 115:301–307, 1975.
26. Meyers, M. A., Volberg, F., Katzen, B., et al.: Haustral anatomy and pathology: a new look. II. Roentgen interpretation of pathological alterations. Radiology 108:505–512, 1973.
27. Moertel, C. G., Hill, J. R., and Adson, M. A.: Surgical management of multiple polyposis. Arch. Surg., 100:521–526, 1970.
28. Morson, B. C.: Some peculiarities in the histology of intestinal polyps. Dis. Colon Rectum 5:337–344, 1962.
29. Morson, B. C.: Precancerous lesions of the colon and rectum. J.A.M.A. 179:316–321, 1962.
30. Ottenjann, R.: Colonic polyps and coloscopic polypectomy. Endoscopy 4:212, 1972.
31. Rider, J. A., Kirsner, J. B., Moeller, H. C., et al.: Polyps of the colon and rectum. Their incidence and relationship to carcinoma. Am. J. Med. 16:555–564, 1954.
32. Sachatello, C. R., Pickren, J. W., and Grace, J. T.: Generalized juvenile gastrointestinal polyposis. Gastroenterology 58:699–708, 1970.
33. Silverberg, S. G.: "Juvenile" retention polyps of the colon and rectum. J. Dig. Dis. 15:617, 1970.
34. Smith, W. G.: Desmoid tumors in familial multiple polyposis. Mayo Clin. Proc. 34:31–38, 1959.
35. Spratt, J. S., and Ackerman, L. V.: Small primary adenocarcinomas of the colon and rectum. J.A.M.A. 179:337–346, 1962.

36. Spratt, J. S., and Ackerman, L. V.: Pathological significance of polyps of the rectum and colon. Dis. Colon Rectum 3:330–335, 1960.
37. Spratt, J. S., Ackerman, L. V., and Moyer, C. A.: Relationship of polyps of the colon to colonic CA. Ann. Surg. 148:682–696, 1958.
38. Turell, R., and Brodman, H. R.: Adenomas of the colon and rectum. In Turell, R. (ed.): Diseases of the Colon and Anorectum. Vol. 1. Philadelphia, W. B. Saunders Company, 1959.
39. Veale, A. M. O.: Intestinal Polyposis. Cambridge, Cambridge University Press, 1965.
40. Wheat, M. W., and Ackerman, L. V.: Villous adenomas of the large intestine. Ann. Surg. 147:476–487, 1958.
41. Williams, C. B., Hunt, R. H., Loose, H., et al.: Colonoscopy in the management of colon polyps. Br. J. Surg. 61:673–682, 1974.
42. Wolf, B. S.: Roentgen diagnosis of villous tumors of the colon. Am. J. Roentgenol. 84:1093–1104, 1960.
43. Wolff, W. I., and Shinya, H.: Polypectomy via the fiberoptic colonoscope. N. Engl. J. Med. 288:329–332, 1973.
44. Yonemoto, R. H., Slayback, J. B., Byron, R. L., et al.: Familial polyposis of the entire gastrointestinal tract. Arch. Surg. 99:427–434, 1969.

Part V
The Rectum and Anal Canal

GEORGE N. STEIN, M.D.
GERALD M. KLEIN, M.D.

RECTAL PROLAPSE

Rectal prolapse is usually a clinical diagnosis but can be confirmed by barium enema examination. It occurs most frequently in children and elderly females. In children, it may be associated with excessive straining at stool; treatment is generally conservative. In adults, associated laxity of the anal sphincters leading to fecal incontinence occurs in up to two thirds of the patients.[9] On barium enema, in the normal patient, straining pushes the rectum and rectosigmoid backward into the hollow of the sacrum. In marked rectal prolapse, the rectum moves anteriorly and downward with straining, forming a straight tube, perhaps owing to a congenital mesorectum or an abundance of loose areolar connective tissue in the presacral space that prevents fixation of the rectum to the sacrum posteriorly.

Several forms of therapy are available, from abdominal rectopexy, as described by Ripstein,[10] to a Thiersch wire operation,[7] in which a ring of wire is inserted around the anal canal, thus making the anal opening smaller and preventing prolapse. The Thiersch operation is reserved for those who are poor risks for abdominal surgery.

FECAL INCONTINENCE

Primary incontinence of feces is probably secondary to chronic stretching of the anal sphincter muscles over a period of many years.[7] Secondary incontinence may be seen in patients with colitis and associated diarrhea and, in some instances, may be due to trauma to the rectal sphincters, such as may occur during delivery. Radiographic findings are those of the primary disease causing the fecal incontinence.

FECAL IMPACTION

Fecal impaction is an accumulation of large, hard fecal masses in the colon that resist natural efforts of expulsion. Some workers think that as these masses increase in size the colon dilates, causing reflex relaxation of the external and sphincter with associated diarrhea and fecal incontinence.[7] Others believe that diarrhea is secondary to bowel wall inflammation resulting from the large fecal masses.[3] Etiologic factors include the loss of the normal defecation reflex, which is especially common in the aged and in psychotics; the loss of normal colonic peristaltic activity, as seen following spinal cord trauma or tertiary syphilis; or lesions in the anus causing painful defecation secondary to anal spasm, such as hemorrhoids, fissures, or fistulas. In the case of ordinary fecal impaction, one must always carefully rule out an anatomic cause for colonic obstruction, such as carcinoma, diverticulitis, or Hirschsprung's disease.

Radiographically, regions most frequently involved include the rectum (in approximately 60 per cent of cases), sigmoid (in approximately 15 per cent of cases), and cecum (in approximately 10 per cent of cases).[3] On survey abdominal films, the outline of the involved colon filled with the mottled radiolucencies of fecal debris and perhaps dilatation of the colon proximally can be noted (Fig. 13–140). Barium enema shows the irregular fecal masses surrounded by the barium. With increased hydrostatic enema pressure, some movement of these fecal masses may be observed. Difficulty in filling the colon is often encountered, and after evacuation, some clearing of the fecal debris may be noted, although nonopaque residue remains. Residual dilatation of the colon also persists after evacuation. With these findings, upper gastrointestinal barium examination should not be performed, for fear of worsening the impaction. Treatment generally consists of stool softeners, laxatives, enemas, and in severe cases, manual fragmentation of the impaction under anesthesia, if necessary. A reported complication of manual disimpaction is acute massive low rectal bleeding.[6]

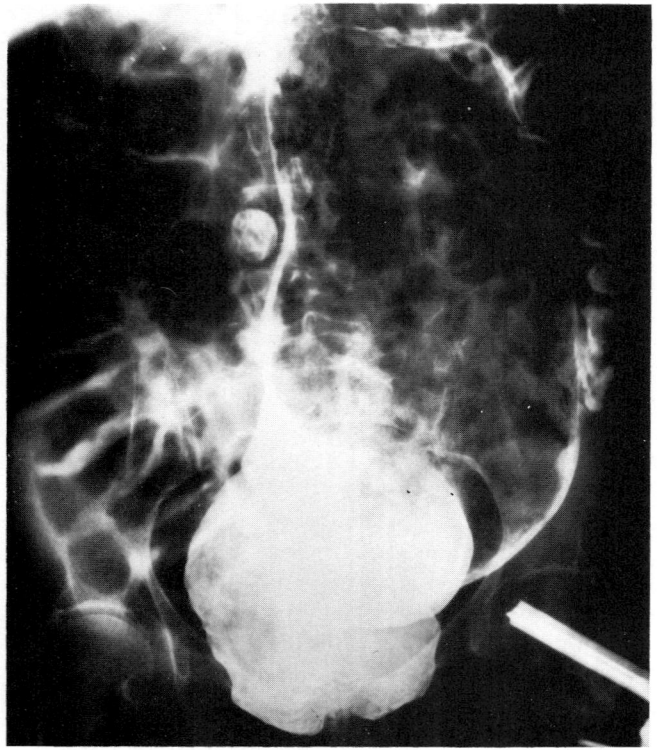

Figure 13–140. Fecal impaction with functional megacolon. Anteroposterior film of the barium-filled rectosigmoid colon reveals marked colonic dilatation with large irregular filling defects, almost conglomerate in appearance, filling most of the bowel. Marked difficulty was encountered in filling the rest of the colon with barium. (Courtesy of the Philadelphia General Hospital and the Mutter Museum of the Philadelphia College of Physicians.)

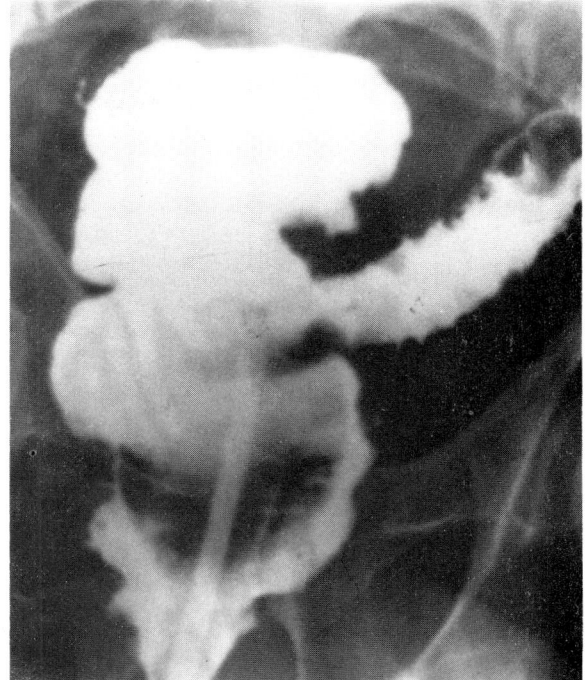

Figure 13–141. Acute ulcerative proctitis. Posteroanterior film of the barium-filled rectosigmoid reveals multiple marginal irregularities secondary to small ulcerations. (Courtesy of the Philadelphia General Hospital and the Mutter Museum of the Philadelphia College of Physicians.)

PROCTITIS

Proctitis refers to an inflammation of the rectal ampulla. Its causes may be idiopathic, traumatic, or infectious, or it may follow irradiation or be a part of a more extensive colitis.

Ulcerative proctitis, or "granular proctitis," is the most common form of proctitis in Western countries.[7] Actually, this is a localized form of ulcerative colitis that may present in the second decade as rectal bleeding, left-sided abdominal cramps, or constipation secondary to rectal spasm. Some may have symptoms of the irritable bowel syndrome. The disease usually remains localized to the rectum over a period of many years. In two thirds or more of patients the changes localize permanently to the rectum; in the remainder they may progress to involve more of the colon and result in the characteristics of ulcerative colitis. Acute attacks may be followed by long periods of remission. Grossly, the mucosa has a granular appearance, and histologic examination reveals mucosal inflammation and ulceration. The barium enema examination may be normal or may show a lack of definition of the mucosal outline and small ulcerations (Fig. 13–141). One may also see an increase in the presacral space, and late in the course of the disease a rectal stricture may develop (Fig. 13–142). Treatment is local, and complications from proctitis per se are rare.

Crohn's proctitis is a localized form of granulomatous colitis. The disease involves the mucosa, the submucosa, the muscularis, and to varying degrees, the serosa. An irregular nodularity, or "cobblestone" appearance, of the rectum and colon is common and results from the intersection of longitudinal and transverse ulcers with swollen intervening mucosa. Anal fissures or fistulas occur in a vast majority of these patients. Disease in the rectum is almost always associated with diseases elsewhere in the colon and is more progressive than ulcerative proctitis. Histologic examination reveals marked edema of the mucosa and submucosa with hypertrophy of the muscularis; infiltration with chronic inflammatory cells predominates. Clinically, these patients

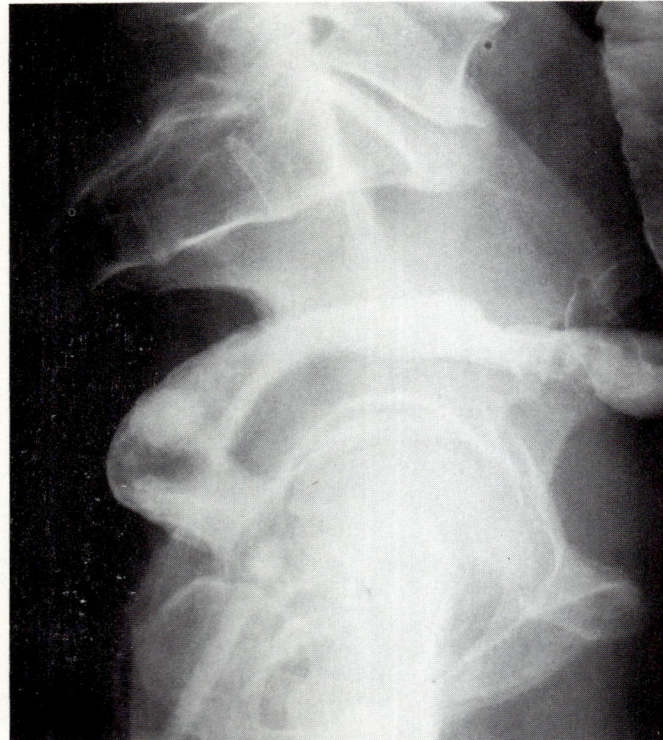

Figure 13–142. Chronic ulcerative proctitis. Lateral view of the barium-filled rectum shows a marked increase in the presacral space as well as smooth narrowing of the rectum and distal sigmoid. The remainder of the colon appeared normal on the barium enema examination.

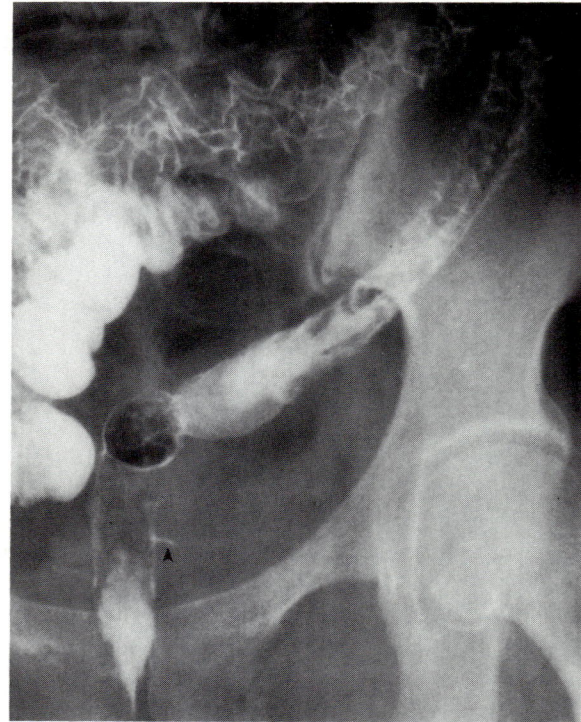

Figure 13–143. Crohn's disease. Postevacuation film from a barium enema shows narrowing of the rectum with a fixed tubular configuration. A fistulous tract (arrowhead) is seen arising from the diseased rectum. The sigmoid colon is also noted to be abnormal.

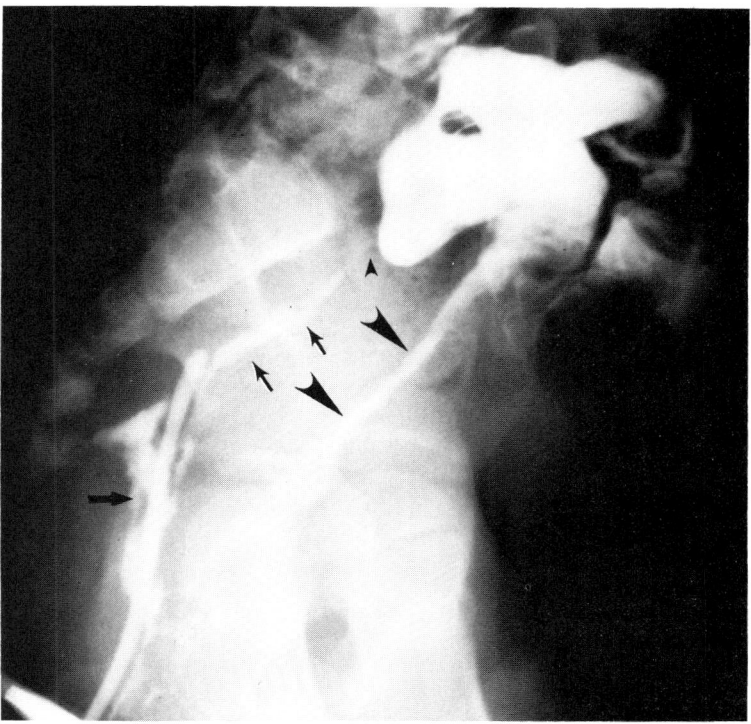

Figure 13–144. Perirectal abscess and fistula. Lateral view of the presacral region following injection of contrast material through a catheter within a perianal fistula (large arrow) demonstrates filling of a presacral abscess (small arrows) as well as filling of the large bowel and rectum through a fistulous tract (small arrowhead). The rectum (large arrowheads) is markedly narrowed and displaced anteriorly by the presacral abscess and marked inflammatory edema. (Courtesy of the Philadelphia General Hospital and the Mutter Museum of the Philadelphia College of Physicians.)

present with abdominal pain and diarrhea. X-ray examination may show a fistulous tract or irregularity and ulceration of the mucosa or both. Evidence of involvement of other portions of the colon with skip areas, associated with small bowel involvement, helps in the differential diagnosis, although when each is limited to the rectum it is difficult to distinguish Crohn's proctitis from ulcerative proctitis. Treatment is usually conservative, unless the symptoms are so severe that surgery is required. Complications of the disease include perirectal abscesses (Figs. 13–143 and 13–144) and strictures, which may require more aggressive treatment.

OTHER COLITIDES WITH RECTAL INVOLVEMENT

Amoebic infestation of the colon must also be considered in the differential diagnosis of proctitis. Clinically, these patients may present with acute infestation, which closely resembles acute ulcerative colitis, with symptoms of bloody diarrhea, abdominal pain, and occasionally megacolon or perforation; on the other hand, chronic infestation is usually associated with the symptoms of irritable bowel syndrome and multiple episodes of diarrhea. The presence of amoebic cysts in the stool is noted more often in the acute form. Additionally, a small percentage of people are known to be asymptomatic cyst carriers. On barium enema examination, the acute changes include contour irregularity of the colon, especially in the cecum; spasm and irritability may produce a funnel-shaped cecum with shaggy margins. Mucosal ulcerations with associated spasm may be seen in any portion of the bowel. These findings are similar to those seen in ulcerative colitis. Changes occurring later in the course of the disease include strictures, which are often multiple and most common in the transverse colon and flexures. Amebomas and fistulas often occur.

Bacillary colitis infestation is secondary to infection with *Shigella*. Transmission is via the fecal-oral route, and the major symptom is diarrhea. Sigmoidoscopy reveals an edematous mucosa, which is usually very friable and covered with pus. The mucosal folds are thickened, and shallow irregular ulcerations are noted (Fig. 13–145). The sites of most frequent involvement as shown by barium enema are the rectosigmoid (particularly in the chronic stage), the flexures, the cecum, and in up to 50 percent of cases, the terminal ileum.[5] During the acute stage, the entire colon and distal ileum may show mucosal edema and irregular areas of spasm, which hinder the complete filling of the colon with barium. In the more severe cases, superficial ulceration may be seen throughout the colon but most commonly in the rectosigmoid area. In chronic cases, strictures, colonic rigidity, and loss of haustration may occur.

Lymphogranuloma venereum is a venereal disease caused by a small filterable virus; it may result in proctocolitis or rectosigmoid stricture. The disease occurs in both males and females, although ulcers and strictures occur almost exclusively in females.[1, 2] The virus is transmitted by sexual contact, and the disease may manifest itself primarily as an indolent inguinal or femoral lymphadenitis with associated vesicles, which may break down, causing superficial ulcerations. In the female, the primary involvement takes place in the vagina and extends into the anorectal lymphatics, causing a retrograde lymphangitis and stasis involving the rectal wall or distal sigmoid. Occasionally, this process may also occur in the male. Infrequently, other areas of the gastrointestinal tract may be involved, including the buccal mucosa. Clinically, these patients may have rectal bleeding or purulent discharge from the anus.[1] Close questioning reveals a history of intercourse followed by the development of a small ulcer or punctate vesicles 3 to 30 days later; the spontaneous disappearance of these lesions occurs over the course of a week, followed in two to three weeks by the

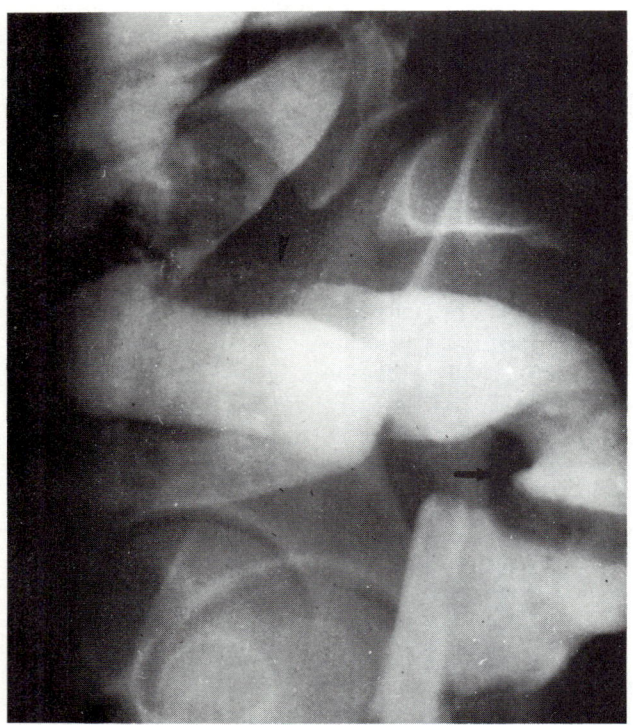

Figure 13–145. Shigellosis. Lateral view of the barium-filled rectosigmoid shows multiple shallow collar-buttoned ulcers (arrowhead) in the sigmoid region. Inflammatory edema is causing widening of the presacral space and thickening of the rectal valves (arrow). (*From* Goldberg, H. I., and Reeder, M. M.: Infections and infestations of the gastrointestinal tract. *In* Margulis, A. R., and Burhenne, H. J. (eds.): Alimentary Tract Roentgenology, Ed. 2. St. Louis, The C. V. Mosby Company, 1973. Reproduced by permission.)

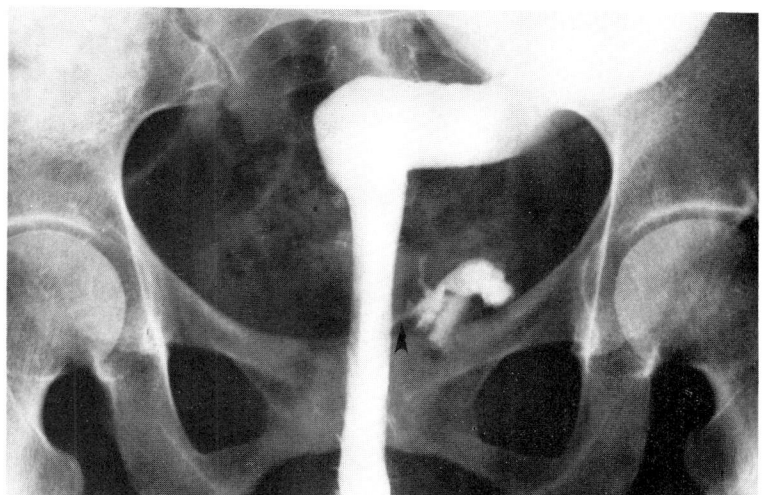

Figure 13–146. Lymphogranuloma venereum. Barium-filled posteroanterior film of the rectosigmoid reveals marked rectal narrowing. Several small ulcerations are noted along the right lateral rectal wall as well as a fistulous tract (arrowhead) to a perirectal abscess. (Courtesy of the Philadelphia General Hospital and the Mutter Museum of the Philadelphia College of Physicians.)

appearance of inguinal lymphadenitis. At this stage, the patient may have malaise, headache, low back pain, excessive perspiration, and chills. Later, as the stricture develops over a period of several months, the symptoms change to constipation and tenesmus. Stool caliber may decrease. Cicatricial changes about the genitalia may also be seen. On sigmoidoscopy, there is a friable granular mucosa, with marked edema of the bowel wall and luminal narrowing. Ulcerations and mucosal destruction with replacement by granulation tissue is often noted.

Roentgen changes depend to a large extent on the stage of the disease. The regions most frequently involved are the rectum and rectosigmoid. In the acute stage, localized irritability with inability to retain the barium enema is seen. The narrowed rectum may show contour irregularity secondary to ulcers (Fig. 13–146), fistulous tracts, perirectal abscesses, and widening of the presacral space (Fig. 13–147) may also be seen. The fistulas may extend to the skin and involve other segments of the colon (Fig. 13–148) or the small bowel, or the vagina. During the chronic phase, strictures of varying length develop. The strictures have smooth or irregular walls; the irregularity is usually secondary to persistent ulceration or fistulous tracts. Strictures may vary in length from 4 to 25 cm.[4, 8] Usually there is only a single stricture, although skip lesions, mimicking those of Crohn's disease, have been reported.[2] The colon proximal to the stricture is often dilated.

The differential diagnosis of this entity includes ulcerative colitis, Crohn's colitis, and tuberculosis (Fig. 13–149); also to be considered are the following: actinomycosis, which rarely causes ulcers and fistulous tracts; schistosomiasis of the rectum, which can cause coarse ulcerations, polypoid lesions, and rectal narrowing; post-traumatic strictures from foreign bodies or repeated rectal prolapse; scirrhous rectal carcinoma; perirectal masses and extrinsic narrowing, secondary to either tumor (Figs. 13–150 and 13–151) or inflammatory masses; or strictures secondary to the treatment of hemorrhoids with sclerosing agents.

Radiation to the pelvis and abdomen for the treatment of carcinoma of the cervix, uterus, or prostate can damage either the rectosigmoid colon or the small bowel loops that are fixed by adhesions in the pelvis within the field of treatment. Clinically, symptoms may present acutely during or immediately after the x-ray treatment, but sometimes they occur several years later. Diarrhea is the usual symptom, associated

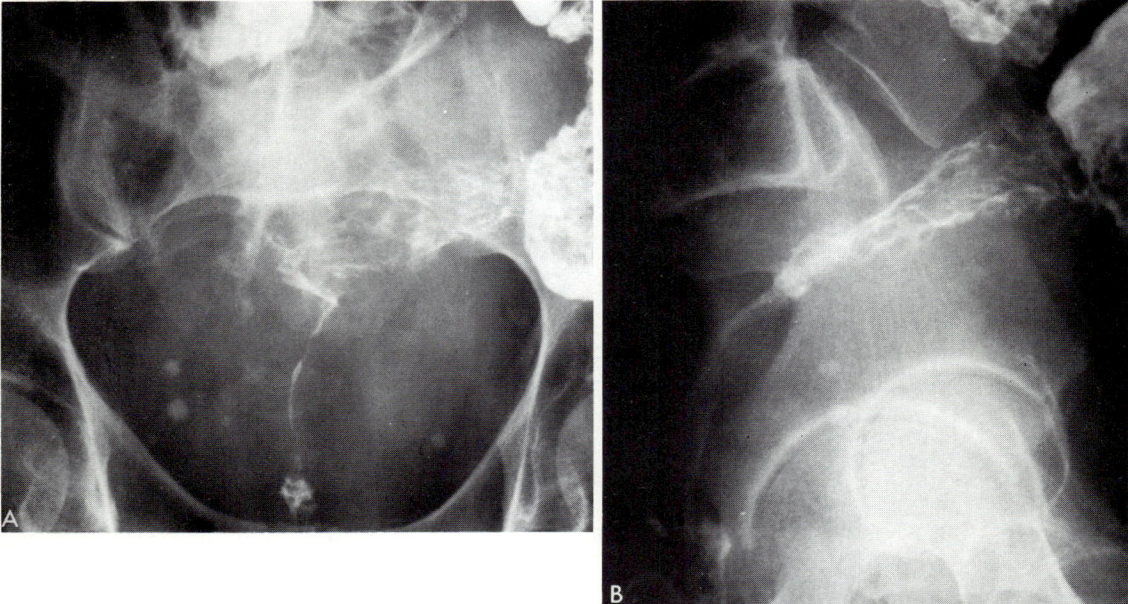

Figure 13–147. Lymphogranuloma venereum. *A*, Posteroanterior film of the barium-filled rectosigmoid region reveals a marked stricture of the rectum. The distal descending colon is seen to be dilated secondary to some obstruction. *B*, Lateral view of the barium-filled rectum shows marked widening of the presacral space secondary to perirectal fibrosis.

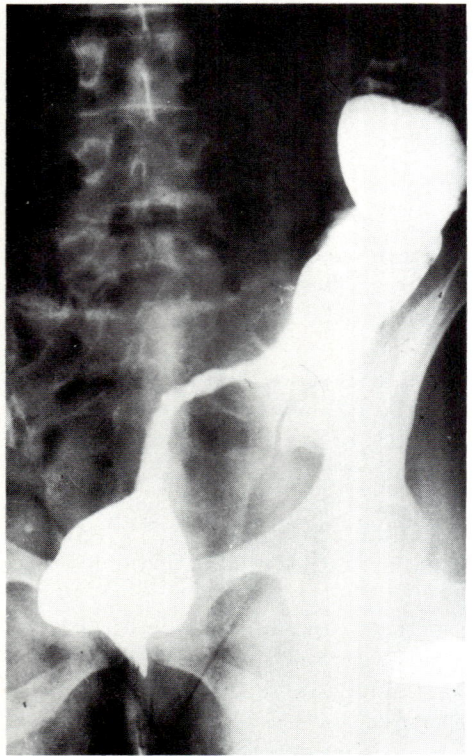

Figure 13–148. Lymphogranuloma venereum. Barium-filled posteroanterior film of the colon reveals a stricture of the distal sigmoid colon with evidence of mucosal irregularity. The mucosal irregularity is secondary to ulcerations. The distal rectum is normal. This is an unusual location for a stricture secondary to lymphogranuloma venereum. (*From* Goldberg, H. I., and Reeder, M. M.: Infections and infestations of the Gastrointestinal Tract. *In* Margulis, A. R., and Burhenne, H. J. (eds.): Alimentary Tract Roentgenology. Ed. 2. St. Louis, The C. V. Mosby Company, 1973. Reproduced by permission.)

Figure 13–149. Rectal tuberculosis. Lateral view of the barium-filled rectum shows multiple superficial ulcerations (white arrow) as well as some widening of the presacral space secondary to edema. This could easily be mistaken for one of the other inflammatory colitides. (Courtesy of Henry I. Goldberg, M.D., San Francisco.)

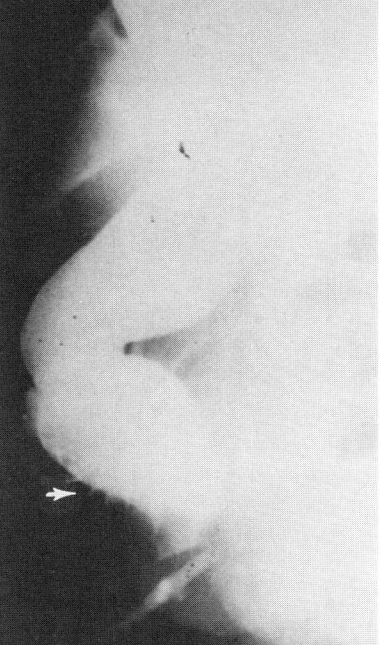

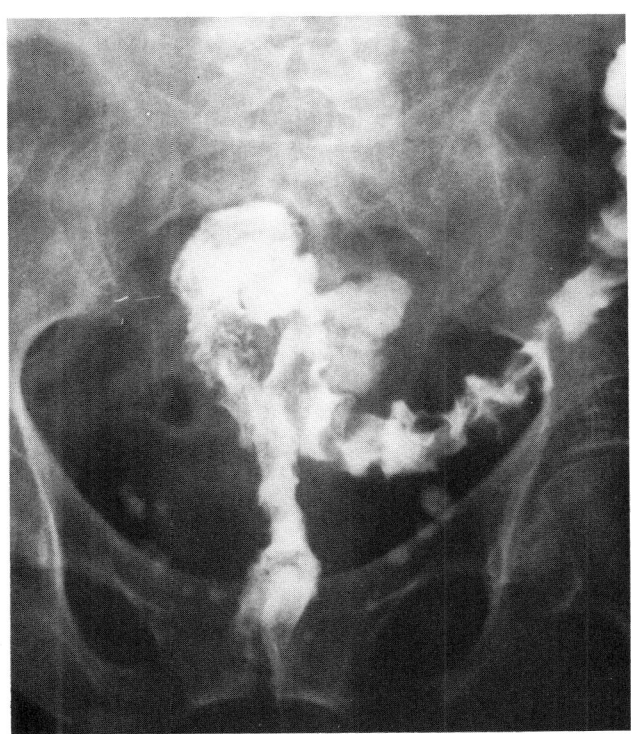

Figure 13–150. Rectal lymphoma. Posteroanterior film of the barium-filled rectosigmoid shows narrowing of the rectum and distal sigmoid associated with marked mucosal distortion and irregularity.

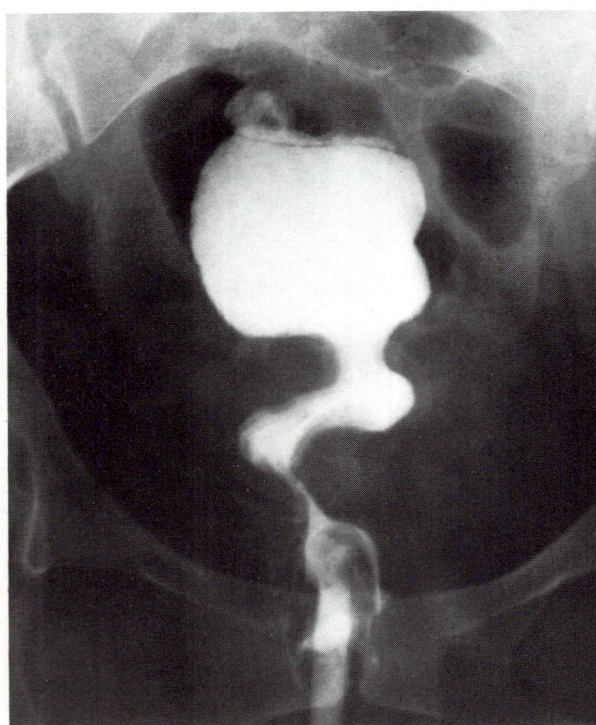

Figure 13–151. Rectal stricture secondary to scleroderma (?). Posteroanterior film of the barium-filled rectosigmoid shows a smooth tapered stricture of the rectum with mild proximal dilatation. The results of rectal biopsy were negative, but a skin biopsy revealed scleroderma.

with rectal bleeding and tenesmus in the more severe acute cases. Rarely, perforation may occur (Fig. 13–152), but more often a fistula (Fig. 13–153) forms between the radiated segment and another portion of the gut or on an adjacent organ, such as the uterus, vagina, or bladder. Chronic manifestations include prolonged diarrhea, with associated malabsorption if the small bowel is involved. Intestinal obstruction may be a late manifestation.

Radiation has a direct effect on the bowel mucosa; histologically, leukocytic infiltration is present in the wall of the rectum, especially with eosinophils, which disappear several weeks after treatment has ceased. Radiation also causes an endarteritis, which results in endothelial proliferation and vascular insufficiency to the involved segments of gut. It is not certain which of these two mechanisms is more important pathophysiologically in the development of radiation enteritis. However, the final result to the bowel is edema, hyperemia, and inflammation that reach their peak in a few weeks and subside, the bowel returning to its normal appearance. If the injury has been too great, however, mucosal ulcerations develop that may perforate or lead to fistulas. When the bowel attempts to heal, it does so imperfectly, resulting in thickening of the wall, matting together of adjacent loops with fibrotic stiff mesentery, and localized strictures.

During the acute phase, barium studies may show thickened edematous folds (Fig. 13–154), ulcerations, spasm, and eventual progression to stricture. In the appropriate clinical setting, this presents no diagnostic problem. In chronic cases, however, there may be a long, narrowed segment that gradually merges with normal bowel (with no overhanging edges) proximally and distally (Figs. 13–155 and 13–156); the involved segment is usually smooth and rigid, and the presacral space may be increased. With these roentgen findings an attempt should be made to learn if the patient has a history

Text continued on page 786

THE LARGE BOWEL — 783

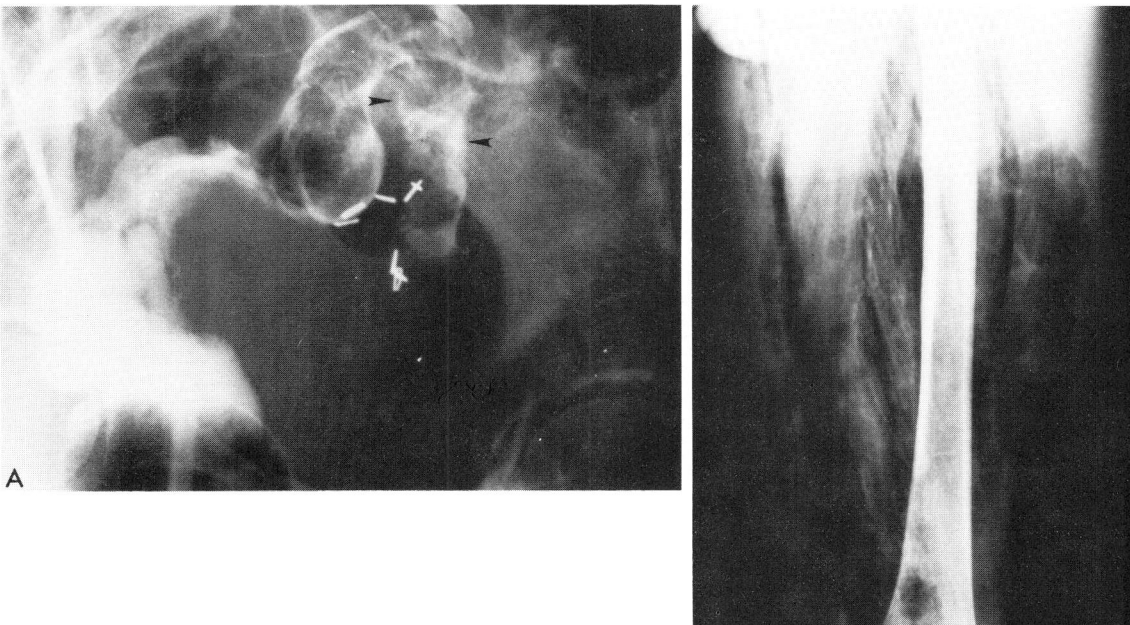

Figure 13–152. Sigmoid perforation secondary to irradiation. *A*, Oblique film of the barium-filled rectosigmoid demonstrating extraluminal barium (arrowheads) at a site of sigmoid perforation following radiation therapy for ovarian carcinoma. This represented an extraperitoneal perforation. *B*, Film of the thigh showing gas dissecting along the soft tissue planes. The gas is arising from the sigmoid perforation and dissecting its way down from the rectoperitoneal areas.

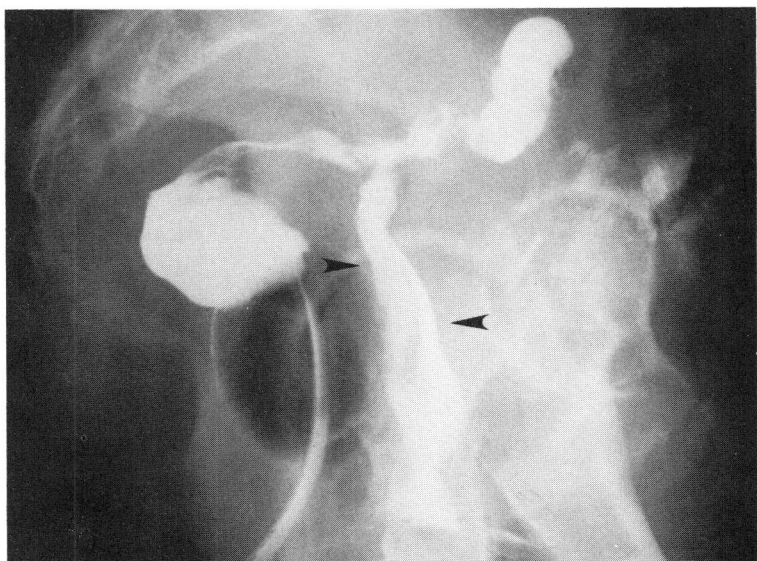

Figure 13–153. Rectovaginal fistula. Lateral view of the barium-filled rectosigmoid showing a rectovaginal fistula in a patient previously irradiated for carcinoma of the cervix. The fistula occurred spontaneously one year after radiation therapy. Note the barium in the vagina (arrowheads). (Courtesy of the Philadelphia General Hospital and the Mutter Museum of the Philadelphia College of Physicians.)

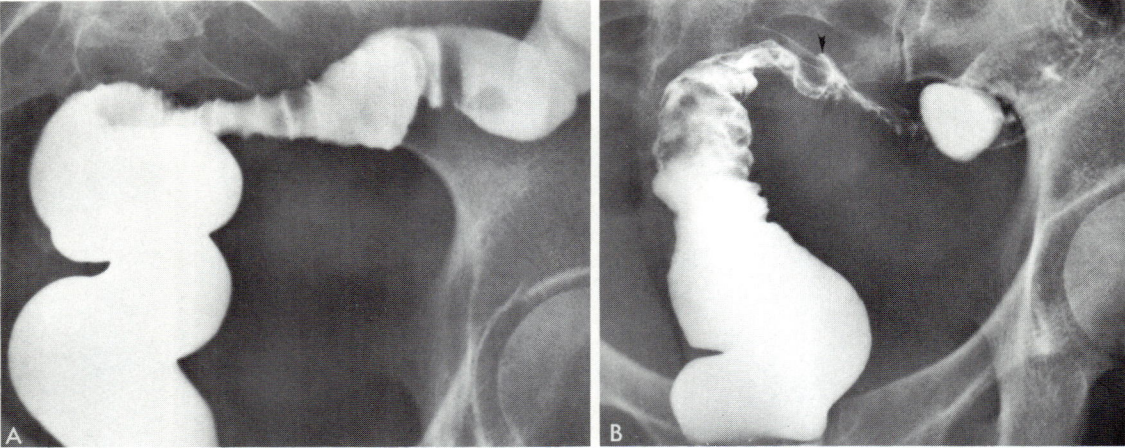

Figure 13–154. Radiation colitis. *A*, Anteroposterior view of the barium-filled rectosigmoid three months after combined internal and external irradiation for carcinoma of the cervix: Note the moderate narrowing of the sigmoid associated with thickened edematous mucosal folds. *B*, Anteroposterior view of the barium-filled rectosigmoid region five months after therapy: Note the marked narrowing of the sigmoid associated with nodular distortion of the mucosa. A gradual tapering from the normal to the abnormal bowel is seen as well as a short sinus tract (arrowhead) from the stenotic segment. (Courtesy of The American College of Radiology. *From* Stein, G. N., and Finkelstein, A. K.: Atlas of Tumor Radiology: The Duodenum, Small Intestine and Colon. Chicago, Year Book Medical Publishers, 1973. Reproduced by permission.)

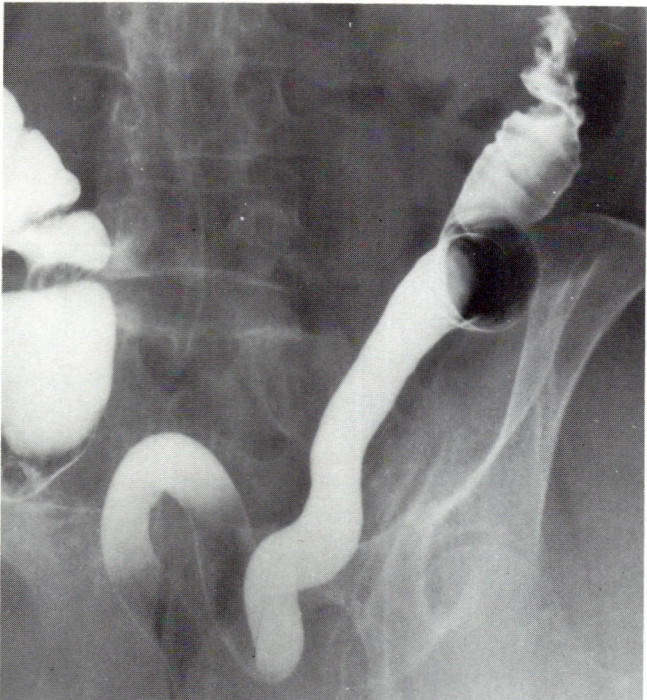

Figure 13–155. Radiation colitis. Angled view of the rectum and sigmoid colon reveals smooth narrowing of the rectum and distal sigmoid three months after radiation therapy for carcinoma of the cervix. (*From* Templeton, F. E.: Colonic malignancy. *In* Margulis, A. R., and Burhenne, H. J. (eds.): Alimentary Tract Roentgenology. Ed. 2. St. Louis, The C. V. Mosby Company, 1973. Reproduced by permission.)

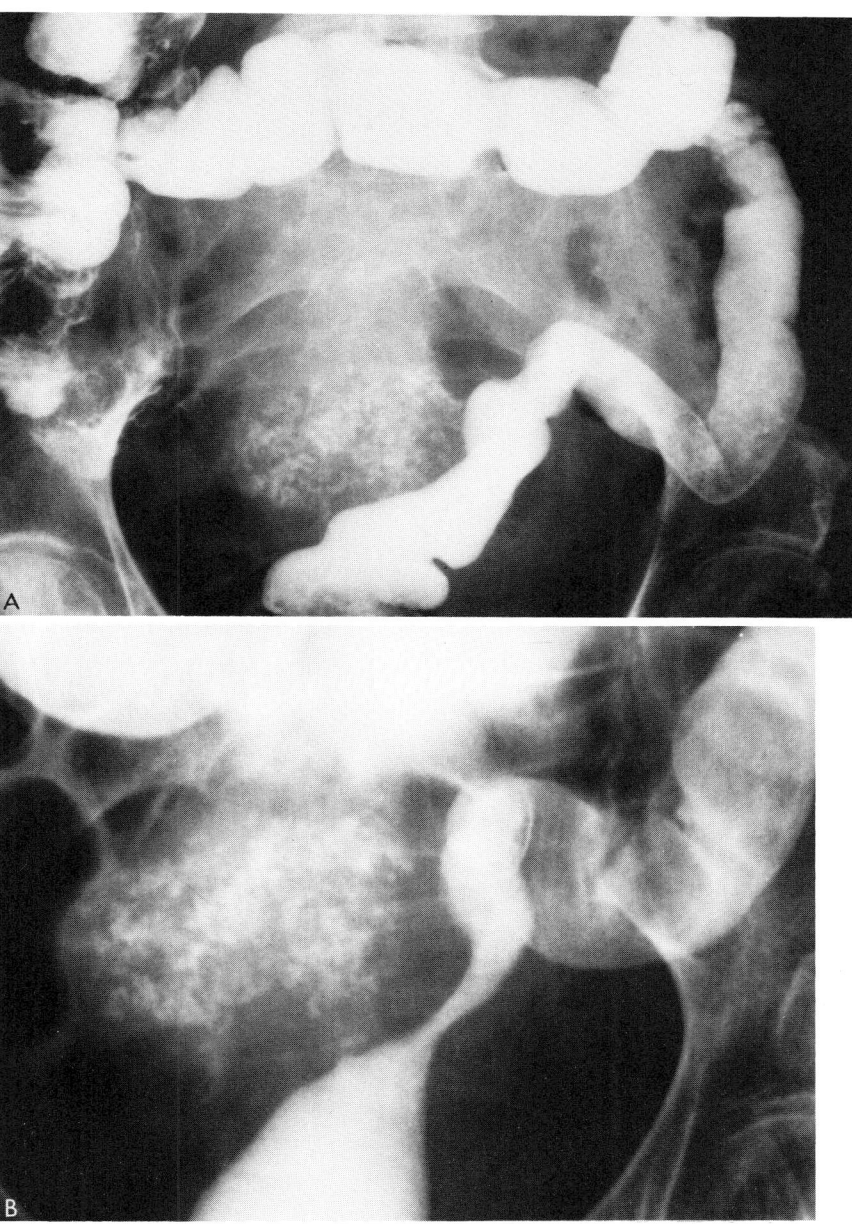

Figure 13–156. Radiation colitis. *A,* Anteroposterior film of the barium-filled colon showing mild narrowing of the rectosigmoid following radiation therapy for carcinoma of the cervix. A large calcified fibroid is also seen. *B,* A film of the rectosigmoid 13 months later shows a smoothly tapering stricture in this region secondary to chronic radiation fibrosis. (Courtesy of the Philadelphia General Hospital and the Mutter Museum of the Philadelphia College of Physicians.)

of prior radiation treatment. The differential diagnosis includes ulcerative colitis, diverticulitis, and carcinoma. Carcinoma usually involves a shorter segment, however, with abrupt transition from the normal to the abnormal area, associated with overhanging edges. Treatment in the acute phase is for symptomatic relief—to control the diarrhea. Chronic cases may require removal of the damaged bowel.

Ischemic proctitis is a rare entity owing to the excellent collateral blood supply to this area, but it can occur, especially in people who are old or who have had surgery in the lower abdomen. The sites of ischemic colitis, when localized, are most often around the splenic flexure region, although other areas can be involved. These patients present with abdominal pain and rectal bleeding. The disease process may lead to gangrene of the bowel, with associated perforation or segmental stricture; complete recovery of the bowel is possible, however. Sigmoidoscopically, bizarre polypoid or ulcerated lesions secondary to mucosal necrosis and slough may be evident. The rapidity of change, either to healing or to worsening, is diagnostic of this entity (Fig. 13–157). Barium enema may show early changes of mucosal edema, spasm, thumbprinting, and possibly, bowel wall thickening. Small ulcerations may also be seen early. In the healing phase, restoration of the normal bowel appearance may result; so may strictures similar to those seen secondary to irradiation.

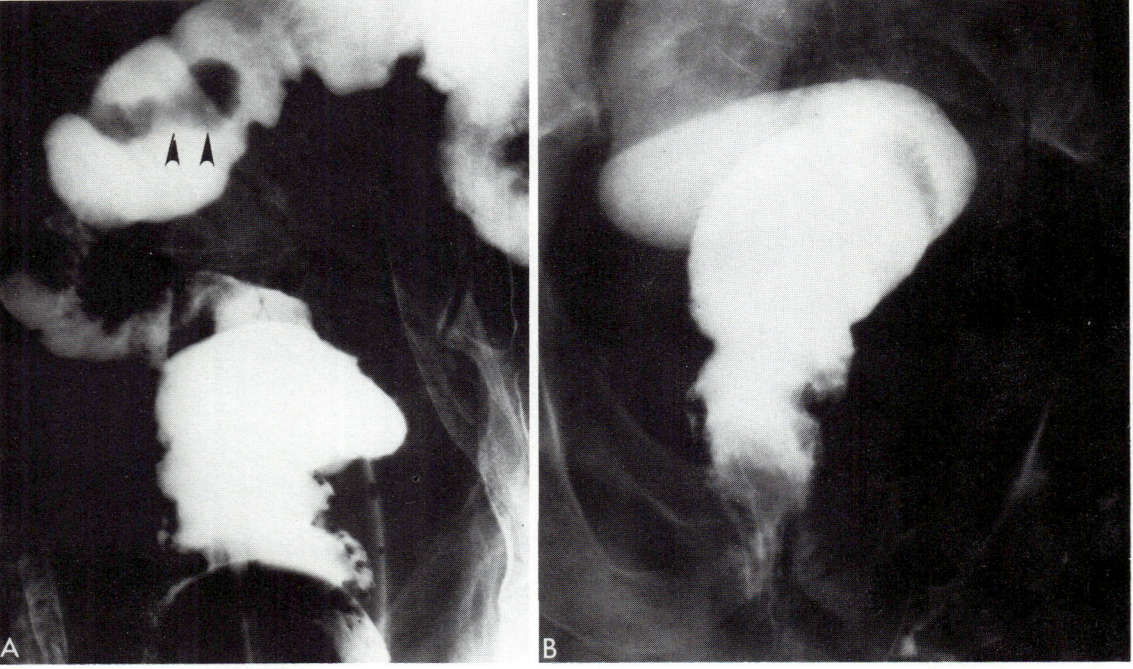

Figure 13–157. Ischemic proctitis. *A,* A film of the barium-filled rectosigmoid in a patient with a two-week history of diarrhea showing multiple collar-button ulcers in the rectum. Note also the pedunculated polyp (arrowheads) in the sigmoid colon. *B,* Repeat study 21 days later shows a marked decrease in the size and number of the rectal ulcers without specific therapy. The rapidity of change is strongly suggestive of the diagnosis of ischemic proctitis. (Courtesy of the Philadelphia General Hospital and the Mutter Museum of the Philadelphia College of Physicians.)

HEMORRHOIDS

Hemorrhoids represent dilatations of the venous plexuses of the lower rectum and are among the most common of afflictions. Clinically they present with either bleeding, protrusion, or thrombosis. The bleeding is usually mild and intermittent, with blood appearing on the stool or toilet paper. Rarely, more marked bleeding can occur, resulting in iron deficiency anemia. Both external and internal hemorrhoids may protrude; the external hemorrhoids are covered with skin and the internal ones with mucous membrane. Therefore, internal hemorrhoids are usually painless. Only internal hemorrhoids can be reduced, since external hemorrhoids originate below the anal sphincter. The external hemorrhoids usually remain small but may thrombose, causing exquisite pain and eventual skin tag formation. Internal hemorrhoids thrombose less often but bleed more frequently. Diagnosis is usually made by palpation and direct visualization. Occasionally, hemorrhoids may be seen on barium enema examination as smooth filling defects with a mural origin (Fig. 13–158).

Conservative treatment includes the use of stool softeners and antiinflammatory agents, scrupulous attention to cleanliness, and applications of heat. When these fail, surgery is often performed. Injection of sclerosing agents around the hemorrhoids to obliterate them or elastic banding of the hemorrhoids may be performed. An unusual, but troublesome, complication of hemorrhoidectomy or injection of sclerosing agents is rectal stricture. This can usually be treated conservatively, by manual dilatation.

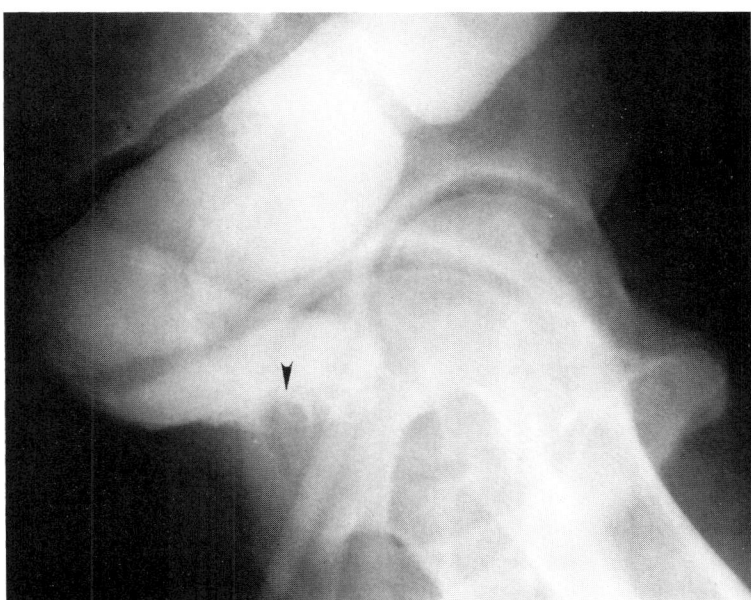

Figure 13–158. Hemorrhoids. Lateral view of the barium-filled rectum reveals a small mural mass arising from the posteroinferior rectal wall (arrowhead). The barium enema was otherwise normal; this mass represented enlarged internal hemorrhoids.

ANORECTAL INFECTION

Perirectal inflammatory disease is a diagnosis often made by clinical examination. These patients may present with pain, fever, and other symptoms of infection. Treatment is usually surgical drainage if the inflammatory mass is large enough. Barium studies may show displacement of bowel loops or extrinsic pressure on the bowel (see Fig. 13–144). Asymmetric bowel wall edema and spasm may be seen if the inflammatory mass actually involves the bowel wall.

ANAL FISTULA

This is an abnormal communication between the mucosa of the rectum and the skin adjacent to the anus. Fistulas are not uncommon and may occur without any predisposing cause other than local infection; their presence should suggest the possibility of Crohn's ileocolitis, however. Treatment is surgical resection when no primary cause is found. If secondary to regional enteritis, the primary disease should be treated, since resection is almost always followed by recurrent fistula. Usually patients can tolerate these fistulas as long as they drain freely and do not become obstructed.

ANAL FISSURE

This is a small tear in the lining of the anus down to, but not through, the circular muscle. Symptoms include pain both during and after defecation in a patient who is usually constipated. Bleeding may also occur. Treatment is given to relieve symptoms. In some cases, however, surgery is required. This consists of excising a chronic fissure and reapproximating the ends of the surgically created acute fissure. More conservative therapy, consisting of anal dilatation and medical treatment of the constipation, is sometimes successful.

References

1. Annamunthodo, H.: Rectal lymphogranuloma venereum in Jamaica. Dis. Colon Rectum 4:17–26, 1961.
2. Annamunthodo, H., and Marryatt, J.: Barium studies in intestinal lymphogranuloma venereum. Br. J. Radiol. 34:53–57, 1961.
3. DeLorimier, A. A., Moehring, H. G., and Hannan, J. R.: Fecal impaction in the colon. *In* Clinical Roentgenology. Vol. 4, Springfield, Illinois, Charles C Thomas, Publisher, 1956, p. 292.
4. DeLorimier, A. A., Moehring, H. G., and Hannan, J. R.: Lymphogranuloma venereum. *In* Clinical Roentgenology. Vol. 4, Springfield, Illinois, Charles C Thomas, Publisher, 1956, p. 333.
5. DeLorimier, A. A., Moehring, H. G., and Hannan, J. R.: Bacillary colitis. *In* Clinical Roentgenology. Vol. 4. Springfield, Illinois, Charles C Thomas, Publisher, 1956, p. 330.
6. Naderi, M. J., and Bookstein, J. J.: Rectal bleeding secondary to fecal disimpaction: angiographic diagnosis and treatment. Radiology 126:387, 1978.
7. Parks, A. G., and Thomson, M. S.: The rectum and anal canal. *In* Sabiston, D. C., Jr.: Davis-Christopher Textbook of Surgery. Ed. 11. Philadelphia, W. B. Saunders Company, 1977, p. 1134.
8. Pessel, J. F.: Lymphogranuloma venereum. *In* Bockus, H. L. (ed.): Gastroenterology. Vol. 2. Ed. 2. Philadelphia, W. B. Saunders Company, 1964, p. 1051.
9. Porter, N. H.: A physiological study of the pelvic floor in rectal prolapse. Ann. R. Coll. Surg. Engl. 31:379–404, 1962.
10. Ripstein, C. B.: Surgical care of massive renal prolapse. Dis. Colon Rectum 8:34–38, 1965.

14

GASTROINTESTINAL HEMORRHAGE: ANGIOGRAPHY AND TRANSCATHETER THERAPY

JOSEPH J. BOOKSTEIN, M.D.
GUERDON D. GREENWAY, M.D.

INTRODUCTION

Like the biologic systems they support, medical procedures evolve through stages of conception, gestation, maturation, and sometimes, senescence. Angiography of gastrointestinal bleeding has reached an early maturation stage. Its conception occurred in 1960, when Margulis noted extravasation from a cecal branch during operative arteriography.[64] Gestation proceeded rapidly, and in 1963, Nusbaum and Baum localized human gastrointestinal bleeding by conventional (nonoperative) selective intestinal arteriography.[72] Their experimental results indicated that bleeding rates of as little as 0.5 ml per minute could be demonstrated angiographically. Others soon confirmed the value of the technique in localizing the source of gastrointestinal bleeding and in indicating its cause.[56, 81]

In 1967, Nusbaum et al. reported the value of superior mesenteric arterial infusion of vasopressin in controlling bleeding from *esophageal varices* and implied that intra-arterial infusion of vasopressin had a more favorable therapeutic ratio than did intravenous infusion.[73] In 1972, Rösch described results of vasopressin and epinephrine, or epinephrine and propranolol in controlling gastrointestinal bleeding from *arteriocapillary* sources.[87] Numerous papers soon confirmed these favorable reports.

The limitations of vasoconstrictor infusion in the treatment of arteriocapillary bleeding were soon appreciated. Bleeding from certain lesions, particularly gastric or duodenal ulcers, often was not alleviated. In 1972, Rösch et al. described a single case in which a blood clot, injected into the gastroepiploic artery, transiently controlled a bleeding ulcer.[88] Because of the problem of clot lysis, other embolic materials have been utilized, including oxidized cellulose (Oxycel*),[19] gelatin sponge (Gelfoam†),[82] and clot modified with aminocaproic acid.[82] Recently polyvinyl alcohol (Ivalon‡)[96] has been advocated as a permanent occlusive agent. Large vessels can be occluded with metallic coils,[43, 44, 47] isobutyl cyanoacrylate,[37, 45] or balloon catheters.[103]

In the therapy of bleeding varices, results after vasopressin infusion were inconstand. Alternative transcatheter methods were sought, and transcatheter embolism of the varices themselves was described by Lunderquist and Vang in 1974.[60] Percutaneous techniques were used to pass a catheter through the upper abdominal wall and liver into the portal system, then into variceal tributaries. After the injection of sclerosing and embolic agents, the varices could be occluded. Sizable series have now been reported indicating short-term, and occasionally long-term, hemostasis.[61, 77]

Thus, within one-and-a-half decades, angiography has matured remarkably, assuming a vital role in the diagnosis and therapy of gastrointestinal bleeding.

ANGIOGRAPHIC DIAGNOSIS

Angiography may be performed for diagnosis of the site and cause of bleeding or for therapy of bleeding or for both. In patients with active upper gastrointestinal bleeding, aggressive management and prompt diagnosis are currently advocated.[15, 59, 76] Endoscopy is the primary diagnostic method in cases of upper gastrointestinal bleeding, where it enables localization of most bleeding sources. In 10 to 20 per cent of cases, however, endoscopy is technically impossible or results are ambiguous.[16, 27, 52, 62, 69, 76] In this subgroup, angiography may be indicated for diagnostic purposes. Barium plays no role in the management of active massive upper gastrointestinal bleeding. Of course, if the bleeding subsides and the vital signs are stabilized, the upper gastrointestinal series assumes high priority as a diagnostic method. Colonoscopy is relatively ineffective in massive active lower gastrointestinal bleeding, rendering angiography the primary diagnostic method after simple rectal examination and sigmoidoscopy.

Technique and Complication

When angiography is indicated for localization of upper gastrointestinal bleeding, celiac and superior mesenteric arteriography are performed initially. Aortography is ordinarily not performed, unless the possibility of aortoenteric fistula must be excluded because of a history of previous aortic surgery.[32] Aortography is also indicated occasionally when active upper gastrointestinal bleeding continues despite negative celiac and superior mesenteric arteriography, in which case bleeding from an anoma-

---

*Oxidized cellulose, Parke Davis, Ann Arbor, Michigan.
†Upjohn Company, Kalamazoo, Michigan.
‡Polyvinyl alcohol, Unipoint Industries, Hi Point, North Carolina.

lous aortic branch supplying the stomach or esophagus should be suspected.[94] Ordinarily, active arteriocapillary bleeding from the upper gastrointestinal tract is demonstrated by celiac or superior mesenteric angiography. If bleeding is variceal in origin, extravasation is not demonstrable by arteriography, although the varices are usually visible during the venous phase. In about 20 per cent of patients with upper gastrointestinal bleeding, selective left gastric or gastroduodenal arteriography is required to demonstrate the bleeding point.[18] Thus, selective catheterizations should be performed when initial studies are indeterminate.

In patients with lower gastrointestinal bleeding, superior mesenteric arteriography is generally performed initially, because lower gastrointestinal bleeding requiring angiography usually arises from the right colon. Care must be exercised to include the entire cecum, ascending colon, and hepatic flexure on the initial study. If the superior mesenteric arteriogram is not diagnostic, then inferior mesenteric arteriography is performed, two injections generally being required to display the entire colon from anus to midtransverse colon. If both superior and inferior mesenteric arteriography are negative, celiac arteriography is performed, because bleeding from an upper gastrointestinal source frequently masquerades clinically as lower gastrointestinal bleeding.[26]

The rates and volume of injection of contrast medium are to some extent dependent on preliminary fluoroscopic estimates of blood flow in the vessel to be injected. Typical volumes and rates are the following: (1) celiac arteriography, 8 to 12 ml/sec for 3½ seconds; (2) for superior mesenteric arteriography 8 to 12 ml/sec for 4 seconds; and (3) for inferior mesenteric arteriography, 5 to 7.5 ml/sec for 2 to 3 seconds. When opacification of the portal system is of primary importance, longer, slower, and larger injections are required. For example, in order to visualize the portal vein after arteriography, we inject 50 mg of tolazoline into the superior mesenteric artery over a period of 30 seconds, following this after another 30 seconds by an injection of 50 ml of contrast medium over a period of 7 seconds.

The major complications during angiography of the actively bleeding patient are shock and exsanguination. It is imperative that a clinician or nurse be in attendance and responsible for monitoring vital signs and supervising blood and fluid replacement. The examination must be performed with alacrity, and if excessive difficulty is encountered in selectively catheterizing any branch it is often wiser to abandon the attempt. The patient is, of course, at risk from the usual complications of retrograde femoral catheterization, particularly thrombosis and hematoma, but these complications do not occur with disproportionate frequency in the gastrointestinal bleeder.

A major diagnostic difficulty is imposed by the intermittent nature of gastrointestinal bleeding. In some cases, bleeding is not visible initially but appears on a repeat study. Alternatively, we have witnessed bleeding initially, to see it disappear on repeat studies. Therefore, we frequently repeat injections in patients who are apparently actively bleeding even though an initial injection was negative. We have on occasion administered tolazoline intra-arterially to encourage recurrent bleeding, with success in three cases. The vasodilatory effect of tolazoline can be reversed by vasopressin infusion. Caution must be exercised in administering a vasodilator to hypovolemic patients, however. Precipitous hypotension commonly occurs, since the vasodilator overcomes the autoregulatory effect of peripheral vasoconstriction. Thus, in general, volume replacement is required prior to the administration of a vasodilator. Rarely, in patients who have had chronic intermittent bleeding and repeatedly normal arteriograms, heparin is administered when bleeding recurs, with the aim of maintaining the bleeding until angiographic diagnosis can be made. So far, we have not encountered a case in which heparin administration was critical for diagnosis.

Interpretation

When the patient is actively bleeding from a focal arteriocapillary source, contrast medium extravasates from the vascular system and can usually be easily recognized within the lumen or upon the mucosa of the bowel after the intravascular contrast has cleared. Occasionally, however, the diagnosis is not so simple. Axial visualization of veins may simulate extravasation, but misdiagnosis can be avoided by noting venous structures leading to or away from the suspicious site. A stain of the normal mucosa, particularly a segment visualized tangentially, may simulate bleeding, but in such instances the stain is diffuse. It is important to remember that extravasated contrast medium may flow within the bowel, simulating venous opacification of an arteriovenous malformation (see Fig. 14–8A). The intraluminal contrast medium may also flow to a site somewhat remote from the actual origin of the bleeding and result in erroneous localization. In diverticular hemorrhage, contrast medium may spill into adjacent diverticula (see Fig. 14–6A), falsely suggesting simultaneous bleeding from multiple adjacent diverticula.

In Table 14–1, some common causes of angiographically demonstrable gastrointestinal bleeding are listed. Angiographic diagnosis of the cause of bleeding is largely based on the site of bleeding and the patient's history. For example, in a patient with a history of sudden onset of bleeding after emesis, extravasation at the esophagogastric junction is most likely secondary to a Mallory-Weiss tear. Bleeding from gastric or duodenal ulcers may produce a very characteristic accumulation in the crater, surrounded by radiating folds. Accumulations within colonic diverticula (see Fig. 14–5) demonstrate the characteristic contours and location of a diverticulum.

Even in patients who are not actively bleeding, the site and cause of a hemorrhage may be suggested angiographically. For example, demonstration of cecal angiodysplasia suggests that this lesion may be the site of chronic gastrointestinal hemorrhage. Diagnostic certainty requires actual demonstration of extravasation from the visualized lesion, however. Clinicians must be forewarned that demonstration of angiodysplasia

TABLE 14–1. COMPILATION OF THE RESULTS OF TRANSCATHETER HEMOSTASIS

Bleeding Source	Treatment Method	Number Treated	Favorable Results		References
			Number	Per Cent	
Exophageal varices	Vasopressin, IA*	169	112	66	10, 31, 50, 54, 58, 66
	Vasopressin, IV†	11	7	64	51
	Embolus	58	39	67	44, 64, 99
Mallory-Weiss	Vasopressin, IA	12	1	92	58, 66, 87
	Embolus	6	6	100	19, 46, 53, 83
Gastritis	Vasopressin, IA	88	65	74	1, 10, 31, 50, 58, 66, 87
	Embolus	17	11	65	19, 46, 53, 63, 83
Gastric ulcer	Vasopressin, IA	3	2	67	58, 66
	Embolus	11	10	91	83
Duodenal ulcer	Vasopressin, IA	24	10	42	10, 31, 50, 58, 87
	Embolus	17	14	82	19, 39, 46, 53, 66
Diverticulae	Vasopressin, IA	36	26	72	3, 39, 50, 66, 87
	Embolus	3	3	100	21

*IA = intra-arterial
†IV = intravenous

does not prove that it has etiologic relationship to gastrointestinal hemorrhage. A diagnostic work-up should include barium studies and endoscopy in a search for other causes of bleeding. The bowel must also be thoroughly inspected for other lesions at the time of surgery.

TRANSCATHETER THERAPY

Vasoconstrictor Infusion

Transcatheter hemostasis may be accomplished through either pharmacologic or mechanical means. Vasopressin is the most frequently used pharmacologic agent. It causes potent vasoconstrictor activity in the stomach and spleen and slightly less activity in the large and small bowels; it has little effect on renal blood flow.[33, 40] In the liver, the arterial vasoconstrictor activity is transient;[8] within a few minutes, compensatory arterial vasodilation occurs in response to decreased portal blood flow. Vasopressin is subject to little or no tachyphylaxis.[73]

The undesirable effects of intra-arterial or intravenous administration include decreased coronary blood flow and cardiac output,[7, 40, 4] an antidiuretic effect,[3] and variable degrees of systemic hypertension.[18] Decreased coronary flow and cardiac output have generally been described[40] in experimental animals and are occasionally of clinical significance.[31, 50] Despite the potent vasoconstrictor activity of vasopressin, hepatic arterial escape occurs,[8, 33, 40] and hepatic necrosis has not been documented as a complication of intra-arterial vasopressin infusion. Vasopressin infusion does not augment gastric mucosal permeability to hydrogen ions, nor does it produce gastritis—two other sequelae that had been anticipated.[36]

Nusbaum et al. originally implied that there was a therapeutic advantage of superior mesenteric arterial infusion over intravenous infusion of vasopressin.[73] This supposed advantage came into serious question after several papers demonstrated equivalent effects on portal pressure, portal flow, cardiac output, and systemic pressure.[7, 33, 55, 93] Furthermore, Johnson et al. described equivalent clinical results of intravenous and intra-arterial vasopressin infusions in patients with bleeding esophageal varices.[51] On the other hand, intra-arterial infusion seems more effective in the control of *arteriocapillary* bleeding. Athanasoulis et al. have demonstrated that selective left gastric infusion reduces left gastric flow more effectively than does intravenous or celiac infusion.[6] Several cases of arteriocapillary bleeding have now been described in which selective arterial infusion of vasopressin controlled bleeding after intravenous infusion had failed.[18, 34]

Early investigators evaluated other vasoconstrictors in addition to vasopressin.[73] Epinephrine infusion into the celiac artery produces marked vasoconstriction capable of controlling hemorrhage.[87] Epinephrine is subject to tachyphylaxis, however, which occurs within five minutes in experimental animals.[73] Furthermore, epinephrine infusion into the superior mesenteric artery does not consistently produce vasoconstriction because of beta (vasodilator) effects, although when combined with a beta blocker (propranolol), it can produce effective constriction of intestinal branches of some duration.[87, 95] Although it may reduce superior mesenteric arterial blood flow, epinephrine raises portal pressure, presumably as a result of portal venular constriction,[73] and thus is not suitable for treatment of bleeding varices. Angiotensin is unsuitable because of the rapid development of tachyphylaxis.[73]

Dose and Administration

Variceal Bleeding. Until recently, vasopressin was generally administered via selective superior mesenteric arterial infusion. The dose is 0.2 to 0.4 U per minute, continued for about 24 hours.[5, 11, 54, 66] The infusion rate is then decreased by half every 12 hours until 0.05 U per minute are infused. The vasopressin infusion is then terminated, but the catheter is left in place and infused with 5 per cent dextrose for 24 hours.

For many years, bolus intravenous injections of vasopressin have been used to control bleeding varices.[91] With the recent demonstration of approximately equivalent effects of intra-arterial and intravenous vasopressin on portal and systemic hemodynamics in dogs,[7, 33, 93] intravenous vasopressin infusion has been increasingly used clinically in the management of variceal bleeding.[51, 55, 89] The dose rate is identical to that used for superior mesenteric arterial infusion *(supra vide)*.

Arteriocapillary Bleeding. If a trial of vasopressin is planned, intra-arterial infusion is recommended; the catheter is positioned as closely to the bleeding site as possible. The infusion is usually begun at 0.2 U per minute; if bleeding is not controlled, the rate may be increased up to 0.4 U per minute. Continued bleeding is generally monitored by repeat arteriography after 20 minutes of infusion. Bleeding from the stomach or esophagus can also be evaluated by frequent examination of the gastric aspirate. If bleeding stops, the infusion is continued for 12 to 24 hours and then tapered off by 50 per cent increments, as described earlier. If bleeding has not stopped after 20 minutes of infusion, transcatheter embolization may be tried for focal arteriocapillary hemorrhage. Some patients, particularly those with gastritis, may require 12 hours of infusion before a satisfactory response occurs.[58] In general, however, we are reluctant to maintain an infusion for 12 hours in the face of continued bleeding and except in cases of gastritis and varices, generally opt for alternative therapeutic measures if bleeding persists after a 20-minute vasopressin infusion.

Although intra-arterial vasopressin has been shown to be more effective,[6, 18, 34] anecdotal reports indicate occasional cessation of lower gastrointestinal arteriocapillary bleeding after intravenous infusion. Considering the frequency of spontaneous cessation of lower gastrointestinal bleeding, the efficacy of the intravenous route remains to be clarified.

Epinephrine has been infused at the rate of 8 to 16 μg per minute into the left gastric, gastroduodenal, or inferior mesenteric artery and at 20 to 30 μg per minute into the celiac or superior mesenteric artery.[88] Prior to its injection into the superior or inferior mesenteric artery, propranolol, in the dose of 3 to 5 mg, should be administered to prevent vasodilator beta-adrenergic effects.[87, 95] Epinephrine infusions have been virtually totally replaced by vasopressin for transcatheter hemostasis of gastrointestinal bleeding.

Care of the Patient During Infusion. The infusion catheter must be sutured to the skin at the puncture site to prevent dislodgment. In order to discourage slippage, the catheter is wrapped with paper adhesive tape, and the anchor suture is passed through the tape. The external aspect of the catheter is cleansed with alcohol daily, and an antibiotic ointment is applied to the puncture site. Fluid infusion through the catheter must be maintained at all times to prevent clotting.

During infusion, the patient should be placed in an intensive care unit. The vital signs must be carefully monitored to detect inappropriate secondary hypertension and temperature, which may suggest infection. A control electrocardiogram should be obtained prior to infusion, and afterwards if symptoms of myocardial ischemia develop. Urine output must be watched, and an excessive antidiuretic effect may be corrected by furosemide.[1]

Transcatheter Embolization

A vast array of agents have been injected through the catheter in an effort to control bleeding, including metal shot,[85] various types of blood clot,[19, 88] gelatin sponge,[82] polyvinyl alcohol,[96] metal coils,[43-45, 47] and various glues.[37, 46] For short-term occlusion, we currently favor ordinary blood clot, or a clot modified with thrombin and aminocaproic acid, to delay lysis.[9, 19, 82, 83] Short-term occlusion may be adequate for clinical purposes when the underlying tissues are healthy and the bleeding stimulus is not likely to be soon repeated—as, for example, in Mallory-Weiss syndrome. When long-term occlusion is desired, we inject gelatin sponge initially, followed by a fragment of compressed polyvinyl alcohol. The initial gelatin sponge plug holds the latter in place until it can expand and set firmly. Although gelatin sponge usually lyses,[9] fibroblasts grow into the nonresorbable polyvinyl alcohol lattice, producing a permanent occlusion.[96]

Isobutyl cyanoacrylate is a liquid adhesive that polymerizes and hardens very rapidly when exposed to water.[37] We have no clinical experience with this agent and are concerned by its tendency to adhere to the catheter.[18, 37] Doppman and Hilal have recently investigated varieties of Silastic glue, with encouraging preliminary results.[35, 49] This agent hardens more slowly and passes into, and occasionally through, the capillary network. For the occlusion of relatively large arteries, Gianturco coils[37, 43] and similar devices have been utilized.

The mechanism by which embolization controls bleeding without impairing tissue viability has not been critically studied. Repeat arteriography after embolization generally demonstrates the immediate development of collateral flow,[17] which explains the absence of tissue injury. Presumably, the reduced quantity of blood flow, reduced blood pressure, and reduced pulse pressure enable natural hemostatic mechanisms to operate effectively.

Complications of Transcatheter Hemostasis

Considering the severity of illness of patients with massive gastrointestinal bleeding and the high risks of surgery,[13, 48, 63, 75, 84, 90, 97] the complication rate of transcatheter hemostasis is acceptable. Complications of vasopressin infusion, although rare, include the following:

1. Intestinal or gastric infarction[14, 25, 80, 86]
2. Cardiac ischemia or arrhythmia[31, 50]
3. Vascular occlusion at the puncture site[31, 58]
4. Sepsis[50, 54]
5. Hypertension[31]
6. Antidiuretic effects[1]

Embolization has rarely resulted in gastric or intestinal infarcts when used with or without vasopressin infusion.[19, 22, 44, 79, 83] In our opinion, embolization is a greater hazard after intestinal surgery because of operative interruption of collateral routes. Infarctions may be minimized by using the least amount of embolic material needed to completely control the hemorrhage. In one of our patients, a mycotic aneurysm formed at the site of a gelatin sponge embolus that had been deposited three months earlier. Whether this aneurysm was due to bacterial contamination of the gelatin sponge or to a sterile arteritis is unknown.

Results

For several reasons, the efficacy of transcatheter hemostasis is difficult to assess. Various investigators have evaluated (1) the frequency of the initial control of bleeding, (2) the frequency of control during the entire time of vasopressin infusion, (3) the frequency of control for five days, and (4) patient survival enabling hospital discharge. Table 14–1 summarizes satisfactory results from representative series published up to July 1977. In general, satisfactory results indicate control of hemorrhage long enough to eliminate the need for an emergency operation or until the patient dies of other causes. Only a few investigators have evaluated efficacy on the basis of patient survival.[3, 19, 31, 50, 58] Analysis of these reports indicates that many patients succumb despite control of their bleeding. Conn, in particular, points out the poor relationship between patient survival and control of hemorrhage in variceal bleeding.[31]

Common Specific Entities

ARTERIOCAPILLARY ESOPHAGEAL BLEEDING. This is most commonly due to the Mallory-Weiss syndrome, esophagitis, or esophageal injury from nasogastric tubes. Mallory-Weiss tears account for about 10 per cent of upper gastrointestinal hemorrhages and are commonly associated with a hiatal hernia.[57] In about 90 per cent of these cases, bleeding stops spontaneously or after conservative measures are taken.[57] Diagnosis is usually accomplished endoscopically.

Mallory-Weiss bleeding arises from branches of the left gastric artery and should be apparent on celiac or left gastric arteriography. The commonly associated hiatus hernia may be indicated by gastric branches projected above the diaphragm. In the minority of cases not responding to conservative measures, transcatheter hemostasis has been effective, and a trial of transcatheter therapy is strongly advocated before resorting to surgery. Vasopressin or embolus has controlled the hemorrhage in 17 of 18 reported cases (see Table 14–1 and Fig. 14–1).

VARICEAL HEMORRHAGE. Variceal hemorrhage may be suspected in a patient with a history of alcoholism or liver disease who has massive bleeding. The presence of varices usually can be diagnosed endoscopically.[16, 27, 52, 62, 69, 76] Several series point out that 10 to 40 per cent of patients with varices and upper gastrointestinal bleeding actually bleed from nonvariceal sources. Gastritis, duodenal ulcers, and Mallory-Weiss tear are particularly common causes.[30, 52, 62] Nevertheless, endoscopic differentiation of variceal and nonvariceal bleeding is said to be quite reliable, although objective confirmation is difficult to obtain.

In those cases in which the bleeding source is equivocal or possibly multiple, diagnostic angiography is indicated. Celiac and superior mesenteric arteriography usually demonstrates varices and collateral portal circulation during the venous phase. Actual venous extravasation is almost never seen after arteriography, although it may be evident after transhepatic portography.[77] The angiographic demonstration of varices, however, does not prove they are the source of bleeding. The absence of evidence of arteriocapillary bleeding elsewhere further supports an etiologic relationship between the varices and hemorrhage.

Varices may develop in and bleed from extraesophageal locations. This most frequently occurs in patients with portal hypertension who have had abdominal surgery resulting in adhesions that allow collateral flow between colonic and retroperitoneal veins.[12] In such cases, endoscopy may be normal or show nonbleeding esophageal varices, and angiography is crucial for diagnosis.

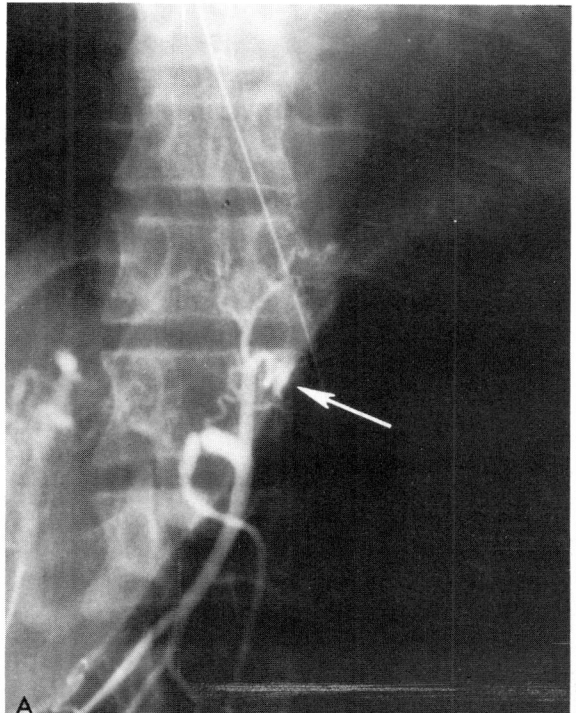
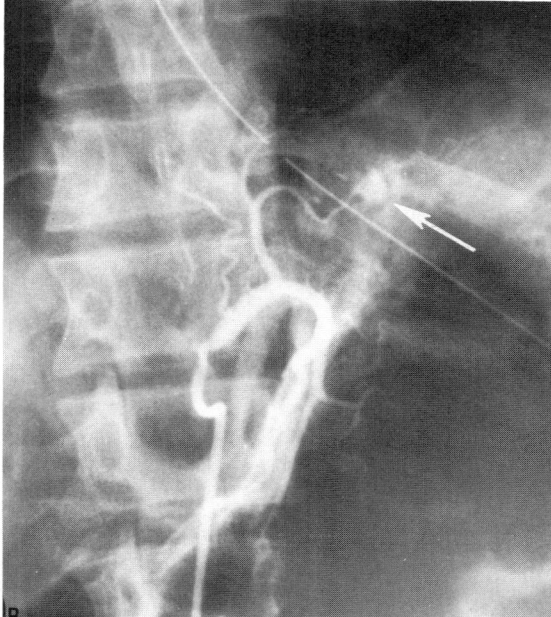
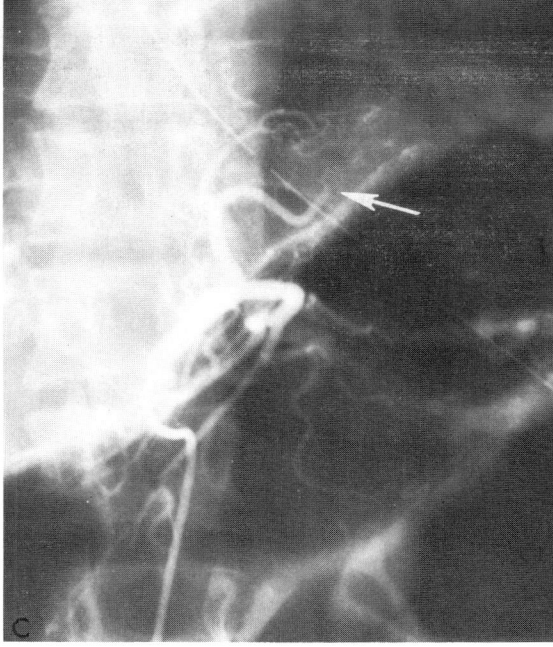

Figure 14–1. Mallory-Weiss tear treated with intravenous and intra-arterial vasopressin and embolization. The young male patient noted hematemesis after 24 hours of vomiting. Endoscopy showed a bleeding site at the esophagogastric junction. *A,* Selective left gastric arteriogram performed during intravenous infusion of 0.2 U/min vasopressin. Minor extravasation (arrow) is evident near the esophagogastric junction. *B,* Arteriogram after 20 minutes of selective left gastric infusion of vasopressin. Bleeding is reduced but continues at esophagogastric junction (arrow). Note further constriction of descending branches of the left gastric artery. *C,* Arteriogram after injection of 0.3 ml of autologous clot. Bleeding branch is occluded (arrow). Bleeding was promptly and permanently controlled, without untoward sequelae.

In variceal bleeding, angiography is frequently performed in order to plan the surgical approach rather than to localize the source of hemorrhage.[98] The venous phase of celiac or superior mesenteric arteriography demonstrates the patency of the portal, splenic, and superior mesenteric veins—critical information in planning portal decompressive surgery. Wedge hepatic manometry and venography indicate the presence and cause of portal hypertension[20] and most clearly demonstrate the direction of flow in the portal vein. Retrograde portal flow contraindicates an end-to-side portacaval shunt, since the portal vein is functioning as an outflow tract of the liver.

Vasopressin has been moderately effective in the temporary control of esophageal bleeding. One hundred twelve of one hundred sixty-nine cases (66 per cent) reported in several series[10, 31, 50, 54, 58, 66] responded favorably to superior mesenteric infusion. Favorable response was more frequent in Child's class-A patients[28] and progressively less favorable in classes B and C.[54] Despite the efficacy of vasopressin in controlling variceal hemorrhage and reducing transfusion requirements, Conn et al. could detect little survival benefit[31]; only 47 per cent and 38 per cent of patients receiving and not receiving vasopressin, respectively, survived that hospitalization.

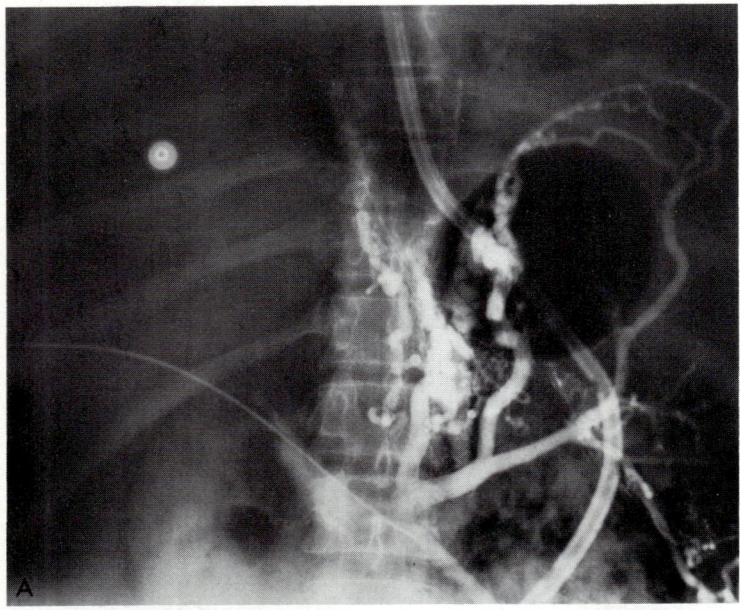

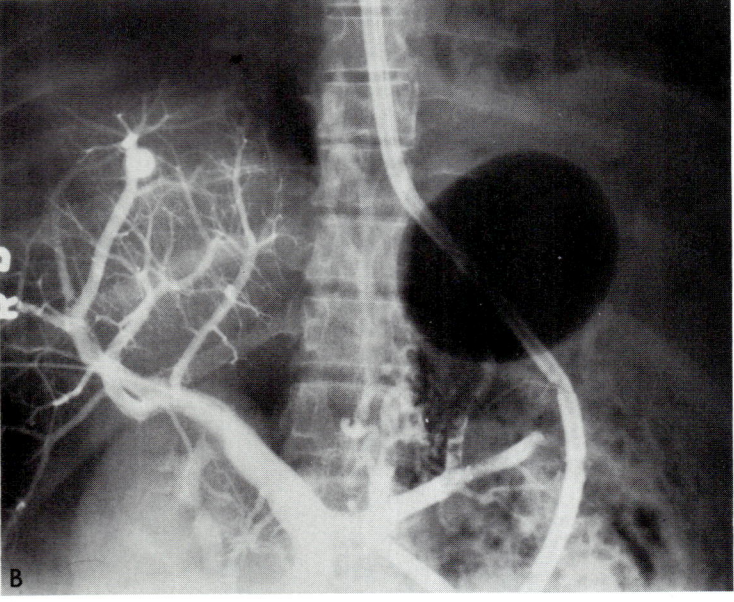

Figure 14–2. Variceal bleeding, treated by embolization. The patient, an alcoholic male with massive hematemesis, was not an operative candidate, and transhepatic embolization was performed. *A,* Splenic venogram performed via transhepatic catheter demonstrates total hepatofugal flow via gastric and esophageal varices. *B,* Repeat venogram after selective catheterization and embolization with polyvinyl alcohol (Ivalon) of short and left gastric veins. Varices are now completely occluded, and hepatofugal flow is re-established. Bleeding stopped for two days and then recurred with fatal results.

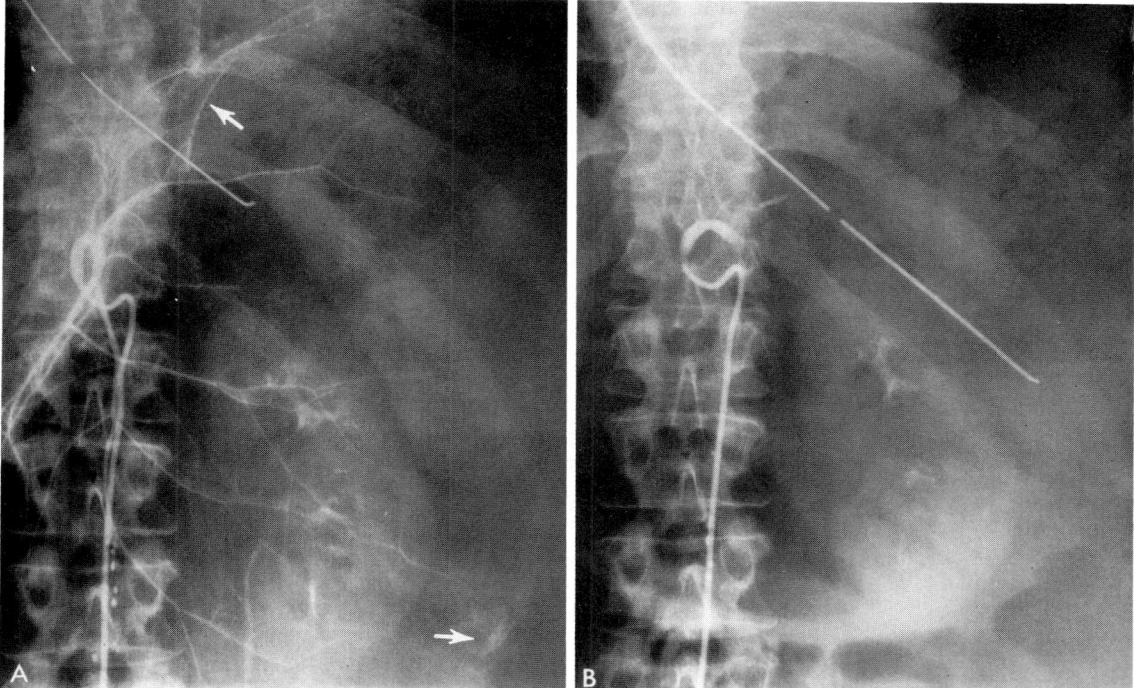

Figure 14–3. Erosive gastritis treated with vasopressin in a young man with post-traumatic quadriplegia. Endoscopy demonstrated gastritis with several erosions. A, Left gastric arteriogram demonstrates bleeding at the esophagogastric junction and along the greater curvature (arrows). Celiac injection (not shown) demonstrated additional supply to both these bleeding sites. The lesion at the esophagogastric junction was also supplied by a short gastric branch from the splenic artery, and the lesion on the greater curvature by a branch of the gastroepiploic artery. B, Arteriogram after 15 minutes of left gastric infusion of vasopressin. Flow in the left gastric artery is almost nil. The nasogastric aspirate cleared shortly after. Bleeding was permanently controlled.

Increasingly, vasopressin is being administered via intravenous infusion (supra vide).[5, 51, 55] In a prospective random study of 25 patients, Johnson et al. found no significant difference in the frequency of control when vasopressin was infused by intravenous or selective intra-arterial routes.[51] Because of its equivalent efficacy, and because of a reduced complication rate, the intravenous route has gained preference.

Within the past several years, techniques for transcatheter variceal embolization have been developed (Fig. 14–2).[60, 61, 77, 99] After lateral transabdominal puncture, a needle-catheter is passed into the liver and slowly withdrawn during continuous aspiration until a portal branch is encountered. A guide wire is then passed into the portal system, over which the catheter tip is advanced into variceal tributaries. Various embolic agents are then injected, particularly gelatin sponge, sometimes combined with a sclerosing agent.

The technique has been used both in patients who are actively bleeding and in those who have recently bled. Preliminary experience is moderately encouraging. Lunderquist reported control of bleeding for over 18 days in 8 of 21 actively bleeding patients.[61] Viamonte et al. reported similar control in 30 of 35 patients.[99] Refinements in catheterization techniques and the utilization of nonresorbable embolic materials, such as polyvinyl alcohol, may further improve the efficacy of this procedure.

ACUTE GASTRIC MUCOSAL BLEEDING. The most common causes of angiographically demonstrable gastric bleeding are hemorrhagic or erosive gastritis, stress ulcer, and ordinary gastric ulcer. In about half of the cases of gastritis, diffuse gastric hypervascularity is evident angiographically (Fig. 14–3). Despite diffuse disease in gastritis, relatively focal bleeding has often been demonstrated to arise from the lesser curvature and fundus.

Gastritis is ordinarily readily diagnosed by endoscopy,[52, 69, 76] and bleeding responds to conservative therapy in over 90 per cent of patients.[76] In the minority not responding to conservative measures, transcatheter vasopressin infusion has been highly effective.[4] Considering both cases of stress ulcer and cases of gastritis, 65 of 88 patients (74 per cent) have responded favorably to intra-arterial infusion of vasopressin (see Table 14–1). Preferably the left gastric artery is infused, but celiac infusions are also efficacious and direct the vasopressin to the left and right gastric, as well as to the gastroepiploic and short gastric, branches. In our experience, bleeding from gastritis may persist up to 24 hours after the onset of vasopressin infusion, and infusion should not be abandoned if hemostasis is not immediately achieved. Because of the diffuse nature of the gastric disease, embolism is not generally recommended.[83]

GASTRIC ULCER. In the minority of cases eluding endoscopic diagnosis, diagnostic angiography demonstrates extravasation from a gastric branch. Not uncommonly, a small aneurysm is evident at the point of bleeding, reflecting arterial destruction by the peptic process.[29] With the patient in a supine position, contrast medium accumulates within posterior ulcers and may demonstrate the crater and radiating mucosal folds characteristic of a benign ulcer.

Transcatheter therapy has not been widely applied in bleeding gastric ulcers, since an operation is usually performed. Evaluation of the role of transcatheter therapy is further limited by the fact that reported results in gastric ulcer, duodenal ulcer, and acute gastric mucosal bleeding are often not distinguished.[87, 89] Of three specifically identified bleeding gastric ulcers treated with vasopressin, two responded.[58, 66] Of 11 treated by embolization, 10 responded. In our own unpublished experience with embolization, however, only two thirds of cases remain controlled for more than 24 hours. In three of our cases, bleeding from the left gastric bed persisted after left gastric occlusion, because of collateral circulation from short gastric arteries. Despite initial control, persistent peptic disease often leads to recurrent hemorrhage. Thus, in our opinion, surgery remains the treatment of choice in most patients with major hemorrhage from chronic gastric ulcer.

DUODENAL ULCER. The cause of bleeding can be directly visualized endoscopically in 80 to 90 per cent of patients,[16, 27, 52, 69] thus usually obviating the need for diagnostic angiography. In the minority of cases requiring angiographic localization, bleeding is usually visualized arising from the posterior-superior pancreaticoduodenal or supraduodenal branches of the gastroduodenal artery. Since the supraduodenal artery also furnishes branches to the gastric antrum, it may be difficult to differentiate duodenal from antral bleeding unless multiple views are obtained. The bleeding arteries often communicate with both superior and inferior pancreaticoduodenal sources (Fig. 14–4).

Transcatheter vasopressin therapy was effective in 10 of 24 cases (42 per cent) collected from several reported series (see Table 14–1); transcatheter embolism was effective in 14 of 17 cases (82 per cent). Thus, transcatheter hemostatic techniques, particularly embolism, provide a viable alternative to emergency operation in selected cases.

BLEEDING FROM THE SMALL INTESTINE. Hemorrhage from the jejunum or ileum cannot usually be diagnosed endoscopically, and angiography is often the key diagnostic procedure. We have observed, or have found reported in the literature, numerous causes demonstrated angiographically, including marginal ulcer,[19, 66] polyps,[18] vascular dysplasia,[18] uremia,[18] regional or typhoid enteritis,[18] metastatic tumor,[41] leiomyoma,[18] jejunal diverticulum,[66] Meckel's diverticulum,[23] and benign ulcer.[18] A few cases have been successfully treated with vasopressin[66] or embolus.[19]

Figure 14–4. Massively bleeding duodenal ulcer temporarily controlled by embolization. *A*, Celiac arteriogram demonstrates extravasation (arrow). *B*, After a 20-minute vasopressin infusion into the gastroduodenal artery, bleeding has slowed but persists. Note communication with inferior pancreaticoduodenal arteries, indicating a dual source of blood supply to the bleeding site. *C*, After embolization with gelatin sponge (Gelfoam) and polyvinyl alcohol (Ivalon), bleeding stopped abruptly. Bleeding remained controlled for one and one half days, then recurred. At surgery, a very large bleeding duodenal ulcer was found, which had eroded the gastroduodenal artery.

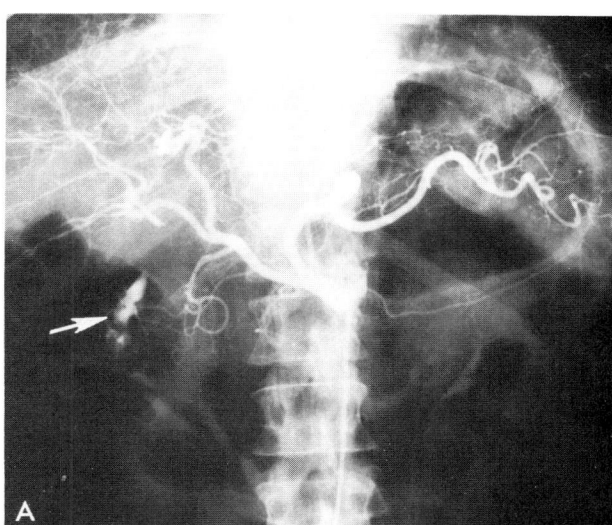
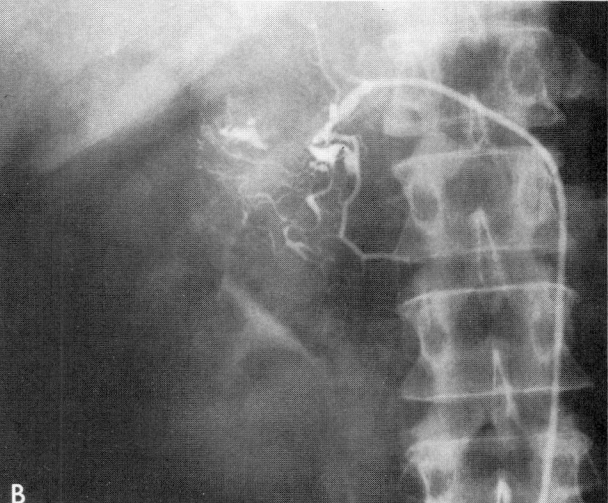
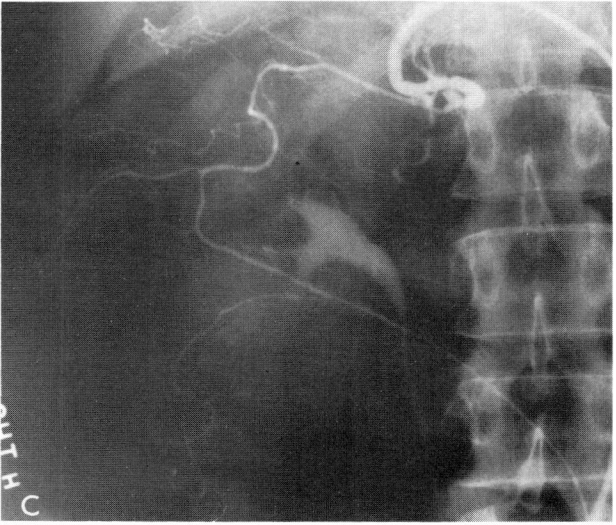

COLONIC DIVERTICULOSIS. This condition is estimated to occur in 25 per cent of patients between the ages of 60 and 70.[65] Hemorrhage of varying degrees occurs in 20 to 30 per cent of these patients, 5 per cent of these requiring hospitalization.[70, 102] Diverticulosis is the most common cause of massive lower gastrointestinal hemorrhage.[71] Although conservative management with bed rest, sedation, and blood replacement is successful in treating 70 to 80 per cent of those hospitalized, operative intervention is frequently necessary. Colonoscopy is generally unrewarding. Prior to the general application of mesenteric angiography, identification of the bleeding diverticulum was infrequent, and when surgery was required there was little alternative to empirical segmental or subtotal colonic resection. Angiography, however, generally enables specific identification of the bleeding diverticulum (Figs. 14–5 and 14–6) and has had a major impact on the management of such cases. Significantly, diverticular hemorrhage arises from the ascending or transverse colon in 75 per cent of cases,[26, 38] despite the predominance of diverticula in the descending and sigmoid colon. Bleeding is probably related to the intimate association between the diverticulum and the perforating colonic branches.[68]

Emergency colectomy for colonic diverticular hemorrhage is associated with a high mortality rate. Of the 99 cases covered in 5 recent reports,[13, 48, 74, 84, 97] the mortality rate was 28 per cent. Morbidity was also significant. Elective colectomy is probably associated with less risk.[3]

Athanasoulis et al. have utilized transcatheter vasopressin infusion of bleeding

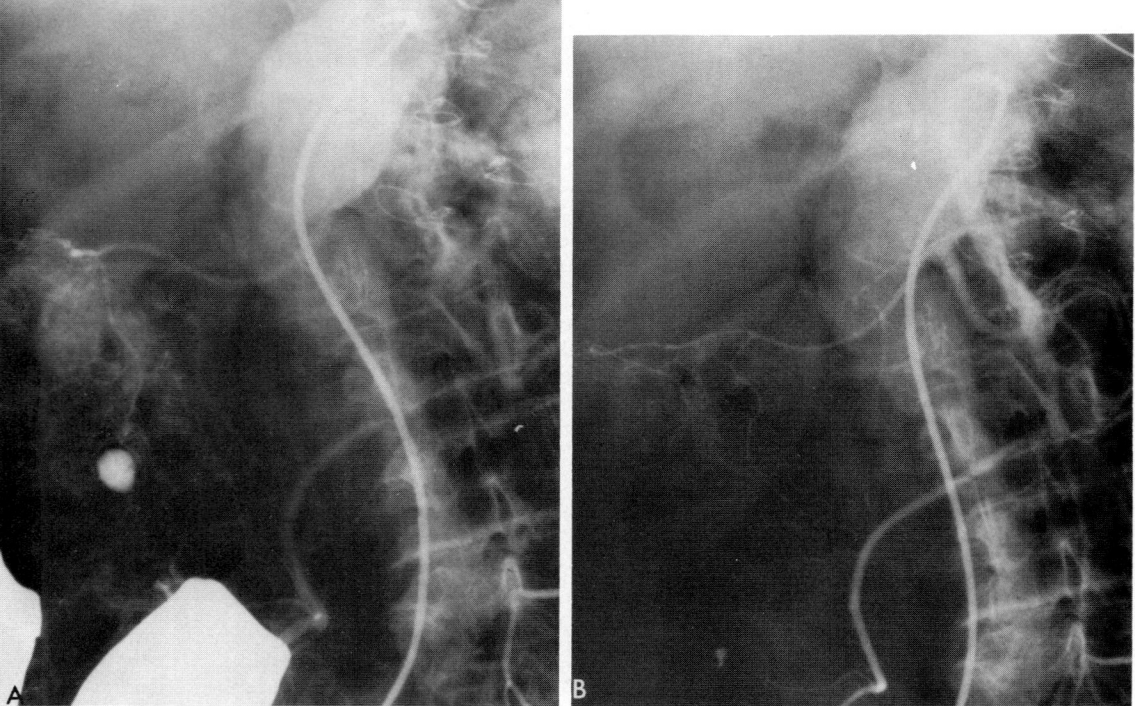

Figure 14–5. Diverticular bleeding temporarily controlled after vasopressin infusion. *A,* Late phase of superior mesenteric arteriogram demonstrates intraluminal accumulation of contrast medium with characteristic position and contours of a diverticulum of the ascending colon. *B,* After a 20-minute infusion of 0.2 U/min vasopressin into the superior mesenteric artery, arterial branches have constricted and bleeding has stopped. Bleeding recurred at 12 hours, and emergency right colectomy was performed.

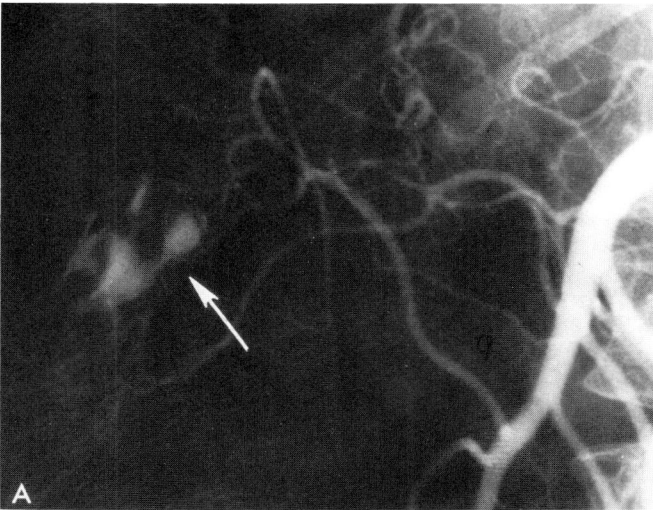

Figure 14–6. Diverticular bleeding permanently controlled by embolization. *A,* Extravasation from a bleeding diverticulum of the ascending colon (arrow) is seen. *B,* After a superior mesenteric arterial infusion of vasopressin, bleeding slows but does not stop. *C,* After embolization, the embolus (arrow) occludes the bleeding artery. Hemorrhage was immediately controlled. No rebleeding has occurred for 18 months.

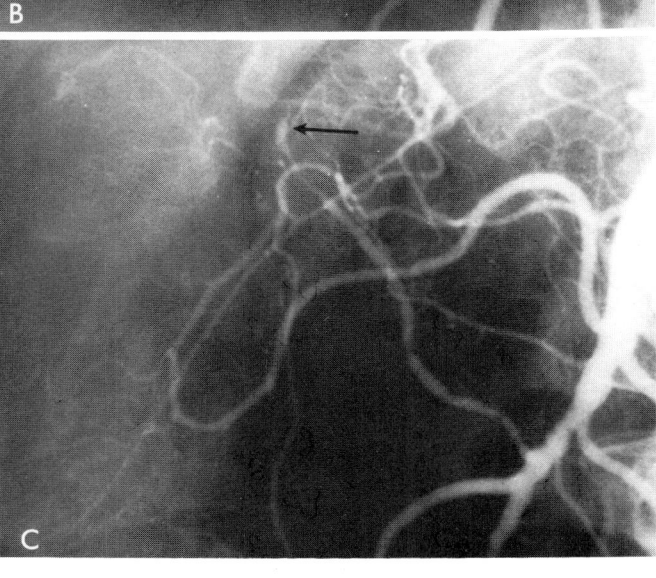

diverticula as an alternative to emergency operation.[3] Immediate control was obtained in 22 of 24 patients. Five patients underwent elective resection a few days after initial control, and 5 of the remaining 17 underwent emergency surgery for rebleeding within a week. Of 12 patients discharged without surgery, 3 had recurrence of bleeding within a year, and 2 underwent resection. Thus, of 24 patients, 14 eventually required some form of colectomy.

On the other hand, we have successfully employed transcatheter embolization in five patients with diverticular bleeding who failed to respond to vasopressin.[18, 21] None of these patients had experienced bleeding from the embolized diverticulum, although one bled from a diverticulum in a remote location. There were no complications.

It is now clear that angiographic localization is generally indicated before surgery for lower gastrointestinal bleeding. Furthermore, transcatheter therapy usually deserves trial in order to avoid the high mortality rate associated with emergency colectomy. Control after vasopressin infusion is often temporary. If transcatheter embolization continues to produce consistent and permanent control, it should become the therapeutic method of choice.

COLONIC ANGIODYSPLASIA. Colonic angiodysplasia is, in our experience, the second most common cause of massive lower gastrointestinal bleeding and the most common cause of chronic lower gastrointestinal bleeding.[5, 12, 17, 26, 92] The lesions may be located anywhere within the colon but most frequently involve the cecum and ascending colon (Fig. 14–7). They are frequently multiple, larger lesions being near the cecum and smaller ones extending to the hepatic flexure. Histologically, they consist of tortuous, dilated submucosal and mucosal vessels. The overlying mucosa may be ulcerated. The lesions may be difficult or impossible to detect at surgery or upon direct inspection of the operative specimen. *In vitro* intravascular injection of colored Silastic facilitates their demonstration.[11]

Angiographically, the lesions appear as tangled vascular networks. Sometimes the vessels are too small to be separately resolved, and the lesion appears as an amorphous blush. Early or dense venous opacification is almost always evident and is usually the first clue to the angiographic diagnosis.[17] Bleeding tends to be less massive than from diverticulosis, and actual extravasation is not usually demonstrable angiographically.[17]

The angiodysplasias are usually treated surgically. Transcatheter therapy has been applied in only five reported cases.[18, 66, 87] Bleeding was controlled initially in each. In one patient treated with vasopressin infusion, bleeding recurred after 48 hours, requiring an emergency operation.[66] The presence or absence of rebleeding was not reported in two other cases treated by vasopressin.[87] In two cases treated with embolus, rebleeding occurred three and four months after embolization.[21]

OTHER CAUSES. Other causes of colonic bleeding have occasionally been diagnosed and treated through the angiographic catheter. Colitis has responded in three cases.[24, 87] In one patient, rectal bleeding secondary to fecal disimpaction was successfully treated by intra-arterial vasopressin after intravenous vasopressin had failed (Fig. 14–8).[34] Other causes of angiographically identified low rectal or anal bleeding have included episiotomy and trauma from a rectal thermometer.

MISCELLANEOUS. Three cases of postbiopsy hematobilia have been treated by transcatheter embolism.[67, 78, 100] Gelatin sponge produced permanent control in each.

Gastrointestinal bleeding may originate from pancreatic disease, most frequently from sequelae of pancreatitis.[101] Transcatheter vasopressin infusion, embolization, and balloon tamponade have been used to control temporarily the bleeding from pseudocysts,[101] with significant benefit in each of our five cases.[18]

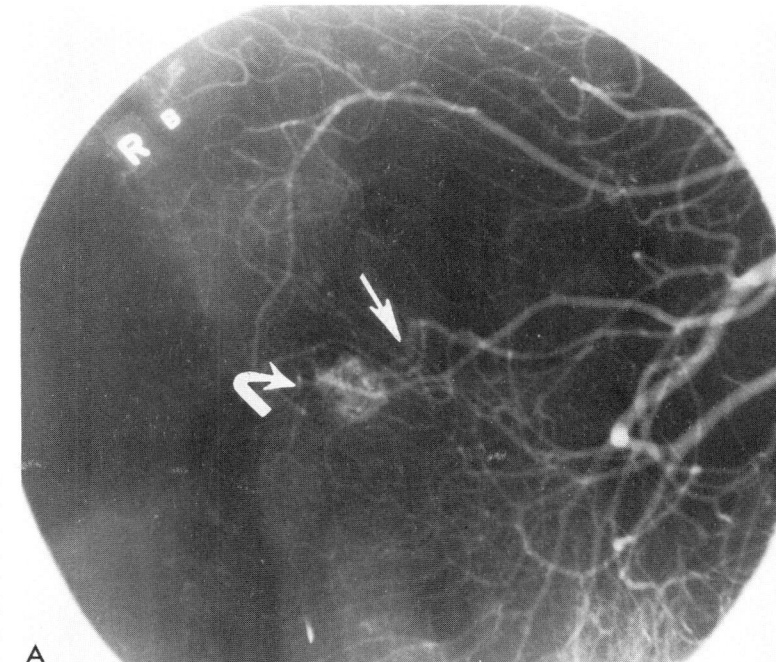

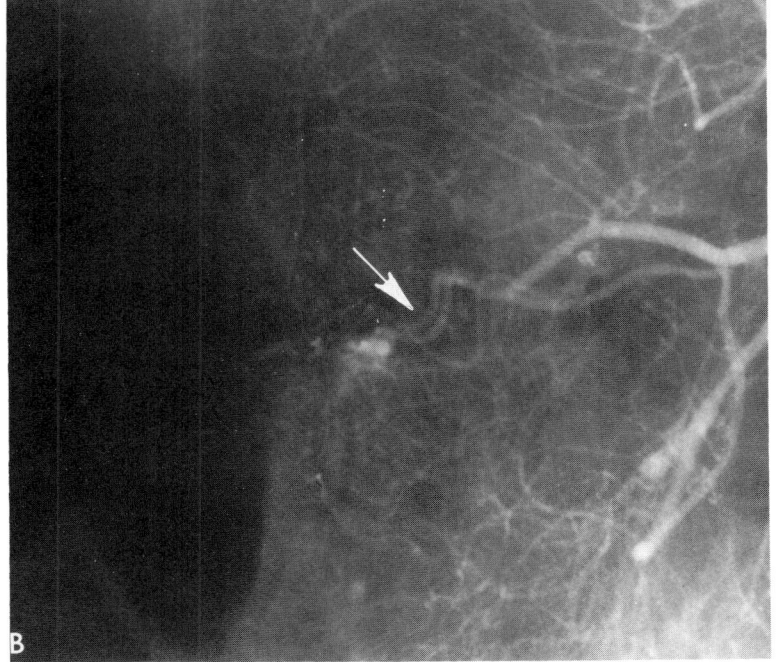

Figure 14–7. Angiodysplasia temporarily controlled by embolization. This woman had five episodes of major lower gastrointestinal bleeding in six months. After embolization, bleeding recurred after four months, and the lesion was surgically excised. *A,* Angiography demonstrates angiodysplasia of the cecum (curved arrow). Note the tangled cluster of vessels and early venous opacification (straight arrow). *B,* After embolization with polyvinyl alcohol (ivalon), the malformation is partially obliterated, although early venous opacification persists (arrow).

Transcatheter hemostasis may be particularly appropriate in instances of bleeding after gastrointestinal surgery. Bleeding may arise from ligated or cauterized arteries or the pedicle of a snared polyp. Once the bleeding is controlled, it is unlikely to recur. Thus, successful transcatheter hemostasis generally obviates the need for a second abdominal operation. Athanasoulis et al. successfully controlled 9 of 11 postoperative bleeders by vasopressin infusion.[2]

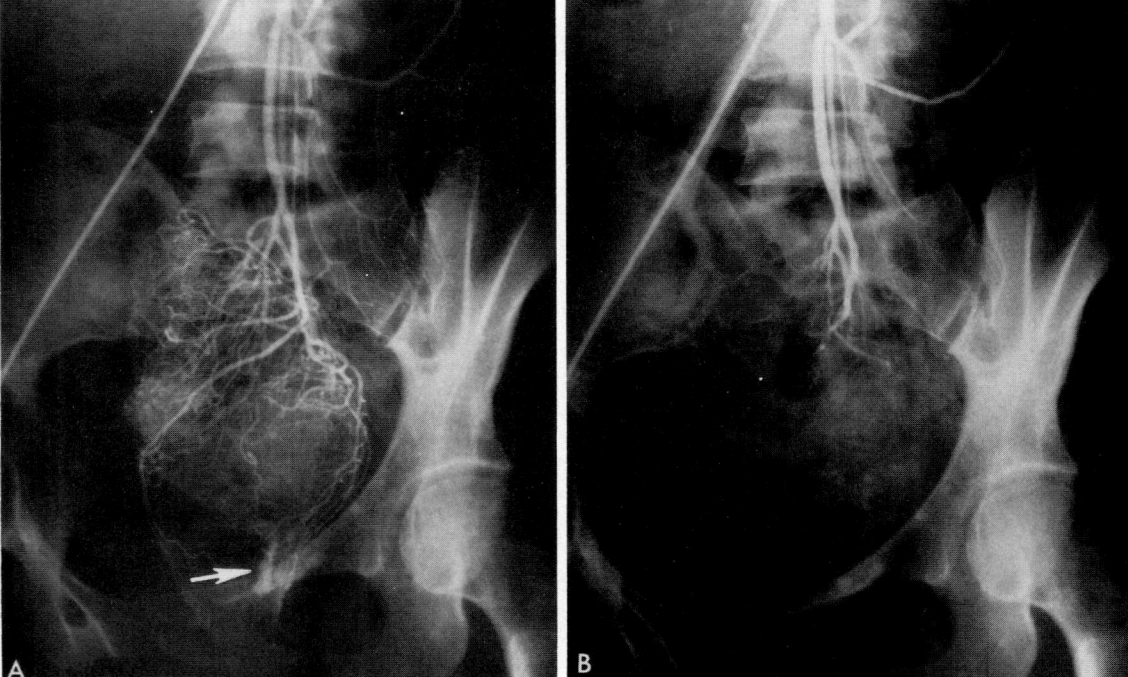

Figure 14-8. Rectal laceration treated with vasopressin. This woman began to bleed rectally several days after fecal disimpaction. Sigmoidoscopy did not demonstrate the bleeding site. *A*, Inferior mesenteric arteriography performed during intravenous infusion of vasopressin at the rate of 0.2 U/min demonstrates extravasation at the rectoanal junction (arrow). *B*, After infusion of the same solution of vasopressin at the same rate into the inferior mesenteric artery, bleeding stopped immediately and permanently.

General Considerations

Transcatheter hemostasis is generally indicated to either (1) avoid an operation or (2) convert an emergency to an elective operation. There is little question regarding the justification for transcatheter hemostasis when it obviates the need for major surgery provided it can be performed expeditiously, safely, and effectively. Thus, a trial of transcatheter hemostasis is preferable to an operation in cases of bleeding resulting from Mallory-Weiss tears, gastritis, diverticulosis, or following gastrointestinal surgery. Transcatheter hemostasis may not permanently control bleeding from chronic duodenal or gastric ulcer, so that risk-benefit ratios must be individually assessed in patients with these ailments.

Even in cases that eventually require surgery, transcatheter hemostasis may be beneficial, because it may enable elective, rather than emergency, surgery. In a large series reported by Schiller, emergency surgery for upper gastrointestinal bleeding was associated with a 20 per cent mortality rate, whereas elective surgery carried only a 7 per cent mortality rate.[90] The study was not prospectively randomized, however, and it can be argued that the more severely bleeding patients required emergency operations, a possibility that would explain the higher mortality rate.

McGinn more directly examined the risk of emergency versus elective surgery.[63] In both controlled animal experiments and uncontrolled clinical data, recent hemorrhage itself appeared to have a significant adverse effect on survival.

In cases of lower gastrointestinal bleeding, emergency operations are associated with a considerably higher mortality rate than elective ones.[3, 13, 97] The opportunity to prepare the bowel with antibiotics and to improve the generally poor condition of these elderly patients makes elective surgery preferable. The efficacy of transcatheter technique in controlling lower gastrointestinal bleeding indicates that emergency colectomy can usually be avoided.[2, 3, 20, 21] Furthermore, transcatheter embolization may obviate the need for an operation altogether.

At what point in the course of a bleeding episode is *diagnostic angiography* indicated? No firm answer is available. Mortality rates rise with increasing transfusion requirements. According to Schiller's report, operations on patients who receive less than 4 U of blood are associated with a significantly lower mortality rate than operations on patients who require 10 U or more.[90] Thus, an aggressive diagnostic and therapeutic approach to gastrointestinal bleeding is generally recommended. If active bleeding persists after transfusion with 2 U of blood and the bleeding source is unknown after endoscopy, diagnostic angiography is recommended. Following angiographic demonstration of the bleeding site, a trial of transcatheter therapy is usually indicated regardless of the source of bleeding, since the catheter is already in place.

Angiography is frequently indicated for therapeutic purposes, even when the source of bleeding is already known. This is particularly true in patients with continued bleeding owing to a Mallory-Weiss tear, gastritis, or diverticulosis, in which cases the efficacy of transcatheter therapy is high. In such patients, transcatheter therapy should generally be initiated if bleeding continued after 2 U of blood have been transfused. Transcatheter therapy is also frequently indicated for cases of bleeding from less favorably responding lesions when patients are poor operative risks.

In summary, angiography has come to play an important role in the management of gastrointestinal bleeding. This role is being constantly revised in keeping with continuing technical development and clinical experience. In properly selected cases, transcatheter therapy offers an effective alternative to surgery.

References

1. Athanasoulis, C. A., Baum, S., Waltman, A. C., et al.: Control of acute gastric mucosal hemorrhage. Intra-arterial infusion of posterior pituitary extract. N. Engl. Med. J. *290:*597–603, 1974.
2. Athanasoulis, C. A., Waltman, A. C., Ring, E. J., et al.: Angiographic management of postoperative bleeding. Radiology *113:*37–42, 1974.
3. Athanasoulis, C. A., Baum, S., Rösch, J., et al.: Mesenteric arterial infusion of vasopressin for hemorrhage from colonic diverticulosis. Am. J. Surg. *129:*212–216, 1975.
4. Athanasoulis, C. A.: Angiographic methods for the control of gastric hemorrhage. Am. J. Dig. Dis. *21:*174–181, 1976.
5. Athanasoulis, C. A., Waltman, A. C., and Novelline, R. P.: Angiography: its contribution to the emergency management of gastrointestinal hemorrhage. Radiol. Clin. North Am. *14:*265–280, 1976.
6. Athanasoulis, C. A., Simmons, J. T., Sheehan, B., et al.: Gastric blood flow alterations during intra-arterial and systemic infusion of vasopressin. Abstract. Assoc. Univ. Radiol. Kansas City, 1977.
7. Barr, J. W., Lakin, R. C., and Rösch, J.: Similarity of arterial and intravenous vasopressin on portal and systemic hemodynamics. Gastroenterology, *69:*13–19, 1975.
8. Barr, J. W., Lakin, R. C., and Rösch, J.: Vasopressin and hepatic artery. Effect of selective celiac infusion of vasopressin on the hepatic artery flow. Invest. Radiol. *10:*200–205, 1975.
9. Barth, K., Standberg, J., and White, R. I.: Long term follow-up of transcatheter embolization with autologous clot, Oxycel, and gelfoam in domestic swine. Invest. Radiol. *12:*273–280, 1977.
10. Baum, S., and Nusbaum, M.: The control of gastrointestinal hemorrhage by selective mesenteric arterial infusion of vasopressin. Radiology *98:*497–505, 1971.
11. Baum, S., Athanasoulis, C. A., Waltman, A. C., et al.: Gastrointestinal hemorrhage. Part II. Angiographic diagnosis and control. Adv. Surg. *7:*149–190, 1973.

12. Baum, S., Athanasoulis, C. A., and Waltman, A. C.: Angiography in the diagnosis and therapy of hemorrhage from the large bowel. Radiology 15:427–433, 1975.
13. Behringer, G., and Albright, N.: Diverticular disease of the colon: a frequent case of massive rectal bleeding. Am. J. Surg. 125:419–423, 1973.
14. Berardi, R. S.: Vascular complications of superior mesenteric artery infusion with pitressin in treatment of bleeding esophageal varices. Am. J. Surg. 127:757–761, 1974.
15. Berkowitz, D.: Fatal gastrointestinal hemorrhage: diagnostic implications from a study of 200 cases. Am. J. Gastroenterol. 40:372–377, 1963.
16. Blumgart, L. A.: Endoscopy of the upper gastrointestinal tract. Adv. Surg. 9:97–138, 1975.
17. Boley, S. J., Sprayregen, S., Sammantano, R. J., et al.: The pathophysiologic basis for the angiographic signs of vascular features of the colon. Radiology 125:615–621, 1977.
18. Bookstein, J. J.: Unreported observations.
19. Bookstein, J. J., Chlosta, E. M., Foley, D., et al.: Transcatheter hemostasis of gastrointestinal bleeding using modified autogenous clot. Radiology 113:277–285, 1974.
20. Bookstein, J. J., Appelman, H. D., Walter, J. F., et al.: Histological venographic correlates in portal hypertension. Radiology 116:565–573, 1975.
21. Bookstein, J. J., Naderi, M., and Walters, J.: Transcatheter embolization for lower GI hemorrhage. Radiology 127:345–349, 1978.
22. Bradley, E. L., and Goldman, M. L.: Gastric infarction after therapeutic embolization. Surgery 79:421–424, 1976.
23. Bree, R. L., and Reuter, S. R.: Angiographic demonstration of bleeding Meckel's diverticulum. Radiology 108:287–288, 1973.
24. Calavaluzzi, J. A., Kaufman, S. L., and White, R. I.: Vasopressin control of massive hemorrhage in chronic ulcerative colitis. Am. J. Roentgenol. 127:672–675, 1976.
25. Campbell, D. R., Mason, W. F., Fraser, D. B., et al.: Angiography in gastrointestinal bleeding. J. Can. Assoc. Radiol. 28:26–32, 1977.
26. Casarella, W. J., Galloway, S. J., Taxin, R. N., et al.: "Lower" gastrointestinal tract hemorrhage: new concepts based on arteriography. Am. J. Roentgenol. 121:357–368, 1974.
27. Cayton, R. M., and Smith, F. W.: Pan-endoscopy in the early diagnosis of acute upper gastrointestinal bleeding. Gastroenterology 65:728–734, 1973.
28. Child, C. G.: The Liver and Portal Hypertension. Philadelphia, W. B. Saunders Company, 1964.
29. Clemens, F.: False aneurysm associated with gastric ulcer. Report of a case. Radiology 101:85–86, 1971.
30. Conn, H. O., and Brodoff, M.: Emergency esophagoscopy in the diagnosis of upper gastrointestinal hemorrhage. Gastroenterology 47:505–512, 1964.
31. Conn, H. O., Ramsby, G. R., Stoher, E. H., et al.: Intra-arterial vasopressin in the treatment of upper gastrointestinal hemorrhage: a prospective, controlled clinical trial. Gastroenterology 68:211–221, 1975.
32. Dalinka, M. K., Gohel, V. K., Schaffer, B., et al.: Gastrointestinal complications of aortic bypass surgery. Clin. Radiol. 27:255–258, 1976.
33. Davis, G. B., Bookstein, J. J., and Hagan, P. L.: The relative effects of selective intra-arterial and intravenous vasopressin infusion. Radiology 120:537–538, 1976.
34. Davis, G. B., Bookstein, J. J., and Cole, M. N.: Advantage of intra-arterial over intravenous vasopressin infusion in gastrointestinal hemorrhage. Am. J. Roentgenol. 128:733–735, 1977.
35. Doppman, J. L., Sapol, W., and Pierce, V.: Transcatheter embolization with a silicone rubber preparation. Invest. Radiol. 6:304–309, 1971.
36. Dorricott, N. H., Eisenberg, H., and Silen, W.: Effect of intra-arterial vasopressin on canine gastric mucosal permeability. Gastroenterology 65:625–629, 1973.
37. Dotter, C. T., Goldman, M. L., and Rösch, J.: Instant selective arterial occlusion with isobutyl 2-cyanoacrylate. Radiology 114:227–230, 1975.
38. Eisenberg, H., Laufer, I., and Skillman, J. V.: Arteriographic diagnosis and management of suspected colonic diverticular bleeding. Gastroenterology 64:1091–1100, 1973.
39. Eisenberg, H., and Steer, M.: The non-operative treatment of massive pyloduodenal hemorrhage by autogenous clot embolization. Surgery 79:414, 1976.
40. Ericsson, B. F.: Hemodynamic effects of vasopressin. An experimental study of normovolemic and hypovolemic anesthetized dogs. Acta Chir. Scand. (Suppl.) 414:1–29, 1971.
41. Evans, T. N., Zuidema, G. D., Anderson, D. G., et al.: Metastatic chorio-adenoma destruens with intestinal hemorrhage. Obstet. Gynecol. 26:570–574, 1965.
42. Fisher, C. V., Sheff, R. N., Novak, G., et al.: The effect of superior mesenteric artery vasopressin infusions on cardiac output and coronary blood flow in dogs. Invest. Radiol. 9:456–461, 1974.
43. Gianturco, C., Anderson, J. H., and Wallace, S.: Mechanical devices for arterial occlusion. Am. J. Roentgenol. 124:425–428, 1975.
44. Goldstein, H. M., Medellin, H., Ben-Menachem, Y., et al.: Transarterial embolization in the management of bleeding in the cancer patient. Radiology 115:603–608, 1975.
45. Goldstein, H. M., Medellin, H., Beydoun, M. T., et al.: Transcatheter embolization of renal cell carcinoma. Am. J. Roentgenol. 123:557–562, 1975.
46. Goldman, M. L., Land, W. C., Bradley, E. L., et al.: Transcatheter therapeutic embolization in the management of massive upper gastrointestinal bleeding. Radiology 120:513–521, 1976.

47. Goldstein, H. M., Wallace, S., and Anderson, J. H., et al.: Transcatheter occlusion of abdominal tumors. Radiology 120:539–545, 1976.
48. Griffin, J. M., Butcher, H. R., and Ackerman, L. V.: Surgical management of colonic diverticulitis. Arch. Surg. 94:619–626, 1967.
49. Hilal, S. K., and Michelsen, J. W.: Therapeutic percutaneous embolization for extra-axial vascular lesions of the head, neck and spine. J. Neurosurg. 43:275–287, 1975.
50. Johnson, W. C., and Widrich, W. C.: Efficacy of selective splenic arteriography and vasopressin perfusion in diagnosis and treatment of gastrointestinal hemorrhage. Am. J. Surg. 131:481–489, 1976.
51. Johnson, W. C., Widrich, W. C., Ansell, J. E., et al.: Control of bleeding varices by vasopressin: a prospective randomized study. Ann. Surg. 186:369–374, 1977.
52. Josen, A. S., Giuliani, E., Voorhees, A. B., et al.: Immediate endoscopic diagnosis of upper gastrointestinal bleeding. Arch. Surg. 111:980–986, 1976.
53. Katzen, B. T., Rossi, P., Passariello, R., et al.: Transcatheter therapeutic arterial embolization. Radiology 120:523–531, 1976.
54. Kaufman, S. L., Harrington, D. P., Barth, K. H., et al.: Control of variceal bleeding by superior mesenteric artery vasopressin infusion. Am. J. Roentgenol. 128:567–569, 1977.
55. Kaufman, S. L., Maddrey, W. C., Harrington, D. P., et al.: Hemodynamic effects of intra-arterial and intravenous vasopressin infusions in patients with portal hypertension. Assoc. Univ. Radiol. Kansas City, 1977.
56. Klein, H. J., Alfidi, R. J., Meaney, T. F., et al.: Angiography in the diagnosis of chronic gastrointestinal bleeding. Radiology 98:83–91, 1971.
57. Knauer, C. M.: Mallory-Weiss syndrome. Characterization of 75 Mallory-Weiss lacerations in 528 patients with upper gastrointestinal hemorrhage. Gastroenterology 71:5–8, 1976.
58. Komaki, S., and Sunday, M. T.: Angiographic management of acute gastrointestinal hemorrhage. Wis. Med. J. 75:50–53, 1976.
59. Logan, R. F. A., and Finlayson, N. D. C.: Death in acute upper gastrointestinal bleeding. Can endoscopy reduce mortality? Lancet 1:1173–1175, 1976.
60. Lunderquist, A., and Vang, J.: Transhepatic catheterization and obliteration of the coronary vein in patients with portal hypertension and esophageal varices. N. Engl. J. Med. 291:646–649, 1974.
61. Lunderquist, A., Simert, G., Tyler, U., et al.: Follow-up of patients with portal hypertension and esophageal varices treated with percutaneous obliteration of gastric coronary vein. Radiology 122:59–63, 1977.
62. McCray, R. S., Martin, F., and Amirahmade, H.: Erroneous diagnosis of hemorrhage from esophageal varices. Am. J. Dig. Dis. 14:755–759, 1969.
63. McGinn, F. P.: Effects of hemorrhage upon surgical operations. Br. J. Surg. 63:742–746, 1976.
64. Margulis, A. R., Heinbecker, P., and Bernard, H. R.: Operative mesenteric arteriography in the search for the site of bleeding in unexplained gastrointestinal hemorrhage. Surgery 48:534–539, 1960.
65. Massive bleeding from diverticular disease of the colon. Editorial. Lancet 1:706–707, 1963.
66. Melson, G. L., Gissie, G., and Stanley, R. J.: Selective intra-arterial infusion of vasopressin for control of gastrointestinal bleeding: experience with 35 cases. Gastrointest. Radiol. 1:59–65, 1976.
67. Merino-deVillasante, J., Alvarez-Rodriquez, R. E., and Hernandez-Ortiz, J.: Management of post-biopsy hemobilia with selective arterial embolization. Am. J. Roentgenol. 128:668–671, 1977.
68. Meyers, M., Alonso, D. R., and Baer, J.: Pathogenesis of massively bleeding colonic diverticulosis: new observations. Am. J. Roentgenol. 127:901–908, 1976.
69. Morris, D. W., Levine, G. M., Soloway, R. D., et al.: Prospective randomized study of diagnosis and outcome in acute upper gastrointestinal bleeding: endoscopy versus conventional radiography. Am. J. Dig. Dis. 20:1103–1109, 1975.
70. Noer, R. J.: Hemorrhage as a complication of diverticulitis. Ann. Surg. 141:674–685, 1955.
71. Noer, R. J.: Rectal hemorrhage. Ann. Surg. 155:794–805, 1962.
72. Nusbaum, M., and Baum, S.: Radiographic demonstration of unknown sites of gastrointestinal bleeding. Surg. Forum 14:374–375, 1963.
73. Nusbaum, M., Baum, S., Sakiyalak, P., et al.: Pharmacologic control of portal hypertension. Surgery 62:299–310, 1967.
74. Olsen, W. R.: Hemorrhage from diverticular disease of the colon. The role of emergency subtotal colectomy. Am. J. Surg. 115:247–263, 1968.
75. Orloff, M. J., Chandler, J. G., Charters, A. C., et al.: Emergency portacaval shunt treatment for bleeding esophageal varices. Arch. Surg. 108:293–299, 1974.
76. Palmer, E. D.: The vigorous diagnostic approach to upper gastrointestinal tract hemorrhage. A 23 year prospective study of 1400 patients. J.A.M.A. 207:1477–1489, 1969.
77. Pereiras, R., Viamonte, M., Russell, E., et al.: New techniques for interruption of gastroesophageal venous blood flow. Radiology 124:313–323, 1977.
78. Perlberger, R.: Control of hemobilia by angiographic embolization. Am. J. Roentgenol. 128:672–673, 1977.
79. Prochaska, J. M., Flye, M. W., and Johnsrude, I. S.: Left gastric embolization for control of gastric bleeding: a complication. Radiology 107:521–522, 1973.
80. Renert, W. A., Button, K. F., Fuld, S. I., et al.: Mesenteric venous thrombosis and small bowel infarction following infusion of vasopressin into the superior mesenteric artery. Radiology 102:299–302, 1972.

81. Reuter, S. R., and Bookstein, J. J.: Angiographic localization of gastrointestinal bleeding. Gastroenterology 54:876–883, 1968.
82. Reuter, S. R., and Chuang, V. P.: Control of abdominal bleeding with autogenous embolized material. Radiology 14:86–91, 1974.
83. Reuter, S. R., Chuang, V. P., and Bree, R. L.: Selective arterial embolization for control of massive upper gastrointestinal bleeding. Am. J. Roentgenol. 125:119–126, 1975.
84. Rigg, B. M., and Ewing, M. R.: Current attitudes on diverticulitis with particular reference to colonic bleeding. Arch. Surg. 92:321–332, 1966.
85. Rizk, G. K.: Successful management of postbiopsy arteriovenous fistula with selective arterial embolization. Radiology 109:535–536, 1973.
86. Roberts, C., and Maddison, F. E.: Partial mesenteric arterial occlusion with subsequent ischemic bowel damage due to pitressin infusion. Am. J. Roentgenol. 126:829–831, 1976.
87. Rösch, J., Dotter, C. T., and Antonovic, R.: Selective vasoconstrictor infusion in the management of arterio-capillary gastrointestinal hemorrhage. Am. J. Roentgenol. 116:279–288, 1972.
88. Rösch, J., Dotter, C. T., and Brown, M. J.: Selective arterial embolization. A new method for control of acute gastrointestinal bleeding. Radiology 102:303–306, 1972.
89. Rösch, J., Antonovic, R., and Dotter, C. T.: Current angiographic approach to diagnosis and therapy of acute gastrointestinal bleeding. Fortschr. Geb. Roentgenstr. Nuklearmed. 125:301–310, 1976.
90. Schiller, K. F. R., Truelove, S. C., and Williams, D. G.: Haematemesis and melena with special reference to factors influencing the outcome. Br. Med. J. 2:7–14, 1970.
91. Shaldon, S., and Sherlock, S.: The use of vasopressin (pitressin) in the control of bleeding from esophageal varices. Lancet 2:222–225, 1960.
92. Sheedy, P. F., Fulton, R. E., and Atwell, D. J.: Angiographic evaluation of patients with chronic gastrointestinal bleeding. Am. J. Roentgenol. 123:338–347, 1975.
93. Sirinek, K., Thomford, N. R., and Pace, W. G.: Adverse cardiodynamic effect of vasopressin not avoided by selective intra-arterial administration. Surgery 81:723–728, 1977.
94. Smith, D. C., and Kidching, G. B.: Angiographic demonstrations of esophagogastric bleeding from the inferior phrenic artery. Radiology 125:613–614, 1977.
95. Steckel, R. J., Ross, G., and Grollman, J. H.: A potent drug combination for producing constriction of the superior mesenteric artery and its branches. Radiology 91:579–581, 1968.
96. Tadavarthy, S. M., Moller, J. H., and Amplatz, K.: Polyvinyl alcohol (Ivalon)—a new embolic material. Am. J. Roentgenol. 125:609–616, 1975.
97. Taylor, F. W., and Epstein, L. I.: Treatment of massive diverticular hemorrhage. Arch. Surg. 98:505–508, 1969.
98. Turcott, J. G., and Lambert, M. J.: Variceal hemorrhage, hepatic cirrhosis and portacaval shunts. Surgery 73:801–817, 1973.
99. Viamonte, M., Pereiras, R., Russell, E., et al.: Transhepatic obliteration of gastro-esophageal varices: results in acute and non-acute bleeders. Am. J. Roentgenol. 129:237–241, 1977.
100. Walter, J. F., Paaso, B. T., and Cannon, W. B.: Successful transcatheter embolic control of massive hematobilia secondary to liver biopsy. Am. J. Roentgenol. 127:847–849, 1976.
101. Walter, J. F., Chuang, V. P., Bookstein, J. J., et al.: Angiography of massive hemorrhage secondary to pancreatic disease. Radiology 124:337–342, 1977.
102. Welch, C. E., and Hedberg, S.: Gastrointestinal hemorrhage. Part I. General considerations of diagnosis and therapy. Adv. Surg. 7:95–148, 1973.
103. Wholey, M. H., Stockdale, R., and Hunt, T. K.: A percutaneous balloon catheter for the immediate control of hemorrhage. Radiology 95:65–71, 1970.

15

THE LIVER

HENRY I. GOLDBERG, M.D.
ROBERT KOEHLER, M.D.

INTRODUCTION

Many radiologic techniques currently exist for imaging the liver. These include plain film radiographs of the abdomen, radionuclide scans for both parenchymal and specific lesions, hepatic arteriography, portal and hepatic venography, ultrasound, and whole-body computed tomographic (CT) scanning. These examinations enable the borders of the liver to be determined and its vasculature, ductal system, and parenchyma to be visualized. Therefore, they are useful both in the preoperative evaluation of liver abnormalities and in the preoperative diagnosis of other disease possibly involving the liver. Radiologic procedures also enable the surgeon to evaluate the postoperative appearance of the liver, alterations in its vasculature, and complications of surgery. This chapter discusses these three roles for radiographic imaging procedures. Techniques of imaging the biliary tract and evaluating cases of jaundice are discussed in Chapter 16.

ANATOMY

As classically presented in anatomy textbooks, the liver is composed of several areas, or divisions, related to the topographic features of the parietal and visceral surfaces. Anatomically, it is divided into a large right and a left lobe by the ligamentum teres and the interlobar fissure. These can occasionally be seen on plain films of the abdomen by detection of the falciform ligament and are almost always seen on ultrasound, CT, and radionuclide scans.

When surgical resection of a portion of the liver is under consideration, it is more important to recognize that the right and left lobes are defined by their portal venous components, hepatic arterial supply, and biliary ductal divisions rather than by topographic features.[31] The anatomy of the right and left lobes of the liver is quite different from the topographic divisions. The true left lobe of the liver is larger than it appears to be on topographic inspection and includes the medial portion of the topographic right lobe (see further on). The vascular divisions are best recognized on

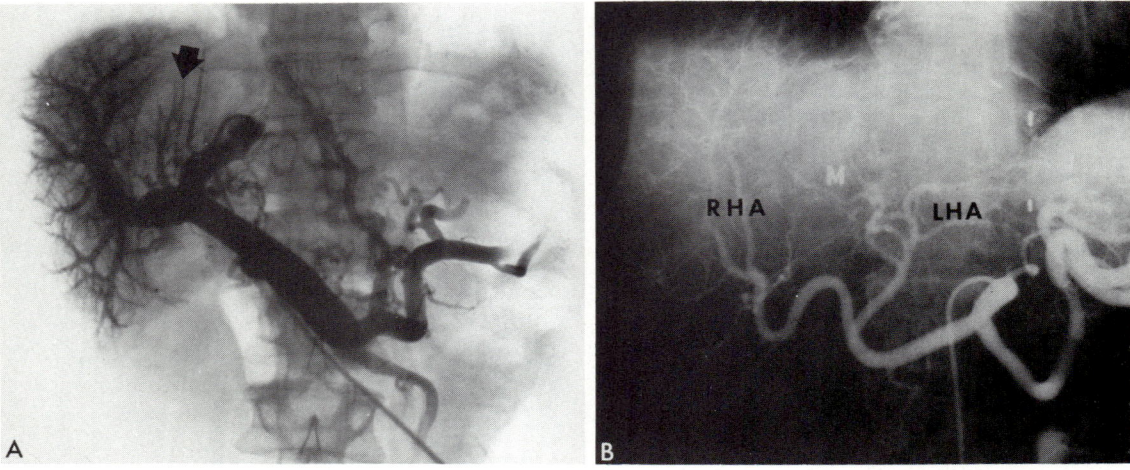

Figure 15–1. *A*, Umbilical venogram in a patient with cirrhosis and varices. Coronary veins are demonstrated arising from the splenic vein. Venous branches from the left portal vein supply the region of the medial segment and the quadrate process of the left lobe (arrow). This vascular study helps to determine the boundaries of the left and right lobes as determined by the portal venous supply. *B*, Hepatic arteriogram showing the most common arterial distribution to the right and left lobes. The right hepatic artery (RHA) supplies the right lobe. The left hepatic artery (LHA) has major branches to the lateral and medial (M) segments.

angiographic studies of portal venous and hepatic arterial systems (Fig. 15–1). On ultrasound and CT scans, the true division between the right and the left hepatic lobes corresponds roughly to a line drawn between the main portal vein in the porta hepatis and the anterior axillary line. Thus, the quadrate lobe is part of the left hepatic lobe and the caudate lobe part of the right (Fig. 15–2).

On supine or erect films of the abdomen, most of the right lobe of the liver is visible in the right upper abdominal quadrant beneath the right hemidiaphragm. The extent of the left lobe of the liver is less easy to appreciate on plain films because it is smaller,

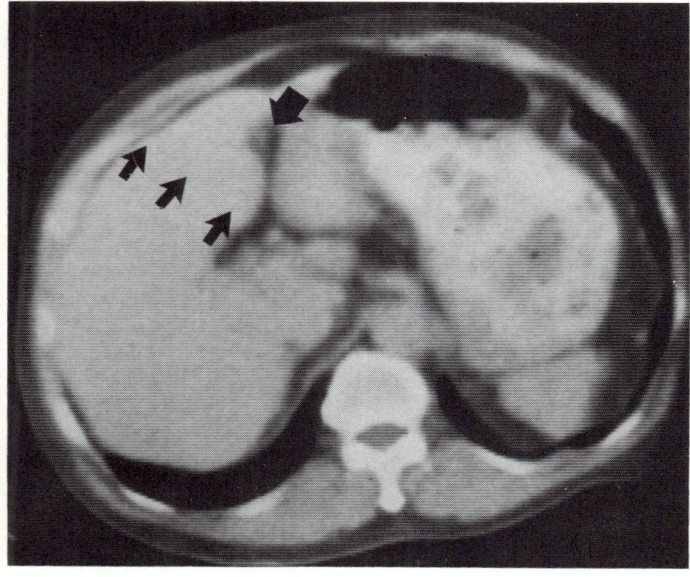

Figure 15–2. Computed tomographic (CT) scan of the liver demonstrating the interlobar fissure (arrow). This topical anatomic feature often separates the lateral from the medial segment of left lobe of the liver. The medial segment of the left lobe is located a variable distance from the fissure, and the true interlobar separation occurs along a line drawn between the porta hepatis and the anterior axillary line (arrows).

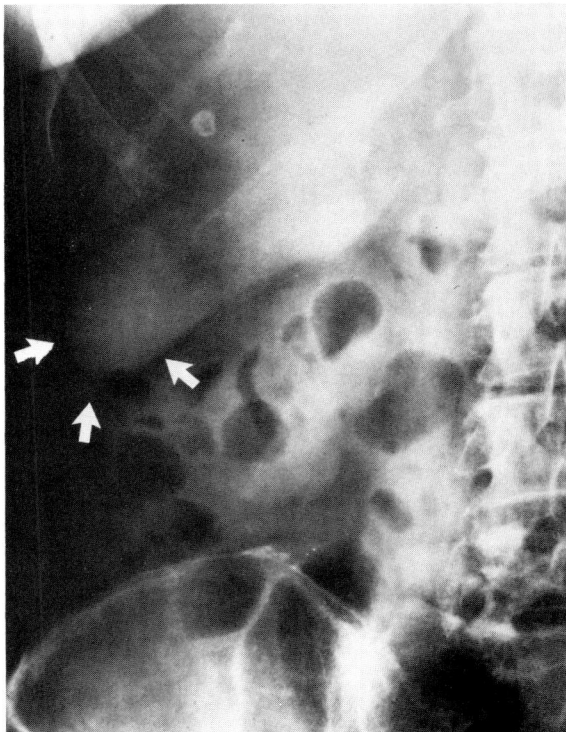

Figure 15–3. Plain film of abdomen (supine), showing hepatic angle formed by the liver tip (arrows) surrounded in part by retroperitoneal fat.

having less depth and width than the right lobe, and its border is difficult to see. The plain film of the abdomen is an unreliable method of determining liver size. Most often, the inferior border of the liver seen on plain films lies posteriorly in the abdomen and is not the edge that is palpable.

On plain films of the abdomen, however, one can estimate the location of the tip of the right lobe. The so-called hepatic angle seen on the plain film (Fig. 15–3) demonstrates the normal relationship of the tip of the right lobe to retroperitoneal fat. The angle is seen on a plain film because this portion of the liver lies in a bed of retroperitoneal fat. When fluid, blood, or any other substance is interposed between the fat and the liver tip, the hepatic angle disappears.[58]

Portal Vein

The most direct techniques for studying the portal venous anatomy are splenoportography, umbilical vein catheterization, and direct transhepatic portography. Splenoportography requires the injection of contrast material into splenic pulp through an 18- to 20- gauge needle with polyethylene oversheath. Contrast material outlines both the splenic vein and the portal vein and its branches. Use of the umbilical vein requires surgical isolation and catheterization of the vein near the umbilicus, with fluoroscopic guidance of the catheter until it reaches the main portal vein. Contrast material can then be injected into the main portal vein to outline its branches (Fig. 15–4). Less direct radiographic methods of opacifying the portal venous system include splenic arteriography and superior mesenteric arteriography.

814 — THE LIVER

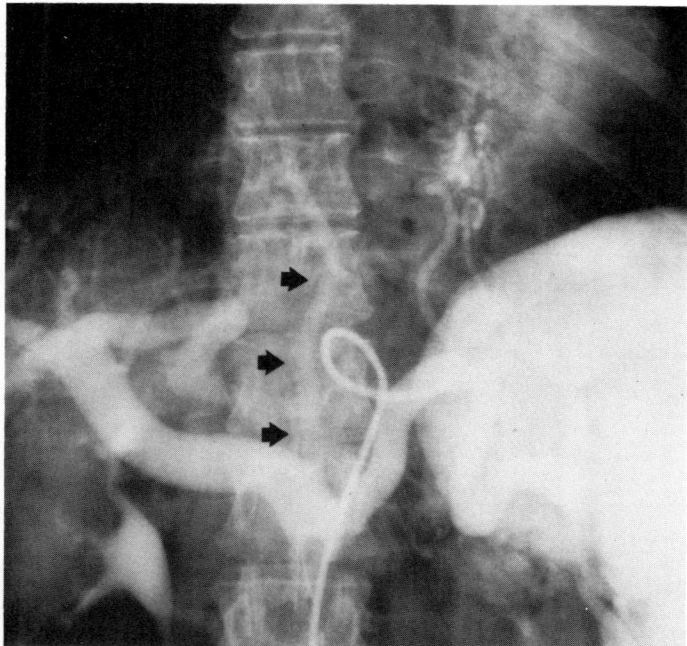

Figure 15–4. Excellent portal vein opacification has been achieved by obtaining a delayed film after injection of 80 ml of iodinated contrast material into the splenic artery. An enlarged coronary vein (arrows) is present in this patient with portal hypertension.

The portal vein, formed by the confluence of the superior mesenteric vein and the splenic vein at the level of the second lumbar vertebral body, courses laterally from just anterior to the inferior vena cava to the porta hepatis. The relationship of the portal vein to the inferior vena cava is a relatively constant one. In the porta hepatis, the main portal vein branches into a horizontally oriented right intrahepatic portal vein and a left portal vein branch, which ascends almost perpendicular to the main portal vein before coursing into the left lobe. This relationship aids in differentiating portal veins from

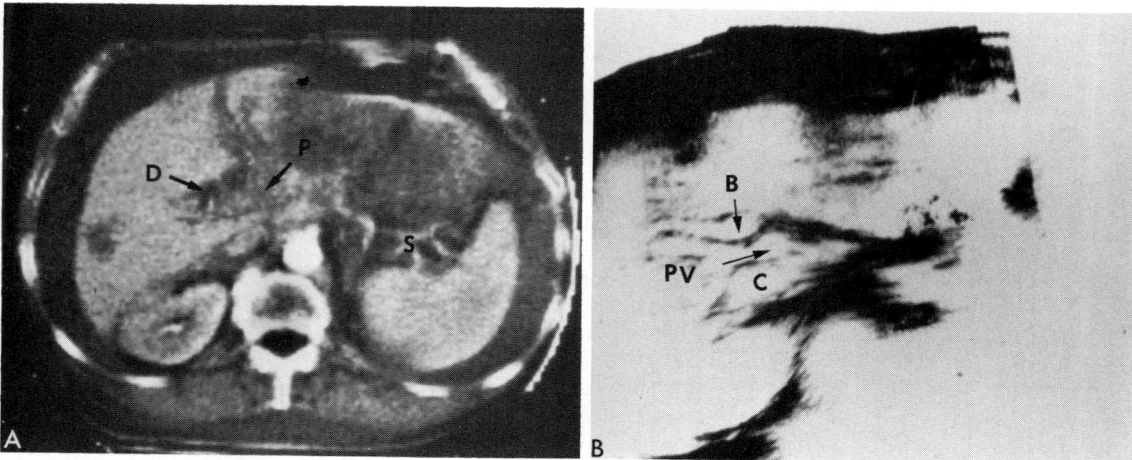

Figure 15–5. *A*, CT scan of the liver in a patient with jaundice. After intravenous infusion of iodinated contrast material, the splenic veins (S) and main portal vein (P) are seen as well as branching of the portal vein into left and right branches. The low-density structures anterior to these veins represent dilated bile ducts (D). This patient also has ascites and liver metastases. *B*, This transverse ultrasonogram shows the constant anatomic relationship between the inferior vena cava (C) and the portal vein (PV) as it crosses over that structure. The third tubular structure paralleling the main portal vein and its right branch is a dilated bile duct (B).

dilated bile ducts in ultrasound and CT scanning, since the bile ducts accompany the portal vein but are always anterior to these structures (Fig. 15–5).[7, 24] The left portal vein, which originates lateral to the interlobar fissure, receives the umbilical vein, which courses in the ligamentum teres.

In planning hepatectomy, it is important to demonstrate the portal venous anatomy. Experimental studies in dogs have shown that if the portal vein is catheterized via the umbilical vein, the catheter selectively placed in either the left or the right portal vein and toluidine blue injected intravenously, the parenchyma will stain with the toluidine blue and this will be seen on the surface of the liver.[18] This method may provide an appraisal of the topographic correlate of the underlying hepatic vascular supply.

Hepatic Arteries

Although the liver receives 70 to 80 per cent of its blood supply from the portal venous sytem, 20 to 30 per cent is supplied by the hepatic arterial system, originating primarily from the celiac artery and to some degree from the superior mesenteric artery. Knowledge of hepatic arterial supply is important for planning a hepatectomy, for directing a perfusion catheter to a specific lesion in chemotherapy, and for planning occlusive therapy for hepatic arterial bleeding (see Figs. 15–1 and 15–6).

There are many variations in the arterial supply to the liver. In about 80 per cent of cases, a common hepatic artery arises from the celiac trunk. In the remaining 20 per cent, the major supply to the right lobe arises as a separate branch from the superior mesenteric artery (Fig. 15–6). After giving off the gastroduodenal artery, the hepatic artery often, but not invariably, gives rise to the right gastric artery, although the latter may also arise from the left hepatic artery.

The common hepatic artery branches in the porta hepatis to form a right hepatic artery to the right lobe of the liver and a left hepatic artery to the left lobe, with a smaller branch to the caudate lobe. There are many intrahepatic variations in supplies of the right and left lobe; in some instances, portions of the left lobe are supplied by branches from the right hepatic artery. The reader is referred to the classic articles on hepatic arterial anatomic variations, such as those by Nebesar[37] and Michaels.[35]

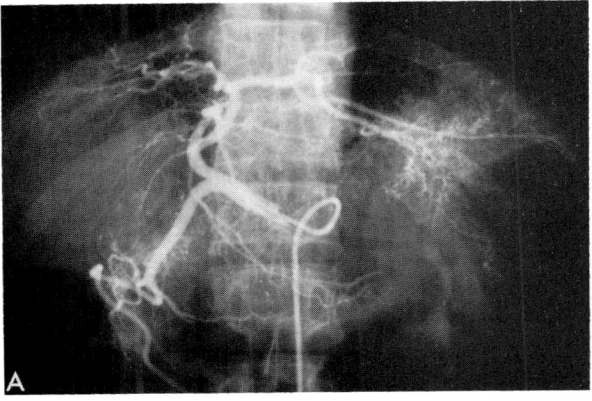
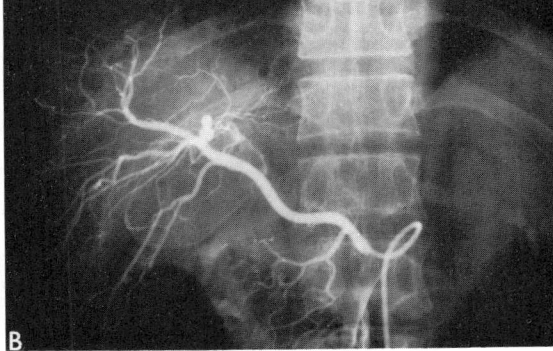

Figure 15–6. *A*, Selective hepatic arteriogram showing an anatomic variant. No right hepatic artery is seen, and both the left hepatic artery and a middle hepatic arterial branch to the left lobe originate from the main hepatic artery trunk. The appearance of the left lobe arteries is abnormal owing to presence of a hepatoma. *B*, Selective superior mesenteric artery injection shows that the right hepatic artery arises from the SMA to supply the right lobe of the liver. No tumor vessels are identified from the right hepatic artery distribution.

Hepatic Veins

The liver sinusoids drain into hepatic venules, which drain into three major hepatic venous channels emptying into the inferior vena cava just below or at the diaphragm. In addition, there is a separate set of small veins draining the caudate lobe of the liver directly into the inferior vena cava. This anatomic characteristic of hepatic vein drainage is important in the diagnosis of hepatic vein thrombosis. Radionuclide imaging may demonstrate only a well-imaged caudate lobe, which because of its alternative venous drainage is sometimes spared the functional abnormalities associated with hepatic vein thrombosis.

Because hepatic venography and hepatic wedge pressures are used for evaluation prior to a portal-systemic shunt procedure, a knowledge of hepatic vein anatomy is required in these cases as well as in the evaluation of patients with the Budd-Chiari syndrome (pp. 834 to 835). Since the hepatic veins do not follow the hepatic arteries or portal veins, hepatic venous drainage is often disrupted during partial hepatectomy when the line of resection follows the portal venous supply rather than the hepatic venous drainage.

Hepatic Lymphatics

The hepatic lymphatics are frequently seen during percutaneous transhepatic cholangiography in patients with cirrhosis and ascites. In these patients, the lymphatics of the liver tend to be dilated and increased in number. In some patients with liver disease, but without ascites, percutaneous transhepatic cholangiography also demonstrates the lymphatics.[15] The network of lymphatics does not parallel the course of the hepatic veins. Lymphatics begin in the perisinusoidal space of Disse and drain into small lymph vessels that converge into larger channels that exit from the liver in the

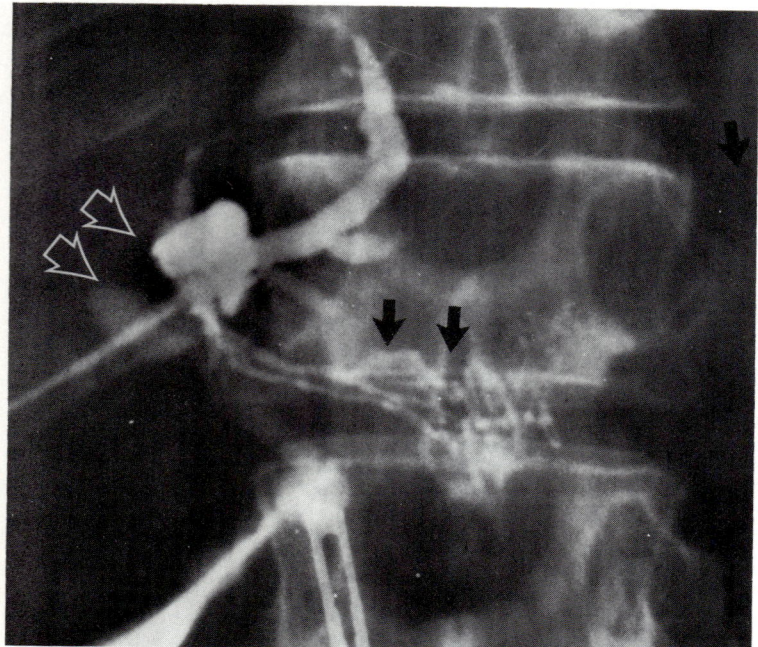

Figure 15–7. Opacified hepatic lymphatics (solid arrows) course along the gastrohepatic ligament and vascular pedicle toward lymph nodes in the region of the celiac axis. These lymphatics have filled from a parenchymal injection of contrast material (open arrows) as part of a percutaneous transhepatic cholangiogram.

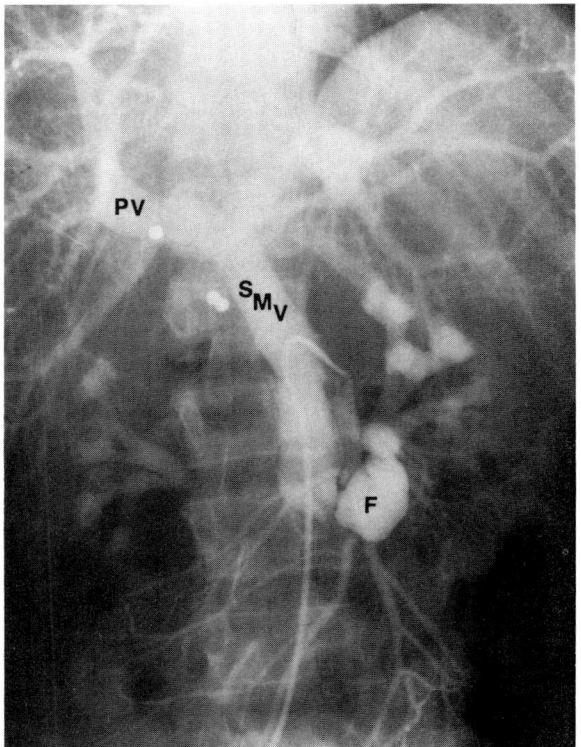

Figure 15–8. Superior mesenteric arteriogram in a young patient with traumatic arteriovenous fistula following an abdominal gunshot wound. Two seconds after the beginning of the arterial injection there is dense opacification of the fistula (F) and the superior mesenteric (SMV) and portal (PV) veins

region of the porta hepatis and extend to the celiac lymph nodes (Fig. 15–7). It is important to recognize these lymphatic vessels radiographically, but at this time no specific disorders are evaluated by opacification of liver lymphatics.

PORTAL HYPERTENSION

Elevation of pressure in the portal venous system results from a number of intrahepatic and extrahepatic pathologic processes. With the rare exception of patients in whom portal hypertension is due to increased portal blood flow through a splanchnic arteriovenous fistula (Fig. 15–8), portal hypertension is caused by obstruction. The level of obstruction is usually intrahepatic and is related to cirrhosis, due to either alcoholism or the aftermath of hepatitis. The obstruction to the hepatic venous outflow of the liver (Budd-Chiari syndrome) is a less common cause of portal hypertension.

Portal Hypertension due to Cirrhosis

Many different radiographic tests may be used to evaluate patients with cirrhosis and portal hypertension. These can effectively assess the stage and severity of the illness and aid in deciding whether surgery should be performed. Plain films of the abdomen often provide clues to the presence of cirrhosis and its complications.

Although liver size is difficult to judge accurately on the abdominal plain film, significant alterations in size and shape can often be ascertained. Patients with acute alcoholic hepatitis and resultant hepatic enlargement may show a large, triangular soft tissue density occupying much of the upper abdomen, with inferior displacement of the gas-filled hepatic flexure of the colon (Fig. 15–9). Gas is often present in the duodenal bulb, which may also be medially and inferiorly displaced. Conversely, the patient with severe, long-standing cirrhosis and extensive hepatic fibrosis may have a shrunken liver, evident on the plain abdominal radiograph as a liver shadow of diminished size, which is retracted up into the right subdiaphragmatic region.

Abdominal plain films in patients with cirrhosis and portal hypertension usually show evidence of splenic enlargement. The size of the spleen usually can be accurately determined from the plain film, particularly if the inferior and medial borders can be demonstrated. The positions of the splenic flexure of the colon and of the gas in the stomach are evident in most patients and are useful in determining splenic size. If the size of the spleen cannot be ascertained from a frontal radiograph, a film in the left anterior oblique position may be helpful.

Ascites is often evident on abdominal plain films, and a number of radiographic signs can be used to detect or confirm its presence. If the volume of fluid within the peritoneal cavity is great, the gas-filled portions of the small bowel tend to float to an anterior central position within the abdomen when the patient is supine. The supine abdominal radiograph will therefore show clustering of bowel gas in the center of the abdomen with little or no gas on the periphery. Because the pelvic portion of the abdominal cavity is dependent when the patient is supine, fluid collects in this area, displaying a homogeneous gray density above and on either side of the urinary bladder.

Another useful sign is an alteration in the normal relationship of the ascending and descending portions of the colon to the adjacent flank stripe. The flank stripe consists of a radiolucent linear shadow produced by a layer of fat surrounding the peritoneum in the right and left flanks, indicating the lateral borders of the peritoneal cavity. Normally, the ascending and descending portions of the colon lie in the posterolateral

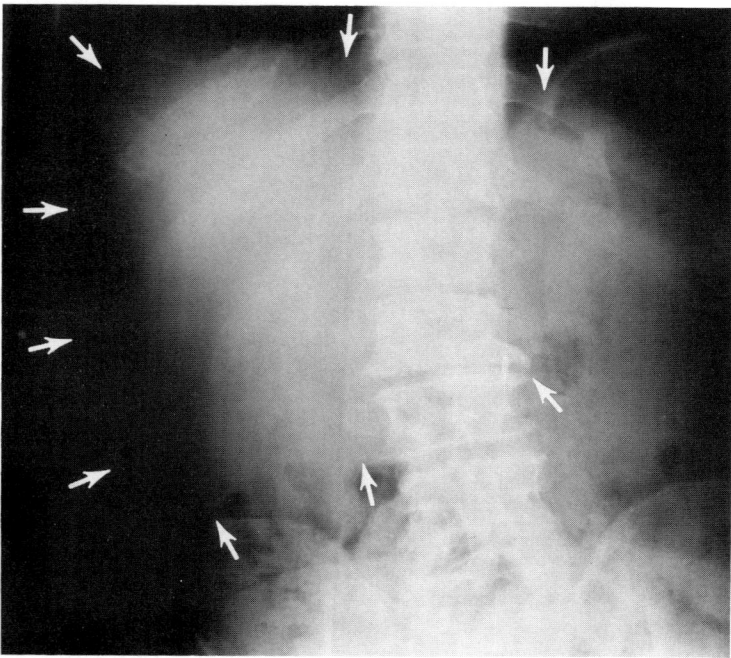

Figure 15–9. Hepatomegaly evident on plain abdominal film. The liver (arrows) occupies most of the upper abdomen.

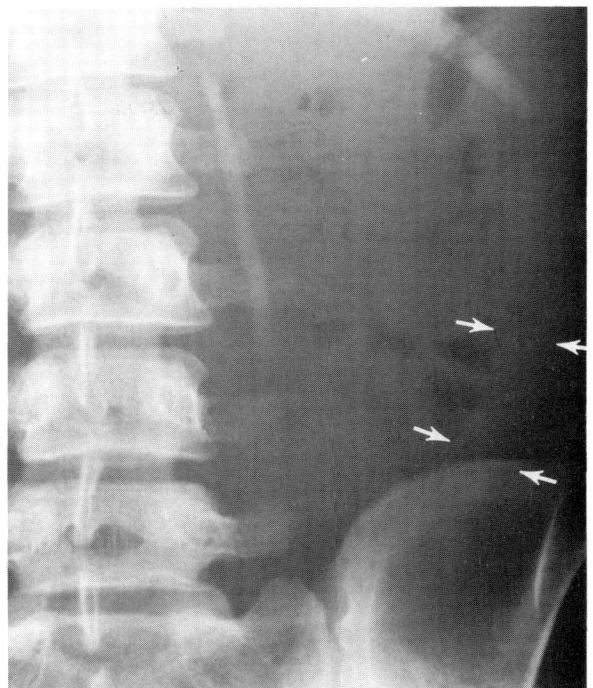

Figure 15–10. Moderate ascites. The fluid appears as a band (arrows) of soft tissue density lying between the descending colon and the adjacent properitoneal fat.

abdominal gutters immediately adjacent to the flank stripes. In ascites, fluid collects in the gutters when the patient is supine, and the shadows of the ascending and descending colon are displaced medially from the flank stripe by fluid that appears as a strip of homogeneous gray density (Fig. 15–10).

It is also helpful to search for the right inferolateral angle of the liver border on the abdominal plain film (Fig. 15–11). This angle is caused by the shadow of the right posteroinferior tip of the liver, which normally lies in direct contact with fat in the posterior abdomen. Ascites collects in this location, displacing the liver medially and anteriorly away from the adjacent fat, and obliterating the radiographic shadow of the inferior liver angle.

A more subtle radiographic finding of ascites is visualization of medial displacement of the lateral edge of the liver from the right abdominal wall. This sign is best appreciated on low-kilovoltage films and with plain film tomography. After the intravenous injection of iodinated contrast material, in an intravenous urogram, a slight increase in the radiographic opacity of the liver occurs, and the border between the medially displaced liver edge and the adjacent ascites may become visible.

Barium studies of the upper gastrointestinal tract may help in assessing the severity of portal hypertension. The lower esophagus is one of the most common sites for dilated collateral veins from portal hypertension. Large esophageal varices are invariably well seen on the barium esophagogram (Fig. 15–12); they appear as linear, wormlike filling defects in the barium-filled esophagus. Small esophageal varices, however, are often difficult to demonstrate by esophagography and are not likely to be seen unless the films of the distal esophagus are obtained with special attention to technique. Even very small esophageal varices can be demonstrated radiographically if views are obtained of the barium-coated, collapsed esophagus (Fig. 15–13). Since peristaltic stripping waves of the esophagus effectively empty the varices, these views

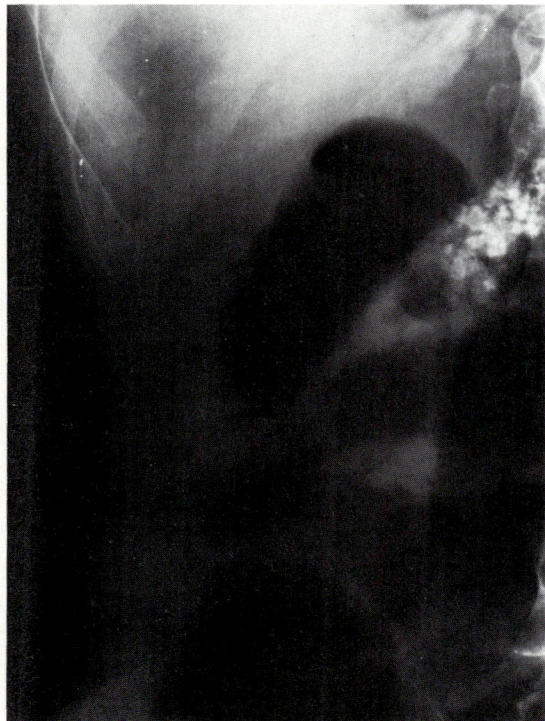

Figure 15–11. The liver angle is obliterated in this patient because of ascites, which has lifted the tip of the right lobe away from the retroperitoneal fat.

Figure 15–12. Large serpiginous varices are demonstrated in the lower half of the esophagus.

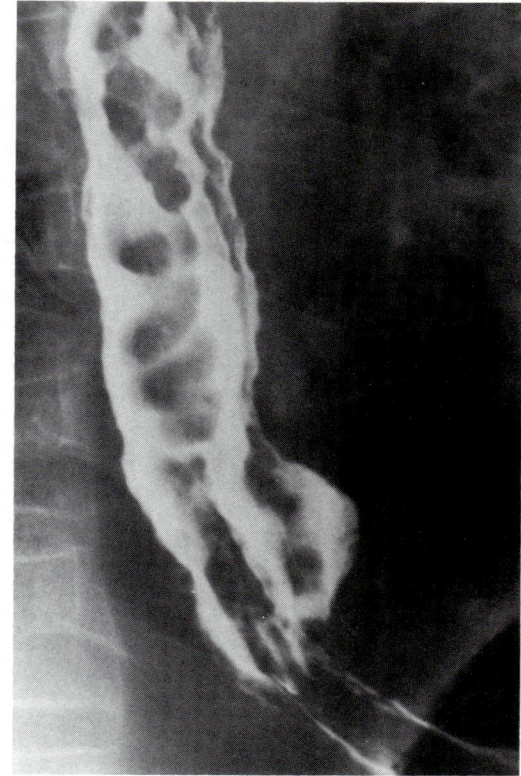

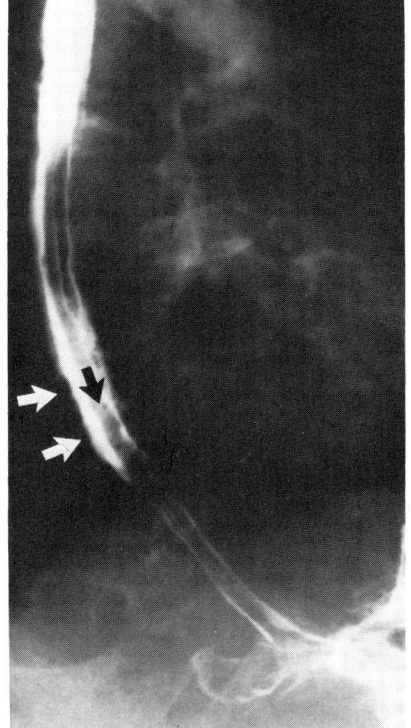

Figure 15–13. Slight tortuosity of the longitudinal filling defects seen in this partially collapsed esophagus denotes the presence of small esophageal varices (arrows). These were verified by endoscopy.

should be obtained after a five- to ten-minute period, during which the patient is asked not to swallow. On collapsed views, the normal, thin, straight mucosal fold pattern of the lower esophagus is replaced by thickened folds with wavy, irregular contours.

Varices demonstrable on barium studies of the upper gastrointestinal tracts are not confined to the esophagus. Not uncommonly, varices of the gastric fundus and cardia are seen in association with esophageal varices. Varices in the proximal stomach appear as multiple rounded or nodular filling defects (Fig. 15–14). Unlike filling defects caused by tumor, however, they change considerably in size and shape from one film to another. Rarely, varices are evident on barium studies of the duodenum. These occur more commonly in persons with extrahepatic portal obstruction or obstruction of the splenic vein.

Radionuclide scanning is a noninvasive, highly sensitive, and moderately specific diagnostic test for the detection and evaluation of cirrhosis.[13] The test is performed after intravenous administration of 8 to 10 mCi of ^{99m}Tc sulphur colloid. The colloid material is cleared from the blood by the reticuloendothelial cells of the liver and, to a lesser extent, by reticuloendothelial cells of the spleen, bone marrow, and other organs. After an interval of approximately 30 minutes, a gamma camera is used to image the upper abdomen from posterior, anterior, and right lateral positions. Normally, the liver takes up the majority of the isotope and is brightly labeled on the images. The spleen takes up a lesser amount of isotope, and the bone marrow is ordinarily not visible.

In patients with cirrhosis, several abnormalities are noted. The most frequent and sensitive finding is the presence of diffuse nonhomogeneous uptake of isotope by the liver (Fig. 15–15). This has been reported to occur in more than 90 per cent of cases. In addition, there is an overall decrease in the uptake of isotope by the liver, accompanied by an increase in isotopic labeling of the spleen and bone marrow. This results both in visibility of the bone marrow on the scan and in a reversal of the normal ratio of hepatic to splenic labeling. Other findings include hepatomegaly and splenomegaly, each of which occurs in about 75 per cent of cases. None of these findings is specific for the diagnosis of cirrhosis, and each is seen to a variable extent in other hepatocellular disease, particularly in cases of fatty metamorphosis of the liver. However, the combination of diffuse inhomogeneity of liver uptake, reversal of the normal liver to spleen ratio, and visible labeling of the bone marrow is specific for cirrhosis if each of these findings is present in a moderate to severe degree.[13]

Ultrasonography is capable of producing highly detailed images of the liver, and is an easy, noninvasive means of assessing liver size and shape. Intrahepatic vessels of both the portal and the hepatic venous systems also are usually well seen. Gray-scale ultrasound equipment, which can selectively amplify low-level echoes produced within the liver, provides information regarding diffuse pathologic changes in the architecture of the liver parenchyma.[54] Normally, there is a nearly homogeneous pattern of finely textured, low-level echoes emanating from the liver parenchyma (Fig. 15–16). On parasagittal scans these internal hepatic echoes are only one half to one third the size of the echoes from the adjacent right hemidiaphragm.

In the presence of cirrhosis, this pattern is considerably altered (Fig. 15–17). In mild to moderate cirrhosis, the sonogram shows numerous high-level echoes scattered unevenly throughout the liver. The echo pattern is much coarser than normal, and many of the individual returning echoes are as large as those from the diaphragm. As fibrotic change in the liver becomes more severe, the attenuation of the ultrasound beam increases, so that transducers of the usual diagnostic frequency (2.5 to 3.5 mHz) may be unable to penetrate to the deeper portions of the liver. In such cases, high-level, irregular echoes may be imaged only in the anterior aspect of the cirrhotic liver, and a lower frequency transducer may be needed to image the posterior aspect of the right hepatic lobe.

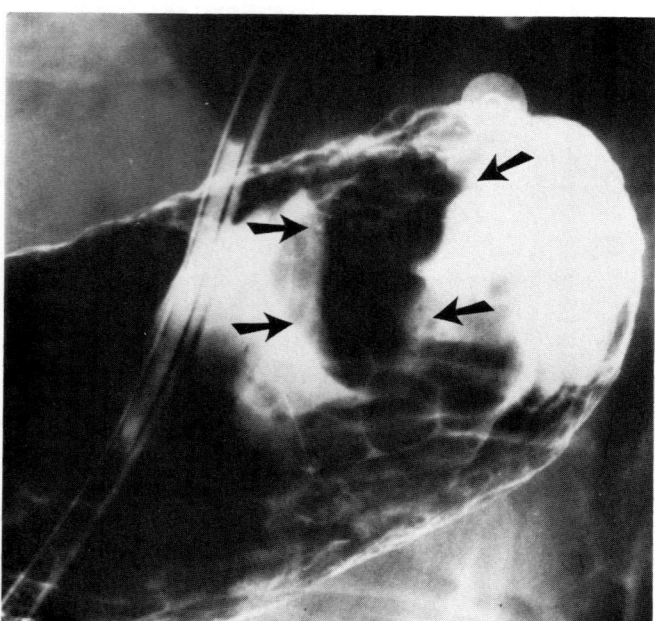

Figure 15–14. A large, thumblike projection into the lumen of the fundus of the stomach was produced by a huge gastric varix (arrows) in a patient with a splenic vein thrombosis.

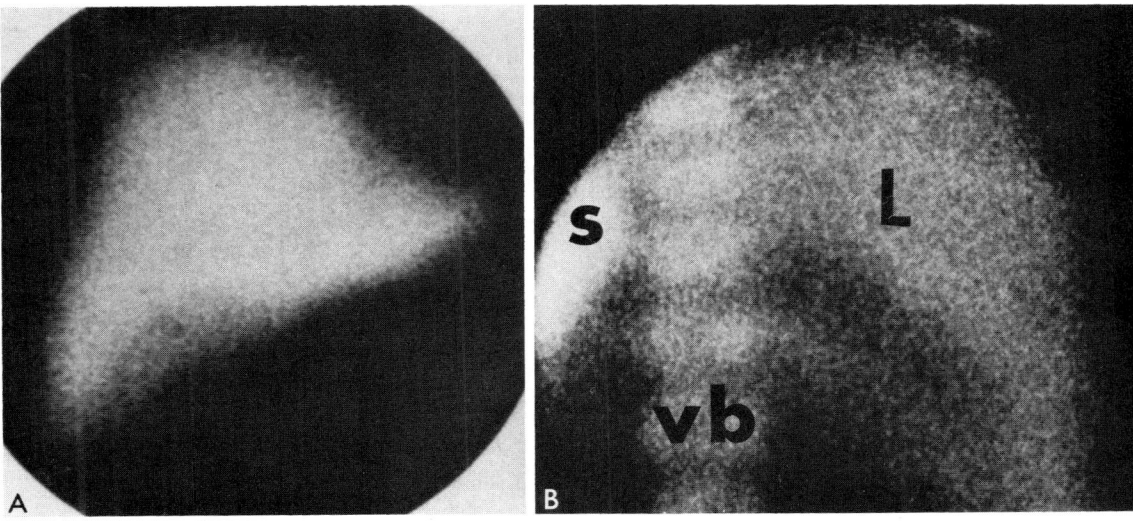

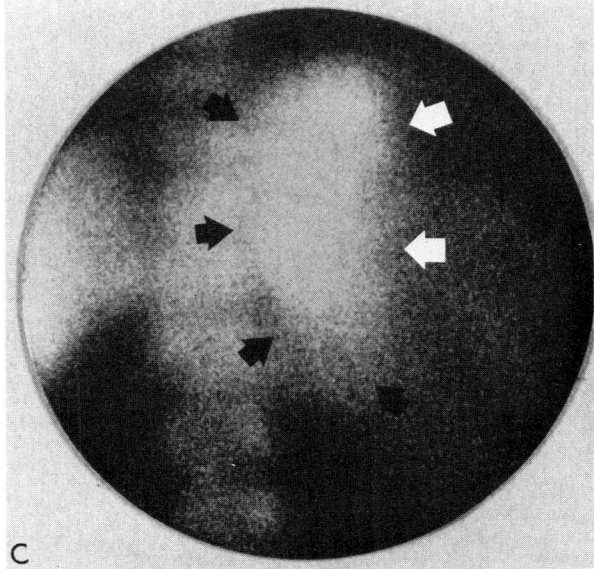

Figure 15–15. *A*, This ^{99m}Tc sulfur colloid liver-spleen scan shows a normal pattern of homogenous hepatic uptake of radionuclide. *B*, Posterior ^{99m}Tc sulfur colloid liver-spleen scan shows diffuse decrease in hepatic uptake (L) but increased splenic uptake (S) and bone marrow uptake in vertebral bodies (vb). *C*, Posterior ^{99m}Tc sulfur colloid liver-spleen scan in a patient with Budd-Chiari syndrome. Note that only the medial segment of the right lobe of the liver, representing the caudate lobe, has normal uptake (arrows). This is because the venous drainage of the caudate lobe is directly into the intrahepatic portion of the inferior vena cava. Therefore, hepatic venous occlusion does not affect this segment.

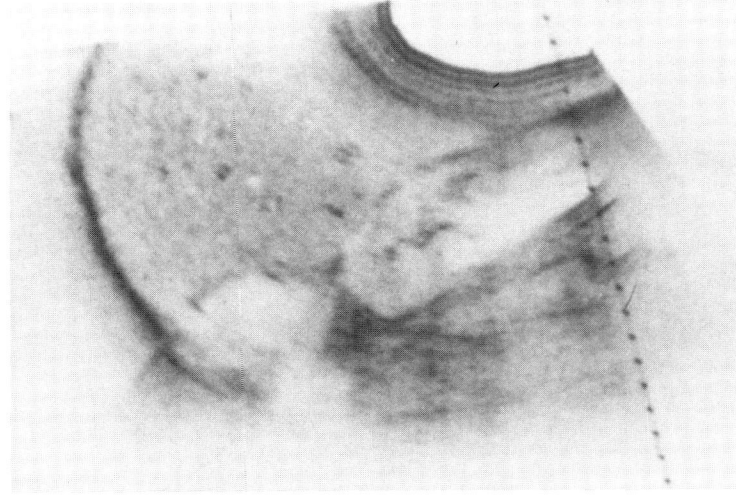

Figure 15–16. Sagittal-section ultrasonogram of normal liver, demonstrating the homogenous, smooth echo texture of the liver parenchyma interrupted by a few vessels of normal caliber.

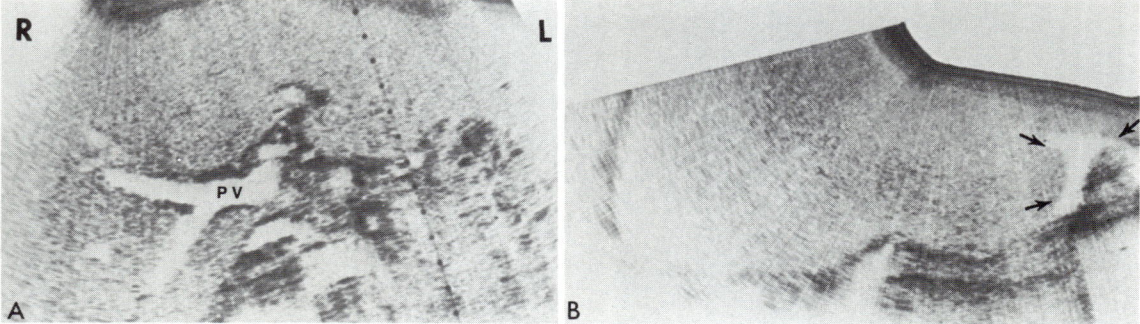

Figure 15–17. Sonogram in a patient with cirrhosis and hepatomegaly. *A*, Transverse scan showing large liver with prominent portal vein (PV) and coarse echo texture within the liver. *B*, Parasagittal scan through the enlarged right hepatic lobe. Echo-free area (arrows) inferior to the liver represents ascites.

In addition to the changes in the parenchymal echo pattern in cirrhosis, dilatation and tortuosity of the portal vein and its intrahepatic branches can be shown in many patients with portal hypertension (Fig. 15–18). The major splanchnic tributaries of the portal vein may be increased in caliber. Ultrasound also provides a very sensitive means for the detection of ascites (Fig. 15–19). Collections of ascitic fluid too small to be seen on plain radiographs or to be detected on physical examination can be seen routinely. Finally, the size of the spleen can be determined by sector scans in the appropriate left intercostal space. The presence of splenomegaly can thus provide supportive evidence for the presence of portal hypertension.

Computed tomography (CT) of the liver is another useful technique for the preoperative evaluation of patients with portal hypertension. The size and shape of the liver and spleen are readily demonstrable with this technique. The detail and resolution of the image are such that an irregular liver outline, due to the nodular surface contour that may accompany cirrhosis, can often be shown (Figs. 15–20 and 15–21).

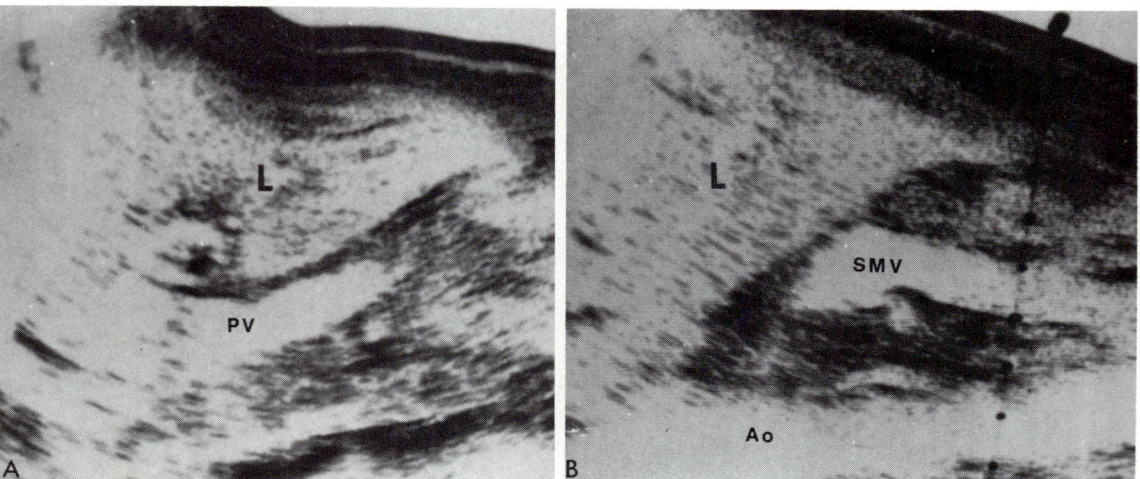

Figure 15–18. Sonogram of middle-aged man with jaundice and cirrhosis. Bile ducts were not dilated. *A*, Parasagittal scan 3 cm right of midline shows dilated portal vein (PV) beneath the liver (L). *B*. Midsagittal scan shows dilated superior mesenteric vein (SMV) between liver and aorta (Ao).

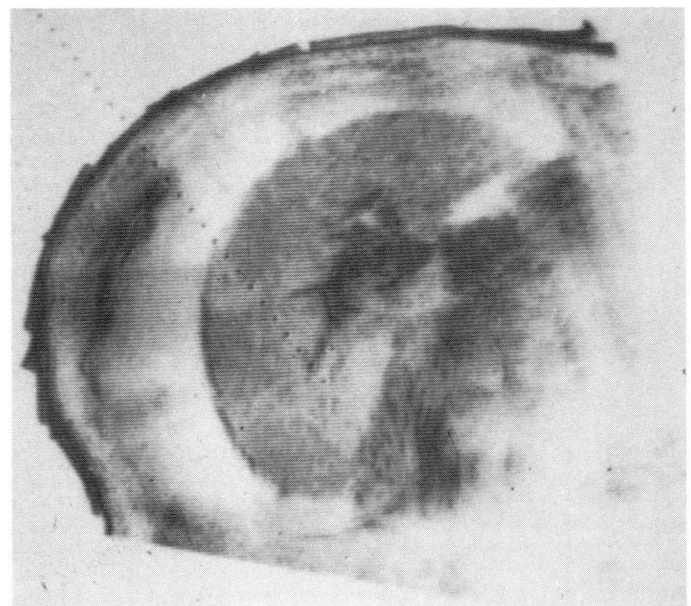

Figure 15–19. Transverse-section ultrasonogram showing a small, shrunken liver surrounded by ascites, appearing here as an echo-free zone.

In the detection of microanatomic changes in the liver parenchyma, however, CT is less useful. CT is insensitive to the physiologic abnormalities detected by radionuclide scanning and the increased fibrous tissue content detectable by ultrasound. However, only the CT scan can detect a decrease in liver density associated with fatty infiltration (Fig. 15–22).

Like the imaging modalities already mentioned, CT can afford indirect evidence of cirrhosis and portal hypertension. Splenomegaly and ascites are easily appreciated (see Fig 15–20). In some patients, dilated umbilical veins are seen in the falciform ligament, representing portosystemic collaterals.

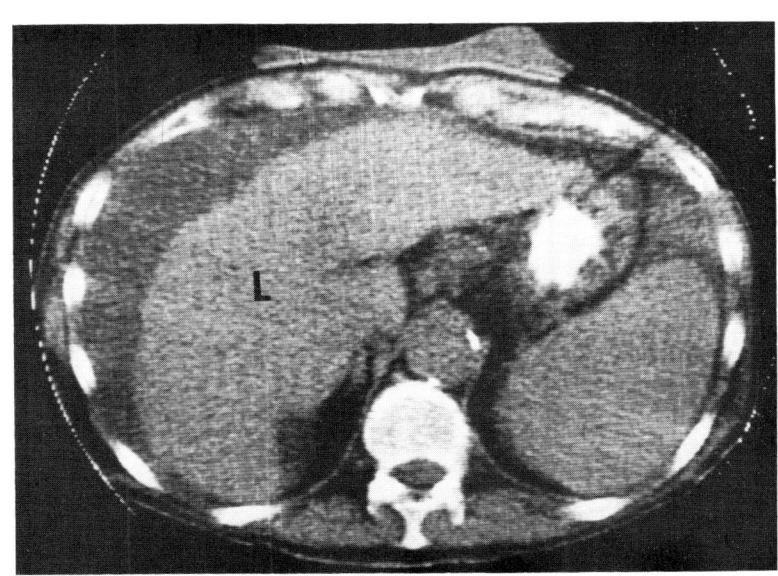

Figure 15–20. CT scan in a patient with cirrhosis. The liver (L) is small and is separated from the right abdominal wall by a crescentic area of fluid density representing ascites. The contour of the liver is slightly nodular. The spleen is enlarged.

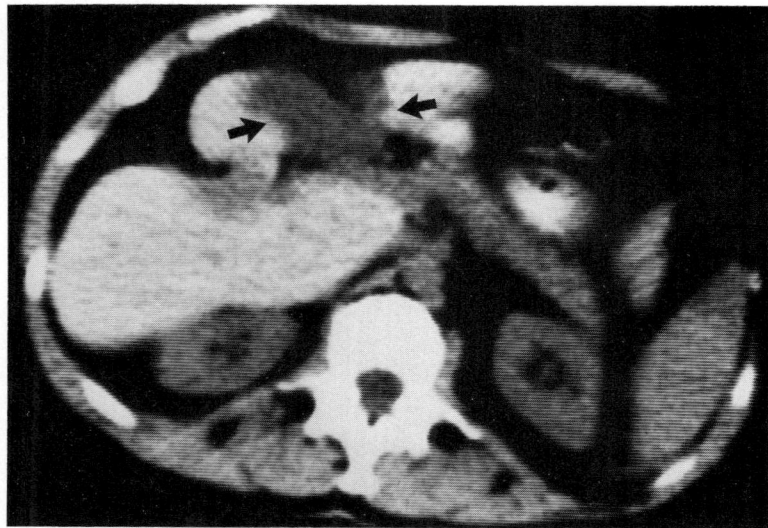

Figure 15–21. The CT scan of the liver in this alcoholic man shows an irregular nodular contour with a decrease in overall liver size. This finding is typical of advanced cirrhosis owing to the presence of hemochromatosis, the liver appears dense when compared with all the other abdominal organs. The homogeneous low-density area in the left lobe (arrows) is a hepatoma.

A variety of angiographic procedures are the most direct radiologic means for evaluating the patient with portal hypertension, both before and after surgery. Angiography also provides information about the amount and direction of the visceral blood flow.[41]

The three major angiographic approaches used to visualize the portal venous system are splenoportography, arterial portography, and percutaneous transhepatic portography. Splenoportography was frequently performed in the past but is no longer widely used. It involves the insertion of a needle into the spleen under fluoroscopic guidance and the injection of contrast material into the splenic pulp. Ideally, the tip of the needle is positioned near the hilus of the spleen, and the contrast material flows directly into the splenic vein. Dense opacification of the portal vein usually results (Fig. 15–23). The major drawback of the technique lies in its complications. Although rare,

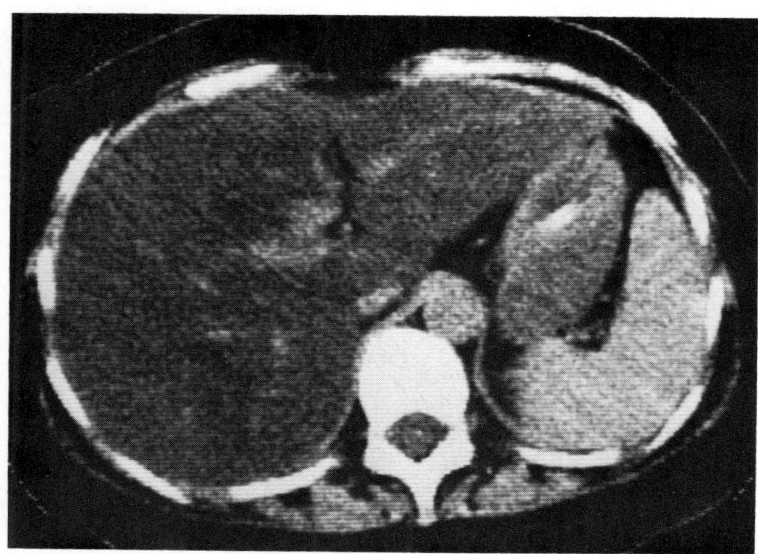

Figure 15–22. Fatty metamorphosis of the liver. The liver appears darker than normal because of diminished density. The spleen is normal.

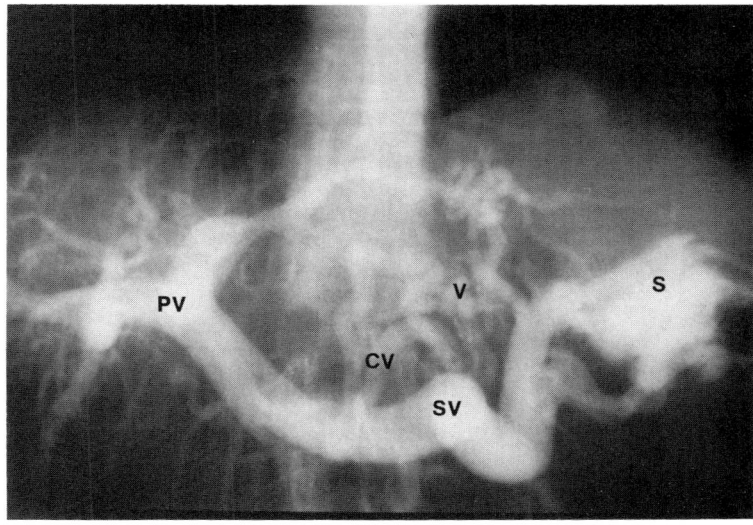

Figure 15–23. Splenoportogram in a patient with cirrhosis. Near the catheter tip there is a stain (S) in the splenic parenchyma. The splenic vein (SV) and portal vein (PV) are both well opacified. A tangled network of collateral varices (V) is visible as opacified blood flows into the coronary vein (CV) in retrograde fashion.

the most notable complication is laceration of the splenic capsule with consequent hemorrhage requiring splenectomy.

Percutaneous transhepatic portography is an alternative means of direct angiographic visualization of the portal venous system. This approach has been recently advocated by Viamonte and coworkers[55] but has not yet been widely adapted. A catheter-trocar assembly is inserted into the liver during suspended respiration under fluoroscopic guidance. The trocar is quickly withdrawn, leaving the flexible catheter tip near the right main portal vein. The catheter is slowly retracted until its tip enters a portal vein branch. A flexible guide wire is then passed through the catheter into the portal vein. With the wire left in place, the catheter is removed and a longer catheter is passed over the guide wire and positioned selective in the vessel to be studied. Portal venography can then be performed (Fig. 15–24).

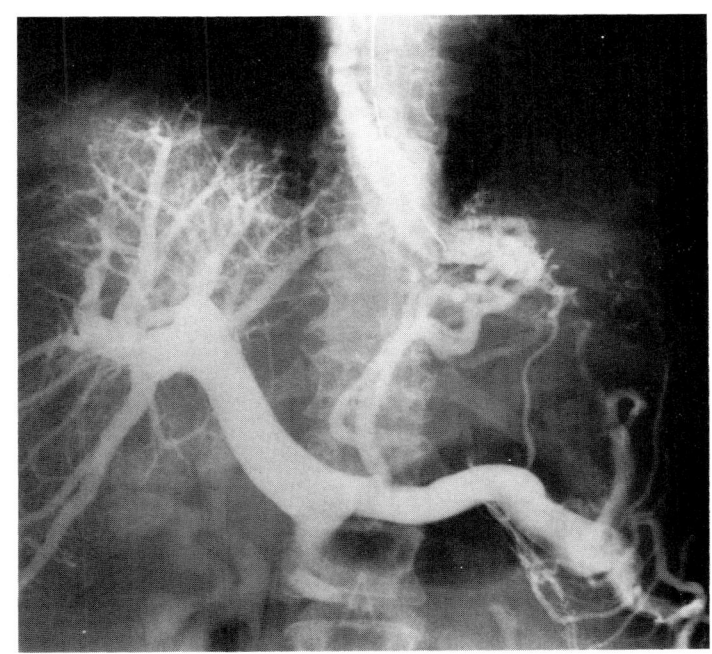

Figure 15–24. Percutaneous transhepatic portal venogram performed on a 50-year-old woman with alcoholic cirrhosis. The portal vein was cannulated via a percutaneous transhepatic approach, and contrast material was injected to fill the intra- and extrahepatic portal venous system as well as the gastroesophageal varices, splenic vein, and confluence with superior mesenteric vein. (Courtesy of Patrick C. Freeny, M.D., Seattle, Washington.)

828 — THE LIVER

This method has also been used to introduce a variety of thrombotic and embolic materials directly into the coronary vein and esophageal varices.[40] This allows the radiologist to selectively interrupt these vessels as a means of stopping or preventing bleeding.

The procedure is technically difficult and entails the risk of bleeding from the liver wound and the passage of embolic material through the azygous system into the lungs. Unlike a surgically produced shunt, this method does not reduce portal venous pressure, and recurrent bleeding from esophageal varices may be a problem.

Arterial portography is the preferred method for evaluating the portal venous anatomy and flow patterns prior to the performance of a shunt procedure. In this technique, a preshaped catheter is introduced into the aorta via percutaneous femoral arteriotomy. The catheter tip is positioned in the celiac artery, and 40 to 60 ml of contrast material are injected. Selective arterial injection of vasodilator drugs, such as tolazoline, is often made just before the contrast injection to enhance venous opacification. Films are obtained during the arterial and venous phases of opacification (Fig. 15–25). This technique is preferable to splenoportography not only from the standpoint of complications but also because it provides an assessment of the arterial supply to the liver. Superior mesenteric arteriography can be performed at the same time, so that the size, configuration, and direction of the flow in the superior mesenteric vein can be studied.

Arteriography in patients with cirrhosis shows several abnormalities. The increase in hepatic arterial blood flow that accompanies intrahepatic portal obstruction is associated with an increase in the diameter of the common hepatic artery and its branches. The diameter of the common hepatic artery averages 7 mm in normal

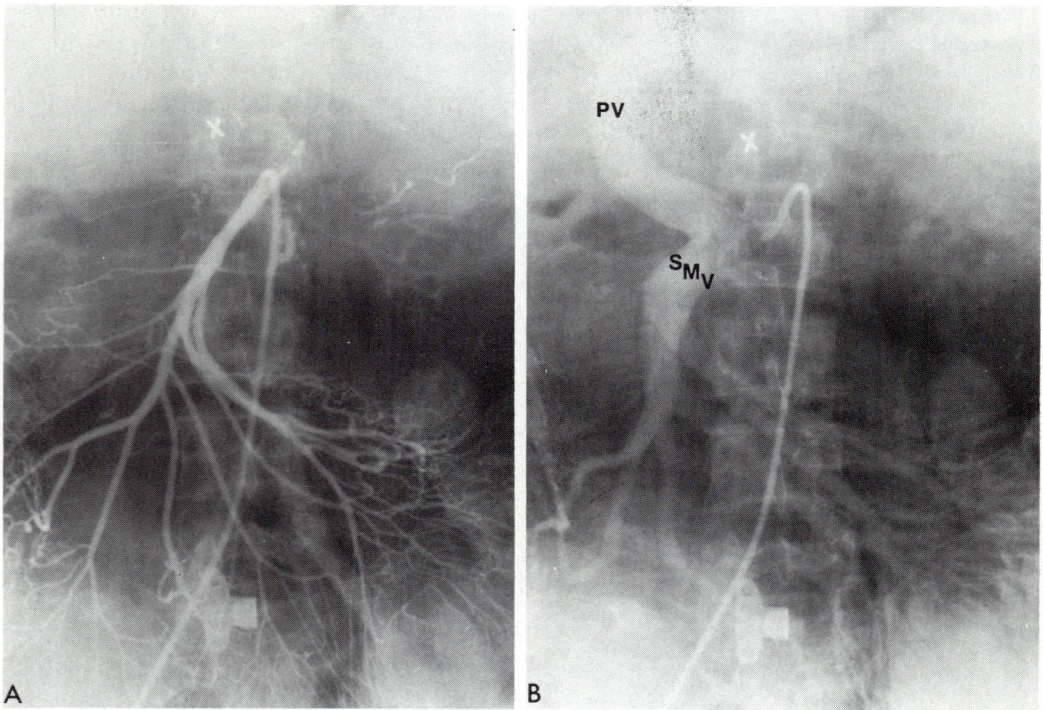

Figure 15–25. Normal superior mesenteric arteriogram. *A*, Arterial phase. *B*, Venous phase with opacification of superior mesenteric vein (SMV) and portal vein (PV). Note the absence of filling of the splenic vein.

Figure 15–26. Hepatic arteriogram in a 65-year-old man with chronic persistent hepatitis. The corkscrew appearance of the arteries in the superior aspect of the right hepatic lobe is consistent with cirrhosis and focal liver shrinkage. The stretching (arrows) of arteries in the inferior portion of the right lobe results from the presence of regenerating nodules.

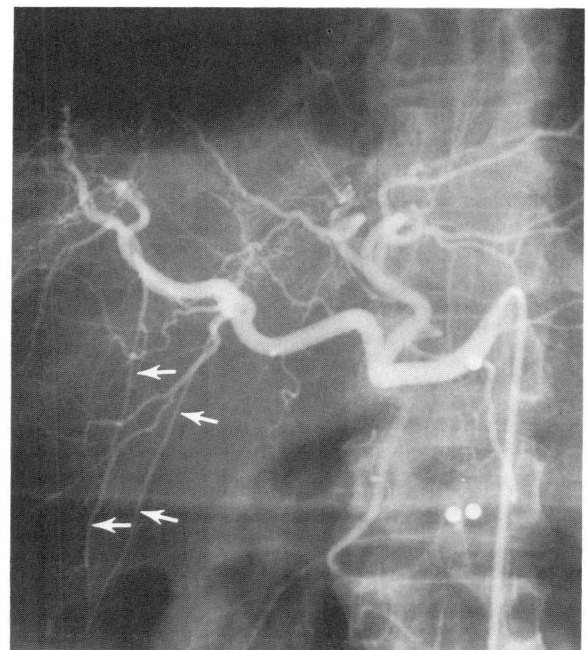

individuals but is often 10 mm or more in those with cirrhosis.[41] An associated finding is tortuosity of the peripheral branches of the hepatic artery. In cirrhotic patients with increased hepatic arterial flow and diminished liver size this tortuosity can be pronounced, producing the so-called corkscrew appearance (Fig. 15–26). One should always be alert to the possibility of a hepatoma, which may be found unexpectedly during celiac arteriography in a cirrhotic patient.

Films obtained 10 to 20 seconds after the onset of the celiac injection ordinarily show opacification of the splenic and portal veins. Opacification of the coronary vein or esophageal varices may be seen, indicating retrograde flow in these vessels (Fig. 15–27).

Figure 15–27. Large varices (V) arising from the coronary vein (CV) are seen in the late phase of the superior mesenteric artery injection. The coronary vein and splenic vein (SV) are dilated, and a small amount of contrast material has entered the portal vein (PV).

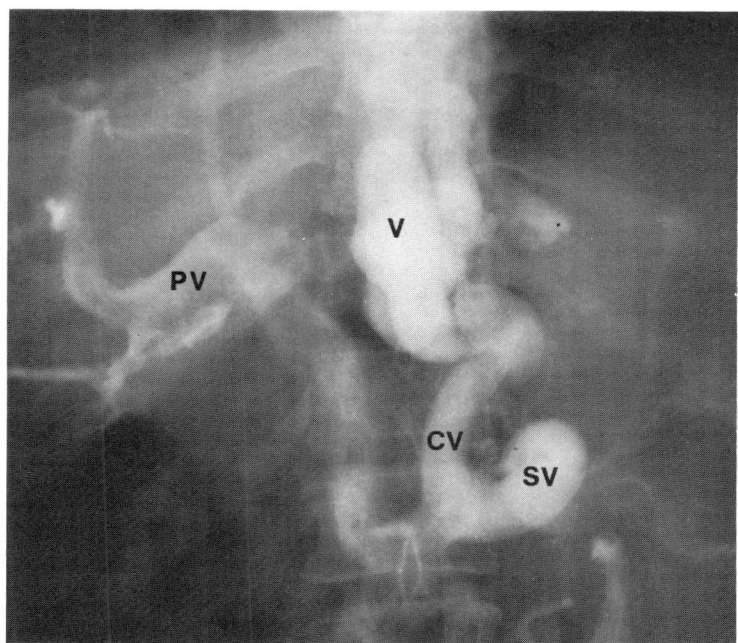

Retrograde filling of either the superior or the inferior mesenteric veins is also abnormal, and portosystemic collaterals may emanate from these vessels. At times, large collateral veins are seen draining splenic venous efflux into the left renal vein. In other cases, a dilated umbilical vein anastomoses the left portal vein to the inferior vena cava (Fig. 15–28).

Patients with portal hypertension often show veins in the bowel wall and mesentery that are increased in size and number. The configuration of the superior mesenteric vein can be studied as an aid in planning a mesocaval shunt procedure. Opacification of the coronary, splenic, or inferior mesenteric veins following injection in the superior mesenteric artery is abnormal and indicates hepatofugal flow in those vessels. Esophageal varices are often visualized by this method.

Hepatic venous catheterization is also useful in the evaluation of patients prior to portosystemic shunt procedures. This technique, which is performed via the femoral or median antecubital vein, enables the radiologist to obtain pressure measurements as well as free or wedged hepatic venograms. In experienced hands, the technique is virtually free of serious complications and provides information not obtainable by the arterial route.

The wedged hepatic vein pressure is obtained by passing an end-hole catheter as far into the hepatic vein as it will go. A saline manometer or pressure strain gauge is then used to record the resultant wedged hepatic vein pressure. It is convenient to place the baseline at the level of the right atrium. The catheter is then withdrawn until it lies freely in the hepatic vein, and the free hepatic vein pressure is recorded. The wedged hepatic vein pressure minus the free hepatic vein pressure is termed the corrected

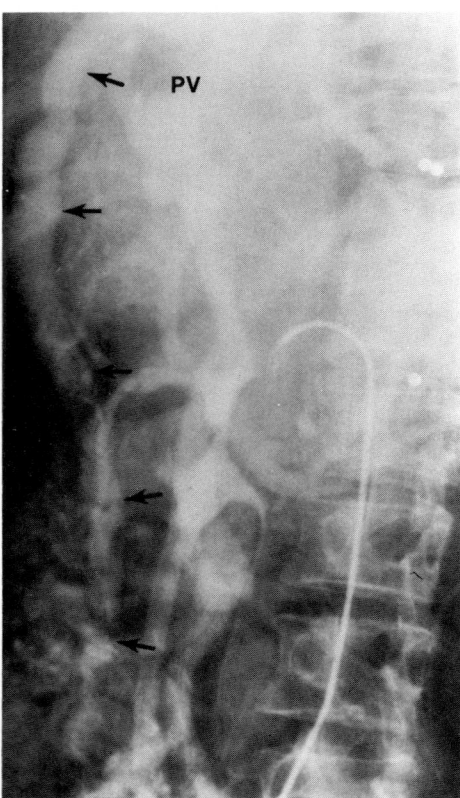

Figure 15–28. Oblique film from the venous phase of a superior mesenteric arteriogram in a young woman with postnecrotic cirrhosis and bleeding varices. A large umbilical vein collateral (arrows) connects the left portal vein (PV) with the lower abdominal branches of the vena cava.

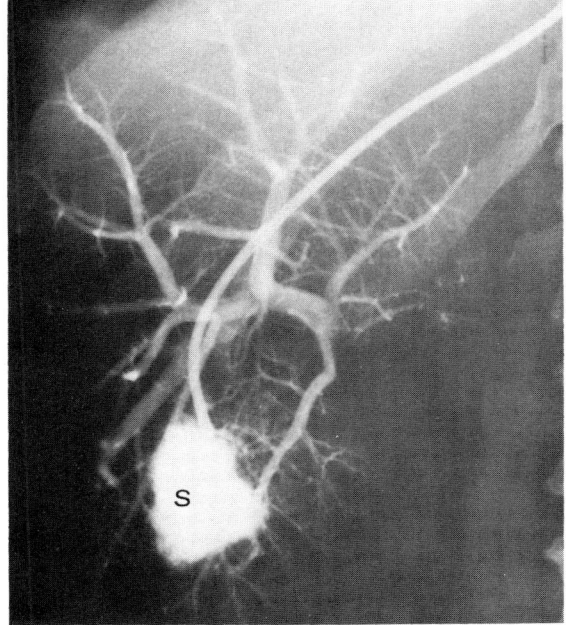

Figure 15–29. Normal wedged hepatic venogram in a patient with hepatomegaly and ascites. A dense parenchymal stain (S) is present at the catheter tip. Collateral flow opacified the portal venous branches which empty in a hepatopetal direction. The corrected hepatic wedged pressure was normal.

hepatic wedge pressure or corrected sinusoidal pressure (because it correlates closely with the pressure in the hepatic sinusoids). This pressure is a fairly accurate reflection of portal venous pressure in patients with cirrhosis. Normally, the corrected hepatic wedge pressure measures 8 mm Hg or less. Values in excess of 10 mm Hg indicate portal hypertension.[5] In cases of severe intrahepatic portal hypertension, the corrected wedge pressure may exceed 20 mm Hg.

Liver sinusoidal pressure may also be estimated by recording intraparenchymal pressure through a needle placed percutaneously into the liver. Pressures recorded in this way agree closely with those measured by the wedged hepatic vein approach. Because the added risk associated with percutaneous liver puncture and the occasional difficulty in recording the intraparenchymal pressure, the wedged hepatic vein catheter is usually the method of choice.

Wedged hepatic venography is performed by injecting 3 to 6 ml of contrast material through a catheter wedged in a hepatic vein. Normally, the contrast material opacifies a small area of hepatic parenchyma, with some entering the portal vein branches in that area (Fig. 15–29). At the end of the injection the contrast material in the portal branches immediately flows back into the liver parenchyma and is carried out of the liver with the hepatic venous flow.

Stenosis and occlusion of small hepatic vein radicals occur in patients with portal hypertension, giving the appearance of a "pruned tree" (Fig. 15–30). The parenchymal opacification takes on an inhomogeneous lobular or nodular pattern. There is often an increased degree of portal venous opacification. In cases of fairly severe portal hypertension, the washout time of the portal venous branches may exceed six seconds.[41] In the most severely affected patients, the flow in the opacified portal veins is hepatofugal (i.e., away from the liver) and the contrast material may outline the coronary vein or other collateral channels.

The hepatic venogram may also be obtained with the catheter tip in a nonwedged or free position (Fig. 15–30). Larger volumes are injected at a more rapid flow rate through a catheter with end and side holes. Normally the free venogram results in

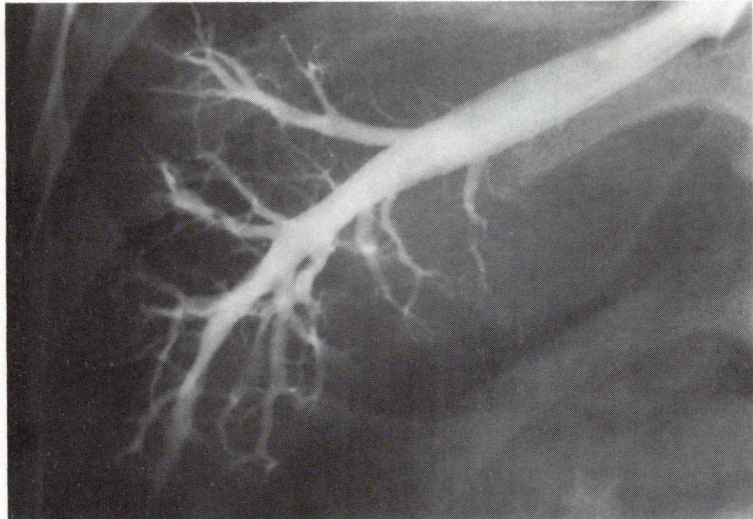

Figure 15–30. Free hepatic venogram in a patient with postnecrotic cirrhosis. Less than the normal number of small venous tributaries are filled, giving a mild form of the "pruned tree" appearance. The corrected hepatic wedged pressure was 17 cm of water, which indicates mild portal hypertension.

opacification of the hepatic vein and an extensive tree of tributaries out to fourth-order branches. Patients with cirrhosis show variable degrees of pruning and irregularity of side branches.

RADIOGRAPHIC EVALUATION AFTER PORTOSYSTEMIC SHUNT. Each of the angiographic techniques described is useful postoperatively for evaluating the results of portosystemic shunt procedures. Corrected hepatic wedge pressure is most helpful and shows a significant return toward normal following side-to-side portacaval or mesocaval shunts or other shunt procedures that effectively decompress the intrahepatic portal veins. Ideally, the postoperative corrected hepatic wedge pressure reflects a pressure gradient insufficient to stimulate the formation of new venous collaterals. Patients studied after end-to-side portacaval shunt in which the portal vein is ligated show less marked reduction in corrected wedge pressure. The hepatic venogram is less helpful in the postoperative period and is not commonly used.

Celiac and superior mesenteric arteriography with arterial portography show several changes after side-to-side portosystemic shunts. The hepatic artery, already larger than normal, may enlarge further after surgery as hepatic arterial flow increases. Both liver and spleen usually decrease in size. Blood flow in the portal vein reverses as the portal vein becomes an outflow tract for hepatic blood. Portal vein opacification is not likely to be seen if the shunt is open and effective. With the subtraction films it is usually possible to demonstrate faint opacification of the inferior vena cava at and above the site of the shunt (Fig. 15–31). Conversely, if the shunt has closed or is ineffective, none of these changes may occur, and celiac and superior mesenteric venous outflow will continue to opacify the portal vein and its abnormal venous collaterals (Fig. 15–31).

Portal Hypertension due to Presinusoidal Portal Obstruction

The radiologic approach to the work-up of portal hypertension resulting from presinusoidal portal obstruction includes the same tests as those used in cirrhosis. The presinusoidal block may be intrahepatic, as in cases of periportal fibrosis or congenital hepatic fibrosis. Because the pressure in the hepatic sinusoids tends to be normal, the

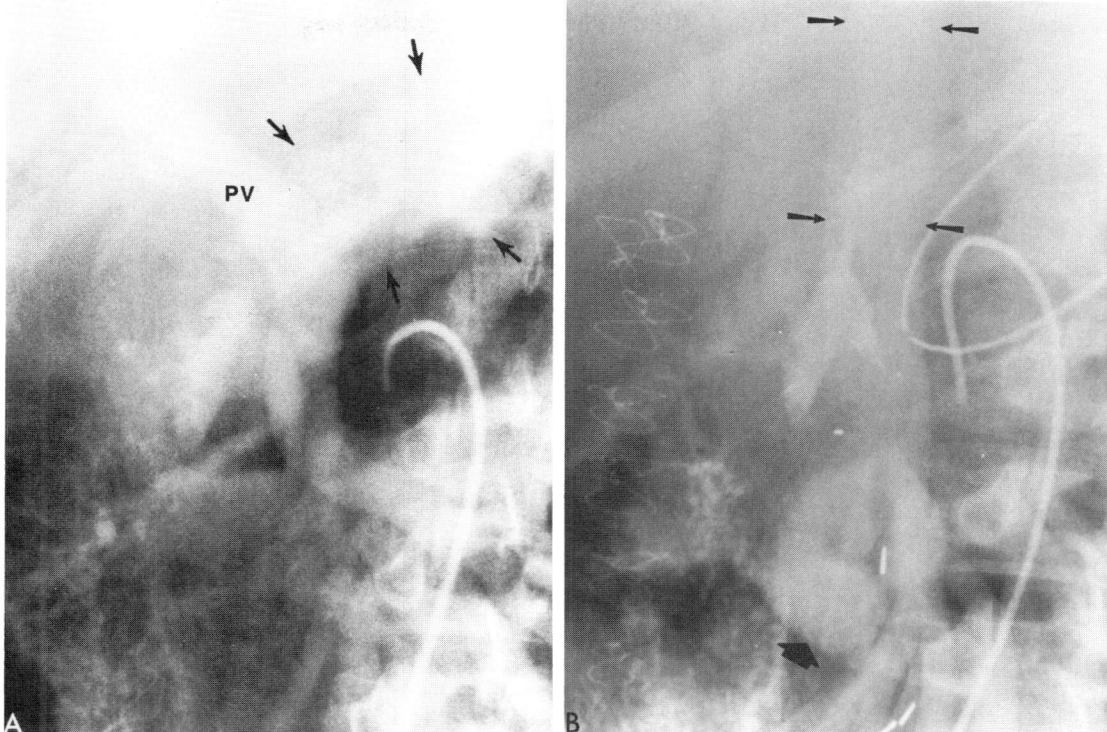

Figure 15–31. Arteriographic appearance after portosystemic shunt. *A*, Film from the venous phase of a superior mesenteric arteriogram performed one day after emergency mesocaval shunt for bleeding esophageal varices. The shunt is closed, as evidenced by lack of opacification of the shunt and persistent opacification of portal vein (PV) and varices (arrows) arising from the coronary vein. *B*, At the second operation, six days later, the shunt was tailored for better fit. Superior mesenteric arteriogram performed after the second operation shows findings typical of a patent and functional shunt. The shunt (large arrow) is opacified, and there is faint visualization of the inferior vena cava (small arrows). No blood is seen flowing from the mesenteric veins into the portal venous system or varices.

corrected hepatic wedge pressure is either normal or only moderately elevated. Hepatic arteriography in patients with congenital hepatic fibrosis shows inhomogeneous staining during the parenchymal or capillary phase of the injection sequence, while the hepatic parenchyma tends to be normal in patients with periportal fibrosis.

Congenital hepatic fibrosis is frequently associated with polycystic disease of the kidney and liver. In these patients the diagnosis can be established by demonstrating the hepatic and renal cysts ultrasonographically or by CT.

When the level of obstruction of the portal vein is outside the liver, the corrected hepatic wedge pressure will be normal, as will the hepatic venogram. Arterial portography is useful to confirm the diagnosis and to show nonfilling of the occluded portion of the venous system. The arteriogram may show pancreatic or other masses compressing the portal vein and causing obstruction. CT and ultrasound are also useful in demonstrating masses in the porta hepatis.

When the portal vein obstruction is long-standing, an appearance known as cavernous transformation may be seen. Patients with this condition usually present in adulthood with signs of portal hypertension due to occlusion of the portal vein that in most cases occurred as an unrecognized event in childhood. Arterial portography demonstrates a tangled network of collateral veins in the porta hepatis and no

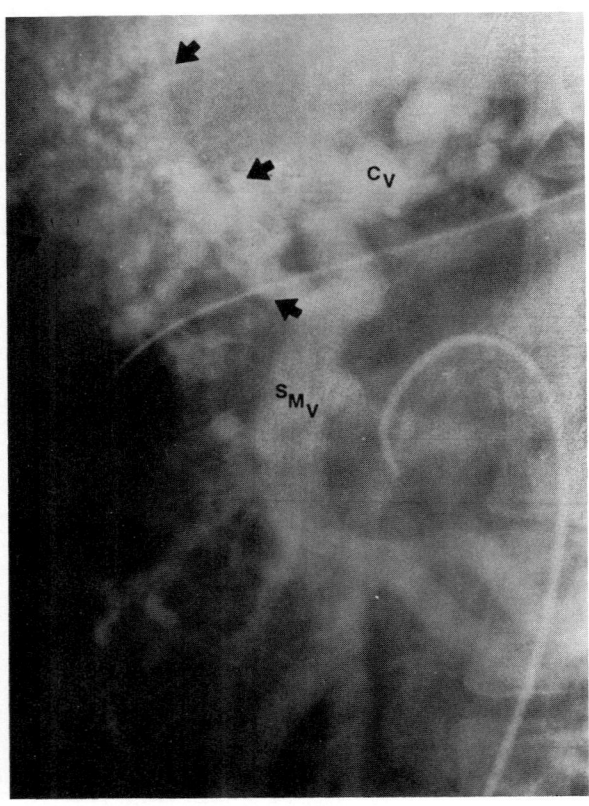

Figure 15-32. Venous phase from a superior mesenteric angiogram performed prior to portacaval shunt in a 31-year-old man with clinical evidence of portal hypertension. There is cavernous transformation of the portal vein manifested by a cluster of collateral veins (arrows) in the porta hepatis. The superior mesenteric vein (SMV) and dilated coronary vein (CV) are well seen.

recognizable main portal vein (Fig. 15–32). Esophageal varices and other portosystemic collaterals are often seen as well.

Portal Hypertension due to Hepatic Venous Obstruction

Hepatic vein obstruction, or the Budd-Chiari syndrome, is an unusual cause of portal hypertension. It may be due to tumor, trauma, or thrombosis. Hepatic vein thrombosis may in turn be a complication of paroxysmal nocturnal hemoglobinuria, polycythemia, or the use of oral contraceptive medication. In many cases, the cause of the Budd-Chiari syndrome cannot be ascertained.

Abdominal plain films or ultrasound are useful in detecting the ascites that is almost always present. ^{99m}Tc sulphur colloid liver-spleen scans show diminished hepatic uptake of the isotope and often diffusely heterogeneous uptake. Since there are usually one or two separate hepatic veins draining the caudate lobe, this area may be partially or completely spared. In such cases the isotopic uptake is normal in the caudate lobe and diminished in the remainder of the liver, giving the appearance of a central "hot spot" (see Fig. 15–15 C).

Angiographic procedures provide the most specific radiologic approach to the diagnosis of hepatic venous occlusion.[33] Venography of the inferior vena cava or hepatic veins may show compression or filling defects in these vessels, representing tumor or thrombus. Wedged venography in a patent or partially occluded hepatic vein often reveals a peculiar and characteristic network of intrahepatic collateral veins, sometimes referred to as a spider web pattern.

Hepatic arteriographic abnormalities are also present in the Budd-Chiari syndrome. The involved portions of the liver atrophy and receive a reduced volume of portal venous blood. This may account for the prolonged dense stain seen in the capillary or parenchymal phase. The portal vein supplying an involved lobe often becomes its venous outflow tract. Shrinkage of the involved portions of the liver leads to crowding and tortuosity of arterial branches in these areas. Conversely, unaffected portions of the liver undergo considerable hypertrophy, with consequent stretching and splaying of hepatic arterial branches that may simulate the appearance of a hepatic neoplasm.[21]

In summary, numerous radiographic examinations are available to aid in the evaluation of patients with portal hypertension. Once the diagnosis is established, however, liver panangiography is usually recommended prior to surgery. This involves celiac arteriography with filming during the venous phase, hepatic venography, and wedged hepatic vein pressure determination. The combination of these procedures usually clarifies the nature and severity of the underlying obstruction to flow. The same angiographic procedures can be performed postoperatively to assess the patency of portosystemic shunts and the degree of reduction in portal venous and portosystemic collaterals.

Never therapeutic approaches to the obliteration of esophageal varices via catheter and without surgery are being tried with varying success and may play an important role in the future.

TRAUMA

Radiologic procedures can be of great help in the evaluation of patients with direct penetrating trauma to the liver and blunt trauma to the abdomen with secondary hepatic abnormalities. When a stab wound or a missile injury to the liver occurs, with resultant severe hemorrhage and shock, the radiologist generally plays only a small role in the preoperative evaluation because the patient immediately undergoes primary surgical repair. However, the patient with closed abdominal blunt trauma affecting the liver and other organs requires diagnostic tests for evaluation of the extent of trauma prior to surgical correction. Patients with fractures of the liver capsule, avulsion of vessels, and hematomas present diagnostic problems needing radiologic evaluation. The radiologist must aid in evaluating both the extent and nature of the trauma and the complications resulting from repair. These include postoperative infection, hematoma, changes related to partial liver resection, and complications resulting from partial hepatectomy.

Radiologic Procedures

PLAIN FILM OF THE ABDOMEN. Often a supine film of the abdomen taken on a fixed or portable radiographic unit is obtained shortly after the patient has arrived in the emergency room, particularly in cases of missile wounds. Many abnormalities may be visible that indirectly indicate the extent of trauma, but these are nonspecific. They include fracture of one or more ribs, elevation of the right hemidiaphragm, and loss of the normal inferior liver angle, indicating the presence of fluid between the liver and the abdominal wall (see Fig. 15–11). Medial displacement of the right lateral surface of the liver and displacement of the colon away from the properitoneal fat can result from either blood or fluid in the peritoneal cavity.[60]

ARTERIOGRAPHY DURING THE ACUTE PHASE OF TRAUMA. The radiologic test most likely to be performed in the early phase of hepatic injury, other than a plain film, is a *selective hepatic arteriogram* to evaluate the status of the vessels inside and outside of the liver. The arteriogram is performed after the patient is relatively stabilized and other more life-threatening injuries have been evaluated. If cerebral trauma has accompanied blunt abdominal trauma and a cerebral angiogram is being done, it is then possible to study simultaneously the abdominal vasculature via a midstream aortogram, followed by selective hepatic arteriography if necessary. Arteriographic findings of liver trauma include:

1. Displacement of intrahepatic arteries around a hematoma or a newly formed collection of extravasated blood. The hematoma can still be identified as a negative defect in the contrast-enhanced parenchymal phase of the angiogram (Figs. 15–33 and 15–34). Later, there may be a contrast-enhanced rim caused by compressed liver tissue.

2. Occasionally a traumatic arteriovenous fistula between the hepatic artery and the portal vein branches may be demonstrated. This can be diagnosed by noting early opacification of a vein during the arterial phase.

3. In most blunt injuries to the liver the liver capsule is fractured.[31] Such fractures and lacerations may appear on the arteriogram as a lucent defect in the capillary phase, with ill-defined contrast collections appearing within them in the venous phase.

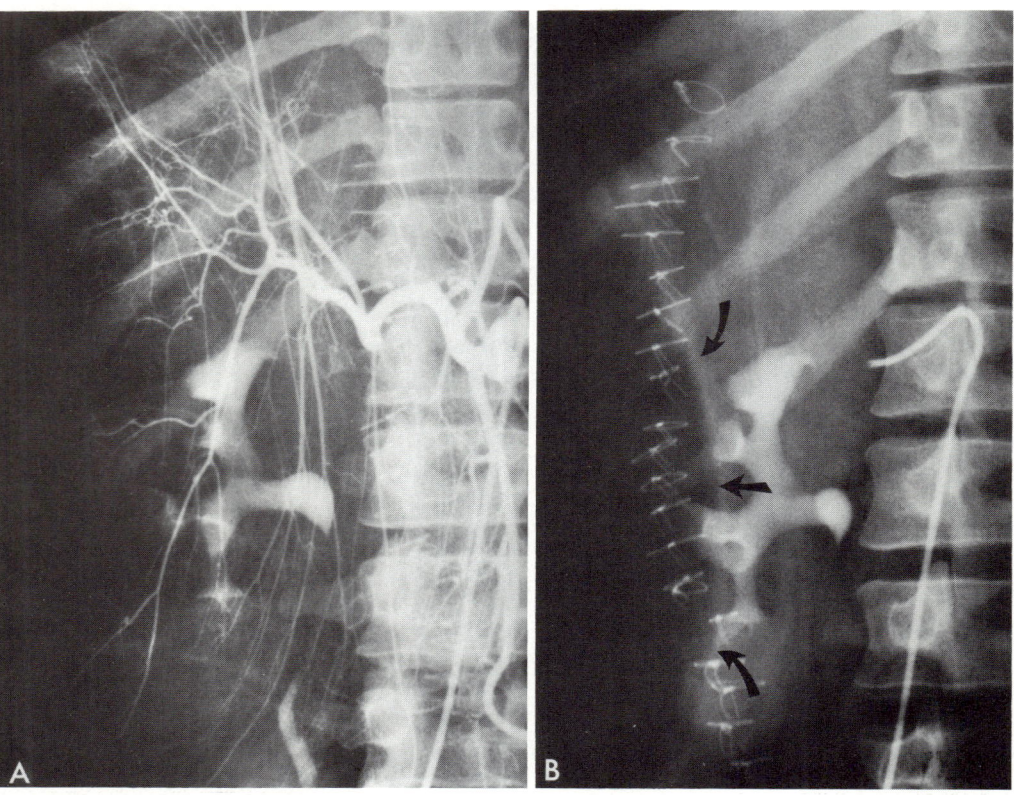

Figure 15–33. *A,* Hepatic arteriogram performed three weeks after blunt abdominal trauma demonstrates stretching of the arteries in the periphery of the right lobe of the liver, with crowding of arterial vessels. *B,* In the venous phase of the arteriogram, the avascular area occupied by the hematoma has compressed normal liver parenchyma, resulting in a sharp demarcation of the hematoma (arrows).

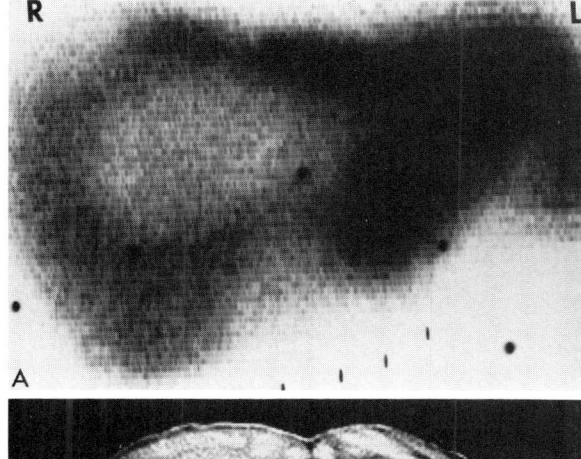
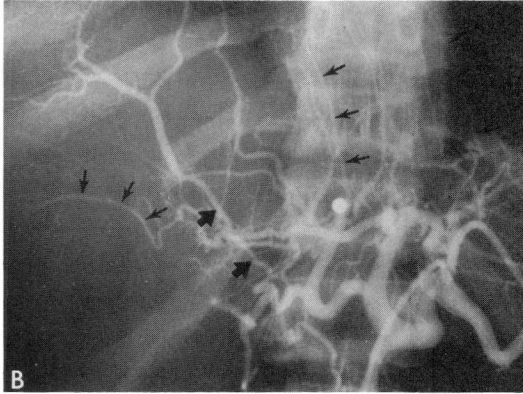
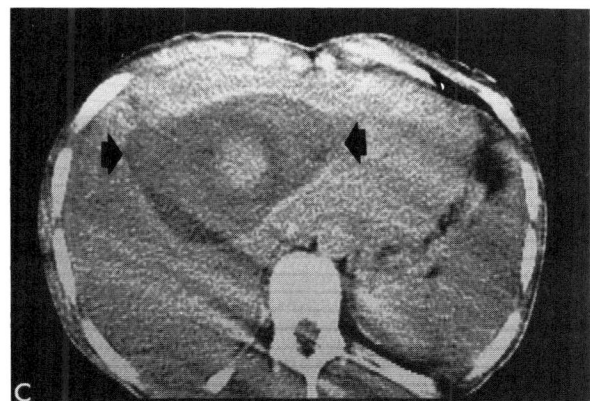

Figure 15–34. An 18-year-old man with a gunshot wound to the liver. The liver wound was debrided and repaired immediately after injury, but the patient later developed fever and weight loss. A, Four months after surgery, ^{99m}Tc sulfur colloid scan shows a large central area of diminished uptake. B, Celiac arteriogram shows compression and displacement of the right hepatic artery by mass (large arrows). Straightening and displacement by smaller arteries in right and left lobes (small arrows) indicate extent of the mass. C, CT scan shows low-density fluid-filled mass (arrows) within the liver, consistent with abscess or hematoma. Dense area in the center of the low-density area probably represents viable liver tissue protruding into the hematoma. At surgery, a large infected hematoma was drained.

Different priorities exist for diagnostic radiographic procedures in evaluating a patient who has received blunt abdominal trauma without the severe and catastrophic consequences of massive abdominal hemorrhage. Arteriography still affords a great deal of information and until recently was the single best test to guide the surgeon in assessing vascular damage and its consequences. However, other imaging modalities now available provide information about the status of the liver parenchyma and obviate subjecting the patient to an arteriogram. These include the radionuclide liver-spleen scan, hepatic ultrasound, and CT (Fig. 15–34).

RADIONUCLIDE SCAN. The *liver-spleen scan* using ^{99m}technetium sulfur colloid can be performed with relatively little difficulty in the injured patient. Since the study provides both static and dynamic flow information, it is possible to demonstrate, shortly after injection of the radionuclide, areas of increased and decreased uptake within the liver. These represent areas of extravasation or arteriovenous fistula (hot spots) and areas of hematoma formation (cold spots). The static scintigram is also capable of demonstrating subcapsular hematomas and marked disruption of the liver parenchyma. This is particularly true if the damage has occurred in the periphery of the liver as the test is less sensitive in the central portion and porta hepatis.[11, 14] However, the radionuclide liver scan is the least specific of the new tests in locating the abnormality and determining its characteristics.

ULTRASOUND. Both transverse and longitudinal *ultrasonic scans* of the liver may reveal disrupted continuity of the liver capsule, subcapsular or intrahepatic hematomas, and displacement of the liver by fluid as well as subhepatic and perihepatic hematoma and abscess formation. Since ultrasonography is noninvasive and relatively easy to perform, it should be considered when damage to the liver is suspected,

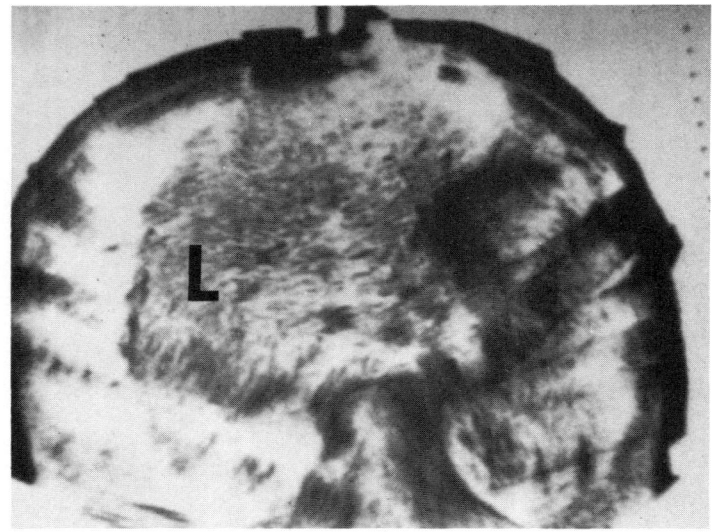

Figure 15–35. Transverse ultrasonogram in a young man with recent abdominal trauma shows an area lateral to the liver margin (L) that is mainly echo-free but contains a few echoes near the liver parenchyma. A large subcapsular hematoma was discovered at surgery.

particularly in the evaluation of possible intrahepatic or subcapsular hematomas. However, in fractured ribs, lacerations of the abdominal wall, or exploratory laparotomy, bandages and operative wounds may interfere with the performance and evaluation of ultrasound. As hematomas form within the liver, they produce a detectable difference in the pattern of echoes compared with the surrounding normal liver. Early in the development of hematoma, an echogenic area representing disruption of the normal parenchymal pattern occurs without clear or sharp margins (Fig. 15–35). As the hematoma organizes and fluid within the hematoma becomes more homogeneous and serous, a more sonolucent center appears within the liver — in some instances resulting in acoustic enhancement of the back wall of this mass, so that the hematoma may take on the sonographic appearance of a cyst or an abscess.

CT SCANNING. Changes in the anatomy of the liver produced by blunt or open trauma, such as the presence of perihepatic fluid displacing the liver or subcapsular and intrahepatic hematomas, can be evaluated by CT. Subcapsular hematomas resulting from needle liver biopsy may also be detected (Fig. 15–36). The appearance of hepatic

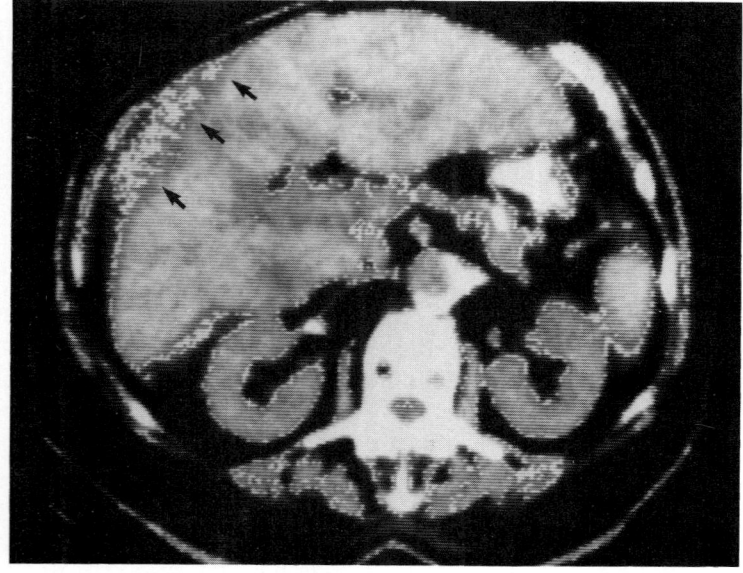

Figure 15–36. A subcapsular hematoma (arrows), the result of a needle biopsy of the liver, produces a peripheral, crescentic low-density area at the periphery of the liver. The CT number of the hematoma is 10.

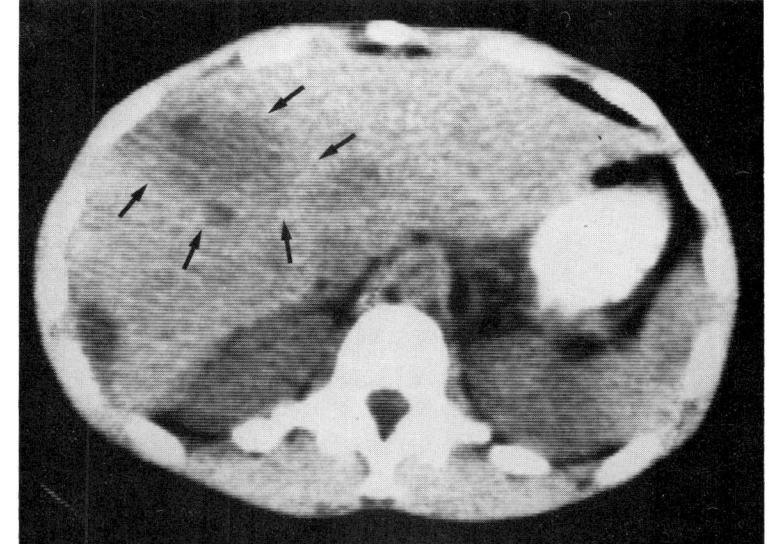

Figure 15–37. Diffuse hepatic parenchymal hemorrhage occurred along the tract of a missile from a gunshot (arrows). The CT appearance is one of an ill-defined low-density area. A second hematoma (low-density area) was found at the periphery of the right lobe.

hematomas is similar to that of splenic hematomas.[48] Initially, disruption of the liver parenchyma results in an area of slightly greater density and higher CT number than the surrounding liver. After several days to weeks, the hematoma organizes further, and the CT number of the center of the hematoma decreases as the fluid becomes more serous (Figs. 15–37 and 15–38). This is partially demonstrated after intravenous infusion of contrast material, enhancing the normal liver parenchyma and raising its CT number, thereby accentuating areas that are not supplied by normal vasculature. In cases of significant arteriovenous connection, it may be possible to image intravenous contrast material in this fistula by CT scanning.[42] The hematoma may compress normal tissue, and when intravenous contrast material is given it may demonstrate a rim similar to that noted with an abscess. Earliest CT findings of intrahepatic hematoma occur a few days after trauma.

Experience with subcapsular and pericapsular renal hematomas has shown that an initial CT number of 36 to 40 occurs when the hematoma is fresh and that it decreases to

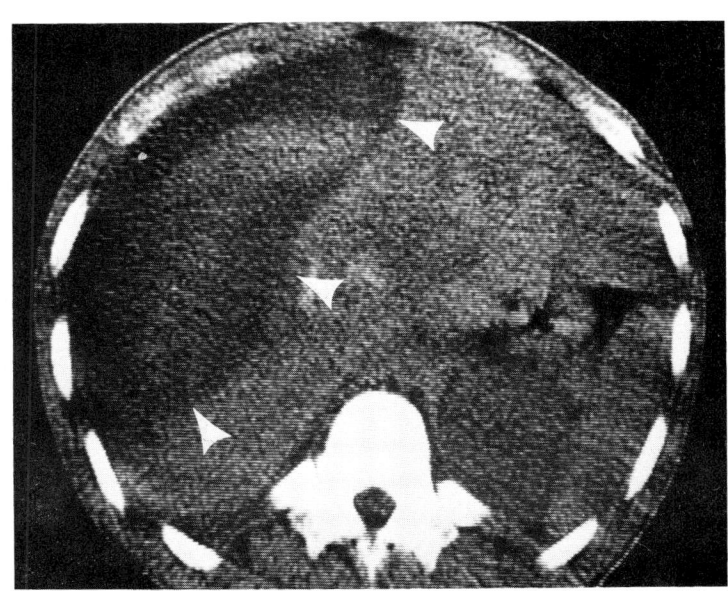

Figure 15–38. CT scan through the liver in a 19-year-old man two weeks after blunt abdominal trauma. The patient had fever, upper abdominal pain, and falling hematocrit. CT showed a large subcapsular hematoma (arrowheads) of the liver, subsequently confirmed at surgery. The periphery of the hematoma is of low density, but the center approaches the same density as the liver parenchyma.

the range of 15 to 25 within five or six days, indicating a change in the nature of the hematoma.[48]

ARTERIOGRAPHY DURING RECOVERY PHASE OF TRAUMA. Selective *hepatic arteriography* can be used to further elucidate the abnormality seen on any of the previously mentioned imaging studies in the later phases of post-traumatic liver damage. When arteriograms are performed several days to weeks after liver trauma, the main findings are usually those resulting from subcapsular or intrahepatic hematomas. These appear as avascular areas that crowd and displace smaller vessels in the arterial phase. The avascular peripheral location of subcapsular hematomas is seen best in the delayed parenchymal or capillary phase (see Fig. 15–33), and the hematoma frequently compresses normal hepatic tissues, producing a vascular blush around its periphery.[42, 52]

Other complications of hepatic trauma can also be detected by arteriography. Pseudoaneurysms and arteriovenous fistulas can be demonstrated.

Portal vein thrombosis may result from blunt trauma to the abdomen, and ascites and esophageal varices may develop over a period of weeks. To evaluate these possibilities a splenic or superior mesenteric arteriogram should be performed, using a large volume of contrast material. The late venous phase would show whether the portal vein is patent. Blunt trauma to the abdomen, particularly in children, is one of the most common causes of isolated portal vein thrombosis. If an inferior venacavagram is performed, compression of the intrahepatic portion of the cava by intrahepatic hematomas may sometimes be seen.

IMAGING PROCEDURES TO EVALUATE THE LIVER AFTER SURGERY. Radiographic procedures are performed after surgery for blunt trauma, drainage of an intrahepatic infection, resection of a lobe for tumor or cyst, evaluation of changes in appearance of the venous, biliary, and arterial systems as a result of surgery, or evaluation of postoperative complications.

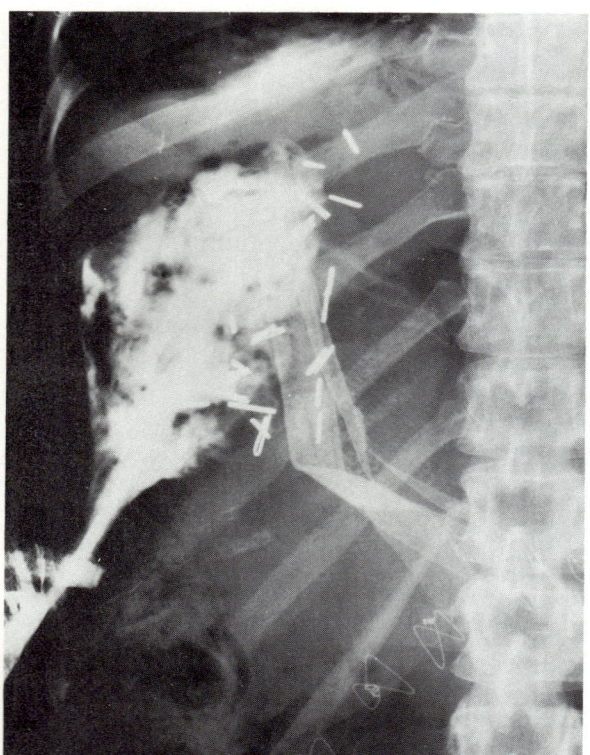

Figure 15–39. As a result of a gunshot wound, a large area of the right lobe of the liver was debrided and drained. Instillation of iodinated contrast material in the partial hepatectomy sinus tract permits evaluation of the size and extent of the remaining cavity.

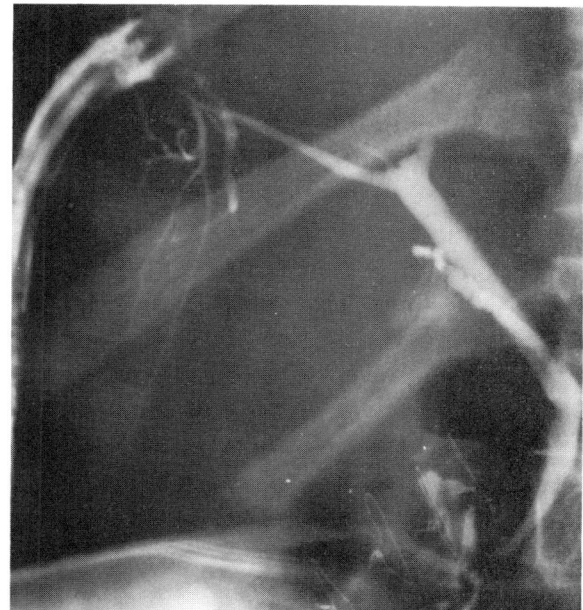

Figure 15–40. A drain was placed in a subcapsular hematoma, the result of blunt abdominal trauma, in this 25-year-old man. Subsequent injection of water-soluble contrast material shows a connection between the drain site and the bile ducts.

After closure of the liver capsule following missile tract injury, drains placed in the liver bed or in the liver parenchyma may be used as conduits for sinus tract injections to follow the resolutions of hematoma or necrotic liver and the development of fistulas (Figs. 15–39 and 15–40). In these instances, water-soluble contrast material may be injected through the drain tubes, or the drainage tracts may be cannulated with soft rubber catheters. The radiographs provide a continuing series of images portraying the resolution of hematomas and fluid collections. Often, when suspected bile duct injury accompanies liver trauma a T-tube is placed in the common bile duct at the time of surgery. T-tube cholangiography, therefore, becomes an important aspect of the postoperative monitoring of the patient with liver injury. A cholangiogram, performed in the conventional manner using diluted water-soluble contrast material, is useful for determining the patency of the biliary tract and for detecting biliary sinus tracts (Fig. 15–41), disruption of the biliary tract, or biliary venous fistulas.

Hepatic arteriography is also useful following surgery for hepatic trauma (Fig. 15–42). Occasionally, the hepatic injuries resulting from blunt abdominal trauma may appear rather minor at the time of emergency exploratory laparotomy. Subsequent arteriography may demonstrate signs of much more severe and extensive liver injury than was initially suspected.[36] These findings may dictate the need for reoperation and removal of portions of devitalized liver.

In other patients, the need may arise to determine whether the occurrence of hemorrhagic shock in the postoperative period is due to recurrent hepatic bleeding. Arteriography can then be useful to demonstrate progressive increase in hepatic or perihepatic hematomas. Extravasation of contrast material from an injured vessel can also be demonstrated.

To control massive hepatic bleeding following trauma, it is sometimes necessary to ligate the common or proper hepatic artery or a major branch. After this type surgery, arteriography can document the site and extent of collateral arterial flow to the liver (Figs. 15–43 and 15–44).[23] It has been shown arteriographically that collateral arterial supply to the liver following hepatic artery ligation arises mainly from branches of the gastroduodenal artery and the right inferior phrenic artery (Fig. 15–45).

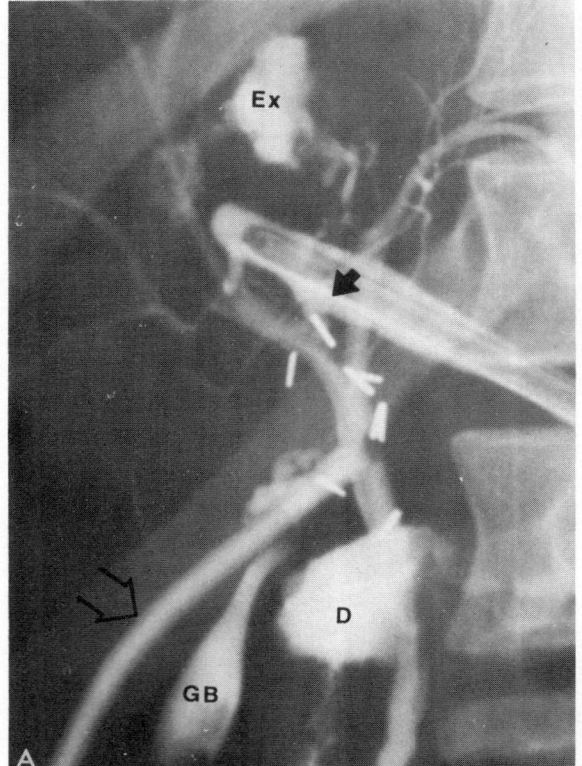
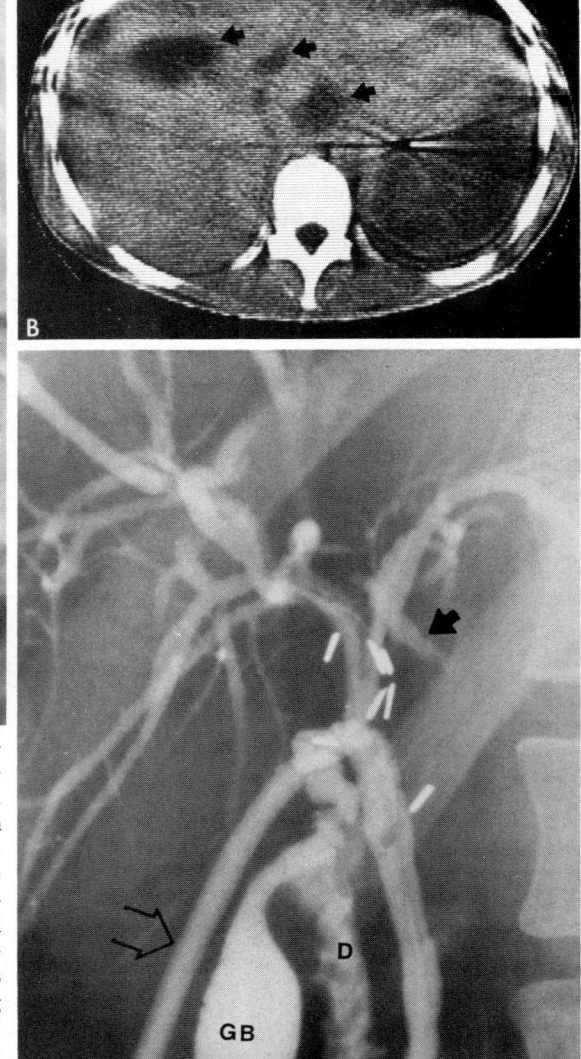

Figure 15–41. Laparotomy revealed a hepatic laceration involving the biliary tree near its main bifurcation in a young man with blunt abdominal trauma. T-tube with split upper limb was put in place, with one portion of upper limb in each main hepatic duct. *A*, Cholangiogram through T-tube (open arrow) shows extravasation (Ex) into the liver and a communication (solid arrow) between the drainage tube and the right hepatic duct (GB = gallbladder; D= duodenum). *B*, CT scan performed the following day shows low-density areas (arrows) in the liver, representing fluid collections (bile leaks, hematomas, or abscess). *C* Two months after surgery, a T-tube (open arrow) cholangiogram shows minimal filling of residual sinus tract (solid arrow) at the site of prior drainage tube. The patient recovered.

Complications of Liver Trauma

Complications of blunt trauma and of surgery to correct trauma or remove tumor are not uncommon. They are related to destruction of large areas of liver parenchyma, leading to intrahepatic hemorrhage, hematoma, and abscess formation. Also, perihepatic, suprahepatic, and subhepatic abscesses may develop, owing to soiling of the peritoneal cavity, which is often associated with leakage of bile. Arteriovenous fistulas, biliary-parenchymal and biliary-venous fistulas, and even hepatic-pulmonary fistulae may develop following surgery.

The three most common complications are infection, respiratory difficulty, and the consequences of hemorrhage.[39] Infection takes the form of abscesses, either around or

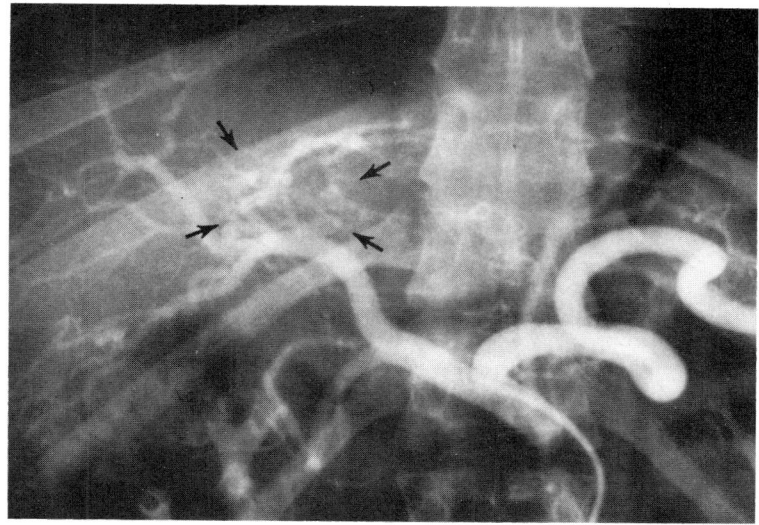

Figure 15-42. Laparotomy revealed liver lacerations and avulsion of the left hepatic artery in a young man with blunt abdominal trauma. The artery was ligated to control bleeding. A celiac arteriogram taken two years later shows well-developed arterial collaterals (arrows) between right and left hepatic arteries.

within the liver. Hepatic and perihepatic abscesses are discussed on page 847. Pneumonia, pulmonary edema, and "shock lung" may all result from severe hepatic injury and hepatic surgery, and each has its distinctive appearance on chest x-ray. Although the radiographic features of pulmonary complications are beyond the scope of this chapter, the radiologist should be aware that fevers following liver surgery do not always indicate infection from the damaged liver. Chest radiographs are an important adjunct in the evaluation of the posthepatectomy patient.

Radiographic features of intrahepatic or perihepatic hemorrhage have been discussed and illustrated (see Figs. 15-33 to 15-39). The selection of particular tests and their sequence depends upon the equipment available and the status of the patient. Certainly a plain film of the abdomen can be obtained in any patient with suspected complication following liver surgery. But unless the resultant hematoma is very extensive or necrotic liver tissue is filled with gas-forming organisms, the plain film has little value. In the postsurgical patient, noninvasive imaging of the liver can be

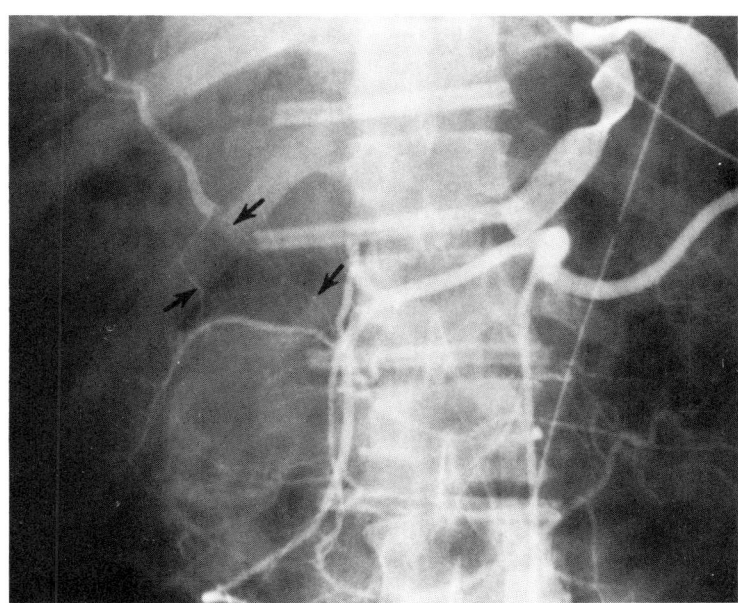

Figure 15-43. Celiac arteriogram taken four hours after proper hepatic artery ligation for control of bleeding due to extensive liver lacerations. Fine arterial collaterals (arrows) from the gastroduodenal and supraduodenal arteries have already reconstituted the flow in the hepatic artery distal to the point of interruption.

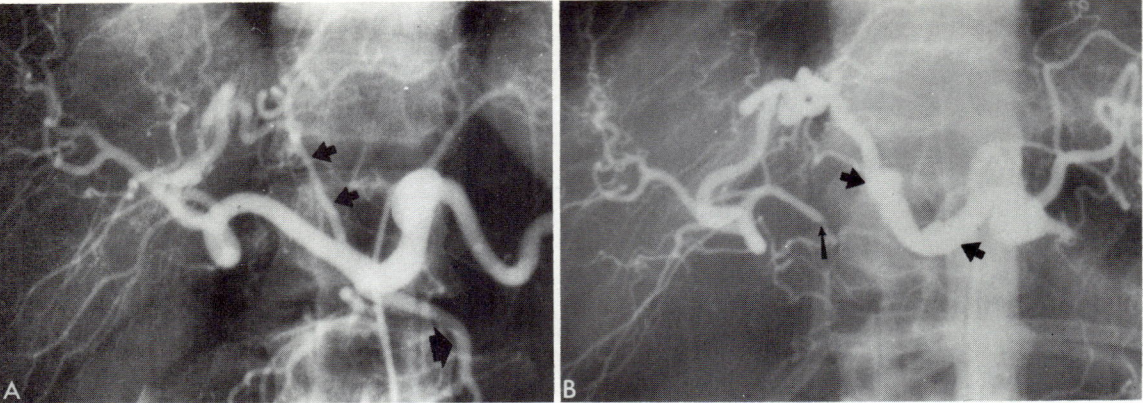

Figure 15-44. *A,* Preoperative celiac arteriogram before total pancreatectomy in a patient with chronic relapsing pancreatitis. The gastroduodenal artery is displaced (large arrow) by an inflmmatory mass in the head of the pancreas. Note the left hepatic branch of the proper hepatic artery (small arrows). At surgery, portions of the common and proper hepatic arteries were incorporated into the resected specimen. *B,* To revascularize the liver, the left hepatic branch was joined to the stump of the common hepatic artery with a saphenous vein graft. Celiac arteriogram two weeks after surgery shows the graft (between large arrows) supplying good flow to both lobes of the liver, with retrograde opacification of the proper hepatic artery back to the point of ligation (small arrow).

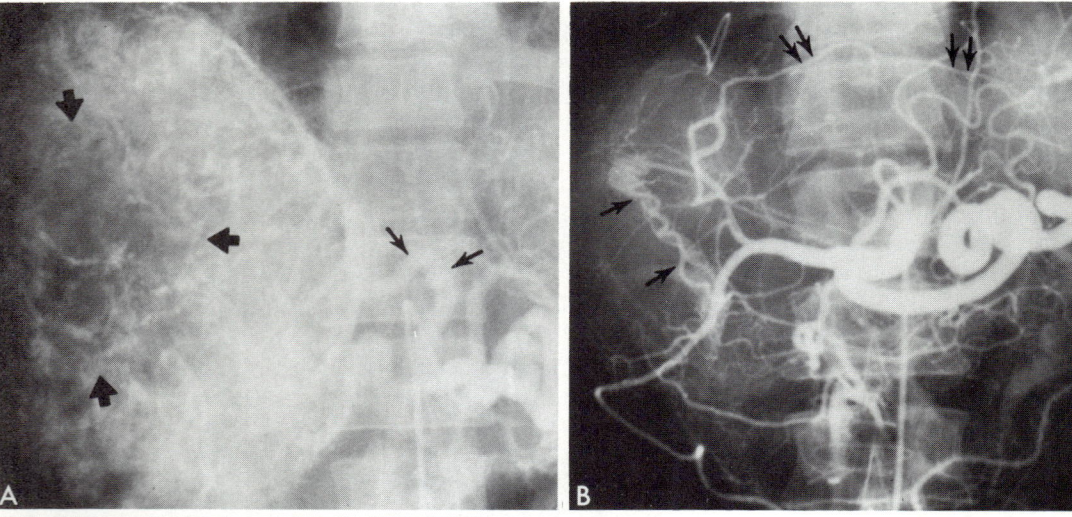

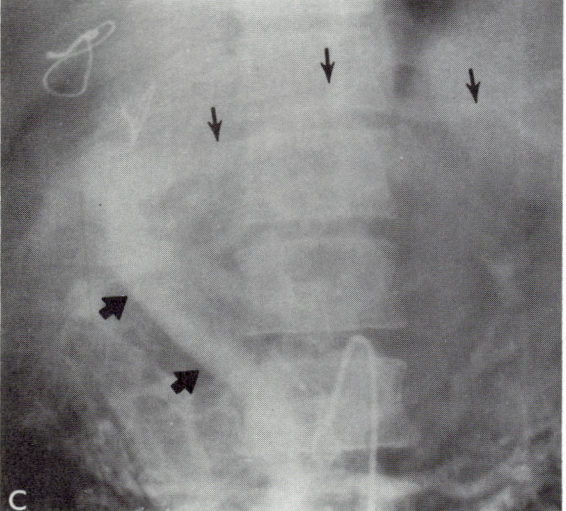

Figure 15-45. Weight loss and a palpable epigastric mass in a middle-aged Chinese male who developed sudden abdominl pain and hypotension. *A,* Celiac arteriogram at the time of the acute illness shows a large, well-circumscribed, hypervascular mass occupying most of the right hepatic lobe. Arterial supply is from the proper hepatic artery (small arrows). A central region of hypovascularity (large arrows) indicates hemorrhage into the tumor. The tumor was resected immediately thereafter. To control bleeding, it was necessary to ligate the proper hepatic and right hepatic arteris. *B,* One month later, celiac arteriography demonstrates collateral branches (arrows) of the gastroduodenal artery entering the liver and good opacificiation of arterial supply in the left hepatic lobe (double arrows). No recurrence of tumor is seen. *C,* Venous phase from a superior mesenteric artery arrows) and left portal vein (small arrows). The right portal vein was surgically removed.

accomplished with radionuclide liver scan, ultrasound, or CT scan. The ^{99m}Tc sulphur colloid liver-spleen scan can be used not only to detect hematomas (see Fig. 15–34) but to follow their regression. However, at the present time, the image provided by radionuclide scan is not as detailed as that obtained by ultrasound or CT. Because the latter afford better images of the liver and perihepatic spaces and show the relationship of other organs to the porta hepatis and liver, they are preferable for evaluating hemorrhage. Resolution or exacerbation of liver bleeding can be followed by either method, and it is not necessary, except in unusually difficult cases, to perform more than one imaging test.

The arteriographic features of liver hemorrhage after surgery have also been discussed (p. 841). Repeated arteriography is not the best way to follow the progress of a liver hematoma, both because of the risk and expense and because it does not delineate the size and nature of the hematoma as well as ultrasound and CT.

The appearance of the liver after partial resection is quite variable and depends upon the nature of the surgery. After a left lobectomy, radiography shows a large oval structure in the right upper abdomen with no evidence of a left lobe. Usually the line of resection in left lobectomy is to the right of the interlobar fissure. A right lobectomy distorts the hepatic anatomy. Large and small bowel loops move in to fill the space previously occupied by the right lobe (Fig. 15–46). As the remaining liver regenerates, its contour may become somewhat nodular and irregular. Serial ultrasound or CT studies can demonstrate regrowth of liver parenchyma, and regenerating nodules may appear as masses on the surface of the liver (Fig. 15–47).

HEMOBILIA. Hemobilia may result from either blunt trauma and liver fracture of stab wounds. Blood in the biliary tract may be caused by rupture of a hepatic artery aneurysm or by an arterial-biliary fistula following needle biopsy of the liver — an increasingly common cause of hemobilia.[47, 50] Spontaneous hemobilia develops when blunt trauma causes a fracture of the liver or avulsion of the duct and vessels.

Clinically, hemobilia may be difficult to detect. Blood may appear in the stool; if hemorrhage is massive, signs and symptoms of blood loss will develop. If these signs and symptoms are associated with recent liver biopsy, bleeding in the biliary tract should be

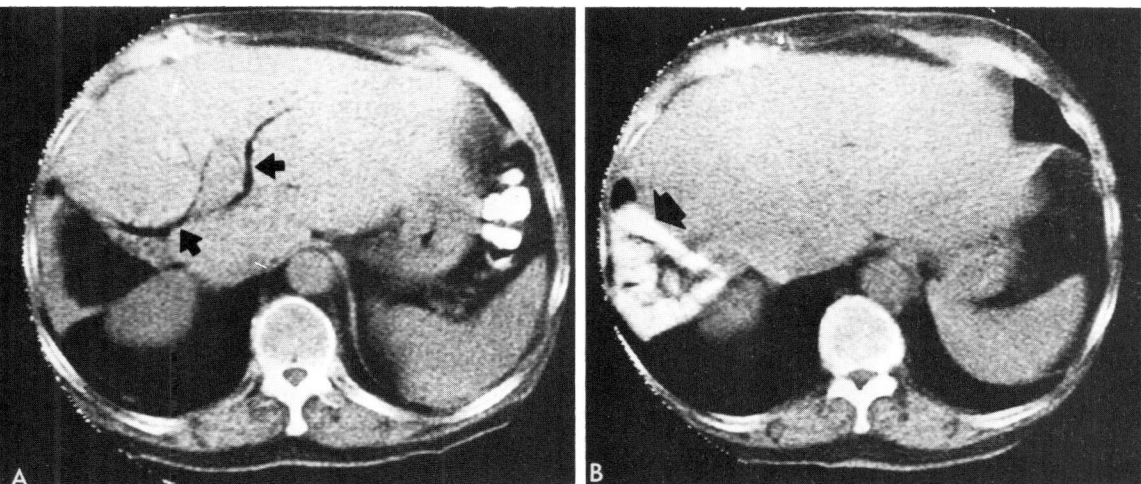

Figure 15–46. CT scan through the liver nine years after right hepatic lobectomy and anastomosis of the jejunum to the left hepatic duct. *A*, The left lobe has undergone compensatory hypertrophy, and there is air in the biliary tree (arrows). *B*, After ingestion of oral contrast material the jejunum (arrow) can be seen in the area previously occupied by the right hepatic lobe.

846 — THE LIVER

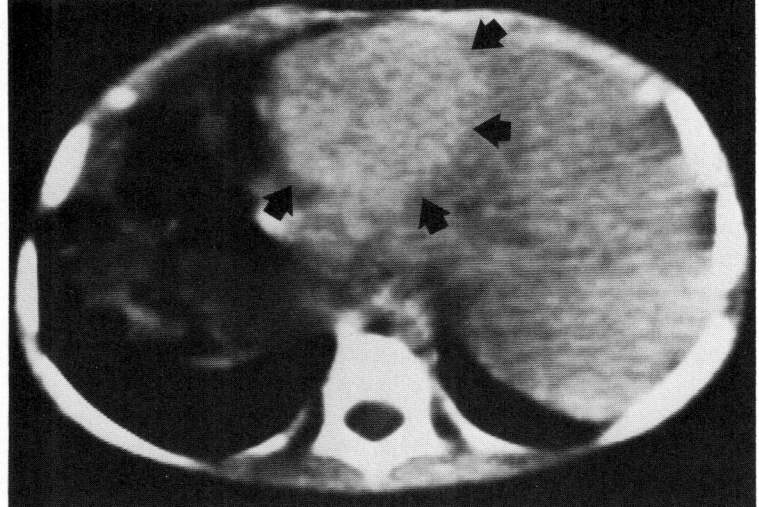

Figure 15–47. This patient had previously undergone a right hepatectomy because of trauma. The remaining left lobe is enlarged. The right side of this hypertrophied lobe is composed of a rounded mass of slightly higher CT number than the left lobe and represents focal nodular hyperplasia (arrows), proven by liver biopsy.

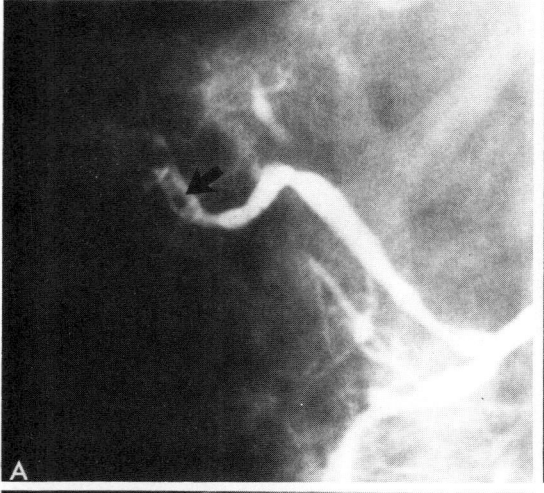
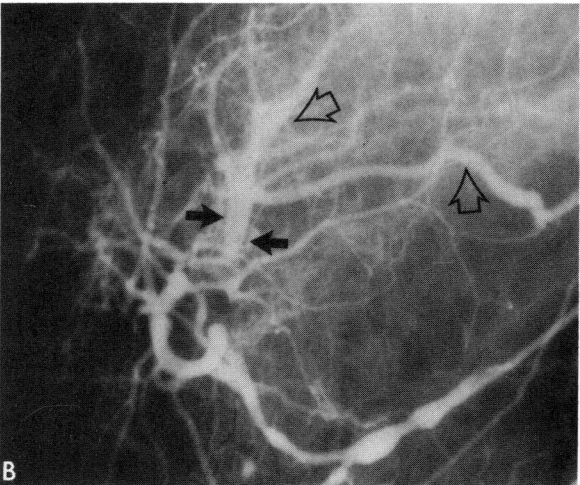
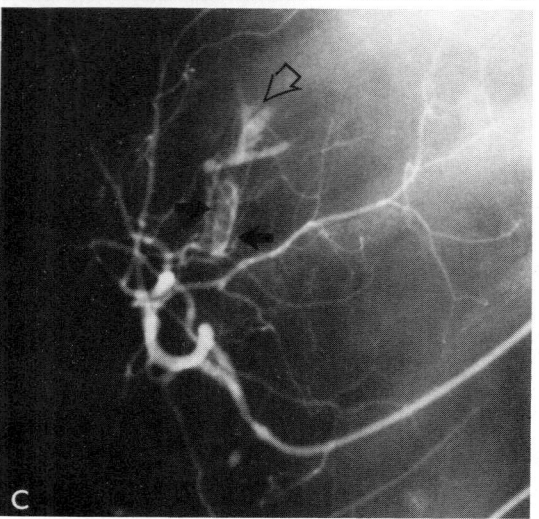

Figure 15–48. *A*, Selective hepatic arteriogram performed in a woman with massive gastrointestinal bleeding and a recent liver biopsy. The contrast material injected into the right hepatic artery appears in an adjacent bile duct which contains clot (arrow). In addition to the arterial-biliary fistula, an arterial-hepatic venous fistual is also present, as indicated by contrast material in the veins. *B*, An x-ray obtained later in the arteriogram shows contrast material in the bile duct (closed arrows) and veins (open arrows). *C*, The arteriogram performed after the instillation of multiple Gelfoam emboli demonstrates that the arterial-biliary fistula has been occluded. Some emboli may be seen in the artery (arrow). (Courtesy of John Barr, M.D., Oakland, California.)

suspected. If hemobilia is associated with recent blunt or penetrating trauma to the abdomen, hemorrhage into a large hematoma with a concurrent biliary fistula must also be considered. The association of melena with intermittent right upper quadrant pain and intermittent jaundice greatly increases the likelihood that the biliary tract is the source of bleeding.[48]

Occasionally, hemobilia can be demonstrated by arteriography. When rapid bleeding into the biliar tract is occurring, selective hepatic arteriography may demonstrate extravasation of contrast material from a hepatic artery branch into the liver parenchyma or into a bile duct (Fig. 15–48).

Treatment usually consists of operative ligation of the bleeding vessel. If this is not possible, lobectomy may have to be done. Transcatheter hepatic artery embolization has also been successful in controlling intrahepatic hemorrhage.[45, 56]

HEPATIC ABSCESSES

Liver abscesses are usually either pyogenic or amoebic. While the clinical signs, symptoms, and history may differ, these two entities can be considered together from the standpoint of radiographic detection.

In a suspected hepatic abscess, the imaging investigation includes plain film radiography, radionuclide scanning, cross-sectional imaging (CT, ultrasound), and occasionally arteriography. Supine and erect radiographs of the abdomen may be helpful; however, plain film findings are usually nonspecific and indirect. For instance, a hepatic abscess situated near the diaphragm results in a right pleural effusion. Liver abscess may also result in hepatic enlargement and may show an abnormal bulge of its border on the plain radiographs. Ascites may occur, with consequent loss of the "liver angle." Gas bubbles overlying the liver suggest an abscess, either with gas-forming organisms or with a connection to the biliary tree and the gastrointestinal tract (Fig. 15–49).

Radionuclide Scanning

The most widely used and best screening method for localization of intrahepatic abscess is the radionuclide scan, using either technetium sulphur colloid (^{99m}Tc-SC) or ^{67}gallium citrate. An abscess will appear as an area of nonuptake of ^{99m}Tc-SC. The limitation of the technetium scan is its inability to detect lesions of less than about 1 cm in diameter. Lesions between 1 and 4 cm in diameter may or may not be detected, depending upon their location. Smaller lesions at the periphery can be detected, but lesions deep in the center of the liver must be larger in order to be visible.

For this reason, imaging with both ^{99m}Tc-SC and ^{67}Ga-citrate is often used. ^{67}Ga-citrate is taken up by most hepatic abscesses, whether pyogenic or amoebic. Therefore, if a lesion is detected on the ^{99m}Tc-SC scan, it may be further defined by a supplementary ^{67}Ga-citrate scan. A focal lesion that accumulates ^{67}Ga-citrate represents either an abscess or a hepatoma. Given the clinical setting of fever, chills, and right upper quadrant pain (particularly in the postoperative patient), a positive gallium scan is most likely to disclose an abscess (Fig. 15–50). Gallium scanning is performed by injection of 5 to 8 mCi of the radionuclide, followed by an abdominal scan six hours later. Although an area of increased uptake in the liver may be seen on this early scan, it must be remembered that the abnormality may show up only on scans obtained at 24

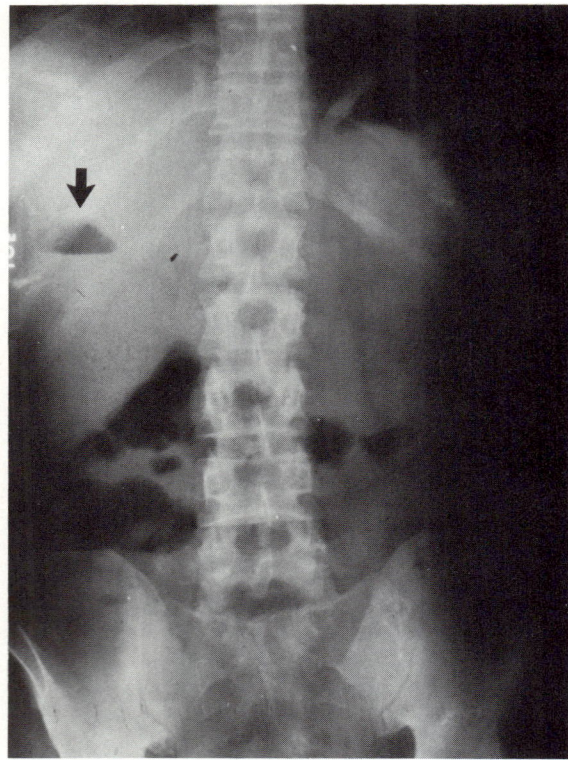

Figure 15-49. This erect abdomen radiograph demonstrates an air-fluid level overlying the midportion of the liver (arrow) in a patient with fever, chills, leukocytosis, and abdominal pain. At surgery, a centrally located liver abscess was discovered.

hours or even as late as 72 hours. Failure to obtain delayed scans may lead to a false negative interpretation.

Although an abscess can be detected by radionuclide scanning, its exact extent and its relationship to the surface of the liver and the porta hepatis are best seen with ultrasound or CT. The reported accuracy of the gallium scan in the detection of hepatic abscesses is quite high. In one series,[20] gallium scan was 93 per cent accurate in detecting an abdominal abscess and 95 per cent accurate in ruling out abscess. In another series,[25] the gallium scan was 100 per cent accurate both in detecting and in excluding abscess. False positive interpretations are sometimes made because of spurious collections of the radionuclide in the intestinal tract.

Ultrasonography

Ultrasound is highly accurate in detecting hepatic masses, particularly fluid-filled masses such as abscess. Most intrahepatic abscesses appear as sonolucent defects within the liver parenchyma with prominent through-transmission of the ultrasound beam (Fig. 15–51). However, they may also contain echogenic elements, caused by tissue or debris, producing an inhomogeneous appearance (see Fig. 15–50). An intrahepatic hematoma[9] or necrotic liver metastasis[65] may resemble an abscess. The ultrasonic appearance of abscesses depends to some degree upon the amount of debris and the thickness of the abscess wall. Some abscesses appear almost like cysts, with smooth walls and sonolucent centers, but most have irregular walls and some echogenicity in the center.

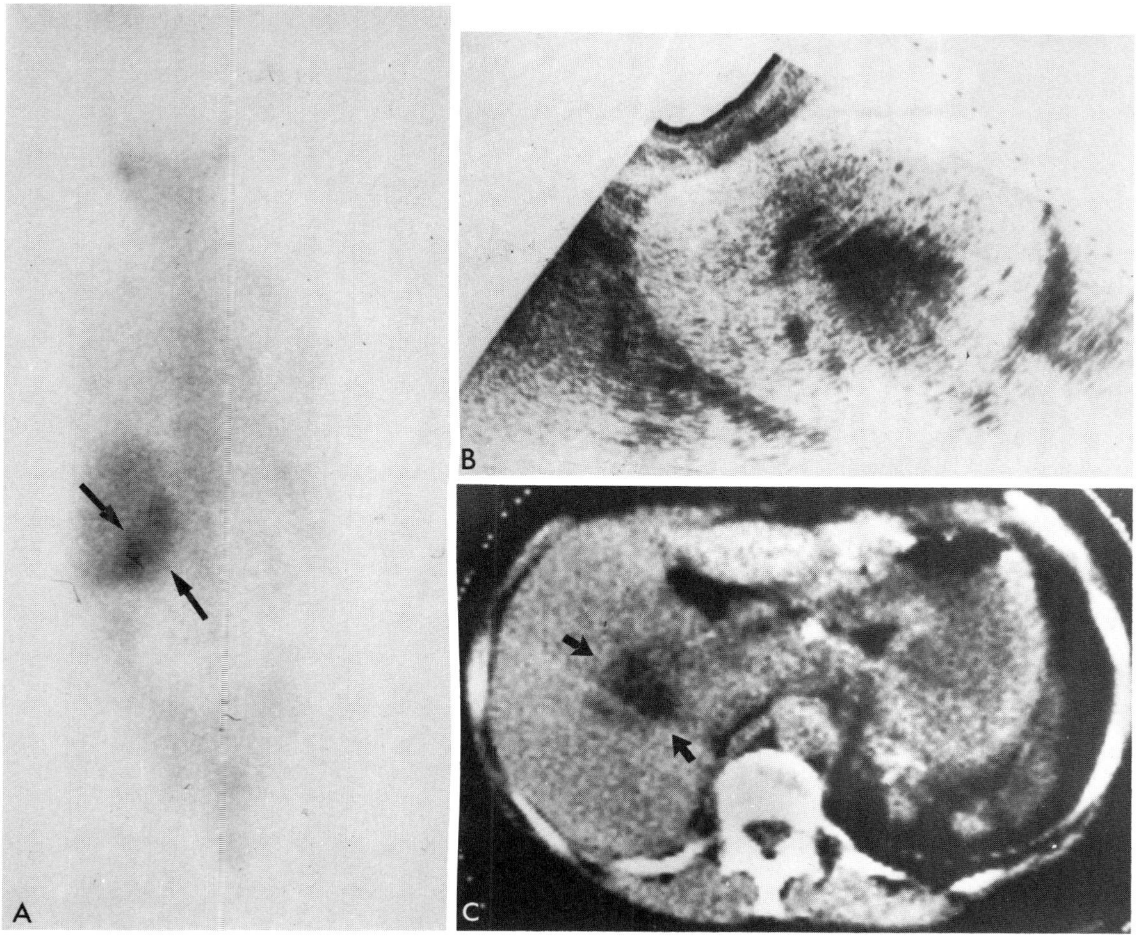

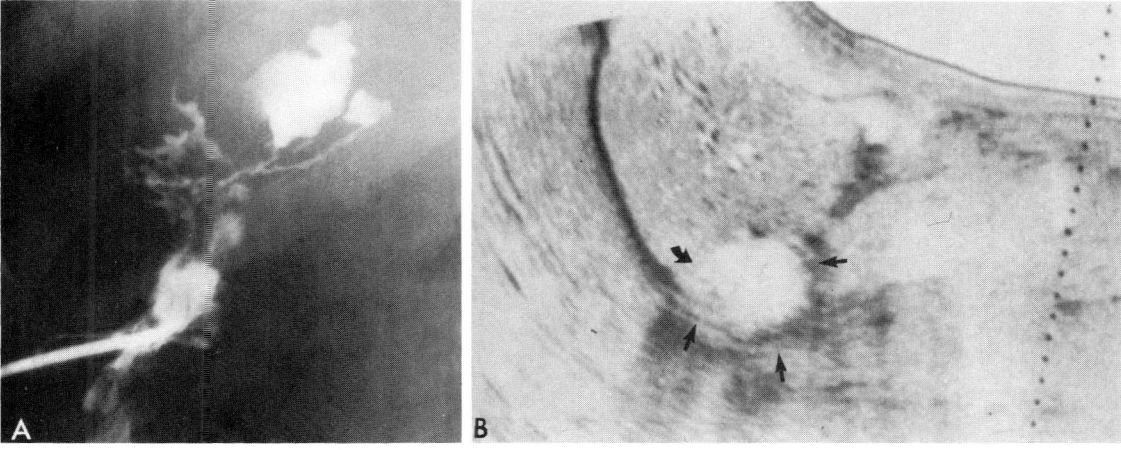

Figure 15–50. *A*, Scan obtained 24 hours after administration of 5 mCi of 67-gallium citrate demonstrates increased uptake of isotope in the area either of the medial portion of the right lobe of the liver or of the gallbladder (arrows). *B*, The sagittal-sector gray-scale ultrasonogram shows a central hepatic lesion of intense echogenicity, consistent with abscess. *C*, CT scan shows a low-density central lesion in the right lobe, also consistent with abscess (arrows). The presence of a pyogenic abscess was confirmed at surgery.

Figure 15–51. *A*, Sinus tract injection demonstrates multiple fine tracts in the liver parenchyma and one larger collection of contrast material in an abscess cavity. *B*, The ultrasonogram demonstrates a sonolucent lesion in the periphery of the right lobe (arrows) with slight acoustic enhancement (shadowing) of the back wall of this abscess.

849

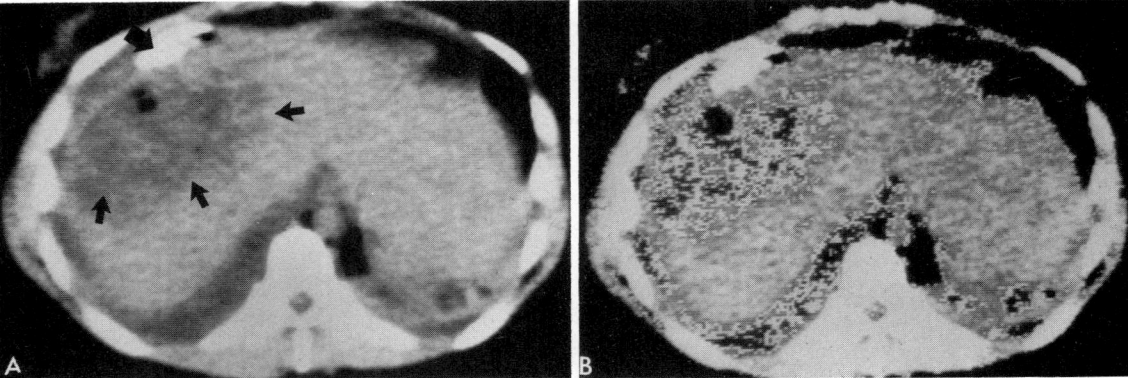

Figure 15–52. *A*, CT scan demonstrates a low-density area (small arrows) in the periphery of the liver. A gas collection (black circle) is present in the low-density area. A portion of a penrose drain (large arrow) is also seen in this section. This lesion demonstrates typical CT features of hepatic abscess. *B*, The CT number of the contents of the abscess averages 10, as indicated by the white squares within the abscess margins.

Intrahepatic abscesses are more easily detected than subphrenic or subhepatic ones, because the liver parenchyma produces a homogeneous background in which abnormal echo patterns are more easily discerned. It has been estimated that abscesses within the liver as small as 2 cm in diameter can be detected by ultrasound.[26] In one series of 17 cases, abscesses were correctly diagnosed by ultrasound in 88 per cent.[57]

CT Scanning

CT body scanning is an alternative to ultrasound in imaging intrahepatic and perihepatic abscesses. The CT diagnosis depends upon demonstration of a low-density mass within or about the liver or upon detection of a gas collection in this region (Fig. 15–52).[19, 32] The abscess mass has a lower CT number than the surrounding liver parenchyma because of the low density of its fluid contents. Ordinarily the CT number

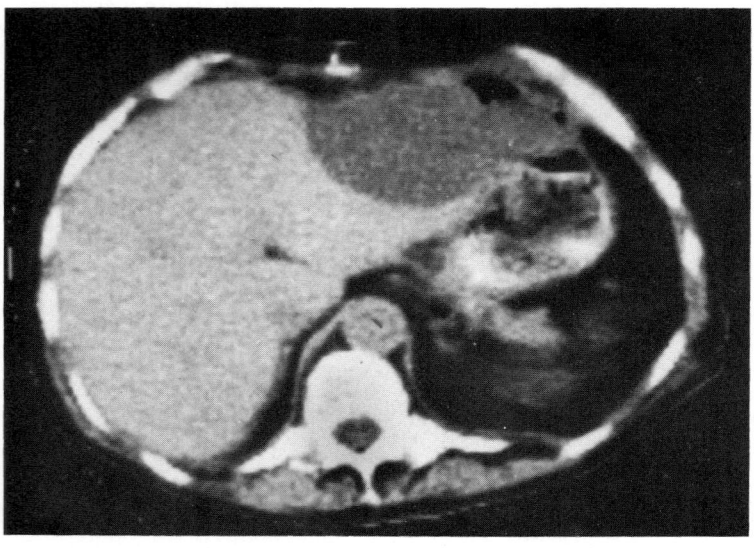

Figure 15–53. The low-density lesion occupying most of the left lobe is clearly separable from normal-appearing liver parenchyma. The CT number of this lesion remained approximately 10, even though the liver parenchyma CT number increased with iodine. Surgical exploration revealed an abscess of the left lobe.

of abscess fluid is 10 and 30 Hounsfield units (5 to 15 EMI units). Intravenous iodinated contrast accentuates the low-density abscess by increasing the CT number of the surrounding liver parenchyma (Fig. 15–53). The walls of the abscess may be irregular. Organized debris in the center may produce inhomogeneity. Small bubbles of gas produced by gas-forming bacteria appear as multiple small structures of very low density. While these occasionally may be seen on plain film radiographs of the abdomen in and around the liver, the CT scan can clearly locate them in relation to the liver parenchyma.

However, all fluid-filled masses detected by CT within or around the liver are not abscesses. Hematomas and cysts also may show findings (see Fig. 15–34). Generally, cysts have a lower CT number. Hematomas may have a higher or a lower CT number depending upon their chronicity, and they may be indistinguishable from abscess. When the CT scan is used to supplement a gallium scan, the diagnosis of abscess can be made with greater certainty.

CT scanning is an excellent method of determining the extent of subhepatic and periphepatic abscesses and is perhaps the best single imaging modality for ascertaining whether the kidney, abdominal wall, or other abdominal organs are involved.

Interaction of Radionuclide Scans, Ultrasound, and CT Scans

At the present stage of technological development, the three major diagnostic imaging modalities for detecting hepatic abscesses (radionuclide scan, ultrasound, and CT) may present the radiologist with a difficult choice. Consequently, the advantages and disadvantages of these techniques must be considered. Radionuclide liver scanning with ^{99m}Tc sulphur colloid is sensitive and noninvasive and can be performed in a short time. Therefore, it is a logical first step in the search for a possible hepatic abscess. If a lesion is seen with this technique, a ^{67}gallium citrate scan can be performed. ^{67}Ga-citrate scanning has the advantage of selectively imaging inflammatory tissue. However, ^{67}Ga-citrate may also be taken up by tumors, notably hepatomas and lymphomas. The major disadvantage of the gallium scan is the long delay between the initiation of the scan and its final interpretation (up to 72 hours). In addition, poorer image resolution follows gallium scanning compared with ultrasound, CT, or ^{99m}Tc-SC scanning.

Ultrasound can detect even small fluid-filled masses and differentiate them from solid masses. In addition, it is performed quickly, is relatively inexpensive, and does not require ionizing radiation. Parasagittal sections of the liver can be obtained, including images of the diaphragm and retrohepatic space for detection of subphrenic and perihepatic abscesses. The ultrasonogram may be degraded, however, by interference from overlying gas-filled bowel. The quality of the examination is closely related to the expertise of the ultrasonographer.

CT is best for showing the retroperitoneal and subhepatic space and the relationship of the liver to other organs. However, like ultrasound, CT often fails to distinguish abscess from hematoma. The evaluation of the subphrenic space by CT is somewhat limited by the inability to obtain scans in the longitudinal orientation. However, sagittal and coronal reconstructions of transverse CT images are obtainable with some CT units. CT can be performed quickly but is more costly than ultrasound.

After these advantages and disadvantages are weighed, the most useful strategy for the problem of possible hepatic abscess is first to utilize the ^{99m}Tc-SC liver scan to localize a hepatic lesion rapidly. Once a lesion is detected in or about the liver, then ^{67}gallium citrate scanning, ultrasound, or CT may be performed to further characterize the lesion. CT and ultrasound are particularly helpful when surgical drainage is considered. The choice between the two depends upon the availability of the equipment, the expertise of the radiologist, and the status of the patient. Ultrasound may be difficult in a patient who has a fresh surgical wound, in which case CT scanning may be preferable. When both procedures are available and there are no contraindications to either one, ultrasound is usually the study of choice, with CT used only to clarify problems not solved by ultrasound. If the clinical situation is such that a ^{99m}Tc-SC scan or a ^{67}Ga-citrate scan cannot be performed, either ultrasound or CT can be utilized as the first diagnostic test.

All three modalities are capable of following the progress of healing of a hepatic or perihepatic abscess. However, CT and ultrasound reveal much more exactly the dimensions of the shrinkage of the abscess than does either ^{99m}Tc-SC or ^{67}Ga-citrate. In the past, abscesses of the liver, particularly amoebic abscesses, were followed by radionuclide scans to determine response to therapy. However, ultrasound and CT provide more accurate information about the abscess.

Arteriography

The role of hepatic arteriography in the evaluation of liver abscesses has been greatly diminished by the advent of nuclear medicine and ultrasound. Nevertheless, it may still play a limited role in the differentiation of abscess from hepatoma. This is particularly true when the gallium scan is positive and CT and ultrasound show a complex mass with both solid and cystic components. In these instances, it is possible for abscess and hepatoma to be confused. Hepatic angiography may show a classic feature of an avascular mass stretching and displaying hepatic arterial vessels. Sometimes a vascular blush or stain may be seen around the periphery of the abscess. The classic features of hepatoma may be demonstrated: hypervascularity, shunt vessels, distorted arteries, and inhomogeneous staining in the capillary phase.

BENIGN AND MALIGNANT HEPATIC TUMORS

Detection of hepatic masses and determination of their location, nature, and extent have improved greatly with the advent of CT and gray-scale ultrasonography. These two imaging modalities have changed the approach to hepatic masses. Radionuclide scans have also improved. Superselective hepatic arteriography has added new dimensions to detection and diagnosis. Lesser roles are played by endoscopic retrograde cholangiography and percutaneous cholangiography, unless the masses have produced jaundice.

Plain Films of the Abdomen

Plain abdominal radiographs may show calcification within the liver. Adenomas and hemangiomas calcify occasionally, but calcification should alert the radiologist to the possibility of a malignant neoplasm, either primary or metastatic. Calcification can occur in hepatomas in adults and in infantile hepatomas and even hemangioendotheliomas. In hepatomas, calcification may appear as rounded densities, as amorphous punctate calcifications forming the so-called sunburst appearance, or as irregular streaks.

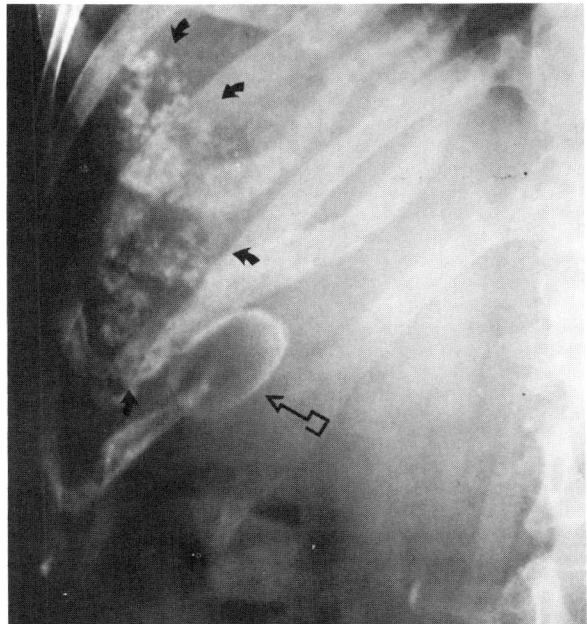

Figure 15–54. Multiple small clusters of calcification are present in the liver on this plain abdominal radiograph (small arrows). A calcified gallstone is also present (single arrow).

Metastatic liver tumors that calcify are usually mucin-secreting adenocarcinomas. These include gastrointestinal neoplasms and breast and ovarian tumors. The calcification in metastases is usually in the form of clusters of tiny punctate densities (Fig. 15–54).

Radionuclide Scan

Radionuclide studies of the liver remain the simplest and most sensitive screen tests for detecting any type of hepatic mass. The technetium sulphur colloid scan (^{99m}Tc-SC) is usually used to detect metastases, which appear as areas of decreased uptake in static scintiphotographs. During the early flow phase of this study, highly vascular lesions, such as hemangiomas and hemangioendotheliomas, may appear as areas of increased radionuclide activity.[30] One of the limitations of radionuclide liver scans is that lesions smaller than 1 cm cannot be resolved unless they are confluent, even with the most sophisticated scintigraphic units. Lesions greater than 1 cm at the periphery of the liver may be demonstrated, but lesions as large as 3 to 4 cm may be difficult to detect if they are situated deep within the liver. A particularly difficult area is the porta hepatis, where false positive and false negative interpretations may be made because of the variability in the normal anatomy of this region.[29] Resolution is relatively good with ^{99m}Tc-SC liver scanning, but the information is nonspecific for vascular lesions and focal nodular hyperplasia. About one third of hepatic masses caused by focal nodular hyperplasia show some ^{99m}Tc-SC uptake owing to the presence of Kupffer cells,[8] whereas hepatic adenomas or carcinomas remain as areas of nonuptake. The isotope scan is least sensitive when there are multiple, very small hepatic metastases studding the liver. In these cases, a decreased patchy uptake of radionuclide material is demonstrated, and it may be impossible to differentiate this pattern from that of a hepatic parenchymal disease.

A less sensitive but more specific radionuclide test is [67]gallium citrate imaging. Most hepatomas have a great avidity for ^{67}Ga-citrate. However, liver abscesses also take up gallium. In a clinical setting of weight loss with an enlarged liver without fever or chills, an area of increased uptake of gallium is more likely to be hepatoma. The gallium scan is particularly useful in patients with advanced cirrhosis who are suspected of having hepatoma. The cirrhotic liver may produce regenerating nodules, which on isotope scans, CT, or ultrasound may be difficult to differentiate from tumor. However, because the gallium scan may permit this distinction, it is a valuable test for cirrhotic patients, who have an increased incidence of hepatomas.

The overall accuracy in detecting metastases by ^{99m}Tc-SC scanning has been reported as 85 per cent[2] and 95 per cent,[10] so that the radionuclide scan is an extremely useful and sensitive method of detecting hepatic masses.[6, 32] False positive rates of 4 per cent,[6] 9.7 per cent,[2] 16 per cent,[32] and 21 per cent[43] have been reported. A false negative rate, based on analysis of 1688 scans, was noted to be 23 per cent.[43]

Ultrasonography

With modern gray-scale equipment, the usefulness of ultrasound in detecting hepatic masses has increased greatly. Single or multiple cysts, seen as nonspecific filling defects on a radionuclide scan, appear on the ultrasonogram as trans-sonic areas with well-demarcated posterior walls (Fig. 15–55). Solid lesions, including primary and metastatic hepatic neoplasms, have variable ultrasonic patterns including (1) sonolucent areas with very little echogenicity but with rather poorly demarcated margins (Fig. 15–56) in contrast to sonolucent cysts;[17, 49] (2) densely echogenic areas (Fig. 15–57) with homogeneous internal architecture and uniform echo pattern, usually in a milieu of normal-appearing liver, a common pattern for metastases;[49] (3) a mass with an echogenic rim and a sonolucent center, thought to represent a necrotic metastasis; (4) a metastasis with an echodense center and a sonolucent rim (Fig. 15–58); and (5) a mixed pattern without any clear-cut characteristics.

A single metastasis as small as 1 or 2 cm can be detected by ultrasound.[31] Multiple small metastases are more easily detected than a solitary lesion because they tend to be

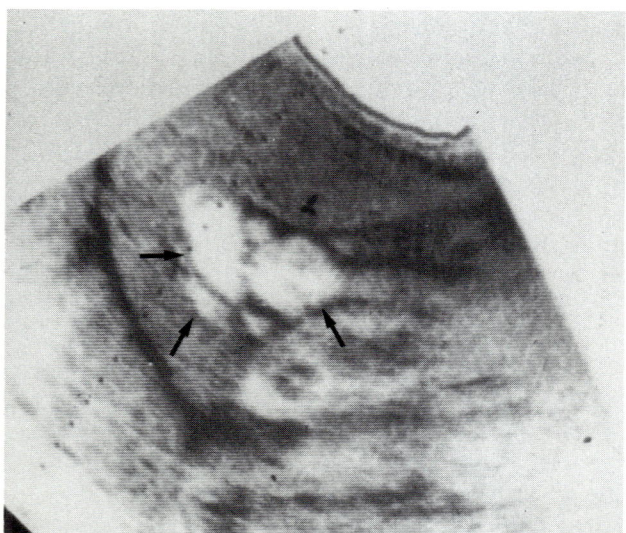

Figure 15–55. This sagittal-section sonogram demonstrates several simple cysts (arrows) that are echo-free and have well-demarcated walls.

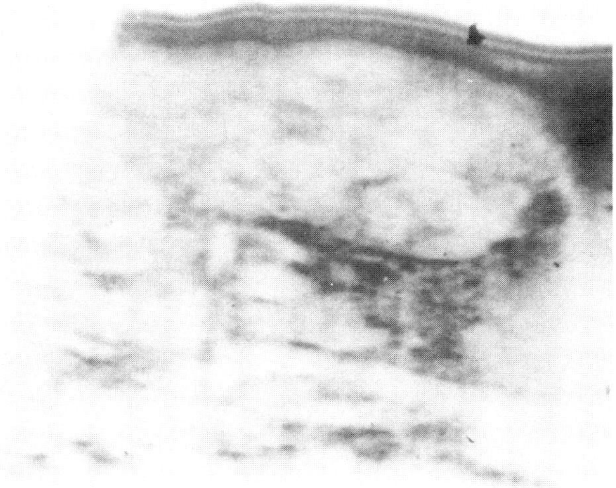

THE LIVER — 855

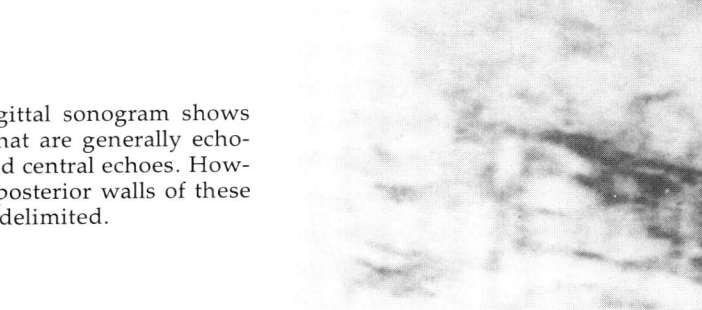

Figure 15-56. This sagittal sonogram shows numerous metastases that are generally echo-free except for some mild central echoes. However, unlike cysts, the posterior walls of these lesions are not sharply delimited.

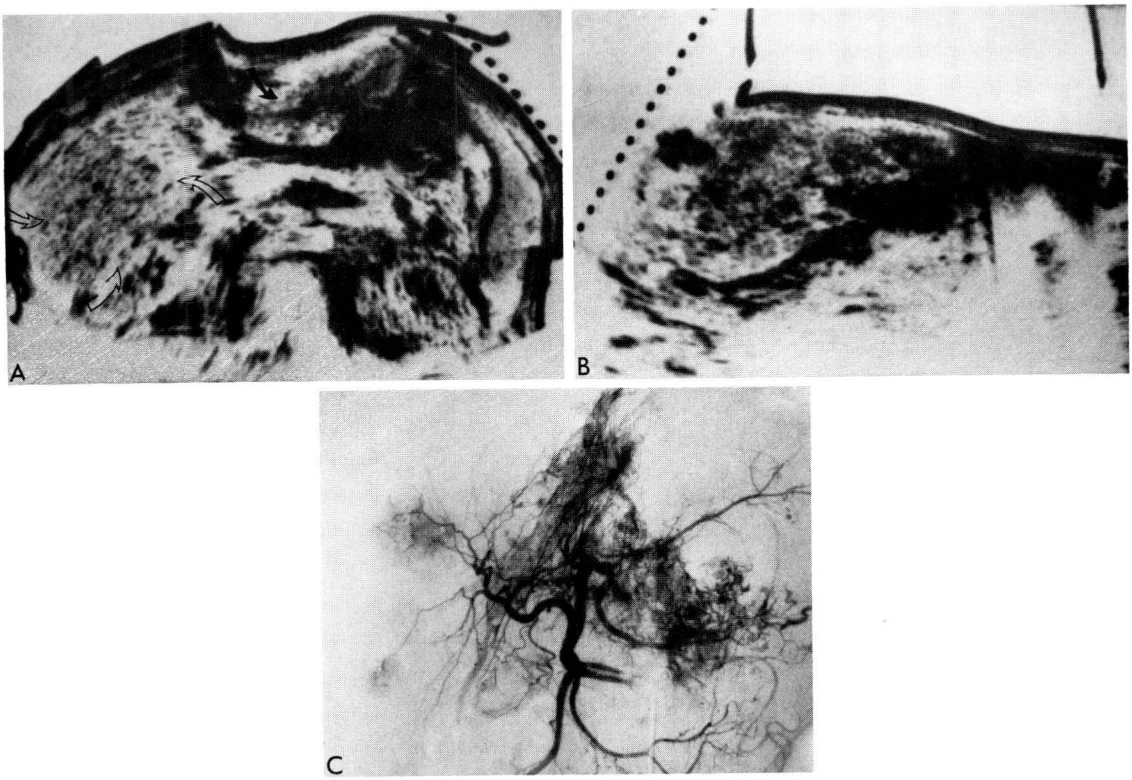

Figure 15-57. *A*, Transverse gray-scale ultrasonogram demonstrates a large echogenic lesion in the right lobe of the liver (open arrows) and one in the left lobe (closed arrows). These were proven to be hepatocellular carcinomas. *B*, Parasagittal section shows the dense echogenic areas in the right and left lobes. *C*, Selective celiac arteriogram demonstrates the irregular contour of vessels feeding hypervascular areas of the right and left lobes. The intense tumor stains and neovascularity are typical of hepatomas.

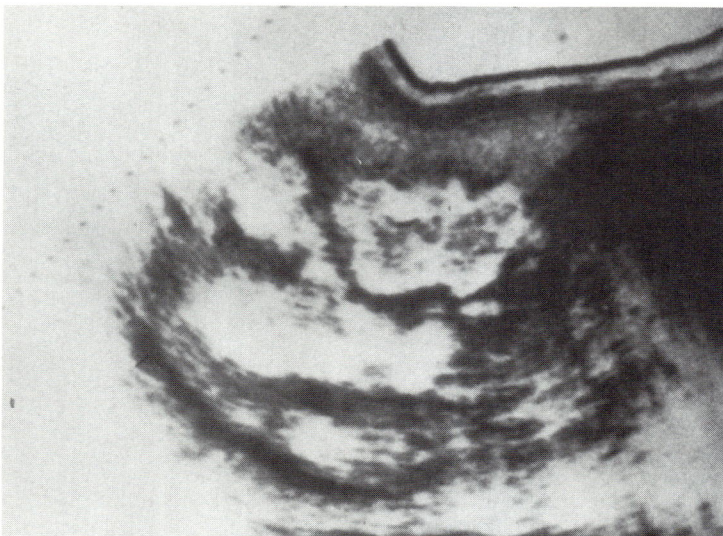

Figure 15–58. These large liver metastases have an ultrasonographic pattern of sonolucent rim and echo-dense centers.

confluent and to distort the hepatic parenchymal pattern. In one series it was shown that echodense lesions were frequently associated with adenocarcinoma,[52] while another report concluded that the ultrasonic pattern offered no predictability of histologic type.[17]

Ultrasound is also useful in evaluating the appearance of the lesion during and after chemotherapy. During chemotherapy the appearance of the lesion may change and the center may become more sonolucent, probably indicating necrosis.

In one series of hepatic masses, gray-scale ultrasonography was reported to provide the most useful information, with a low number of both false positive and false negative results[6] in comparison with either CT or radionuclide scanning. Ultrasound detected 90 per cent of metastases in 350 patients[54] and was 100 per cent accurate in diagnosing hepatic cysts.[51]

CT Scanning

When evaluating a hepatic mass by CT scanning, it is useful to scan first without and then with iodinated intravenous contrast material. Contrast containing blood has a higher CT number. In those areas of the liver with a rich vascular supply, an increased CT number will develop after intravenous contrast infusion. Many primary and metastatic neoplasms of the liver are hypovascular. These will appear as low-density areas in the liver parenchyma. The normal liver parenchyma ordinarily has a CT number between 40 and 80 Hu. Neoplasms have CT numbers in the range of 15 to 50. However, some well-vascularized neoplasms take up a significant amount of an intravenous contrast infusion. Occasionally a liver mass normally distinguishable from the parenchyma on a no-contrast scan may be obscured by the addition of intravenous contrast material. For this reason liver scans should be performed first without contrast material. Most primary and secondary lesions, however, are seen on a noncontrast scan, and intravenous contrast may be helpful when the scan is negative (Fig. 15–59). Some primary and metastatic neoplasms undergo central necrosis, resulting in a lower CT number in the center.[61] However, differentiation between a simple cyst and a cystic

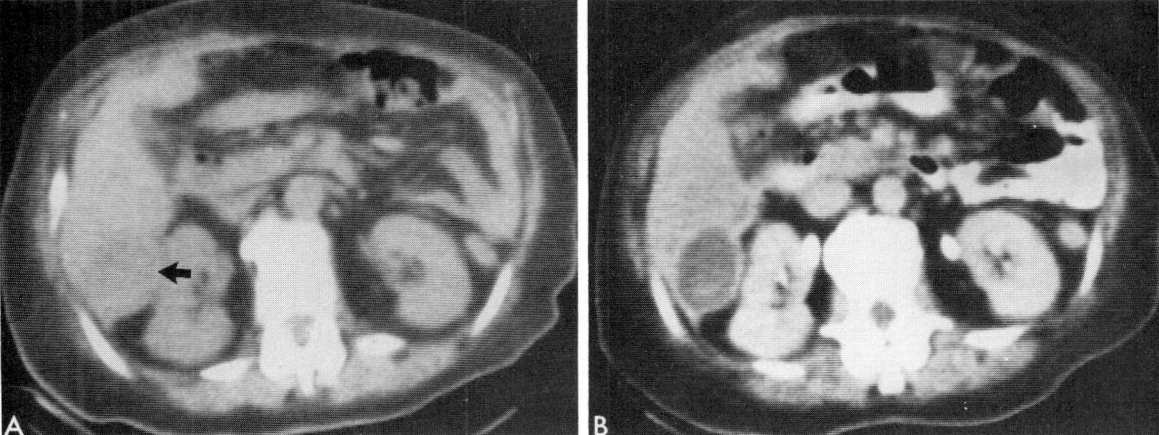

Figure 15–59. *A*, A CT scan of the liver prior to administration of water-soluble iodinated contrast material shows no definite liver lesions, although the bulge in the tip of the right lobe is suspicious (arrow). *B*, After intravenous contrast material was administered, the metastatic lesion in the tip of the right lobe is clearly seen as a low-density area.

neoplasm is usually not difficult. Pure cysts of the liver have an extremely low CT number (between 0 and 5) and can be distinguished from neoplasms by this feature (Fig. 15–60). Furthermore, the cyst walls are well circumscribed and separated from the surrounding parenchyma.

Hepatomas vary in appearance on CT scan. While they may appear as homogeneous low-density lesions, they may also contain isodense areas and even calcifications (Figs. 15–61 and 15–62). Some extrinsic lesions eroding into the liver may be difficult to differentiate from intrahepatic lesions when only a radionuclide scan is used, but the site of origin usually becomes clear with a CT scan. In the evaluation of a patient with hepatic neoplasm for elective surgery and partial hepatectomy, CT scanning, like ultrasound, is useful in determining the exact extent of the lesion and its relationship to

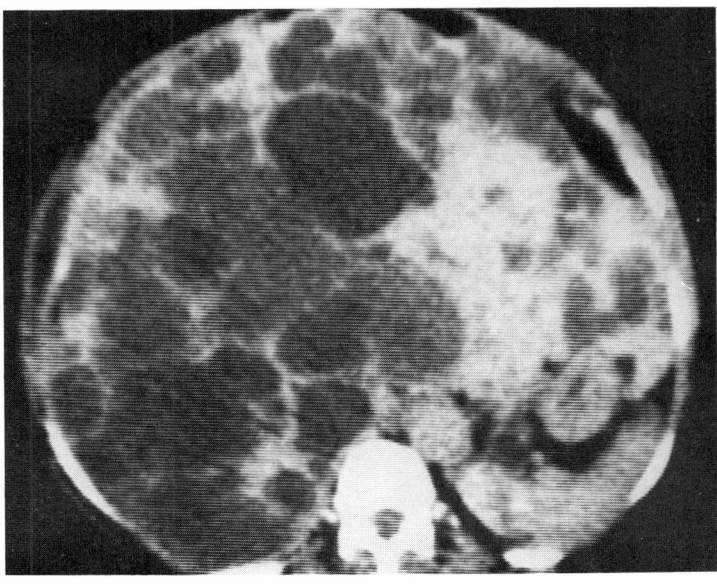

Figure 15–60. Multiple simple cysts of the liver appear as low-density structures surrounded by distinct rims of compressed hepatic parenchyma.

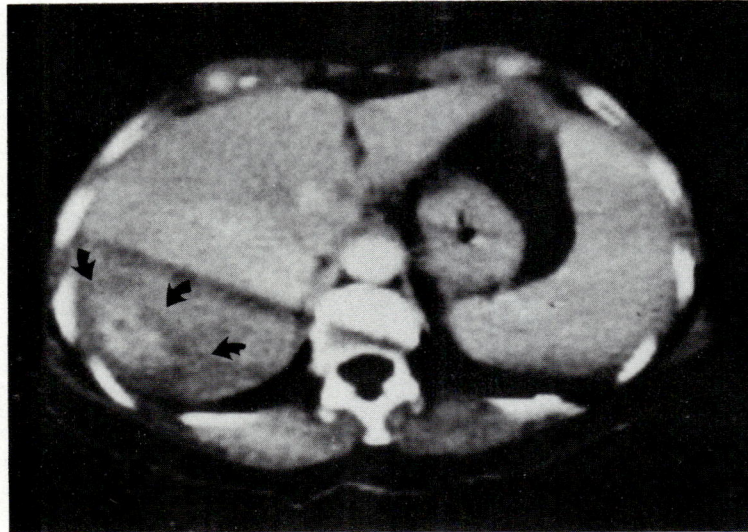

Figure 15–61. Calcification occurring in this hepatoma appears as a dense area occupying most of the lesion in the tip of the right lobe (arrows).

such vital structures as the common bile duct and main portal vein. CT scan of the liver is an accurate method of detecting hepatic masses. In one study,[4] 25 out of 29 solitary liver masses and 49 out of 54 multiple masses were detected by CT. This general range of accuracy has been confirmed by other studies.[27, 32, 53]

Interaction of Radionuclide Scan, Ultrasonography, and CT Scan

In determining the relative roles of the liver-spleen radionuclide scan, ultrasound, and CT, current data indicate that all three methods have comparable sensitivity in detecting hepatic masses, with about 80 to 90 per cent accuracy.[4, 6, 27, 32] All current studies agree that these three methods are not mutually exclusive. As a screening study

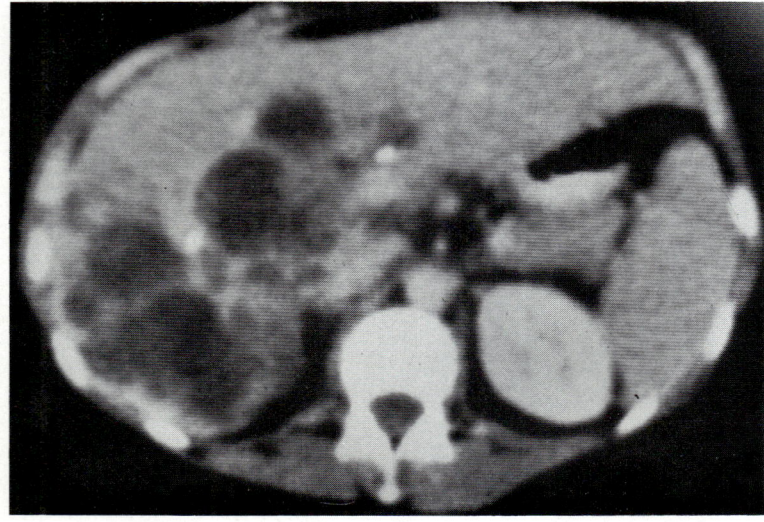

Figure 15–62. The hepatoma present in the right lobe and part of the left lobe of the liver on this CT scan contains areas of low density, areas near the same density of liver, and circular areas of high density due to calcification.

for hepatic mass, the ^{99m}Tc-SC liver scan is the test of choice. If the results are equivocal, CT or ultrasound may clarify the issue. Both studies are useful in evaluating the solitary mass on ^{99m}Tc-SC liver scan by providing information about the nature of its borders and content (fluid or solid material). The use of ultrasound rather than CT as the next study depends upon the expertise of the ultrasonographer and the nature of the gray-scale equipment. Similarly, use of CT scanning may depend upon whether fast scanners are available.

Arteriography

The role of angiography in the evaluation of liver masses has diminished because of improvement in imaging with radionuclide scans, ultrasound, and CT. Nevertheless, arteriography is still the most reliable study for predicting the histologic diagnosis. It is the most specific modality for providing a vascular map and for indicating the extent of the hepatic mass to aid in surgical or chemotherapeutic management. Angiography is usually the final diagnostic test before therapy is instituted.

Complete angiographic evaluation of the liver may include not only conventional celiac or superior mesenteric arteriographic injections but also superselective injections, slow infusion arteriography, and evaluation of the portal venous component of hepatic masses using arterial portography. Vasodilators may be used to increase delivery of contrast material to liver parenchyma, so that avascular lesions will stand out as low-density defects.[16] Vasoconstrictive agents may be used to diminish opacification around a vascular tumor, the vessels in the tumor being relatively unresponsive to the vasoconstrictor. The vascular anatomy of the liver and the type and extent of vascularity of various intrahepatic lesions offers needed information for surgical resection of a mass.

HEPATIC ANGIOGRAPHY IN BENIGN LIVER MASSES. The major role of hepatic angiography in benign liver masses is to evaluate vascular lesions. Cysts and abscesses, which tend to produce avascular areas in the liver, with stretching and displacement of small artery branches (Fig. 15–63), can be evaluated and correctly diagnosed by CT or ultrasound. However, solitary masses in the liver that appear vascular on CT need further arteriographic evaluation for determination of their benign or malignant character.

The most common benign tumor of the liver is the cavernous hemangioma. Occasionally, these hemangiomas may be large and must be differentiated from a malignant tumor. Most often, however, they are small and are detected incidentally. Hemangiomas have a characteristic angiographic appearance. They are fed by normal to slightly enlarged arteries. Vascular lakes or puddles of contrast material appear and persist for up to 30 seconds. This is helpful in differentiating hemangiomas from vascular hepatomas, which tend to show rapid arteriovenous shunting.[42]

Hepatic adenoma is another benign neoplasm that often occurs in young women and seems closely related to the use of oral contraceptives.[3, 34, 42] Although they are usually single lesions in the right lobe, they may be multiple. They have a tendency to occur on the inferior edge of the liver. Large adenomas may be detected on plain abdominal radiographs as rounded masses projecting from the inferior border of the liver (Fig. 15–64). Because these lesions are very vascular, hemorrhage can occur within the tumor, resulting in sudden enlargement. If the tumor is located just beneath the capsule, it may rupture, resulting in a hemoperitoneum.

The angiographic appearance is quite characteristic and includes hypervascularity and well-demarcated margins (Fig. 15–65). The arteries supplying this lesion are normal

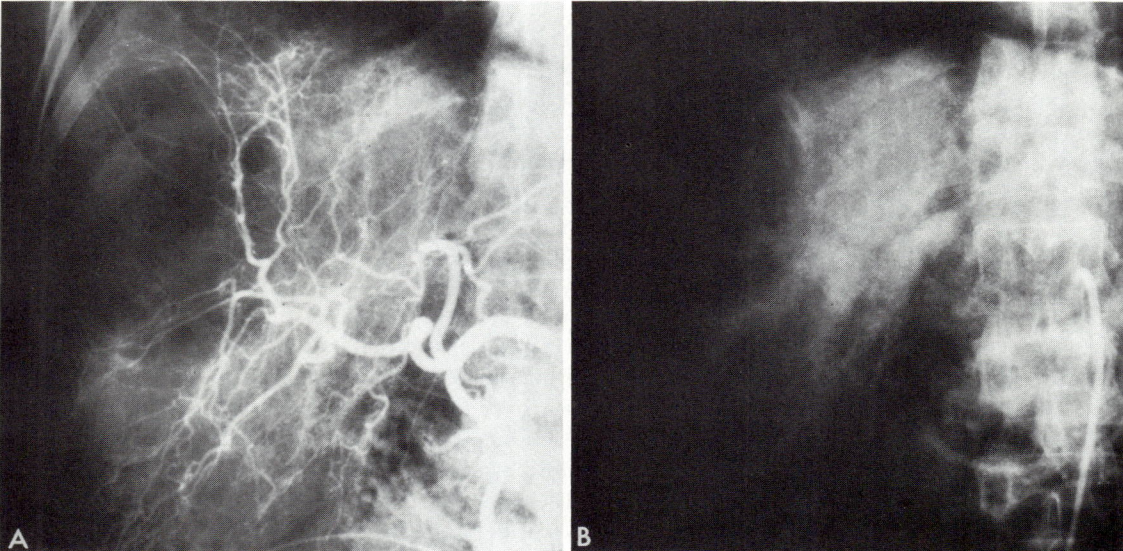

Figure 15–63. *A,* In the arterial phase of this hepatic arteriogram, normal-appearing vessels are draped over an avascular area in the periphery of the right lobe. The lesion is a benign liver cyst. *B,* The cyst is more clearly seen in the parenchymal phase because it compresses normal liver parenchyma, producing a distinct rim.

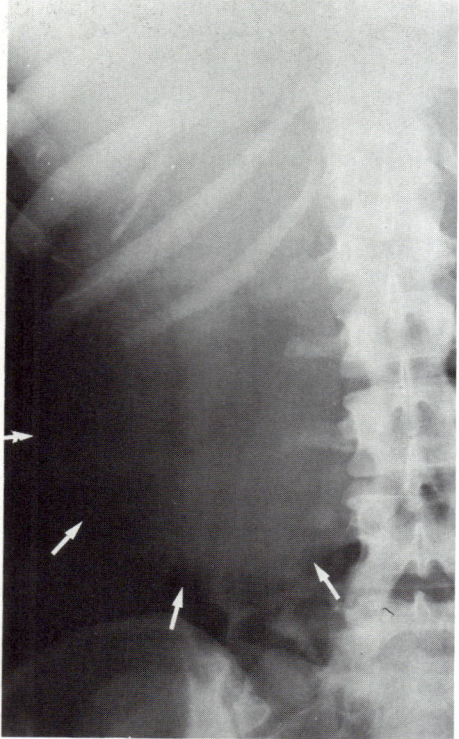

Figure 15–64. A large round mass protrudes from the inferior edge of the liver (arrows) in this young woman. The patient had been taking oral contraceptives and had noted a dull, painful ache in her right side. The lesion is an hepatic adenoma.

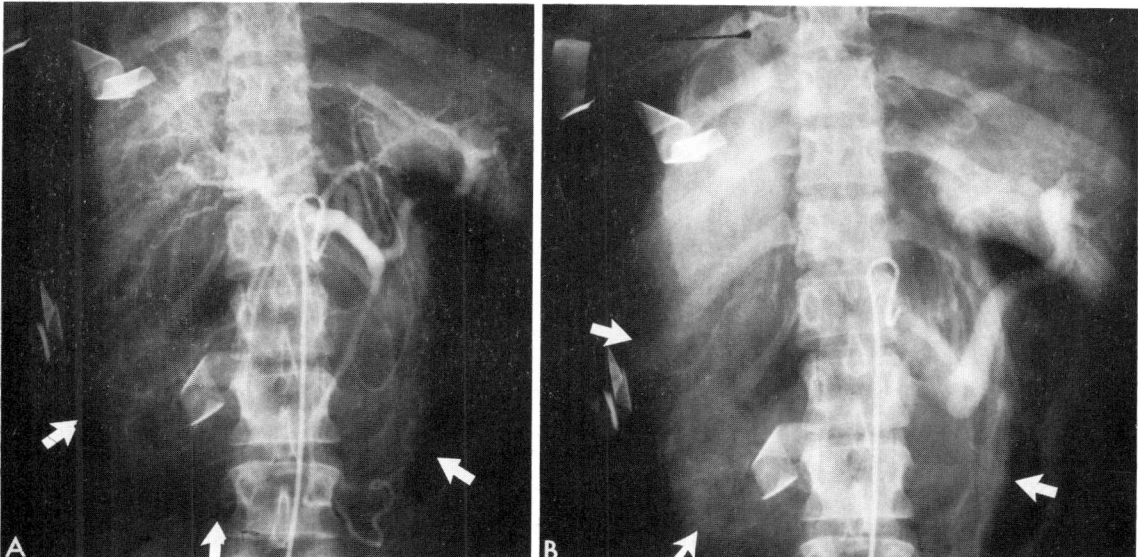

Figure 15–65. *A*, Hepatic adenoma. A large liver mass developed in this young woman. The radiopaque sponges mark the site of prior resection of an adenoma in the right lobe. The celiac arteriogram demonstrates displacement of the celiac, splenic, and gastroduodenal arteries to the left (right and left arrows). The hepatic mass extends inferiorly to the level of the fourth lumbar vertebral body (caudad arrow). Arteries are draped over the mass and are normal in size and appearance. *B*, In the venous phase of the arteriogram, a dense blush is present, outlining the tumor (arrows).

in size and appearance. Small arteries drape over the surface of the tumor and project into its center. In the parenchymal phase, a dense tissue blush is noted, which is homogeneous and lacks the pooling of contrast material that is seen with hemangiomas or hepatomas.

Another benign neoplasm is focal nodular hyperplasia. This lesion is similar to hepatic adenoma and is sometimes labeled as hamartoma. The lesion is usually multiple and smaller than the hepatic adenoma. Most often it occurs in young women, although its relationship to oral contraceptives is not as clear as that of hepatic adenomas. The angiographic features of focal nodular hyperplasia may mimic those of hepatic adenoma, making differentiation extremely difficult. Like adenomas, nodular hyperplastic lesions have normal-appearing feeding arteries and a dense, homogeneous tumor blush. Sometimes multiple septa can be seen within the mass in the parenchymal phase of the injection, and this helps to distinguish the lesion from hepatic adenoma. With multiple areas of focal nodular hyperplasia, it can be difficult to differentiate the arteriographic features from those of vascular metastasis and occasionally from a hepatoma.[1] Some focal nodular hyperplastic lesions show normal uptake of ^{99m}Tc-SC on liver scan, whereas adenomas or hepatomas appear as negative defects.[8, 46]

HEPATIC ANGIOGRAPHY IN MALIGNANT HEPATIC MASSES. The most common malignant mass in the liver is metastatic tumor. Ordinarily an arteriogram is performed after single or multiple masses are detected by a radionuclide study, ultrasound, or CT. When a primary source for metastasis is not known, it may not be recognized that the hepatic mass is metastatic. Angiography may then assist in the differentiation between primary and metastatic tumor, and superselective arteriography may detect additional masses not demonstrated by the other studies. A wide spectrum of arteriographic changes is present, many of which resemble those seen with primary lesions. Metastatic deposits may be hypervascular, hypovascular, or isovascular with the liver.

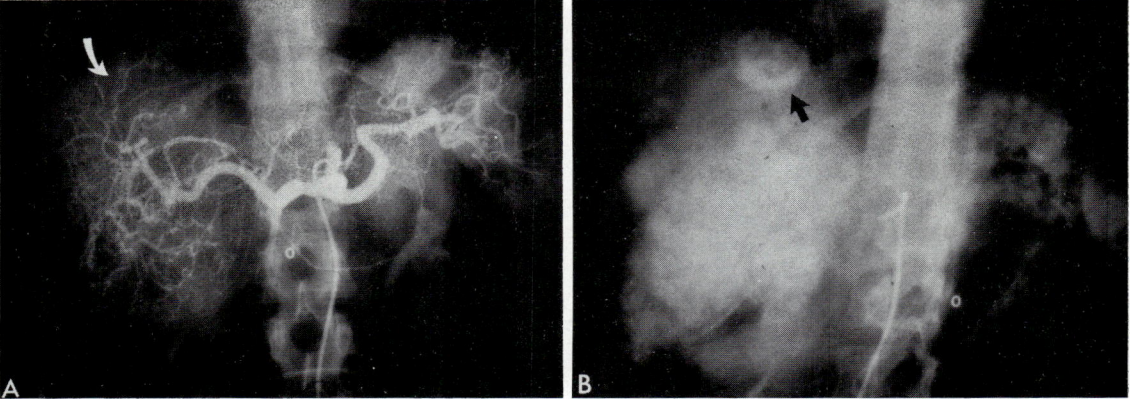

Figure 15–66. *A*, Hepatoma seen in arterial phase of arteriogram. Multiple tortuous irregular vessels arising from the right hepatic arteries produce an arteriographic appearance of a hypervascular mass in the caudal portion of the right lobe. Some vessels are stretched around this mass. In addition, an irregular vessel is seen extending toward the diaphragm (arrow). *B*, Parenchyma seen in the venous phase. A dense irregular tumor stain occupies most of the right lobe. It appears to be made up of multiple lesions; in addition, a large lesion is present just beneath the diaphragm, which has a necrotic center and a hypervascular rim (arrow).

parenchyma. The most vascular metastases occur with renal carcinoma and choriocarcinoma. However, hypervascular metastases have been reported from carcinoid tumors, pancreatic carcinoma, adrenal carcinomas, melanomas, and breast carcinomas. Occasionally, metastases from the stomach or colon are hypervascular, although usually these are hypovascular.[57]

Hypervascular hepatic neoplasms are identified by the increased amount of contrast material within the tumor. With proper superselective catheterization technique and modern radiographic equipment, hypervascular lesions ½ to 1 cm in diameter can be detected.[42] Frequently, the arteries feeding the metastasis widen as they near the lesion. Tumor hypervascularity may take the form of multiple small arteries or even arteriovenous shunting (see Figs. 15–57 and 15–66). A dense tumor stain may be seen in the parenchymal phase.

Hypovascular and avascular masses are more difficult to detect angiographically. Their identification is dependent upon sufficient opacification of the normal liver parenchyma during the capillary or parenchymal phase, when hypovascular lesions appear as relative lucencies. Hypovascular metastases are probably the most common, arising from the majority of gastrointestinal neoplasms and from the breast. As a rule, a hypovascular metastasis must be larger than a hypervascular metastasis in order to be detected. The lower limit of detectability is 2 to 3 cm.[42] Superselective hepatic arteriography with slow infusion of large volumes of contrast material may enhance detection of both hypovascular and hypervascular lesions by providing a longer and denser parenchymal phase.[44, 59]

Some metastases have a vascular supply similar to that of the normal surrounding parenchyma, and these cannot be discerned by a tumor blush or by relative lucency. These can be detected only by noting changes in the large or small arteries, such as obstruction, invasions, or displacement.

Hepatocellular carcinoma or hepatoma is usually visualized by ultrasound, CT scan, or liver-spleen scan as a large solitary lesion within the liver, although some hepatomas are isodense and may not be evident on CT. Hepatic arteriography then becomes the primary method of confirming the diagnosis. If the lesion appears to be unresectable on the basis of the CT scan, only a biopsy is needed and arteriography is not done. These tumors can usually be recognized by their characteristic hypervascular angiographic pattern. Unlike metastases, which rarely invade either the portal vein or the inferior vena cava, hepatomas frequently invade the portal vein and compress the vena cava. The angiographic evaluation of primary liver tumor prior to surgery should include inferior venacavography and portal venography by superior mesenteric artery injection. Information about the status of these major veins is vital to the surgeon who is considering resection of a liver tumor.[28]

The vascular pattern in hepatomas may be variable. Most often, however, the tumor is fed by hepatic arteries that dilate as they approach the tumor. The arteries may be tortuous, beaded, and irregular throughout the tumor (see Figs. 15–57 and 15–66). Amorphous irregular collections can be seen within the tumor in the parenchymal phase owing to pooling of contrast material (Fig. 15–66). Arteriovenous shunting between hepatic arteries and portal venous system frequently occurs.[38] The most vascular hepatomas have been found to be well differentiated, while those with less prominent vascularity tend to be more anaplastic.[22] When hepatoma undergoes central necrosis, the center may be quite avascular with a hypervascular rim (see Fig. 15–45), a feature easily confused with abscesses or hemorrhagic adenomas. The presence of arterioportal shunting aids in the distinction. Hypervascular metastases, particularly if they are confluent, and regenerating nodules in the liver may both mimic hepatoma arteriographically. A positive ^{67}Ga-citrate scan, however, may be of help in the diagnosis.

Although radionuclide scanning, ultrasound, CT, and arteriography can provide information about the presence and nature of hepatic masses, a rational and orderly use of these tests should be followed depending on the clinical situation. In patients with a palpable epigastric or right subcostal mass, the first test should be either CT or ultrasound. Both of these will not only confirm the intrahepatic location of the mass but also provide some information about its character (fluid-filled versus solid), multiplicity, and extent. If, however, the major clinical problem is weight loss, slightly abnormal liver function tests, and suspicion of a primary neoplasm elsewhere, then a ^{99m}Tc-SC liver scan may be the first test employed. In a patient with a known primary tumor of the gastrointestinal tract, the ^{99m}Tc-SC scan may also be used to evaluate the liver for the presence of metastases. If the scan discloses multiple focal lesions, further diagnostic testing may not be necessary. If selective arterial infusion of chemotherapeutic agents in the liver is being considered, hepatic arteriography must be performed. If the patient's major clinical problem raises suspicion of liver abscess, ^{67}Ga-citrate scan should be the primary test, followed by CT or ultrasound to disclose the size and nature of the mass.

In patients with long-standing cirrhosis the problem is more difficult. The firm, palpable, right subcostal mass in a patient with cirrhosis and possibly jaundice may represent a dilated gallbladder, a regenerating liver nodule, or hepatoma. An ultrasonogram, an easy and rapid test to perform, will help to confirm the presence of one or more masses, will give information about the general shape and size of the liver, and may help differentiate a mass from gallbladder. Ultrasound will also indicate whether or not bile ducts are dilated. ^{67}Ga-citrate scanning may be of use in identifying a hepatoma. A more specific diagnosis can usually be obtained by hepatic arteriography.

When surgical intervention is being considered, arteriography should be the last diagnostic test. It affords the most information about the vascular anatomy and the likelihood of resectability based on the extent of tumor and involvement of the portal vein and the inferior vena cava.[12] Specialized arteriographic techniques may detect multiple small masses in addition to a single large hepatic mass seen on the other studies, thereby influencing decisions regarding resectability.

References

1. Alpert, E., Ferrucci, J., Athanasoulis, C., et al.: Primary hepatic tumor. Gastroenterology 74:759–769, 1978.
2. Ariel, I. M., and Molander, D.: Hepatic gamma scanning: an aid in determining treatment policies for cancer involving the liver. Am. J. Surg. 118:5–14, 1969.
3. Baum, J. K., Holtz, F., Bookstein, J. J., et al.: Possible association between benign hepatomas and oral contraceptives. Lancet 2:926–929, 1973.
4. Biello, D. R., Levitt, R. G., Siegel, B. A., et al.: Computed tomography and radionuclide imaging of the liver: a comparative evaluation. Radiology 127:159–163, 1978.
5. Bookstein, J. J., Appelman, H. D., Walter, J. F., et al.: Histological-venographic correlates in portal hypertension. Radiology 116:565–573, 1975.
6. Bryan, P. J., Denn, W. M., Grossman, Z. D., et al.: Correlation of computed tomography, grey scale ultrasonography, and radionuclide imaging of the liver in detecting space-occupying processes. Radiology 124:387–393, 1977.
7. Carlsen, E. N., and Filly, R. A.: Newer ultrasonographic anatomy in the upper abdomen. I. The portal and hepatic venous anatomy. J. Clin. Ultrasound 4:85–90, 1976.
8. Casarella, W. J., Knowles, D. M., Wolff, M., et al.: Focal nodular hyperplasia and liver cell adenoma: radiologic and pathologic differentiation. Am. J. Roentgenol. 131:393–402, 1978.
9. Doust, B. D., Quivos, F., and Stewart, M. B.: Ultrasonic distinction of abscesses from other intraabdominal fluid collections. Radiology 125:213–218, 1977.
10. Felix, R. L., Bagley, D. H., Sindelar, W. F., et al.: The value of the liver scan in preoperative screening of patients with malignancies. Cancer 38:1137–1141, 1976.
11. Friedman, G. S.: Radionuclide imaging of the injured patient. Radiol. Clin. North Am. 9:461–477, 1973.
12. Gammell, S. L., Takahashi, M., Kawanami, M., et al.: Hepatic angiography in the selection of patients with hepatomas for heptic lobectomy. Radiology 101:549–554, 1971.
13. Geslien, G. E., Pinsky, S. M., Poth, R. K., et al.: The sensitivity and specificity of ^{99m}Tc-sulfur colloid liver imaging in diffuse hepatocellular disease. Radiology 118:115–119, 1976.
14. Gilday, D. L., and Alderson, P. O.: Scintigraphic evaluation of liver and spleen injury. Semin. Nucl. Med. 4:357–370, 1974.
15. Goldberg, H. I., Dodds, W. J., Lawson, T. L., et al.: Hepatic lymphatics demonstrated by percutaneous transhepatic cholangiography. Am. J. Roentgenol. 123:415–419, 1975.
16. Goldstein, H. M., Thoggard, A., Wallace, S., et al.: Priscoline-augmented hepatic angiography. Radiology 119:275–279, 1976.
17. Green, B., Bree, R. L., Goldstein, H. M., et al.: Grey scale ultrasound evaluation of hepatic neoplasms: patterns and correlations. Radiology 124:203–208, 1977.
18. Gross, G., Goldberg, H. I., and Schrock, T. R.: Use of selective intrahepatic portal venography and in vivo coloration in planning segmental hepatic resection. Am. J. Roentgenol. 122:327–332, 1974.
19. Haaga, J. R., Alfidi, R. J., Havrilla, T. R., et al.: CT detection and aspiration of abdominal abscesses. Am. J. Roentgenol. 128:465–474, 1977.
20. Hopkins, G. G., Kan, M., and Mendex, C. W.: Early ^{67}gallium scintigraphy for the localization of abdominal abscesses. J. Nucl. Med. 16:990–992, 1975.
21. Hungerford, G. E., Hamlyn, A. N., Lunzer, M. R., et al.: Pseudo-metastases in the liver; a presentation of the Budd-Chiari syndrome. Radiology 120:627–628, 1976.
22. Kido, C., Susaki, T., and Kaneko, M.: Angiography of primary liver cancer. Am. J. Roentgenol. 113:70–81, 1971.
23. Koehler, R. E., Korobkin, M., and Lewis, F.: Arteriographic demonstration of collateral arterial supply to the liver after hepatic artery ligations. Radiology 117:49–53, 1975.
24. Kressel, H. V., Korobkin, M., Goldberg H. I., et al.: The portal venous tree simulating dilated biliary ducts on computed tomography of the liver. J. Comput. Assist. Tomog. 1:169–175, 1977.
25. Kuwar, B., Alderson, P. O., and Geisse, G.: The role of Ga-67 citrate imaging and diagnostic ultrasound in patients with suspected abdominal abscesses. J. Nucl. Med. 18:534, 1977.
26. Lawson, T. L.: Hepatic abscess: ultrasound as an aid to diagnosis. Am. J. Digest. Dis. 22:33–37, 1977.
27. Levitt, R. G., Sagel, S. S., Stanly, R. J., et al.: Accuracy of computed tomography of the liver and biliary tract. Radiology 124:123–128, 1977.
28. McBride, C. M., and Wallace, S.: Cancer of the right lobe of the liver: a variety of operative procedures. Arch. Surg. 105:289–295, 1972.
29. McClelland, R. R.: Focal porta hepatis scintiscan defects. What is their significance? J. Nucl. Med. 16:1007–1012, 1976.
30. McCready, V. R.: Scintigraphic studies of space-occupying liver disease. Semin. Nucl. Med. 2:108–127, 1972.
31. McNulty, J. G.: Radiology of the Liver. Chapters 1, 4 and 7. Philadelphia, W. B. Saunders Company, 1977.
32. MacCarty, R. L., Wahner, H. W., Stephens, D. H., et al.: Retrospective comparison of radionuclide scans and computed tomography of the liver and pancreas. Am. J. Roentgenol. 129:23–28, 1977.

33. Maguire, R., and Doppman, J.: Angiographic abnormalities in partial Budd-Chiari syndrome. Radiology 122:629–635, 1977.
34. Mays, E., Christopherson, W. M., Mahr, M. M., et al.: Hepatic changes in young women ingesting contraceptive steroids. Hepatic hemorrhage and primary hepatic tumors. J.A.M.A. 235:730–732, 1976.
35. Michels, N. A.: Blood Supply to the Upper Abdominal Organs with a Descriptive Atlas. Philadelphia, J. B. Lippincott Company, 1955.
36. Nahum, H., and Levesque, M.: Arteriography in hepatic trauma. Radiology 109:557–563, 1973.
37. Nebesar, R. A., Kornblith, P. L., Pollard, J. J., et al.: Celiac and Superior Mesenteric Arteries: A Correlation of Angiograms and Dissections. Boston, Little, Brown & Company, 1969.
38. Okuda, K., Musha, H., Yamasaki, T., et al.: Angiograhic demonstration of intrahepatic arterio-portal anastamosis in hepatocellular carcinoma. Radiology 122:53–58, 1977.
39. Orloff, M. J.: The liver. In Sabiston, D. C. (ed.): Davis-Christopher Textbook of Surgery. Ed. 11. Chapter 35. Philadelphia, W. B. Saunders Company, 1977.
40. Pereiras, R., Viamonte, M., Russell, E., et al.: New techniques for interruption of gastroesophageal venous blood flow. Radiology 124:313–323, 1977.
41. Reuter, S. R., Berk, R. N., and Orloff, M. J.: An angiographic study of pre- and postoperative hemodynamics in patients with side-to-side portacaval shunts. Radiology 116:33–39, 1975.
42. Reuter, S. R., and Redman, H. C.: Gastrointestinal Angiography, Ed. 2. Chapters 4 and 5. Philadelphia, W. B. Saunders Company, 1977.
43. Rosenthal, S.: Are hepatic scans overused? Am. J. Digest. Dis. 21:659–663, 1976.
44. Rösch, J., Freeny, P., Antonovic, R., et al.: Infusion hepatic angiography in diagnosis of liver metastases. Cancer 38:2278–2286, 1976.
45. Ruben, B. E., and Katzen, B. T.: Selective hepatic artery embolization to control massive hepatic hemorrhage after trauma. Am. J. Roentgenol. 129:253–256, 1977.
46. Salvo, A. F., Schiller, A., Athanasoulis, C. A. et al.: Hepatoadenoma and focal nodular hyperplasia: pitfalls in radiocolloid imaging. Radiology 125:451–455, 1977.
47. Sandblom, P. H.: Hemobilia. Springfield, Illinois, Charles C Thomas Publisher, 1972.
48. Schaner, E. G., Balow, J. E., and Doppman, J. L.: Computed tomography in the diagnosis of subcapsular and perirenal hematoma. Am. J. Roentgenol. 129:83–88, 1977.
39. Scheible, W., Gosink, B. B., and Leopold, G. R.: Grey scale echographic patterns of hepatic metastatic disease. Am. J. Roentgenol. 129:983–987, 1977.
50. Seltzer, R. A., Rossiter, S. B., Cooperman, L. R., et al.: Hemobilia following needle biopsy of the liver. Am. J. Roentgenol. 127:1035–1036, 1976.
51. Spiegel, R. M., Kin, D. L., and Green, W. M.: Ultrasonography of primary cysts of the liver. Am. J. Roentgenol. 131:235–238, 1978.
52. Steichen, F. M.: Hepatic trauma in adults. Surg. Clin. North Am. 55:387–407, 1975.
53. Stephens, D. H., Sheedy, P. F., II, Hattery, R. R., et al.: Computed tomography of the liver. Am. J. Roentgenol. 128:579–590, 1977.
54. Taylor, K. J. W., Carpenter, D. A., Hill, C. R., et al.: Gray scale ultrasound imaging. Radiology 119:415–523, 1976.
55. Viamonte, M., LePage, J., Lunderquist, A., et al.: Selective catheterization of the portal vein and its tributaries. Radiology 114:457–460, 1975.
56. Walter, J. F., Passo, B. T., and Cannon, W. B.: Successful transcatheter embolic control of massive hematobilia secondary to liver biopsy. Am. J. Roentgenol. 127:847–849, 1976.
57. Watson, R. C., and Baltaxe, H. A.: The angiographic appearance of primary and secondary tumors of the liver. Radiology 101:539–548, 1971.
58. Whalen, J. P., Berne, A. S., and Riemenschneider, P.: The extraperitoneal perivisceral fat-pad. I. Its role in the roentgenological visualization of abdominal organs. Radiology 92:466–472, 1969.
59. Wirtanen, G. W.: A new angiographic technique in the diagnosis of liver tumor. Radiology 108:51–54, 1973.
60. Wixson, D., Kazam, E., and Whalen, J. P.: Displaced lateral surface of the liver (Hellmer's sign) secondary to extraperitoneal fluid collection. Am. J. Roentgenol. 127:679–682, 1976.
61. Wooten, W. B., Bernardino, M. D., and Goldstein, H. M.: Computed tomography of necrotic hepatic metastases. Am. J. Roentgenol, 131:839–842, 1978.
62. Wooten, W. B., Green, B., and Goldstein, H. M.: Ultrasonography of necrotic metastases. Radiology 128:447–450, 1978.

16

THE BILIARY SYSTEM

Part I

Biliary Tract Investigation by Imaging Modalities

STEVEN K. TEPLICK, M.D.

ANATOMY AND ANATOMIC VARIANTS

Biliary tract surgery is one of the most common forms of surgery performed in this country. Anatomic variations of the gallbladder and bile ducts are encountered frequently. To avoid serious surgical complications, it is imperative that the radiologist and surgeon be aware of these variations.

Normally, the gallbladder is covered by peritoneum and attached to the inferior surfaces of the right and quadrate lobes of the liver. In about 80 per cent the gallbladder is in close proximity to the superior medial aspect of the hepatic flexure of the colon. It is often in close relationship with the duodenal bulb and proximal descending duodenum (Fig. 16–1). Because of these relationships, cholecystitis may cause inflammatory changes of the colon or duodenum, falsely suggesting primary gastrointestinal disease (Fig. 16–2).[4]

In about 95 per cent, the cystic artery, which supplies the gallbladder, arises from the right hepatic artery in the triangle of Calot (Fig. 16–3).[8] However, the cystic artery may arise outside the triangle of Calot from a major branch of the celiac trunk or superior mesenteric artery and cross anterior to the common hepatic duct or common bile duct. Occasionally there is a double cystic artery. Both arteries can arise from the right hepatic artery, or one may originate anomalously outside the triangle. The common bile duct is supplied by branches of the gastroduodenal artery. The venous drainage of the extrahepatic biliary tract is through the portal system.

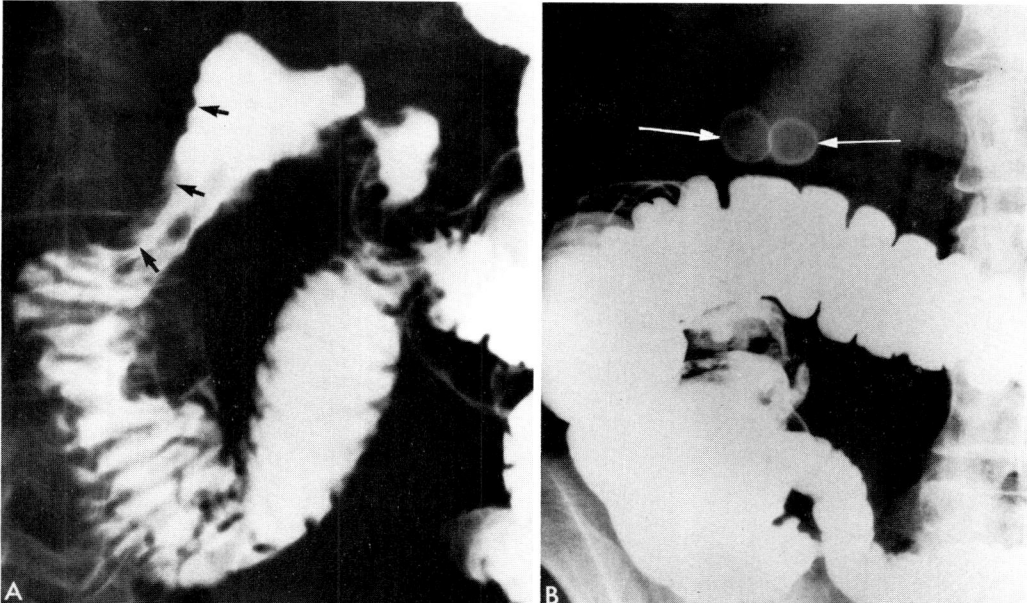

Figure 16–1. Relationship of the gallbladder to the duodenum and colon. *A*, The impression on the duodenal bulb and the second part of the duodenum (arrows) is from a normal gallbladder. *B*, The opaque gallstones (arrows) demonstrate the intimate relationship between the gallbladder and the hepatic flexure of the colon.

The right and left hepatic ducts usually join to form the common hepatic duct in the porta hepatis. The cystic duct, which has spiral mucosal folds (valves of Heister), joins the common hepatic duct to form the common bile duct. The common bile duct empties into the duodenum at the papilla of Vater, which is frequently located in the middle of the descending limb of the duodenum. Often the distal common bile duct is joined by the pancreatic duct just before the papilla to form a common channel, the ampulla of Vater (Fig. 16–4).

The cystic duct usually inserts into the right lateral margin of the common bile duct 2 to 8 cm distal to the bifurcation of the common hepatic duct. The insertion is often perpendicular, but not uncommonly the cystic duct runs parallel and closely adherent to the common bile duct for a variable distance before joining. This can result in a long cystic duct remnant after cholecystectomy, a potential site of recurrent stone formation and infection (see the section on postcholecystectomy syndromes). The cystic duct may insert into the anterior, posterior, or left lateral borders of the common bile duct. Rarely, it empties separately into the duodenum or joins the right or left hepatic ducts. There are many other variations of ductal anatomy. For example, anomalous ducts from the liver may insert into the bladder or into one of the extrahepatic ducts. Failure to recognize these variations can result in serious postsurgical complications, such as bile fistulas and bile peritonitis (Fig. 16–5).

The common bile duct and pancreatic ducts empty separately into the duodenum in about 30 to 40 per cent of patients. The papilla of Vater is usually found in the posteromedial border of the midpoint of the descending limb of the duodenum (75 per cent), but it may be located at the junction of the second and third portions of the duodenum (17 per cent) or even in the third portion of the duodenum (8 per cent).[5,7]

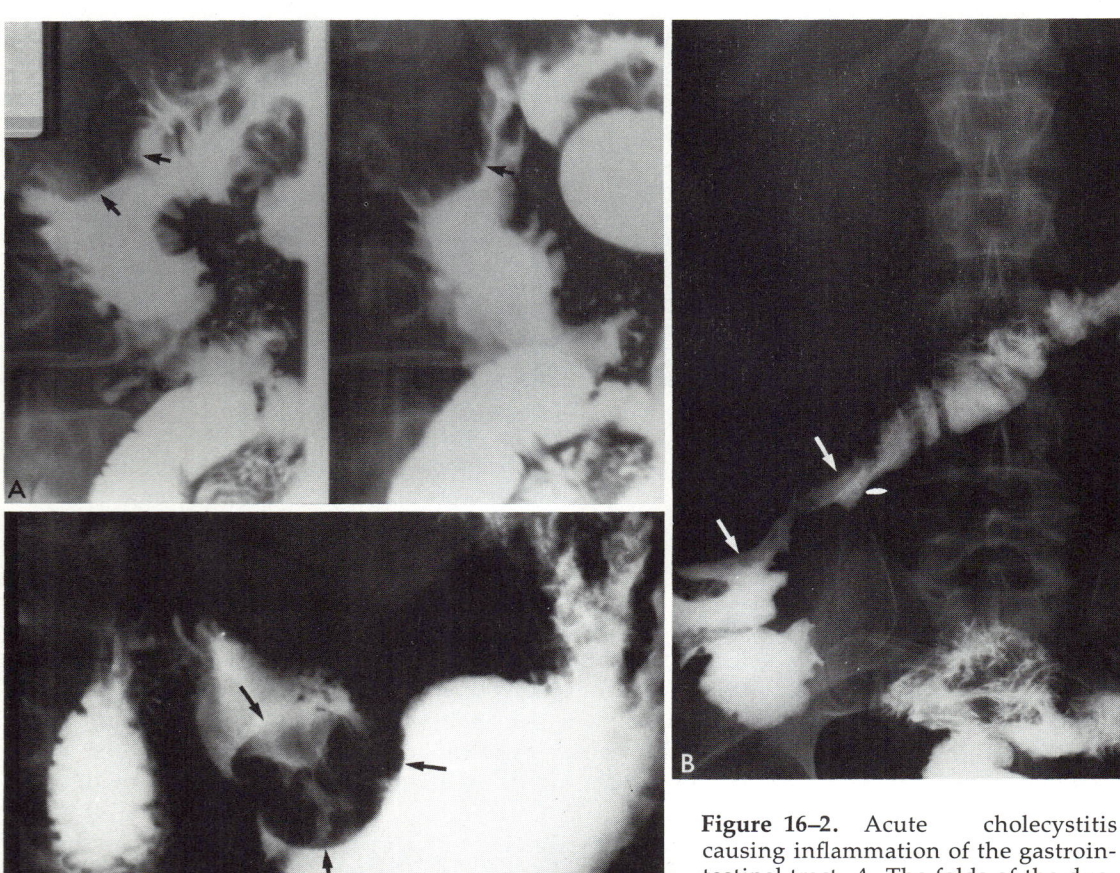

Figure 16–2. Acute cholecystitis causing inflammation of the gastrointestinal tract. *A*, The folds of the duodenal bulb and postbulbar areas are thickened. There is a mass indenting the superolateral aspect of the duodenal sweep (arrows). *B*, There is a right upper quadrant soft tissue mass from an enlarged gallbladder. Inflammatory changes of the transverse colon (arrows) are caused by adjacent cholecystitis. *C*, Edema of the distal stomach and bulb (arrows) from cholecystitis simulates a polypoid mass.

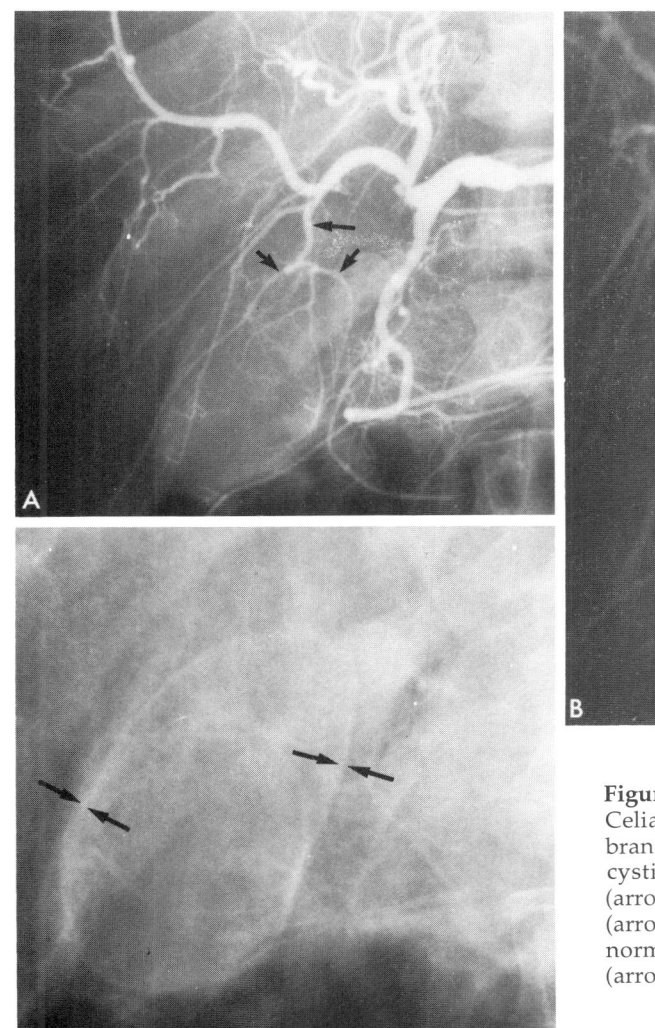
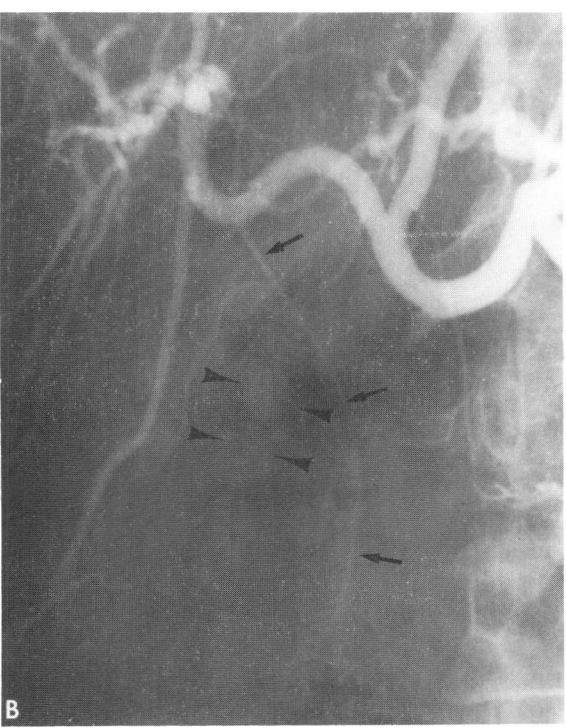

Figure 16-3. Normal angiographic anatomy. *A*, Celiac angiogram showing cystic artery and branches in the triangle of Calot (arrows). *B*, The cystic artery outlines an enlarged gallbladder (arrows), which contains faintly opaque calculi (arrowheads). *C*, Venous phase, showing the normal thickness of the gallbladder wall (arrows).

870 — THE BILIARY SYSTEM

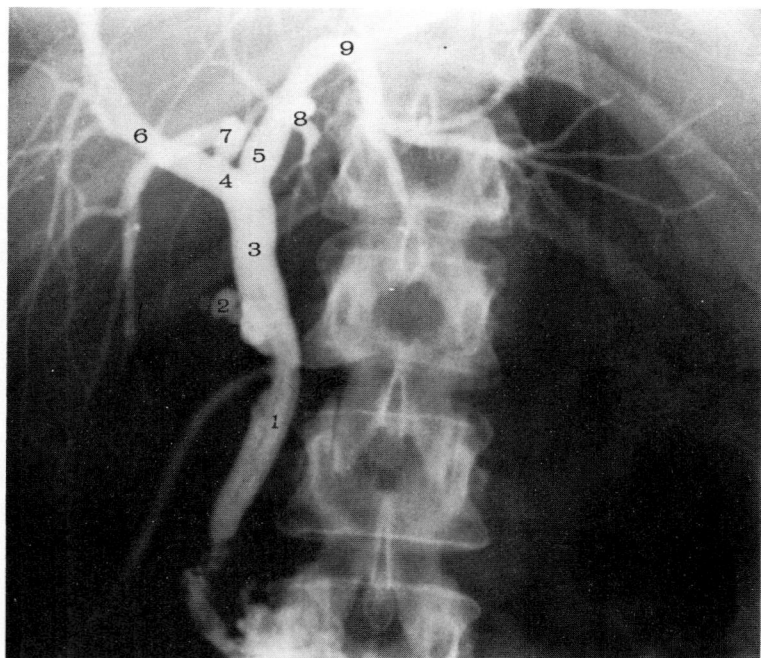

Figure 16–4. Normal bile duct anatomy. 1. common bile duct; 2. cystic duct; 3 common hepatic duct; 4. main right hepatic duct; 5. main left hepatic duct; 6. anterior division right lobe; 7. posterior division right lobe; 8. duct to quadrate lobe; 9. characteristic curve at level of umbilical fissure (which divides the left lobe into medial and lateral divisions).

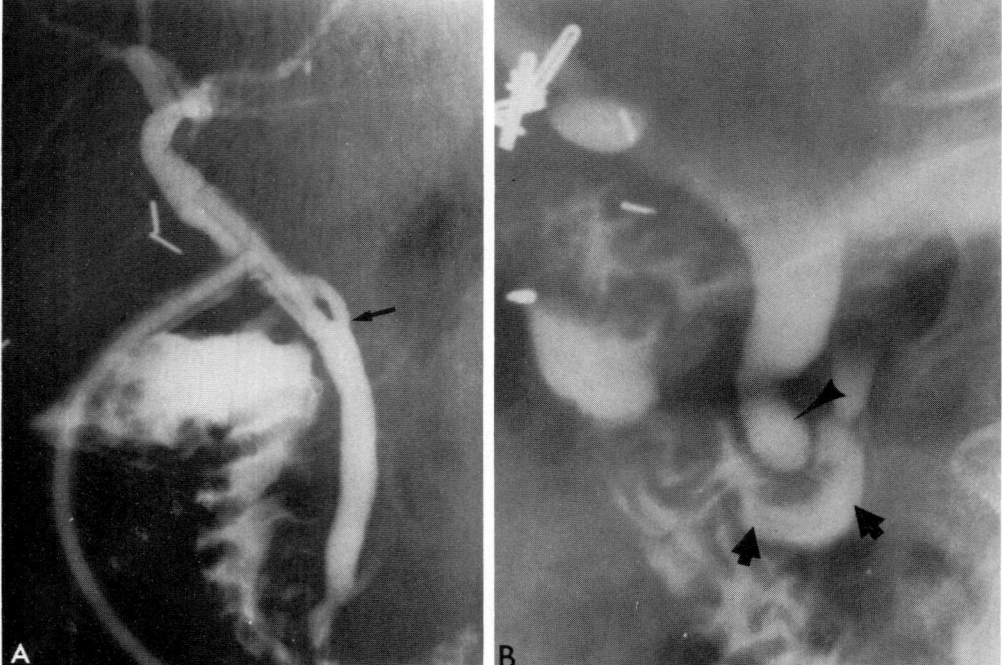

Figure 16–5. Anatomic variations of the bile ducts. *A*, The cystic duct inserts into the left lateral border of the common bile duct (arrow). *B*, The common bile duct (arrowhead) inserts into a duodenal diverticulum (large arrows.) This is probably of no clinical significance even though bile may reflux into the pancreatic duct (small arrow).

Rarely, there is dilatation of part of the intraduodenal segment of the common bile duct (choledochocele). This anomaly is proably congenital and most likely represents a form of choledochal cyst. On the upper gastrointestinal series, choledochoceles are seen as smooth, polypoid filling defects in the duodenal loop (Fig. 16–6). Their shape may be altered by peristalsis or compression. They may be indistinguishable from other duodenal lesions, such as intraluminal diverticula or adenomatous polyps. When visualized during cholangiography, they appear as an opaque, rounded dilatation of the distal common bile duct surrounded by a radiolucent rim (similar to ureterocele).[9]

On occasion the gallbladder is not in its usual location. It may be entirely covered with peritoneum and attached to the liver by a long mesentery (floating gallbladder), allowing considerable mobility. Rarely, a mobile gallbladder herniates through the foramen of Winslow into the lesser sac (Fig. 16–7). Other positional anomalies include left-sided gallbladder, pelvic gallbladder, infra- or suprahepatic gallbladder, or gallbladder in the falciform ligament[2, 3, 5, 10] (Fig. 16–8). Because of positional variations, it is imporant on oral cholecystography to obtain a radiograph of the entire abdomen and not just of the right upper quadrant before deciding that the gallbladder does not visualize.

A partially or completely intrahepatic gallbladder may make cholecystectomy more difficult and increase surgical complications. The diagnosis is difficult to ascertain on oral cholecystography but should be considered when a radionuclide scan shows a single filling defect in the liver (Fig. 16–9). The diagnosis of intrahepatic gallbladder can usually be confirmed by ultrasound. The "liver mass" will be cystic, and no gallbladder will be identified elsewhere.

Agenesis, or congenital absence of the gallbladder and cystic duct, is a rare anomaly usually discovered at autopsy or during surgery for a "nonvisualized gallblad-

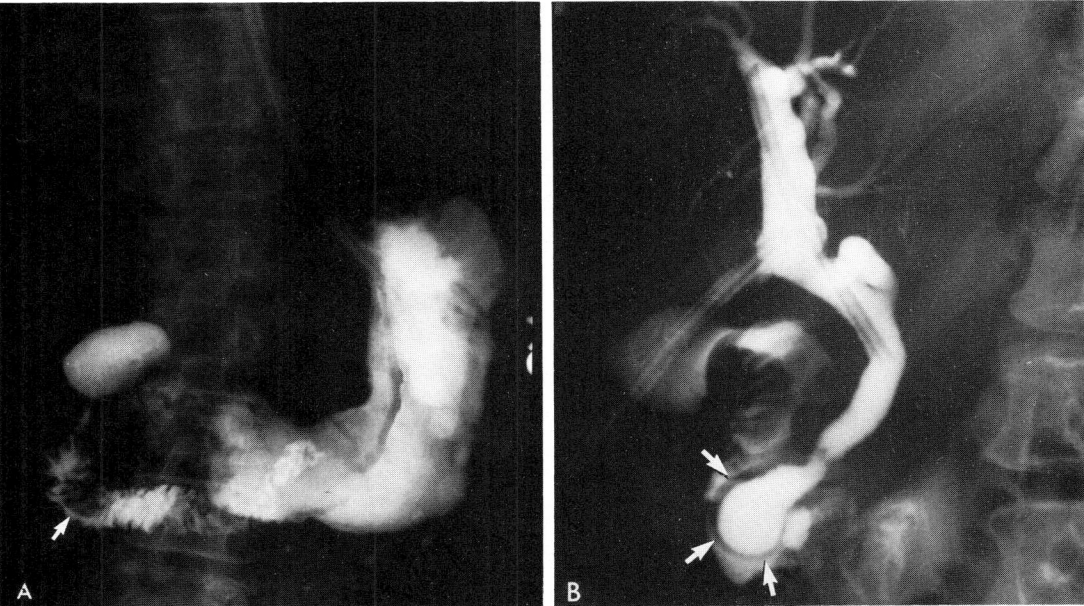

Figure 16–6. Choledochocele. *A*, Mass in the region of duodenal ampulla (arrow). *B*, T-tube cholangiogram showing dilatation of the distal common bile duct surrounding a thin radiolucent rim (arrows). (Courtesy of Carl R. Larsen, M.D.)

872 — THE BILIARY SYSTEM

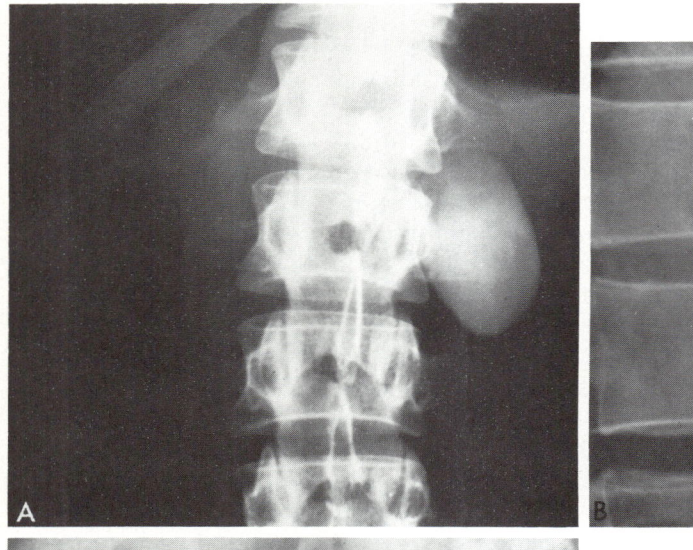
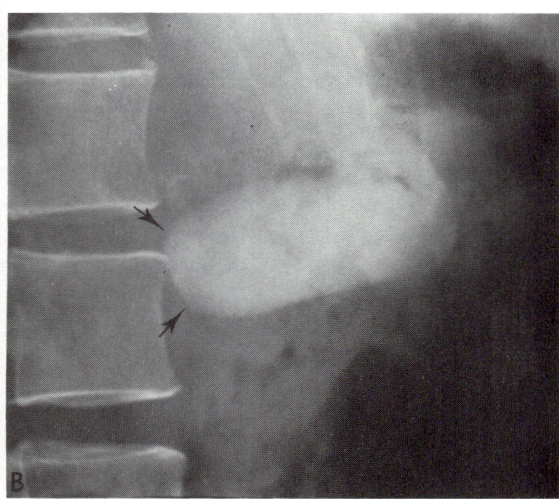
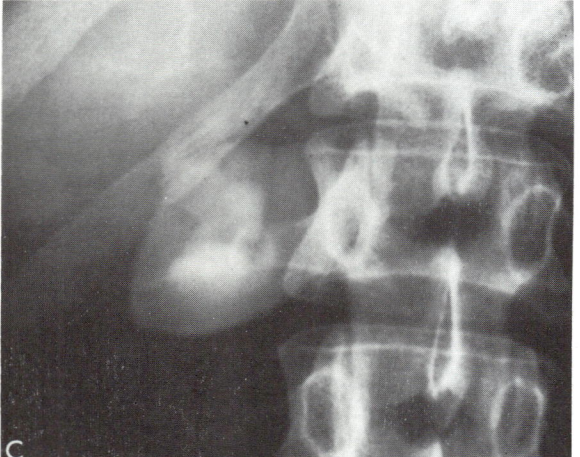

Figure 16–7. Gallbladder in lesser sac. *A,* The gallbladder has herniated through the foramen of Winslow into the lesser sac and lies to the left of the spine. *B,* Lateral view of herniated gallbladder showing the fundus facing posteriorly (arrows). *C,* When the hernia is reduced the gallbladder returns to its normal location in the right upper quadrant.

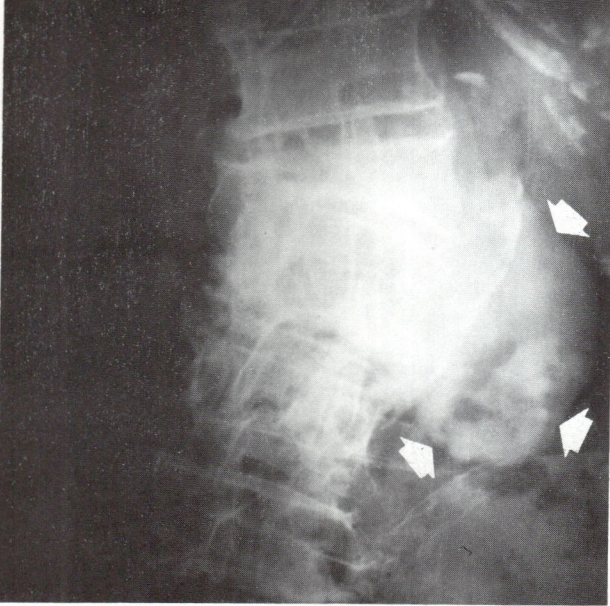

Figure 16–8. Left-sided gallbladder. The gallbladder (arrows) is displaced to the left side by an enlarged liver and tumor mass on the right.

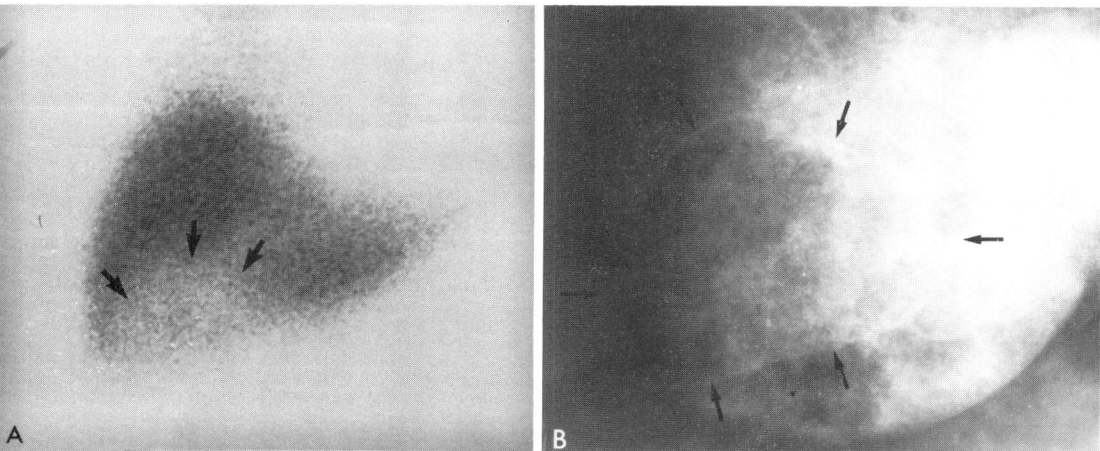

Figure 16–9. Intrahepatic gallbladder. *A*, ^{99m}Technetium liver scan shows a filling defect at the inferior margin of the right lobe (arrows). *B*, Late phase of angiogram showing the gallbladder (arrows) entirely within the liver parenchyma.

der" on oral cholecystography. The diagnosis is rarely made preoperatively but should be suspected when the patient has other congenital abnormalities, particularly rectovaginal fistula, imperforate anus, intracardiac shunts, and hypoplasia of one or more bones.[6] Computerized transaxial tomography or ultrasound may confirm the diagnosis without the need to resort to laparotomy. When no gallbladder is found at surgery, an operative cholangiogram should be performed to confirm the diagnosis and to exclude a gallbladder in an anomalous location.[1] A double or even triple gallbladder occurs rarely (Fig. 16–10).

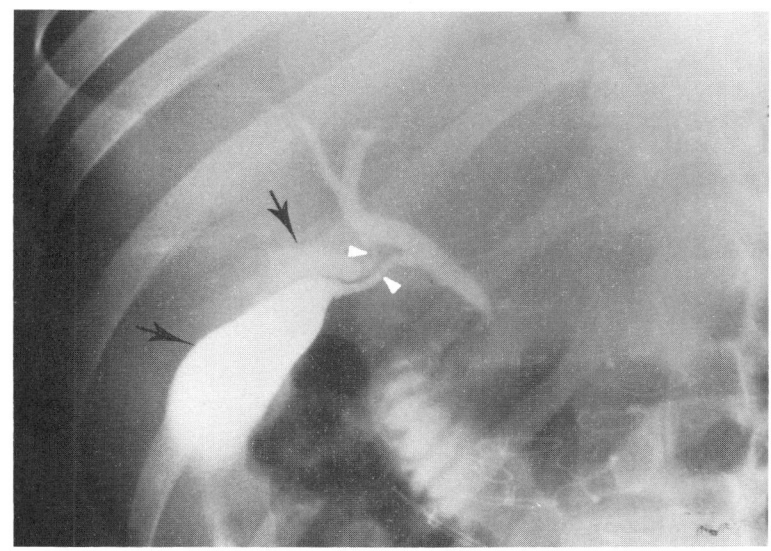

Figure 16–10. Double gallbladder. Oral cholecystogram shows two separate gallbladders (arrows). Each cystic duct is inserted separately into the common bile duct (arrowheads).

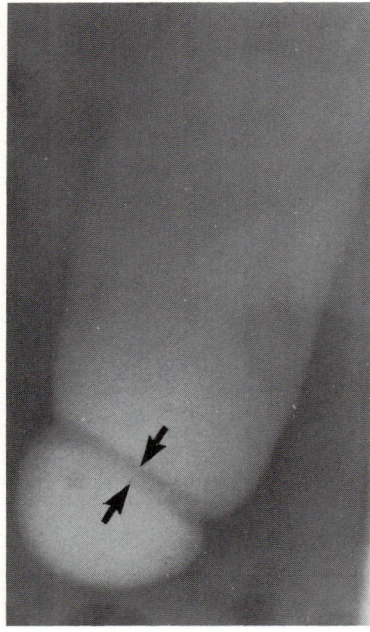

Figure 16–11. Phrygian cap. A thin radiolucent line partially encircles the fundus of the gallbladder (arrows).

Developmental variations of the gallbladder are interesting radiologically but are usually of no clinical significance (Figs. 16–11 and 16–12). The phrygian cap deformity is caused by a transverse septum traversing part of the fundus of the gallbladder. Other bands or septa are occasionally demonstrated on cholecystography but are much less common than the phrygian cap. Congenital variations should be differentiated from segmental adenomyomatosis (see the section on the cholecystoses).

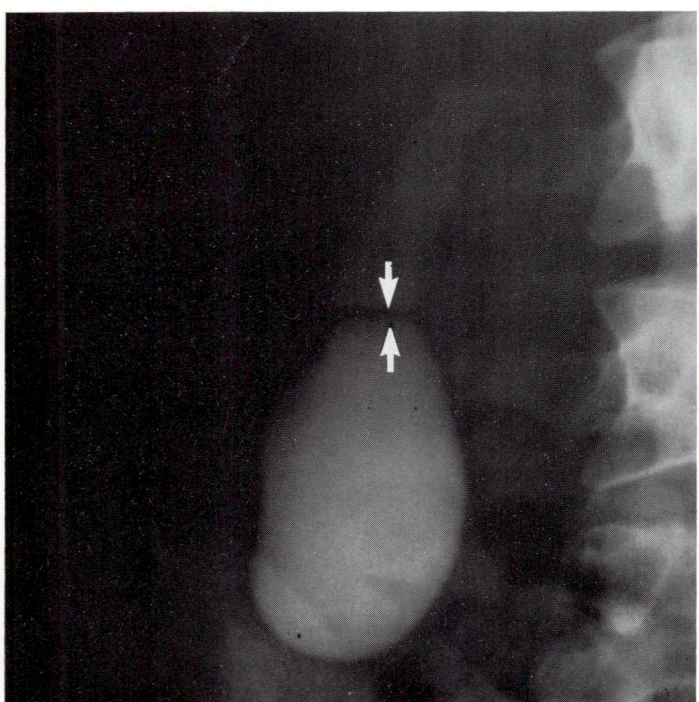

Figure 16–12. Gallbladder septum. A radiolucent band surrounds the proximal third of the gallbladder (arrows). The post-fatty meal film did not show any evidence of adenomyomatosis.

TABLE 16–1. IMAGING MODALITIES USEFUL FOR EVALUATION OF THE BILIARY SYSTEM

Plain films
Oral cholecystography
Intravenous cholangiography
UGI and hypotonic duodenography
Isotopes
Ultrasound
Computed Tomography (CT scan)
Percutaneous transhepatic cholangiography
Endoscopic retrograde cholangiopancreatography (ERCP)
Infusion tomography
Angiography
Operative and postoperative tube cholangiography

MODALITIES TO EVALUATE THE BILIARY TRACT

The imaging modalities available to evaluate the biliary tract are listed in Table 16–1. An understanding of the use of each procedure facilitates diagnosis and treatment.

Plain Films

Plain films of the abdomen are often helpful in diagnosing biliary tract disease. The demonstration of radiopaque gallstones can obviate the time and expense of oral cholecystography. Occasionally, opaque gallstones are obscured on oral cholecystography, and the diagnosis will be missed if a plain abdominal film is not available (Fig. 16–13).

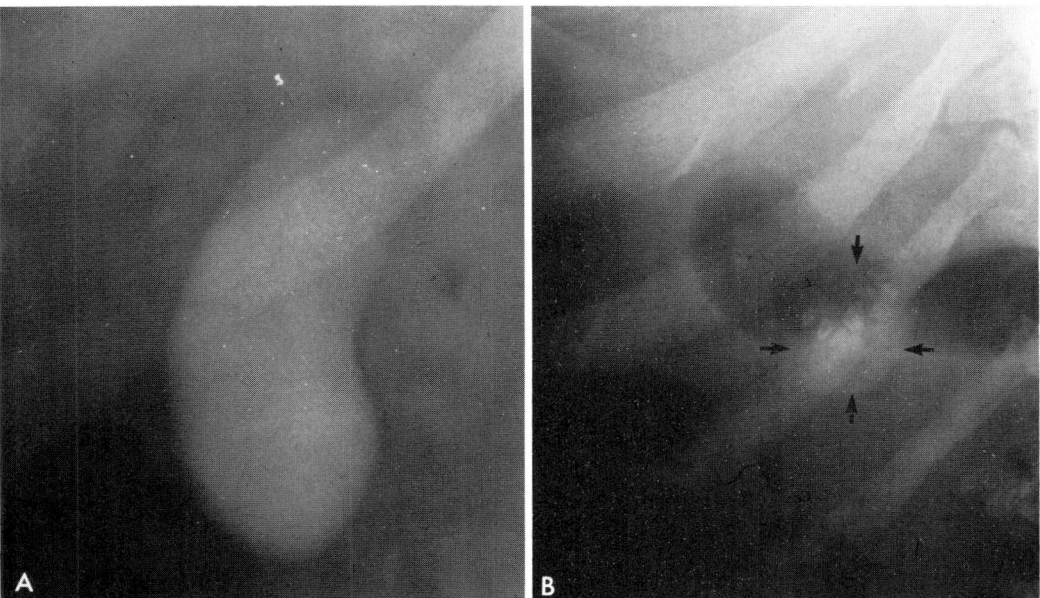

Figure 16–13. False negative oral cholecystogram. *A,* The oral cholecystogram is normal. *B,* A previous abdominal film shows small, faintly opaque gallstones (arrows).

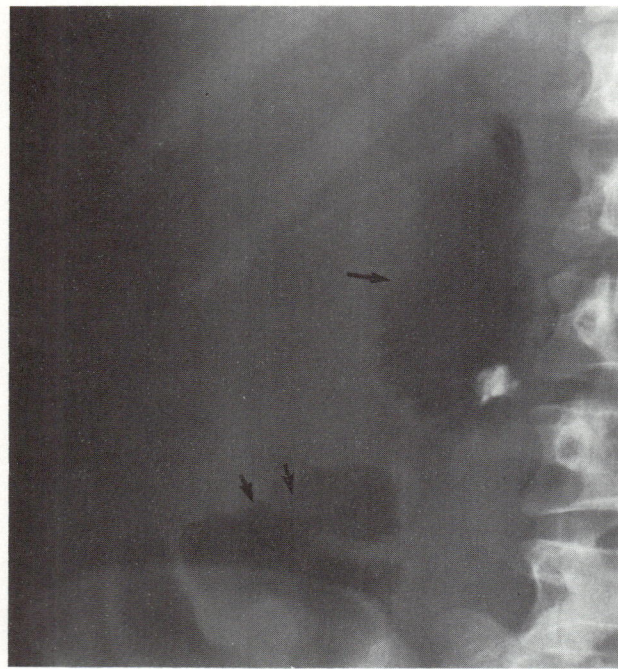

Figure 16–14. Localized ileus. There is an atonic dilated segment of small bowel (arrow) adjacent to an inflamed gallbladder. Inflammatory changes are also present on the hepatic flexure of the colon (arrows).

The sentinel loop, which represents a localized ileus adjacent to an area of inflammation, is usually nonspecific. Occasionally it is a useful indication of cholecystitis when located in the right upper abdomen adjacent to an inflamed gallbladder (Fig. 16–14).

Only 10 to 15 per cent of gallstones contain enough calcium to be radiopaque (Fig. 16–15). Consequently, it is usually necessary to opacify the gallbladder in order to visualize the calculi. On occasion, however, gas-containing fissures within radiolucent stones are visible on plain abdominal radiographs (the "Mercedes-Benz" sign).[14] *In*

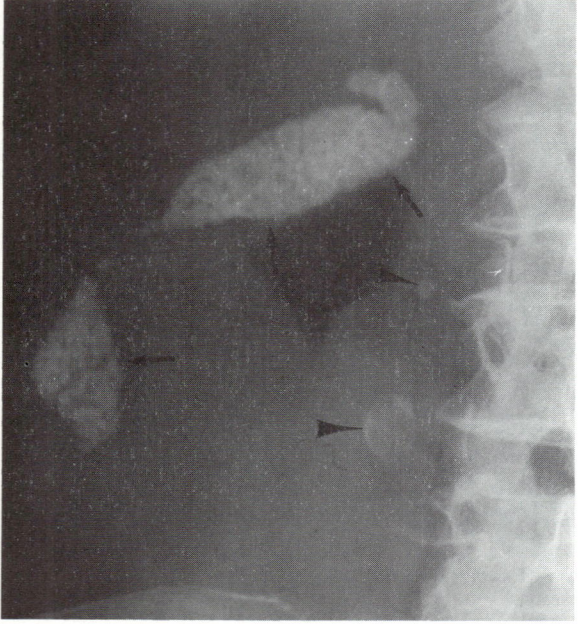

Figure 16–15. Radiopaque gallstones. The gallbladder is packed with small opaque stones (arrows). Calculi are present in the common bile duct (arrowheads). An oral cholecystogram would add little additional information.

vitro, radiographs show that fissures in gallstones are common, especially in the mixed type of stone containing predominantly cholesterol. The gas within these fissures is a mixture of carbon dioxide, oxygen, and nitrogen. The fissures are usually seen as triradiating, thin, fairly symmetric radiolucencies in the region of the gallbladder just above the hepatic flexure of the colon (Fig. 16–16). Sometimes a faintly discernible rim of calcium surrounds the fissures. The "Mercedes-Benz" sign is easily overlooked but when recognized is diagnostic for gallstones.

When the gallbladder contains bile with a high concentration of calcium carbonate, it becomes radiopaque (milk of calcium bile) (Fig. 16–17). In this circumstance an oral cholecystogram can be misinterpreted as normal if a preliminary film is not available. In most instances, however, the cystic duct is occluded by a radiopaque calculus and discrete calculi are visible within the gallbladder lumen so that the diagnosis is easily established. Milk of calcium bile has the same clinical significance as gallstones, and if the symptoms warrant, a cholecystectomy is usually indicated.

Calcification in the gallbladder wall presents a characteristic x-ray appearance, often referred to as a porcelain gallbladder (Fig. 16–18). Its incidence is difficult to determine but is estimated at 0.06 to 0.8 per cent. The calcifications occur both in the muscularis and in the glandular elements of the mucosa. In many cases there are associated gallstones, and the cystic duct is usually occluded. Chronic cholecystitis can nearly always be demonstrated histologically. The porcelain gallbladder is thought to be a precursor of carcinoma of the gallbladder. The frequency of cancer in porcelain gallbladder is estimated to be as high as 22 per cent. Therefore, prophylactic cholecystectomy may be warranted in younger persons even in the absence of any gallbladder symptoms.[11, 16]

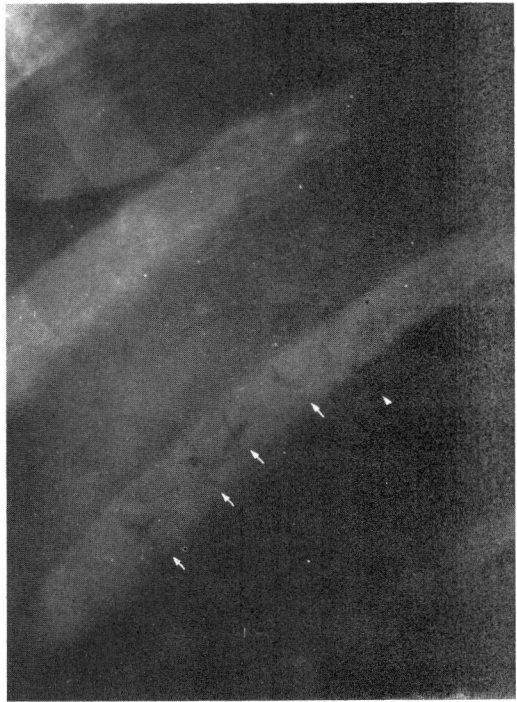

Figure 16–16. "Mercedes-Benz" sign. Thin, radiolucent X-shaped lines are visible over the eleventh rib (arrows).

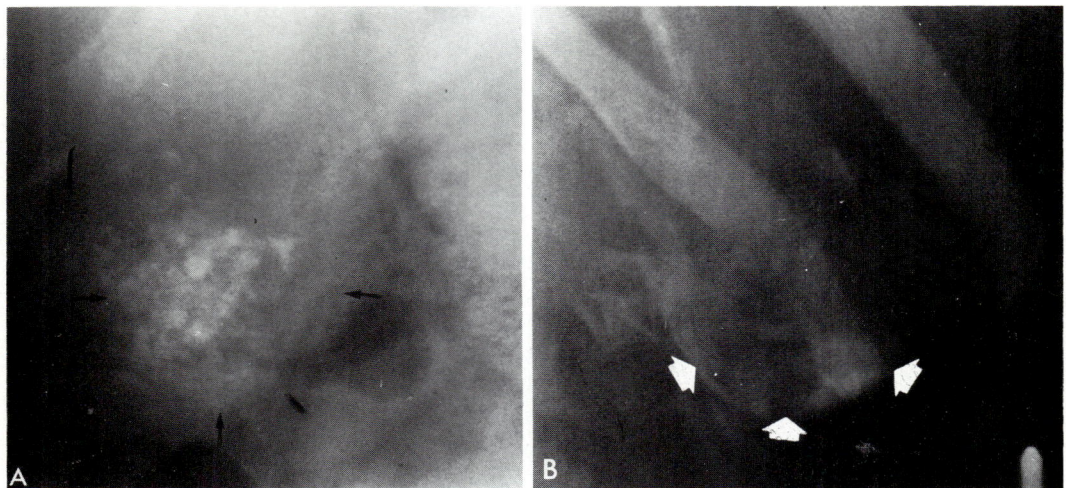

Figure 16–17. Milk of calcium bile. *A,* There is calcified sludge and small stones in the gallbladder (arrows). *B,* On the upright film, the sludge has shifted to the fundus of the gallbladder (arrows).

Emphysematous cholecystitis[12, 13] is a severe form of acute cholecystitis frequently associated with stones obstructing the cystic duct. The diagnosis can be made on the plain film of the abdomen. Twenty-four to 48 hours after the onset of acute cholecystitis, gas can be seen in the lumen of the gallbladder and subsequently in the gallbladder wall (Fig. 16–19). Less frequently, gas is also seen in the bile ducts. The gallbladder is often considerably distended. The formation of intraluminal gas is related to blockage of the

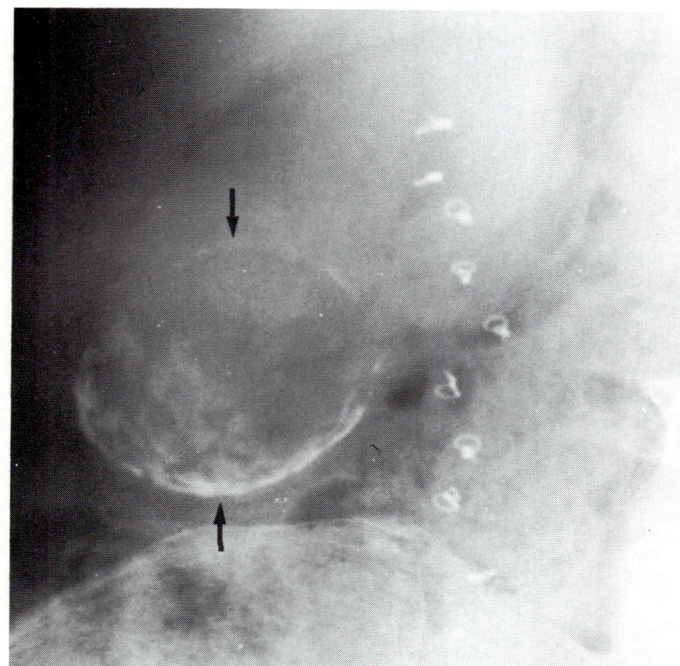

Figure 16–18. Porcelain gallbladder. The gallbladder wall is calcified (arrows). Often, but not in this example, an opaque stone can be seen in the cystic duct.

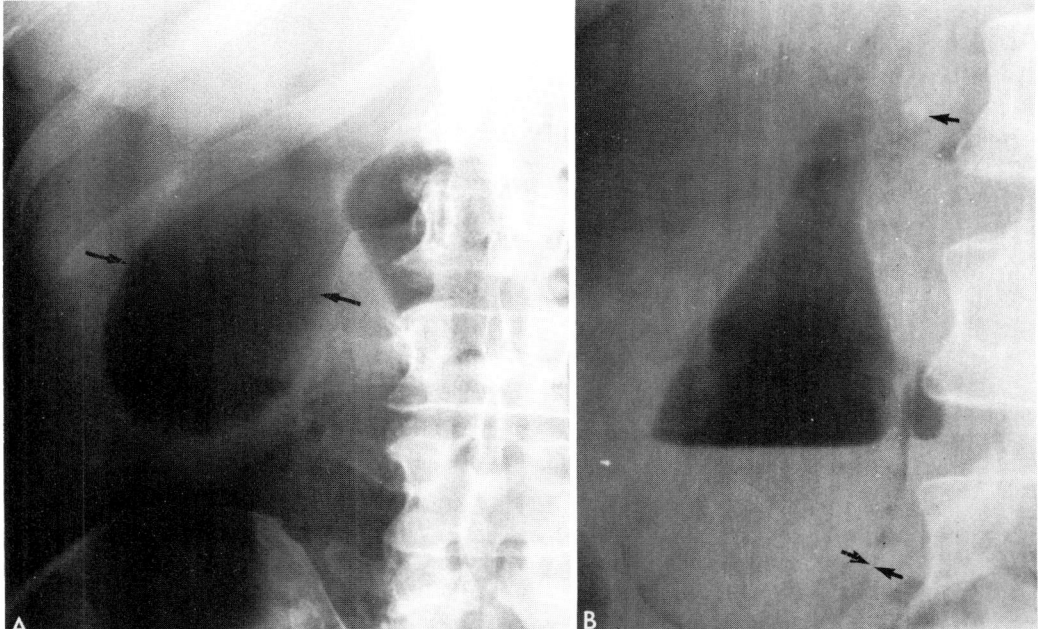

Figure 16–19. Emphysematous cholecystitis. *A,* Air in the gallbladder lumen (arrows). *B,* An upright radiograph in a different patient shows air in the gallbladder wall (arrows) and an intraluminal air-fluid level. There is a stone in the cystic duct (arrow).

cystic duct and subsequent overgrowth of gas-producing organisms, usually *Clostridium welchii* and *Escherichia coli*. Ischemic necrosis of the gallbladder seems to have a role in the process and is probably the mechanism for the development of intramural gas.

Emphysematous cholecystitis occurs more commonly in males, in contrast to the usual form of cholecystitis. Approximately one third of the cases occur in diabetics, and the peak incidence is in the sixth and seventh decades. Patients with emphysematous cholecystitis are often severely ill. Treatment consists of intensive antibiotic therapy and early surgery, either a cholecystectomy or a cholecystotomy. Rarely, a patient recovers without surgery. The amount of gas gradually diminishes over several weeks and eventually disappears.

Gas in the biliary system can be caused by a variety of conditions. Biliary-enteric bypass and drainage procedures are the most common causes. Intestinal contents, including gas and contrast material, reflux freely into the biliary system after this type of surgery. In fact, failure to reflux gas or barium into the biliary tract should raise the suspicion of either recurrent disease or faulty surgical anastomosis. Reflux of intestinal contents or contrast agents does not seem to predispose to biliary tract infection. Gas in the gallbladder and bile ducts also occurs in emphysematous cholecystitis and any condition producing a fistula between the gastrointestinal tract and biliary system, such as gallstone ileus, perforation of a duodenal ulcer, and tumor (Fig. 16–20).

Gas in the biliary tract must be distinguished from gas in the portal venous system. Gas in the portal system usually signifies extensive bowel necrosis and is associated with a high mortality. It can, however, be seen in more benign conditions, such as inflammatory bowel disease. With gas in the portal vein, linear streaks of intrahepatic

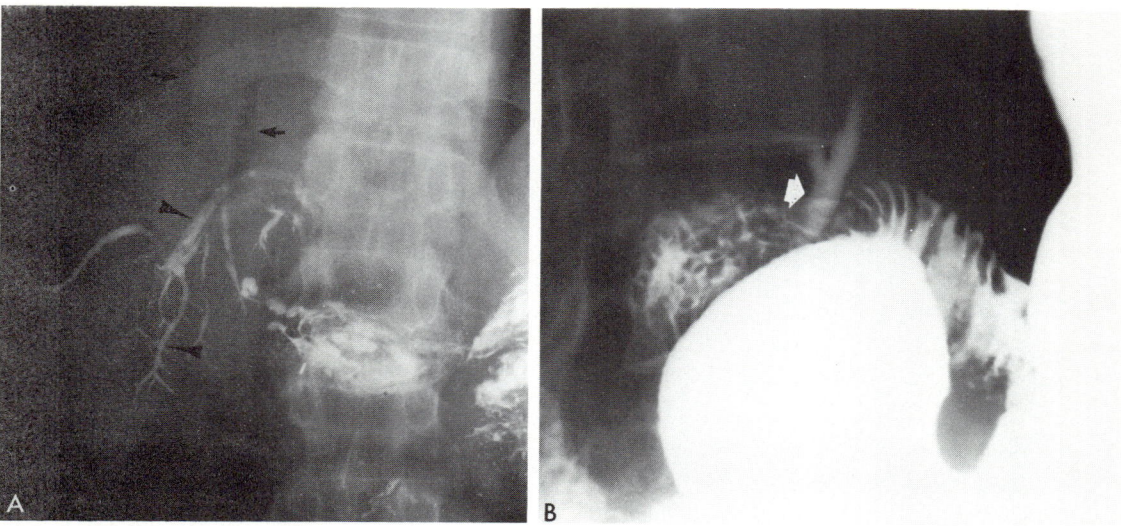

Figure 16–20. Biliary-enteric communications. *A,* Choledochoduodenostomy. Barium refluxed freely into the bile ducts (arrowheads) during the upper gastrointestinal series. Other ducts contain gas (arrows). *B,* Choledochoduodenal fistula secondary to duodenal ulcer disease. During the upper gastrointestinal series, the common bile duct filled with barium (arrow).

portal venous gas extend toward the periphery of the liver. Sometimes the main portal vein can be seen (Fig. 16–21). In contrast, gas in the bile ducts appears closer to the porta hepatis, and usually the extrahepatic bile ducts and the gallbladder are visualized.

The extrahepatic bile ducts are surrounded by a variable amount of fat, which may be seen on x-ray as linear or branching lucencies in the right upper abdomen.[17] These must be distinguished from biliary or portal vein gas. Occasionally the width of the common bile duct can be determined by the periductal fat lines.

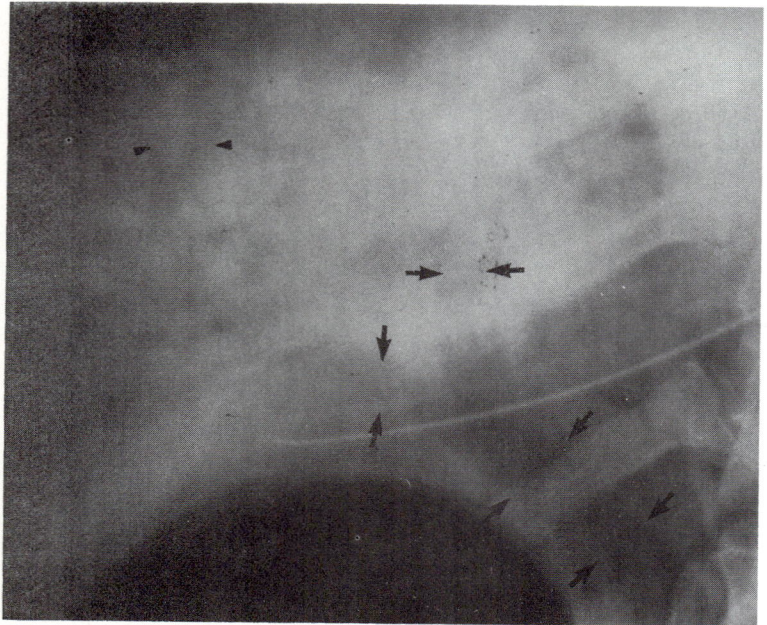

Figure 16–21. Portal vein gas. Radiolucencies near the periphery of the liver (arrowheads) represent gas in the small portal vein radicals. The main portal vein as well as its right and left branches contain gas (arrows). The patient died from extensive bowel infarction.

THE BILIARY SYSTEM — 881

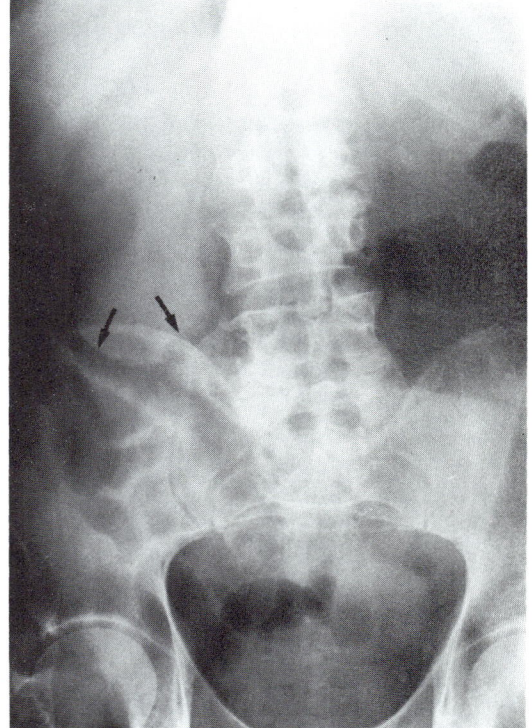

Figure 16–22. Hydrops of the gallbladder. The soft tissue density in the right abdomen represents a moderately enlarged gallbladder. The fundus of the gallbladder indents the superior border of the hepatic flexures (arrows).

Hydrops of the gallbladder can occur if the cystic duct remains occluded after an episode of acute cholecystitis. The gallbladder becomes filled with clear mucoid fluid and enlarges. The abdominal plain film shows a soft tissue density in the right upper abdomen and an extrinsic soft tissue mass pressing on the superior border of the hepatic flexure (Fig. 16–22).

Oral Cholecystography

Properly performed oral cholecystography is a reliable diagnostic test for gallbladder disease. In 1924, Graham and Cole first produced x-ray visualization of the gallbladder using iodinated organic compounds. Today, many such compounds are available. The two most frequently used in the United States are iopanoic acid (Telepaque) and ipodate (Oragrafin). Fortunately, toxic reactions from these drugs are uncommon.[20, 23] Toxicity from intravenous iodinated contrast agents is much more common than with oral agents. Meglumine iodipamide (Cholografin), which is used for intravenous cholangiography, has the highest incidence of toxic reactions. Side effects range from mild reactions, such as skin rashes, sweating, nausea, vomiting, and diarrhea, to the more severe problems of anaphylaxis and acute renal insufficiency. The minor side effects of nausea, vomiting, and diarrhea are probably dose-related. Diarrhea occurs most commonly with Telepaque, and care should be taken when using this agent in patients with inflammatory bowel disease.

Urticaria occurs frequently with both the oral and the intravenous drugs. Skin rashes are uncomfortable but pose no serious danger and can be treated with antihistaminic agents. Possibly, pretreatment with an antihistamine decreases the incidence of hives. Anaphylaxis with cardiovascular collapse is fortunately rare. Immediate recognition and treatment is usually necessary to prevent death.

Acute renal insufficiency has been reported following oral and intravenous cholecystocholangiography. It usually occurs within 24 hours after administration of the drugs. Patients often complain of back pain. Oliguria with proteinuria are characteristic findings. A dense and persistent nephrogram may be seen on serial abdominal films owing to persistence of contrast in the renal parenchyma. Most patients recover. Proposed mechanisms of acute renal failure include the potent uricosuric properties common to all biliary contrast agents, a direct cellular toxicity on the kidney, idiosyncratic reaction, and reduced renal blood flow. All organic iodinated contrast agents elevate the serum protein-bound iodine levels for as long as several years, and therefore interferes with evaluation of thyroid function.

Patients with a history of previous reaction to iodinated contrast material are more likely to develop a reaction if given contrast a second time. Unfortunately, the nature of the first reaction does not predict the severity of future reactions. A patient with an initial mild reaction may have a life-threatening complication the second time. Those who are likely to develop reactions should be given steroids prior to the examination; this will usually reduce the incidence of complications.

An initial dose of 3 gm of Telepaque or Oragrafin is generally adequate for oral cholecystography. Unfortunately, as many as 30 per cent of patients with a normal gallbladder require a second dose to produce adequate gallbladder opacification. About 10 per cent of those with nonvisualization and about 60 per cent of those with faint visualization, prove to have a normal gallbladder following the second dose.[18, 19, 31] The second dose should be given on the next day, again using 3 gm. A double dose (6 gm) has not been demonstrated to increase the chance of opacification and adds to the toxicity. Repeating the examination after more than two consecutive days usually does not yield additional information.[31]

A probable explanation for the frequent necessity of a second dose is diminished intestinal absorption of the contrast due to a decreased bile volume. The low volume is caused by a reduction in circulating bile salts in fasting patients or patients on a low-fat and protein diet. This mechanism is mainly applicable to the more fat-soluble agents, such as Telepaque, which require bile for intestinal absorption. The more water-soluble agents, such as Bilopaque, are less affected by decreased bile volume.[27] Another possible cause is stagnation of nonopaque bile in the gallbladder, preventing the influx of opaque bile (cholecystocholectasis),[32] but this mechanism is disputed by Loeb et al.[26] Whatever the mechanism, if the gallbladder is not opacified after a single dose of contrast material, a second-dose study is necessary before the gallbladder can be considered diseased.

Possible alternatives to a second-dose study include the preliminary use of cholecystogogue, such as a fatty meal, in order to increase intestinal bile, or the use of a more water-soluble contrast agent.[21] In many institutions, an ultrasound examination has replaced the second-dose study.

In order for the gallbladder to opacify, the contrast agent must be ingested, absorbed from the gastrointestinal tract, excreted by the liver, and concentrated in the gallbladder. A number of conditions unrelated to gallbladder disease can cause faint visualization or nonvisualization. These must be excluded before making a diagnosis of cholecystitis and considering surgery. Table 16–2 lists the causes of non-visualization. Several of these merit discussion.

Retention of the contrast material in the stomach is usually obvious and may

THE BILIARY SYSTEM — 883

TABLE 16–2. CAUSES OF NONVISUALIZATION OF THE GALLBLADDER WITH ORAL CHOLECYSTOGRAPHY

Failure to take pills
Failure of contrast to enter small bowel (e.g., gastric or esophageal retention)
Malabsorption
Previous cholecystectomy
Cholecysto- or choledochoenterostomy (adequate visualization often indicates abnormal anastomosis)
Congenital anomalies (e.g., absent gallbladder, left-sided gallbladder)
Liver disease
Obstructive jaundice
Acute pancreatitis and fasting (transient)
Cholecystitis (cystic duct obstruction or rapid absorption of contrast)

indicate gastroduodenal abnormalities (Fig. 16–23). On rare occasions, contrast can be sequestered in the esophagus owing to a stricture or a diverticulum (Fig. 16–24). The appearance of the Telepaque in the small or large bowel can help determine the cause of a nonopacified gallbladder. A coarse, granular, or particulate appearance in the bowel indicates that the contrast was not conjugated either because it had not been absorbed from the gastrointestinal tract or because of liver disease. Conjugated dye that has passed through the bile ducts appears smooth and homogeneous. The presence of conjugated contrast in the bowel and an unopacified gallbladder usually indicates blockage of the cystic duct (Fig. 16–25).[28]

Opacification of the gallbladder and bile ducts usually does not occur with either oral cholecystography or intravenous cholangiography if an abnormal communication exists between the biliary and the gastrointestinal tracts.[27] Such communications may be the result of surgery, for example, choledochojejunostomy, or of a pathologic fistula. In these circumstances the bile flows directly into the intestine, resulting in nonopacification or poor opacification of the bile ducts and gallbladder. Gas in the biliary system on a plain film suggests the presence of a biliary-enteric communication and indicates that oral or intravenous biliary studies will generally be unsuccessful. If adequate visualization does occur after a bypass procedure, the possibility of recurrent disease at the anastomosis should be considered. Probably the best way to evaluate the biliary

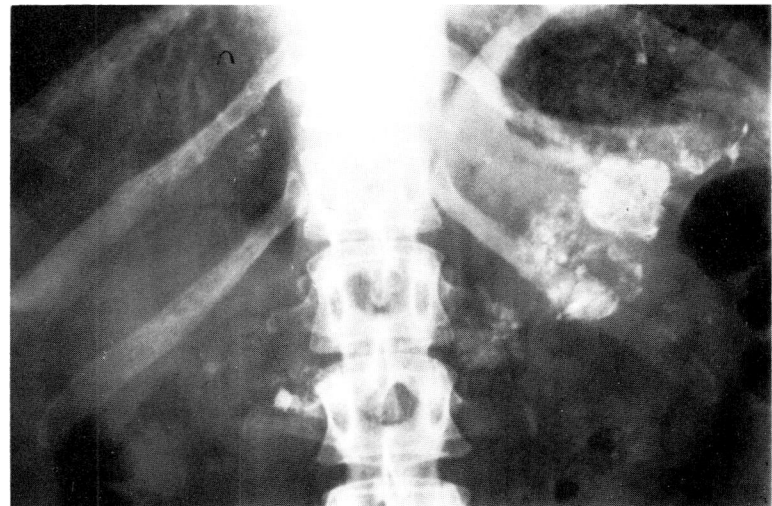

Figure 16–23. Retention of contrast in the stomach. There was no discernible reason for the gastric retention. Note the coarse appearance of unconjugated contrast that has not passed through the liver.

884 — THE BILIARY SYSTEM

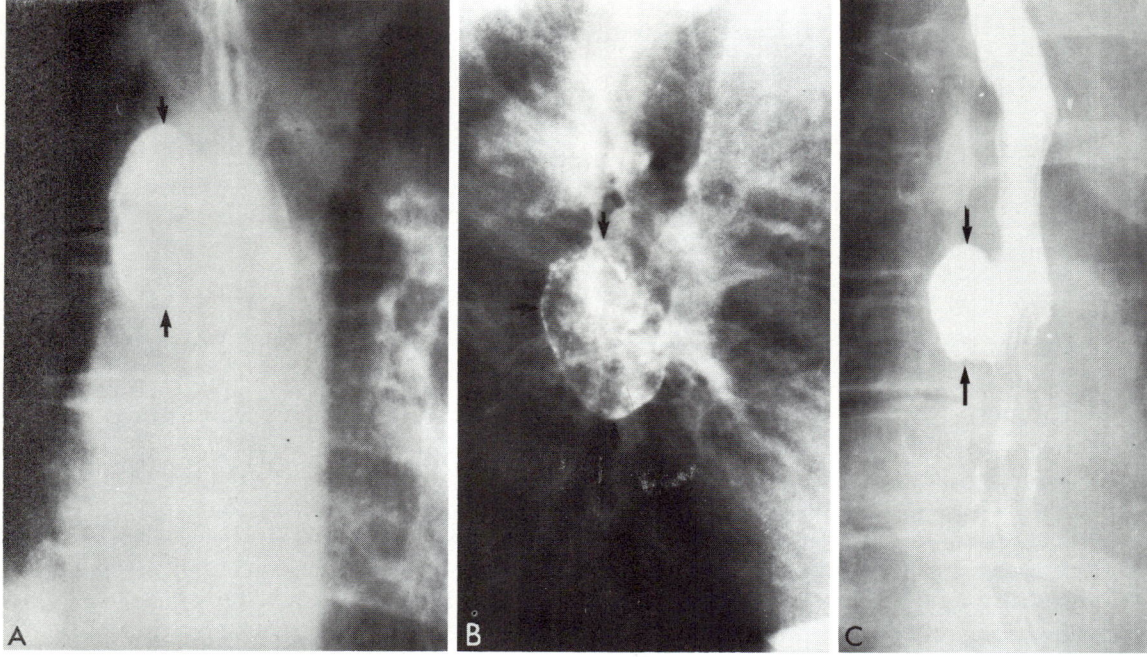

Figure 16–24. Retention of contrast in the esophagus. *A* and *B*, Posteroanterior and lateral chest views. The Telepaque is sequestered in an esophageal diverticulum (arrows). *C*, Barium swallow better demonstrates the diverticulum (arrows).

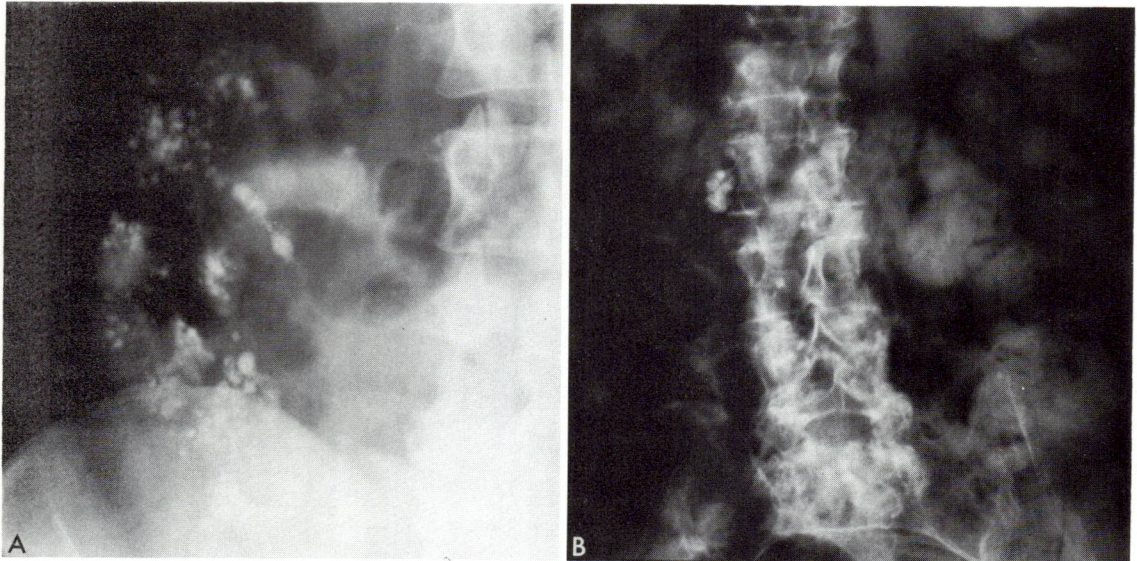

Figure 16–25. The appearance of Telepaque in the bowel. *A*, The coarse, granular appearance indicates that the contrast is unconjugated and has not passed through the liver (see Fig. 16–23). *B*, The homogeneous appearance of the contrast indicates that it has been conjugated in the liver and excreted in the bile.

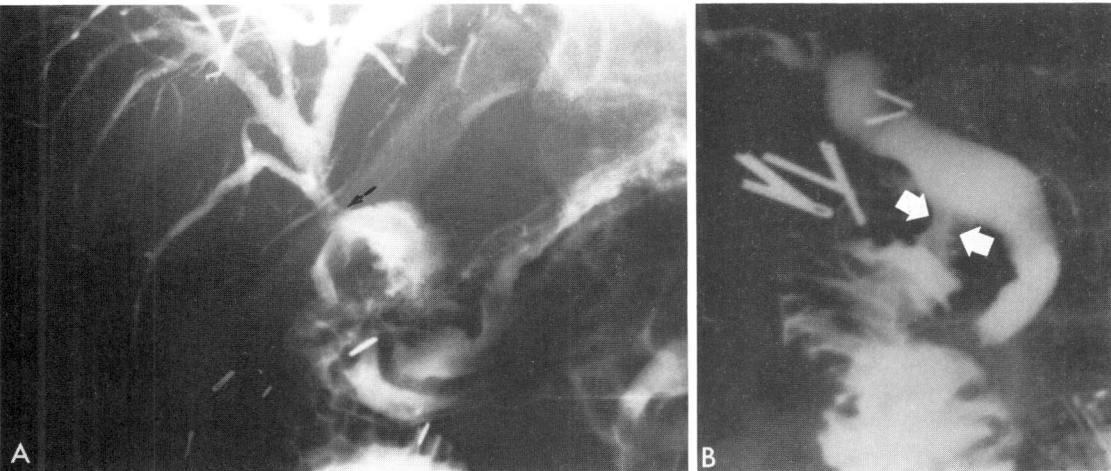

Figure 16–26. Barium cholangiogram. *A*, There is excellent opacification of the choledochoduodenal anastomosis (arrow) and the bile ducts. A prior intravenous cholangiogram showed very faint ductal visualization. *B*, Excellent demonstration of a normal choledochoduodenal anastomosis (arrows) filling from the afferent limb in a patient who had a Billroth II procedure and a distal common bile duct stricture.

system under these conditions is from barium refluxed through the anastomosis during an upper gastrointestinal series (Fig. 16–26).

Table 16–3 shows the relationship of the bilirubin values to visualization of the biliary tract with oral or intravenous biliary studies. The probability of opacifying the biliary system is better if the serum bilirubin level is decreasing rather than increasing. However, the quality of the examination (the degree of opacification) is usually unsatisfactory with even minimal abnormalities in liver function. It is best, when possible, to wait until the bilirubin levels have returned to normal before performing cholecystography or intravenous cholangiography. Not uncommonly, the serum alkaline phosphatase is elevated in patients with intrinsic liver disease or bile duct obstruction. With an elevated alkaline phosphatase, even if the bilirubin is normal or near-normal, the oral and intravenous studies often fail to opacify the biliary tract. At present, there are few precise data for alkaline phosphatase levels to help predict when satisfactory opacification will not occur (Table 16–4).

Nonvisualization with oral cholecystography often occurs in patients with acute alcoholic pancreatitis. Up to 60 per cent of normal gallbladders in these patients may not opacify when the study is performed during the acute episode. A recent study by Roller

TABLE 16–3. RELATION OF SERUM BILIRUBIN CONCENTRATION TO VISUALIZATION OF THE BILIARY TRACT*

Oral Cholecystography
Bilirubin 2–3 mg%-considerably decreased incidence of adequate visualization
Bilirubin >3 mg%-near 0% visualization

Intravenous Cholangiography
Bilirubin 1–2 mg%-about 80% visualization
        2–3 mg%-about 40% visualization
Bilirubin 3–4 mg%-about 30% visualization
Bilirubin >4 mg%-near 0% visualization

*These figures do not apply to prehepatic jaundice.

TABLE 16–4. RELATION OF SERUM ALKALINE PHOSPHATASE TO VISUALIZATION BY INTRAVENOUS CHOLANGIOGRAPHY*

Alkaline Phosphatase	Total	Visualized	Nonvisualized	Visualized (1%)
Normal	469	452	17	96
Abnormal	270	107	163	39

*From Wise, R. E.: Intravenous Cholangiography. Charles C Thomas, Publishers, Springfield, Illinois, 1962.

et al.[30] showed that the vast majority of these normal gallbladders (90 per cent) opacify if the oral cholecystogram is performed after the patient has resumed a regular diet. Fasting reduces the bile volume, which decreases the intestinal absorption and the hepatic excretion of Telepaque. Therefore, it is important not to presume that cholelithiasis is the cause of the pancreatitis if the gallbladder does not opacify in fasting patients with acute pancreatitis.

Faulty methodology and radiographic techniques can result in misinterpretation of the oral cholecystogram. When possible, a preliminary film of the abdomen should be obtained before contrast is given. Demonstration of opaque gallstones can obviate the need for oral cholecystography. The routine radiographs should be taken 14 to 18 hours after administration of the contrast medium, since maximal opacification occurs at 17 hours.[18] A 14- by 17-inch prone abdominal film should be included in case the gallbladder is not in its usual location. Upright spot-filming with and without compression is recommended. Compression helps show small stones that may be obscured by excessive contrast in the gallbladder. On the upright or lateral decubitus view, stones change position and, if multiple, may form a layer in the opaque bile (Fig. 16–27). Since stones changes position, they can be distinguished from polyps, which remain fixed. Occasionally, the radiopaque bile in the gallbladder forms a layer with the nonopaque bile on upright films. This is caused by poor mixing and must be distinguished from small stones or sludge. A fatty meal usually mixes the bile and

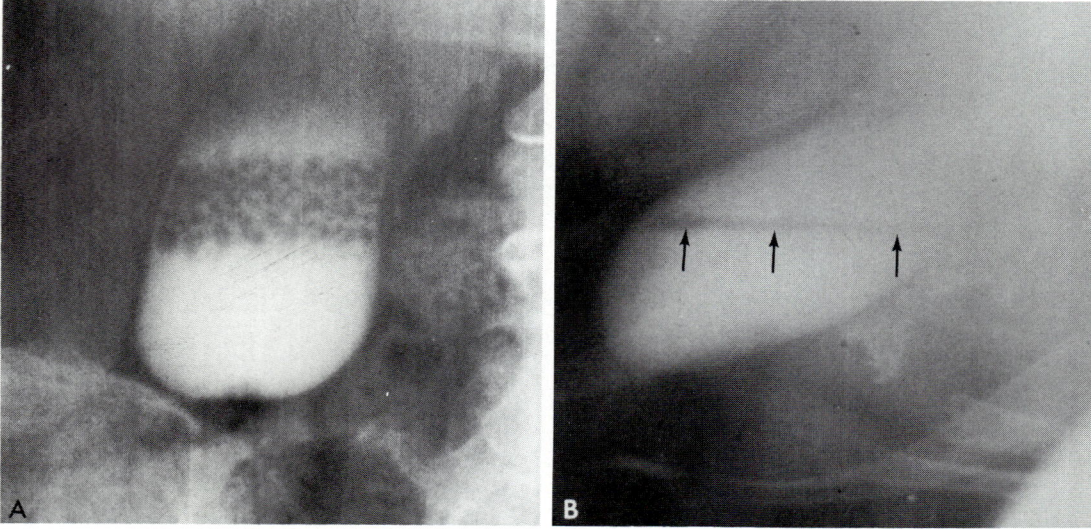

Figure 16–27. Layering of gallstones. A, A thick band of stones has layered in the body of the gallbladder. Layering can occur in any part of the gallbladder and depends on the weight of the stones relative to the specific gravity of the bile and contrast. B, A thin layer of gallstones (arrows) was barely discernible on the recumbent films.

eliminates layering.[22] Layering of opaque bile is seen more frequently during intravenous cholangiography (Fig. 16–28).[29] Rarely, the contrast medium is deconjugated in the gallbladder and precipitates in small clumps of radiopaque densities resembling stones (Fig. 16–29). A scout film will show that there are no opaque calculi.[18]

The routine use of a fatty meal or cholecystokinin during oral cholecystography is of limited value. Its major importance is in the diagnosis of adenomyomatosis and cholesterolosis. Occasionally, however, it may be helpful in differentiating a polyp from a stone and in separating the gallbladder from overlying bowel gas. Rarely, small stones that were not seen on the pre-fatty meal films can be demonstrated. It is now generally agreed that the response of the gallbladder to fat or cholecystokinin is too variable to permit reliable conclusions concerning gallbladder function or "biliary dyskinesia."[24, 25]

The radiographic findings of cholecystitis on oral cholecystography consist of the demonstration of gallstones in an opacified gallbladder or nonvisualization of the gallbladder. Faint visualization implies gallbladder disease but is less reliable. When the nonbiliary causes are excluded, an unopacified gallbladder is highly diagnostic of gallbladder disease. Nonvisualization in acute or chronic cholecystitis may be the result of obstruction of the cystic duct. However, when the cystic duct is patent, failure to opacify the gallbladder is probably due to the reabsorption of the contrast material through the inflamed gallbladder mucosa. A less accepted explanation is the inability of the diseased gallbladder to transport water and concentrate bile.

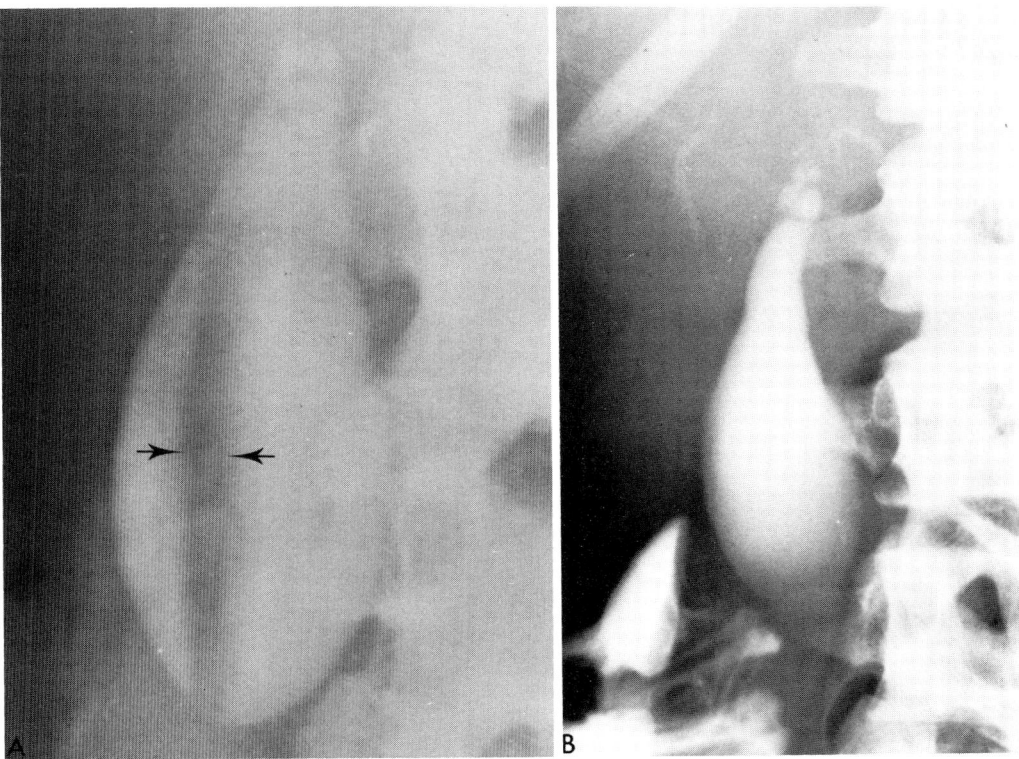

Figure 16–28. Incomplete mixing of bile and contrast. *A,* Right lateral decubitus film of the gallbladder during intravenous cholangiography. The radiolucent band (arrows) resembles gallstones but is actually a layer of bile that has not mixed with the contrast. *B,* A delayed decubitus view shows a normal gallbladder.

Illustration and legend continued on the following page

888 — THE BILIARY SYSTEM

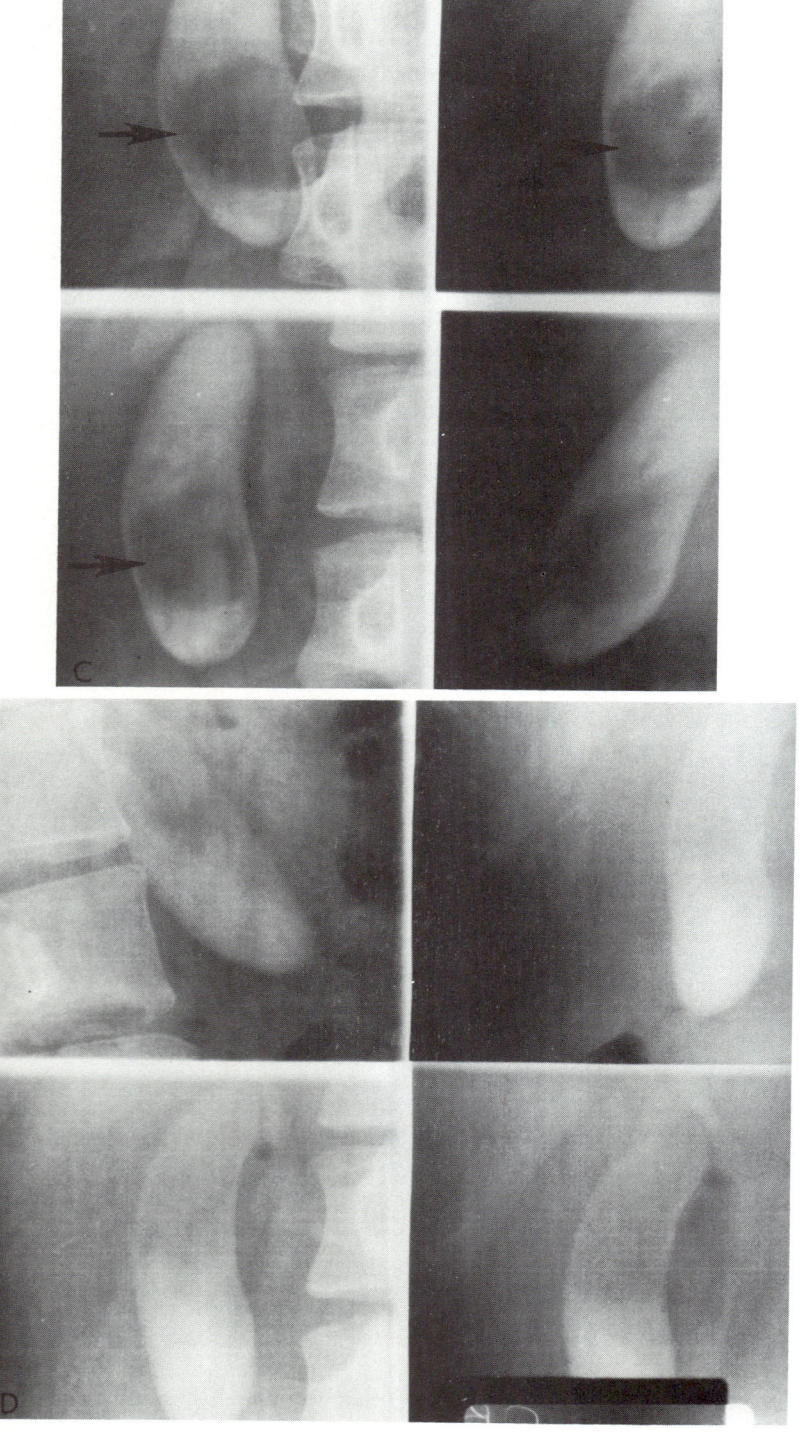

Figure 16–28 *Continued. C,* In a different patient, the filling defect (arrows) in the gallbladder during intravenous cholangiography resembles a large calculus but is caused by incomplete mixing of bile and contrast. *D,* After a fatty meal there is adequate mixing. The gallbladder is normal.

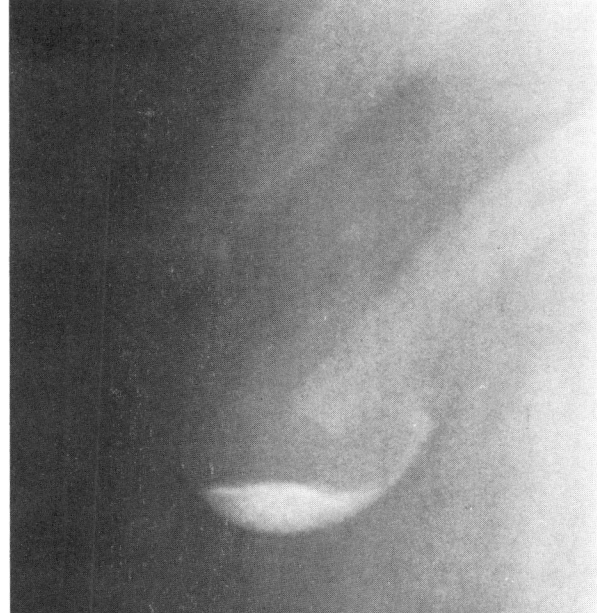

Figure 16–29. Precipitated Telepaque. Telepaque has precipitated in the gallbladder, resembling opaque sludge or mild of calcium bile. A repeat oral cholecystogram several weeks later demonstrated a normal gallbladder.

Intravenous Cholangiography

Most of the indications for intravenous cholangiography are listed in Table 16–5. The intravenous cholangiogram can be helpful in acute abdomianl conditions, particularly in the distinction of acute cholecystitis from pancreatitis.[44] They cystic duct is occluded in nearly every case of acute cholecystitis. Adequate visualization of the extrahepatic bile ducts without visualization of the gallbladder is reliable evidence of acute cholecystitis (Fig. 16–30). Conversely, opacification of the gallbladder virtually excludes acute cholecystitis.

Unfortunately, in 30 to 50 per cent of patients with acute abdominal disorders, particularly pancreatitis, the biliary system is not visualized. When neither bile ducts nor gallbladder are opacified, no conclusions can be made regarding the biliary system. If the bile ducts are faintly opacified, and occasionally even if they are not visualized, delayed radiographs at 4 and sometimes at 24 hours may slow opacification of the gallbladder, proving patency of the cystic duct and therefore excluding acute cholecystitis.

With the utilization of ultrasound, intravenous cholangiography is less necessary when the gallbladder is not opacified by oral cholecystography. If nonbiliary factors, such as malabsorption (see Table 16–2), are thought to be responsible for nonopacification on oral cholecystography, then perhaps evaluation by intravenous cholangiogra-

TABLE 16–5. INDICATIONS FOR INTRAVENOUS CHOLANGIOGRAPHY

Previous cholecystectomy with recurrent symptoms
Inability to take oral medication
Known conditions that decrease intestinal absorption, e.g., malabsorption
Suspected acute cholecystitis
Symptoms referable to bile ducts
Likelihood of failure with oral cholecystography, e.g., mild elevation of serum bilirubin
Nonvisualization of the gallbladder on oral cholecystography (controversial)

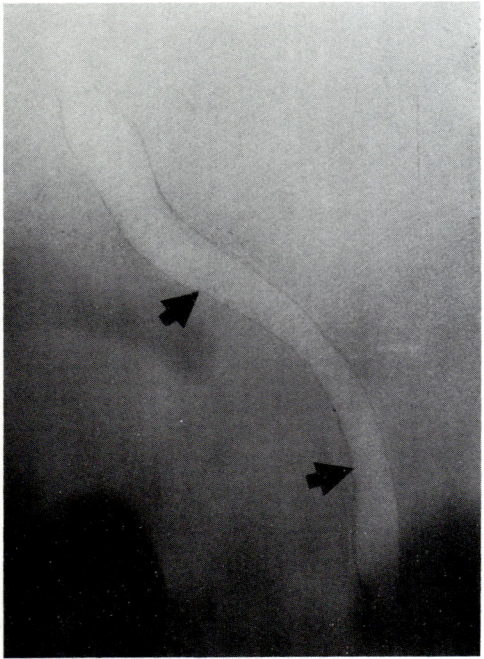

Figure 16–30. Intravenous cholangiogram in acute cholecystitis. There is visualization of the extrahepatic bile ducts (pencilied) (arrows) but not of the gallbladder.

phy is warranted. The intravenous cholangiogram may elucidate the reason for the diseased gallbladder by demonstrating cystic duct obstruction or gallstones. Probably, however, this additional information is not worth the time spent or the risk involved.

If the gallbladder does not opacify on oral cholecystography and no calculi are found on intravenous cholangiography, which test is more accurate for calculous cholecystitis? Scholz et al.[40] feel strongly that adequate visualization of an acalculous gallbladder by intravenous cholangiography indicates a normal gallbladder. Mujahed et al.[58] found that in 17 per cent of 80 intravenous cholangiograms the opacified gallbladder appeared normal but at surgery was found to have gallstones. They concluded that oral cholecystography is a much more reliable study for pathologic conditions of the gallbladder than intravenous cholangiography. If the gallbladder is not opacified on oral cholecystography, ultrasound is the procedure of choice for demonstrating calculi. It is far safer than intravenous cholangiography and, undoubtedly, much more accurate.

There are probably no absolute contraindications to intravenous cholangiography. Cholografin (meglumine iodipamide), the contrast agent used in this country, incurs more toxic reactions than any of the other iodinated contrast media. The death rate from intravenous cholangiography may be as high as 1 in 5000 compared with 1 in 60,000 deaths from the diatrizoate agents used for renal or angiographic studies. A previous allergic reaction to any iodinated contrast agent is good reason to avoid their reuse. If the study must be performed, the patient should be treated with steroids for three days prior to the examination. Cholografin should be used cautiously in individuals with impaired renal and hepatic function. In these high-risk patients, other diagnostic tests should replace the cholangiogram when possible.

Mild toxic reactions, such as nausea, vomiting, and hives, are fairly common and much more frequent than in oral cholecystography. The slow administration of the contrast agent and pretreatment with antihistamines will probably minimize the mild side effects. The contrast agent is mildly hepatotoxic, and transient elevations in SGOT may occur.[40]

Cholografin can be given only intravenously. It is excreted unchanged into the biliary system. Unlike oral preparations, it need not be concentrated in the gallbladder to produce opacification. The recommended dose of Cholografin is 20 ml or 0.3 ml per kg. Forty ml (0.6 ml per kg) has been shown to give better ductal opacification.[46] Doses higher than 0.6 ml per kg cause increased toxicity without significantly improving ductal opacification. The drug is usually administered either by direct injection over 10 minutes or by drip infusion usually lasting 30 to 60 minutes. Controversy exists as to which is the better method, but probably there is no significant difference.[34, 37, 45] Some advocate prolonged infusions, even up to ten hours, to increase the possibility of opacifying the bile ducts in jaundiced patients.[34] Our animal studies have indicated that the interval between administration of the contrast agent and opacification of bile ducts is prolonged in the presense of bile duct obstruction.[43] It appears, therefore, that the time at which the films are taken is more important for obtaining ductal opacification than is the method of administering the contrast agent.

Films are usually taken at 20-minute intervals until the ductal system is adequately visualized. Tomograms are often helpful for better anatomic delineation. Pharmacologic agents, such as morphine or cerulein, occasionally produce better ductal opacification. When the gallbladder is visualized, supine and upright films should be obtained to look for stones. Delayed films at 4 hours and even up to 24 hours may demonstrate a previously unopacified gallbladder. Occasionally, the duodenal bulb is mistaken for an opacified gallbladder, but radiographs in different obliquities usually clarify the anatomy. If necessary, gas or other contrast material can be put into the duodenum (Fig. 16–31).

Wise et al.[36, 40] have emphasized the importance of the time-density retention concept for diagnosing partial common bile duct obstruction. Ordinarily, the common bile duct should be less densely opacified at two hours than at one hour. If the duct is denser on the two-hour film, it is likely to be partially obstructed, even though no anatomic abnormality has been seen. Use of the time-density concept has substantially increased the diagnostic accuracy of intravenous cholangiography (Fig. 16–32). Opacification of the intrahepatic ducts before the common bile duct is also considered a sign of partial obstruction.[33]

Interpretation of intravenous cholangiography can be difficult, because the ducts often opacify poorly and because a normal common bile duct varies in size. A common bile duct 8 mm or less in diameter is not likely to be obstructed. At 15 mm or greater, partial obstruction is probable.[40] Between 8 and 15 mm, no definite conclusions can be made. The common bile duct should not enlarge after cholecystectomy; an increase in size should suggest partial obstruction. The biliary tract may not opacify during intravenous cholangiography in as many as 7 per cent of patients with normal serum bilirubin levels;[40] nonvisualization is a totally inconclusive finding. Since the incidence of missed common bile duct calculi by intravenous cholangiography is high,[35, 39] more invasive procedures, such as transhepatic cholangiography, often are required. Intrahepatic ductal stones are practically never seen on intravenous cholangiography.

In addition to demonstrating calculi, intravenous cholangiography may show other types of ductal disorders. For example, strictures from chronic pancreatitis may be visualized as well as displacement of the ducts by a mass, such as a pancreatic pseudocyst (Figs. 16–33 and 16–34).

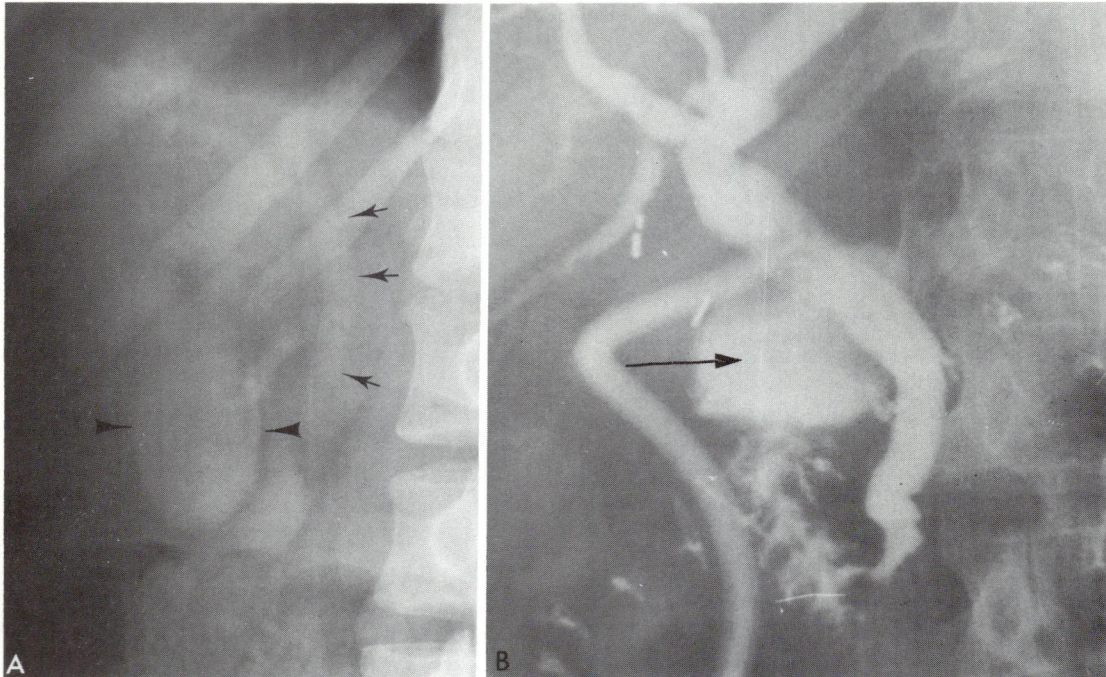

Figure 16–31. Duodenal bulb mimicking gallbladder. *A*, Intravenous cholangiogram in a cholecystectomized patient. The bile ducts are normal (arrows). The duodenal bulb (arrowheads) is faintly opacified and could be mistaken for the gallbladder. *B*, T-tube cholangiogram in a different patient showing how opacification of the duodenal bulb (arrow) can mimic the gallbladder on intravenous cholangiography.

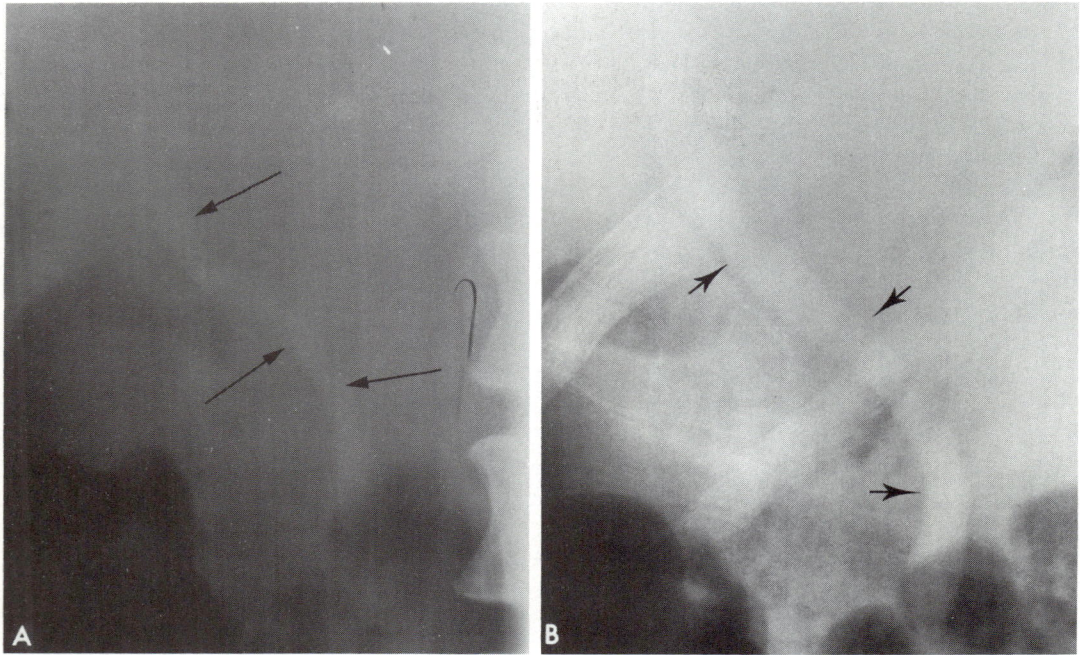

Figure 16–32. Intravenous cholangiogram showing time-density retention concept. *A*, Bile ducts at one hour (arrows). *B*, Bile ducts are more opaque at two hours (arrows), indicating partial obstruction even though the ducts are of normal size.

Figure 16–33. Choledocholithiasis. Intravenous cholangiogram showing large ductal stone (arrows) and proximal obstruction.

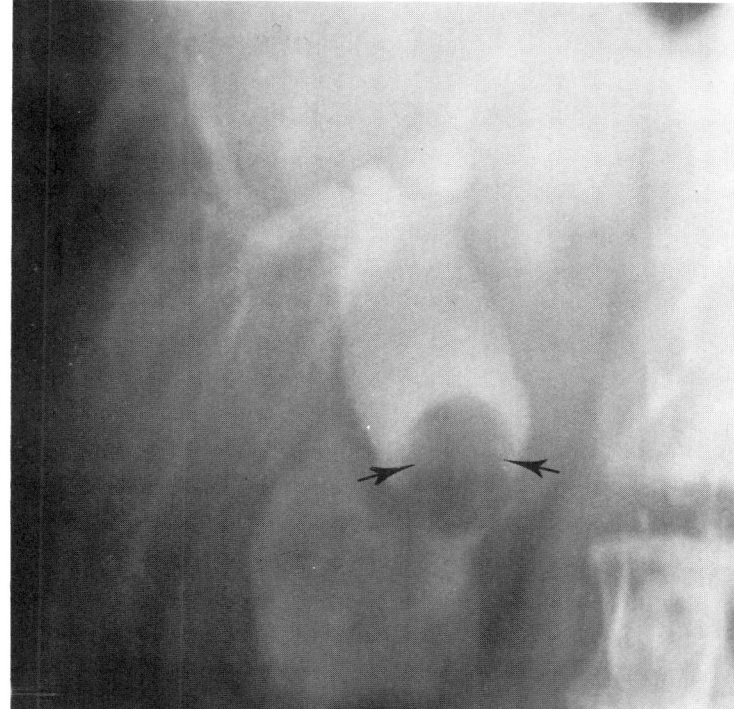

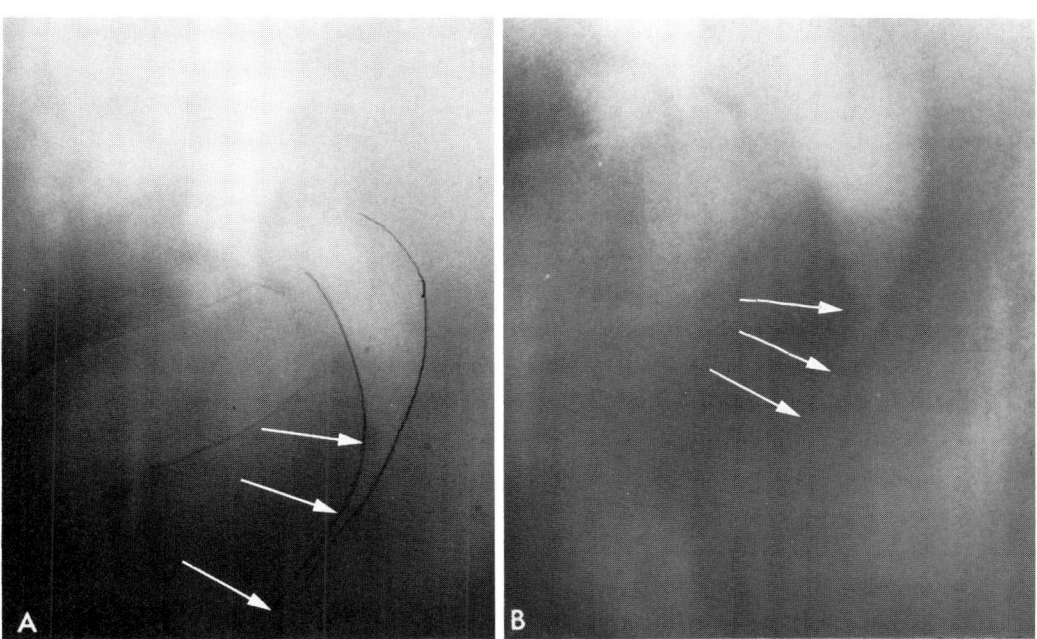

Figure 16–34. *A* and *B*, Chronic pancreatitis. There is a long tapered narrowing of the distal common bile duct (arrows) (penciled) with proximal dilatation. The appearance is typical of chronic pancreatitis.

894 — THE BILIARY SYSTEM

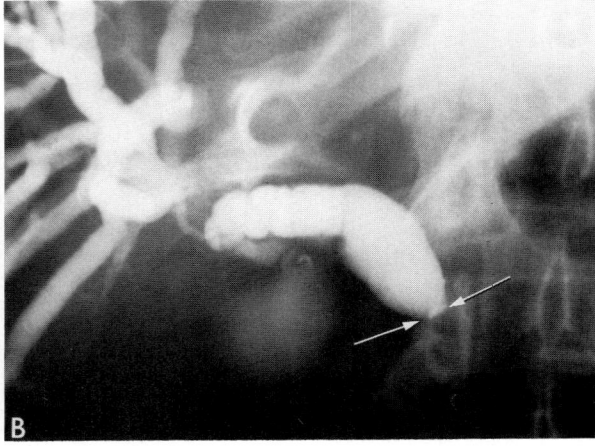

Figure 16–35. Common bile duct crossing the duodenum. *A*, Jaundiced patient. Extrinsic defect on the duodenum (arrows) is due to a dilated common bile duct. *B*, Transhepatic cholangiogram showing obstruction of the common bile duct (arrows) from pancreatic carcinoma.

Barium Studies of the Gastrointestinal Tract

The upper gastrointestinal series is an important study if gallbladder disease is suspected. Frequently, the signs and symptoms of other gastrointestinal disorders, such as peptic ulcer disease, pancreatitis, and hiatus hernia, mimic biliary tract disease. Occasionally, concurrent abnormalities such as gallstones and peptic ulcers are present. The patient's symptoms may be caused by either or both conditions. Cholecystectomy should be deferred at least until the associated disease has resolved. Failure to appreciate that symptoms suggestive of biliary disease may be due to other abdominal

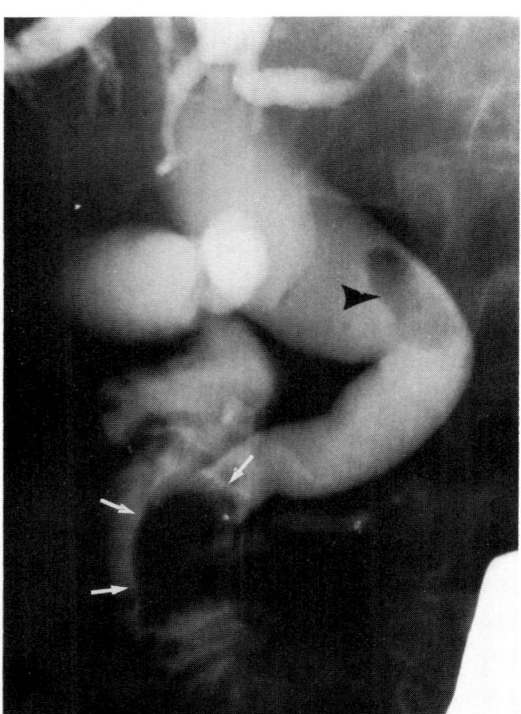

Figure 16–36. Ampullary carcinoma. Transhepatic cholangiogram demonstrating a mass in the ampulla of Vater extending into the distal common bile duct (arrows). The proximal ducts are dilated. There is a stone in the mid-common bile duct (arrowhead).

or chest disorders results in a high incidence of recurrent symptoms after cholecystectomy.

Because of the proximity of the two organs, cholecystitis can sometimes cause inflammation of the duodenum. The upper gastrointestinal series may show localized inflammation and an extrinsic duodenal mass. As discussed previously, similar changes can occur on the hepatic flexure of the colon (see Fig. 16–2). Occasionally a dilated common bile duct can be seen crossing under the duodenum, thus helping to confirm the diagnosis of obstructive jaundice (Fig. 16–35). A mass in the region of the ampulla is important diagnostic information in evaluating jaundiced patients (Fig. 16–36).

In as many as 80 per cent of patients with pancreatitis, abnormalities are disclosed on the upper gastrointestinal series.[44] Abdominal masses, such as pancreatic pseudocysts or edema of the pancreas, are often demonstrated (Fig. 16–37). However, because

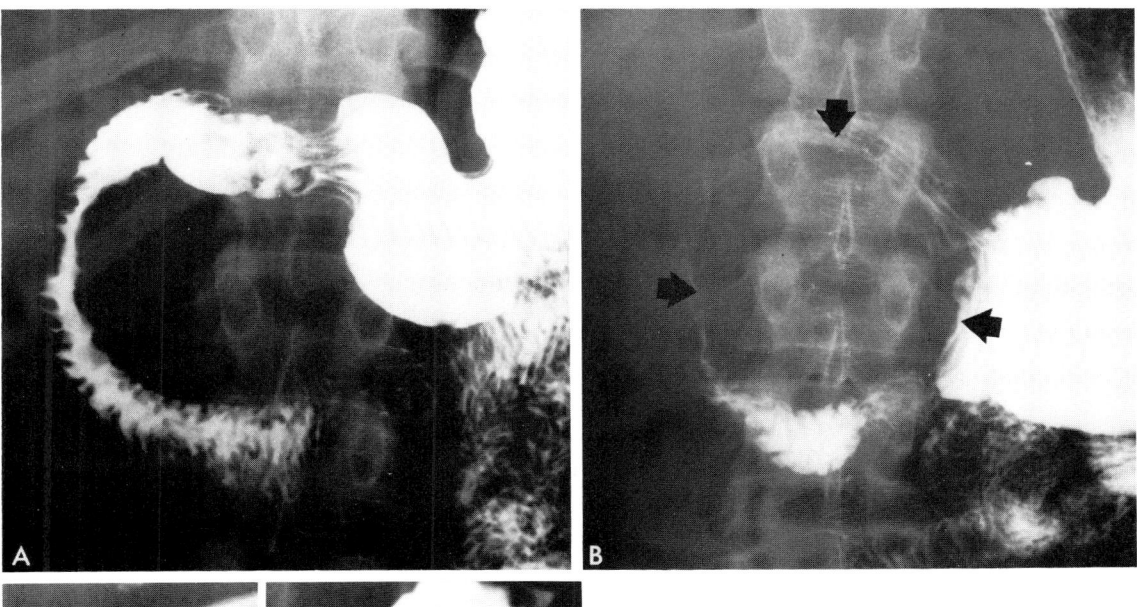

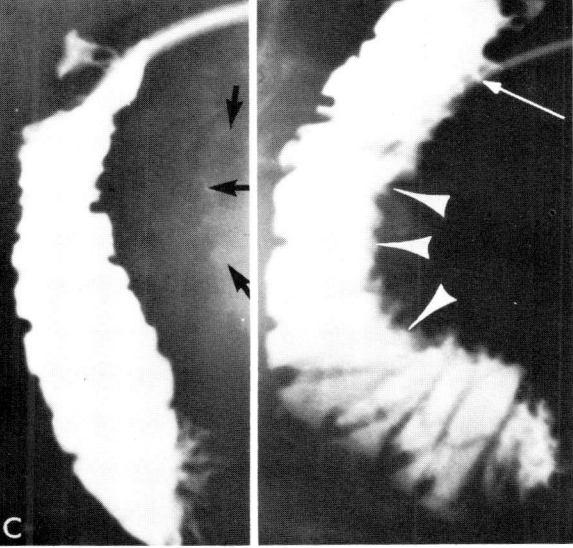

Figure 16–37. Pancreatitis (three patients). *A*, Acute pancreatitis. The duodenal sweep is enlarged owing to swelling of the head of the pancreas. Narrowing of the lumen and coarse folds are consistent with inflammation of the pancreas. *B*, Pancreatic pseudocyst. The duodenal sweep is enlarged by an extrinsic mass, which is also pressing on the distal stomach (arrows). The diagnosis was confirmed by ultrasound. *C*, Hypotonic duodenogram in a patient with chronic pancreatitis. A tube is in the duodenal sweep (long arrow). A mass in the head of the pancreas is impressing on the medial aspect of the descending duodenum (arrowheads), causing an irregular border. There are pancreatic calcifications (short arrows). The study does not distinguish chronic pancreatitis from pancreatic carcinoma.

the upper gastrointestinal series frequently cannot differentiate a pseudocyst, pancreatitis, or pancreatic carcinoma, other studies, such as ultrasound, CT scanning, and angiography, are required.

Hypotonic duodenography[41, 42] can be a useful supplement to the upper gastrointestinal series in the evaluation of pancreatic or duodenal disease (see Fig. 16–37C). The study consists of temporarily inhibiting the peristaltic activity of the duodenum with an anticholinergic agent, such as Pro-Banthine. More recently, glucagon, a safer smooth muscle relaxant, has been used. The flaccid duodenum can then be maximally distended with air and barium through a tube positioned at the junction of the second and third portions. The examination enhances the demonstration of lesions of the pancreatic head and duodenum. Perhaps its most important use is to verify the presence of questionable duodenal abnormalities seen on the standard upper gastrointestinal series.

Radionuclide Studies

Nuclear medicine procedures can be useful in the diagnosis of disorders of the biliary tract and in the differential diagnosis when the clinical situation is confusing. The nuclide examinations most commonly employed are liver scans, using technetium (Tc) and rose bengal, and gallium studies.

^{99m}Tc sulfur colloid is taken up by the reticuloendothelial system and is very helpful for demonstrating the gross morphology of the liver and spleen. Lesions 2 cm or larger can usually be detected. Technetium scans are helpful in evaluating jaundiced patients and can demonstrate the presence of cirrhosis and metastatic disease.

The ^{131}I rose bengal scan[49] is more specific for the biliary system than is the sulfur colloid scan. However, ultrasound and computerized tomography are more reliable than rose bengal studies, and consequently the latter are now infrequently used. Rose bengal is cleared from the blood by the polygonal cells of the liver and excreted in the biliary system in a manner probably similar to bile excretion. Its main use is in the distinction of hepatocellular jaundice from extrahepatic biliary tract obstruction. The normal rose bengal scan shows the gallbladder, duodenum, and small bowel. An absence of radioactivity in the small bowel on sequential scans indicates complete bile duct obstruction (Fig. 16–38). Occasionally the width of the ducts can be demonstrated.

More recently, the isotope ^{67}gallium has been used to diagnose and localize areas of inflammation. Unfortunately, gallium is also taken up by tumor masses and therefore cannot differentiate a neoplasm from an abscess. However, gallium studies are useful in confirming suspected abdominal abscesses. There are several reports showing that ^{67}gallium accumulates in diseased gallbladders with either acute or chronic cholecystitis and in empyema of the gallbladder (Fig. 16–39).[47, 50] The procedure can be used when the diagnosis of cholecystitis is uncertain. The main disadvantage is that optimal uptake does not occur for 18 to 72 hours after injection.

A new agent, ^{99m}Tc-HIDA and its derivatives, are currently being evaluated in patients with hepatobiliary disease. Cystic duct patency can be determined rapidly (in as little as 30 minutes), as well as hepatocellular disease and bile duct obstruction in patients with considerably elevated bilirubin levels.

Ultrasonography

The technical improvements in ultrasonography, particularly the development of gray-scale B-scan equipment, have vastly improved its usefulness in evaluating the

THE BILIARY SYSTEM — 897

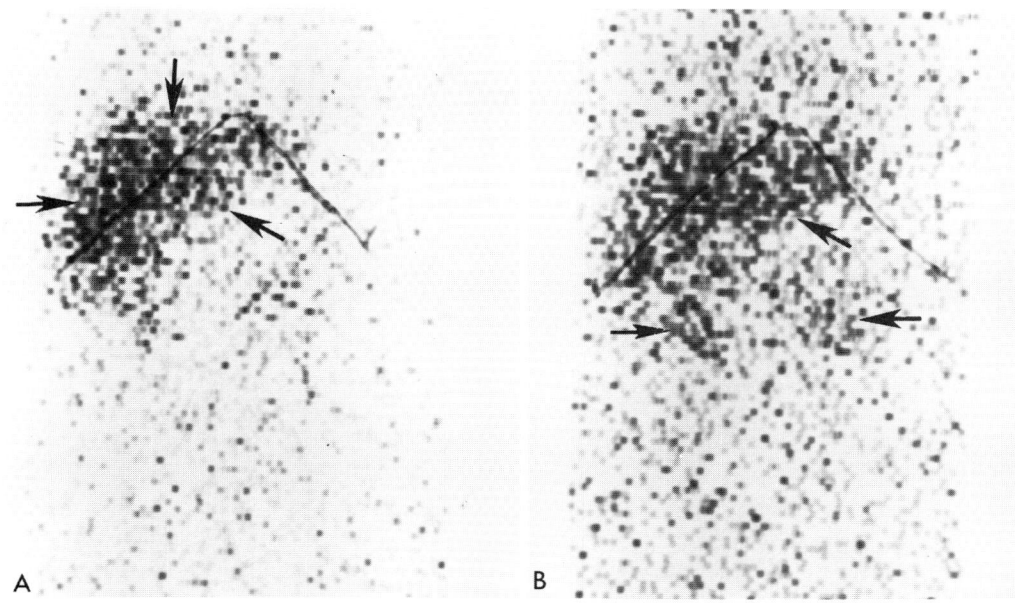

Figure 16–38. Rose bengal scan. Child with biliary atresia. *A*, A four-hour scan shows activity in the liver (arrows) but none in the gallbladder or bowel. *B*, At 48 hours, the isotope is located in the liver and kidneys (arrows). The absence of isotope in the small bowel is consistent with biliary obstruction.

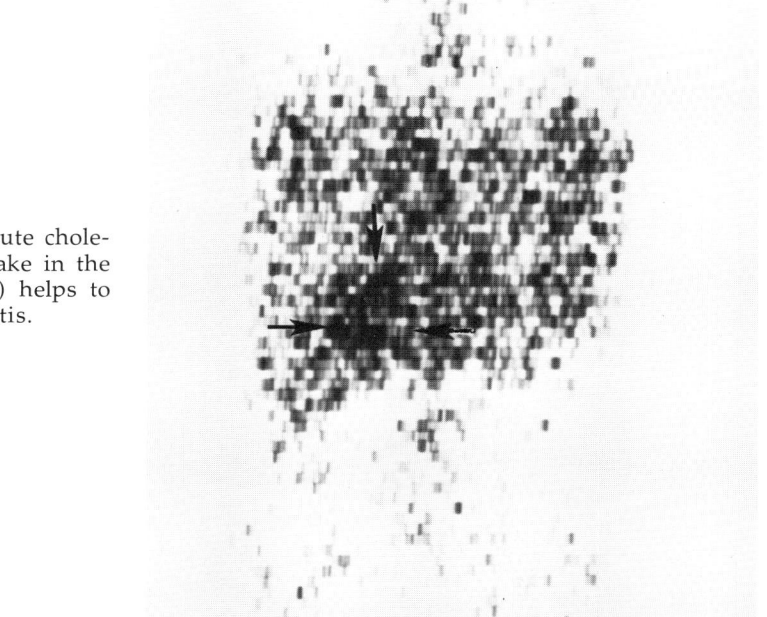

Figure 16–39. Gallium scan in acute cholecystitis. An area of increased uptake in the region of the gallbladder (arrows) helps to confirm the diagnosis of cholecystitis.

898 — THE BILIARY SYSTEM

biliary system. It provides information rapidly and at relatively low cost. It is noninvasive, readily tolerated even by critically ill patients, and has no known contraindications or complications. In addition to providing data on the biliary tract, ultrasound can usually evaluate the pancreas and other abdominal organs at the same time. Since there is no radiation hazard, ultrasound can be used without risk during pregnancy.

In most instances, the gallbladder is easily visualized. Its size as well as the presence of calculi can be determined reliably and rapidly. The normal gallbladder is an echo-free structure usually near the inferior surface of the liver. Gallstones produce echoes within the gallbladder and create echo-free zones located behind the calculi (shadowing) (Fig. 16–40). The stones move when the position of the patient is changed.

Carefully performed ultrasound has an accuracy of 90 per cent in the diagnosis of gallstones.[53] Gosnik et al.[52] routinely use ultrasound when the gallbladder is not visualized or poorly visualized on oral cholecystography. This is particularly applicable when extrabiliary tract disease, such as malabsorption, decreases the reliability of oral cholecystography. Bartrum et al.[51] find that ultrasound can replace the second-dose oral cholecystogram when the gallbladder fails to opacify satisfactorily on the first dose. Moreover, if the ultrasound examination can be performed on the same day as the initial oral cholecystogram, the cost and inconvenience of a second visit is eliminated.

False negative ultrasound studies account for most of the errors; false positive studies are rare. Reasons for false negative results include an incomplete series of scans, for example, failure to obtain a lateral decubitus view, and rapid respiratory motion in a restless, uncooperative patient. One frequent problem is the inability to visualize the gallbladder when there is excessive adjacent bowel gas or when barium is in the gastrointestinal tract.

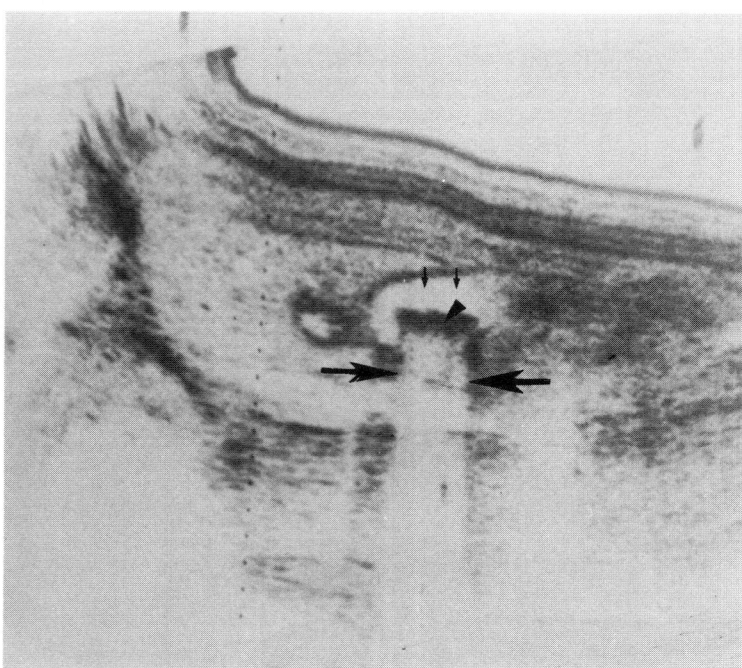

Figure 16–40. Ultrasound of gallbladder with stone. The echo-free gallbladder (small arrows) contains a large stone (arrowhead), which produces the characteristic shadowing effect (large arrows).

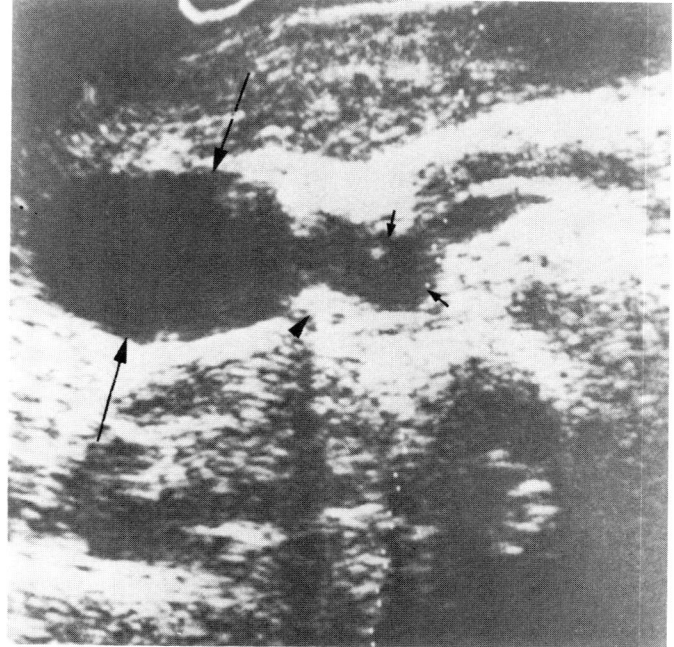

Figure 16–41. Ultrasound in obstructive jaundice. The gallbladder (large arrows) and the common bile duct (small arrows) are enlarged. There is a stone in the common bile duct (arrowhead), with shadowing effect. (White and black are reversed on this sonogram; cf. Fig. 16–40. Many ultrasonographers prefer this "white on black" form).

In addition to detecting gallstones, ultrasound is useful in accessing the bile ducts. Although normal-sized ducts are not often visualized, dilated ducts are more readily seen (Fig. 16–41), permitting differentiation between intrahepatic cholestasis and bile duct obstruction. Unfortunately, the location etiology of the ductal obstruction frequently cannot be determined by ultrasound, and more invasive studies, such as endoscopic retrograde cholangiopancreatography or transhepatic cholangiography, are necessary.

Computerized Tomography

In recent years, there have been numerous reports on the use of computed tomography for evaluating pathologic conditions of the abdomen. Considerable information is emerging comparing CT body scanning to other imaging modalities, such as ultrasound and radionuclide studies. At present, the consensus of opinion seems to be that the information on the biliary tract that is obtained from CT studies is not greater than that from ultrasound. The radiation dose for CT scanning is about the same as that for conventional x-ray studies. Both CT and ultrasound are good noninvasive screening procedures for biliary tract disease. In a high percentage of cases they both can distinguish obstructive jaundice from hepatocellular disease by the presence or absence of dilated ducts (Fig. 16–42).[55] Gallstone identification is less reliable by CT than by ultrasound.

CT is superior to radionuclide imaging in examining the biliary system but is probably no more sensitive in detecting intrahepatic lesions. It is, however, more accurate in determining the type of hepatic mass than is the liver scan. Liver scans, however, are considered more reliable for diagnosing hepatocellular disease as well as diffuse infiltrative liver processes.[54, 56]

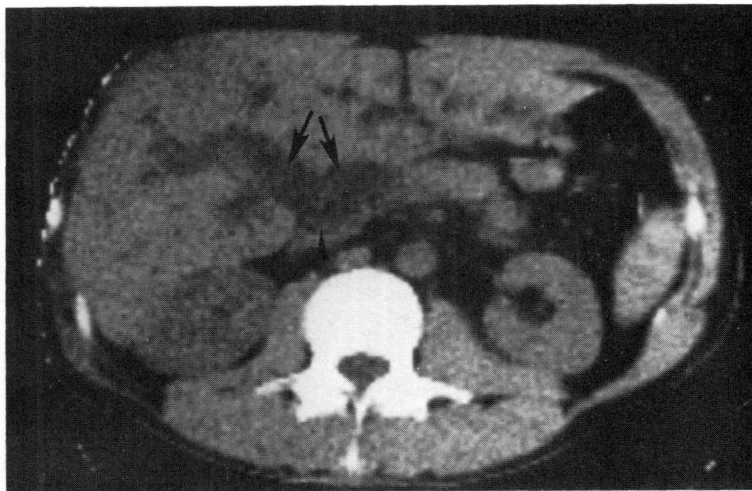

Figure 16–42. CT scan in obstructive jaundice. A 38-year-old man with a pancreatic pseudocyst obstructing the distal common bile duct. There is dilatation of the right and left intrahepatic ducts (arrows) and the common bile duct (arrowhead). (Courtesy of Hebert Y. Kressel, M.D. *From* Radiology *126*:153–157, 1978. Reproduced by permission.)

An important advantage of both CT and ultrasound compared with isotope scanning is that information concerning other abdominal organs (such as the pancreas) is provided at the same time. However, the quality of CT scans is considerably reduced when patients cannot suspend respiration during the scan exposure. Respiratory motion does not usually interfer with ultrasound studies. Currently, scanners have shorter exposure times (six seconds or less) and improved spatial and contrast resolution. These technical advances will undoubtedly increase the usefulness of CT scanning and help establish guidelines for the optimal utilization of the various imaging modalities.

Transhepatic Cholangiography

Percutaneous transhepatic cholangiography is in most instances the procedure of choice for evaluating the biliary system in the presence of jaundice. Since the popularization of the "skinney needle" (Chiba) by Okuda et al.,[60] the incidence of serious complications has been reduced and the need for surgical stand-by largely eliminated.[64] The previous methods using Teflon-sheathed needles, ranging in size from 18 to 20 gauge, incurred about a 5 per cent incidence of significant complications, mainly bile peritonitis and hemorrhage.[58] This rate increased significantly if the ducts were dilated, and surgery to alleviate the obstruction was usually performed shortly after the cholangiogram.

The skinny needles now used for percutaneous cholangiography have a diameter of 22 or 23 gauge and are 6 to 8 inches long. They are made of flexible steel and have a thin inner core. Cannulation of very small bile ducts is frequently successful, but aspiration of bile is usually difficult.

The most common technique is puncture of the liver from the midaxillary line at about the tenth intercostal space. Anterior abdominal and transjugular approaches are alternative methods but have certain disadvantages and are used less frequently. Usually, the needle is aimed at the eleventh or twelfth vertebral body and inserted under fluoroscopic guidance so the point is just to the right of the vertebral body. The direction and depth of insertion vary according to the size of the liver. Once the needle is in place and the stylet removed, the patient is instructed to breathe normally.

However, even deep respirations do not seem to cause complications. Under fluoroscopic monitoring, contrast is injected as the needle is slowly withdrawn. Once a duct is cannulated, the entire biliary tree can usually be opacified. Care should be taken not to inject contrast outside the liver parenchyma. This can be painful and may require premature termination of the procedure. Sometimes as many as 10 to 15 passes are needed to opacify nondilated bile ducts. Attempts to remove bile before injecting contrast are usually unsuccessful. Hepatic and portal veins are easily distinguished from bile ducts by the rapid washout of the contrast material. Hepatic lymphatics empty slowly but appear as tortuous beaded channels extending to the hilum and out over the spine (Fig. 16–43).

Transhepatic cholangiography should be employed early in the evaluation of jaundiced patients.[57, 58] It readily distinguishes intrahepatic cholestasis from obstruction of the bile ducts. Usually the location and cause of the obstruction can be accurately determined (Fig. 16–44). If the obstruction is considered inoperable, as in tumor near the porta hepatis, a large catheter can be inserted percutaneously through the liver into a bile duct and left in place for external drainage. A catheter can often be manipulated past the site of obstruction for long-term internal biliary drainage (Fig. 16–45).[59, 61, 63] Temporary bile duct decompression can be used prior to surgery to reduce the incidence of cholangitis and to simplify the operative procedure.

There are few contraindications to transhepatic cholangiography. A hemorrhagic diathesis is probably the only absolute contraindication. Others, such as sensitivity to the contrast medium, ascites, septicemia, and lack of cooperation by the patient, are relative contraindications that usually can be manged, and will not necessarily obviate the study.

The success rate of transhepatic cholangiography depends on the number of passes made with the needle. In most series, dilated ducts are visualized in 95 to 100 per cent of cases; normal-sized ducts are visualized from 60 to 80 per cent of the time.[62]

Serious complications, such as bile peritonitis and hemorrhage, are less frequent

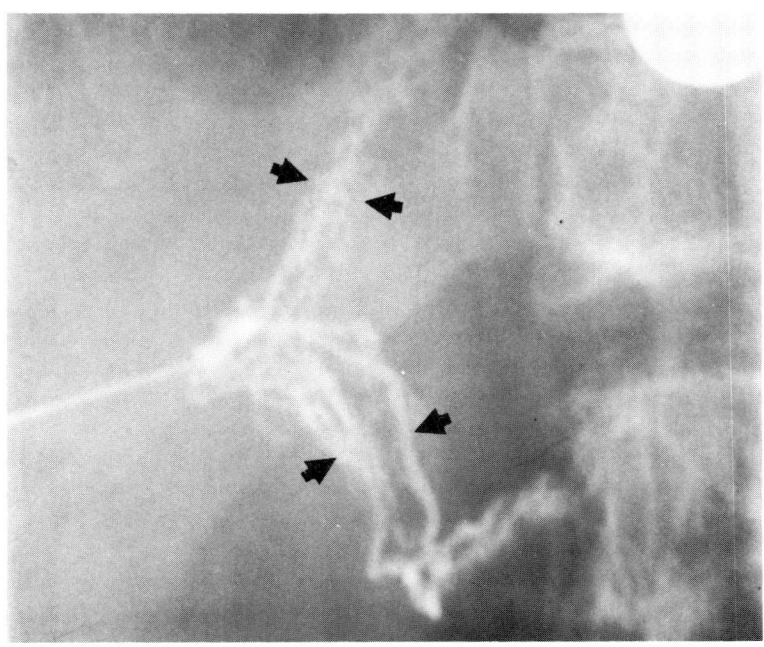

Figure 16–43. Hepatic lymphatics. The tortuous, beaded channels (arrows) empty slowly but are easily distinguished from bile ducts.

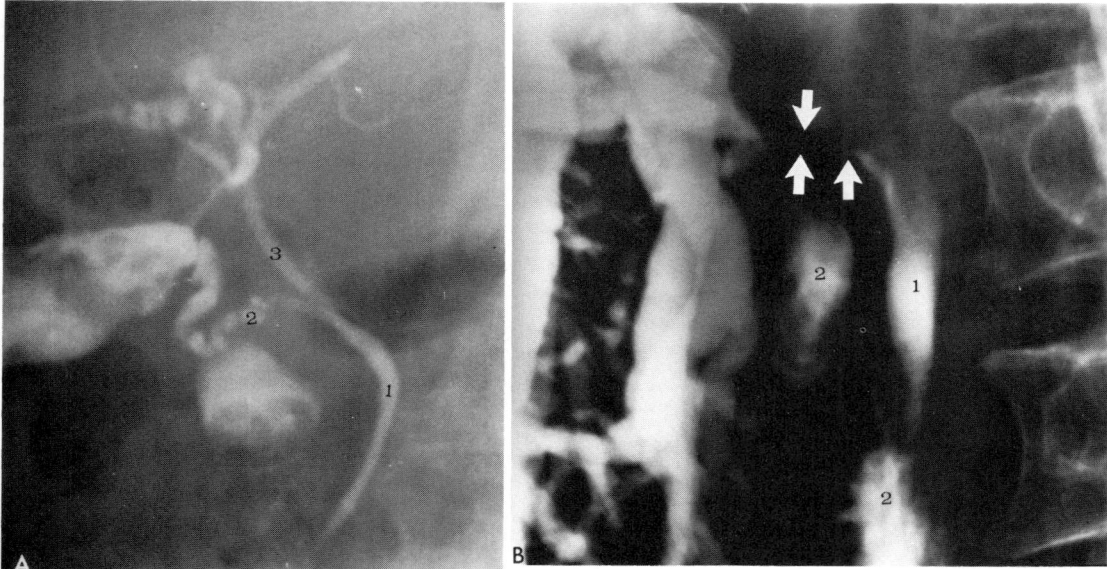

Figure 16–44. Transhepatic cholangiography. *A*, A normal transhepatic cholangiogram in this deeply jaundiced patient established the diagnosis of intrahepatic cholestasis. 1. common bile duct; 2. cystic duct; 3. common hepatic duct. *B*, Obstructive jaundice. Transhepatic cholangiogram showing a stricture in the porta hepatis region (arrows) from metastatic tumor and markedly dilated proximal ducts. 1. common bile duct; 2. duodenum.

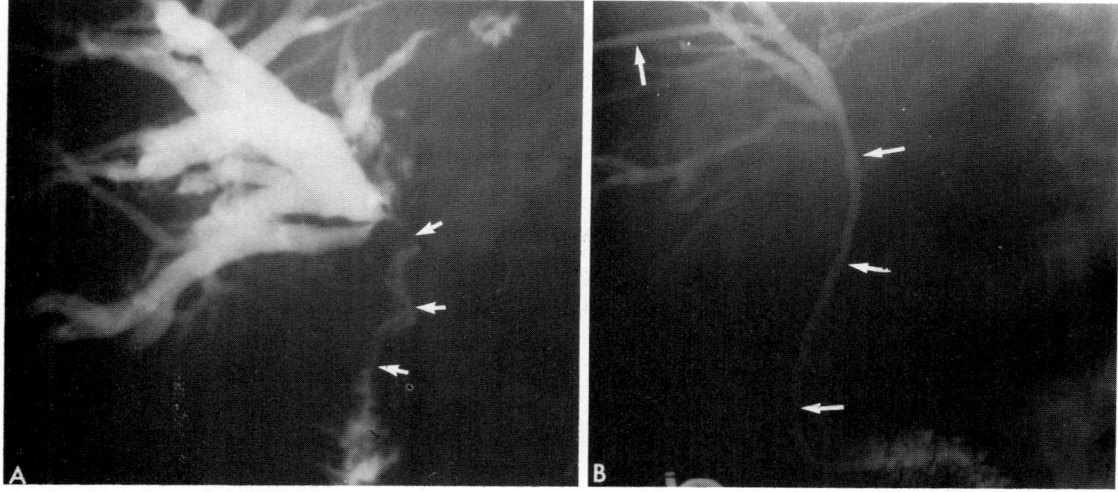

Figure 16–45. Biliary obstruction and drainage. A 70-year-old male with a previous choledochojejunostomy for bile duct carcinoma. *A*, Transhepatic cholangiogram showing a stricture at the surgical anastomosis (arrows). The proximal ducts are dilated. *B*, A large catheter (arrows) was manipulated through the stricture. Multiple side holes in the catheter allow for both internal and external decompression. The catheters can be left in place for long periods. Maintenance care consists of flushing to prevent clogging and periodic replacement.

with the skinny needle. Bile leakage can be reduced by avoiding overdistention of the ducts with contrast and, if possible, removing bile prior to injecting contrast. Fever and chills are the most common complications of transhepatic cholangiography and probably result from the introduction of bacteria into the bile. These occur most commonly when the ducts are obstructed and the bile drainage is poor. Antibiotics, such as ampicillin, are nearly always effective. Prophylactic antibiotics given 24 hours prior to the procedure appear to reduce the incidence of cholangitis.

Endoscopic Retrograde Cholangiopancreatography (ERCP)

The development of the flexible fiberoptic duodenoscope has made possible cannulization of the pancreatic and biliary ducts through the papilla of Vater. These ducts can then be visualized radiographically by the injection of contrast material through the endoscope (Fig. 16–47).

Endoscopic retrograde cholangiopancreatography (ERCP) is an important procedure for evaluating the pancreas. An experienced operator can cannulate the pancreatic duct in about 75 per cent of patients. Visualization of a normal pancreatic duct usually excludes pancreatic disease. Not infrequently, the radiographic appearance of the duct permits differentiation between chronic pancreatitis and pancreatic carcinoma, but in a substantial number of cases the x-ray findings overlap and this distinction cannot be made (Fig. 16–46).

Disagreement exists about whether to use ERCP or transhepatic cholangiography for primary biliary tract problems.[65-67] Both procedures have comparable complication rates, but ERCP requires more experience and technical skill than transhepatic cholangiography. The success rate for visualizing the biliary system is about the same for both procedures (60 to 80 per cent) when the ducts are normal-sized. Transhepatic cholangiography, however, approaches a success rate of 100 per cent when the ducts are dilated.

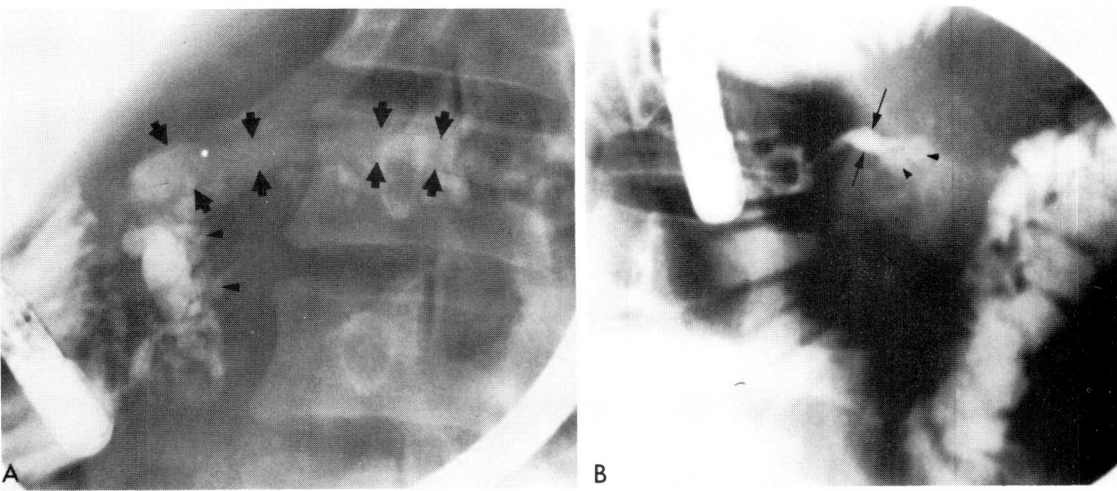

Figure 16–46. ERCP, chronic pancreatitis. *A*, The main pancreatic duct (arrows) is markedly dilated. The side branches (arrowheads) aer also dilated and beaded. These findings are characteristic of chronic pancreatitis. *B*, The main pancreatic duct (arrows) is completely obstructed by intraductal calculi (arrowheads).

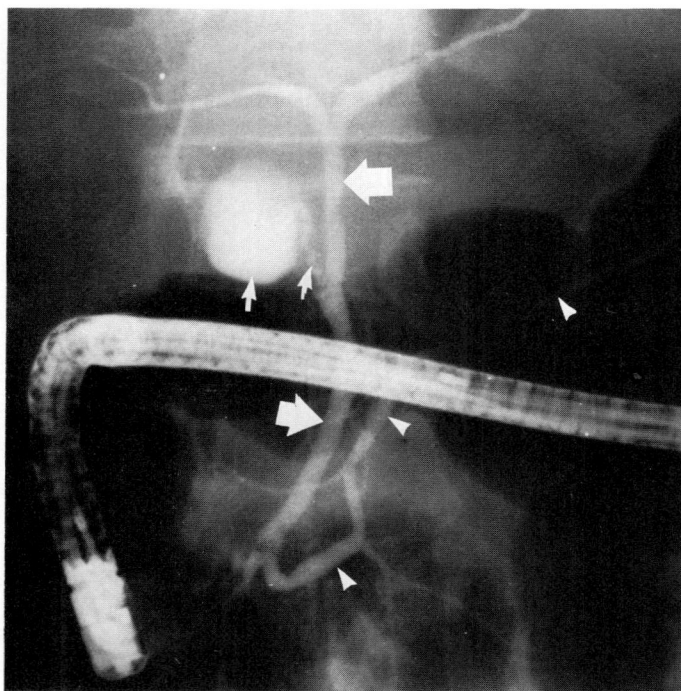

Figure 16–47. Normal ERCP. There is good opacification of the normal bile ducts (large arrows) including the cystic duct and gallbladder (small arrows). A normal pancreatic duct (arrowheads) is also visualized. ERCP is the best procedure to visualize both ductal systems.

ERCP is frequently used to evaluate patients with unexplained abdominal pain. In addition to evaluating the pancreatic and bile ducts, it permits endoscopic evaluation of the upper intestinal tract, biopsy of suspicious areas, and removal of fluid for cytologic studies. Contraindications are few and inlcude acute pancreatitis, infectious hepatitis, and allergy to contrast media. The major disadvantage of ERCP is that it is a costly and sometimes time-consuming procedure. It also requires a highly trained endoscopist as well as the use of a fluoroscopic unit and additional personnel.

The complications of this imaging modality are infrequent and usually minor. In many instances there is a transient elevation of serum amylase following injection of contrsat into the pancreatic duct, but clinical pancreatitis is not common.[68] Sepsis, the most serious complication, can occur from cannulation of either the biliary or the pancreatic ducts and is usually related to injecting sizable amounts of contrast through a stenotic or partially obstructed duct. Other complications include instrument injuries, aspiration pneumonia, and drug reactions. The death rate is less than 0.2 per cent.[60, 67]

Infusion Tomography of the Gallbladder

Infusion tomography of the gallbladder is a rapid, safe, and accurate procedure for the evaluation of patients with acute cholecystitis.[69] The study is based on demonstrating the actual gallbladder wall rather than relying on opacification of the lumen and visualization of stones.

The examination consists of the rapid intravenous infusion of any one of the iodinated contrast agents that are used for arteriography or intravenous pyelography. Antero-posterior tomograms of the right upper quadrant are then immediately obtained to visualize the gallbladder wall. The test is considered positive for cholecystitis when a thickened gallbladder wall (greater than 1 mm) is demonstrated (Fig. 16–48). In the normal gallbladder, the wall is 1 mm or less or is not opacified at all.

The reported accuracy rate in acute cholecystitis is as high as 95 per cent.[69] The procedure is also useful in patients with acute acalculous cholecystitis, since it relies on the presence of a thickened gallbladder wall and not on the demonstration of gallstones. The thickened gallbladder wall is opacified during acute inflammation probably as a result of the hypervascularity from hyperemia and the leakage of the contrast material into the edematous tissues.[70]

In Moncada's series,[69] infusion tomography was useful in patients with acute cholecystitis, chronic cholecystitis with an acute exacerbation, empyema of the gallbladder, and acute acalculous cholecystitis. In chronic cholecystitis, however, only 64 per cent of patients had a positive test.

Angiography

Angiography is rarely used as a primary means to evaluate the gallbladder. It is, however, often an important part of the work-up of jaundiced patients. Detailed angiography of the pancreas frequently can differentiate pancreatic carcinoma from chronic pancreatitis and pseudocysts, all of which can cause obstruction of the common bile duct. Angiography provides information about various hepatic disorders, such as liver metastases and cirrhosis, and therefore may help to differentiate obstructive jaundice from intrahepatic cholestasis.

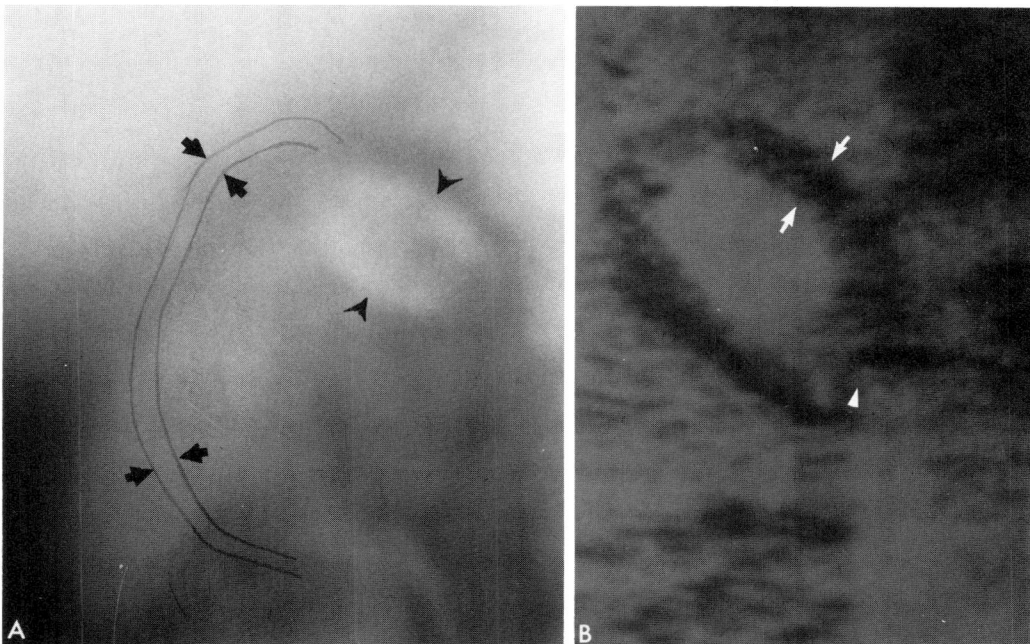

Figure 16–48. Infusion tomography of the gallbladder. *A*, Tomographic section showing a thickened gallbladder wall (penciled) (arrows) in a patient with suspected acute cholecystitis. Note the large gallstone (arrowheads). *B*, An ultrasound in the same patient confirms the thickened gallbladder wall (arrows) and the calculus in the gallbladder neck (arrowhead).

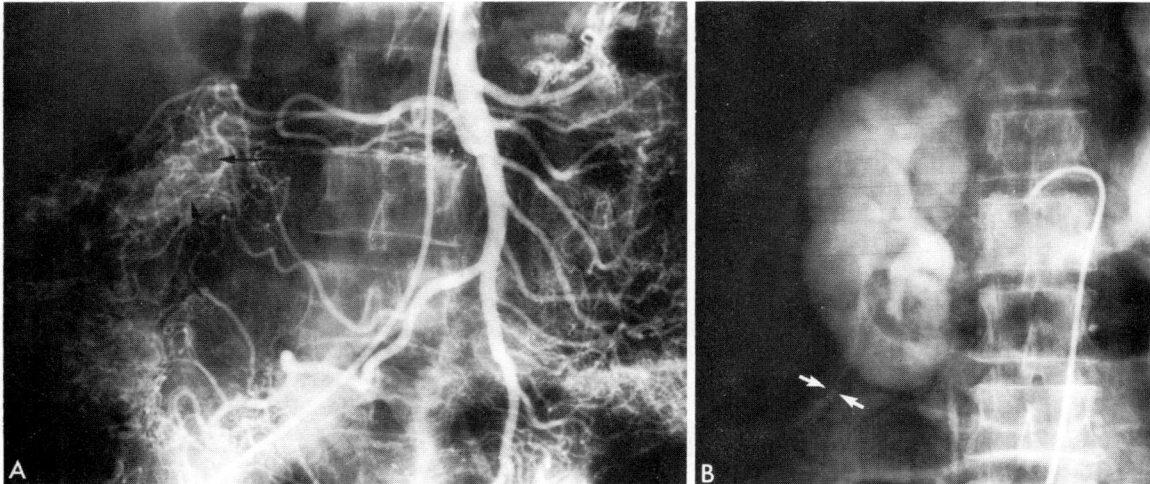

Figure 16–49. Angiographic demonstration of acute cholecystitis. *A*, Superior mesenteric arteriogram suggesting hyperemia of the hepatic flexure of the colon (arrows). *B*, Late phase of celiac arteriogram showing thickened gallbladder wall (arrows).

The cystic artery is often not visualized on hepatic arteriograms, but usually the gallbladder wall is opacified. The angiogram, therefore, provides information about the size and location of the gallbladder as well as the thickness of the wall. An enlarged gallbladder may be the cause of an unexplained right-sided abdominal mass or may indicate common bile duct obstruction. The normal gallbladder wall is seen as a thin rim of contrast, measuring 1 mm or less, during the middle and late phases of the angiogram.[71] A thickened gallbladder wall indicates cholecystitis. Occasionally, unsuspected acute cholecystitis is diagnosed by angiography performed for unexplained abdominal symptoms (Fig. 16–49).

Operative and Postoperative Tube Cholangiography

Since the introduction of operative cholangiography by Mirizzi in 1931,[77] the indicence of retained biliary tract stones following surgery and the need for surgical exploration of the common bile duct, have been considerably reduced. Without operative cholangiography, the incidence of overlooked common bile duct stones is as high as 10 to 25 per cent, this is reduced to 1 to 5 per cent when cholangiography is employed.[74, 78] The cholangiogram also demonstrates calculi in the intrahepatic bile ducts. Surgically important anatomic variations and unsuspected ductal disease can be demonstrated as well (Fig. 16–50). Operative cholangiography is extremely valuable and it is used routinely by many surgeons.

The cholangiogram should be performed prior to common duct exploration in order to avoid changes due to manipulation, such as spasm of the sphincter of Oddi. A water-soluble contrast agent, such as one of the diatrizoates, should be used. It is best to dilute the contrast agent, such as one of the diatrizoates, should be used. It is best to dilute the contrast by at least 50 per cent, especially if the ducts are dilated, to reduce the risk of obscuring small calculi. The contrast can be administered in several ways. Injection through the cystic duct is perhaps the most popular method, but contrast can be injected directly into the gallbladder (used most often in infants and children), or into the common duct. A slow injection, using minimal pressure or simple gravity, is best to avoid overdistention and spasm. High-pressure injections increase the incidence of septicemia and may rupture the ducts. One or more films should be obtained to evaluate the extrahepatic ducts, and then additional contrast should be given to fill the intrahepatic ducts. If possible, films should be taken with the patient in a slight right posterior oblique projection (about 15 degrees), so that the common bile duct is projected away from the spine. The radiographs should be interpreted immediately by a radiologist and the results communicated to the surgeon. The radiologist should insit on a technically adequate study. Improper x-ray technique and inadequate filling of the ducts are common reasons for failure to detect calculi.

The overall accuracy of operative cholangiography is about 90 per cent. In about 1 to 5 per cent of studies, there is a false negative result (calculi missed), an in about 6 per cent a false positive result (stones diagnosed but not found).[72, 74-76] The most common causes for error are improper x-ray technique, incomplete and inadequate opacification of the ducts, air bubbles mimicking stones, and spasm of the sphincter of Oddi. Careful technique should eliminate air bubbles in most instances. Bubbles are spherical, usually multiple and may change position with each injection (Fig. 16–51). Occasionally, the study should be repeated after flushing with saline in order to distinguish air bubbles from stones.

Spasm of the muscle fibers of the sphincter of Oddi is caused by many factors, including drugs such as morphine sulfate and narcotic analogs, surgical manipulation, and rapid forceful injection of contrast into the duct. The typical radiographic appearance of spasm is a gradual smooth tapered narrowing of the distal common bile

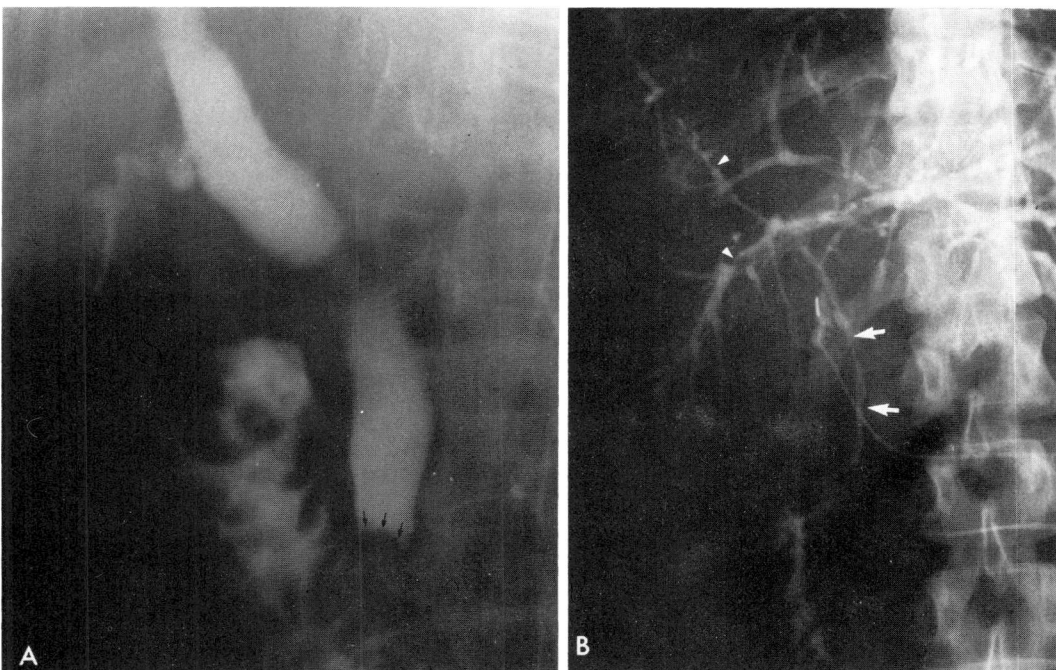

Figure 16–50. Operative cholangiograms. Bile duct stones and sclerosing cholangitis. *A*, Bile duct stone. The stone is in the distal end of the common bile duct (arrows). The filling defect in the mid-common bile duct was artifactual. *B*, Unsuspected sclerosing cholangitis in another patient. The preoperative clinical diagnosis was chronic cholecystitis. The cholangiogram demonstrates a markedly narrow common bile duct (arrows). Many intrahepatic ducts are narrowed and beaded (arrowheads).

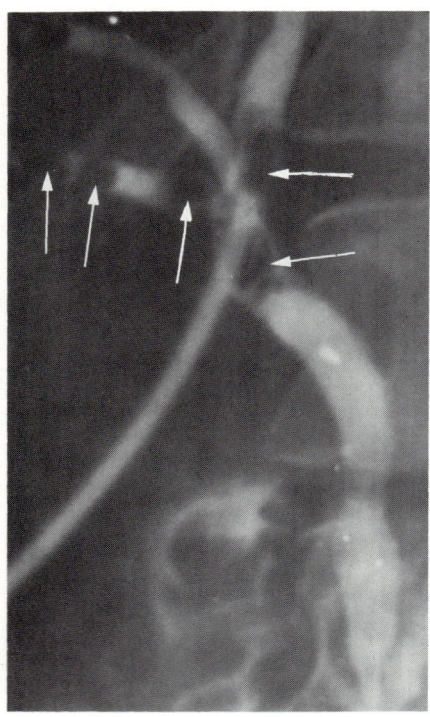

Figure 16–51. Air bubbles. The cholangiogram shows multiple radiolucencies (arrows) resembling calculi. A repeat study (not shown) was normal.

duct with little or no contrast entering the duodenum. Spasm does not cause dilatation of the proximal bile ducts (Fig. 16–52). Usually, serial films show relaxation or a change in the configuration of the distal common bile duct and contrast emptying into the duodenum, thus confirming the diagnosis of spasm. Occasionally, antispasmodic agents are necessary to relax the sphincter. Numerous drugs have been used, including amyl nitrate, nitroglycerine, Pro-Banthine, and magnesium sulfate infused into the duodenum. Glucagon, 0.5 to 1 mg intravenously, also is frequently empolyed. It is a safe and effective smooth muscle relaxant.

On occasion, contraction of the circular muscle fibers of the sphincter of Boyen (a part of the sphincter of Oddi) causes a meniscus-like configuration of the distal common bile duct resembling a stone. This "pseudocalculous" defect is probably caused by asynchronous contraction of the spincter muscles rather than by actual spasm. Antispasmodic agents are usually not helpful, but serial films will eventually demonstrate a normal distal common bile duct (Fig. 16–53).

Postoperative T-tube cholangiograms are usually obtained seven to ten days after surgery. The procedure can be performed in a more leisurely fashion than the operative cholangiogram, permitting a more detailed study. The contrast used is a diatrizoate, which should be diluted (usually by 50 per cent) to reduce its radiodensity and to avoid obscuring small stones. Care should be taken to avoid injecting air bubbles. The contrast should be administered under minimal pressure to avoid both distention of the ducts and distal common bile duct spasm. If spasm occurs, antispasmodics, such as glucagon, are often helpful. If the interpretation remains uncertain, a repeat examination should be performed at a later date, before removal of the T-tube.

THE BILIARY SYSTEM — 909

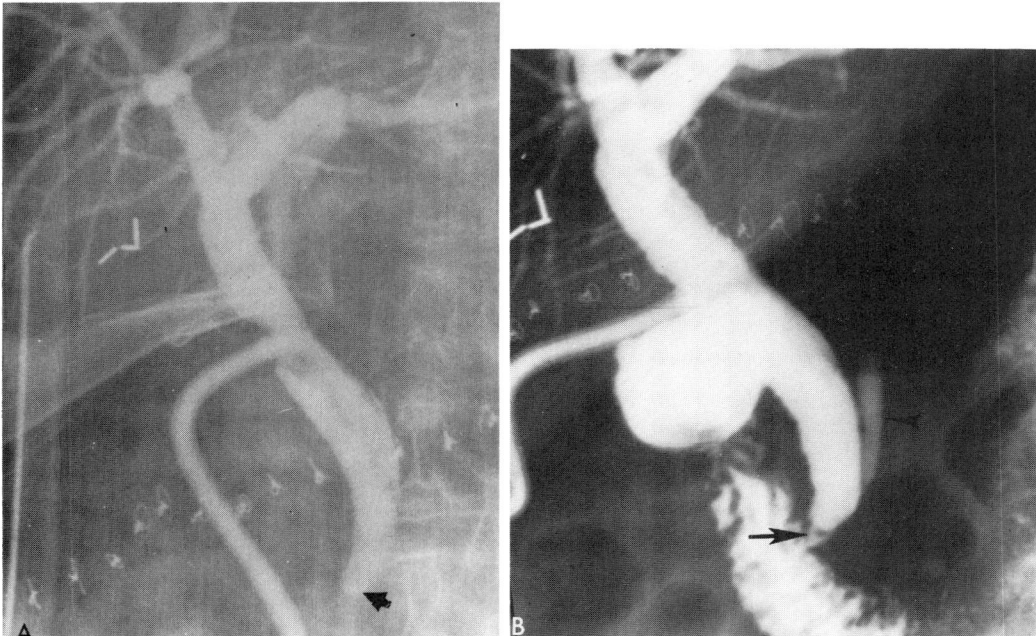

Figure 16–52. Common bile duct spasm. *A*, Operative cholangiogram showing "obstruction" of the distal common bile duct (arrow) and no contrast in the duodenum. The proximal ducts are not dilated. *B*, A repeat cholangiogram after the use of antispasmodics shows that the distal common bile duct is normal (arrow). The pancreatic duct is opacified (arrowhead).

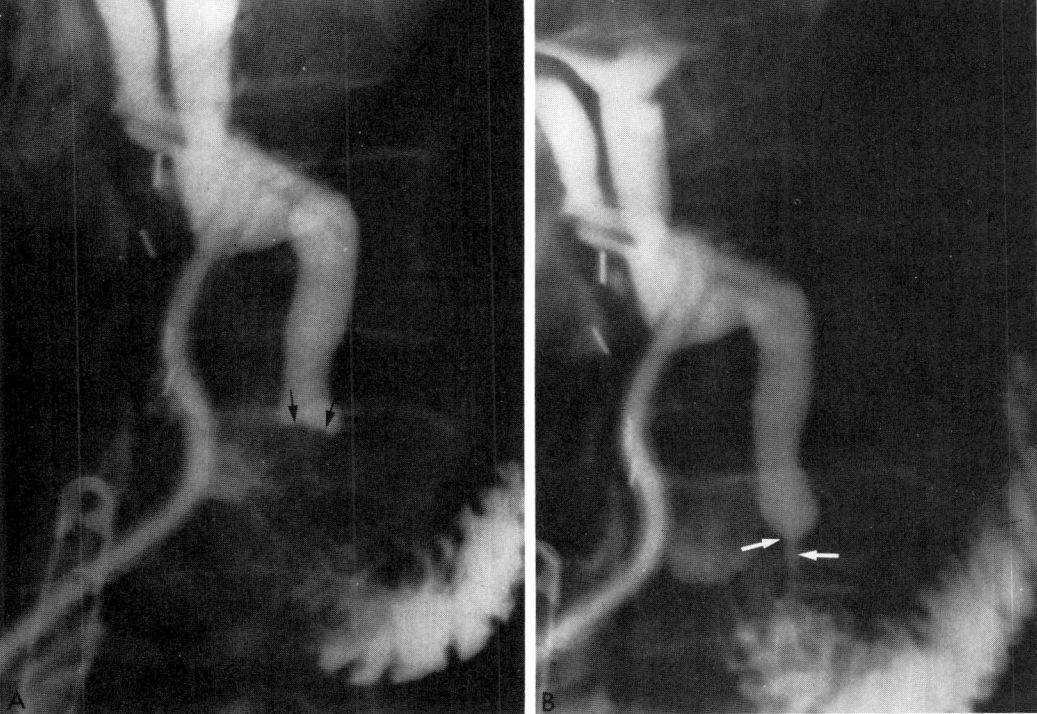

Figure 16–53. Pseudocalculous defect. *A*, There is a meniscus-like configuration of the distal common bile duct (arrows) resembling a stone. Previous exploration of the common bile duct was normal. *B*, A repeat cholangiogram shows a normal distal common bile duct (arrows).

References

Anatomy and Anatomic Variants

1. Bartone, N. F., and Grieco, R. V.: Absent gallbladder and cystic duct. Am. J. Roentgenol. *110*:252–255, 1970.
2. Blanton, D. E., Bream, C. A., and Mandel, J. R.: Gallbladder ectopia; a review of anomalies of position. Am. J. Roentgenol. *121*:396–400, 1974.
3. Chiavarini, R. L., Chang, S. F., and Westerfield, J. D.: The wandering gallbladder. Radiology *115*:47–48, 1975.
4. Ghahremani, G. G., and Meyers, M. A.: The cholecysto-colic relationships. Am. J. Roentgenol. *125*:21–34, 1975.
5. Hatfield, P. M., and Wise, R. E.: Anatomic variation in the gallbladder and bile ducts. Semin. Roentgenol. *11*:157–164, 1976.
6. Haughton, V., and Lewicki, A. W.: Agenesis of the gallbladder. Radiology *106*:305–306, 1973.
7. Nelson, J. A., and Burhenne, H. J.: Anomalous biliary and pancreatic duct insertion into duodenal diverticula. Radiology *120*:49–52, 1976.
8. Redman, H. C., and Reuter, S. R.: The angiographic evaluation of gallbladder dilatation. Radiology *97*:367–370, 1970.
9. Scholz, F. J., Carrera, G. F., and Larsen, C. R.: The choledochocele: correlation of radiological, clinical, and pathological findings. Radiology *118*:25–28, 1976.
10. Southan, J. A.: Left-sided gallbladder. Ann. Surg. *182*:135–137, 1975.

Plain Films

11. Berk, R.N., Armbuster, T. G., and Saltzstein, S. L.: Carcinoma in the porcelain gallbladder. Radiology *106*:29–31, 1973.
12. Campbell, E. W., and Rogers, C. L.: Submucosal gallbladder emphysema. J.A.M.A. *227*:790–791, 1974.
13. Keller, H. L., Ferstl, M., and Rupp, N.: Roentgenographic and clinical findings in emphysematous cholecystitis. Fortschr. Roentgenstr. *115*:475–482, 1971.
14. Meyers, M. A., and O'Donohue, N.: The Mercedes-Benz sign: insight into the dynamics of formation and disappearance of gallstones. Am. J. Roentgenol. *119*:63–70, 1973.
15. Moadel, E., and Byrk, D.: Obscuration of opaque gallstones in oral cholecystography. J. Can. Assoc. Radiol. *25*:55–57, 1974.
16. Polk, H. C., Jr.: Carcinoma and the calcified gallbladder. Gastroenterology *50*:582–585, 1966.
17. Shaub, M. S., Birnbaum, W. W., and Meyers, H. I.: Peribiliary fat. A new roentgenographic finding. Am. J. Roentgenol. *123*:330–337, 1975.

Oral Cholecystography

18. Berk, R. N.: The consecutive dose phenomena in oral cholecystography. Am. J. Roentgenol. *110*:230–234, 1970.
19. Berk, R. N.: The problem of impaired first-dose visualization of the gallbladder. Am. J. Roentgenol. *113*:186–188, 1971.
20. Berk, R. N., and Clemett A. R.: *Radiology of the Gallbladder and Bile Dcuts.* Philadelphia, W. B. Saunders Company, 1977, pp. 88–90.
21. Berk, R. N., Loeb, P. M., Goldberger, L. E., et al.: Oral cholecystography with iopanoic acid. N. Engl. J. Med. *290*:204–210, 1974.
22. Byrk, D., and Moadel, E.: Layering of contrast material in oral cholecystography. Dig. Dis. *20*:727–734, 1975.
23. Duggan, F. J., and Rohner, T. J.: Acute renal insufficiency following oral cholecystography. J. Urol. *109*:156–159, 1973.
24. Harvey, I. C., Thwe, M., and Low-Beer, T. S.: The value of the fatty meal in oral cholecystography. Clin. Radiol. *27*:117–121, 1976.
25. Laufer, I., and Gledhill, L.: The value of the fatty meal in oral cholecystography. Radiology *114*:525–527, 1975.
26. Loeb, P. M., Berk, R. N., Janes, J. O., et al.: The effect of fasting on gallbladder opacification during oral cholecystography: a controlled study in normal volunteers. Radiology *126*:395–401, 1978.
27. Mujahed, Z.: Nonopacification of the gallbladder and bile ducts. A previously unreported cause. Radiology *112*:297–298, 1974.
28. Nathan, M. H., and Newman, A.: Conjugated iopanoic acid (Telepaque) in the small bowel. An aid in the diagnosis of gallbladder disease. Radiology *109*:545–548, 1973.
29. Preuss, H. J.: Layering phenomena of the gallbladder with intravenous cholecystography. Expression of the reabsorptive mucosal function? Fortschr. Roentgenstr. *112*:219–230, 1970.

30. Roller, J., Mallory, A., Caruthers, S., et al.: Oral cholecystography after alcoholic pancreatitis. Gastroenterology 73:218–221, 1977.
31. Rosenbaum, H. D.: an evaluation of oral cholecystography. J.A.M.A. 229:76–79, 1974.
32. Zaboralski, F. F., and Amberg, J. R.: Cholecysto-cholestasis: a cause of cholecystographic error. Am. J. Dig. Dis. 7:339–346, 1962.

Intravenous Cholangiography

33. Black, E. B., and Ferrucci, J. T.: New cholangiographic sign of common bile duct obstruction: initial opacification of intrahepatic ducts. Am. J. Roentgenol. 130:61–65, 1978.
34. Fuchs, W. A., and Preisig, R.: Prolonged drip-infusion cholangiography. Br. J.Radiol. 48:539–544, 1975.
35. Grundy, D. J., King, P. A., and Lloyd, G.: Comparative evaluation of preoperative and operative radiology in biliary-tract disease. Br. J. Surg. 59:205–208, 1972.
36. Hatfield, P. M., and Wise, R. E.: Radiology of the Gallbladder and Bile Ducts. Baltimore, The Williams & Wilkins Company, 1976 pp. 63–65.
37. Maida, J. W., Kratz, G., Martinez, L. O., et al.: The utilization of intravenous cholangiography in the demonstration of common duct foreign bodies. Br. J. Radiol. 44:388–392, 1971.
38. Mujahed, Z., Evans, J. A., and Whalen, J. P.: The nonopacified gallbladder on oral cholecystography. Radiology 112:1–3, 1974.
39. Salzman, E.: Opacification of bile duct calculi. Radiol. Clin. North Am. 4:525–533, 1966.
40. Scholz, F. J., Larsen, C. R., and Wise, R. E.: Intravenous cholangiography: recurring concepts. Semin. Roentgenol. 11:197–201, 1976.
41. Solomon, A.: Hypotonic duodenography. S. Afr. Med. J. 42:1039–1040, 1968.
42. Stage, P., and Banke, L.: Hypotonic duodenography. Gut 10:428–432, 1969.
43. Teplick, S. K., Maturi, R., Wittenberg, J., et al.: Intravenous cholangiography during acute common bile duct obstruction in the Rhesus monkey. In press.
44. Weens, H. S., and Walker, L. A.: The radiologic diagnosis of acute cholecystitis and pancreatitis. Radiol. Clin. North Am. 2:89–106, 1964.
45. Wittenberg, J., Maturi, R. A., Teplick, S. K., et al.: Intravenous cholangiography in the Rhesus monkey. II: Determination of the optimal iodipamide delivery time. Invest. Radiol. In press.
46. Wittenberg, J., Maturi, R. A., Williams, L., et al.: Iodipamide infusion cholangiography in Rhesus monkeys-determination of dose. Invest. Radiol. 11:45–53, 1976.

Isotopes

47. Lomas, F., and Wagner, H. N.: Accumulation of ionic ^{67}Ga in empyema of the gallbladder. Radiology 105:689–692, 1972.
48. Rosenthal, L., Shaffer, E. A., Lisbona, R., et al.: Diagnosis of hepatobiliary disease by 99m TC-HIDA cholescintigraphy. Radiology 126:467–474, 1978.
49. Verow, P. W., and Wisbey, M.: Sequential liver and biliary tract scanning with ^{131}I labelled rose bengal. Clin. Radiol. 26:499–504, 1975.
50. Waxman, A. D., and Siemsen, J. K.: Gallium gallbladder scanning in cholecystitis. J. Nucl. Med. 16:148–150, 1974.

Ultrasound

51. Bartrum, R. J., Jr., Crow, H. C., and Foote, S. R.: Ultrasonic and radiographic cholecystography. N. Engl. J. Med. 296:538–541, 1977.
52. Gosnik, B. B., and Leopold, G. R.: Ultrasound and the gallbladder. Semin. Roentgenol. 11:185–189, 1976.
53. Leopold, G. R., Amberg, J., Gosnik, B. B., et al.: Gray scale ultrasonic cholecystography: a comparison with conventional radiographic techniques. Radiology 121:445–448, 1976.

Computed Tomography

54. Biello, D. R., Levitt, R. G., Siegel, B. A., et al.: Computed tomography and radionuclide imaging of the liver: a comparative evaluation. Radiology 127:159–163, 1978.
55. Levitt, R. G., Sagel, S. S., Stanley, R. J., et al.: Accuracy of computed tomography of the liver and biliary tract. Radiology 124:123–128, 1977.
56. MacCarty, R. L., Wahner, H. W., Stephens, D. H., et al.: Retrospective comparison of radionuclide scans and computed tomography of the liver and pancreas. Am. J. Roentgenol. 129:23–28, 1977.

Transhepatic Cholangiography

57. Fazel, I., and Finley, R. K., Jr.: Experience with percutaneous transhepatic cholangiography in a community hospital. Ohio State Med. J. 66:1193–1200, 1970.
58. Göthlin, J., and Tranberg, K-G.: Complications of percutaneous transhepatic cholangiography (PTC). Am. J. Roentgenol. 117:426–431, 1973.
59. Molnar, W., and Stockum, A. E.: Relief of obstructive jaundice through percutaneous transhepatic catheter-a new therapeutic method. Am. J. Roentgenol.22:356–367, 1974.
60. Okuda, K., Tanikawa, K., Emura, T., et al.: Nonsurgical percutaneous transhepatic cholangiography-diagnostic significance in medical problems of the liver. Am. J. Dig. Dis. 19:21–36, 1974.
61. Pereiras, P. V., Jr., Rheingold, O. J., Hutson, D., et al.: Relief of malignant obstructive jaundice by percutaneous insertion of a permanent prosthesis in the biliary tree. Ann. Intern. Med. 89:589–593, 1978.
62. Pereiras, P. V., Jr., White, P., Dusol, M., Jr., et al.: Percutaneous transhepatic cholangiography utilizing the Chiba University needle. Radiology 121:219–221, 1976.
63. Ring, E. J., Oleaga, J. A., Freiman, D. B., et al.: Therapeutic applications of catheter cholangiography. Radiology 128:333–338, 1978.
64. Tabrisky, J., Lindstrom, R. L., Hanelin, L. G., et al.: Chiba percutaneous transhepatic cholangiography. A valuable method for visualizing the nondilated biliary tract. Am. J. Roentgenol. 126:755–760, 1976.

Endoscopic Retrograde Cholangiopancreatography (ERCP)

65. Ferrucci, J. T., and Wittenberg, J.: Refinements in Chiba needle transhepatic cholangiography. Am. J. Roentgenol. 129:11–16, 1977.
66. Kessler, R. E., Falkenstein, D. B., Clemett, A. R., et al.: Indications, clinical value and complications of endoscopic retrograde cholangiopancreatography. Surg. Gynecol. Obstet. 142:865–870, 1976.
67. Paul, R. E.: Endoscopic retrograde cholangiography. Semin. Roentgenol. 11:233–225, 1976.
68. Vennes, J. A., Jacobson, J. R., and Silvis, S. E.: Endoscopic cholangiography for biliary system diagnosis. Ann. Intern. Med. 80:61–64, 1974.

Infusion Tomography

69. Moncada, R., Cardoso, M., Danley, R., et al.: Acute cholecystitis: 137 cases diagnosed by infusion tomography of the gallbladder Am. J. Roentgenol.129:583–585, 1977.
70. Moncada, R., Cardoso, M., Danley, R., et al.: Infusion tomography of the gallbladder: mechanism of gallbladder wall opacification in experimental acute cholecystitis. Am. J. Roentgenol. 129:587–590, 1977.

Angiography

71. Kaude, J. V., and Hawkins, I. F., Jr.: Angiography of the gallbladder and biliary tract. Semin. Roentgenol. 11:191–195, 1976.

Operative Cholangiography

72. Faris, I., Thomson, J. P. S., Grundy, D. J., et al.: Operative cholangiography: a reappraisal based on a review of 400 cholangiograms. Br. J. Surg. 62:966–972, 1975.
73. Ferrucci, J. T., Jr., Wittenberg, J., Stone, L. B., et al.: Hypotonic cholangiography with glucagon. Radiology 118:466–467, 1976.
74. Goldberg, H. I.: Operative and postoperative cholecystocholangiography. Semin. Reoengenol. 11:203–211, 1976.
75. Grundy, D. J., King, P. A., and Lloyd, G.: Comparative evaluation of preoperative and operative radiology in biliary-tract disease. Br. J. Surg. 59:205–208, 1972.
76. Marks, C. G., and Kelvin, F. M.: Operative cholangiography: criteria which make exploration of the common bile duct desirable. Br. J. Surg. 63:51–54, 1976.
77. Mirizzi, P. L., and Quiroga Losada, C.: La exploracion de las vias billiares principales en el curso de la operacion. Proc. 3rd Argentinian Congr. Surg. 1:694–703, 1931.
78. Sachs, M. D.: Routine cholangiography, operative and postoperative. Radiol. Clin. North. Am. 4:547–569, 1966.

PART II
Cholecystitis, Calculi, and Miscellaneous Conditions

STEVEN K. TEPLICK, M.D.

CHOLECYSTITIS

Acute Cholecystitis

Acute cholecystitis is most often precipitated by obstruction of the cystic duct. Usually the obstruction is caused by a gallstone, but acute acalculous cholecystitis occurs in 5 to 10 per cent of cases. Initially, the gallbladder wall is edematous and the lumen distended with sterile bile. As the disease progresses, the bile frequently becomes infected. The common bacterial organisms are *Escherichia coli, Klebsiella, Aerobacter*, enterococci, and staphylococci.[5] In the majority of cases (about 85 per cent), the stone in the cystic duct disimpacts, and the inflammatory process spontaneously subsides. If the obstruction persists, the illness may worsen and complications, such as perforation of the gallbladder, may develop.

The most typical clinical manifestations of acute cholecystitis are pain and tenderness in the right upper quadrant or epigastrium. The pain may radiate to the inferior tip of the right scapula via the seventh intercostal nerve. The pain may begin as colic but usually becomes constant, and nausea is often present. Peritoneal irritation causes guarding, rebound tenderness, and a positive Murphy sign. The temperature and white blood cell count are usually mildly elevated. If jaundice is present a common bile duct stone should be suspected.[1] However, mild jaundice can occur without ductal obstruction due to narrowing of the common bile duct from the adjacent distended and inflamed gallbladder.[3] The gallbladder is palpable as a right upper quadrant mass in less than 50 per cent of cases.

The diagnosis of acute cholecystitis on the basis of clinical symptoms alone may be difficult. The differential diagnosis can be extensive and includes pancreatitis, perforated peptic ulcer, appendicitis, right renal stone or pyelonephritis, acute hepatitis, salpingitis with perihepatitis (Fitz-Hugh–Curtis syndrome), and chest disorders, such as right lower lobe pneumonia or myocardial infarction. Many of these conditions can be readily eliminated by appropriate laboratory tests and radiographs.

The radiographic evaluation of patients with suspected acute cholecystitis should begin with upright films of the chest and abdomen and a supine film of the abdomen. Sometimes the findings on the plain films are quite diagnostic, eliminating the need for further tests. For example, gas in the gallbladder wall is diagnostic of emphysematous cholecystitis (see Fig. 16–19). If radiopaque gallstones are present, there is often no need for oral cholecystography. Other findings, such as a soft tissue mass in the right upper quadrant, a subphrenic or right upper abdominal abscess, and a localized right-sided ileus, are somewhat less specific but nevertheless useful (Fig. 16–54).

Ultrasound and, more recently, computerized tomography of the abdomen are very useful in patients with acute abdominal problems. They are rapid and noninvasive and provide information about the gallbladder, pancreas, liver, and other abdominal organs. They are being used increasingly to confirm the diagnosis of acute cholecystitis. In some institutions, the ultrasound study is replacing second-dose oral cholecystog-

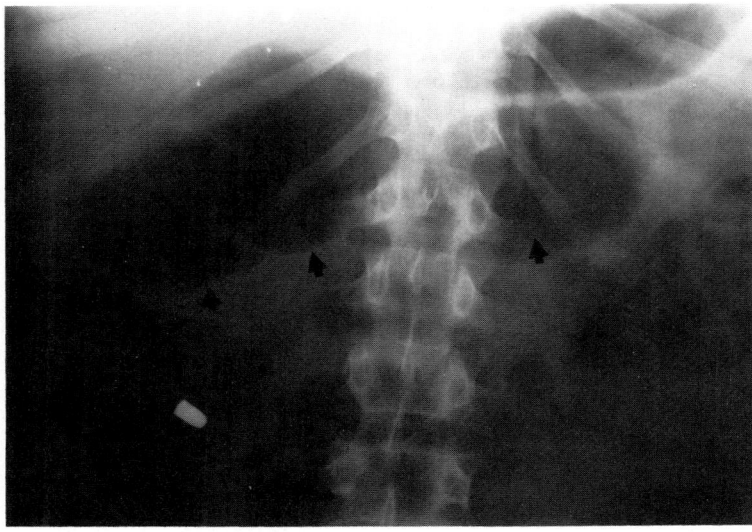

Figure 16–54. Localized ileus from cholecystitis. There is distended, atonic small bowel in the upper abdomen (arrows). This is nonspecific and could be due to a variety of disorders. A bullet from an old gunshot wound is an incidental finding.

raphy and often is the first procedure in evaluating patients with suspected acute cholecystitis.

The ultrasound or CT scan in acute cholecystitis often shows a distended gallbladder with stones. Acute inflammation of the gallbladder with pericholecystic edema appears as thickening of the wall and loss of the normally discrete outline of the gallbladder on the ultrasound study (Fig. 16–55). The CT scan may also demonstrate a thickened gallbladder wall.

Intravenous cholangiography is often employed in patients with suspected acute cholecystitis.[6] It is a reasonably rapid procedure, and when the bile ducts are adequately opacified, highly reliable. Unfortunately, in many acute abdominal conditions, including acute cholecystitis, the bile ducts often are not visualized. This may occur in up to 50 per cent of patients with acute abdomen. The absence of ductal

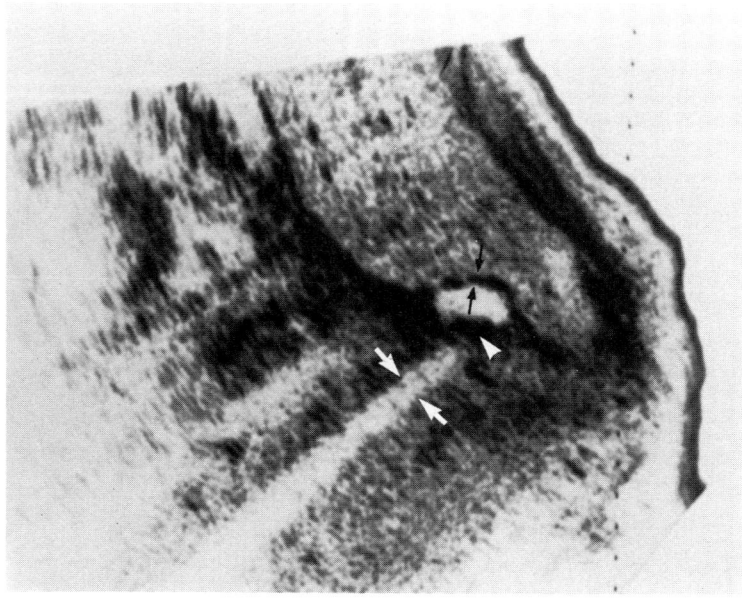

Figure 16–55. Ultrasound in acute cholecystitis. The gallbladder wall is thickened (small arrows). A gallstone (arrowhead) casts an echo-free zone (large arrows).

THE BILIARY SYSTEM — 915

opacification is not helpful in diagnosing or excluding biliary tract disease. It is simply an indication of diminished hepatic excretion of contrast. The cholangiogram should be performed as described previously (see p. 889–893). Serial films, including tomograms if necessary, should be taken to visualize the bile ducts and gallbladder. Delayed films at 4, 8, and 24 hours may be helpful, since occasionally the gallbladder opacifies even though no ducts are seen.

The purpose of the intravenous cholangiogram in suspected acute cholecystitis is to demonstrate patency or occlusion of the cystic duct. When the bile ducts and gallbladder or the gallbladder alone are visualized, the cystic duct is patent and acute cholecystitis can be excluded. If the bile ducts are opacified and the gallbladder is not, then the cystic duct is probably obstructed, a finding consistent with acute cholecystitis. If the biliary system is not visualized, no valid conclusion can be drawn concerning cystic duct obstruction. On occasion, the delayed films show an opacified gallbladder even in the absence of bile duct visualization, indicating a patent cystic duct (Fig. 16–

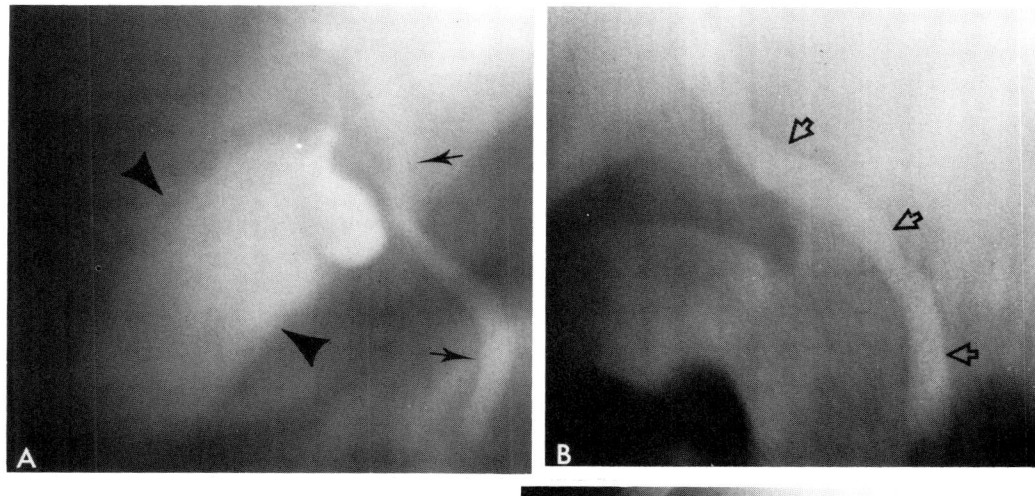
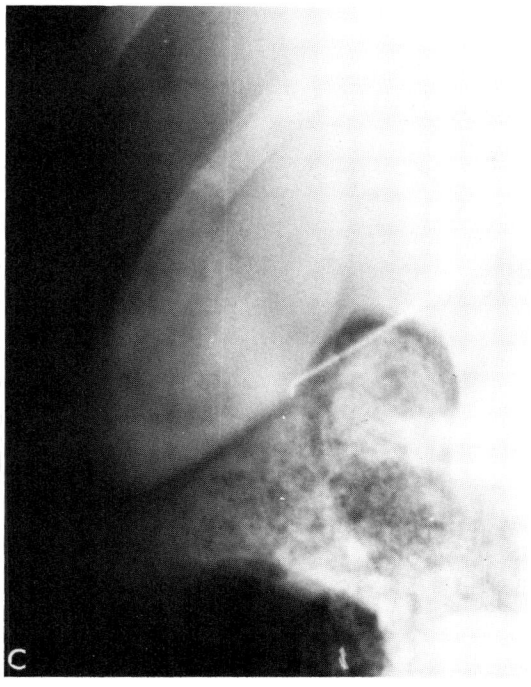

Figure 16–56. Suspected acute cholecystitis. A, Intravenous cholangiogram showing normal bile ducts (arrows) and gallbladder (arrowheads). Visualization of gallbladder virtually excludes the diagnosis of acute cholecystitis. Incidentally noted was a kink near the gallbladder neck. B, If the common bile duct (arrows) and not the gallbladder is opacified, the diagnosis of acute cholecystitis is probable. C, In this patient, neither ducts nor gallbladder was visualized up to eight hours. On the 24-hour film, the gallbladder was opacified. This implies cystic duct patency and argues against the diagnosis of acute cholecystitis.

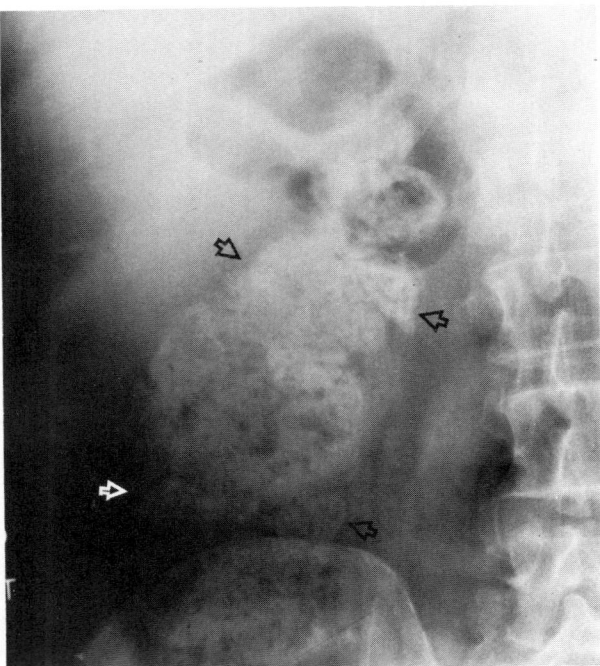

Figure 16–57. Intravenous cholangiography in acute cholecystitis. A delayed film shows homogeneous contrast in the colon (arrows) and no opacification of the gallbladder. This indicates that contrast was excreted through the bile ducts and that the cystic duct is occluded.

57), which means that the contrast was excreted by the liver and, in the absence of gallbladder filling, implies cystic duct obstruction.

Oral cholecystography has several disadvantages in patients with acute cholecystitis. Many hospitalized patients are kept NPO or are too ill to take or retain the tablets. In addition, many with normal gallbladders (about 25 per cent) require a repeat dose of contrast before the gallbladder is adequately opacified. A gallbladder should not be considered abnormal until it has failed to visualize after two consecutive doses (see the section on oral cholecystography). This, of course, causes a delay in diagnosis.

Gallium scans of the abdomen can demonstrate inflammation of the gallbladder and have been used to diagnose acute cholecystitis. The main disadvantage of using gallium is that often several days are needed to complete the study (see Fig. 16–39). An experimental nuclear agent, ^{99m}Tc HIDA and its derivatives, will soon be available for evaluation of patients with suspected acute cholecystitis. The isotope rapidly enters the biliary system, and cystic duct patency can be determined in as little as 15 to 30 minutes. It promises to be extremely accurate.

Infusion tomography of the gallbladder has been popularized recently and has been reported to be a rapid, accurate means to diagnose acute cholecystitis.[2] Tomographic sections in the region of the gallbladder are obtained during intravenous infusion of a diatrizoate contrast medium. A positive study for cholecystitis occurs when a thickened gallbladder wall (greater than 1 mm) is demonstrated (see Fig. 16–48). In Moncado's series,[2] the overall accuracy of infusion tomography in the diagnosis of acute cholecystitis was 95 per cent.

The initial treatment of acute cholecystitis is nonsurgical and consists of supportive measures. Unless the patient is critically ill with, for example, signs of generalized peritonitis, emergency surgery is not indicated. Cholecystectomy is usually performed electively either during the initial hospitalization or at a future date.

In most instances, acute cholecystitis subsides, probably because the cystic duct obstruction is relieved. If the inflammatory process progresses, complications may occur; they are most frequent in the elderly and in diabetic patients. The most serious complication is perforation of the gallbladder, which is precipitated by distention of the lumen and occlusion of the blood vessels. Perforations may be free, extending into the peritoneal cavity, or confined.

Most often the perforation is contained by adjacent tissues that have become adherent to the gallbladder wall, resulting in a pericholecystic abscess. Free perforation causes generalized peritonitis, necessitating emergency surgery. Sometimes there is transient relief of symptoms as the gallbladder decompresses itself into the peritoneal cavity. Occasionally, the gallbladder ruptures into an adjacent organ, resulting in a fistula. This occurs most commonly into the duodenum and less often into the hepatic flexure of the colon. Rarely, the gallbladder perforates into the thorax or renal pelvis. Fistulous communication to the duodenum is best demonstrated by an upper gastrointestinal series. Many cholecystoenteric fistulas are of little clinical significance. However, if gallstones remain the patient may develop recurrent gallbladder symptoms, or a stone may later enter the gastrointestinal tract producing intestinal obstruction (gallstone ileus) (Fig. 16–58).

Other complications of acute cholecystitis include gangrene of the gallbladder, which is probably due to occlusions of branches of the cystic artery; pneumonia, cerebrovascular and cardiovascular complications, which account for much of the mortality during acute cholecystitis; and infrequently, empyema or hydrops of the gallbladder.[4]

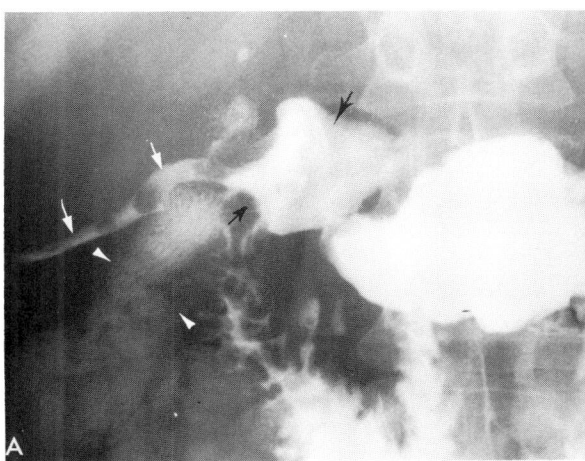
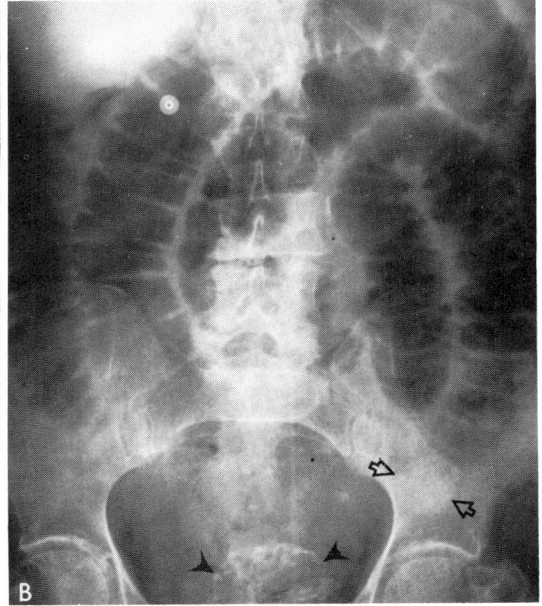

Figure 16–58. Complications of cholecystitis. *A,* Fistula. An upper gastrointestinal series shows a deformed duodenal bulb (black arrows), which communicates with the gallbladder (arrowheads) and bile ducts (white arrows). *B,* Gallstone ileus in an elderly patient with intestinal obstruction. The small bowel loops are dilated. A faint gallstone is seen in the left lower quadrant (arrows). A review of previous films showed that the same gallstone was visible in the gallbladder area prior to the obstruction. Incidentally noted is a uterine fibroid (arrowheads).

Illustration and legend continued on the following page

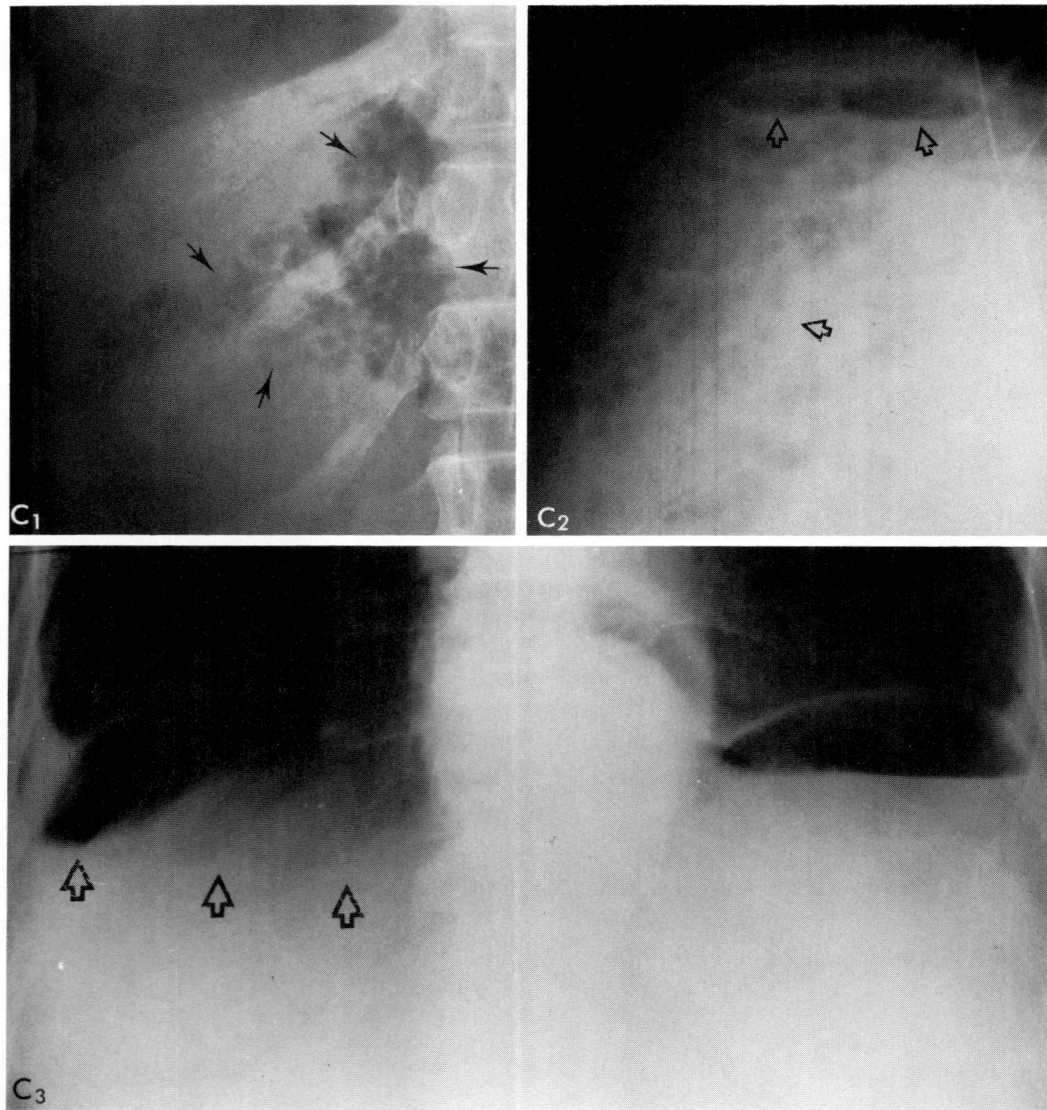

Figure 16–58 *Continued.* C, Several examples of perforation of the gallbladder. 1. Perforation confined to the region of the gallbladder bed. Multiple gas bubbles (arrows) delineate the extent of the abscess. 2. There is an extensive subphrenic abscess with multiple gas pockets (arrows). 3. A generalized peritonitis resulted from gallbladder perforation. There is free peritoneal gas and a fluid level, best demonstrated in the right upper quadrant (arrows).

Gallstones

The overall incidence of gallstones may be increasing. In the United States alone, approximately 15 million people have gallstones, 800,000 develop stones annually, and about 300,000 require cholecystectomy each year.

Gallstones are rare before the age of ten, after which the incidence rises with advancing age. About 10 per cent of the adult population harbor gallstones. This figure increases to about 30 per cent by the eighth or ninth decade. The highest incidence is in American Indians, of whom 50 percent of adults have cholelithiasis. In general, women are affected at least twice as often as men, and there seems to be a direct relationship with pregnancy.[7, 15]

The incidence of gallstones is thought to be higher than usual in a wide variety of diseases. In some, the association with gallstones has not been statistically validated, including coronary artery disease, peptic ulcer, and hiatus hernia with associated colonic diverticulosis, vagotomy and gastric resection.[11] Conditions known to have a higher than normal incidence of gallstones include hemolytic anemias and cirrhosis, in which the incidence of pigment gallstones is increased; pancreatitis, which is frequently related to gallbladder or bile duct stones; diseases of the terminal ileum, such as Crohn's disease, in which the incidence is three to five times higher than in the general population; drugs, such as oral contraceptives and clofibrate; pregnancy; obesity; and diabetes.[11, 12]

The simplest classification of gallstones is the division into cholesterol stones and pigment stones. Since the introduction of chenodeoxycholic acid for the dissolution of gallstones, it is of some importance to distinguish these two types clinically and radiographically. Cholesterol stones dissolve or become smaller with oral chenodeoxycholic acid therapy, whereas pigment stones are unaffected.

In the United States most calculi (70 to 90 per cent) are composed predominantly of cholesterol. Cholesterol stones can be subclassified as (a) mixed, which are composed of at least 70 per cent cholesterol, light tan in color, and smooth or faceted; and (b) pure cholesterol stones, which are often large, round, and solitary. The latter type is much less common.

Pigment stones are thought to constitute nearly 30 per cent of gallstones in the United States, rather than 10 per cent as previously thought.[14] Pigment stones contain much less cholesterol (less than 25 per cent). They are dark brown or black, usually small and multiple, and often irregular in shape.

Varying amounts of calcium salts are found in all types of stones. The degree of radiopacity of the calculi is directly proportional to their calcium content.[8, 9, 12, 14, 16] Determination of the chemical composition is important for medical treatment of cholelithiasis, since only cholesterol-rich stones can be dissolved by chenodeoxycholic acid.

The radiologic appearance of the stone is a clue to its chemical composition. Eighty to ninety per cent of all gallstones are radiolucent, and the majority of these are cholesterol stones. Most radiopaque calculi are of the pigment variety and do not contain sufficient cholesterol to be dissolved. Recent studies, however, have shown that 15 to 20 per cent of pigment calculi are radiolucent.[8] Therefore, a significant number of radiolucent stones will not dissolve. These are usually small, multiple stones that are irregularly shaped, nonfaceted and do not float. Large, round, radiolucent stones are apt to have a high cholesterol content and may respond to chenodeoxycholic acid (Fig. 16–59).

It is generally accepted that the liver is the source of lithogenic bile. However, the role of the gallbladder in stone formation is also important. Stasis of bile in the gallbladder is probably a factor in the development of macroscopic stones. In addition, the gallbladder probably provides the nidus for stone development. The formation of

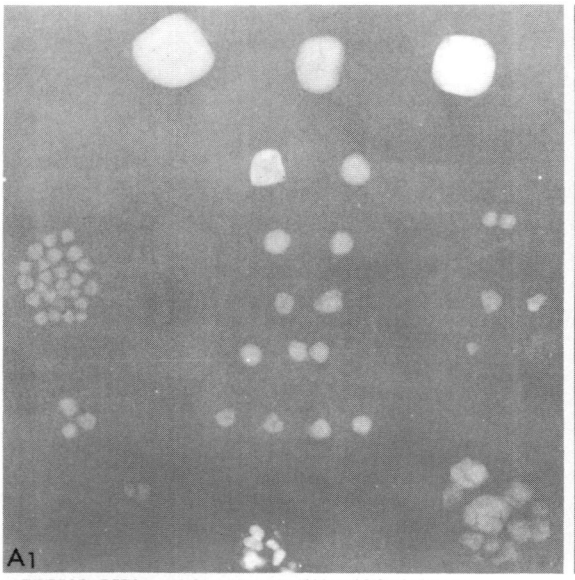
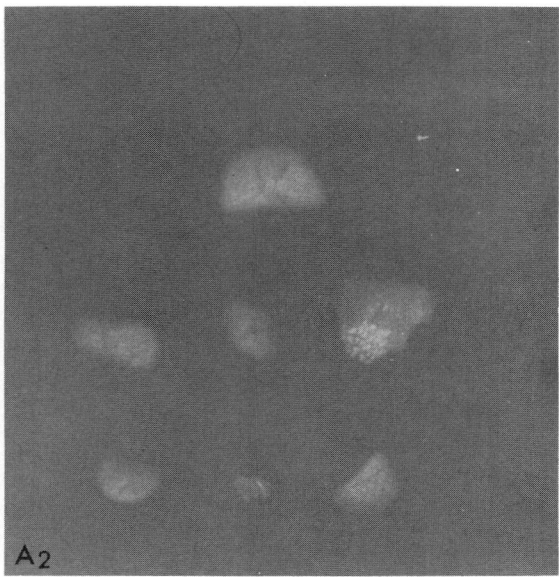
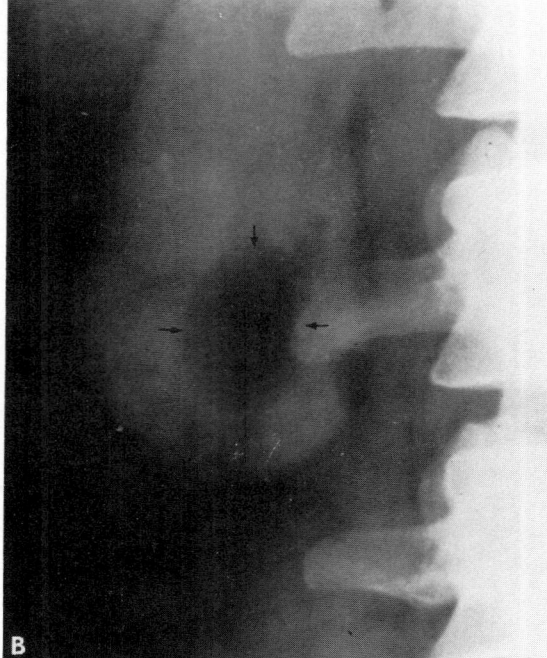

Figure 16–59. Radiologic appearance of gallstones. A_1 and A_2, *In vitro* radiographs showing a variety of calculi. The large uncalcified stones are likely to be composed predominantly of cholesterol. Note how often radiolucent fissures are present (A_2). *B,* Oral cholecystogram demonstrating a functioning gallbladder with a single large calculus (arrows). Chenodeoxycholic acid is most effective in these circumstances. *C,* A variety of opaque gallstones in cholecystogram. The calcifications in C_4 and C_5 are unusual because they are located in the center of the calculi.

Illustration continued on the opposite page

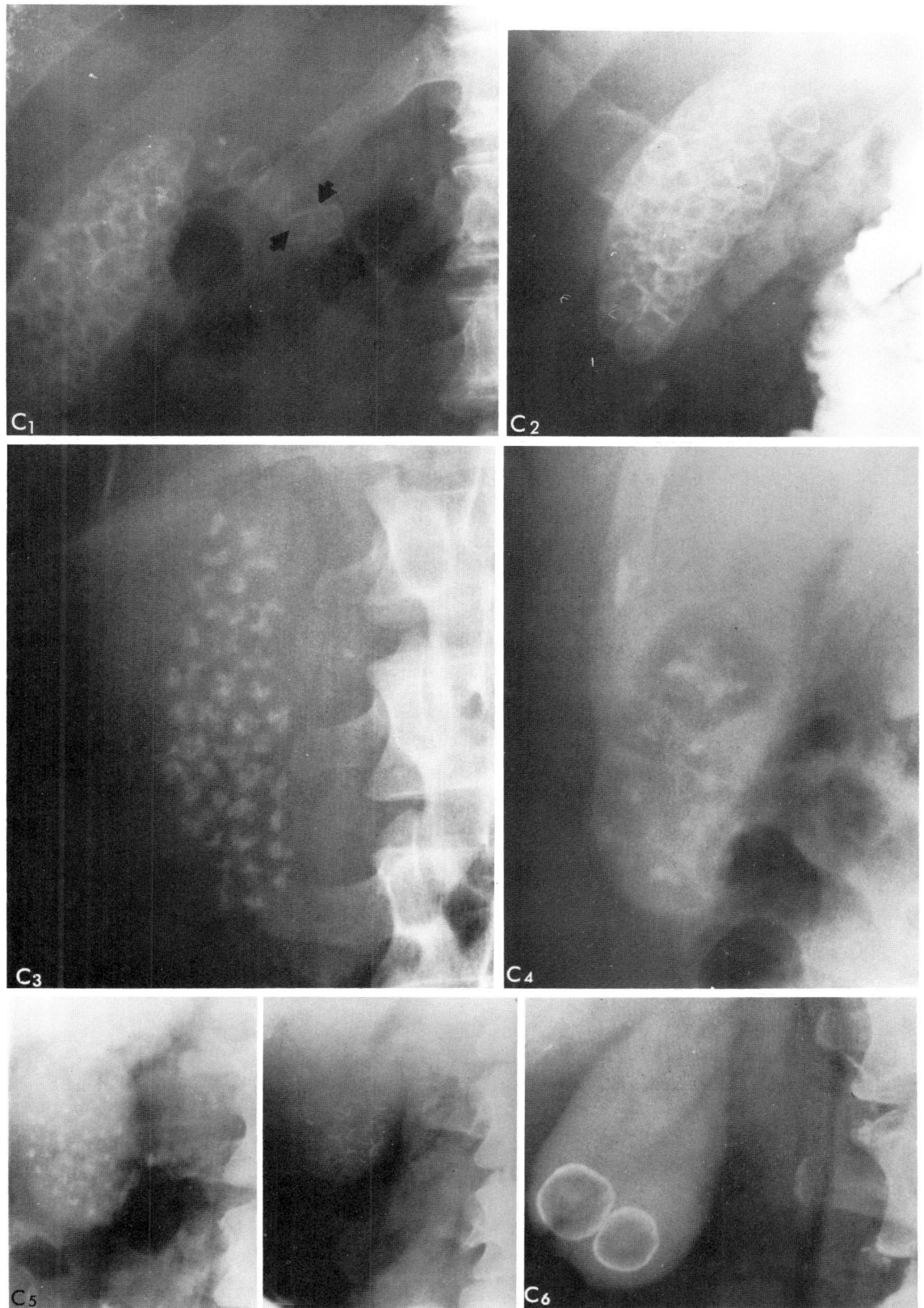

Figure 16–59 Continued.

cholesterol gallstones is thought to proceed through several stages; saturation of bile with cholesterol, crystallization of cholesterol, and finally stone growth.[8, 9, 12] The cause of pigment stone formation is unknown. In Japan, *Escherichia coli* is found in the bile of most patients with pigment stones. Parasites are the nidus for pigment stones in many Oriental countries, and it is possible that infection is an etiologic factor. The role of infection is probably not important in cholesterol gallstones. In this country, only 5 to 10 per cent of bile cultured at cholecystectomy contains bacteria.

At present, the standard treatment for symptomatic gallstones is cholecystectomy. However, dissolving cholesterol gallstones with drugs is now possible in some cases. Chenodeoxycholic acid (a bile acid) given orally for months to several years can completely dissolve cholesterol gallstones or reduce their size sufficiently to allow spontaneous passage into the duodenum. Periodic oral cholecystography can monitor the efficacy of the treatments. Radiopaque and pigment stones are not affected by this drug. Results are poor if the gallbladder is nonfunctioning radiologically. Results with ductal stones also have been disappointing. Chenodeoxycholic acid treatment is usually reserved for patients who refuse surgery or who are poor operative risks. Side effects have been mainly diarrhea, abnormal hepatic enzymes, and possible liver damage. There are no data on the value or necessity of long-term maintenance therapy to prevent recurrence after successful dissolution.

Opinions vary concerning prophylactic cholecystectomy in patients with asymptomatic gallstones. However, the risk of developing carcinoma of the gallbladder is probably not sufficient to warrant prophylactic surgery.

Chronic Cholecystitis

Chronic cholecystitis is usually associated with gallstones. It often presents as recurrent episodes of biliary colic or bouts of acute cholecystitis. The pain is usually in

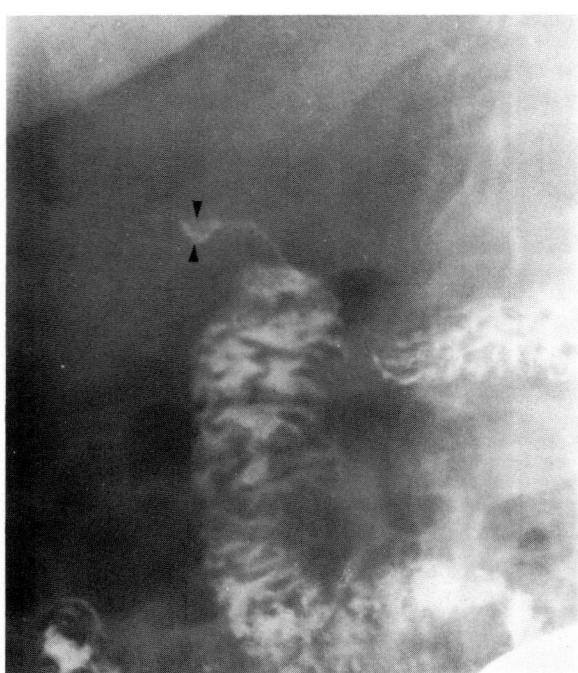

Figure 16–60. Scarred, shrunken gallbladder. Patient with chronic cholecystitis and a nonfunctioning gallbladder on oral cholecystography. The upper gastrointestinal series shows a fistula from the duodenum to the tiny gallbladder (arrowheads).

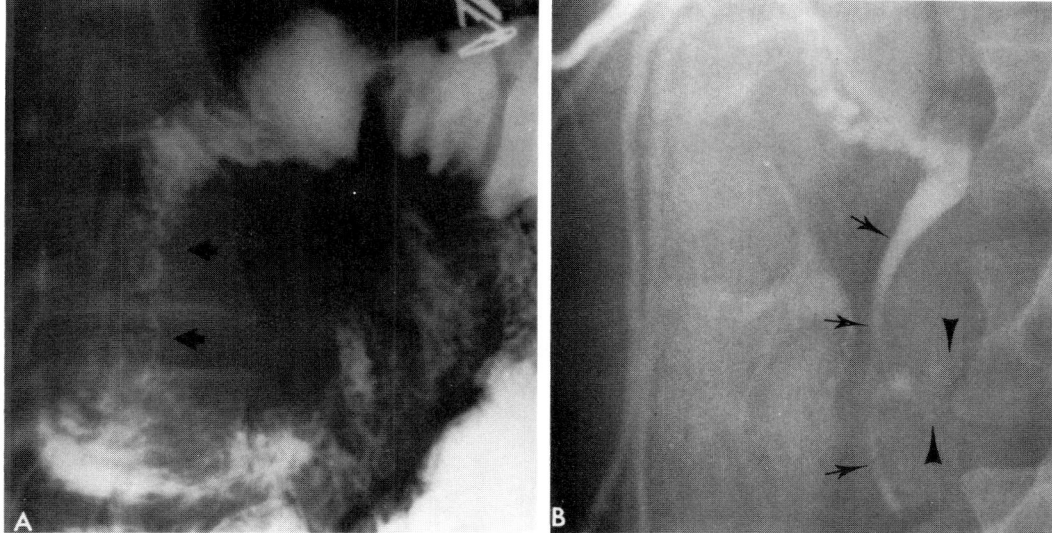

Figure 16-61. Gallstone pancreatitis. *A*, An upper gastrointestinal series showing spasm of the descending duodenum (arrows) in a patient with acute recurrent pancreatitis. *B*, Transhepatic cholangiogram showing a smoothly tapered, long, narrowed common bile duct (arrows) characteristic of chronic pancreatitis. This patient also had pancreatic calcifications (arrowheads) and a pseudocyst displacing the common bile duct away from the spine. These latter features are much more frequently seen in alcoholic than in gallstone pancreatitis.

the right upper abdomen or epigastrium and may radiate to the back. Right upper quadrant tenderness is frequently the only physical finding. The presence of icterus suggests obstruction from a common duct stone. Repeated attacks result in gradual loss of gallbladder function. The end result is a shrunken, scarred gallbladder (Fig. 16-60). Many disorders, including gastritis, ulcers, hiatus hernia, pancreatitis, and colon or kidney lesions, may mimic chronic cholecystitis.

In many individuals, chronic "dyspepsia" is the major complaint. Dyspepsia usually refers to indigestion, discomfort relieved by belching, and intolerance to fatty foods. Dyspepsia is not specific for gallbladder disease, and after cholecystectomy there is a relatively high rate of recurrence of these symptoms (see the section on postcholecystectomy syndrome).

These complications of chronic calculous cholecystitis include pancreatitis, obstructive jaundice, gallstone ileus, and possibly carcinoma of the gallbladder. In England, approximately two thirds of patients with acute pancreatitis have gallstones (Fig. 16-61). Removal of the stones usually prevents recurrent attacks.[10]

The diagnosis of chronic cholecystitis is based largely on radiography, which is about 95 per cent accurate. In most instances the diagnosis is made by oral cholecystography. The cholecystogram shows either a functioning gallbladder with calculi or a nonopacified gallbladder. Failure to visualize the gallbladder is due either to cystic duct obstruction or to absorption of the contrast through the gallbladder wall. Oral cholecystography may not be necessary if the plain films show gallstones, milk of calcium bile, or a porcelain gallbladder. Ultrasound will confirm the presence of gallstones in a nonopacified gallbladder, and will reveal the size of the gallbladder. Enlarged gallbladders from cystic duct obstruction, whether hydrops, mucocele, or empyema, are best demonstrated by ultrasound (Fig. 16-62). Intravenous cholangiography can be used to uncover common bile duct stones. Opacification of the ducts with failure to

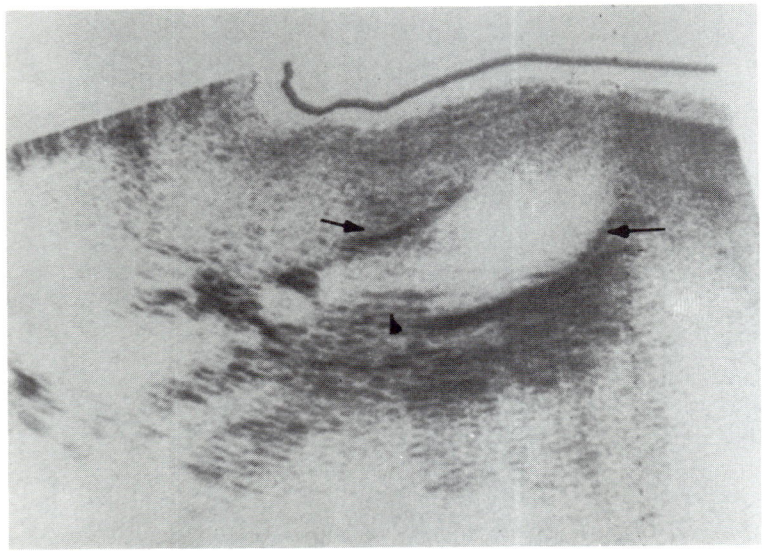

Figure 16–62. Hydrops of the gallbladder. The gallbladder (arrows) is enlarged from chronic cystic duct obstruction. There is a history of previous cholecystitis. Some sediment is seen within the lumen (arrowhead).

visualize the gallbladder on intravenous cholangiography confirms cystic duct obstruction. Opacification of the gallbladder may demonstrate the calculi in a gallbladder that did not visualize on oral cholecystography. Acalculous chronic cholecystitis, which occurs in 2 to 10 per cent of patients, is a more difficult clinical and radiologic diagnosis, and most physicians are reluctant to remove gallbladders that do not contain stones (see the section on acalculous cholecystitis).

Duodenal drainage for bile analysis has been used for a presumptive diagnosis of cholelithiasis. The presence of cholesterol crystals indicates cholesterol stones. This method is infrequently used today but could be helpful in patients who are allergic to iodinated contrast material.

The definitive treatment for chronic cholecystitis is cholecystectomy. Dissolving cholesterol gallstones with oral chenodeoxycholic acid may be useful for aged or inoperable patients. Unfortunately, months to years of treatment are usually needed for dissolution, and lifetime maintenance therapy may be necessary to prevent recurrence.

Acalculous Cholecystitis

Acute and chronic cholecystitis are not always associated with gallstones. In the past, bacterial infection was implicated as a cause of cholecystitis, especially in patients with typhoid fever, but today primary infection of the gallbladder is rare. About 1 per cent of cases of cholecystitis are caused by neoplasms of the gallbladder obstructing the cystic duct (Fig. 16–63). Other causes of acalculous cholecystitis include major abdominal surgery, abdominal trauma, severe burns, chronic renal failure, and compromised blood supply to the gallbladder from arteritis or collagen disease. A substantial number of patients with emphysematous chlecystitis do not have gallstones. The suggested etiology of this condition is compromise of the cystic artery.

In most cases of acalculous cholecystitis, however, no cause can be determined. This condition has been referred to as acalculous cholecystitis, biliary dyskinesia, and cystic duct syndrome.

Several radiographic tests are used to help diagnose acalculous cholecystitis. Regardless of the etiology, a nonopacified gallbladder on oral cholecystography is indicative of cholecystitis. However, in patients with chronic acalculous cholecystitis and a functioning gallbladder, the diagnosis is very difficult. Various radiographic studies have been recommended for this group, and their value is controversial. These tests are based on the contractibility of the gallbladder. In the United States, very little significance is attributed to the function of the gallbladder, and a fatty meal stimulus is frequently not a routine part of oral cholecystography.

Adams and Foxley[17] state that persistent opacification of the gallbladder 36 hours or longer after oral cholecystography is diagnostic of acalculous cholecystitis but this is refuted by recent reports.[18] Prolonged visualization possibly is due to enterohepatic recirculation of the contrast agent or to a lack of stimulus for gallbladder contraction.[19]

Cholecystokinin cholecystography[19, 21] is a test designed to diagnose acalculous cholecystitis or biliary dyskinesia. Cholecystokinin (CCK) is a hormone, activated by fat in the small intestine, that causes gallbladder contraction. The test is performed by injecting CCK intravenously and obtaining serial radiographs of the opacified gallbladder from 1 to 15 minutes. There is no unanimity as to what constitutes a positive study, but most believe it should include two components: (1) reproduction of the patient's symptoms, and (2) emptying of the gallbladder less than 20 to 50 per cent, the presence of irregular spastic contractions, or both (Fig. 16–64).

Several authors[21, 23] have reported good results when CCK cholecystography was used to select patients for surgery. On the other hand, Dunn et al.[20] concluded that the CCK test is of little value in diagnosis.

Another procedure for diagnosing acalculous chronic cholecystitis is infusion tomography of the gallbladder. Although quite reliable in acute cholecystitis, this study is much less accurate in chronic cholecystitis. A thickened gallbladder wall (greater than 1 mm) on one or more radiographs following the intravenous injection of a water-soluble contrast agent is considered a positive result.

Fat in the gallbladder wall has been described as a radiographic sign of chronic cholecystitis. This is an uncommon finding, since there is rarely sufficient fat to be visualized radiographically.[22]

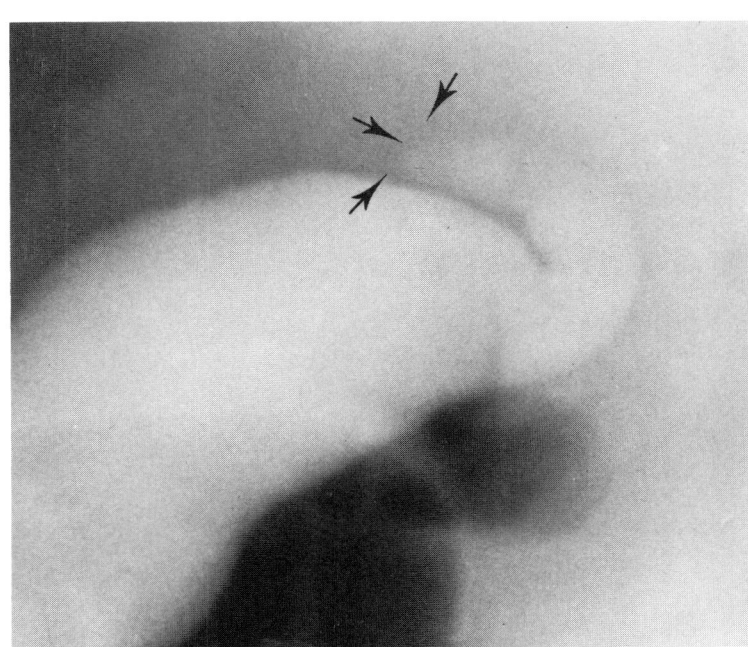

Figure 16–63. Tumor in cystic duct. Chronic cystic duct obstruction (arrows) is caused by a hepatoma invading the cystic duct. The contrast entered the gallbladder during a transhepatic cholangiogram, and shortly thereafter the cystic duct became obstructed. At autopsy one month later, the gallbladder was filled with semisolid bile and contrast.

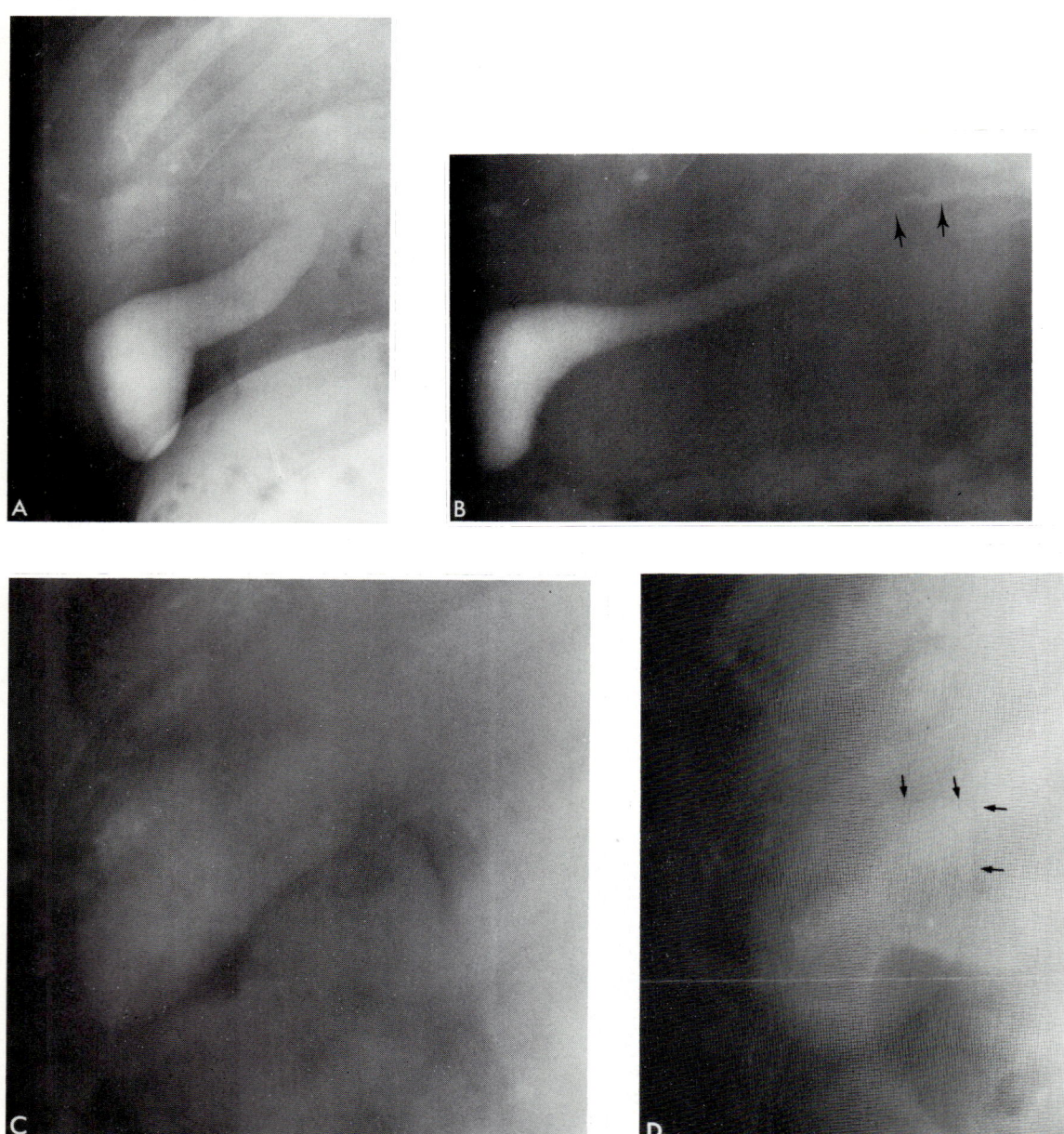

Figure 16–64. Cholecystokinin (CCK) cholecystography. *A* and *B*, Normal CCK test. *A*, Prior to CCK. *B*, Five minutes after cholecystokinin, the gallbladder contracted symmetrically and emptied greater than 50 per cent of its volume. The cystic duct (arrows) is normal. *C* and *D*, Positive CCK test. *C*, Prior to CCK (arrows). After the administration of CCK, the patient's symptoms recurred. *D*, The gallbladder did not empty but assumed a "fighting" or "football" configuration (arrows); that is, it appeared to be trying to empty against a closed cystic duct.

CHOLEDOCHOLITHIASIS

In the United States, 12 to 15 per cent of persons with gallstones also have calculi in the bile ducts. The incidence of choledocholithiasis is considerably higher in patients whose gallbladders do not opacify during oral cholecystography. Only rarely (less than 1 per cent of cases) in Western countries are stones found in the bile ducts and not in the gallbladder. In the Far East, however, primary ductal calculi are common. Possibly the high incidence of parasitic infestation in the Far East is responsible.[26, 29, 31, 33]

In 2 to 10 per cent of patients after cholecystectomy, bile duct stones are found. The vast majority are retained stones that formed in the gallbladder, passed through the cystic duct, and were overlooked during surgery. In patients with T-tubes, retained calculi discovered on the tube cholangiogram can usually be removed without reoperation by basket extraction. Patients without T-tubes may develop symptoms from retained stones from several days to several years after cholecystectomy and usually need reoperation. Occasionally, stones in intrahepatic radicles are difficult to remove at surgery and are intentionally left in place with the hope that they can be removed by basket extraction at a later date.

There is no doubt that stones can also form in the bile ducts after removal of the gallbladder. These primary bile duct stones are also termed stasis or earthly stones. They are ovoid, light brown, very soft, and easily fragmented.

The incidence of retained bile duct stones following cholecystectomy has been significantly reduced by the routine use of operative cholangiography. This procedure uncovers unsuspected duct stones in 3 to 8 per cent of cases. However, despite common duct exploration and operative cholangiography, the incidence of retained calculi remains significant. A major cause is over-reliance on technically poor operative cholangiograms. Rapid communication between the surgeon and the radiologist, good quality films, adequate filling of the ducts, and use of diluted contrast material all contribute to a good cholangiogram and will keep the number of retained stones to a minimum.

In the absence of an indwelling T-tube the choice of radiographic studies to confirm the presence of bile duct stones depends on several factors, including the facilities available, the patient's clinical status, and the liver function tests. Plain films of the abdomen are rarely helpful, since only about 5 per cent of the bile duct stones contain enough calcium to be radiopaque.[30]

Intravenous cholangiography is frequently used to uncover ductal calculi, but is often unrewarding. Demonstration of common bile duct stones is successful in only 50 to 70 per cent. The diagnostic accuracy can be improved if indirect signs of partial ductal obstruction, such as the time-density retention concept, are appreciated (see the section on intravenous cholangiography). Even under optimal circumstances, intrahepatic ductal stones are only rarely visualized by this modality. In addition, even mildly abnormal liver function substantially reduces ductal opacification.

The four-day cholecystographic (Telepaque) test (Fig. 16–65) has been used with moderate success to demonstrate bile duct calculi.[28, 30] Three gms of Telepaque are given daily for four days. On the fifth day, radiographs of the right upper quadrant may show opacification of ductal stones. The calculi become visible because the Telepaque coats the surface, probably as a result of a chemical reaction between the surface biliverdin and the contrast medium. The advantages of this test over intravenous cholangiography are that ductal calculi may opacify even when the patient is moderately jaundiced (serum bilirubin level of up to 5 mg) and that stones in the intrahepatic ducts can also be visualized. However, the major percentage of bile duct calculi are not visualized by this technique.

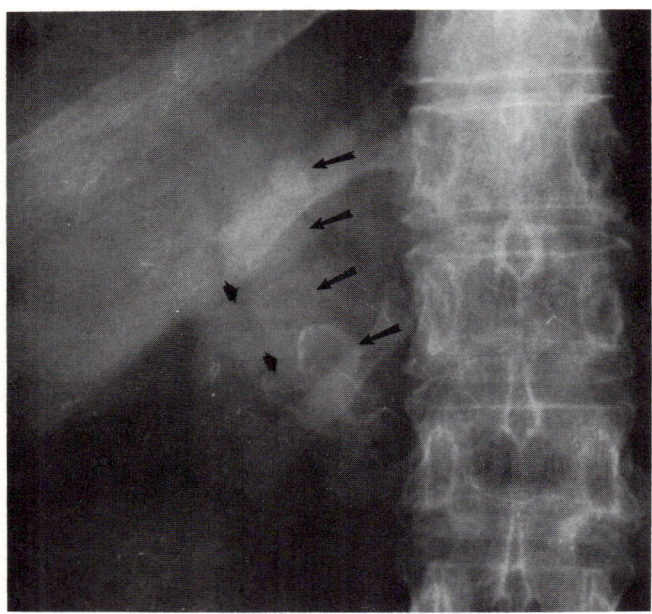

Figure 16–65. Four-day Telepaque test. The preliminary film (not shown) of the right upper quadrant was normal. The patient had a previous cholecystectomy. After four days of Telepaque ingestion, three stones are visible in the common bile duct and one in the left hepatic duct (long arrows). There is faint visualization of the common bile duct (short arrows). (Courtesy of Emanuel Salzman, M.D. *From* Semin. Roentgenol. *11*:171–173, 1976.)

Ultrasound and CT scanning can sometimes demonstrate bile duct stones (see Fig. 16–41), and infrequently an upper gastrointestinal series may suggest a stone impacted in the ampulla of Vater (Fig. 16–66).

The most reliable and definitive preoperative tests to demonstrate ductal calculi are transhepatic cholangiography and to a lesser extent endoscopic retrograde cholangiopancreatography (Fig. 16–67). The complication rate with these procedures has

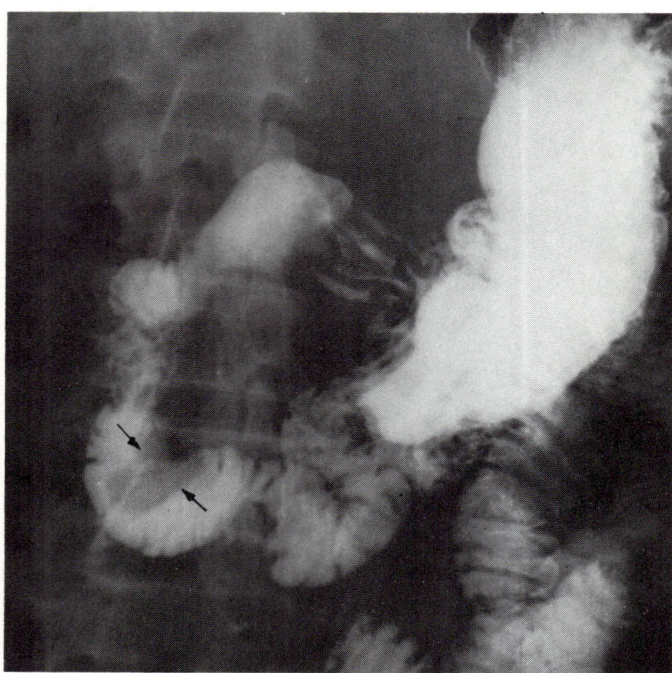

Figure 16–66. Impacted stone. An upper gastrointestinal series on a jaundiced patient shows a filling defect in the region of the ampulla of Vater (arrows) dur to an impacted stone. Other ampullary lesions, such as carcinoma, may have a similar appearance.

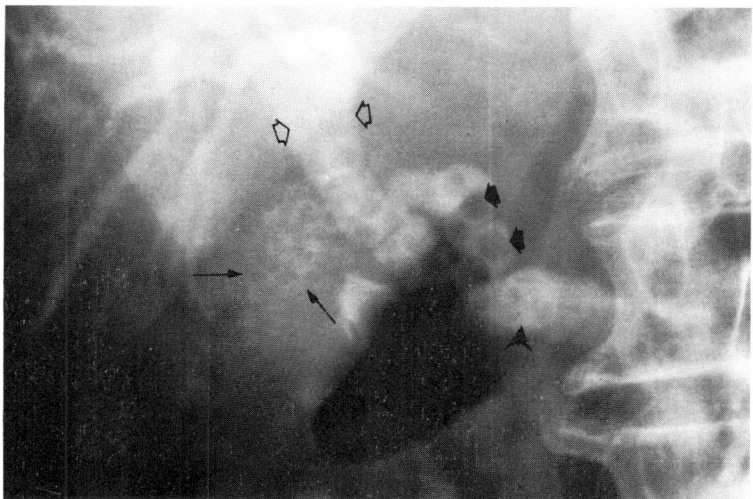

Figure 16–67. Bile duct calculi. Transhepatic cholangiogram demonstrating multiple calculi in the extrahepatic bile ducts (arrowhead), including the cystic duct (short arrows), and the gallbladder (long arrows) and extending into the main intrahepatic ducts (open arrows). The patient was only mildly symptomatic and had slightly abnormal liver function tests. Visualization of calculi in the cystic and intrahepatic ducts is quite uncommon by less invasive procedures, such as intravenous cholangiography.

become minimal. Either of these tests should be employed when clinically suspected calculi are not demonstrated by the less invasive studies and when abnormal liver function tests preclude intravenous cholangiography.

Stones in the bile ducts can remain asymptomatic for many years, and sometimes may pass spontaneously into the duodenum. However, the incidence of complications is sufficiently high to warrant surgical removal.[27] The complications of choledocholithiasis include cholangitis (both nonsuppurative and suppurative), pancreatitis, hepatic abscesses, secondary biliary cirrhosis with portal hypertension, and fistulas to the duodenum or colon (Fig. 16–68).[27, 31, 32]

Ascending cholangitis can result from partial obstruction of bile drainage by calculi. The symptoms vary considerably. In nonsuppurative cholangitis (the most common type), Charcot's triad of abdominal pain (biliary colic), fever, and jaundice is usual. The patient is not very toxic, and symptoms usually subside with antibiotics in 24 to 48 hours. Recurrent attacks of cholangitis can result in fibrosis and stenosis of the sphincter of Oddi. If superimposed purulent bacterial infection develops in the obstructed bile ducts (acute suppurative cholangitis), the patient is extremely ill with systemic symptoms, septicemia, and possibly septic shock. Emergency surgery is required to decompress the biliary system.

Multiple hepatic abscesses may develop from prolonged ascending cholangitis. Once established, neither surgical nor antibiotic treatment is very successful. Often, progressive deterioration from persistent sepsis ends in death.

Secondary biliary cirrhosis is a rare complication of bile duct calculi, usually developing over several years of intermittent obstruction. Once present, it can progress to hepatic failure, portal hypertension and bleeding esophageal varices.

An unusual complication is Mirizzi's syndrome, which is partial common hepatic duct obstruction due to a stone impacted in the cystic duct or gallbladder neck (Fig. 16–91G). The chronic inflammatory reaction from the stone causes shortening of the cystic duct and eventual compression and partial obstruction of the adjacent common hepatic duct. Episodes of cholangitis can occur. Eventually the stone erodes into the common hepatic duct, creating a single cavity and obstructive jaundice. Cholangiographic findings include narrowing and displacement of the common hepatic duct. The duct is usually displaced medially, but the direction varies depending on the anatomic

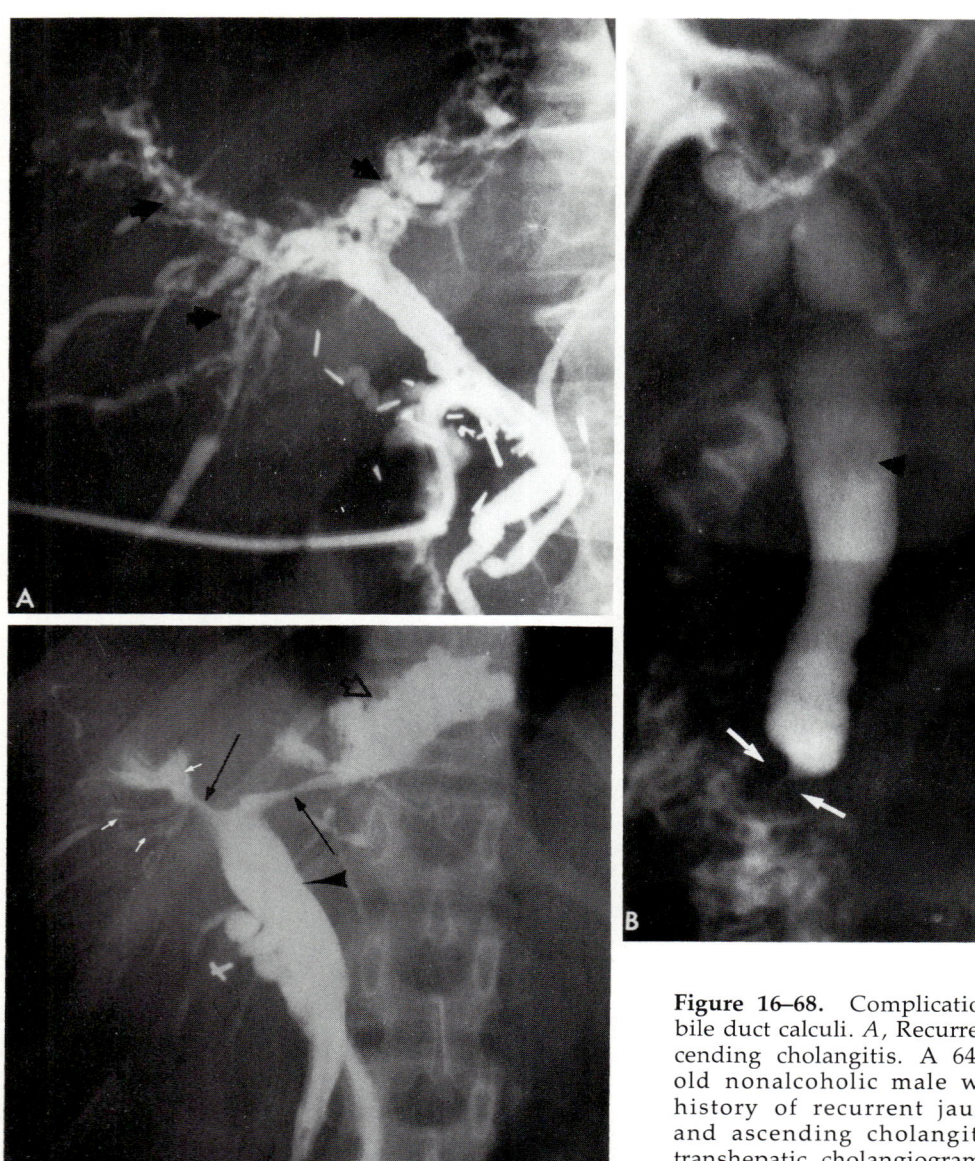

Figure 16–68. Complications of bile duct calculi. *A,* Recurrent ascending cholangitis. A 64-year-old nonalcoholic male with a history of recurrent jaundice and ascending cholangitis. A transhepatic cholangiogram (not shown) demonstrated normal-caliber extrahepatic ducts, poor visualization of the intrahepatic ducts, and gallstones. At surgery, there were gallstones. and a common bile duct stone. The operative cholangiogram showed marked distortion and beading of the intrahepatic ducts (arrows). The pathologic report confirmed the diagnosis of chronic cholangitis. *B,* Fibrosis of the sphincter of Oddi. The patient had recurrent bouts of cholangitis from stones. There is narrowing of the distal common bile duct (arrows) as it enters the duodenum. The proximal ducts are dilated. There is a calculus in the mid-common bile duct (arrowhead). *C,* Pyogenic cholangitis in a patient with recurrent episodes of fever, chills, and jaundice. There are several strictures (long arrows), and the common hepatic duct is enlarged (arrowhead). The intrahepatic branches opacify poorly. There are calculi in the right intrahepatic ducts (short arrows). The irregular collection of contrast at the distal left hepatic duct (open arrow) may represent an abscess or extravasation, possibly caused by manipulation with a Fogarty catheter. (Courtesy of Seth Glick, M.D.)

location of the cystic duct. Because of the distorted anatomy and the chronic inflammation, serious ductal injury may result if the condition goes unrecognized at surgery. The common hepatic duct may be mistaken for the cystic duct and ligated.

Biliary tract calculi can cause pancreatitis, but the exact pathogenesis of gallstone pancreatitis has not been established. Obstruction of the pancreatic duct by a stone in the common bile duct is a possible explanation but most patients do not have ductal stones at the time of surgery. Possibly, repeated passage of gallstones through the common bile duct into the duodenum is responsible. Whatever the mechanism, removal of the stones is curative in 95 per cent of cases.

In patients without T-tubes, surgery is the usual method for removal of bile duct stones.

Endoscopic retrograde sphincterotomy (ERS) is a new procedure for removing common bile duct stones.[32] ERS is used mainly in European countries but is gaining popularity in the United States. An endoscope is passed into the duodenum to the ampulla of Vater. The ampullary and sphincter tissues are incised, allowing the calculus to pass into the duodenum. The procedure is reported to be successful in 92 per cent of patients. The major use of ERS at present is in patients who are poor surgical risks.

Medical therapy for common bile duct stones has not proved beneficial. Oral chenodeoxycholic acid is the only dissolving agent available and is more effective for gallstones than for ductal calculi. Dissolution takes six months to several years.

The treatment of choice in patients with T-tubes is the nonoperative basket extraction technique under fluoroscopic guidance, popularized by Burhenne.[24, 25] It is a safe and highly reliable procedure that can be performed on an outpatient basis, usually without premedication. Successful removal of calculi ranges from 75 to 95 per cent. Intrahepatic stones may be more difficult to extract. However, basket extraction of intrahepatic calculi is more successful and safer than the blind instrumentation techniques used in surgery.

Nearly all retained stones can be extracted if the surgeon creates a short, direct path for the externalized limb of the T-tube. Preferably, the limb should be brought out through a lateral stab wound as nearly perpendicular to the common bile duct as possible. Also important is the use of a large-bore T-tube (if smaller than 14F, extraction is more difficult). Objections to using large T-tubes could be overcome if tubes were specially manufactured with small-diameter intraductal limbs and an exteriorized limb of 14F or larger.

A variety of instruments are available for removing stones. The basic equipment consists of a steerable catheter that can be directed to the site of the calculi and a basket or forceps to grip the stone (Fig. 16–69).

Basket extractions should be performed four to six weeks after surgery to allow time for a fibrous tract to form around the T-tube. The initial step is to repeat the cholangiogram to ascertain the presence and location of the calculi. The T-tube is then removed, and a steerable catheter is guided through the sinus tract into the bile duct. The catheter can be directed cephalad into the intrahepatic ducts or caudad toward the ampulla. The tip of the catheter should be positioned just beyond the stone. A collapsible basket is then inserted through the catheter and opened near the stone. In most instances, the stone readily engages in the basket. The entire unit with the entrapped stone is then withdrawn through the sinus tract (Fig. 16–70). The procedure can be repeated as often as necessary to remove all the stones. A soft rubber catheter is then left in place for one or more days until the edema resulting from the procedure has subsided.

To date, no fatalities have been reported (compared with a 3 per cent mortality for reoperation). Morbidity occurs in about 5 per cent of patients. Reported complications

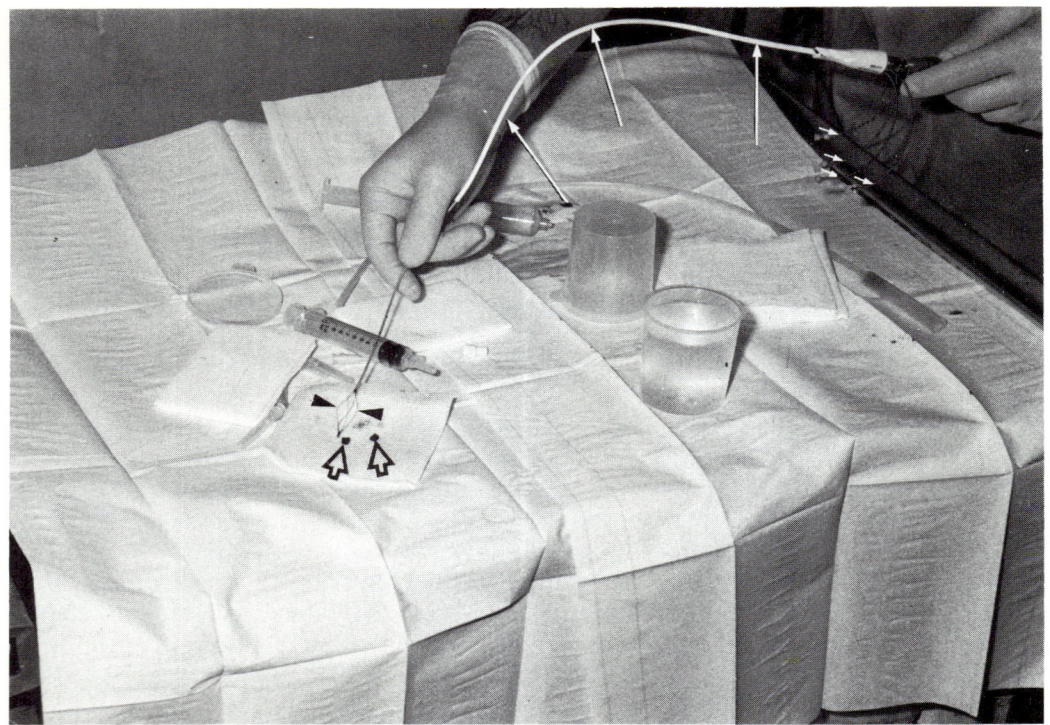

Figure 16–69. Equipment for basket extraction of bile duct calculi. The white, steerable catheter (arrows) is inserted through the T-tube tract can be directed to any part of the biliary tree by pulling the wires on the end (small arrows). Once positioned, the basket (arrowheads) is inserted through the catheter to entrap the stones. The whole unit is then removed. In this patient, two common bile duct calculi (open arrows) were extracted.

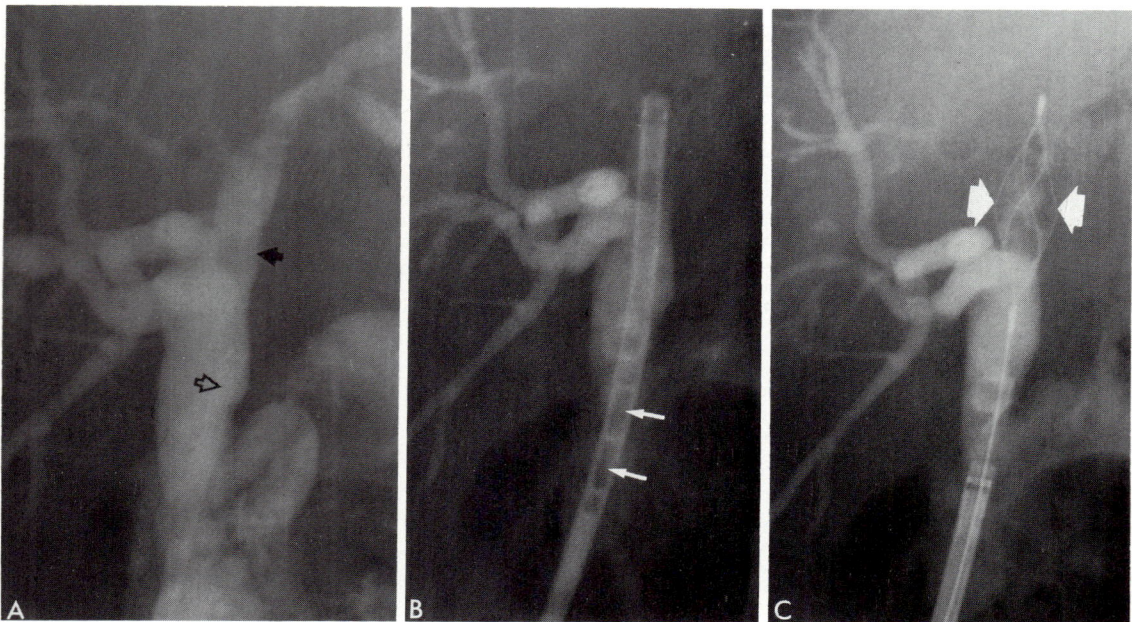

Figure 16–70. Basket extraction of bile duct stones. Patient with multiple intraductal calculi. All eight to ten stones were successfully removed. A, Extraction of calculus in proximal left hepatic duct (arrow). The T-tube was removed and the steerable catheter inserted (open arrow). B, The catheter is positioned just beyond the stone. There are multiple air bubbles in the catheter (arrows). C, The basket (arrows) is inserted through the catheter, and the stone is engaged and removed.

include fever from instrumentation, perforation of the sinus tract, pancreatitis, sepsis, and vagotonic shock.[25] In most instances, the complications are not severe and resolve in several days.

Attempts to dissolve ductal stones by infusing various agents through indwelling T-tubes have had only limited success. Several drugs, such as chloroform, ether, heparin, and chenodeoxycholic acid, have been tried. Cholic acid is currently considered the best dissolving agent. Unfortunately, one to six weeks of hospitalization are usually necessary for dissolution. In addition, cholic acid often causes uncomfortable side effects, such as right upper quadrant pain, mild pancreatitis, and diarrhea. The use of dissolving agents probably should be reserved for those patients in whom basket extraction is unsuccessful.

SCLEROSING CHOLANGITIS

Sclerosing cholangitis is an uncommon disease of unknown etiology.[34-40] It is usually classified as primary or secondary, depending on whether it occurs alone or in association with other diseases, such as ulcerative colitis. The characteristic feature is multiple areas of fibrosis causing extensive narrowing of the bile ducts. The extrahepatic ducts are almost always involved. The intrahepatic ducts are affected somewhat less often, although, rarely, the disease is limited to the intrahepatic ducts. Sclerosing cholangitis is more common in males and has been reported in all age groups except infancy.

The clinical manifestations are variable. Obstructive jaundice is the main feature. The jaundice may be intermittent initially but usually becomes progressive. Recurrent episodes of bacterial cholangitis are common. The liver may be enlarged and occasionally tender. Chronic biliary obstruction may result in secondary biliary cirrhosis with portal hypertension. Pathologically, there is inflammation and fibrosis of the wall of the involved bile ducts. The outer diameter of the ducts is often normal, but the inner diameter is narrowed or even obliterated. At surgery, the ducts are described as cordlike, resembling thrombosed veins. The ductal mucosa is usually normal. Lymph nodes in the region of the porta hepatis are often hyperplastic from the chronic inflammatory process. The cause of sclerosing cholangitis is unknown. Bacterial, viral, and autoimmune origins have been proposed but not substantiated.

Secondary sclerosing cholangitis may be associated with ulcerative colitis, scleroderma, regional enterocolitis, thrombocytopenia purpura, Riedel's struma, retro-orbital tumors, retroperitoneal fibrosis, and mediastinal fibrosis. The most commonly associated condition is ulcerative colitis. About 1 per cent of patients with ulcerative colitis develop sclerosing cholangitis, and about 25 per cent of patients with sclerosing cholangitis have a history of ulcerative colitis.

The diagnosis of sclerosing cholangitis is based on the radiographic appearance of the bile ducts and on the following prerequisites: absence of previous biliary surgery, abscence of biliary calculi, diffuse involvement of the extrahepatic ducts, and exclusion of bile duct carcinoma by follow-up studies of sufficient duration. Occasionally, widespread fibrosis of the bile ducts occurs after cholecystectomy or even from pancreatitis. Some authorities feel that the presence of calculi should not exclude the diagnosis.

The characteristic x-ray appearance is the presence of strictures, which are of varying length and usually multiple. Between the strictures the ducts may be of normal caliber or slightly dilated, producing a beaded appearance. Marked dilatation proximal to a stricture is quite uncommon and if present should suggest a different etiology, such as carcinoma. There is often diminished branching of the intrahepatic radicles.

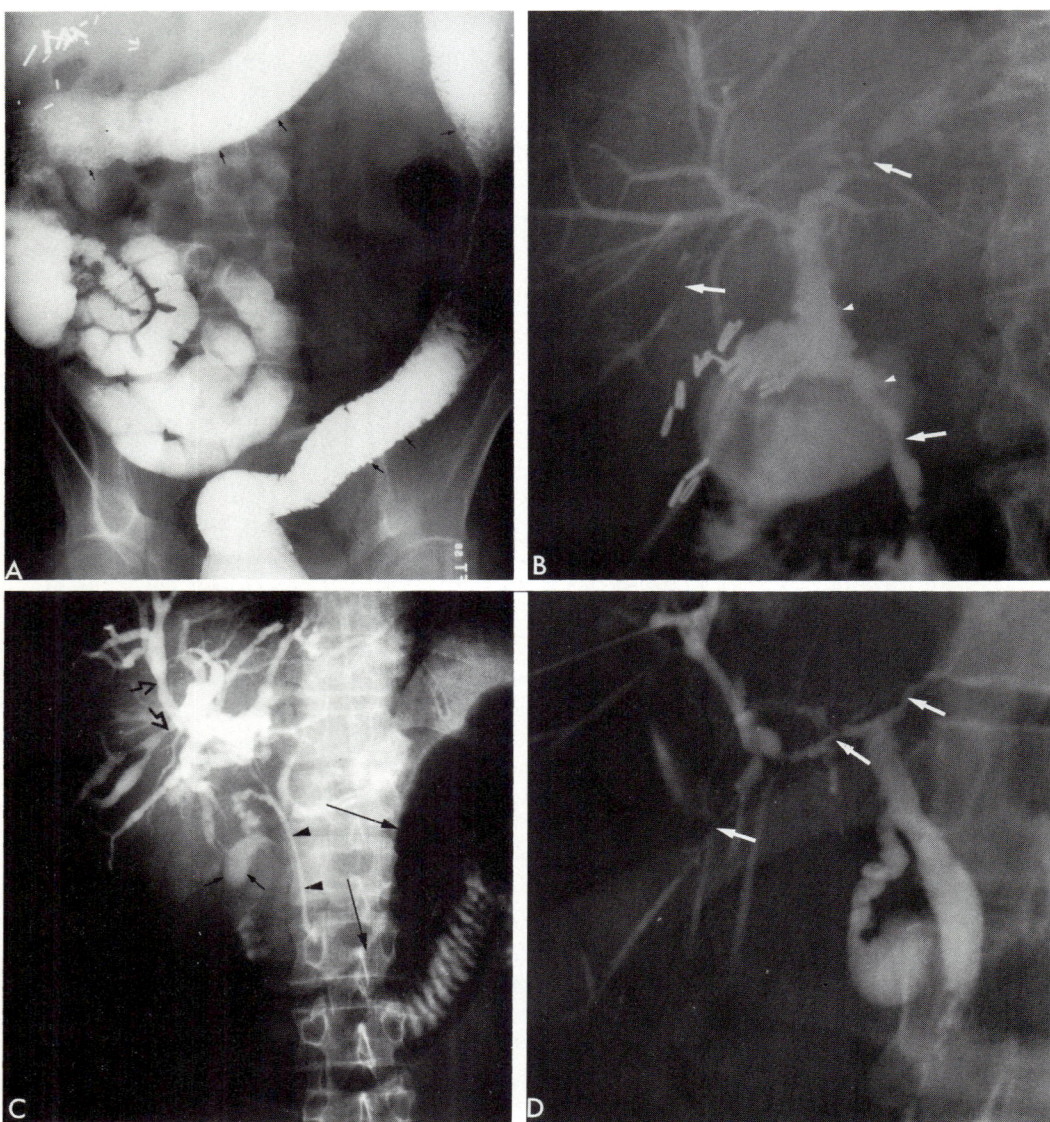

Figure 16–71. Sclerosing cholangitis. *A*, 36-year-old male with panulcerative colitis. The normal haustrations are absent, and there are small ulcerations (arrows). *B*, Operative cholangiogram in the same patient, showing typical features of sclerosing cholangitis. The intra- and extrahepatic ducts are involved. There are multiple strictures (arrows), causing a beaded appearance. Marginal irregularities of the extrahepatic ducts are prominent (arrowheads). *C*, Different patient with ulcerative colitis. The haustrations are absent on the transverse colon (large arrows). The common bile duct is markedly narrowed (arrowheads), and the gallbladder is tiny (small arrows). The typical beaded configuration is seen in the intrahepatic ducts (open arrows). (Courtesy of Carl Larsen, M.D.) *D*, Transhepatic cholangiogram in a 20-year-old male shows the typical strictures (arrows) of sclerosing cholangitis. The case is unusual because of the patient's age.

resulting in a "pruned tree" configuration. Superimposition of cirrhosis causes additional distortion of the intrahepatic ducts. Marginal irregularities of the extrahepatic ducts have also been described and are probably due to small areas of mucosal invaginations (Figs. 16–71 and 16–72).

Oral cholecystography and intravenous cholangiography are usually not useful for diagnosing sclerosing cholangitis because of the elevated serum bilirubin levels and abnormal liver function tests. Preoperatively, the radiologic procedure of choice is ERCP. Usually, the ducts can be opacified and the extent of the disease determined. Transhepatic cholangiography can be diagnostic, but because of the marked narrowing of the intrahepatic ducts it is often technically unsuccessful. If the biliary tract has not been adequately evaluated preoperatively, an operative cholangiogram is essential to determine the extent of disease and to find an optimal site for surgical decompression of the biliary system.

The differential diagnosis of sclerosing cholangitis includes other causes of benign and malignant strictures. A solitary short stricture is usually not due to sclerosing chol-

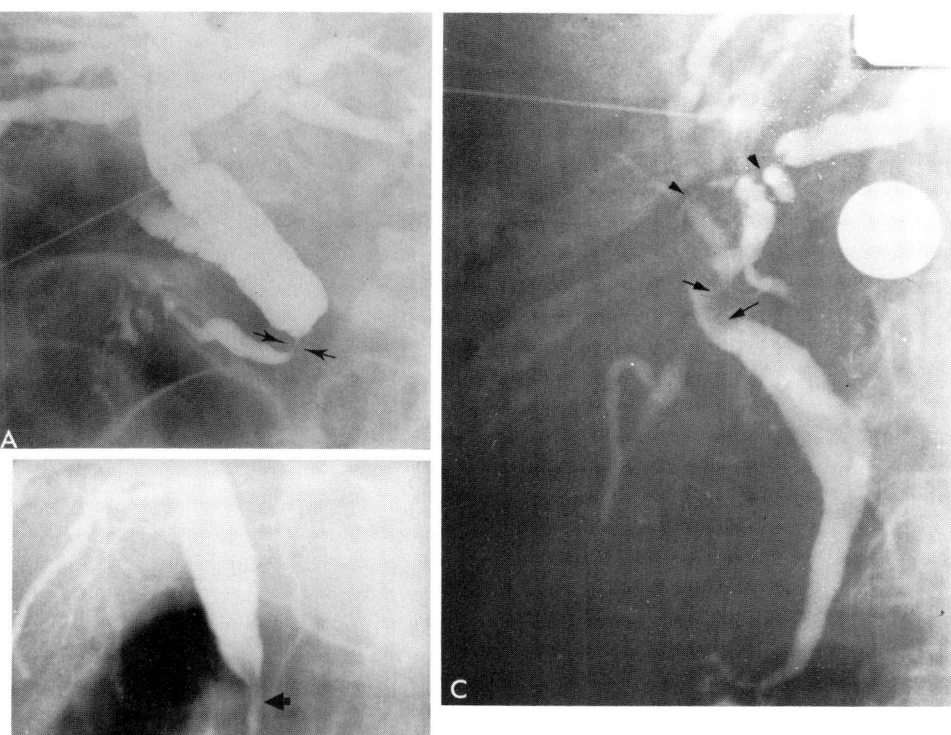

Figure 16–72. Carcinomas simulating stricture or sclerosing cholangitis. *A*, Bile duct carcinoma. Transhepatic cholangiogram showing single stricture of the mid-common bile duct (arrows) caused by a primary bile duct carcinoma. The ducts proximal to the stricture are uniformly dilated. Radiographically, this could be a benign stricture but is unlikely to be sclerosing cholangitis. *B*, Transhepatic cholangiogram. There is a stricture of the common bile duct (arrows) due to pancreatic carcinoma. The proximal ducts are dilated. *C*, Primary bile duct carcinoma. The transhepatic cholangiogram shows narrowing of the proximal common hepatic duct (arrows) as well as many of the intrahepatic ducts (arrowheads). The appearance is similar to that of sclerosing cholangitis.

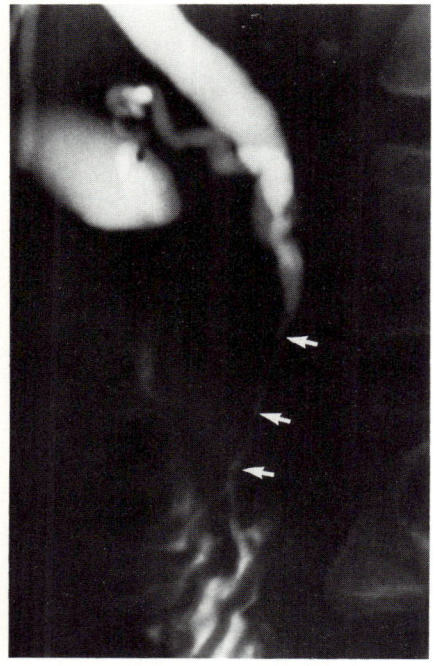

Figure 16–73. Benign stricture of the common bile duct. In a patient with chronic pancreatitis and jaundice, the transhepatic cholangiogram shows a long stricture of the pancreatic portion of the common bile duct (arrows) and proximally dilated ducts. This type of stricture is typically benign.

angitis. Dilatation of the ducts proximal to a short stricture tends to favor other diseases, since the diffuse fibrosis in sclerosing cholangitis usually prevents significant dilatation.

Benign strictures of the biliary tract are most often due to surgical trauma. Other causes include congenital stenoses and inflammatory conditions such as recurrent pancreatitis and gallstones (Fig. 16–73). Rarely, duodenal ulcers that penetrate into the

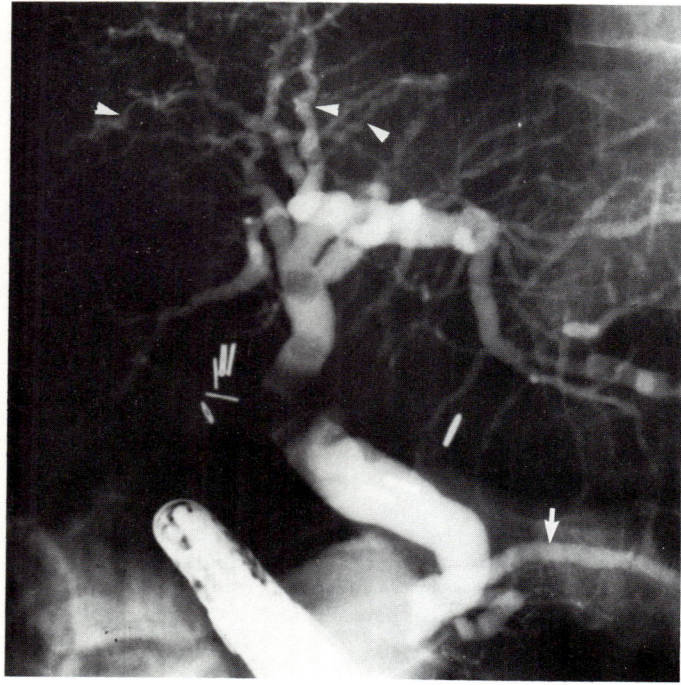

Figure 16–74. Cirrhosis. ERCP in a patient with cirrhosis shows a beaded, tortuous configuration of the intrahepatic ducts (arrowheads). The extrahepatic ducts appeared slightly dilated, but there were no strictures. The radiolucencies are due to air bubbles. The pancreatic duct is also opacified (arrow).

common bile duct can lead to strictures. Occasionally, cirrhosis (especially primary biliary cirrhosis) may cause beading and pruning of the intrahepatic ducts similar to that of sclerosing cholangitis. However, the extrahepatic ducts are normal (Fig. 16–74). Ductal involvement from pancreatic carcinoma can occasionally simulate a benign stricture. Primary adenocarcinoma of the bile ducts commonly appears as a single stricture (see Fig. 16–72).

Occasionally, a primary tumor involves the ducts diffusely, making the radiologic differentiation from sclerosing cholangitis impossible (see Fig. 16–72C). In fact, differentiation in these cases may be difficult surgically and even histologically. There is no reliable evidence that sclerosing cholangitis predisposes to carcinoma of the bile ducts. However, in ulcerative colitis there is a higher incidence of both ductal carcinoma and sclerosing cholangitis. In some patients, these conditions coexist. The prognosis of primary sclerosing cholangitis is uncertain. However, it is generally agreed that attempted treatment is warranted because a number of patients respond to therapy and have prolonged remissions.

Treatment is aimed at decompressing the biliary tract. The feasibility of restoring bile flow depends on the location and extent of the diseases. A bypass procedure should be attempted when possible, otherwise, prolonged T-tube drainage is recommended. Occasionally the lumen of the ducts increases following T-tube decompression, and the T-tube can eventually be removed. Medical management should include the long-term use of steroids. Prolonged administration of antibiotics is generally not recommended. Antibiotics should be given only during episodes of acute cholangitis.

Treatment of secondary sclerosing cholangitis is the same as for the primary form. Coexistent diseases, such as ulcerative colitis, are treated independently. The course and prognosis of sclerosing cholangitis is not affected by the treatment for ulcerative colitis, and even proctocolectomy apparently does not afford protection.

STENOSIS OF THE SPHINCTER OF ODDI, SPASM, AND THE PSEUDOCALCULOUS DEFECT

Stenosis or fibrosis of the sphincter of Oddi[41, 43] is a controversial but probably real entity, resulting in obstruction to the flow of bile and pancreatic secretions (Fig. 16–75; see Fig. 16–68B). It is an uncommon condition, with a two to one female preponderance.

The fibrosis, in the majority of cases, is thought to result from inflammation caused by the passage of biliary stones through the ampulla of Vater. Gallbladder and ductal calculi may or may not be present when the diagnosis is established. Other probable causes of firbosis include inflammation from pancreatitis and injury from surgical manipulation of the sphincter region.

Stenosis of the sphincter of Oddi is thought to be one of the causes of the postcholecystectomy syndrome (the persistence or recurrence of symptoms following cholecystectomy). In addition, stenosis may be a cause of recurrent attacks of pancreatitis. The most common clinical manifestations are episodes of obstructive jaundice with attacks of biliary colic. The serum bilirubin and alkaline phosphatase values are usually elevated.

The preoperative diagnosis can be suggested when cholangiography demonstrates a dilated common bile duct, with abnormal persistent narrowing in the region of the ampulla. If the bilirubin is elevated, intravenous cholangiography will probably not be useful and more invasive studies, such as transhepatic cholangiography, should be used. At surgery, the diagnosis can be made by operative cholangiography or by mea-

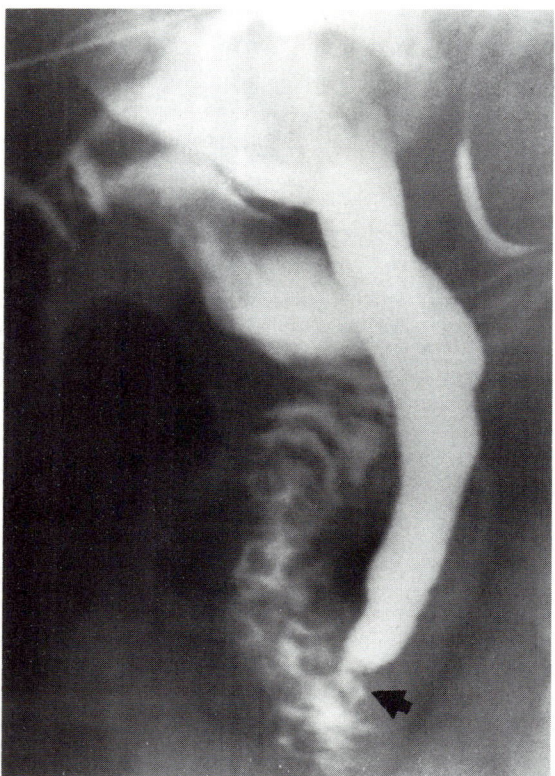

Figure 16–75. Stenosis of the sphincter of Oddi. The patient is a 68-year-old male who had had a cholecystectomy 25 years earlier. He presented with recurrent symptoms and jaundice. A transhepatic cholangiogram showed dilatation of the bile ducts down to the level of the ampulla (arrow). There were no calculi. At surgery, the sphincter was narrowed with considerable fibrosis.

surement of the width of the ampulla with calibrated probes. Treatment consists of biliary bypass procedure. It is important to distinguish spasm of the sphincter of Oddi and the pseudocalculous defect of the distal common duct from actual fibrosis in order to avoid unnecessary surgery.

Spasm of the sphincter[42] may be precipitated by a variety of agents, including morphine sulfate and other narcotic analogs, certain anesthetic agents, operative manipulation of the ampulla, and rapid injection of cold contrast agents. Spasm is usually seen on operative cholangiography but may also be seen on post- or preoperative cholangiography.

The radiographs show tapered narrowing or abrupt termination of the distal common bile duct. If the spasm is severe, no bile enters the duodenum (Fig. 16–76; see Fig. 16–152). A significant feature is the absence of proximal bile duct dilatation. Spasm is temporary and disappears on subsequent examinations, or it can frequently be dissipated by antispasmodics, such as parenteral glucagon or intraductal xylocaine. Spasm and edema from excessive surgical manipulations sometimes result in permanent fibrosis of the sphincter.

The psudocalculous defect[44] is a peculiar roentgenographic appearance that mimics a stone at the distal end of the common bile duct. It is an anatomic variation probably due to prominence or an unusual arrangement of the smooth muscle fibers of the sphincter of Oddi. During contraction, these muscle fibers bulge into the common bile duct, simulating a radiolucent stone. There is no obstruction to bile flow and no proximal ductal dilatation. Antispasmodics do not change the x-ray appearance.

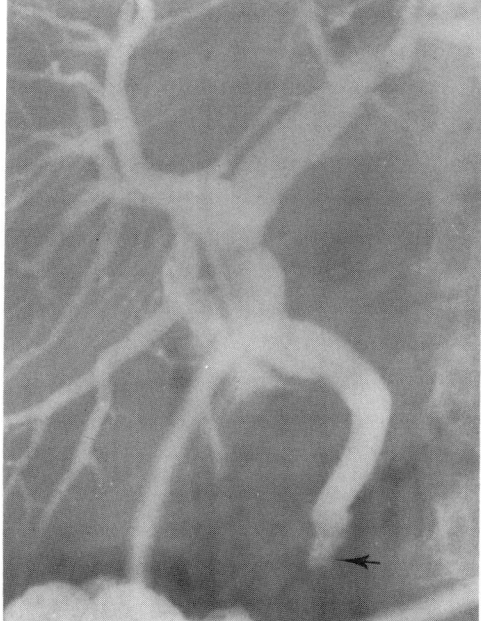

Figure 16–76. Spasm of the sphincter of Oddi. A T-tube cholangiogram shows the typical narrowing of the distal common bile duct (arrow) due to spasm. No contrast entered the duodenum. The distal duct opened normally on the prior operative cholangiogram and a subsequent T-tube study (not shown).

Characteristic of the pseudocalculous defect is its cyclic nature. During the cholangiogram, it appears as the distal common bile duct contracts and disappears as it relaxes. The changing appearance of the distal duct is diagnostic and is usually readily observed fluoroscopically or on cineradiography (Fig. 16–77).

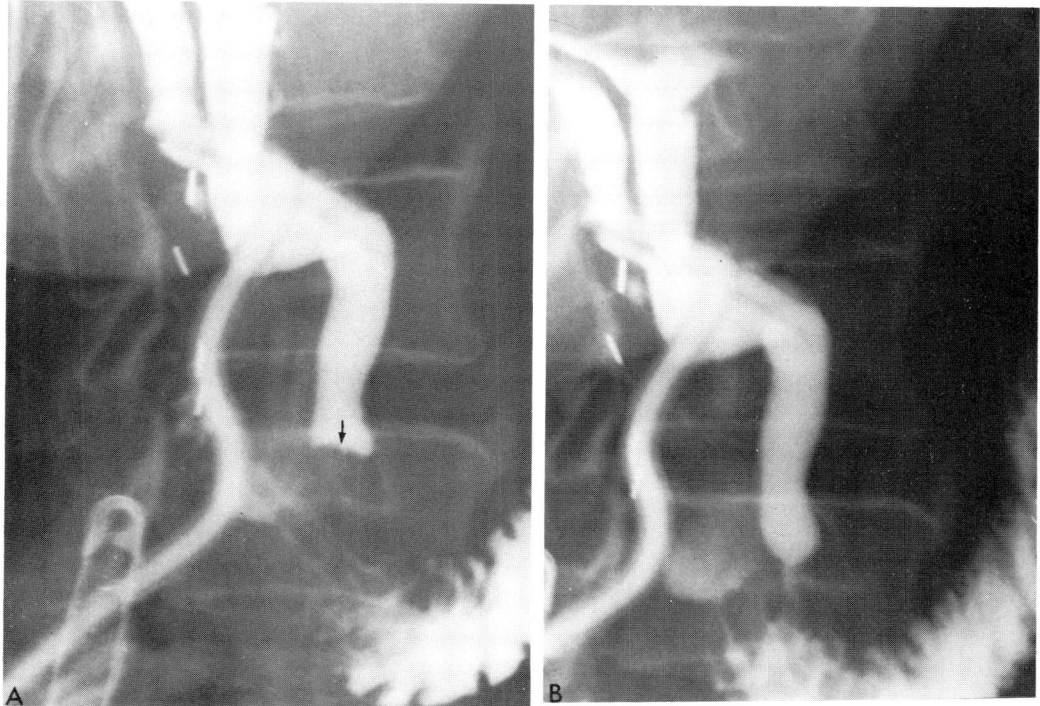

Figure 16–77. Pseudocalculous defect A, The meniscus-like configuration of the distal common bile duct (arrow) resembles a stone. B, The distal duct several seconds later is normal.

HYPERPLASTIC CHOLECYSTOSES

The hyperplastic cholecystoses, or simply cholecystoses, are a group of associated disorders of the gallbladder that appear to be distinct from cholecystitis and gallstones. They are benign, degenerative conditions characterized by excessive proliferation of various components of the gallbladder wall. The cholecystoses include adenomyomatosis, cholesterolosis, neuromatosis, lipomatosis, fibromatosis, and calcified gallbladder wall. The predominant tissues involved determine which of these pathologic conditions is present. Histologically, two or more of the cholecystoses frequently coexist. Adenomyomatosis and cholesterolosis are by far the most common of these entities.[45, 46, 48, 52]

The etiology is unknown, but the disease is presumed to be acquired rather than congenital since no pediatric cases have been reported. The cholecystoses are found in about 5 per cent of cholecystograms,[46, 49] and the incidence increases with age. A high percentage of cases are associated with gallstones.

Adenomyomatosis[45-48, 50, 52] is the most common of the cholecystoses. It is characterized by hyperplasia of the epithelium, thickening of the muscular layer of the gallbladder wall, proliferation of the Rokitansky-Aschoff sinuses (RAS), and strictures. Adenomyomatosis can be classified into three types: generalized, segmental, and fundal. The fundal variety is frequently referred to as an adenomyoma or adenoma of the gallbladder. This terminology is confusing, since it is not a neoplasm. The segmental form is characterized by one or more strictures with a central ostium. The strictures divide the gallbladder into two or more segments. The loculus distal to the stricture is usually the smaller compartment, and often contains calculi. In generalized adenomyomatosis, the entire gallbladder may be surrounded by Rokitansky-Aschoff sinuses.

The radiographic findings in adenomyomatosis include both functional and morphologic alterations. The former consist of hypercontractility of the gallbladder, possibly caused by the increased musculature, and hyperconcentration of the contrast medium, which may be due to the hyperplasia of the mucosa (Fig. 16–78). Associated cholecystitis, however, decreases the hypercontractility and hyperconcentrating ability of the gallbladder. Because the functional changes are largely subjective, alone they are not adequate to establish the diagnosis.

The definitive radiographic findings in all types of adenomyomatosis are the Rokitansky-Aschoff sinuses. On cholecystography, these are seen as oval collections of contrast material adjacent to the gallbladder. They vary from pinpoint dots to 10 mm in size. The Rokitansky-Aschoff sinuses are separated from the gallbladder lumen by a radiolucent line that represents the thickness of the gallbladder wall. In the generalized form, these sinuses form a ring around the entire gallbladder. In segmental adenomyomatosis, the Rokitansky-Aschoff sinuses are seen adjacent to the stricture and often around the distal loculus (Fig. 16–79). They are often best, and occasionally only, visualized after contraction of the gallbladder. Consequently, a fatty meal is indicated in suspected cases. Occasionally, the Rokitansky-Aschoff sinuses are filled with bile or calculi and do not opacify. Rarely, the calculi in the sinuses are opaque and can be seen on plain films.

In the fundal type of adenomyomatosis (adenomyoma), a circumscribed nodule, resembling a tumor mass, develops in the fundus of the gallbladder. The radiologic features are variable and depend on the degree of projection into the gallbladder lumen. Typically, the nodule is visualized as a rounded, fixed filling defect in the fundus of the opacified gallbladder. There may be one or more opaque dots near the center of the mass owing to umbilication of the mucosa. If the adenomyoma is entirely extraluminal, the gallbladder may appear normal or have a somewhat angular fundus. Diagnosis in

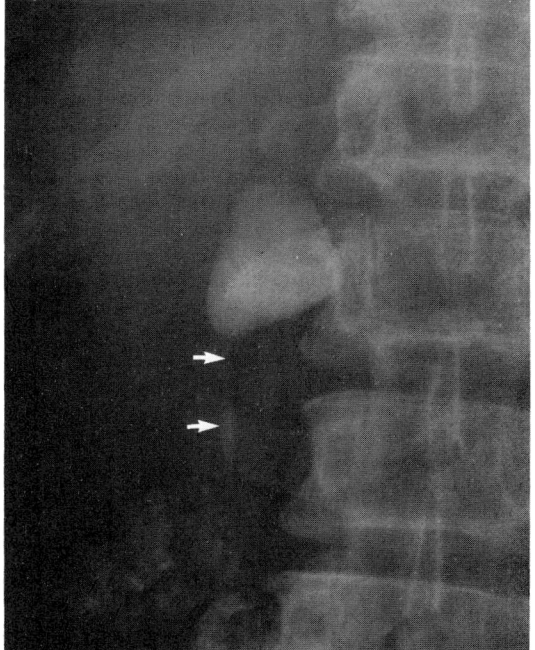

Figure 16–78. Segmental adenomyomatosis—hypercontractility. The post-fatty meal film shows extreme hypercontractility of the distal half of the gallbladder (arrows). Prior to the fatty meal, both segments of the gallbladder were nearly equal in size.

these circumstances depends on demonstrating the Rokitansky-Aschoff sinuses (Fig. 16–80).

Segmental adenomyomatosis should be susepcted when strictures, septa or bands, and nonpostural kinks are demonstrated on cholecystography (Fig. 16–81). The use of a fatty meal usually better delineates these findings and often results in visualization of the Rokitansky-Aschoff sinuses.

Cholesterolosis[45, 51-53] or "strawberry gallbladder" is characterized by abnormal deposits of cholesterol in fat-laden macrophages located in the lamina propria of the gallbladder. The mucosa of the gallbladder may be studded with these small yellowish deposits and resemble the surface of a strawberry. The cholesterol deposits may coalesce to form one or more polyps. However, cholesterol polyps can also occur independently of the diffuse form. Gallstones develop in 50 to 70 per cent of patients, possibly because the cholesterol deposits may act as a nidus.

As in all the cholecystoses, in cholesterolosis there is usually excellent concentration on oral cholecystography and hypercontractility after a fatty meal. Numerous small fixed filling defects due to the cholesterol deposits can sometimes be seen. These are best demonstrated by compression spot films. The small cholesterol deposits may produce an unsharp, finely irregular outline of the gallbladder wall. An irregular contour can also be seen in adenomyomatosis, presumably caused by areas where the wall is thickened and projecting into the lumen (Fig. 16–82).

When the cholesterol deposits are larger, they present as one or more radiolucent filling defects on cholecystography (Fig. 16–83). These cholesterol polyps resemble gallstones, are variable in size, and may involve any portion of the gallbladder. Unlike stones, the polyps remain fixed when the patient's position is changed, a diagnostic feature.

The other forms of hyperplastic cholecystoses, such as neuromatosis and lipomatosis, are much less common; their radiographic appearance is identical to that of adenomyomatosis. The diagnosis is made histologically.

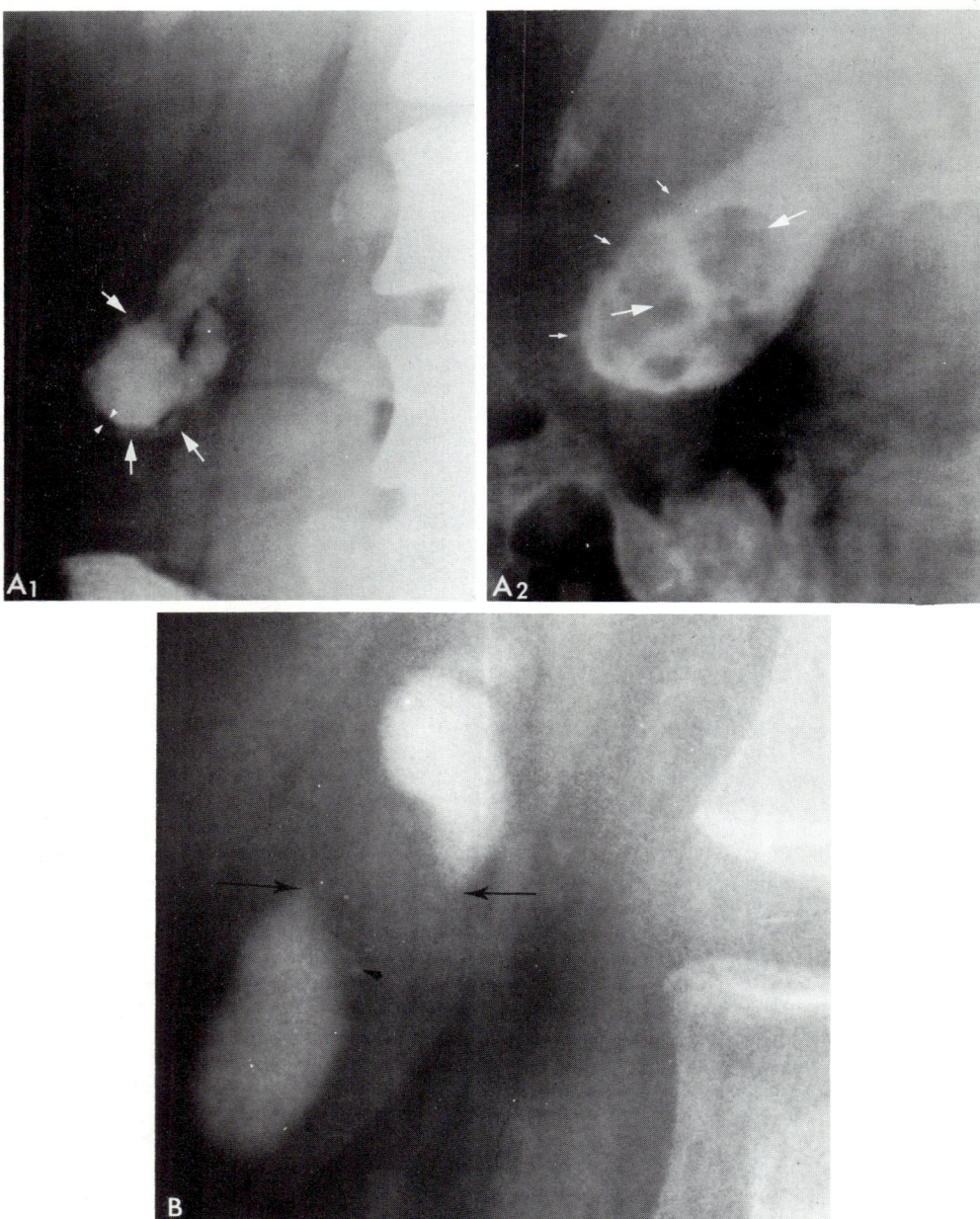

Figure 16–79. Rokitansky-Aschoff sinuses. *A*, 1. Generalized form. There are small collections of contrast (arrows) surrounding the gallbladder. The thin radiolucent line between the Rokitansky-Aschoff sinuses and the gallbladder lumen (arrowheads) represents the thickness of the gallbladder wall. 2. Rokitansky-Aschoff sinuses (small arrows) surround most of the gallbladder. These are multiple gallstones (large arrows). *B*, Segmental adenomyomatosis with a stricture (arrows) and adjacent Rokitansky-Aschoff sinuses (arrowhead).

THE BILIARY SYSTEM — 943

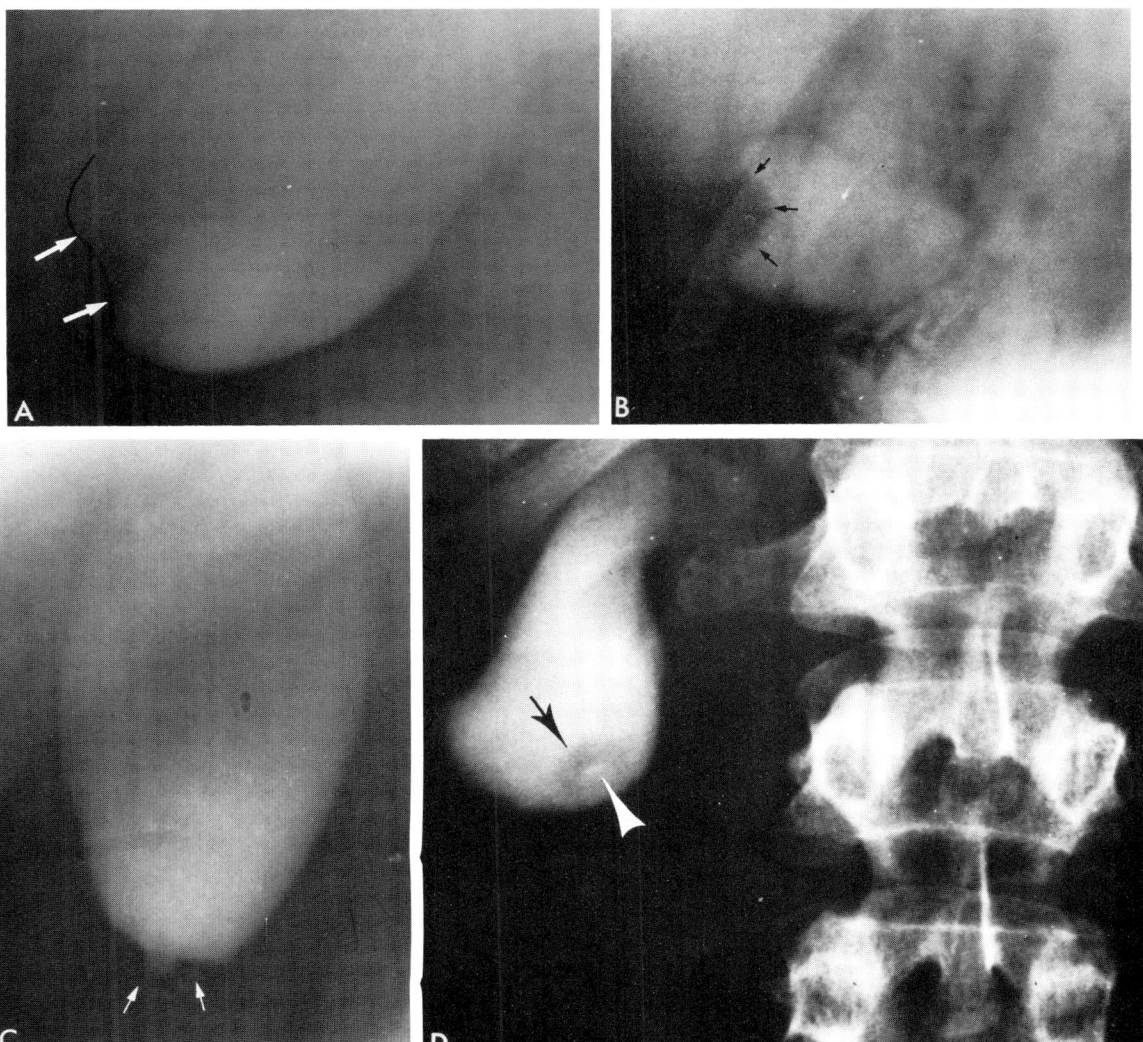

Figure 16–80. Fundal adenomyomatosis. *A*, There is a fixed indentation at the fundus of the gallbladder (arrows). No Rokitansky-Aschoff sinuses were demonstrated. *B*, This fundal filling defect (arrows) has a more malignant appearance. *C*, The beak-shaped fundus is surrounded by Rokitansky-Aschofff sinuses (arrows). *D*, There is a fixed radiolucent filling defect in the fundus (arrow) with a central umbilication (arrowhead).

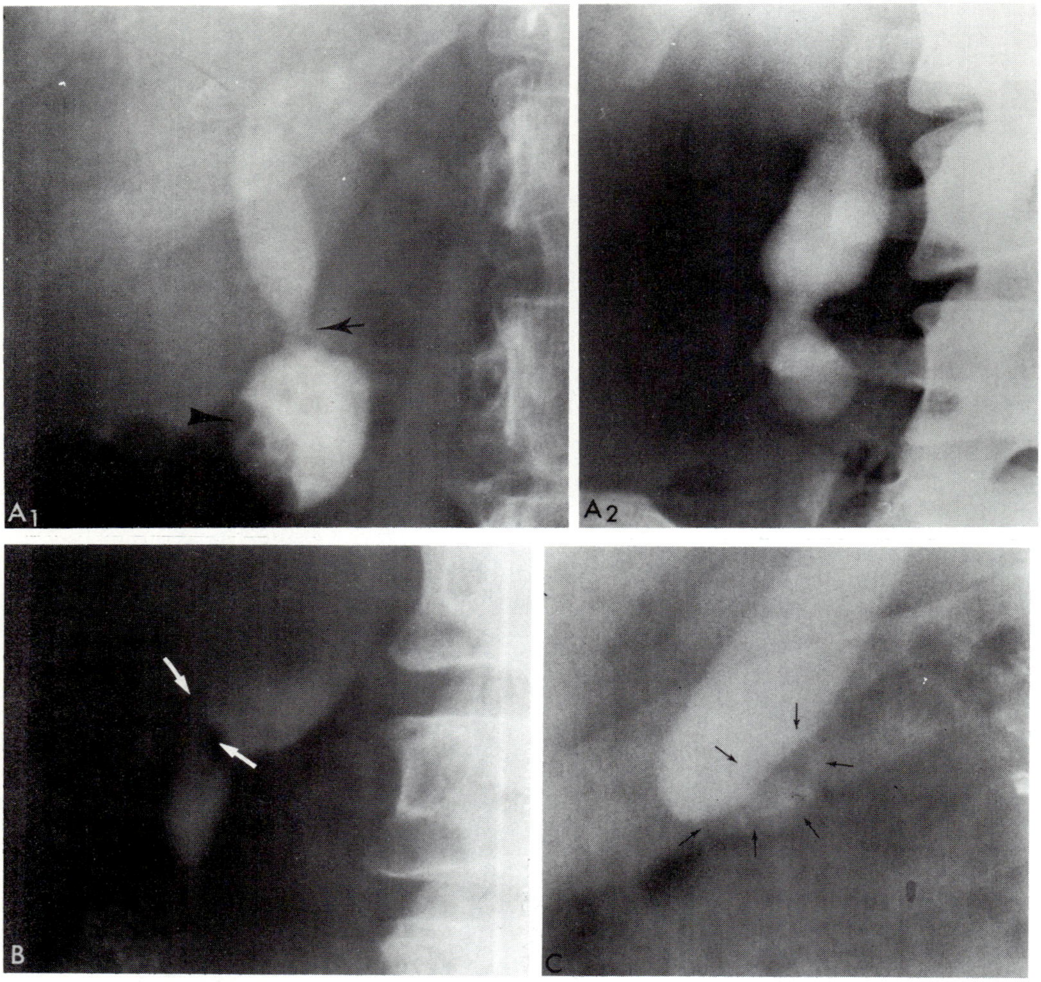

Figure 16–81. Segmental adenomyomatosis. *A*, 1. The stricture in the midgallbladder (arrow) was due to segmental adenomyomatosis. There are gallstones in the distal loculus (arrowhead). 2. Different patient with a constriction in the midgallbladder (arrow). *B*, The entire distal half of the gallbladder is small, and there is an eccentrically located stricture (arrows) that resembles a kink. *C*, There is a single large calculus (arrows) situated in the fundus of the gallbladder, which was kinked owing to adenomyomatosis.

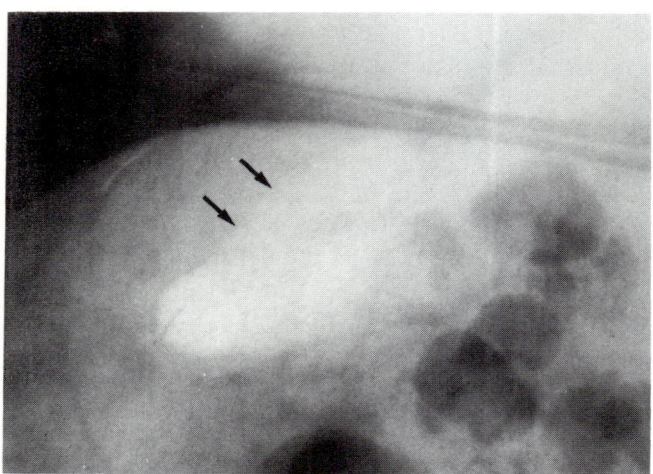

Figure 16–82. Diffuse cholesterolosis. The multiple tiny filling defects are due to cholesterol deposits. The gallbladder wall lacks sharpness (arrows).

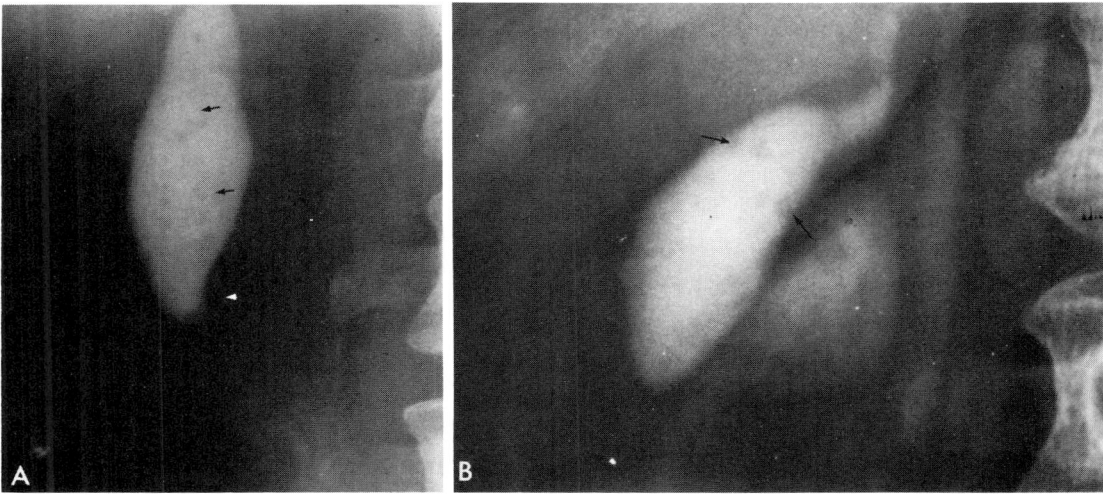

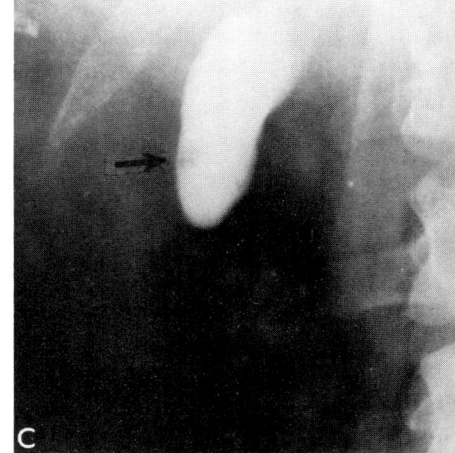

Figure 16–83. Cholesterol polyps. *A*, There are multiple round radiolucencies (arrows) that remain fixed when the patient's position is changed. *B*, Different patient with several cholesterol polyps (arrows). *C*, Solitary fixed filling defects (arrow) are usually cholesterol polyps.

The differential diagnosis of cholesterolosis includes a variety of uncommon entities. Fixed filling defects of the gallbladder wall may also be due to embedded stones, inflammatory polyps, and benign neoplasms. Their radiographic appearances may be similar, but the great majority of "polypoid" lesions are due to cholesterol polyps. Benign epithelial tumors (true polyps), inflammatory polyps, and mesodermal neoplasms are very rare.

The differential diagnosis of adenomyomatosis inlcudes a phrygian cap, postural kinks, and mucosal septa and bands. Congenital anomalies are probably less common than adenomyomatosis. The most common congenital anomaly is the phrygian cap (see Fig. 16–11), which is a fold of tissue extending partly across the lumen of the gallbladder. It is visulized on cholecystography as a smooth, narrow radiolucent line with parallel surfaces traversing part of the lumen and located near the fundus. There are no Rokitansky-Aschoff sinuses, and after a fatty meal both segments of the gallbladder contract equally. In segmental adenomyomatosis the stricture produces a wider radiolucent line with a phrygian cap. In addition, the adjacent surfaces of the stricture line in adenomyomatosis are not parallel, and there is disparate contraction of the affected gallbladder segment. Rokitanksy-Aschoff sinuses are usually visualized (see Fig. 16–1*A*). Postural kinks in the gallbladder are common and superficially resemble the fixed angular deformities of adenomyomatosis. Oblique views of the gallbladder and a change in the patient's position readily distinguish postural kinks from true disease. Congenital bands or septa probably exist but are quite rare. The gallbladder can occasionally be contricted by extrinsic bands. These may be congenital or caused by acquired adhesions from previous inflammatory disease (Fig. 16–84).

Opinions differ concerning the significance of the hyperplastic cholecystoses. There is no evidence that they are premalignant. In asymptomatic patients no treatment seems necessary. When they are associated with gallstones, the decision to operate is based on the same criteria as in other cases of calculous gallbladder disease. There is controversy over the treatment of cases of cholecystoses without gallstones but with gallbladder symptoms. Many recommend cholecystectomy when the symptoms strongly suggest gallbladder disease. When the symptoms are vague, as is not infrequent, the value of surgery is questionable, since the incidence of recurrent symptoms following cholecystectomy is high.

EXTERNAL TRAUMA

Because of its well-protected location, injuries to the extrahepatic biliary system are uncommon.[55] Blunt trauma, as from automobile accidents, as well as missile wounds may damage the biliary tract but is nearly always associated with serious injuries to other abdominal viscera, chest, or skull, which usually dominate the clinical picture. Hence, damage to the gallbladder or the extrahepatic bile ducts is rarely suspected prior to surgical exploration. Mortality is nearly always due to damage to other organs. If the patient recovers, however, the injury to the biliary system may result in a bile duct stricture.

Probably the most common causes of injury to the extrahepatic biliary tract are iatrogenic lacerations from percutaneous transhepatic cholangiograms and liver biop-

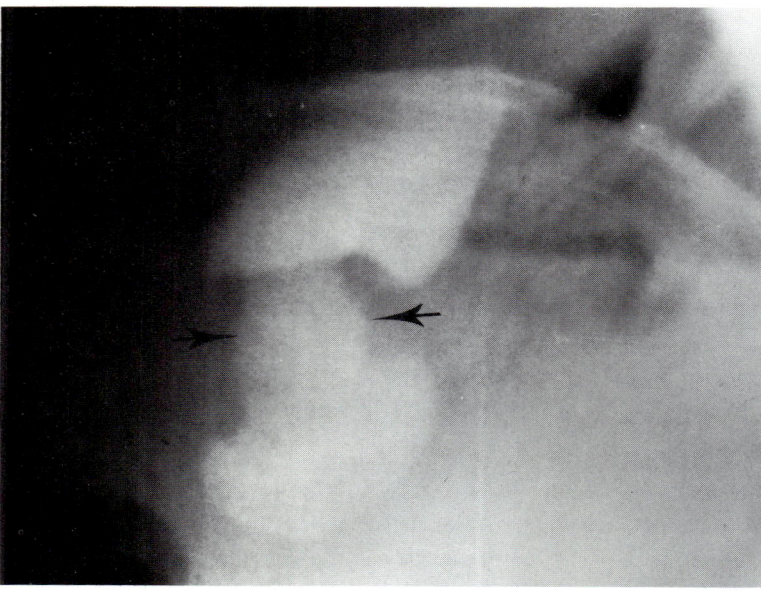

Figure 16–84. Peritoneal adhesion. There is a broad radiolucent band across the gallbladder (arrows) due to a peritoneal band. The appearance resembles that of segmental adenomyomatosis.

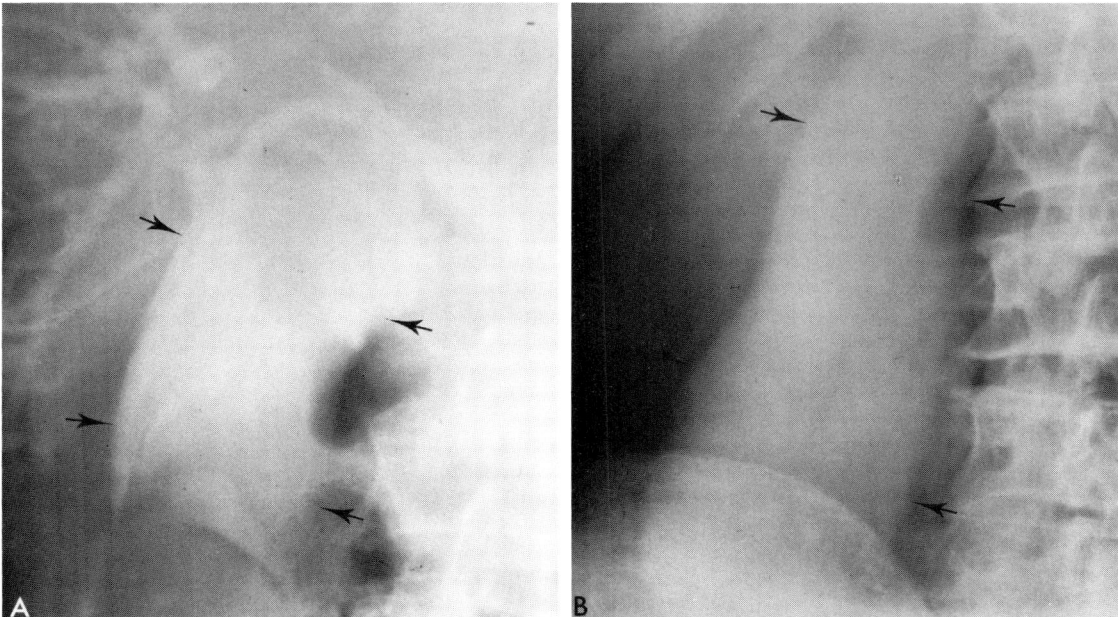

Figure 16–85. Puncture of the gallbladder during percutaneous transhepatic cholangiography. *A,* A 75-year-old male with jaundice due to metastatic tumor to the bile ducts. During the transhepatic cholangiogram, the gallbladder was accidentally punctured and injected with contrast (arrows). *B,* Two days later the contrast is seen in the distended gallbladder (arrows). There were no complications of the procedure.

sies. There is little published information regarding the incidence and subsequent complication rate of iatrogenic perforation of the gallbladder. DeMasi et al.[54] described seven cases of unintentional puncture of the gallbladder during percutaneous transhepatic cholangiography. They used large-bore needles for their studies. Only one patient developed bile leakage into the peritoneum; there were no deaths. These authors advocate decompressing the gallbladder to reduce the chance of bile leakage when it is inadvertently entered, especially in cases of distal bile duct obstruction. Their technique was to leave a polyethylene catheter in the gallbladder for drainage prior to surgery.

The skinny needle (22- or 23-gauge) is now used for most percutaneous transhepatic cholangiography, and the complication rate from accidental puncture of the gallbladder or extrahepatic bile ducts is probably small (Fig. 16–85). Our own experience in five cases and the unpublished experience of others indicate a low incidence of complications from puncture of the gallbladder.

The clinical manifestations of injury to the extrahepatic biliary system are due to bile leakage and hemorrhage. Sterile bile in the peritoneum frequently causes only mild inflammation. However, if the bile is infected, severe generalized peritonitis or localized abscesses may develop.

Surgical intervention is usually unnecessary when the gallbladder or extrahepatic bile ducts are iatrogenically punctured, unless complications develop. A cholecystectomy is recommended for lacerations of the gallbladder. Every attempt should be made to repair lacerations of the bile ducts. If this is not possible, a biliary-enteric bypass procedure may be necessary.

SURGICAL INJURIES AND COMPLICATIONS

Following cholecystectomy and other types of biliary tract surgery, there are several significant complications in which radiography or other imaging techniques have a role in diagnosis and management. These include the development of localized abscesses, generalized peritonitis, biliary fistulas, hemorrhage, drainage tube difficulties, lacerations of intrahepatic ducts, and bile duct strictures.[56-64]

After cholecystectomy, small collections of bile and blood often accumulate transiently in the subhepatic space near the gallbladder bed. Drains are normally placed in this location and usually are effective in preventing significant fluid accumulations. Occasionally, however, large subhepatic collections develop that can become infected and result in an abscess. Significant subhepatic fluid collections occur in 5 to 6 per cent of postcholecystectomy patients and are the most frequent major surgical complication.

Clinically, there is fullness or a mass in the right upper quadrant, tenderness, fever, and a leukocytosis. Radiographs of the abdomen and chest may show an elevated right hemidiaphragm and extraluminal gas bubbles characteristic of an abscess. An upper gastrointestinal series or barium enema examination can be useful to demonstrate the mass, and there may be focal inflammation of the duodenum or colon from the adjacent abscess (Fig. 16–86). Ultrasound is a rapid and easy method to delineate a subhepatic fluid collection or abscess. The diagnosis can be confirmed by percutaneously tapping the abscess with a skinny needle, using ultrasound or CT as a guide for the needle placement. Once the diagnosis is established, a large catheter can be inserted for percutaneous drainage.[59] This procedure is gaining popularity and may obviate the need for surgery. Without prompt attention, these abscesses may extend to other areas of the abdomen or cause generalized peritonitis.

Bile leakage and the development of bile peritonitis after cholecystectomy is usually caused by a slipped cystic duct ligature or by accidental laceration of the liver or extrahepatic bile duct. Failure to recognize anatomic variations of the ducts increases the risk of laceration. Rarely, the routine removal of a T-tube seven to ten days after surgery results in significant bile extravasation. In general, the amount of bile leakage depends on the size of the injured duct and the presence or absence of distal obstruction.

Bile in the peritoneum causes a variable clinical picture. Some patients have only minor discomfort, while others develop severe acute peritonitis. Sepsis is most likely to occur if the bile is infected. In addition, the bile may irritate the peritoneum, causing massive ascites. Treatment consists of supportive therapy, prompt surgical drainage of the abdomen, and correction of the leak.

Fistulas from the bile ducts to the skin surface may develop as a result of any of the previously mentioned causes of bile leakage. External fisutlas are of less immediate danger than internal fistulas, which can cause bile peritonitis or localized abscess. If the duct distal to the site of the fistula is obstructed, the fistula will not close and will require surgical correction. The amount of bile that drains from the fistula is proportional to the degree of obstruction of the distal bile duct. Fistulography is often useful to delineate the site of the fistula as well as the presence of bile duct obstruction (Fig. 16–87).

Hemorrhage can be a serious complication of biliary surgery. It is usually caused by direct injury to vessels but occasionally is due to an unrecognized bleeding diathesis. Damage to the hepatic artery, especially the right hepatic artery, occurs because of its variable anatomic course; in addition to major bleeding, it may cause liver infarction. In uncertain cases, selective hepatic angiography may disclose the presence and site of bleeding.

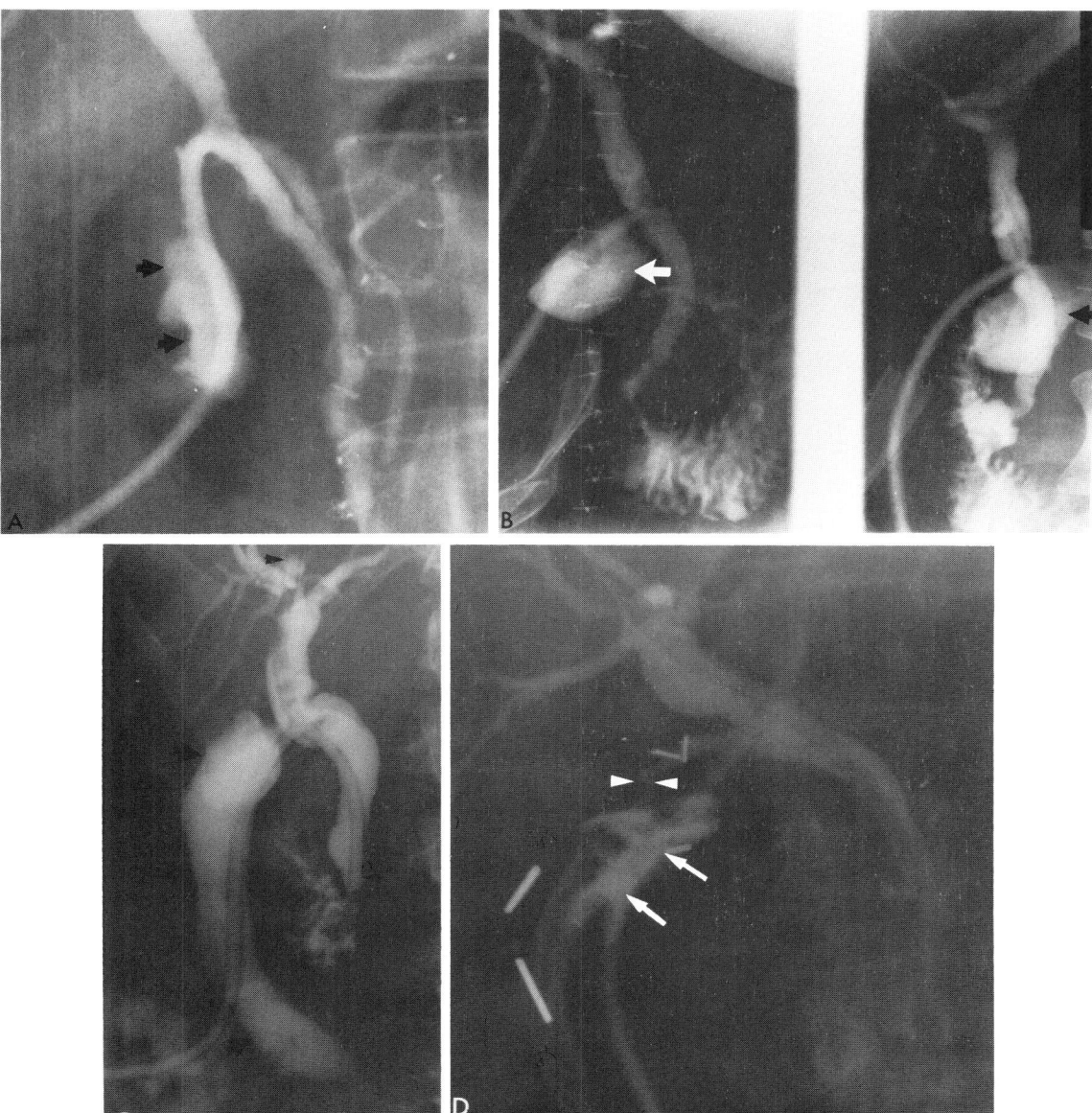

Figure 16–86. Bile leakage. *A*, A tube cholangiogram two weeks after cholecystectomy shows a small collection of contrast around the tube (arrows). The subhepatic drain has been removed. These collections occur frequently and are usually of no concern. They are often caused by excessive pressure of injection. *B*, Duodenal bulb resembling bile leakage. Normal T-tube cholangiogram seven days postcholecystectomy. The duodenal bulb (arrows) simulates extravasation around the tube (left). This is easily clarified by changing the position of the patient (right). *C*, Extensive extravasation (arrows) around the T-tube. Possible consequences include abscess or fistula formation. Note the excessively long T-tube (arrowheads). If the T-tube extends into the duodenum, it may obstruct the pancreatic duct and cause pancreatitis. *D*, T-tube cholangiogram one week after cholecystectomy shows extravasation (arrows) from the end of the cystic duct remnant (arrowheads) into the subhepatic space. Because of adequate drainage, the leak eventually closed.

Illustration and legend continued on the following page

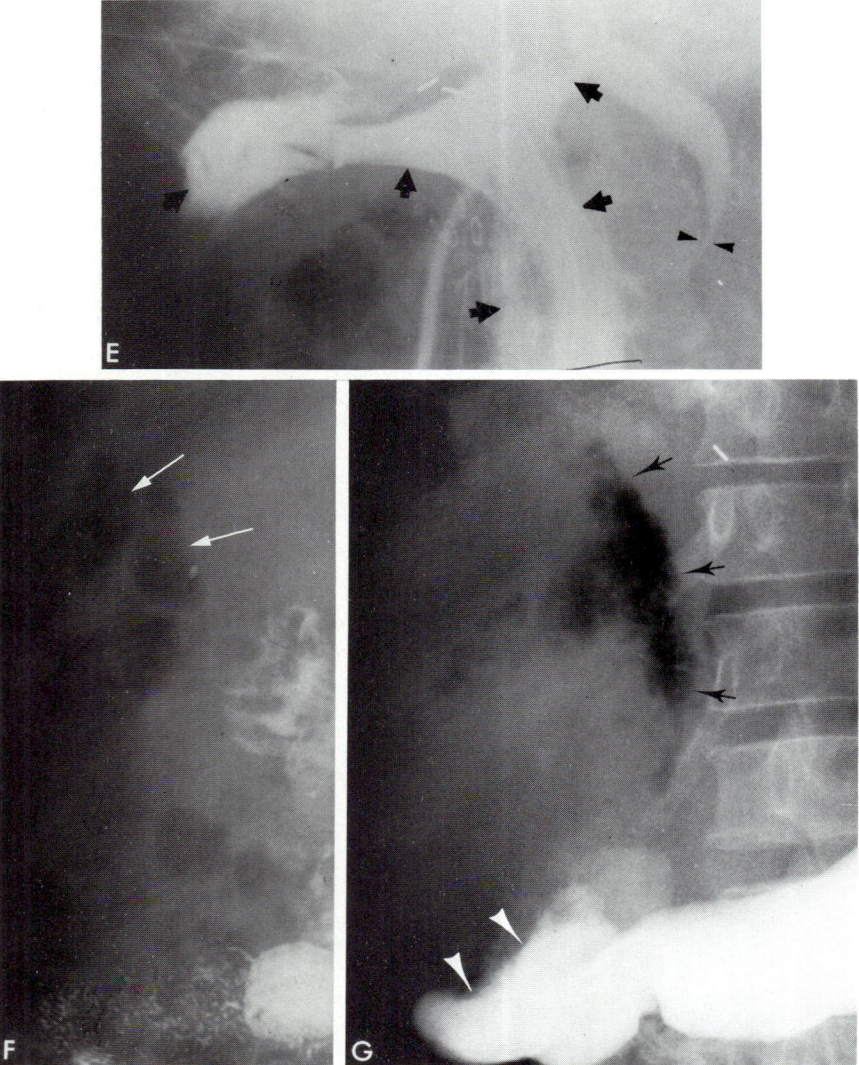

Figure 16–86 *Continued.* *E*, There is extensive leakage from the cystic duct stump (arrows). The contrast is filling a large abscess cavity. The leak is not likely to heal because the distal common bile duct is partially obstructed (arrowheads). *F*, The air bubbles (arrows) represent a subhepatic abscess that became clinically apparent one month after cholecystectomy. *G*, A different patient with a postcholecystectomy abscess (arrows). The abscess is large and distorts the duodenal bulb (arrowheads).

The use of T-tubes after biliary tract surgery is common, and only rarely causes complications. Occasionally the tube may become occluded from blood clots or gravel (Fig. 16–88). The frequency of occlusion is related to the length of time the tube is left in place. Flushing with saline usually relieves the obstruction. In the vast majority of patients with T-tubes are removed without incident, but occasionally, extraction is difficult. Continuous mild traction usually succeeds in dislodging the tube. Very rarely, the tube breaks and a fragment is left in the duct. Foreign bodies in the ducts can act as a nidus for stone formation and cause obstruction to the flow of bile. The T-tube can sometimes become prematurely dislodged from the bile duct. If the amount of draining bile is

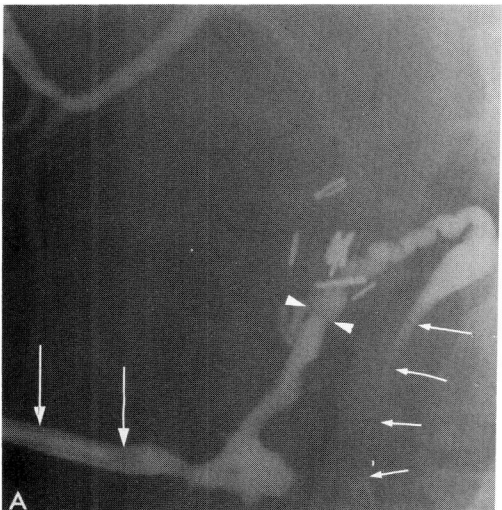 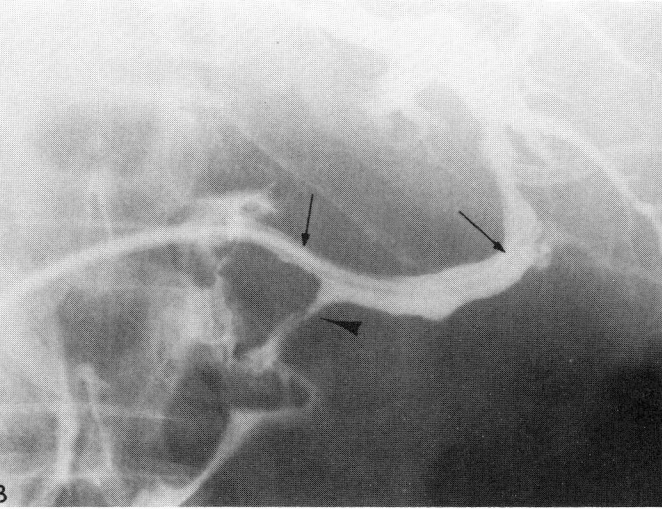

Figure 16–87. Biliary cutaneous fistula. *A*, A patient with chronic pancreatitis. A tube was inserted through the skin fistula (large arrows) and contrast injected, filling first a small cavity and then communicating with the cystic duct stump (arrowheads). The long, smooth, tapered narrowing of the common bile duct (small arrows) is typical of chronic pancreatitis. The fistula will not close as long as the common bile duct is partially obstructed. *B*, A patient with obstruction just proximal to the main right and left hepatic ducts. A tube was inserted through a cutaneous sinus tract (arrows) which communicates with the right ductal system. There is also leakage into the peritoneal cavity (arrowhead).

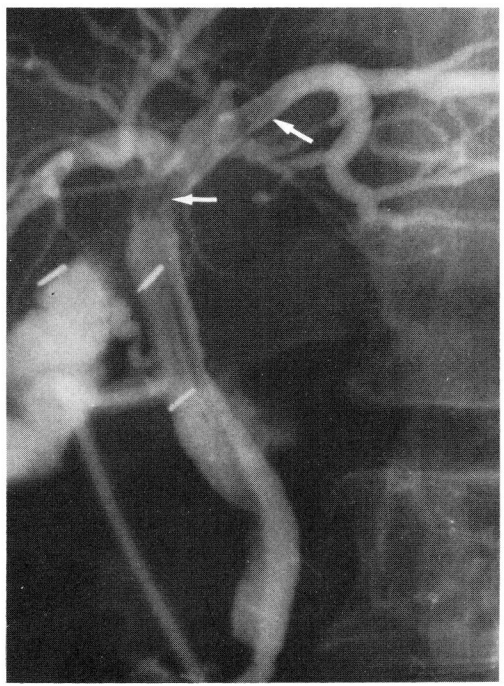

Figure 16–88. Blood clots in the bile ducts. A T-tube cholangiogram seven days postcholecystectomy in a patient with a bleeding disorder shows several radiolucent filling defects (arrows) resembling stones. The operative cholangiogram was normal as was a follow-up T-tube cholangiogram.

minimal, the tube can be left in the sinus tract. This provides a temporary route for the escape of bile until the tube can be removed. When the bile drainage is large, implying ductal obstruction, it is necessary to replace the T-tube in the duct. Although this can be done surgically, the T-tube often can be reinserted under fluoroscopic guidance. Alternatively, a straight tube can be positioned in the bile duct, eliminating the need for reoperation (Fig. 16–89).

Exploration of the intrahepatic ducts during surgery in an attempt to remove calculi with Fogarty balloon catheters and other instruments can cause rupture of one or more of the ducts. Ductal perforations are readily visualized on operative or postoperative cholangiography (Fig. 16–90). The radiologic appearance resembles that of intrahepatic abscesses that communicate with the biliary system or cystic disease of the liver. However, in most instances there is no difficulty in establishing the diagnosis.

Most of the reported complications from lacerations of the intrahepatic ducts have not been very significant clinically and in general require no treatment. The most frequent complication is transient hemobilia. More serious problems, however, are

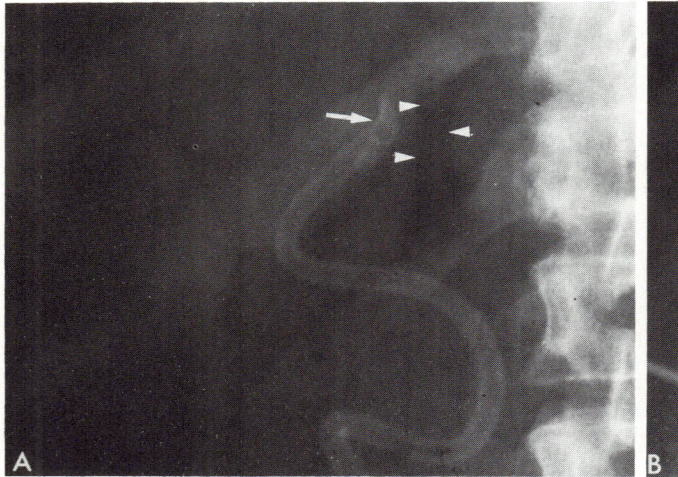
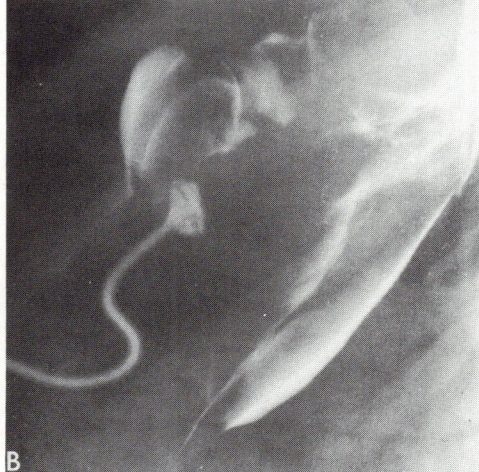
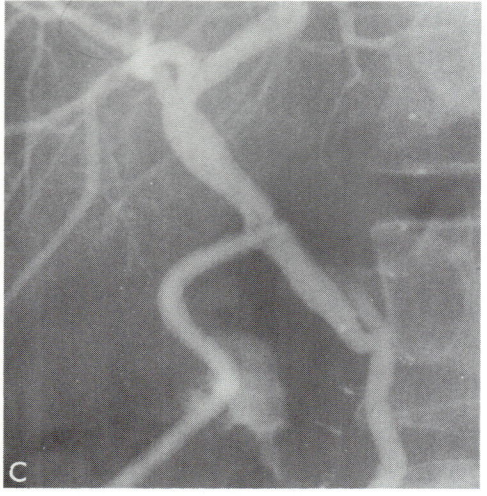

Figure 16–89. Dislodged T-tube. *A,* Scout film for a T-tube cholangiogram shows that the end of the T-tube (arrow) is out of the common bile duct (arrowheads). *B,* A small amount of injected contrast accumulated in the perihepatic area. *C,* A different patient in whom the T-tube was removed accidentally several days after surgery.

Illustration and legend continued on the opposite page

persistent or severe bleeding, intraductal strictures, and possibly infection. The rate of healing probably depends on the size of the tear. In some instances, follow-up cholangiograms show complete healing in one week.

Perhaps the most serious surgical complication is injury to the extrahepatic bile ducts, resulting in obstruction. Over 90 per cent of benign biliary strictures are caused by surgical trauma. The common hepatic duct is most frequently affected. Bile duct injuries are most often seen after cholecystectomy and gastrectomy. Often the reason for injury is unknown. Obscuration of the surgical anatomy due to chronic inflammatory changes, such as occurs with Mirizzi's syndrome, and anatomic variations such as a short cystic duct result in a higher incidence of surgical trauma.

Occasionally, injury to the ducts is recognized and repaired during surgery. Unfortunately, in most cases the damage is not appreciated until later. The common clinical manifestations are obstructive jaundice, often without signs of cholangitis, and excessive bile drainage from the T-tube. About 60 per cent of strictures develop during the first postoperative week. The remaining 40 per cent are not symptomatic until months or occasionally years after surgery.

Radiographic evaluation is essential (Fig. 16–91). Transhepatic cholangiography or endoscopic retrograde cholangiopancreatography is the best procedure to demonstrate strictures. Intravenous cholangiography is rarely successful. If an external fistula

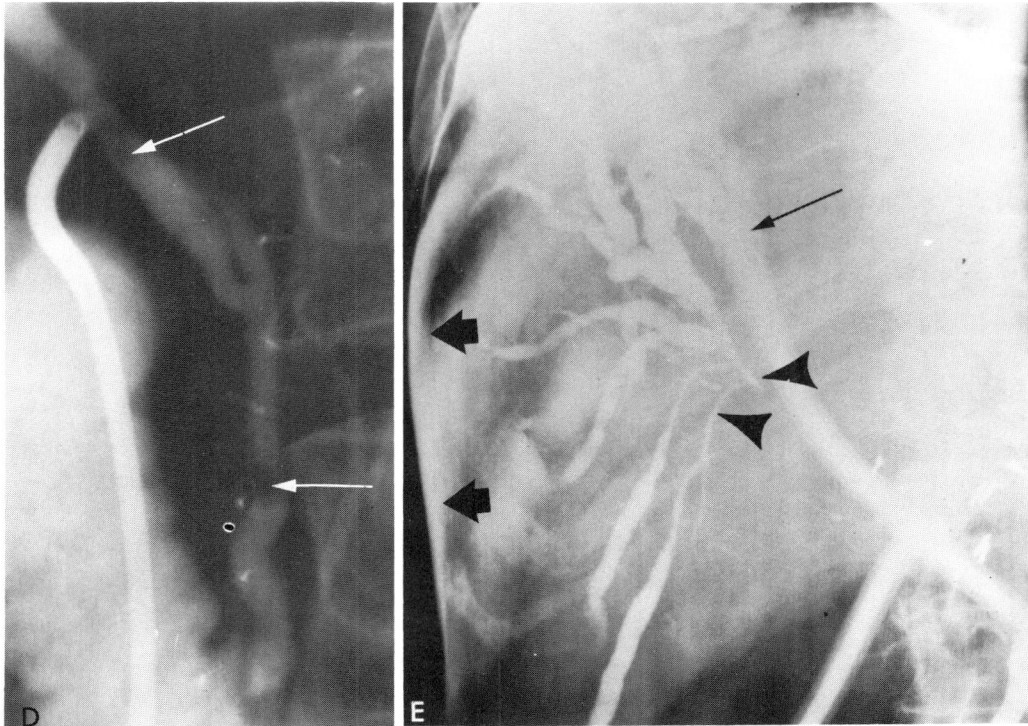

Figure 16–89 *Continued.* *D,* A soft rubber catheter was successfully manipulated through the T-tube tract. The round radiolucencies (arrows) are air bubbles. In the early postoperative period, the tract closes quickly and prompt reinsertion is necessary. *E,* Surgically malpositioned T-tube in a patient with extensive cholangiocarcinoma (arrowheads). The proximal end of the tube (small arrow) is only partially in the ductal system. Contrast has extravasated around the liver (large arrows).

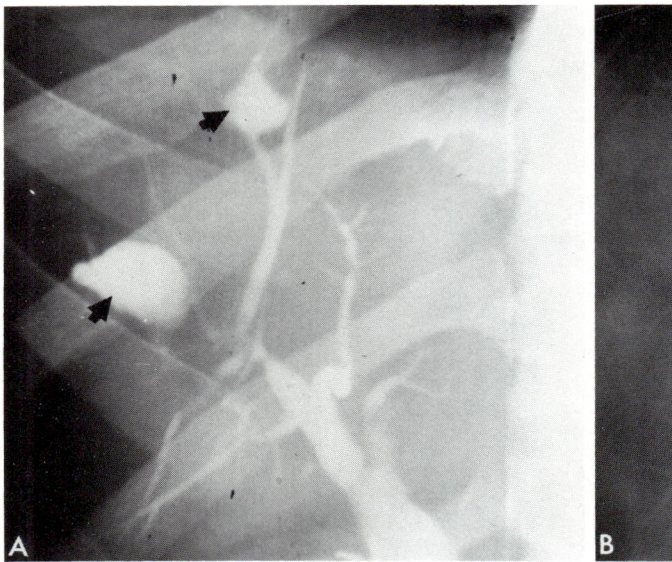 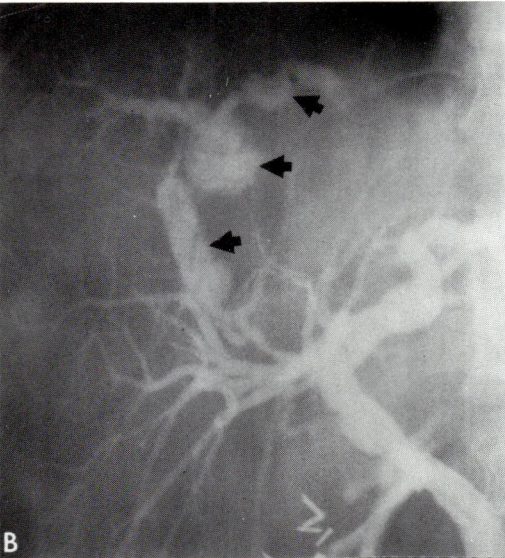

Figure 16–90. Bile duct tears from instrumentation. *A,* Extravasated contrast (arrows) from lacerated ducts was caused by probing with a Fogarty catheter during surgery. The appearance resembles that of abscesses or cysts. *B,* Different example of ruptured ducts (arrows) from a Fogarty catheter. The tears usually have no clinical consequences.

is present, fistulography should be performed. Strictures that occur after biliary-enteric anastomoses are often best demonstrated by barium cholangiography. If left untreated, bile duct strictures are often fatal. Chronic liver damage occurs, and can lead to biliary cirrhosis, portal hypertension, and their sequelae. There may be recurrent cholangitis with hepatic abscesses. Bile duct injuries should be treated by surgery as early as possible. The overall success rate in the repair of injuries is about 60 to 80 per cent. Failure is usually due to recurrent stricture formation. Biliary surgery can occasionally deform the duodenal bulb, simulating chronic ulcer disease.

POSTCHOLECYSTECTOMY SYNDROMES

The term "postcholecystectomy syndrome" is applied to the persistence or recurrence of symptoms after cholecystectomy that are similar to the symptoms prior to surgery.[65-69] The term is a misnomer, since there is no well-defined clinical syndrome and since symptoms may be due to a number of different etiologies.

The causes of recurrent symptoms after cholecystectomy can be classified as follows.

1. Errors in initial diagnosis. This group represents the most frequent cause of recurrent symptoms and includes such diverse conditions as hiatus hernia, peptic ulcer disease, pancreatitis, coronary insufficiency, and renal and colon disease.
2. Inadequate surgery. Examples include retained bile duct stones as well as gallbladder and cystic duct remnants.
3. Overlooked malignancies.
4. Surgical injuries causing bile duct fistulas and ductal stenosis.
5. Fibrosis of the sphincter of Oddi.
6. Biliary dyskinesia.

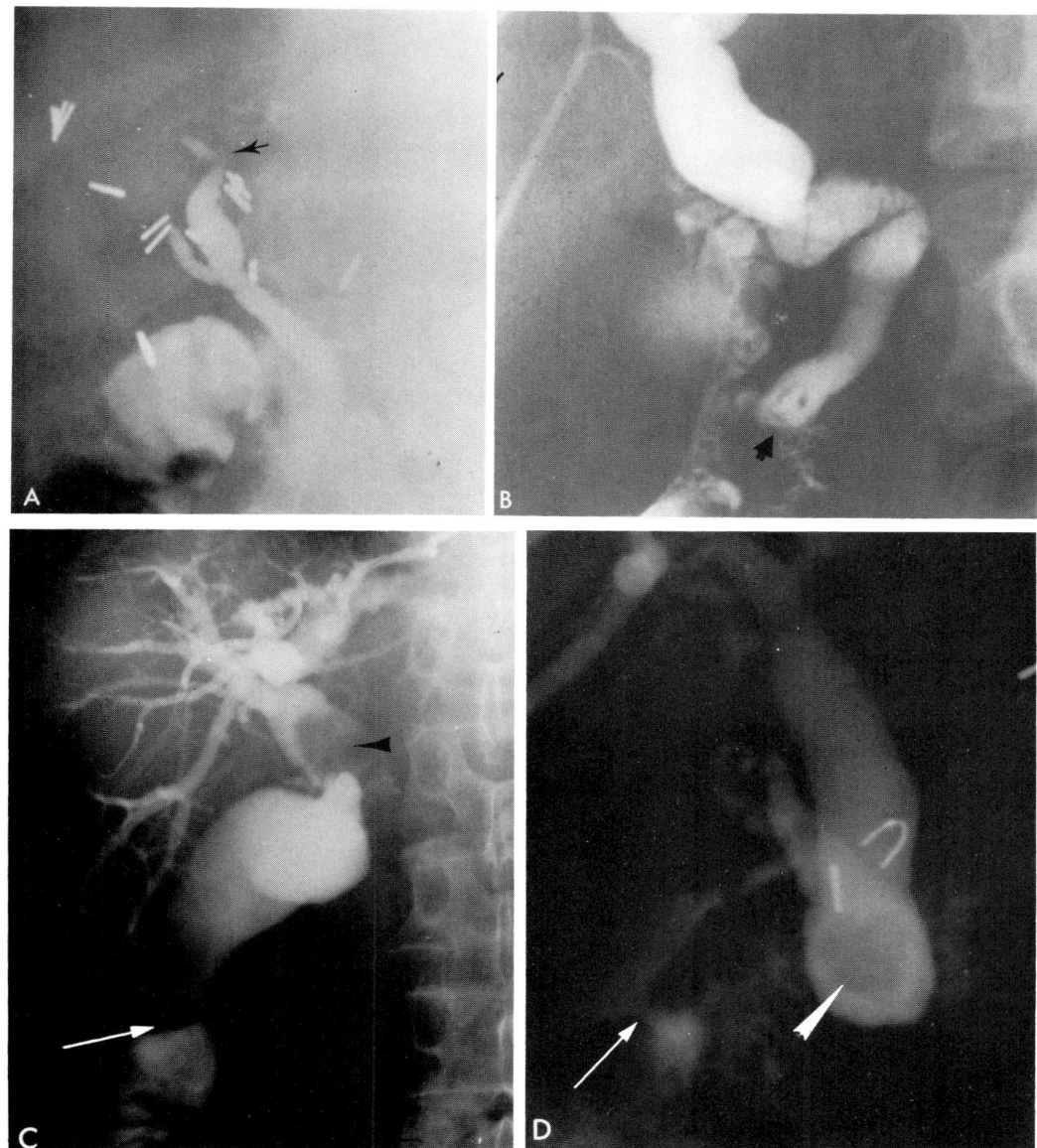

Figure 16–91. Surgical bile duct injuries. *A,* ERCP demonstrating a tight stricture of the proximal common hepatic duct (arrow) from a surgical injury several months previously. *B,* The distal common bile duct was occluded by staples (arrow) during a difficult surgical procedure. A choledochojejunostomy successfully relieved the obstruction. *C,* A narrow cholecystoduodenal anastomosis (arrow) resulted in stasis and the formation of a bile duct stone (arrowhead). *D,* As in *C,* there is a narrow cholecystojejunostomy opening (arrow), with recurrent stone formation (arrowhead) and proximal bile duct dilatation.

Illustration and legend continued on following page

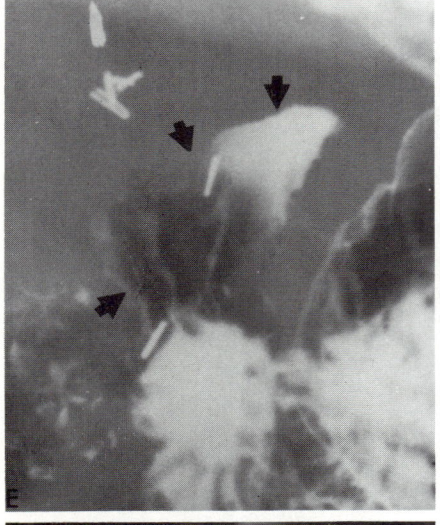
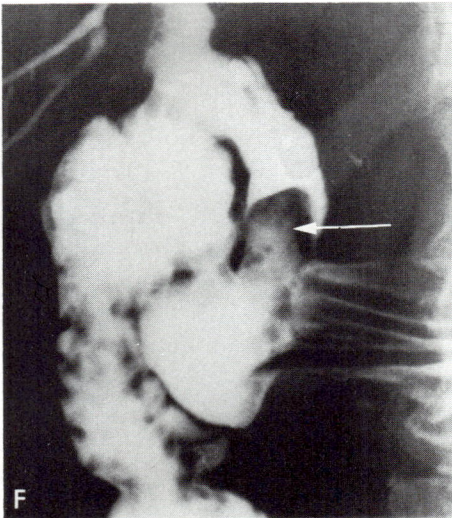
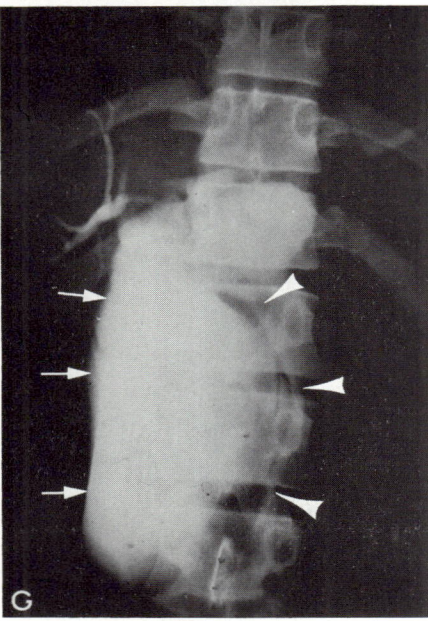

Figure 16–91 *Continued.* *E,* Deformed duodenal bulb (arrows) due to a prior cholecystectomy. *F,* Following a choledochoduodenostomy, food particles (arrow) resembling calculi were intermittently found in the common bile duct. *G,* Mirizzi's syndrome. Patient with recurrent jaundice and ascending cholangitis. A dilated gallbladder (arrows) was inadvertently punctured during the transhepatic cholangiogram. The gallbladder is impressing on and displacing the extrahepatic ducts (arrowheads) to the left.

In published reports, the incidence of recurrent symptoms varies greatly. About 90 per cent of patients are cured or have substantially reduced symptoms following cholecystectomy for chronic cholecystitis. Patients with more severe and definite symptoms of cholecystitis, such as episodes of colic or recurrent bouts of cholangitis, have a lower incidence of recurrent symptoms. The amount of inflammation and scarring of the gallbladder wall also correlates fairly well with symptomatic relief following cholecystectomy. Patients with minimal scarring of the gallbladder are more likely to develop recurrent symptoms.

The postcholecystectomy syndrome can occur at any time following cholecystectomy, but most often symptoms tend to recur within the first several months. The syndrome is more common in females, and the incidence tends to decrease with increasing age.

The role of cystic duct and gallbladder remnants as a cause for the postcholecystectomy syndrome is controversial. Lewicki et al.[69] defined a potentially symptomatic cystic duct remnant as one longer than 5 mm. Often, long remnants are left when the cystic duct inserts low near the ampulla of Vater and runs parallel to the common hepatic duct. In these circumstances, a remnant longer than 5 mm may be intentionally retained in order to avoid damage to the common bile duct.

In general, the length of the cystic duct stump correlates poorly with the recurrence of symptoms. Most probably, acalculous cystic duct and gallbladder remnants are of no clinical importance. However, when they contain stones they can be the cause of recurrent symptoms. Stones in the remnant occasionally migrate into the common bile duct and cause obstruction. Surgical excision of remnants containing calculi is indicated in symptomatic patients. Removal of acalculous stumps often fails to relieve the symptoms. Inflammation of cystic duct remnants without stones as well as cysts and neuromas at the sutured end of the remnants has also been implicated as a cause of the postcholecystectomy syndrome.

Cystic duct or gallbladder remnants are best demonstrated on postoperative T-tube cholangiography but often can be seen on the operative cholangiogram (Fig. 16–92). Intravenous cholangiography usually shows the remnant, but demonstration of calculi in the stump is often unsuccessful. Occasionally a cystic duct or gallbladder remnant may become considerably dilated. This condition has been erroneously referred to as a reformed gallbladder.

Contrary to popular belief, the common bile duct does not enlarge after cholecystectomy. When the common bile duct does dilate after surgery, ductal obstruction should be suspected. Unfortunately, the range of normal size is quite variable. A width of between 8 and 15 mm is a gray zone, in which the duct may be normal-caliber or enlarged from partial obstruction. If over 15 mm, obstruction is invariably present, if under 8 mm, obstruction is unlikely. Once an obstructed duct becomes chronically dilated, it usually remains dilated for an indefinite time even after the obstruction has been relieved. If repeat cholangiography after relief of obstruction shows persistent dilatation, it may be difficult to determine if there is recurrent mechanical obstruction (Fig. 16–93). Acute common bile duct obstruction (at least experimentally in monkeys) can result in considerable dilatation of the extrahepatic ducts, and after relief of the obstruction the ducts rapidly return to normal size (Fig. 16–94).

Biliary dyskinesia, referring to inadequate emptying of bile into the duodenum, has been suggested as a cause of the postcholecystectomy syndrome. Data supporting this entity are at present circumstantial. The diagnosis is suggested in patients who have postcholecystectomy symptoms but no demonstrable anatomic abnormality or who have had a second operation without relief of their symptoms.

Biliary dyskinesia is believed to be due to a dysfunction of the sphincter of Oddi that intermittently interferes with the flow of bile into the duodenum. This presumably results in increased ductal pressure and symptoms. The diagnosis is difficult to establish. Attempts have been made to try to correlate the common bile duct pressure at the time of surgery with the patient's symptoms. Often the common bile duct pressures are normal; even if elevated, the increase could be attributed to surgical manipulation and/or general anesthesia. Biliary drainage procedures are advocated by those who believe this to be a clinical entity.

Finally, it should be emphasized that many cases of postcholecystectomy syndrome can be managed medically with choleretic agents and without surgical intervention. Some patients with severe symptoms respond well to progesterone medications.

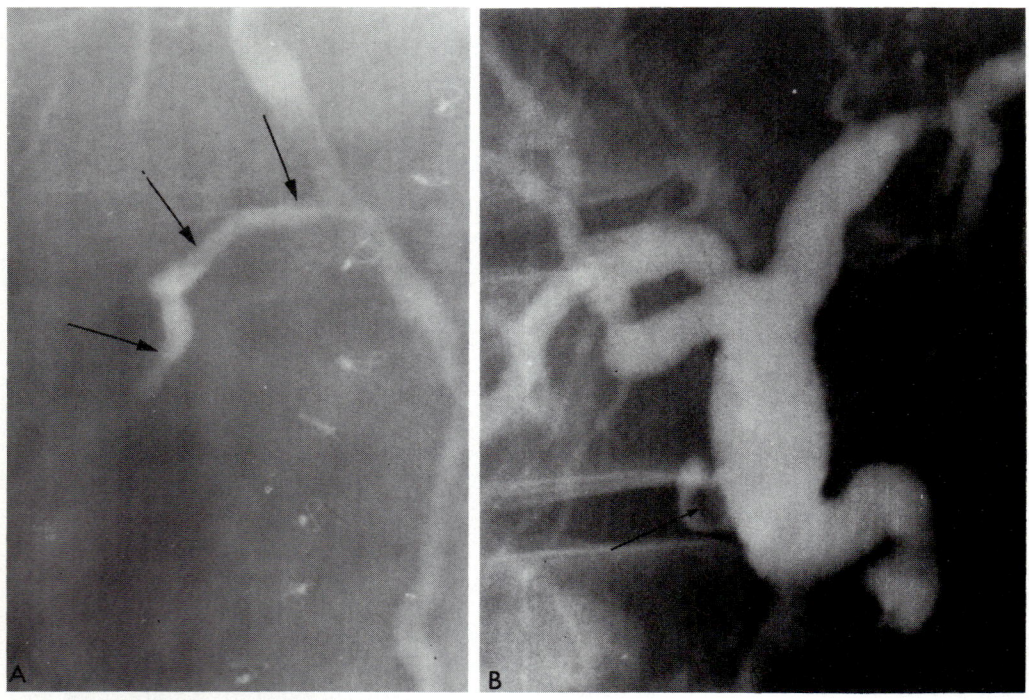
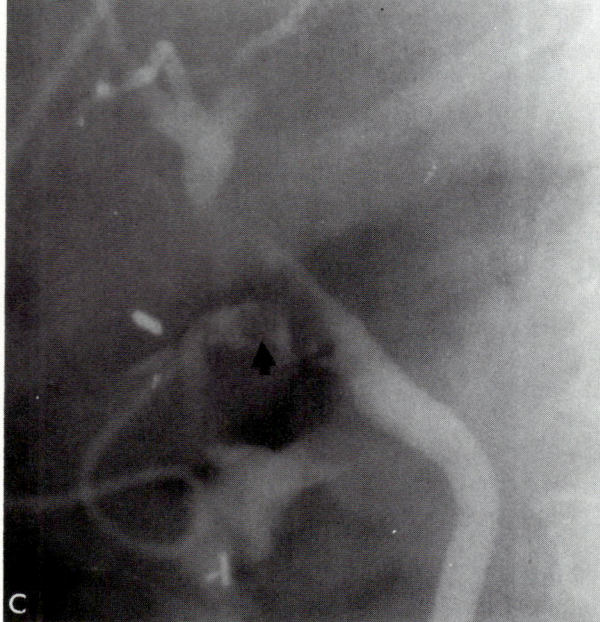

Figure 16–92. "PCS" cystic duct remnant. *A,* Postoperative cholangiogram shows a long cystic duct remnant (arrows) in an asymptomatic patient. *B,* Calculus in a cystic duct remnant (arrow). The patient had recurrence of her symptoms. The bile ducts are chronically dilated from previous ductal stones. *C,* Operative cholangiogram demonstrating a calculus in the cystic duct (arrow).

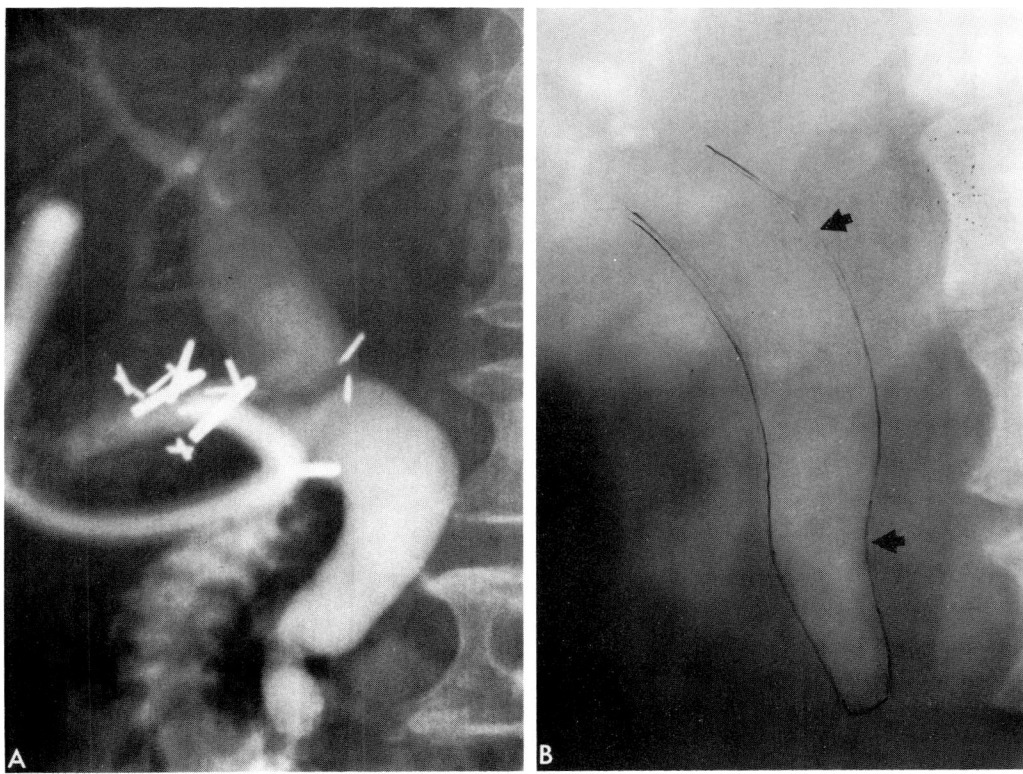

Figure 16–93. Chronic bile duct enlargement. *A,* The common bile duct is dilated and has not changed in size for six months. There is no mechanical obstruction. The patient had a previous cholecystectomy. *B,* The common bile duct (arrows) has been enlarged for four years. There is no obstructing lesion. Without the knowledge that the bile duct is chronically dilated, this intravenous cholangiogram would have been interpreted as common bile duct obstruction, and the patient would needlessly have been subjected to further work-up.

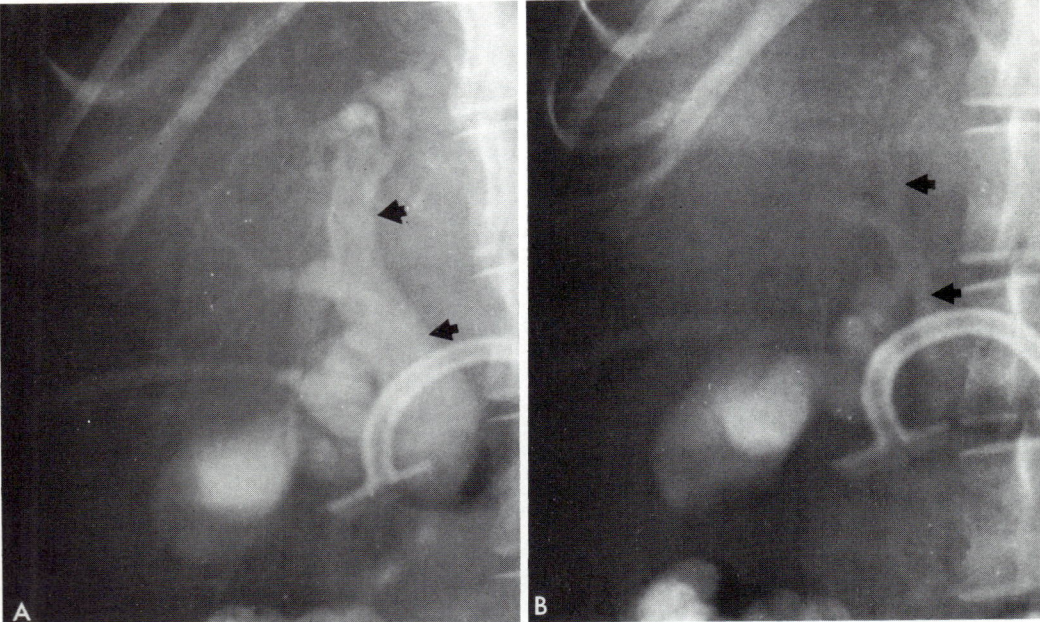

Figure 16–94. Experimental acute common bile duct obstruction. *A,* A cholangiogram in a Rhesus monkey done several hours after the common bile duct pressure was mechanically elevated shows dilated extrahepatic and intrahepatic ducts (arrows). *B,* Five minutes following return of the common bile duct pressure to normal, a repeat cholangiogram shows normal-sized ducts (arrows).

References

Acute Cholecystitis

1. Dawson, J. L.: Cholecystitis and cholecystectomy. Clin. Gastroenterol. 2:85–102, 1973.
2. Moncada, R., Cardoso, M., Danley, R., et al.: Acute cholecystitis: 137 patients studied by infusion tomography of the gallbladder. Am. J. Roentgenol. 129:583–585, 1977.
3. Nolan, D. J., and Espiner, H. J.: Compression of the common bile duct in acute cholecystitis. Br. J. Radiol. 45:821–824, 1972.
4. Sleisenger, M. H., and Fordtran, J. S.: Gastrointestinal Disease. Pathophysiology, Diagnosis, Management. Philadelphia, W. B. Saunders Company, 1973, p. 1125.
5. Thorbjarnarson, B.: Surgery of the Biliary Tract. Philadelphia, W. B. Saunders Company, 1975, pp. 39–98.
6. Weens, S. H., and Clements, J. L., Jr.: The radiologic diagnosis of acute cholecystitis. Semin. Roentgenol. 11:245–247, 1976.

Gallstones and Chronic Cholecystitis

7. Berk, R. N., Loeb, P. M., Goldberger, L. E., et al.: Oral cholecystography with iopanoic acid. N. Engl. J. Med. 290:204–210, 1974.
8. Bouchier, I. A. D.: Gallstones. Proc. R. Soc. Med. 70:597–599, 1977.
9. Bouchier, I. A. D.: The biochemistry of gallstone formation. Clin. Gastroenterol. 2:49–65, 1973.
10. Dawson, J. L.: Cholecystitis and cholecystectomy. Clin. Gastroenterol. 2:85–102, 1973.
11. Heaton, K. W.: The epidemiology of gallstones and suggested etiology. Clin. Gastroenterol. 2:67–81, 1973.
12. Palayew, M. J.: Chronic cholecystitis and cholelithiasis. Semin. Roentgenol. 11:249–257, 1976.
13. Rosenbaum, H. D.: The cholecystogram as a yardstick of gallbladder pathology. Radiology 111:737–739, 1974.
14. Soloway, R. D., Trotman, B. W., and Ostrow, J. D.: Pigment gallstones. Gastroenterology 72:167–182, 1977.

15. Thorbjarnarson, B.: Surgery of the Biliary Tract. Philadelphia, W. B. Saunders Company, 1975, pp. 35–38.
16. Whitney, B., and Sutor, D. J.: The value of radiology in predicting gallstone type when selecting patients for medical treatment. Gut 16:359–364, 1975.

Acalculous Cholecystitis

17. Adams, T. W., and Foxley, E. G.: A diagnostic technique for acalculous cholecystitis. Surg. Gynecol. Obstet. 142:168–170, 1976.
18. Banner, M. P., Bleshman, M. H., and Speckman, J. M.: Persistent gallbladder opacification after iopanoic acid cholecystography: diagnostic implications for acalculus cholecystitis. Am. J. Roentgenol. 132:51–54, 1979.
19. Berk, R. N.: Cholecystokinin cholecystography in the diagnosis of chronic acalculus cholecystitis and biliary dyskinesia. Gastrointest. Radiol. 1:325–330, 1977.
20. Dunn, F. H., Christensen, E. C., Reynolds, J., et al.: Cholecystokinin cholecystography. J.A.M.A. 228:997–1003, 1974.
21. Goldstein, F., Grunt, R., and Margulies, M.: Cholecystokinin cholecystography in the differential diagnosis of acalculus gallbladder disease. Dig. Dis. 19:835–849, 1974.
22. Russell, J. G. B., Keddie, N. C., Gough, A. L., et al.: Radiology of acalculus gall-bladder disease — a new sign. Br. J. Radiol. 49:420–424, 1976.
23. Valberg, L. S., Jabbari, M., Kerr, J. W., et al.: Biliary pain in young women in the absence of gallstones. Gastroenterology 60:1020–1026, 1971.

Choledocholithiasis

24. Bean, W. J., Smith, S. L., and Mahorner, H. R.: Equipment for nonoperative removal of biliary tract stones. Radiology 107:452–453, 1973.
25. Burhenne, H. J.: Nonoperative extraction of stones from the bile ducts. Semin. Roentgenol. 11:213–217, 1976.
26. Caroli, J.: Diseases of the intrahepatic biliary tree. Clin. Gastroenterol. 2:147–161, 1973.
27. George, P.: Disorders of the extrahepatic bile ducts. Clin. Gastroenterol. 2:127–146, 1973.
28. Grundy, D. J., King, P. A., and Lloyd, G.: Comparative evaluation of preoperative and operative radiology in biliary tract disease. Br. J. Surg. 59:205–208, 1972.
29. Larsen, C. R., Scholz, F. J., and Wise, R. E.: Diseases of the biliary ducts. Semin. Roentgenol. 11:259–267, 1976.
30. Salzman, E.: Opacification of bile duct calculi. Radiol. Clin. North Am. 4:525–533, 1966.
31. Thorbjarnarson, B.: Surgery of the Biliary Tract. Philadelphia, W. B. Saunders Company, 1975, pp. 39–98.
32. Wilson, I. D., Delaney, J. P., Duane, W. C., et al.: Choledocholithiasis. Gastroenterology 75:120–128, 1978.
33. Woolam, G. L., Freeman, F. J., and Priestley, J. T.: Relationship of cholecystographic visualization of the gallbladder to incidence of cholelithiasis. Surgery 61:699–671, 1967.

Sclerosing Cholangitis

34. Dockler, L.: Primary sclerosing cholangitis. Radiology 95:377–378, 1970.
35. Geisse, G., Melson, G. L., Tedesco, F. J., et al.: Stenosing lesions of the biliary tree. Evaluation with endoscopic retrograde cholangiography and percutaneous transhepatic cholangiography. Am. J. Roentgenol. 123:378–385, 1975.
36. Kriegler, J., Seaman, W. B., and Porter, M. R.: The roentgenologic appearance of sclerosing cholangitis. Radiology 95:367–375, 1970.
37. Larsen, C. R., Scholz, F. J., and Wise, R. E.: Diseases of the biliary ducts. Semin. Roentgenol. 11:259–267, 1976.
38. Scully, R. E., Galdabini, J. J., and McNeely, B. U.: Case records of Massachusetts General Hospital. N. Engl. J. Med. 295:492–499, 1976.
39. Thorbjarnarson, B.: Surgery of the Biliary Tract. Philadelphia, W. B. Saunders Company, 1975, pp. 39–98.
40. Whelton, M. J.: Sclerosing cholangitis. Clin. Gastroenterol. 2:163–173, 1973.

Stenosis of the Sphincter of Oddi

41. Anacker, H., Weiss, H-D., and Kramann, B.: Normal and pathological emptying of the pancreatic duct, particularly in the presence of papillary stenosis. Fortschr. Roentgenstr. 118:391–399, 1973.

42. Chessick, K. C., Black, S., and Hoye, S.: Spasm and operative cholangiography. Arch. Surg. *110*:53–57, 1975.
43. Larsen, C. R., Scholz, F. J., and Wise, R. E.: Diseases of the biliary ducts. Semin. Roentgenol. *11*:259–267, 1976.
44. Mujahed, Z., and Evans, J. A.: Pseudocalculus defect in cholangiography. Am. J. Roentgenol. *116*:337–341, 1972.

Cholecystoses

45. Aguirre, J. R., Boher, R. O., and Guraieb, S.: Hyperplastic cholecystoses; a new contribution to the unitarian theory. Am. J. Roentgenol. *107*:1–13, 1969.
46. Colquhoun, J.: Adenomyomatosis of the gallbladder. Br. J. Radiol. *34*:101–112, 1961.
47. Cynn, W-S., Forbes, T., and Schreiber, M.: Unusual radiographic manifestations of adenomyomatosis of the gallbladder. Radiology *113*:577–579, 1974.
48. Jutras, J. A., and Lévesque, H-P.: Adenomyoma and adenomyomatosis of the gallbladder. Radiologic and pathologic correlations. Radiol. Clin. North Am. *4*:483–500, 1966.
49. Mujahed, Z., Evans, J. A., and Whalen, J. P.: The nonopacified gallbladder on oral cholecystography. Radiology *112*:1–3, 1974.
50. Ochsner, S. F.: Intramural lesions of the gallbladder. Am. J. Roentgenol. *113*:1–9, 1971.
51. Ochsner, S. F.: Solitary polypoid lesions of the gallbladder. Radiol. Clin. North Am. *4*:501–510, 1966.
52. Shapiro, R.: Fixed defects of the gallbladder wall and adenomyomatosis. Surg. Gynecol. Obstet. *136*:745–752, 1973.
53. Thorbjarnarson, B.: Surgery of the Biliary Tract. Philadelphia, W. B. Saunders Company, 1975, pp. 39–98.

Trauma

54. DeMasi, C. J., Akdamar, K., Sparks, R. D., et al.: Puncture of the gallbladder during percutaneous transhepatic cholangiography. J.A.M.A. *201*:79–82, 1967.
55. Diethrich, E. B., Beall, A. C., Jr., Jordon, G. L., Jr., et al.: Traumatic injuries to the extrahepatic biliary tract. Am. J. Surg. *112*:756, 1966.

Surgical Complications

56. Dawson, J. L.: Cholecystitis and cholecystectomy. Clin. Gastroenterol. *2*:85–102, 1973.
57. Eaton, S. B., Wirtz, R. D., Eyck, J. R. T., et al.: Iatrogenic liver injury resulting from ductal instrumentation with the Fogarty biliary balloon catheter. Radiology *100*:581–584, 1971.
58. Geisse, G., Melson, G. L., Tedesco, F. J., et al.: Stenosing lesions of the biliary tree. Am. J. Roentgenol. *123*:378–385, 1975.
59. Gerzof, S. G., Robbins, A. H., and Birkett, D. H.: Computed tomography in the diagnosis and management of abdominal abscesses. Gastrointest. Radiol. *3*:287–294, 1978.
60. Goldman, S. M., Diamond, A., and Salik, J. O.: Intrahepatic rupture secondary to duct exploration demonstrated by cholangiography. Radiology *118*:13–17, 1976.
61. Larsen, C. R., Scholz, F. J., and Wise, R. E.: Diseases of the biliary ducts. Semin. Roentgenol. *11*:259–267, 1976.
62. Tabrisky, J., and Pollack, E. L.: The aberrant divisional bile duct. Radiology *99*:537–538, 1971.
63. Thorbjarnarson, B.: Surgery of the Biliary Tract. Philadelphia, W. B. Saunders Company, 1975, pp. 99–118.
64. Thorbjarnarson, B.: Surgery of the Biliary Tract. Philadelphia, W. B. Saunders Company, 1975, pp. 145–162.

Postcholecystectomy Syndrome

65. Berk, J. E. Postcholecystectomy syndrome. Am. J. Dig. Dis. *6*:1002, 1961.
66. Bodvall, B.: The postcholecystectomy syndromes. Clin. Gastroenterol. *2*:103–126, 1973.
67. Dawson, J. L.: Cholecystitis and cholecystectomy. Clin. Gastroenterol. *2*:85–102, 1973.
68. Hatfield, P. M., and Wise, R. E.: Radiology of the Gallbladder and Bile Ducts. Baltimore, The Williams & Wilkins Company, 1976, pp. 234–247.
69. Lewicki, A. M., Kleinhaus, U., and Ozer, H.: Remnant cystic duct in T-tube cholangiography. Am. J. Roentgenol. *119*:52–56, 1973.

Part III
Acute Suppurative Cholangitis

CARL R. LARSEN, M.D.
ROBERT E. WISE, M.D.

Bacterial contamination of the biliary system may be secondary to hematogenous or lymphatic dissemination or to direct reflux into the bile duct.[9] Although bacteria enter the bile from regurgitation, particularly in bypass biliary surgery, suppuration rarely occurs unless biliary stasis is present.[9, 10] Ductal obstruction most frequently is caused by calculi, although it may result from stricture, neoplasm, ampullary fibrosis, congenital anomalies, pancreatic disorders, and parasites.[8, 9, 15] Clinically, suppurative or pyogenic cholangitis presents with intermittent or persistent pain the right upper quadrant, fever, chills, or jaundice. Septicemia, shock, and possibly death may result from complete obstruction.

RADIOGRAPHIC EVALUATION

Radiographically, little information can be obtained in patients with acute obstructive suppurative cholangitis. Air may be present in the biliary system from incompetence of the sphincter or from a fistula. Patients with complete biliary obstruction with suppuration require immediate surgical intervention. Preoperative radiographic evaluation, although not performed in patients with complete obstruction, is a necessary part of the evaluation of patients with recurrent or intermittent cholangitis. Oral or intravenous cholangiography is rarely helpful, particularly in patients with complete biliary obstruction and elevated levels of bilirubin.[1, 3, 18, 23] Depending on the degree of obstruction, intravenous cholangiography may be successful in demonstrating calculi. Percutaneous transhepatic cholangiography can readily identify the cause of obstruction and any communication with abscess cavities.

Sepsis is a major complication of percutaneous transhepatic cholangiography,[7] particularly since bile cultures are positive for infectious organisms in more than 50 per cent of patients who have surgical obstruction of the bile ducts.[2] Use of the Chiba needle or the skinny needle lessens complications, although the possibilities of infection and septicemia remain. The needle tract, which causes the fistula between the biliary and the vascular systems, seals more quickly with the use of the Chiba needle than with the sheathed needle.[6] In patients with obstruction and high intraductal pressure, the venous pressure may be exceeded. It is therefore important to aspirate and not overly distend the ducts so that the high pressure will not force bacteria into the circulatory system.[2] In contrast to percutaneous cholangiography with a sheathed needle, immediate operation is not necessary with the skinny needle. Antibiotic prophylaxis is recommended.[1, 2]

Endoscopic retrograde cannulation of the biliary tract can also offer information regarding the status of the pancreatic duct and the duodenum. Although this procedure is less invasive, it is not as widely available and is generally more costly than percutaneous transhepatic cholangiography. Contraindications to endoscopic retrograde cannulation include recent acute pancreatitis, sepsis, and acute intestinal obstruction.[2]

Ultrasonography and computerized tomographic (CT) scanning can demonstrate a dilated biliary system in addition to an obstructing mass or calculus. Ultrasound is capable of showing a nonopaque calculus, whereas CT scanning of the biliary system requires the use of contrast agents. Abscess cavities are better demonstrated by CT scans than by ultrasonography. Ultrasound and CT studies are not as accurate when a significant degree of biliary tract obstruction occurs without dilation of the biliary system.[3] Nonspecific defects from abscess cavities or a dilated biliary system may appear on isotope liver scan. Angiography offers information about vascular changes of the liver, pancreas, and biliary tree that may be caused by infection or neoplasm.

The timing of these procedures in the diagnosis of biliary obstruction and their relationship to each other are not fully defined. The various procedures are complementary, but the choice depends on availability, expertise, cost, risk, and information desired. Operative and T-tube cholangiography in the postoperative period may demonstrate all the radiologic features, and frequently these are the only direct cholangiograms available, particularly in patients requiring immediate operative intervention.

Recurrent or chronic cholangitis can present a variety of patterns in the biliary tree. The bile ducts can be dilated with an abnormal branching pattern caused by stretching, elongation, or compression, depending on the degree of hepatic congestion or atrophy.[8, 11, 13] The number of biliary radicles may be decreased owing to fibrosis associated with recurrent disease. Communication with abscess cavities (Fig. 16–95) may be demonstrated. Calculi, neoplasm, stricture, or parasites can be seen by direct cholangiography.

Roentgen signs of parasitic infestations of the biliary system vary from direct visualization of the parasites to changes caused by parasites in the adjacent liver parenchyma. The abscess cavities can be confirmed by nuclear scans, arteriography, ultrasound, or CT scan.[17] *Ascaris lumbricoides* may migrate from the intestinal tract to obstruct the bile ducts either partially or completely (Fig. 16–96).[5, 13, 19] The parasite may

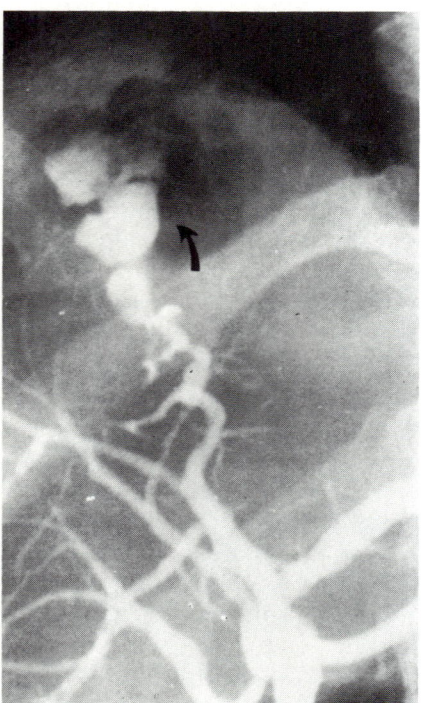

Figure 16–95. Abscess of liver. T-tube cholangiogram. Communication of an abscess cavity (arrow) with an intrahepatic duct.

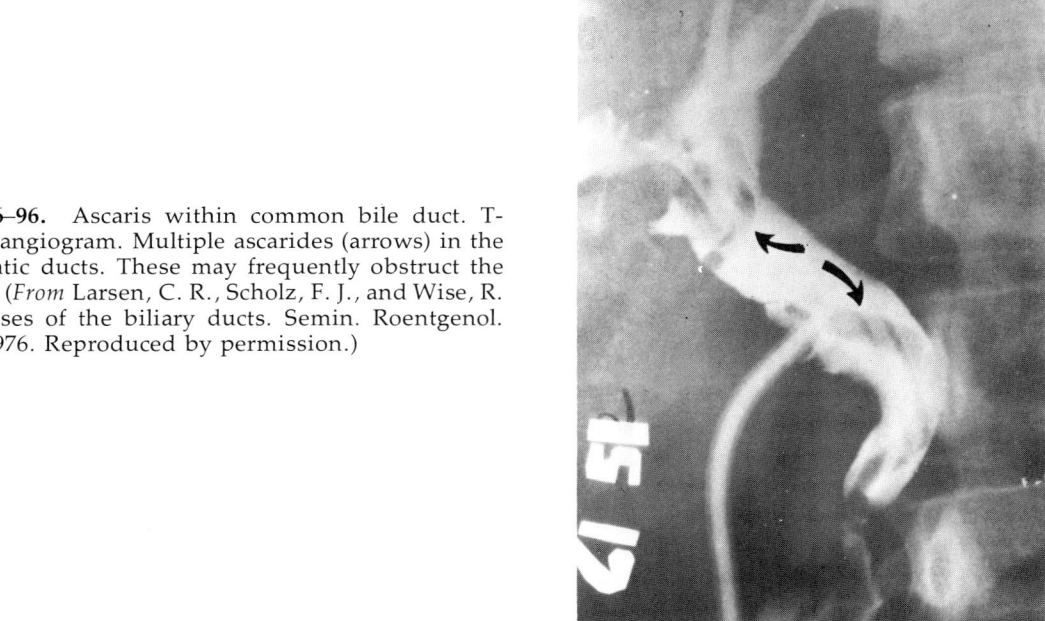

Figure 16–96. Ascaris within common bile duct. T-tube cholangiogram. Multiple ascarides (arrows) in the extrahepatic ducts. These may frequently obstruct the bile duct. (*From* Larsen, C. R., Scholz, F. J., and Wise, R. E.: Diseases of the biliary ducts. Semin. Roentgenol. *11*:259, 1976. Reproduced by permission.)

give rise to cholangitis, hepatic abscess, cholecystitis, stricture, jaundice, or choledocholithiasis.[19] The Chinese liver fluke *Clonorchis sinensis* inhabits the peripheral small intrahepatic ducts and occasionally the larger ducts.[8] These flukes appear as small curved or crescentic filling defects or as semilunar mounds fixed to the wall of the duct (Fig. 16–97).[16,17] They rarely occur in the extrahepatic ducts. Soft pigmented calculi,

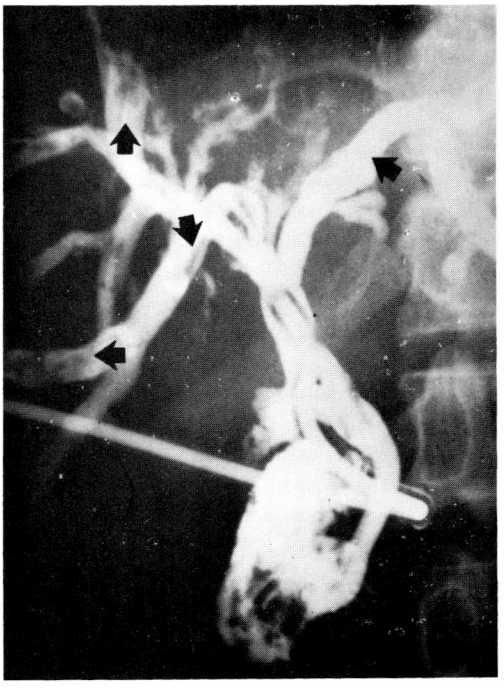

Figure 16–97. Clonorchis infestation of bile ducts. T-tube cholangiogram. *Clonorchis sinensis* infestation producing small lucent defects (arrows) in the intrahepatic ducts. (*From* Hatfield, P. M., and Wise, R. E., Radiology of the Gallbladder and Bile Ducts. Baltimore, The Williams & Wilkins Company, 1976, p. 253. Reproduced by permission.)

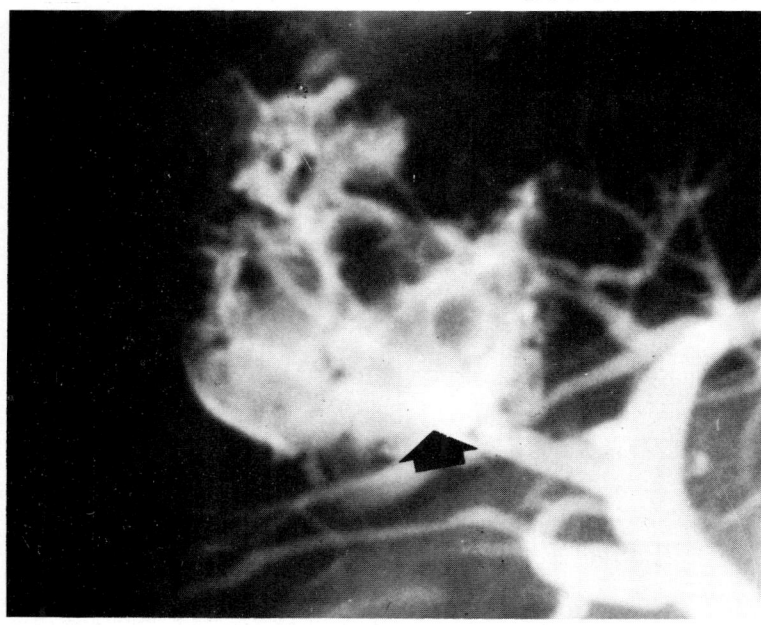

Figure 16–98. Echinococcal abscess. Endoscopic retrograde cholangiogram. Filling of an echinococcal abscess communicating with the bile ducts (arrow).

sludge, pus, and flukes may migrate with bile to cause biliary obstruction.[8, 17] Periductal abscesses and strictures are common. *Fasciola hepatica* and *Opisthorchis viverrini* produce similar radiographic findings.[13]

Parasites may indirectly affect the bile ducts. Fibrosis of the periportal connective tissue is caused by schistosomiasis.[13] Amebiasis and echinococcal infection may cause pressure changes in the bile ducts or may communicate with a biliary radicle (Fig. 16–98).[13, 17, 21]

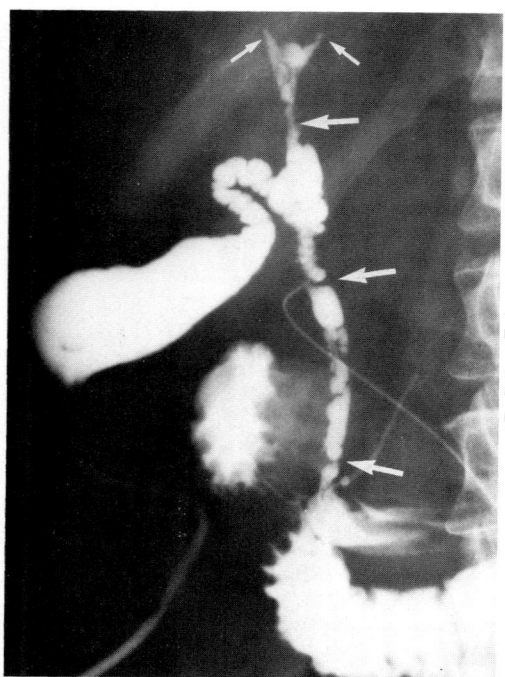

Figure 16–99. Sclerosing cholangitis. Cholangiogram through cholecystostomy tube. Irregular stenosis of the extrahepatic bile ducts (large arrows). Obstruction at the level of the hepatic ducts (small arrows). (*From* Larsen, C. R., Scholz, F. J., and Wise, R. E.: Diseases of the biliary ducts. Semin. Roentgenol. *11*:263, 1976. Reproduced by permission.)

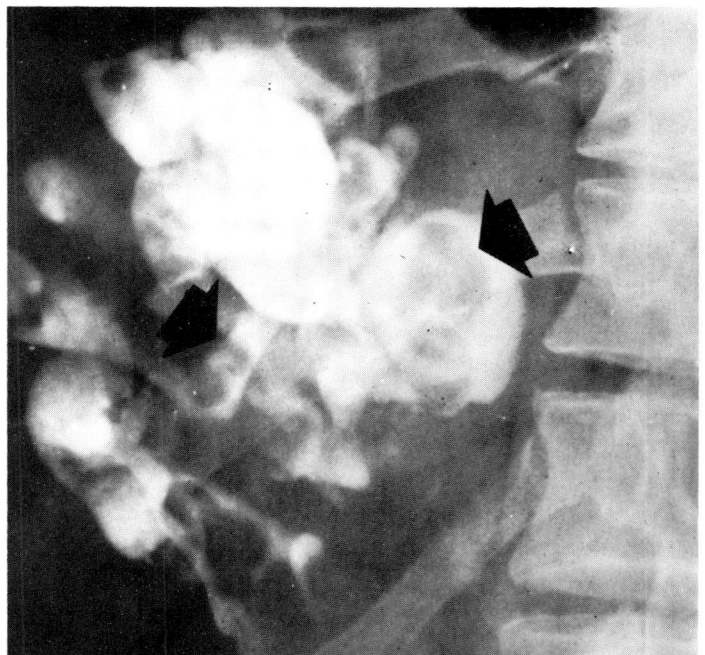

Figure 16–100. Caroli's disease. T-tube cholangiogram. Marked intraductal ectasia with calculi (arrows).

The differential diagnosis of cholangitis includes sclerosing cholangitis, a rare disease of unknown origin characterized by multiple areas of diffuse fibrous narrowing with partial or complete obstruction.[12,13] Primary sclerosing cholangitis has been attributed to bacterial infection, hypersensitivity, and an autoimmune response.[20] In 1966 Warren et al.[22] reviewed 42 patients with sclerosing cholangitis at the Lahey Clinic and found 12 (28 per cent) with associated ulcerative colitis. Radiographically (Fig. 16–99), strictures are usually multiple and of variable length. The extrahepatic ducts almost always are involved in the sclerosing process. The intrahepatic ducts may become involved later in many patients. Beading may be present between the narrowed segments.[12,20]

Segmental saccular dilatation of the intrahepatic ducts, frequently associated with biliary calculi, liver abscess, and cholangitis, is a disease described by Caroli (Fig. 16–100).[4,14] Jaundice, cirrhosis, and portal hypertension do not occur.[8] Symptoms are intermittent and are usually preceded by the formation of stones secondary to bile stasis. Intravenous cholangiography with tomography may show accumulation of contrast material within the ectatic ducts, but the disease is most often detected by direct cholangiography of some type.[8] Liver scanning with radiopharmaceutical agents may show nonspecific cold areas, whereas ultrasound and CT scanning show the cystic nature of the ectatic ducts without necessarily determining that they originate from the biliary system. Arteriography is of little value in the diagnosis.

References

1. Berk, R. N., and Clemett, A. R.: Radiology of the Gallbladder and Bile Ducts, Philadelphia, W. B. Saunders Company, 1977, p. 294.
2. Berk, R. N., Ferrucci, J. T., Goldstein, H. M., et al.: Progress in clinical radiology: diagnostic imaging of the liver and bile ducts. Invest. Radiol. 13:265–278, 1978.

3. Blumgart, L. H.: Biliary tract obstruction: new approaches to old problems. Am. J. Surg. 135:19–31, 1978.
4. Caroli, J.: Diseases of the intrahepatic biliary tree. Clin. Gastroenterol. 2:147–161, 1973.
5. Cremin, B. J., and Fisher, R. M.: Biliary ascariasis in children. Am. J. Roentgenol. 126:352–357, 1976.
6. Elias, E., Hamlyn, A. N., Jain, S., et al.: A randomized trial of percutaneous transhepatic cholangiography with the Chiba needle versus endoscopic retrograde cholangiography for bile duct visualization in jaundice. Gastroenterology 71:439–443, 1976.
7. Evans, J. A., and Mujahed, Z.: Percutaneous transhepatic cholangiography. Semin. Roentgenol. 11:219–222, 1976.
8. Hatfield, P. M., and Wise, R. E.: Radiology of the Gallbladder and Bile Ducts. Baltimore, The Williams & Wilkins Company, 1976, pp. 201–204, 213–221.
9. Hinshaw, D. B.: Acute suppurative cholangitis. In Sabiston, D. C., Jr. (ed.): Davis-Christopher Textbook of Surgery. Vol. 1 Ed. 11. Philadelphia, W. B. Saunders Company, 1977, pp. 12–14.
10. Hinshaw, D. B.: Acute obstructive suppurative cholangitis. Surg. Clin. North Am. 53:1089–1094, 1973.
11. Ho, C. S., and Wesson, D. E.: Recurrent pyogenic cholangitis in Chinese immigrants. Am. J. Roentgenol. 122:368–374, 1974.
12. Krieger, J., Seaman, W. B., and Porter, M. R.: The roentgenologic appearance of sclerosing cholangitis. Radiology 95:369–375, 1970.
13. Larsen, C. R., Scholz, F. J., and Wise, R. E.: Disease of the biliary ducts. Semin. Roentgenol. 11:259–267, 1976.
14. Mujahed, Z., Glenn, F., and Evans, J. A.: Communicating cavernous ectasia of the intrahepatic ducts (Caroli's disease). Am. J. Roentgenol. 113:21–26, 1971.
15. Nardi, G. L.: Acute suppurative cholangitis due to ampullary fibrosis. Surg. Clin. North Am. 50:1137–1140, 1970.
16. Okuda, K., Emura, T., Morokuma, K., et al.: Clonorchiasis studied by percutaneous cholangiography and a therapeutic trial of toluene-2,4-diiosothiocyanate. A case report. Gastroenterology 65:457–461, 1973.
17. Reeder, M. M.: Tropical diseases of the liver and bile ducts. Semin. Roentgenol. 10:229–243, 1975.
18. Scholz, F. J., Larsen, C. R., and Wise, R. E.: Intravenous cholangiography: recurring concepts. Semin. Roentgenol. 11:197–202, 1976.
19. Schulman, A.: Biliary ascariasis presenting in the United States. Am. J. Gastroenterol. 68:167–170, 1977.
20. Schwartz, S. I. Primary sclerosing cholangitis: a disease revisited. Surg. Clin. North Am. 53:1161–1167, 1973.
21. Tuttle, R. J.: Cause of recurring obstructive jaundice revealed by percutaneous cholangiography — hydatid cyst. N. Engl. J. Med. 283:805–806, 1970.
22. Warren, K. W., Athanassiades, S., and Monge, J. I.: Primary sclerosing cholangitis: a study of forty-two cases. Am. J. Surg. 111:23–28, 1966.
23. Wise, R. E.: Radiology of the liver and biliary tract. Gastroenterology 53:312–325, 1967.

Part IV
Gallstone Ileus and Fistula

CARL R. LARSEN, M.D.
ROBERT E. WISE, M.D.

A biliary fistula, which may occur spontaneously or after operation, is an abnormal passage or communication from the biliary system to an organ, cavity, or free surface. Fistulas are classified as external (biliary cutaneous) or internal (biliobiliary, bronchobiliary, or biliary enteric). Most internal fistulas are spontaneous, whereas most external fistulas arise after a surgical procedure.[15] Of the spontaneous internal biliary fistulas, 90 per cent result from calculi of the gallbladder or bile ducts. Peptic ulcer disease causes fistulas in 6 per cent of patients, and neoplasm of the stomach, gallbladder, pancreas, duodenum, colon, or bile duct is the causative factor in the remaining 4 per cent.[11] Transient anastomotic leaks are the most common cause of postsurgical biliary fistula.

Whereas external fistulas are easily recognized (Fig. 16–101) and are not a

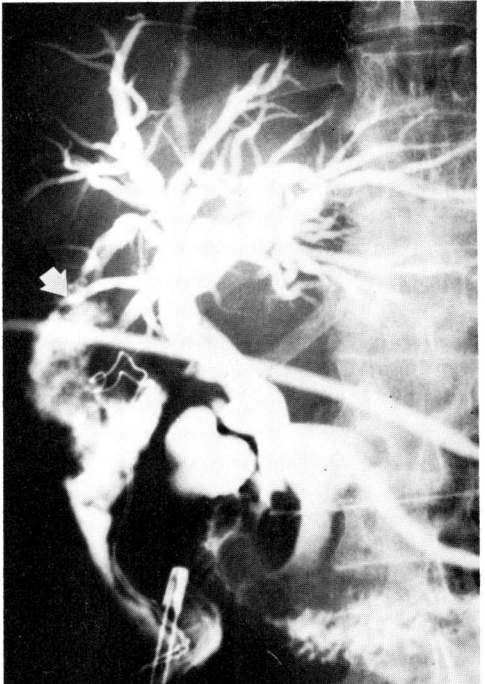

Figure 16–101. Biliary cutaneous fistula. T-tube cholangiogram. These usually follow an anastomotic leak or dislodgment of the T-tube. A fistulous tract extends from a right hepatic duct to the skin (arrow).

diagnostic problem, the presence of an internal fistula can be difficult to establish, as symptoms often are not distinguishable from the antecedent disease. A clinical presentation of recurrent upper abdominal distress, jaundice, colic, and fever, which is suddenly relieved, is typical but not diagnostic of a spontaneous biliary fistula.[13, 15] Bile-tinged, bitter-tasting, or malodorous sputum suggests the presence of a bronchobiliary fistula.[11] The passage of a gallstone may cause symptoms of mechanical bowel obstruction (gallstone ileus). Hyponatremia, inanition, weight loss, and infection are critical complications of biliary fistulas regardless of the cause.[9, 15]

RADIOGRAPHIC EVALUATION

Internal Biliary Fistula

The radiographic evaluation of a biliary tract fistula can be accomplished with plain films of the abdomen and with contrast studies (Fig. 16–102). Unless a surgical bypass procedure has been performed or an incompetent sphincter of Oddi (Fig. 16–103) is present, air within the bile ducts or gallbladder indicates an abnormal connection or biliary fistula. Pneumobilia in the absence of a fistula may also be the result of a disturbance of the sphincter from peptic ulcer disease, local tumors (pancreas, duodenum, or bile ducts), marked antiperistalsis of the duodenum, drug effects, ascending infection with gas-forming organisms, or passage of biliary calculi. Entry of the common bile duct into a duodenal diverticulum anatomic variant may be associated with hypoplasia of the sphincteric musculature allowing passage of air into the bile ducts.[16] Plain film diagnosis of fistula or its cause is the exception rather than the rule. The presence of air within the bile ducts associated with an ectopic calculus (gallstone ileus) or seen simultaneously with air in the wall of the gallbladder (emphysematous cholecystitis)[10] may permit a probable diagnosis after plain film examination of the abdomen.

970 — THE BILIARY SYSTEM

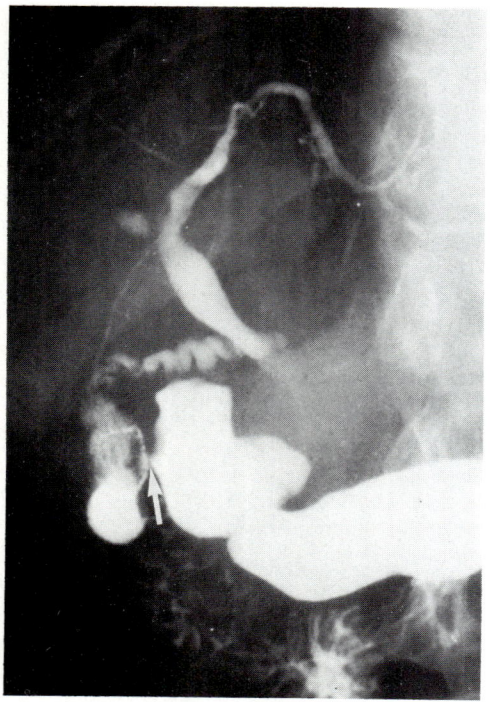

Figure 16–102. Cholecystoduodenal fistula. Upper gastrointestinal series. Asymptomatic, incidentally demonstrated, spontaneous cholecystoduodenal fistula (arrow), presumably secondary to a previous ulcer of the duodenal bulb.

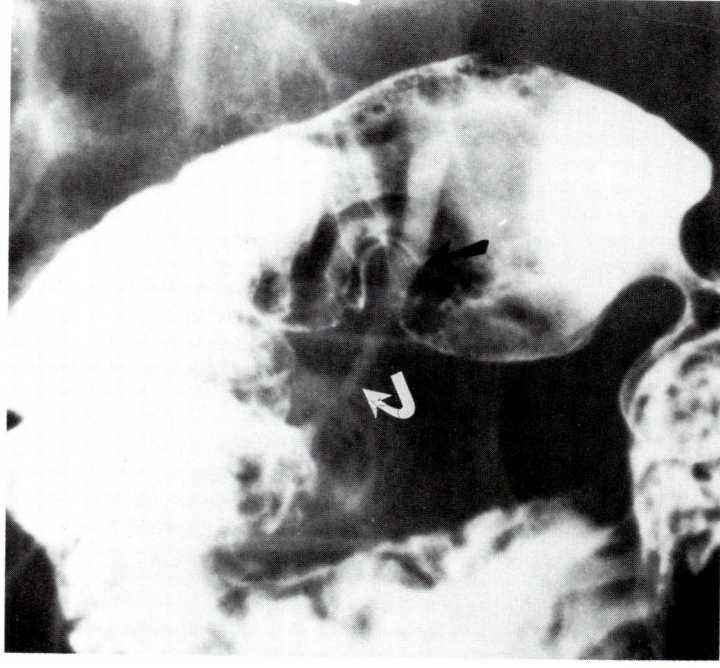

Figure 16–103. Incompetent sphincter of Oddi. Upper gastrointestinal series. Incompetent sphincter with reflux of barium into the common bile duct (arrows).

Opacification of the bile ducts on intravenous cholangiography with undisturbed liver function depends on intermittent delay in emptying of the common bile duct caused by the normal action of the sphincter.[20] As with the poor opacification that is obtained owing to rapid drainage (Fig. 16–104) in patients with hepaticojejunostomy, a large fistulous tract rarely allows opacification of the bile ducts. A narrow fistula may permit visualization of the bile ducts, although the fistula itself is rarely demonstrated.[11]

Barium cholangiography is an essential study in evaluating the site of anastomosis and the biliary ducts after bypass surgery.[14, 21] When a fistula is suspected, barium studies may clearly show the site of communication if the fistulous tract has not been walled off. The passage of barium in and out of the bile ducts depends on the size and location of the fistula, and in the majority of patients the fistula is not demonstrated by barium examination.[11, 13] Fistulas secondary to peptic ulcer disease (Fig. 16–105) affect different locations of the biliary system depending on the site of ulceration. Duodenal ulcers, especially those that frequently occur in the second (Fig. 16–106) and third segments of the duodenum, connect with the common bile duct, whereas gastric ulcers communicate with the gallbladder.[11] Communication with the biliary tree may be seen in Crohn's disease of the duodenum (Fig. 16–107) either secondary to small communicating fistulas or to a disturbance of the sphincter caused by localized inflammation.

Ultrasonography may reveal biliary calculi or dilated bile ducts; however, air within the biliary tract, like air within the intestine, reflects the sound beam to the transducer, preventing satisfactory visualization. Computerized body tomography shows air within the biliary system and the presence of an opaque calculus. Unlike ultrasonography, computerized scanning requires the use of a contrast agent to visualize a nonopaque calculus. Computerized scanning may also demonstrate the presence of an eroding mass or abscess.

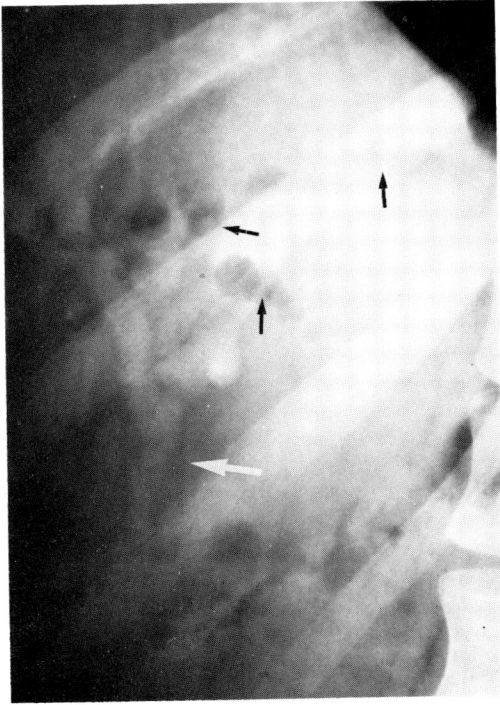

Figure 16–104. Postoperative biliary bypass. Intravenous cholangiogram. Air in intrahepatic ducts (black arrows) after bypass for choledochal cyst. Minimal opacification of other bile ducts (white arrow).

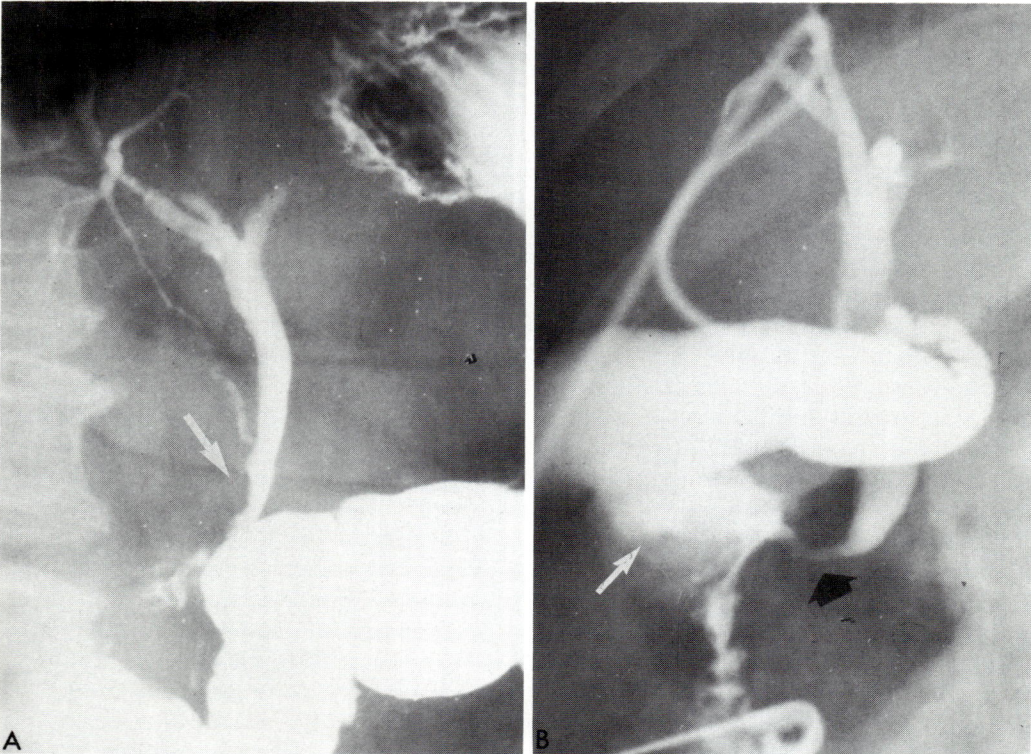

Figure 16–105. Choledochoduodenal fistula. Upper gastrointestinal series. Reflux of barium into the common bile duct (arrow) secondary to an ulcer in the duodenal bulb — an infrequent complication of duodenal ulcer disease. *B*, Choledochoduodenal fistula. Operative cholangiogram. Drainage of contrast medium into the duodenum through the fistula (black arrow) and into the duodenal bulb (white arrow).

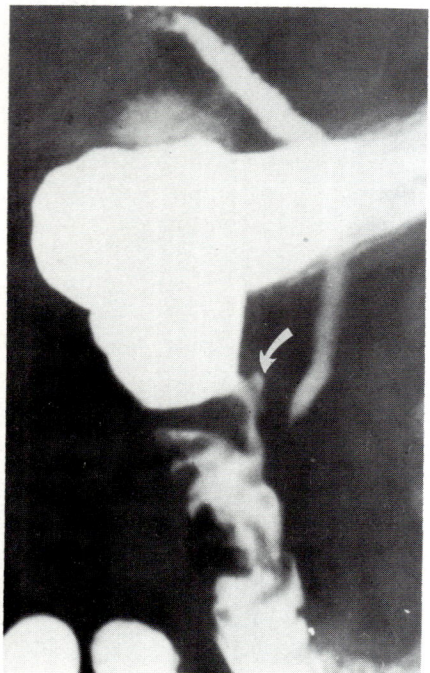

Figure 16–106. Duodenal ulcer with biliary reflux. Upper gastrointestinal series. Reflux of barium into the common bile duct secondary to an ulcer (arrow) in the second portion of the duodenum. This is caused by inflammation disturbing the sphincter. (*From* Hatfield, P. M., and Wise, R. E.: Radiology of the Gallbladder and Bile Ducts. Baltimore, The Williams & Wilkins Company, 1976, p. 211. Reproduced by permission.)

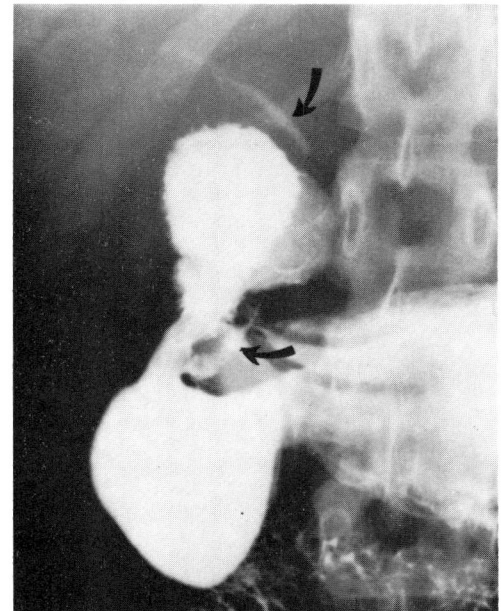

Figure 16–107. Crohn's disease with biliary reflux. Upper gastrointestinal series. Reflux of barium into the common bile duct (arrows) secondary to Crohn's disease of the second part of the duodenum.

Biliobiliary and Bronchobiliary Fistulas

Biliobiliary and bronchobiliary fistulas occur infrequently. Biliobiliary fistula, a complication of cholelithiasis, is an abnormal communication between the accessory biliary tract (gallbladder or cystic duct) and the extrahepatic ducts.[6] The symptoms are nonspecific but include the abrupt onset of jaundice in patients with known gallbladder calculi. Retrograde cholangiography is the only preoperative study that demonstrates the abnormality.[19]

Bronchobiliary fistulas (Fig. 16–108) may be congenital[3] or acquired.[22] Hydatid disease of the liver is the most frequent cause, although a communication between the biliary and the bronchial systems (Fig. 16–109) may result from any inflammatory disease of the liver associated with a subcapsular or subphrenic abscess. An inflammatory process that extends from the liver to a point adjacent to the diaphragm associated with increased biliary pressure secondary to obstruction may lead to perforation into a bronchus.[11] Congenital bronchobiliary fistulas are demonstrated more frequently by bronchography than by direct cholangiography.[3] Inflammation or a pleural effusion may be evident on radiographs of the chest. T-tube cholangiography or tube cholangiography from the drainage site of an abscess frequently demonstrates the communication.

Gallstone Ileus

Spontaneous biliary enteric fistulas occur in approximately 3 to 5 per cent of all patients with gallstones,[12] and asymptomatic passage of the calculus into the gastrointestinal tract occurs in the majority (Fig. 16–110). In 90 per cent of patients, a fistula between the biliary tract and the intestine is caused by the erosion of a gallstone.[3] The incidence of cholecystoenteric fistulas exceeds that of gallstone ileus by a ratio of six to

974 — THE BILIARY SYSTEM

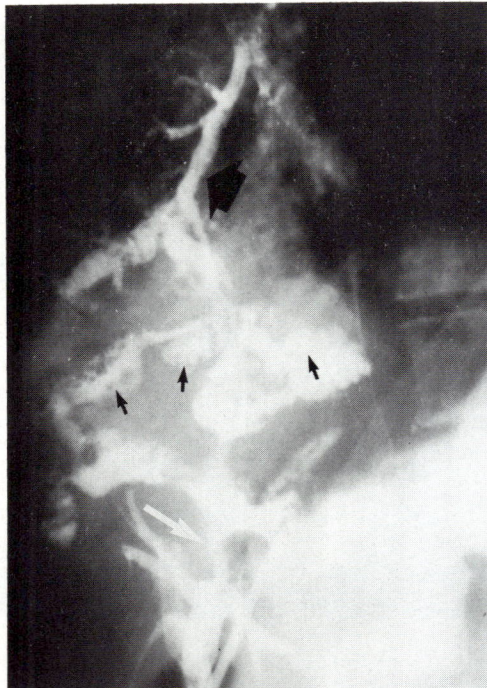

Figure 16–108. Bronchobiliary fistula from subphrenic abscess. Lateral view of fistulogram shows communication of contrast in the abscess (small arrows) with a bronchus (large black arrow) and the biliary tree (large white arrow).

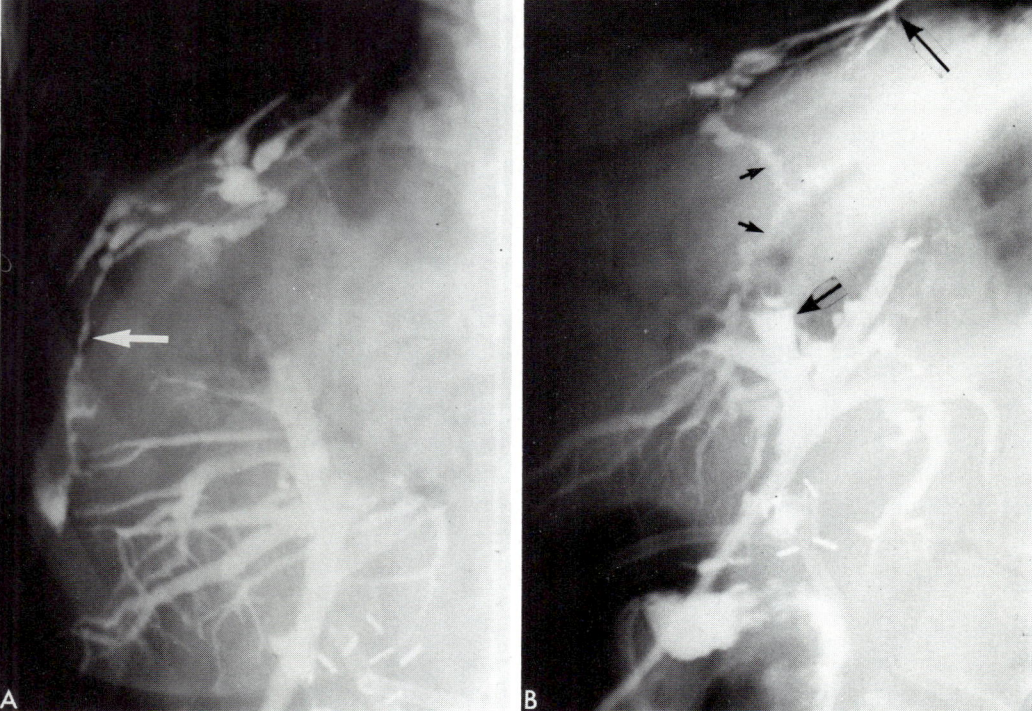

Figure 16–109. *A*, Bronchobiliary fistula. Fistulogram, anteroposterior projection. Bronchobiliary fistula (arrow) in a patient with persistent cough and pleural effusions after operation. *B*, Bronchobiliary fistula. Fistulogram, lateral projection. The fistulous tract (small arrows) is communicating with a bronchus above and the biliary tree below (large arrows).

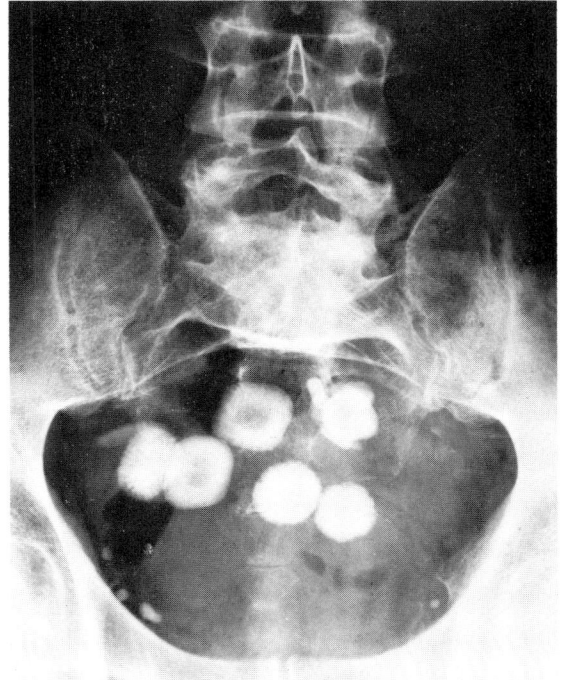

Figure 16–110. Gallstones in intestine. Plain film. Multiple opaque calculi are in the pelvis. A small bowel series showed them to be in the ileum. The patient was asymptomatic and had had a cholecystectomy several months before this film was taken.

one.[11] Biliary calculi account for 1 to 2 per cent of all instances of mechanical obstruction of the small intestine.[1, 3, 13]

The duodenal bulb is by far the most common site of the fistula; the postbulbar duodenum or, rarely, the gastric antrum may be the entry point. Fistulization to the colon (hepatic flexure) is not rare, but obstructive ileus, of course, will not result.

Gallstone ileus occurs frequently in the elderly and accounts for 20 per cent of intestinal obstruction in patients over the age of 65 and for 24 per cent in those over 70 years.[13] Symptoms frequently are minimal; 20 to 30 per cent of patients give a history consistent with acute cholecystitis within ten days of bowel obstruction.[11] Symptoms of bowel obstruction may be intermittent as the calculus passes through the intestine (tumbling obstruction).[3, 13] Obstruction from impaction of the calculus occurs most often in the terminal ileum (60 per cent). The proximal ileum (24 per cent), the distal jejunum (9 per cent), and the colon (3 to 5 per cent) represent the other sites of obstruction.[3] The sigmoid is the most common colonic site because it is the narrowest segment; however, obstruction usually occurs in association with diverticulitis, neoplasm, or other causes of constriction.[13]

The triad of radiographic findings of biliary enteric fistulas with gallstone ileus is (1) air in the biliary system, (2) ectopic calculus or calculi, and (3) small bowel obstruction.[1] A correct preoperative diagnosis has been made in 4 to 48 per cent of patients in published series.[11, 13] Both plain film studies (Fig. 16–111A) and barium examinations (Fig. 16–111B) contribute to the diagnosis.

Closure of the biliary fistula, in some instances before the onset of intestinal obstruction, accounts for the absence of air in the gallbladder[2] or bile ducts in one-third of patients.[3] Air within the biliary tree tends to be present in the major branches near the porta hepatis and can be differentiated from gas in the portal venous system which is present in the peripheral regions of the liver. Peribiliary fat (pseudopneumobilia)[8]

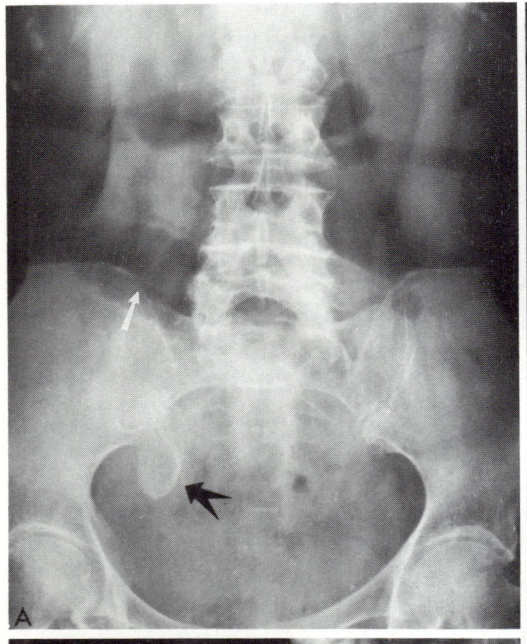
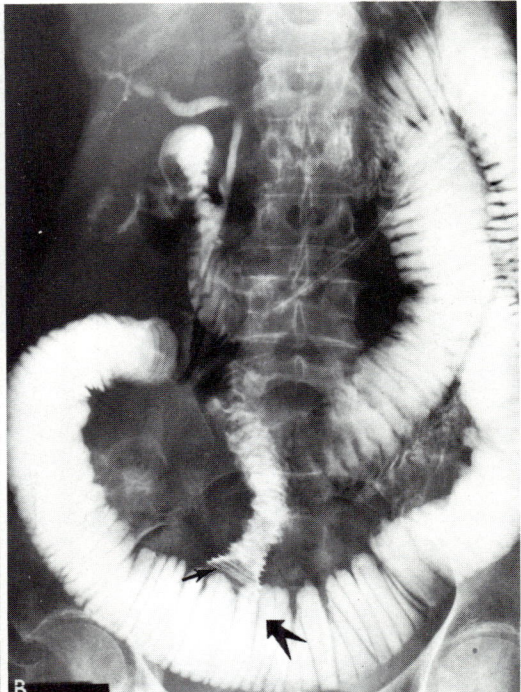
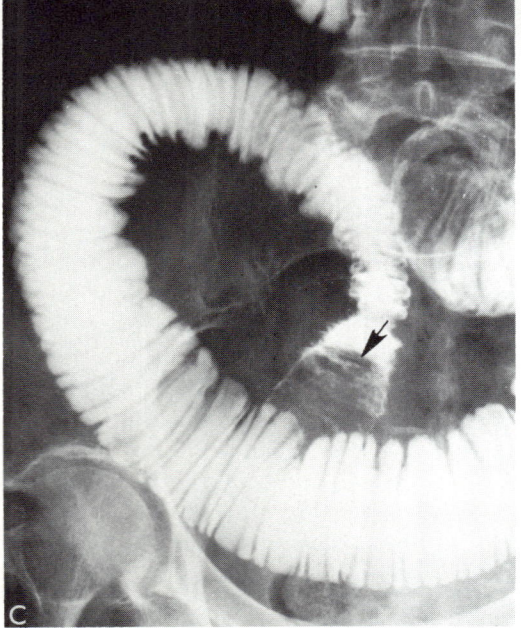

Figure 16–111. *A*, Gallstone ileus. Plain film. Gallstone ileus with ectopic gallstone (black arrow). Minimal air was present in the bile duct. Small bowel distention was present with fluid-filled loops and relatively little air (white arrow). *B*, Gallstone ileus. Upper gastrointestinal series. Reflux of barium into the bile duct. Obstructed small bowel (large arrow) is secondary to ectopic calculus (small arrow). *C*, Gallstone ileus. Small bowel series. Ectopic gallstone (arrow) obstructing small intestine.

appears as branching or linear lucencies on plain films and may be confused with air in the bile ducts.[18] Pseudopneumobilia can be confirmed by intravenous cholangiography.

An ectopic gallstone (see Fig. 16–110) is not always associated with obstruction; it may be seen migrating through the intestine on serial abdominal plain films. The majority (80 to 90 per cent)[3] pass unnoticed or may lodge within the intestine,[11] perhaps within a diverticulum, without causing symptoms. These stones eventually may cause symptoms if they continue to grow while retained in the small intestine.[3] Infrequently, ectopic calculi have been reported in the stomach,[4] lung,[17] urinary tract, and aorta.[3]

Small bowel obstruction from impaction of a calculus (Fig. 16–111B and C) is difficult to diagnose and is associated with a mortality rate five times greater than that of small bowel obstruction from other causes.[13] The "loop obturation pattern,"[7] as seen on the plain film, consists of minimal to moderate degrees of gaseous distention of the fluid-filled loops of bowel with prominent valvulae conniventes without extreme effacement. Fluid-filled loops of intestine are well delineated with gas-containing segments frequently assuming a radial configuration. Rarely, this pattern occurs with other forms of mechanical obstruction, but most of these patients have moderate to severe degrees of gaseous distention. Fluid accumulation with lesser amounts of air (loop obturation pattern) is predominant in patients with gallstone ileus; it occurred in 86 per cent of these patients in one series.[7] Contrast examination is necessary if only one or two parts of the triad of radiographic findings are present. A barium enema or retrograde small bowel series may dislodge the calculus and cause its spontaneous passage.[11] The upper gastrointestinal series may show the fistulous site in addition to outlining an unsuspected obstructing calculus (particularly if the calculus is non-opaque).

External Biliary Fistula

External fistulas most frequently develop after operation (Fig. 16–112), with persistent drainage through the T-tube tract.[11, 15] They may occur after trauma or may

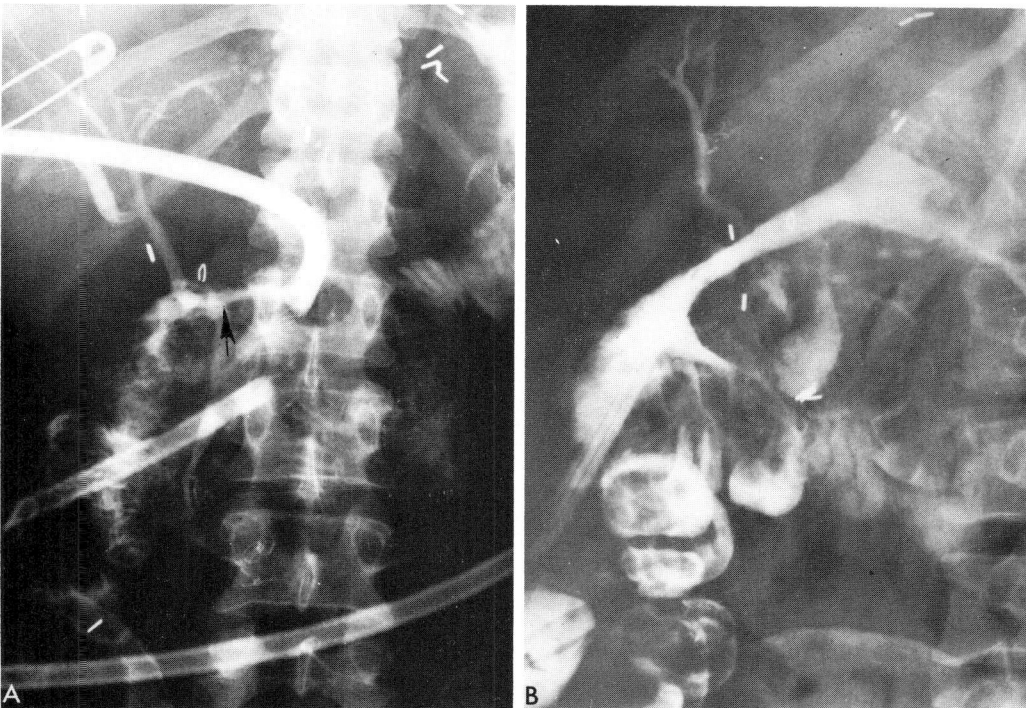

Figure 16–112. Biliary duodenocolocutaneous fistula. Fistulogram, anteroposterior projection. Patient had had a Billroth II procedure. Contrast material in the cutaneous fistulous tract (arrow) is opacifying the biliary tree and duodenum. B, Fistulogram, lateral projection. The right colon is also opacified a short time later. Postsurgical fistula may occur after anastomotic leaks, dislodgment of the T-tube, or injury to bile ducts.

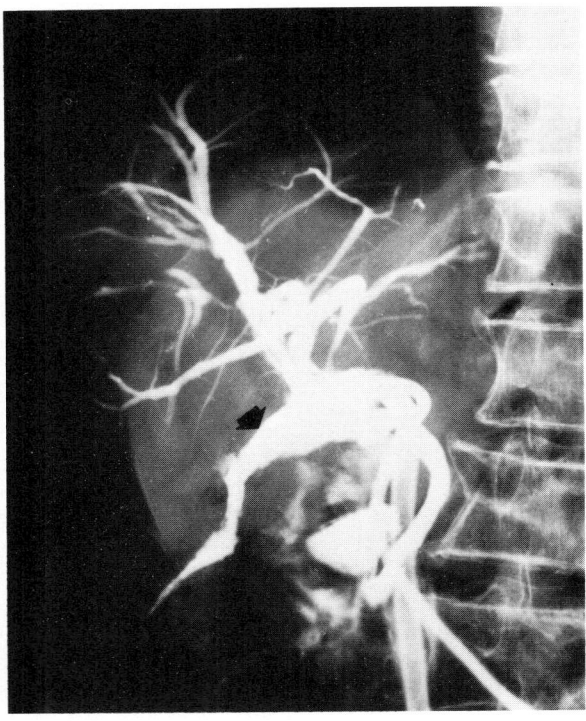

Figure 16–113. Biliary fistula. T-tube cholangiogram. Leak (arrow) from insertion site of T tube in the common duct.

result from a spontaneous external communication caused by rupture of an acutely inflamed gallbladder.[19] Postsurgical fistulas (Fig. 16–113) usually follow anastomotic leakage, incomplete closure of the cystic duct remnant (Fig. 16–114), or dislodgment of the T-tube (Fig. 16–115). In the absence of distal obstruction, the fistulous tract may close spontaneously without surgical intervention. Considerable drainage from a T-tube during the initial two to seven postoperative days suggests the possibility of injury to the bile ducts.[14] Injury often occurs when excessive bleeding at the time of

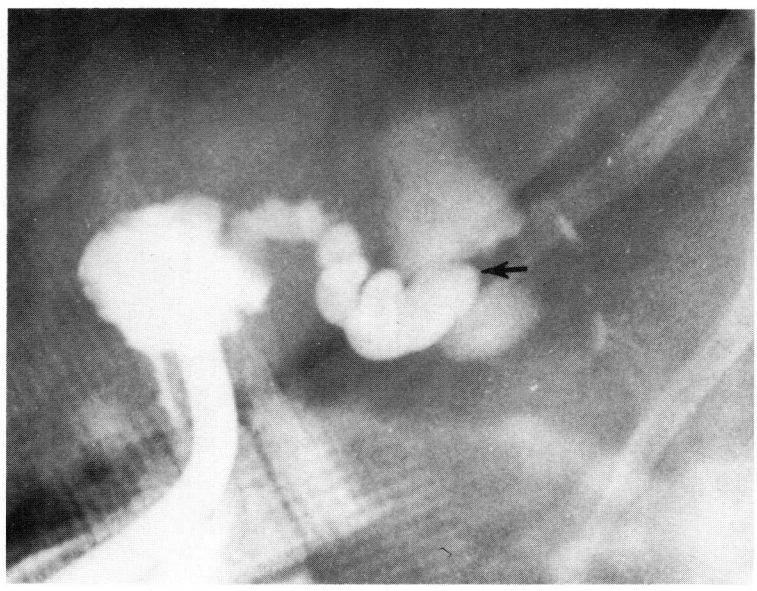

Figure 16–114. Biliary fistula. Tube cholangiogram. Cholecystostomy was performed at time of operation because of severe inflammation. Necrosis of cystic duct developed with formation of fistula (arrow) at the posterior margin of the common bile duct at insertion of the cystic duct. (*From* Hatfield, P. M., and Wise, R. E.: Radiology of the Gallbladder and Bile Ducts. Baltimore, The Williams & Wilkins Company, 1976, p. 213. Reproduced by permission.)

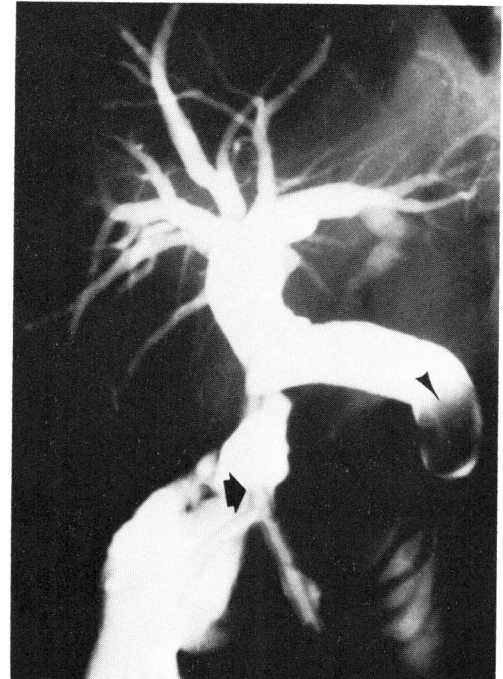

Figure 16–115. Biliary fistula with distal bile duct obstruction. T-tube cholangiogram. Calculus in distal common bile duct (arrowhead). Displaced T tube (arrow) with large leak from bile duct.

operation necessitates blind application of hemostats or when an anomalous right hepatic duct is inadvertently severed.

External fistulas are evaluated by inserting a French catheter into the fistulous tract if a T-tube is not present and injecting contrast material. Fistulas from ductal damage at the time of operation, slippage of the T-tube, or persistent obstruction (Fig. 16–116) can

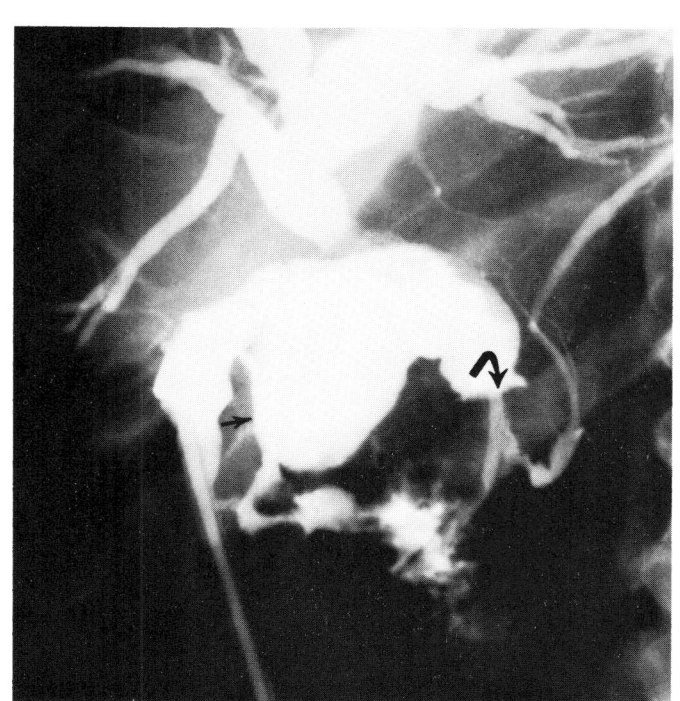

Figure 16–116. Biliary fistula with distal bile duct obstruction. T-tube cholangiogram. Fistula between cystic duct remnant and duodenum (straight arrow) secondary to a retained calculus (curved arrow) in the distal common bile duct. (*From* Hatfield, P. M., and Wise, R. E.: Radiology of the Gallbladder and Bile Ducts. Baltimore, The Williams & Wilkins Company, 1976, p. 213. Reproduced by permission.)

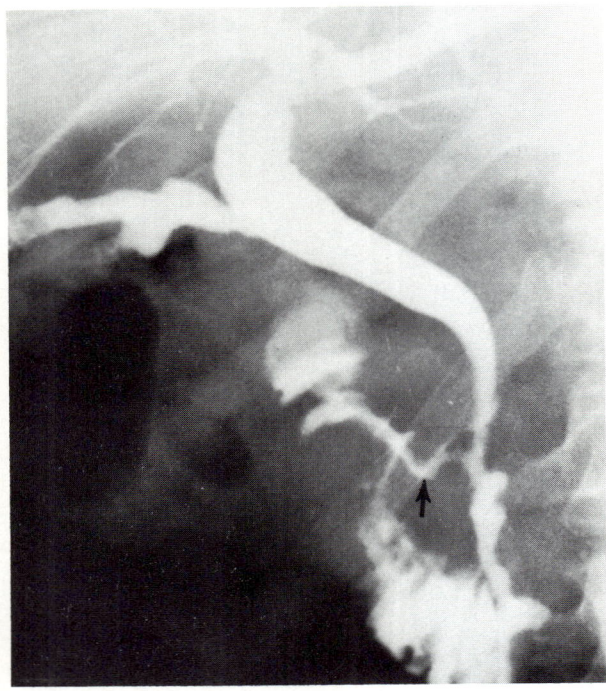

Figure 16–117. Choledochoduodenal fistula. T-tube cholangiogram. Fistula (arrow) between the distal common bile duct and the second portion of the duodenum. (*From* Hatfield, P. M., and Wise, R. E.: Radiology of the Gallbladder and Bile Ducts. Baltimore, The Williams & Wilkins Company, 1976, p. 208. Reproduced by permission.)

be demonstrated using T-tube cholangiography. In patients with persistent drainage from a fistulous tract caused by a retained calculus, the calculus can be removed via the tract avoiding a second surgical procedure.[5] Monitoring of transient anastomotic leaks of transient fistulas (Figs. 16–117 and 16–118) can be performed easily with cholangiography via a T-tube. Frequently, several fistulas (see Fig. 16–112) may communicate with

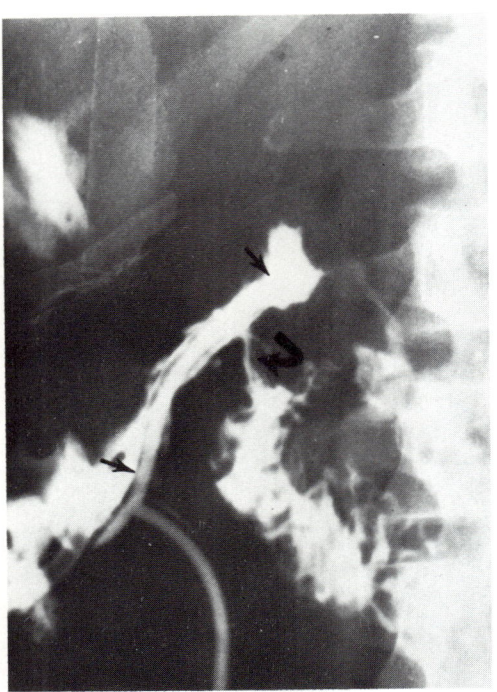

Figure 16–118. Dislodged T-tube (straight arrows). T-tube cholangiogram. A fistula (curved arrow) is present between the T-tube tract and the duodenum. (*From* Hatfield, P. M., and Wise, R. E.: Radiology of the Gallbladder and Bile Ducts. Baltimore, The Williams & Wilkins Company, 1976, p. 213. Reproduced by permission.)

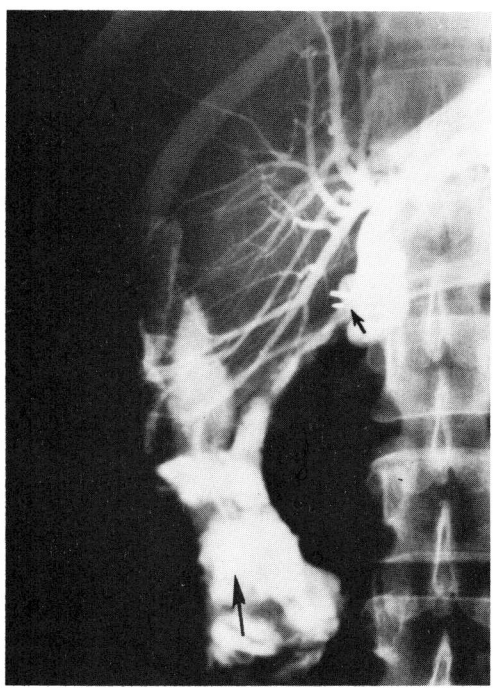

Figure 16–119. Subhepatic abscess. Fistulogram, anteroposterior projection. Leak from cystic duct remnant (small arrow) is extending into a large subhepatic collection (large arrow). (*From* Hatfield, P. M., and Wise, R. E.: Radiology of the Gallbladder and Bile Ducts. Baltimore, The Williams & Wilkins Company, 1976, p. 212. Reproduced by permission.)

the external surface, the peritoneum, or the intestine. Occasionally, a bronchobiliary fistula may be demonstrated through the external drain site (see Figs. 16–108 and 16–109). Communications with the peritoneum may form a walled-off collection of bile (Fig. 16–119), producing a chemical peritonitis.

Ultrasonography and CT scan are useful, quick, and noninvasive procedures for establishing the presence of an abnormal fluid collection. Nuclear scanning techniques may help localize the presence of intrahepatic or subphrenic abscesses (Fig. 16–120).

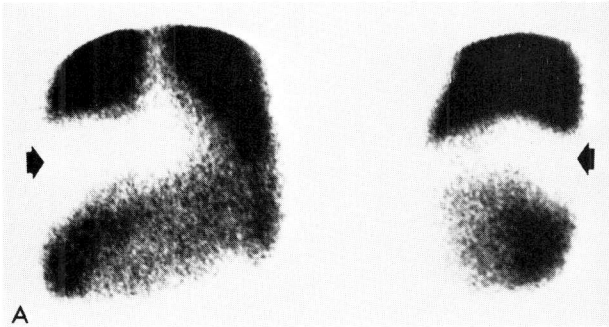

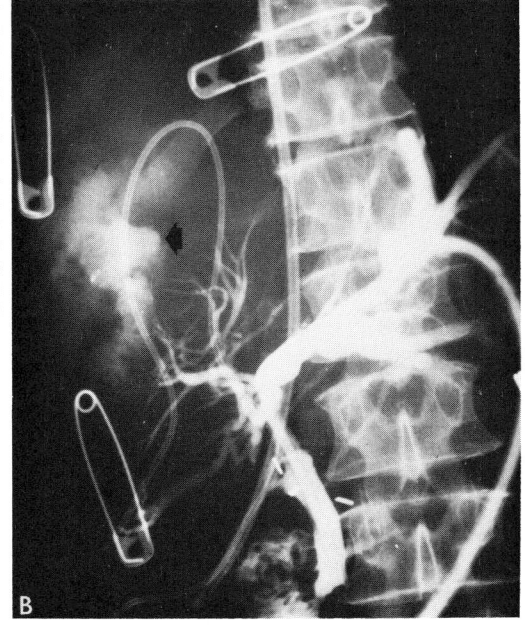

Figure 16–120. Subphrenic abscess. Liver-lung scan, anteroposterior and lateral projections. A large area of no activity (arrows) between the right lung and the liver. A large subphrenic abscess was present. *B*, Communication with intrahepatic abscess. Tube cholangiogram. Communication of right intrahepatic ducts with intrahepatic abscess (arrow). This is the same patient as seen in *A*.

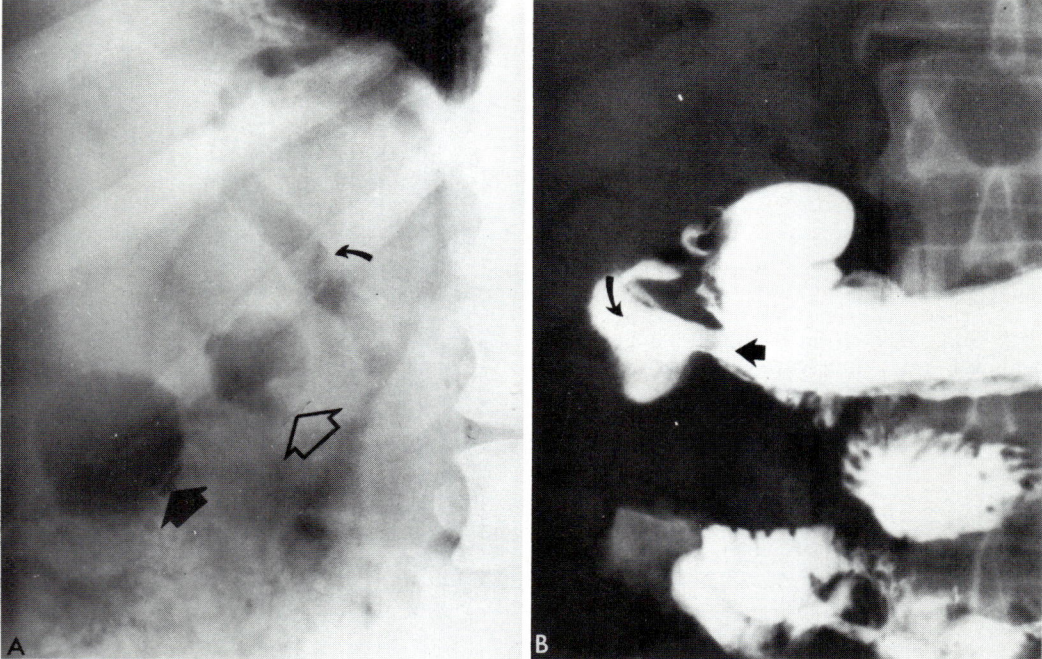

Figure 16–121. *A*, Pneumobilia. Preliminary film for intravenous cholangiogram. Patient had had a cholecystoduodenal bypass procedure. Air is present in the common bile duct (curved arrow), duodenal bulb (opened arrow), and gallbladder (solid arrow). *B*, Cholecystoduodenal bypass. Upper gastrointestinal series. Cholecystoduodenal fistula (straight arrow) of surgical origin; gallbladder (curved arrow) fills with barium.

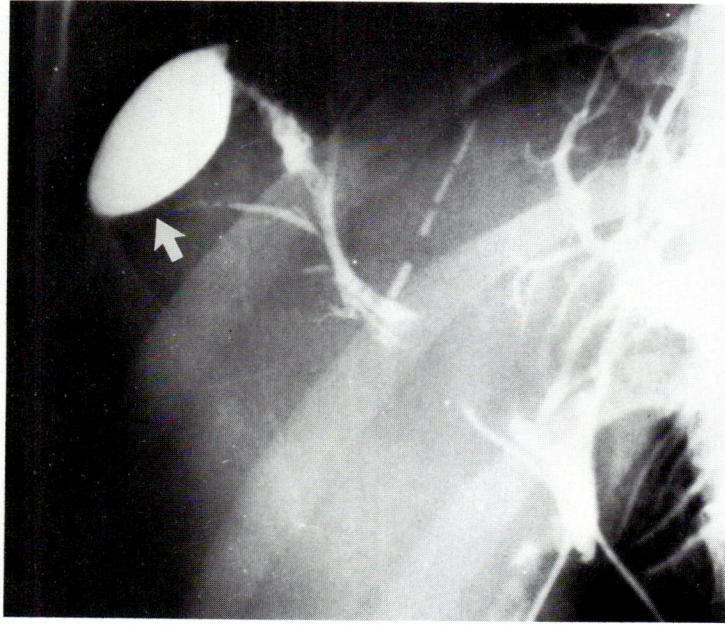

Figure 16–122. Subcapsular hematoma. Operative cholangiogram. Subcapsular hematoma (arrow) with mild hemobilia. Communication of bile ducts with hematoma is post-traumatic in origin.

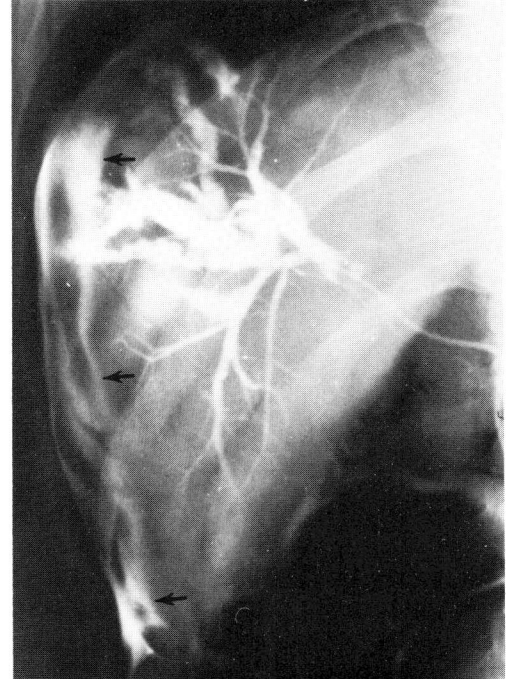

Figure 16–123. Subcapsular hematoma. Operative cholangiogram. Subcapsular extravasation (arrows). (*From* Hatfield, P. M., and Wise, R. E.: Radiology of the Gallbladder and Bile Ducts. Baltimore, The Williams & Wilkins Company, 1976, p. 227. Reproduced by permission.)

Postsurgical fistulas may also be demonstrated on barium series of the upper gastrointestinal tract after bypass surgery (Fig. 16–121). Operative cholangiography occasionally demonstrates communication with an abscess, hematoma (Fig. 16–122), or subcapsular extravasation (Fig. 16–123). Angiography may demonstrate a fistula between the biliary tree and the vascular system as an incidental finding (Figs. 16–124 and 16–125).

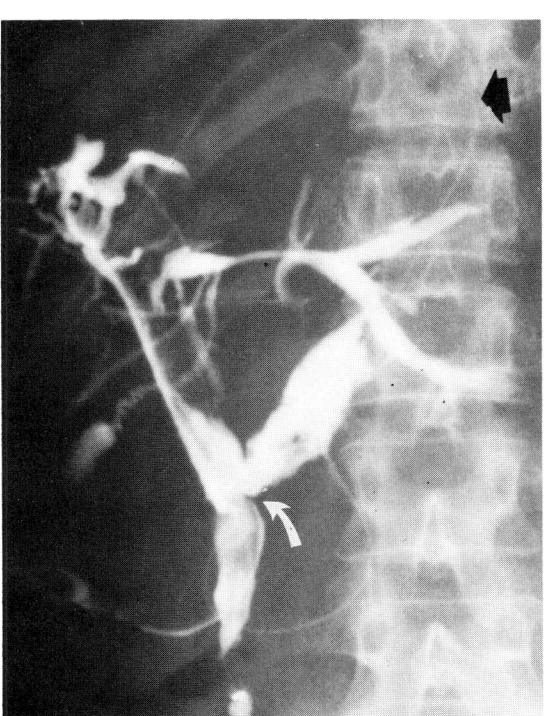

Figure 16–124. Arterial biliary fistula. Infusion hepatic arteriogram. Arterial biliary fistula (curved arrow) in a patient with carcinoma of the common hepatic duct. Contrast material injected through indwelling arterial catheter (large arrow) has opacified the biliary tree.

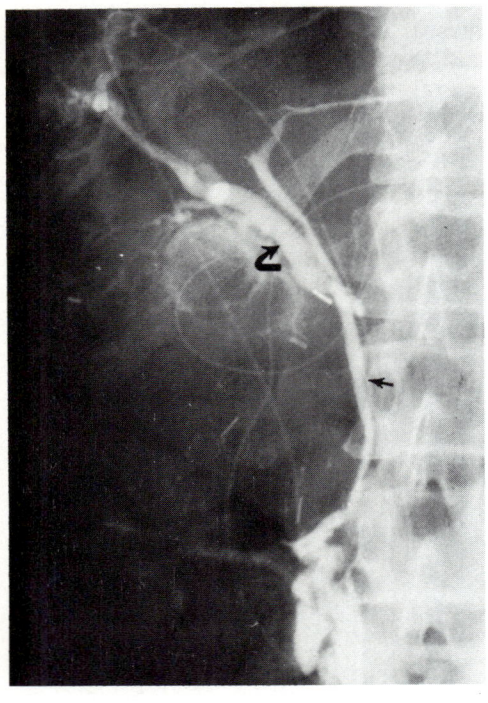

Figure 16–125. Arterial biliary fistula. Infusion hepatic arteriogram. Arterial (curved arrow) biliary (straight arrow) fistula in a patient with metastatic carcinoma of the pancreas (*From* Hatfield, P. M., and Wise, R. E.: Radiology of the Gallbladder and Bile Ducts. Baltimore. The Williams & Wilkins Company, 1976, p. 88. Reproduced by permission.)

References

1. Balthazar, E. J., and Schecter, L. S.: Gallstone ileus: the importance of contrast examinations in the roentgenographic diagnosis. Am. J. Roentgenol. 125:374–379, 1975.
2. Balthazar, E. J., and Schechter, L. S.: Air in gallbladder: a frequent finding in gallstone ileus. Am. J. Roentgenol. 131:219–222, 1978.
3. Berk, R. N., and Clemmett, A. R.: Radiology of the Gallbladder and Bile Ducts. Philadelphia, W. B. Saunders Company, 1977, pp. 27–70.
4. Braxton, M., and Jacobson, G.: Intragastric gallstone. Am. J. Roentgenol. 78:631–632, 1957.
5. Burhenne, H. J.: Nonoperative retained biliary tract stone extraction: a new roentgenologic technique. Am. J. Roentgenol. 117:388–399, 1973.
6. Corlette, M. B., and Bismuth. H.: Biliobiliary fistula: a trap in the surgery of cholelithiasis. Arch. Surg. 110:377–383, 1975.
7. Eisenman, J. I., Finck, E. J., and O'Loughlin, B. J.: Gallstone ileus: a review of the roentgenographic findings and report of a new roentgen sign. Am. J. Roentgenol 101:361–366, 1967.
8. Govoni, A. F., and Meyers, M. A.: Pseudopneumobilia. Radiology 118:526, 1976.
9. Hardy, J. D.: Some lesions of the biliary tract: idiopathic retroperitoneal fibrosis and other problems. Am. J. Surg. 103:457–468, 1962.
10. Harley, W. D., Kirkpatrick, R. H., and Ferrucci, J. T., Jr.: Gas in the bile ducts (pneumobilia) in emphysematous cholecystitis. Am. J. Roentgenol. 131:661–663, 1978.
11. Hatfield, P. M., and Wise, R. E.: Radiology of the Gallbladder and Bile Ducts. Baltimore, The Williams & Wilkins Company, 1976, pp. 140–143, 206–216.
12. Hricak, H., and Vander Molen, R. L.: Duodenocolonic fistula with gallstone ileus. Am. J. Gastroenterol. 69:711–715, 1978.
13. Hudspeth, A. S., and McGuirt, W. F., Gallstone ileus: a continuing surgical problem. Arch. Surg. 100:668–672, 1970.
14. Larsen, C. R., Scholz, F. J., and Wise, R. E.: Diseases of the biliary ducts. Semin. Roentgenol. 11:259–267, 1976.
15. Rosato, F. E.: Gallstone ileus and fistula. *In* Sabiston, D. C., Jr. (ed.): Davis-Christopher Textbook of Surgery. Vol. I. Ed. 11. Philadelphia, W. B. Saunders Company, 1977, pp. 1277–1281.
16. Schechner, S. A., Miller, I. D., Ehrlich, F. E., et al.: "Innocent" pneumobilia: report of a case and review of the literature. Arch. Surg. 108:118–120, 1974.
17. Schwegler, N., and Endrei, E.: Gallstone in the lung. Radiology 115:541–542, 1975.
18. Shaub, M. S., Birnbaum, W. W., and Meyers, H. I.: Peribiliary fat: a new roentgenographic finding. Am. J. Roentgenol. 123:330–337, 1975.

19. Shehadi, W. H.: Roentgenologic observations in cases of fistulae of the biliary tract. J.A.M.A. 174:2204–2208, 1960.
20. Wise, R. E.: Intravenous Cholangiography. Springfield, Ill., Charles C Thomas, Publisher, 1962.
21. Wise, R. E., and Keefe, J. P.: Radiologic evaluation of hepaticojejunal anastomoses. Surg. Clin. North Am. 48:579–584, 1968.
22. Wise, R. E., and O'Keeffe, A. P.: The Accessory Digestive Organs. Chicago, Year Book Medical Publishers, Inc., 1975.

Part V

Carcinoma of the Gallbladder and Biliary Ducts

CARL R. LARSEN, M.D.
ROBERT E. WISE, M.D.

CARCINOMA OF THE GALLBLADDER

Primary carcinoma of the gallbladder, an uncommon tumor with a poor prognosis, occurs most frequently in patients in the sixth and seventh decades and is three times more frequent in women than in men.[37] It accounts for approximately 1 per cent of all neoplasms and 3 per cent of all neoplasms of the gastrointestinal tract.[10] Cancer of the gallbladder is associated with calculi in 50 to 90 per cent of patients;[14, 37] however, postmortem data indicate only a 0.5 per cent incidence of carcinoma in all patients with gallstones.[1] Because of this association, some authorities recommend prophylactic cholecystectomy to prevent cancer in patients with cholelithiasis. However, the incidence of carcinoma associated with gallstones approaches the mortality rate of cholecystectomy, indicating a low benefit-to-risk ratio for cholecystectomy performed solely to prevent development of cancer.

Carcinoma of the gallbladder may be associated with a calcified gallbladder (porcelain gallbladder).[3] Porcelain gallbladder (Fig. 16–126) is a descriptive term for the blue discoloration and brittle consistency of the gallbladder wall.[2] The frequency of carcinoma in calcified gallbladders is estimated to be 22 per cent.[25] Cholelithiasis exists in nearly all patients who have calcification of the wall of the gallbladder. Histologically, two forms of calcification occur: a broad continuous band of calcification in the muscularis or multiple punctate calcifications in the glandular spaces of the mucosa.[3] Porcelain gallbladder, like cholelithiasis, is frequently present in elderly women.

Despite advances in radiologic and surgical techniques, the dismal cure rate in carcinoma of the gallbladder can be attributed to the lack of distinguishing symptoms. Most patients present with abdominal pain, anorexia, weight loss, nausea, or fever and are usually diagnosed at the time of operation for suspected cholelithiasis or cholecystitis. Correct preoperative diagnosis has been reported to range from 0 to 19 per cent.[24] Jaundice, usually painless, occurs in 33 to 66 per cent of patients and usually indicates the neoplastic process has extended to the extrahepatic ducts. At the time of operation only 10 to 25 per cent of cancers of the gallbladder are resectable with a five-year survival rate of less than 5 per cent.[24] Usually patients who survive are those whose disease is discovered incidentally as *in situ* carcinoma during histologic examination after cholecystectomy for cholelithiasis or cholecystitis.

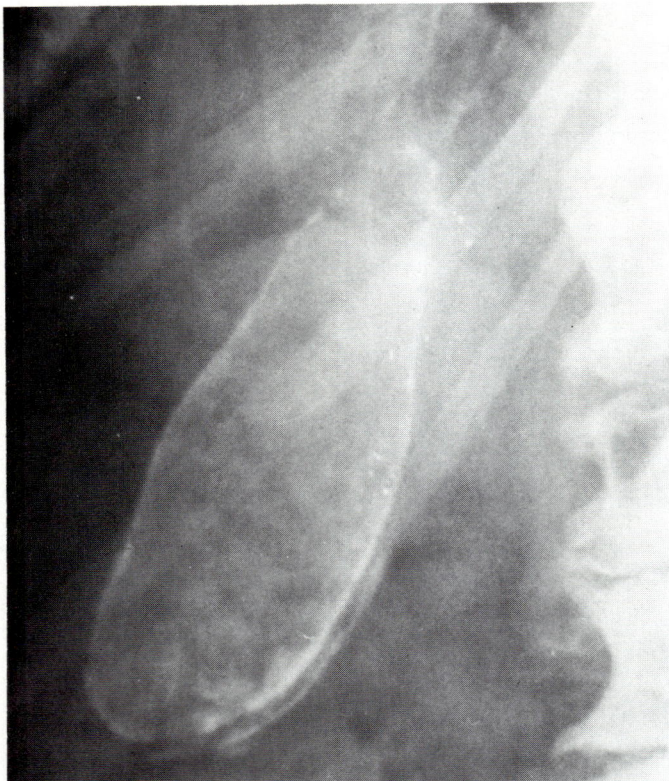

Figure 16–126. Calcification of wall of the gallbladder. Plain film of abdomen. Porcelain gallbladder. Extensive calcification throughout wall of the gallbladder is indicative of disease of the gallbladder and a high probability of cancer.

Adenocarcinomas represent 85 to 95 per cent of carcinomas of the gallbladder;[10, 21, 37] the remainder consist primarily of anaplastic carcinomas, squamous cell carcinomas, and adenoacanthomas. Occasionally, but extremely rarely, lymphomas, basal cell carcinomas, sarcomas, and carcinoid tumors may be discovered in the gallbladder.[10] Secondary tumors of the gallbladder may be blood borne or disseminated through the lymphatics, although in most instances these are direct extensions from cancers of a nearby organ. Implants from metastatic melanoma were found in 11 of 78 patients with melanoma (11 per cent) in one series.[32] In the early stages of primary cancer, the fundus and neck of the gallbladder are the most commonly involved areas; however, in the majority of patients, metastasis has already occurred. These tumors metastasize most often by direct extension or lymphatic spread; distant metastases, vascular dissemination, or neural spread are relatively rare.[21]

Radiographic examination has been of limited value because of the nonspecific presentation of carcinoma of the gallbladder. Conventional or plain films of the abdomen may suggest evidence of a soft-tissue mass in the right upper quadrant or the presence of an irregular punctate gas collection within the mass,[14] which results from lack of decompression after fistulization. Opaque calculi or calcification of the wall of the gallbladder, both of which have a predilection for carcinoma, may be present.

Oral cholecystography is not generally effective in patients with elevated levels of bilirubin. In a study at the Lahey Clinic,[10] oral cholecystography was performed in 34 patients with gallbladder cancer but without jaundice. The gallbladder was not visualized in 27, 2 had normal studies, and 5 had calculi. A preoperative diagnosis of gallbladder carcinoma was not made in any of the patients. The presence of jaundice precludes intravenous cholangiography for visualization of the biliary ducts.

Barium studies frequently are performed after the neoplasm has become widespread, yielding nonspecific changes that are suggestive of a more frequently occurring neoplasm of the pancreas or duodenum. An eccentric pressure defect displacing and stretching the duodenum or mucosal changes suggesting infiltration (Fig. 16–127) may be present. Ulceration may occur late in the disease.[14]

Selective celiac or superior mesenteric arteriography displays characteristic changes associated with carcinoma of the gallbladder; however, the diagnosis is rarely made before the disease reaches an unresectable stage. When the lesion is localized to the gallbladder, angiographic findings include tumor blush, neovascularity, enlargement, or displacement (Fig. 16–128B) of the cystic artery or its branches, arterial encasement, and uneven thickness of the gallbladder wall.[10, 29, 33] Because of the propensity of gallbladder carcinoma to infiltrate the liver, regional lymph nodes, stomach, duodenum, and abdominal wall, the most frequent angiographic findings are associated with the vascular supply to these structures. The common and right hepatic artery (Fig. 16–129A) and gastroduodenal and cystic artery or their branches are most commonly involved.[37] Portal vein obstruction and thrombosis may also occur.

Carcinoma of the gallbladder is usually associated with biliary calculi, bile stasis, and bile duct obstruction, enabling a high success rate for percutaneous cholangiography (Fig. 16–129B).[19] The tumor may be identified in the gallbladder or, as is more frequently the case, tumor infiltration obstructing the extrahepatic biliary or cystic ducts (Fig. 16–130) will be evident. Endoscopic retrograde cholangiography may incidentally show a few small lesions in the gallbladder. When advanced disease obstructs the extrahepatic ducts, endoscopic cholangiography permits visualization of only the distal bile ducts without revealing the extent of involvement. Percutaneous transhepatic cholangiography is the procedure of choice in patients with jaundice secondary to biliary tumors.

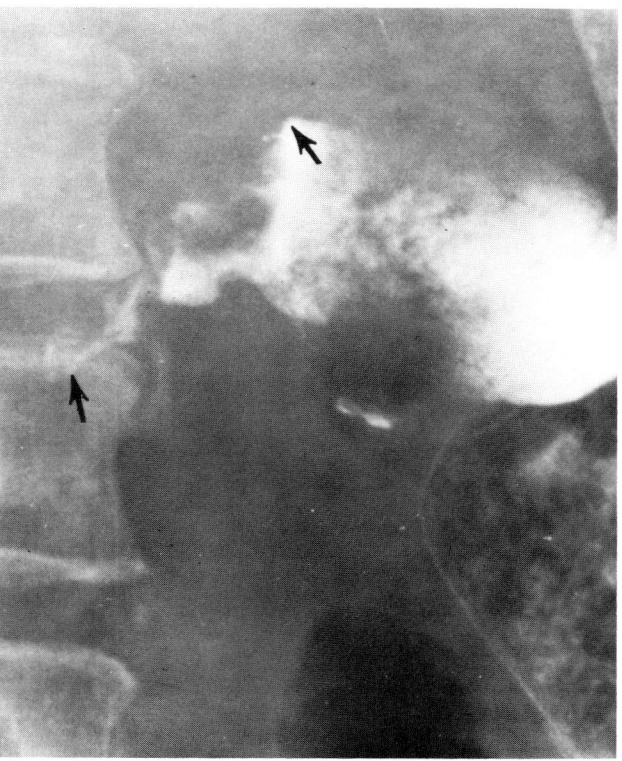

Figure 16–127. Carcinoma of gallbladder. Upper gastrointestinal examination. Advanced infiltration of the postbulbar segment of the duodenum (arrows) from direct extension of a cancer of the gallbladder with obstruction of the duodenum. (*From* Hatfield, P. M., and Wise, R. E.: Radiology of the Gallbladder and Bile Ducts. Baltimore, The Williams & Wilkins Company, 1976, p. 148. Reproduced by permission.)

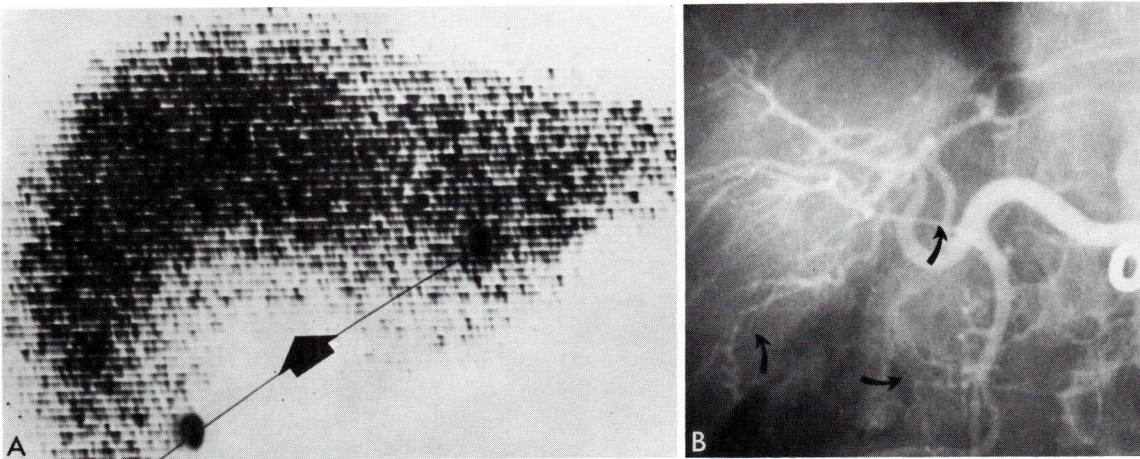

Figure 16–128. Carcinoma of gallbladder. Liver scan. Defect in hilum of liver (arrow) from infiltrating carcinoma of gallbladder. B, Selective celiac arteriogram in the same patient. Stretching of cystic artery and irregular branching of right hepatic artery (curved arrows) in association with infiltrating carcinoma.

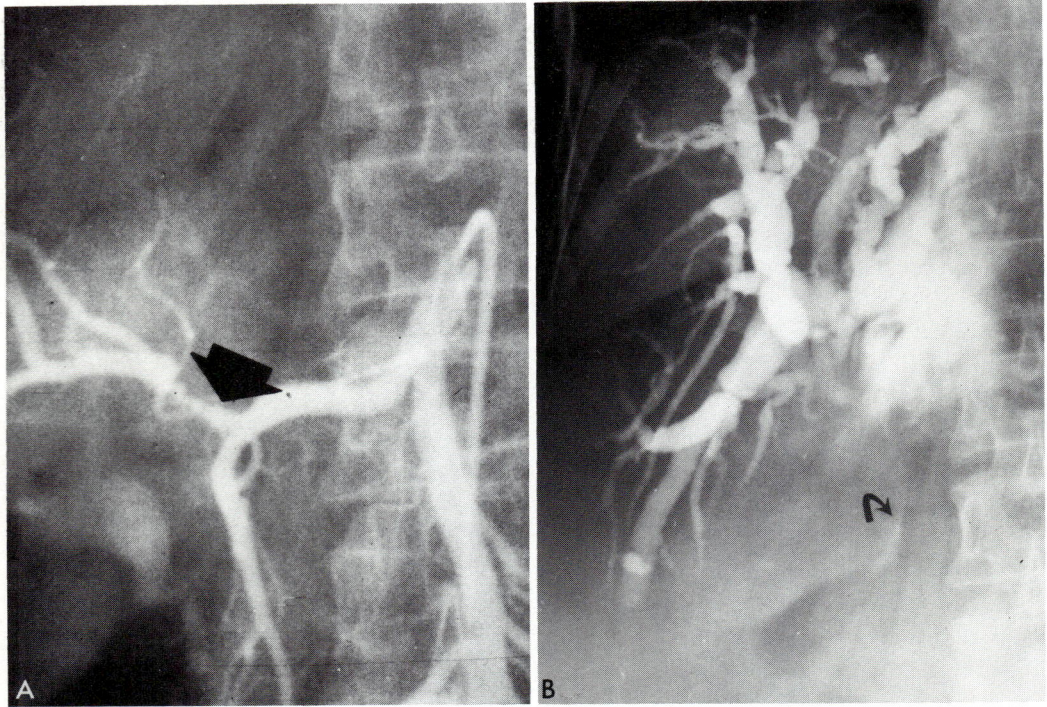

Figure 16–129. Carcinoma of gallbladder. Selective superior mesenteric arteriogram. Encasement of right hepatic artery (arrow). B, Percutaneous transhepatic cholangiogram. Obstruction of the hepatic ducts with dilated intrahepatic ducts. Minimal contrast material has passed into the extrahepatic ducts (arrow).

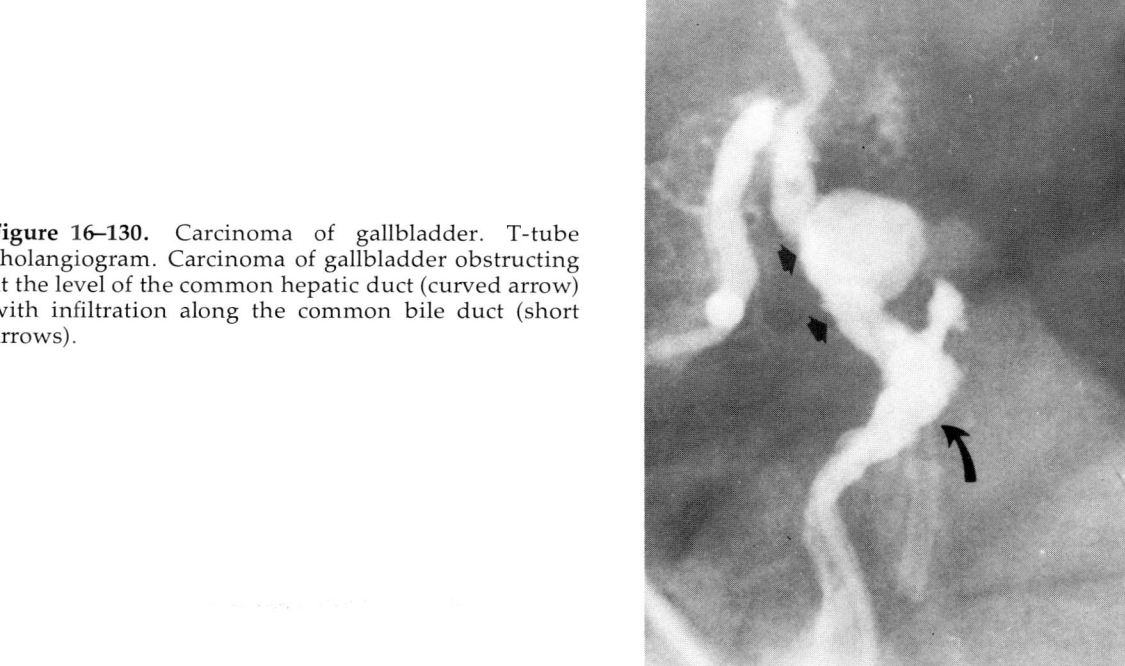

Figure 16–130. Carcinoma of gallbladder. T-tube cholangiogram. Carcinoma of gallbladder obstructing at the level of the common hepatic duct (curved arrow) with infiltration along the common bile duct (short arrows).

Biliary obstruction can be identified with an accuracy of approximately 85 to 97 per cent[11, 23, 28, 35] with either ultrasonography or computerized body tomography. Both studies can show a mass or calculi in association with the obstruction; these techniques, however, have not provided early demonstration of gallbladder cancer before extension. Liver scanning (see Fig. 16–128A) may also show evidence of the dilated intrahepatic ducts or local metastases, but an early cancer is rarely detected because of the nonspecific symptoms and a low index of suspicion on the part of the clinician.

Benign neoplasms of the gallbladder (Fig. 16–131) are fixed filling defects seen with oral cholecystography and occasionally seen after filling of the gallbladder during intravenous cholangiography or endoscopic retrograde cholangiography. These neoplasms may be papillomas, adenomas, cholesterol polyps, adenomyomas, or inflammatory polyps. They are usually asymptomatic and measure 2 to 3 mm in diameter. Whether these lesions have a malignant potential and require prophylactic cholecystectomy is an unsettled question.[37]

CARCINOMA OF THE BILE DUCTS

Primary carcinoma of the bile ducts, an uncommon lesion, has an autopsy incidence ranging from 0.01 to 0.46 per cent.[10] The peak incidence of bile duct carcinoma is similar to that for gallbladder carcinoma (sixth and seventh decades), but, unlike carcinoma of the gallbladder, it shows a male predominance.[1, 4, 15] Approximately one-third of patients have a history of calculi, and 5 per cent have an association with

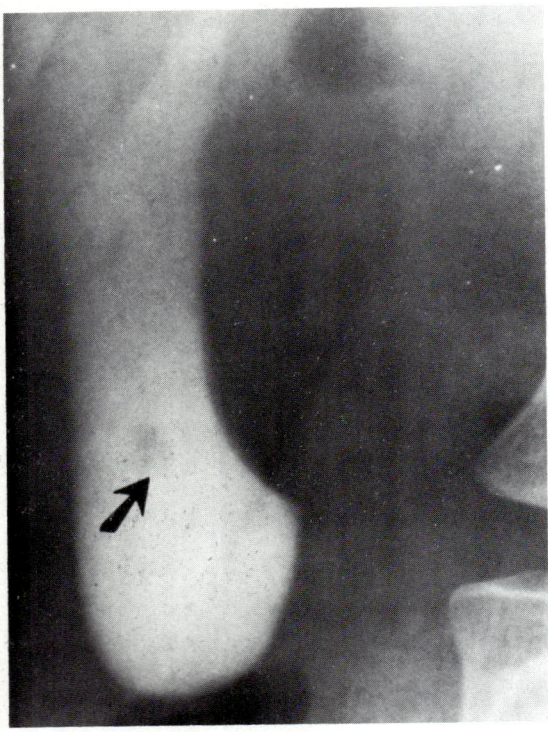

Figure 16–131. Benign gallbladder polyp (arrow). Oral cholecystogram. These are usually asymptomatic and fixed in position unlike calculi which change position when the patient is erect.

ulcerative colitis.[4] A similar relationship exists between sclerosing cholangitis and ulcerative colitis.[15] Cancer of the bile ducts develops at an earlier age when it is associated with ulcerative colitis. In a Lahey Clinic series[27] of 103 patients with bile duct carcinoma, 8 had ulcerative colitis, and 6 of the 8 patients were 50 years of age or younger.

Jaundice, usually intermittent and painless in the early stages, is the presenting complaint of approximately 95 per cent of patients.[1] Nausea, pruritus, anorexia, weight loss, and fever occur less frequently. Detection of a palpable mass (gallbladder) depends on the relationship of the tumor to the cystic duct. Carcinomas may obstruct the cystic duct, causing pain mimicking calculous obstruction or acute cholecystitis.[4] A five-year survival rate of more than 30 per cent is obtainable when the tumor involves the distal common bile duct compared with the survival rate of frequently undetected neoplasms of the more proximal ducts.[17]

Adenocarcinomas, either undifferentiated or moderately well differentiated, are the most common neoplasm, with the differentiated type occurring more often.[15] Melanomas, leiomyosarcomas, papillary adenomatosis, squamous cell carcinoma, and mucoepidermoid tumors are less frequently seen.[4, 37] Benign tumors of the bile ducts are rare, with an incidence one tenth to one twelfth that of malignant tumors.[10, 37] The most frequent benign neoplasms are papillomas, adenomas, and fibromas. Benign tumors appear as small, rounded filling defects with or without ductal obstruction.

Carcinoma may occur at any site along the bile duct; however, the majority arise in the common hepatic duct near the carina (Fig. 16–132) or in the common bile duct (Fig. 16–133). In a series of 570 carcinomas[29] the common bile duct was the most frequent site. Tumors of the common bile duct accounted for 36 per cent of the cases, with 24 per cent occurring at the junction of the common hepatic, cystic, and common bile ducts,

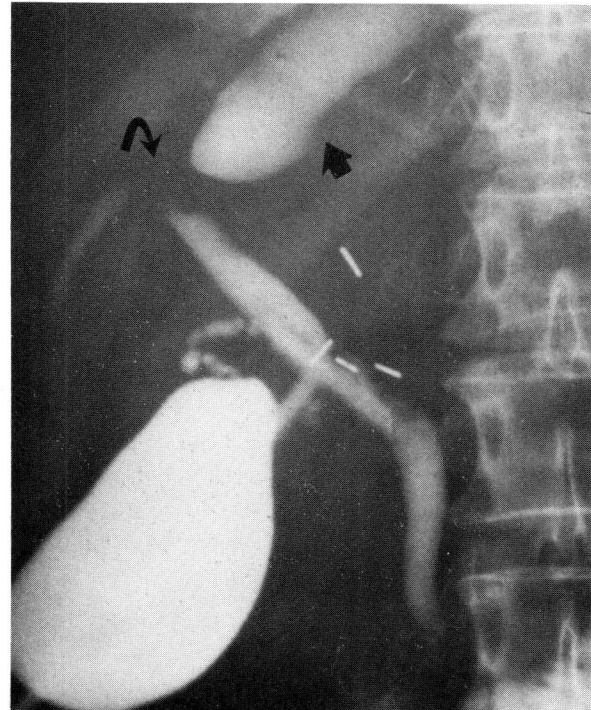

Figure 16–132. Carcinoma of common hepatic duct. T-tube cholangiogram. Carcinoma of common hepatic duct bifurcation (curved arrow) with dilated left intraheptic duct (straight arrow).

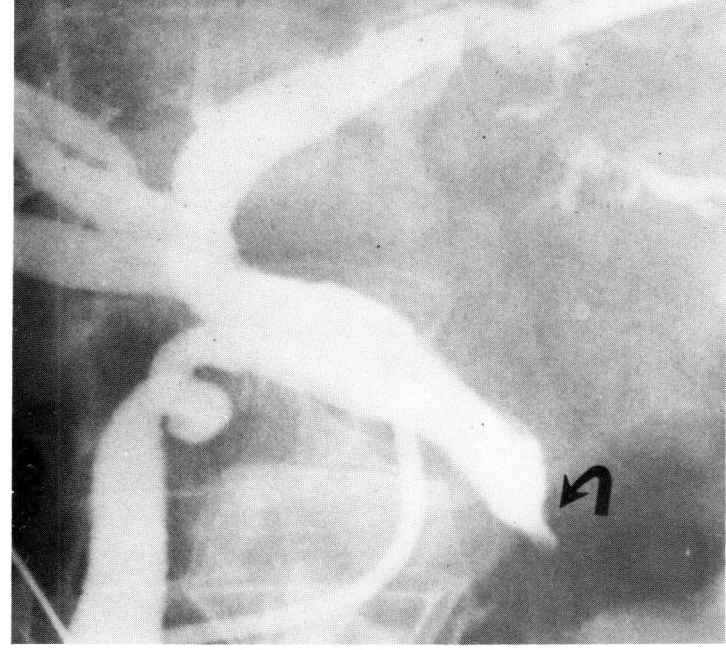

Figure 16–133. Cancer of common bile duct. T-ube cholangiogram. Carcinoma of common bile duct with abrupt occlusion (curved arrow). This appearance may also be seen with cancer of the pancreas.

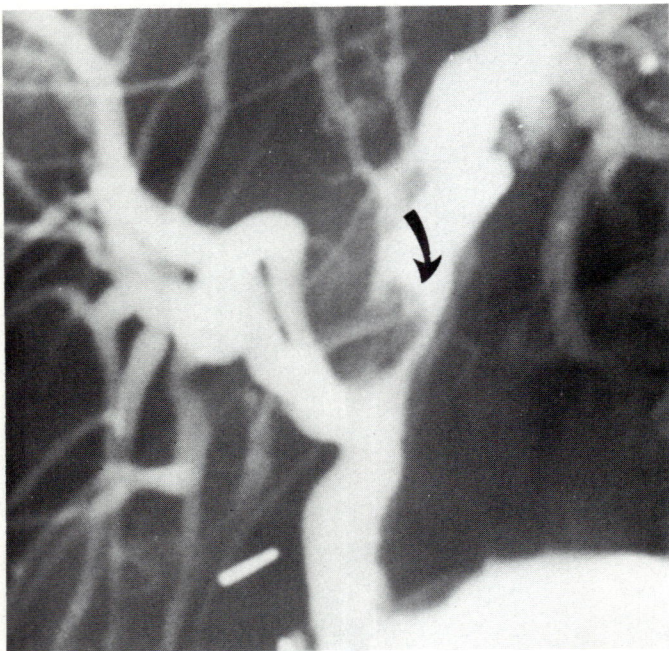

Figure 16–134. Polypoid carcinoma of hepatic duct. T-tube cholangiogram. These tumors may grow to obstruct the duct completely. (*From* Larsen, C. R., Scholz, F. J., and Wise, R. E.: Diseases of the biliary ducts. Semin. Roentgenol. 11:260, 1976. Reproduced by permission.)

14 per cent from the hepatic duct, 8 per cent from the intrahepatic ducts, and 6 per cent from the cystic duct.[10] Three major patterns of growth are described. Papillary tumors (Fig. 16–134), the least common, grow intraluminally and may obstruct the lumen of the bile duct. They may have a multicentric origin. Scirrhous or diffuse infiltrating carcinoma occurs with slightly greater frequency, involving single or multiple sites (Fig. 16–135); it may resemble sclerosing cholangitis. The most frequent pattern is an annular infiltrating mass or nodule that causes a short stricture, frequently with overhanging margins (Fig. 16–136).[37] The majority of bile duct tumors are slow growing and metastasize by local extension.[17] Metastasis occurs earlier in the polypoid and annular infiltrating types and late in the scirrhous type.[37] Metastatic disease to the porta hepatis and bile ducts (Fig. 16–137) is frequently from malignant neoplasms of the gastrointestinal tract and less frequently from the breast or lung or from a lymphoma. Tumors of the pancreas or duodenum may involve the common bile duct. Ampullary or periampullary tumors (Fig. 16–138) are the most common cancers involving the biliary tract.[5, 20] The site of origin of periampullary tumors is often difficult to determine histologically or at the time of operation.

The preoperative radiographic evaluation of biliary tumors may be pursued with a plethora of diagnostic techniques, which include plain film of the abdomen, oral or intravenous cholangiography, barium examinations, nuclear scanning, percutaneous transhepatic cholangiography, endoscopic retrograde cholangiography, and angiography. Transjugular cholangiography, splenic portography, and percutaneous transhepatic venography are other studies that are available, although not as frequently used. Recently, ultrasonography and computerized body scanning have been added to this battery of examinations.

Plain radiographs of the abdomen may show liver enlargement, possibly a mass effect displacing air shadows, or calcification — a rare occurrence in ductal cancers. Because many of the patients have advanced disease, barium studies may display

THE BILIARY SYSTEM — 993

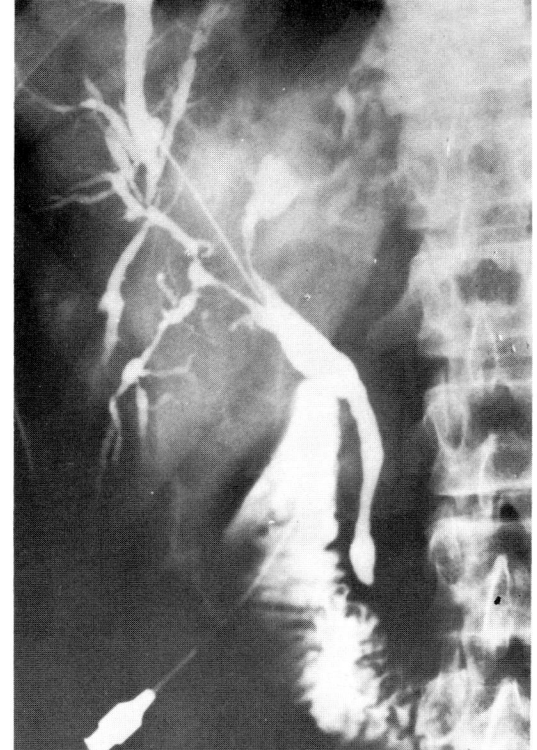

Figure 16–135. Carcinoma of common hepatic duct. Transhepatic percutaneous cholangiogram. Carcinoma of common hepatic duct bifurcation with infiltration and narrowing of intrahepatic ducts. (*From* Hatfield, P. M., and Wise, R. E.: Radiology of the Gallbladder and Bile Ducts. Baltimore, The Williams & Wilkins Company, 1976, p. 187. Reproduced by permission.)

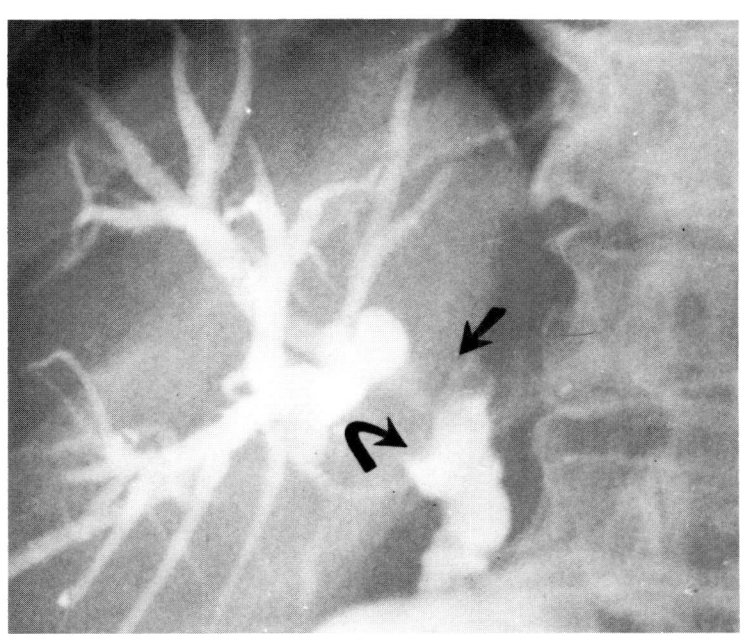

Figure 16–136. Carcinoma (applecore) of common hepatic duct. T-tube cholangiogram. Napkin-ring carcinoma (straight arrow) with overhanging margin (curved arrow) in common hepatic duct occluding left hepatic duct. (*From* Larsen, C. R., Scholz, F. J., and Wise, R. E.: Diseases of the biliary ducts. Semin. Roentgenol. 11:261, 1976. Reproduced by permission.)

994 — THE BILIARY SYSTEM

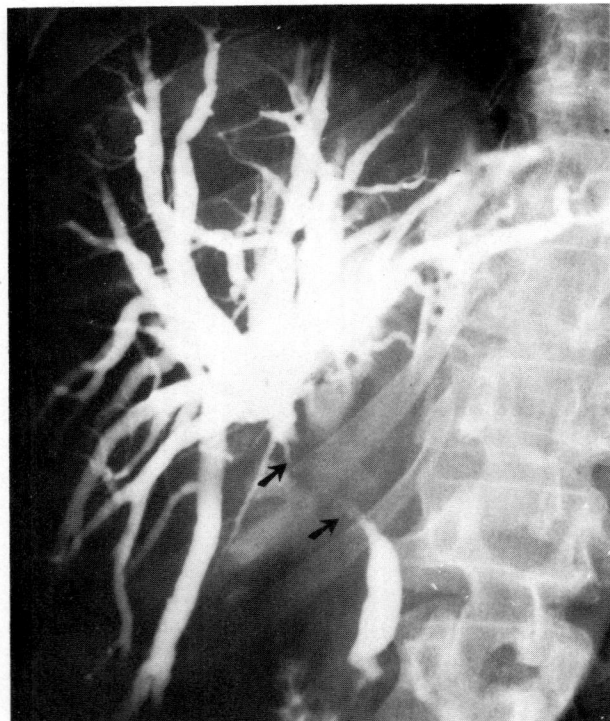

Figure 16–137. Metastatic carcinoma of extrahepatic ducts. Transhepatic percutaneous cholangiogram. Metastatic carcinoma of breast to porta hepatis (arrows) with obstruction of extrahepatic duct and dilatation of intrahepatic ducts.

Figure 16–138. Ampullary carcinoma. T-tube cholangiogram. Ampullary carcinoma (straight arrow) with infiltration of duodenum (curved arrows). Common bile duct is partially obstructed above the carcinoma.

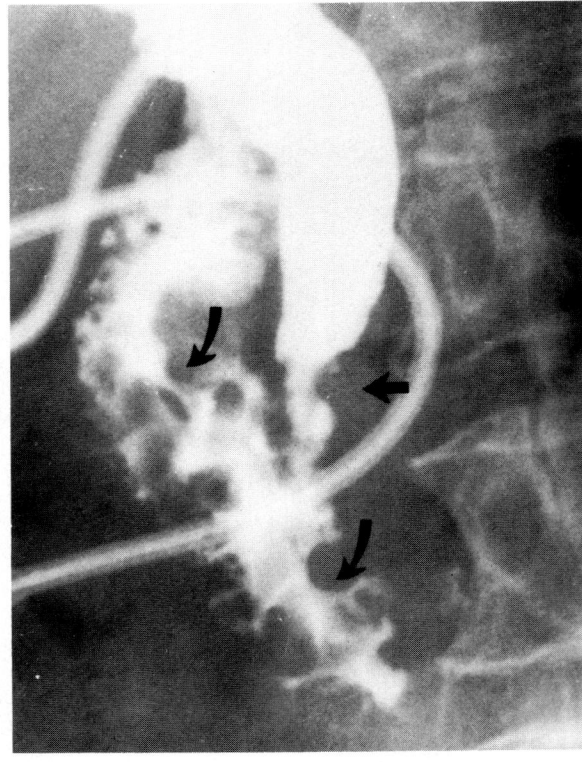

evidence of extrinsic pressure or infiltration of the stomach or duodenum (Fig. 16–139) or a crossing defect of the duodenum caused by a dilated bile duct. A periampullary tumor may be perceptible as a nodular intraluminal mass projecting from the medial wall of the second segment of the duodenum. Oral or intravenous cholangiography is not indicated in the jaundiced patient, particularly if the level of serum bilirubin is above 4 mg per dL.[30] Angiography[34] may demonstrate tumor vessels, tumor blush, vascular displacement or encasement, arterioarterial collaterals,[36] or venous obstruction, or it may outline an obstructed gallbladder. Unless carcinoma of the bile duct is well vascularized, arteriography may be of no aid in diagnosis. It may, however, help establish the presence of a pancreatic tumor or hepatoma as the cause of symptoms.

Percutaneous cholangiography (see Fig. 16–135) is the radiologic procedure of choice for the diagnosis of biliary carcinoma. It indicates the probable cause of obstruction as well as the level and extent of involvement, offering the surgeon information for determining the type of operation that may be required. Transhepatic cholangiography performed with the fine-caliber Chiba needle has a high rate of success in ductal opacification with few complications.[6] Palliation in obstructive jaundice secondary to malignancy may be achieved with percutaneous transhepatic intubation of the bile ducts (Fig. 16–140). Nonsurgical biliary decompression (Fig. 16–141) reduces the risk of septicemia and the need for immediate operation after cholangiography.[13, 22]

Cholangiographic findings are variable (see Figs. 16–132 to 16–134, 16–137, and 16–138). An abrupt occlusion is present in the majority of patients, although delayed or upright studies may allow sufficient contrast material to trickle beyond the obstruction to indicate the type of neoplasm and its extent. The point of obstruction usually has an irregular, eccentric, abrupt, or bluntly tapered appearance. Carcinomas of the porta hepatis appear frequently as an area of diffuse narrowing (Fig. 16–142) or total occlusion.[16] Diffuse narrowing of the hepatic ducts and segmental narrowing of the common bile duct can coexist. The extent to which a polypoid mass is demonstrated depends on the degree of obstruction of the duct. Annular or constricting carcinomas

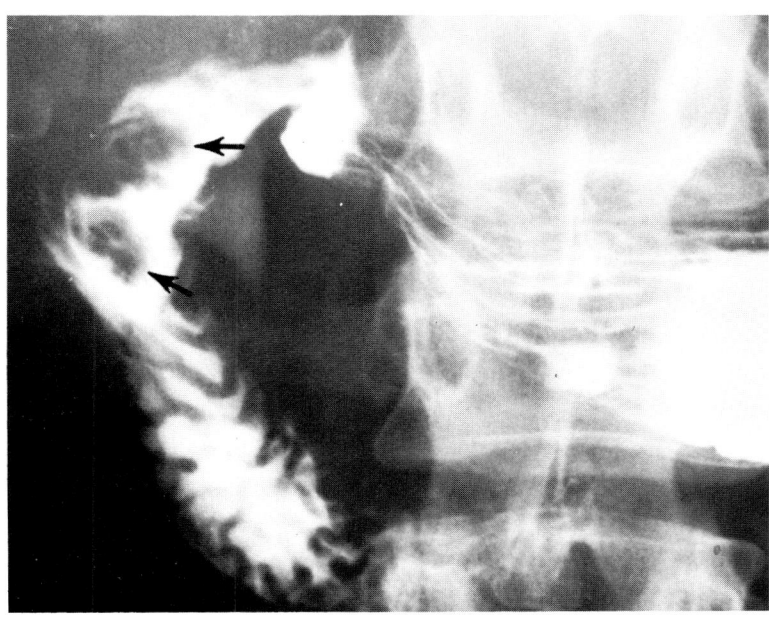

Figure 16–139. Carcinoma of common bile duct. Upper gastrointestinal series. Bilobed metastasis in the duodenum (arrows) from carcinoma of common bile duct. (*From* Hatfield, P. M., and Wise, R. E.: Radiology of the Gallbladder and Bile Ducts. Baltimore. The Williams & Wilkins Company, 1976, p. 175. Reproduced by permission.)

996 — THE BILIARY SYSTEM

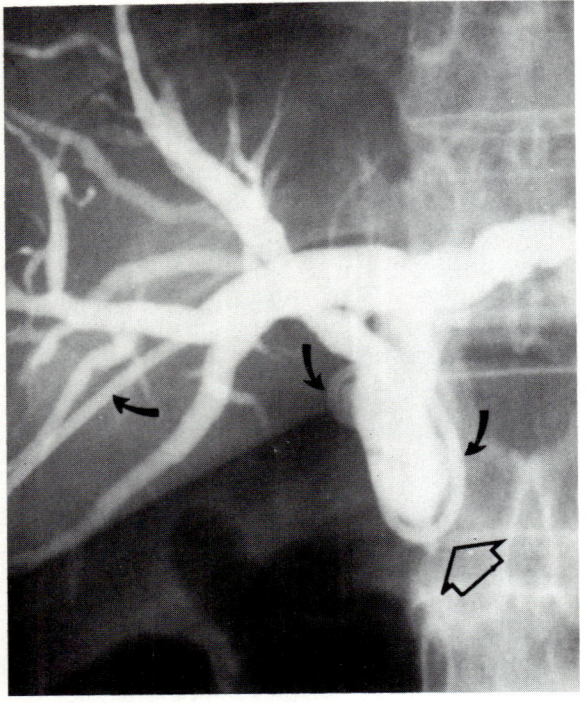

Figure 16–140. Carcinoma of common bile duct. Percutaneous cholangiogram with catheter drainage. Carcinoma of common duct with complete obstruction (open arrow) and drainage catheter (curved arrows).

(see Fig. 16–136) with a napkin-ring type of defect may be observed. These may progress to complete obstruction and may mimic carcinoma of the pancreas.

Endoscopic retrograde cannulation of the bile duct (Figs. 16–143 and 16–144) permits evaluation of the duodenum and pancreatic duct and biopsy of an intraluminal mass. The information may be limited to visualization of the bile duct distal to the

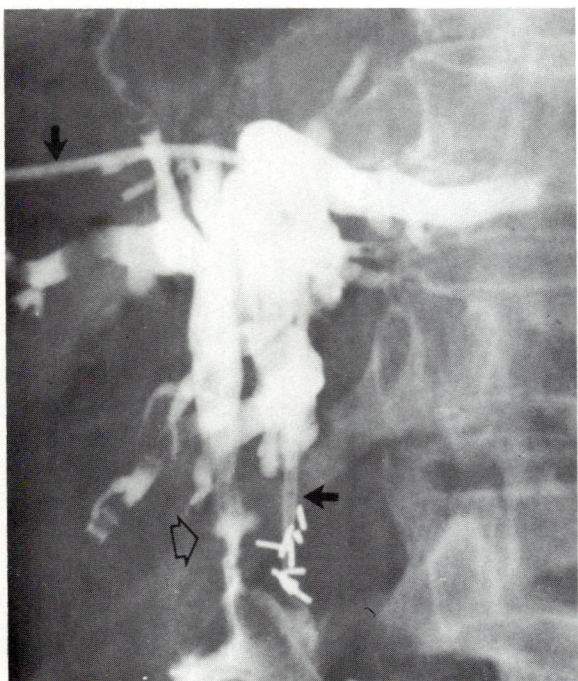

Figure 16–141. Carcinoma of common bile duct. Percutaneous cholangiogram with catheter drainage. Carcinoma of distal common bile duct (open arrow) with palliative drainge (straight arrows).

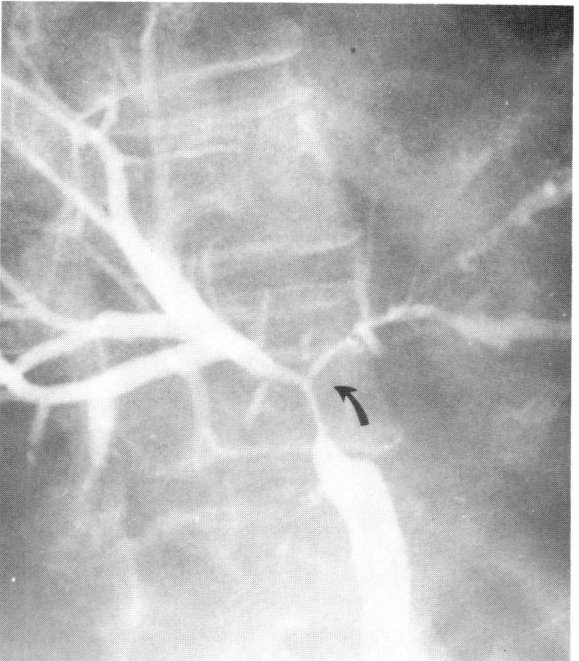

Figure –142. Carcinoma of common hepatic duct. T-tube cholangiogram. Carcinoma of common hepatic duct with narrowing of hepatic ducts near bifurcation (arrow). (*From* Hatfield, P. M., and Wise, R. E.: Radiology of the Gallbladder and Bile Ducts. Baltimore, The Williams & Wilkins Company, 1976, p. 187. Reproduced by permission.)

neoplasm if the obstruction is complete. Retrograde cholangiography does not offer evidence of the extent of disease if the bile duct is completely occluded or ascertain the availability of the bile ducts for a possible bypass procedure. The accessibility of experienced endoscopists and the expense of equipment are other limiting factors.[6]

Radiopharmaceuticals that localize within the biliary system have been useful in

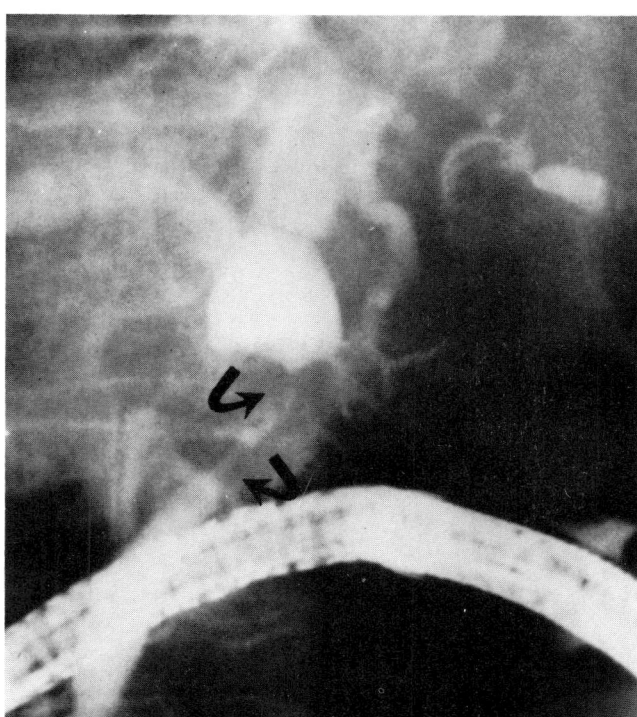

Figure 16–143. Carcinoma of common hepatic duct (arrows). Endoscopic retrograde cholangiogram. Marked narrowing with overhanging margins.

998 — THE BILIARY SYSTEM

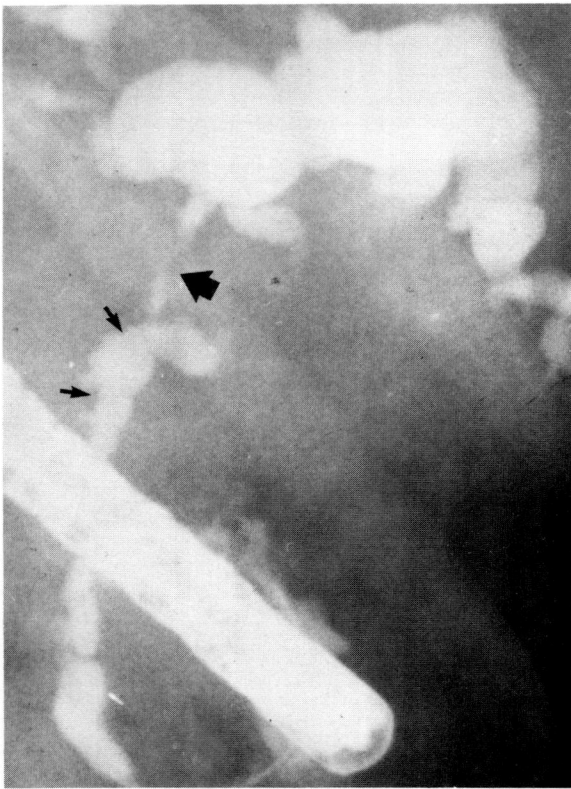

Figure 16–144. Carcinoma of common hepatic duct. Endoscopic retrograde cholangiogram. Carcinoma of common hepatic duct (large arrow) infiltrating along common bile duct (small arrows) and obstructing intrahepatic ducts.

the assessment of biliary drainage in the jaundiced patient. Rose bengal I^{131} scanning is limited by the occurrence of false positive and false negative results.[8] Recently, a new pharmaceutical (^{99m}Tc-HIDA) has been developed for cholescintigraphy,[26] but its role is still to be determined. Dilated bile ducts can be identified on liver scans (Fig. 16–145).[12]

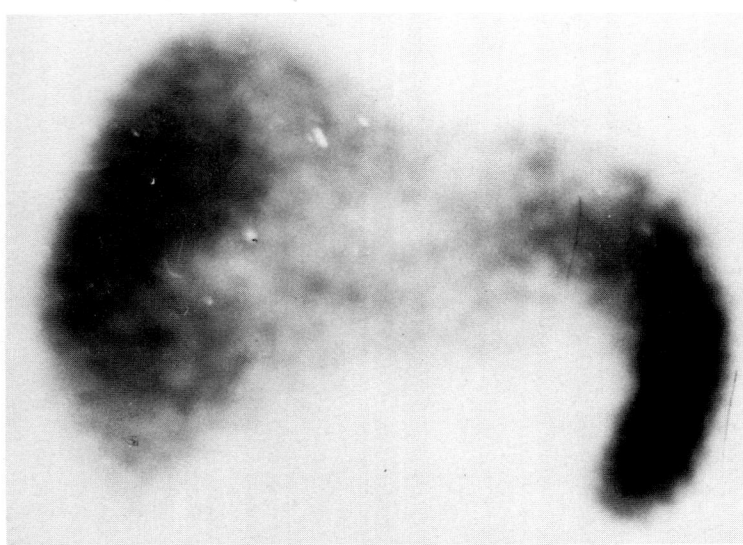

Figure 16–145. Carcinoma of common hepatic duct. Liver scan. Demonstration of defects secondary to dilated bile ducts in a patient with cancer of the common hepatic duct.

Dynamic scintigraphic studies offer the possibility of distinguishing partially obstructed but not dilated biliary ducts — an advantage over ultrasound.[28]

Ultrasonography offers a safe, noninvasive, inexpensive, quick, and relatively accurate method of determining the caliber of the bilary system (Fig. 16–146). Its accuracy in demonstrating dilated intrahepatic bile ducts ranges from 85 to 97 per cent.[7, 18, 28, 35] Ultrasonography is of limited value in patients with sclerosing cholangitis who have surgical jaundice but do not have a dilated biliary system. Excessive bowel gas in the porta hepatis, particularly in the patient who has had bypass surgery, limits the visualization of the extrahepatic system. Frequently the extrahepatic ducts may be

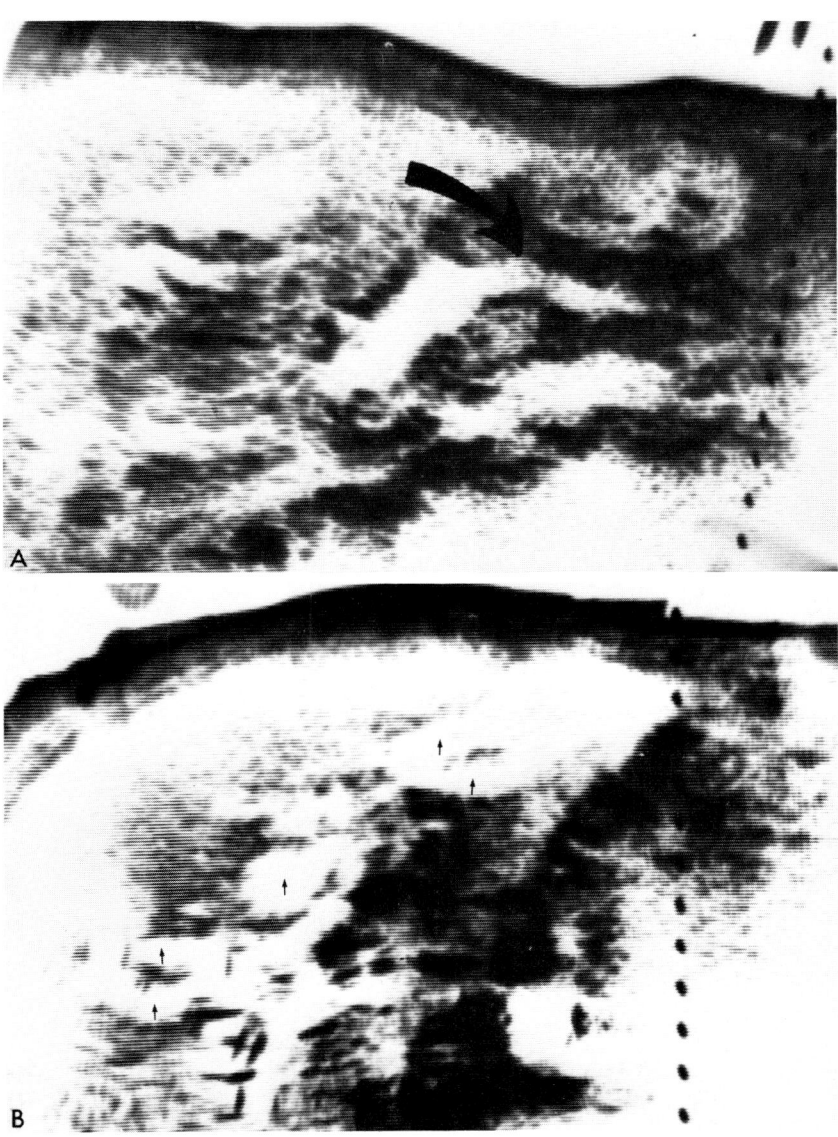

Figure 16–146. *A*, Carcinoma of common bile duct. Ultrasound examination. Sagittal scan shows a dilated extrahepatic duct with irregular narrowing (arrow) in a patient with carcinoma of the distal common bile duct. *B*, Transverse plane. Dilated intrahepatic ducts (arrows) in patient with cancer of common bile duct.

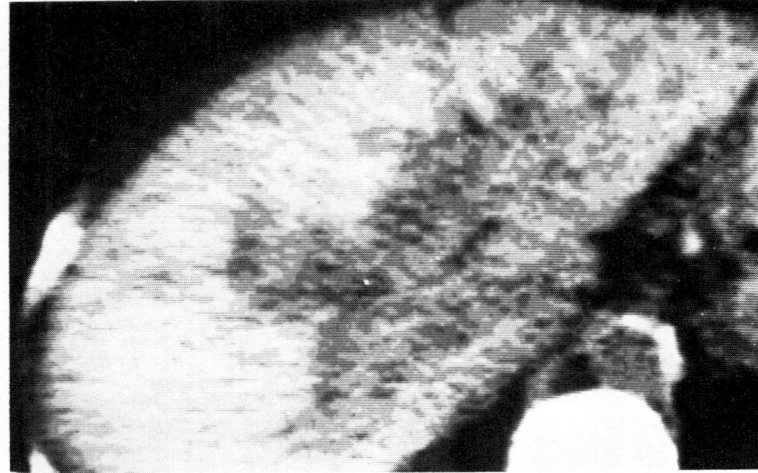

Figure 16–147. Carcinoma of common bile duct. Computerized body tomography. Liver with dilated intrahepatic ducts (relatively lucent areas) secondary to carcinoma of common bile duct.

obstructed with a delay in distention of the intrahepatic ducts. Demonstration of the extrahepatic ducts was successful in 38 per cent cent of patients in one series,[28] and frequently the cause of extrahepatic obstruction can be determined.

Computerized scanning, like ultrasonography, can demonstrate the dilated biliary tree (Fig. 16–147) and the cause of obstruction with comparable diagnostic accuracy.[9, 31]

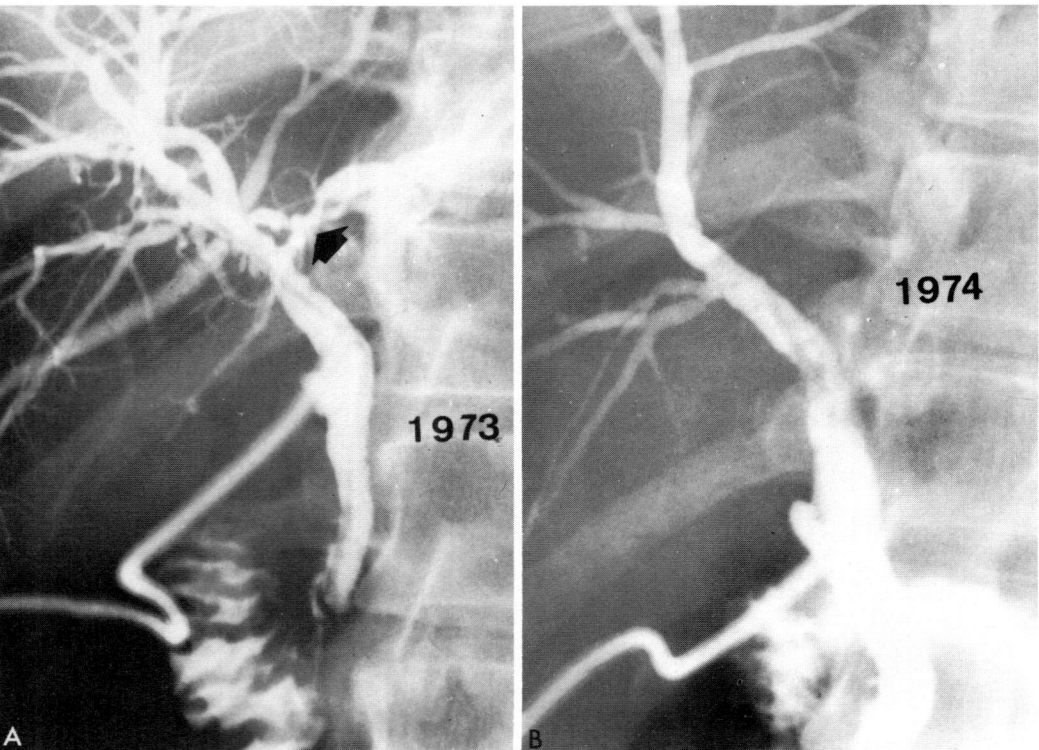

Figure 16–148. Carcinoma of left hepatic duct (arrow). T-tube cholangiogram. *B*, Carcinoma has progressed to occlude completely the left ducts within ten months of the examination shown in *A*.

Disadvantages include limited availability, higher cost, radiation exposure, and need for contrast material. Computerized scanning is not affected by the presence of bowel gas and therefore has an advantage over ultrasonography in evaluating patients who have had bypass surgery. Ultrasound, however, is the screening procedure of choice.

Operative cholangiography is extremely important in the evaluation of those patients in whom preoperative cholangiograms were not obtained or in whom the study was unsuccessful. Cooperation between radiologist and surgeon ensures that operative cholangiography is technically and diagnostically acceptable. T-tube cholangiography should be obtained whenever possible to ensure that complete visualization of the biliary system has been obtained and to monitor the progression of disease (Fig. 16–148).

References

1. Abbruzzese, A. A., Braasch, J. W., and Shipley, W. U.: Cancer of the pancreas and biliary tract. *In* Cady, B. (ed.): Cancer: A Manual for Practitioners. Ed. 5. Boston, American Cancer Society, Massachusetts Division, Inc., 1978, pp. 167–174.
2. Ashur, H., Siegal, B., Oland, Y., et al.: Calcified gallbladder (porcelain gallbladder). Arch. Surg. *113*:594–596, 1978.
3. Berk, R. N., Armbuster, T. G., and Saltzstein, S. L.: Carcinoma in the porcelain gallbladder. Radiology *106*:29–31, 1973.
4. Braasch, J. W.: Carcinoma of the bile duct. Surg. Clin. North Am. *53*:1217–1227, 1973.
5. Braasch, J. W., and Camer, S. J.: Periampullary carcinoma. Med. Clin. North Am. *59*:309–314, 1975.
6. Ferrucci, J. T., Jr., Wittenberg, J., Sarno, R. A., et al.: Fine needle transhepatic cholangiography: a new approach to obstructive jaundice. Am. J. Roentgenol. *127*:403–407, 1976.
7. Goldberg, H. I., Filly, R. A., Korobkin, M., et al.: Capability of CT body scanning and ultrasonography to demonstrate the status of the biliary ductal system in patients with jaundice. Radiology *129*:731–737, 1978,
8. Handmaker, H.: Nuclear medicine in the evaluation of the patient with jaundice. J.A.M.A. *231*:1172–1176, 1975.
9. Harell, G. S., Marshall, W. H., Jr., Breiman, R. S., et al.: Early experience with the Varian Six Second body scanner in the diagnosis of hepatobiliary tract disease. Radiology *123*:355–360, 1977.
10. Hatfield, P. M., and Wise, R. E.: Radiology of the Gallbladder and Bile Ducts. Baltimore. The Williams & Wilkins Company, 1976.
11. Havrilla, T. R., Haaga, J. R., Alfidi, R. J., et al.: Computed tomography and obstructive biliary disease. Am. J. Roentgenol. *128*:765–768, 1977.
12. Heck, L. L., and Gottschalk, A.: The appearance of intrahepatic biliary duct dilatation on the liver scan. Radiology *99*:135–140, 1971.
13. Hoevels, J., Lunderquist, A., and Ihse, I.: Percutaneous transhepatic intubation of bile ducts for combined internal-external drainage in preoperative and palliative treatment of obstructive jaundice. Gastrointest. Radiol. *3*:23–31, 1978.
14. Khilnani, M. T., Wolf, B. S., and Finkel, M.: Roentgen features of carcinoma of the gallbladder on barium-meal examination. Radiology *79*:264–273, 1962.
15. Larsen, C. R., Scholz, F. J., and Wise, R. I.: Diseases of the biliary ducts. Semin. Roentgenol. *11*:259–267, 1976.
16. Legge, D. A., and Carlson, H. C.: Cholangiographic appearance of primary carcinoma of the bile ducts. Radiology *102*:259–266, 1972.
17. Longmire, W. P., Jr., McArthur, M. S., Bastounis, E. A., et al.: Carcinoma of the extrahepatic biliary tract. Ann. Surg. *178*:333–345, 1973.
18. Malini, S., and Sabel, J.: Ultrasonography in obstructive jaundice. Radiology *123*:429–433, 1977.
19. McNulty, J. G.: Preoperative diagnosis of carcinoma of the gallbladder by percutaneous transhepatic cholangiography. Am. J. Roentgenol. *101*:605–607, 1967.
20. Menuck, L., and Amberg, J.: The bile ducts. Radiol. Clin. North Am. *14*:499–525, 1976.
21. Meyers, R. T.: Carcinoma of the gallbladder. *In* Sabiston, D. C. (ed.): Davis-Christopher Textbook of Surgery. Vol. 1. Ed. 11. Philadelphia, W. B. Saunders Company, 1977, pp. 1281–1286.
22. Nakayama, T., Ikeda, A, and Okuda, K.: Percutaneous transhepatic drainage of the biliary tract: technique and results in 104 cases. Gastroenterology *74*:554–559, 1978.
23. Olken, S. M., Bledsoe, R., and Newmark, H., III: The ultrasonic diagnosis of primary carcinoma of the gallbladder. Radiology *129*:481–482, 1978.
24. Piehler, J. M., and Crichlow, R. W.: Primary carcinoma of the gallbladder. Arch. Surg. *112*:26–30, 1977.
25. Polk, H. C., Jr.: Carcinoma and the calcified gall bladder. Gastroenterology *50*:582–585, 1966.

26. Rosenthall, L., Shaffer, E. A., Lisbona, R., et al.: Diagnosis of hepatobiliary disease by ^{99m}Tc-HIDA cholescintigraphy. Radiology *126*:467–474, 1978.
27. Ross, A. P., Braasch, J. W., and Warren, K. W.: Carcinoma of the proximal bile ducts. Surg. Gynecol. Obstet. *136*:923–928, 1973.
28. Sample, W. F., Sarti, D. A., Goldstein, L. I., et al.: Gray-scale ultrasonography of the jaundiced patient. Radiology *128*:719–725, 1978.
29. Sato, T., Watanabe, K., Saitoh, Y., et al.: Selective arteriography for gallbladder diseases: evaluation with reference to carcinoma of the gallbladder. Arch. Surg. *99*:598–605, 1969.
30. Scholz, F. J., Larsen, C. R., and Wise, R. E.: Intravenous cholangiography recurring concepts. Semin. Roentgenol. *11*:197–202, 1976.
31. Shanser, J. D., Korobkin, M., Goldberg, H. I., et al.: Computed tomographic diagnosis of obstructive jaundice in the absence of intrahepatic ductal dilatation. Am. J. Roentgenol. *131*:389–392, 1978.
32. Shimkin, P. M., Soloway, M. S., and Jaffe, E.: Metastatic melanoma of the gallbladder. Am. J. Roentgenol. *116*:393–395, 1972.
33. Sprayregen, S., and Messinger, N. H.: Carcinoma of the gallbladder: diagnosis and evaluation of regional spread by angiography. Am. J. Roentgenol. *116*:382–392, 1972.
34. Sprayregen, S., and Messinger, N. H.: Angiography of the jaundiced patient: with emphasis upon the angiographic appearance of biliary duct dilatation. Am. J. Roentgenol. *122*:335–355, 1974.
35. Taylor, K. J. W., and Rosenfield, A. T.: Grey-scale ultrasonography in the differential diagnosis of jaundice. Arch. Surg. *112*:820–825, 1977.
36. Walter, J. F., Bookstein, J. J., and Bouffard, E. V.: Newer angiographic obstructions in cholangiocarcinoma. Radiology *118*:19–23, 1976.
37. Wise, R. E., and O'Keeffe, A. P.: The Accessory Digestive Organs. Chicago, Year Book Medical Publishers, Inc., 1975.

17

THE PANCREAS

Part I
Nonhormonal Diseases of the Pancreas

JAMES L. CLEMENTS, JR., M.D.
ANTONIO C. GONZALEZ, M.D.
H. STEPHEN WEENS, M.D.

INTRODUCTION

Formerly evaluation of the pancreas was based on secondary or indirect signs seen on plain films of the abdomen and barium-contrast studies of the upper gastrointestinal (UGI) tract. The development of angiography, diagnostic ultrasound, computed tomography of the abdomen, endoscopic retrograde cholangiopancreatography, and percutaneous transhepatic cholangiography have led to more sophisticated evaluation of the pancreas and more accurate diagnosis.

Currently we depend on CT and ultrasound, rather than on nuclear studies, for direct imaging of the pancreas. This appears to be a general trend but it may change with increasing experience in the use of positron emission-computed tomography of the pancreas.[20, 21] This technique promises superior anatomic resolution and etiologic specificity. Its use is currently limited because of the relative unavailability and expense of the imaging equipment, and the limited access of short-lived, cyclotron-generated, positron-emitting radionuclides.

NORMAL ANATOMY

Computed Tomographic and Ultrasonographic Anatomy

An appreciation of cross-sectional anatomy is necessary for interpreting pancreatic abnormalities in both B-mode ultrasonography (US) (Fig. 17–1) and computed tomography (CT) (Fig. 17–2). Five vessels are used for identification; in order of ease and con-

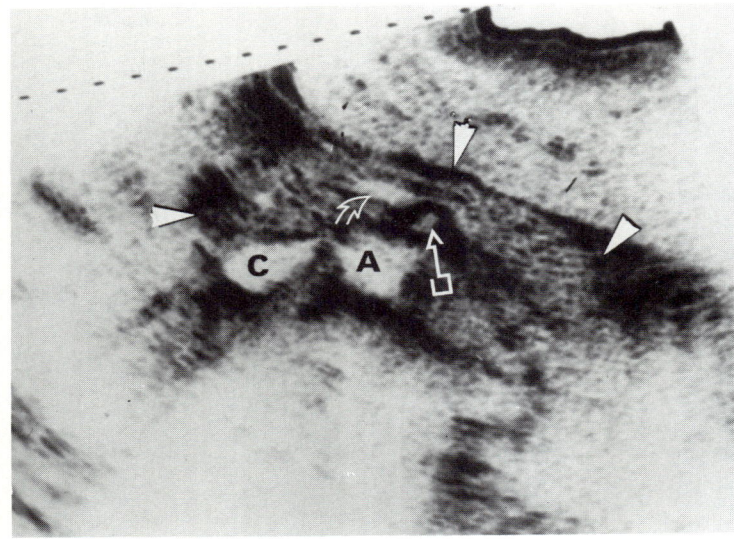

Figure 17–1. Normal transverse pancreatic ultrasonogram. Solid white arrows point to the head, body, and tail of the pancreas, from left to right. The square-based arrow points to the superior mesenteric artery and the curved arrow to the portal vein at its junction with the splenic vein. The latter passes between the body of the pancreas and the superior mesenteric artery. Notice the difference in sonographic texture between the normal pancreas and the liver immediately above it. C = vena cava; A = aorta.

sistency of localization, they are (1) the superior mesenteric artery (SMA); (2) the portal vein (PV); (3) the splenic vein (SV); (4) the vena cava (VC); and (5) the left renal vein (LRV).

The superior mesenteric artery identifies the midportion of the gland, or the body; the portal vein identifies the junction of head and body above and the uncinate process below. The anastomosis of the portal and splenic veins marks the midbody as does the superior mesenteric artery, which is immediately beneath these two veins. The splenic vein continues under the organ and is the landmark for the more lateral body and the tail. The vena cava lies immediately beneath the head of the pancreas, where it is joined by the left renal vein. The head is therefore best localized at the junction of the vena cava and the left renal vein: The latter vessel is variably prominent, but its course

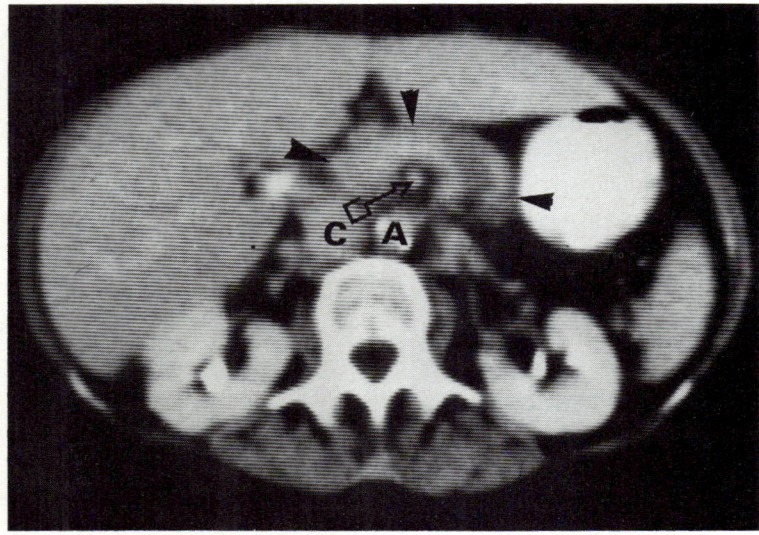

Figure 17–2. Normal pancreatic CT scan. Black arrowheads point to the head, body, and tail of the pancreas, from left to right. The open arrow points to the superior mesenteric artery. C = vena cava; A = aorta. The stomach, to the left, is filled with contrast medium. The slight variations in density within the pancreas are normal and reflect differences in content and distribution of fat and mucin. This is the scan of a young individual. Compare it with Figure 17–3, the scan of a normal pancreas in an old, obese person.

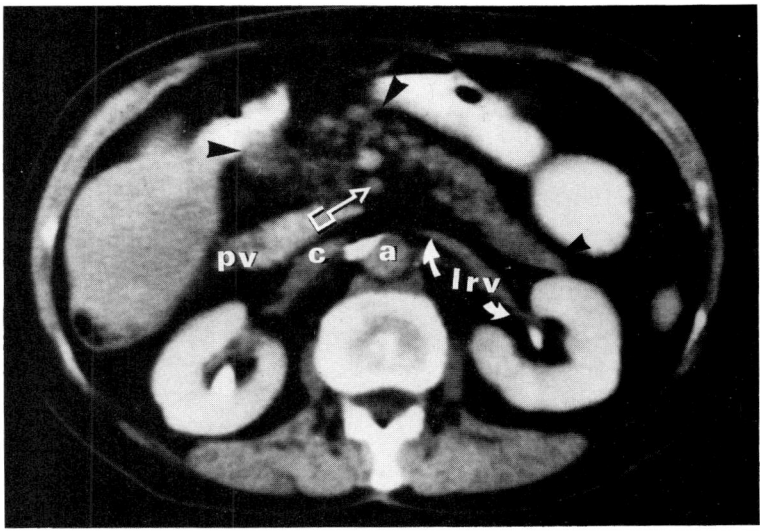

Figure 17–3. Normal pancreatic CT scan in advanced age. Notice the preponderance of fat density within and around a significantly thinner pancreas. Black arrowheads identify the organ. There is a small subcapsular cyst in the liver. Sizable amounts of peripancreatic and pancreatic fat interfere with ultrasound demonstration of the pancreas because of the marked echogenicity of fatty tissue. pv = portal vein; lrv (curved arrows) = left renal vein, passing between the aorta (a) and the superior mesenteric artery (open arrow).

between the superior mesenteric artery and the aorta (A) accurately identifies the pancreatic head.

Other vessels and structures are used to advantage in axial pancreatic localization. These are, however, often smaller than 0.5 cm in diameter and are less consistently demonstrated by US and CT. The gastroduodenal artery (GDA) is seen superior, and the common bile duct (CD) inferior, to the head of the pancreas. The tail of the pancreas borders the superior and anteromedial portion of the upper pole of the left kidney. The pancreas is a bilobular organ, perched centrally and at variable obliquity over the spine and aorta. The head lies more caudal than the body and tail.

The dimensions of the normal pancreas vary depending on patient size, fat content, and age (Fig. 17–3). Obese and young individuals have a larger and thicker pancreas than do smaller, thinner, and older persons. The average measurement given for the organ varies with the type of axial tomography used (US or CT). Ultrasonographic anteroposterior measurements suggested for the head, body, and tail are 2.8 to 3.5 cm, 1.5 to 3.0 cm, and 2.8 to 3.5 cm, respectively.[31] In computed tomograms, anteroposterior values of 3.0, 2.5 and 2.0 cm, respectively, are given for head, body, and tail measurements.[31] The ratio to vertebral bodies has also been used to evaluate size of the pancreatic head, body, and tail.[37] Normal estimates of these ratios are 0.6 ± 0.1 for the head and 0.5 ± 0.1 for the body and tail.

The ultrasonographic texture of pancreatic parenchyma also varies with individual anatomy and to a lesser degree with the type of equipment used. The normal pancreas is usually seen as an organ of intermediate echogenicity, being equally or more, but never less, echogenic than the normal liver.[13]

The CT density of the normal pancreas is less than that of the liver and nearly doubles after contrast administration; specific Hounsfield values quoted for normal area are 30 to 45 H without, and 60 to 85 H with, contrast.[37] Detection of pancreatic disease by CT scanning is based mainly on recognition of size and shape alterations and detection of major density changes and focal masses.

Radiographic contrast is important in the CT examination of the pancreas. Diluted Gastrografin is given orally to profile the stomach, antrum, duodenum, and jejunum and to distinguish the head, body, and tail of the pancreas from bowel densities. Intravenous contrast medium enhances the outline of pancreatic parenchyma and also helps by contrasting the kidney and ureter. Contrast aids in differentiating the body and tail of the pancreas from the adjacent splenic vein or dilated pancreatic duct or both.

The normal anatomic details of the pancreatic duct are described in the section on endoscopic retrograde cholangiopancreatography.

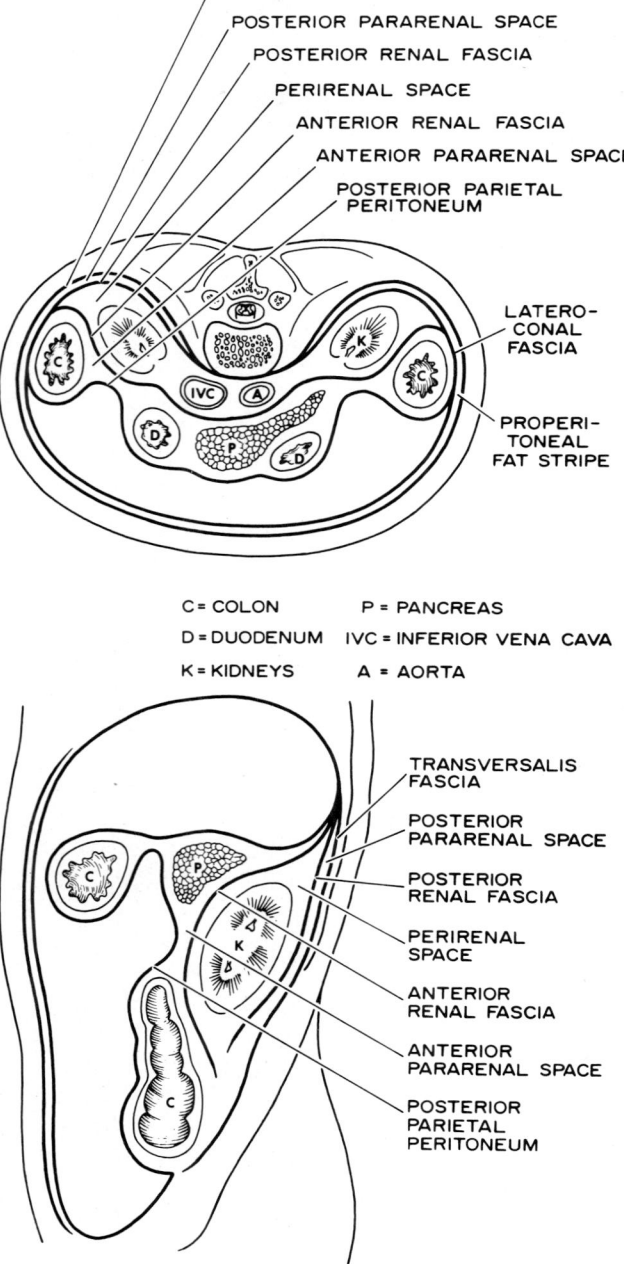

Figure 17–4. Fascial anatomy of the pancreas. Many pancreatic effusions, such as pseudocysts and hematomas, are contained within the anterior pararenal space. Indirect evidence of their pancreatic origin can be deduced from x-rays, by an understanding of the extension and connections of this fascial plane. (*From* Hunziker, R. J.: Pathologic effusions localized to the anterior pararenal space. Gastrointest. Radiol. 3:411–414, 1978. Reproduced by permission.)

Fascial Anatomy

The pancreas is contained, unencapsulated, in a potential fascial plane within the retroperitoneum. This plane is known as the anterior pararenal (APR) space.[22] Two other retroperitoneal fascial planes, the posterior pararenal (PPR) and the perirenal space (PR), lie posterior to the anterior pararenal space (Fig. 17–4). The APR also contains the vertical retroperitoneal portions of the colon and duodenum. The posterior pararenal space contains the properitoneal fat. The perirenal space contains the kidneys, adrenals, abdominal aorta, cava, and surrounding fat. The anterior pararenal space is surrounded by peritoneum anteriorly and the anterior renal fascia posteriorly. The distribution of these retroperitoneal compartments can determine the route of spread of many effusions. The predominant vector of displacement by pancreatic masses is also closely related to these fascial landmarks.

The anterior pararenal space extends from side to side across the midline, from the line of fusion of the anterior and posterior renal fascia, termed the lateroconal fascia. The lateroconal fascia runs up and down the abdomen along the lateral walls of the ascending and descending colon, fusing anteriorly with the posterior parietal peritoneum. The most superior border of the anterior pararenal space is the fusion line of the diaphragmatic fascia, renal fascia, and transversalis fascia, in that order, from anterior to posterior. The anterior pararenal space opens inferiorly into the pararenal space at the iliac fossa.

Angiographic Anatomy (Figs. 17–5 to 17–7)

The pancreas receives a dual blood supply from the branches of the celiac and superior mesenteric arteries. Accordingly, very often both the celiac and the superior mesenteric arteries must be selectively injected for complete angiographic demonstration of the

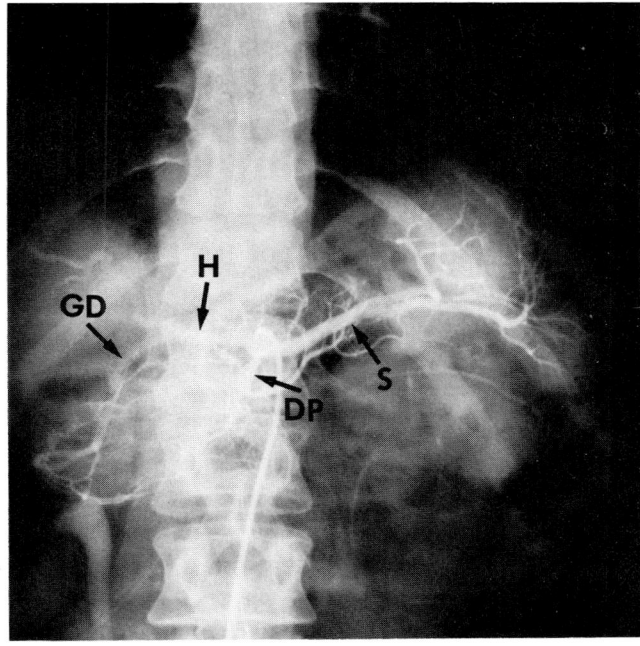

Figure 17–5. Angiographic anatomy of the normal pancreas. In order to demonstrate the entire blood supply of the pancreas, both the celiac artery (tip of catheter, not labeled) and the superior mesenteric artery (not shown) should be opacified. The gastroduodenal artery (GD) branches from the hepatic (H) and the dorsal pancreatic (DP) arteries to form the pancreaticoduodenal arcade, the arterial supply to the head and the right portions of the body of the pancreas. S = splenic artery.

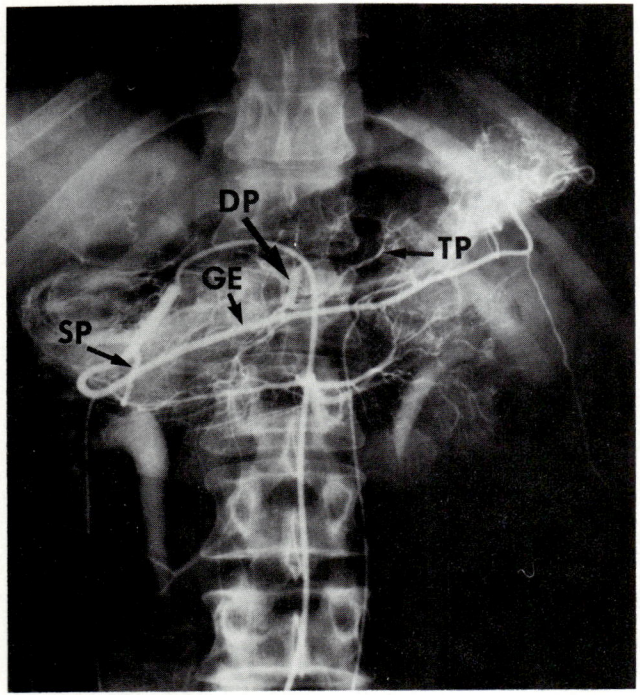

Figure 17–6. Angiographic anatomy of the normal pancreas. Selective catheter injection of the gastroduodenal artery demonstrates the blood supply of the inferior pancreas and the rest of the body and tail. This type of injection can also be performed by injecting the superior mesenteric artery. SP = superior pancreaticoduodenal artery; GE = gastroepiploic artery; DP = dorsal pancreatic artery; TP = transverse pancreatic artery.

Figure 17–7. Angiographic anatomy of the normal pancreas. Capillary phase of contrast injection showing the outline of the pancreas (arrowheads). This excellent visualization is not always possible because of superimposition of capillary stains by adjacent viscera.

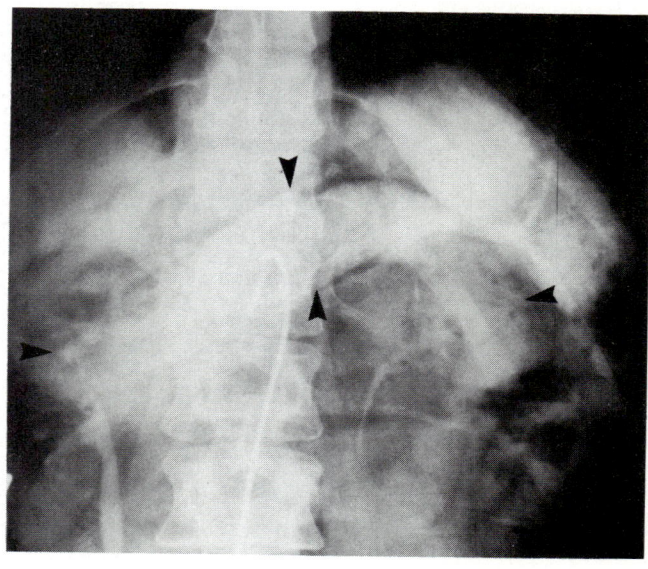

pancreas. Enhancement of pancreatic capillary contrast visualization has been attempted with simultaneous injection of vasodilator or vasoconstrictor pharmacologic agents. Vasoconstrictors have proved more useful in demonstrating pancreatic tumor vessels, but tumor staining has been less consistently observed.[5]

DISEASES OF THE PANCREAS

Pancreatic Cysts

True cysts of the pancreas are extremely rare and undistinguishable from pseudocysts by imaging modalities. They share the same radiographic and sonographic characteristics of pseudocysts.

Cystadenomas are also very rare lesions of the pancreas and can be very difficult to distinguish from cystadenocarcinomas. They usually occur in the tail of the pancreas. Visible radiographic calcifications may be present in 10 per cent of cases.[25] These tumors are angiographically hypervascular (Fig. 17–8). Their sonographic appearance is variable; some are reported as transonic (cystic) (Fig. 17–9), and others are echogenic (Fig. 17–10).[25] The role of CT in the diagnosis and differentiation of pancreatic adenomas has not yet been clearly defined.

Acute Pancreatitis

The specific metabolic accident that precipitates pancreatitis in humans is unknown. Multiple causative factors are recognized to cause an attack or exacerbation;[32] these include block of exocrine flow, toxic cellular damage, and parenchymal trauma.

The most common complication of acute pancreatitis is pseudocyst formation. Nearly 90 per cent of all pseudocysts associated with pancreatitis occur during the acute

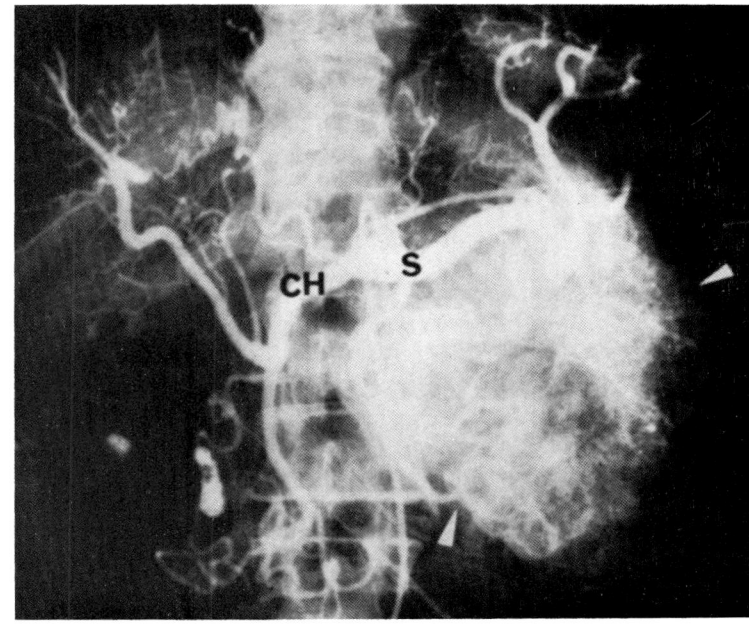

Figure 17–8. Pancreatic cystadenoma. Celiac arteriogram demonstrates a well-defined hypervascular mass in the body and tail of the pancreas (arrowheads). S = splenic artery; CH = common hepatic artery. (*From* Floyd, T. V., Antonmattei, S., and Freimanis, A. K.: Gray scale sonography of cystadenoma of the pancreas: report of two cases. J. Clin. Ultrasound 7:149–151, 1979. Reproduced by permission.)

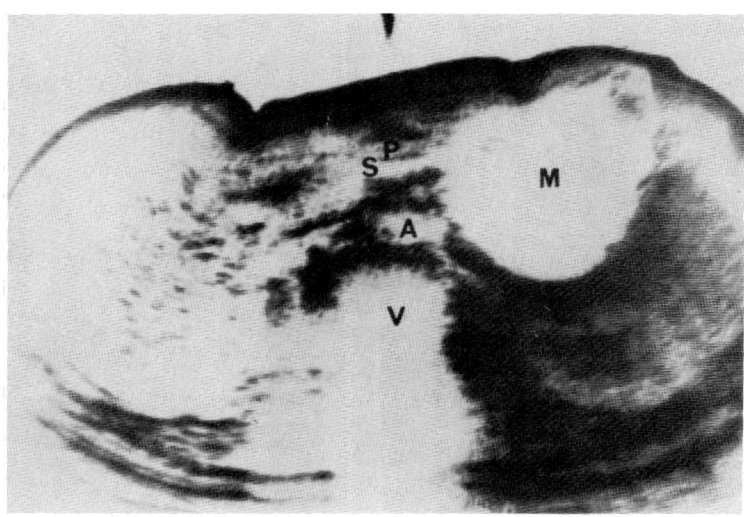

Figure 17–9. Pancreatic cystadenoma. Transverse sonogram demonstrating a large, well-defined sonolucent mass (M) in the tail of the pancreas. P = pancreas; S = splenic vein; A = aorta; V = vertebra. Compare with Figure 17–10. (*From* Floyd, T. V., Antonmattei, S., and Freimanis, A. K.: Gray scale sonography of cystadenoma of the pancreas: report of two cases. J. Clin. Ultrasound 7:149–151, 1979. Reproduced by permission.)

episode.[17] As many as 52 of 99 patients admitted to a general hospital with the diagnosis of acute pancreatitis developed pseudocysts,[17] approximately 20 per cent of which resolved spontaneously. However, reported experience has shown that persisting pseudocysts are best managed by surgical drainage.[6, 7] The risk of rupture was high when treatment was delayed, the probability of spontaneous resolution in chronic pseudocysts was low, and the morbidity and mortality of spontaneous intraperitoneal rupture was significant.[6]

PLAIN FILMS OF THE ABDOMEN. Radiographic examination of the abdomen with the patient in supine, erect, and decubitus positions should be used when there is any clinical evidence of an acute intra-abdominal condition. There are a number of plain film findings in patients with acute pancreatitis; however, none of these is specific.

A generalized adynamic or paralytic ileus may be observed in varying degrees, but marked intestinal distention is uncommon. A localized segmental small bowel dilata-

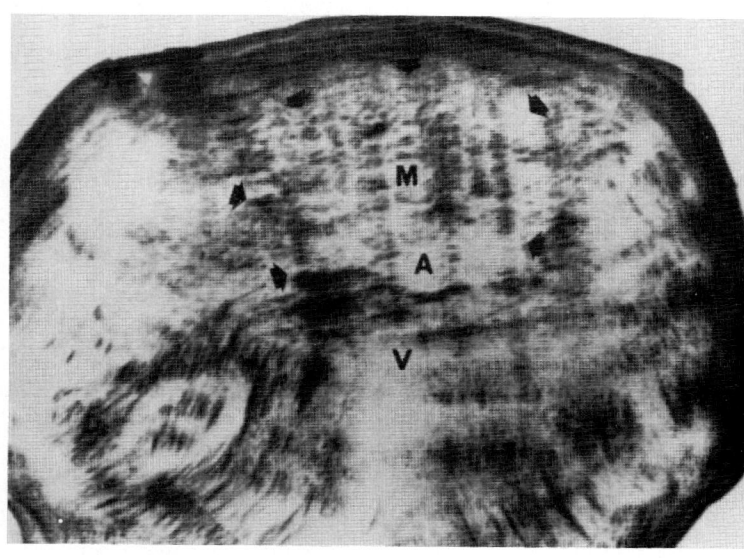

Figure 17–10. Pancreatic cystadenoma. Transverse sonogram showing an echogenic mass in the body and tail of the pancreas (arrows). M = mass; A = aorta; V = vertebra. (*From* Floyd, T. V., Antonmattei, S., and Freimanis, A. K.: Gray scale sonography of cystadenoma of the pancreas: report of two cases. J. Clin. Ultrasound 7:149–151, 1979. Reproduced by permission.)

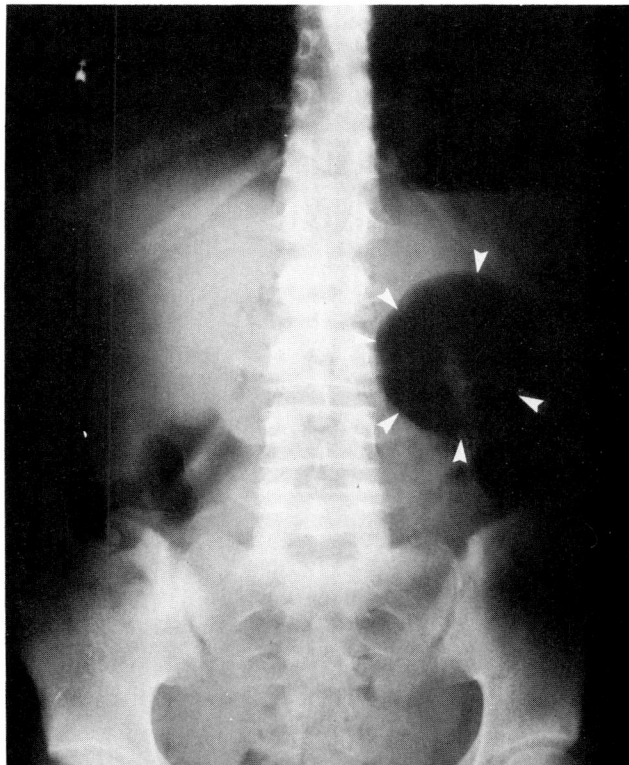

Figure 17–11. Acute pancreatitis. Plain radiograph of the abdomen showing a sentinel loop (arrowheads) near the midbody the tail of the pancreas. This is a nonspecific finding, since it can be seen in many acute intraabdominal conditions, such as cholecystitis, intestinal infarction, and others.

tion, referred to as the sentinel loop sign (Fig. 17–11), is considered more characteristic of pancreatitis than is generalized distention but has been observed in less than 10 per cent of these patients.[42] The distended loops are usually localized to the left upper abdomen in the region of the proximal jejunum. However, localized small intestinal distention in the left upper quadrant cannot be considered specific for acute pancreatitis; it may be observed in patients with acute cholecystitis and early mechanical ileus as well as other acute intra-abdominal conditions.

Adynamic duodenal ileus, the gaseous distention of the descending limb of the duodenum, may be considered a more characteristic finding of acute pancreatitis. This distention of the duodenal segment, however, may also occur with acute cholecystitis and may even occur normally from aerophagia.

The "colon cut-off sign" has been considered highly suggestive of acute pancreatitis. This consists of gaseous distention of the right and transverse colon with sudden transition, or cut-off, to a collapsed distal colon.[27] The site of the cut-off may vary from the proximal transverse colon to the splenic flexure. This sign may be significant but, it is, unfortunately, infrequently observed. In addition, the same pattern of colon cut-off may be associated with acute cholecystitis and colonic ischemia.

A rarely encountered plain film finding of acute pancreatitis is evidence of fat necrosis within the abdomen. It appears as mottled areas of decreased and increased density in the peritoneal fat due to edema and saponification. Fat necrosis does not appear to affect the posterior pararenal plane, so that the retroperitoneal fat outline of kidneys and psoas muscles is not distorted.

Enlargement of the pancreas and thickening of peripancreatic tissues may produce a mass effect in the upper abdomen, appreciable on plain films. However, such mass effect is more characteristic of pseudocyst formation.

The presence of opaque biliary calculi in the right upper quadrant has implications for both acute cholecystitis and biliary pancreatitis.

The presence of pancreatic calculi (See Fig. 17–39) also has diagnostic importance. These calculi are associated with chronic pancreatitis, and their visualization in patients with acute symptoms strongly suggests recurrent acute pancreatitis superimposed on chronic pancreatitis.

Detection of extraluminal gas in the upper abdomen in a patient with the clinical diagnosis of acute pancreatitis is an ominous finding, indicating emphysematous infection or abscess of the pancreas.[42] The gas pattern has a finely reticulated or a coarse, bubbly configuration. Whenever extraluminal gas is suspected on plain films, contrast studies are indicated to confirm the extraluminal location of the gas.

INTRAVENOUS CHOLANGIOGRAPHY (IVC). Intravenous cholangiography is often used to screen patients presenting with acute abdominal pain. In the acute abdomen it is often quite difficult to differentiate acute cholecystitis from acute pancreatitis. IVC is a method of assessing the patency of the cystic duct; patency is almost never present in acute cholecystitis.[41, 42]

After the intravenous injection of 20 ml of contrast medium, the common hepatic and common bile ducts are normally visualized within 20 to 30 minutes. If the cystic duct is patent, gallbladder opacification can be expected in 30 to 60 minutes.

If the gallbladder is not opacified within several hours after injection and there is visualization of the bile duct, cystic duct obstruction is indicated. These findings probably represent acute cholecystitis in patients with acute abdominal symptoms. If, on the other hand, the common bile duct fails to opacify and the gallbladder is not opacified, the procedure must be considered nondiagnostic. However, if a film of the abdomen taken 12 to 24 hours after the injection of contrast material reveals opacification of the colon and nonopacification of the gallbladder, this is indicative of cystic duct obstruction.

BARIUM-CONTRAST STUDIES OF THE UPPER GASTROINTESTINAL TRACT. Contrast examination of the upper gastrointestinal tract was once considered the most definitive procedure in the diagnosis of acute pancreatitis. Today, it has been superseded by diagnostic ultrasound and computerized tomography of the abdomen.

The stomach and duodenum may demonstrate changes secondary to pancreatic masses and inflammation (Figs. 17–12, and 17–13). The most prominent findings are in the duodenal loop, which is situated close to the head of the pancreas. Swelling and masses of the pancreatic head consequently enlarge in the duodenal loop. The swelling of the gland and peripancreatitis are in turn reflected in the mucosal pattern of the duodenum by thickening and spiculization of its folds. The distal body of the stomach and antrum are in apposition to the pancreatic body and head. Enlargement in these areas of the pancreas results in anterior and superior displacement of the gastric antrum ("pad sign") (Figs. 17–12 and 17–13). Similarly located pancreatic swelling and accumulation of extravasated enzymes (pseudocysts) may produce an increase in the size of the retrogastric space, with anterior displacement of the distal stomach. The retrogastric space is difficult to evaluate because of its variability. Obesity, the presence of ascitic fluid, or obstructive pulmonary disease with depression of the diaphragm can result in anteroposterior increases in this space.

Effacement and stretching of the posterior contours of the stomach in association with a large retrogastric space are more definitive indications of mass formation. Peripancreatic inflammation may result in thickening and hyper-rugosity of the adjacent mucosal folds of the stomach. On occasion the degree of inflammatory

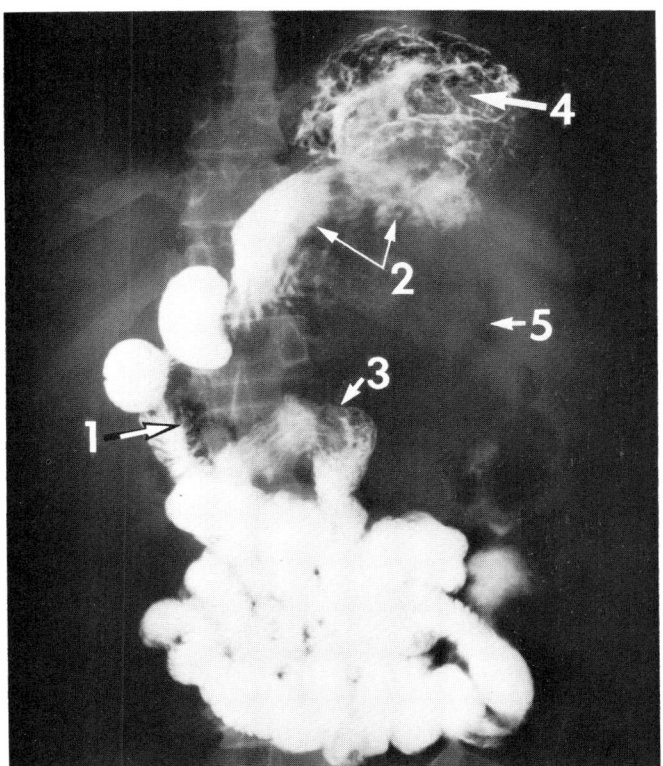

Figure 17–12. Barium-contrast study of the upper gastrointestinal tract in a patient with acute pancreatitis demonstrates a number of radiographic signs of pancreatitis. 1. Spiculated mucosal pattern on the medial margin of the descending duodenum. 2. Extrinsic pressure on the greater curvature of the body and antrum of the stomach by the pancreatic swelling and peripancreatic edema. The so-called pad sign. 3. Downward and medial displacement of the duodenojejunal junction (ligament by Treitz) by the pancreatic and peripancreatic swelling. 4. Mucosal swelling in the fundus of the stomach secondary to the adjacent inflammatory mass. 5. Gas formation in the region of the pancreatic mass, indicating early evidence of emphysematous infection.

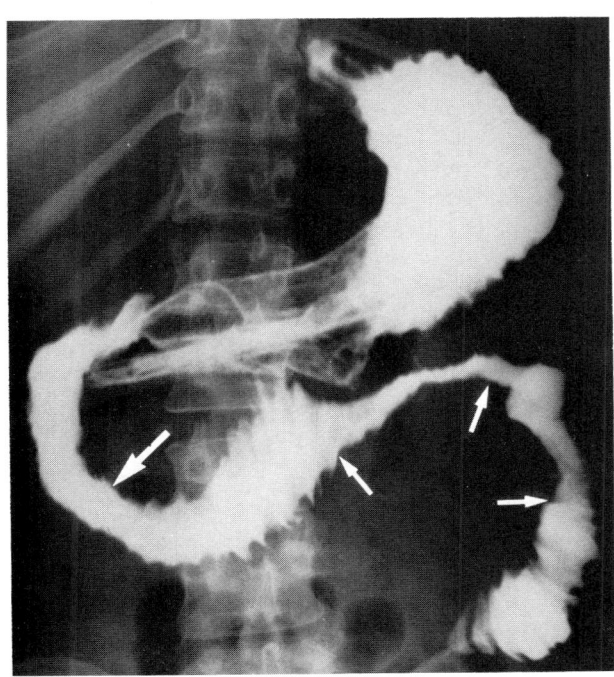

Figure 17–13. Barium-contrast study of the upper gastrointestinal tract in a patient with acute pancreatitis, demonstrating mass effect and mucosal effacement involving the duodenal loop (large arrow). Inflammatory changes are also present, involving the jejunum with narrowing secondary to transmural inflammation (small arrows).

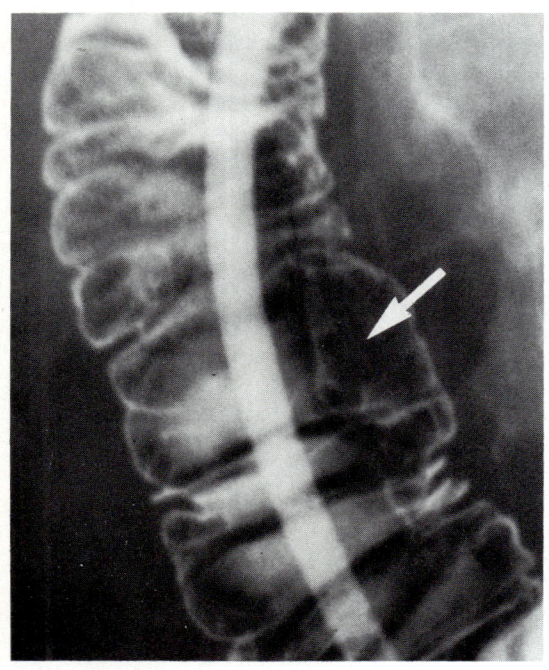

Figure 17–14. Hypotonic duodenogram in a patient with acute pancreatitis. The film of the mid-descending duodenum demonstrates a swollen papilla of Vater (arrow) secondary to acute pancreatic inflammation.

response and thickening of the mucosal folds may suggest the possibility of gastric neoplasm or some other submucosal infiltrative process.

Pancreatic enlargement and peripancreatitic fluid accumulation can cause downward displacement of the duodenojejunal junction (ligament of Treitz).[22] Mucosal edema may also be observed at this level. Inflammatory changes in the jejunum distal to this point may occur but only with extensive peripancreatic response.

BARIUM-CONTRAST EXAMINATION OF THE COLON. Barium enema examination plays a minor role in the radiologic evaluation of acute pancreatitis. More importantly, changes secondary to pancreatitis that are inadvertently encountered in the colon can frequently be a source of diagnostic confusion. They can simulate primary segmental colonic disease, such as neoplasm, inflammation, or ischemia (Figs. 17–15 to 17–17).

Changes in the large bowel associated with acute pancreatitis are most often seen in the splenic and hepatic flexures and the transverse colon. This is because of the anatomic continuity of the pancreatic bed with the root of the transverse mesocolon and the proximity of the tail of the pancreas to the phrenocolic ligament in the anterior pararenal space.[27] This mesenteric plane provides a route of spread of extravasated pancreatic enzymes to the transverse colon and its flexures.

Pericolitis secondary to pancreatitis (Figs. 17–15 to 17–17) is most easily detected in the region of the splenic flexure, where narrowing of the lumen and thickening and distortion of the mucosal pattern are observed. Pericolitis can produce partial obstruction to the colon, accounting for the plain film finding of the colon cut-off sign.

Less commonly, segmental narrowing may be encountered anywhere along the course of the transverse colon and the hepatic flexure. Spread of enzymes and exudate may extend into the retroperitoneal areolar tissue and through both flanks, producing mucosal thickening and irregularity of the cecum and the ascending and descending colon. This spread may eventually extend along the retroperitoneal paracolic gutters to the pelvis, where secondary radiographic changes may be visualized in the sigmoid colon.

THE PANCREAS — 1015

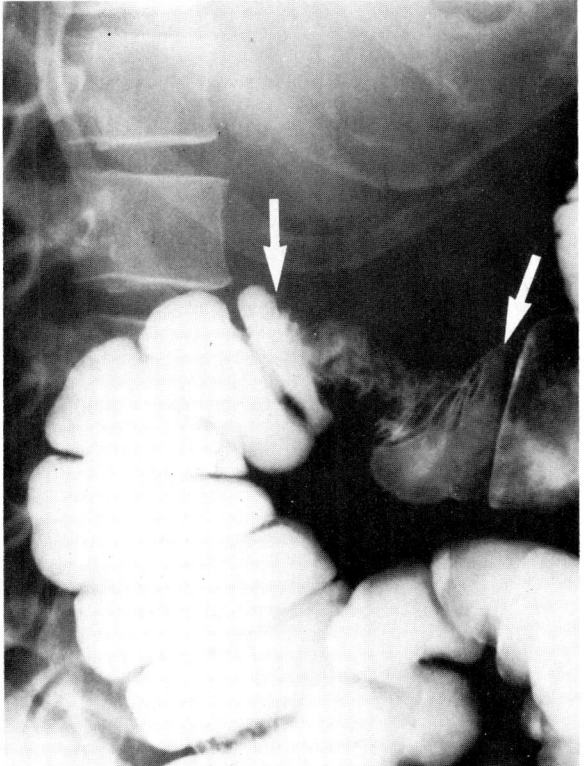

Figure 17–15. Barium enema in a case of peripancreatitis that produced pericolitis (arrows) in the transverse hepatic flexure. These changes are virtually undistinguishable from those of carcinoma of the colon.

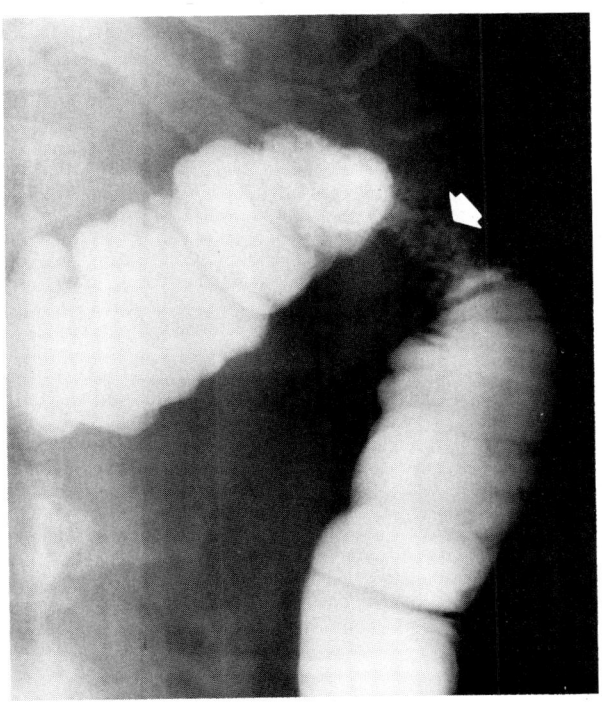

Figure 17–16. Barium enema demonstration of pericolitis involving the splenic flexure (arrow) secondary to acute pancreatitis. The mucosal pattern is thickened and irregular but appears intact. On occasion radiographic differential diagnosis between constricting carcinoma and pericolitis is difficult without a history of pancreatitis.

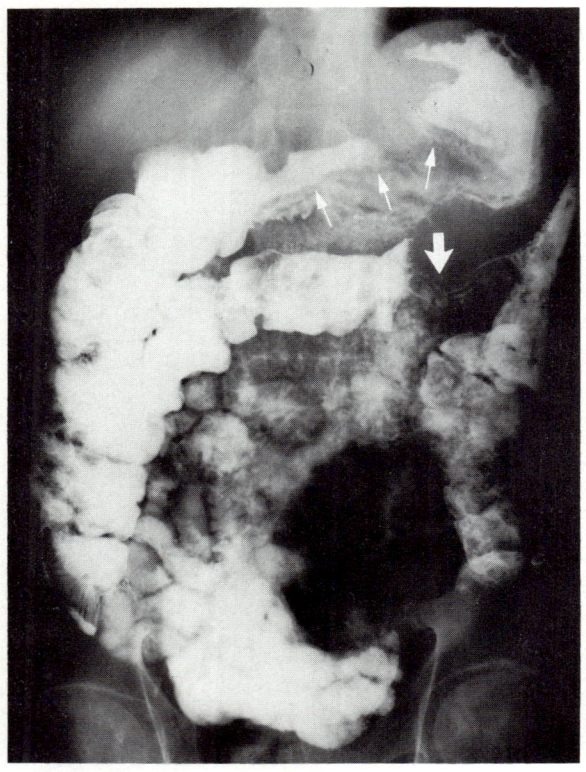

Figure 17–17. Acute pancreatitis. Later film of a small intestinal study demonstrates evidence of pericolitis in the distal transverse colon (large arrow) secondary to acute pancreatitis. The sharp shelving margin at the proximal extent of the narrowed colon suggests the possibility of carcinoma of the colon; however, there are changes of extrinsic pressure on the body of the stomach (small arrows) produced by the pancreatic mass. The displacement of small intestinal loops in the left lower quadrant is fortuitous and is not evidence of a mass in this area.

ENDOSCOPIC RETROGRADE CHOLANGIOPANCREATOGRAPHY (ERCP). Endoscopic retrograde cholangiopancreatography is a method of evaluating the ductal system of both the biliary tree and the pancreas.[12, 28, 34, 36] This procedure requires a cooperative effort by the endoscopist and the radiologist, since it involves the cannulation of the pancreatic and bile ducts by a fiberoptic endoscope and radiographic filming of retrograde injection of contrast. In general, the clinical diagnosis of acute pancreatitis is a relative contraindication for ERCP.[34, 36] On occasion the procedure must be carried out because of strong suspicion of obstructing bile duct stones as a cause of pancreatitis or pancreatic pseudocyst undocumented by ultrasound.

The majority of patients with acute pancreatitis have minimal or no demonstrable abnormality of the pancreatic duct by ERCP.[36] Displacement of the main pancreatic duct is not specific, since it can be secondary to pancreatic swelling, peripancreatitis, or pseudocyst.

PSEUDOCYST: PLAIN FILMS OF THE ABDOMEN (Fig. 17–18). The mass effect of large pseudocysts may be appreciated on plain films of the abdomen. Gas within the stomach, duodenal loop, and transverse colon may show displacement. Such findings on plain film do not necessarily indicate a pseudocyst in patients with pancreatic disease. The pancreas itself can enlarge with edema, hemorrhage, or intense peripancreatitis.[33]

PSEUDOCYST: BARIUM-CONTRAST STUDIES OF THE UPPER GASTROINTESTINAL TRACT. A large pseudocyst extending from the pancreatic bed to the region of the lesser omental sac can produce marked distortion in all segments of the stomach and duodenum (Figs. 17–19 and 17–20). The most characteristic finding is marked displacement of the stomach anteriorly, with stretching and effacement of the posterior aspect of

Figure 17–18. Pseudocyst. Erect plain film of the abdomen in a patient with a large upper abdominal pseudocyst. There is a mass displacing inferiorly the middle and distal transverse colon. The gas in the proximal descending colon shows a fusiform narrowing (arrow) from pressure effect from the pseudocyst.

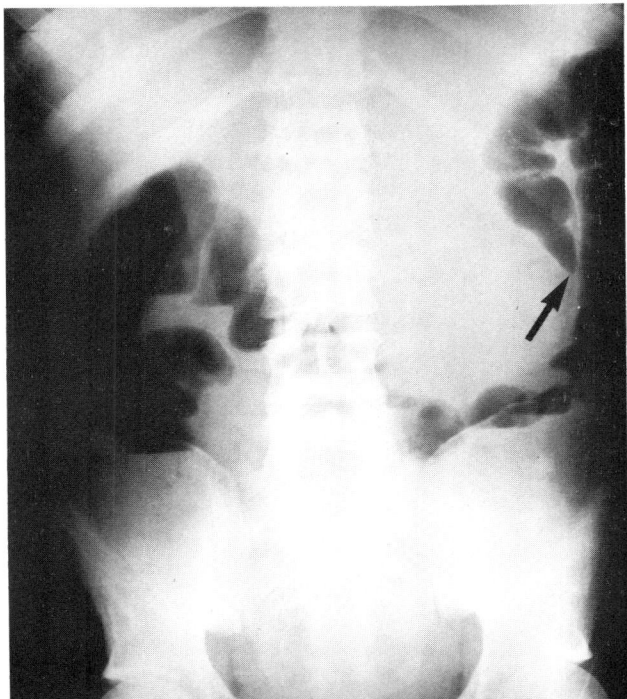

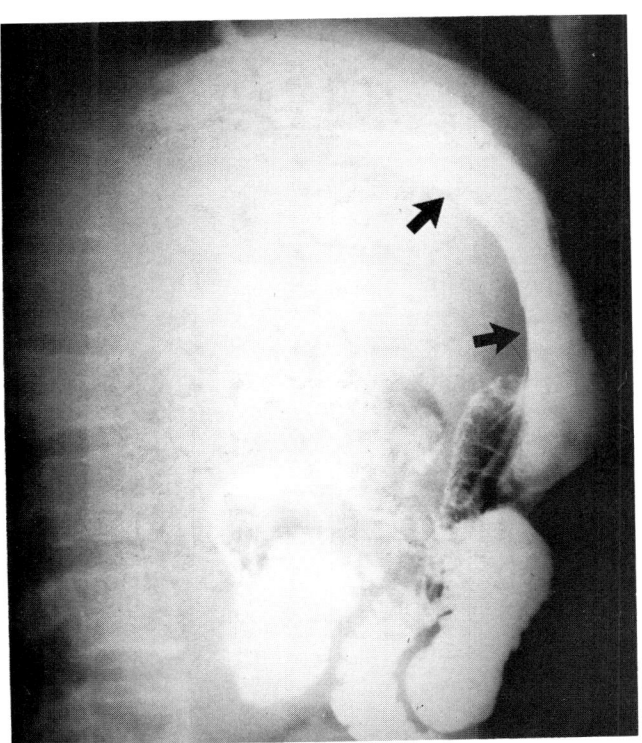

Figure 17–19. Barium-contrast study of the upper gastrointestinal tract in the lateral projection demonstrates a marked increase in the retrogastric space, with stretching and effacement of the posterior aspect of the barium-filled stomach (arrows). This finding is quite characteristic of pseudocyst formation.

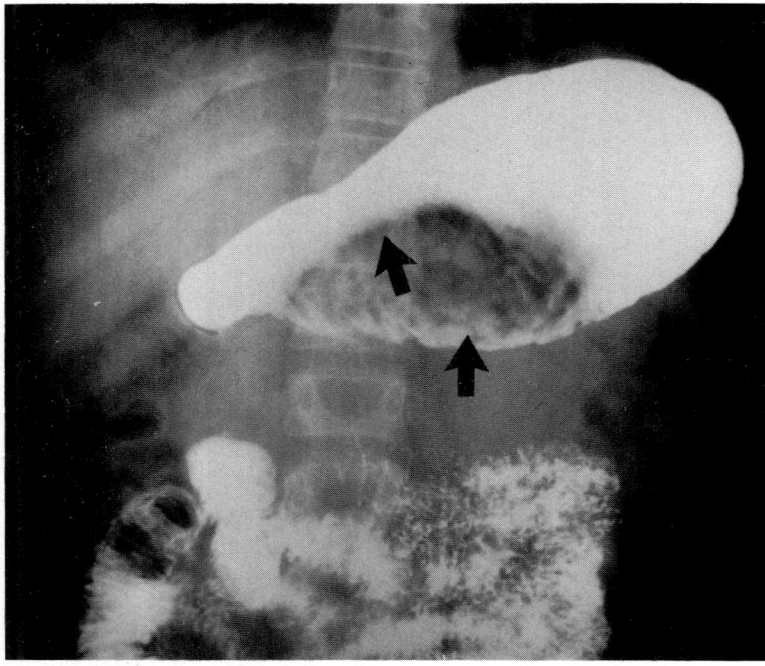

Figure 17–20. Barium-contrast study of the upper gastrointestinal tract in a patient with epigastric pseudocyst. Extrinsic pressure on the inferior aspect of the stomach is apparent (arrows). On the lateral film, the mass producing this defect was noted to encroach upon the posterior aspect of the stomach.

the stomach. Mucosal hyper-rugosity, as seen in acute pancreatitis, may be obvious in the stomach, duodenal loop, and proximal jejunum. Loculation of the pseudocyst in the left subphrenic area can produce marked displacement of the fundus of the stomach from the diaphragmatic margin.

Less commonly, mass effects of pancreatic pseudocysts can be seen distant from the pancreatic bed. The anatomic continuity of the pancreatic gland with the base of the transverse mesocolon allows loculation of extravasated effusion through the entire gastrocolic region, effecting marked separation of the stomach from the transverse colon. The relationship of the small intestinal mesentery to the transverse mesocolon can lead to pseudocyst formation in the right lower quadrant; such masses displace small intestinal loops in this area (Fig. 17–21).

Pseudocyst: Barium-Contrast Studies of the Colon. On barium enema examination, the presence of a pseudocyst is most often revealed by distortion of the transverse colon and splenic flexure (Fig. 17–22).[33] When the pseudocyst is localized to the gastrocolic area there may be marked stretching and displacement of the transverse colon.[27] Pseudocysts following the route of spread via the root of the mesentery of the small intestine distort the distal ileum, cecum, and ascending colon.[27, 33] Pseudocysts in the pelvis produce evidence of pelvic masses with extrinsic distortion of the rectosigmoid and sigmoid colon (Fig. 17–23).

Pseudocyst: ERCP. Cannulation of the pancreatic duct and pancreatogram may demonstrate contrast material in pseudocysts that communicate with the ductal system (Fig. 17–24). Pseudocysts that do not communicate (Fig. 17–25) may be demonstrated by their mass effect.[12, 36] There is a definite risk of infection from retrograde filling of large pseudocysts (Figs. 17–26 and 17–27); therefore, other methods of diagnosis, such as ultrasound and computerized axial tomography, are preferable.[36] If ERCP is carried out with the knowledge that a cyst is present, it should be planned close to the time of anticipated surgery for drainage.[36]

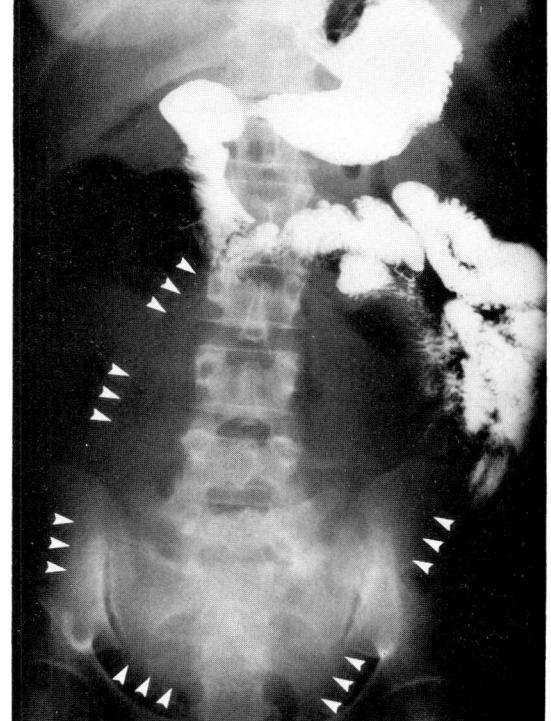

Figure 17–21. Large pseudocysts occupying the lower abdominal quadrants. The upper gastrointestinal series shows displacement of the jejunum to the left upper quadrant and a soft tissue mass effect (arrowheads).

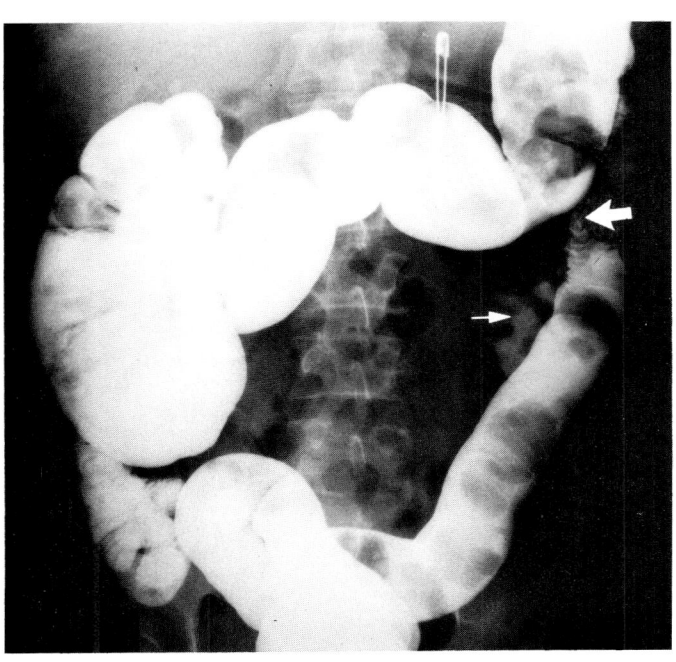

Figure 17–22. Barium enema examination demonstrating pericolitis involving the proximal descending colon (large arrow) secondary to pancreatic pseudocyst. There was spontaneous communication with this pseudocyst. The small arrow demonstrates barium extravasated from the colon into a portion of the pancreatic pseudocyst.

1020 — THE PANCREAS

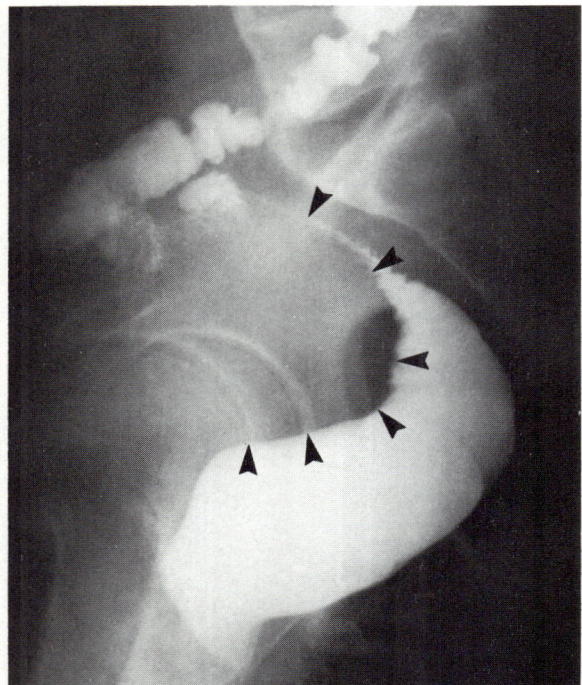

Figure 17–23. Lateral view of the rectosigmoid colon in barium enema examination showing pelvic pancreatic pseudocyst. There is anterior indentation of the sigmoid (arrowheads) by the pseudocyst.

Figure 17–24. Filling of a pancreatic pseudocyst on ERCP examination. The cyst (C) is seen to fill from the duct in the region near the junction of the body and tail of the pancreas. This cyst drained completely on follow-up films.

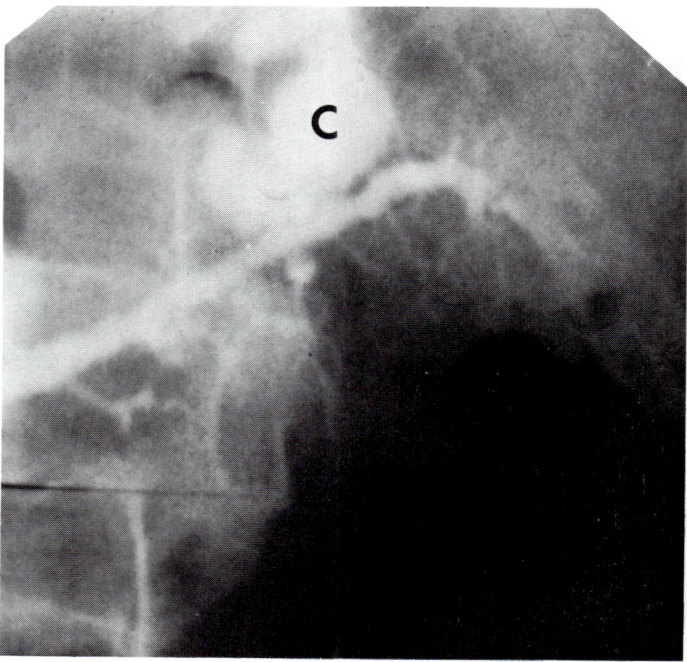

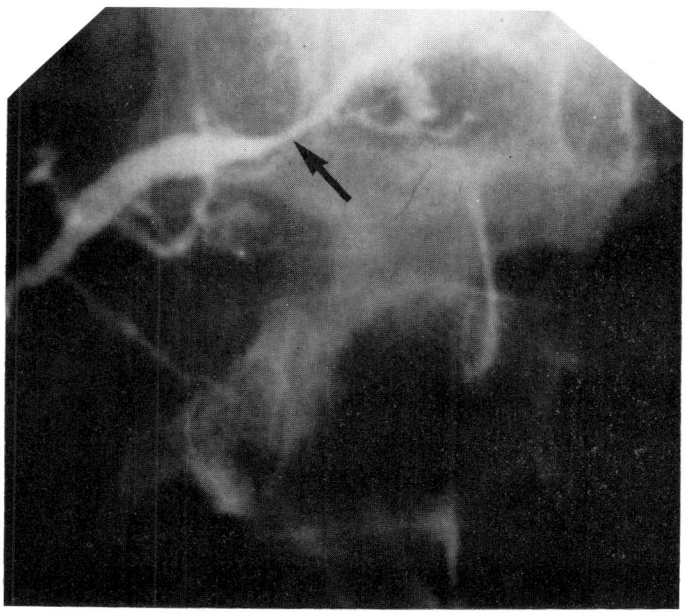

Figure 17–25. Endoscopic retrograde pancreatogram (ERP) in a patient with pancreatitis and pseudocyst. The pseudocyst was not filled on the retrograde injection of the pancreatic duct; duct narrowing and extrinsic pressure are demonstrated on the superior aspect of the duct in the region of the body of the pancreas (arrow). Pancreatic tumor could not be excluded without the aid of ultrasound, which demonstrated the cystic nature of the nonfilling pseudocyst.

Small pseudocysts, usually within the gland, may be filled on cannulation studies. The contrast in these pseudocysts usually promptly drain back into the ductal system.

ANGIOGRAPHY: ACUTE PANCREATITIS AND PSEUDOCYST. Angiography is indicated when the diagnosis of pancreatitis is not clearly established by fluoroscopically guided percutaneous pancreatic aspiration biopsy and for the presurgical demonstration of blood supply.[16, 20] The technique is valuable because it may help exclude lesions in the peripancreatic organs, such as the kidney, liver and spleen, that are associated

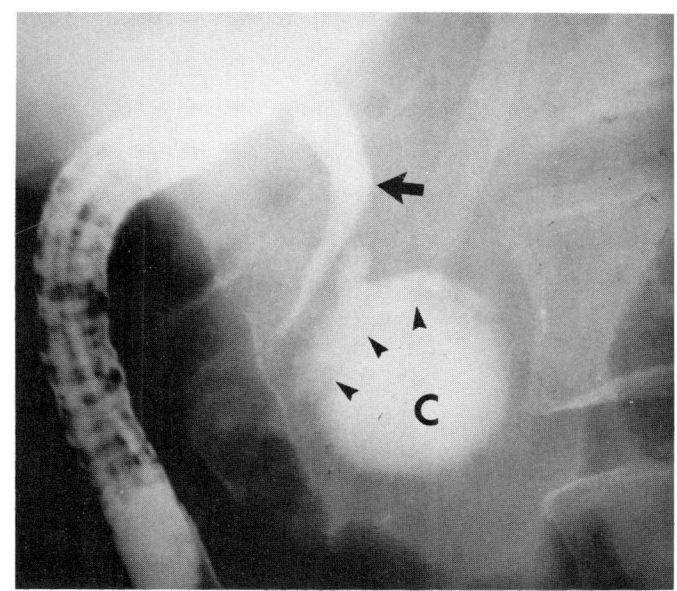

Figure 17–26. Endoscopic retrograde cholangiopancreatogram demonstrating filling of a pancreatic pseudocyst in the head of the pancreas (C). The arrowheads indicate displacement of the pancreatic duct in the head of the pancreas. There is mild fusiform narrowing of the distal common bile duct (arrow) secondary to pancreatic swelling.

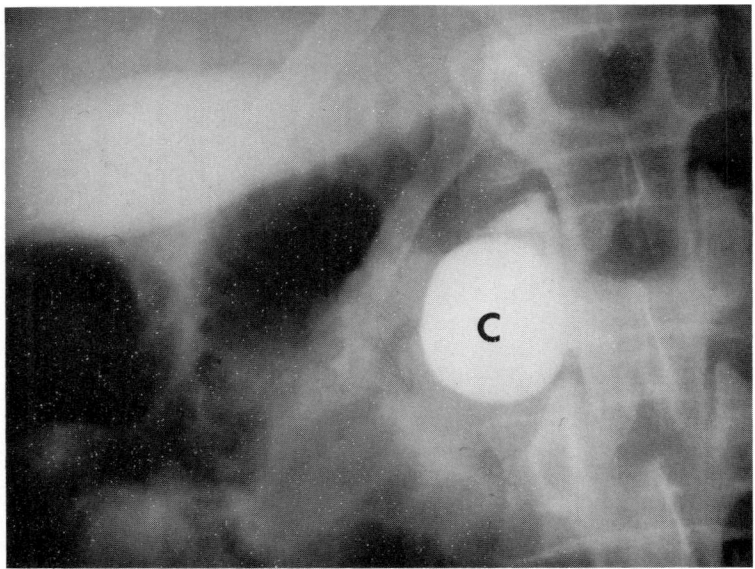

Figure 17–27. A delayed film of the abdomen following the cannulation study shown in Figure 17–26 demonstrates retention of the contrast material in the pancreatic syst (C), indicating failure of the cyst to drain. There is a high risk of infection in this situation.

with trauma, malignancy, or abscess. Its use has diminished considerably because US and particularly CT are increasingly helpful. Angiography nevertheless remains a most important diagnostic procedure in other types of pancreatic disease, particularly in the evaluation of hormonally active pancreatic tumors, such as insulinoma and glucagonoma.

The angiographic changes in pancreatitis vary with the stage of the disease. Basically, two major changes are seen in acute pancreatitis; hypervascularization of the pancreas and uniform displacement of peripancreatic vessels. Chronic pancreatitis, on the other hand, is characterized by localized constriction of major arterial suppliers, focal and conical deformities, or complete avascularization of major portions of the pancreas. Aneurysm formation in the large pancreatic arteries has also been reported.[5] The milder forms of pancreatitis, chronic or acute, may have no demonstrable angiographic abnormalities.

Pseudocysts cause vessel displacement and in some instances pericystic angiographic stain. There are conflicting reports on the accuracy of identifying a pseudocyst angiographically (Fig. 17–28).[17]

ULTRASONOGRAPHY: ACUTE PANCREATITIS AND PSEUDOCYST. Ultrasonography is valuable in the evaluation of acute pancreatitis because of its sensitivity in detecting pseudocysts.[17] Visualization of the pancreas itself in the acute stage is often inadequate because of the frequency of gas-containing bowel loops in the peripancreatic region. Typically, the acutely inflamed pancreas is diffusely enlarged and more sonolucent than normal (Figs. 17–29 and 17–30). Some cases, however, may show no significant ultrasonic abnormality.[31]

Pancreatic pseudocysts characteristically present as round, purely cystic (transonic, devoid of internal echoes) masses (Fig. 17–31). They have well-defined walls and strong through-transmission of sound, denoted by prominent echoes posteriorly; these echoes generally reflect their fluid content. Occasionally, internal debris produces echoes within the cysts. Floating pancreatic tissue or an adjacent organ on which the cyst encroaches, such as the liver or bowel, may also produce intracystic defects. Gas in infected pseudocysts may make them undetectable. Ultrasonography is significantly less accurate

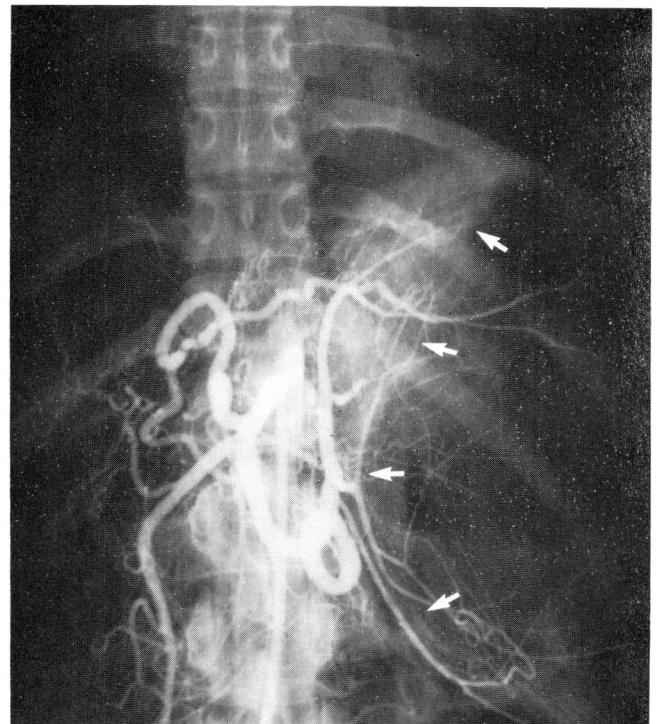

Figure 17–28. Celiac angiogram in a patient with acute pancreatitis and pseudocyst formation which is stretching the adjacent vessels (arrows). There was only minimal capillary stain in the pancreatic bed and the wall of the pseudocyst.

in discerning lesions smaller than 5 cm,[17] although pseudocysts as small as 2 cm often have been detected presurgically. Pseudocysts located in the left upper quadrant are particularly hard to detect because of the overlying gas in the stomach. Pseudocysts in ectopic locations, such as the pelvis, are also easily overlooked in the routine abdominal ultrasound study. Clinical or radiologic suspicion of such a location must be presented when the ultrasound study is ordered.

COMPUTED TOMOGRAPHY: ACUTE PANCREATITIS AND PSEUDOCYST. Changes

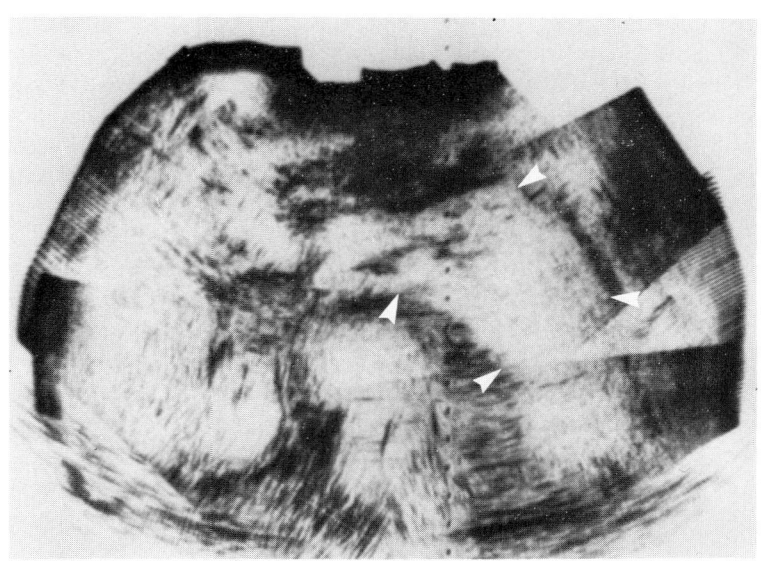

Figure 17–29. Ultrasonogram in acute pancreatitis. Portions of the body and tail are shown (arrowheads). There is a generalized increase in the size and sonolucency of the pancreas. The head and parts of the body are not shown because they lie in a different plane and also, as is often the case in acute pancreatitis, they were surrounded by gas in the bowel. Similar changes may be seen in pancreatic hemorrhage or abscess.

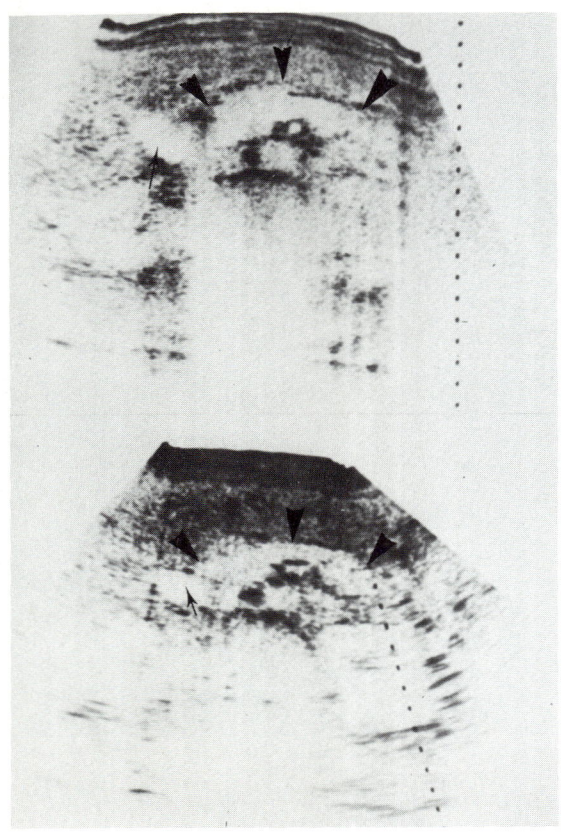

Figure 17–30. Acute pancreatitis. Transverse ultrasound scan of the level of the pancreas. The upper figure is done at normal sound output, the lower one at higher output. Notice the persistent transonic echo response of the pancreas (arrowheads) in contrast to the liver (immediately above). The gallbladder (arrow) is seen to the right of the head of the pancreas.

detected ultrasonographically in acute pancreatitis and pseudocyst formation are corroborated and enhanced by CT studies (Figs. 17–32 and 17–33). Mild cases of pancreatitis may show a variable degree of generalized pancreatomegaly. The pancreas itself shows minimal, patchy decrease of x-ray attenuation, but in some instances it may have a normal density. At times a peripancreatic halo of radiolucency is detected. More severe pancreatitis presents a variegated pattern of internally distributed radiolucent lakes. These differ in both size and degree of attentuation. Intrapancreatic gas formation and segmental or generalized dilatation of the pancreatic duct may be present.

In fulminant hemorrhagic pancreatitis, all these changes may occur within a very large pancreas. These phlegmons may expand and produce effusions that spread along nonconventional fascial planes, such as the pararenal and perirenal spaces.[18] The overall pattern of x-ray attentuation in these instances is also more variegated in degree and distribution.[18, 31]

Pseudocysts are readily detected by CT regardless of their location. The thickness of their walls and fascial plane localization is also more accurately demonstrated by CT. Infected pseudocysts can be accurately diagnosed, since gas and inhomogeneous fluid densities are clearly shown.

PULMONARY COMPLICATIONS OF ACUTE PANCREATITIS. Supradiaphragmatic manifestations of acute pancreatitis are usually the consequence of direct spread of

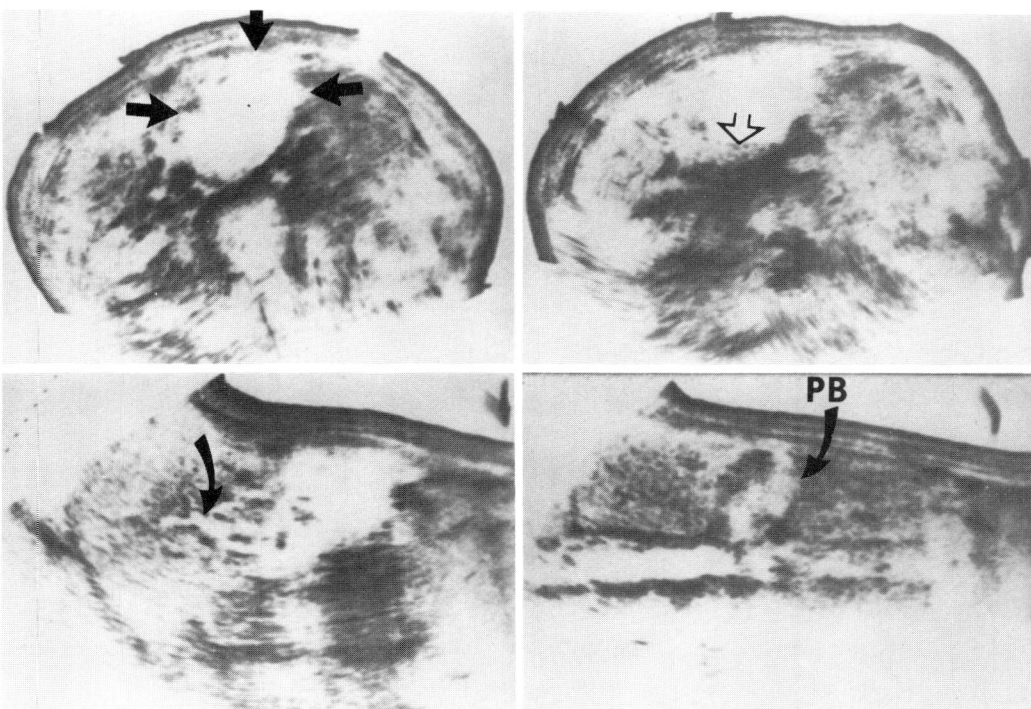

Figure 17–31. Ultrasonogram of pancreatic pseudocyst. A pseudocyst approximately 6 cm in diameter is seen transversely in the area of the head of the pancreas (upper left frame, solid arrows). Notice the purely transonic (cystic) characteristics of the mass. The right upper frame shows debris-like sediment at the bottom of the same pseudocyst (open arrow), a not unusual finding. The lower frames show the pseudocyst longitudinally (left lower frame) and the enlarged pancreatic body (PB) (left right frame). The arrow in the lower left frame points to the dilated tertiary and secondary biliary radicles. The pseudocyst is compressing the common duct, which is not shown.

Figure 17–32. CT scan in acute pancreatitis. This CT scan was taken in the same patient studied in Figure 17–29. The pancreatic head, body, and tail (arrowheads) are nearly three times normal size and their CT density is diminished. The entire extent of the pancreatic head is not seen because it lies slightly more caudal than the tomographic section. The open arrow points to the superior mesenteric artery.

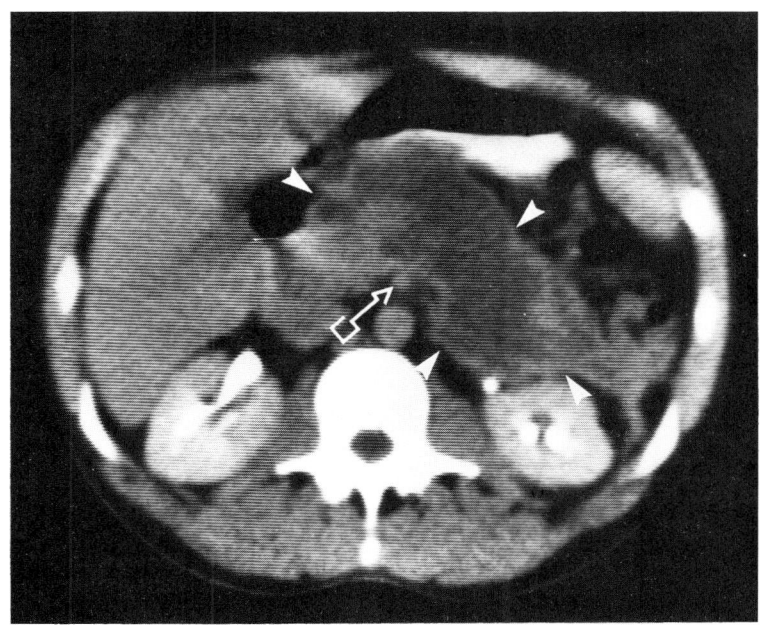

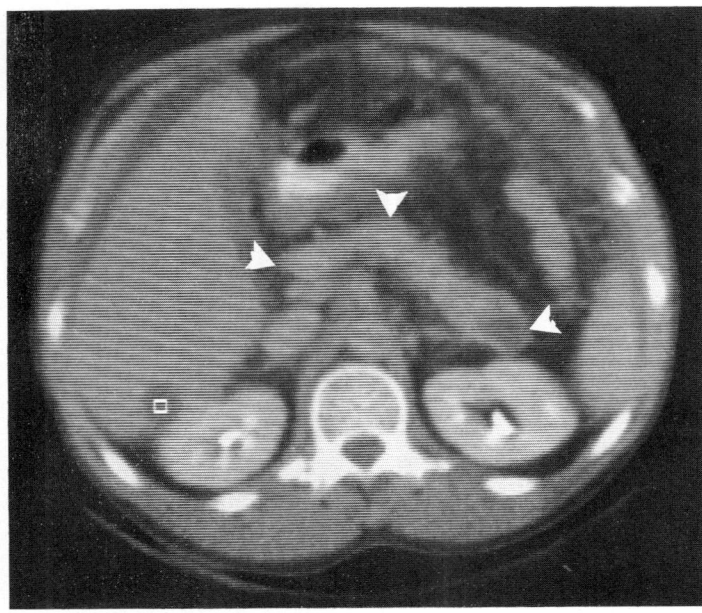

Figure 17–33. Transverse CT scan of the pancreas (arrowheads) in acute pancreatitis. There is an inhomogeneous decrease in density throughout the organ, most noticeably in the enlarged tail. The area-of-interest square marker points to an incidental intrahepatic cyst.

pancreatic enzymes into the pleural space and, rarely, into the mediastinum. The most common resulting complication is pleural effusion. Mediastinal pseudocyst formation can occur but is extremely rare.

Pleural effusions usually develop in the left hemithorax and are nonspecific radiographically. Analysis of their fluid usually shows a high amylase level as well as polymorphonuclear leukocytes or hemorrhage. Effusions may be associated with pancreatic ascites or mediastinal pseudocyst formation (Fig. 17–34). The latter presents as a nonspecific mediastinal mass and is best evaluated by a CT scan.

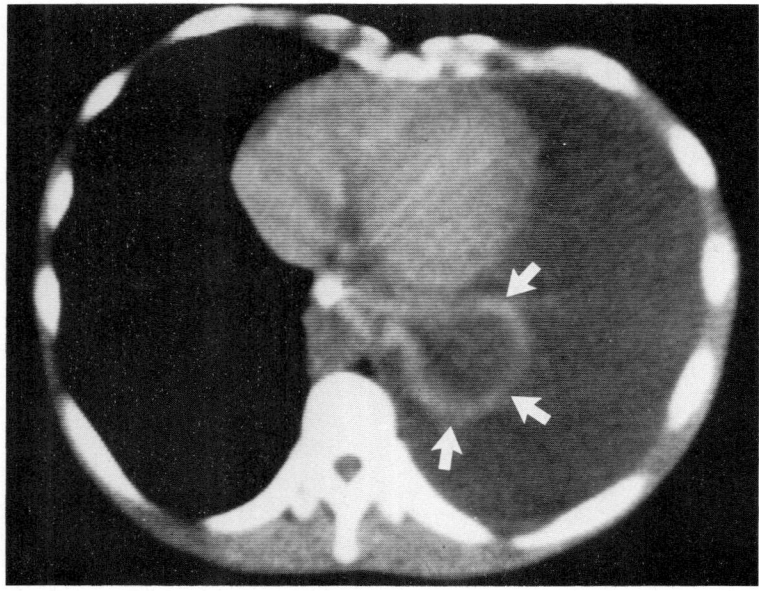

Figure 17–34. Computerized axial tomograph of a mediastinal pseudocyst associated with left pleural effusion. Pseudocysts of the pancreas may develop in the mediastinum. Arrows indicate the pseudocyst, behind the heart. There is fluid density in the left thorax and normal air density in the right. Pleural effusions in acute pancreatitis usually occur on the left.

Pancreatic Abscess

The findings of pancreatic abscess on the plain film and contrast studies have already been detailed in the discussion of acute pancreatitis (Figs. 17–35 and 17–36). The most common setting for pancreatic abscess is postoperative pancreatitis.[29, 30, 32, 40] Pancreatic abscess can occur spontaneously in acute pancreatitis but seldom before the third week after onset and usually in hemorrhagic or severe pancreatitis; it is very rare in chronic pancreatitis.[19] The mortality rate of the complications of pancreatic abscess can be nearly 100 per cent.[40]

RADIONUCLIDE STUDIES. The utility of gallium 67–labeled citrate for localization of abscesses is well established (Fig. 17–37).[3, 8, 19] However, this type of scan is not practical as an initial imaging procedure in cases with acute localizing signs and symptoms. CT or US usually provides a diagnosis more rapidly. On the other hand, a ^{67}gallium scan can be positive when other imaging modalities, such as CT and US, fail to specifically identify an abscess. Therefore, it may be used as first imaging study when there are no localizing signs and symptoms or when CT and US are inconclusive.

ULTRASONOGRAPHY. Ultrasonographic findings in pancreatic abscess are not specific. There may be evidence of a cystic mass with or without debris, which often cannot be differentiated from fluid witin the bowel, pseudocyst, or hemorrhage. Furthermore, an abscess containing gas may alter sound transmission and appear as a nonspecific echo-forming focus or be completely obscured by echoes from overlying

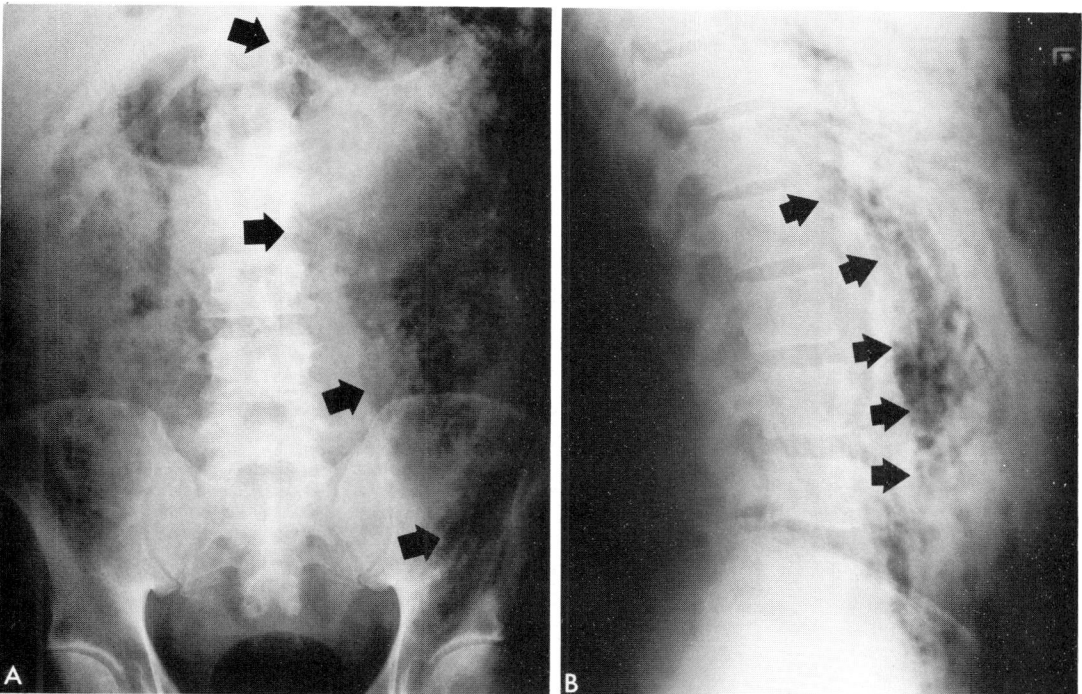

Figure 17–35. *A*, Pancreatic abscess with extensive gas formation (arrows). The significance of this moth-eaten or flocculent pattern of gas distribution can be difficult to assess on a single view. *B*, Lateral radiograph of the same patient. The patient is supine, and the gas collections (arrows) follow the curve of the psoas muscles, giving a more characteristic radiographic pattern.

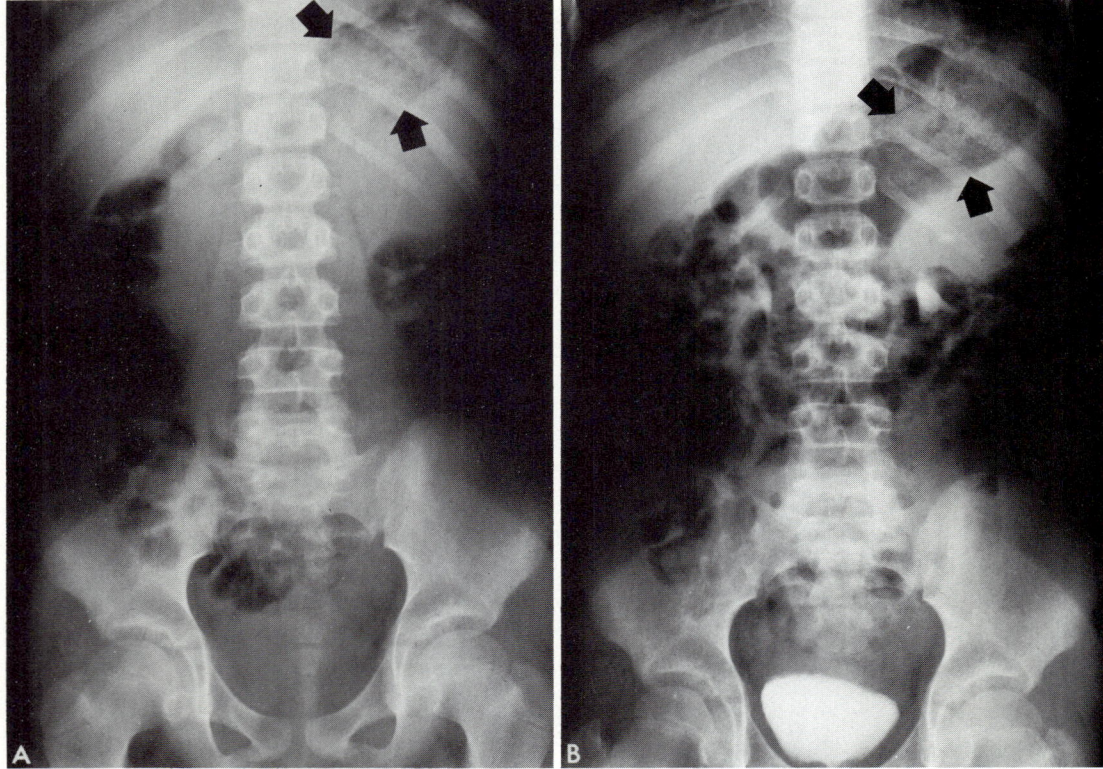

Figure 17–36. *A,* Pancreatic abscess (arrows) simulating gas within the stomach in a scout abdominal radiograph taken before an excretory urogram. *B,* The unchanging gas pattern in a film done during the urogram suggests an abscess. A static or persistent gas pattern is a useful radiographic sign for detection of intra-abdominal abscess formation.

gas. Despite claims of the high accuracy of ultrasound diagnosis of abdominal abscesses,[39] our experience indicates that it is most helpful in the corroboration of other clinical and imaging evidence.

COMPUTERIZED TOMOGRAPHY. Pancreatic abscesses may localize anywhere in the abdomen. Predicted extension through the pancreatic retroperitoneal routes does not necessarily occur. Psoas, intrarenal and paracolic, retroperitoneal, and intra- and

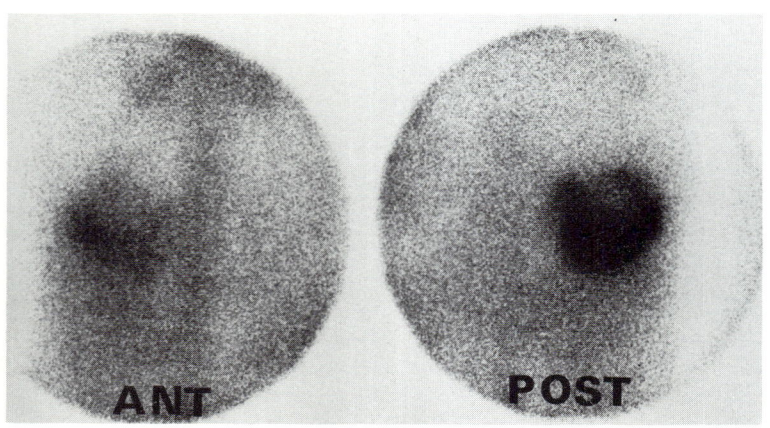

Figure 17–37. Infected pseudocyst. A gallium-67 scintiscan 48 hours after injection shows an infected pseudocyst near the head of the pancreas. The high concentration of activity in the pseudocyst is more easily appreciated in the posterior view. Pseudocysts do not normally concentrate gallium. (Courtesy of Oliver A. Sorsdahl, M.D., Atlanta, Georgia.)

parapancreatic localizations may develop. Gas and fluid within a mass are the most diagnostic CT findings.[26] With its ability to penetrate bone and gas, CT can uncover abscesses (Fig. 17–38) that are not seen on US, and it may be the more reliable method for investigation of these lesions.

Chronic Pancreatitis

PLAIN FILMS. One of the most characteristic findings of chronic pancreatitis on plain film examination is the presence of pancreatic calculi (Fig. 17–39). This finding is indicative of chronic relapsing pancreatitis that has been present for a number of years. The presence of pancreatic calculi strongly suggests that the pancreatitis is alcoholic in origin. Infrequently, pancreatitis may be idiopathic or have a nonalcoholic etiology.

Radiographically detectable pancreatic calcifications rarely occur in other conditions. Pancreatic carcinomas, pseudocysts, and the rare pancreatic cystadenomas occasionally produce visible calcium deposits but these are usually focal and not "calculous" in appearance. Bony abnormalities may be found in patients with chronic pancreatitis. These include bony infarcts and aseptic necrosis of the femoral head (Figs. 17–40 and 17–41).

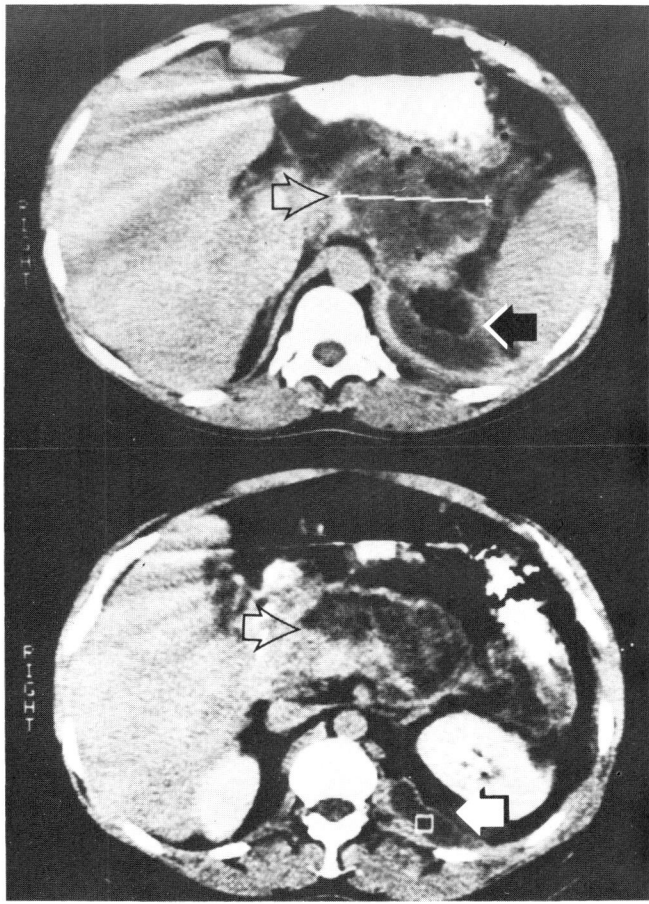

Figure 17–38. Computerized tomogram of pancreatic abscess. There is contrast in the stomach and bowel. The upper arrows point to the pancreatic bed, the lower ones to its extension into the psoas muscle. Notice the wide range of attentuation densities. The presence of air within the abscess is confirmed by the CT density number.

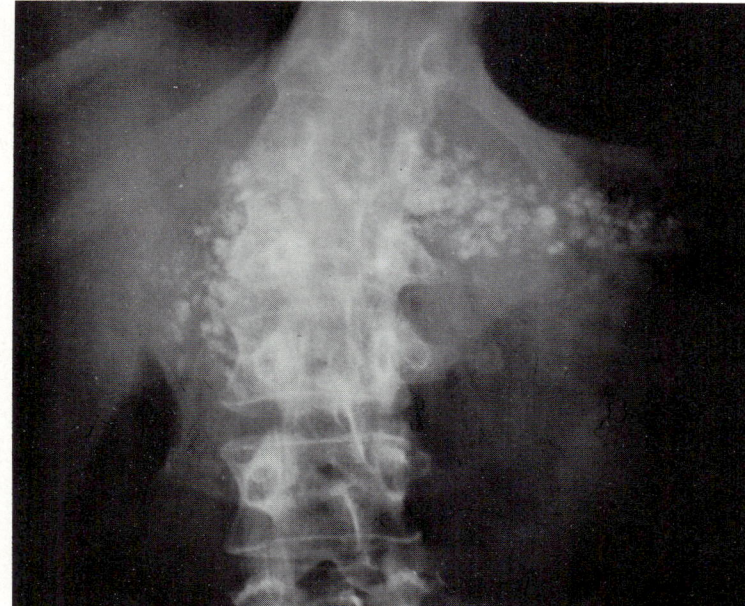

Figure 17-39. Plain film of the abdomen in a patient with chronic relapsing alcoholic pancreatitis demonstrates the characteristic pattern of pancreatic calculi in the head, body, and tail of the pancreas.

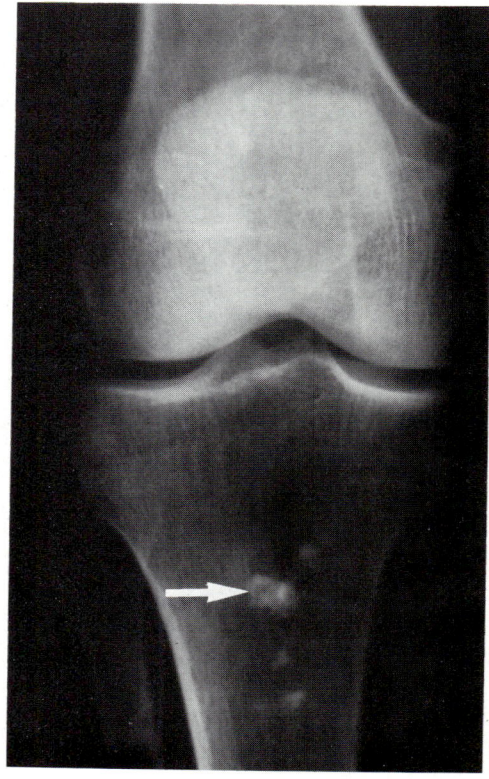

Figure 17-40. Calcified bony infarct (arrow) associated with chronic pancreatitis.

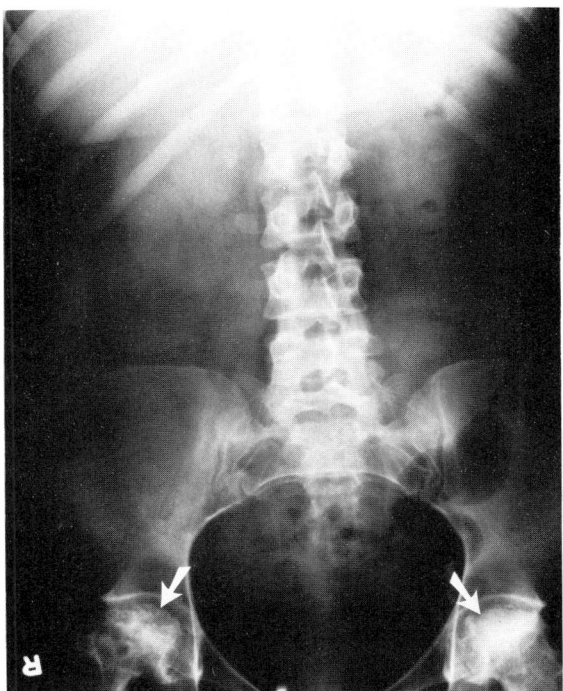

Figure 17–41. Chronic pancreatitis; aseptic necrosis. The aseptic necrosis is associated with osteosclerosis of the femoral head (arrows). These changes are not specific, since they can be found in other diseases in which the vascular supply to the epiphyses is compromised.

BARIUM CONTRAST STUDIES OF THE UPPER GASTROINTESTINAL TRACT. In chronic pancreatitis there may be thickening and spiculization of the mucosal pattern of the inner aspect of the descending duodenum, often associated with a mass pressure effect upon this loop (Fig. 17–42). Occasionally, the enlarged pancreas may also produce a pressure defect on the inferior aspect of the distal stomach ("pad sign"). In the

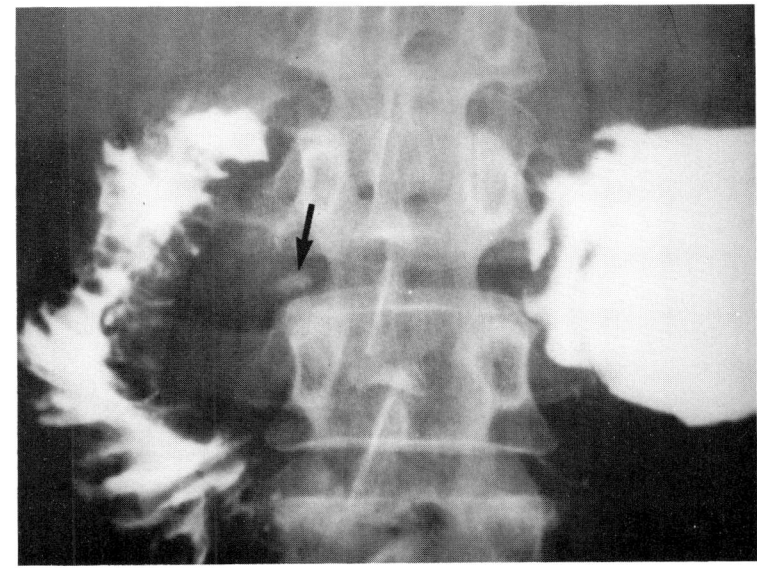

Figure 17–42. Barium-contrast study of the upper gastrointestinal tract in a patient with chronic relapsing pancreatitis. The descending duodenum shows a mass effect on its medial margin, with a coarse thickening of the mucosal pattern. The arrow indicates a pancreatic calculus in the region of the pancreatic duct.

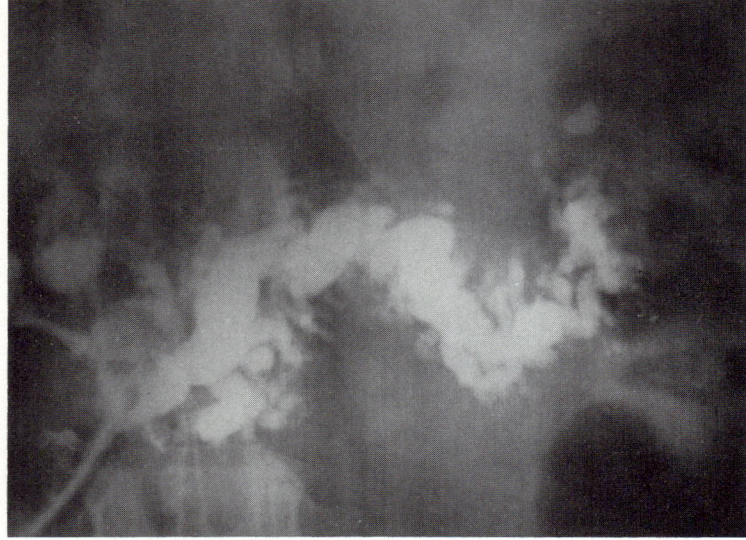

Figure 17–43. A pancreatogram in a patient with chronic pancreatitis demonstrates numerous areas of short strictures and dilatation, the "chain-of-lakes" pattern characteristic of chronic pancreatitis. This is in contrast to Figure 17–44, which demonstrates the appearance of a normal pancreatic duct.

absence of pancreatic calcifications, these changes are virtually indistinguishable from those of pancreatic head carcinoma. A severe acute pancreatitis can produce somewhat similar findings but in a distinctly different clinical setting.

ENDOSCOPIC RETROGRADE CHOLANGIOPANCREATOGRAPHY (ERCP). This procedure is recommended in all patients being considered for surgery or when the cause of recurrent pancreatitis is being sought. Abnormalities of the pancreatic duct are evident in the vast majority of patients with chronic pancreatitis on retrograde cannulation studies.[36] The most characteristic findings are dilatation and tortuosity of the main pancreatic duct and dilatation and distortion of its lateral branches (Figs. 17–43 and 17–44).[12, 36] Other abnormalities include strictures that alternate with dilated areas of the duct ("chain of lakes"). Areas of inflammatory stricture are usually less than 1 cm in length, and longer segments of narrowing suggest the possibility of malignant

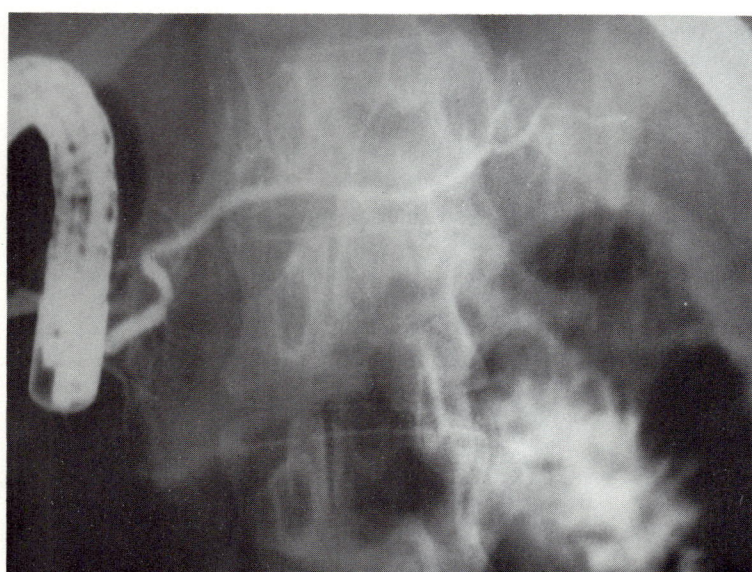

Figure 17–44. Normal pancreatic duct on ERCP (endoscopic retrograde pancreatogram). The entire duct is filled showing smooth margins and gradual tapering. Normal secondary ducts are outlined.

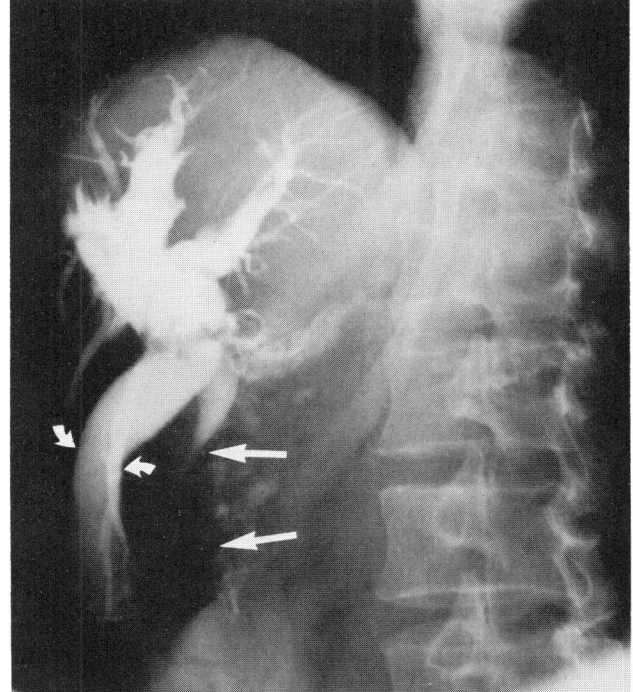

Figure 17-45. Percutaneous cholangiogram in a case of chronic pancreatitis shows dilatation of the tertiary biliary radicles, ductus hepaticus, and proximal common duct. Note the smooth compression on the distal common duct (straight arrows). The gallbladder (curved arrows) is seen to the right of the common duct.

change. Narrowing of the distal portion of the common bile duct secondary to pancreatic scarring is at times associated with chronic pancreatitis. Occasionally, nonopaque calculi are seen within the duct.

In cases in which jaundice is present, a transhepatic cholangiogram will show the site of common bile duct narrowing (Figs. 17-45 and 17-46). Distinction from pancreatic carcinoma is usually not possible on the basis of the cholangiogram alone.

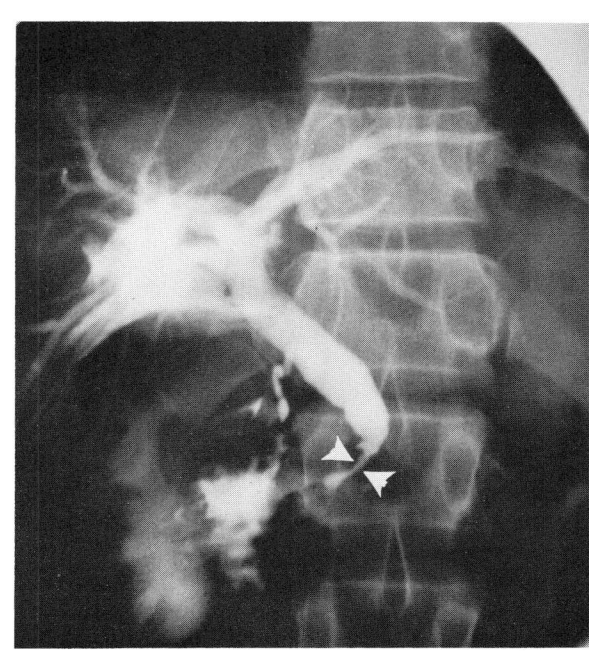

Figure 17-46. Percutaneous cholangiography in a case of chronic pancreatitis. The lower end of the common duct is narrowed (arrowheads), and the proximal duct is moderately dilated. The appearance is indistinguishable from that of carcinoma of the pancreas.

1034 — THE PANCREAS

ULTRASONOGRAPHY. Chronic pancreatitis can be arbitrarily classified by size into three sonographic types: atrophic, normal, and hypertrophic. All three types may be associated with pancreatic calcifications, which present as high-amplitude echogenic foci, with or without sonic shadowing (Fig. 17–47).

Atrophic pancreatitis shows a small, highly echogenic pancreas. The pancreas may not be distinguishable from peripancreatic connective tissue and fat.[31] Unless calcifications are seen, the diagnosis of chronic atrophic pancreatitis may be very difficult to establish ultrasonographically.

If the pancreas is of normal size and shape, only diffuse or focally increased echogenicity from its increased fibrous tissue and fat may be seen. If calcifications or dilatation of the pancreatic duct are apparent sonographically, the diagnosis of chronic pancreatitis becomes more definite.[31]

Hypertrophic chronic pancreatitis presents as diffuse or focal single or multiple intrapancreatic masses.[11, 23, 31, 32] The echo formation of these masses is usually lower than that of the normal pancreas. Scattered calcifications, fat, and mucin increase the amplitude of echo response. The gland may have a "salt-and-pepper" gray-scale appear-

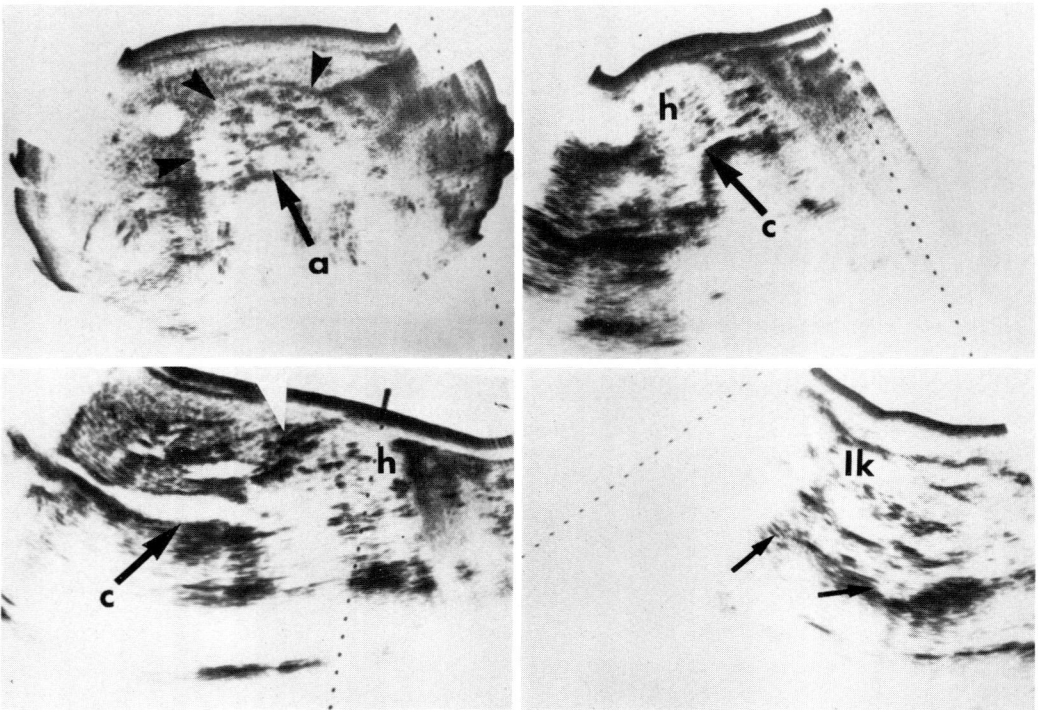

Figure 17–47. Ultrasonogram of chronic pancreatitis. The left upper frame (transverse view) shows a diffusely enlarged pancreas (arrowheads) with internal high- and low-amplitude echoes. This range of echo formation is strongly suggestive of chronic pancreatitis when associated with generalized pancreatomegaly. The circular cystic structure next to the head of the pancreas is the gallbladder (a = aorta). The right upper frame (transverse view) shows the enlarged head of the pancreas (h) at a more caudal level, compressing the vena cava (c). The gallbladder is seen once again adjacent to the pancreatic parenchyma. The left lower frame (sagittal view) shows the area of the pancreatic head (h) overlying the vena cava. The white arrowhead indicates an area of strong echoes and a sonic shadow (clear area immediately beneath); these findings are indicative of calcifications or gas. Abdominal x-ray examination confirmed the presence of calculi. The right lower frame (prone sagittal view) shows the enlarged tail of the pancreas (arrows) anterior to the left kidney (lk). This prone view is often used to see the tail of the pancreas, which cannot be demonstrated in the supine position because of the superimposed gas bubble in the stomach.

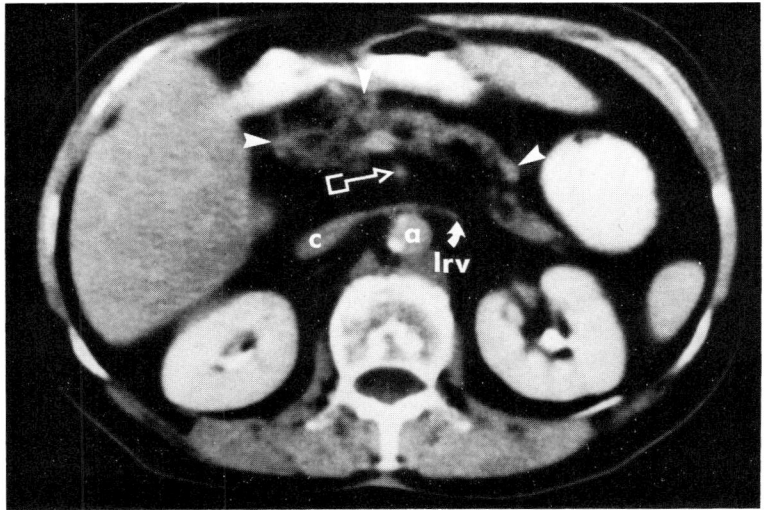

Figure 17–48. CT scan of chronic atrophic pancreatitis. The pancreas (arrowheads) appears shriveled and thin. The low-density areas are fatty deposits and probably lakes of mucin concentration; the overall appearance is moth-eaten. In the absence of calcifications, this appearance could well be that of a normal fatty infiltrated pancreas in an older individual (see Fig. 17–3). The open arrow points to the superior mesenteric artery. a = aorta; c = vena cava; lrv = left renal vein.

ance much different from that of other pancreatic lesions. Because pancreatic carcinomas are also associated with low-amplitude echogenic masses, the focal enlargement of pancreatitis may be virtually undistinguishable from that of cancer. Dilatation of the pancreatic duct, focal or generalized, is common in hypertrophic chronic pancreatitis. Chronic inflammatory masses may enlarge, become smaller, or remain unchanged during the course of the illness.

COMPUTED TOMOGRAPHY (Fig. 17–48). CT accurately demonstrates focal defects as well as generalized parenchymal involvement in chronic pancreatitis. The quality of the examination is better in individuals with more abundant intra-abdominal fat. Thin persons may be best studied by ultrasound. Dilatation of the duct and pancreatic calcifications, the latter often not easily demonstrable by standard x-rays or US, are readily seen on CT scans. However, like US, CT is unable to distinguish an atrophic or normal gland with a high mucin or fat content from the atrophic or fibrofatty variety of chronic pancreatitis. Distinction between some malignant and focal inflammatory pancreatic masses is also very difficult by CT. As in the case of US, x-ray attenuation density for both malignancy and pancreatitis may be the same. CT, however, resolves focal changes more sharply, particularly with the adjuvant use of contrast medium. The tail of the pancreas, specifically, is better seen and enhanced on CT. Finally, both CT and US can be used advantageously for topographic localization of pancreatic masses in percutaneous aspiration for diagnosis.[14, 16]

Newer current scanners, with short (a few seconds) scanning time an higher resolution have considerably improved pancreatic detail and diagnosis.

ANGIOGRAPHY. In suspected chronic pancreatitis, angiography is employed only when distinction from carcinoma is equivocal on ultrasound and CT studies. However, even angiographic distinction is sometimes difficult or impossible.

The most common angiographic findings in chronic or recurrent pancreatitis are focal or diffuse pancreatic blush and irregularity and beading of the smaller arteries (Figs. 17–49 and 17–50). The splenic vein may be occluded in cases with severe body or tail involvement. In about 10 per cent, one or more aneurysms of the peripancreatic arteries is uncovered (Fig. 17–51), a finding not seen in pancreatic carcinoma. In many cases, however, angiography fails to make an unequivocal distinction from carcinoma (Fig. 17–52).

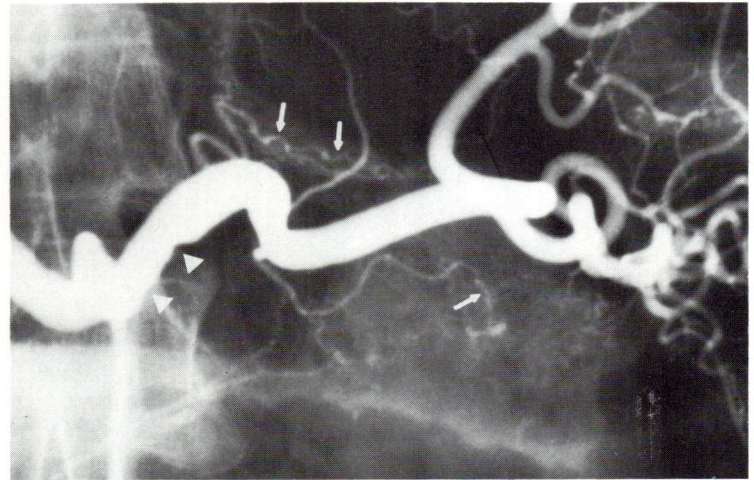

Figure 17–49. Celiac angiogram in chronic pancreatitis showing irregularities in the branches of the arteria magna (arrows) and encasement of the proximal portion of the splenic artery (arrowheads). These changes are frequent in chronic pancreatitis but are nonspecific. (Modified from Reuter, S. R., and Redman, H. C.: *Gastrointestinal Angiography.* Ed. 2. Philadelphia, W. B. Saunders Company, 1977.)

Trauma

Penetrating injuries to the pancreas usually require prompt abdominal exploration to control hemorrhage and to repair damage inflicted by the wound to adjacent organs. Blunt trauma, on the other hand, may not require immediate exploration unless there is evidence of internal bleeding. In many instances of blunt trauma, focal or generalized acute pancreatitis may develop, and pseudocyst formation is common. In addition, a localized hematoma and abscess may form and may dissect along the anterior pararenal space in the same route of spread as pseudocysts.

The radiographic evaluation of these patients should consist of plain abdominal films, upper gastrointestinal tract studies, US, and CT, as indicated.

PLAIN FILMS OF THE ABDOMEN. The plain abdominal film in abdominal trauma may reveal a mass effect, metallic or other type of foreign body, evidence of retroperitoneal or intraperitoneal blood, or gas extravasation. These radiographic changes are discussed elsewhere (see Chapter 5).

BARIUM-CONTRAST STUDIES OF THE UPPER GASTROINTESTINAL TRACT. When clinical circumstances permit, an upper gastrointestinal tract series is helpful in detecting mass effect (Fig. 17–53), fistulas, and possible obstruction. In addition, this study can demonstrate the intraluminal duodenal spread of a hematoma (Fig. 17–54).[21]

ULTRASONOGRAPHY. The ultrasound findings in focal or generalized traumatic pancreatitis are those of increased transonic response that is essentially indistinguishable from acute pancreatic changes of other origin. The same can be said of traumatic pseudocysts. On the other hand, hematomas, duodenal intramural hematomas in particular, can be confused with solid pancreatic masses in their subacute stages. This is caused by the proximity of the duodenum to the pancreatic head and by the echogenicity of subacute hematomas. Acutely, hematomas are quite transonic but as the clots organize they become echogenic (see Fig. 17–54). Within seven to ten days these hematomas break up and become transonic (cystic) once again. Therefore, the acute and chronic hematomas may be indistinguishable from pseudocysts or an abscess. As indicated, the upper gastrointestinal study can be very helpful in differentiating the intramural duodenal hematoma from these two types of pancreatic masses (see Fig. 17–54). The characteristic coiled-spring appearance and the extraluminal intramural mass effect are diagnostic. Nevertheless, US is the optimal method for following hematomas for serial estimate of size, healing, and disappearance.

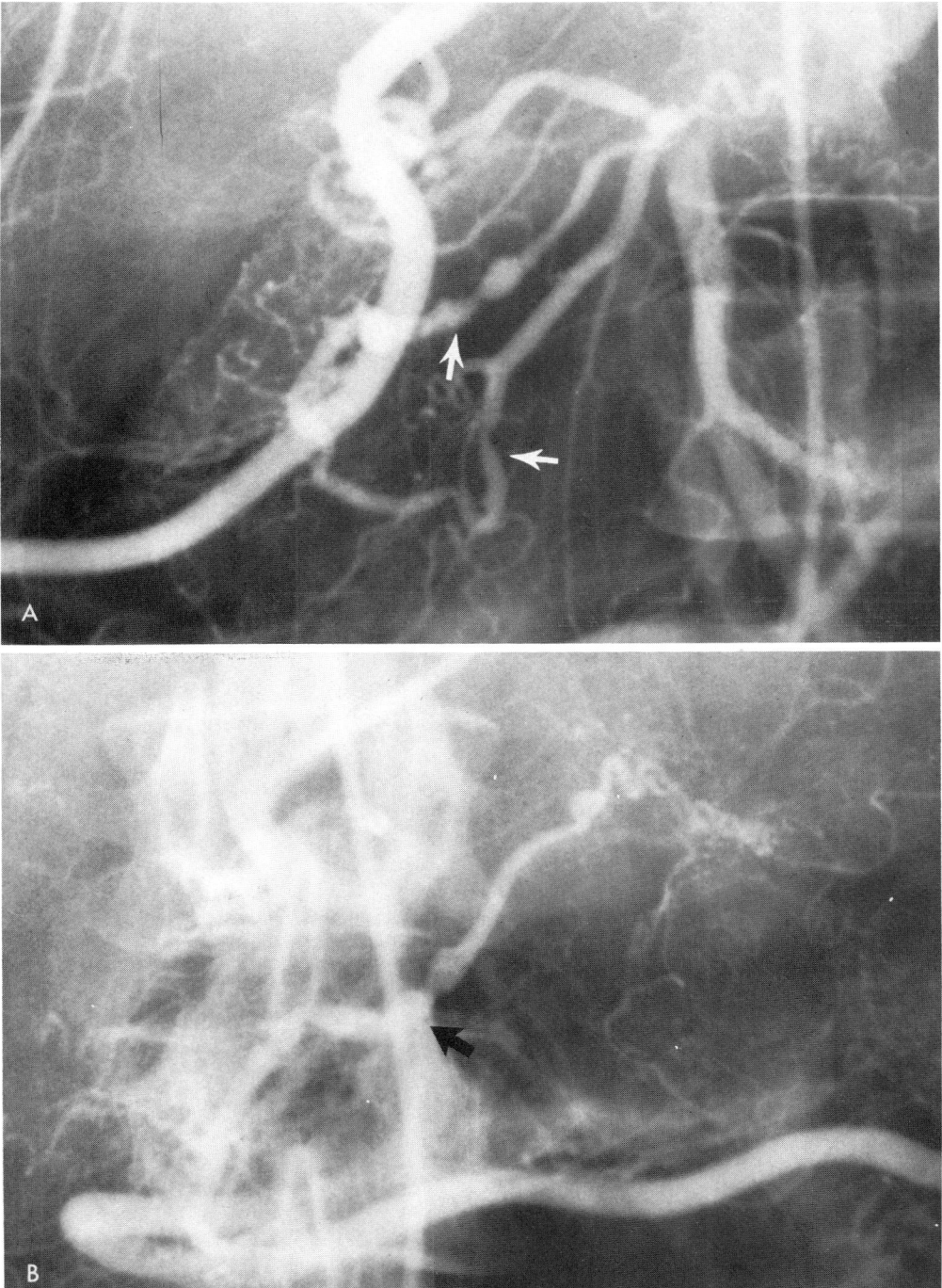

Figure 17–50. *A*, Early arterial phase. Typical beaded arterial changes of pancreatitis (arrows) involving the pancreaticoduodenal arcades, which are markedly dilated. *B*, Late arterial phase, showing beading and aneurysmal dilatation of the transverse pancreatic artery (arrow). (Modified from Reuter, S.R., and Redman, H.C.: Gastrointestinal Angiography. Ed. 2. Philadelphia, W. B. Saunders Company, 1977.)

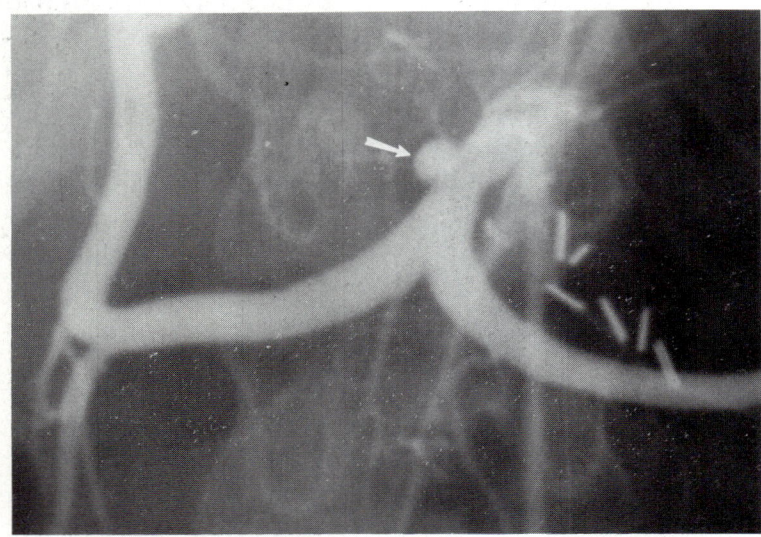

Figure 17–51. Proximal celiac artery aneurysm (arrow) in celiac angiogram in a case of chronic pancreatitis. (Modified from Reuter, S. R., and Redman, H. C.: Gastrointestinal Angiography. Ed. 2. Philadelphia, W. B. Saunders Company, 1977.)

Figure 17–52. Chronic pancreatitis simulating neoplastic encasement. An anastomotic branch from the anterior pancreaticoduodenal arcade is abruptly angulated at its midportion (arrow) and narrowed. These changes may also be seen in early carcinoma of the pancreas. (Modified from Reuter, S. R., and Redman, H. C.: Gastrointestinal Angiography. Ed. 2. Philadelphia, W. B. Saunders Company, 1977.)

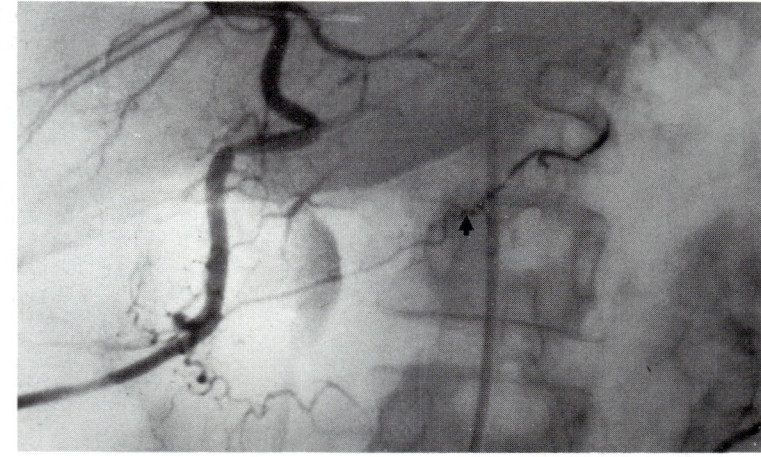

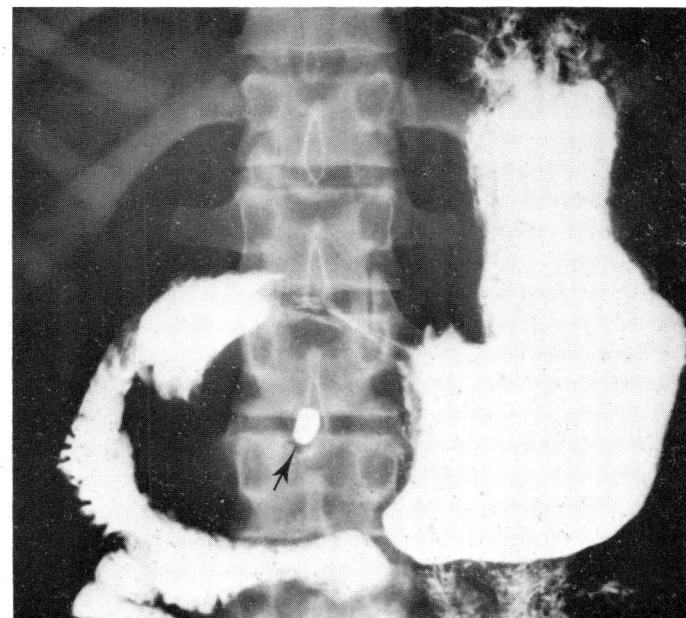

Figure 17–53. Traumatic pseudocyst. This patient was shot in the midabdomen, and the bullet (arrow) passed through the head of the pancreas. The patient developed focal pancreatitis and a pseudocyst. The pseudocyst is clearly outlined by barium-contrast in the stomach and duodenal loop.

COMPUTERIZED TOMOGRAPHY. In cases of trauma the CT findings corroborate and expand ultrasound findings. The retroperitoneal extravasation of minor amounts of blood or pancreatic effusions, however, is better detected by CT. Therefore, the latter technique is more useful when minimal or slow bleeding is suspected. In addition, damage to other organs, such as chronic subcapsular splenic, hepatic, or muscular hematomas, may become clearly evident on CT. At present, CT service is not immediately available, particularly in busy emergency services. As the number of CT scanners increases, it is not unreasonable to anticipate that their emergency use will help to sort out surgical and nonsurgical cases following abdominal trauma.

Pancreatic Carcinoma

Despite the contributions of modern imaging to the visualization of the pancreas, when the diagnosis of pancreatic carcinoma is made there is already advanced disease. Detection of resectable cancer of the pancreas is quite infrequent. Conversely, demonstration of normal pancreas by US and CT criteria shows a high index of reliability.[10, 38] A useful algorithm for the imaging work-up of pancreatic carcinoma has been presented by Weingarten et al.[43]

PLAIN FILMS OF THE ABDOMEN, UPPER GASTROINTESTINAL STUDIES, AND BARIUM ENEMA. Plain films of the abdomen and barium-contrast studies of the upper and lower gastrointestinal tract play a minor role in the diagnosis of pancreatic cancer. The more sophisticated imaging modalities, such as angiography, ultrasound, computed axial tomography, ERCP, and transhepatic cholangiography, give considerably more specific and complete information. As a general rule, any pancreatic neoplasm identifiable on plain films or barium-contrast studies is far advanced and usually inoperable.

1040 — THE PANCREAS

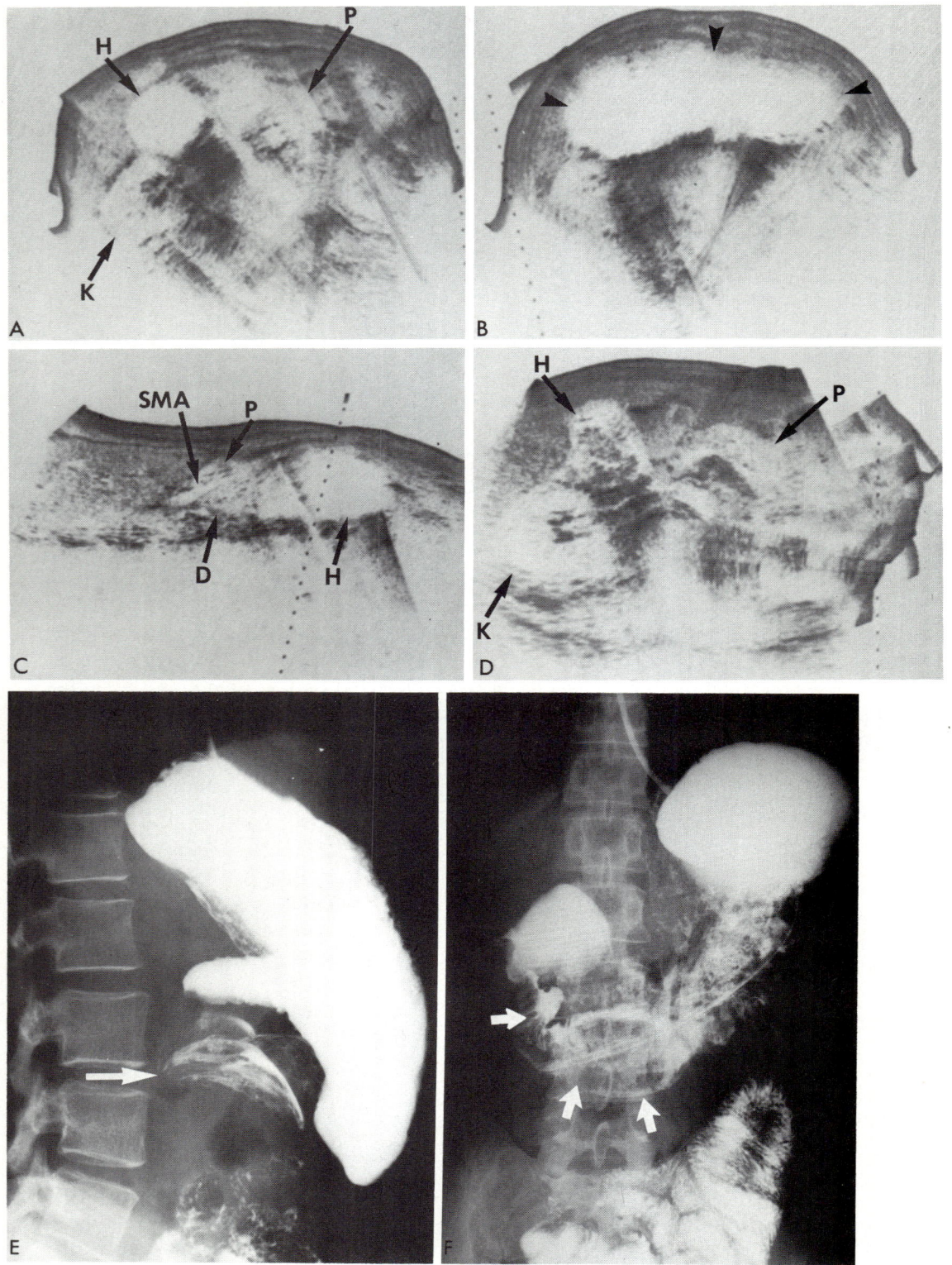

See legend on the opposite page.

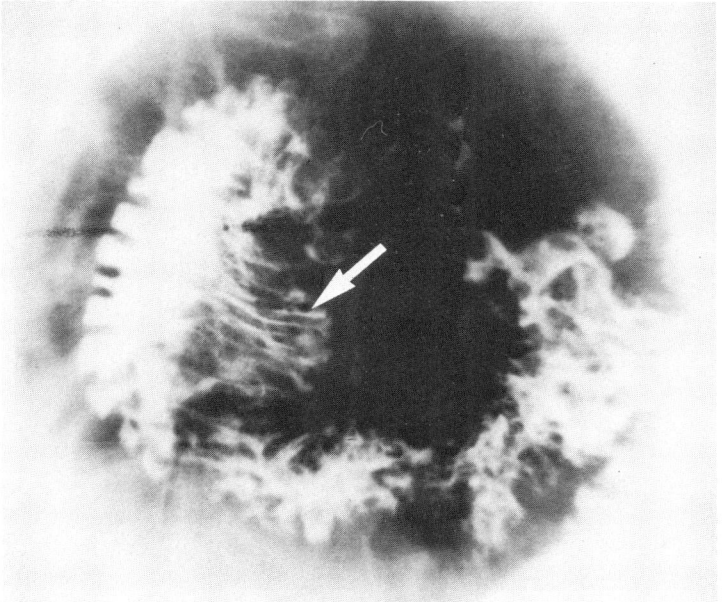

Figure 17–55. Barium-contrast study of the duodenum in patient with pancreatic carcinoma. There is marked spiculization and distortion of the medial portion of the descending duodenum (arrow) secondary to invasion by pancreatic carcinoma.

Plain films of the abdomen may show a nonspecific mass effect. Evidence of upper gastrointestinal obstruction by cancer invasion is shown as gastric dilatation. Encasement of the gastric outlet or the transverse colon may be discernible from study of the gas pattern.

Carcinoma of the head of the pancreas may produce a mass effect by pressure and mucosal distortion (Figs. 17–55 and 17–56) by invasion of the duodenal wall. On barium studies, the "reverse-3 sign," or defect in the region of the papilla, is seen in carcinoma as well as in acute pancreatitis and thus is nonspecific. This sign consists of two or more fixed adjacent invaginations of the mucosa of the duodenum.

Hypotonic duodenography is a useful technique to study the mucosal pattern. By means of air-barium contrast, mucosal detail of the duodenum is obtained after the intravenous administration of glucagon or an anticholinergic drug to relax the duodenal wall. With this technique it is possible to demonstrate minimal or early changes in the mucosa suggestive of infiltration of its wall. This may not be appreciated on the routine duodenal barium-contrast study.

Figure 17–54. Post-traumatic intramural duodenal hematoma resembling pancreatic pseudocyst ultrasonographically. A, The transonic mass (H) is adjacent to the pancreas (P) and lies above the right kidney (K). B, At a lower level, the hematoma (arrowheads) is seen extending across the abdomen. Actually, it is following the course of the duodenum. C, On the longitudinal scan, the hematoma (H) lies below the pancreas (P). SMA= superior mesenteric artery; D = compressed duodenum. On these scans, the transonic mass could not be distinguished from a pseudocyst. D, Over a week later, the transverse scan shows that the hematoma (H) has become echogenic (compare with the same level early scan in A). P = pancrease; K = kidney. E, Gastrointestinal series shows the characteristic coiled-spring appearance (arrow) of an intramural duodenal mass. F, Later film shows the typical appearance of an extraluminal intramural mass (hematoma, arrows). In this post-traumatic case, the upper gastrointestinal tract series was quite definitive, while the ultrasonographic studies were nonspecific and somewhat misleading.

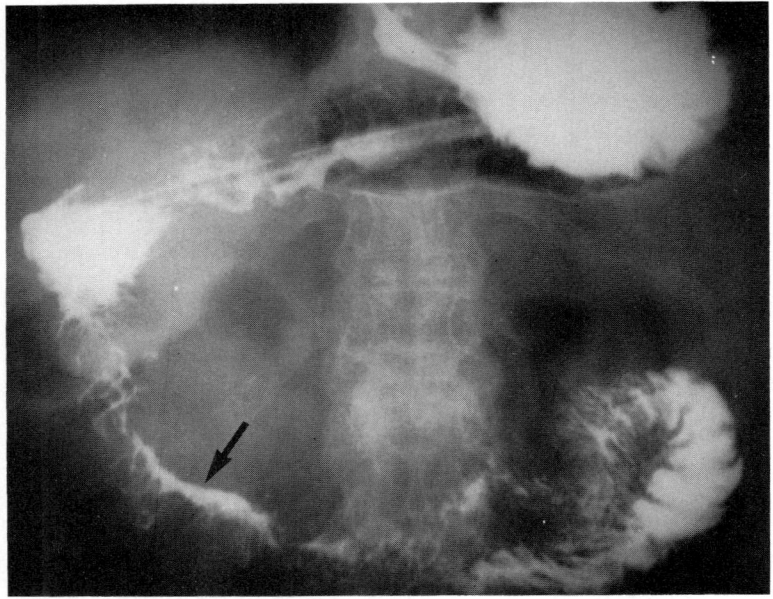

Figure 17–56. Barium-contrast study of the upper gastrointestinal tract in a patient with far advanced pancreatic carcinoma. There is marked enlargement of the duodenal loop secondary to the neoplastic mass. The arrow points to a longitudinal ulceration secondary to neoplastic invasion of the duodenum.

Pancreatic carcinoma rarely produces structural changes in the distal small bowel or colon. Far advanced pancreatic carcinoma, however, can distort the transverse colon and splenic flexure or any portion of the bowel by direct extension, encasement, and invasion.

ENDOSCOPIC RETROGRADE CHOLANGIOPANCREATOGRAPHY (Figs. 17–57 to 17–60). This technique is rapidly becoming an important tool for the detection of pancre-

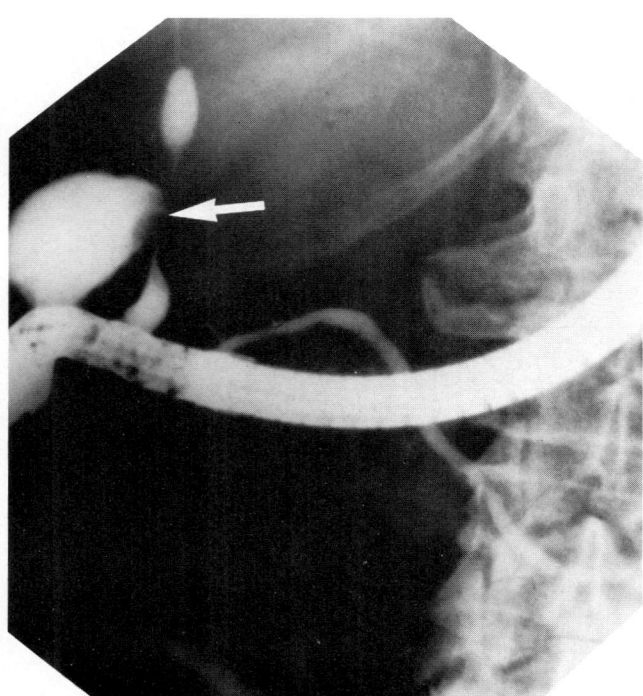

Figure 17–57. ERCP demonstrating involvement by pancreatic carcinoma of the common bile duct and the common hepatic bile duct at the site of origin of the cystic duct (arrow). The pancreatic duct in the region of the head of the pancreas shows only minimal mass effect.

Figure 17–58. ERCP in carcinoma of the pancreas. The large arrow demonstrates the narrowing of the common bile duct near the papilla, with marked proximal dilatation. The small arrow points to the origin of the very compressed pancreatic duct. The open arrow shows filling of a tumor cavitation within the pancreatic neoplasm. A dilated pancreatic segment of normal pancreatic duct can also produce this latter type of contrast collection.

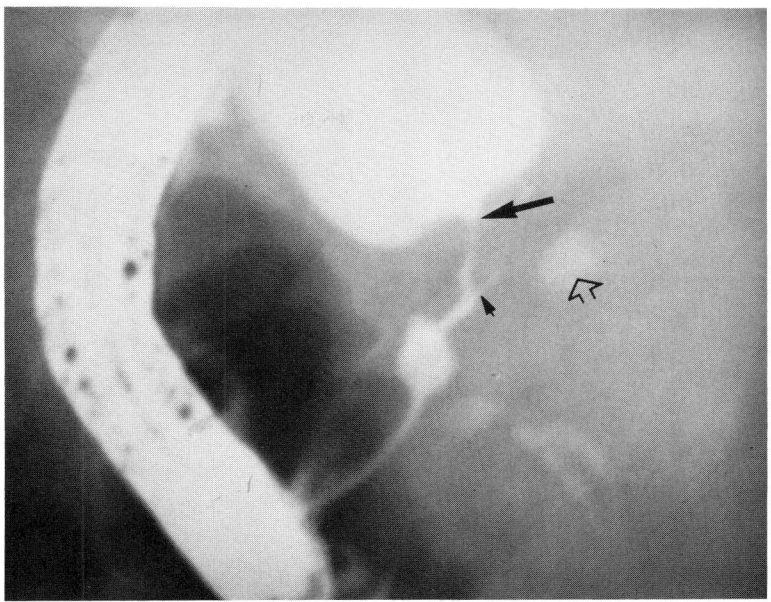

atic carcinoma.[1, 4, 12, 35] It may be of particular help in discerning small lesions.[1] The most characteristic changes are seen in the main pancreatic duct. Abrupt obstruction with a normal-appearing distal lumen suggests cancer. Stenosis that is long and tapering or stenosis with ectasia of the duct proximal to the narrowing is also characteristic.[1, 4] Extravasation of contrast material into dilated ducts or into the tumor itself is suggestive of carcinoma.[4] Finally, combined obstruction or stenosis of the main pancreatic duct and

Figure 17–59. ERCP of carcinoma of the pancreas. Double duct sign. There is obstruction of both the common bile duct and the pancreatic duct near the papilla of Vater (large arrow). The dilated pancreatic duct is displaced inferiorly by the mass (small arrows). This is the "double duct sign" considered quite characteristic of carcinoma of the pancreas.

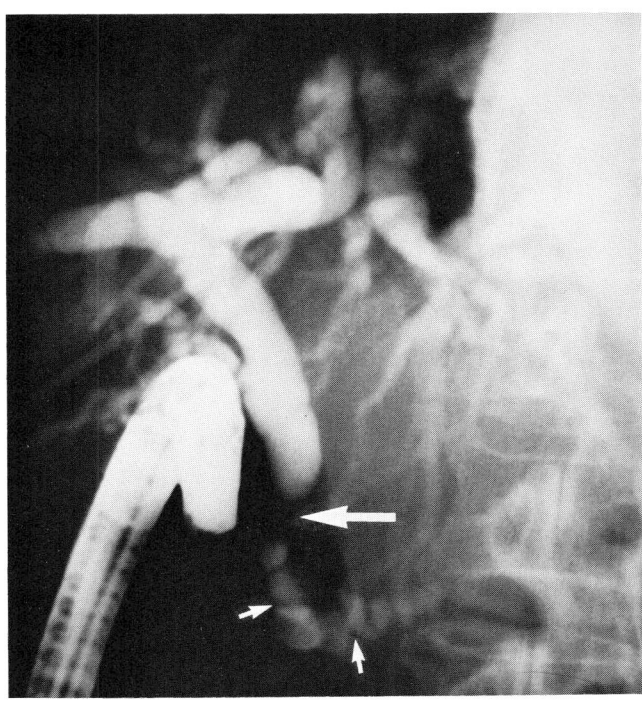

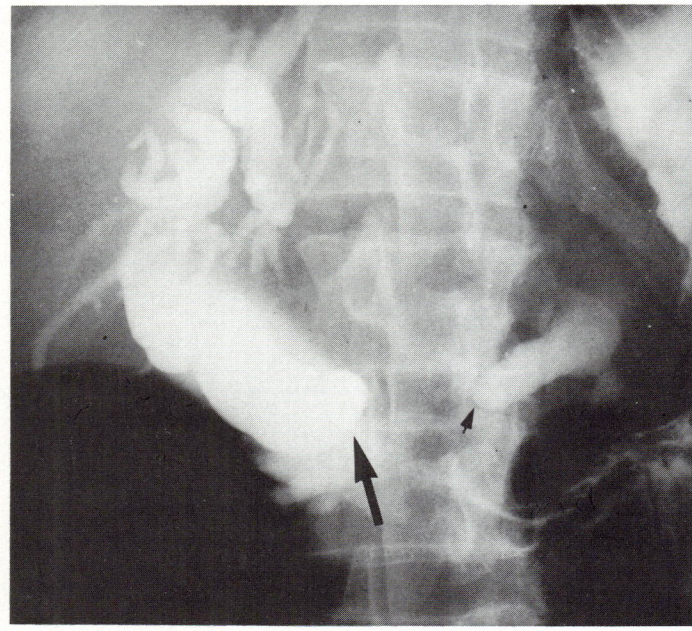

Figure 17–60. ERCP of carcinoma of the pancreas. The "double duct sign" is evident, with obstruction of the common bile duct (large arrow) and obstruction of the pancreatic duct near the junction of the head and body of the pancreas (small arrow).

the common bile duct is considered characteristic of malignancy ("double-duct sign") (Fig. 17–59).[4, 15] Small cancers that do not involve the pancreatic duct are more difficult to detect. However, these may be sometimes identified by filling of distorted secondary pancreatic ducts and their smaller branches.

PERCUTANEOUS TRANSHEPATIC CHOLANGIOGRAPHY. This is an effective method for evaluation of the common bile duct in jaundiced patients with suspected carcinoma of the head of the pancreas.[15] Dilated tertiary bile ducts enhance the

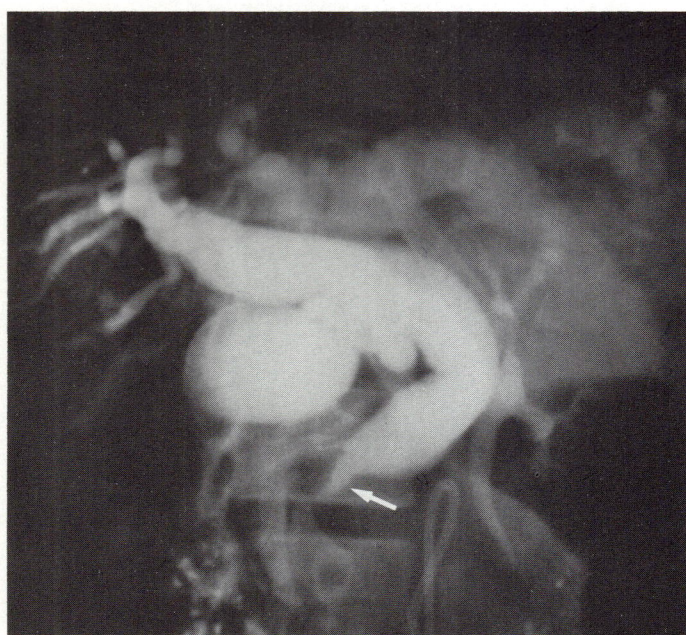

Figure 17–61. Percutaneous transhepatic cholangiography in a patient with carcinoma of the pancreas. The sites of encasement and obstruction of the common bile duct are demonstrated (arrow).

probability of successful percutaneous cannulation of the system. Stenotic or obstructed common bile ducts can be optimally demonstrated in this way (Fig. 17–61).

This technique can also be therapeutic by draining the obstructed bile ducts and reducing jaundice. A percutaneous approach has an advantage over retrograde cannulation in that it may demonstrate more proximal obstructions secondary to metastases. Carcinomas involving the body and tail of the pancreas cannot be evaluated by percutaneous transhepatic approach unless they have extended to obstruct the common bile duct. Finally, demonstration of the obstruction itself can be highly suggestive but not diagnostic of cancer; pancreatitis and even cholelithiasis may mimic cancer and vice versa.

ANGIOGRAPHY. Pancreatic carcinomas are usually avascular. Their demonstration depends on indirect evidence of a mass effect, such as vessel encasement (Fig. 17–62), compression, displacement, or intrapancreatic capillary stain. The accuracy of detection varies with a reported range of 60 to 95 per cent.[5, 32] Since many of these angiographic signs can be seen in arteriosclerosis, chronic pancreatitis, and congenital variants (Fig. 17–62), close diagnostic correlation and angiographic experience are necessary for proper interpretation and diagnosis. Angiography is extremely useful in mapping the parenchymal and collateral blood supply of the pancreas prior to tumor resection or pancreatoduodenotomy. In addition, angiography is used adjunctively with CT and US in tumor localization for percutaneous aspiration biopsy.[16] Because it is an invasive procedure, angiography does not lend itself to screening for cancer. Its use is thus relegated to those cases with definitive clinical evidence of this disease.

Obstructive jaundice in suspected carcinoma requires demonstration of the com-

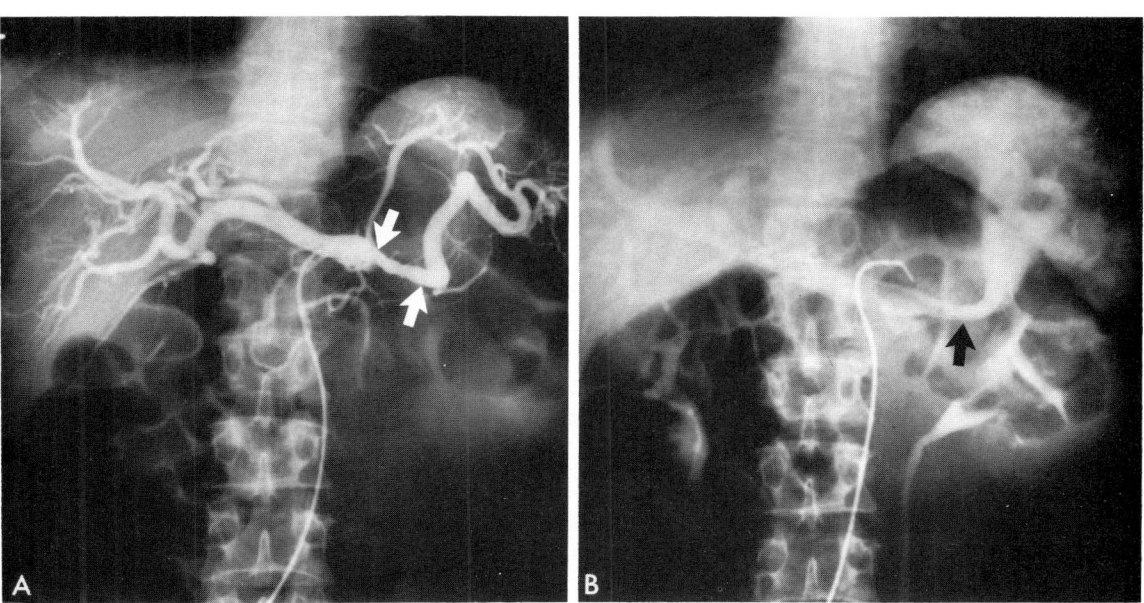

Figure 17–62. Angiogram of pancreatic carcinoma. *A,* The arterial phase of the celiac injection shows encasement deformity of the proximal splenic artery (arrows). Similar arteriographic findings could be produced by chronic pancreatitis. Therefore, clinical and imaging correlation must be achieved in the interpretation of an angiogram with these findings. *B,* The venous phase shows focal compression (arrow) of the splenic vein near its take-off from the spleen. These changes are also nonspecific and could be caused by other mass lesions in this area, such as those of chronic pancreatitis.

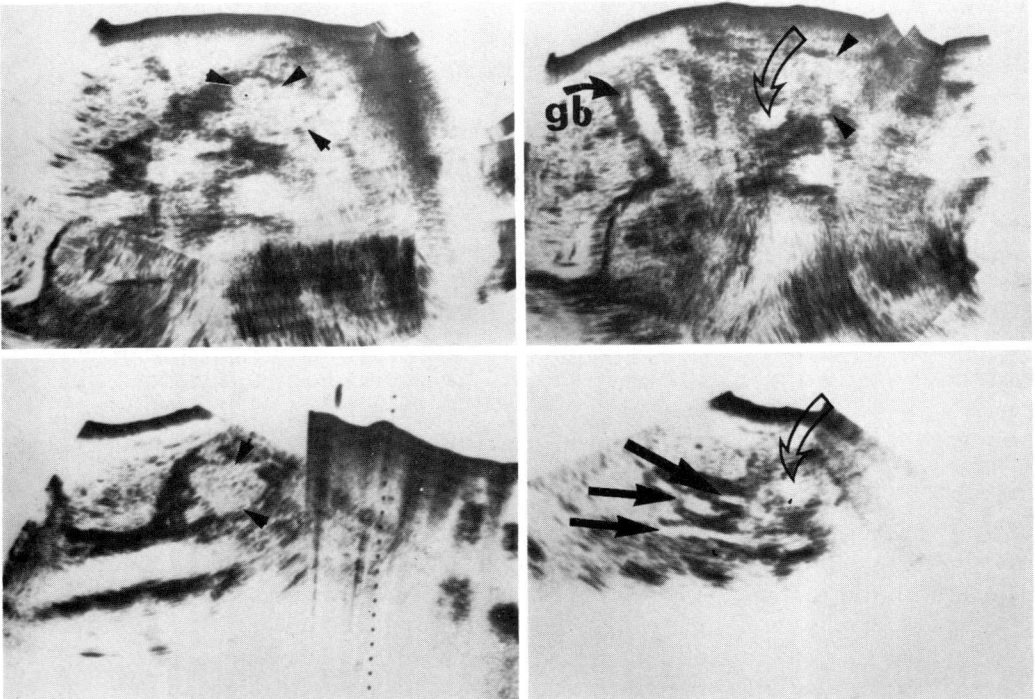

Figure 17–63. Ultrasonogram in pancreatic carcinoma. Transverse scan (left upper frame) shows a focal, low-amplitude area of pancreatic enlargement near the midbody (arrowheads). At a slightly lower level (right upper frame), an area of tumor necrosis (curved open arrow) is shown. The gallbladder (gb) is seen to the right; notice its thick, densely echoed wall. These findings in the gallbladder are characteristically associated with ascites. A small collection of ascitic fluid is seen to the immediate left of the gallbladder.

Longitudinal (sagittal) scan (lower left) shows the tumor mass (arrowheads). Oblique parasagittal view (lower right) again shows the tumor (curved arrow). Solid arrows point to the vena cava below, the portal vein above, and a slightly dilated common duct (largest solid arrow). These three structures are identified on scans by their relationship to each other, which is fairly constant.

mon duct through transhepatic or transjugular cholangiography. The degree of invasion of the duct by tumor determines the type of surgical ductal anastomosis.

ULTRASONOGRAPHY (Fig. 17–63). Pancreatic cancers present as focal masses of variable size, slightly less echogenic than the normal pancreas.[14, 31, 37] Calcifications can occur but are rarely detectable by ultrasound. Cancers in the head of the pancreas are commonly associated with pancreatic duct and common bile duct obstruction and dilatation. Demonstration of metastases to other organs and retroperitoneum strongly supports the diagnosis of malignancy. Hemorrhage and accumulation of debris may occur within a pancreatic tumor and be essentially indistinguishable from a pseudocyst, abscess, or the rarely encountered pancreatic adenoma.[25]

COMPUTERIZED TOMOGRAPHY. Pancreatic carcinomas characteristically present as focal parenchymal masses of variable size and location.[14, 24, 31] Their CT attentuation is lower than that of the normal pancreas (Fig. 17–64). X-ray density alone cannot be used as a criterion for diagnosis because the masses of chronic pancreatitis and cancers may have equal attenuation values. Calcifications, cystic focal degenerations, pancreatic duct dilatation, or gas formation, although readily detectable, are nonspecific. Evidence of common duct dilatation is also a nonspecific finding. Enhancement of tumor density by

THE PANCREAS — 1047

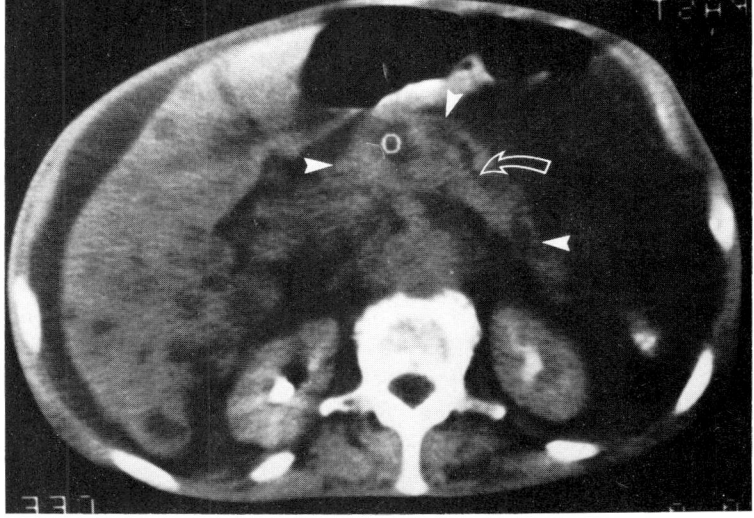

Figure 17-64. CT scan in pancreatic carcinoma. The pancreas is indicated by arrowheads; the curved arrow points to the dilated pancreatic duct. The area of interest marker (white central circle) overlies the area of cystic necrosis within the tumor; CT densities of near-water equivalent were obtained. All these changes could be mimicked by pancreatitis.

intravenous contrast administration has not been reliably demonstrated by CT[31] but appears much more promising with the newer, shorter-time scanners. Infiltration of fascial planes is also not definitively indicative of malignancy, since it can be seen in abscesses. Liver and retroperitoneal metastases strongly reinforce the diagnosis of cancer (Fig. 17-65).

Radiology of the Postoperative Patient

After definitive or palliative surgery for pancreatic disease, complications such as abscess, anastomotic leaks or strictures, obstructions, recurrent disease, and so forth, are investigated by various imaging techniques. These studies may be confusing and difficult to interpret unless the radiologist obtains information about the specific anatomic alterations produced by the surgery. Ultrasound or CT studies usually are the most informative when abscess, hematoma, or recurrent disease is suspected.

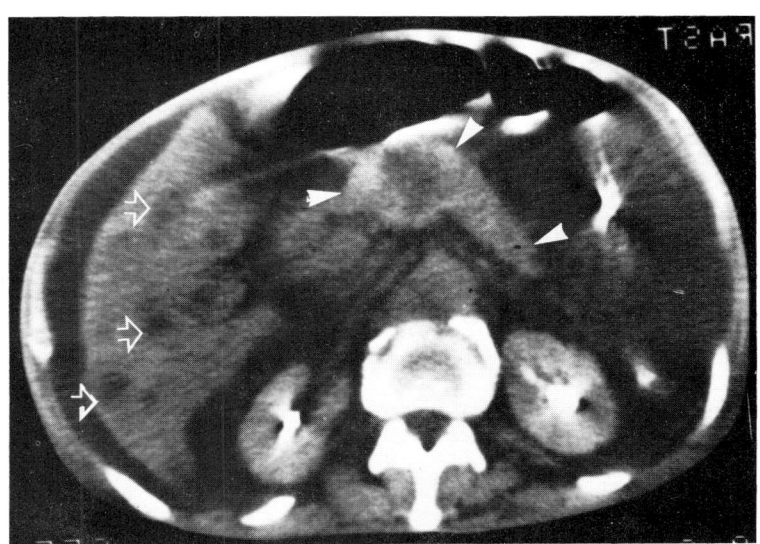

Figure 17-65. CT scan in pancreatic carcinoma. The pancreas (arrowheads) shows focal enlargement of the midbody with decreased density. Metastases (open arrows) are readily seen in the hepatic parenchyma. The presence of metastases strongly corroborates the diagnosis of malignancy. The pancreatic mass as shown could otherwise just as well be caused by pancreatitis.

In this section, only contrast studies of the upper gastrointestinal tract or biliary tree are considered, depending upon the type of surgical procedure.

SPHINCTEROTOMY. It is not uncommon for patients who have undergone sphincterotomy to show free reflux of barium into the common bile duct. This barium usually empties back into the duodenum in a short time, and the event is most often of no clinical significance.

ROUX-EN-Y RECONSTRUCTIONS FOR DIRECT PANCREATIC DUCT DRAINAGE (PUESTOW PROCEDURE) (Fig. 17–66). These patients may show no discernible abnormalities of the stomach, duodenum, or upper jejunum unless there is reflex of barium or air into the afferent loop. This occurs very rarely and shows the barium filling in reverse direction to normal flow into the left upper quadrant. Unless there is considerable delay in emptying of the afferent loop or fistula formation, these changes carry little clinical significance. The only prospective way of studying this type of anastomosis is through cannulation of pancreatic duct, by means of ERCP, in instances in which the proximal duct is sufficiently patent to allow a retrograde injection (Fig. 17–67).

PSEUDOCYST DRAINAGE. Drainage of pseudocyst by enteric anastomosis may occasionally be demonstrable radiographically. The anastomotic site is most easily recognized when the stomach or proximal small bowel is used for anastomosis (Figs. 17–68 to 17–70).

EXTIRPATIVE PROCEDURES. The two basic approaches to pancreatectomy are Whipple's procedure, or pancreaticoduodenectomy, and caudal or distal pancreatectomy. The former is used in cases of chronic pancreatitis or malignancy. The latter is usually indicated for relief of intractable pain in chronic pancreatitis or segmental carcinoma in the tail of the pancreas.

The radiographic changes in these instances depend on the type and extent of pancreatectomy. Distal pancreatectomies are usually handled through a Roux-en-Y,

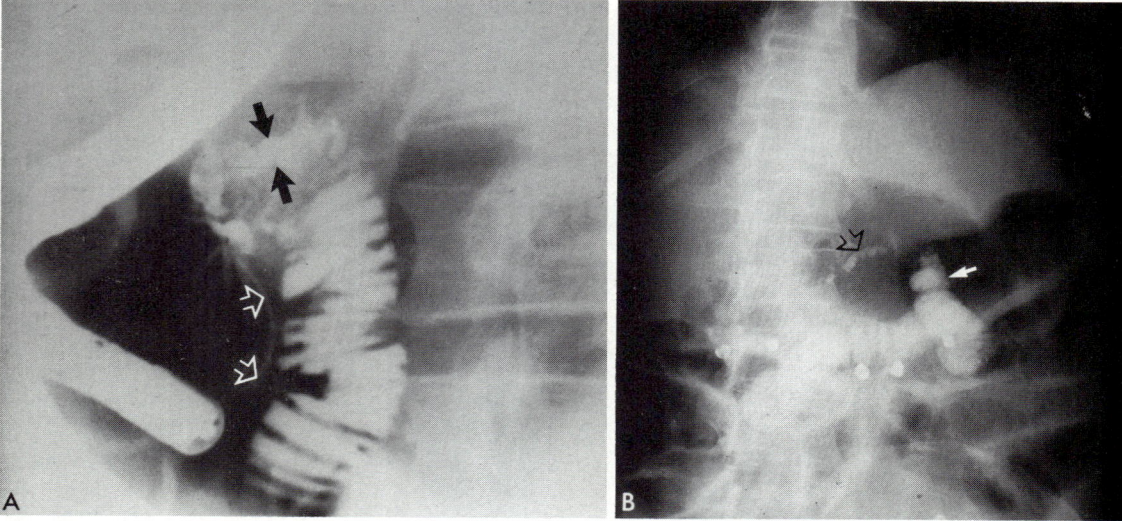

Figure 17–66. *A*, Endoscopic retrograde pancreatogram performed on a patient following the Puestow procedure for chronic pancreatitis. The open arrows indicate the cannula extending into the pancreatic duct. The closed arrows demonstrate the irregular dilated pancreatic duct indicating chronic pancreatitis. There is opacification of the Roux-en-Y jejunal loop. *B*, A drainage film following the retrograde injection of the pancreatic duct again demonstrates retention in the irregular pancreatic duct (open arrow) and opacification of the Roux-en-Y jejunal segment (closed arrow).

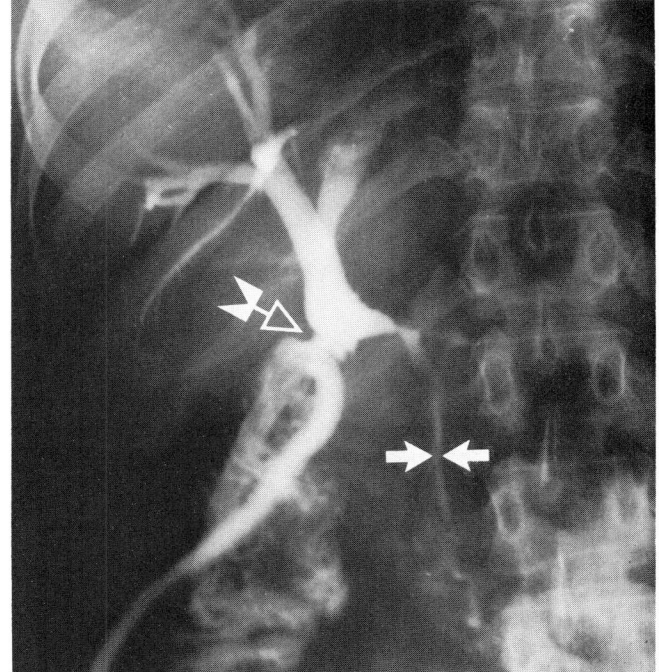

Figure 17–67. T-tube cholangiogram following choledochojejunostomy performed by bypass of a stricture of the common bile duct secondary to chronic pancreatitis. The common hepatic bile duct and the intrahepatic radicals are well defined. The site of choledochojejeunostomy is demonstrated (double-tailed arrow). In addition, the strictured common bile duct secondary to chronic pancreatitis is demonstrated (solid arrows).

end-to-end jejunal anastomosis, with the stomach and duodenum left in place. These show little changes on upper gastrointestinal tract studies. The radiographic changes are essentially similar to those described for the Puestow procedure.

Pancreatoduodenectomy (Whipple's procedure), on the other hand, produces significant anatomic alteration by the removal of the distal stomach and duodenum as well as portions of the proximal jejunum. The contrast radiographic examination in these

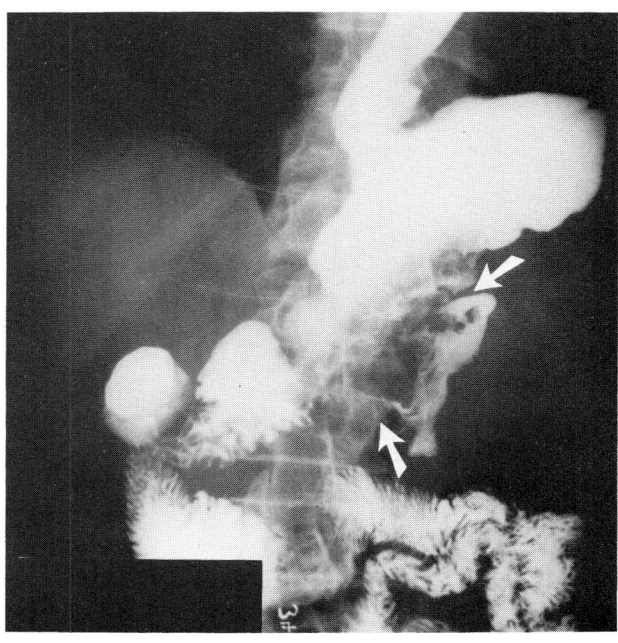

Figure 17–68. Cystogastrotomy for drainage of pseudocyst. The upper gastrointestinal series shows the area of anastomosis between the pseudocyst and the greater curvature to the stomach (arrows). The cyst, seen to the left of the stomach, contains air and barium.

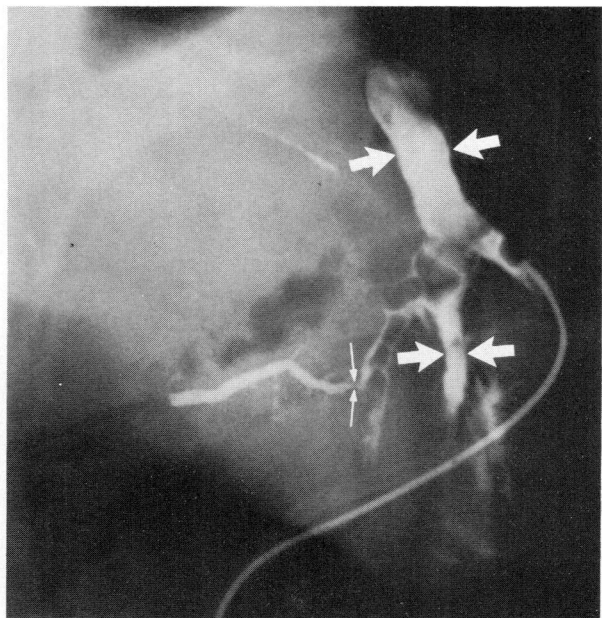

Figure 17–69. Sinogram demonstrating a left upper quadrant pseudocyst that developed following surgery for traumatic rupture of the tail of the pancreas. The tail was resected. The pseudocyst is outlined by injection of contrast material into the drainage tube (large arrows). Communication of the pseudocyst with the pancreatic duct at the site of resection is seen (small arrows).

cases predictably shows considerable structural and dynamic alteration to the passage of barium. The usual type of reconstruction after Whipple's procedure (Fig. 17–71) consists of a Billroth II gastrojejunostomy in additon to end-to-side anastomosis of the common duct and end-to-end anastomosis of the pancreatic duct to the afferent jejunal loop. Inthese instances the initial passage of barium is very similar to that in a patient

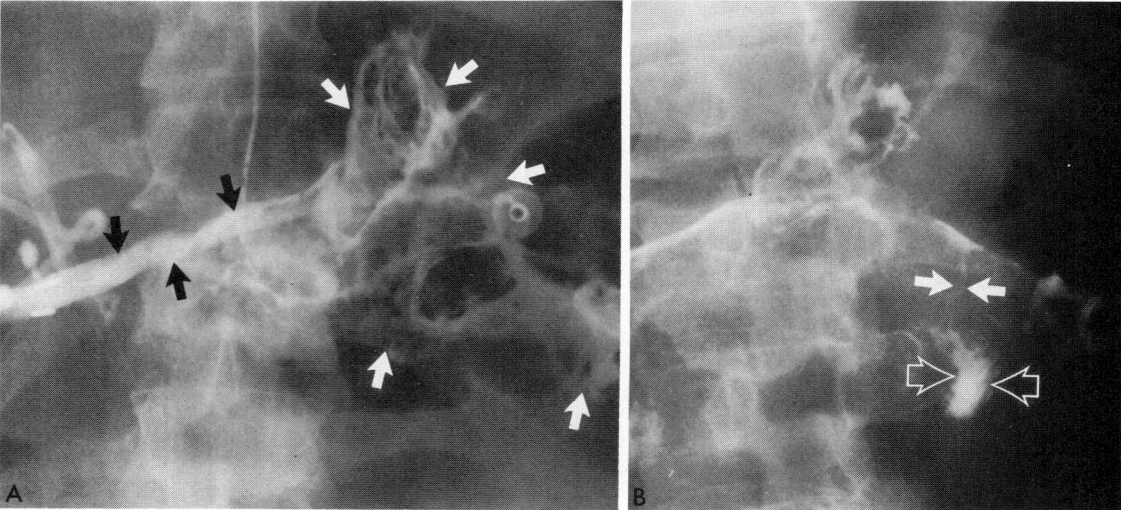

Figure 17–70. Spontaneous pseudocyst, jejunal fistula. A, A pancreatic duct injection performed in a patient who developed pancreatitis and a pseudocyst following biliary tract surgery. The black arrows demonstrate the pancreatic duct. The white arrows outline the extent of a large pseudocyst communicating with the pancreatic duct. B, A later film made to determine drainage of the cyst demonstrates a fistulous communication between the pseudocyst and the jejunum. Fistulous tract = solid arrows; jejunal filling = open arrows.

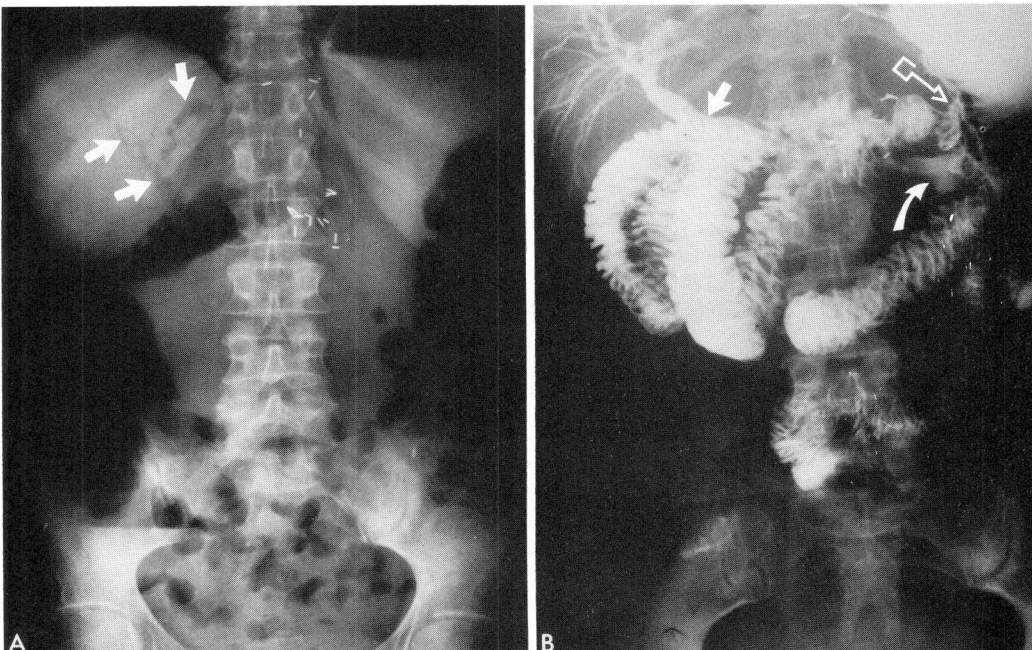

Figure 17–71. Plain radiograph of the abdomen in a patient who has had a Whipple anastomosis for carcinoma of the pancreas. There is air in the biliary tree (arrows). This is a nonspecific finding commonly seen after surgical exploration or reanastomosis of the common bile duct. However, air in the biliary tree may indicate rupture, fistula, abscess formation, or recent passing of large biliary calculi. B, Early phase of the upper gastrointestinal series shows the gastrojejunal end-to-side anatomosis (open arrow), the common duct end-to-side anastomosis (straight arrow), and the jejunopancreatic end-to-end anastomosis (curved arrow). Barium partly fills the pancreatic duct and the biliary tree.

who has had a Billroth II anastomosis. In the absence of significant tumor recurrence or other complications, there may be rapid filling of both jejunal afferent and efferent loops with resultant overlying of the proximal bowel by distal bowel. Therefore, early films without significant distal small bowel filling are the most diagnostic. The common duct and its branches also often fill with barium. Mass effects as well as fistulas and significant mucosal abnormalities, such as spiculization and partial obstruction, should be sought, since tumor recurrence is probable.

BILIARY DRAINAGE PROCEDURES. Obstructive jaundice secondary to chronic pancreatitis or carcinoma requires surgical palliative relief. The extent of disease determines the type of biliary anastomosis. The kind of drainage provided in Whipple's procedure is not possible in patients with evidence of unresectable cancer. In that case, relief of biliary stasis can be accomplished by anastomosing the gallbladder to the stomach, duodenum, or jejunum (end-to-side or Roux-en-Y anastomosis) (Fig. 17–72). The cystic duct has to be shown patent by preoperative percutaneous or operative cholangiogram.

As with other biliary-enteric anastomoses, air or barium may reflux into the gallbladder and opacify the intrahepatic biliary radicles. This reflux is clinically of no significance, and re-emptying into the bowel is usually prompt. Identification of the anastomosis is best seen in early films before the distal small bowel fills. The Roux-en-Y type of correction is usually not fully filled by refluxing barium.

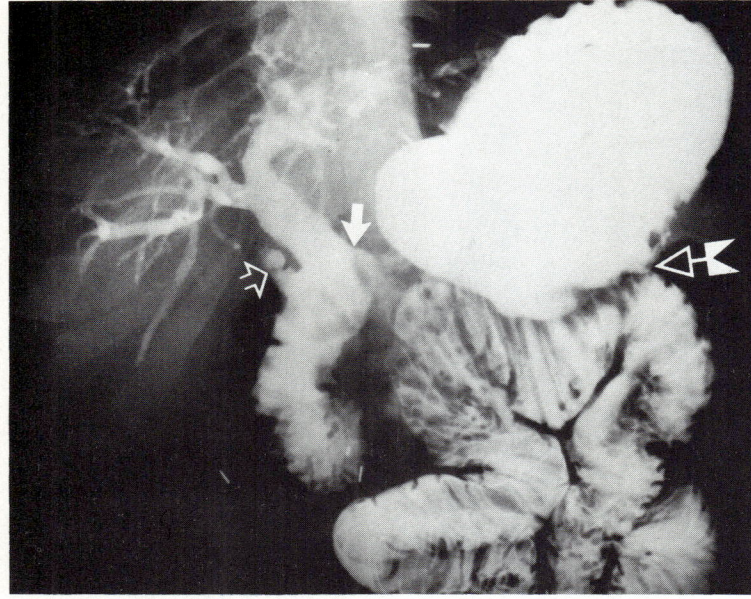

Figure 17–72. Pancreatic carcinoma, postoperative. Upper gastrointestinal study demonstrates a gastrojejunostomy (double-tailed arrow) and choledochoduodenostomy (solid arrow), performed because of a pancreatic mass obstructing the gastric outlet and the distal common bile duct. The open arrow demonstrates the cystic duct remnant from prior cholecystectomy.

References

1. Ariyama, J., Shirakabe, H., Ikenobe, H., et al.: The diagnosis of the small resectable pancreatic carcinoma. Clin. Radio., 28:437–444, 1977.
2. Benedetto, P. W.: Pancreatic pseudocyst. John Hopkins Med. J. 143:109–113, 1978.
3. Biello, D. R., Levitt, R. G., and Melson, G. L.: The roles of gallium-67 scintigraphy, ultrasonography and computed tomography in the detection of abdominal abscesses. Semin. Nucl. Med. 19:58–65, 1979.
4. Bilbao, M. K., and Katon, R. M.: Neoplasms of the pancreas. In Stewart, E. T. et al. (eds.): Atlas of Endoscopic Retrograde Cholangiopancreatography. St. Louis, The C. V. Mosby Company, 1977, pp. 181–235.
5. Boijsen, E.: Pancreatic angiography. In Abrams, H. (ed.): Angiography Ed. 2. Boston, Little, Brown and Company, 1971, pp. 953–981.
6. Bradley, E. L., Clements, J. L., and Gonzalez, A. C.: The natural history of pancreatic pseudocysts: a unified concept of management. Am. J. Surg. 137:135–141, 1979.
7. Bradley, E. L., Gonzalez, A. C., and Clements, J. L.: Acute pancreatic pseudocysts. Ann. Surg. 184:734–737, 1976.
8. Carretta, R. F., Weiland, F. L., Harvey, W. C., et al.: The diagnostic efficacy of gallium-67 in the localization of abscesses or inflammatory processes: a review of 300 consecutive cases. J. Nucl. Med. 734, 1978.
9. Eaton, S. B., and Ferrucci, J. T.: Radiology of the Pancreas and Duodenum. Philadelphia, W. B. Saunders Company, 1973, pp. 95–124.
10. Feinberg, S. B., Schreiber, D. R., and Goodale, R.: Comparison of ultrasound pancreatic scanning and endoscopic retrograde cholangiopancreatograms: a retrospective study. J. Clin. Ultrasound 5:96–100, 1977.
11. Ferrucci, J. T., Jr.: Body ultrasonography. N. Engl. J. Med. 300:590–602, 1979.
12. Ferrucci, J. T., Jr.: Radiology of the pancreas, 1976. Sonography and ductography. Radiol. Clin. North Am. 16:543–561, 1976.
13. Filly, R. A., and London, S. S.: The normal pancreas: acoustic characteristics and frequency of imaging. J. Clin. Ultrasound 7:121–124, 1979.
14. Freeny, P. C., and Ball, T. J.: Rapid diagnosis of pancreatic carcinoma: an algorithmic approach. Radiology 127:627–633, 1978.
15. Freeny, P. C., Bilbao, M. K., and Katon, R. M.: "Blind" evaluation of endoscopic retrograde cholangiopancreatography (ERCP) in the diagnosis of pancreatic carcinoma: the "double duct" and other signs. Radiology 119:271–274, 1976.
16. Goldman, M. L., Naib, Z. M., Galambos, J. T., et al.: Preoperative diagnosis of pancreatic carcinoma by percutaneous aspiration biopsy. Am. J. Dig. Dis. 22:1076–1082, 1977.
17. Gonzalez, A. C., Bradley, E. L., and Clements, J. L.: Pseudocyst formation in acute pancreatitis: ultrasonographic evaluation of 99 cases. Am. J. Roentgenol. 127:315–317, 1976.

18. Haertel, M., Tillmann, U., and Fuchs, W. A.: Die akute pankreatitis im computertomogramm. Fortschr. Rontgenstr. *130*(5):525–530, 1979.
19. Harvey, W. C., Podoloff, D. A., and Kopp, D. T.: ^{67}Gallium in 68 consecutive infection searches. J. Nucl. Med. *16*:2–4, 1975.
20. Henkin, R. E.: Selected topics in intra-abdominal imagining via nuclear medicine techniques. Radiol. Clin. North Am. *17*:39–54, 1979.
21. Hubner, K. F., Buonocore, W. D., Gibbs, S., et al.: Differentiation of pancreatic and other retroperitoneal tumors by positron emission computerized tomography (ECT). Paper presented at the 25th Annual Meeting Society of Nuclear Medicine, Atlanta, 1979.
22. Hunziker, R. J.: Pathologic effusions localized to the anterior pararenal space. Gastrointest. Radiol. *3*:411–414, 1978.
23. Lawson, T. L.: Sensitivity of pancreatic ultrasonography in the detection of pancreatic disease. Radiology *128*:733–736, 1978.
24. Lee, J. K. T., Stanley, R. J., Melson, G. L., et al.: Pancreatic imaging by ultrasound and computed tomography: A general review. Radiol. Clin. North Am. *16*:105–117, 1979.
25. Lloyd, T. V., Antonmattei, S., and Freimanis, A. K.: Gray scale sonography of cystadenoma of the pancreas: report of two cases. J. Clin. Ultrasound *7*:149–151, 1979.
26. Mendez, G., and Isikoff, M. B.: Significance of intrapancreatic gas demonstrated by CT: a review of nine cases. Am. J. Roentgenol. *132*:59–62, 1979.
27. Meyers, M. A., and Evans, J. A.: Effect of pancreatitis on the small bowel and colon: spread along mesenteric planes. Am. J. Roentgenol. *119*:151–165, 1973.
28. Moss, A. A., Goldberg, H. I., and Stewart, E. T.: Radiographic technique. In Stewart, E. T. et al. (eds.), Atlas of Endoscopic Retrograde Cholangiopancreatography. St. Louis, The C. V. Mosby Company, 1977, pp. 19–28.
29. Pollak, E. W., Michas, C. A., and Wolfman, E. G.: Pancreatic pseudocyst: management in fifty-four patients: Am. J. Surg. *135*:199–201, 1978.
30. Ranson, J. H. C., and Spencer, F. C.: Prevention, diagnosis and treatment of pancreatic abscess. Surgery *82*:99–106, 1977.
31. Sample, W. F., and Sorti, D. A.: Diagnosis of pancreatic disease by ultrasound and computed tomography. In Taylor, K. J. W. (Ed.): Clinics in Diagnostic Ultrasound. New York, Churchill Livingstone, 1979, pp. 85–101.
32. Schmidt, H., and Creutzfeldt, W.: Etiology and pathogenesis of pancreatitis. In Bockus, H. L. (ed.): Gastroenterology. Ed. 3. Philadelphia, W. B. Saunders Company, 1976, pp. 1005–1069.
33. Shafer, R. B., and Silvis, S. E.: Pancreatic pseudo-pseudocysts. Am. J. Surg. *127*:320–325, 1974.
34. Shaffer, R. D.: Indications and contraindications for the use of endoscopic retrograde cholangiopancreatography. In Stewart, E. T. et al. (eds.): Atlas of Endoscopic Retrograde Cholangiopancreatography. St. Louis, The C. V. Mosby Company, 1977, pp. 1–3.
35. Silvis, S. E., Rohrmann, C. A., and Vennes, J. A.: Diagnostic accuracy of endoscopic retrograde cholangiopancreatography in hepatic, biliary and pancreatic malignancy. Ann. Intern. Med. *84*:438–440, 1976.
36. Silvis, S. E., and Schuman, B. M.: Benign conditions of the pancreas. In Stewart, E. T. et al. (eds.): Atlas of Endoscopic Retrograde Cholangiopancreatography. St Louis, The C. V. Mosby Company, 1977, pp. 124–180.
37. Simeone, J. F., and Simonds, B. D.: Normal anatomy of the pancreas by computed tomography and diagnostic ultrasound. In Taylor, K. J. W. (ed.): Clinics in Diagnostic Ultrasound. New York, Churchill Livingstone, 1979, pp. 73–84.
38. Stanley, R. J., Sagel, S. S., and Levitt, R. J.: Computed tomographic evaluation of the pancreas. Radiology *124*:715–722, 1977.
39. Taylor, K. J. W., McWasson, J. F., deGraaff, C. S., et al.: Accuracy of grey-scale ultrasound diagnosis of abdominal and pelvic abscesses in 220 patients. Lancet *1*:83–84, 1978.
40. Warshaw, A. L.: Pancreatic abscesses. N. Engl. J. Med. *287*:1234–1236, 1972.
41. Weens, H. S., and Clements, J. L.: The radiologic diagnosis of acute cholecystitis. Semin. Roentgenol. *21*:245–247, 1976.
42. Weens, H. S., and Walker, L. A.: The radiologic diagnosis of acute cholecystitis and pancreatitis. Radiol. Clin. North Am. *2*:89–106, 1964.
43. Weingarten, L., Gelb, A. M., and Fischer, M. G.: Dilemma of pancreatic ductal carcinoma. Am. J. Gastroenterol. *71*:473–476, 1979.

Part II
Endocrine Tumors

JOHN DOPPMAN, M.D.

Islet cell tumors of the pancreas are capable of producing a variety of peptide hormones and are consequently associated with a spectrum of clinical presentations (Table 17–1).[16] In all instances except for the case of the rare nonfunctional tumors, the initial diagnosis is a clinical one, confirmed by demonstrating elevated circulating levels of the specific hormone. The radiologist's contribution to the care of patients with islet cell tumors is usually to localization of these often small and elusive adenomas. Arteriography is the most successful localizing technique, adenomas appearing as foci of homogeneous staining during the capillary phase.[1, 6-8] Neither abnormal vessels nor arteriovenous shunting is demonstrated in the small benign lesions, but adenomas larger than 2.0 cm and islet cell carcinomas may demonstrate abnormal vessels and prominent draining veins. Arteriography should include celiac and superior mesenteric artery injections followed, if nondiagnostic, by selective gastroduodenal, splenic, and dorsal pancreatic arteriograms.[2, 4] Recently, the localization of glucagonomas and gastrinomas by the assaying of pancreatic vein samples for hormone gradients, using a percutaneous transhepatic approach to the portal venous bed, has been reported by Lunderquist et al.[10, 11] This technique holds considerable promise for patients with a negative arteriographic work-up, but experience is still limited.

INSULINOMAS

The most common islet cell tumor is an insulin-producing adenoma of beta cell origin. These tumors are rarely malignant (10 per cent) and can usually be treated by simple enucleation. They are often small (less than 2 cm in diameter), however, and because of their soft consistency, difficult to palpate within the pancreas. For these reasons, preoperative arteriographic localization should always be attempted to avoid the necessity for blind distal pancreatic resection. Insulinomas appear as discrete areas of diffuse homogeneous staining during the late arterial-capillary phase (Fig. 17–73). Abnormal vasculature or vessel displacement is rarely seen in benign insulinomas, and early venous filling is absent. Occasionally, a circumferential arterial pattern with centrally converging branches, like the spokes of a wheel, is seen in the arterial phase

TABLE 17–1. PRESENTATION OF ISLET CELL TUMORS

Cell	Hormone	Syndrome	Malignant Potential	Arteriographic Localization
Beta	Insulin	Hypoglycemia	10%	75–80%
Alpha$_1$	Gastrin	Zollinger-Ellison	60–70%	10–20%
Alpha$_2$	Glucagon	Diabetes, rash	90%	90%
Non-Beta	VIP, GIP, prostaglandins	Pancreatic cholera, WDHA syndrome	50%	Too little data
Non-Beta	Nonfunctioning	Abdominal mass	80–90%	Too little data

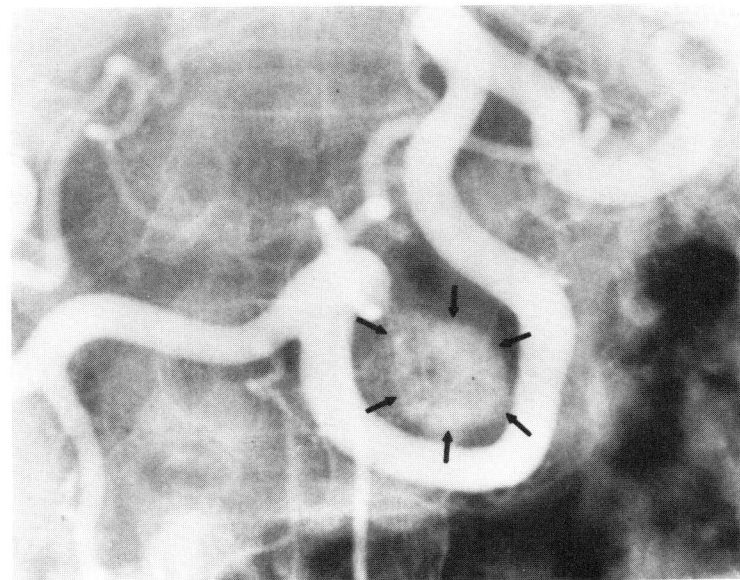

Figure 17–73. Insulinoma of the body of the pancreas presenting as a well-circumscribed homogeneous stain (arrows) without abnormal vessels or arteriovenous shunting.

(Fig. 17–74) and may be helpful when the adenoma is obscured by a densely staining pancreas (Fig. 17–75). A focal area of staining just to the left of the spine at the junction of the body and the tail of the pancreas may occasionally be seen in patients with dense filling of a large pancreatica magna artery (Fig. 17–76). Reuter has cautioned against confusing this stain with an islet cell tumor. It probably represents a normal pancreas projected semiaxially as the gland courses posteriorly just lateral to the vertebral column.[14] A redundant splenic vein, staining of gastric and duodenal mucosa, accessory spleens, and granulations about peptic ulcers may occasionally mimic the stain of an

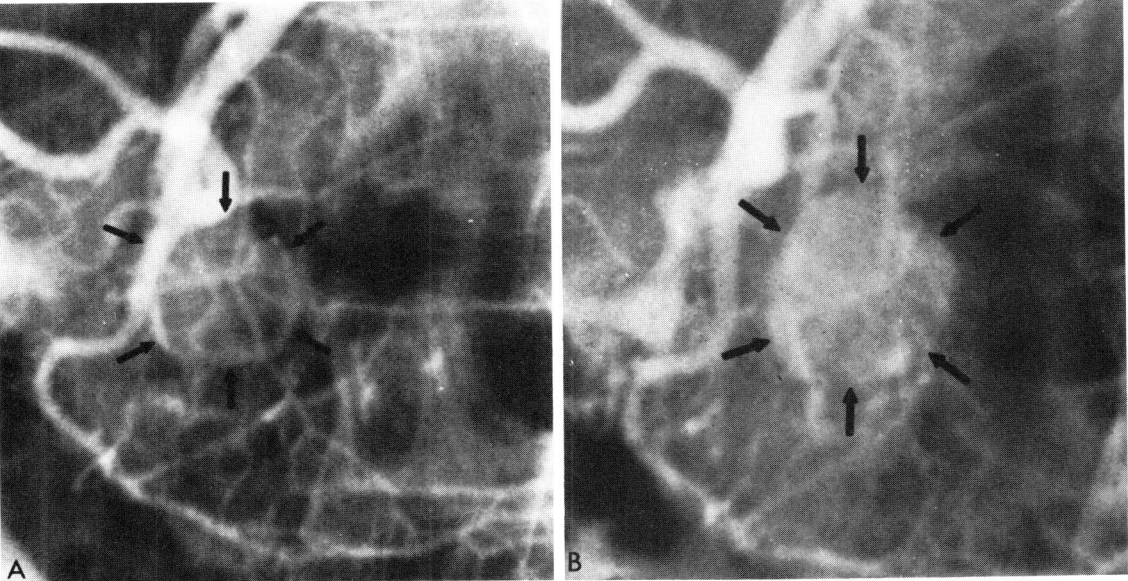

Figure 17–74. Insulinoma. A, A selective gastroduodenal arteriogram shows the typical circumferential arterial pattern (arrows), with multiple, centrally converging branches, of insulinoma of the pancreatic head. B, The capillary phase reveals diffuse homogeneous staining (arrows).

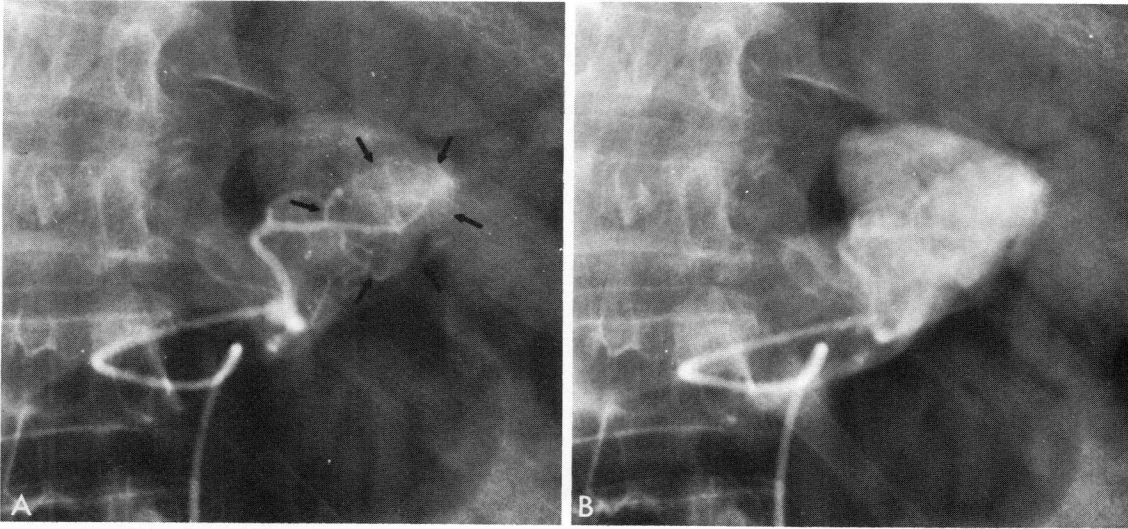

Figure 17–75. Insulinoma. *A,* A selective dorsal pancreatic arteriogram reveals a circumferential arterial pattern (arrows) and permits the localization of the insulinoma even though the area of staining is lost within the densely staining pancreas during capillary phase. *B,* Adenoma was not visualized on a celiac or a selective splenic arteriogram.

islet cell tumor,[13] but these can usually be distinguished by oblique projections and air insufflation of the stomach. Subtraction is often helpful, particularly for adenomas overlying the spine.

The incidence of successful arteriographic localization of insulinomas varies from 90 per cent down to 30 per cent.[7, 8, 15] Although islet cell hyperplasias rather than discrete adenomas account for some of the failures in localization, all angiographers having any experience with islet cell tumors have been called to the operating room to view a 3-cm lesion in the tail of the pancreas not detected on good preoperative arteriographic studies. Histologic differences do not satisfactorily account for these

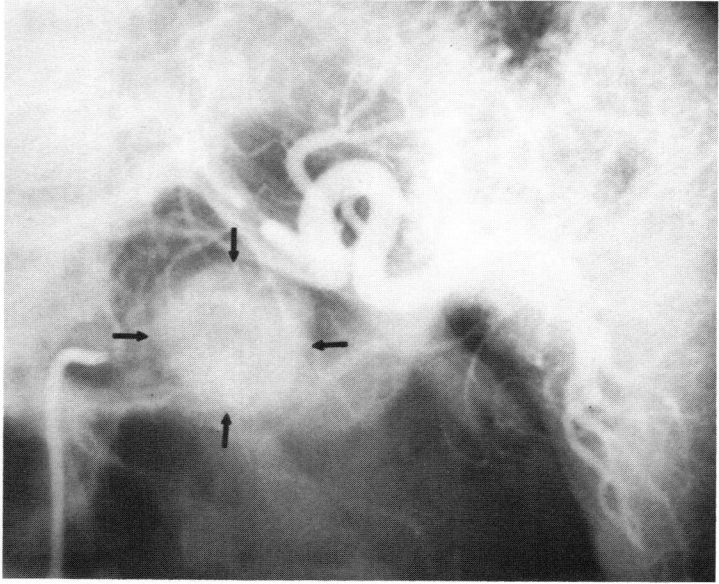

Figure 17–76. Pseudostain simulating tumor. Note the pseudostain (arrows) just to the left of the spine due to the body of the pancreas; it is usually distinguishable by its location and diameter. (*From* Reuter, S.: Potential overdiagnosis of pancreatic islet cell adenomas. J. Can. Assoc. Radiol. 22:184–186, 1971.)

occasional false negative studies. In arteriographic failures, selective sampling of the pancreatic veins may make its major contribution.[10, 11]

Malignant insulinomas metastasize to peripancreatic lymph nodes and to the liver. Even if the primary tumor is not demonstrated arteriographically, liver metastases invariably are, and a selective hepatic arteriogram should always be included in the work-up of patients with hypoglycemia. Dense hepatic staining may obscure hypervascular metastases (Fig. 17–77), but these will become apparent during epinephrine (15 to 20 μg) arteriography.

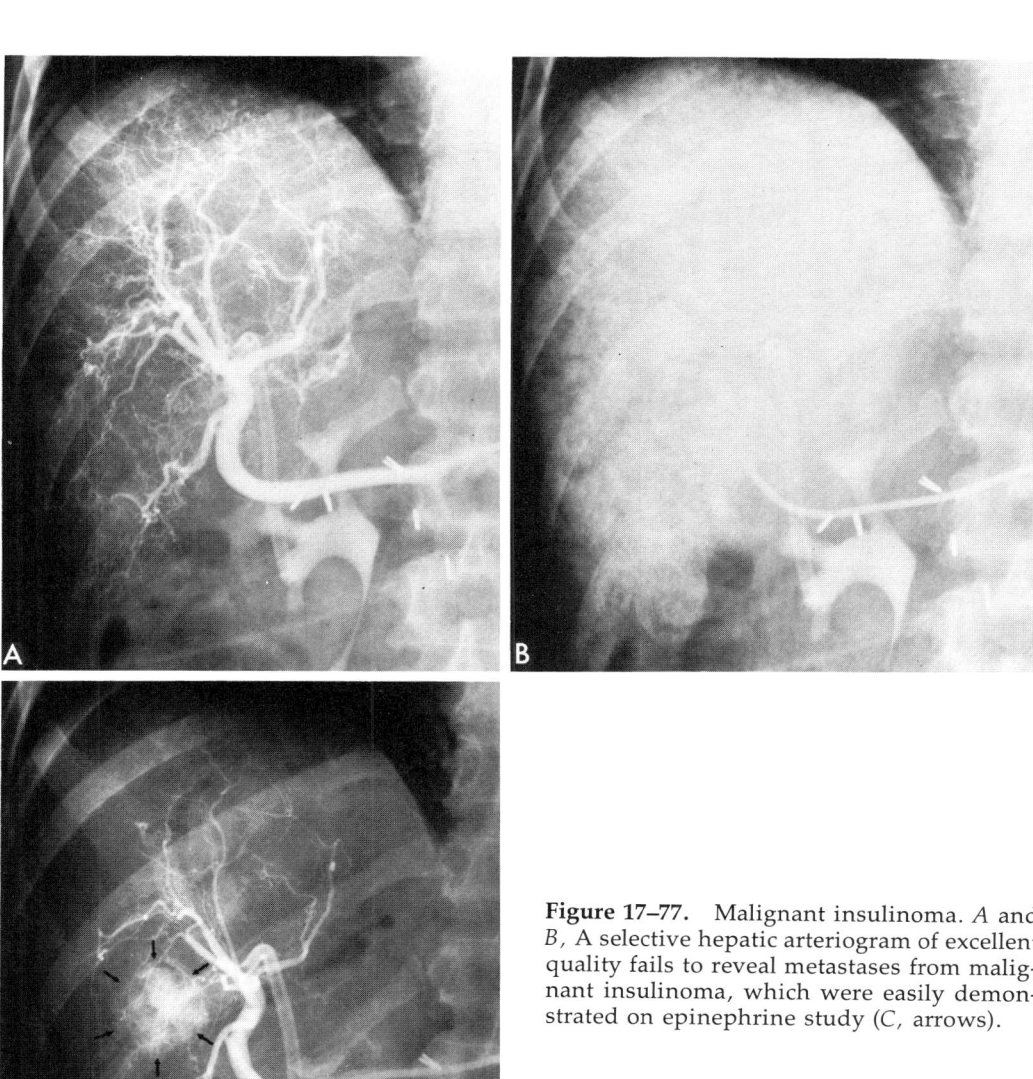

Figure 17–77. Malignant insulinoma. A and B, A selective hepatic arteriogram of excellent quality fails to reveal metastases from malignant insulinoma, which were easily demonstrated on epinephrine study (C, arrows).

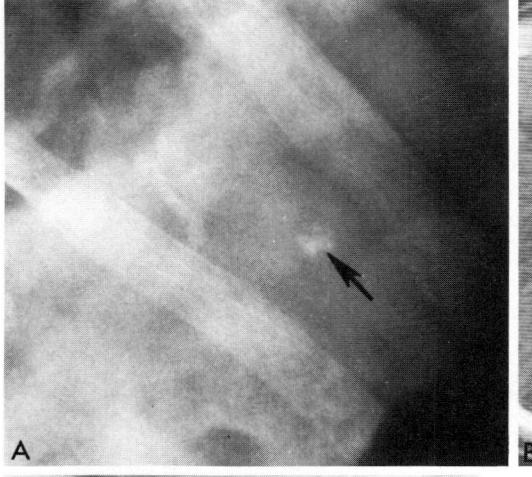
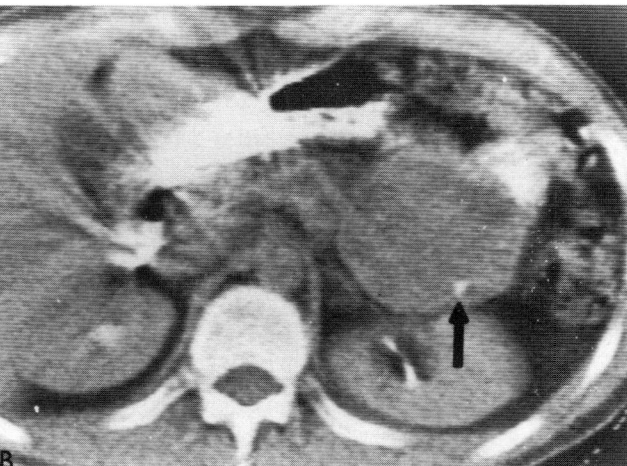
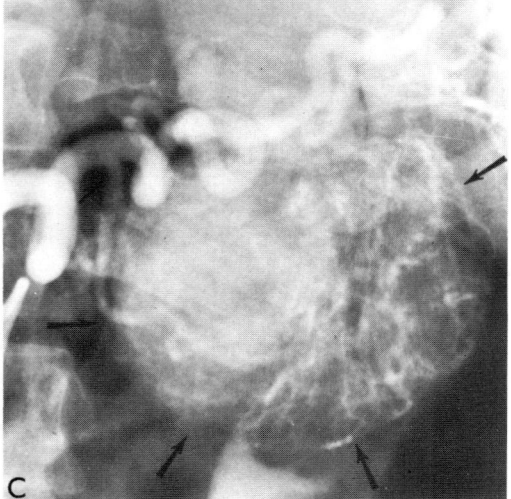

Figure 17–78. Malignant insulinoma. *A*, A dense benign-appearing calcification in the left upper abdomen (arrow). This is confirmed on the CT scan (*B*, arrow) to be lying within the insulinoma of the pancreatic tail. A selective splenic arteriogram demonstrates abnormal vessels within this malignant insulinoma (*C*, arrows).

Although the presence of calcification has not been reported in cases of benign insulinomas, malignant insulinomas sometimes contain small foci of dense benign-appearing calcifications.[9] Figure 17–78 demonstrates such calcifications on both plain abdominal films and CT scans.

Computerized tomography does not demonstrate islet cell tumors totally confined within the pancreas. We have succeeded in demonstrating only adenomas large enough to distort the pancreatic outline (see Fig. 17–78*B*). CT scanning following contrast-medium infusion has not improved the detection rate of small adenomas.

GASTRINOMAS

Zollinger and Ellison in 1955 described the association of non-beta islet cell tumors of the pancreas with a particularly virulent peptic ulcer diathesis.[18] Gastrin was later identified as the responsible hormone; the development of a radioimmunoassay for gastrin has greatly simplified the diagnosis of the Zollinger-Ellison syndrome. The diagnosis can be suggested radiologically by the demonstration of hypertrophied gastric mucosa, multiple or distal duodenojejunal ulcerations, and a prominent hypersecretory small bowel pattern.[17] Figure 17–79 demonstrates typical upper gastrointestinal findings. Anastomotic ulcers are common following subtotal gastric resection; total gastrectomy was the treatment of choice before the development of an effective acid antisecretory agent, cimetidine (Tagomet). Although the diagnosis may be suggested by gastrointestinal findings, an elevated serum gastrin level is essential to establish the diagnosis of Zollinger-Ellison syndrome. As in the case of insulinomas, localization of the gastrinoma, rather than diagnosis, is the major contribution of the radiologist. Unlike insulinomas, gastrinomas are not likely to be demonstrated by arteriography. Multiple small tumors or islet cell hyperplasia is more common than single, discrete adenomas. In addition, gastrin is also produced by G cells of the antral and proximal duodenal mucosa, a fact that accounts for the frequent location of gastrinomas in the wall of the antrum or duodenum. Hypervascularity of gastric and duodenal mucosa, and the granulation tissue associated with gastrectomies and marginal ulcers, produce spurious stains that are difficult to distinguish from gastrinomas. In our experience, arteriography usually fails to demonstrate a discrete resectable adenoma in cases of the

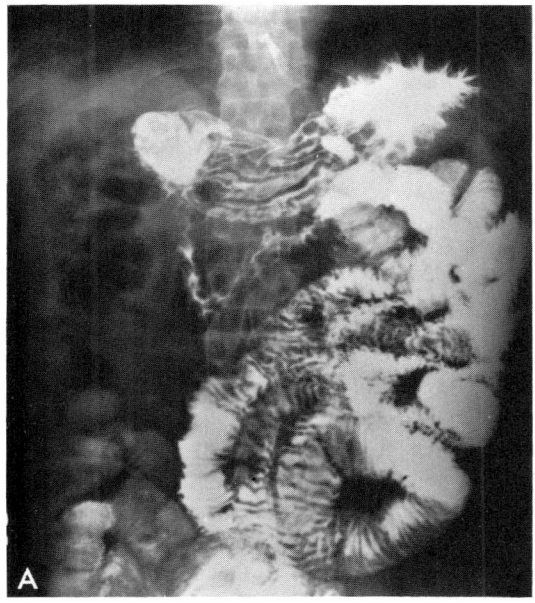
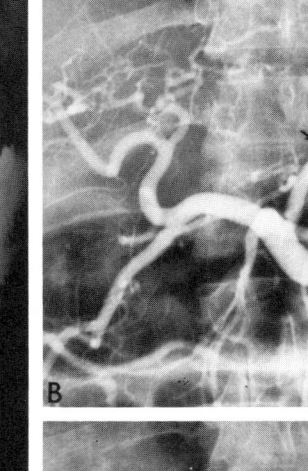
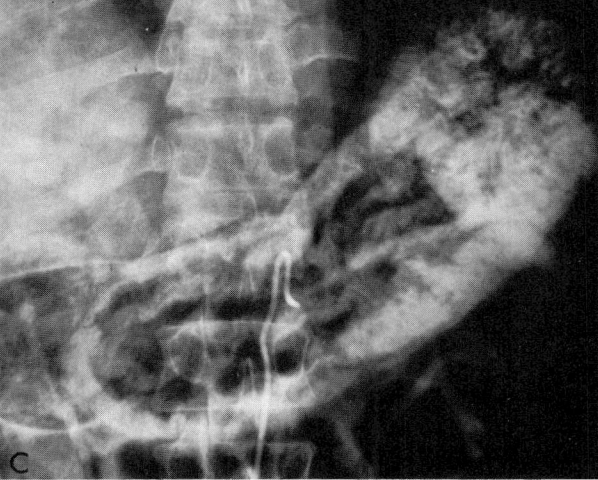

Figure 17–79. Zollinger-Ellison syndrome. *A,* Note the striking mucosal hyperplasia, which gives the stomach a cerebroid appearance. Ulcerations of the stomach and the duodenum were present. *B,* The left gastric artery (arrow) is enlarged in patients with the Zollinger-Ellison syndrome, often to the same diameter as splenic or common hepatic arteries. *C,* Note the intense staining of gastric mucosa, obscuring small gastrinomas of antral or duodenal G cells.

Zollinger-Ellison syndrome, although there are exceptions (Fig. 17–80). Lunderquist et al. have reported the successful localization of a gastrin-producing tumor in the tail of the pancreas through the sampling of multiple pancreatic veins.[11] Since 60 per cent of the gastrinomas are malignant, liver metastases are often demonstrated even when the primary lesion cannot be shown angiographically. Such hepatic metastases grow slowly and may respond dramatically to hepatic artery ligation or to intra-arterial infusion of streptozotocin; thus, their demonstration is critical in these cases.

GLUCAGONOMAS

Fewer than 25 glucagon-producing islet cell tumors have been reported.[5] These patients present with diabetes and a characteristic rash (migrating necrolytic erythema). The tumors are generally discrete adenomas and are demonstrable at arteriography. Figure 17–81 illustrates a particularly large glucagonoma that was totally resected, resulting in an apparent cure. Most glucagon-secreting tumors are malignant, however, and the patient returned seven years after pancreatectomy with a recurrence in the pancreatic bed and hepatic metastases. Slow growth rates and delayed recurrence are common to all islet cell tumors.

PANCREATIC CHOLERA

Diarrhea frequently occurs in patients with the Zollinger-Ellison syndrome, and is the result of the excessive outpouring of gastric secretions into the small bowel. It responds to total gastrectomy or medical control of acid secretion with cimetidine. A

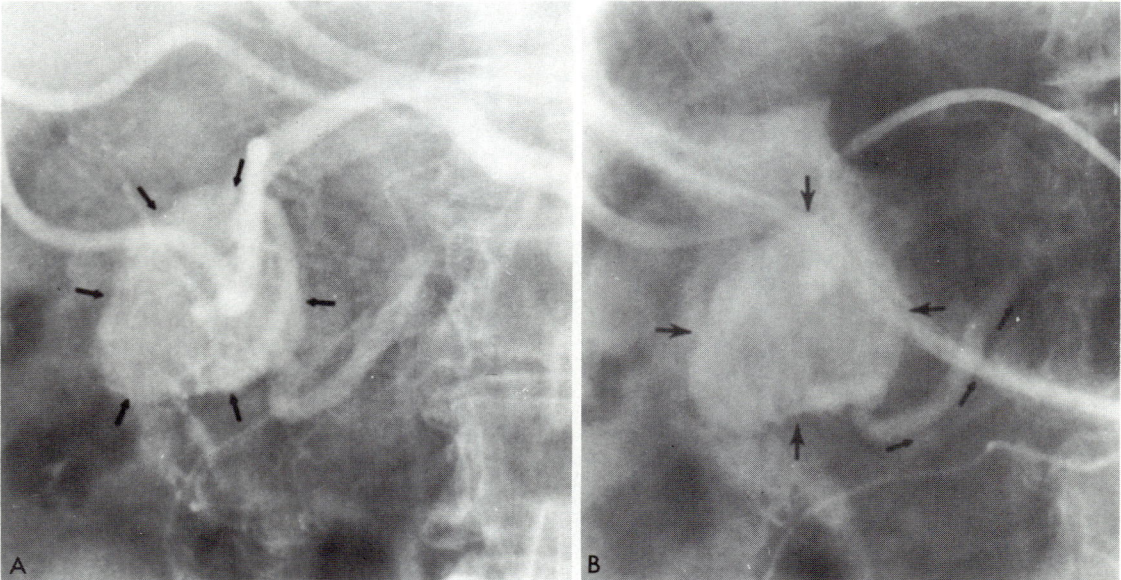

Figure 17–80. Gastrinoma. *A* and *B*, Selective gastroduodenal arteriogram demonstrates a large gastrinoma of the pancreatic head (arrows). Note the dense opacification in the capillary phase of the vein of the pancreatic head (*B*, arrows), from which high gastrin levels could be obtained.

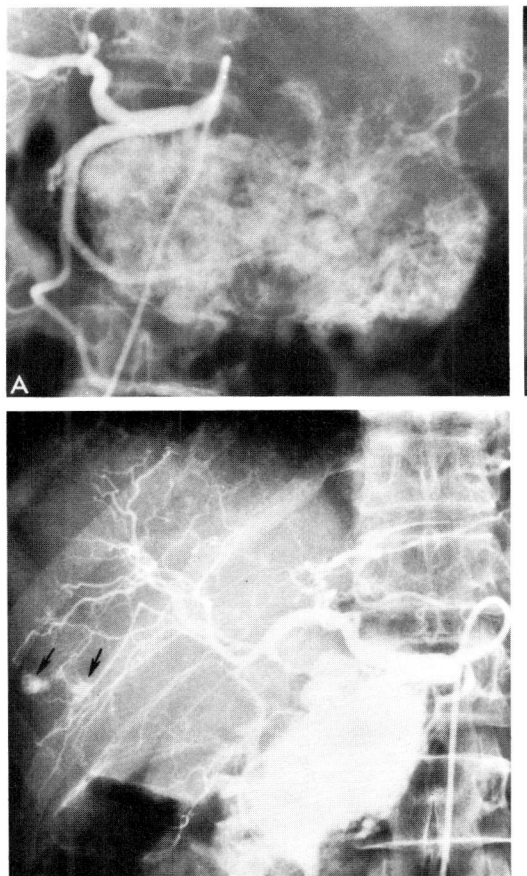

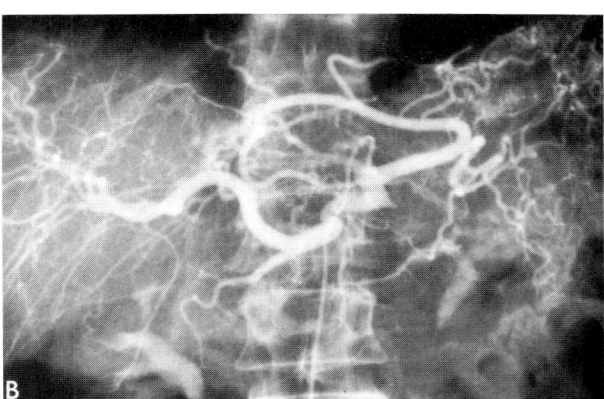

Figure 17–81. Glucagonoma: arteriography. *A,* Large glucagonoma replacing the head and the body of the pancreas. *B,* Following complete resection, the glucagon syndrome remitted and periodic celiac arteriograms were normal for six years. *C,* Tumor recurred in the pancreatic head and liver (arrows) seven years after resection.

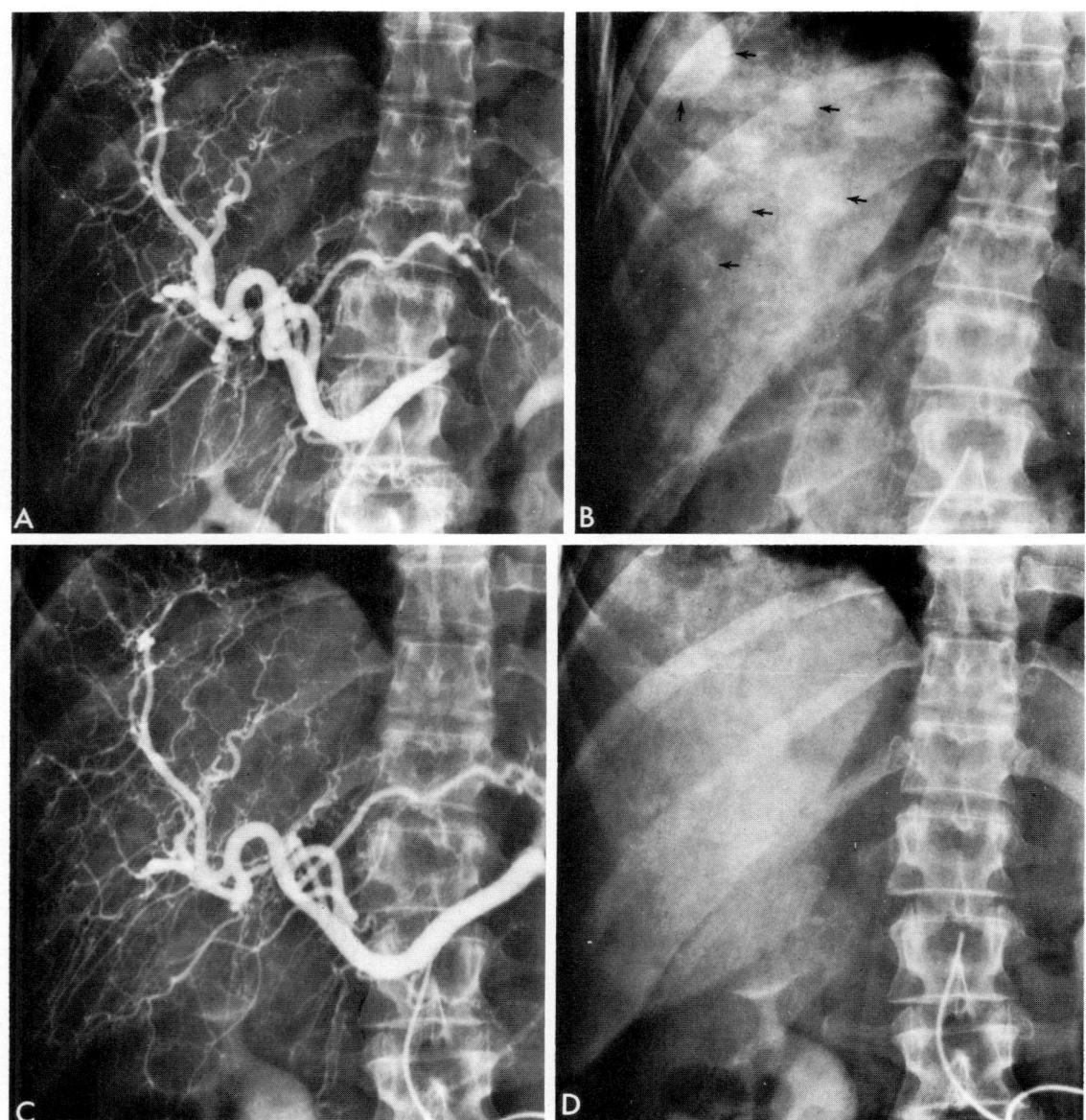

Figure 17–82. Pancreatic cholera: infusion therapy. Selective hepatic arteriograms before (*A* and *B*) and eight weeks after (*C* and *D*) intra-arterial streptozotocin infusion. Hypervascular hepatic metastases (*B*, arrows) disappeared and diarrhea remitted for more than one year.

few patients with non-beta islet cell tumors present with life-threatening diarrhea, basal achlorhydria, and hypokalemia — hence, the designation WDHA (watery diarrhea, hypokalemia, achlorhydria) syndrome. The specific hormone responsible for this syndrome has not been definitely identified, but vasoactive intestinal polypeptide (VIP), gastric inhibitory polypeptide (GIP), and various prostaglandins have been implicated. Aside from displaying signs of intestinal hypersecretion, barium studies are usually negative. Since more than 50 per cent of these tumors are malignant, hypervascular hepatic metastases are frequently demonstrated and may respond dramatically to intra-arterial streptozotocin (Fig. 17–82).[12] Since this drug can be infused as a discrete bolus and is rapidly fixed by the liver, the radiologist may be requested to periodically catherize the hepatic artery for streptozotocin infusion in these patients. Gratifying palliation of a distressing and life-threatening case of diarrhea can be achieved for significant periods of time by this technique.

References

1. Auerbach, R. C., and Koehler, P. R.: Many faces of islet cell tumors. Am. J. Roentgenol. *119*:113–140, 1973.
2. Boijsen, E., and Samuelson, L.: Angiographic diagnosis of tumors arising from pancreatic islets. Acta Radiol. (Diagn.) *10*:161–176, 1970.
3. Bookstein, J. J., and Oberman, H. A.: Appraisal of selective angiography in localizing islet cell tumors of the pancreas. Radiology *86*:682–685, 1966.
4. Clouse, M. E., Costello, P., Legg, M. A., et al.: Subselective angiography in localizing insulinomas of the pancreas. Am. J. Roentgenol. *128*:741–746, 1977.
5. Danforth, D. A., Triche, R., Doppman, J. L., et al.: Elevated plasma proglucagon-like component with a glucagon secreting tumor: Effect of streptozotocin. N. Engl. J. Med. *295*:242–245, 1976.
6. Deutsch, V., Adar, R., Jacob, E. T., et al.: Angiographic diagnosis and differential diagnosis of islet cell tumors. Am. J. Roentgenol. *119*:121–132, 1973.
7. Fulton, R. E., Sheedy, P. F., McGrath, D. C., et al.: Preoperative angiographic localization of insulin producing tumors of the pancreas. Am. J. Roentgenol. *123*:367–377, 1975.
8. Gray, R. K., Rösch, J., and Grollman, J. H., Jr.: Arteriography in the diagnosis of islet cell tumors. Radiology *97*:39–44, 1970.
9. Imhof, H., and Frank, P.: Pancreatic calcifications in malignant islet cell tumors. Radiology *122*:333–357, 1977.
10. Ingemansson, S., Lunderquist, A., and Holst, J.: Selective catheterization of the pancreatic vein for radioimmunoassay in glucagon secreting carcinoma of the pancreas. Arch. Surg. *119*:555–556, 1976.
11. Ingemansson, S., Larsson, L., Lunderquist, A., et al.: Pancreatic vein catheterization with gastrin assay in normal patients and in patients with the Zollinger-Ellison syndrome. Am. J. Surg. *134*:558–563, 1977.
12. Kahn, R. C., Levy, A. G., Gardner, J. D., et al.: Pancreatic cholera: beneficial effects of treatment with streptozotocin. N. Engl. J. Med. *292*:941, 1975.
13. Korobkin, M. T., Palubinskas, A. J., and Glickman, M. G.: Pitfalls in arteriography of islet cell tumors of pancreas. Radiology *100*:319, 1971.
14. Reuter, S. R.: Potential overdiagnosis of pancreatic islet cell adenomas. J. Can. Assoc. Radiol. *22*:184–186, 1971.
15. Robins, J. M., Bookstein, J. J., Oberman, H. A., et al.: Selective angiography in localizing islet cell tumors of pancreas: Further appraisal. Radiology *106*:525–528, 1973.
16. Schein, P. S., De Lellis, R. A., Kahn, R. C., et al.: Islet cell tumors. Current concepts and management. Ann. Intern. Med. *79*:239–257, 1973.
17. Zboralski, F. F., and Amberg, J. R.: Detection of Zollinger-Ellison syndrome: the radiologist's responsibility. Am. J. Roentgenol. *104*:529–543, 1968.
18. Zollinger, R. M., and Ellison, E. H.: Primary peptic ulcerations of the jejunum associated with islet cell tumors of the pancreas. Ann. Surg. *142*:709–728, 1955.

18

THE SPLEEN

ROBERT E. KOEHLER, M.D.
RONALD G. EVENS, M.D.

When confronted with the problem of evaluating splenic disease, the surgeon finds that diagnostic radiology offers several possible ways to obtain information. The size, shape, and position of the spleen can be easily demonstrated by a number of methods. In addition, radionuclide scanning provides information related to a number of physiologic aspects of splenic function. Selective angiography demonstrates the vascular anatomy of the spleen and, in some cases, provides information regarding lesions within the spleen. The newer modalities of ultrasound and computed tomography offer noninvasive means of investigating diffuse or focal pathologic processes. A clear understanding of the relative usefulness of these different radiologic modalities is needed in order to obtain the most diagnostic information with the least risk and cost to the patient.

A number of radiographic techniques are also applicable to the study of complications following splenectomy. Here again, the appropriate choice of diagnostic procedure depends on familiarity with the relative usefulness of each imaging modality in a variety of situations.

HISTORICAL ASPECTS

Radiology has played a role in the evaluation of diseases involving the spleen since the early twentieth century.[13] The earliest techniques consisted of plain film examinations of the abdomen for evaluation of the size and shape of the spleen. Insufflation of air into the stomach or large intestine was sometimes used to obtain better delineation of the spleen. Soon thereafter, diagnostic pneumoperitoneum came into use as an aid in the radiographic diagnosis of abnormalities of the spleen and other abdominal organs; pneumoretroperitoneum was applied as a method in subsequent years. Although these techniques afford good images of the splenic contour, they have been supplanted by newer and less invasive methods and are no longer in common use.

These early methods were limited to providing information on splenic size and shape and were not useful in detecting focal lesions within the spleen or abnormalities in splenic function. In 1930, intravenous Thorotrast (colloidal thorium dioxide) was first used for hepatosplenography. This procedure provided excellent opacification of the spleen and liver and demonstrated focal mass lesions as filling defects. By 1950, Thorotrast studies were all but completely abandoned, since the permanent deposition of radioactive thorium dioxide in the reticuloendothelial tissues proved to be carcinogenic. In the 1950's splenoportography and selective celiac and splenic arteriography provided means of determining the factors responsible for splenomegaly. Splenoportography evaluates the morphologic condition and blood flow patterns of the portal venous system and delineates the site and severity of obstruction to portal venous blood. Selective splenic arteriography determines the existence, size, and distribution of lesions within the spleen and has been very helpful in the evaluation of patients with possible splenic trauma.

The first radionuclide images of the spleen were performed in the early 1960's after the discovery that "heat-treated" red cells previously labeled with chromium-51 (^{51}Cr) localized in the normal spleen. This technique was based on earlier findings that erythrocytes could be labeled with ^{51}Cr for quantifying red cell volume and red cell survival *in vivo*. In 1964, it was noted that treating red cells with isotopes of mercury resulted in both isotopic labeling of the red cells and damage to the cell membrane, causing the labeled cells to localize in the spleen. Splenic imaging by mercurial alteration of red cells, although technically easier than heat treating, resulted in a relatively high radiation dose to the patient, particularly to the kidneys. As colloidal agents that could be easily tagged with various isotopes became available in the late 1960's, spleen scanning became a routine procedure in most centers. Technetium-99m (^{99m}Tc) sulfur colloid is currently the most commonly used radiopharmaceutical for splenic imaging.

The most recent developments in the radiologic evaluation of the spleen have been ultrasound and computed tomography. Ultrasound has proved to be particularly suitable for the evaluation of cysts and other fluid-filled masses of the spleen. At this time, experience with computed tomography (CT) of the spleen is limited, but this modality has already been shown to be useful in the evaluation of splenic trauma and focal pathologic conditions within the spleen. Splenic size can be determined by either CT or ultrasound, and additional applications are expected to be developed in the future.

RADIOLOGY OF THE NORMAL SPLEEN

The spleen is normally surrounded by a considerable amount of retroperitoneal and intra-abdominal fat. For this reason, many of the borders of the spleen may be visible on plain radiographs of the left upper abdomen (Fig. 18–1). Films obtained for the evaluation of spleen size and position are best taken in the frontal and left posterior oblique projections. On films of this type the lateral and inferior margins of the spleen are usually well seen, and splenic length can often be measured. Normally the spleen does not exceed 14 cm in length. The medial border of the spleen, particularly its upper half, is more difficult to visualize on plain films.

Plain film tomography can be used as an adjunct for the evaluation of the spleen when its size and shape cannot be assessed from standard radiographs. The medial border and the structures around the splenic hilus can often be seen on tomograms of the left upper abdomen (Fig. 18–2).

The upper half of the spleen often lies adjacent to the gastric fundus or the greater curvature of the body of the stomach. An indentation on the gastric air shadow or a barium-filled stomach on upper gastrointestinal examination sometimes indicates the

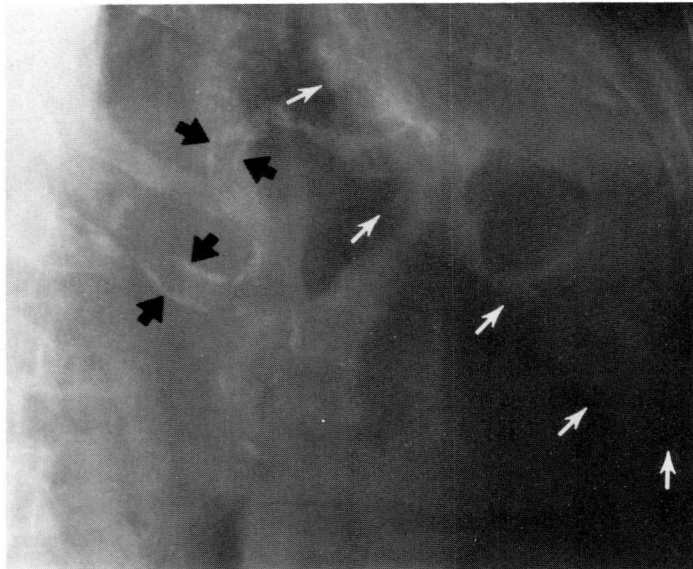

Figure 18–1. Normal spleen (white arrows) visible on a plain radiograph of the left upper abdomen. There is calcification in the wall of the splenic artery (black arrows).

position of the upper pole of the spleen (Fig. 18–3). This is also true of the barium enema examination, in which the position and size of the spleen in some patients may be accurately inferred from the position of the splenic flexure of the colon.

The splenic artery is frequently involved with calcific atherosclerotic disease in older patients and therefore is often visible on plain films as a series of curvilinear calcifications in the left upper abdomen (see Fig. 18–1). The splenic vein is often identifiable at the time of nephrotomography (Fig. 18–4) but is rarely seen on plain films. Confusion sometimes arises on intravenous urography regarding the differentia-

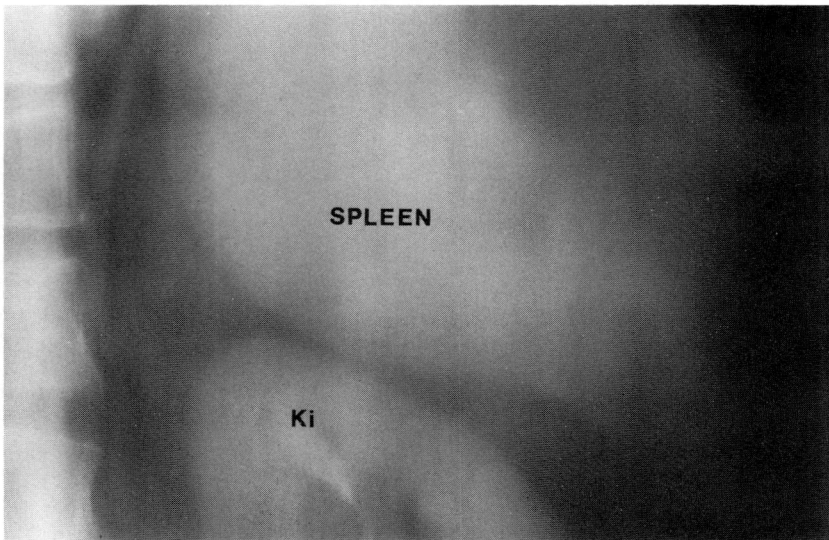

Figure 18–2. The spleen is well seen on this tomogram of the left upper abdomen obtained during intravenous urography. (Ki = left kidney.)

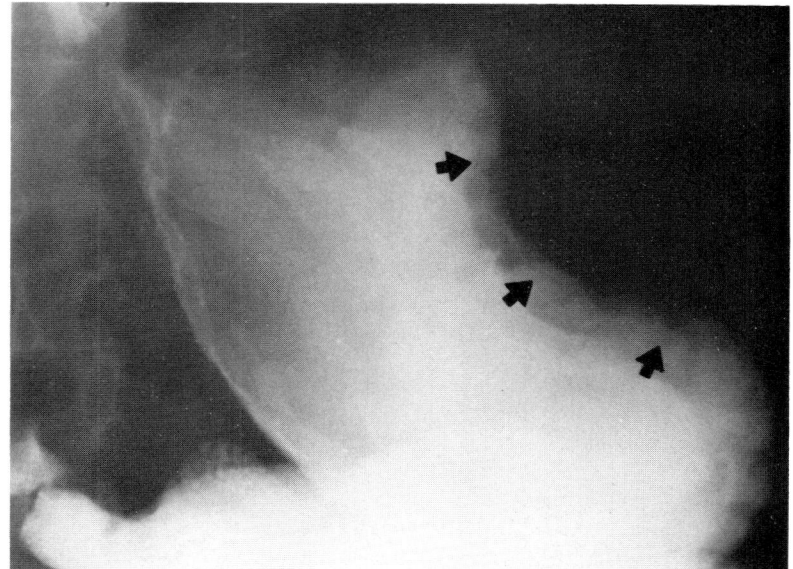

Figure 18–3. Normal splenic impression (arrows) on the barium-filled stomach seen on upper gastrointestinal examination.

tion of a tortuous splenic vein from a mass in the region of the upper pole of the left kidney.

A much better image of the spleen and its vessels can be obtained angiographically. In most centers, splenic angiography is performed via a percutaneous femoral arteriotomy with a preshaped catheter. The tip of the catheter is positioned in the splenic artery, and iodinated contrast material is injected while films are taken in rapid succession. Films obtained during the arterial phase show the splenic artery and its short gastric branches to the greater curvature of the stomach (Fig. 18–5A). The splenic artery is normally tortuous, particularly in older patients. Films taken during the capillary phase show a uniform parenchymal blush as the contrast passes through the

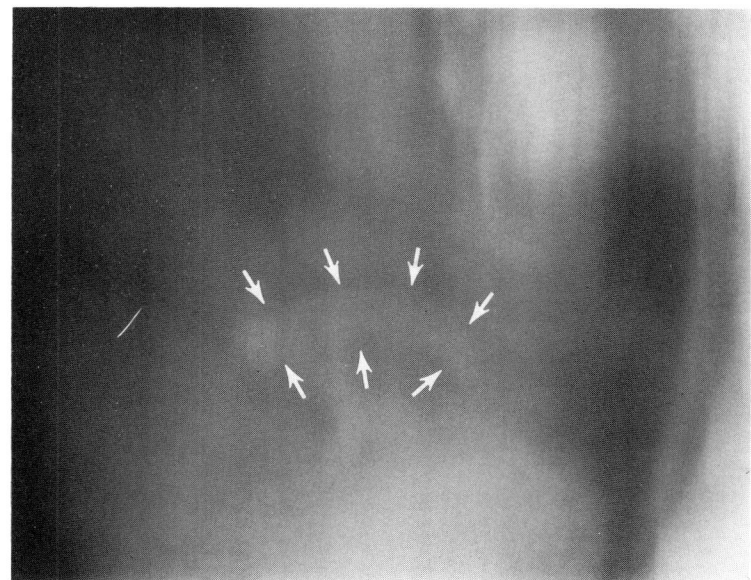

Figure 18–4. The splenic vein (arrows) is often faintly visualized at the time of nephrotomography and should not be confused with a suprarenal mass.

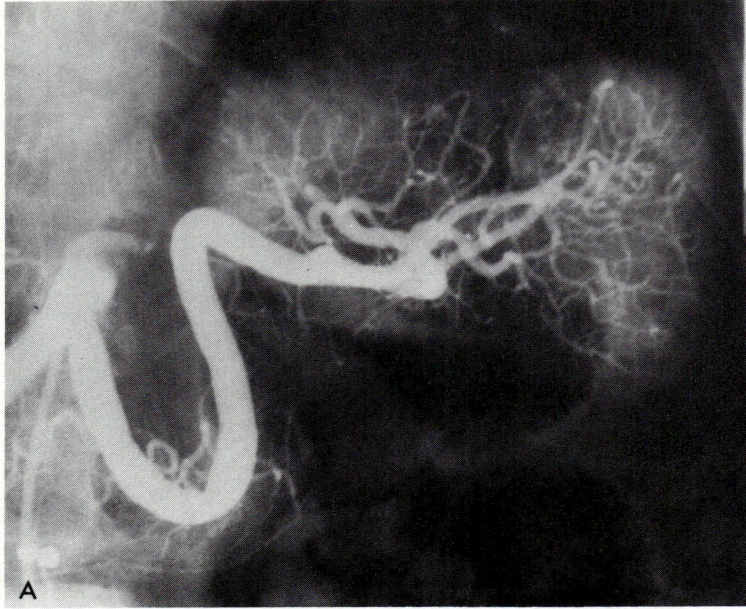
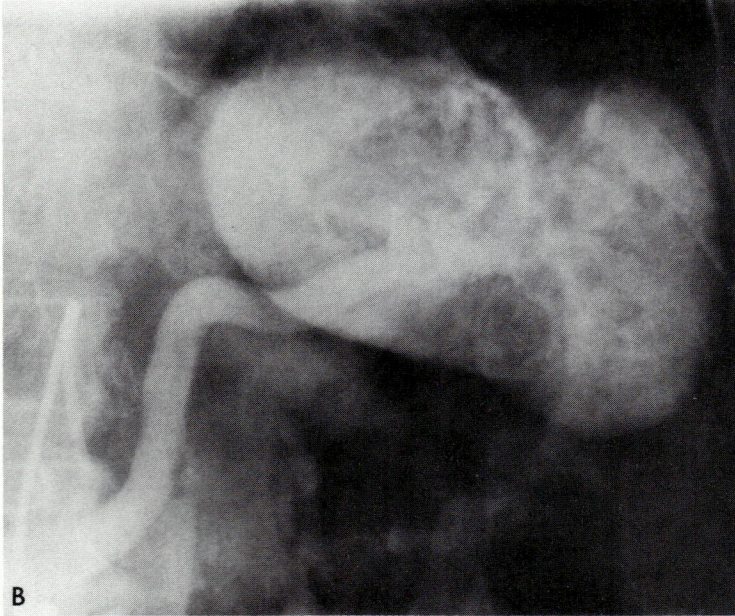

Figure 18–5. Normal splenic arteriogram. *A*, Film taken during the arterial phase shows the splenic artery and its branches. *B*, Film taken during the venous phase shows relatively uniform opacification of the splenic parenchyma and a well-opacified splenic vein.

splenic pulp, demonstrating clearly the size, shape, and position of the spleen. Films taken during the venous phase of the injection show the size and position of the splenic vein (Fig. 18–5B). The patterns and direction of flow of splenic venous blood can also be ascertained.

There are two major methods of obtaining radionuclide images of the spleen.[15] Either colloidal radiopharmaceuticals, for example, ^{99m}Tc sulfur colloid, or damaged red cells labeled with ^{51}Cr or ^{99m}Tc can be used. Both are trapped by reticuloendothelial cells in the spleen. Satisfactory diagnostic images can be obtained with a gamma camera or retilinear scanner. The normal spleen is visualized as an oval structure with blunted

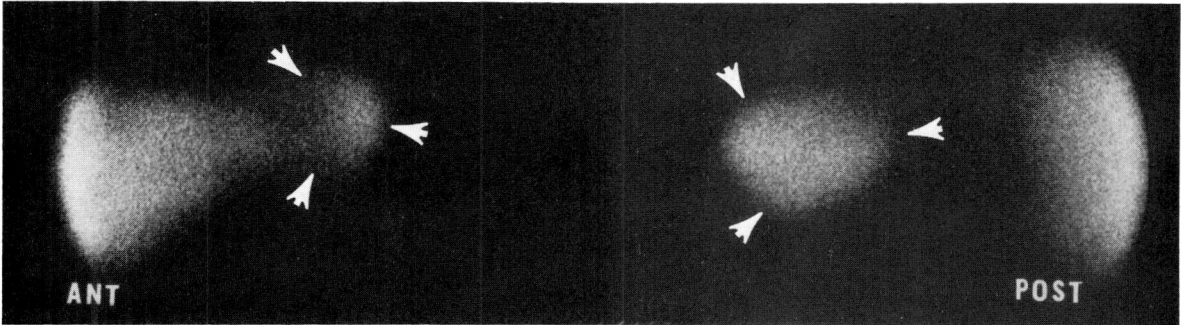
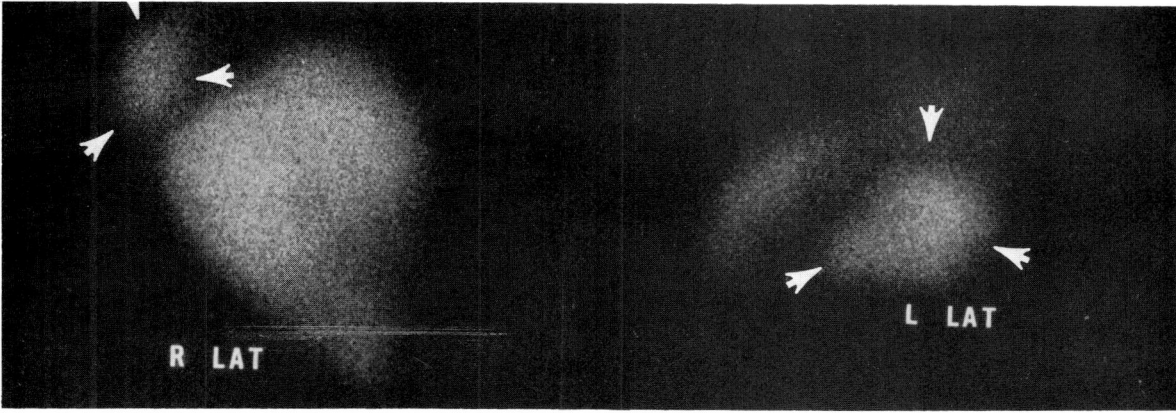

Figure 18–6. A normal spleen scan utilizing technetium sulfur colloid and a gamma camera. Both the spleen (arrows) and the liver are visualized; the spleen is best seen on the posterior and left lateral views.

ends lying directly beneath the diaphragm, its lateral margin adjacent to the left lateral abdominal wall (Fig. 18–6). The spleen is best identified in the posterior and left lateral views, on which it is closest to the imaging instrument. The splenic hilus is usually identified as an indentation on the medial margin, but there is great variability in its position and size.

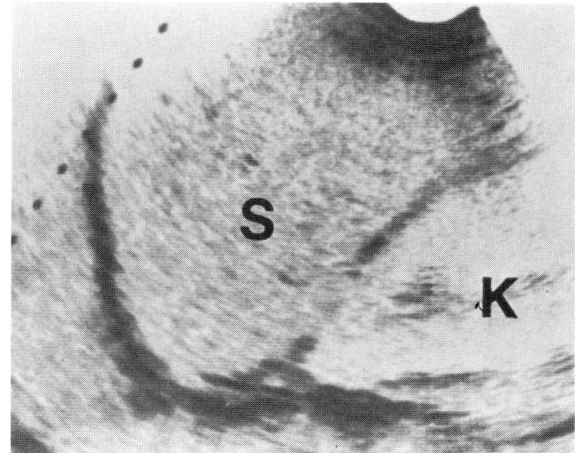

Figure 18–7. Sonogram of a normal spleen (S) and the upper pole of adjacent left kidney (K). The scan was performed along the axis of the ninth intercostal space.

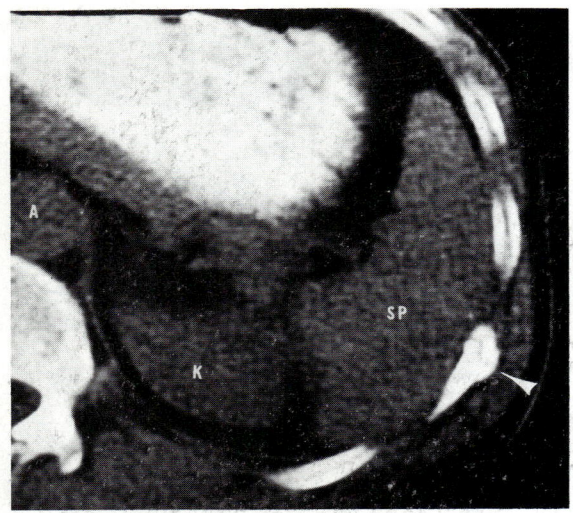

Figure 18–8. Computed tomographic scan of a normal spleen (SP). The thickened area of the adjacent rib (arrowhead) represents a healed fracture. Note the close relationship of the spleen to the adjacent ribs. (K = kidney; A = aorta.)

Several methods for quantifying splenic volume from radionuclide scans have been suggested, but these are subject to considerable error because of the wide range of normal splenic shapes. The most widely used measure of splenic size is the splenic length in the posterior or left lateral view. A length exceeding 15 cm is good evidence of splenomegaly, and a measurement of 13 to 15 cm is considered borderline. The spleen is a relatively mobile and pliable organ, and its position and shape can be modified by the position of the patient and the location and size of the surrounding structures. This mobility can be useful in evaluating the spleen. For example, if the patient is placed in a right lateral decubitus position, the spleen can be made to fall medially so that it can be separated from the left lobe of the liver on the scan.

On ultrasonographic examination the spleen appears as an ovoid area with relatively few internal echoes, and its borders can often be well delineated. By increasing the gain on modern gray-scale ultrasound equipment, however, it is possible to bring out a homogeneous pattern of fine internal echoes and to demonstrate the vascular structures within the spleen (Fig. 18–7). Ultrasound can also be used to determine spleen size. Scans are often best obtained by placing the patient in the right lateral decubitus position. The technique usually employed involves scanning the spleen longitudinally along the overlying rib interspaces. Sector scans through these interspaces can give a transverse image of the spleen as well. Transverse scans obtained in the supine position are less useful, because gas in the stomach or splenic flexure of the colon casts a shadow over the area of the spleen.

Computed tomography invariably produces excellent images of the spleen. The normal spleen is imaged as an ovoid shadow in the left upper abdomen with sharply defined borders and homogeneous soft tissue density (Fig. 18–8). CT scans of the spleen also demonstrate the splenic artery and vein in many patients (Fig. 18–9). The close relationship between the splenic vein and the posterior aspect of the body and tail of the pancreas is particularly well seen. In some cases, the splenic vein and adjacent pancreas are clearly distinguishable by CT, whereas in other cases they are inseparable and appear as one structure. In such cases, one must avoid overestimating the thickness of the body and tail of the pancreas. Occasionally, the lucent line caused by the thin layer of fat lying between the splenic vein and the posterior aspect of the pancreas mimics the CT appearance of a dilated pancreatic duct.

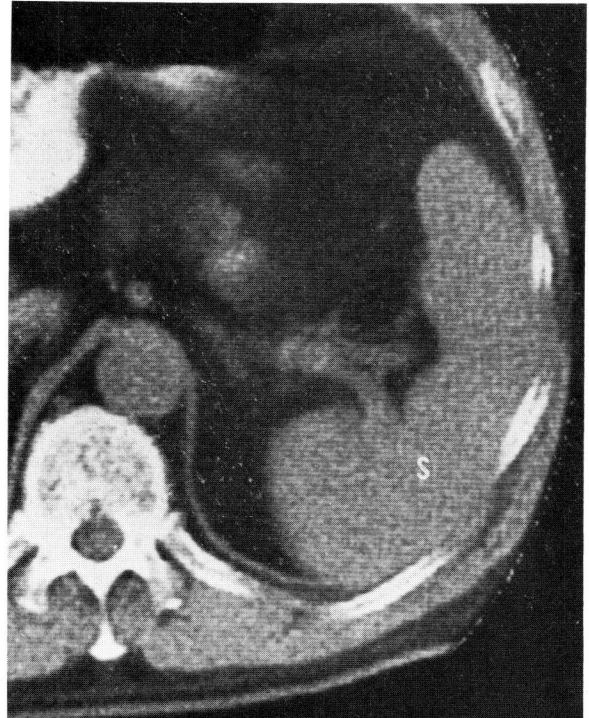

Figure 18–9. CT scan of a normal spleen (S) showing splenic vein branches in the splenic hilus.

Anatomic Variants

In some patients, a lobulation of the spleen projects medially and may lie between the tail of the pancreas and the anterior aspect of the left kidney. In such cases, this splenic morphologic variant can simulate a retroperitoneal mass. On intravenous urography, spleens of this configuration may mimic a mass arising from the upper pole of the kidney (Fig. 18–10). Nephrotomography usually permits distinction between an upper-pole renal mass and a splenic lobulation or mass by demonstrating the continuity of the presumed mass shadow with the remainder of the splenic outline. Problems of this nature also arise in the interpretation of ultrasound scans of the left upper abdomen (Fig. 18–11).[6] Because of the transonic nature of the spleen, a portion of the spleen lying between the pancreas and kidney can mimic the appearance of a pancreatic pseudocyst. By the use of computed tomography, it is usually a simple matter to distinguish masses of the kidney or pancreas from variations in splenic location and shape.

When the ligamentous attachments of the spleen are deficient or very lax, the spleen may assume an unusual position and may mimic an abdominal mass. This condition, sometimes referred to as floating or wandering spleen, is rare and occurs most often in women of childbearing age. Splenic enlargement may also be a predisposing factor, since many patients have had associated splenomegaly from various causes. Although most cases of wandering spleen are probably asymptomatic, some patients experience intermittent abdominal discomfort, apparently related to tension on splenic ligaments and possibly to splenic congestion. Torsion of the vascular pedicle has been reported and can lead to splenic congestion or infarction, causing acute abdominal pain.[7]

The diagnosis of wandering spleen is seldom made preoperatively, but there are

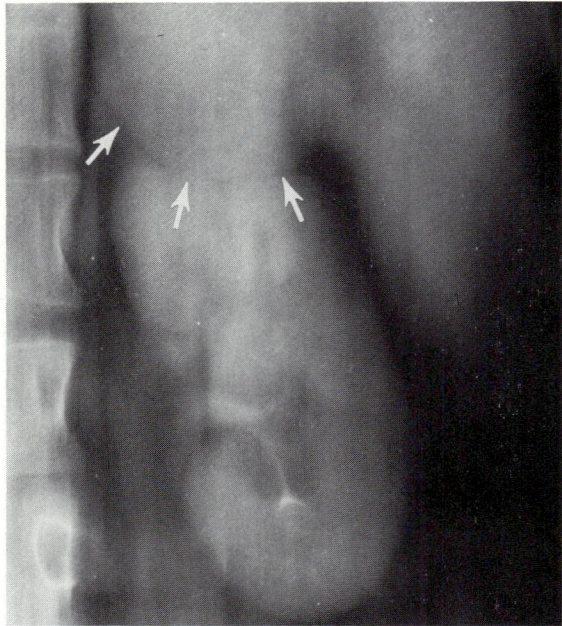

Figure 18–10. Tomogram taken during intravenous urography shows an impression on the left kidney suggestive of a suprarenal mass (arrows). On CT is was evident that this represented a medial lobulation of the spleen and not a mass.

several radiographic findings that may suggest the diagnosis. On the plain film the normal splenic shadow is absent, and a central abdominal or left flank mass may be seen. On intravenous urography the left kidney may be elevated. A barium enema may show a mass extrinsic to the gastrointestinal tract and medial displacement of the

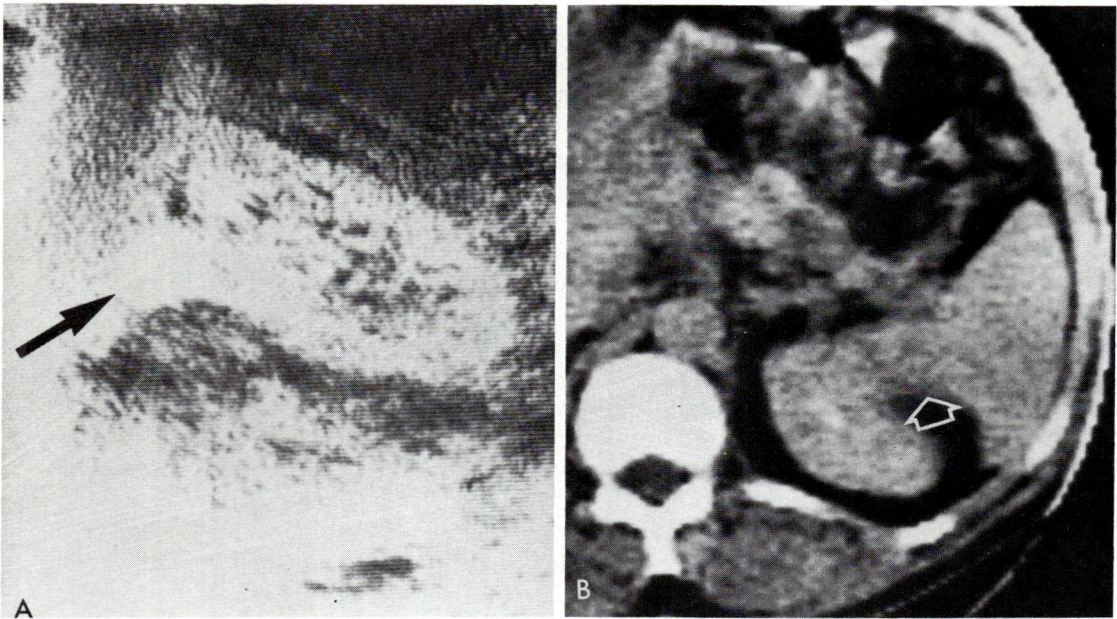

Figure 18–11. Prone longitudinal sonogram of a 49-year-old man. *A*, A sonolucent mass (arrow) anterosuperior to the left kidney that was thought to represent a cyst in the tail of the pancreas. *B*, CT scan of the same patient shows a lobulation of the spleen (arrow) lying immediately adjacent to the left kidney, which simulated a mass on ultrasound examination. (*From* Gooding, G. A. W.: The ultrasonic and computed tomographic appearance of splenic lobulations. Radiology 126:719–720, 1978.)

splenic flexure of the colon. A characteristic bandlike impression on the splenic flexure by the elongated splenic pedicle is sometimes present. The stomach may be inverted, its greater curvature lying under the left hemidiaphragm. Radionuclide scan shows inferomedial displacement of the spleen, but if torsion of the splenic pedicle has occurred there may be no splenic uptake. Arteriography has been employed only rarely but can be used to establish the diagnosis.[14]

Anomalous orientation of the spleen can also occur without ligamentous laxity. The term "upside-down spleen" denotes an anatomic variant in which the splenic hilus is directed superiorly or laterally and the convex splenic border is adjacent to the kidney. In this position the spleen often mimics a suprarenal mass on intravenous urography. A radionuclide scan shows concave superior and convex inferior borders of the spleen and often resolves the problem. Arteriography can be diagnostic but is seldom necessary. CT is helpful in demonstrating a high transverse spleen and the absence of a separate suprarenal mass.

ACCESSORY SPLEENS

Embryologically, the spleen forms by a coalescence of multiple buds of splenic tissue in the dorsal mesogastrium. Accessory spleens, thought to result from the failure of one or more of these buds to fuse, are found in 10 to 30 per cent of individuals and are often multiple. Accessory spleens vary in size from microscopic deposits of splenic tissue to well-defined spheric or ovoid structures as large as 4 cm in diameter. They are most commonly found in the splenic hilus near the course of the splenic artery or one of its major branches. Occasionally, accessory spleens occur in the tail of the pancreas or in the suspensory ligaments of the spleen. Rarely, they are found in the wall of the stomach or in more distant locations, such as the greater omentum, the mesentery, the bowel, the pelvis, or even the scrotum.[8]

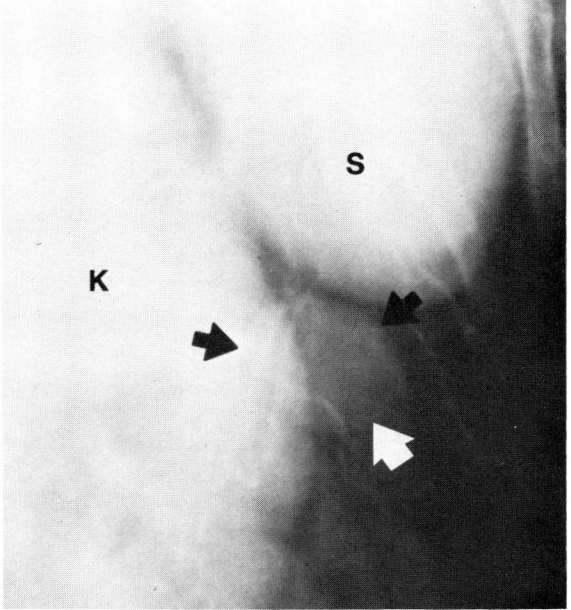

Figure 18–12. Small accessory spleen (arrows) between the lower pole of the spleen (S) and the kidney (K) that was found incidentally during abdominal arteriography.

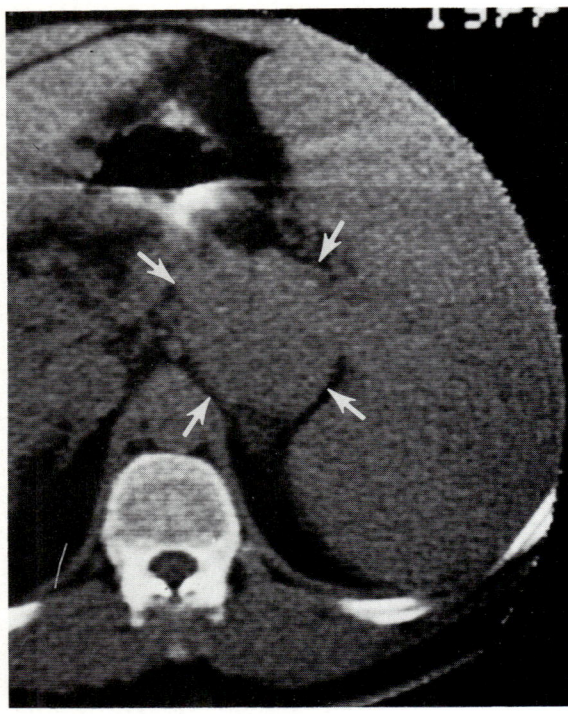

Figure 18–13. CT scan of a patient with malignant lymphoma and splenomegaly. The rounded mass (arrows) adjacent to the splenic hilus is an accessory spleen enlarged by lymphomatous involvement.

While accessory spleens are usually of no clinical significance, their recognition and detection become important in certain situations. When they are large or occur in an unusual location, accessory spleens can simulate an abdominal or retroperitoneal mass. They may be mistaken for pancreatic, adrenal, or retroperitoneal tumors on angiography. Enlargement usually occurs in patients with systemic diseases that lead to splenomegaly. After splenectomy, accessory spleens can enlarge and take on the function of the normal spleen. It is particularly important to identify accessory spleens in patients who have had splenectomies for hematologic disorders resulting in hypersplenism. In these cases the accessory spleen may take on the pathologic activity of the previously removed spleen, leading to a relapse of the patient's disease.

Accessory spleens can be difficult to diagnose, particularly when they are atypical in location or smaller than 2 cm in size. Radionuclide images may be helpful in identifying the location of the accessory splenic tissue. The usual approach is to scan initially with ^{99m}Tc sulfur colloid. If the ^{99m}Tc sulfur colloid scan is not successful, scanning should be performed with red cells, a method that is particularly useful in identifying accessory splenic tissue that lies adjacent to the liver. This is because normal liver uptake of the ^{99m}Tc sulfur colloid can obscure the adjacent small focus of splenic tissue.

Angiography can also be used to locate accessory spleens.[5] Typically, accessory spleens receive their blood supply from a branch of the splenic artery. During the capillary phase, the accessory spleen develops a homogeneous blush similar to that seen in the normal spleen (Fig. 18–12). Occasionally, even the accessory splenic vein may be visualized.

There is a growing amount of experience with the detection of accessory spleens by computed tomography (Fig. 18–13). This may be particularly useful following splenectomy or when the accessory spleen is enlarged by systemic disease.

HYPERSPLENISM

Hypersplenism may be defined as an abnormal increase in the destruction of blood elements by the spleen. The causes of hypersplenism are many,[12] and the radiologic evaluation of various body systems is often helpful in the differential diagnosis.

Splenomegaly usually, but not always, accompanies hypersplenism. There are no rigid radiographic criteria for the diagnosis of splenic enlargement, since the dimensions of normal spleens in some persons overlap those of mildly enlarged spleens in others. Splenic length exceeding 14 cm should raise the suspicion of splenomegaly, however. It may be helpful to look at the shape of the spleen. The normal spleen is elongated and flattened from its medial to lateral aspects. Splenomegaly should be considered when the spleen takes on a more globular configuration. The appearance of medial displacement of the gas-filled splenic flexure of the colon is usually displaced inferiorly and medially (Fig. 18–14). Barium studies of the gastrointestinal tract may confirm these findings or make them more obvious (Fig. 18–15). Ultrasound and CT offer direct, noninvasive means of evaluating the extent of splenomegaly. Arteriography can also be used but is rarely necessary to define splenic size, except in problematic cases (Fig. 18–16).

Imaging with ^{99m}Tc sulfur colloid may be of value in identifying an enlarged spleen (greater than 14 cm in length), but this does not identify the spleen as a source of blood element destruction. The functional degree of hypersplenism can be evaluated by the injection of ^{51}Cr-labeled damaged red cells and daily measurements of isotope levels over the spleen, liver, and precordium (blood pool). If the ratio of counts of spleen to liver or precordium exceeds 2:1, then hypersplenism is said to be present. This counting technique is subject to several possible errors involving, among other things,

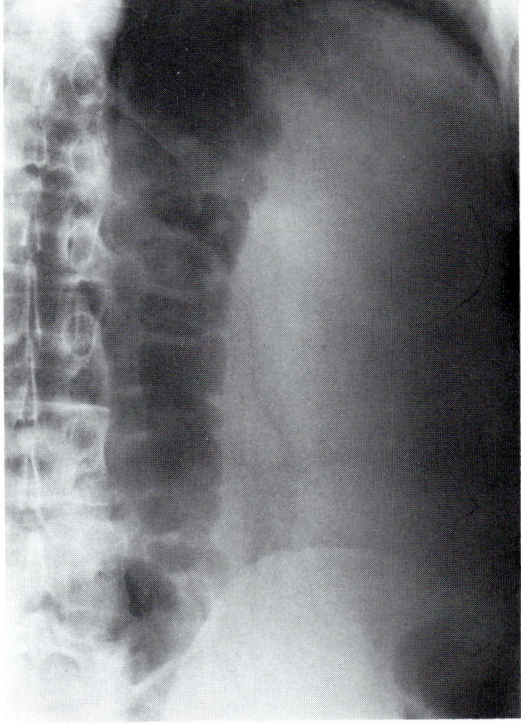

Figure 18–14. Massive splenomegaly in a patient with polycythemia vera. The spleen appears as a large soft tissue mass displacing the gas-filled splenic flexure medially.

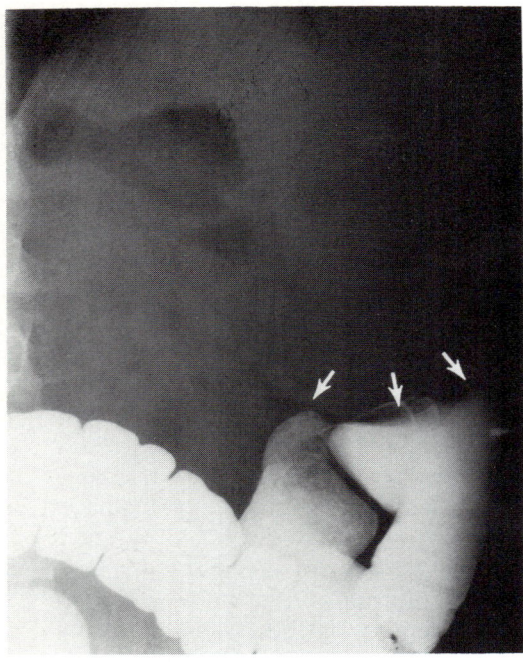

Figure 18–15. Enlarged spleen causing inferior displacement of the splenic flexure of the colon (arrows) demonstrated with a barium enema.

the positioning of the counting probes and the relative sizes of the liver and the spleen. For example, a markedly enlarged spleen has increased isotope accumulation even without increased splenic destruction of red cells. This technique should not be considered strictly quantitative.

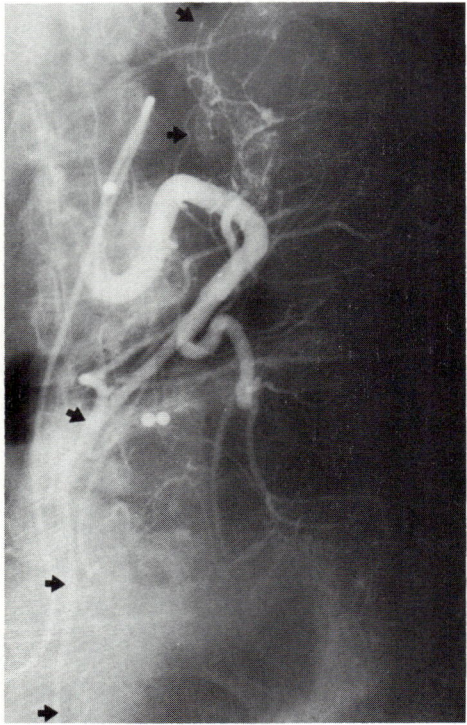

Figure 18–16. Selective splenic arteriogram of an elderly woman with a large left abdominal mass originally thought not to represent the spleen, since it showed no uptake on a ^{99m}Tc sulfur colloid liver-spleen scan. Splenic artery branches (arrows) are draped around the huge spleen, which was subsequently found to be involved with chronic lymphocytic lymphoma.

TRAUMA

The spleen is a common site of injury in cases of blunt or penetrating abdominal trauma. Massive splenic rupture is a surgical emergency that has a significant mortality rate. Even seemingly minor injuries to the spleen may be the site of significant bleeding and are potentially dangerous. Splenectomy has usually been performed in all cases of splenic injury to stop bleeding or to prevent the occurrence of delayed rupture. Recently, however, it has been learned that after splenectomy, young children are susceptible to severe sepsis caused by *Diplococcus pneumoniae* or other bacteria. For this reason, some surgeons now recommend the avoidance of splenectomy in children younger than five whenever possible.[4] Splenic injury in this age group is sometimes managed by partial splenectomy or by suturing the laceration.[2]

In cases of extensive injury to the spleen, abdominal plain films usually show highly specific abnormalities. Splenomegaly is often present (Fig. 18–17). In the appropriate clinical setting the appearance of progressive splenic enlargement on serial films is suggestive of splenic hematoma. The margins of the spleen may be indistinct owing to the presence of blood in the left upper abdomen. There may be obliteration of the margins of the left kidney and the psoas muscle for the same reason. Fractures of one or more of the left lower ribs should raise the suspicion of splenic injury (see Fig. 18–8).

Free blood in the peritoneal cavity produces the same plain film abnormalities as are seen with ascites. Blood displaces the liver edge from the fat of the posterior abdomen, so that the right inferolateral hepatic angle becomes invisible on the radiograph. Blood collects in the posterolateral abdominal gutters and displaces the ascending and descending portions of the colon from the adjacent properitoneal fat stripes. Blood also collects in the pelvis and may produce a homogeneous gray density above the urinary bladder.

Radionuclide scanning can be used to good advantage in the evaluation of patients with possible splenic injury. A rate of diagnostic accuracy as high as 90 per cent has

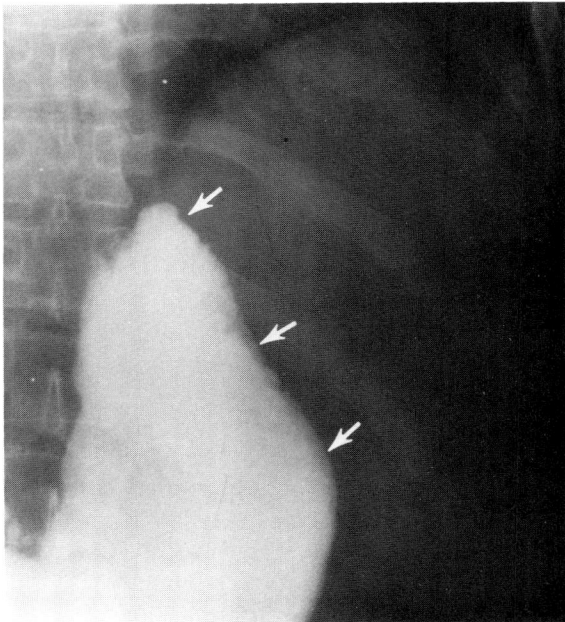

Figure 18–17. Upper gastrointestinal series taken of a patient with fullness in the left upper quadrant two weeks after he fell from a horse. The splenic shadow is enlarged and displaces the stomach medially (arrows). A subcapsular splenic hematoma was found at surgery.

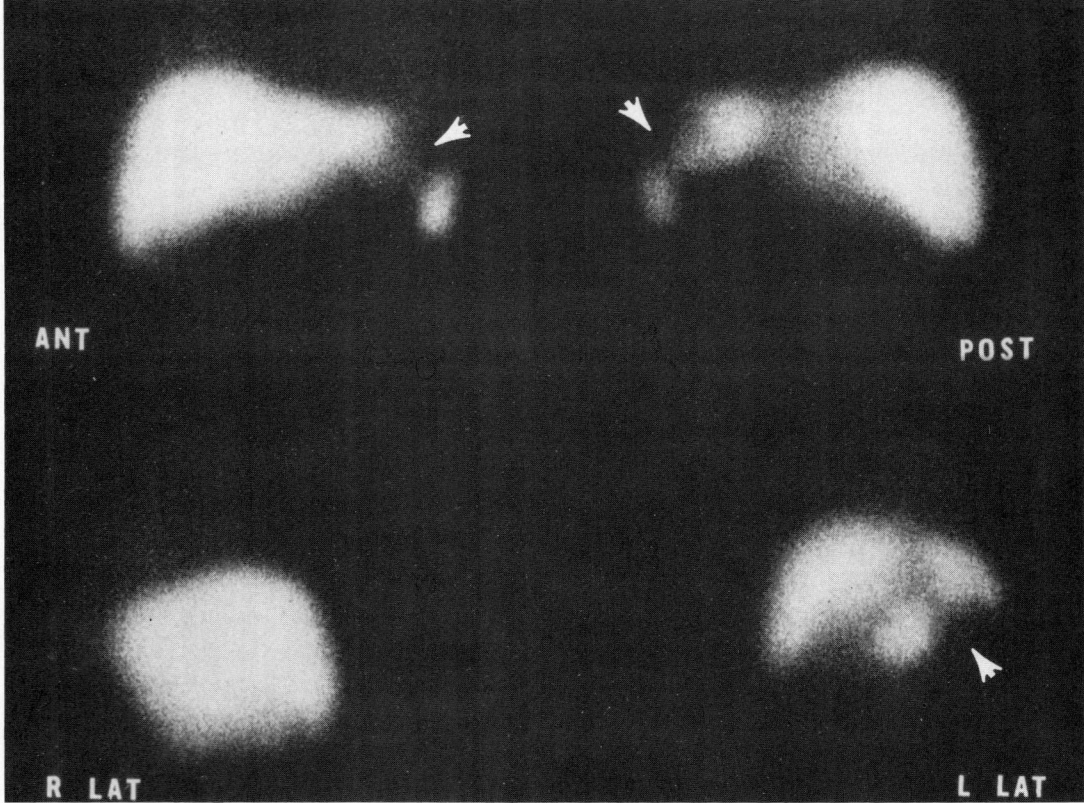

Figure 18–18. Splenic laceration and subcapsular hematoma. The patient was involved in a bicycle accident the day before this scan was performed and noted increasing left upper quadrant pain. The spleen was not palpable. The large filling defect (arrows) is in the superior portion of the spleen.

been found in some centers.[12] Negative defects are seen at sites of splenic lacerations (Fig. 18–18). Concave or wedge defects may occur with subcapsular hematomas. Care must be exercised in interpreting the results of a positive radionuclide spleen study, however, since abnormalities of the scan are not specific for trauma and may reflect other types of splenic disease.

Selective splenic arteriography can be used to evaluate possible splenic trauma when the clinical findings and the results of other radiographic studies are equivocal. The demonstration of disruption of arteries or of extravasation of contrast material is highly specific for splenic injury. Arteriovenous shunting also may take place and cause early venous opacification (Fig. 18–19). Arterial displacement and stretching around an avascular intrasplenic or subcapsular mass suggest the presence of hematoma (Fig. 18–20). Occasionally, the arteriogram shows only displacement of the spleen from the abdominal wall and diaphragm; this sign is less specific.

Ultrasound is rarely used for the preoperative evaluation of possible splenic trauma, but it has been helpful in a few reported cases.[1]

Clear images of subcapsular splenic hematomas can sometimes by produced by computed tomography (Fig. 18–21). At the time of this writing, however, there is too little experience with this modality to indicate its overall usefulness in the evaluation of possible splenic trauma. It seems reasonable to examine the spleen by CT in cases not resolved by radionuclide scan before resorting to arteriography.

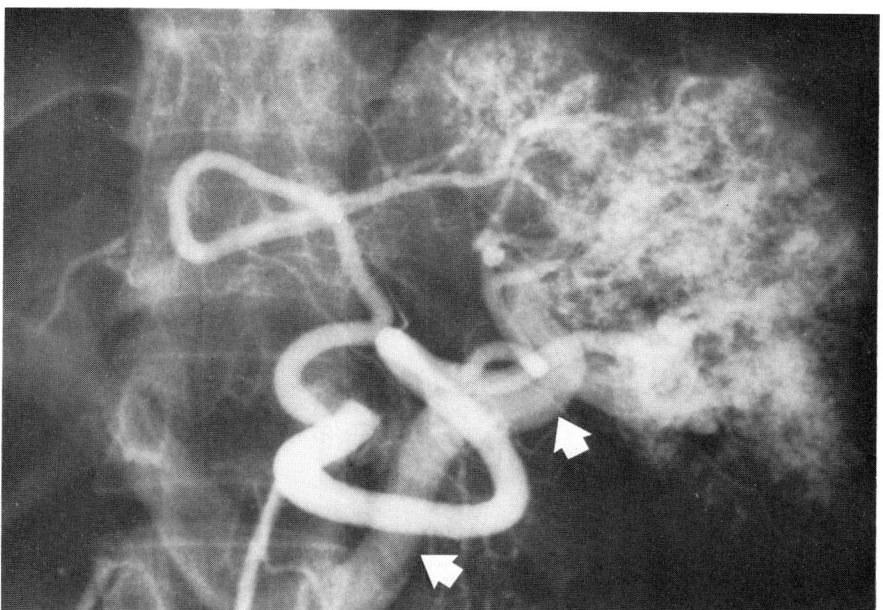

Figure 18–19. Arterial phase film from a splenic arteriogram taken after splenic trauma shows multiple areas of extravasation throughout the splenic pulp. Early filling of the splenic vein (arrows) indicates arteriovenous shunting in the spleen.

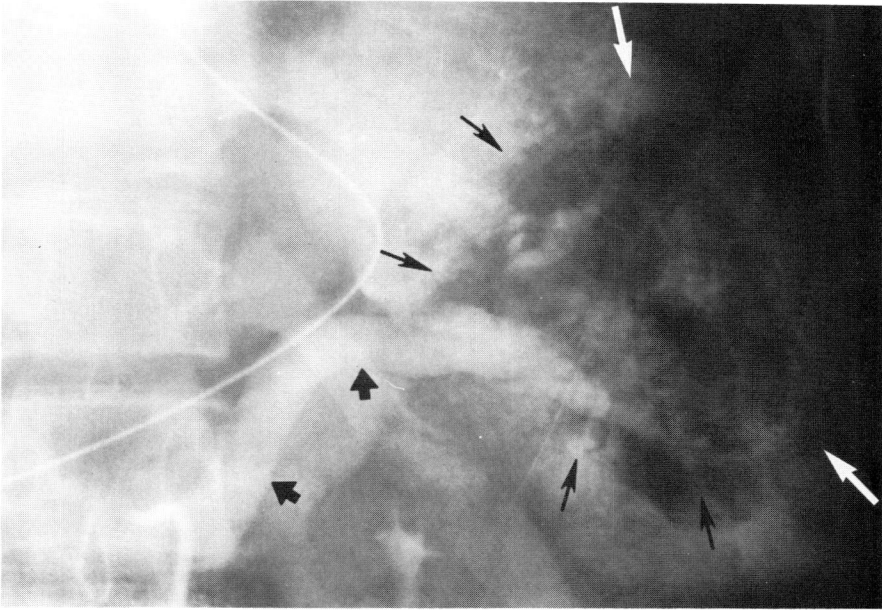

Figure 18–20. Capillary-venous phase film from a splenic arteriogram of a young man with multiple trauma. The defect in the midportion of the spleen (large arrows) corresponds to a large splenic laceration. The splenic vein (small arrows) is intact.

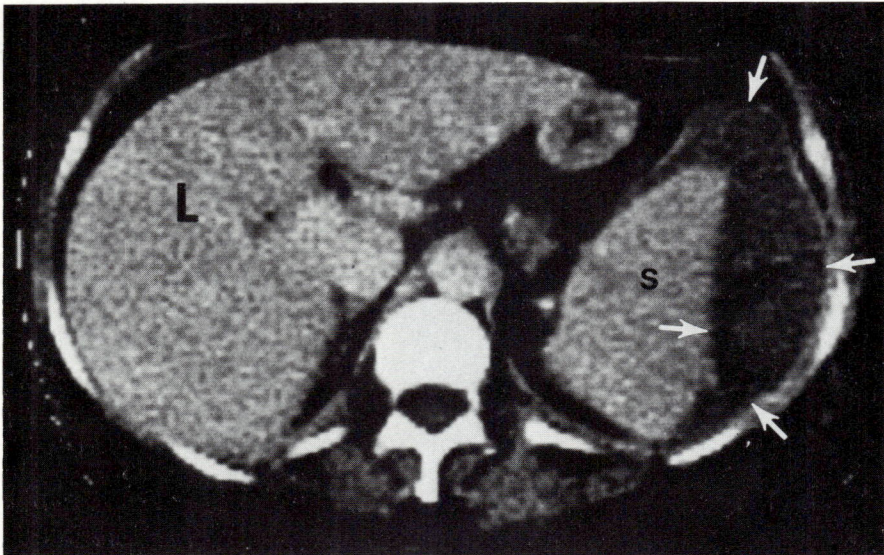

Figure 18–21. CT scan of the upper abdomen of a patient suspected of having splenic trauma. Contrast material given intravenously has produced spleen (S) and liver (L) opacification. A large subcapsular hematoma (arrows) appears as low-density area enveloping the spleen. (Courtesy of Melvyn Korobkin, M.D.)

Splenosis

Splenosis is a rare condition that can occur after surgical or traumatic injury to the spleen. Multiple small implants of splenic tissue occur throughout the abdomen, apparently as a result of autotransplantation by the peritoneal seeding of splenic tissue. The condition is usually asymptomatic, but the spleen implants can lead to intestinal obstruction or the appearance of one or more abdominal masses. If splenosis is suspected, it can sometimes be demonstrated by radionuclide scanning.[9]

FOCAL DISEASES OF THE SPLEEN

Splenic Cysts

Three types of cystic lesions — echinococcal, epidermoid, and pseudocysts — occur in the spleen. Echinococcal cysts are rare even in patients with echinococcal disease elsewhere in the body. Epidermoid cysts, which are thought to be congenital in origin, are encountered occasionally, usually in persons younger than age 15. Splenic pseudocysts, the most common of the three types, do not have an epithelial lining and probably arise from old hematomas or infarcts.

These three types of cysts have similar radiographic features. Plain films usually show splenomegaly. Curvilinear calcification may be present in the cyst wall (Fig. 18–22). Radionuclide scans can detect lesions greater than 2 cm in diameter. Cysts appear as well-demarcated focal areas of diminished uptake (Fig. 18–23). Ultrasound is a simple way to confirm the cystic nature of such a finding on a radionuclide scan.[3] Cysts appear sonographically as well-circumscribed, echo-free areas with enhanced through-transmission of sound. CT also accurately defines cystic lesions that appear as round or oval areas of water density. It is not rare for a cystic lesion of the spleen to turn up incidentally on a CT study of the pancreas or liver (Fig. 18–24). Finally, angiography can be used to delineate splenic cysts. Stretching and draping of arteries around an avascular mass are the typical features (Fig. 18–25).

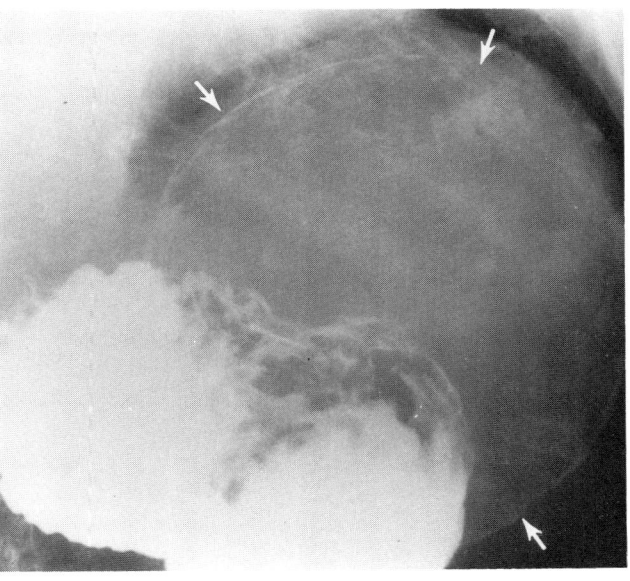

Figure 18–22. Left upper quadrant mass with a thin calcified rim (arrows). The appearance of the mass remained unchanged for several years and is typical of a splenic cyst. At the time of a cholecystectomy, the surgeon found a hard, calcified mass adherent to the left hemidiaphragm and stomach. The mass presumably arose post-traumatically; it was not removed.

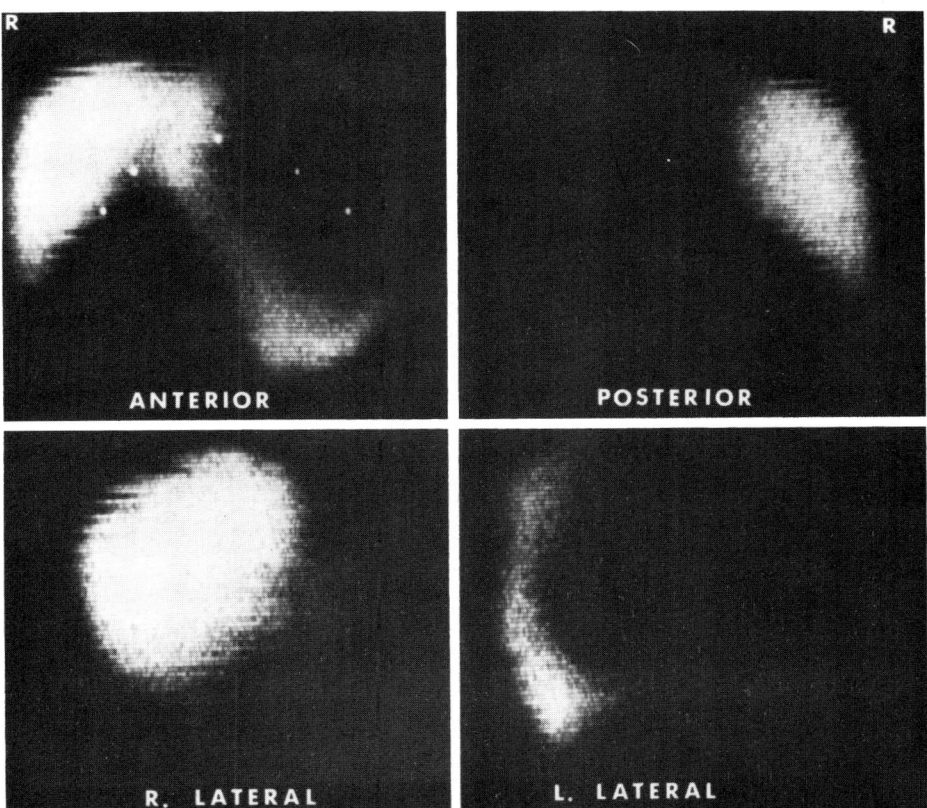

Figure 18–23. Radionuclide scan of a patient with a post-traumatic splenic pseudocyst seen as a large defect on anterior and left lateral views. Six months prior to this scan, the patient had been involved in an automobile accident without sustaining a recognizable major injury. The scan was obtained because of an enlarging left upper quadrant mass.

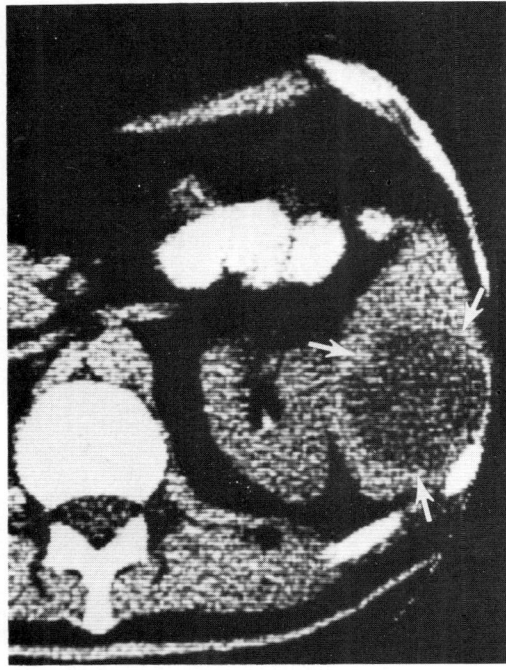

Figure 18–24. Abdominal CT scan performed for the evaluation of pancreatic disease shows a well-defined, spheric mass within the spleen (arrows). The water density of the mass indicates that it is cystic. The spleen felt normal at a subsequent cholecystectomy and was not removed.

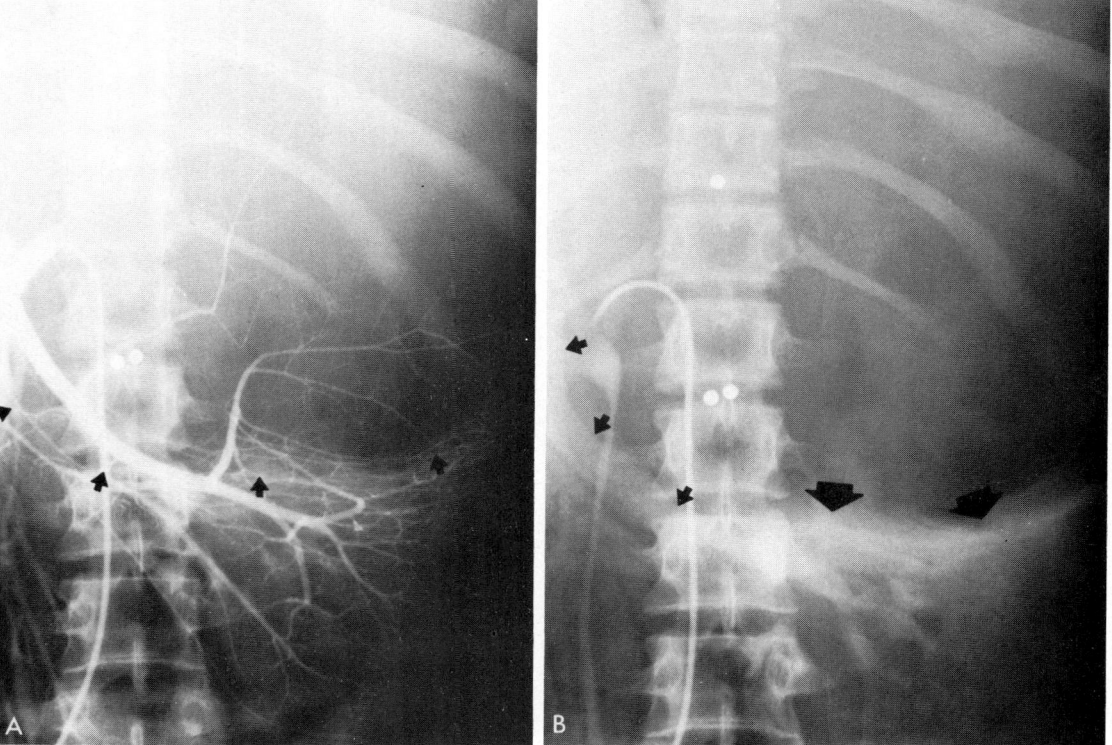

Figure 18–25. Superior mesenteric arteriogram of a 15-year-old girl with an epidermoid cyst of the spleen. The splenic artery in this patient arises from the superior mesenteric artery (lienomesenteric trunk). *A,* The arterial phase shows draping of splenic artery branches (arrows) around the avascular mass, which fills entire left upper quadrant. *B,* The capillary phase shows splenic parenchymal tissue (large arrows) compressed inferiorly by the avascular splenic mass. Note the displacement of the splenic vein (small arrows) as well.

Neoplasms

Lymphoma tends to involve the spleen by diffuse infiltration, but some forms, particularly histiocytic lymphoma, may produce focal tumors. Unfortunately, splenic radionuclide imaging is not a good screening test, because approximately 25 per cent of the spleens involved with lymphoma are normal in size and relatively few have focal defects. In diffuse splenic lymphoma, angiography may show nothing more than slight hypovascularity. On ultrasound, there may be considerably increased transonicity, sometimes resembling a cystic lesion.

Primary tumors consist essentially of sarcomas. Radioisotope scanning shows a focal defect. There is as yet little experience with CT or ultrasound. Angiography is useful to define the nature of a focal defect that does not appear to be cystic on CT or ultrasound examination. In addition to the displacement of arterial branches by the mass, abnormal tumor vessels may be seen. The multicystic tumor of splenic lymphangiomatosis has a characteristic "Swiss cheese" appearance on arteriography.

Metastatic tumors may also occur in the spleen and are found at autopsy in 2 to 4 per cent of patients with primary tumors elsewhere. Nathanson reported metastases to the spleen in 36 per cent of patients with melanoma.[11] Single or multiple focal defects may be seen on radionuclide scan. CT shows focal low-density lesions or heterogeneity of splenic density (Fig. 18–26). Isodense metastases may be overlooked on CT studies.

Abscess

The radionuclide spleen scan is probably the best screening test when the presence of a splenic abscess is considered a possibility. As such, it is useful in evaluating patients with clinical signs of upper abdominal infection who may have bacteremia resulting from bacterial endocarditis or drug abuse. Focal areas of diminished isotope

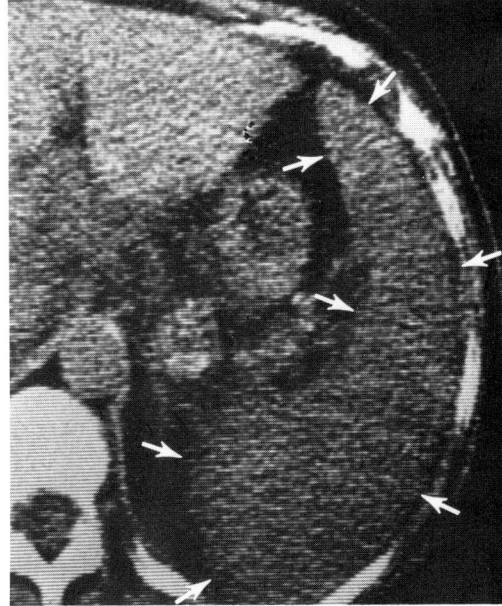

Figure 18–26. CT scan of a patient with widespread metastatic disease involving the liver and the spleen (arrows). The spleen is enlarged, and there is subtle but definite heterogeneity in its density.

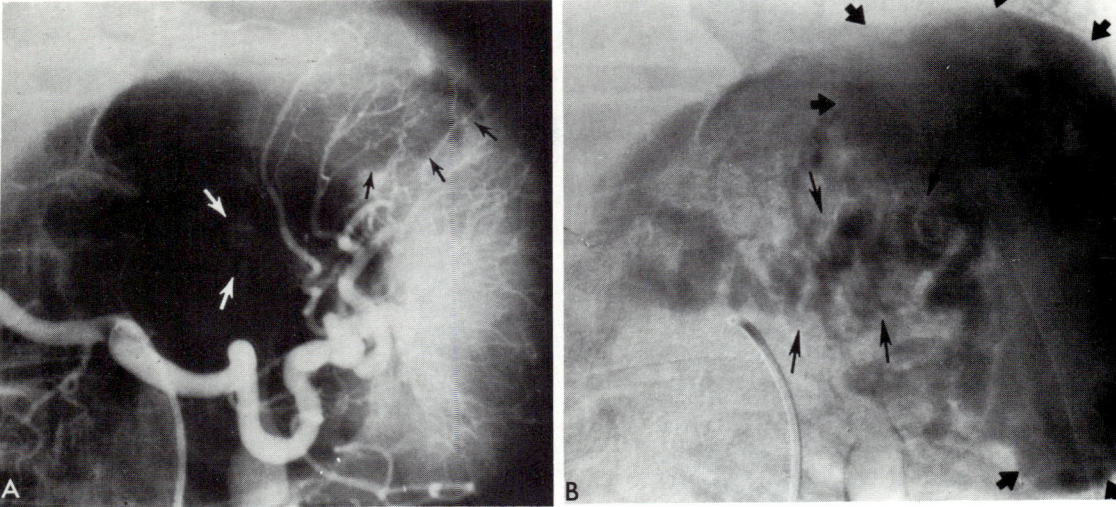

Figure 18–27. Celiac arteriogram of an elderly man with an idiopathic abscess in the superior pole of the spleen and the splenic hilus. He presented with vague left upper abdominal pain of two months' duration. *A*, The arterial phase shows displacement of the arteries around a mass in the upper pole of the spleen. Diminished parenchymal opacification (black arrows) is seen in the same area. A small area of fine neovascularity is barely visible near the splenic hilus (white arrows). *B*, A subtraction film taken during the venous phase shows splenic vein obstruction with a cluster of venous collaterals (small arrows) in the splenic hilus. Large arrows outline the spleen. The radiographic findings also are consistent with those of tumor, such as pancreatic carcinoma with splenic involvement.

uptake are seen. As with other focal diseases of the spleen, however, the findings on radionuclide scan are not specific. Ultrasound may show a transonic area in the spleen, which may contain some internal echoes representing debris within the abscess cavity. CT shows a focal lesion, the density of which usually lies between that of cyst fluid and that of the splenic parenchyma. Arteriography, if needed, shows displacement of vessels by the abscess and variable degrees of hypervascularity in the abscess wall (Fig. 18–27).

Infarction

Like splenic abscesses, infarcts of the spleen cause focal areas of diminished uptake on radionuclide scan (Fig. 18–28). Splenic arteriography shows one or more defects in the parenchymal blush. These may be wedge-shaped, with the apex directed toward the hilus. Arterial occlusions are sometimes seen. The repeated splenic infarctions that occur in persons with sickle cell anemia result in a progressive decrease in splenic size. The small, shrunken spleen may calcify and thus become evident on plain films.

SPLENIC ARTERY ANEURYSMS

Calcification in the splenic artery is common in adults (see Fig. 18–1), and calcium in the wall of a splenic artery aneurysm often appears on plain abdominal films as a thin curvilinear density in the left upper abdomen. Arteriography is, of course, the definitive radiographic means of evaluating this lesion and is usually performed if surgery is contemplated (Fig. 28–29).

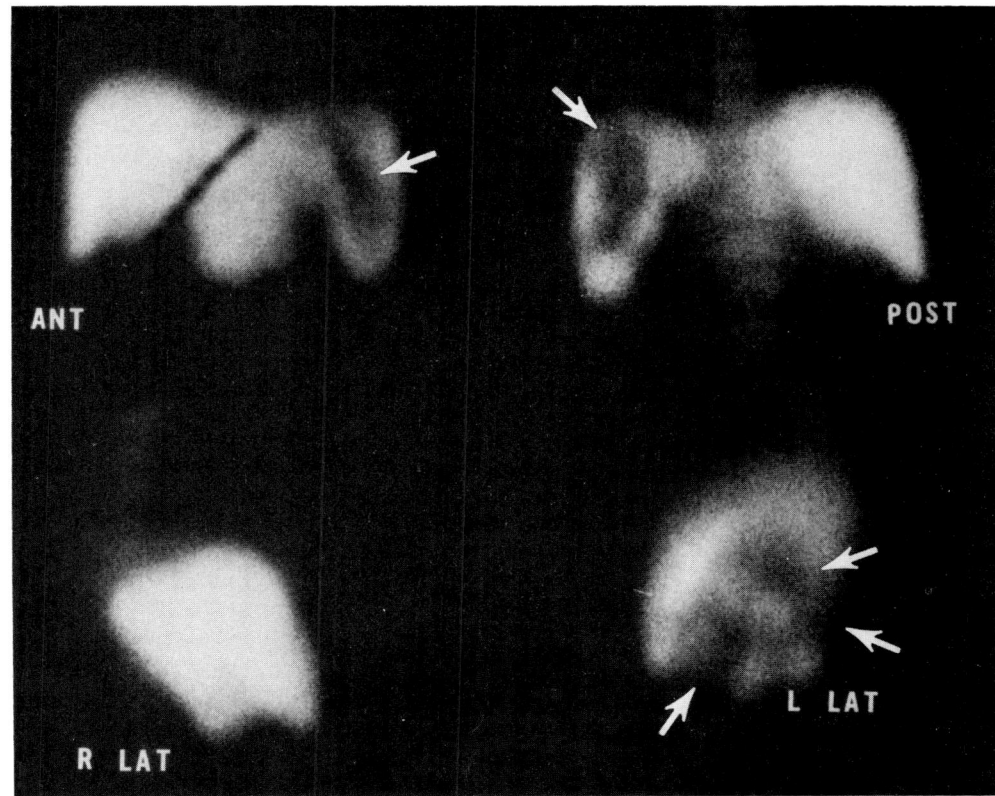

Figure 18–28. Multiple splenic infarcts. This patient had multiple clinical problems, including chronic pancreatitis, fever, and splenomegaly. The scan demonstrates multiple filling defects (arrows), which were thought to represent multiple splenic abscesses or infarcts. Note radiopharmaceutical uptake in the spinal arrow, indicating hepatic disease.

FINDINGS FOLLOWING SPLENECTOMY

Some radiographic findings are common after splenectomy but are of no clinical significance. Free air in the peritoneum is always present for a few days and is occasionally seen in trace amounts for as long as two or three weeks after surgery. A small left pleural effusion and left basilar atelectasis are common and are usually of no significance if transient (Fig. 18–30). Changes in the position of the gas-filled stomach and colonic splenic flexure reflect the fact that these organs take up some of the space formerly occupied by the spleen.

The most common major complication following splenectomy is left subphrenic abscess. In this condition, there may be elevation of the left hemidiaphragm and fluoroscopy may demonstrate diminished diaphragmatic mobility. Left upper quadrant extracolonic gas collections are suggestive of infection in the operative area (Fig. 18–31A), especially if air-fluid levels are seen on upright views. Barium studies of the upper gastrointestinal tract may show irregularity and thickening of rugal folds in the portion of the stomach adjacent to the abscess (Fig. 18–31B). Both ultrasound and CT may be useful in demonstrating a fluid collection (Fig. 18–32) although ultrasound examination of this area is often hampered by the presence of gas in the adjacent stomach and colon. Radionuclide scanning with gallium-67 citrate may localize an abscess as an area of accumulation of the isotope 6 to 72 hours after injection. Recent experimental work indicates that technetium-labeled white blood cells may prove to be useful in defining inflammatory masses.[16]

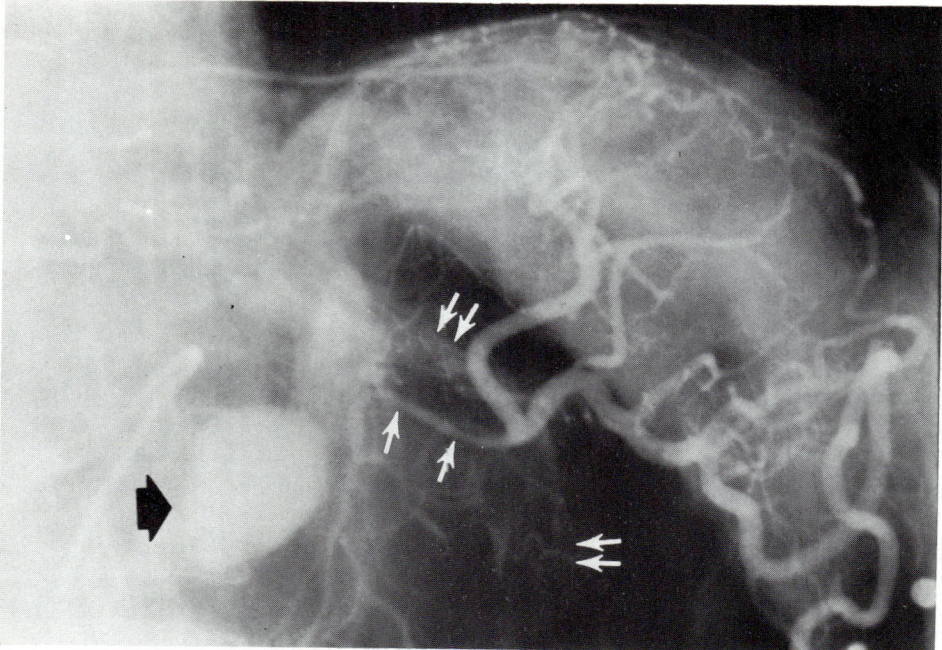

Figure 18–29. Celiac arteriogram demonstrating a splenic artery aneurysm (black arrow) in a man with chronic relapsing pancreatitis. Leakage of blood from the aneurysm has caused spasm of the adjacent splenic artery (single white arrows) and draping of vessels around a hematoma (double white arrows).

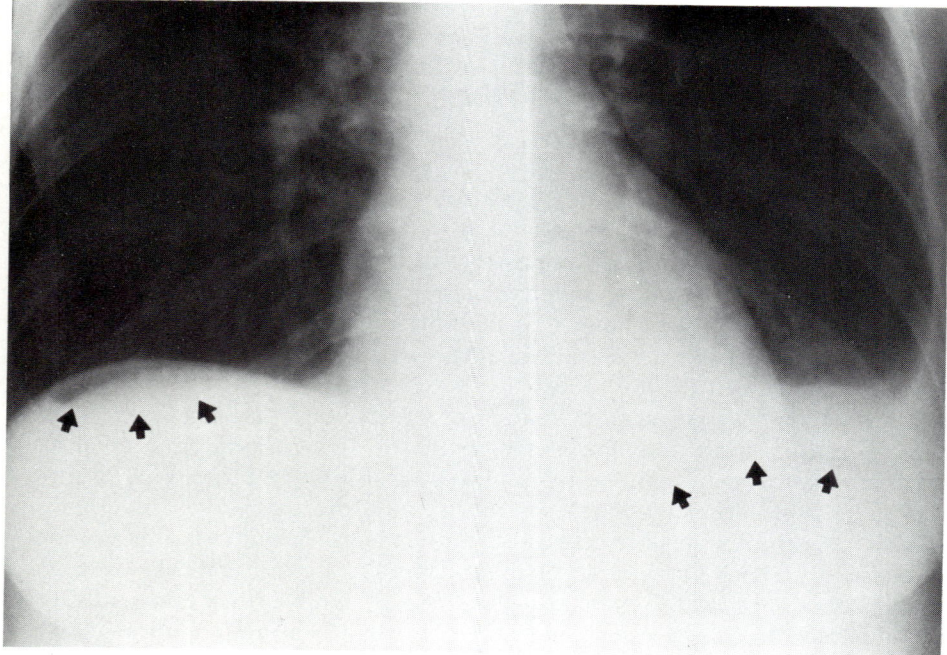

Figure 18–30. Chest film taken one day after splenectomy for chronic myelogenous leukemia. Free air (arrows) is present beneath both hemidiaphragms and there is a left pleural effusion. The postoperative recovery was uneventful, and free air and pleural fluid were no longer present one week after surgery.

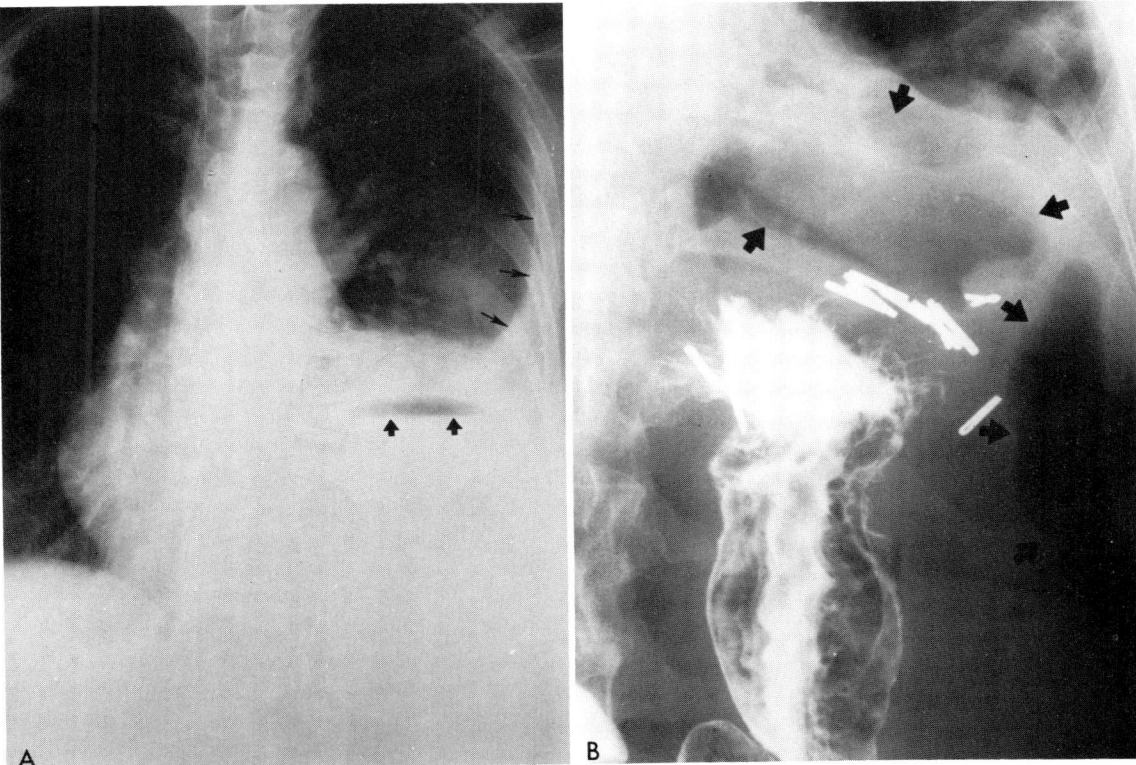

Figure 18–31. Persistent fever following splenectomy for lymphoma. *A*, A chest film taken ten days after surgery showing left pleural effusion (small arrows), marked elevation of the left hemidiaphragm, and an air-fluid level in the left subdiaphragmatic area (large arrows), all of which are indicative of left subphrenic abscess. *B*, The abscess was drained, but upper gastrointestinal examination 20 days after splenectomy shows residual abdominal air (arrows) and deformity of the proximal stomach, indicating persistent infection.

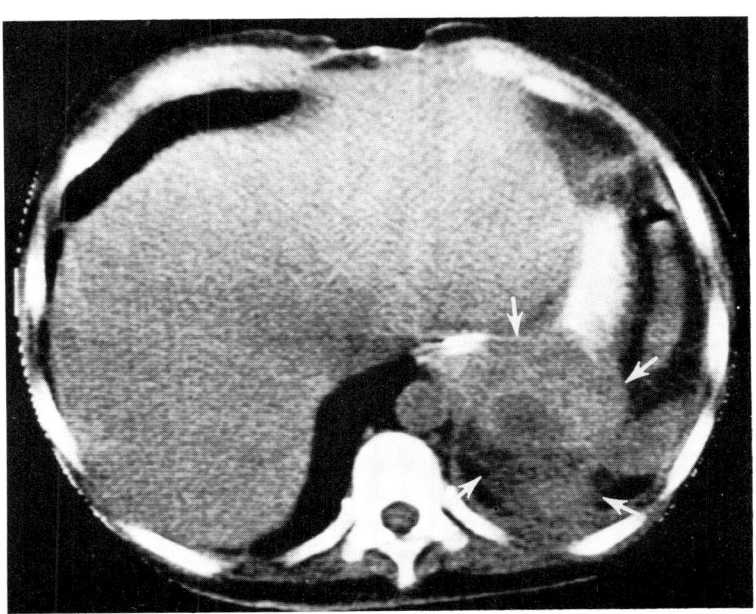

Figure 18–32. Abdominal abscess following splenectomy. The CT scan shows an ill-defined left upper quadrant mass (arrows) containing low-density, fluid-filled areas within it. Contrast material is present in the proximal stomach, and a radiopaque tube is in the esophagus.

References

1. Asher, W. M., Parvin, S., Virgilio, R. W., et al.: Echographic evaluation of splenic injury after blunt trauma. Radiology *118*:411–415, 1976.
2. Belfanz, J. R., Nesbit, M. E., Jarvis, C., et al.: Overwhelming sepsis following splenectomy for trauma. J. Pediatr. *88*:458–460, 1976.
3. Bhimji, S. D., Cooperberg, P. L., Naiman, S., et al.: Ultrasound diagnosis of splenic cysts. Radiology *122*:787–789, 1977.
4. Claret, I., Morales, L., and Montaner, A.: Immunologic studies in the post splenectomy syndrome. J. Pediatr. Surg. *10*:59–64, 1975.
5. Clark, R. E., Korobkin, M., and Palubinskas, A. J.: Angiography of accessory spleens. Radiology *102*:41–44, 1972.
6. Gooding, G. A. W.: The ultrasonic and computed tomographic appearance of splenic lobulations: a consideration in the ultrasonic differential of masses adjacent to the left kidney. Radiology *126*:719–720, 1978.
7. Gordon, D. H., Brurell, M. I., Levin, D. C., et al.: Wandering spleen — the radiological and clinical spectrum. Radiology *125*:38–46, 1977.
8. Halpert, B., and Gyorkey, F.: Lesions observed in accessory spleens of 311 patients. Am. J. Clin. Pathol. *32*:165–168, 1959.
9. Jacobson, S. J., and DeNardo, D. L.: Splenosis demonstrated by splenic scan. J. Nucl. Med. *12*:570–572, 1971.
10. Koga, T., and Morikawa, Y.: Ultrasonographic determination of the splenic size and its clinical usefulness in various liver diseases. Radiology *115*:157–161, 1975.
11. Nathanson, L., Hall, T. C., and Farber, S.: Biological aspects of human malignant melanoma. Cancer *20*:650–655, 1967.
12. Philpott, G. W., and Ballinger, W. F.: The spleen. *In* Sabiston, D. C.: Davis-Christopher Textbook of Surgery. Ed. 2. Philadelphia, W. B. Saunders Company, 1977, pp. 1321–1322.
13. Rösch, J.: Roentgenology of the Spleen and Pancreas. Springfield, Illinois, Charles C Thomas, Publisher, 1967, pp. 5–6.
14. Smulewicz, J. J., and Clemett, A. R.: Torsion of the wandering spleen. Am. J. Dig. Dis. *20*:274–279, 1975.
15. Spencer, R. P., and Pearson, H. A.: Radionuclide Studies of the Spleen. Cleveland, CRC Press, 1975.
16. Thakur, M. L., Coleman, R. E., and Welch, M. J.: Indium-111-labeled leukocytes for the localization of abscesses: Preparation, analysis, tissue distribution and comparison with gallium-67 citrate in dogs. J. Lab. Clin. Med. *89*:217–228, 1977.

INDEX

Page numbers in *italics* refer to illustrations; (t) indicates tabular material.

A-mode scanning, 56, *56*
Abdomen, abscess, 156–158, *157*
  after gastric surgery, 492, *492*
  acute, 169–247. See also *Acute abdomen*.
  anatomic considerations, *170*, 171, *171–173*, *174–175*, *174–175*
  computed tomography of, 126, *127*, *128–133*
    vs. ultrasound, 165–166
  mass, in children, 112
  pain in, evaluation of, endoscopic retrograde cholangiopancreatography in, 904
  trauma to, 835
Abdominal hernias, 287–318. See also *Hernia(s)*.
  internal, 306–316
Abdominal wall, 248–261
  congenital abnormalities, 248–249, *250*, 251–252, *251–253*
  disorders of, ultrasound in, 101, *101*
  hematoma, 255, *256*
  hernias, 302–304, *303–306*, 306
  pneumoperitoneum, 256, *257*, 258, *258–259*, 260–261
  tumors, 253–254, *254–255*
Aberrant pancreatic rests, 469–472, *469–472*
Abnormalities, congenital, abdominal wall, 248–249, *250*, 251–252, *251–253*
Abortion, incomplete, ultrasound in, 91
Abruptio placentae, ultrasound in, 53
Abscess(es), abdominal, 105, *106*, 156–158, *157*
  after gastric surgery, 492, *492*
  acute abdomen due to, 232–234, 233(t)
  appendiceal, 200, 226–227, *227*, 583, 584–587, *584–587*
  in children, 114
  biliary, 69
  diverticular, *106*, 669, *670*
  echinococcal, effect on bile ducts of, 966, *966*
  esophageal perforation with, 372
    due to radiotherapy, 413
  evaluation of, 164
    ultrasound in, 104–108, *105–108*
  extraperitoneal, postoperative, 246, 246(t)
  following appendectomy, *176*
  following cholecystectomy, 948, *950*
  following colotomy, *759*
  following radical pelvic surgery, 93

Abscess(es) (*Continued*)
  following splenectomy, 1085, *1087*
  imaging techniques, 50–51
  liver, 137–138, 847–848, *848–850*, 850–852
    cholangitis and, 929, 964, *964*
    following trauma, 837, 842–843
    scintigraphy in, 41–42, *41*
    ultrasound in, 61–63, *61*, *64*
  localization, radiation dose from, 24(t)
  mediastinal, with esophageal perforation, 378
  of male genitals, 88
  of pancreas, 1027–1029, *1027–1029*
    vs. pseudocyst, 143, *143*
  of spleen, 82, *82*, 1083–1084, *1084*
  paracolic, *193*
  pelvic, 92, *94*, *95*, 107, *107*
  perinephric, *78*, 106
  perirectal, *777*
  postoperative, acute abdomen due to, 240, *241*, *241–244*, 243, 244(t)
  renal, 77, *78*, *79*, 146, *146*
    transplant and, 81, *81*
  retroperitoneal, 84–85, 106, *107*
  small bowel, with radiation enteritis, 593
  subhepatic, *64*, 105, 981
  subphrenic, 104–105, *105*, 981
    bronchobiliary fistula from, 974
    following hiatus hernia repair, 366, 367
    with cholecystitis, 918
  tubo-ovarian, 91, *91*, 92, 107
  versus esophageal diverticula, 335
  versus ileus of right colon, *215*
  visceral, *61*, 105
  with Crohn's disease, 554, *555–557*, 557
  wound, 108, *108*
Acalculous cholecystitis, 924–925, *925–926*
Acanthosis nigricans vs. herpes esophagitis, 346
Achalasia, 323–326, *324*, *326–328*, 359
  esophageal tumor with, *388*, 389
  versus carcinoma, *397*, 398
  versus diffuse spasm, *328*
  versus metastatic disease, 401, *402*
Acid ingestion, corrosive gastritis due to, 473
  corrosive strictures of esophagus due to, 379
  esophageal perforation and, 369
Actinomycosis of cecum, *674*, 675

i

Acute abdomen, 169–247
  due to abscesses, 232–234, 233(t)
  due to biliary tract disease, 201–203, *203–204*
  due to blunt trauma, 205, 207–209, *208*, 208(t), 209(t), 210(t)
  due to emphysematous pyelonephritis, 231
  due to extraperitoneal hemorrhage, 231–232, 232(t), *232–233*
  due to gynecologic disorders, 228–230
  due to large bowel disorders, 212–228, *213–229*, 217(t), 226(t)
  due to obstructive uropathy, 230–231, *230–231*
  due to pancreatitis, 205–207, 207(t)
  due to perforated gastric and duodenal ulcer, 201, *201–202*
  due to small bowel disease, 209–212, *210–214*, 211(t)
  due to uriniferous perirenal pseudocysts, 231
  in emergency room, 177, 177(t)
  intravenous cholangiography in, 889
  postoperative, 177, 234–246
  radiologic findings in, abnormal calcification, 194, *196–198*, 198, *199–200*, 200(t)
    abnormal gas collections, *190*, 191, *191–194*, 194, *195*
    abnormal gas pattern, 183, 187, 187(t)
    extraperitoneal effusion, 181, 183, *184–186*, 186(t)
    intraperitoneal effusion, 180–181, *181–183*, 184(t)
    intraperitoneal free air, 178, *178–180*, 180, 245
    loss of visualization of structures normally seen, 178
    mass densities, 189, *189–190*, 206
    organ enlargement, 187, *188*
  vs. rectus sheath hematoma, 255
Acute care unit, 1–22
Adenocarcinoma(s), adrenal, 151
  cecal, 742
  in Barrett's esophagus, *388*
  of bile ducts, 937
  of duodenum, 463–466, *464–465*, 604
  of large intestine, 726, 758
  of liver, 853, 856
  of small intestine, 608–609, *608–610*
    vs. radiation enteritis, 591
  of stomach, 455–457, *455–461*, 461
  ovarian, omental metastases from, *157*
  rectal, after surgical resection, *747*
  with Crohn's disease, 558–559
Adenoma(s), adrenal, 151, *152*, 165
  of Brunner's glands, 503, *504*
  of duodenum, 502, 503, *502–503*
  of liver, 852, 859, *860–861*, 861
  parathyroid, 109, *109*
  thyroid, 109, *109*
  villous. See *Villous adenoma*.
Adenomatous polyp, of colon, 751, 756, *757*
  carcinoma with, *731*, 758
  of stomach, 448, *449–450*
Adenomyomatosis, of gallbladder, 940–941, *941–944*
  differential diagnosis, 945–946, *946*
  oral cholecystography in, 887
Adhesions, ascites and, 102
  following jejunoileal bypass, *642*
  pelvic, 92
  peritoneal, across gallbladder, *946*, *946*
  peritonitis and, 264–265

Adhesions (*Continued*)
  pleural, 15
  small bowel obstruction due to, *192*, 209, *237*, *238*, 267, *539*, 544, *546*, *547*
  with incisional hernias, 304
  with lye ingestion, 379
  with radiation enteritis, 592, 593
  with serosal metastases, *269*, 270
  with umbilical hernia, 303
Adrenal glands, computed tomography of, 132, 150–152, *151–152*
  disorders of, evaluation of, 165
  ultrasound in, 83–84, *83*
  imaging of, 52–53
Adrenalectomy, 53
Adult respiratory distress syndrome (ARDS), 17, 20–21, *21*
  conditions leading to, 20(t)
  synonyms for, 20(t)
Adynamic ileus vs. mechanical small bowel obstruction, 543–544, *543*
Aerophagy, 541
Afferent loop syndrome, 498, *499*
  malabsorption with, 566, *567*
Agenesis, abdominal muscle, 249, *250*
  renal, 112
  splenic, with congenitally short esophagus, 354
Air, extra-alveolar, 5, 12–13, *13–14*, 15–16, *15–16*
  intraperitoneal, 234, 239, *239*
Air-contrast study of colon, *650*, 651
Alcoholism, cirrhosis in, *826*, 827
  gastritis in, 473, *474*
  hepatitis in, hepatomegaly with, 818, *818*
  pancreatitis in, calculi in, 1029, *1030*
    nonvisualization with oral cholecystography in, 885–886
  variceal hemorrhage in, 796
Aldosteronism, 53
Alkali ingestion, corrosive gastritis due to, 473
Ambiguous genitalia, 114
Amebiasis, 673, 675, *675*
  effect on bile ducts of, 966
Amniocentesis, ultrasound with, 118–119, *118*
Amoebic infestation of colon, 777
Ampulla of Vater, carcinoma of, 510, 894
  impacted stone in, 928, *928*
Ampullary carcinoma, biliary tract in, *139*, 992, 994
Ampullary disconnection, with Billroth procedures, 530, *531*
Amyloidosis, malabsorption with, 572, *573*
Anastomosis, breakdown, with radiation enteritis, 593
  choledochoduodenal, *885*
  esophagogastric, for carcinoma, 404, 405, *406*
    complications of, 411, 414, *415–416*
  ileotransverse, 743, *743–746*
  leakage, 239, *239*, 243
    after gastric surgery, 492, *492*
  postgastrodiverticular, 339, *339*
  rectal, perforation of, 743, *746*
  rectosigmoid, villous adenoma with, *747*
  sigmoid, 743, *744–745*
Anemia, pernicious, atrophic gastritis with, 474, *475*
Anesthesia, pneumoperitoneum with, 260
Aneurysm(s), aortic. See *Aortic aneurysm*.
  iliac artery, 97, *98*
  intra-abdominal, 97

Aneurysm(s) (*Continued*)
  popliteal artery, 98, *98*
  splenic artery, 1084, *1086*
Angiodysplasia, cecal, bleeding with, 792–793
  colonic, bleeding with, angiography and transcatheter therapy for, 804, *805*
Angiography, in acute gastric mucosal bleeding, 799, *799*
  in biliary system disorders, 905–906, *906*
  in cirrhosis with portal hypertension, 826–830, *827–830*
  in colonic angiodysplasia, 804
  in colonic diverticulosis, 802
  in duodenal ulcer, 800
  in gastric ulcer, 800
  in gastrointestinal hemorrhage, 789–793
    indications for, 807
    interpretation of, 792–793, 792(t)
  in liver tumors, 859, *860–862*, 861–863
  in small intestine bleeding, 800
  in variceal hemorrhage, 796
  of pancreas, normal anatomy, 1007, *1007, 1008,* 1009
    with acute pancreatitis and pseudocyst, 1021–1023, *1023*
    with carcinoma, 1045–1046, *1045*
    with chronic pancreatitis, 1035, *1036–1038*
  radionuclide, 36
    cerebral, 25, *26–27*
Angioneurotic edema of colon, 685
Anisakiasis, vs. tuberculosis, 675
Annular pancreas, duodenum in, 520, *522,* 523
Anorectal infection, 787
Anticoagulant therapy, abdominal hematoma with, *159*
Antral carcinoma vs. gastritis, 476
Anus, bleeding from, transcatheter therapy for, 804
  fissure, 788
  fistula, 788
Aorta, 95–96, *95–96*
  abdominal, 159
  computed tomography of, 127
Aortic aneurysm, 95, *96,* 159
  computed tomography of, *135*
  duodenal obstruction due to, 526, 527
  evaluation of, radionuclide angiography in, 36
  leaking, 275
  ruptured, 158, *158*
    acute abdomen due to, 231–232, *232–233*
  vs. renal colic, *198*
Aortic-superior mesenteric angle, 97
Aortoenteric fistula, 527, 529–530, 790
Aortography in gastrointestinal bleeding, 790
Aphthoid ulcers in Crohn's disease, 551, *552*
Appendectomy, complications of, *588,* 589
  sepsis following, ultrasound in, *64*
Appendicitis, *176,* 198, *199–200,* 226–228, 226(t), *226–227,* 587–589
  abscess with, *200,* 583, 584–587, *584–587*
  in children, 114
  appendicoliths in, 577–578, *578*
  barium enema in, 580–582, *581–582*
  cecal and terminal ileum dilatation in, 579, *579*
  fistula with, *588,* 589
  free fluid with, 583–584
  lumbar scoliosis in, 579–580, *580*
  obliteration of flank stripe in, 580
  perforation and pneumoperitoneum with, 582–583

Appendicitis (*Continued*)
  peritonitis with, 583
  vs. Crohn's disease, *715*
  vs. Meckel's diverticulum, 627
  vs. salpingitis, 229
Appendicoliths, 198, *199–200,* 577–578, *578*
Appendix, epiploica, 685
  gas in, 578
  perforation of, 258
  retrocecal, 228, *228*
  ruptured, abscesses secondary to, 107
Arrhythmias, central venous pressure catheter and, 3
Arterial biliary fistula, 983, *983–984*
Arterial portography in cirrhosis, 828–830, *828–830*
Arteriocapillary gastrointestinal bleeding, transcatheter therapy for, 793, 794, 796, 797
Arteriography, of liver, with abscess, 852
  with trauma, 836–837, 840, 841, *836–837, 843–844*
  with tumors, 859, *860–862,* 861–863
Arteriovenous fistula, hepatic, traumatic, 836, 837
  splanchnic, traumatic, 817, *817*
Arteriovenous malformation, cerebral radionuclide angiography in, *26–27*
  of cecum, 676, *678*
Artery(ies), hepatic, *812,* 815, *815*
  intra-abdominal, 96–97, *97–98*
  patency of, evaluation of, radionuclide angiography in, 36
  peripheral, 98, *98*
Arthritis, following jejunoileal bypass, 644
  with Crohn's disease, 557, 705
Asbestos exposure, 137
Ascariasis, of bile duct, 964–965, *965*
  of large intestine, 675, *676*
Ascites, hepatic lymphatics in, 816
  hepatomegaly and, *831*
  in acute abdomen, *182*
  in Budd-Chiari syndrome, 834
  jaundice and, *814*
  peritoneal, 262, *262–263*
  pneumoperitoneum and, *257*
  serosal metastases with, 270, *270*
  ultrasound in, 102–103, *102*
  with cirrhosis, *62,* 63
    and portal hypertension, 818–819, *819, 820,* 824, 825, *824–825*
  with liver abscess, 847
  with pelvic masses, 89
  with retroperitoneal lymphoma, 277
Aspiration, due to upper esophageal sphincter disorders, 320, *321,* 323
  postoperative, 17, *17*
  with corrosive ingestion, 380
  with esophageal carcinoma, 404, *404*
Aspiration biopsy procedures, ultrasound in, 115–119, 115(t), *116–118*
Aspiration pneumonia, 17, 18
  with Zenker's diverticula, 337
Asplenia, 43
Atelectasis, 10, 16–17, *17*
Atresia, biliary, *68,* 69, 113
  of colon, 653, *657*
Atrophic gastritis, 474–475, *475*

B-mode scanning, 56, *56*
Backwash ileitis, 690, *693*

Bacterial overgrowth in small intestine, malabsorption and, 565–567, *567–568*, 569
Baker's cyst, *110*
Bands, in gallbladder, 946, *946*
  Ladd's duodenal stenosis with, 523
Barium-contrast examination, in appendicitis, 580–582, *581–582*
  in biliary tract disease, 894–896, *894–895*
  in small intestine obstruction, 544–545
  of colon, 647
    in acute pancreatitis, 1014, *1015–1016*
    in pancreatic pseudocysts, 1018, *1019–1020*
  of upper gastrointestinal tract, in acute pancreatitis, 1012, *1013–1014*, 1014
    in chronic pancreatitis, 1031–1032, *1031*
    in pancreatic pseudocysts, 1016, *1017–1019*, 1018
Barotrauma, pulmonary, 12, *13*, 16
Barrett's esophagus, 52, 354–355, *356–357*, 358
  adenocarcinoma in, *388*
  vs. carcinoma, 400, *400*
Bascule, cecal, 218, 653, *654*
Basket extraction of bile duct stones, 931, *932*
Beagle-ear sign, 486, *490*
Behçet's disease, 686
Belsey-Mark IV operation, 361, *363*
Bezoar, postoperative, 496, *498*
  vs. gastric adenocarcinoma, 457
Bifid genitalia, 249
Bile, insufficiency, malabsorption with, 569
  leakage, detection of, scintigraphy in, 43
    following cholecystectomy, 948, *949–950*
  milk of calcium, 877, *878*
  peritonitis, following cholecystectomy, 948
Bile ducts, anatomy and variants of, 867, *870*, 1005
  benign stricture of, 936, *936*
  blood clots in, following cholecystectomy, 951
  calculi in. See *Choledocholithiasis*.
  carcinoma of, *935*, 937, 989–990, *991–1000*, 992, 995–1001
  computed tomography of, 129, *130*
  enlargement, 959
  injury, with liver trauma, 841, *842*
  obstruction of, 201
    biliary fistula with, 978–979, *979*
    experimental, *960*
    vs. intrahepatic cholestasis, 901, *902*
  pseudocalculus defect, 908, *909*
  spasm, 908, *909*
Biliary atresia, *68, 69*, 113
  radionuclide study in, *897*
Biliary bypass, postoperative, 971, *971*
Biliary cirrhosis with choledocholithiasis, 929
Biliary drainage procedures, 1051, *1052*
Biliary dyskinesia, 924–925, *926*
  postcholecystectomy syndrome and, 957
Biliary-enteric communication, *880*, 883, 885
Biliary fistula, arterial, 983, *983–984*
Biliary system, air in, 969
  anatomy and variants, 866–867, *867–874*, 871, 873–874
  bypass procedures, 43
  calculi, 1012
  carcinoma of, 985–1002
  Caroli's disease, 967, *967*
  cholangitis, acute suppurative, 963–968, *964–967*
    sclerosing, 933, *934*, 935–937, *966*, 967

Biliary system (*Continued*)
  cholecystitis, acalculous, 924–925, *925–926*
    acute, 913–917, *914–918*
    chronic, 922–924, *922–924*
  choledocholithiasis, 927–929, *928–930*, 931, *932*, 933
  disorders, 201–203, *203–204*
  evaluation of, angiography in, 905–906, *906*
    barium studies in, 894–896, *894–895*
    computerized tomography in, 138–140, *139*, 899–900, *900*
    endoscopic retrograde cholangiopancreatography in, 903–904, *903–904*
    imaging modalities for, 875(t)
    infusion tomography of gallbladder in, 904–905, *905*
    intravenous cholangiography in, 889–891, *890*, *892–893*
      indications for, 889(t)
    operative and postoperative tube cholangiography in, 906–908, *907–909*
    oral cholecystography in, 881–883, *883–889*, 885–887
    plain films, 875–881, *875–881*
    radionuclide studies in, 896, *897*
    transhepatic cholangiography in, 900–901, *901–902*, 903
    ultrasonography in, 64–69, *65–69*, 898–899, *898–899*
  fistula, 968–985
    external, 968, *969*, 977–981, *977–984*, 983
    internal, 968, *969*, *970–973*, 971
    with gallstone ileus, 973, *975–977*, *975–976*
  gallstones, 919, *920–921*, 922
  gas in, 879–880, *880*, 883
  hyperplastic cholecystoses, 940–941, *941–945*, 945–946
  postcholecystectomy syndromes, 954, 956–957, *958–960*
  pseudocalculus defect, 938–939, *939*
  spasm of sphincter of Oddi, 938, *939*
  stenosis of sphincter of Oddi, 937–938, *938*
  surgical injuries and complications, 948, *949–956*, *950, 952–954*
  trauma to, 847, 946–947, *947*
  visualization of, bilirubin concentration and, 885, 885(t)
Biliobiliary fistula, 973
Bilirubin concentration, visualization of biliary tract and, 885, 885(t)
Billroth I procedures, 484–489, *485, 486*
  ampullary disconnection following, 530
  complications of, 493, *493–495*, 497
Billroth II procedures, ampullary disconnection following, 530
  biliary duodenocolocutaneous fistula following, 977
  complications of, 492, *492*, 493, 496, *496*, 498, 499, *499*, 500
  malabsorption with, 566, *566*, 567
  stump leak following, 531–532, *532*
Biopsy, percutaneous needle, computed tomography in, 137
  renal, hematoma following, *150*
  ultrasound in, 115–119, 115(t), *116–118*
Bladder, disorders, ultrasound in, 87, *87*
  enlarged, *189*

Bladder (*Continued*)
  extrophy of, 249
  fistula, due to pelvic irradiation, 593
    with Crohn's disease, *555*
  herniation of, 294
  in prune belly syndrome, 249, *250*
  urinary, computed tomography of, 132
Blalock-Taussig operation, radionuclide methods with, 38
Bleaches, corrosive strictures of esophagus due to, 379
Bleeding. See *Hemorrhage*.
Blind loop syndrome, malabsorption with, 565–566, 593
Blood, cerebral flow, abnormalities of, 25, *26–27*
  disorders, 45
  intraperitoneal, *181*
  sampling, fetal, 119
Blood clots in bile ducts, following cholecystectomy, *951*
Blood pool studies, 33, *33*
Blood vessels, abdominal, 159
  computed tomography of, 127
  disorders, ultrasound in, 95–100, *95–100*
Bochdalek hernia, 288, *289*, 290, *290*
  vs. traumatic diaphragmatic hernia, 293
Bodies, foreign. See *Foreign bodies*.
Body-cast syndrome, 478, *479*
Bone, evaluation of, 165
  fractures, with celiac disease, 571
  in Crohn's disease, 560, *560*
  scintigraphy, 48–50, *49–50*
    radiation dose from, 24(t)
  tumors, computed tomography in, 163
Bone islands vs. appendicoliths, 578
Bone marrow imaging, 53
Bougienage, esophageal, for carcinoma, 407–408
Bowels. See *Intestine(s)*.
Brain, disorders of, 27(t)
  scintigraphy, 25, *26–27*, 27(t), 28–29, *28–29*
    radiation dose from, 24(t)
Breast, carcinoma of, metastatic to porta hepatis, 992, *994*
  lesions, ultrasound in, 111
Bromsulphalein (BSP) test, radioactive, 43
Bronchobiliary fistulas, 973, *974*, 981
Bronchoesophageal fistula with esophageal carcinoma, 404, *404*
Bronchogenic carcinoma, adrenal metastasis with, 83
Brunner's glands, hamartoma, 602, *603*
  hyperplasia of, 503, *504*
Budd-Chiari syndrome, 834–835
  hepatic vein anatomy in, 816
Burns, corrosive, of esophagus, 379–387, *380–386*
Bypass malabsorption, 493
Bypass procedures for morbid obesity, 563, 565, *565*, 637–641, *638–640*, 642–644, *643–644*

Calcification, abdominal, 194, *196–198*, 198, *199–200*, 200(t)
  of pulmonary nodule, 136, *136*
  pancreatic, 144
  with liver tumors, 852–853, *858*
Calculi, in bile ducts. See *Choledocholithiasis*.
  in gallbladder. See *Gallstone(s)*.

Calculi (*Continued*)
  pancreatic, 1012
    in chronic pancreatitis, 1029, *1030*, *1031*
  renal, 77, *78*, 197
    with Crohn's disease, 559
  ureteral, ileus with, 230–231, *230–231*
    postoperative, 246
  with Meckel's diverticulum, 628, 633
Camera, gamma, 24–25
Candidiasis, esophageal, *377*
Carcinoid syndrome, 624
Carcinoid tumors, of large intestine, 680, *683*
  of small intestine, 620–622, *622–623*, 624–625
Carcinoma. See also *Tumor(s)*.
  achalasia and, 325
  adrenal cortical, imaging of, 53
  ampullary, *894*
    biliary tract in, 992, *994*
  antral, vs. gastritis, 476
  bone, scintigraphy in, 49, *49*
  breast, 111
    metastatic to porta hepatis, 992, *994*
    serosal metastases from, *269*
  bronchogenic, 136
    adrenal metastasis with, *83*
  colorectal, 722, 730–731, *730–733*, 733, *734–738*, *738*, *739–742*, *740–741*, *743*, *743–747*
    clinical features, 730
    differential diagnosis of, 738, *740–741*, 740(t)
    polypoid tumors and, 752, *755–756*, 756
    postoperative features, 741, *742–747*, 743
    villous adenoma and, 725, *726*, 727
  cortical, 83
  diverticulitis with, 672, *672*
  embryonal cell, 155
    undescended testicle and, *162*
  esophageal, 394, *395–400*, 397–400
    complications of, 404, *404*
    vs. Barrett's esophagitis, 355, *357*
    vs. corrosive stricture, 383
    with corrosive ingestion, 385–386
  fundal, vs. mass created by bundoplication procedure, 490, *491*
  gastric, adenomatous polyps and, 448
    ulcerating, 427–428, *428–430*
    vs. lymphoma, 462, 463
    vs. varices, *403*, 404
  hepatocellular, *855*, 862–863
  hiatus hernia repair and, 367, *367*
  ileocecal valve, *725*, *736*
  metastatic follicular, *110*
  of bile ducts, *935*, *937*, 989–990, *991–1000*, 992, 995–1001
  of cecum, *757–758*
  of colon, 216, *217*
    hepatomegaly and, ultrasound in, *60*
    metastatic to duodenum, 511, *514*
    rectal villous adenoma with, *729*
    vs. pericolitis with pancreatitis, *1015*
  of duodenum, 508–509, *510–511*
  of gallbladder, *190*, 985–987, *986–989*, 989
    metastatic to duodenum, 511, *513*
    porcelain gallbladder and, 877
  of gastric stump, 500–501, *501*
  of gastroesophageal junction, *358*
  of hepatic duct, arterial biliary fistula with, *983*
  of liver, ultrasound in, *62*

Carcinoma (*Continued*)
  of lung, gallium imaging in, 51
  of pancreas, 71, 73–74, *73*, 96, *117*, 140–142,
      140–142, 1039, 1041–1047, *1041–1047*, 1052
    arterial biliary fistula with, *984*
    bile duct stricture due to, *935*
    metastasis with, *466*, *467*
    metastatic to duodenum, 511, *512–513*
    obstruction of common bile duct with, *894*
    vs. pancreatitis, 903
      and pseudocysts, 905
      with obstructive jaundice, *68*
  of prostate, 88
    bone metastases with, *49*
    metastatic, *163*
  of small intestine, 209
    strictures due to, 546
  of uterine cervix, 269
  rectal, in tubulovillous adenoma, *729*
    in villous adenoma, *728*
  renal, 147, *147*, *148*
  sigmoid, in tubulovillous adenoma, *728*
  splenic flexure, small bowel obstruction due to, *540*
  thyroid, imaging in, 30, 31, *32*
  vs. hiatus hernia, 351, *354*
  with esophageal webs, 340–341
  with familial polyposis, 765
  with ulcerative colitis, 694, 696, *696–699*
Carcinosarcoma of esophagus, *388*, 400
Cardiac tamponade, central venous pressure catheter and, 3
Cardiopulmonary disorders, 12–13, *13–14*, 15–21, *15–17*, *19*, 20(t), *21*
Cardiovascular system, imaging procedures, radiation dose from, 24(t)
  malformations, 248–249
  scintigraphy, 32–36, *33–35*
Carman's meniscus sign, 428, *429*, *430*
Caroli's disease, 967, *967*
Carotid artery, ultrasound in, 98
Cathartic colon, 684, *685*
Catheter(s), intravascular, 2–6, *3–8*
  pulmonary capillary wedge pressure, 5–6, *7–8*
Catheterization, hepatic venous, in cirrhosis with portal hypertension, 830–832, *831–832*
Caustic strictures, esophageal perforation and, 369
Cavernous transformation, of portal vein, 833
Cecum. See also *Large intestine*.
  actinomycosis of, *674*, 675
  adenocarcinoma in, *742*
  air-fluid level in, in appendicitis, 579, *579*
  amebiasis of, *675*
  angiodysplasia, bleeding with, 792–793
  arteriovenous malformation of, 676, *678*
  bascule, 218, 653, *654*
  carcinoid tumors of, 680
  carcinoma of, *757–758*
  ileus of, 227
  malakoplakia in, 685
  pseudovolvulus, *216*
  redundant or mobile, 653, *653*
  roentgen anatomy, 652–653, *653–654*
  spasm of, 264
  villous adenoma, *726–727*, 727
  volvulus of, 218, *220*, 663, 664
Celestin tube for esophageal carcinoma, 408–409, *410*, *416*, 417

Celiac arteriography in gastrointestinal bleeding, 791
Celiac artery, ultrasound in, 96, *97*
Celiac disease, after vagotomy, 564
  malabsorption with, 570–571, *570–571*
Celosomia, 248
Central nervous system, scintigraphy, 25, *26–27*, 27(t), 28–29, *28–29*
Central venous pressure catheters, 2–5, *3–6*
Cerebral blood flow abnormalities, 25, *26–27*
Cerebral radionuclide angiography, 25, *26–27*
Cerebrospinal fluid, leaks, cisternography in, 29
  pseudocysts, 103
Cerebrovascular disease, scintigraphy in, *26*, *28*
Chagas disease, 686
  vs. achalasia, 324
Chain of lakes in chronic pancreatitis, 1032, *1032*
Chemical peritonitis due to leak from cystic duct remnant, 981, *981*
Chemical pneumonitis, 18
Chenodeoxycholic acid for gallstones, 919, 922
Chest, lesions, computed tomography of, 126, *127–128*, 133–137, *134–136*
  ultrasound in, 111, *111*
Chest wall, computed tomography of, 136–137
  congenital defects, 248
Chilaiditi's syndrome vs. free peritoneal air, 261
Children, ultrasound in, 112–114
  umbilical hernia in, 302
Cholangiography, intravenous, 881–882, 883, 885, 889–891, *890*, *892–893*
  in acute abdomen, 202
  in acute pancreatitis, 1012
  in cholecystitis, 914–916, *915–916*
  operative, 1001
  percutaneous transhepatic, 140, 900–901, *901–902*, 903, 995–996
  postoperative and operative tube, 906–908, *907–909*
  visualization by, alkaline phosphatase and, 885, 886(t)
Cholangiopancreatography, endoscopic retrograde, in acute pancreatitis, 1016, *1021*
  in biliary system disorders, 903–904, *903–904*
  in chronic pancreatitis, 1032–1033, *1032–1033*
  in pancreatic carcinoma, 1042–1044, *1042–1044*
  in pancreatic pseudocysts, 1018, *1020–1021*, 1021
Cholangitis, acute suppurative, 963–968, *964–967*
  ascending, with choledocholithiasis, 929, *930*
  sclerosing, *907*, 933, *934*, 935–937, *966*, 967
  with Crohn's disease, 559
Cholecystectomy, complications following, 948, *949–950*
  persistence of symptoms following, 954, *956–957*, *958–960*
Cholecystitis, 196, *197*
  acalculous, 924–925, *925–926*
  acute, 189, 201–202, *203*, 913–917, *914–918*
    adynamic duodenal ileus in, 1011
    angiography in, 906, *906*
    biliary calculi in, 1012
    colon cut-off sign in, 1011
    complications of, 917, *917–918*
    computed tomography in, 913–914
    infusion tomography of gallbladder in, 904–905, *905*, 914–916, *915–916*
    intravenous cholangiography in, *890*
    scintigraphy in, *42*, *43*

Cholecystitis (*Continued*)
  acute, ultrasound in, 913–914, *914*
    vs. pancreatitis, 889
  chronic, 922–924, *922–924*
  emphysematous, *195*, 878–879, *879*, 913
    pneumobilia with, 969
  gastrointestinal tract disease due to, 866, *868*
  ileus with, *914*
  oral cholecystography in, 887
  radionuclide studies in, 896, *897*, 916
  ultrasound in, 64–66, *66*
Cholecystocholectasis, 882
Cholecystoduodenal fistula, *203*, *970*, *982*
Cholecystoenteric fistulas, 973
Cholecystography, oral, 64, 881–883, *883–889*, 885–887
  nonvisualization of gallbladder with, causes of, 882, 883(t)
Cholecystokinin cholecystography in acalculous cholecystitis, 925, *926*
Cholecystoses, hyperplastic, 940–941, *941–945*, 945–946
Choledochal cyst, 68
  in infants, 112
Choledochocele, 517–518, *517*, 871, *871*
Choledochoduodenal anastomosis, 885
Choledochoduodenal fistula, *880*, *972*, *980*
Choledochoduodenostomy, *880*
Choledochojejunostomy, T-tube cholangiogram following, *1049*
Choledocholithiasis, 64–66, *65–66*, 69, *69*, 202–203, *204*, 518, *876*, *907*, 927–929, *928–930*, 931, *932*, 933, *1012*
  basket extraction in, 931, *932*
  complications of, 929, *930*, 931
  edema of papilla of Vater with, 515, *516*
  intravenous cholangiography in, *893*
Cholelithiasis. See *Gallstone(s)*.
Cholera, pancreatic, 1060, *1062*, *1063*
Cholestasis, intrahepatic, vs. obstruction of bile ducts, 901, *902*
Cholesterol polyps, 941, 945, *945*
Cholesterol stones, 919, 922
Cholesterolosis, 941, *944*, 945
  oral cholecystography in, 887
Cholic acid for bile duct stones, 933
Cholografin, toxic reactions of, 881–882
Chondrosarcoma, computed tomography of, 163
Chordoma, computed tomography of, recurrent, *160*
Chronic obstructive pulmonary disease (COPD), edema and, 19, *19*
  embolus with, scintigraphy in, *37*
  pneumonia and, 18
Cirrhosis, 62, 63, *812*, 854
  ascites with, *182*
  biliary, *936*, 937
    with choledocholithiasis, 929
  cryptogenic, *263*
  hepatic lymphatics in, 816
  liver tumor and, 863
  portal hypertension due to, 817–819, *818–821*, 821–822, *822–833*, 824–832
  scintigraphy in, 43
Cisternography, 29, *29*
  radiation dose from, 24(t)
Clinitest tablet, corrosive stricture due to, 379, 383, *384*
Clonorchis sinensis in bile ducts, 965, *965*

Cobblestoning, of esophagus, 345
Coils for transcatheter embolization, 795
Colitis, acute bacterial, vs. pseudomembranous enterocolitis, *673*
  cystica profunda, 680, *684*
  granulomatous, 224
  ischemic, 218, 222–223, 223(t), 676, *677–678*
    vs. pneumatosis cystoides intestinalis, *679*
  nonspecific or infective, 226
  radiation, 784–785
  ulcerative, 224, 224(t), 224–225, 689–690, *689–695*, 694, 696, *696–701*. See also *Ulcerative colitis.*
Collar-button ulcer, 421, 425, *425*
Colon. See also *Large intestine.*
  amoebic infestation of, 777
  angiodysplasia, bleeding with, angiography and transcatheter therapy for, 804, *805*
  angioneurotic edema of, 685
  atresia of, 653, *657*
  barium-contrast examination of, in acute pancreatitis, 1014, *1015–1016*
    in pancreatic pseudocysts, 1018, *1019–1020*
  blunt trauma to, 658, 663, *663*
  carcinoid tumors of, 680, *683*
  carcinoma of, 216, *217*, 731–735
    clinical features, 730
    hepatomegaly and, ultrasound in, *60*
    metastasis with, 466, *467*, 468
    rectal villous adenoma with, *729*
    vs. pericolitis with pancreatitis, *1015*
  cathartic, 684, *685*
  computed tomography of, 132, *133*
  congenital diaphragm in, 653, *656*
  Crohn's disease of, 555. See also *Crohn's disease.*
  dilatation of, following jejunoileal bypass for morbid obesity, 639, *640*
  diverticulosis, bleeding with, angiography and transcatheter therapy for, 802, *802–803*, 804
  in ganglioneuromatosis, 685
  double-contrast examination of, 688
  duplication of, 653, *655*
  extramedullary plasmacytoma in, 686
  high, simulating free air, *190*, 191, *191–192*
  ileus of, 202, *203*, 212–213, 215–216, 217(t), 235
  in gastric adenocarcinoma, 461, *461*
  in herpes zoster, 686
  incomplete rotation or nonrotation of, 523
  indentation or stenosis of, with appendix epiploica, 685
  inflammatory changes, cholecystitis and, 866, *868*
  intussusception of, *221*
  lipoma of, 680, *681*
  obstruction, 187, 187(t)
  peritonitis, 663, *664–665*
  polyps of, 604, *605*, 751–753, *752–758*, 761, *762–764*, 764–765
    familial, 765, *766*, 767
    in Gardner's syndrome, 748, *749–751*, 750–751
    syndromes in, 722
  postoperative, 653, *657–662*, 658
  preparation of, 652
  pseudotumors of, 685
  radiation changes in, 594–595, *595*
  rupture of, 209(t), 230
  standard imaging studies of, 647, *648–651*, 651
  ulcer of, benign, 685
  urticaria of, 685
  vascular lesions, 676, *677–678*
  volvulus, 663–664, *665–666*

Colon cut-off sign in acute pancreatitis, 1011
Colonic interposition for esophageal carcinoma, 405–406, *407*, 408
   complications of, 417
Colonoscopic polypectomy, 756, 761
Colorectal carcinoma, 722, 730–731, *730–733*, 733, *734–738*, 738, *739–742*, 740–741, 743, *743–747*
   clinical features, 730
   differential diagnosis of, 738, 740–741, 740(t)
   polypoid tumors and, 752, *755–756*, 756
   postoperative features, 741, *742–747*, 743
   villous adenoma and, 725, *726*, 727
Colostomy, postoperative studies, 653, *657–662*, 658
Colotomy, complications of, 756, *759–760*
Common bile duct. See *Bile ducts.*
Computed tomography, 125–168
   general principles of, 125–126
   in cholecystitis, 913–914
   of abdomen, 128–133
   of adrenal glands, 150–152, *151–152*
   of biliary system, 138–140, *139*, 899–900, *900*, 1000–1001
   of kidneys, 144–148, *146–150*
   of large intestine, 652
   of liver, 137–138, *137–138*
      with abscess, 850–851, *850*, 852
      with cirrhosis with portal hypertension, 824–825, *825–826*
      with trauma, 838–840, *838–839*
      with tumors, 856–858, *857–858*, 859
   of musculoskeletal system, 162–163, *162–163*
   of pancreas, 140–144, *140–145*
      in acute pancreatitis and pseudocyst, 1023–1024, *1025–1026*, 1026
      normal anatomy, 1003–1006, *1004–1005*
      with abscesses, 1028, *1028–1029*, 1029
      with carcinoma, 1046–1047, *1047*
      with chronic pancreatitis, 1035, *1035*
      with traumatic pancreatitis, 1039
   of normal anatomy, 127–133
   of pelvis, 160–162, *160–162*
   of pleura and chest wall, 136–137
   of retroperitoneum and peritoneal cavity, 153–159, *153–155*, *157–159*
   of thorax, 133–137, *134–136*
      normal anatomy, 127–128
   techniques for, 126–127
   vs. radionuclide imaging, 164–165
   vs. ultrasound, 165–166
Congenital abnormalities, abdominal wall, 248–249, *250*, 251–252, *251–253*
Congenitally short esophagus, 348, 354, *355*
Congestive heart disease, *11*, 19–20, *19*
   intracardiac shunts in, radiocardiography in, 32
Connective tissue disorders, esophagus in, 331, *332–333*, 334
Conn's syndrome, 165
Contusion, traumatic, to kidney, *185*
Corpus luteum cyst, hemorrhagic, *93*
Corrosive gastritis, 473, *474*
Corrosive strictures of esophagus, 379–387, *380–386*
Crescent sign, in peptic ulcer, 421, 425, *425*
Cricopharyngeal muscles, abnormal function of, 322–323, *323*
Crohn's disease, 210, *211*
   anal fistula in, 788

Crohn's disease (*Continued*)
   differential diagnosis, 560–561
   gastroduodenal, *525*
   intra-abdominal abscess with, *106*
   malabsorption with, 573
   of duodenum, 532, *533*
   of esophagus, 346, *346*
   of large intestine, 673, 675, 701–702, *702–705*, 705, *706–711*, 711, *712–717*, 717, *718–720*
      extent and spread of, *704–711*, 705
      post-therapy changes, *716–720*, 717
      radiologic appearance, 701–702
      types of examination, 711
      vs. amebiasis, 675
      vs. ulcerative colitis, 720–721
   of small intestine, 550–561, *552–560*
      strictures due to, 546
   with biliary reflux, 971, *973*
Crohn's proctitis, 775, *776*
Cronkhite-Canada syndrome, 770
Cushing's disease, 165
   imaging of, 53
Cyst(s), adrenal, 83, 151
   Baker's, *110*
   breast, 111
   choledochal, 68
      in infants, 112
   hemorrhagic, of thyroid gland, *109*
   hemorrhagic corpus luteum, *93*
   in abdominal wall and mesentery, 101
   liver, 854, *854*, 856–857, *857*, 859, *860*
      computed tomography of, 137
      ultrasound of, *60*, 61
      vs. abscesses, 851
   mediastinal, 133, *134*
   mesenteric, 267
   of duodenum, 514–515, *515*
   of male genitals, 88
   ovarian, 93
      acute abdomen due to, 229
   pancreatic, *206*, 1009, *1009–1010*
   renal, 76, *76*, 96, 145–147, *146*, 148
      aspiration, 115, *116*
      vs. subhepatic abscess, 105
   splenic, 82, *1081–1082*
   subcapsular, in liver, *1005*
   theca lutein, 91
   ultrasound of, *56*, 57
   urachal, 249, *251*
   vs. visceral abscess, 105
Cystadenocarcinoma of pancreas, *73*, 74
Cystadenoma, of pancreas, 74, 144, *145*, 1009, *1009–1010*
   ovarian, 89–90, *89*, *90*
Cystic duct, obstruction of, 202
   remnant, postcholecystectomy syndrome and, 957, *958*
   tumor in, cholecystitis due to, 924, *925*
Cystic duct syndrome, 924–925, *926*
Cystic hygroma, *114*
Cystic lymphangioma, 267
Cystic vs. solid superficial lesions, ultrasound in, 110, *110*
Cystitis, 87

Dacryocystography, 51
Death, brain, scintigraphy in, *26*

Dermatomyositis, esophageal, 334
Detergents, corrosive strictures of esophagus due to, 379
Dextrocardia, 249
Diabetes mellitus, gastropathy in, *479*, 480
　hypotonic gastric state in, 52
Diaphrgam, congenital, in colon, 653, *656*
　congenital defects, 248, 249
Diaphragmatic hernias, 288, *289*, 290–291, *290–292*, 293
Diarrhea, in Zollinger-Ellison syndrome, 1060, 1063
　with radiation enteritis, 590
Diffuse esophageal spasm, 328–329, *328–329*
Dilatation, gastric, 478, *478–479*, 480
Dissection of aorta, 95
Diverticular abscess, *106*
Diverticular disease, 216
　bleeding with, angiography in, 722, 792(t)
　colonic, bleeding with, angiography and transcatheter therapy for, 802, *802–803*, 804
　　in ganglioneuromatosis, 685
　duodenal, 532–536, *534–535*
　epiphrenic, *338*, 339, *339*, 350
　esophageal, 335–340
　　retention of contrast in, 883, *884*
　intraluminal, 340, *341*
　　duodenal, 523–524, *524*
　intramural, 339–340, *340*
　　vs. esophageal moniliasis, 345
　　with corrosive stricture, 383, *385*
　left ventricular, 249
　Meckel's, 210–211, *212*, 251, *251*, 252, 625–629, *626–633*, 633, *634–635*, *636–637*
　　imaging of, 52, *52*
　midthoracic, 337, *338*
　of large intestine, 669, *669–672*, 672
　of small intestine, malabsorption with, 567, *568*, 569
　perforation in, *180*, 258
　pharyngeal, 335
　pharyngoesophageal, 335, *336–337*, 337
　subphrenic, 339
　urachal, 251
　vs. colorectal carcinoma, 738
　vs. diffuse esophageal spasm, 329
　vs. salpingitis, 229
　vs. sigmoid colon carcinoma, *735*
Double duct sign in pancreatic carcinoma, 1043–1044, *1044*
Doughnut sign, in brain scintigraphy, 25, 28, *28*
Drugs, corrosive strictures of esophagus due to, 379
　erosive gastritis due to, 473
Dumping vs. retroanastomotic hernias, 315
Duodenal bulb mimicking gallbladder, 891, *892*
Duodenal cap, simulation of, 433, *437*
　superimposition of pyloric canal in, 433, *435*
Duodenal-colic fistula, 548
Duodenal ulcer, 419, 432–433, *433–441*
　biliary fistulas with, 971, *972*
　bleeding with, angiography and transcatheter therapy for, 792, 792(t), 800, *801*
　choledochoduodenal fistula with, *880*
　gastric outlet obstruction due to, *446*
　perforation of, *178*, 201, *201–202*, 444, *445*
　　pneumoperitoneum with, *259*
　postbulbar, 440, *442–443*
Duodenitis, edema of papilla of Vater with, 515

Duodenography, hypotonic, *895*, 896
Duodenotomy, pseudotumor following, 518, *518–519*
Duodenum, 502–537. See also *Small intestine*.
　adenocarcinoma of, 463–466, *464–465*, 608–609, *609–610*
　adynamic ileus, in acute pancreatitis, 1011
　ampullary disconnection, 530, *531*
　atresia, 523, *523*
　bands, 249
　carcinoid tumors of, 621
　choledochocele, 517–518, *517*
　computed tomography of, 129, *130–131*
　Crohn's disease of, 532, *533*
　　biliary reflux with, 971, *973*
　cysts of, 514–515, *515*
　disorders of, barium studies in, *894*, 895
　　hypotonic duodenography in, 896
　diverticular disease, 532–536, *534–535*
　edema of papilla of Vater, 515, *516*, 517
　fistulas, 527, 529–530, *530*
　flexure pseudotumors of, 519–520, *520–521*
　gastric polyps prolapsed into, 448, *450*
　hematomas, 527, *528–529*
　　post-traumatic, 1036, *1040–1041*
　ileus of, *196*, *197*, 202, *207*
　in annular pancreas, 520, *522*, 523
　in superior mesenteric artery syndrome, 524, *525*, 526–527
　in Zollinger-Ellison syndrome, 477, *478*
　intraluminal diverticulum, 523–524, *524*
　intussusception pseudotumors, 518–519, *519*
　leiomyosarcoma of, *600*
　lipomas in, 605
　lymphoma of, 466, *466*
　　malignant, 611, *614*, *616*
　metastatic disease, 466, *467–468*, 468, 511, *512–514*, 513, *617*
　obstruction of, 520
　　due to aortic aneurysm, *526*, 527
　paralytic ileus of, 526
　polyps in, 602, *603*, 604
　postoperative pseudotumor, 518, *518–519*
　rupture of, *208*, 208, 209(t), 230, 483, *483*
　stump leak, 531–532, *532*
　tumors of, benign, 502–507, *502–509*
　　malignant, 507–513, *510–514*
Duplication, bowel, scintigraphy in, 52
　of colon, 653, *655*
Duplication cyst of duodenum, 514–515, *515*
Dysphagia, sideropenic, 340–341, *342*
　with achalasia, *324*, 326
　with Barrett's esophagitis, 354, *356*
　with connective tissue disorders, 331, *333*, 334
　with diffuse esophageal spasm, 328–329
　with double esophageal lumen, *362*
　with epiphrenic diverticulum, *339*
　with esophageal perforation, *358*, *372*, *374*
　with esophageal tumor, 387, *392*
　with esophageal webs, *343*
　with gastroesophageal carcinoma, *367*, 367
　with hiatus hernia, 351, *353–354*
　with intramural diverticulosis, 340
　with upper esophageal sphincter disorders, 320
　with Zenker's diverticula, 337
Dysplastic kidney in children, ultrasound in, 112
Dystrophy, myotonic, dysphagia due to, 322, *322*

Echinococcal abscess, effect on bile ducts, 966, *966*
Echocardiography, 56
Ectasias, vascular, of large intestine, 676
Ectopia cordis, 248
Ectopic pancreas in duodenum, 506–507, *507*
Ectopic pregnancy, ultrasound in, 92–93, *92*
    acute abdomen due to, 228–229
    paracolic abscess following, *193*
    vs abscesses, 107
Edema, of papilla of Vater, 515, *516*, 517
    pulmonary, *5*, *11*, 18–20, *19*
      with liver trauma, 843
    stomal, vs. retroanastomotic hernias, 315
Effusion, extraperitoneal, 181, 183, *184–186*, 186(t)
    intraperitoneal, 180–181, *181–183*, 184(t)
    pleural, 111, *111*, 118, 136
      vs. subphrenic abscess, 104
      with esophageal perforation, 374, *377*
Embolization, transcatheter, 795
Embolus(i), central venous pressure catheter, 3–4, *6*
    pulmonary, 17
      edema and, 19
      scintigraphy in, 36–37, *37*
      vs. pneumonia, 51
      with Swan-Ganz catheterization, *6*, *7*
Embryonal cell carcinoma, 155
    undescended testicle and, *162*
Emergency room, acute abdomen in, 177, 177(t)
Emphysema, *12*, *13*, 16
    with esophageal perforation, 358, 370, 371, *371–373*, 373
Emphysematous cholecystitis, *195*, 878–879, *879*, 913
    pneumobilia with, 969
Emphysematous pancreatitis, 233
Emphysematous pyelonephritis, 231
Empyema, following hiatus hernia repair, *365*, 367
    with appendicitis, 586
Endarteritis, radiation, 782
Endocrine tumors, 1054–1060, *1055–1062*, 1063
    in duodenum, 509
Endometriosis, 91, 229
    in large intestine, 679, *681*
Endoscopic retrograde cholangiopancreatography,
    in acute pancreatitis, 1016, *1021*
    in biliary system disorders, 903–904, *903–904*
    in chronic pancreatitis, 1032–1033, *1032–1033*
    in pancreatic carcinoma, 1042–1044, *1042–1044*
    in pancreatic pseudocysts, 1018, *1020–1021*, 1021
Endoscopic retrograde pancreaticocholangiography, 140
Endoscopic retrograde sphincterotomy (ERS) for bile duct stones, 931
Endotracheal tube, 8–9, *9–10*, 11
Enteritis, bypass, 641
    radiation, 550–561, *552–560*, 590–596, *591*, *592*, *594–595*
      malabsorption with, 573
Enterocele, partial, 301, *301*
    with obturator hernia, 302
Enterocolitis, pseudomembranous, 673, *673*
    vs. pneumatosis cystoides intestinalis, 679
Enteroliths, 554
    with Meckel's diverticulum, 628, *633*
Enteropathy, bypass, 641
Eosinophilic gastritis, 475–476, *476*
Eosinophilic gastroenteritis, malabsorption with, 572–573

Epididymitis, ultrasound in, *47*, 48
Epigastric hernia, 303–304
Epinephrine in gastrointestinal bleeding, 789, 793
Epiphrenic diverticula, *338*, 339, *339*, 350
Erosive gastritis, 473, *473*
Esophageal dilatation, 358, *359–362*, 360–361
Esophageal hiatus hernia, *135*, 288, *289*
Esophageal sphincter, upper, disorders of, 320, *321–323*, 322–323
Esophagitis, Barrett's, 354–355, *356–357*, 358
    bleeding with, transcatheter therapy for, 796
    corrosive, 379
    herpes, 345–346, *345*
    reflux, 325, 330–331, *330–331*
      vs. carcinoma, *400*
      with hiatus hernia, 351, *354*
      with intramural diverticulosis, 339
Esophagobronchial fistula, 346, *346*
Esophagocutaneous fistula following hiatus hernia repair, *366*, 367
Esophagogastric anastomosis for carcinoma, 404, *405*, *406*, *408*
    complications of, 411, 414, *415–416*
Esophagomyotomy, Heller, 326, *327*, *328*
Esophagoscopy, complications of, 358, *358–362*, 360–361
Esophagram, normal, components of, 390–391, *390–391*
Esophagus, achalasia, 323–326, *324*, *326–328*
    Barrett's, 52
      vs. carcinoma, 400, *400*
    candidiasis, *377*
    carcinoma of, *357*
      with corrosive ingestion, 385–386
    congenitally short, 348, *354*, *355*
    connective tissue disorders, 331, *332–333*, *334*
    corrosive strictures of, 379–387, *380–386*
    Crohn's disease, 346, *346*
    diverticula, 335, *336*, 337, *337–339*, 339–340, *340–341*
    double lumen, *362*
    foreign body in, vs. carcinoma, *396*, 397
    moniliasis of, *344*, 345
    motility disorders, 319–335
    peptic stricture of, vs. carcinoma, *396*, 397
    perforation, 358, *358–361*, 360, 368–378, *371–377*
      causes of, 369(t)
      clinical features, 370
      contrast examination, 375–376, *375–377*, 378
      pathophysiology, 368–369
      plain film examination in, 370–371, *371–374*, 373–374
      with corrosive ingestion, 379, 380, 381
      with radiotherapy, *413*
    radiation changes in, 593–594
    retention of contrast in, 883, *884*
    ripple, 329, *329*
    spasm, 334
      diffuse, 328–329, *328–329*
      vs. achalasia, 325
      with moniliasis, *344*, 345
      with scleroderma, *333*
    tumors of, 387–418, *388–389*, *392–405*, *416*
      treatment of, 404–409, *405–410*
        complications of, 409, 411, 411(t), *412–416*, 414, 417
    ulcers, vs. intramural diverticulosis, 339

Esophagus (*Continued*)
  varices, bleeding with, 789
    angiography in, 792(t)
    with cirrhosis and portal hypertension, 819,
      820–821, 821
  webs, 340–341, *342–343*, 344
Extra-alveolar air, 5, 12–13, *13–14*, 15–16, *15–16*
Extraperitoneal effusion, 181, 183, *184–186*, 186(t)
Extraperitoneal hemorrhage, 231–232, 232(t),
  232–233
Extrophy of bladder, 249
Eyes, ultrasound examination of, 111

Familial polyposis, 765, *766*, 767
Fasciola hepatica, in bile ducts, 966
Fat simulating pneumatosis and
  pneumoperitoneum, *192, 193*
Fecal impaction, 667, *667–668*, 774, *774*
Fecal incontinence, 773
Feces vs. villous adenoma, *723*, 727
Female genital system, disorders of, ultrasound in,
  88–94, *89–95*
Femoral hernia, 300–301, *300–301*
Fetus, blood sampling of, 119
Fibrinogen uptake test, scintigraphy in, 38
Fibroid, uterine, ultrasound in, *91*
Fibromatosis of gallbladder, 940
Fibrosis, congenital hepatic, 832–833
  due to pyloric ulcer, 446
  mediastinal, with corrosive ingestion, 385
  of sphincter of Oddi, 937–938, *938*
    with cholangitis, *929, 930*
  pelvic, 92
  retroperitoneal, 284–285, *284*
Fibrous peritonitis, 265, *267*, 267
"First pass" radiocardiography, 32
Fissure, anal, 788
Fistula(s), anal, 788
  aortoenteric, 790
    and paraprosthetic-enteric, 527, 529–530, *530*
  appendiceal, *588*, 589
  bile, 867
  biliary, 968–985
    arterial, 983, *983–984*
    duodenocolocutaneous, *977*
    external, 968, *969*, 977–981, *977–984*, 983
    internal, 968, 969, 970–973, *971*
    with gallstone ileus, 973, 975–977, *975–976*
  biliobiliary, 973
  bronchobiliary, 973, *974*, 981
  cholecystoduodenal, *203, 970, 982*
  cholecystoenteric, 917, *917*, 973
  choledochoduodenal, *880, 972, 980*
  duodenal-colic, *548*
  esophageal, 360, *362*
  esophagobronchial, 346, *346*
  following cholecystectomy, 948, *951*
  following hiatus hernia repair, *365, 366*, 367
  gastrojejunocolic, postoperative, 493, *495*
  ilioumbilical, 249
  in Crohn's disease, *554–556*, 554, 557, *559*, 702,
    703, 710–711
  jejunal, *1050*
  jejunocolic, transverse colon carcinoma with, *738*
  malabsorption with, 565, *566*
  of small bowel, with radiation enteritis, *592*, 593
  perirectal, *777*

Fistula(s) (*Continued*)
  post-colotomy, *759*
  postoperative, acute abdomen due to, 241
  rectovaginal, following irradiation, 679, *679, 783*
  renal arteriovenous, *149*
  splanchnic arteriovenous, traumatic, 817, *817*
  tracheoesophageal, due to radiotherapy for
    esophageal carcinoma, *412*
  vesicoumbilical, 251
  with diverticular disease of large intestine, 669,
    670–672
  with esophageal carcinoma, 404, *404*, 408
  with liver trauma, 842, *846*
Flexure pseudotumors of duodenum, 519–520,
  520–521
Floating spleen, 1071–1073
Fluid(s), collections of, evaluation of, 165
  following cholecystectomy, 948
  ectopic infusion of, central venous pressure
    catheter and, 3, *3*
  extraperitoneal, 181, 183, *184–186*, 186(t)
  free, with appendicitis, 583–584
  intra- or retroperitoneal, 180–181, *181–183*
  intra-abdominal, 102–104, *102–104*
  intraperitoneal, 261–262, *261–263*, 264
Focal nodular hyperplasia, liver, 861
Foramen of Winslow hernias, 309, *311–312*, 312
Foreign bodies, esophageal perforation due to, 369,
  371
  in esophagus, vs. carcinoma, *396*, 397
  in eye, 111
Four-day cholecystographic (Telepaque) test in bile
  duct calculi, 927, *928*
Fractures, computed tomography of, 163
  liver capsule, 836
  scintigraphy in, 49, *50*
  with celiac disease, 571
Fundal adenomyomatosis, 940, *943*
Fundoplication procedures, 490, *491*
  Nissen, 361–362, *363–364*, 384

Gallbladder. See also *Biliary system*.
  absence of, 113
  adenomyomatosis of, 940–941, *941–944*
    differential diagnosis, 945–946, *946*
  agenesis, 871, 873
  anatomy and variants, 866, *867*
  benign polyp, 989, *990*
  calcified, 940
  calculus of, *196, 197*, 202, *204*
  carcinoma of, 190, 985–987, *986–989*, 989
    metastatic to duodenum, 511, *513*
  cholesterolysis, 941, *944*, 945
  computed tomography of, 129, *130*
  congenital bands or septa, 946
  disease, *196, 197*
    oral cholecystography in, 881–883, *883–889*,
      885–887
  distended, vs. subhepatic abscess, 105
  double, 873, *873*
  duodenal bulb mimicking, 891, *892*
  enlarged, 652
  evaluation of, angiography in, 905–906, *906*
    scintigraphy in, *42*, 43
  following jejunoileal bypass for morbid obesity,
    640
  herniated, 871, *872*

Gallbladder (*Continued*)
  hydrops of, 189, *189, 190,* 201, 881, *881*
    with cystic duct obstruction, 923, *924*
  hyperplastic cholecystoses, 940–941, *941–945,* 945–946
  infusion tomography of, 904–905, *905*
    in cholecystitis, 916, 925
  normal, ultrasound of, *65*
  perforation of, cholecystoduodenal fistula secondary to, *203*
    with cholecystitis, 917, *918*
  phrygian cap deformity, 874, *874*
  porcelain, 877, *878*
    carcinoma with, 985, *986*
  positional anomalies, 871, *872–873*
  postural kinks, 945–946
  role of, in stone formation, 919, 922
  septum, 874, *874*
  shrunken, scarred, *922,* 923
  strawberry, 941, *944,* 945
  trauma to, 946–947, *947*
Gallium scanning, 164. See also *Radionuclide scanning*.
Gallium-67 scanning, in appendicitis, 586–587, *587*
  in tumor and abscess imaging, 50–51
Gallstone(s), 64–66, *65–66,* 196, *197,* 919, *920–921,* 922
  biliobiliary fistula with, 973
  carcinoma of gallbladder and, 985
  oral cholecystography of, 886–887, *886*
  plain film of, 875–879, *875–879*
  ultrasound of, *66,* 898, *898*
  vs. appendicoliths, 578
  with Crohn's disease, 559
Gallstone ileus, *194,* 212, 214(t), *548,* 549, 917, *917,* 973, 975–977, *975–976*
Gallstone pancreatitis, 923, *923*
Gamma camera, 24–25
Ganglioneuromatosis, intestinal, 685
Gangrenous closed loop obstruction, *213*
Gardner's syndrome, 748, *749–751,* 750–751
  duodenal carcinoma with, 509
  polyps in, 602, 604, *605*
Gas, abnormal collections, *190,* 191, *191–194,* 194, *195*
  abnormal pattern, 183, 187, 187(t)
  bowel, absence of, 543
  free peritoneal, abdominal wall disorders and, 256, *257,* 258, *258–259,* 260–261
  in appendix, 578
  in biliary system, 879–880, *880,* 883
  in portal venous system, 879–880, *880*
Gastrectomy, malabsorption following, 563, *564*
Gastric. See also *Stomach.*
Gastric antrum, contraction of, postoperative, 498–499, *499*
Gastric mucosa, imaging of, 52, *52*
  prolapse of, postoperative, 493, *496–497*
Gastric ulcer, 419, *420,* 421
  benign, 421, *422–427,* 425–427
    scar from, *428,* 431
    vs. adenocarcinoma, 457
  biliary fistulas with, 971
  bleeding with, angiography in, 792, 792(t)
    and transcatheter therapy for, 800
  malignant, 421, 427–428, *428–430*
  perforation of, 201, 444, *444*
  vs. outpouching, 490, *491*

Gastrinomas, 1058–1060, *1059–1060*
Gastritis, 472–477, *473–476*
  bleeding with, angiography in, 792(t)
    transcather therapy for, 794
  erosive, bleeding with, angiography and transcatheter therapy for, 799–800, *799*
  with Crohn's disease, *709*
Gastrocolic fistula, malabsorption with, 565
Gastroduodenal artery, normal anatomy, 1005, *1007*
Gastroduodenostomy, Billroth I, 485–486
Gastroenteritis, eosinophilic, malabsorption with, 572–573
  versus obstruction or ileus, 541
  viral, 226
Gastroesophageal junction, carcinoma of, *358*
Gastroesophageal reflux, 52, 334
  peptic stricture of esophagus due to, 396, *397*
  with corrosive ingestion, 385
  with sliding hiatus hernia, 349
Gastroileostomy, malabsorption with, 565
Gastrointestinal hemorrhage, angiography in, 789–793
  interpretation of, 792–793, 792(t)
  in Crohn's disease, 558
  in Mallory-Weiss syndrome, 480–481
  transcatheter therapy for, 789–790, 793–807
  with aortoenteric and paraprosthetic-enteric fistula, 529
  with esophageal tumors, 393
  with Meckel's diverticulum, 626–627, *626, 628–632, 634–635,* 636
  with peptic ulcer, 444
Gastrointestinal tract, barium-contrast studies of, in acute pancreatitis, 1012, *1013–1014,* 1014
  in biliary tract disease, 894–896, *894–895*
  in chronic pancreatitis, 1031–1032, *1031*
  in pancreatic pseudocysts, 1016, *1017–1019,* 1018
  changes, with radiation enteritis, 593–595, *594–595*
  computed tomography of, 126
  congenital abnormalities, 249
  disease, due to cholecystitis, 866, *868*
  metastasis, from esophageal carcinoma, 392
  polyposis, 602–604, *603–605*
  tumor, evaluation of liver with, 863
Gastrojejunocolic fistula, malabsorption with, 565, *566*
  postoperative, 493, *495*
Gastrojejunostomy, 485, 486, *486–489*
  afferent loop syndrome following, 566, *567*
  complications of, 498–499, *499*
  intussusception following, 496, *497*
  retroanastomotic hernia with, 314, 315, *315*
Gastropexy, posterior, 362, *365*
Gastropleural fistula following hiatus hernia repair, *365, 366,* 367
Gastrostomy tube, removal of, outpouches after, 490, *491*
Gated blood pool studies, 33, *33*
Genitalia, ambiguous, 114
  bifid, 249
  female, disorders of, ultrasound in, 88–94, *89–95*
  male, evaluation of, ultrasound in, 88, *88*
Genitourinary organs, pelvic, computed tomography of, 161–162, *161, 162*
  scintigraphy of, 45–46, *46–47,* 48
Giardiasis, malabsorption with, 575–576, *575*

Glioblastoma multiforme, scintigraphy in, 28
Glioma, malignant, 25, 27(t), 28
Glucagonomas, 1060, 1061
Goiter, nodular, 109
Graft patency, evaluation of, radionuclide angiography in, 36
Granular proctitis, 775, 776
Granulomatous colitis, 211, 224. See also *Crohn's disease*.
  inflammatory polyps in, 768
Granulous cell tumor, 89, 90
Graves' disease, 109
Groin, hernias of, 293–302, 294–302
  inguinal, 293–295, 294–296, 297–300, 297–300
Gynecologic disorders, acute abdomen due to, 228–230

Hamartoma, liver, 861
  of small intestine, 602, 603–604
Hampton's line, 421, 424
Heart, arrhythmias, central venous pressure catheter and, 3
  computed tomography of, 128
  congenital abnormalities of, 248–249
    shunts in, 32
  enlarged, esophageal displacement by, 319, 320
  evaluation of, radionuclide tests in, 32–36, 33–35
  failure of, congestive, 11, 19–20, 19
  perforation, central venous pressure catheter and, 3
  shunts, radionuclide methods with, 38
Heller esophagomyotomy, 326, 327, 328
Hemangioendothelioma, liver, 852, 853
Hemangioma, liver, 852, 853, 859
  of large intestine, 684
  of small intestine, 605, 606, 607
Hematobilia, postbiopsy, transcatheter therapy for, 804
Hematologic disorders, evaluation of, scintigraphy in, 45
Hematoma(s), abdominal, ultrasound in, 102, 103
  adrenal, 83
  biliary tract, 983
    with hemobilia, 982
  duodenal, 527, 528–529
    post-traumatic, 1036, 1040–1041
  extraperitoneal, 158–159, 158–159, 232
  extrapleural, central venous pressure catheter and, 3, 4
  following radical pelvic surgery, 93
  in perirenal and pararenal spaces, 185, 186
  intramural, esophageal obstruction due to, 361
  liver, following trauma, 836–843, 836–839, 841–842
    ultrasound in, 62, 63, 63
    vs. abscesses, 851
  of scrotum, 88
  pancreatic, 1006
  perinephric, 116, 117, 158
    vs. abscess, 106
  post-renal biopsy, 150
  rectus sheath, 101, 101, 255, 256
  renal, 78, 81
  retroperitoneal, 84–85, 85, 100, 100, 158–159, 158–159
  splenic, 43, 44, 45, 188, 1077, 1078, 1078, 1080
  subcapsular and perirenal, with kidney trauma, 185

Hematoma(s) (*Continued*)
  thigh, chronic, 162
  vs. pelvic abscesses, 107
  with pancreatitis, 144
Hemigastrectomy, Billroth I, 484–485
  complications of, 493, 493–495, 497
  Billroth II, complications of, 492, 492, 493, 496, 496, 498, 499, 499, 500
Hemobilia, 845, 847
  subcapsular hematoma with, 982
Hemoglobinuria, paroxysmal nocturnal, hepatic vein thrombosis with, 834
Hemophilia, chronic thigh hematoma in, 162
Hemorrhage, diverticular, of large intestine, 669
  extraperitoneal, 158–159, 231–232, 232(t), 232–233
    postoperative, 246
  following biliary surgery, 948
  following surgery for tumors of small intestine, 618
  gastrointestinal. See *Gastrointestinal hemorrhage*.
  hepatic, following trauma, 841
  in duodenal diverticulum, 534–535, 535
  in postoperative abdomen, 244
  large bowel, 218
  post-appendectomy, 588, 589
  pulmonary, with Swan-Ganz catheterization, 6, 8
  retroperitoneal, 158–159
  with liver trauma, 843, 845
  with pancreatitis, 143–144
  with radiation enteritis, 590, 592
Hemorrhagic cyst, thyroid, 109
Hemorrhoids, 787, 787
  vs. rectal carcinoma, 741, 741
Henoch-Schönlein purpura vs. Crohn's disease, 561
Hepatectomy, 816
  planning of, 815
Hepatic. See also *Liver*.
Hepatic arteries, 812, 815, 815
Hepatic duct, carcinoma of, 992, 992–993, 998, 1000
  arterial biliary fistula with, 983
Hepatic lymphatics, 816–817, 816, 901
Hepatic veins, 816
  catheterization, in cirrhosis with portal hypertension, 830–832, 831–832
  obstruction, portal hypertension due to, 834–835
  thrombosis, 816, 834
Hepatitis, alcoholic, hepatomegaly with, 818, 818
  chronic, 829
  scintigraphy in, 43
Hepatoma, 826, 829, 852, 854, 855, 857, 858, 862, 862–863
  in cystic duct, 925
Hepatomegaly, 831
  alcoholic hepatitis with, 818, 818
  colon carcinoma and, ultrasound in, 60
  with cirrhosis, 822, 824
Hepatosplenomegaly with ascites, 263
Hernia(s), 88, 287–318
  diaphragmatic, 288, 289, 290–291, 290–292, 293
  femoral, 300–301, 300–301
  foramen of Winslow, 309, 311–312, 312
  hiatus, 348–368. See also *Hiatus hernia*.
  inguinal, 293–295, 294–296, 297–300, 297–300
  peritoneography in, 261
  internal, 306–316
    location and relative incidence of, 307
  intersigmoid, 313, 314
  obturator, 301–302, 302
  of anterior abdominal wall, 248

Hernia(s) (*Continued*)
  of small bowel, 212, 546
  omental fat, *135*
  paraduodenal, 308–309, *309–311*
  pericecal, 312–313, *313*
  retroanastomotic, 315–316, *316*
  sciatic, 302
  transmesenteric, 313, *314*, 315
  umbilical, 302–303, *303–304*
  ventral, 303–304, *305–306*, 306
Herpes esophagitis, 345–346, *345*
Herpes zoster, colon in, 686
Hesselbach's hernia, 301
Heterotopic pancreatic rests, 469–472, *469–472*
Hiatus hernia, 348–368
  esophageal, *135*
  fundoplication procedures for, 490, *491*
  paraesophageal, 348–349, *348–350*
  peptic strictures with, *396*
  repair, 361–362, *363–365*
    complications of, 365–367, *367*
  sliding, 349, 351, *351–354*
  volvulus of stomach with, 482, *482*
  with Barrett's esophagitis, 354
  with congenitally short esophagus, 355
  with corrosive ingestion, *384*, 385
  with diffuse esophageal spasm, 329
  with esophageal scleroderma, 334
  with esophageal webs, 341
  with Mallory-Weiss syndrome, 796
  with midthoracic diverticulum, *338*
  with reflux esophagitis, 330, *330*, 400
Hill procedure, 362, *365*
Hirschsprung disease, 652
  fecal impaction in, 667
Histiocytoma, fibrous, retroperitoneal, 282
Histoplasmosis of large intestine vs. tuberculosis, 675
Hodgkin's disease, 153, *153*, 154
  gastric lymphoma in, 462
  lymphography in, 275, *276*
  malignant lymphoma in, *615*
  with pulmonary involvement, 377
Hofmeister defect, 486
Hofmeister type Billroth II hemigastrectomy, 486, *487–489*
Hydatid disease of liver, bronchobiliary fistulas with, 973
Hydatid mole, 91
Hydrocele, 88, 294, *295*
Hydrocephalus, 113, *114*
  cisternography in, 29
Hydronephrosis, 76, 77, *94*, *100*, 149
  in children, 112, *113*
  transplant, 79, *80*
  with appendicitis, 584, *586*
  with retroperitoneal fibrosis, *284*, 285
Hydropneumothorax with esophageal perforation, 373, *374*, *375*
Hydrops of gallbladder, 189, *189*, *190*, 201, 881, *881*
  with cystic duct obstruction, 923, *924*
Hydrosalpinx, 92
Hygroma, cystic, *114*
Hyperaldosteronism, *151*
Hypernephroma, 75–76, *75*
  tumor thrombus with, 98
Hyperplasia, adrenal, 151, 165
  lymphoid, vs. Crohn's disease, 560
  of Brunner's glands, 503, *504*

Hyperplastic cholecystoses, 940–941, *941–945*, 945–946
Hyperplastic polyps, 765
Hypersplenism, 1075–1076, *1075–1076*
Hypertension, portal, 99, *100*, 817–835
  due to cirrhosis, 817–819, *818–821*, 821–822, *822–833*, 824–832
Hypoperistalsis with reflux esophagitis, 330
Hypotonic duodenography, *895*, 896

^{131}I-radioactive iodinated serum albumin (RISA), 53
Iatrogenic peritonitis, 265, *266*
Ileal disease, 716–717
Ileitis, 712
  backwash, 673, 690, *693*
Ileocecal hernias, 312
Ileocecal tuberculosis, 673, 675
Ileocecal valve, carcinoma of, 725
    intussuscepting, *736*
  lipoma of, 680, *682*
Ileocolic hernia, 312
Ileocolic intussusception, 666, 667
Ileocolitis, granulomatous, 211. See also *Crohn's disease*.
Ileosigmoid fistula in Crohn's disease, 554
Ileotransverse anastomosis, 743, *743–746*
Ileum. See also *Small intestine*.
  adenocarcinoma of, *608*
  bleeding from, angiography in, 800
  carcinoid tumors of, 621, *622–623*
  Crohn's disease, 550, 551, *552*, 710
  gallstones in, *975*
  hemangioma of, 605, *606*, *607*
  leiomyosarcoma of, *601–602*
  lipomas in, 605
  malignant lymphoma of, 611, *611–612*, *615*
  metastatic tumor of, *617*
  obstruction in, *544*, 545
  terminal, air-fluid level in, in appendicitis, 579
  volvulus of, *298*
Ileus, adynamic vs. mechanical bowel obstruction, 183, 187, *187*(t), 209, 543–544, *543*
  gallstone, 194, 212, 214(t), *548*, 549, 917, *917*, 969, 973, 975–977, *975–976*
  in cholecystitis, 876, 914
  of cecum, 227
  of duodenum, 196, *197*, *207*, 526
  of large bowel, 202, *203*, 212–213, *215–216*, 217(t)
  postoperative, 234, *234–236*
  vs. intestinal obstruction due to adhesions, 265
  with appendicitis, 583
  with peritonitis, 264
  with ureteral calculi, 230–231, *230–231*
Iliac artery aneurysm, ultrasound in, *97*, *98*
Ilioumbilical fistula, 249
Impaction, fecal, 667, *667–668*, *774*, 774
Incisional hernia, 304, 306, *306*
Indium-111 chloride, 53
Infants, ultrasound in, 112–114
Infarcts, myocardial, scintigraphy of, 35–36, *35*
  pulmonary, with Swan-Ganz catheterization, 6, *7*
  sickle cell, 50, 53
  small bowel, perforation of, 245
  splenic, 1084, *1085*
Infection(s), anorectal, 787
  esophageal, 344–346, *344–345*
  imaging techniques in, 51
  malabsorption with, 575–576

Infection(s) (*Continued*)
  pelvic, 91–92, *91*
  renal, 77, *78*
  Trypanosoma cruzi, vs. achalasia, 324
Inferior mesenteric arteriography in gastrointestinal bleeding, 791
Inferior vena cava, 97, 98, *99*, 100
Inflammation, peritoneal, 264–265, *264–267*, 267
Inflammatory disease, esophageal, 344–346, *344–346*
  of large bowel, 52, 224–228, *224–228*, 224(t), 673–676, 688–721
  pelvic, 91–92, *91*, 229
Infusion tomography of gallbladder, in acute cholecystitis, 904–905, *905*, 916
  in acalculous cholecystitis, 925
Inguinal hernia, 212, 293–295, *294–296*, 297–300, *297–300*
  peritoneography in, 261
Injury. See *Trauma*.
Insulinomas, 1054–1058, *1055–1058*
Intensive care unit, 1–22
Intersigmoid hernias, 313, *314*
Intestine(s), appearance of contrast in, 883, *884*
  disease, imaging of, 52, *52*
  gallstones in, 973, *975*
  ileus vs. mechanical obstruction, 183, 187, 187(t)
  ischemia, postoperative, 244, *245*
  large, 647–788. See also *Large intestine*.
  obstruction, due to adhesions, vs. postoperative ileus, 265
    due to gallstone ileus, 973, *975*
    malrotation with, 249
  perforation of, 258
  small, 538–646. See also *Small intestine*.
Intra-abdominal abscess, 105, *106*
Intra-abdominal air, 16
Intra-abdominal arteries, ultrasound in, 96–97, *97–98*
Intra-abdominal fluid collections, 102–104, *102–104*
Intraluminal diverticulosis, 340, *341*
Intramesosigmoid hernia, 313
Intramural diverticulosis, 339–340, *340*
  vs. esophageal moniliasis, 345
Intraperitoneal abscess, *242*
Intraperitoneal air, *12*, 16, 178, *178–180*, 180, 234, 239, *239*, *245*
Intraperitoneal effusion, 180–181, *181–183*, 184(t)
Intraperitoneal fluid, 261–262, *261–263*, 264
Intraperitoneal gas, 256, *257*, 258, *258–259*, 260–261
Intraperitoneal masses, 652
  inferior vena cava displacement by, 98
Intrauterine transfusion, ultrasound in, 119
Intravascular catheters, 2–6, *3–8*
Intravenous cholangiography, in acute abdomen, 202
  in acute pancreatitis, 1012
  in biliary system disorders, 881–882, 883, 885, 889–891, *890*, *892–893*
    indications for, 889(t)
  in cholecystitis, 914–916, *915–916*
Intravenous vasopressin for gastrointestinal hemorrhage, 793, *793*
Intubations, endotracheal, 8–9, *9–10*, 11
Intussusception, 52
  following gastrojejunostomy, 496, *497*
  jejunojejunal, following bypass surgery for morbid obesity, 565
  of large intestine, 218, *220*, *666*, 667
  of small intestine, 211, 549, *549*

Intussusception (*Continued*)
  with colorectal carcinoma, 733, *736*
  with Meckel's diverticulum, 627, 628, *632*
  with tumors of small intestine, 598
Intussusception pseudotumors of duodenum, 518–519, *519*
Iodine-123, 52
Iodine-131, 52
Iopanoic acid (Telepaque), toxic reactions to, 881–882
Ipodate (Oragrafin), toxic reactions to, 881–882
Iron deficiency, dysphagia with, 340–341, *342*
Ischemia, of large bowel, 218, 222–223, 223(t)
  of small bowel, *204*, 210, 211(t)
  postoperative, 244, *245*
Islet cell tumors of pancreas, 1054, 1054(t)

Jabolay pyloroplasty, ulcer following, *494*
Jaundice, *814*
  angiography with, 905
  barium studies with, *894*, 895
  bile duct stricture with, *936*
  computed tomography with, 138–139, *900*
  due to impacted stone in ampulla of Vater, *928*
  evaluation of, 164
  in cholecystitis, 913
  in infants, 112
  in pancreatic carcinoma, 1045–1046
  in sclerosing cholangitis, 933
  transhepatic cholangiography with, 900–901, *902*
  ultrasound in, 66–69, *67–69*, *899*
  with cirrhosis, *824*
  with stenosis of sphincter of Oddi, 937, *938*
Jejunal interposition for esophageal carcinoma, complications of, 417
Jejunocolic fistula, transverse colon carcinoma with, *738*
Jejunoileal bypass for morbid obesity, 637–641, *639–640*, *642–644*, 643–644
Jejunojejunal intussusception following bypass surgery for morbid obesity, 565
Jejunum. See also *Small intestine*.
  adenocarcinoma of, 608–609, *608–609*
  bleeding from, angiography in, 800
  carcinoid tumors of, 621
  fistula, *1050*
  hemangioma of, 605, 607
  leiomyosarcoma of, *600*
  lipoma of, *606*
  lymphangioma of, *607*
  malignant lymphoma of, 611, *612–615*
  metastatic tumor of, *616*
  obstruction, with adhesion, 547
  polyp in, *603*
Joints in Crohn's disease, 560, *560*
Juvenile polyps, 764–765, *764*

Kidney(s), abscess vs. hematoma, ultrasound in, 106
  absent or ectopic, 249
  biopsy, ultrasound in, 115–116, *117*
  calculi, ultrasound in, 77, *78*, 197
  computed tomography of, 127, 128, 129, 131, 144–148, *146–150*
  cyst, ultrasound in, *96*
    aspiration, ultrasound in, 115, *116*

Kidney(s) (*Continued*)
    disorders, in children, 112, *113*
        ultrasound in, 74–79, *75–80*, 81, *81*
    enlarged, 187
    evaluation of, ultrasonic, 164
        scintigraphy in, 45–46, *46*, 48
    failure, ultrasound in, 70, *76*, 77, *77*
    hydronephrosis, ultrasound in, *94*, 100
    in prune belly syndrome, 249
    mass in, 652
    normal, ultrasound in, 74
    polycystic disease of, congenital hepatic fibrosis with, 833
    scan, radiation dose from, 24(t)
    traumatic contusion of, *185*

Laceration, hepatic, *842*
    splenic, *1078*, *1079*
Lacrimal duct obstruction, scintigraphy of, 51
Ladd's bands, duodenal stenosis with, 523
Large intestine, 647–788
    amoebic infestation, 777
    angioneurotic edema of, 685
    blunt trauma, 658, 663, *663*
    carcinoid tumors of, 680, *683*
    carcinoma, differential diagnosis of, 738, 740–741, 740(t)
    cathartic colon, 684
    Chagas disease, 686
    colitis cystica profunda, 680, *684*
    computed tomography of, 652
    Crohn's disease, 701–702, *702–705*, 705, *706–711*, 711, *712–717*, 717, *718–720*. See also *Crohn's disease*.
    Cronkhite-Canada syndrome, 770
    disorders of, acute abdomen due to, 212–228, *213–229*, 217(t), 226(t)
    diverticular disease, 669, *669–672*, 672
    endometriosis in, 679, *681*
    extramedullary plasmacytoma in, 686
    familial polyposis, 765, *766*, 767
    fecal impaction, 667, *667–668*
    ganglioneuromatosis, 685
    Gardner's syndrome, 748, *749–751*, 750–751
    hemangioma of, 684
    in Behçet's disease, 686
    in herpes zoster, 686
    in lymphogranuloma venereum, 778–779, *779–780*
    indentation or stenosis of, with appendix epiploica, 685
    inflammatory disease, 673, *673–676*, 675, 688–721
    intussusception, *666*, 667
    isotope studies of, 652
    lipoma of, 680, *681–682*
    malakoplakia in, 685
    nonfamilial multiple polyps, 767, *767–768*
    non-neoplastic lesions, 647–688
    peritonitis in, 663, *664–665*
    Peutz-Jeghers syndrome, 767, *769–770*, 770
    pneumatosis cystoides intestinalis, 679, *680*
    polyps of, 751–753, *752–758*, 761, *762–764*, 764–765
    postoperative, 653, *657–662*, 658
    precancerous and malignant lesions, 722–748
        examination techniques, 722–723
    preparation of, 652
    pseudotumors of, 685
    radiation injury, 676, 679, *679*, 779, 782, *783–785*

Large intestine (*Continued*)
    roentgen anatomy, 652–653, *653–657*
    schistosomiasis, 685
    shigellosis, 778, *778*
    standard imaging studies, 647, *648–651*, 651
    ulcer of, benign, 685
    ultrasound of, 652
    urticaria of, 685
    vascular lesions of, 676, *677–678*
    volvulus of, 663–664, *665–666*
Left renal vein, normal anatomy, 1004, *1005*
Left ventricular failure, 18–19
Legg-Perthes disease, 49
Leiomyoblastoma of stomach, 452–453, *453*
Leiomyoma(s), esophageal, 393, *393*
    of duodenum, 504–505, *505–506*
    of small intestine, 599
    of stomach, 451, *451–452*
    of uterus, 90, *91*
Leiomyosarcoma, in retroperitoneum or peritoneal cavity, 156
    of abdominal wall, *101*
    of duodenum, 504–505, *506*
    of esophagus, 400, *401*
    of inferior vena cava, 98
    of small intestine, 599, *600–602*
    of stomach, 461–462, *462*
    retroperitoneal, *280–281*
Lipoma, in retroperitoneum or peritoneal cavity, 156
    of abdominal wall, 101
    of duodenum, 503, *505*
    of large intestine, 680, *681–682*
    of small intestine, 605, *606*
    of stomach, 451, 453, *454*
Lipomatosis, of gallbladder, 940, *941*
    pelvic, 160
Liposarcoma, retroperitoneal, 84, *84*, 156, 271, 274
    duodenum and, 468, *468*
Littre's hernia, 301
Liver, 811–865
    abscesses, 847–848, *848–850*, 850–852
        with cholangitis, 929, 964, *964*
    anatomy, 811–817, *812–816*
    angiography of, 905
    ascites, 102, *102*, *814*, 816. See also *Ascites*.
    cirrhosis, *812*, 816, 854. See also *Cirrhosis*.
    computed tomography of, 128–129, *128*, 137–138, *137–138*
    disease, bronchobiliary fistulas with, 973
        ultrasound in, 58, *59*, 60–64, *60–64*
    enlarged, 652
    evaluation of, by ultrasound, 164
    hemangioma of, 606
    jaundice, *814*. See also *Jaundice*.
    lymphatics, *901*
    metastases, *814*
    polycystic disease, 77
    portal hypertension. See *Portal hypertension*.
    ruptured, 208(t)
    scintigraphy, 41, *41–42*, 43
        radiation dose from, 24(t)
    subcapsular cyst in, *1005*
    trauma, 835–843, *836–846*, 845, 847
        arteriography in, 836–837, *836–837*
        complications of, 842–843, 845, 847
        ultrasound in, 63, *63*
    tumors, *844*, 852–854, *853–858*, *856–859*, *860–862*, *861–863*
    varices, *812*

Loop obturation pattern in gallstone ileus, 977
Lumbar hernia, 304, *305*
Lumbar scoliosis in appendicitis, 579–580, *580*
Lung(s), barotrauma to, 12, *13*, 16
  computed tomography of, 127, 134–136, *136*
  disease, with scleroderma, *332*
  edema, *5*, *11*, 18–20, *19*
  embolus, 17
    edema and, 19
  hemorrhage, with Swan-Ganz catheterization, 6, 8
  Hodgkin's disase and, *377*
  scintigraphy, 36–38, *37*, 51
    radiation dose from, 24(t)
  shock, with liver trauma, 843
Lupus erythematosus, peristaltic activity with, 331, *334*
Lye ingestion, *380*, *382*, *384*, *385*, *386*
  corrosive gastritis due to, *474*
  corrosive strictures of esophagus due to, 379
  double esophageal lumen and, *362*
  esophageal perforation and, 369
Lymph nodes, evaluation of, ultrasound in, 84–87, *84–86*
Lymphadenopathy, computed tomography in, 153–155, *153–155*
  in children, evaluation of, 114
  retroperitoneal, 86–87, *86*
Lymphangiectasia, congenital, malabsorption with, 574, *574*
Lymphangiography, 87, 154–155
Lymphangioma, cystic, 267
  of small intestine, 607, *607*
Lymphangiomatosis of spleen, 1083
Lymphatics, hepatic, 816–817, *816*, *901*
  obstruction of, malabsorption with, 573–575, *574*
Lymphocele, 78, *80*, 81, 103, *103*
  following radical pelvic surgery, 93
Lymphocyst, 88
Lymphogranuloma venereum, 673, *674*, 778–779, *779–780*
Lymphography, 54
  in retroperitoneal lymphoma, 275, *276*
Lymphoid hyperplasia vs. Crohn's disease, 560
Lymphoma, 153–154, *154*
  bone, scintigraphy in, 49
  gallium imaging in, 51
  gastric, 462–463, *463*
  intraperitoneal, 267–268, *268*
  malignant, of small intestine, 611, *611–616*
    splenomegaly and, *1074*
  of duodenum, 466, *466*, 511, *512*
  of esophagus, 401, *401*
  of small intestine, malabsorption with, 574–575
    with celiac disease, 570–571
  of spleen, 1083
  rectal, *781*
  retroperitoneal, 84, 86–87, *86*, 273, 275, *277–279*
    vs. pancreatic tumor, 73–74
    vs. aneurysm, 96, *96*
    vs. colorectal carcinoma, 741
Lymphosarcoma, of duodenum, *466*
  of small bowel, *210*
  of stomach, 462, *463*
  vs. Crohn's disease, 560–561

M-mode scanning, 56, *57*
Malabsorption, 562–577
  bypass, 493

Malabsorption (*Continued*)
  causes of, 562(t)
  due to idiopathic pseudo-obstruction, 569
  due to partial or total gastrectomy, 563, *564*
  short bowel syndrome, 563, *564*
  with afferent loop syndrome, 566, *567*
  with amyloidosis, 572, *573*
  with bile acid insufficiency, 569
  with blind loops, 565–566
  with bypass surgery for morbid obesity, 563, 565, *565*
  with celiac disease, 570–571, *570–571*
  with Crohn's disease, 557–558, 573
  with eosinophilic gastroenteritis, 572–573
  with giardiasis, 575–576, *575*
  with lymphatic obstruction, 573–575, *574*
  with pancreatic insufficiency, 569, *569*
  with radiation enteritis, 573, 593
  with scleroderma, 566–567, *568*
  with small bowel diverticula, 567, *568*, 569
  with strongyloides stercoralis, 576
  with tropical sprue, 576
  with Whipple's disease, 571, *572*
Malakoplakia in cecum, 685
Male genitals, evaluation of, ultrasound in, 88, *88*
Malformations, arteriovenous, scintigraphy in, *26–27*
  of cecum, 676, *678*
Mallory-Weiss syndrome, 480–481, *480–481*
  bleeding with, angiography in, 792, 792(t)
  transcatheter therapy for, 795, *796*, *797*
Malrotation with intestinal obstruction, 249
Mass(es), abdominal, in children, ultrasound in, 112
  orbital, ultrasound in, 111
  superficial, ultrasound in, 110, *110*
  with acute abdomen, 189, *189–190*, 206
Meckel's diverticulum, 52, *52*, 210–211, *212*, 251, *251*, 252, 625–629, *626–633*, 633, *634–635*, *636–637*
Meconium peritonitis, 264, *265*
Mediastinitis from corrosive ingestion, 380
Mediastinum, computed tomography of, 127, 133, *134–135*
  fibrosis with corrosive ingestion, 385
  pseudocyst, 1026, *1026*
Megacolon, fecal impaction with, *774*
  following jejunoileal bypass for morbid obesity, 639, *640*
  idiopathic, 667, *667*
  in Chagas disease, 686
  in ulcerative colitis, 689, *689*
  toxic, *225*
    in Crohn's disease, 558
Megaesophagus, due to achalasia, *328*
  in Chagas disease, 686
Meglumine iodipamide (Cholografin), toxic reactions of, 881–882, 890
Melanoma, metastatic, to adrenal gland, *152*
  spleen in, 1083
Melanosarcoma of esophagus, 401, *401*
Ménétrier's disease, *476*, 477
Meningioma, scintigram of, 25, 27(t)
Meningomyelocele, sacral, 249
Mercedes-Benz sign, 876–877, *877*
Mesenteric cysts, 267
Mesenteric nodes vs. appendicoliths, 578
Mesentery, disorders of, ultrasound in, 100
  metastases to, *154*, 156
  tumors of, 267–270, *268–270*

Metal coils for transcatheter embolization, 795
Microatelectasis, 17
Midthoracic diverticula, 337, *338*
Milk of calcium bile, 877, *878*
Mirizzi's syndrome, 929, 931, 953, *956*
Moniliasis, esophageal, 344, *345*
  vs. herpes esophagitis, 346
  with intramural diverticulosis, 339
Morbid obesity, bypass procedures for, 563, 565, *565*, 637–641, *638–640*, 642–644, *643–644*
Morgagni hernia, 290–291, *291*
Motility, esophageal, disorders of, 319–335
Mouth ulcers with Crohn's disease, 346
Mucocele of umbilicus, 251
Multicystic kidney in infant, ultrasound in, 112, *113*
Multiple endocrine adenoma syndrome, 477
Musculoskeletal system, computed tomography of, 162–163, *162–163*
  evaluation of, 165
Myasthenia gravis, decreased peristalsis in, 325
  thymoma in, 133–134
Myelolipoma, adrenal, computed tomography in, 151
  retroperitoneal, ultrasound in, 84, *85*
Myeloma, multiple, 49
Myocardial infarct imaging, 35–36, *35*
Myocardial perfusion imaging, 33–35, *34*
Myositis ossificans, 50, 163
Myotonic dystrophy, dysphagia due to, 322, *322*

Nasogastric tubes, esophageal injury from, 796
Neck mass, in children, 114
  ultrasound examination of, 110
Neonate, esophageal perforation in, 369, *370*
  pneumoperitoneum in, *258–259*
Nervous system disorders, dysphagia with, 320
Neural arch defects, 249
Neuroblastoma, ultrasound in, 53
Neurofibroma of stomach, 451, 453, *454*
Neurofibromatosis, 255
  vs. polyposis, *771*
Neurolemmoma of stomach, 452
Neuromatosis of gallbladder, 940, 941
Neuromuscular disorders, upper esophageal sphincter disorders with, 322, *327*
Nissen fundoplication, 361–362, *363–364*, 384
Nodules, thyroid, imaging in, 30, *31*

Obesity, morbid, bypass procedures for, 563, 565, *565*, 637–641, *638–640*, 642–644, *643–644*
Obstruction, bile duct, 139–140, *139*, 201–202
    biliary fistula with, 978–979, *979*
  colon, roentgen signs of, 187, 187(t)
  esophageal, due to carcinoma, 404, 406–408
    from pneumatic dilatation, 361
    scleroderma with, *333*
  following jejunoileal bypass, 641
  following surgery for tumors of small intestine, 618
  gangrenous closed loop, acute abdomen due to, *213*
  hepatic venous, portal hypertension due to, 834–835
  intestinal, adhesions and, *192*
    due to gallstone ileus, 973, 975
    malrotation with, 249
    mechanical, vs. ileus, 183, 187, 187(t), 209

Obstruction (*Continued*)
  large bowel, 212–213, 216, 218
  lymphatic, malabsorption with, 573–575, *574*
  of duodenum, 520
    due to aortic aneurysm, *526*, 527
  of ureter, postoperative, 246
  presinusoidal portal, 832–834, *834*
  pseudo-, idiopathic, malabsorption with, 569
  pyloric, *244*
    vs. diabetic gastropathy, 480
  renal, 148, *149*
  small intestine, 538–550
    after pelvic surgery, 544
    contrast examinations, 544–546, *544–547*
    postoperative, *237–238*
    simple mechanical, 538–539, *539–540*, 541
    strangulation, 541, *542*, 543
    types of, 546, *547–549*, 549
    vs. adynamic ileus, 543–544, *543*
    with radiation enteritis, 592, *592*
    with tumors, 596. See also *Small intestine, tumors of.*
  with Meckel's diverticulum, 627
  with paraesophageal hiatus hernia, 349, *350*
Obstructive jaundice, ultrasound in, *899*
Obstructive uropathy, 230–231, *230–231*
Obturator hernia, 301–302, *302*
Oddi, sphincter of, dysfunction of, 957
  incompetent, 969, *970*
  spasm of, 938, *939*
  stenosis or fibrosis of, 937–938, *938*
  with cholangitis, 929, *930*
Omental fat herniation, 133, *135*
Omentum, metastases of, 156, *157*
  tumors of, 267–270, *268–270*
Omphalocele, 248, 249, 302
Omphalomesenteric duct anomalies, 249, 251–252, *251*
Operative cholangiography, 1001
Opisthorchis viverrini in bile ducts, 966
Oragrafin, toxic reactions to, 881–882
Oral cholecystography, 881–883, *883–889*, 885–887
  nonvisualization of gallbladder with, causes of, 882, 883(t)
Oral contraceptives, hepatic vein thrombosis with, 834
Orbits, ultrasound examination of, 111
Organ enlargement, acute abdomen and, 187, *188*
Osteochondroma, computed tomography in, 163
Osteoma in Gardner's syndrome, 748, *749–750*, 750
Osteomalacia with celiac disease, 571
Osteomyelitis, computed tomography in, 163
  scintigraphy in, 49
  with Crohn's disease, 557
Osteosclerosis in chronic pancreatitis, *1031*
Outpouches in gastric wall after removal of gastrostomy tube, 490, *491*
Ovary(ies), adenocarcinoma, omental metastases from, computed tomography in, *157*
  cyst, ultrasound in, 93
    acute abdomen due to, 229
  cystadenoma, ultrasound in, 89, *89*
  tumors, acute abdomen due to, 228

Pad sign, in acute pancreatitis, 1012, *1013*
  in chronic pancreatitis, 1031
Pain, abdominal, evaluation of, endoscopic retrograde cholangiopancreatography in, 904

Pancreas, abscess of, 1027–1029, *1027–1029*
  angiography of, 905
  annular, duodenum in, 520, *522*, 523
  aspiration biopsy techniques, 117, *117*
  calculi, 1012
  carcinoma of, 71, 73–74, *73*, 96, 1039, 1041–1047, *1041–1047*, 1052
    arterial biliary fistula with, *984*
    bile duct stricture due to, *935*
    metastasis with, 466, *467*, 468
      to duodenum, 511, *512–513*
    obstruction of common bile duct with, *894*
    vs. pancreatitis, 903
    with obstructive jaundice, ultrasound in, *68*
  cholera, 1060, *1062*, 1063
  computed tomography of, 126, 127, 130, *131*, 140–144, *140–145*
  cysts, 1009, *1009–1010*
  disorders of, 230
    bleeding from, transcatheter therapy for, 804
    hypotonic duodenography in, *895*, 896
    postoperative radiology with, 1047–1051, *1048–1052*
    ultrasound in, 69–74, *70–73*
  effusions, *1006*
  endocrine tumors, 1054–1060, *1055–1062*, 1063
  evaluation of, endoscopic retrograde cholangiopancreatography in, 903, *903*, 904
  gastrinomas, 1058–1060, *1059–1060*
  glucagonomas, 1060, *1061*
  imaging techniques, 51
  injury to, with duodenal rupture, 483
  insulinomas, 1054–1058, *1055–1058*
  islet cell tumors of, presentation of, 1054, 1054(t)
  laceration of, 208–209, 210(t)
  localization of, by ultrasound, 97
  mass in, 652
  nonhormonal diseases of, 1003–1053
  normal anatomy, *70*, 1003–1009, *1004–1008*
  pseudocyst, 68, 71, *71*, *72*, 141–144, 1022–1023
    dilated biliary radicles secondary to, *67*
    obstructive jaundice with, *900*
    vs. splenic morphologic variants, 1071, *1072*
  trauma to, 1036, 1039, *1039–1041*
  tumors of, in Zollinger-Ellison syndrome, 477
Pancreatectomy, 1048–1051, *1051*
Pancreatic insufficiency, malabsorption with, 569, *569*
Pancreatic rests, aberrant, 469–472, *469–472*
  in duodenum, 506–507, *507*
Pancreaticocholangiography, endoscopic retrograde, 140
Pancreatitis, acute, 1009–1012, *1011*, *1013–1026*, 1014, 1016, 1018, 1021–1024, 1026
  angiography in, 1021–1023, *1023*
  barium-contrast examination of colon in, 1014, *1015–1016*
  barium-contrast examination of upper gastrointestinal tract in, 1012, *1013–1014*, 1014
  computed tomography in, 1023–1024, *1025–1026*, 1026
  endoscopic retrograde cholangiopancreatography in, 1016, *1021*
  intravenous cholangiography in, 1012
  plain films in, 1010–1012, *1011*
  pseudocyst with, 1009–1010, 1016, *1017–1026*, 1018, 1021–1024, 1026

Pancreatitis (*Continued*)
  acute, pulmonary complications of, 1024, 1026, *1026*
    ultrasonography in, 1022–1023, *1023–1024*
  acute abdomen due to, 205–207, 207(t)
  alcoholic, nonvisualization with oral cholecystography in, 885–886
  barium studies in, 895–896, *895*
  bile duct stricture with, *936*
  Billroth II procedures for, stump leak following, *532*
  calcific, 198, *199*
  chronic, 1029, *1030–1038*, 1031–1035
    angiography in, 1035, *1036–1038*
    barium studies of upper gastrointestinal tract in, 1031–1032, *1031*
    biliary cutaneous fistula with, *951*
    computed tomography in, 1035, *1035*
    endoscopic retrograde cholangiopancreatography in, 903, 1032, *1032*
    plain films in, 1029, *1030–1031*
    ultrasonography in, 1034–1035, *1034*
  chronic relapsing, 844
  computed tomography in, 142–144, *143*, 145
  due to biliary tract calculi, 931
  duodenal obstruction due to, 520, *522*
  edema of papilla of Vater with, 515, *516*
  effusion from, 183
  emphysematous, 233
  gallstone, 923, *923*
  intravenous cholangiography in, 891, *893*
  pseudocysts with, 189
  small bowel ileus and, 543
  stenosis of sphincter of Oddi and, 937
  ultrasound in, 69–71, *70*
  vs. adenocarcinoma of papilla of Vater, 466
  vs. carcinoma and pseudocysts, 905
  vs. cholecystitis, 202, 889
  vs. retroanastomotic hernias, 315
  with perforation of duodenal ulcer, 445
  with postbulbar duodenal ulcers, 440, *442*, 443
Pancreatoduodenectomy, 1048–1051, *1051*
Pantaloon hernia, 299–300
Papilla of Vater, adenocarcinoma of, 465–466, *465*
  edema of, 515, *516*, 517
Papilloma, esophageal, 393, *394*
Paracecal hernia, 312
Paracolic abscess, *193*
Paraduodenal hernia, 308–309, *309–311*
Paraesophageal hiatus hernia, 348–349, *348–350*
Paralytic ileus, of duodenum, 526
  postoperative, *234*, 236
Paraprosthetic-enteric fistula, 527, 529–530, *530*
Pararenal abscess, *241*
Parasitic infestations of biliary system, 964–966, *965–966*
Parathyroid gland, imaging techniques, 51
  ultrasound of, 109, *109*
Paravertebral abscess, 233
Paroxysmal nocturnal hemoglobinuria, hepatic vein thrombosis with, 834
Patent vaginal process, 294
Paterson-Kelly syndrome, 340–341, *342*
Pelvis, abnormalities, with gynecologic disorders, 228
  abscess, 94, 95, 107, *107*
    with appendicitis, 584, *585–586*
  computed tomography of, 132–133, *132*, 160–162, *160–162*

Pelvis (*Continued*)
  hernias of, 293–302, *294–302*
    inguinal, 293–295, *294–296*, 297–300, *297–300*
  inflammatory disease, 91–92, *91*
  irradiation, small bowel injury due to, 590–596, *591*, *592*, *594–595*
  lymph nodes, 155
  mass in, *189*
    postoperative, 103, *103*
    ultrasound in, 89–91, *89–91*
  studies, in children, 114
  surgery, small bowel obstruction after, 544
Penicillin, gastritis due to, 473–474, *475*
Peptic stricture of esophagus vs. carcinoma, *396*, 397
Peptic ulcer, 419–447
  biliary fistulas with, 968, 971, *972*
  complications of, 444, *444–446*
  in Zollinger-Ellison syndrome, 477, 478
  intraperitoneal free air in, 178
  perforation of, *202*
    pneumoperitoneum with, 258, *259*, 260
    with Meckel's diverticulum, 626–627
Percutaneous needle biopsy, 137
Percutaneous transhepatic cholangiography, 140
  in biliary carcinoma, 995–996
  in cirrhosis, 827–828, *827*
  in pancreatic carcinoma, 1044–1045, *1044*
Perforation(s), bile duct, following surgery, 952–953, *954*
  esophageal, 358, *358–361*, 360, 368–378, *371–377*
    causes of, 369(t)
    clinical features, 370
    contrast examination, 375–376, *375–377*, 378
    pathophysiology, 368–369
    plain film examination in, 370–371, *371–374*, 373–374
    with corrosive ingestion, 379, 380, 381
    with radiotherapy, 413
  gastric, pneumoperitoneum following, *257*
  heart, central venous pressure catheter and, 3
  in Crohn's disease, 558
  of bowel, 258
  of colorectal carcinoma, 733, *737*
  of diverticulum, *180*, 258
  of gallbladder, cholecystoduodenal fistula secondary to, *203*
    with cholecystitis, 917, *918*
  of ulcers, 201, *201–202*, 244, 444, *444*, *445*
    abscesses and, 243, *244*
  of uterine cervix, 266
  rectal anastomotic, 743, *746*
  sigmoid, secondary to irradiation, *783*
  with appendicitis, 258, 582–583
  with colonoscopic polypectomy, 761, *762–763*
  with radiation enteritis, 593
  with Zenker's diverticula, 337
Periampullary cancer, 509
Periappendiceal abscess, *583*, 584, *584–587*
Pericardial effusion, radiocardiography in, 32
Pericecal hernia, 312–313, *313*
Pericolitis with pancreatitis, 1014, *1015–1016*
Pericolonic fat, simulating pneumatosis, *192*
Perinephric abscess, *78*, 106
Perinephric hematoma, 116, *117*, 158
Peripheral arteries, on ultrasound, 98, *98*
Peripheral vascular disease, evaluation of, radionuclide angiography in, 36

Perirectal fistula with Crohn's disease, *555*
Peristalsis, decreased, 325
  simple tertiary, 329, *329*
Peritoneum, abnormalities of, 261–270
  computed tomography of, 153–159, *153–155*, *157–159*
  fluid in, 261–262, *261–263*, 264
  inflammation of, 264–265, *264–267*, 267
  tumors of, 267–270, *268–270*
Peritonitis, 264–265, *264–267*, 267
  bile, 867
    following cholecystectomy, 948
  chemical, due to leak from cystic duct remnant, 981, *981*
  diffuse, with appendicitis, 583
  in large intestine, 663, *664–665*
  with cholecystitis, *918*
Pernicious anemia, atrophic gastritis with, 474, *475*
Pertechnetate, 53
Peutz-Jeghers syndrome, 767, *769–770*, 770
  duodenal carcinoma with, 509
  polyps in, 602–603, *604*
  small bowel obstruction in, 549, *549*
Pharyngoesophageal diverticula, 335, *336–337*, 337
Pharyngoesophageal muscles, abnormal function of, 322
Pharynx, abnormal function of, 322
  burns, 380
  diverticula, 335
  pseudodiverticula, 335, *336*
Pheochromocytoma, 53, 83, *83*, 151
Phlebography, 38, *39–40*
Pheboliths vs. appendicoliths, 578
Phrygian cap, deformity, 874, *874*
  vs. adenomyomatosis, 945
Pigment stones, 919, 922
Placenta, aspiration, 119
  imaging, 53
Plain films, in acute pancreatitis, 1010–1012, *1011*
  in biliary tract disease, 875–881, *875–881*
  in chronic pancreatitis, 1029, *1030–1031*
  in pancreatic pseudocyst, 1016, *1017*
Plasmacytoma, extramedullary, in colon, 686
Pleura, computed tomography of, 136–137
Pleural effusion, 111, *111*, *118*
  vs. subphrenic abscess, 104
  with acute pancreatitis, 1026
  with esophageal perforation, 374, *377*
Plication defects, 486, *487–489*
Plummer-Vinson syndrome, 340–341, *342*
Pneumatocele, rupture of, 12, *12*
Pneumatosis, pericolonic fat simulating, *192*
Pneumatosis cystoides intestinalis, 228, *229*, 261, 679, *680*
  following jejunoileal bypass, 641, *643*
  vs. polyposis, *771*
  with scleroderma, 567
Pneumaturia, pelvic irradiation and, 593
Pneumobilia, 969
  with postsurgical fistulas, *982*
Pneumomediastinum, 15–16
  endotracheal intubation and, 9
  ventilatory support and, 12
Pneumonectomy, radionuclide methods with, 38
Pneumonia, 18, *377*
  aspiration, *17*, 18
    with Zenker's diverticula, 337
  with liver trauma, 843

Pneumonitis, chemical, 18
Pneumoperitoneum, 256, *257*, 258, *258–259*, 260–261
    postoperative, 234
    with appendicitis, 582–583
    with esophageal perforation, 358
Pneumothorax, 12–13, *14*, 15–16, *15–16*
    in neonate, *259*
    tension, 15, *16*
        endotracheal intubation and, 9
    ventilatory support and, 12, *12*, *13*
    with central venous pressure catheter, 3, 5
    with esophageal perforation, *373*, 374
Pólya procedure, 486
Polycystic disease, 77, *77*
    of kidney and liver, congenital hepatic fibrosis with, 833
Polycythemia, hepatic vein thrombosis with, 834
    vera, splenomegaly in, *1075*
Polyp(s), adenomatous, of stomach, 448, *449–450*
        sigmoid colon carcinoma with, *731*
    cholesterol, 941, 945, *945*
    hyperplastic, 765
    in ulcerative colitis, 689, *689*, 690, *692–694*, 694, 696–697
    juvenile, 764–765, *764*
    nonfamilial multiple, 767, *767–768*
    of colon and rectum, 751–753, *752–758*, 761, *762–764*, *764–765*
    of gallbladder, 989, *990*
    of small intestine, 602–604, *603–605*
Polypectomy, colonoscopic, 756, 761
Polyposis, colonic, in Gardner's syndrome, 748, *749–751*, 750–751
    familial, 765, *766*, 767
    multiple, vs. pneumatosis cystoides intestinalis, 679
Polysplenia, 45
Polyvinyl alcohol for transcatheter embolization, 795
Popliteal artery aneurysms, ultrasound in, 98, *98*
Popliteal space, ultrasound examination of, 110
Poppel's sign, 466
Porcelain gallbladder, 877, *878*
    carcinoma with, 985, *986*
Portable radiography, 1–2
Portal hypertension, 99, *100*, 817–835
    due to arteriovenous fistula, 817, *817*
    due to cirrhosis, 817–819, *818–821*, 821–822, *822–833*, 824–832
    due to hepatic venous obstruction, 834–835
    due to presinusoidal portal obstruction, 832–834, *834*
Portal systemic shunt procedure, 816
Portal vein, 99, 813–815, *814*
    normal anatomy, 1004, *1004*, *1005*
    preduodenal, 523
    thrombosis, 840
Portal venous system, gas in, 879–880, *880*
Portacaval shunting, ultrasound following, 63
Portography, arterial, in cirrhosis, 828–830, *828–830*
    percutaneous transhepatic, in cirrhosis, 827–828, *827*
Portosystemic shunt procedures, evaluation of, 832, *833*
Positive end-expiratory pressure (PEEP), effects of, 11–12, *11–13*
Postbulbar duodenal ulcers, 440, 442–443
Postbulbar ring strictures vs. annular pancreas, 523

Postcholecystectomy syndromes, 937, 954, 956–957, 958–960
Postgastrodiverticular anastomosis, 339, *339*
Postoperative acute abdomen, 234–246
Postoperative aspiration, 17, *17*
Postoperative colon, 653, *657–662*, 658
Postoperative complications of radical pelvic surgery, 88
Postoperative pseudotumors, following duodenotomy, 518, *518–519*
Postoperative stomach, 484–501
    anatomy of, 485, 486, *486–491*, 490
    complications of, 492–493, *492–501*, 496, 498–501
    technique of examination, 484–485, *484–485*
Postoperative studies of biliary system, 69
    of blood vessels, 99–100, *100*
    of female genital tract, 93–94, *94*, *95*
    of liver, 63, *64*
    renal, in, 78, *79*
    ultrasound in, 58, 59(t)
        limitations of, 57
Practolol, peritonitis due to, 265
Precocious puberty, 114
Pregnancy, complications of, ultrasound in, 93, *93*, *94*
    ectopic, 92–93, *92*
        acute abdomen due to, 228–229
        paracolic abscess following, *193*
        vs. abscesses, 107
Preoperative studies, ultrasound in, 58
Prepyloric ulcers, 430, *431–432*, 432
Presbyesophagus, 329. *329*
Presinusoidal portal obstruction, portal hypertension due to, 832–834, *834*
Pressure, central venous, catheter for, 2–5, *3–6*
    liver sinusoidal, 831
    positive end-expiratory (PEEP), effects of, 11–12, *11–13*
    pulmonary capillary wedge, increase in, 19
    monitoring of, 5–6, *7–8*
    pulmonary venous, increase in, 18–19
    wedged hepatic vein, 830–831
Proctitis, 775, *775–777*, 777
    following therapeutic irradiation, 590
    ischemic, 786, *786*
    ulcerative, 690, *690–692*
Proctocolitis, due to lymphogranuloma venereum, 778–779, *779–780*
Prolapse, of gastric mucosa, postoperative, 493, *496–496*
    rectal, 773
Propranolol in gastrointestinal bleeding, 789
Prostate, carcinoma, metastatic, 49, *163*
    computed tomography of, 132, *133*
    ultrasound of, 88, *88*
Prune belly syndrome, 249, *250*
Pseudoabscesses, intra-abdominal, 244(t)
Pseudocalculus defect, 908, *909*, 938–939, *939*
Pseudocyst(s), cerebrospinal fluid, 103
    mediastinal, 1026, *1026*
    pancreatic, *1006*
        angiography in, 1021–1023, *1023*
        barium studies in, 895–896, *895*
        computed tomography in, 141–144, *144*, 1023–1024, 1026, *1026*
        dilated biliary radicles secondary to, *67*
        drainage following, 1048, *1049–1050*
        obstructive jaundice with, *900*

Pseudocyst(s) (*Continued*)
  pancreatic, traumatic, 1036, *1039*
    ultrasound in, 71, *71, 72, 1022–1023, 1025*
    vs. choledochal cysts, 68
    vs. pancreatitis and carcinoma, 905
    vs. splenic morphologic variants, 1071, *1072*
    with acute pancreatitis, 189, 1009–1010, 1012, 1016, *1017*–1026, *1018, 1021*–*1024, 1026*
  splenic, 1080, *1081*
  uriniferous perirenal, 231
Pseudodiverticula, following pyloroplasty, 486, *490*
  in Crohn's disease, 702
  pharyngeal, 335, *336*
Pseudomembranous enterocolitis, 673, *673*
Pseudomucinous cystadenomas, ultrasound in, 89–90, *90*
Pseudo-obstruction, idiopathic, malabsorption with, 569
Pseudopneumobilia, 975–976
Pseudopolyps in ulcerative colitis, 694, 767, *768–769*
Pseudosacculations of scleroderma, 567, 569
Pseudosarcoma of esophagus, 401
Pseudotumor, of colon, 685
  of duodenum, 514–527, *515–527*
  of Nissen fundoplication, *364*
  small bowel obstruction and, 541, *542*
  volvulus of small bowel with, *213*
  with jejunoileal bypass, 641
Pseudovolvulus, *216*, 218
Psoas abscess, *157*
Puberty, precocious, ultrasound in, 114
Pubis, deficient, 249
Puestow procedure, 1048, *1048*
Pulmonary. See also *Lung(s)*.
Pulmonary artery thrombosis, Swan-Ganz catheterization and, 6, *7*
Pulmonary capillary wedge pressure monitoring, 5–6, *7–8*
Pulmonary edema with liver trauma, 843
Pulmonary embolus vs. pneumonia, 51
Pulmonary infarction with Swan-Ganz catheterization, 6, *7*
Pulmonary stenosis, 249
Purpura, Henoch-Schönlein, vs. Crohn's disease, 561
Pyelonephritis, emphysematous, 231
  scintigraphy, in, 48
  xanthogranulomatous, 148
Pyloric obstruction, *244*
  vs. diabetic gastropathy, 480
Pyloric ulcer, gastric obstruction with, *446*
Pyloroplasty, charges following, 485, 486, *490*
  ulcer following, *494*
Pylorus, gastric adenocarcinoma into, 456, *456*
Pyogenic cholangitis, 963–968, *964–967*

Radiation dose from imaging procedures, 24(t)
Radiation endarteritis, 782
Radiation enteritis, 590–596, *591, 592, 594–595*
  malabsorption with, 573
Radiation injury to large intestine, 676, 679, *679, 779, 782, 783–785*
Radioactive tracer, 23
  localization of 23, 23(t)
Radiocardiography, "first pass," 32
Radiocolloid, 53
Radioisotope techniques, 23–54
Radiology, intensive care unit, 1–22

Radionuclide angiography, 36
Radionuclide dacryocystography, 51
Radionuclide phlebography or venography, 38, *39–40*
Radionuclide scanning, bone, 48–50, *49–50*
  cardiovascular, 32–36, *33–35*
  central nervous system, 25, *26–27*, 27(t), 28–29, *28–29*
  genitourinary tract, 45–46, *46–47*, 48
  in biliary system disorders, 896, *897*
  in cholecystitis, 916
  in pancreatic abscess, 1027, *1028*
  liver, 41, *41–42*, 43
    with abscess, 847–848, *849*, 851, 852
    with cirrhosis, 821–822, *823*
    with trauma, 837
    with tumors, 61, 853–854, 859
  lung, 36–38, *37*
  radiation dose from, 24(t)
  spleen, 43, *44*, 45
  venous system, 38, *39–40*
  versus computed tomography, 164–165
Radiotherapy for esophageal tumors, 404, *405*, 406
  complications of, 409, 411, *412–414*
Raynaud's phenomenon, peristaltic activity with, 331
Rectilinear scanner, 24–25
Rectosigmoid anastomosis, villous adenoma with, 747
Rectosigmoid stricture due to lymphogranuloma venereum, 778–779, *779–780*
Rectovaginal fistula following irradiation, 679, *679*, 783
Rectum, adenocarcinoma, after surgical resection, 747
  anastomosis, perforation of, 743, *746*
  bleeding from, transcatheter therapy for, 804, *806*
  carcinoma, 730
    clinical features, 730
    in tubulovillous adenoma, *729*
    in villous adenoma, *728*
  colitis cystica profunda, 680, *684*
  computed tomography of, 133
  familial polyposis, 765, *766*, 767
  hemorrhoids, 787, *787*
  lymphogranuloma venereum, 673, *674*
  lymphoma, *781*
  polyp of, *754*
  proctitis, 775, *775–777*, 777
  prolapse, 773
  stone, 685
  stricture, secondary to scleroderma, *782*
  tuberculosis, *781*
  ulcerative colitis of, 690, *690–692*
  villous adenoma, 725, *726*
    with colon carcinoma, *729*
    with rectosigmoid anastomosis, *747*
Rectus sheath hematomas, 101, *101*, 255, *256*
Reduplication, intestinal, 249
Reflux esophagitis, 325, 330–331, *330–331*
  vs. carcinoma, *400*
  with Barrett's esophagitis, 354
  with hiatus hernia, 351, *354*
  with intramural diverticulosis, 339
Regional enteritis, 550–561, *552–560*. See also *Crohn's disease*.
  anal fistula with, 788
  differential diagnosis, 560–561
Renal. See also *Kidney(s)*.

Renal artery, ultrasound in, 96, *97*
Rendu-Osler-Weber syndrome, 607
Residual urine determinations in children, 114
Respiratory distress, neonatal, due to esophageal perforation, 370
　with liver trauma, 843
Respiratory distress syndrome, adult, 17, 20–21, 20(t), *21*
Respiratory support, 8–9, *9–10*, 11
Rests, pancreatic, aberrant, 469–472, *469–472*
　in duodenum, 506–507, *507*
Retinal detachments, ultrasound in, 111
Retroanastomotic hernia, 315–316, *316*
Retrocecal hernia, 312
Retroperitoneal fat, kidney displacement by, *150*
Retroperitoneal nodes in malignant lymphoma, 611, *611*, *613–616*
Retroperitoneum, abnormalities of, 270–285
　abscesses, 106, *107*
　air, 13, 16
　computed tomography of, 126, 132, 153–159, *153–155*, *157–159*
　evaluation of, 165
　fibrosis, 284–285, *284*
　hematomas, 103
　masses, 652
　　inferior vena cava displacement by, 98, *99*
　　vs. splenic morphologic variants, 1071
　postoperative changes in, 99–100, *100*
　tumors of, 271, *271–274*, 274–275, 276—283
　　duodenum and, 468, *468*
　ultrasound of, 84–87, *84–86*
Richter's hernia, 301, *301*
Ring sign, 433, *440*
Rings, esophageal, 341, *343*, 344
Ripple esophagus, 329, *329*
Rokitansky-Aschoff sinuses in adenomyomatosis, 940–941, *942–943*
Rose bengal scan in biliary system disorders, 896, *897*
Roundworms, 675, *676*
Roux-en-Y reconstruction, 1048, *1048*
Rupture, esophageal, 368, 369, 370, 373, 374, 376
　of aortic aneurysm, 158, *158*
　of aneurysm, acute abdomen due to, 231–232, *232–233*
　of colon, 209(t), 230
　of duodenum, 208, *208*, 209(t), 230, 483, *483*
　of ectopic pregnancy, *92*, 93
　of liver, 208(t)
　of pneumatocele, 12, *12*
　of small bowel, 209(t)
　of spleen, 82, 208, 209(t), 1077
　pulmonary, with Swan-Ganz catheterization, 6, *8*

Sacral meningomyelocele, 249
Saddlebag hernia, 299–300
Salivary gland imaging, 53
Salpingitis, 229
Sarcoma, abdominal wall, 101, *101*
　in retroperitoneum or peritoneal cavity, 84, 156, *283*
　of spleen, 1083
　parosteal, 163
　Schatzki's ring, *343*
　Schistosomiasis, 685
　　effect on bile ducts of, 966
Sciatic hernia, 302

Scintiangiography, 25
Scintigraphy. See *Radionuclide scanning.*
Scirrhous carcinoma of duodenum, 511
Scleroderma, 190
　malabsorption with, 566–567, *568*
　peristaltic activity with, 331, *332–333*, 334
　rectal stricture secondary to, *782*
　reflux esophagitis with, 330
　vs. achalasia, 325
Sclerosing cholangitis, 933, *934*, *935–937*, *966*, 967
Scoliosis, lumbar, in appendicitis, 579–580, *580*
Scott procedure. See *Jejunoileal bypass.*
Scrotum imaging of, *47*, 48
　ultrasound of, 88
Segmental adenomyomatosis, 940, *941–942*, *944*
Selenium-75-selenomethionine, 51
Seminal vesicle, computed tomography of, 132
　cystic dilatation of, *161*
Seminoma, 155, *155*
Sentinel loop sign in acute pancreatitis, 1011, *1011*
Septa, congenital, in gallbladder, 946
Serosal metastases, 269, *269*, 270
　pneumoperitoneum with, *257*
Shigellosis, 778, *778*
Shock lung with liver trauma, 843
Short bowel syndrome, 563, *564*
　malabsorption with, 593
Shunt(s), cardiac, radionuclide methods with, 38
Shunt procedures, portosystemic, evaluation of, 816, 832, *833*
　radionuclide methods with, 38
　ventricular, 113
Sickle cell disease, asplenia in, 43
　bone marrow imaging in, 53
　infarcts in, 50
Sideropenic dysphagia, 340–341, *342*
Sigmoid. See also *Large intestine.*
　anastomosis, 743, *744–745*
　carcinoid of, *683*
　carcinoma, in tubulovillous adenoma, 728
　　perforating, *737*
　　vs. diverticulitis, *735*
　　with adenomatous polyp, *731*
　endometriosis of, *681*
　lymphogranuloma venereum, 673, *674*
　perforation, secondary to irradiation, *783*
　ulcerative colitis of, *691–694*
　villous adenoma, 725
　volvulus of, *218–219*, 541, *542*, 663–664, *665*
Sinus tracts in Crohn's disease, 702, *703*, *709*
Sjögren's syndrome, 53
Sliding hiatus hernia, 349, 351, *351–354*
Small intestine, 538–646
　absence of gas, 543
　appendicitis, 577–589
　bleeding from, angiography and transcatheter therapy for, 800
　bypass procedures for morbid obesity, 637–641, *638–640*, *642–644*, *643–644*
　carcinoma of, strictures due to, 546
　disorders of, 209–212, *210–214*, 211(t)
　distended loop, vs. abscess, 104
　ileus, 235
　ischemia, *204*, 210, 211(t)
　lumen, obturation of, *548–549*, 549
　malabsorption syndromes in, 562–577. See also *Malabsorption syndromes.*
　Meckel's diverticulum, 625–629, *626–633*, 633, *634–635*, *636–637*

Small intestine (*Continued*)
  obstruction, 538–550
    after pelvic surgery, 544
    contrast examinations, 544–546, *544–547*
    due to adhesions, *192, 267*
    postoperative, *237–238*
    simple mechanical, 538–539, *539–540*, 541
    strangulation, 541, *542*, 543
    types of, 546, *547–549*, 549
    vs. adynamic ileus, 543–544, *543*
    with appendicitis, 227
  perforation, *245*
  radiation enteritis, 590–596
  regional enteritis, 550–561, *552–560*. See also *Crohn's disease.*
  rupture of, 209(t)
  tuberculosis, vs. Crohn's disease, 560
  tumors of, 596–619
    adenocarcinoma, 608–609, *608–610*
    angiography in, 597
    benign glandular, 602–604, *603–605*
    carcinoid, 620–622, *622–623*, *624–625*
    computerized tomography and ultrasound in, 597
    contrast examination in, 597
    hemangioma, 605, *606*, 607
    incidence of, 596
    leiomyoma and leiomyosarcoma, 599, *600–602*
    lipomas, 605, *606*
    lymphangioma, 607, *607*
    malignant lymphoma, 611, *611–616*
    metastatic, 616–618, *616–618*
    postoperative complications, 618, *619*
    roentgenologic signs, 598
    symptoms and signs, 598
Sodium hydroxide. See *Lye*
Soft tissue tumor, 110, *110*
Spasm, bile duct, 908, *909*
  esophageal, 334
    diffuse, 328–329, *328–329*
    vs. achalasia, 325
    with moniliasis, *344*, 345
    with scleroderma, *333*
  large intestine, vs. colorectal carcinoma, 740, *740*
  of cecum, 264
  of sphincter of Oddi, 938, *939*
  with duodenal ulcer, 433, *436*
Spermatic cord, computed tomography of, 133
Sphincter, upper esophageal, disorders of, 320, *321–323*, *322–323*
Sphincter of Oddi, dysfunction of, 957
  incompetent, 969, *970*
  spasm of, 938, *939*
  stenosis or fibrosis of, 937–938, *938*
  with cholangitis, 929, *930*
Sphincterotomy, endoscopic retrograde, for bile duct stones, 931
  for pancreatic disease, 1048
Spider telangiectasias, 607
Spider web pattern in Budd-Chiari syndrome, 834
Spigelian hernia, 304, *305*
Spine, congenital anomalies, 249
Spleen, 1064–1088
  abscess of, 1083–1084, *1084*
  accessory, 1073–1074, *1073–1074*
  agenesis, with congenitally short esophagus, 354
  anatomic variants, 1071–1073, *1072*
  computed tomography of, 128–129
  cysts. 1080, *1081–1082*

Spleen (*Continued*)
  enlarged. See *Splenomegaly.*
  floating or wandering, 1072–1073
  historical aspects, 1064–1065
  hypersplenism, 1075–1076, *1075–1076*
  in malignant lymphoma, 611, *615*
  infarction of, 1084, *1085*
  neoplasms, 1083, *1083*
  normal, 1065–1073, *1066–1072*
  rupture of, 208, 209(t)
  scintigraphy, 43, *44*, 45
    radiation dose from, 24(t)
  trauma to, 1077–1078, *1077–1080*, 1080
  ultrasound of, 82, *82*
  upside-down, 1073
Splenectomy, 1077, 1085, *1086–1087*
Splenic artery, aneurysms, 1084, *1086*
  calcific atherosclerotic disease in, 1066, *1066*
Splenic vein, 97, 1066–1067, *1067*
  normal anatomy, 1004, *1004*
Splenomegaly, 82, *82*, 187, *188*, 652, 1075, *1075–1076*
  following trauma, 1077, *1077*
  lymphoma and, *279*, *1074*
  with cirrhosis and portal hypertension, 818, 822, 824, 825
  with retroperitoneal tumors, 271
Splenoportography, 813
  in cirrhosis, 826, *827*
Splenosis, 45, 1080
Sprue, malabsorption with, 576
  vs. radiation enteritis, 593
  vs. scleroderma, 567
Staphylococcal enterocolitis, 673
Stenosis, of sphincter of Oddi, 937–938, *938*
  with cholangitis, 929, *930*
  pulmonary, 249
Stomach, aberrant pancreatic rests, 469–472, *469–472*
  adenocarcinoma of, 455–457, *455–461*, 461
  adenomatous polyps, 448, *449–450*
  bypass, for morbid obesity, 637, *638*, 641
  carcinoma of, adenomatous polyps and, 448
    vs. lymphoma, 462, *463*
    vs. varices, *403*, 404
  computed tomography of, 128
  Crohn's disease, *553*, *709*
  dilatation of, 478, *478–479*, 480
  edema of, cholecystitis and, *868*
  gastritis, 472–477, *473–476*
  imaging of, 52, *52*
  in Mallory-Weiss syndrome, 480–481, *480–481*
  in Zollinger-Ellison syndrome, 477–478, *477*
  leiomyosarcoma, 461–462, *462*
  lymphoma of, 462–463, *463*
  metastatic involvement of, 466, *467*, 468
    from esophageal carcinoma, *392*
  obstruction, due to duodenal ulcer, *446*
    with hiatus hernia, *350*
    with pyloric ulcer, *446*
  perforation, pneumoperitoneum following, *257*
  postoperative, 484–501
    anatomy of, 485–486, *486–491*, 490
    complications of, 492–493, *492–501*, 496, 498–501
    technique of examination, 484–485, *484–485*
  prepyloric region, ulcers of, 430, *431–432*, 432
  radiation changes in, 594, *594*
  radiographic study of, 419, *420*, 421

Stomach (Continued)
  remnant, carcinoma of, 500–501, *501*
  retention of contrast in, 882–883, *883*
  rupture of, 208
  tumors of, 448–463, *449–463*
    benign mesenchymal, 451–453, *451–454*
  ulcers, 419
    benign, 421, *422–427*, 425–427
      scar from, 428, *431*
      vs. adenocarcinoma, 457
    malignant, 421, 427–428, *428–430*
  volvulus of, 482, *482*
Stomal edema vs. retroanastomotic hernias, 315
Stones, bile duct. See *Choledocholithiasis*.
  gallbladder. See *Gallstone(s)*.
  pancreatic, 1012
    in chronic pancreatitis, 1029, *1030*, *1031*
  rectal, 685
  renal, 77, *78*, 197
    with Crohn's disease, 559
  ureteral, ileus with, 230–231, *230–231*
    postoperative, 246
  urinary tract, following jejunoileal bypass, 644, *644*
  with Meckel's diverticulum, 628, *633*
Strangulation obstruction of small intestine, 541, *542*, 543
Strawberry gallbladder, 941, *944*, 945
Stress ulcer, bleeding with, angiography and transcatheter therapy for, 799, 800
  perforation of, 244
Stricture(s), Barrett's esophagitis with, *356*, 357
  caustic, esophageal perforation and, 369
  corrosive, of esophagus, 379–387, *380–386*
  due to postbulbar ulcer, vs. annular pancreas, 523
  esophageal, radiation-induced, *414*
  gastroesophageal, due to carcinoma, *367*
  hiatus hernia with, 351, *353*
  ischemic colon and, *678*
  midesophageal, *359*
  of biliary tract, 935–937, *934–936*
    due to carcinoma, *935*
    due to surgical trauma, 953–954, *955*
  of small intestine, 546
    malabsorption with, 565
    with radiation enteritis, 592
  peptic, of esophagus, vs. carcinoma, *396*, 397
  post-colotomy, 760
  rectal, secondary to scleroderma, *782*
  reflux esophagitis with, *400*
  with congenitally short esophagus, 354, *355*
  with Crohn's disease, 554, *556*
  with sclerosing cholangitis, *933*, 934
String sign, in Crohn's disease, 554, 702, *708*
Strongyloides stercoralis, malabsorption with, 576
Subcapsular cyst, *1005*
Subcapsular hematoma, *983*
  with hemobilia, *982*
Subcutaneous tissues, air in, 16
Subdiaphragmatic abscess, *242–243*
Subhepatic abscess, *64*, 105, *981*
Subphrenic abscess, 104–105, *105*, *981*
  bronchobiliary fistula from, *974*
  following hiatus hernia repair, *366*, 367
Subphrenic diverticulum, 339
Superior mesenteric arterial infusion of vasopressin for gastrointestinal hemorrhage, 789–790, 793, 794
Superior mesenteric arteriography in gastrointestinal bleeding, 790–793

Superior mesenteric artery, 96, *97*
  normal anatomy, 1004, *1004*
  occlusion of, 676
  syndrome, 524, *525*, 526–527
Suppurative cholangitis, 963–968, *964–967*
Suprapubic aspiration, with ultrasound, 87
Surgical disorders, computed tomography in, 125–168
Surgical injuries to biliary system, 948, *949–956*, 950, 952–954
Swallowing disorders, 320, 322–323
Swan-Ganz catheterization, 5–6, *7–8*
Systemic lupus erythematous, peristaltic activity with, 331, 334

T-tubes, following biliary tract surgery, complications with, 950, 952, *952–953*, 977–981, *977–979*
Tamponade, cardiac, central venous pressure catheter and, 3
^{99m}Tc-albumin, 53
Telangiectasis, spider, 607
Telepaque, four-day cholecystographic test, in bile duct calculi, 927, *928*
  toxic reactions, 881–882
Tension pneumothorax, 15, *16*
  with esophageal perforation, *373*
Teratocarcinoma, 155
Teratodermoid, retroperitoneal, 271, *272*
Teratoma, retroperitoneal, *271*
Testis, epididymitis, 47, *48*
  torsion, 47, *48*
  tumors, 155, *155*
  undescended, 161, *161*, *162*, 294, *295*
    in prune belly syndrome, 249
Thal fundal patch technique, 362
Theca lutein cysts, 91
Thigh, hematoma, chronic, *162*
Thoracentesis, 109
  ultrasound with, *118*, 119
Thoracic aorta, 96
Thorax, computed tomography of, 126, *127–128*, 133–137, *134–136*
  ultrasound of, 111, *111*
Thromboangiitis obliterans, 676
Thrombophlebitis, Baker's cyst with, *110*
  scintigraphy in, 38, *39–40*
Thrombosis, central venous pressure catheter and, 2, 3, 4
  detection of, fibrinogen uptake test, 38
  venous system scintigraphy, 38, *39–40*
  hepatic vein, 816, 834
  portal vein, 840
  pulmonary artery, Swan-Ganz catheterization and, 6, *7*
  renal, 148
  tumor, with hypernephromas, 98
  with aortic aneurysm, 95, *96*
Thymoma, *134*
Thyroid gland, imaging, 30–31, *31*, *32*
  radiation dose from, 24(t)
  ultrasound of, 108–109, *108–109*
Thyroiditis, subacute, 109
Tomography, computed, 125–168. See also *Computed tomography*.
  infusion, of gallbladder, 904–905, *905*
    in cholecystitis, 916

Toxic megacolon, 225
  in Crohn's disease, 558
  vs. megacolon following jejunoileal bypass, 639
Tracer, radioactive, 23
  localization of, 23, 23(t)
Tracheoesophageal fistula due to radiotherapy for esophageal carcinoma, 412
Transcatheter therapy, for arteriocapillary esophageal bleeding, 796, 797
  for colonic angiodysplasia, 804, 805
  for colonic diverticulosis, 802, 802–803, 804
  for gastrointestinal hemorrhage, 787–790, 793–807
    complications of, 795
    dose and administration, 794
    due to duodenal ulcer, 800, 801
    due to erosive gastritis, 799–800, 799
    due to gastric ulcer, 800
    due to Mallory-Weiss tears, 804, 805
    due to stress ulcer, 799, 800
    due to varices, 796–799, 798
    from small intestine, 800
    indications for, 806
Transfusion, intrauterine, 119
Transhepatic cholangiography in biliary system disorders, 900–901, 901–902, 903
Transmesenteric hernia, 313, 314, 315
Transmesosigmoid hernia, 313, 314
Transplant kidney, 79, 79–81, 81
  function, evaluation of, 46, 48
Trauma, acute abdomen due to, 205, 207–209, 208, 208(t), 209(t), 210(t)
  biliary, 841, 842, 946–947, 947
    surgical, 948, 949–956, 950, 952–954
  bone, 49, 50
  diaphragmatic hernia due to, 291, 292, 293
  duodenal, 483, 483
  liver, 835–843, 836–846, 845, 847. See also under *Liver*.
  pneumoperitoneum due to, 260
  to duodenum, 527–532, 528–532
  to kidney, 78, 185
    scintigraphy in, 46
  to large intestine, 658, 663, 663
  to pancreas, 208–209, 210(t), 1036, 1039, 1039–1041
  to right flank, 186
  to spleen, 82, 1077–1078, 1077–1080, 1080
    scintigraphy in, 43, 44, 45
Trophoblastic disease, 90
Tropical sprue, malabsorption with, 576
Trypanosoma cruzi infection vs. achalasia, 324
Tuberculosis, gallium-67 citrate imaging in, 51
  ileocecal, 673, 675
  intestinal, vs. Crohn's disease, 560
  rectal, 781
Tuberculous peritonitis, 264, 268
Tubo-ovarian abscess, 91, 91, 92, 107
Tubulovillous adenoma, 725
  rectal carcinoma in, 729
  sigmoid colon carcinoma in, 728
Tumor(s). See also *Carcinoma*.
  abdominal wall, 253–254, 254–255
  adrenal gland, 83–84, 151, 151
    imaging in, 53
  ampullary, 139
  bladder, 87
  bone, computed tomography in, 163
  carcinoid, of large intestine, 680, 683
  cystic duct, cholecystitis due to, 924, 925

Tumor(s) (*Continued*)
  endocrine, 1054–1060, 1055–1062, 1063
  eye, 111
  genitourinary, 162
  imaging techniques, 50–51
    radiation dose from, 24(t)
  in Gardner's syndrome, 748, 749–750, 750
  liver, 137–138, 138, 844, 852–854, 853–858, 856–859, 860–862, 861–863
    ultrasound in, 60–61, 60
  lung, computed tomography in, 134–136, 136
  of bile ducts, benign, 990
  of duodenum, benign, 502–507, 502–509
    malignant, 507–513, 510–514
  of esophagus, 387–418, 388–389, 392–405, 416
    treatment of, 404–409, 405–410
      complications of, 409, 411, 411(t), 412–416, 414, 417
  of gallbladder, benign, 989, 990
  of pancreas, 71, 73–74, 73, 144, 145
    computed tomography of, 130
    in Zollinger-Ellison syndrome, 477
  of peritoneum, mesentery, and omentum, 267–270, 268–270
  of pleura and chest wall, 136–137
  of scrotum, 88
  of small intestine, 209, 210, 210, 596–619. See also under *Small intestine*.
  of spleen, 1083, 1083
  of stomach, 448–463, 449–463
    benign mesenchymal, 451–453, 451–454
  ovarian, acute abdomen due to, 228
  pelvic, 89, 161
  renal, 147–148, 147, 148
    with cyst, 116
  retroperitoneal, 84, 84, 85, 155–156, 157, 271, 271–274, 274–275, 276–283
    duodenum and, 468, 468
  soft tissue, 110, 110
  testicular, 155, 155
  vs. cyst, ultrasound of, 57
  vs. radiation enteritis, 591
Tumor thrombus, inferior vena cava, with hypernephromas, 98

Ulcer(s), anastomotic, 415
  aphthoid, in Crohn's disease, 551, 552
  benign, of colon, 685
  bleeding, in duodenal diverticulum, 534–535, 535
  duodenal, 419, 432–433, 433–441. See also *Duodenal ulcer*.
  esophageal, vs. intramural diverticulosis, 339
    with corrosive ingestion, 382
  following gastric surgery, 493, 493–495
  gastric. See *Gastric ulcer*.
  hiatus hernia with, 351, 352–353
  in Behçet's disease, 686
  in Crohn's disease, 702, 702, 704–705, 707, 709
  mouth, with Crohn's disease, 346
  of small bowel, with radiation enteritis, 592
  peptic, 419–447. See also *Peptic ulcer*.
  perforation of, 201, 201–202
    abscesses and, 243, 244
  postbulbar, strictures from, vs. annular pancreas, 523
  prepyloric, 430, 431, 432, 432
  pyloric, gastric obstruction with, 446
  radiation, 594, 595

Ulcer(s) (*Continued*)
  stress, bleeding with, angiography and transcatheter therapy for, 799, 800
    perforation of 244
  vs. pancreatic rests, 507
  with Barrett's esophagitis, 355, *356, 400*
  with corrosive stricture, *384*
  with esophageal carcinoma, *398, 399*
  with duodenal carcinoma, 509, *510*
  with esophageal moniliasis, *344,* 345
  with herpes esophagitis, 345
  with lye ingestion, 379
  with reflux esophagitis, 330–331, *330–331, 400*
  with Zenker's diverticula, 337
Ulcer collar, 421, *422, 424*
Ulcerative colitis, 224, 224(t), 224–225, 673, 689–690, *689–695, 694,* 696, *696–701*
  barium enema, 690, *690–693*
  plain-film appearance, 689, *289*
  polypoid changes and carcinoma, *692–694, 694,* 696, *696–701,* 722, 733, *733–734,* 990
  post-therapy changes, 696, *698–701*
  pseudopolyposis in, *767, 769*
  sclerosing cholangitis and, 933, *934*
  vs. amebiasis, 675
  vs. cathartic colon, 684
  vs. Crohn's disease, 560, *714,* 720–721
  vs. pseudomembranous enterocolitis, *673*
  vs. strongyloides stercoralis, 576
Ulcerative proctitis, 775, *776*
Ultrasonography, 55–124
  in abdominal wall disorders, 101, *101*
  in adrenal gland disorders, 83–84, *83*
  in aspiration biopsy procedures, 115–119, 115(t), *116–118*
  in bladder disorders, 87, *87*
  in blood vessel disorders, 95–100, *95–100*
  in breast lesions, 111
  in chest lesions, 111, *111*
  in cholecystitis, 913–914, *914*
  in female genital system disorders, 88–94, *89–95*
  in kidney disorders, 74–79, *75–80,* 81, *81*
  in mesenteric disorders, 100
  in parathyroid gland disorders, 109, *109*
  in pericardial effusion, 32
  indications for, 58, 59(t)
  limitations of, 57
  of abscess, 104–108, *105–108*
  of biliary system, 64–69, *65–69,* 896, 898–899, *898–899,* 999–1000
  of eye and orbit, 111
  of large intestine, 652
  of liver, 53, 60–64, *60–64*
    with abscess, 848, *849,* 850, 851, 852
    with cirrhosis, 822, *823–825,* 824
    with trauma, 837–838, *838*
    with tumors, 854, *854–856,* 856, 859
  of male genitals, 88, *88*
  of pancreas, 69–74, *70–73*
    normal anatomy, 1003–1006, *1004*
    with abscess, 1027–1028
    with acute pancreatitis and pseudocyst, 1022–1023, 1023, *1023–1025*
    with carcinoma, 1046, *1046*
    with chronic pancreatitis, 1034–1035, *1034*
    with trauma, 1036, *1040–1041*
  of retroperitoneum and lymph nodes, 84–87, *84–86*
  of spleen, 82, *82*

Ultrasonography (*Continued*)
  of thyroid gland, 108–109, *108–109*
  of thyroid nodules, 30
  pediatric considerations, 112–114, *112–114*
  physical principles, 55–57, *56, 57*
  resolution, 58
  safety of, 57
  vs. computed tomography, 165–166
Umbilical defect, congenital, 249
Umbilical discharge, 251, *253*
Umbilical hernia, 302–303, *303–304*
Umbilical vein catheterization, 813
Undescended testes, 161, *161, 162,* 294, *295*
  in prune belly syndrome, 249
Upside-down spleen, 1073
Urachal anomalies, 249, 251–252, *252–253*
Ureter, dilatation of, with Crohn's disease, 559
  herniation of, 294
  in prune belly syndrome, 249, *250*
  obstruction of, 230–231, *230–231*
    postoperative, 246
Urethra in prune belly syndrome, 249, *250*
Urinary bladder, computed tomography of, 132
  enlarged, *189*
Urinary tract, anomalies, in prune belly syndrome, 249, *250*
  congenital anomalies, 249
  disorders, with Crohn's disease, 559
  in appendicitis, 584, *586*
  obstruction, 78
  stones, following jejunoileal bypass, 644, *644*
Urine, residual, 87
  determinations, in children, 114
Uriniferous perirenal pseudocysts, 231
Urinoma, 78, 81, 88, 103, *104*
  following radical pelvic surgery, 93
Uropathy, obstructive, 230–231, *230–231*
Urticaria of colon, 685
Uterine cervix, carcinoma of, *269*
  perforation of, *266*
Uterus, computed tomography of, 133
  fibroid, *91*

Vagotomy, malabsorption following, 563, *564*
Varices, bleeding with, 789, 791
  angiography in, 792(t)
  and transcatheter therapy for, 794, 796–799, *798*
  vs. gastric carcinoma, *403,* 404
  with cirrhosis, *812,* 830, *830*
  and portal hypertension, 819, *820–822,* 821
Varicoceles, 88
Vascular disease, of large intestine, 676, *677–678*
  peripheral, evaluation of, radionuclide angiography in, 36
  retroperitoneal and peritoneal, 159
Vasopressin infusion. See *Transcatheter therapy.*
Vater, ampulla of, carcinoma of, *894*
  impacted stone in, *928, 928*
Vein(s), hepatic, 816
  portal, 813–815, *814*
    thrombosis, 840
  ultrasound of, 98–99, *99–100*
Vena cava, normal anatomy, 1004, *1004*
Venography, radionuclide, 38, *39–40*
  wedged hepatic, in cirrhosis with portal hypertension, 831, *831*
Venous system scintigraphy, 38, *39–40*

Ventilation, assessment of, scintigraphy in, 36–37, *37*
  endotracheal tube for, 8–9, *9–10*, 11
Ventilatory support, 11–12, *11–13*
Ventral hernia, 212, 303–304, *305–306*, 306
Ventricular size, evaluation of, 113, *114*
Vesicoumbilical fistula, 251
Vesicoureteral reflux, 48
Villous adenocarcinoma, *758*
Villous adenoma, of colon, 751, 753, *755–756*
  of duodenum, 507, *508–509*
  of large intestine, *724–729*, 725, 727
  rectal, with colon carcinoma, *729*
    with rectosigmoid anastomosis, *747*
    rectal carcinoma in, *728*
    vs. retained feces, *723*, 727
Viral gastroenteritis, 226
Visceral abscess, *61*, 105
Volvulus, from Meckel's diverticulum, 627, 628
  of ileum, *298*
  of large intestine, 216, 218, *218–220*, 663–664, *665–666*
  of small bowel, 211, *213*, *214*
  of stomach, 482, *482*
  sigmoid, 541, *542*

von Recklinghausen's neurofibromatosis, 453

Wandering spleen, 1071–1073
Waterston operation, radionuclide methods with, 38
WDHA syndrome, 1063
Webs, esophageal, 340–341, *342–343*, 344
Wedged hepatic vein pressure, 830–831
Wedged hepatic venography, in cirrhosis with portal hypertension, 831, *831*
Whipple's procedure, 486, *487*, 1048–1051, *1051*
  malabsorption with, 571, *572*
Worms, 675, *676*
Wound abscess, 108, *108*

Xanthogranulomatous pyelonephritis, 148

Zenker's diverticula, 335, *336–337*, 337
Zollinger-Ellison syndrome, 477–478, *477*, 1058–1060, *1059–1060*
  diarrhea in, 1060, 1063